WH149

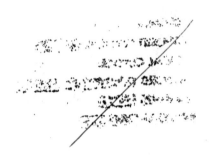

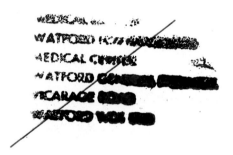

# CLINICAL MALIGNANT HEMATOLOGY

## Notice

Medicine is an ever-changing science. As new research and clinical experience broaden our knowledge, changes in treatment and drug therapy are required. The authors and the publisher of this work have checked with sources believed to be reliable in their efforts to provide information that is complete and generally in accord with the standards accepted at the time of publication. However, in view of the possibility of human error or changes in medical sciences, neither the editors nor the publisher nor any other party who has been involved in the preparation or publication of this work warrants that the information contained herein is in every respect accurate or complete, and they disclaim all responsibility for any errors or omissions or for the results obtained from use of the information contained in this work. Readers are encouraged to confirm the information contained herein with other sources. For example and in particular, readers are advised to check the product information sheet included in the package of each drug they plan to administer to be certain that the information contained in this work is accurate and that changes have not been made in the recommended dose or in the contraindications for administration. This recommendation is of particular importance in connection with new or infrequently used drugs.

# CLINICAL MALIGNANT HEMATOLOGY

*Editors*

## Mikkael A. Sekeres, MD, MS
*Assistant Professor of Medicine*
*Cleveland Clinic Lerner College of Medicine*
*Department of Hematologic Oncology and Blood Disorders*
*Taussig Cancer Center*
*Cleveland Clinic*
*Cleveland, Ohio*

## Matt E. Kalaycio, MD, FACP
*Director, Chronic Leukemia and Myeloma Program*
*Department of Hematologic Oncology and Blood Disorders*
*Taussig Cancer Center*
*Cleveland Clinic*
*Cleveland, Ohio*

## Brian J. Bolwell, MD
*Chairman, Department of Hematologic Oncology and Blood Disorders*
*Professor of Medicine, Cleveland Clinic Lerner College of Medicine*
*Taussig Cancer Center*
*Cleveland Clinic*
*Cleveland, Ohio*

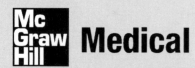 **Medical**

New York   Chicago   San Francisco   Lisbon   London   Madrid   Mexico City   Milan
New Delhi   San Juan   Seoul   Singapore   Sydney   Toronto

The *McGraw·Hill* Companies

# Clinical Malignant Hematology

1 2 3 4 5 6 7 8 9 0   CCW/CCW  0 9 8 7

**ISBN-13:**     **978-0-07-143650-2**
**ISBN-10:**     **0-07-143650-2**

This book was set in Stone Serif 9.5/12 by Aptara Inc., New Delhi, India.
The editors were Joe Rusko, Robert Pancotti, and
Regina Y. Brown.
The production supervisor was Sherri Souffrance.
The cover designer was Eve Siegel
Cover Photo: Leukemia blood cells
Credit: SPL/Photo Researchers, Inc.
The indexer was Pooja Naithani, Aptara Inc., New Delhi, India.
Courier Westford was printer and binder.

This book is printed on acid-free paper.

**Library of Congress Cataloging-in-Publication Data**

Clinical malignant hematology / editors, Mikkael A. Sekeres, Matt E. Kalaycio, Brian J, Bolwell.
    p. ; cm
Includes bibliographical references and index.
ISBN 0-07-143650-2 (alk. paper)
  1. Blood—Diseases. 2. Cancer. 3. Hematology. I. Sekers, Mikkael A. II. Kalaycio,
Matt. III. Bolwell, Brian J.
  [DNLM: 1. Hematologic Neoplasms. 2. Hematologic Neoplasms—therapy.
3. Hematopoietic Stem Cell Transplantation. WH 525 C6415 2007]
RC261.C555 2007
616.99'4—dc22                   2006046249

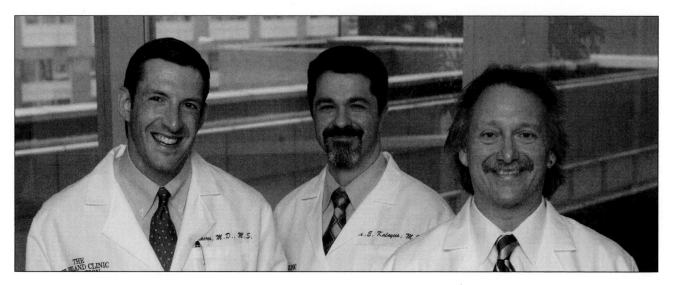

**Mikkael A. Sekeres**     **Matt E. Kalaycio**     **Brian J. Bolwell**

*To my children, Gabriel and Samantha, and to Jennifer, for their unwavering support and unremitting love, and for putting my life in perspective. To my parents and teachers, my inspirations. And always to my patients, for what they have taught me.*

Mikkael A. Sekeres

*To my wife Linda for all her love and support.*

Matt E. Kalaycio

*To all members of the Cleveland Clinic Bone Marrow Transplant Program, past and present; to our patients and their caregivers; to the Elisabeth Severance Prentiss Foundation for their continued support; and to Nina, Brian, Greg, and Augusta.*

Brian J. Bolwell

# CONTENTS

**THE COLOR INSERT CAN BE FOUND BETWEEN PAGES 554 AND 555**

| | |
|---|---|
| Contributors | xiii |
| Preface | xxi |
| Acknowledgments | xxii |

## PART I LEUKEMIA

### SECTION 1 ACUTE MYELOID LEUKEMIA

1. Epidemiology, Risk Factors, and Classification — 1
   Leonard T. Heffner Jr.

2. Molecular Biology, Pathology, and Cytogenetics of Acute Myeloid Leukemia — 9
   Krzysztof Mrózek, Claudia D. Baldus, and Clara D. Bloomfield

3. Clinical Features and Making the Diagnosis — 25
   Anjali S. Advani and Karl S. Theil

4. Treatment for Acute Myeloid Leukemia in Patients Under Age 60 — 41
   Richard M. Stone

5. Treatment Approach to Acute Myeloid Leukemia in Older Adults — 51
   Mikkael A. Sekeres

6. Treatment Approach to Acute Promyelocytic Leukemia — 63
   James L. Slack

7. Approaches to Treatment of Secondary Acute Myeloid Leukemia and Advanced Myelodysplasia — 73
   Elihu Estey

8. Definition of Remission, Prognosis, and Follow-up — 83
   Mikkael A. Sekeres and Matt E. Kalaycio

9. Treatment of Relapsed or Refractory Acute Myeloid Leukemia and New Frontiers in Acute Myeloid Leukemia Therapy — 91
   Frederick R. Appelbaum

### SECTION 2 ACUTE LYMPHOBLASTIC LEUKEMIA

10. Epidemiology, Risk Factors, and Classification — 103
    Joseph O. Moore

11. Molecular Biology, Pathology, and Cytogenetics of Acute Lymphoblastic Leukemia — 111
    Meir Wetzler, Krzysztof Mrózek, and Clara D. Bloomfield

12. Clinical Features and Making the Diagnosis — 121
    Ronald M. Sobecks

13. Treatment Approach to Adult Acute Lymphoblastic Leukemia — 127
    Elizabeth S. Rich, Cara A. Rosenbaum, and Wendy Stock

14. Definition of Remission, Prognosis, and Follow-up — 143
    Meir Wetzler

15. Treatment of Relapsed or Refractory Acute Lymphoblastic Leukemia and New Frontiers in Therapy — 151
    Nicole Lamanna and Mark A. Weiss

### SECTION 3 CHRONIC MYELOGENOUS LEUKEMIA

16. Epidemiology, Risk Factors, and Classification of Chronic Myeloid Leukemia — 159
    Tariq I. Mughal and John M. Goldman

17. Molecular Biology, Pathology, and Cytogenetics — 163
    Michael Deininger

18. Treatment Approach to Chronic-Phase Chronic Myelogenous Leukemia — 177
    Jorge E. Cortes

19. Treatment Approach to Accelerated-Phase or Blast-Crisis Chronic Myelogenous Leukemia — 189
    Eric J. Feldman

20. Definition of Remission, Prognosis, and    195
    Follow-up
    Matt E. Kalaycio and Ilka Warshawsky

21. New Frontiers in the Treatment of    203
    Relapsed or Refractory Chronic
    Myelogenous Leukemia
    Seema Gupta, Javier Pinilla-Ibarz,
    Peter Maslak, and David A. Scheinberg

SECTION 4 CHRONIC LYMPHOCYTIC LEUKEMIA

22. Molecular Biology, Pathology, and    213
    Cytogenetics of Chronic Lymphocytic
    Leukemia
    Martin J.S. Dyer and Randy D. Gascoyne

23. Clinical Features and Making the Diagnosis    225
    William G. Wierda, Joan H. Admirand,
    and Susan M. O'Brien

24. Indications for Treatment and Treatment    235
    Approach for Chronic Lymphocytic Leukemia
    Kanti R. Rai and Bhoomi Mehrotra

25. Response Criteria, Prognosis, and Follow-Up    239
    in Chronic Lymphocytic Leukemia
    Emili Montserrat

26. Treatment of Chronic Lymphocytic    245
    Leukemia
    Matt E. Kalaycio

27. Aggressive Transformation and    251
    Paraneoplastic Complications of
    Chronic Lymphocytic Leukemia
    Terry J. Hamblin

SECTION 5 HAIRY CELL LEUKEMIA

28. Epidemiology, Risk Factors, and    265
    Classification of Hairy Cell Leukemia
    Diane M. BuchBarker

29. Molecular Biology, Pathology, and    269
    Cytogenetics in Hairy Cell Leukemia
    Mirko Zuzel and John C. Cawley

30. Clinical Features and Making the Diagnosis    277
    of HCL
    Olga Frankfurt, Martin S. Tallman, and
    LoAnn C. Peterson

31. Indications for Treatment and Initial    285
    Treatment Approach to Hairy Cell Leukemia
    Alan Saven, Andrew P. Hampshire and
    Lyudmila Bazhenova

32. Definition of Remission, Prognosis, and    295
    Follow-up in Hairy Cell Leukemia
    Eric H. Kraut

33. Treatment of Relapsed or Refractory    301
    Hairy Cell Leukemia and New Frontiers
    in Hairy Cell Leukemia Therapy
    Robert J. Kreitman

SECTION 6 SPECIAL TOPICS IN LEUKEMIA

34. Management of Fever and Neutropenia in    311
    Leukemia
    Robin K. Avery

35. Autologous Stem Cell Transplantation for    321
    Leukemia
    Alexander E. Perl, Selina M. Luger, and Edward A.
    Stadtmauer

36. Allogeneic Hematopoietic Stem Cell    337
    Transplantation for the Acute Leukemias
    in Adults
    Corey Cutler and Joseph H. Antin

37. Transplantation in Chronic Leukemia    355
    Thomas S. Lin and Edward A. Copelan

PART II MYELODYSPLASTIC SYNDROMES
AND MYELOPROLIFERATIVE DISEASES

SECTION 1 MYELODYSPLASTIC SYNDROMES

38. Myelodysplastic Syndromes: Molecular    367
    Biology, Pathology, and Cytogenetics
    Rami Komrokji and John M. Bennett

39. Clinical Features and Making the    377
    Diagnosis of Myelodysplastic Syndromes
    Lewis R. Silverman

40. Treatment Approach to Early    385
    Myelodysplastic Syndromes
    Virginia M. Klimek and Stephen D. Nimer

41. Aplastic Anemia and Stem Cell Failure    397
    Jaroslaw P. Maciejewski

42. Allogeneic Stem Cell Transplantation for    415
    Myelodysplastic Syndrome and Aplastic
    Anemia
    Vikram Mathews and John F. DiPersio

43. Definition of Response, Prognosis, and    425
    Follow-up of Myelodysplastic Syndromes
    Miguel A. Sanz and Guillermo F. Sanz

44. Treatment of Relapsed or Refractory    435
    Myelodysplastic Syndromes and New
    Frontiers in Myelodysplastic Syndrome
    Therapy
    Huma Qawi, Naomi Galili, and Azra Raza

## SECTION 2 CHRONIC MYELOPROLIFERATIVE DISEASES

45. Epidemiology, Risk Factors, and Classification    445
    Hanspreet Kaur, Deepjot Singh, and Alan Lichtin

46. Molecular Biology, Pathology, and Cytogenetics    449
    Claire N. Harrison

47. Clinical Features and Making the Diagnosis    461
    Richard T. Silver

48. Treatment Approach to Polycythemia Vera and Essential Thrombocythemia    469
    Steven M. Fruchtman and Celia L. Grosskreutz

49. Approach to Chronic Idiopathic Myelofibrosis (with Extramedullary Hematopoiesis)    475
    Ruben A. Mesa and Ayalew Tefferi

50. Management of Chronic Myelomonocytic Leukemia and Other Rare Myeloproliferative Disorders    487
    Miloslav Beran

## PART III LYMPHOMA

### SECTION 1 NON-HODGKIN'S LYMPHOMA

51. The Classification of Non-Hodgkin's Lymphoma    503
    P.G. Isaacson

52. Pathology and Molecular Genetics of Non-Hodgkin's Lymphoma    513
    James R. Cook and Eric D. Hsi

53. Treatment Approach to Follicular Lymphomas    531
    Bruce D. Cheson

54. Treatment Approach to Diffuse Large B-Cell Lymphomas    543
    Sonali M. Smith and Koen van Besien

55. Treatment Approach to Mantle Cell Lymphoma    555
    Ellie Guardino, Kristen N. Ganjoo, and Ranjana Advani

56. Treatment Approach to High-Grade Non-Hodgkin's Lymphomas    565
    John W. Sweetenham

57. Treatment Approach to Marginal Zone and MALT Lymphomas    577
    Emanuele Zucca

58. Treatment Approach to Primary Central Nervous System Lymphomas    589
    Tamara N. Shenkier and Joseph M. Connors

59. Treatment Approach to Cutaneous Lymphomas    601
    Christiane Querfeld, Timothy M. Kuzel, Joan Guitart, and Steven T. Rosen

60. Mature T-Cell Non-Hodgkin's Lymphoma: Diagnosis and Therapy    613
    Nam H. Dang and Fredrick Hagemeister

61. Treatment Approach to HIV-Related Lymphomas    631
    Mark Bower

62. Posttransplant Lymphoproliferative Disorders    645
    Terrance Comeau and Thomas Shea

63. Treatment Approach to Adult T-Cell Lymphoma/Leukemia    657
    Karen W.L. Yee and Francis J. Giles

64. Autologous Hematopoietic Cell Transplantation for Non-Hodgkin's Lymphoma    671
    Ginna G. Laport and Robert S. Negrin

65. Allogeneic Hematopoietic Stem Cell Transplantation for Non-Hodgkin's Lymphoma    689
    Hillard M. Lazarus

66. Definition of Remission, Prognosis, and Follow-up in Follicular Lymphoma and Diffuse Large B-Cell Lymphoma    701
    John W. Sweetenham

67. Treatment of Transformed Non-Hodgkin's Lymphoma    711
    Philip J. Bierman

68. New Frontiers in Non-Hodgkin's Lymphoma Therapy    723
    Eric Winer, Sridar Pal, and Francine Foss

### SECTION 2 HODGKIN'S LYMPHOMA

69. Hodgkin's Lymphoma: Epidemiology and Risk Factors    733
    Brian J. Bolwell

70. Prognostic Factors in Hodgkin's Lymphoma    739
    Michel Henry-Amar

71. Classification, Pathology, and Molecular Genetics of Hodgkin's Lymphoma    751
    James R. Cook and Eric D. Hsi

72. Clinical Features and Making the Diagnosis    759
    Kristie A. Blum and Pierluigi Porcu

73. **Treatment Approach to Classical Hodgkin's Lymphoma**    767
Brian J. Bolwell and Toni K. Choueiri

74. **Treatment Approach to Nodular Lymphocyte-Predominant Hodgkin's Lymphoma**    783
Brad Pohlman

75. **Autologous Stem Cell Transplantation for Hodgkin's Lymphoma**    793
Craig Moskowitz and Daniel Persky

76. **Hodgkin's Lymphoma: Follow-up Care**    801
Omer N. Koç

77. **Treatment of Relapsed or Refractory Hodgkin's Lymphoma and New Frontiers in Hodgkin's Lymphoma Therapy**    807
Angelo M. Carella, Angela Congiu, Sandro Nati, and Ercole Brusamolino

### SECTION 3  SPECIAL TOPICS IN LYMPHOMA

78. **Epidemiology of Second Malignancies Following Lymphoma Therapy and Screening Recommendations**    815
Jonathan W. Friedberg and Andrea K. Ng

79. **The Appropriate Use of PET and Gallium Scans in Lymphoma**    823
Rebecca Elstrom

## PART IV  MULTIPLE MYELOMA AND RELATED DISORDERS

### SECTION 1  MULTIPLE MYELOMA

80. **Epidemiology and Risk Factors of Multiple Myeloma: Insights Into Incidence and Etiology**    833
Ashraf Badros

81. **Molecular Biology, Pathology, and Cytogenetics**    847
Silvia Ling, Lynda Campbell, Phoebe Joy Ho, John Gibson, and Douglas E. Joshua

82. **Clinical Features and Making the Diagnosis of Multiple Myeloma**    859
Yi-Hsiang Chen

83. **Initial Treatment Approach to Multiple Myeloma**    873
Jeffrey A. Zonder

84. **Treatment of Multiple Myeloma**    889
Robert A. Kyle and S. Vincent Rajkumar

85. **Allogeneic Stem Cell Transplantation for Multiple Myeloma**    901
Edwin P. Alyea

86. **Definition of Remission, Prognosis, and Follow-up**    913
S. Vincent Rajkumar and Angela Dispenzieri

87. **Treatment of Relapsed or Refractory Multiple Myeloma and New Frontiers in Multiple Myeloma Therapy**    927
Manmeet Ahluwalia and Mohamad A. Hussein

### SECTION 2  SPECIAL TOPICS IN MULTIPLE MYELOMA

88. **Hyperviscosity Syndrome**    937
Marcel N. Menke and Steve P. Treon

89. **Monoclonal Gammopathy of Undetermined Significance**    943
Shaji Kumar, Philip R. Greipp

90. **Amyloidosis**    955
Madhav V. Dhodapkar

91. **Treatment of Complications in Multiple Myeloma**    963
Paul Masci

## PART V  STEM CELL TRANSPLANTATION

92. **Principles of Hematopoietic Stem Cell Transplantation to Treat Hematologic Malignancies**    975
Michael R. Bishop

93. **Principles of HLA Matching and the National Marrow Donor Program**    985
Edward J. Ball

94. **Stem Cell Mobilization**    1001
Auayporn Nademanee

95. **Stem Cell Transplantation for Solid Tumors and Nonmalignant Conditions**    1013
E. Randolph Broun

96. **Nonmyeloablative Conditioning Regimen for Allogeneic Hematopoietic Cell Transplantation**    1025
Frédéric Baron, Marie-Thérèse Little, and Rainer Storb

97. **Umbilical Cord Blood Transplantation**    1039
Ian Horkheimer and Nelson Chao

98. **Graft-Versus-Host Disease: New Perspectives on Pathobiology and Therapy**    1051
Thomas R. Spitzer and Robert Sackstein

99. **Infectious Complications Following Stem Cell Transplantation**    1063
David L. Longworth

100. Noninfectious Complications of 1077
     Stem Cell Transplantation
     *Scott I. Bearman*

# PART VI SPECIAL TOPICS IN NEOPLASTIC HEMATOLOGY

101. Pharmacology of Traditional Agents 1089
     Used to Treat Hematologic Malignancies
     *Jennifer L. Shamp*

102. Biological Response Modifying Agents 1105
     in the Treatment of Hematologic
     Malignancies
     *Christopher J. Lowe and Jennifer Fisher Lowe*

103. Pharmacology of Monoclonal Antibodies 1115
     *Jennifer L. Shamp*

104. Blood Product Transfusions in the 1127
     Hematologic Malignancies
     *Ronald E. Domen*

105. Growth Factor Support in the 1139
     Hematologic Malignancies
     *George Somlo*

106. Treatment Approach to Pregnant Women 1147
     *Revathi Suppiah, Joanna Brell, and
     Matt E. Kalaycio*

107. Tumor Lysis Syndrome, Disseminated 1159
     Intravascular Coagulopathy, and
     Other Non-Infectious Complications of
     Leukemia and Lymphoma
     *Rajesh Kukunoor and Mikkael A. Sekeres*

108. Fertility Issues in the Hematologic 1171
     Malignancies
     *Ashok Agarwal and Tamer M. Said*

109. Palliation of Symptoms Associated with 1179
     Hematologic Malignancies
     *Mellar P. Davis*

Index 1191

# CONTRIBUTORS

**Joan H. Admirand,** MD
*Assistant Professor of Medicine, Department of
Hematopathology, Division of Laboratory Medicine
The University of Texas M.D. Anderson Cancer Center
Houston, Texas*

**Anjali S. Advani,** MD
*Assistant Professor, The Cleveland Clinic Lerner College of
Medicine, Department of Hematology and Medical
Oncology, The Cleveland Clinic Foundation
Cleveland, Ohio*

**Ranjana Advani,** MD
*Assistant Professor of Medicine, Department of Medicine
Division of Oncology, Stanford University Medical Center
Clinical Cancer Center, Stanford, California*

**Ashok Agarwal,** PhD, HCLD
*Director, Center for Advanced Research in Human
Reproduction, Infertility and Sexual Function
Glickman Urological Institute
Department of Obstetrics and Gynecology
The Cleveland Clinic Foundation, Cleveland, Ohio*

**Manmeet Ahluwalia**
*Myeloma Multidisciplinary Clinical Research Program
Taussig Cancer Center, The Cleveland Clinic Foundation
Cleveland, Ohio*

**Edwin P. Alyea,** MD
*Assistant Professor of Medicine, Harvard Medical School
Division of Adult Oncology, Dana-Farber Cancer Institute
Boston, Massachusetts*

**Joseph H. Antin,** MD
*Professor of Medicine, Harvard Medical School
Department of Medical Oncology, Chief, Stem Cell
Transplantation Program, Dana-Farber Cancer Institute,
Brigham and Women's Hospital, Boston, Massachusetts*

**Frederick R. Appelbaum,** MD
*Professor and Head, Division of Medical Oncology
University of Washington School of Medicine
Director, Clinical Research Division
Fred Hutchinson Cancer Research Center
Seattle, Washington*

**Robin K. Avery,** MD
*Head, Department of Infectious Disease and Transplant
Center, The Cleveland Clinic Foundation, Cleveland, Ohio*

**Ashraf Badros,** MD
*Associate Professor of Medicine, Greenebaum Cancer
Center, University of Maryland, Baltimore, Maryland*

**Claudia D. Baldus,** MD
*Clinical Instructor in Hematology, Charité,
Universitätsmedizin Berlin, Campus Benjamin Franklin
Medizinische Klinik III, Abteilung für Hämatologie,
Onkologie und Transfusionsmedizin, Berlin, Germany*

**Edward J. Ball,** PhD
*Associate Director, Allogen Laboratories
The Cleveland Clinic Foundation, Cleveland, Ohio*

**Frédéric Baron,** MD,PhD
*Postdoctoral Fellow, Fred Hutchinson Cancer Research
Center, Seattle, Washington*

**Lyudmila Bazhenova,** MD
*Division of Hematology/Oncology, University of California
at San Diego, La Jolla, California*

**Scott I. Bearman,** MD
*U.S. Oncology, Denver, Colorado*

**John M. Bennett,** MD
*Professor of Medicine and Pathology and Laboratory
Medicine, Emeritus, University of Rochester School of
Medicine and Dentistry, Department of Medicine and the
James P. Wilmot Cancer Center, Strong Memorial Hospital
Rochester, New York*

**Miloslav Beran,** MD, PhD, DVM
*Professor of Medicine, Department of Leukemia
The University of Texas M.D. Anderson Cancer Center
Houston, Texas*

**Philip J. Bierman,** MD
*Associate Professor
Department of Internal Medicine
Section of Hematology/Oncology
University of Nebraska Medical Center
Omaha, Nebraska*

**Michael R. Bishop**, MD
*Investigator and Clinical Head, Experimental Transplantation and Immunology Branch, National Cancer Institute, National Institutes of Health Bethesda, Maryland*

**Clara D. Bloomfield**, MD
*William G. Pace III Professor of Cancer Research Cancer Scholar and Senior Advisor, Division of Hematology and Oncology, Department of Internal Medicine, Comprehensive Cancer Center and James Cancer Hospital and Solove Research Institute, The Ohio State University, Columbus, Ohio*

**Kristie A. Blum**, MD
*Assistant Professor of Internal Medicine The Ohio State University, The Arthur G. James Cancer Hospital, Division of Hematology and Oncology Columbus, Ohio*

**Brian J. Bolwell**, MD
*Chairman, Department of Hematologic Oncology and Blood Disorders, Professor of Medicine, Cleveland Clinic Lerner College of Medicine, Taussig Cancer Center, Cleveland Clinic, Cleveland, Ohio*

**Mark Bower**, PhD, FRCP
*Honorary Reader, Imperial College School of Medicine Consultant and Medical Oncologist, Department of Oncology, Chelsea & Westminster Hospital, London, United Kingdom*

**Joanna Brell**, MD
*Department of Hematology and Medical Oncology Case Western Reserve University, Cleveland, Ohio*

**E. Randolph Broun**, MD
*Director, Blood and Marrow Transplant Program Jewish Hospital of Cincinnati, Cincinnati, Ohio*

**Ercole Brusamolino**, MD
*Clinica Ematologica, Policlinico San Matteo IRCCS Università di Pavia, Pavia, Italy*

**Diane M. BuchBarker**, MD
*West Penn/Allegheny Health System Department of Hematology and Medical Oncology Richard Laube Cancer Center, Kittanning, Pennsylvania*

**Lynda Campbell**, MB BS, FRCPA, FHGSA
*Associate Professor, Director, Victorian Cancer Cytogenetics Service, St. Vincent's Hospital Melbourne, Fitzroy, Victoria, Australia*

**Angelo M. Carella**, MD
*Director and Professor, Divisione di Ematologia Centro Trapianti di Midollo, Azienda Ospedaliera e Cliniche Universitaria, Convenzionate Ospedale San Martino, Genova, Italy*

**John C. Cawley**, MD, PhD
*Professor, Department of Haematology Royal Liverpool and Broadgreen University Hospitals NHS Trust, Professor and Head of Department*

*Department of Haematology, University of Liverpool Liverpool, United Kingdom*

**Nelson Chao**, MD
*Division of Cellular Therapy, Duke University Medical Center, Durham, North Carolina*

**Yi-Hsiang Chen**, MD, PhD
*Associate Professor of Medicine Section of Hematology and Medical Oncology Department of Medicine, University of Illinois at Chicago Chicago, Illinois*

**Bruce D. Cheson**, MD
*Professor of Medicine and Oncology Head of Hematology, Georgetown University Hospital Lombardi Comprehensive Cancer Center Washington, D.C.*

**Toni K. Choueiri**, MD
*Department of Hematology and Medical Oncology The Cleveland Clinic Foundation, Cleveland, Ohio*

**Terrance Comeau**, MD, FRCP(C)
*Director of BMT Quality Assurance Blood and Marrow Stem Cell Transplantation Program Division of Hematology and Medical Oncology The School of Medicine, University of North Carolina at Chapel Hill, Chapel Hill, North Carolina*

**Angela Congiu**, MD
*Coordinator of Clinical Studies, Divisione di Ematologia Centro Trapianti di Midollo, Azienda Ospedaliera San Martino, Genova, Italy*

**Joseph M. Connors**, MD
*Clinical Professor, Department of Medicine University of British Columbia, Medical Oncologist British Columbia Cancer Agency, Vancouver British Columbia, Canada*

**James R. Cook**, MD, PhD
*Staff Pathologist, Department of Clinical Pathology Assistant Professor of Pathology, Cleveland Clinic Lerner College of Medicine, Case Western Reserve University The Cleveland Clinic Foundation, Cleveland, Ohio*

**Edward A. Copelan**, MD
*Professor of Internal Medicine, Director, Bone Marrow Transplantation, Medical Director of Inpatient Hematology/ Oncology Division, Arthur G. James Cancer Hospital and Richard J. Solove Research Institute Ohio State University Columbus, Ohio*

**Jorge E. Cortes**, MD
*Department of Leukemia, The University of Texas M.D. Anderson Cancer Center Houston, Texas*

**Corey Cutler**, MD, MPH, FRCP(C)
*Instructor in Medicine, Harvard Medical School Department of Medical Oncology, Dana-Farber Cancer Institute, Boston, Massachusetts*

**Nam H. Dang**, MD, PhD
*Associate Professor of Medicine, Department of Lymphoma/Myeloma, The University of Texas M.D. Anderson Cancer Center, Houston, Texas*

**Mellar P. Davis**, MD, FCCP
*Director of Research*
*The Harry R. Horvitz Center for Palliative Medicine*
*Taussig Cancer Center, The Cleveland Clinic Foundation*
*Cleveland, Ohio*

**Michael Deininger**, MD, PhD
*Assistant Professor, Center for Hematologic Malignancies*
*Oregon Health and Science University, Portland, Oregon*

**Madhav V. Dhodapkar**, MD
*Hematology Service, Memorial Sloan-Kettering Cancer Center, Irene Diamond Associate Professor and Head of Laboratory, Laboratory of Tumor Immunology and Immunotherapy, Rockefeller University*
*New York, New York*

**John F. DiPersio**, MD, PhD
*Chief, Division of Oncology, Deputy Director, Siteman Cancer Center, Barnes-Jewish Hospital*
*Washington University School of Medicine*
*St. Louis, Missouri*

**Angela Dispenzieri**, MD
*Associate Professor of Medicine*
*Mayo Clinic College of Medicine, Rochester, Minnesota*

**Ronald E. Domen**, MD
*Professor of Pathology, Medicine, and Humanities*
*Associate Dean for Graduate Medical Education*
*Medical Director, Blood Bank and Transfusion Medicine*
*Penn State University College of Medicine*
*Milton S. Hershey Medical Center*
*Hershey, Pennsylvania*

**Martin J. S. Dyer**, MA, DPhil, FRCP, FRCPath
*Professor of Haemato-Oncology and Honorary Consultant Physician, MRC Toxicology Unit, University of Leicester*
*Leicester, United Kingdom*

**Rebecca Elstrom**, MD
*Assistant Professor of Hematology/Oncology*
*University of Michigan, Ann Arbor, Michigan*

**Elihu Estey**, MD
*Professor of Leukemia*
*Department of Leukemia, The University of Texas M.D. Anderson Cancer Center, Houston, Texas*

**Eric J. Feldman**, MD
*Professor of Medicine, Division of Hematology and Medical Oncology, Weill Medical College of Cornell University, New York, New York*

**Jennifer Fisher Lowe**, PharmD
*Oncology/Hematology Pharmacotherapy Specialist*
*Akron General Medical Center, Akron, Ohio*

**Francine Foss**, MD
*Associate Professor of Medicine*
*Hematology/Oncology and Bone Marrow Transplantation*
*Tufts New England Medical Center*
*Boston, Massachusetts*

**Olga Frankfurt**, MD
*Division of Hematology/Oncology*
*Feinberg School of Medicine, Northwestern University*
*Robert H. Lurie Comprehensive Cancer Center*
*Chicago, Illinois*

**Jonathan W. Friedberg**, MD
*Associate Director, Lymphoma Clinical Research*
*Assistant Professor of Medicine, James P. Wilmot Cancer Center, University of Rochester, Rochester, New York*

**Steven M. Fruchtman**, MD
*Associate Professor of Medicine, Division of Hematology/Oncology, Mount Sinai Medical Center*
*New York, New York*

**Naomi Galili**, PhD
*Associate Professor, Division of Hematology and Oncology*
*University of Massachusetts Medical School*
*Worcester, Massachusetts*

**Kristen N. Ganjoo**, MD
*Assistant Professor of Medicine, Department of Medicine*
*Division of Oncology, Stanford University Medical Center*
*Clinical Cancer Center, Stanford, California*

**Randy D. Gascoyne**, MD, FRCPC
*Clinical Professor of Pathology, University of British Columbia, Department of Pathology*
*British Columbia Cancer Agency, Vancouver, British Columbia, Canada*

**John Gibson**, MB BS, PhD(Syd), FRACP, FRCPA
*Associate Professor, Faculty of Medicine, University of Sydney, Senior Staff Specialist, Institute of Haematology*
*Royal Prince Alfred Hospital, Camperdown, New South Wales, Australia*

**Francis J. Giles**, MD
*Professor of Medicine, Department of Leukemia*
*The University of Texas M.D. Anderson Cancer Center*
*Houston, Texas*

**John M. Goldman**, DM, FRCP
*Department of Haematology, Hammersmith Hospital*
*Imperial College School of Medicine, London United Kingdom*

**Philip R. Greipp**, MD
*Professor of Medicine, Mayo Clinic College of Medicine*
*Consultant, Division of Hematology and Internal Medicine, Hematology Research, Mayo Clinic*
*Rochester, Minnesota*

**Celia L. Grosskreutz**, MD
*Assistant Professor of Medicine, Division of Hematology/Oncology, Mount Sinai Medical Center*
*New York, New York*

**Ellie Guardino,** MD, PhD
*Clinical Instructor, Department of Medicine*
*Division of Oncology, Clinical Cancer Center*
*Stanford University Medical Center, Stanford, California*

**Joan Guitart,** MD
*Associate Professor, Department of Dermatology*
*Feinberg School of Medicine, Northwestern University*
*Chicago, Illinois*

**Seema Gupta,** MD
*Clinical Assistant Physician, Leukemia Service*
*Department of Medicine, Memorial Sloan-Kettering*
*Cancer Center, New York, New York*

**Fredrick Hagemeister,** MD
*Professor of Medicine, Department of*
*Lymphoma/Myeloma, The University of Texas M.D.*
*Anderson Cancer Center, Houston, Texas*

**Terry J. Hamblin,** DM, FRCP, FRCPath, FMedSci
*Professor of Immunohaematology*
*Department of Cancer Studies, University of Southampton*
*Consultant Haematologist, Department of Haematology*
*Royal Bournemouth Hospital, Bournemouth*
*United Kingdom*

**Andrew P. Hampshire,** MD
*Former Fellow, Division of Hematology/Oncology*
*Scripps Clinic, Staff Physician/Oncologist*
*Scripps Mercy Hospital, San Diego, California*

**Claire N. Harrison,** DM, MRCP, MRCPath
*Consultant Haematologist, Department of Haematology*
*Guy's and St. Thomas' NHS Foundation Trust*
*London, United Kingdom*

**Leonard T. Heffner Jr.,** MD
*Associate Professor of Medicine, Emory University School*
*of Medicine, Winship Cancer Institute*
*Atlanta, Georgia*

**Michel Henry-Amar,** MD, PhD
*Head, Clinical Research Unit, Centre François Baclesse*
*Caen, France*

**Phoebe Joy Ho,** MB BS(Syd), DPhil(Oxon), FRACP, FRCPA
*Associate Professor of Medicine, University of Sydney*
*Senior Staff Specialist, Institute of Haematology*
*Centenary Institute of Cancer Medicine and Cell Biology*
*Royal Prince Alfred Hospital, Camperdown, New South*
*Wales, Australia*

**Ian Horkheimer,** MD
*Fellow, Departments of Hematology/ Oncology/ Cellular*
*Therapy, Division of Hematology-Oncology*
*Duke University Medical Center*
*Durham, North Carolina*

**Eric Hsi,** MD
*Professor of Pathology, Department of Clinical Pathology*
*Cleveland Clinic Lerner College of Medicine*
*The Cleveland Clinic Foundation, Cleveland, Ohio*

**Mohamad A. Hussein,** MD
*Director, Myeloma Multidisciplinary Clinical Research*
*Program, Taussig Cancer Center, The Cleveland Clinic*
*Foundation, Cleveland, Ohio*

**Peter G. Isaacson**
*Professor Emeritus, University College London*
*Consultant Histopathologist, Department of Pathology*
*UCL Hospitals NHS Trust, London, United Kingdom*

**Douglas E. Joshua,** BSc, MB BS(Syd), DPhil(Oxon), FRACP, FRCPA
*Clinical Professor in Medicine, University of Sydney*
*Head, Institute of Haematology, Royal Prince Alfred*
*Hospital, Camperdown, New South Wales, Australia*

**Matt E. Kalaycio,** MD, FACP
*Director, Chronic Leukemia and Myeloma Program*
*Department of Hematologic Oncology and Blood Disorders*
*Taussig Cancer Center, Cleveland Clinic Cleveland, Ohio*

**Hanspreet Kaur,** MD
*Fellow, Taussig Cancer Center, The Cleveland Clinic*
*Foundation, Cleveland, Ohio*

**Virginia M. Klimek,** MD
*Assistant Attending Physician*
*Memorial Hospital for Cancer and Allied Diseases*
*Memorial Sloan-Kettering Cancer Center*
*New York, New York*

**Omer N. Koç,** MD
*Associate Professor of Medicine, Hematology/Oncology*
*Division, Case Western Reserve University*
*Case Comprehensive Cancer Center, University Hospitals*
*of Cleveland, Cleveland, Ohio*

**Rami Komrokji,** MD
*Senior Instructor in Medicine*
*Department of Medicine and the James P. Wilmot Cancer*
*Center, University of Rochester School of Medicine and*
*Dentistry, Rochester, New York*

**Eric H. Kraut,** MD
*Professor of Medicine, Director, Benign Hematology*
*The Ohio State University and Arthur G. James and Richard*
*J. Solove Hospital and Research Institute, Columbus, Ohio*

**Robert J. Kreitman,** MD
*Chief, Clinical Immunotherapy Section, Laboratory of*
*Molecular Biology, National Cancer Institute*
*National Institutes of Health, Bethesda, Maryland*

**Rajesh Kukunoor,** MD
*Fellow in Hematology and Oncology*
*The Cleveland Clinic Foundation*
*Cleveland, Ohio*

**Shaji Kumar,** MD
*Assistant Professor of Medicine, Mayo Clinic College of*
*Medicine, Senior Associate Consultant*
*Division of Hematology and Internal Medicine*
*Mayo Clinic, Rochester, Minnesota*

**Timothy M. Kuzel**, MD
*Associate Professor, Department of Medicine*
*Division of Hematology/Oncology, Feinberg School of*
*Medicine, Northwestern University, Chicago, Illinois*

**Robert A. Kyle**, MD
*Consultant, Division of Hematology and Internal*
*Medicine, Professor of Medicine and of Laboratory*
*Medicine, Mayo Clinic College of Medicine*
*Rochester, Minnesota*

**Nicole Lamanna**
*Leukemia Service, Memorial Sloan-Kettering Cancer*
*Center, New York, New York*

**Ginna G. Laport**, MD
*Assistant Professor*
*Division of Blood and Marrow Transplantation*
*Stanford University Medical Center, Stanford, California*

**Hillard M. Lazarus**, MD, FACP
*Professor of Medicine and General Medical Sciences*
*(Oncology), Case Western Reserve University*
*Department of Medicine, University Hospitals of*
*Cleveland, Cleveland, Ohio*

**Alan Lichtin**, MD
*Staff Hematologist-Oncologist, The Cleveland Clinic*
*Foundation, Cleveland, Ohio*

**Thomas S. Lin**, MD, PhD
*Assistant Professor of Internal Medicine*
*Ohio State University, Arthur G. James Cancer Hospital*
*and Richard J. Solove Research Institute, Columbus, Ohio*

**Silvia Ling**, MB BS
*Centenary Institute of Cancer Medicine and Cell Biology*
*University of Sydney, Camperdown*
*New South Wales, Australia*

**Marie-Térèse Little**, PhD
*Staff Scientist, Fred Hutchinson Cancer Research Center*
*Seattle, Washington*

**David L. Longworth**, MD
*Deputy Chairman, Department of Medicine*
*Tufts University School of Medicine, Boston,*
*Massachusetts, Chairman, Department of Medicine*
*Baystate Medical Center, Springfield, Massachusetts*

**Christopher J. Lowe**, PharmD
*Hematology/Oncology Clinical Specialist*
*The Cleveland Clinic Foundation, Cleveland, Ohio*

**Selina M. Luger**, MD
*Associate Professor of Medicine, Director, Leukemia*
*Program, Attending Physician*
*Division of Hematology/Oncology, Abramson Cancer*
*Center, University of Pennsylvania Medical Center*
*Philadelphia, Pennsylvania*

**Jaroslaw P. Maciejewski**, MD
*Head, Experimental Hematology and Hematopoiesis*
*Section, Taussig Cancer Center, The Cleveland Clinic*

*Foundation, Associate Professor of Medicine*
*Cleveland Clinic College of Medicine, Case Western*
*Reserve University, Cleveland, Ohio*

**Paul Masci**, DO
*Division of Regional Practice, The Cleveland Clinic*
*Foundation, Wooster, Ohio*

**Peter Maslak**, MD
*Chief, Hematology Laboratory Service, Memorial*
*Sloan-Kettering Cancer Center, New York, New York*

**Vikram Mathews**, MD
*Division of Oncology*
*Section of Bone Marrow Transplantation and Leukemia*
*Siteman Cancer Center, Washington University School of*
*Medicine, St. Louis, Missouri*

**Bhoomi Mehrotra**, MD
*Assistant Professor of Medicine, Albert Einstein College of*
*Medicine, Bronx, New York, Director, Oncology Unit*
*Departments of Medicine and Hematology/Oncology*
*Long Island Jewish Medical Center*
*New Hyde Park, New York*

**Marcel N. Menke**, MD
*Schepens Retina Associates Foundation*
*Boston, Massachusetts*

**Ruben A. Mesa**, MD
*Assistant Professor of Medicine, Division of Hematology*
*Mayo Clinic, Rochester, Minnesota*

**Emili Montserrat**, MD
*Professor of Medicine, Institute of Hematology and*
*Oncology, Department of Hematology, Hospital Clínic*
*University of Barcelona, Barcelona, Spain*

**Joseph O. Moore**, MD
*Professor of Medicine, Division of Medical Oncology and*
*Cell Therapy, Duke University Medical Center*
*Durham, North Carolina*

**Craig Moskowitz**, MD
*Associate Professor of Medicine, Cornell University*
*Medical College, Associate Member, Lymphoma Service*
*Memorial Sloan-Kettering Cancer Center*
*New York, New York*

**Krzysztof Mrózek**, MD, PhD
*Research Scientist, Division of Hematology and Oncology*
*Department of Internal Medicine, Comprehensive Cancer*
*Center, The Ohio State University, Columbus, Ohio*

**Tariq I. Mughal**
*Department of Haematology, Hammersmith Hospital*
*Imperial College School of Medicine*
*London, United Kingdom*

**Auayporn Nademanee**, MD
*Associate Clinical Director, Division of Hematology and*
*Bone Marrow Transplantation, City of Hope National*
*Medical Center and Beckman Research Institute*
*Duarte, California*

**Sandro Nati, MD**
*Divisione di Ematologia, Centro Trapianti di Midollo*
*Azienda Ospedaliera Universitaria San Martino*
*Genova, Italy*

**Robert S. Negrin, MD**
*Professor, Division of Blood and Marrow Transplantation*
*Stanford University Medical Center, Stanford, California*

**Andrea K. Ng, MD**
*Assistant Professor of Radiation Oncology*
*Brigham and Women's Hospital, Dana-Farber Cancer*
*Institute, Harvard Medical School, Boston, Massachusetts*

**Stephen D. Nimer, MD**
*Head, Division of Hematologic Oncology, Memorial*
*Sloan-Kettering Cancer Center, New York, New York*

**Susan M. O'Brien, MD**
*Professor of Medicine, Department of Leukemia*
*The University of Texas M.D. Anderson Cancer Center*
*Houston, Texas*

**Sridar Pal, MD**
*Hematology Oncology and Bone Marrow Transplantation*
*Tufts New England Medical Center*
*Boston, Massachusetts*

**Alexander E. Perl, MD**
*Instructor in Medicine, Attending Oncologist*
*Division of Hematology/Oncology, Hospital of the*
*University of Pennsylvania, Philadelphia, Pennsylvania*

**Daniel Persky**
*Fellow in Hematology/Oncology, Memorial Sloan-Kettering*
*Cancer Center, New York, New York*

**LoAnn C. Peterson, MD**
*Division of Pathology, Feinberg School of Medicine*
*Northwestern University, Chicago, Illinois*

**Javier Pinilla-Ibarz, MD, PhD**
*Resident in Medicine, New York Presbyterian*
*Hospital/Weill Cornell Medical Center*
*Clinical Hematology/Oncology Fellow*
*Memorial Sloan-Kettering Cancer Center*
*New York, New York*

**Brad Pohlman, MD**
*Director, Lymphoma Program*
*Department of Hematology and Medical Oncology*
*The Cleveland Clinic Foundation*
*Cleveland, Ohio*

**Pierluigi Porcu, MD**
*Assistant Professor of Internal Medicine*
*The Ohio State University, Division of Hematology and*
*Oncology, The James Cancer Hospital and University*
*Hospital East, Columbus, Ohio*

**Huma Qawi, MD**
*Fellow, Division of Hematology and Oncology*
*Rush University Medical Center, Chicago, Illinois*

**Christiane Querfeld, MD**
*Postdoctoral Fellow, Department of Dermatology*
*Feinberg School of Medicine, Northwestern University*
*Chicago, Illinois*

**Kanti R. Rai, MD**
*Professor of Medicine, Joel Finkelstein Cancer Foundation*
*Albert Einstein College of Medicine, Bronx, New York*
*Chief, Division of Hematology/Oncology*
*Long Island Jewish Medical Center*
*New Hyde Park, New York*

**S. Vincent Rajkumar, MD**
*Associate Professor of Medicine, Mayo Clinic College of*
*Medicine, Consultant, Division of Hematology and*
*Internal Medicine, Mayo Clinic*
*Rochester, Minnesota*

**Azra Raza, MD**
*Chief, Division of Hematology and Medical Oncology*
*Associate Clinical Director of the Cancer Center*
*University of Massachusetts Medical Center*
*Worcester, Massachusetts*

**Elizabeth S. Rich, MD, PhD**
*Assistant Professor, Department of Medicine*
*Section of Hematology/Oncology, The University of*
*Chicago, Chicago, Illinois*

**Steven T. Rosen, MD**
*Geneviève Teuton Professor of Medicine*
*Director, Robert H. Lurie Comprehensive Cancer Center*
*Feinberg School of Medicine, Northwestern University*
*Chicago, Illinois*

**Cara A. Rosenbaum, MD**
*Resident, Department of Medicine*
*Section of Hematology/Oncology, The University of*
*Chicago, Chicago, Illinois*

**Robert Sackstein, MD, PhD**
*Associate Scientific Director, Bone Marrow*
*Transplant Program, Massachusetts General*
*Hospital, Associate Professor of Dermatology and of*
*Medicine, Harvard Medical School*
*Boston, Massachusetts*

**Tamer M. Said, MD**
*Center for Advanced Research in Human Reproduction,*
*Infertility and Sexual Function, Glickman Urological*
*Institute, The Cleveland Clinic Foundation*
*Cleveland, Ohio*

**Guillermo F. Sanz, MD, PhD**
*Attending Physician, Clinical Hematology Section*
*Hospital Universitario La Fe, Valencia, Spain*

**Miguel A. Sanz, MD, PhD**
*Assistant Professor of Medicine, University of Valencia*
*Head, Clinical Hematology Section, Hospital Universitario*
*La Fe, Valencia, Spain*

**Alan Saven**, MD
*Head, Division of Hematology/Oncology*
*Director, Ida M. and Cecil H. Green Cancer Center*
*Scripps Clinic/ Scripps Green Hospital, La Jolla, California*

**David A. Scheinberg**, MD, PhD
*Attending Physician, Department of Medicine, Leukemia,*
*and Clinical Immunology Services and Hematology*
*Laboratory Service, Department of Clinical Laboratories*
*Memorial Hospital, Chairman, Molecular Pharmacology*
*and Chemistry Program and Experimental Therapeutics*
*Center, Memorial Sloan-Kettering Cancer Center*
*Professor and Co-Chairman, Pharmacology Program*
*Cornell University–Weill Graduate School of Medical*
*Sciences, New York, New York*

**Mikkael A. Sekeres**, MD, MS
*Assistant Professor of Medicine*
*Cleveland Clinic Lerner College of Medicine*
*Department of Hematologic Oncology and Blood*
*Disorders Taussig Cancer Center, Cleveland Clinic,*
*Cleveland, Ohio*

**Jennifer L. Shamp**
*Department of Pharmacy, James Cancer Hospital, The*
*Ohio State University Medical Center, Columbus, Ohio*

**Thomas Shea**, MD
*Professor of Medicine, Department of Medicine*
*Division of Hematology and Oncology*
*University of North Carolina at Chapel Hill*
*Chapel Hill, North Carolina*

**Tamara N. Shenkier**, MD
*Clinical Assistant Professor, University of British*
*Columbia, Medical Oncologist, British Columbia Cancer*
*Agency, Vancouver, British Columbia, Canada*

**Richard T. Silver**, MD
*Professor of Medicine, Weill Cornell Medical College*
*New York Presbyterian Hospital, New York, New York*

**Lewis R. Silverman**, MD
*Associate Professor of Medicine, Director of the*
*Myelodysplastic Syndrome and Myeloproliferative Disease*
*Program, Division of Hematology/Oncology*
*Mount Sinai School of Medicine*
*New York, New York*

**Deepjot Singh**, MD
*Fellow, Case Comprehensive Cancer Center*
*University Hospitals of Cleveland, Cleveland, Ohio*

**James L. Slack**, MD
*Senior Associate Consultant, Mayo Clinic Scottsdale*
*Phoenix, Arizona*

**Sonali M. Smith**, MD
*Assistant Professor of Medicine, Section of*
*Hematology/Oncology, Department of Medicine*
*Division of Biological Sciences, The University of Chicago*
*Chicago, Illinois*

**Ronald M. Sobecks**, MD
*Assistant Professor of Medicine*
*Department of Hematology and Medical Oncology*
*The Cleveland Clinic Lerner College of Medicine*
*Case Western Reserve University, The Cleveland Clinic*
*Foundation, Cleveland, Ohio*

**George Somlo**, MD
*Associate Director for High-Dose Therapeutics*
*Divisions of Medical Oncology and Therapeutic Research*
*and Hematology and Hematopoietic Cell Transplantation*
*City of Hope National Medical Center, Duarte, California*

**Thomas R. Spitzer**, MD
*Professor of Medicine, Harvard Medical School*
*Director, Bone Marrow Transplant Program*
*Massachusetts General Hospital, Boston, Massachusetts*

**Edward A. Stadtmauer**, MD
*Associate Professor of Medicine, University of*
*Pennsylvania School of Medicine, Director, Bone Marrow*
*and Stem Cell Transplant Program, Hospital of the*
*University of Pennsylvania, Philadelphia, Pennsylvania*

**Wendy Stock**, MD
*Associate Professor, Department of Medicine*
*Section of Hematology/Oncology, The University of Chicago*
*Hospital and Pritzker School of Medicine, Chicago, Illinois*

**Richard M. Stone**, MD
*Associate Professor of Medicine, Harvard Medical School*
*Clinical Director, Adult Leukemia Program*
*Dana-Farber Cancer Institute, Boston, Massachusetts*

**Rainer Storb**, MD
*Professor of Medicine, University of Washington*
*Head, Transplantation Biology Program, Member, Fred*
*Hutchinson Cancer Research Center, Seattle, Washington*

**Revathi Suppiah**, MD
*Fellow, Division of Hematology/Oncology, The Cleveland*
*Clinic Foundation, Cleveland, Ohio*

**John W. Sweetenham**, MD
*Professor of Medicine, Cleveland Clinic Lerner College of*
*Medicine, Department of Hematologic Oncology and*
*Blood Disorders, Taussig Cancer Center, Cleveland Clinic*
*Cleveland, Ohio*

**Martin S. Tallman**, MD
*Division of Hematology/Oncology, Feinberg School of*
*Medicine, Northwestern University*
*Robert H. Lurie Comprehensive Cancer Center*
*Chicago, Illinois*

**Ayalew Tefferi**, MD
*Professor of Medicine, Division of Hematology*
*Mayo Clinic, Rochester, Minnesota*

**Karl S. Theil**, MD
*Staff Pathologist, The Cleveland Clinic Foundation*
*Cleveland, Ohio*

**Steven P. Treon,** MD, MA, PhD
*Bing Program for Waldenström's Macroglobulinemia*
*Dana Farber Cancer Institute, Boston, Massachusetts*

**Koen van Besien,** MD
*Professor of Medicine*
*Director, Stem Cell Transplantation and Lymphoma*
*Section of Hematology/Oncology, Department of Medicine*
*Division of Biological Sciences, The University of Chicago*
*Chicago, Illinois*

**Ilka Warshawsky,** MD, PhD
*Departments of Hematology and Medical Oncology and*
*Clinical Pathology, The Cleveland Clinic Foundation*
*Cleveland, Ohio*

**Mark A. Weiss,** MD
*Leukemia Service, Memorial Sloan-Kettering Cancer*
*Center, New York, New York*

**Meir Wetzler,** MD
*Associate Professor of Medicine, Leukemia Section*
*Roswell Park Cancer Institute, Buffalo, New York*

**William G. Wierda,** MD, PhD
*Assistant Professor of Medicine*
*Department of Leukemia, Division of Cancer Medicine*
*The University of Texas M.D. Anderson Cancer Center*
*Houston, Texas*

**Eric Winer,** MD
*Division of Hematology/Oncology and Bone Marrow*
*Transplantation, Tufts New England Medical Center*
*Boston, Massachusetts*

**Karen W. L. Yee,** MD
*Department of Medical Oncology and Hematology*
*Princess Margaret Hospital*
*Toronto, Ontario, Canada*

**Jeffrey A. Zonder,** MD
*Assistant Professor of Medicine*
*Division of Hematology-Oncology, Karmanos Cancer*
*Institute, Assistant Professor of Medicine*
*Department of Internal Medicine, Wayne State University*
*School of Medicine, Detroit, Michigan*

**Emanuele Zucca,** MD
*Privatdozent of Oncology/Haematology, University of Bern*
*Bern, Head, Lymphoma Unit*
*Oncology Institute of Southern Switzerland*
*Department of Medical Oncology*
*Ospedale San Giovanni, Bellinzona, Switzerland*

**Mirko Zuzel,** MD
*Reader, Department of Haematology*
*University of Liverpool, Department of Haematology*
*Royal Liverpool and Broadgreen University Hospital NHS*
*Trust, Liverpool, United Kingdom*

# PREFACE

The clinical aspects of hematologic malignancies have changed dramatically over the past decade. The development of targeted therapies, based on years of advanced understanding of basic scientific mechanisms of disease, has led to their widespread use and ultimately to the first decrease in cancer-related mortality not attributable to screening programs. The impact of these advances will be fully felt over the next two decades, when the population of older adults in the United States is expected to double, and continued evolution of intensive therapy and supportive measures will make approaches such as bone marrow transplantation available to more patients than ever before.

Resources available to clinical oncologists or hematologists who treat patients with hematologic malignancies are limited. With this in mind, we planned a textbook devoted solely to this topic. Recognizing, also, that oncologists and hematologists are busier than ever and require accessible information about specific topics, we asked our authors to write focused chapters that address different aspects of a disease, and that would be useful to both general and disease-specific practicing oncologists and hematologists, physicians-in-training, researchers, and nurses. We are proud of the end-product.

Sections of *Clinical Malignant Hematology* are divided by disease, and each disease is further divided into specialty areas where applicable. These areas include epidemiology, risk factors, and classification; molecular biology, pathology, and cytogenetics; clinical features and making the diagnosis; treatment approach to all disease subtypes; and treatment of relapsed or refractory disease, including new frontiers in therapy. In addition, we have included chapters about specialty topics within hematologic malignancies, both within disease sections and in the last part of the book. These topics range from disease-specific indications for bone marrow transplantation and management of infections to treatment of the pregnant patient with a hematologic malignancy and fertility issues in this patient population.

Chapter authors are world experts in their fields. We asked them to use evidence-based findings in the presentation of their material but not at the expense of offering practical information about managing these complicated and often very sick patients. We are grateful to our authors for rising to this challenge and helping us to produce the first definitive textbook on hematologic malignancies. We welcome your feedback about the content and about any areas you would want to see expanded for future editions, particularly as some material may not keep pace with the rapid change in therapy. We ask you to e-mail comments to our editor at McGraw-Hill, Robert Pancotti: robert_pancotti@mcgraw-hill.com.

Mikkael A. Sekeres, MD, MS
Matt E. Kalaycio, MD
Brian J. Bolwell, MD
*February, 2007*

# ACKNOWLEDGMENTS

A book of this magnitude cannot be accomplished without the help of a number of people at every step of the way. We would like to thank our editors at McGraw-Hill, first Marc Strauss and later Robert Pancotti, whose keen intellect, gentle guidance, sound judgment, and good sense of humor made this project possible. We are grateful for the administrative assistance we received from Bridget Rini, Victoria Mineff, and Fran Palasek, whose help in coordinating the receipt and editing of over 100 chapters was invaluable. Finally, we are deeply appreciative of our chapter authors, who provided us with outstanding information.

# Section 1
# ACUTE MYELOID LEUKEMIA

# Chapter 1
# EPIDEMIOLOGY, RISK FACTORS, AND CLASSIFICATION

*Leonard T. Heffner Jr*

## ACUTE MYELOCYTIC LEUKEMIA

### EPIDEMIOLOGY AND RISK FACTORS

Acute myelocytic leukemia (AML) is a clonal expansion of any one of several nonlymphoid hematopoietic progenitors that retain the capacity of self-renewal, but are severely limited in their ability to differentiate into functional mature cells. These various progenitors include cells of granulocytic, monocyte/macrophage, erythroid, and megakaryocytic lineage.

Leukemia is not a common malignancy relative to many other forms of cancer, comprising 3% of all new cancers in males and less than 2% in females. Deaths from leukemia comprised 4.3% of all cancer deaths in males in 2006 and 3.3% in females. In 2006, it was estimated there were 11,930 new cases of AML, representing 34% of all forms of leukemia. An estimated 9040 deaths due to AML occurred in 2006—40.6% of deaths from all leukemias. Both the incidence and the number of deaths are slightly greater in males versus females.[1] Surveillance, epidemiology, and end-results (SEER) data over a 25-year period from 1973 to 1998 show that the incidence rates by age groups have been stable, other than a slight increase in the age group above or equal to 65 years old.[2] As per the SEER data (1996–2000), 86% of acute leukemia in adults (>20 years old) is AML.

Although there are several well-recognized risk factors for the development of AML, little is known about the etiology of most cases. Like most malignancies, there is no recognized factor common to most cases of AML. While there is little reason to assume that adult and childhood leukemia do not have a common etiology, differences in tumor biology and outcomes suggest that these disorders are significantly different. Proven or possible risk factors for AML can be categorized as genetic, environmental, and therapy-related. At this time, the proven risk factors include only radiation, benzene exposure, and chemotherapeutic agents.[3–9]

Studies of leukemia in identical twins have shed considerable light on the pathogenesis of this disease. While concordance rates for monochorionic, monozygotic twin childhood leukemia is less than 25%, concordance in infants (<1-year old) is nearly 100%.[10–15] This implies that events occurring in utero are sufficient for the rapid development of acute leukemia and that clonal progeny spread from the initially affected fetus to the other fetus via shared placental circulation. Yet, in older twin children the discordance rate is 90%, indicating the prenatal event is insufficient for leukemogenesis and a second postnatal event is required, probably involving genes regulating a proliferation or survival function. In adult twins there is no evidence of concordance.[16]

Familial acute leukemia outside of a recognized medical syndrome is rare, but there are documented familial clusters of specific subtypes of AML.[17,18] There are also a number of medical syndromes in which AML is a component feature, including Down syndrome, Bloom syndrome, Fanconi anemia, neurofibromatosis I, ataxia-telangiectasia, Schwachman syndrome, and dyskaratosis congenita.[19–25] Many of these disorders have been associated with both AML and acute lymphocytic leukemia (Table 1.1).

**Table 1.1    Conditions associated with an increased incidence of AML**

| Genetic | Environmental |
|---|---|
| Identical twin with leukemia | Radiation |
| Familial leukemia | Ionizing |
| Down syndrome | Nonionizing |
| Bloom syndrome | Chemicals |
| Fanconi anemia | Benzene |
| Neurofibromatosis I | Pesticides |
| Schwachman syndrome | Smoking |
| Dyskrytosis congenital | |
| Ataxia-telangiectasia | |
| Acquired hematologic diseases | Therapy related |
| Chronic myelocytic leukemia | Alkylating agents |
| Myelofibrosis | Topoisomerase II Inhibitors |
| Essential thrombocythemia | DNA intercalating agents |
| Polycythemia rubra vera | |
| Aplastic anemia | |
| Paroxysmal noctural hemoglobinuria | |

The effects of acute high-dose exposure from the nuclear explosions at Hiroshima and Nagasaki as well as the nuclear accident at Chernobyl demonstrate the leukemogenic potential of ionizing radiation.[3,26] Follow-up of the atomic bomb survivors through 1990 identified 249 leukemic deaths, with 53.7% attributable to radiation exposure. In this population, there is an excess relative risk of leukemia (ERR) per sievert of 4.62 compared with an ERR of 0.40 for other cancers.[27] The risk appears to be greatest at 5–10 years after exposure.[28] Evaluation of the specific types of leukemia in the life span study (LSS) of atomic bomb survivors showed the highest ERR for acute lymphocytic leukemia (Table 1.2), although those exposed to gamma irradiation at Nagasaki more commonly had AML.[28,29] Leukemogenic risks for lower doses of ionizing radiation are less clear, and are complicated by the need to distinguish acute versus protracted low-dose exposure. Table 1.3 outlines the levels of exposure to radiation in routine daily activity compared to the episodes of more acute exposure. Among the cohort in the LSS study with exposure of 5–100 mSv (mean for entire study 200 mSv), there is a statistically significant increased incidence of solid organ cancer compared to the population exposed to less than 5 mSv.[30] Chronic low-dose exposure studies in workers in nuclear plants have found an increased risk of leukemia, although these studies have some limitations and are not all statistically significant.[31] A greater than expected risk of AML has been reported in the use of low doses of radiation for benign medical conditions, such as menorrhagia, ankylosing spondylitis, rheumatoid arthritis, tinea capitis, and peptic ulcer disease.[32–36] Exposure to the chronic low dose a-particles of thorium dioxide in Thorotrast has been associated with an increased incidence of the acute erythroleukemia subtype of AML.[37] However, there is no evidence that diagnostic X-rays are causally related to leukemia.[38,39] The contribution of nonionizing radiation to the development of leukemia is unclear, as there have been conflicting results and criticism of the methodologies in some studies. At this time, there is no evidence of a major contribution of either occupational or residential electromagnetic field exposure resulting in an increased incidence of leukemia.[40–42] Cosmic radiation exposure has been shown to increase slightly the risk of AML in commercial jet pilots.[43,44]

Among environmental factors associated with an increased risk of leukemia, benzene has been studied extensively. Occupational benzene exposure in the leather, petrochemical, rubber, and printing industries has been linked to an excess incidence of leukemia.[8,45,46] Ethylene oxide, butadiene, and styrene are industrial chemicals that have been associated with leukemia, but studies have been somewhat inconsistent or inconclusive in establishing a direct link.[47–51] Pesticide use has been suggested as a possible explanation for the increased risk of dying from leukemia among farmers and other agricultural workers.[52] However, other case-control and cohort studies have

**Table 1.2    Leukemia incidence by cell type and corresponding model-based risk estimates for LSS cohort or atomic bomb survivors**

| Leukemia subtype | Number of cases | Excess relative risk per Sv | Attributable risk (%) | Excess absolute risk (cases per $10^4$ person years at 1 Sv) |
|---|---|---|---|---|
| ALL | 38 | 9.1 | 70 | 0.62 |
| AML | 117 | 3.3 | 46 | 1.1 |
| CML | 62 | 6.2 | 62 | 0.9 |
| All leukemias (includes unspecified types, CLL, etc.) | 231 | 3.9 | 50 | 2.7 |

Reprinted from Zeeb H, Blettner M: Adult leukemia: what is the role of currently known risk factors? *Radiat Environ Biophys* 36:217–228, 1998, copyright 1998 Springer.

**Table 1.3** Approximate mean doses relevant to societal low-dose radiation exposures and to low-dose radiation risk estimation

|  | Approx. mean individual dose (mSv) |
|---|---|
| Round trip flight, New York to London | 0.1 |
| Single screening mammogram (breast dose) | 3 |
| Background dose due to natural radiation exposure | 3/year |
| Dose (over a 70-year period) to 0.5 million individuals in rural Ukraine in the vicinity of the Chernobyl accident | 14 |
| Dose range over 20-block radius from hypothetical nuclear terrorism incident (FASEB scenario 1: medical gauge containing cesium) | 3–30 |
| Pediatric CT scan (stomach dose from abdominal scan) | 25 |
| Radiation worker exposure limit | 20/year |
| Exposure on international space station | 170/year |
| A-bomb survivors (mean dose in LSS cohort) | 200 |
| Medical X-rays (breasts dose in scoliosis study) | 100 |
| Nuclear workers (mean dose from major studies) | 20 |
| Individuals diagnostically exposed in utero | 10 |

Modified from Brenner DJ, et al.: Cancer risks attributable to low doses of ionizing radiation: assessing what we really know. *PNAS* 100:13761–13766, 2003, copyright 2003 National Academy of Sciences, U.S.A.

failed to show an association between pesticide exposure and leukemia.[53,54] Indeed, there has been no evidence for an increased risk of AML related to pesticide exposure, although studies have implicated an increased risk of childhood leukemia.[55] Cigarette smoking has been found in several studies to produce a mild increased risk of leukemia, especially AML, possibly related to the presence of benzene in tobacco smoke.[46,56–58] Indeed, the International Agency for Research on Cancer (IARC) recently reviewed eight cohort studies, with six showing a greater than expected risk of myeloid leukemia.[59] Interestingly, it appears the smoking-associated risk for AML may be restricted to the t(8;21) subgroup.[60] Despite these data, a large prospective cohort study of 334,957 construction workers failed to show evidence that smoking bears any major relationship to the occurrence of leukemia.[61] The use of hair dyes known to contain animal carcinogens has been associated with a slight increased risk of acute leukemia of both myeloid and lymphoid type. This risk seems to be greatest for the use of permanent dyes and for longer and more frequent usage, with no increased risk for nonpermanent dyes.[62] However, two other cohort studies failed to find any consistent association between hair dye use

and hematopoietic cancers.[63,64] Viruses have long been suspected as a causal agent in leukemia, and the retrovirus HTLV-1 has been linked to adult T-cell leukemia/lymphoma.[65] However, there has as yet been no convincing evidence of a viral etiology of adult AML.

The development of acute leukemia in long-term survivors of Hodgkin's lymphoma raised the awareness of a relationship of leukemia to prior chemotherapy.[66,67] An increased incidence of treatment-related AML (tAML) has been found in both benign and malignant diseases for which alkylating agents have been a major part of the therapy, and it is felt that 10–15% of all leukemias are therapy-related.[6,9,68] Secondary disease following treatment may occur in 0–20% of cases.[69] All of the commonly used alkylating agents have been associated with an increased risk of AML, including busulfan, chlorambucil, BCNU, CCNU, cyclophosphamide, mechlorethamine, and procarbazine.[6,9] Typically, in Hodgkin's lymphoma treated with the MOPP (mechlorethamine, vincristine, procarbazine, prednisone), the incidence of AML peaks at 7 years, but may occur even in the first 2 years post-treatment.[70,71] A common characteristic of these therapy-related leukemias is the loss of all or part of chromosomes 5 and/or 7, occurring in 50–90% of cases, often with a complex karyotype.[72,73] There is also an increased risk of AML following treatment with the topoisomerase II inhibitors, notably etoposide and tenoposide. In contrast to the other forms of tAML, this group of leukemias typically show translocations involving the *mixed-lineage leukemia (MLL)* gene on chromosome 11 (band 11q23) or the *AML1* gene on chromosome 21 (band q22). Most commonly, there is a shorter interval between drug exposure and diagnosis of AML, without a preceding myelodysplastic syndrome (MDS) phase.[74,75] Phenotypically, these cases are usually myelomonocytic or monocytic. Additionally, the DNA intercalating agents, such as doxorubicin, are associated with a type of AML similar to that associated with the topoisomerase II inhibitors.[76] The natural history of some hematologic disorders, such as polycythemia vera, essential thrombocythemia, myelofibrosis, and aplastic anemia, is associated with a slightly increased risk of AML, but that risk increases with the use of chemotherapeutic agents, radiotherapy, or immunosuppressive therapy.[77–80] High-dose chemotherapy followed by autologous stem cell transplantation (ASCT) for lymphoma can be complicated by the development of tAML/MDS.[81] The actuarial risk in multiple series has varied from 3% to 24%. Median time from ASCT to development of tAML/MDS is 47–50 months, and has been variably influenced by pretransplant therapy, the conditioning regimen, and stem cell mobilization.[82] As the mechanisms by which leukemia develops as a consequence of these environmental exposures are learned, the burgeoning field of molecular epidemiology will further allow the determination of the risk of subsequent leukemia in these exposed populations.

## AML: CLASSIFICATION

Although acute leukemia has long been recognized as a hematologic malignancy, it has been only in the last 50 years that AML has been looked at as a distinct entity. Indeed, classification of the acute leukemias was primarily based on age and cell morphology, with the adult form being predominately granulocytic with some variants based primarily on the cell type, such as promyelocytic, monocytic (Schilling), myelomonocytic (Naegli), or erythroleukemia of DiGuglielmo. However, there was considerable difficulty at times distinguishing between lymphoid and myeloid acute leukemias other than by age at onset. The development of reliable histochemical staining by Hayhoe and colleagues in the 1960s improved our diagnostic accuracy, but did not produce a clear system of classification.

In 1976, some order was introduced into the classification of the morphologically heterogeneous acute leukemias with the establishment of the French-American–British (FAB) system.[83] The FAB classification was based on morphology, cellularity, blast percentage, and cytochemistry, and was modified over the next several years with the recognition of AML of megakaryocytic lineage (AML-M7) and of minimally differentiated leukemia (AML-M0).[84,85] A limitation of the FAB classification has been the clinical diversity of AML, as well as the emerging genetic diversity of the disease and the lack of correlation to improvement in treatment outcomes. In addition, over the past several decades there has been an increasing recognition of a group of hematologic disorders variously designated as preleukemia or myelodysplasia, which preceded the diagnosis of AML in many, but clearly not all cases. It is important to know and remember the FAB system both for historical purposes and because many important clinical trials still being followed and reported are based on that system.

Beginning in 1995, a project was begun by the World Health Organization (WHO) involving an international group of pathologists, assisted by a clinical advisory committee of expert hematologists, to establish a classification of hematologic malignancies. AMLs are recognized as one of the three main categories of myeloid neoplasms, along with MDSs and myeloproliferative disorders. This classification draws on the combination of morphology, immunophenotype, genetic features, and clinical syndromes. In particular, this system also more formally incorporates the relationship of AML to the MDSs.

The major goal of the WHO classification was to develop a clinically relevant system that could incorporate the genetic and clinical features of AML with the morphology and newer biological information about the disease. An attempt was made to discriminate between distinct disease entities as opposed to

prognostic factors, especially with the increasing information on genetic abnormalities in AML. This has led to recognition of four main groups within the category of AML: (1) AML with recurrent cytogenetic translocations, (2) AML with multilineage dysplasia, (3) AML and MDSs, therapy-related, and (4) AML not otherwise categorized. Within each group are several subcategories, as outlined in Table 1.4.

In addition to placing patients with AML into unique clinical and biological subgroups, the other major departure with the FAB system was the lowering of the threshold for the number of blasts in the blood or bone marrow to 20% rather than 30%. This is based on the data showing similar outcomes and biological features in the patients with 20–29% blasts, who were previously classified as having MDS compared to those patients with traditional AML.

Approximately 30% of patients with newly diagnosed AML will have one of the four well-defined cytogenetic abnormalities listed in Table 1.4. Because patients with these abnormalities have a somewhat distinctive phenotype and a relatively favorable response to treatment, they can be considered distinct clinicopathological entities. While other balanced translocations are considered recurring genetic abnormalities, it is felt that these abnormalities have more prognostic import. Undoubtedly, as we learn more

| Table 1.4   WHO classification of AMLs |
| --- |
| A. AML with recurrent cytogenetic translocations |
|   ■ AML with t(8;21)(q22;q22), AML1(CBFα)/ETO |
|   ■ AML with t(15;17)(q22;q11–12) and variants (PML/RARα) |
|   ■ AML with abnormal bone marrow eosinophils Inv(16)(p13q22) or t(16;16)(p13;q11), (CBFβ/MYH11X) |
|   ■ AML with 11q23(MLL) abnormalities |
| B. AML with multilineage dysplasia |
|   ■ with prior myelodysplastic syndrome |
|   ■ without prior myelodysplastic syndrome |
| C. AML and myelodysplastic syndromes, therapy-related |
|   ■ alkylating agent-related |
|   ■ epipodophyllotoxin-related (some may be lymphoid) |
|   ■ other types |
| D. AML not otherwise categorized |
|   ■ AML minimally differentiated |
|   ■ AML without differentiation |
|   ■ AML with maturation |
|   ■ acute myelomonocytic leukemia |
|   ■ acute monocytic leukemia |
|   ■ acute erythroid leukemia |
|   ■ acute megakaryocytic leukemia |
|   ■ acute basophilic leukemia |
|   ■ acute panmyelosis with myelofibrosis |
| E. Acute biphenotypic leukemia |

Modified from Jaffe ES, et al.: World Health Organization Classification of Tumors: Pathology and Genetics of Tumors of Haematopoietic and Lymphoid Tissues. Lyon, France: IARC Press; 2001:45–107, Copyright 2001 International Agency for Research on Cancer.

about the significance of these and other genetic abnormalities, the WHO classification will need to be modified.

While many cases of AML present with a well-documented history of myelodysplasia, often there are dysplastic changes in the blood and bone marrow at the time of diagnosis of AML without an antecedent history of MDS. The WHO attempts to resolve this dilemma of the relationship between these two entities by establishing the classification of AML with multilineage dysplasia. The recognition of AML in this category without prior MDS requires at least 20% blasts in the blood or bone marrow and dysplastic changes in at least 50% of cells in 2 or more myeloid lineages. It is actually felt by some that AML should be divided into the two large categories of true de novo AML and myelodysplasia-related AML.

Exposure to certain therapies, such as alkylating agents and topoisomoerase II inhibitors, has long been known to increase the risk of the subsequent development of AML. The WHO classification places these cases in a separate category, divided into two groups, based on the known agents associated with this risk. While there are common features between these groups, there is sufficient difference to justify each. The topoisomerase II inhibitor-related AML generally has a shorter latency period between exposure to the mutagen and development of AML. This may be as little as 6 months, but can be as long as 6 years, with a median time of 2–3 years compared to 4–7 years for alkylating agent-related AML. In addition, topoisomerase II inhibitor-related AML typically presents without MDS features, often has a monocytic component, and includes balanced translocations as the genetic abnormality.

Unfortunately, no classification system will be entirely inclusive, and the WHO recognizes this with the group of AML, not otherwise categorized. This group corresponds in most cases to the same morphologic entity as is delineated in the FAB schema. Indeed, this is pointed out as a limitation of the system, one which gives the clinician no help in planning therapy for a given case of AML. However, those who developed the WHO classification point out that the system is meant to be of worldwide application, and that there will be places where the diagnostic facilities are not yet sophisticated enough to provide information to make a more specific categorization. This last category of AML does include the entity of acute erythroid leukemia, and recognizes that there are two subtypes. Pure erythroid leukemia has at least 80% immature erythroid precursors with minimal differentiation and no significant myeloblastic component, as distinguished from the second subtype, which has at least 50% immature erythroid precursors and 20% myeloblasts in the nonerythroid population.

Modifications of the WHO classification will continue to be made with advances in our knowledge of the biology and treatment of AML. An International Working Group has recently recommended some definitions of terminology. Thus, de novo AML is defined as "AML in patients with no clinical history of prior MDS, myeloproliferative disorder, or exposure to potentially leukemogenic therapies or agents." Secondary AML is defined as those patients with AML who do have prior MDS or exposure to leukemogenic therapies and should be categorized as "AML secondary to prior existing MDS, myeloproliferative disorder, or the development of AML secondary to proven leukemogenic exposure."[86]

## REFERENCES

1. Jemal A, Tiwari RC, Murray T, et al.: Cancer statistics. *CA Cancer J Clin* 54(1):8–29, 2004.
2. Xie Y, Davies SM, Xiang Y, et al.: Trends in leukemia incidence and survival in the United States (1973–1998). *Cancer* 97(9):2229–2235, 2003.
3. Kato H, WJ Schull: Studies of the mortality of A-bomb survivors. 7. Mortality, 1950–1978. Part I: Cancer mortality. *Radiat Res* 90(2):395–432, 1982.
4. Adamson RH, SM Seiber: Chemically induced leukemia in humans. *Environ Health Perspect* 39:93–103, 1981.
5. Bernard J: The epidemiology of leukemias (past, present, future). *Nouv Rev Fr Hematol* 31(2):103–109, 1989.
6. Levine EG, Bloomfield CD: Leukemias and myelodysplastic syndromes secondary to drug, radiation, and environmental exposure. *Semin Oncol* 19(1):47–84, 1992.
7. Thirman MJ, Larson RA: Therapy-related myeloid leukemia. *Hematol Oncol Clin North Am* 10(2):293–320, 1996.
8. Austin H, Delzell E, Cole P: Benzene and leukemia. A review of the literature and a risk assessment. *Am J Epidemiol* 127(3):419–439, 1988.
9. Kyle RA: Second malignancies associated with chemotherapeutic agents. *Semin Oncol* 9(1):131–142, 1982.
10. Keith L, Brown E: Leukemia in twins: world-wide review of clinical cases. *Acta Genet Med Gemellol (Roma)* 19(1):66–68, 1970.
11. Hitzig WH, Rampini S: Leukemia in twins; 4 case reports & review of literature. *Helv Paediatr Acta* 14(1):67–97, 1959.
12. Macmahon B, Levy MA: Prenatal origin of childhood leukemia. Evidence from twins. *N Engl J Med* 270:1082–1085, 1964.
13. Keith L, Brown E: Epidemiologic study of leukemia in twins (1928–1969). *Acta Genet Med Gemellol (Roma)* 20(1):9–22, 1971.
14. Miller RW: Deaths from childhood leukemia and solid tumors among twins and other sibs in the United States, 1960–1967. *J Natl Cancer Inst* 46(1):203–209, 1971.
15. Greaves MF, Maia AT, Wiemels, JL, et al.: Leukemia in twins: lessons in natural history. *Blood* 102(7):2321–2333, 2003.

16. Harnden DG: Inherited factors in leukaemia and lymphoma. *Leuk Res* 9(6):705–707, 1985.

17. Horwitz M: The genetics of familial leukemia. *Leukemia* 11(8):1347–1359, 1997.

18. Novik Y, Marino P, Makower DF, et al.: Familial erythroleukemia: a distinct clinical and genetic type of familial leukemias. *Leuk Lymphoma* 30(3/4):395–401, 1998.

19. Zipursky A, Poon A, Doyle J: Leukemia in Down syndrome: a review. *Pediatr Hematol Oncol* 9(2):139–149, 1992.

20. Morrell D, Cromartie E, Swift M: Mortality and cancer incidence in 263 patients with ataxia-telangiectasia. *J Natl Cancer Inst* 77(1):89–92, 1986.

21. Butturini A, Gale RP, Verlander PC, et al.: Hematologic abnormalities in Fanconi anemia: an international Fanconi anemia registry study. *Blood* 84(5):1650–1655, 1994.

22. Largaespada DA, Brannan CI, Shaughnessy JD, et al.: The neurofibromatosis type 1 (NF1) tumor suppressor gene and myeloid leukemia. *Curr Top Microbiol Immunol* 211:233–239, 1996.

23. German J, Bloom D, Passarge E: Bloom's syndrome. VII: progress report for 1978. *Clin Genet* 15(4):361–367, 1979.

24. Woods WG, Roloff JS, Lukens JN, et al.: The occurrence of leukemia in patients with the Shwachman syndrome. *J Pediatr* 99(3):425–428, 1981.

25. Filipovich AH, Heinitz KJ, Robison LL, et al.: The immunodeficiency cancer registry. A research resource. *Am J Pediatr Hematol Oncol* 9(2):183–184, 1987.

26. Noshchenko AG, Zamostyan PV, Bondar OY, et al.: Radiation-induced leukemia risk among those aged 0–20 at the time of the Chernobyl accident: a case-control study in the Ukraine. *Int J Cancer* 99(4):609–618, 2002.

27. Pierce DA, Shimizu Y, Preston DL, et al.: Studies of the mortality of atomic bomb survivors. Report 12, Part I: Cancer: 1950–1990. *Radiat Res* 146(1):1–27, 1996.

28. Preston DL, Kusumi S, Tomonaga M, et al.: Cancer incidence in atomic bomb survivors. Part III: Leukemia, lymphoma and multiple myeloma, 1950–1987. *Radiat Res* 137(suppl 2):S68–S97, 1994.

29. Ishimaru T, Otake M, Ischimaru M: Dose-response relationship of neutrons and gamma rays to leukemia incidence among atomic bomb survivors in Hiroshima and Nagasaki by type of leukemia, 1950–1971. *Radiat Res* 77(2):377–394, 1979.

30. Pierce DA, Preston DL: Radiation-related cancer risks at low doses among atomic bomb survivors. *Radiat Res* 154(2):178–186, 2000.

31. Gilbert ES: Invited commentary: studies of workers exposed to low doses of radiation. *Am J Epidemiol* 153(4):319–322, 2001; discussion: 323–324.

32. Inskip PD, Kleinerman RA, Stovall M, et al.: Leukemia, lymphoma, and multiple myeloma after pelvic radiotherapy for benign disease. *Radiat Res* 135(1):108–124, 1993.

33. Darby SC, Doll R, Gill SK, et al.: Long term mortality after a single treatment course with X-rays in patients treated for ankylosing spondylitis. *Br J Cancer* 55(2):179–190, 1987.

34. Urowitz MB, Rider WD: Myeloproliferative disorders in patients with rheumatoid arthritis treated with total body irradiation. *Am J Med* 78(1A):60–64, 1985.

35. Hempelmann LH, Hall WJ, Phillips M, et al.: Neoplasms in persons treated with X-rays in infancy: fourth survey in 20 years. *J Natl Cancer Inst* 55(3):519–530, 1975.

36. Griem ML, Kleinerman RA, Boice JD Jr, et al.: Cancer following radiotherapy for peptic ulcer. *J Natl Cancer Inst* 86(11):842–849, 1994.

37. Andersson MB, Carstensen B, Visfeldt J: Leukemia and other related hematological disorders among Danish patients exposed to Thorotrast. *Radiat Res* 134(2):224–233, 1993.

38. Boice JD Jr, Morin MM, Glass AG, et al.: Diagnostic X-ray procedures and risk of leukemia, lymphoma, and multiple myeloma. *JAMA* 265(10):1290–1294, 1991.

39. Davis FG, Boice JD Jr, Hrubec Z, et al.: Cancer mortality in a radiation-exposed cohort of Massachusetts tuberculosis patients. *Cancer Res* 49(21):6130–6136, 1989.

40. Savitz DA: Overview of epidemiologic research on electric and magnetic fields and cancer. *Am Ind Hyg Assoc J* 54(4):197–204, 1993.

41. Feychting M: Occupational exposure to electromagnetic fields and adult leukaemia: a review of the epidemiological evidence. *Radiat Environ Biophys* 35(4):237–242, 1996.

42. Li CY, Theriault G, Lin RS: Epidemiological appraisal of studies of residential exposure to power frequency magnetic fields and adult cancers. *Occup Environ Med* 53(8):505–510, 1996.

43. Gundestrup M, Storm HH: Radiation-induced acute myeloid leukaemia and other cancers in commercial jet cockpit crew: a population-based cohort study. *Lancet* 354(9195):2029–2031, 1999.

44. Band PR, Le ND, Fang R, et al.: Cohort study of Air Canada pilots: mortality, cancer incidence, and leukemia risk. *Am J Epidemiol* 143(2):137–143, 1996.

45. Brandt L, Nilsson PG, Mitelman F: Occupational exposure to petroleum products in men with acute non-lymphocytic leukaemia. *Br Med J* 1(6112):553, 1978.

46. Rinsky RA, Smith AB, Hornung R, et al.: Benzene and leukemia. An epidemiologic risk assessment. *N Engl J Med* 316(17):1044–1050, 1987.

47. Shore RE, Gardner MJ, Pannett B: Ethylene oxide: an assessment of the epidemiological evidence on carcinogenicity. *Br J Ind Med* 50(11):971–997, 1993.

48. Cole P, Delzell E, Acquavella J: Exposure to butadiene and lymphatic and hematopoietic cancer. *Epidemiology* 4(2):96–103, 1993.

49. Santos-Burgoa C, Matanoski GM, Zeger S, et al.: Lymphohematopoietic cancer in styrene-butadiene polymerization workers. *Am J Epidemiol* 136(7):843–854, 1992.

50. Kogevinas M, Ferro G, Andersen A, et al.: Cancer mortality in a historical cohort study of workers exposed to styrene. *Scand J Work Environ Health* 20(4):251–261, 1994.

51. Kolstad HA, Lynge E, Olsen J, et al.: Incidence of lymphohematopoietic malignancies among styrene-exposed workers of the reinforced plastics industry. *Scand J Work Environ Health* 20(4):272–278, 1994.

52. Richardson S, Zittoun R, Bastuji-Garin S, et al.: Occupational risk factors for acute leukaemia: a case-control study. *Int J Epidemiol* 21(6):1063–1073, 1992.

53. Kristensen P, Andersen A, Irgens LM, et al.: Incidence and risk factors of cancer among men and women in

Norwegian agriculture. *Scand J Work Environ Health* 22(1):14–26, 1996.

54. Figa-Talamanca I, Mearelli I, Valente P, et al.: Cancer mortality in a cohort of rural licensed pesticide users in the province of Rome. *Int J Epidemiol* 22(4):579–583, 1993.

55. Alavanja MC, Hoppin JA, Kamel F: Health effects of chronic pesticide exposure: cancer and neurotoxicity*3. *Annu Rev Public Health* 25:155–197, 2004.

56. Siegel M: Smoking and leukemia: evaluation of a causal hypothesis. *Am J Epidemiol* 138(1):1–9, 1993.

57. Brownson RC, Novotny TE, Perry MC: Cigarette smoking and adult leukemia. A meta-analysis. *Arch Intern Med* 153(4):469–475, 1993.

58. Korte JE, Hertz-Picciotto I, Schulz MR, et al.: The contribution of benzene to smoking-induced leukemia. *Environ Health Perspect*, 108(4):333–339, 2000.

59. Vineis P, Alavanja M, Buffler P, et al.: Tobacco and cancer: recent epidemiological evidence. *J Natl Cancer Inst* 96(2):99–106, 2004.

60. Moorman AV, Roman E, Cartwright RA, et al.: Smoking and the risk of acute myeloid leukaemia in cytogenetic subgroups. *Br J Cancer* 86(1):60–62, 2002.

61. Adami J, Nyren O, Bergstrom R, et al.: Smoking and the risk of leukemia, lymphoma, and multiple myeloma (Sweden). *Cancer Causes Control* 9(1):49–56, 1998.

62. Rauscher GH, Shore D, Sandler DP: Hair dye use and risk of adult acute leukemia. *Am J Epidemiol* 160(1):19–25, 2004.

63. Altekruse SF, Henley SJ, Thun MJ: Deaths from hematopoietic and other cancers in relation to permanent hair dye use in a large prospective study (United States). *Cancer Causes Control* 10(6):617–625, 1999.

64. Grodstein F, Hennekens CH, Colditz GA, et al.: A prospective study of permanent hair dye use and hematopoietic cancer. *J Natl Cancer Inst* 86(19):1466–1470, 1994.

65. Tajima K, Cartier L: Epidemiological features of HTLV-I and adult T cell leukemia. *Intervirology* 38(3–4):238–246, 1995.

66. Rowley JD, Golomb HM, Vardiman J: Acute leukemia after treatment of lymphoma. *N Engl J Med* 297(18):1013, 1977.

67. Kaldor JM, Day NE, Clarke EA, et al.: Leukemia following Hodgkin's disease. *N Engl J Med* 322(1):7–13, 1990.

68. Kantarjian HM, Keating MJ: Therapy-related leukemia and myelodysplastic syndrome. *Semin Oncol* 14(4):435–443, 1987.

69. Rowley JD, Olney HJ: International workshop on the relationship of prior therapy to balanced chromosome aberrations in therapy-related myelodysplastic syndromes and acute leukemia: overview report. *Genes Chromosomes Cancer* 33(4):331–345, 2002.

70. Cadman EC, Capizzi RL, Bertino JR: Acute non-lymphocytic leukemia: a delayed complication of Hodgkin's disease therapy: analysis of 109 cases. *Cancer* 40(3):1280–1296, 1977.

71. Pedersen-Bjergaard J, Philip P, Pedersen NT, et al.: Acute non-lymphocytic leukemia, preleukemia, and acute myeloproliferative syndrome secondary to treatment of other malignant diseases. II: Bone marrow cytology, cytogenetics, results of HLA typing, response to antileukemic chemotherapy, and survival in a total series of 55 patients. *Cancer* 54(3):452–462, 1984.

72. Le Beau MM, Albain KS, Larson RA, et al.: Clinical and cytogenetic correlations in 63 patients with therapy-related myelodysplastic syndromes and acute nonlymphocytic leukemia: further evidence for characteristic abnormalities of chromosomes no. 5 and 7. *J Clin Oncol* 4(3):325–345, 1986.

73. Heim S, Mitelman F: Cytogenetic analysis in the diagnosis of acute leukemia. *Cancer* 70(suppl 6):1701–1709, 1992.

74. Ratain MJ, Rowley JD: Therapy-related acute myeloid leukemia secondary to inhibitors of topoisomerase II: from the bedside to the target genes. *Ann Oncol* 3(2):107–111, 1992.

75. Sandoval C, Pui CH, Bowman LC, et al.: Secondary acute myeloid leukemia in children previously treated with alkylating agents, intercalating topoisomerase II inhibitors, and irradiation. *J Clin Oncol* 11(6):1039–1045, 1993.

76. Larson RA, LeBeau MM, Vardiman JW, et al.: Myeloid leukemia after hematotoxins. *Environ Health Perspect* 104(suppl 6):1303–1307, 1996.

77. Bloomfield CD, Brunning RD: Acute leukemia as a terminal event in nonleukemic hematopoietic disorders. *Semin Oncol* 3(3):297–317, 1976.

78. Bolanos-Meade J, Lopez-Arvizu C, Cobos E: Acute myeloid leukaemia arising from a patient with untreated essential thrombocythaemia. *Eur J Haematol* 68(6):397–399, 2002.

79. van den Anker-Lugtenburg PJ, SizooW: Myelodysplastic syndrome and secondary acute leukemia after treatment of essential thrombocythemia with hydroxyurea. *Am J Hematol* 33(2):152, 1990.

80. Devine DV, Gluck WL, Rosse WF, et al.: Acute myeloblastic leukemia in paroxysmal nocturnal hemoglobinuria. Evidence of evolution from the abnormal paroxysmal nocturnal hemoglobinuria clone. *J Clin Invest* 79(1):314–317, 1987.

81. Traweek ST, Slovak ML, Nademanee AP, et al.: Myelodysplasia and acute myeloid leukemia occurring after autologous bone marrow transplantation for lymphoma. *Leuk Lymphoma* 20(5–6):365–372, 1996.

82. Gilliland DG, Gribben JG: Evaluation of the risk of therapy-related MDS/AML after autologous stem cell transplantation. *Biol Blood Marrow Transplant* 8(1):9–16, 2002.

83. Bennett JM, Catovsky D, Daniel MT, et al.: Proposals for the classification of the acute leukaemias. French–American–British (FAB) Cooperative Group. *Br J Haematol* 33(4):451–458, 1976.

84. Bennett JM, Catovsky D, Daniel MT, et al.: Criteria for the diagnosis of acute leukemia of megakaryocyte lineage (M7). A report of the French–American–British Cooperative Group. *Ann Intern Med* 103(3):460–462, 1985.

85. Bennett JM, Catovsky D, Daniel MT, et al.: Proposal for the recognition of minimally differentiated acute myeloid leukaemia (AML-MO). *Br J Haematol* 78(3):325–329, 1991.

86. Cheson BD, Bennett JM, Kopecky KJ, et al.: Revised recommendations of the international working group for diagnosis, standardization of response criteria, treatment outcomes, and reporting standards for therapeutic trials in acute myeloid leukemia. *J Clin Oncol* 21(24):4642–4649, 2003.

# Chapter 2

# MOLECULAR BIOLOGY, PATHOLOGY, AND CYTOGENETICS OF ACUTE MYELOID LEUKEMIA

## Krzysztof Mrózek, Claudia D. Baldus, and Clara D. Bloomfield

## INTRODUCTION

The term acute myeloid leukemia (AML) is used to describe several neoplastic blood disorders characterized by clonal expansion of immature myeloid cells in the bone marrow (BM), blood, or other tissue,[1,2] as a result of increased cell proliferation, prolonged survival, and/or disruption of differentiation of hematopoietic progenitor cells. Although the etiology of AML is still unknown, the risk of developing AML is increased by exposure to ionizing radiation and chemical mutagens such as alkylating agents, benzene, and topoisomerase II inhibitors. The risk of AML is also considerably greater in patients suffering from Down syndrome and rare genetic disorders such as Bloom syndrome, neurofibromatosis, Schwachman syndrome, ataxia-telangiectasia, Klinefelter syndrome, Fanconi anemia, and Kostmann granulocytic leukemia.[3] The aforementioned associations suggest a role of genetic factors in initiating leukemogenesis. Indeed, advances in basic and clinical research have revealed that malignant transformation in all patients with AML, the vast majority of whom do not suffer from inherited genetic disorders, is associated with acquisition of somatic mutations and/or epigenetic events, such as hypermethylation, that affect and change expression of genes involved in hematopoiesis.

Many AML-associated genetic rearrangements can be detected cytogenetically as nonrandom chromosome abnormalities, while others are submicroscopic and detectable only by molecular genetic techniques [e.g., a reverse transcription polymerase chain reaction (RT-PCR)].[4-6] A single genetic abnormality is usually not sufficient to cause overt leukemia, but multiple alterations of different pathways within the same cell are involved in the process of leukemogenesis. It appears that at least two different kinds of mutations

must occur in the hematopoietic progenitor cell to transform it into a malignant cell, initiating development of a clonal AML blast population. These are (1) mutations that activate genes involved in signal transduction of proliferation pathways and thereby confer a survival advantage and increase the rate of cell proliferation (referred to as "class I mutations"), and (2) mutations of genes encoding hematopoietic transcription factors, in the form of either gene fusions generated by reciprocal chromosome translocations or intragenic mutations, which disrupt the process of normal cell differentiation ("class II mutations").[7]

A number of cytogenetic and molecular genetic rearrangements correlate well with the morphology and/or immunophenotype of leukemic marrow and blood, as well as the patients' clinical characteristics, and are therefore incorporated into the World Health Organization (WHO) Classification of Tumors of Hematopoietic and Lymphoid Tissues.[1] In other instances, such correlations are less clear, and subtypes of AML are identified primarily on the basis of morphological and cytochemical criteria. In this chapter, we will review major types of AML with an emphasis on cytogenetic and molecular genetic findings.

## PATHOLOGY

Diagnosis of AML is primarily made by experienced hematopathologists on the basis of light microscopic examination of blood and BM smears stained with Romanowsky stains, such as May–Grünwald–Giemsa or Wright–Giemsa stains. Myeloid lineage of leukemic blasts can be confirmed using cytochemical reactions, such as a reaction using o-tolidine or amino-ethyl carbazole as substrates to detect the presence of myeloperoxidase (MPO), an enzyme present in primary granules of myeloblasts and some monoblasts; a reaction employing Sudan black B (SBB) to detect intracellular lipids that has reactivity similar to MPO but with less specificity for the myeloid lineage; and reactions detecting nonspecific esterase (NSE) that employ alpha-naphthyl butyrate and alpha-naphthyl acetate (ANA). Moreover, in the case of minimally differentiated leukemia, a distinction between AML and acute lymphoblastic leukemia (ALL) can be made with the help of immunophenotypic analysis by flow cytometry or immunohistochemical reactions on slides. Immunophenotyping is also helpful in the identification of acute megakaryoblastic leukemia (AMKL), and in suggesting or excluding particular subtypes of AML within the WHO classification.[1] This classification divides AML into several entities based on morphological and cytochemical criteria, which predominated in the previous French–American–British (FAB) classification, but also takes into account cytogenetic, molecular genetic, immunophenotypic, and clinical features. The major categories and subcategories of the WHO classification are presented in Table 2.1.

One of the most important changes introduced by the WHO classification is that the blast percentage in the marrow required for the diagnosis of AML has been reduced from 30% in the FAB classification to 20% in the WHO classification. Moreover, in patients positive for t(8;21)(q22;q22) and the *AML1(RUNX1)-ETO(CBFA2T1)* fusion gene, inv(16)(p13q22)/t(16;16)(p13;q22) and *CBFB-MYH11*, and t(15;17)(q22;q12-21) and *PML-RARA*, AML can be diagnosed even if the percent of blasts in the marrow is less than 20.[1,2]

## CYTOGENETICS

Leukemic blasts of the majority of patients with AML at diagnosis carry at least one clonal chromosome abnormality, i.e., an identical structural aberration or gain of the same, structurally intact chromosome (trisomy) found in at least two metaphase cells or the same chromosome missing (monosomy) from a minimum of three cells. Abnormal karyotypes are more frequent in children with de novo AML, being detected in 70–85% of patients compared with 55–60% of adults.[8–13] Therapy-related (secondary) AML is usually characterized by a high proportion, 80–90%, of both adult and pediatric patients who carry chromosome abnormalities.[12] Among AML patients with an abnormal karyotype, slightly more than one-half harbor only one chromosome aberration, whereas the remaining patients have two or more aberrations, including 10–15% of patients whose karyotype is complex, i.e., contains three or more aberrations.[12,13]

From the cytogenetic standpoint, AML is heterogeneous, with more than 200 different structural and numerical aberrations identified as recurring in this disease.[5] While many of the recurring aberrations are rare, being thus far detected in a few patients worldwide, others are more common (Table 2.2). Notably, cytogenetic findings at diagnosis constitute one of the most important independent prognostic factors for attainment of complete remission (CR), risk of relapse, and survival.[8–14] Recent large collaborative studies[8–10] have proposed cytogenetic risk systems categorizing AML patients into one of three risk groups (favorable, intermediate, or adverse) based upon cytogenetic findings at diagnosis (Table 2.2). Although some differences among the three prioritization schemata exist, pretreatment cytogenetic results are being used to stratify therapy.[15,16] Moreover, a recent report advocates the use of cytogenetic remission as one of the criteria of CR in AML.[17] This is based on a recent study that demonstrated a significantly worse outcome for patients whose marrow on the first day of morphologically documented CR contained cytogenetically abnormal cells than those whose marrow showed an entirely normal karyotype.[18]

Major cytogenetic studies of AML agree that the prognosis of patients with inv(16)/t(16;16), t(8;21), and t(15;17) is relatively favorable (these subtypes of AML are discussed below), whereas the clinical outcome of patients with inv(3)(q21q26) or t(3;3) (q21;q26), −7, and a complex karyotype is adverse (Table 2.2). Complex karyotype has been defined as either greater than or equal to five unrelated cytogenetic abnormalities or greater than or equal to three abnormalities. However, Byrd et al.[10] have shown that although patients with three or four abnormalities [other than t(8;21), inv(16)/t(16;16), or t(9;11) (p22;q23)] had significantly better survival and a lower probability of relapse than those with greater than or equal to five abnormalities, their probabilities of achieving a CR, or obtaining prolonged CR and survival, were significantly worse than those of patients with a normal karyotype. These data seem to justify combining patients with three or four abnormalities with those with greater than or equal to five abnormalities into one complex karyotype category with greater than or equal to three abnormalities if three clinical prognostic groups are going to be used. Of note, patients with inv(16)/t(16;16), t(8;21), t(15;17), or t(9;11) and greater than or equal to three abnormalities are usually not included in this prognostically unfavorable complex karyotype category, because in these patients, the presence of a complex karyotype does not influence prognosis adversely.[8,10]

Patients with a normal karyotype of marrow cells at diagnosis constitute the largest cytogenetic subset of AML and are classified in the intermediate prognostic category by all major classification schemata.[8–10] However, despite the absence of microscopically detectable chromosome aberrations, these patients can harbor submicroscopic genetic abnormalities discernible only by molecular genetic techniques, such as RT-PCR or direct sequencing. Among several such

**Table 2.1    The WHO classification of AMLs[a]**

| WHO category of AML | Postulated cell origin | Morphology and cytochemistry | Cytogenetics | Immunophenotype |
|---|---|---|---|---|
| *AML with recurrent genetic abnormalities* | | | | |
| AML with t(8;21)(q22;q22), [AML1(RUNX1)/ETO(CBFA2T1)] | Myeloid stem cell with predominant neutrophil differentiation | BM contains large blasts with abundant basophilic cytoplasm often with azurophilic granulation and/or single Auer rods, smaller blasts, promyelocytes, myelocytes, and mature neutrophils with variable dysplasia and homogeneous pink cytoplasm. There is an increase in eosinophil precursors, which do not have abnormalities seen in AML with inv(16)/t(16;16) | t(8;21), variant translocations, or insertions | CD34+, CD13+, CD33+, MPO+; frequently, CD19 present on a subset of the blasts; often CD56+; some cases are TdT+, with dim expression |
| AML with abnormal BM eosinophils and inv(16) (p13q22) or t(16;16) (p13;q22). (CBFB/MYH11) | Hematopoietic stem cell with potential to differentiate to granulocytic and monocytic lineages | In addition to myelomonocytic features (see below), marrow contains an increased number of abnormal eosinophils, with immature, large purple-violet eosinophil granules and faint positivity to naphthol ASD chloroacetate esterase reaction. Myeloblasts can have Auer rods. MPO activity is seen in 3% or more of blasts; monoblasts and promonocytes are usually NSE positive | inv(16) or t(16;16) | CD13+, CD33+, MPO+; often positive for some or all of the following: CD14, CD4, CD11b, CD11c, CD64, CD36, and lysozyme; may be CD2+ |
| AML with t(15;17)(q22; q12-21). (PML/RARA) and variants | Myeloid stem cell with potential to differentiate to granulocytic lineage | Hypergranular APL: Abnormal promyelocytes of variable size and irregular shape, often kidney-shaped or bilobed, with cytoplasm packed with pink, red, or purple large granules. Cells containing multiple Auer rods, which are usually larger than in other types of AML, are called Faggot cells. Myeloblasts with single Auer rods may be present. Strongly positive MPO reaction; NSE weakly positive in 25% of cases. Microgranular (hypogranular APL): predominantly bilobed promyelocytes with the apparent absence of or a few large granules. Rare Faggot cells and/or abnormal promyelocytes with visible granules. Higher than in hypergranular APL leukocyte count with numerous abnormal microgranular promyelocytes. Strongly positive MPO reaction | t(15;17), variant translocations, or insertions | CD33+ homogeneously and brightly; CD13+ heterogeneously; CD34 and HLA-DR generally absent, if expressed then only on a subset of cells; CD15− or dimly expressed; frequent coexpression of CD2 and CD9 |

*table continues*

**Table 2.1** continued

| WHO category of AML | Postulated cell origin | Morphology and cytochemistry | Cytogenetics | Immunophenotype |
|---|---|---|---|---|
| AML with 11q23 (MLL) abnormalities | Hematopoietic stem cell with multilineage potential | Mostly monocytic and myelomonocytic morphology, although a minority of cases have morphological features of AML with or without maturation | t(9;11)(p22; q23),t(6;11)(q27;q23), t(11;19)(q23;p13.1) and other translocations, inversions, and insertions involving band 11q23 | No specific immunophentoypic features; variable expression of CD13 and CD33; cases with monoblastic morphology are CD34− and CD14+, CD4+, CD11b+, CD11c+, CD64+, CD36+, and/or lysozyme+ |
| *AML with multilineage dysplasia* | | | | |
| May develop de novo or following an MDS/ myeloproliferative disease | Hematopoietic stem cell | Dysplasia present in at least 50% of the cells of two or more myeloid lineages | Aberrations similar to those occurring in MDS, mostly unbalanced: −5/del(5q), −7/del(7q), +8, +11, −18, +19, +21, del(11q), del(12p), del(20q). Less often der(1;7)(q10;p10), inv(3)/t(3;3), t(3;5)(q25;q34) | Blasts, which often constitute a subpopulation of cells, are CD34+, CD13+, and CD33+. Frequent aberrant expression of CD56 and/or CD7; increased expression of MDR1 on the blasts |
| *AML and MDS, therapy related* | | | | |
| Alkylating agent/radiation-related type | Hematopoietic stem cell | Panmyelosis, dysplastic changes, ringed sideroblasts in up to 60% of cases | Often complex karyotypes with −5/del(5q), −7/del(7q), and del(17p) | Blasts, which often constitute a subpopulation of cells, are CD34+, CD13+, and CD33+. Aberrant expression of CD56 and/or CD7 is frequent, and expression of MDR1 on the blasts increased |
| Topoisomerase II inhibitor-related type (some may be lymphoid) | Hematopoietic stem cell | A significant monocytic component, most cases have acute myelomonocytic or monoblastic leukemia. APL also reported | Balanced translocations involving 11q23 [t(9;11), t(6;11), t(11;19), etc.], t(8;21), t(3;21)(q26;q22), inv(16), t(8;16)(p11;p13), t(6;9)(p23;q34), and, in therapy-related APL, t(15;17) | |

*AML not otherwise categorized*

| | | | | |
|---|---|---|---|---|
| AML, minimally differentiated | Hematopoietic stem cell at the earliest stage of myeloid differentiation/maturation | Medium-size blasts with round or slightly indented nuclei with dispersed chromatin and 1 or 2 nucleoli, and agranular cytoplasm with a varying degree of basophilia. Less often blasts are small and resemble lymphoblasts, with more condensed chromatin, inconspicuous nucleoli, and scanty cytoplasm. MPO, SBB, and naphthol ASD chloroacetate esterase reactions are negative | There is no consistent abnormality; recurrent aberrations include +4, +8, +13, −7, and complex karyotypes | CD13+, CD33+, and/or CD117+; cCD3−; cCD79a−, and cCD22−; often MPO−; most cases are CD34+, CD38+, and HLA-DR+; CD11b−, CD14−, CD15−, CD65−; TdT+ in ≥ one-third cases; CD7, CD2, and CD19 may be expressed but with lower intensity than in lymphoid leukemias |
| AML without maturation | Precursor hematopoietic cell at the earliest stage of myeloid differentiation | In a proportion of cases, myeloblasts with azurophilic granulation and/or Auer rods are present. Other cases have blasts similar to lymphoblasts, without azurophilic granulation. Variable (but always in ≥3% of blasts) MPO and SBB positivity | There is no consistent abnormality | Expression of at least two of the following: CD13, CD33, CD117, and/or MPO. Often CD34+. CD11b− and CD14− |
| AML with maturation | Hematopoietic precursor cell at the earliest stage of myeloid development | Myeloblasts with azurophilic granulation and/or Auer rods are present, and myelocytes, promyelocytes, and mature neutrophils constitute ≥10% of BM cells. There is variable degree of dysplasia. Blasts and maturing neutrophils are lysozyme and MPO positive | Deletions and translocations involving 12p, t(6;9)(p23;q34), t(8;16)(p11;p13) | Expression of one or more of the following: CD13, CD33, and CD15. CD117, CD34, and HLA-DR also may be expressed |
| Acute myelomonocytic leukemia | Hematopoietic precursor cell with potential to differentiate into neutrophil and monocytic lineages | The BM contains ≥20% neutrophils and their precursors and ≥20% monocytes, monoblasts, and promonocytes | The majority of cases are cytogenetically abnormal, but no specific aberration has been identified | Variable expression of CD13 and CD33, CD4, CD14, CD11b, CD11c, CD36, CD64, and/or lysozyme may be expressed. Residual population of less differentiated myeloblasts expresses CD34 and panmyeloid markers |
| Acute monoblastic and monocytic leukemia | BM stem cell with some commitment to monocytic differentiation | 80% or more of the leukemic cells are monoblasts, promonocytes, and monocytes; a neutrophil component is minor (<20%). In acute monoblastic leukemia, monoblasts constitute ≥80% of monocytic cells, whereas in acute monocytic leukemia, promonocytes predominate. Both monoblasts and promonocytes usually display NSE activity; monoblasts are MPO negative and promonocytes may show scattered MPO positivity | In cases with hemophagocytosis by leukemic cells, t(8;16)(p11;p13) is often detected | Variable expression of CD13, CD33, and CD 117. CD4, CD14, CD11b, CD11c, CD36, CD64, CD68, and/or lysozyme may be expressed. CD34 often negative |

*table continues*

**Table 2.1** continued

| WHO category of AML | Postulated cell origin | Morphology and cytochemistry | Cytogenetics | Immunophenotype |
| --- | --- | --- | --- | --- |
| *Acute erythroid leukemias (erythroid/myeloid and pure erythroleukemia)* | | | | |
| Erythroleukemia (erythroid/myeloid) | Multipotent stem cell with wide myeloid potential | Dysplastic erythroid precursors at all maturation stages may be present. There may be large multinucleated erythroid cells. The myeloblasts are similar to those in AML with and without maturation | Complex karyotypes with −5/del(5q) and −7/del(7q) are frequent | Erythroblasts lack myeloid-associated antigens, are MPO−, and react with antibodies to hemoglobin A and glycophorin A. Myeloblasts are usually CD13+, CD33+, CD117+, and MPO+. CD34 and class II HLA-DR expression are variable |
| Pure erythroleukemia | Primitive (BFU-E/CFU-E) stem cell with some degree of commitment to the erythroid lineage | Erythroblasts are medium to large in size and have basophilic cytoplasm. Infrequently, the blasts are smaller and resemble lymphoblasts. Erythroblasts are negative for MPO and SBB, but show reactivity with ANA esterase, acid phosphatase, and periodic acid Schiff | Complex karyotypes with −5/del(5q) and −7/del(7q) are frequent | In more differentiated forms, glycophorin A and hemoglobin A are expressed but MPO and other myeloid antigens are not. Glycophorin A is usually not expressed in more immature forms, which are positive for carbonic anhydrase 1, CD36, and Gero antibody against the Gerbuch blood group |
| Acute megakaryoblastic leukemia | Hematopoietic precursor cell committed to the megakaryocytic lineage and possibly erythroid lineage and/or able to differentiate into these lineages | More than 50% of the blasts are of megakaryocyte lineage. Megakaryoblasts are usually medium to large in size but small blasts resembling lymphoblasts may also be present. Marrow fibrosis may occur in some patients | Translocation t(1;22)(p13;q13) is recurrent in children younger than 2 years. In some adults, inv(3) or t(3;3) is found, but they also may occur in other AML types | Megakaryoblasts express CD36 and one or more of the following: CD41, CD61, and/or CD42 (less often). CD13 and CD33 may be positive, and CD34, CD45, and HLA-DR are often negative |
| Acute basophilic leukemia | Early myeloid cell committed to the basophil lineage | Medium-size blasts with moderately basophilic cytoplasm containing coarse basophilic granules. Characteristically, blasts are positive for cytochemical reaction with toluidine blue, and usually stain diffusely with acid phosphatase, but are negative for SBB, MPO, and NSE by light microscopy | No consistent abnormality | CD13+, CD33+, CD34+, class II HLA-DR+; usually, CD9+, some cases TdT+; negative for specific lymphoid markers |

| | | | | |
|---|---|---|---|---|
| Acute panmyelosis with myelofibrosis | Myeloid hematopoietic stem cell. The fibroblastic proliferation is an epiphenomenon | Marked pancytopenia in the blood. BM aspirations often unsuccessful. BM biopsy hypercellular with variable hyperplasia of the granulocytes, megakaryocytes, and erythroid precursors. Variable degree of fibrosis, with increase in reticulin fibers | If analysis successful, the karyotype is usually complex, with −5/del(5q) and/or −7/ del(7q) | Phenotypic heterogeneity, with expression of one or more of the following: CD13, CD33, CD117, and MPO |
| Myeloid sarcoma | Primitive myeloid hematopoietic cell | Granulocytic sarcoma, the most common type, consists of myeloblasts, neutrophils, and neutrophil precursors, and is divided into three types based upon degree of maturation. The blastic type contains mainly myeloblasts, the immature type myeloblasts and promyelocytes, and the differentiated type promyelocytes and more mature neutrophils. Less frequent monoblastic sarcoma is composed of monoblasts | In some cases of myeloid sarcoma, t(8;2) or inv(16)/ t(16;16); in monoblastic sarcoma 11q23 translocations | Most myeloid sarcomas express CD43. Granulocytic sarcoma myeloblasts are CD13+, CD33+, CD117+, and MPO+. The monoblasts in monoblastic sarcoma are CD14+, CD116+, CD11c+, and react with antibodies to lysozyme and CD68 by immunohistochemistry |
| *Acute leukemia of ambiguous lineage* | | | | |
| Undifferentiated acute leukemia | Multipotent progenitor stem cell | The leukemic cells lack any differentiating features | Frequently abnormal cytogenetically. Recurrent aberrations include del(5q) and +13, often as a sole abnormality | Often HLA-DR+, CD34+, CD38+, and may be TdT+ and CD7+. Negative for markers specific for a given lineage, such as cCD79a, cCD22, CD3, and MPO. Generally, do not express more than one lineage-associated marker. |
| Bilineal acute leukemia | Multipotent progenitor stem cell | May present as monoblastic or poorly differentiated myeloid leukemia, or as ALL. In some cases, blasts are morphologically undifferentiated; in others, populations of small blasts resembling lymphoblasts may coexist with larger blasts | Typically abnormal cytogenetically. Cases with B lymphoid component often have t(9;22) (q34;q11.2), t(4;11), or other 11q23 aberrations; these aberrations are not found in cases with T lymphoid component | Coexistence of two populations of blasts, each of which expresses antigens of a distinct lineage, which is myeloid and lymphoid or B and T |
| Biphenotypic acute leukemia | Multipotent progenitor stem cell | May present as monoblastic or poorly differentiated myeloid leukemia, or as ALL. In some cases, blasts are morphologically undifferentiated; in others, populations of small blasts resembling lymphoblasts may coexist with larger blasts | Usually abnormal cytogenetically. Cases with B lymphoid component often have t(9;22), t(4;11), or other 11q23 aberrations; these aberrations are not found in cases with T lymphoid component | Blasts coexpress myeloid and T- or B-lineage-specific markers or, concurrently, T- and B-specific antigens |

a Data from Jaffe et al.[1] and Mitelman et al.[36]

| Table 2.2 Prognostic significance of the more common chromosome aberrations in AML | |
|---|---|
| Chromosome aberration[a] | Cytogenetic risk category |
| **inv(16)(p13q22)/t(16;16) (p13;q22); t(8;21)(q22;q22); t(15;17)(q22;q12–21)** | Favorable |
| **none (normal karyotype);** −Y; del(7q)[b]; del(9q)[b]; del(11q)[c]; del(20q)[d]; isolated +8[e]; +11, +13, +21, t(9;11)(p22;q23)[c] | Intermediate |
| **complex karyotype with ≥3 abnormalities; inv(3) (q21q26)/t(3;3)(q21;q26);** −7; del(5q)[f]; −5; t(6;9) (p23;q34)[g]; t(6;11)(q27;q23)[h]; t(11;19)(q23;p13.1)[h] | Unfavorable |

[a] Chromosome aberrations whose prognostic impact is agreed on by major studies[8–10] are indicated by bold type.
[b] Classified in the adverse-risk category by SWOG/ECOG.[9]
[c] Would be included in "abn 11q" group and classified in the adverse-risk category by SWOG/ECOG.[9]
[d] Would be included in "abn 20q" group and classified in the adverse-risk category by SWOG/ECOG.[9]
[e] Classified in the adverse-risk category with regard to overall survival by CALGB.[10]
[f] Classified in the intermediate-risk category with regard to probability of achievement of CR and survival by CALGB if not part of a complex karyotype.
[g] Classified in the intermediate-risk category by virtue of being "other structural" abnormality by MRC[8] and by CALGB (but intermediate only with regard to probability of achievement of CR).[10]
[h] Would be included in "abnormal 11q23" group and classified in the intermediate-risk category by MRC[8] and by CALGB (but only with regard to probability of achievement of CR).[10]

mutations associated with AML, internal tandem duplication (ITD) of the *FLT3* gene (*FLT3* ITD), partial tandem duplication (PTD) of the *mixed lineage leukemia* (*MLL*) gene (*MLL* PTD), and point mutations of the *CCAAT/enhancer-binding protein* α (*CEBPA*) gene have been recently found to be of prognostic significance in patients with AML and a normal karyotype (Table 2.3). Likewise, adverse prognosis has been associated with overexpression of the *brain and acute leukemia, cytoplasmic* (*BAALC*) gene.[19–21]

Later in the chapter we will discuss in greater detail the four AML categories delineated primarily because of cytogenetic and molecular genetic findings, followed by data on major molecular genetic rearrangements relevant to AML pathogenesis, some of which are associated with clinical outcome.

### CORE-BINDING FACTOR LEUKEMIA

Two categories in the WHO classification of AML, namely AML with t(8;21)(q22;q22)/*AML1(RUNX1)-ETO(CBFA2T1)* and AML with abnormal BM eosinophils and inv(16)(p13q22) or t(16;16)(p13;q22)/*CBFB-MYH11*, are characterized by chromosomal aberrations that rearrange genes encoding different subunits of core-binding factor (CBF). These AML types are collectively referred to as CBF AML. The CBF complex is a heterodimeric transcription factor, composed of α and β subunits, which regulates transcription of several genes involved in hematopoietic differentiation, including cytokines such as interleukin-3 (*IL-3*), granulocyte-macrophage colony-stimulating factor (*GM-CSF*), and the macrophage colony-stimulating factor receptor (*M-CSFR*). The CBFα subunit, encoded by the *RUNX1* gene (also known as *AML1* and *CBFA2*), harbors a DNA-binding domain, whereas the CBFβ subunit does not directly bind DNA, but physically associates with CBFα and stimulates its DNA-binding activity, thereby regulating transcription.[22] The intact CBF complex is critical for normal hematopoiesis; disruption of either of its subunits directly contributes to leukemic transformation.

### AML with t(8;21)(q22;q22)/*AML1 (RUNX1)-ETO(CBFA2T1)*

This type of CBF AML is associated with t(8;21) and its relatively rare variants, such as insertions ins(8;21) (q22;q22q22) or ins(21;8)(q22;q22q22), and complex translocations involving three or four different chromosomes that invariably include chromosomes 8 and 21 with breaks in bands 8q22 and 21q22. The t(8;21) represents one of the most frequent chromosomal aberrations in AML, occurring in approximately 6% of adult and 12% of childhood patients.[13] Interestingly, most patients, approximately 70%, carry at least one additional (secondary) chromosome abnormality, the most frequent of which are loss of one sex chromosome (−Y in male and −X in female patients), del(9q), and trisomy of chromosome 8 (+8).[23,24]

Both t(8;21) and its variants lead to fusion of the DNA-binding domain of the *RUNX1* gene, located at 21q22, with the *CBFA2T1* gene at 8q22 and creation of a chimeric gene *RUNX1-CBFA2T1*. The chimeric fusion protein impairs normal hematopoiesis through a dominant-negative inhibition of the wild-type RUNX1. In addition, it has been shown that RUNX1-CBFA2T1 itself recruits nuclear corepressor complexes, which includes the histone deacetylase enzyme HDAC1, and is responsible for transcriptional repression of RUNX1 target genes, and thus generates novel signals that alter normal transcription. These observations have prompted studies attempting to reverse the block of differentiation using histone deacetylase (HDAC) inhibitors.[25]

Morphologically, the presence of t(8;21)/*RUNX1-CBFA2T1* is strongly (but not exclusively) associated with AML with maturation in the neutrophil lineage. Characteristic pink-colored cytoplasm of neutrophils and an increased number of eosinophil precursors [without abnormalities typical for AML with inv(16)] appear to distinguish patients with t(8;21) from other patients with AML with maturation but without t(8;21)/*RUNX1-CBFA2T1*.[26,27]

Notably, the clinical outcome of patients with t(8;21) is relatively favorable,[8–10,12–14] especially when regimens containing repetitive cycles of high-dose cytarabine are used as postremission therapy.[28,29] The favorable outcome does not seem to be influenced by the presence of secondary chromosome aberrations, although one recent study reported loss of the Y chromosome in male patients to be associated with shorter overall survival,[23] but this has not been corroborated by another large study.[24]

### AML with inv(16)(p13p22)/*CBFB-MYH11*

This type of CBF AML is characterized by the presence of inversion of chromosome 16, inv(16)(p13q22), or, less commonly, a reciprocal translocation between homologous chromosomes 16, t(16;16)(p13;q22), in leukemic blasts. These chromosome aberrations can be detected in about 7% of adult and 6% of pediatric AML patients.[10,13] Notably, secondary aberrations [e.g., +22, +8, del(7q), or +21] are less common in patients with inv(16)/t(16;16) than in patients with t(8;21), being detected in approximately one-third of patients with inv(16)/t(16;16).[23,24]

Both the inv(16) and the t(16;16) fuse the myosin, heavy chain 11, smooth muscle gene (*MYH11*) with the C terminus of the *CBFB* gene. The chimeric protein retains the ability to interact with the RUNX1 and has been suggested to block CBF-dependent transcription.[22]

The marrow of patients with inv(16)/t(16;16)/*CBFB-MYH11* shows monocytic and granulocytic differentiation and abnormal eosinophils, a hallmark of this disease. These eosinophils are essentially always present, albeit sometimes scarce, constituting as little as 0.2% of marrow cells.

The prognosis of CBF AML patients with inv(16)/t(16;16) is favorable,[8–14] and can be improved by regimens with multicourse high-dose cytarabine.[30] Two large recent studies demonstrated that patients who carry a secondary +22 in addition to inv(16) or t(16;16) have a significantly reduced risk of relapse compared with patients with an isolated inv(16)/ t(16;16).[23,24] The reasons for this difference in outcome and the molecular consequences of trisomy 22 remain to be elucidated.

### ACUTE PROMYELOCYTIC LEUKEMIA—A DISEASE WITH RETINOIC ACID RECEPTOR α REARRANGEMENTS

Acute promyelocytic leukemia (APL) is the third category in the WHO classification that is characterized by specific cytogenetic and molecular genetic rearrangements as well as unique marrow morphology, presenting clinical features, and responsiveness to targeted therapy with all-*trans*-retinoic acid (ATRA). APL comprises from 8% (adults) to 10% (children) of AML cases.[13] Essentially, all patients with APL carry a gene fusion of the *retinoic acid receptor α* (RARA) gene, located at 17q12-21, with one of several partner genes, the most common of which is the *promyelocytic leukemia* (PML) gene, mapped to 15q22. In the vast majority (>90%) of APL patients, the *PML-RARA* fusion gene is created by a subtle but detectable microscopically reciprocal translocation t(15;17)(q22;q12–21); in an additional 4%, the *PML-RARA* gene is generated by an insertion of a small segment from 17q, with the *RARA* gene into the locus of the *PML* gene.[31] Most of these insertions are cryptic, i.e., not detectable by routine cytogenetic study, and associated with a normal karyotype; they can be identified only using RT-PCR or fluorescence in situ hybridization (FISH). Approximately one-third of APL patients with t(15;17) carry at least one secondary aberration, the most common of which is trisomy 8 or 8q. Additionally, in a small proportion of APL cases, other, rather infrequent, chromosomal aberrations are found, including t(11;17)(q23;q12–21), t(11;17)(q13;q12–21), t(5;17) (q35;q12–21), and dup(17)(q21.3q23). Each of these rearrangements results in a fusion of the *RARA* gene with, respectively, the *PLZF* gene at 11q23, *NUMA1* gene at 11q13, *NPM* gene at 5q35, and *STAT5b* gene at 17q21.1–21.2.[32,33]

The *RARA* gene is a member of the nuclear hormone receptor gene family and contains transactivation, DNA-binding, and ligand-binding domains. As a consequence of the t(15;17) or ins(15;17), the DNA- and ligand-binding domains of *RARA* are fused to the *PML* gene. The chimeric PML-RARA fusion protein binds to corepressor/HDAC complexes with higher affinity than does the wild-type RARA, leading to aberrant chromatin acetylation and alterations of chromatin conformation that inhibit the normal transcription of genes regulated by RARA. This blocks cell differentiation and leads to the accumulation of leukemic blasts at the promyelocytic stage. Importantly, therapeutic doses of ATRA, but not physiological ATRA levels, are capable of changing conformation of the PML-RARA protein and releasing corepressor/HDAC complexes that lead to transcriptional activation of downstream target genes. Moreover, both ATRA and arsenic trioxide, another compound used in targeted APL treatment, also induce proteolysis of the PML-RARA protein. This leads to granulocytic differentiation of the leukemic blasts.[34]

A strong correlation exists between t(15;17)/*PML-RARA* and its variants and marrow morphology in which abnormal promyelocytes dominate. There are two major morphologic subtypes of APL, hypergranular (or typical) and microgranular (or hypogranular), and both are associated with the presence of t(15;17)/*PML-RARA* or variants. The microgranular variant, which sometimes can be misdiagnosed morphologically as acute monocytic leukemia, is associated with very high leukocyte counts with abundant abnormal microgranular promyelocytes.[1]

It is important to determine which of the APL-associated translocations and gene fusions are present, because patients with t(11;17)(q23;q12–21)/*PLZF-RARA* are resistant to standard ATRA-based therapy. Although it has been reported that t(11;17)(q23;q12–21)/*PLZF-RARA*-positive APL displays distinguishing morphological and immunophenotypic characteristics, such as prevalence of blasts with regular nuclei, an increased number of Pelger-like cells, and CD56 positivity,[35] the diagnosis should always be supported by results of cytogenetic, FISH, and/or RT-PCR analyses.

### AML WITH REARRANGEMENTS OF BAND 11Q23 AND THE MLL GENE

This category represents approximately 4% of cases of adult AML, but rearrangements involving band 11q23 and the *MLL* gene (also known as *ALL1*, *HRX*, and *HTRX*) are three to four times more common in children with AML, being especially frequent among infants aged 12 months or less, 43–58% of whom carry an 11q23/*MLL* abnormality.[13] At both the cytogenetic and molecular genetic level, AML with the 11q23/*MLL* rearrangements is extremely heterogeneous. Well over 30 different balanced chromosome abnormalities, mostly translocations but also inversions, insertions, and interstitial deletions, involving band 11q23 and another chromosome locus have been reported.[5,36] The most common of these is t(9;11)(p22;q23), resulting in the *AF9-MLL* gene fusion; other more frequent recurrent translocations and fusion genes in AML include t(6;11)(q27;q23)/*AF6-MLL*, t(11;19)(q23;p13.1)/*MLL-ELL*, and t(11;19)(q23;p13.3)/*MLL-MLLT1*.

In some studies, patients with various 11q23/*MLL* rearrangements have been included in the same cytogenetic category and classified as having either adverse[9] or intermediate[8] prognosis. However, increasing evidence suggests that prognosis of patients with 11q23/*MLL* rearrangements depends on the partner chromosome/gene involved, with t(9;11)-positive patients having a better prognosis,[37,38] which places them in the intermediate cytogenetic risk group.[10] The survival of adults with t(6;11) and t(11;19)(q23;p13.1) studied by Cancer and Leukemia Group B (CALGB) was significantly shorter than that of the cytogenetically normal group, and consequently they were assigned to the adverse-risk group for survival.[10]

The *MLL* gene is a homeotic regulator that shares homology to sequences of the *Drosophila* trithorax gene. It encodes a nearly 430-kd protein. The C-terminus of *MLL* positively regulates *HOX* gene expression during development of hematopoietic stem cells. The N-terminus contains an AT hook region functioning as a DNA-binding domain and a region similar to the noncatalytic domain of methyltransferases.

Additionally, amplification of the *MLL* gene, without rearrangements of the gene, has been recently recognized as a recurrent aberration in patients with AML and myelodysplastic syndromes (MDS), a complex karyotype, and results in an adverse prognosis.[39–41] *MLL* amplification was shown to result in overexpression of the gene and MLL gain of function because it was associated with increased expression of one of its physiologic downstream targets, *HOXA9*.[42]

In addition to rearrangements generated by chromosome translocations, the *MLL* gene can also be

**Table 2.3** Genetic anomalies that impact prognosis of AML patients with normal cytogenetics

| Genetic rearrangement | Prognostic significance |
|---|---|
| Internal tandem duplication of the *FLT3* gene | CRD, DFS, and survival significantly shorter for patients with *FLT3* ITD compared with patients without *FLT3* ITD; especially, poor outcome for *FLT3* ITD patients with no expression of an *FLT3* wild-type allele or a high *FLT3* mutant/wild-type allele ratio |
| Loss-of-function mutations of the *CEBPA* gene | CRD and survival significantly longer for patients with the *CEBPA* gene mutations compared with patients without mutated *CEBPA* |
| Partial tandem duplication of the *MLL* gene | CRD and EFS significantly shorter for patients with *MLL* PTD compared with patients without *MLL* PTD |
| Overexpression of the *BAALC* gene | DFS, EFS, and survival significantly shorter for patients with high expression of *BAALC* compared with low *BAALC* expression patients |
| Mutations of the *NPMI* gene | CR rates, EFS, RFS, DFS, and OS significantly better for patients with *NPMI* mutations who do not harbor *FLT3* ITD |

CRD, CR duration; DFS, disease-free survival; EFS, event-free survival; RFS, relapse-free survival; OS, overall survival.

rearranged in AML patients without structural chromosome abnormalities involving band 11q23. These *MLL* rearrangements occur in the majority of patients with isolated trisomy 11[43] and in 8–11% of karyotypically normal adults with de novo AML,[44,45] and result from a PTD spanning exons 5 through 11 or, less frequently, exons 5 through 12.[43–46] Among patients with normal cytogenetics, the *MLL* PTD confers poor prognosis (Table 2.3), and represents an independent adverse prognostic factor for remission duration.[45]

## MOLECULAR GENETICS

### MUTATIONS IN AML-ASSOCIATED TRANSCRIPTION FACTORS
### CEBPA

The *CEBPA* gene encodes a transcription factor expressed mainly in myelomonocytic cells that is essential for granulopoiesis, showing cell-type-specific and differentiation-stage-specific expression patterns. Mutations in *CEBPA* have been reported in 7–11% of AML patients.[47,48] These include N-terminal nonsense mutations resulting in a premature termination of the full-length protein with dominant-negative properties, and C-terminal in-frame mutations resulting in a decrease of DNA-binding potential. Interestingly, *CEBPA* mutations have been found predominantly in AML FAB subtypes M1 or M2, suggesting the induction of a stage-specific block in the differentiation pathway. Clinical studies have revealed that mutations in *CEBPA* confer a favorable prognosis in AML patients with normal cytogenetics,[49] and among those classified in the intermediate-risk cytogenetic group.[47,48]

## RUNX1

In addition to its involvement in the translocation t(8;21), *RUNX1* is also dysregulated by mutations found in patients with AML and MDS, as well as by amplification in patients with ALL. Germline mutations resulting in *RUNX1* haploinsufficiency have been reported in cases of familial platelet disorder, an autosomal-dominant disease with quantitative and qualitative platelet defects and progressive pancytopenia, with a predisposition to development of AML.[50] In de novo AML, somatic point mutations occur in up to 10% of cases. Interestingly, *RUNX1* mutations are mainly found in minimally differentiated AML (FAB M0), with a frequency of up to 22%, reflecting the importance of RUNX1 in the earliest stages of hematopoiesis.

## GATA1

The *gata-binding protein 1* (*GATA1*) gene, located at Xp11.23, encodes a lineage-specific zinc-finger transcription factor required for normal development of erythroid and megakaryocytic lineages. Inherited missense mutations within the zinc-finger domain inhibiting the interaction with the essential cofactor, Friend of GATA1 (FOG1), have been found in familial dyserythropoietic anemia and thrombocytopenia. Somatic mutations leading to production of an alternative protein that retains its intact zinc-finger interaction domain have been identified exclusively in patients with Down syndrome suffering from AMKL or transient myeloproliferative disorder.

## SIGNAL TRANSDUCTION PATHWAYS

Signal transduction pathways control the transmission of extracellular signals (e.g., growth factors, including G-CSF, GM-CSF, and FLT3 ligand) via the receptor-tyrosine-kinase-RAS cascade into intracellular response mechanisms (proliferation, differentiation, and apoptosis). In AML, mutations, epigenetic changes and aberrant expression of genes involved in these pathways, result in increased proliferation and/or dysregulated differentiation and apoptosis.

## RECEPTOR TYROSINE KINASE AND DOWNSTREAM SIGNALING PATHWAYS

Members of the *RTK-RAS* signaling pathway, including receptor tyrosine kinases (RTKs) such as *FLT3*, *FMS*, *KIT*, and *VEGFR*, and the *NRAS* and *KRAS* genes, are frequently (in more than 50% of patients) mutated in AML; as a result, this pathway appears to play a central role in leukemogenesis. The identification of these specific molecular alterations has not only helped in elucidating the mechanisms involved in leukemogenesis, but also has resulted in targeted therapies, such as FLT3 inhibitors for AML patients with *FLT3* ITD or *FLT3* overexpression, RTK inhibitors for patients with *KIT* mutations or overexpression, as well as RAS inhibitors including farnesyltransferase inhibitors.[51]

## FLT3

The *FLT3* gene encodes a class III RTK, which plays an important role in cell proliferation, differentiation, and survival. The *FLT3* receptor is preferably expressed on hematopoietic stem cells, and activation by its ligand (FLT3 ligand) induces oligomerization leading to phosphorylation and activation of downstream pathways (mainly via phosphorylation of intracellular substrates). Mutations of the *FLT3* gene are found in up to 40% of AML patients. These mutations include *FLT3* ITD, affecting exons 14 and 15, in up to 30% of patients, and activating point mutations of D835 within the activation loop in the tyrosine kinase domain (TKD; Asp835 mutation), in about 5–10% of AML cases. The *FLT3* ITD, as well as mutations in the TKD, promote autophosphorylation of FLT3, and the constitutively active receptor confers ligand-independent proliferation.[52]

Clinical studies have demonstrated that both adults and children with AML and *FLT3* ITD have a significantly inferior clinical outcome.[53–60] In some analyses, the worst outcome has been bestowed by *FLT3* ITD coupled with lack of an *FLT3* wild-type allele or a high *FLT3* mutant/wild-type allele ratio.[59,60] In one study, relatively infrequent patients with simultaneous presence of both the *FLT3* ITD and the Asp835 mutation had the least favorable outcome.[61] However, although *FLT3* ITD is also common in APL patients with t(15;17), it has thus far not been shown to predict prognosis in these patients.[55,57,62] Likewise, *FLT3* Asp835 mutations have not hitherto been correlated with inferior prognosis, but because they are relatively infrequent, larger clinical studies are necessary to determine their prognostic importance.

## KIT

Asp816 substitution mutations that result in constitutive activation of KIT have been found in about 5% of AML patients.[63] *KIT* exon 8 mutations have been found in 24% of patients with inv(16) and 2% of t(8;21)-positive patients, whereas *KIT* Asp816 mutations were present in 8% of patients with inv(16) and in 11% of those with t(8;21) AML.[64] In patients with inv(16), *KIT* mutations were associated with a significantly higher relapse rate.[64]

## RAS

The small membrane-associated G protein RAS and its relatives are signal transduction components connecting various classes of receptors (including RTK) to cytoplasmic pathways. Mutations of the GTPase oncogene *NRAS* occur in about 15% of AML patients, *KRAS* mutations occur in fewer than 5% of cases, and *HRAS* mutations are rare. *NRAS* mutations (primarily point mutations in codons 12, 13, and 61) occur at specific positions that are critical for guanine triphosphate (GTP) hydrolysis, thereby preventing the conversion of the active RAS-GTP to the inactive RAS-GDP.

### OVEREXPRESSION OF THE BAALC GENE

The *BAALC* gene, mapped to band 8q22.3, encodes a protein with no homology to any known proteins or functional domains. *BAALC* is expressed mainly in neuroectoderm-derived tissues and hematopoietic precursors, with no expression in mature BM or blood mononuclear cells.[65] High expression of *BAALC* mRNA in circulating blasts is an independent adverse prognostic factor in uniformly treated adults younger than 60 years with de novo AML and normal cytogenetics.[19,20] In another, smaller study, high expression of *BAALC* predicted shorter disease-free survival (DFS) and overall survival in patients with a normal karyotype who did not carry *FLT3* ITD or mutations in the *CEBPA* gene.[21]

### COOPERATION BETWEEN MUTATIONS

It has been hypothesized that at least two somatic mutations with differing consequences collaborate to induce AML, as each alone is incapable of fully transforming a normal into a leukemic cell. These include mutations in the signal transduction pathways conferring a proliferation stimulus and mutations in genes encoding hematopoietic transcription factors that impair cell differentiation. This concept is consistent with Knudson's two-hit hypothesis, which proposes that at least two events are necessary to promote cancer.[66] This concept is important for the understanding of the mechanisms involved in leukemogenesis as well as for the development of novel treatment strategies that may have to target several dysregulated molecules in different pathways. Interestingly, simultaneous mutations of two genes cooperating in the same pathway (e.g., *FLT3* and *RAS*) are rare.

### CBF AML and additional mutations

Neither *RUNX1-CBFA2T1* nor *CBFB-MYH11* alone are capable of inducing overt AML. These fusion genes dictate the phenotype of the disease, but additional abnormalities are required for the leukemic transformation. Recent studies have demonstrated that 40% of AML patients with inv(16) acquire either *KIT* exon 8, *KIT* Asp816, *FLT3* ITD, or FLT3 Asp835 mutations.[63,64]

Mutations of the *KIT* gene were less common in t(8;21) AML, with a frequency of about 13% and were absent in non-CBF AML.[64] Mutations of the *FLT3* and *KIT* gene were mutually exclusive.

### t(15;17)/*PML-RARA* and *FLT3* ITD

*PML-RARA* contributes to the development of APL. However, incomplete penetrance and long latency observed in *PML-RARA* transgenic mice suggest that additional events are required for complete leukemic transformation. The observation that *FLT3* mutations are found in about one-third of patients with t(15;17) has led to the hypothesis that the primary translocation event might impair differentiation and a second hit, such as the *FLT3* ITD, confers the proliferation stimulus for the leukemic cells.[67] Indeed, experimental data demonstrate that *PML-RARA* and *FLT3* ITD cooperate and that the two events lead to an ATRA-responsive APL-like disease with a short latency and 100% penetrance.[68]

### GENE EXPRESSION PROFILING

Gene expression profiling using DNA microarray technology is a powerful tool allowing analysis of expression of thousands of genes in one experiment. Early studies demonstrated that it is possible to correctly distinguish AML from ALL based on gene expression profiles. This proof of principle underscored the accuracy and power of analyzing mRNA expression levels of thousands of genes simultaneously.[69] Subsequent studies have shown that several cytogenetically and molecularly defined AML subtypes, such as t(15;17)/*PML-RARA*, t(8;21)/*AML1(RUNX1)-ETO(CBFA2T1)*, and inv(16)/t(16;16)/*CBFB-MYH11*, display characteristic gene expression signatures and that these gene expression signatures, not surprisingly, correlate with clinical outcome.[70] Moreover, novel gene clusters, apparently not corresponding to cytogenetic aberrations, have also been identified; some have had prognostic significance.[70] These studies have identified numerous genes selectively over- or underexpressed within particular subtypes of AML, which may provide important insights into the molecular pathways involved.

## EPIGENETIC CHANGES—GENE SILENCING THROUGH DNA HYPERMETHYLATION

Expression of genes involved in hematopoiesis may be affected both by gene fusions and point mutations and by epigenetic mechanisms such as DNA methylation. Hypermethylation of cytosine nucleotide residues within CpG-rich regions (CpG islands) in the gene promoters leads to gene inactivation. CpG island hypermethylation has been detected in almost all types of solid tumors and leukemia, but patterns of aberrant DNA methylation appear to differ among particular types of neoplasia, with AML displaying a relatively high number of methylation targets, some of which are not found in solid tumors.[71] There seems to be an overrepresentation of methylated CpG islands on chromosome 11 relative to its size.[72]

Most studies correlating clinical outcome with methylation of other genes have linked CpG island methylation with poor prognosis. Patients with APL and *CDKN2B* methylation had a significantly shorter 5-year DFS than those without *CDKN2B* methylation.[73] In another study,[74] *CDKN2B* methylation was frequently detected in therapy-related AML and MDS patients with deletion or loss of 7q and was shown to confer a poor prognosis. More recently, *EXT1* hypermethylation, which is more common in APL than in other types of AML, has been reported to increase the likelihood of resistance to treatment with ATRA in a relatively small series of patients.[75] Importantly, clinical trials of low-dose hypomethylating agents, such as 5-azacytidine and 5-aza-2'-deoxycytidine (decitabine), in AML and MDS have yielded promising results, especially in elderly patients.

## CONCLUSIONS AND FUTURE DIRECTIONS

Significant progress in unraveling the genetic basis of AML has been made during the last 30 years. First, cytogenetic analyses have identified a great number of recurrent chromosome abnormalities, many of which have been dissected molecularly, leading to identification of novel genes involved in leukemogenesis. More recently, submicroscopic mutations and epigenetic changes affecting other genes have been described, and gene expression profiling has uncovered characteristic molecular signatures of some AML subtypes. Both cytogenetic and molecular findings are associated with specific laboratory and clinical characteristics, and are being used as diagnostic and prognostic markers, guiding the clinician in selecting effective therapies. Clinical trials have begun testing the effectiveness of treatments, using compounds targeting specific molecular defects in leukemic blasts. Ongoing research will likely help resolve differences among the major cytogenetic risk-assignment schemata in prognostic categorization of more frequent chromosome aberrations, and will shed light on the currently unknown prognostic significance of less common aberrations. Likewise, novel molecular genetic rearrangements suitable for therapeutic targeting will continue to be discovered. Standardization of microarray assays will likely enable meaningful comparison of results obtained in different laboratories and may eventually lead to application of gene expression profiling in individual patients, with the goal of predicting their response to therapy and tailoring treatment to specific molecular lesions acquired by the leukemic blasts. These advances will hopefully result in improved clinical outcome of patients with AML.

## ACKNOWLEDGMENTS

This work was supported in part by grant 5P30CA16058 from the National Cancer Institute, Bethesda, MD, and the Coleman Leukemia Research Fund.

## REFERENCES

1. Jaffe ES, Harris NL, Stein H, et al. (eds.): *World Health Organization Classification of Tumours: Pathology and Genetics of Tumours of Haematopoietic and Lymphoid Tissues.* Lyon, France: IARC Press; 2001.
2. Vardiman JW, Harris NL, Brunning RD: The World Health Organization (WHO) classification of the myeloid neoplasms. *Blood* 100:2292–2302, 2002.
3. Sandler DP, Ross JA: Epidemiology of acute leukemia in children and adults. *Semin Oncol* 24:3–16, 1997.
4. Look AT: Oncogenic transcription factors in the human acute leukemias. *Science* 278:1059–1064, 1997.
5. Mrózek K, Heinonen K, Bloomfield CD: Clinical importance of cytogenetics in acute myeloid leukaemia. *Best Pract Res Clin Haematol* 14:19–47, 2001.
6. Marcucci G, Mrózek K, Bloomfield CD: Molecular heterogeneity and prognostic biomarkers in adults with acute myeloid leukemia and normal cytogenetics. *Curr Opin Hematol* 12:68–75, 2005.
7. Kelly L, Clark J, Gilliland DG: Comprehensive genotypic analysis of leukemia: clinical and therapeutic implications. *Curr Opin Oncol* 14:10–18, 2002.
8. Grimwade D, Walker H, Oliver F, et al.: The importance of diagnostic cytogenetics on outcome in AML: analysis of 1,612 patients entered into the MRC AML 10 trial. *Blood* 92:2322–2333, 1998.
9. Slovak ML, Kopecky KJ, Cassileth PA, et al.: Karyotypic analysis predicts outcome of preremission and postremission therapy in adult acute myeloid leukemia: a Southwest Oncology Group/Eastern Cooperative Oncology Group study. *Blood* 96:4075–4083, 2000.
10. Byrd JC, Mrózek K, Dodge RK, et al.: Pretreatment cytogenetic abnormalities are predictive of induction success, cumulative incidence of relapse, and overall survival in adult patients with de novo acute myeloid leukemia: results from Cancer and Leukemia Group B (CALGB 8461). *Blood* 100:4325–4336, 2002.
11. Raimondi SC, Chang MN, Ravindranath Y, et al.: Chromosomal abnormalities in 478 children with acute myeloid leukemia: clinical characteristics and treatment outcome in a cooperative Pediatric Oncology Group study—POG 8821. *Blood* 94:3707–3716, 1999.
12. Schoch C, Kern W, Schnittger S, et al.: Karyotype is an independent prognostic parameter in therapy-related acute myeloid *leukemia* (t-AML): an analysis of 93 patients with t-AML in comparison to 1091 patients with *de novo* AML. *Leukemia* 18:120–125, 2004.
13. Mrózek K, Heerema NA, Bloomfield CD: Cytogenetics in acute leukemia. *Blood Rev* 18:115–136, 2004.
14. Bloomfield CD, Goldman A, Hossfeld D, et al.: Fourth International Workshop on Chromosomes in Leukemia,

1982: clinical significance of chromosomal abnormalities in acute nonlymphoblastic leukemia. *Cancer Genet Cytogenet* 11:332–350, 1984.

15. Schlenk RF, Benner A, Hartmann F, et al.: Risk adapted postremission therapy in acute myeloid leukemia: results of the German multicenter AML HD93 treatment trial. *Leukemia* 17:1521–1528, 2003.

16. Kolitz JE, George SL, Dodge RK, et al.: Dose escalation studies of cytarabine, daunorubicin, and etoposide with and without multidrug resistance modulation with PSC-833 in untreated adults with acute myeloid leukemia younger than 60 years: final induction results of Cancer and Leukemia Group B study 9621. *J Clin Oncol* 22: 4290–4301, 2004.

17. Cheson BD, Bennett JM, Kopecky KJ, et al.: Revised recommendations of the International Working Group for diagnosis, standardization of response criteria, treatment outcomes, and reporting standards for therapeutic trials in acute myeloid leukemia. *J Clin Oncol* 21:4642–4649, 2003.

18. Marcucci G, Mrózek K, Ruppert AS, et al.: Abnormal cytogenetics at date of morphologic complete remission predicts short overall and disease-free survival, and higher relapse rate in adult acute myeloid leukemia: results from Cancer and Leukemia Group B study 8461. *J Clin Oncol* 22:2410–2418, 2004.

19. Baldus CD, Tanner SM, Ruppert AS, et al.: *BAALC* expression predicts clinical outcome of de novo acute myeloid leukemia patients with normal cytogenetics: a Cancer and Leukemia Group B Study. *Blood* 102:1613–1618, 2003.

20. Baldus CD, Thiede C, Soucek S, et al.: *BAALC* expression and *FLT3* internal tandem duplication mutations in acute myeloid leukemia patients with normal cytogenetics: prognostic implications. *J Clin Oncol* 24:790–797, 2006.

21. Bienz M, Ludwig M, Oppliger Leibundgut E, et al.: Risk assessment in patients with acute myeloid leukemia and a normal karyotype. *Clin Cancer Res* 11:1416–1424, 2005.

22. Speck NA, Gilliland DG: Core-binding factors in haematopoiesis and leukaemia. *Nat Rev Cancer* 2:502–513, 2002.

23. Schlenk RF, Benner A, Büchner T, et al.: Individual patient data based meta-analysis on 410 patients 16 to 60 years of age with core binding factor acute myeloid leukemia: a survey of the German AML Intergroup. *J Clin Oncol* 22:3741–3750, 2004.

24. Marcucci G, Mrózek K, Ruppert AS, et al.: Prognostic factors and outcome of core binding factor acute myeloid leukemia patients with t(8;21) differ from those of patients with inv(16): a Cancer and Leukemia Group B study. *J Clin Oncol* 23:5705–5717, 2005.

25. Wang J, Saunthararajah Y, Redner RL, et al.: Inhibitors of histone deacetylase relieve ETO-mediated repression and induce differentiation of AML1-ETO leukemia cells. *Cancer Res* 59:2766–2769, 1999.

26. Bitter MA, Le Beau MM, Rowley JD, et al.: Associations between morphology, karyotype, and clinical features in myeloid leukemias. *Hum Pathol* 18:211–225, 1987.

27. Nakamura H, Kuriyama K, Sadamori N, et al.: Morphological subtyping of acute myeloid leukemia with maturation (AML-M2): homogeneous pink-colored cytoplasm of mature neutrophils is most characteristic of AML-M2 with t(8;21). *Leukemia* 11:651–655, 1997.

28. Bloomfield CD, Lawrence D, Byrd JC, et al.: Frequency of prolonged remission duration after high-dose cytara-

bine intensification in acute myeloid leukemia varies by cytogenetic subtype. *Cancer Res* 58:4173–4179, 1998.

29. Byrd JC, Dodge RK, Carroll A, et al.: Patients with t(8;21)(q22;q22) and acute myeloid leukemia have superior failure-free and overall survival when repetitive cycles of high-dose cytarabine are administered. *J Clin Oncol* 17:3767–3775, 1999.

30. Byrd JC, Ruppert AS, Mrózek K, et al.: Repetitive cycles of high-dose cytarabine benefit patients with acute myeloid leukemia and inv(16)(p13q22) or t(16;16)(p13;q22): results from CALGB 8461. *J Clin Oncol* 22:1087–1094, 2004.

31. Grimwade D, Biondi A, Mozziconacci M-J, et al.: Characterization of acute promyelocytic leukemia cases lacking the classic t(15;17): results of the European Working Party. *Blood* 96:1297–1308, 2000.

32. Zelent A, Guidez F, Melnick A, et al.: Translocations of the *RARα* gene in acute promyelocytic leukemia. *Oncogene* 20:7186–7203, 2001.

33. Arnould C, Philippe C, Bourdon V, Grégoire MJ, Berger R, Jonveaux P. The signal transducer and activator of transcription STAT5b gene is a new partner of retinoic acid receptor α in acute promyelocytic-like leukaemia. *Hum Mol Genet* 8:1741–1749, 1999.

34. Jing Y: The PML-RARα fusion protein and targeted therapy for acute promyelocytic leukemia. *Leuk Lymphoma* 45:639–648, 2004.

35. Sainty D, Liso V, Cantu-Rajnoldi A, et al.: A new morphologic classification system for acute promyelocytic leukemia distinguishes cases with underlying *PLZF/RARA* gene rearrangements. *Blood* 96:1287–1296, 2000.

36. Mitelman F, Johansson B, Mertens F (eds.): Mitelman Database of Chromosome Aberrations in Cancer. Available at: http://cgap.nci.nih.gov/Chromosomes/Mitelman; 2005.

37. Martinez-Climent JA, Lane NJ, Rubin CM, et al.: Clinical and prognostic significance of chromosomal abnormalities in childhood acute myeloid leukemia de novo. *Leukemia* 9:95–101, 1995.

38. Mrózek K, Heinonen K, Lawrence D, et al.: Adult patients with de novo acute myeloid leukemia and t(9;11) (p22;q23) have a superior outcome to patients with other translocations involving band 11q23: a Cancer and Leukemia Group B study. *Blood* 90:4532–4538, 1997.

39. Avet-Loiseau H, Godon C, Li JY, et al.: Amplification of the 11q23 region in acute myeloid leukemia. *Genes Chromosomes Cancer* 26:166–170, 1999.

40. Cuthbert G, Thompson K, McCullough S, et al.: MLL amplification in acute leukaemia: a United Kingdom Cancer Cytogenetics Group (UKCCG) study. *Leukemia* 14:1885–1891, 2000.

41. Mrózek K, Heinonen K, Theil KS, et al.: Spectral karyotyping in patients with acute myeloid leukemia and a complex karyotype shows hidden aberrations, including recurrent overrepresentation of 21q, 11q, and 22q. *Genes Chromosomes Cancer* 34:137–153, 2002.

42. Poppe B, Vandesompele J, Schoch C, et al.: Expression analyses identify *MLL* as a prominent target of 11q23 amplification and support an etiologic role for *MLL* gain of function in myeloid malignancies. *Blood* 103: 229–235, 2004.

43. Caligiuri MA, Strout MP, Schichman SA, et al.: Partial tandem duplication of *ALL1* as a recurrent molecular

defect in acute myeloid leukemia with trisomy 11. *Cancer Res* 56:1418–1425, 1996.

44. Caligiuri MA, Strout MP, Lawrence D, et al.: Rearrangement of *ALL1* (*MLL*) in acute myeloid leukemia with normal cytogenetics. *Cancer Res* 58:55–59, 1998.

45. Döhner K, Tobis K, Ulrich R, et al.: Prognostic significance of partial tandem duplications of the *MLL* gene in adult patients 16 to 60 years old with acute myeloid leukemia and normal cytogenetics: a study of the Acute Myeloid Leukemia Study Group Ulm. *J Clin Oncol* 20: 3254–3261, 2002.

46. Schichman SA, Caligiuri MA, Gu Y, et al.: ALL-1 partial duplication in acute leukemia. *Proc Natl Acad Sci USA* 91: 6236–6239, 1994.

47. Preudhomme C, Sagot C, Boissel N, et al.: Favorable prognostic significance of *CEBPA* mutations in patients with de novo acute myeloid leukemia: a study from the Acute Leukemia French Association (ALFA). *Blood* 100: 2717–2723, 2002.

48. Barjesteh van Waalwijk van Doorn-Khosravani SB, Erpelinck C, Meijer J, et al.: Biallelic mutations in the *CEBPA* gene and low CEBPA expression levels as prognostic markers in intermediate-risk AML. *Hematol J* 4: 31–40, 2003.

49. Fröhling S, Schlenk RF, Stolze I, et al.: *CEBPA* mutations in younger adults with acute myeloid leukemia and normal cytogenetics: prognostic relevance and analysis of cooperating mutations. *J Clin Oncol* 22:624–633, 2004.

50. Song WJ, Sullivan MG, Legare RD, et al.: Haploinsufficiency of CBFA2 causes familial thrombocytopenia with propensity to develop acute myelogenous leukaemia. *Nat Genet* 23:166–175, 1999.

51. Stirewalt DL, Meshinchi S, Radich JP: Molecular targets in acute myelogenous leukemia. *Blood Rev* 17:15–23, 2003.

52. Stirewalt DL, Radich JP: The role of FLT3 in haematopoietic malignancies. *Nat Rev Cancer* 3:650–665, 2003.

53. Kottaridis PD, Gale RE, Frew ME, et al.: The presence of a FLT3 internal tandem duplication in patients with acute myeloid leukemia (AML) adds important prognostic information to cytogenetic risk group and response to the first cycle of chemotherapy: analysis of 854 patients from the United Kingdom Medical Research Council AML 10 and 12 trials. *Blood* 98:1752–1759, 2001.

54. Fröhling S, Schlenk RF, Breitruck J, et al.: Prognostic significance of activating *FLT3* mutations in younger adults (16 to 60 years) with acute myeloid leukemia and normal cytogenetics: a study of the AML Study Group Ulm. *Blood* 100:4372–4380, 2002.

55. Kainz B, Heintel D, Marculescu R, et al.: Variable prognostic value of *FLT3* internal tandem duplications in patients with de novo AML and a normal karyotype, t(15;17), t(8;21) or inv(16). *Hematol J* 3:283–289, 2002.

56. Meshinchi S, Woods WG, Stirewalt DL, et al.: Prevalence and prognostic significance of Flt3 internal tandem duplication in pediatric acute myeloid leukemia. *Blood* 97:89–94, 2001.

57. Liang DC, Shih LY, Hung IJ, et al.: Clinical relevance of internal tandem duplication of the FLT3 gene in childhood acute myeloid leukemia. *Cancer* 94:3292–3298, 2002.

58. Zwaan CM, Meshinchi S, Radich JP, et al.: FLT3 internal tandem duplication in 234 children with acute myeloid leukemia: prognostic significance and relation to cellular drug resistance. *Blood* 102:2387–2394, 2003.

59. Whitman SP, Archer KJ, Feng L, et al.: Absence of the wild-type allele predicts poor prognosis in adult de novo acute myeloid leukemia with normal cytogenetics and the internal tandem duplication of *FLT3*: a Cancer and Leukemia Group B study. *Cancer Res* 61:7233–7239, 2001.

60. Thiede C, Steudel C, Mohr B, et al.: Analysis of FLT3-activating mutations in 979 patients with acute myelogenous leukemia: association with FAB subtypes and identification of subgroups with poor prognosis. *Blood* 99:4326–4335, 2002.

61. Beran M, Luthra R, Kantarjian H, et al: FLT3 mutation and response to intensive chemotherapy in young adult and elderly patients with normal karyotype. *Leuk Res* 28:547–550, 2004.

62. Noguera NI, Breccia M, Divona M, et al.: Alterations of the FLT3 gene in acute promyelocytic leukemia: association with diagnostic characteristics and analysis of clinical outcome in patients treated with the Italian AIDA protocol. *Leukemia* 16:2185–2189, 2002.

63. Gari M, Goodeve A, Wilson G, et al.: c-kit proto-oncogene exon 8 in-frame deletion plus insertion mutations in acute myeloid leukaemia. *Br J Haematol* 105:894–900, 1999.

64. Care RS, Valk PJM, Goodeve AC, et al.: Incidence and prognosis of c-KIT and FLT3 mutations in core binding factor (CBF) acute myeloid leukaemias. *Br J Haematol* 121:775–777, 2003.

65. Tanner SM, Austin JL, Leone G, et al.: BAALC, the human member of a novel mammalian neuroectoderm gene lineage, is implicated in hematopoiesis and acute leukemia. *Proc Natl Acad Sci USA* 98:13901–13906, 2001.

66. Knudson AG: Hereditary cancer: two hits revisited. *J Cancer Res Clin Oncol* 122:135–140, 1996.

67. Kiyoi H, Naoe T, Yokota S, et al.: Internal tandem duplication of *FLT3* associated with leukocytosis in acute promyelocytic leukemia. *Leukemia* 11:1447–1452, 1997.

68. Kelly LM, Kutok JL, Williams IR, et al.: PML/RARα and FLT3-ITD induce an APL-like disease in a mouse model. *Proc Natl Acad Sci USA* 99:8283–8288, 2002.

69. Golub TR, Slonim DK, Tamayo P, et al.: Molecular classification of cancer: class discovery and class prediction by gene expression monitoring. *Science* 286:531–537, 1999.

70. Bullinger L, Döhner K, Bair E, et al.: Use of gene-expression profiling to identify prognostic subclasses in adult acute myeloid leukemia. *N Engl J Med* 350:1605–1616, 2004.

71. Costello JF, Frühwald MC, Smiraglia DJ, et al.: Aberrant CpG-island methylation has non-random and tumour-type-specific patterns. *Nat Genet* 24:132–138, 2000.

72. Rush LJ, Dai Z, Smiraglia DJ, et al.: Novel methylation targets in de novo acute myeloid leukemia with prevalence of chromosome 11 loci. *Blood* 97:3226–3233, 2001.

73. Chim CS, Liang R, Tam CY, et al.: Methylation of p15 and p16 genes in acute promyelocytic leukemia: potential diagnostic and prognostic significance. *J Clin Oncol* 19:2033–2940, 2001.

74. Christiansen DH, Andersen MK, Pedersen-Bjergaard J: Methylation of *p15INK4B* is common, is associated with deletion of genes on chromosome arm 7q and predicts a poor prognosis in therapy-related myelodysplasia and acute myeloid leukemia. *Leukemia* 17:1813–1819, 2003.

75. Ropero S, Setien F, Espada J, et al.: Epigenetic loss of the familial tumor-suppressor gene exostosin-1 (EXT1) disrupts heparan sulfate synthesis in cancer cells. *Hum Mol Genet* 13:2753–2765, 2004.

# Chapter **3**
# CLINICAL FEATURES AND MAKING THE DIAGNOSIS
## *Anjali S. Advani and Karl S. Theil*

## HISTORY OF ACUTE MYELOGENOUS LEUKEMIA

Acute myelogenous leukemia (AML) is a clonal disorder of the bone marrow that is characterized by abnormal proliferation of immature myeloid cells and arrested stem cell differentiation.[1] The history of AML dates back to the middle of the nineteenth century, when Virchow described the clinical disease as "the direct cause for the increase in the number of colorless particles in the blood."[2] In 1868, Neumann related AML to changes in the bone marrow.[2]

## CLINICAL FEATURES IN AML

Patients usually present with symptoms secondary to cytopenias, as the leukemia suppresses normal hematopoiesis. Patients may have pallor, fatigue, and shortness of breath secondary to anemia; bleeding, bruising, and ecchymoses secondary to thrombocytopenia/coagulation defects; and infections secondary to neutropenia.[3] Fifteen to twenty percent of patients will present with fevers, which can result from infection or from the leukemia itself.[4] Fewer than 20% of patients will have bone pain.[4]

### *EXTRAMEDULLARY INVOLVEMENT*
More uncommonly, patients present with symptoms secondary to leukemic infiltration of various tissues, leading to hepatomegaly, splenomegaly, leukemia cutis (2–10% of patients), gingival involvement, tumorous nodules (myeloid sarcoma) (3–5% of patients), lymphadenopathy, bone, or central nervous system (CNS) involvement (1% of patients).[3,5] Occasionally, patients may present with pericardial effusions.[2] Pulmonary infiltrates may also represent leukemia. Leukemic infiltrates in the lungs occur more commonly in patients presenting with high white blood counts and a monocytic component to their leukemia. Computed tomographic scan and bron-choscopy may be needed to make a definitive diagnosis and to rule out other etiologies, such as infection and pulmonary hemorrhage.

Extramedullary involvement is more common with the monocytic or myelomonocytic subtypes of AML, and may be associated with a worse prognosis. The cytogenetic abnormality most commonly associated with extramedullary leukemia is t(8;21)(q22;q22).[5,6] The incidence of extramedullary leukemia appears to be particularly high in patients who relapse, and may be decreasing with the use of intensive high-dose cytarabine as consolidation.[5] The most common site of extramedullary leukemia in patients with the t(8;21)(q22;q22) abnormality is paraspinal disease.[5] The presence of CD56, an adhesion molecule expressed in a variety of tissues including neural tissues, may be an additional risk factor for extramedullary leukemia in patients with t(8;21) or monocytic AML.[5,7–9]

### *MYELOID SARCOMAS*
Also known as granulocytic sarcomas, chloromas, and extra-medullary myeloid tumors, myeloid sarcomas are tumors of immature myeloid precursors.[10] They may precede or occur concurrently with another hematologic condition, such as chronic myelogenous leukemia (CML), AML, or other myeloproliferative disorders.[10,11] They also may be a sign of relapsed disease.[12] These patients should be treated with systemic induction therapy, regardless of whether or not the bone marrow is involved. On physical examination, myeloid sarcomas frequently have a purplish hue, and may be associated with itching.[12] When placed in dilute acid, myeloid sarcomas turn green, because of their increased content of myeloperoxidase.[4] The diagnosis should be suspected if eosinophilic myelocytes are present in a hematoxylin—eosin-stained biopsy.[4] If Auer rods are present or a myeloid origin detected, the diagnosis is confirmed.[4,13,14] CD43 positivity in the absence of CD3 is a nonspecific but sensitive marker for myeloid sarcoma.[10] Three types of myeloid sarcomas are described in the World Health Organization (WHO) classification:

(1) blastic granulocytic sarcoma, which is composed almost exclusively of myeloblasts; (2) immature form of granulocytic sarcoma, composed of a mixture of promyelocytes and myeloblasts; and (3) differentiated granulocytic sarcoma, composed of maturing neutrophils and promyelocytes.[10,11]

Granulocytic sarcomas occur commonly in subcutaneous tissues, but can affect any organ.[12] Patients presenting with an extramedullary chloroma causing spinal cord compression benefit from adequate local spine radiation (in addition to chemotherapy), and have a higher chance of neurologic recovery.[5]

### OTHER SKIN MANIFESTATIONS
Leukemia cutis usually presents as itchy papules or nodules that may be single or multiple.[2] Skin biopsy demonstrates myeloblasts. Numerical abnormalities of chromosome 8 may be more common in patients with leukemia cutis.[15] There is also a trend toward a shorter remission duration in patients with leukemia cutis.[15]

Unlike myeloid sarcomas and leukemia cutis, Sweet syndrome involves a benign dermal infiltration by neutrophils.[2] Sweet syndrome occurs most commonly in advanced myelodysplastic syndrome and AML, and is characterized by fevers and painful red raised lesions.[2] This syndrome responds well to steroids.[4,16]

### CNS LEUKEMIA
CNS leukemia associated with AML is not very common, and CNS prophylaxis is not routine [unlike with acute lymphoblastic leukemia (ALL)].[17] The incidence of meningeal disease has been reported to be as high as 15% in adults.[4,18] It tends to occur more commonly with the monocytic and myelomonocytic subtypes and is associated with higher white blood counts, t(8;21), and the inv (16).[4,12] Symptoms typically occur secondary to elevated intracranial pressure and include headache, blurred vision, and vomiting.[12] Cranial nerve palsies, secondary to infiltration of cranial nerve roots, particularly abducens palsy leading to a lateral strabismus, may occur.[12] Ophthalmologic examination may reveal retinal infiltration and/or papilledema.[12] Cerebral masses are rare, but may occur in patients with M4eo and inv(16).[4]

### HYPERLEUKOCYTOSIS
Patients with high white blood counts and blast counts can present with symptoms of leukostasis secondary to hyperleukocytosis.[3] Hyperleukocytosis is defined as a blast count of greater than $100,000/mm^3$ and occurs more commonly in patients with acute monocytic or myelomonocytic leukemia.[2,4] A high early mortality is observed in patients with hyperleukocytosis.[2] With hyperleukocytosis, inelastic myeloblasts pack and plug blood vessels, leading to leukostasis and thrombus formation.[12] Specific signs and symptoms can include shortness of breath, hypoxia, diffuse pulmonary infiltrates, headache,

blurred vision, heart failure, myocardial infarction, and priapism.[2,4,12] Leukostasis more commonly occurs with a rapidly rising blast count.[12] Blasts can also invade and disrupt arterioles, leading to hemorrhage.[12,19] Although there are no randomized controlled trials, patients with hyperleukocytosis should be leukapheresed to help bring the blast count down. Cytotoxic therapy should be initiated as soon as possible. If a definitive diagnosis has not been made, hydroxyurea can be used in conjunction with (or in place of) a pheresis until a diagnosis is made and definitive chemotherapy is started. A single dose of cranial radiation may also have some benefit in patients presenting with CNS symptoms and high white blood counts.[19,20] Patients with hyperleukocytosis should not be transfused with packed red cells until they have received appropriate cytoreductive treatment, since transfusion can increase blood viscosity and worsen symptoms.

### LABORATORY ABNORMALITIES IN HYPERLEUKOCYTOSIS
Pseudohyperkalemia can be present in patients with a high white blood count secondary to breakdown of white cells in vitro with subsequent release of potassium.[2] Other spurious laboratory data that can be seen in association with hyperleukocytosis include a falsely elevated platelet count (secondary to white cell fragments), pseudohypoxemia (secondary to oxygen consumption by leukocyte cells), falsely prolonged coagulation tests, and pseudohypoglycemia.[4,21–24] Pseudohypoxemia and pseudohypoglycemia can be avoided by placing samples on ice and performing tests immediately.[4,14]

### TUMOR LYSIS
Tumor lysis syndrome is usually seen 1–5 days after the initiation of chemotherapy in patients with AML and high circulating blast counts.[25] In response to chemotherapy, leukemic cells lyse, leading to hyperphosphatemia, hyperkalemia (or hypokalemia), hypocalcemia, an elevated lactate dehydrogenase (LDH), and hyperuricemia. Hyperuricemia results from breakdown of nucleotide precursors in leukemic cells to hypoxanthine and xanthine, and subsequent conversion to uric acid.[25] Renal failure can occur secondary to precipitation of calcium phosphate crystals or uric acid in the renal tubules.[25–28] Patients at risk for tumor lysis should be aggressively hydrated and started on allopurinol. Allopurinol, an inhibitor of xanthine oxidase, decreases the production of uric acid.[25] Rasburicase, a novel recombinant form of urate oxidase, converts uric acid to allantoin.[25] Allantoin is five to ten times more soluble than uric acid, thus allowing for more rapid urinary excretion.[25,29] Rasburicase should be considered for patients with renal dysfunction or high serum uric acid (i.e., >10).[25] The drug should not be administered to patients with G6PD deficiency, as an

additional by-product of the drug is hydrogen peroxide, which can lead to hemolytic anemia or methemoglobinemia in these patients.[25] Alkalinizing the urine may also increase the solubility of uric acid.[25,30] Electrolytes, uric acid, and LDH should be monitored carefully in tumor lysis syndrome.[25] Any electrolyte abnormalities should be corrected appropriately.

## CLINICAL FEATURES ASSOCIATED WITH SPECIFIC AML SUBTYPES AND/OR CYTOGENETIC ABNORMALITIES

### ACUTE MYELOID LEUKEMIA WITH INV(16) OR VARIANT

AML with inv(16) is characterized by abnormal bone marrow eosinophilic precursors. Most will be associated with a pericentric inversion of chromosome 16.[31] Less commonly, patients will have a translocation between two homologous of chromosome 16.[31] CD2 is often aberrantly expressed.[17] Associated clinical features include a good prognosis with high-dose cytarabine, hyperleukocytosis, young age at diagnosis, and an increased risk for CNS involvement.[17,32–34] Extramedullary sites of disease, including cervicotonsillar involvement and generalized lymphadenopathy, are particularly common, with a 33% incidence.[17] An increased incidence of acute pulmonary syndrome (pulmonary infiltrates, hypoxia, fever, and impending respiratory failure) has also been reported in patients with AML and inv(16) (54%) versus patients with the same diagnosis but without inv(16) (9%).[35]

### ERYTHROLEUKEMIA

Erythroleukemia can occasionally be familial.[36–38] Signs or symptoms which occur more commonly with this subtype include synovitis, serositis, effusions, bone pain, and immunologic abnormalities.[4,36,39] Rheumatologic symptoms tend to respond to anti-inflammatory agents.[36,39] Specific immunologic abnormalities include hypergammaglobulinemia, a positive Coombs test, a positive antinuclear antibody test, and an elevated rheumatoid factor titer.[36,39] Cytogenetics demonstrate aneuploidy in almost two-thirds of patients.[4,40,41]

### ACUTE MEGAKARYOCYTIC LEUKEMIA

Patients with acute megakaryocytic leukemia rarely present with high blast counts or extramedullary involvement.[36] Platelet counts are often normal or elevated at presentation,[36] while LDH levels are usually markedly elevated, with an isomorphic pattern.[36,42] Osteosclerotic and osteolytic lesions may be present.[4,43,44] Acute megakaryocytic leukemia in infants is associated with a t(1;22)(p13;q13) abnormality.[4,45] This translocation involves fusion of OTT on chromosome 1 with MAL on chromosome 22, thus leading to activation of platelet-derived growth factor.[4,46] This activation may lead to the megakaryocytic proliferation and fibrosis seen in acute megakaryocytic leukemia.[4,46] These infants present with extensive organomegaly.[4] Acute megakaryocytic leukemia is also the most common acute leukemia seen in patients with Down syndrome[47,48] and may be transient, resolving spontaneously.

### ACUTE BASOPHILIC LEUKEMIA

This leukemia often arises from a blast crisis of CML.[36,49] Patients may present with increased histamine levels and urticaria.[36] By flow cytometry, many cases will express CD9 and some will express CD7 or CD10.[10,50]

### SECONDARY LEUKEMIAS

Secondary leukemias are classified as a distinct type of AML in the new WHO classification. They may develop in patients with a preceding hematologic disorder [including myelodysplasia (MDS)], inherited genetic disorder (Bloom or Fanconi anemia), or history of exposure to radiation or chemotherapy.[3] Leukemias secondary to chemotherapy fall into two major categories: those associated with topoisomerase inhibitors and those associated with alkylating agents. Chromosomal translocation 6, involving the mixed lineage leukemia (MLL) gene at 11q23 are significantly associated with secondary leukemias.[51] Eighty-five percent of AML cases with 11q23 abnormalities develop after exposure to topoisomerase II inhibitors, such as etoposide.[3] The leukemias are most often monocytic or myelomonocytic in lineage, occur shortly after chemotherapy (2–3 years), and usually are not preceded by MDS.[3] Three to ten percent of patients who receive alkylating agents as part of their therapy for Hodgkin's disease, non-Hodgkin's lymphoma, ovarian cancer, breast cancer, or multiple myeloma develop secondary AML.[3,52] The incidence of this leukemia peaks at 5–10 years after treatment, is often preceded by MDS, and is characterized by deletions of chromosomes 5 and/or 7.[3,53–55]

### NATURAL KILLER CELL ACUTE LEUKEMIA

This form of leukemia typically falls under M0 [in the French—American—British (FAB) classification] or AML minimally differentiated (WHO classification). It is characterized by a unique immunophenotype, with both myeloid and natural killer cell markers, suggesting that it arises from a precursor common to both natural killer cell and myeloid lineages.[56] The typical immunophenotype is CD33+, CD56+, CD11a+, CD13lo, CD15lo, CD34±, HLA-DR−, CD16−.[56] Morphologically, the cells have deep invaginations in the nuclear membrane, scant cytoplasm, and fine azurophilic granules.[56] These granules often stain positive for myeloperoxidase and Sudan black B.[56] Because of the morphology and absence of HLA-DR on flow cytometry, this entity can sometimes be confused with the microgranular variant of acute promyelocytic leukemia (APL).[56] However, it lacks the characteristic translocation [t(15;17)] and patients tend to have a poor prognosis.[56]

### DIABETES INSIPIDUS

Diabetes insipidus is a rare complication of AML.[57] Patients present with polyuria, polydipsia, and a low-serum antidiuretic hormone (ADH) level.[58] Cytogenetic abnormalities associated with cases in the literature include monosomy 7, deletions of chromosome 7, and chromosome 3 abnormalities.[57,59] The reason for these specific associations is unknown.[57] However, the proposed mechanism involves leukemic infiltration of the neurohypophysis. Magnetic resonance imaging (MRI) demonstrates a "bright spot" in the neurohypophysis prior to treatment.[59] Both MRI findings and ADH release subsequently resolve after chemotherapy.[59]

### THROMBOCYTOSIS

Thrombocytosis is rare in AML, and when seen it is usually associated with chromosome 3q abnormalities.[60] Platelet counts as high as 1 million/mm$^3$ have been reported.[60–62] Typically, patients are asymptomatic,[60] and may have a preceding history of MDS.[4] Expression of the EVI 1 gene (3q26.2) is thought to be involved.[4,63,64]

### COAGULOPATHY

Coagulopathy is most commonly associated with APL, which is characterized by the cytogenetic abnormality t(15;17) or varient. Although APL is the most curable subtype of AML in adults, it needs to be recognized and treated immediately because of the risks of significant bleeding.[65] Patients with coagulopathy should be transfused to keep their platelets above 50,000/mm$^3$ and transfused with cryoprecipitate to keep their fibrinogen within the lower limits of normal. Fresh frozen plasma should be used to correct an abnormal prothrombin time or partial thromboplastin time. Heparin and antifibrinolytics, such as amicar, do not have a standard role in the treatment of APL-induced coagulopathy, as trials have demonstrated a similar rate of hemorrhagic death in patients with APL treated with heparin, antifibrinolytics, or supportive care.[66,67] Initially, it was thought that the coagulopathy in APL was secondary to release of granules from the leukemic promyelocytes.[36,68,69] However, it is more likely that the coagulopathy is secondary to release of plasminogen activator from leukemic cells; while there is no increase in platelet turnover, there is an increase in fibrinogen turnover and an increase in fibrin/fibrinogen degradation products with a decrease in $\alpha_2$-antiplasmin levels, suggesting activation of plasmin.[36,70–74] Recent data suggest that annexin II, a receptor for fibrinolytic proteins, is increased in patients with APL.[75]

High levels of annexin increase the production of plasmin.[75] All-*trans*-retinoic acid (ATRA) should be initiated concurrent with chemotherapy in patients with APL. ATRA induces differentiation of leukemic cells into mature granulocytes and decreases the incidence of coagulation and bleeding.[76] In addition, ATRA blocks annexin II messenger RNA production through a transcriptional mechanism.[75] Patients with the microgranular variant of APL tend to present with hyperleukocytosis in addition to coagulopathy.[77] Coagulopathy can also occur in the other subtypes of AML, especially the monocytic forms and patients with high white blood cell counts.[36]

### HYPOKALEMIA

Hypokalemia occurs more frequently in patients with monocytic and monoblastic leukemias.[36] The mechanism involves excess lysozyme (muramidase) production, which may damage the proximal renal tubule, leading to proximal renal tubular acidosis and hypokalemia.[4]

## MAKING THE DIAGNOSIS

On a routine complete blood count (CBC), most patients with AML are anemic and thrombocytopenic.[78] The white blood count is variable, with 20% of patients having white blood counts less than 5000/mm$^3$ and 20% of patients with white blood counts greater than 100,000/mm$^3$.[78] High white blood counts and hyperleukocytosis are more common in the monocytic leukemias.[36,79] Although blasts are usually present in the peripheral blood, a subset of patients present with "aleukemic leukemia."

A review of the peripheral blood film and a bone marrow aspirate/biopsy is part of the initial diagnostic work-up and is essential for distinguishing AML from other hematologic disorders such as ALL, MDS, or AML arising in the setting of MDS (Table 3.1).[3] Occasionally, immature blasts can be confused with metastatic carcinoma, plasma cell neoplasms, or lymphoma.[77] The peripheral blood film and bone marrow slides should be air-dried and stained with a polychrome dye such as Wright–Giesma.[12]

Based on the new WHO criteria, the diagnosis of AML is made when at least 20% of nucleated cells in the bone marrow or peripheral blood are myeloid blasts.[11] The previous FAB classification system required 30% blasts to make a diagnosis of AML. The major reason for lowering the blast threshold is that patients with 20–30% blasts (previously considered as RAEB-t, refractory anemia with excess blasts in transformation) have an identical prognosis to those with 30% blasts.[2] The percentage of blasts should be determined on a 500 cell count on well-stained bone marrow aspirate slides or a 200 cell differential on peripheral blood smears.[10,11] In certain

**Table 3.1** Specimen submission requirements and diagnostic utility

| Diagnostic study | Specimen requirements | Tests performed | Diagnostic utility | Comments |
|---|---|---|---|---|
| CBC and differential | 2.5 mL whole blood in 4 mL (EDTA) lavender top tube. Fill tube to at least half of fill volume | Automated CBC with differential; manual review of smear | Determine absolute leukocyte count and blast count; assess for anemia and thrombocytopenia; evaluate blast morphology; rule out quantitative or qualitative abnormalities in other cell types, including dysplastic features, presence of nucleated red blood cells, and/or microangiopathic changes | Blood remaining after CBC may be used for cytochemistry, flow cytometry, and molecular analysis |
| Bone marrow aspirate | Bone marrow aspirate smears with extra unstained smears for cytochemistry, iron stain, or other studies as necessary | Wright–Giemsa stain for routine morphology and cell differential count | Determine blast percentage and evaluate blast morphology; assess quantitative and qualitative abnormalities in myeloid, erythroid, and megakaryocytic lineages | High quality smears are essential for accurate diagnosis; iron stain useful to assess iron stores and presence of ringed sideroblasts; make touch preps of biopsy if dry tap |
| Bone marrow biopsy | Bone marrow core biopsy ideally >1 cm in length. Place in appropriate fixative (B5, acid zinc formalin, or buffered formalin) | Hematoxylin–eosin stain for routine histologic examination with immunostains (CD34, TdT, CD79a, Hgb, CD20, CD3, MPO, CD61, CD10, and CD31) as necessary | Determine overall cellularity and percentage and lineage of blasts; assess residual normal hematopoietic elements; evaluate for associated fibrosis and/or dysplastic features; rule out associated disorders that mimic leukemia | Immunostains may aid in diagnosis, especially in the absence of flow cytometry (dry tap) |
| Cytochemical stains | Unfixed, fresh air-dried bone marrow aspirate smears | May include MPO, nonspecific esterase, chloroacetate esterase, PAS, and Sudan black B | Assess lineage and differentiation of blasts. MPO and Sudan black B are used as sensitive markers of myeloid differentiation (positive defined as staining ≥3% blasts). Nonspecific esterase is a marker of monocytic differentiation. Abnormal erythroid precursors show "block-like" cytoplasmic staining with PAS | Negative MPO and/or SBB stains do not exclude a diagnosis of AML; enzyme activity degrades over time, so fresh unfixed material is necessary |

*table continues*

**Table 3.1**    continued

| Diagnostic study | Specimen requirements | Tests performed | Diagnostic utility | Comments |
|---|---|---|---|---|
| Flow cytometry | 4 mL bone marrow in 4 mL (EDTA) lavender top tube; 4 mL whole blood in 4 mL (EDTA) lavender top tube, 7 mL (ACD) yellow top tube or 4 mL heparinized (sodium or lithium) green top tube; or 4 mL bone marrow in a heparinized syringe or heparinized green top tube. Store at room temperature. Samples should be <30 h old | Usually includes CD45 with myeloid markers CD13, CD33, CD117, and CD65; monocytic marker CD14; T-cell markers CD2, CD5, and CD7; B-cell markers CD19, and CD20; non-lineage-specific markers HLA-DR, CD10, CD34, and TdT; NK cell marker CD56; megakaryocytic marker CD61; may also include CD79a, cCD22, cCD3, cIgM, sIgM, and MPO | Determine lineage of blasts and evaluate for aberrant antigen expression; rule out precursor T or precursor B acute lymphoblastic leukemias and acute leukemia of ambiguous lineage. Baseline phenotype of blasts may be helpful for excluding relapse or monitoring minimal residual disease following treatment | Bone marrow aspirate is preferred. Helps in recognition of minimally differentiated AML; immunophenotypic patterns can help identify AML with t(8;21) and t(15;17). Blast percentage by flow cytometry may not correlate with aspirate smear if hemodilute sample submitted |
| Cytogenetics | 2–3 mL bone marrow in 4 mL heparinized (sodium) green top tube. Peripheral blood may be alternate sample if circulating immature cells present (>1,000/μL). Store at room temperature; do not refrigerate or freeze | GTG-banded chromosome analysis; minimum 20 metaphases analyzed (when available) | Gives global information about cell karyotype; identifies nonrandom abnormalities with prognostic significance | First pull of aspirate preferred. Do not collect specimen in lithium heparin or EDTA. Excess cells from cytogenetics may be used for FISH analysis |
| Molecular analysis by FISH | 8 mL whole blood in two 4 mL (EDTA) lavender top tubes; 4 mL bone marrow from (EDTA) lavender top tube | May include BCR-ABL, t(15;17), t(8;21), inv(16), MLL rearrangement, and RARα rearrangement | Gives specific information about presence or absence of a particular genetic abnormality | Helpful at diagnosis, especially when cytogenetic sample not submitted or no growth |
| Molecular analysis by polymerase chain reaction (PCR) | 5 mL whole blood in (EDTA) lavender top tube; 2–3 mL bone marrow in (EDTA) lavender top tube; refrigerate | May include t(9;22), t(15;17), inv(16), t(8;21), MLL rearrangement, and FLT3 rearrangement, as necessary | Gives specific information about presence or absence of a particular genetic abnormality. Helpful for minimal residual disease monitoring | Heparinized tube unacceptable due to interference with PCR |

circumstances, 20% blasts are not needed for the diagnosis. For example, cases with inv(16), t(r,21) or t(15;17) are diagnosed as acute myeloid leukemia regardless of blast percentage according to WHO guidelines. In acute monocytic and myelomonocytic leukemias, promonocytes are also counted as monoblasts for the diagnosis.[10,11,81] In acute erythroleukemia, blasts are counted as a percentage of non-erythroid cell if erythroid precursors marrow comprise >50% of the differential count.

On morphologic review, myeloblasts in patients with AML typically have delicate nuclear chromatin, three to five nucleoli, and a variable number of fine myeloperoxidase granules in the cytoplasm[82] (Figure 3.1). Auer rods (azurophilic granules within lysozymes) are pathognomonic for AML[3] (Figure 3.2). "Faggot cells," blast with bundles of Auer rods, are also characteristic in certain AML subtypes (AML with maturation and APL).[36] Phi bodies, fusiform or spindle-shaped rods, which are similar to Auer rods and stain with myeloperoxidase, may also be present.[4,83]

Other AML subtypes may have distinct morphologic features in the blood and bone marrow. In the monocytic/monoblastic subtype of AML, the nucleus of the monoblasts is often indented and contains one to four large nucleoli.[36] A moderate amount of cytoplasm is present (Figure 3.3). Patients with acute myelomonocytic leukemia often have a significant monocytosis in the peripheral blood.[10] Acute myeloid

leukemia with inv(16), is characterized by abnormal eosinophils.[36,84,85] In acute erythroleukemia, abnormal erythroblasts with giant multinucleate forms, nuclear budding, and nuclear fragmentation are found in the bone marrow.[36] (Figure 3.4). On review of a peripheral blood film, nucleated red blood cells are often present.[36,86,87] Bone marrow fibrosis, which can make bone marrow aspiration difficult, is typical of acute megakaryoblastic leukemia and acute panmyelosis with myelofibrosis.[10,47] Megakaryoblasts in acute megakaryoblastic leukemia typically have a high nuclear/cytoplasmic ratio, varying size, and pale agranular cytoplasm.[36] Malignant proliferation of all three myeloid cell lines is present in acute panmyelosis with myelofibrosis.[10] Finally, acute basophilic leukemia is characterized by striking basophilic granularity in myelocytes, and cells stain strongly with toluidine blue.[36]

MDS is differentiated from AML on the basis of percentage of blasts in the bone marrow. AML arising from MDS is characterized by dysplastic maturation of the hematopoietic precursors and certain chromosomal abnormalities (such as loss of part or all of chromosome 5 or 7).[3] In addition, patients may have a preceding history of low blood counts. AML can often be differentiated from ALL on morphologic grounds. Lymphoblasts tend to be smaller in size, with little cytoplasm and indistinct nucleoli.[77]

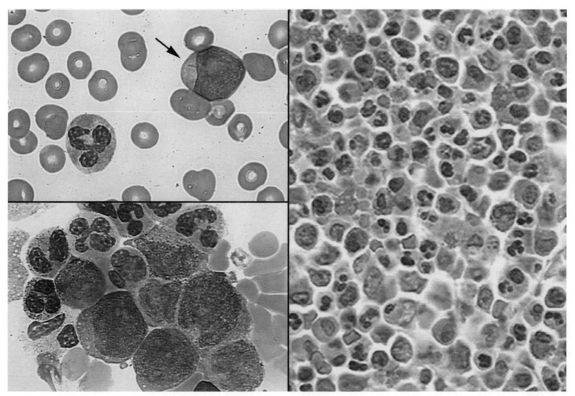

**Figure 3.1**  *Acute myeloid leukemia with t(8;21)(q22;q22): Peripheral blood smear shows a blast with an Auer rod (arrow) and a neutrophil with characteristic salmon-colored cytoplasmic granules (upper left); bone marrow aspirate shows blasts admixed with maturing myeloid cells (bottom left); and bone marrow biopsy is hypercellular with blasts admixed with maturing myeloid cells and eosinophils. (Wright–Giemsa stain, left panels; hematoxylin–eosin stain, right panel)*

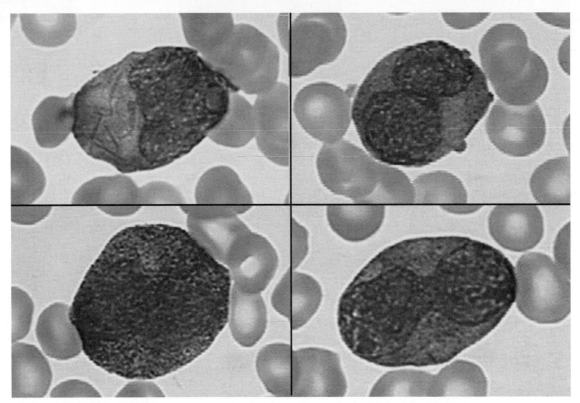

**Figure 3.2** *Acute myeloid leukemia with t(15;17)(q22;q21): Features of blasts include multiple Auer rods (upper left), hypergranular cytoplasm (lower left), and bilobed nuclei (upper and lower right panels). This leukemia is often associated with a low white blood cell count, and characteristic blasts containing multiple Auer rods may require a careful search to identify. (Wright–Giemsa stain)*

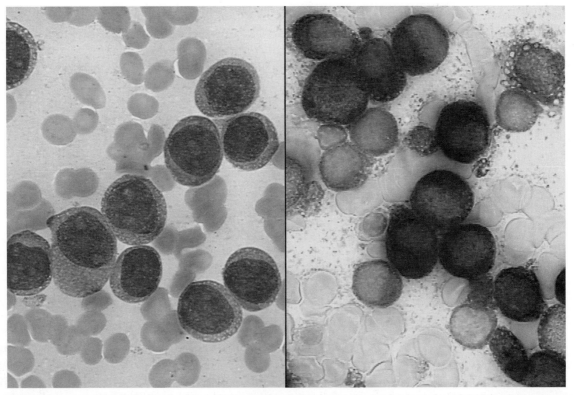

**Figure 3.3** *Acute monoblastic leukemia: Blasts have moderate amounts of cytoplasm and nuclei with one to two nucleoli (left panel). Monocytic differentiation is demonstrated in the blasts by positive cytochemical stain for nonspecific esterase as shown by red-brown cytoplasmic staining (right panel). (Wright–Giemsa stain, left panel; nonspecific esterase stain [α-naphthyl butyrate], right panel)*

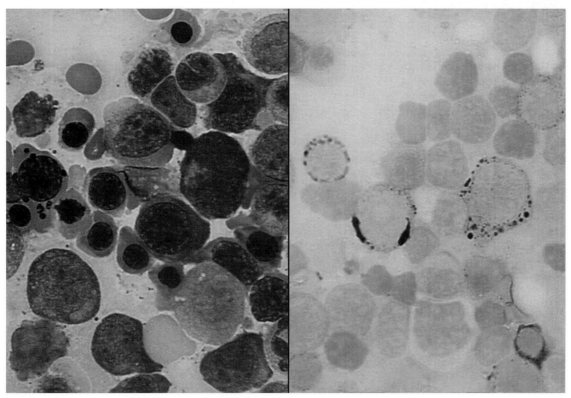

**Figure 3.4**    *Acute erythroleukemia: An increase in erythroid elements with dysplastic features including megaloblastoid chromatin and nuclear fragmentation is evident in this bone marrow aspirate smear (left panel). PAS stain is useful to identify abnormal "blocklike" cytoplasmic staining in immature erythroid precursors (right panel). (Wright–Giemsa stain, left panel; PAS stain, right panel)*

However, immunophenotyping and immunohisto-chemistry are used to make a definitive diagnosis. By flow cytometry, myeloblasts usually express the cell surface antigen markers CD13 and CD33. Cells of myeloid origin usually will be myeloperoxidase positive by cytochemical or immunostains.[10] In minimally differentiated AML (M0), blasts do not express myeloperoxidase cytochemically; however, they are myeloid antigen positive (CD13 and CD33) based on flow cytometry.[82]

When performing a bone marrow aspirate, a small amount of the first pull of the aspirate should be placed on a slide, as hemodilution may make it difficult to interpret the aspirate. At least 5 mL of aspirate should be sent in heparinized tubes for flow cytometry and cytogenetics. If an aspirate cannot be obtained secondary to fibrosis or a "packed" marrow, these studies can be performed on the peripheral blood if enough peripheral blasts are present. Flow cytometry can also be attempted on a biopsy specimen by performing an extra biopsy, placing the sample in saline, and "teasing" the cells from the marrow. Although bone marrow aspirates are usually obtained from the posterior iliac crest, a sternal aspirate can be performed if a sample cannot be obtained. Immunophenotyping by flow cytometry is helpful in diagnosing and subclassifying AML.[88] The most commonly used monoclonal

antibodies in the diagnosis of AML are CD13, CD14, CD15, CD33, CD34, and HLA-DR[47]: CD13 and CD33 both are myeloid markers; CD34 and HLA-DR both are stem cell markers; CD14, monocytic; and CD15, myeloid-granulocytic.[89] Myeloid antigens such as CD14, CD15, and CD11b expressed on more differentiate myeloid cells may be found in AMLs with myeloid or monocytic maturation.[90] CD14 and CD64 are the best markers for monocytic differentiation.[10,91] The platelet glycoproteins CD41, CD42, and CD61 are usually present in acute megakaryocytic leukemia.[47,92] Flow cytometry may be particularly helpful in diagnosing the microgranular variant of APL. With the microgranular variant, granules are not readily seen by light microscopy[77] (Figure 3.5). However, unlike the other AMLs, APL is both CD34 negative and HLA-DR negative by flow cytometry.[47] In certain instances, flow cytometry may also provide prognostic information. The presence of CD56 in both M2 and M3 AML appears to correlate with adverse prognosis.[88,93–96]

Immunostains used in evaluating bone marrow biopsies include myeloperoxidase (myeloid), hemoglobin A (erythroid), and CD34, CD79a, CD61, TdT (PAS, non-specific esterase are cytochemical stains, not immunostains). Biopsies can be stained for these markers if an aspirate for flow cytometry cannot be obtained to better subclassify the AML.

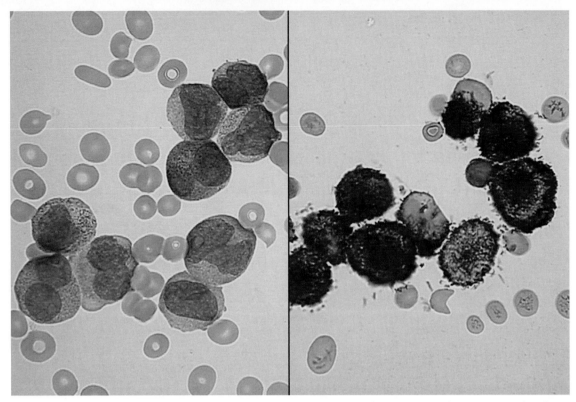

**Figure 3.5** *Acute myeloid leukemia with t(15;17)(q22;q21): The hypogranular variant is often associated with an elevated white blood count with most blasts having lightly granular to almost agranular cytoplasm, but still retaining the typical bilobed nucleus (left panel). A cytochemical stain for myeloperoxidase (right panel) demonstrates intense cytoplasmic positivity as shown by blue-black granules. (Wright–Giemsa stain, left panel; myeloperoxidase stain, right panel)*

Cytogenetics are needed to assess prognosis, risk-adapt therapy, as well as to subclassify the AML. Cytogenetic abnormalities most commonly involve translocations and inversions of genes encoding transcription regulators.[97] Particular cytogenetic abnormalities are associated with specific clinical features and prognosis. Based on the new WHO classification, AML with specific cytogenetic abnormalities [t(8;21) (q22;q22), t(15;17)(q22;q21), 11q23 abnormalities, and variants inv(16)(p13q22) and t(16;16)(p13;q22)] are classified as AML independently of the proportion of blasts in the bone marrow[12] (Figure 3.6). Fluorescence in situ hybridization (FISH) for t(15;17) inv(16), t(8;21) or 11q23 rearrangement should be performed if there is suspicion for one of these rearrangements, especially if cytogenetics are normal or unsuccessful since identification of an abnormality can affect both prognosis and therapy. FISH can be more rapid and sensitive than routine cytogenetics. In the future, other molecular markers, such as the presence or absence of fms-like tyrosine kinase 3 (FLT3) and assessment of multidrug resistance markers may become a standard part of the initial evaluation.

## THE FAB AND WHO CLASSIFICATION OF AML

The FAB classification was composed of eight AML subtypes: M0–M7. These subtypes were distinguished based on both the degree of differentiation and the cell lineage.[3] Cytochemical stains, including myeloperoxidase, nonspecific esterase, and sudan black B, were used in conjunction with morphology to identify the subtype.[47] This classification system did not require immunophenotyping to make a diagnosis, except in the M0 subtype (minimally differentiated AML subtype). Cytogenetics were also not incorporated into this classification system. The WHO classification system differs from the FAB classification in several aspects. The blast percentage for AML is decreased from 30 to 20%. In addition, biological, clinical, and prognostic markers (such as cytogenetics) are incorporated into the classification. Such factors allow us to better define the disease and risk-adapt therapy. The new WHO classification for AML recognizes four distinct entities: (1) AML with specific cytogenetic abnormalities, (2) AML with multilineage dysplasia

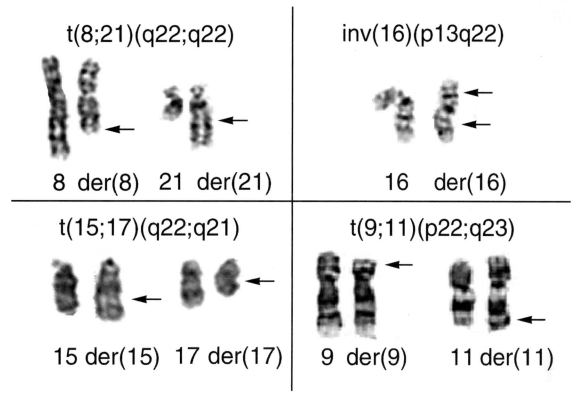

**Figure 3.6** *Critical nonrandom chromosome abnormalities that define disease subtypes included in the WHO entity "acute myeloid leukemia with recurrent genetic abnormalities" include t(8;21), t(15;17) and variants, inv(16) and variants, and 11q23 abnormalities. For each pair of GTG-banded chromosomes shown, the normal homologues are shown on the left, and abnormal homologues on the right; arrows mark chromosome breakpoints. These abnormalities can also be detected by molecular methods, including RT-PCR and FISH*

(with or without prior MDS), (3) therapy-related AML and MDS (alkylating-agent-related or epipodophyllo-toxin-related), and (4) AML not otherwise classifiable.[1,12,98,99]

## OTHER ACUTE LEUKEMIA ENTITIES

In addition to diagnosing and subclassifying AML, flow cytometry is needed to recognize the entities of undifferentiated acute leukemia, bilineage leukemia, and biphenotypic leukemia.[10] Lineage-specific antigens include myeloperoxidase (myeloid), cytoplasmic CD3 (T-lymphoblasts), cytoplasmic CD22 (B-lymphoblasts), cytoplasmic IgM (B-lymphoblasts) and cytoplasmic CD79a (B-cell lymphoblasts).[12] In undifferentiated acute leukemias, no lineage-specific antigen is detected,[10] and often only one lineage-associated antigen (such as CD13 or CD33) is positive by flow.[10] Non-lineage specific primitive stem cell markers, such as CD34, CD38, and HLA-DR, may be present.[90]

Bilineage leukemia occurs when blasts derive from two distinct lineages.[10] These leukemias are sometimes associated with the Philadelphia chromosome, t(9;22), or the MLL gene, 11q23.[90]

In biphenotypic leukemias, blasts are positive for two or three distinct lineages on the same cell.[10] Specific criteria are used to make this diagnosis. One commonly used scoring system is the Royal Marsden criteria.[12,100] Blasts with greater than two points for two or more lineages are considered biphenotypic,[12] and are considered distinct from AML with aberrant coexpression of lymphoid markers.[88] CD7 is the most frequent lymphoid-associated antigen expressed in such cases.[88]

## CLINICAL WORK-UP

A full history and physical examination should be performed with special attention to any preceding history of blood disorder or malignancy, past chemotherapy or radiation treatments, occupational exposure, family history, general performance status, age of the patient, signs/symptoms of infection, and extramedullary signs of leukemia involvement. Risk factors associated with adverse outcome in AML include age greater than 60 years, poor performance status, secondary AML, white blood count greater than 30,000/mm³ and an elevated LDH.[1,3,101] Tests performed at diagnosis should include a CBC with differential, comprehensive metabolic panel, uric acid, LDH, prothrombin time, partial thromboplastin time, fibrinogen, and chest X-ray (with posterior anterior and lateral views). HLA typing (serology) should also be performed in case a patient becomes alloimmunized to random donor platelet transfusions and requires HLA-matched platelets during his or her treatment course. HLA typing at the DNA level should be performed on any patient who may be a stem cell transplant candidate in the future. It is best for HLA typing to be done prior to the initiation of chemotherapy, when more cells are present. A multiple gated acquisition scan should be done to assess cardiac function, as induction chemotherapy regimens for AML include an anthracycline. In addition, an indwelling venous catheter (i.e., Hickman catheter) should be placed for blood draws, blood product transfusions, fluid management, and antibiotic administration.[2] A lumbar puncture is not a routine part of the work-up unless there is clinical suspicion for CNS leukemia.

Patients who are neutropenic and febrile should have blood cultures drawn and should be started on appropriate broad-spectrum antibiotics. Most patients will also require transfusions of packed red cells and platelets because of their anemia and thrombocytopenia. Blood products should be leukoreduced to prevent transmission of cytomegalovirus, alloimmunization, and to decrease the risk of nonhemolytic febrile transfusion reactions.[78] Products should be irradiated to prevent the risk of graft-versus-host disease from the blood products themselves, especially if the patient is a potential stem cell transplant candidate.[78] Pooled random donor platelets (with exposure to six to eight donors per transfusion) are used initially, and single donor or HLA-matched platelets are used if patients become refractory to pooled platelets.[102] Patients who are not bleeding and are not having procedures done should be transfused for platelet counts less than or equal to 10,000/mm$^3$.[102,103] Hydration and allopurinol should be initiated to decrease the risk of tumor lysis syndrome in patients with high circulating blast counts. It is important to have a frank discussion with the patient prior to treatment regarding the diagnosis, prognosis, tests needed for work-up, length of hospitalization, potential complications of treatment, need for transfusions, and treatment plan.

## REFERENCES

1. Stone RM: Treatment of acute myeloid leukemia: state-of-the-art and future directions. *Semin Hematol* 39:4–10, 2002.
2. Rohatiner A, Lister T: Acute myelogenous leukemia. In: Henderson E, Lister T, Greaves M (eds.) *Leukemia.* Philadelphia: Saunders; 2002:485–517.
3. Lowenberg B, Downing JR, Burnett A: Acute myeloid leukemia. *N Engl J Med* 341:1051–1062, 1999.
4. Greer J, Baer MR, Kinney MC: Acute myelogenous leukemia. In: Lee GR, Foerster J, Lukens J, Paraskevas F, Greer JP, Rodgers GM (eds.) *Wintrobe's Clinical Hematology.* Baltimore: Williams and Wilkins; 1998:2272–2319.
5. Byrd JC, Weiss RB, Arthur DC, et al.: Extramedullary leukemia adversely affects hematologic complete remission rate and overall survival in patients with t(8;21)(q22;q22): results from Cancer and Leukemia Group B 8461. *J Clin Oncol* 15:466–475, 1997.
6. Byrd JC, Edenfield WJ, Shields DJ, et al.: Extramedullary myeloid cell tumors in acute nonlymphocytic leukemia: a clinical review. *J Clin Oncol* 13:1800–1816, 1995.
7. Byrd JC, Weiss RB: Recurrent granulocytic sarcoma. An unusual variation of acute myelogenous leukemia associated with 8;21 chromosomal translocation and blast expression of the neural cell adhesion molecule. *Cancer* 73:2107–2112, 1994.
8. Scott AA, Kopecky KJ, Grogan TM, et al.: CD56: a determinant of extramedullary and central nervous system involvement in acute myeloid leukemia. *Mod Pathol* 7:120A, 1994.
9. Seymour JF, Pierce SA, Kantarjian HM, et al.: Investigation of karyotypic, morphologic and clinical features in patients with acute myeloid leukemia blast cells expressing the neural cell adhesion molecule (CD56). *Leukemia* 8:823–826, 1994.
10. Todd WM: Acute myeloid leukemia and related conditions. *Hematol Oncol Clin North Am* 16:301–319, 2002.
11. Jaffe ES, Harris NL, Stein H, Vardiman JW (eds.): *World Health Organization Classification of Tumours: Pathology and Genetics of Tumour of Haematopoietic and Lymphoid Tissues.* Lyon, France: International Agency for Research on Cancer; 2001.
12. Henderson ES, McArthur J: Diagnosis, classification, and assessment of response to treatment. In: Henderson ES, Lister T, Greaves M (eds.) *Leukemia.* Philadelphia: Saunders; 2002:227–248.
13. Goagsguen JE, Bennett JM, Henderson E: Biological diagnosis of leukemias. In: Henderson ES, Lister T, Greaves M (eds.) *Leukemia.* 6th ed. Philadelphia: WB Saunders; 1996:8–33.
14. Baer MR: Management of unusual presentations of acute leukemia. *Hematol Oncol Clin North Am* 7:275–292, 1993.
15. Agis H, Weltermann A, Fonatsch C, et al.: A comparative study on demographic, hematological, and cytogenetic findings and prognosis in acute myeloid leukemia with and without leukemia cutis. *Ann Hematol* 81:90–95, 2002.
16. Cohen PR, Talpaz M, Kurzrock R: Malignancy-associated Sweet's syndrome: review of the world literature. *J Clin Oncol* 6:1887–1897, 1988.
17. Billstrom R, Ahlgren T, Bekassy AN, et al.: Acute myeloid leukemia with inv(16)(p13q22): involvement of cervical lymph nodes and tonsils is common and may be a negative prognostic sign. *Am J Hematol* 71:15–19, 2002.

18. Rohatiner A, Lister T: The general management of the patient with leukemia. In: Henderson ES, Lister T, Greaves M (eds.) *Leukemia.* 6th ed. Philadelphia: WB Saunders; 1996:247–255.

19. Davies A, Rohatiner A: General management of the patient with leukemia. In: Henderson ES, Lister T, Greaves M (eds.) *Leukemia.* 6th ed. Philadelphia: WB Saunders; 2002:285–296.

20. Wiernik PH, Serpick AA: Factors effecting remission and survival in adult acute nonlymphocytic leukemia (ANLL). *Medicine (Baltimore)* 49:505–513, 1970.

21. Abe R, Umezu H, Uchida T, et al.: Myeloblastoma with an 8;21 chromosome translocation in acute myeloblastic leukemia. *Cancer* 58:1260–1264, 1986.

22. Fox MJ, Brody JS, Weintraub LR: Leukocyte larceny: a cause of spurious hypoxemia. *Am J Med* 67:742–746, 1979.

23. Field JB, Williams HE: Artifactual hypoglycemia associated with leukemia. *N Engl J Med* 265:946–948, 1961.

24. Hess CE, Nichols AB, Hunt WB, et al.: Pseudohypoxemia secondary to leukemia and thrombocytosis. *N Engl J Med* 301:361–363, 1979.

25. Holdsworth MT, Nguyen P: Role of i.v. allopurinol and rasburicase in tumor lysis syndrome. *Am J Health Syst Pharm* 60:2213–2222, 2003; quiz: 2223–2224.

26. Jeha S: Tumor lysis syndrome. *Semin Hematol* 38:4–8, 2001.

27. Altman A: Acute tumor lysis syndrome. *Semin Oncol* 28:3–8, 2001.

28. Annemans L, Moeremans K, Lamotte M, et al.: Pan-European multicentre economic evaluation of recombinant urate oxidase (rasburicase) in prevention and treatment of hyperuricaemia and tumour lysis syndrome in haematological cancer patients. *Support Care Cancer* 11:249–257, 2003.

29. Pui CH, Jeha S, Irwin D, et al.: Recombinant urate oxidase (rasburicase) in the prevention and treatment of malignancy-associated hyperuricemia in pediatric and adult patients: results of a compassionate-use trial. *Leukemia* 15:1505–1509, 2001.

30. Klinenberg JR, Goldfinger SE, Seegmiller JE: The effectiveness of the xanthine oxidase inhibitor allopurinol in the treatment of gout. *Ann Intern Med* 62:639–647, 1965.

31. Biondi A, Rambaldi A: Molecular diagnosis and monitoring of acute myeloid leukemia. *Leuk Res* 20:801–807, 1996.

32. Le Beau MM, Larson RA, Bitter MA, et al.: Association of an inversion of chromosome 16 with abnormal marrow eosinophils in acute myelomonocytic leukemia. A unique cytogenetic-clinicopathological association. *N Engl J Med* 309:630–636, 1983.

33. Holmes R, Keating MJ, Cork A, et al.: A unique pattern of central nervous system leukemia in acute myelomonocytic leukemia associated with inv(16)(p13q22). *Blood* 65:1071–1078, 1985.

34. Haferlach T, Gassmann W, Loffler H, et al.: Clinical aspects of acute myeloid leukemias of the FAB types M3 and M4Eo. The AML Cooperative Group. *Ann Hematol* 66:165–170, 1993.

35. Perez-Zincer F, Juturi JV, Hsi ED, et al.: A pulmonary syndrome in patients with acute myelomonocytic leukemia and inversion of chromosome 16. *Leuk Lymphoma* 44:103–109, 2003.

36. Lichtman M: Acute myelogenous leukemia. In: Beutler E, Lichtman M, Coller B, Kipps T (eds.) *Williams Hematology.* 5th ed. New York: McGraw-Hill; 1995:272–298.

37. Stanley M, McKenna RW, Ellinger G, Brunning RD: Classification of 358 cases of acute myeloid leukemia by FAB criteria: analysis of clinical and morphological features. In: Bloomfield CD (ed.) *Chronic and Acute Leukemias in Adults.* Boston: Martinus Nijhoff; 1985:147.

38. Lee EJ, Schiffer CA, Misawa S, et al.: Clinical and cytogenetic features of familial erythroleukaemia. *Br J Haematol* 65:313–320, 1987.

39. Copelli M: Di una emopatia sistemizzata rapresentata de una iperplasia eritronastosis. *Pathologica* 4:460, 1912.

40. Rowley JD, Golomb HM, Vardiman JW: Nonrandom chromosome abnormalities in acute leukemia and dysmyelopoietic syndromes in patients with previously treated malignant disease. *Blood* 58:759–767, 1981.

41. Stamberg J: Chromosome abnormalities in erythroleukemia. *Cancer* 60:2649–2653, 1987.

42. Breton-Gorius J, Daniel MT, Flandrin G, Kinet-Deouel C: Fine structure and peroxidase activity of circulating micromegakaryoblasts and platelets in a case of acute myelofibrosis. *Br J Haematol* 25:331, 1973.

43. Peterson BA, Levine EG: Uncommon subtypes of acute nonlymphocytic leukemia: clinical features and management of FAB M5, M6 and M7. *Semin Oncol* 14:425–434, 1987.

44. Dharmasena F, Wickham N, McHugh PJ, et al.: Osteolytic tumors in acute megakaryoblastic leukemia. *Cancer* 58:2273–2277, 1986.

45. Jenkins RB, Tefferi A, Solberg LA Jr, et al.: Acute leukemia with abnormal thrombopoiesis and inversions of chromosome 3. *Cancer Genet Cytogenet* 39:167–179, 1989.

46. Carroll A, Civin C, Schneider N, et al.: The t(1;22) (p13;q13) is nonrandom and restricted to infants with acute megakaryoblastic leukemia: a Pediatric Oncology Group study. *Blood* 78:748–752, 1991.

47. Ghaddar HM, Estey EH: Acute myelogenous leukemia. In: Pazdur R (ed.) *Medical Oncology: A Comprehensive Review.* New York: PRR; 1997:27–34.

48. Kojima S, Matsuyama T, Sato T, et al.: Down's syndrome and acute leukemia in children: an analysis of phenotype by use of monoclonal antibodies and electron microscopic platelet peroxidase reaction. *Blood* 76:2348–2353, 1990.

49. Goh KO, Anderson FW: Cytogenetic studies in basophilic chronic myelocytic leukemia. *Arch Pathol Lab Med* 103:288–290, 1979.

50. Fergdal M, Astrom M, Tidefelt U, Karlsson MG: Differences in CD14 and alpha-napthyl acetate esterase positivity and relation to prognosis in AML. *Leuk Res* 22:25–30, 1998.

51. Viniou N, Terpos E, Rombos J, et al.: Acute myeloid leukemia in a patient with ataxia-telangiectasia: a case report and review of the literature. *Leukemia* 15:1668–1670, 2001.

52. van Leeuwen FE: Risk of acute myelogenous leukaemia and myelodysplasia following cancer treatment. *Baillieres Clin Haematol* 9:57–85, 1996.

53. Kyle RA, Pierre RV, Bayrd ED: Multiple myeloma and acute myelomonocytic leukemia. *N Engl J Med* 283:1121–1125, 1970.

54. Levine EG, Bloomfield CD: Leukemias and myelodysplastic syndromes secondary to drug, radiation, and environmental exposure. *Semin Oncol* 19:47–84, 1992.

55. Pedersen-Bjergaard J: Radiotherapy- and chemotherapy-induced myelodysplasia and acute myeloid leukemia. A review. *Leuk Res* 16:61–65, 1992.

56. Scott AA, Head DR, Kopecky KJ, et al.: HLA-DR-, CD33+, CD56+ CD16- myeloid/natural killer cell acute leukemia: a previously unrecognized form of acute leukemia potentially misdiagnosed as French—American—British acute myeloid leukemia-M#. *Blood* 84:244–255, 1994.

57. Slater SE, Maccallum PK, Birjandi F, et al.: Acute myelogenous leukemia (AML) and diabetes insipidus (DI): further association with monosomy 7. *Hematol Oncol* 10:221–223, 1992.

58. Nakamura F, Kishimoto Y, Handa T, et al.: Myelodysplastic syndrome with central diabetes insipidus manifesting hypodipsic hypernatremia and dehydration. *Am J Hematol* 75:213–216, 2004.

59. Muller CI, Engelhardt M, Laubenberger J, et al.: Myelodysplastic syndrome in transformation to acute myeloid leukemia presenting with diabetes insipidus: due to pituitary infiltration association with abnormalities of chromosomes 3 and 7. *Eur J Haematol* 69:115–119, 2002.

60. Chang VT, Aviv H, Howard LM, et al.: Acute myelogenous leukemia associated with extreme symptomatic thrombocytosis and chromosome 3q translocation: case report and review of literature. *Am J Hematol* 72:20–26, 2003.

61. Jotterand Bellomo M, Parlier V, Muhlematter D, et al.: Three new cases of chromosome 3 rearrangement in bands q21 and q26 with abnormal thrombopoiesis bring further evidence to the existence of a 3q21q26 syndrome. *Cancer Genet Cytogenet* 59:138–160, 1992.

62. Sweet DL, Golomb HM, Rowley JD, Vardiman JM: Acute myelogenous leukemia and thrombocythemia associated with an abnormality of chromosome no. 3. *Cancer Genet Cytogenet* 1:33–37, 1979.

63. Fichelson S, Dreyfus F, Berger R, et al.: Evi-1 expression in leukemic patients with rearrangements of the 3q25-q28 chromosomal region. *Leukemia* 6:93–99, 1992.

64. Levy ER, Parganas E, Morishita K, et al.: DNA rearrangements proximal to the EVI1 locus associated with the 3q21q26 syndrome. *Blood* 83:1348–1354, 1994.

65. Tallman MS, Nabhan C, Feusner JH, et al.: Acute promyelocytic leukemia: evolving therapeutic strategies. *Blood* 99:759–767, 2002.

66. Barbui T, Finazzi G, Falanga A: Management of bleeding and thrombosis in acute leukemia and chronic myeloproliferative disorders. In: Henderson ES, Lister T, Greaves M (eds.) *Leukemia*. Philadelphia: Saunders; 2002:363–383.

67. Rodeghiero F, Avvisati G, Castaman G, et al.: Early deaths and anti-hemorrhagic treatments in acute promyelocytic leukemia. A GIMEMA retrospective study in 268 consecutive patients. *Blood* 75:2112–2117, 1990.

68. Bauer KA, Rosenberg RD: Thrombin generation in acute promyelocytic leukemia. *Blood* 64:791–796, 1984.

69. Falanga A, Alessio MG, Donati MB, et al.: A new procoagulant in acute leukemia. *Blood* 71:870–875, 1988.

70. Bennett B, Booth NA, Croll A, et al.: The bleeding disorder in acute promyelocytic leukaemia: fibrinolysis due to u-PA rather than defibrination. *Br J Haematol* 71:511–517, 1989.

71. Velasco F, Torres A, Andres P, et al.: Changes in plasma levels of protease and fibrinolytic inhibitors induced by treatment in acute myeloid leukemia. *Thromb Haemost* 52:81–84, 1984.

72. Avvisati G, ten Cate JW, Sturk A, et al.: Acquired alpha-2-antiplasmin deficiency in acute promyelocytic leukaemia. *Br J Haematol* 70:43–48, 1988.

73. Chan TK, Chan GT, Chan V: Hypofibrinogenemia due to increased fibrinolysis in two patients with acute promyelocytic leukemia. *Aust N Z J Med* 14:245–249, 1984.

74. Takahashi H, Tatewaki W, Wada K, et al.: Fibrinolysis and fibrinogenolysis in disseminated intravascular coagulation. *Thromb Haemost* 63:340–344, 1990.

75. Menell JS, Cesarman GM, Jacovina AT, et al.: Annexin II and bleeding in acute promyelocytic leukemia. *N Engl J Med* 340:994–1004, 1999.

76. Appelbaum FR, Rowe JM, Radich J, et al.: Acute myeloid leukemia. *Hematology Am Soc Hematol Educ Program* 62–86, 2001.

77. Cripe LD: Adult acute leukemia. *Curr Probl Cancer* 21:1–64, 1997.

78. Rizzieri DA, Long G, Chao N: Acute leukemia. In: Wachter R, Goldman L, Hollander H (eds.) *Hospital Medicine*. 1st ed. Baltimore: Williams and Wilkins; 2000:765–772.

79. Cuttner J, Conjalka MS, Reilly M, et al.: Association of monocytic leukemia in patients with extreme leukocytosis. *Am J Med* 69:555–558, 1980.

80. Bennett JM, Catovsky D, Daniel MT, et al.: Proposals for the classification of the acute leukaemias. French—American—British (FAB) Co-Operative Group. *Br J Haematol* 33:451–458, 1976.

81. Bennett JM, Catovsky D, Daniel MT, et al.: Proposed revised criteria for the classification of acute myeloid leukemia. A report of the French—American—British Cooperative Group. *Ann Intern Med* 103:620–625, 1985.

82. Cotran RS, Kumar V, Robbins SL: Disease of white cells, lymph nodes, and spleen. In: Cotran RS, Kumar V, Robbins SL, Schoen FJ (eds.) *Robbins Pathologic Basis of Disease*. 5th ed. Philadelphia: WB Saunders; 1994: 629–672.

83. Hanker JS, Laszlo J, Moore JO: The light microscopic demonstration of hydroperoxidase-positive phi bodies and rods in leukocytes in acute myeloid leukemia. *Histochemistry* 58:241, 1978.

84. Hamamoto K, Yoshioka A, Taniguchi H, et al.: Acute myelomonocytic leukemia with marrow eosinophilia showing 5q- and 16q22 mosaicism. *Cancer Genet Cytogenet* 58:130–133, 1992.

85. Berger R, Dombret H: New variant translocation in acute myelomonocytic leukemia with bone marrow eosinophilia. *Cancer Genet Cytogenet* 58:204–245, 1992.

86. Hetzel P, Gee TS: A new observation in the clinical spectrums of erythroleukemia. A report of 46 cases. *Am J Med* 64:765–772, 1978.

87. Roggli VL, Saleem A: Erythroleukemia: a study of 15 cases and literature review. *Cancer* 49:101–108, 1982.

88. Bahia DM, Yamamoto M, Chauffaille Mde L, et al.: Aberrant phenotypes in acute myeloid leukemia: a high frequency and its clinical significance. *Haematologica* 86:801–806, 2001.

89. Van Dongen JJM, Szczepanski T, Adriaansen HJ: Immunobiology of leukemia. In: Henderson ES, Lister T, Greaves M (eds.) *Leukemia.* Philadelphia: Saunders; 2002:85–129.

90. Weir EG, Borowitz MJ: Flow cytometry in the diagnosis of acute leukemia. *Semin Hematol* 38:124–138, 2001.

91. Krasinskas AM, Wasik MA, Kamoun M, et al.: The usefulness of CD64, other monocyte-associated antigens, and CD45 gating in the subclassification of acute myeloid leukemias with monocytic differentiation. *Am J Clin Pathol* 110:797–805, 1998.

92. Olopade OI, Thangavelu M, Larson RA, et al.: Clinical, morphologic, and cytogenetic characteristics of 26 patients with acute erythroblastic leukemia. *Blood* 80:2873–2882, 1992.

93. Orfao A, Chillon MC, Bortoluci AM, et al.: The flow cytometric pattern of CD34, CD15 and CD13 expression in acute myeloblastic leukemia is highly characteristic of the presence of PML-RAR alpha gene rearrangements. *Haematologica* 84:405–412, 1999.

94. Baer MR, Stewart CC, Lawrence D, et al.: Expression of the neural cell adhesion molecule CD56 is associated with short remission duration and survival in acute myeloid leukemia with t(8;21)(q22;q22). *Blood* 90:1643–1648, 1997.

95. Murray CK, Estey E, Paietta E, et al.: CD56 expression in acute promyelocytic leukemia: a possible indicator of poor treatment outcome? *J Clin Oncol* 17:293–297, 1999.

96. Ferrara F, Morabito F, Martino B, et al.: CD56 expression is an indicator of poor clinical outcome in patients with acute promyelocytic leukemia treated with simultaneous all-trans-retinoic acid and chemotherapy. *J Clin Oncol* 18:1295–1300, 2000.

97. Alcalay M, Orleth A, Sebastiani C, et al.: Common themes in the pathogenesis of acute myeloid leukemia. *Oncogene* 20:5680–5694, 2001.

98. Harris NL, Jaffe ES, Diebold J, et al.: The World Health Organization classification of neoplasms of the hematopoietic and lymphoid tissues: report of the Clinical Advisory Committee meeting—-Airlie House, Virginia, November, 1997. *Hematol J* 1:53–66, 2000.

99. Haferlach T, Schoch C: WHO classification of acute myeloid leukaemia (AML) and the myelodysplastic syndrome (MDS). *Dtsch Med Wochenschr* 127:447–450, 2002.

100. Matutes E, Morilla R, Farahat N, et al.: Definition of acute biphenotypic leukemia. *Haematologica* 82:64–66, 1997.

101. Sekeres MA, Stone RM: The challenge of acute myeloid leukemia in older patients. *Curr Opin Oncol* 14:24–30, 2002.

102. Webb IJ, Anderson KC: Transfusion support in acute leukemias. *Semin Oncol* 24:141–146, 1997.

103. Aderka D, Praff G, Santo M, et al.: Bleeding due to thrombocytopenia in acute leukemias and reevaluation of the prophylactic platelet transfusion policy. *Am J Med Sci* 291:147–151, 1986.

# Chapter 4

# TREATMENT FOR ACUTE MYELOID LEUKEMIA IN PATIENTS UNDER AGE 60

*Richard M. Stone*

## INTRODUCTION

Acute myeloid leukemia (AML) is a disorder characterized by a malignancy of the bone marrow stem cell at either a pluripotent or committed stage of development, which leads to an overproliferation of leukemic cells (blasts), which can be shown to have either cytochemical and/or immunophenotypic features of myeloid (including monocytoid, erythroid, or megakaryocytic) lineage. A brief list of the pathophysiologic abnormalities leading to this malignancy include unbridled proliferation, failure to undergo normal maturation, the inability to undergo programmed cell death, and overreliance on angiogenic mechanisms. The disordered growth in the myeloid stem cell compartment leads to the patient's death from bone marrow failure, unless a successful therapeutic strategy is employed. The fundamental differences in disease biology and clinical response between AML arising in younger (generally considered to be less than 60 years in age) verses older adults have lead to different therapeutic approaches in these groups. This chapter deals with the therapeutic strategies available for those younger adults who are by and large able to withstand (and benefit from) intensive chemotherapy and stem cell transplantation.

The major challenge in the management of the adult, age 18–60 years, with AML is to employ the available therapies in a fashion that will maximize the chance of a cure for any individual. The chance of long-term disease-free survival for an adult in this age group today is approximately 33%.[1,2] However, our recent knowledge of risk at presentation, largely due to chromosome findings at diagnosis, suggests that some patients with AML can expect long-term disease-free survival rates in the range of 70%, while others are rarely cured.[3] These vastly different prior probabilities of success with available therapy suggest that, with appropriate use of so-called risk-adapted approaches,

one could prevent overtreatment in the good prognosis groups and maximize treatment in those destined to do poorly. Moreover, increasing knowledge about the specific pathophysiological events at the genetic level[4] also gives rise to the hope that therapy could target the specific genetic lesion or lesions in a given patient's leukemic cells, thereby improving the therapeutic index and leading to a higher cure rate with less toxicity.

## DIAGNOSIS AND CLASSIFICATION

Once the diagnosis of acute leukemia is suspected on the basis of abnormal blood counts, immature cells appearing in the peripheral blood differential, or the finding of extramedullary leukemia (especially in central nervous system, gums, or meninges, particularly in patients with monocytic subtypes), one should undertake a full diagnostic work-up that includes delineation of the AML subtype, as well as the definition of the risk group. In fact, the classification system for AML is evolving from the cytochemical and morphologically based French—American—British scheme[5] to the cytogenetically centered World Health Organization (WHO) system.[6] The WHO classification system acknowledges the critical impact of cytogenetics on prognosis as well as our improved pathophysiological understanding based on genes at balanced translocation breakpoints.

Although most subtypes of AML are treated in a similar fashion at least initially, it is important to recognize the 10–15% of AML patients who have acute promyelocytic leukemia (APL),[7] characterized by malignant cells that appear as heavily granule-laden malignant promyelocytes with frequent Auer rods. These heavily myeloperoxidase-positive APL cells generally possess the characteristic t(15;17) cytogenetic abnormality, with a resultant PML-RARA rearrangement detectable on reverse transcription polymerase chain reaction analysis. APL is treated in a distinct fashion (see Chapter 6).

In addition to the definition of the AML subtype and risk strata, it is imperative to assess the underlying medical state of the patient, determining if any issues such as cardiac, renal, or pulmonary dysfunction might compromise the ultimate therapeutic plan. Finally, given the possibility that the patient might become a candidate for allogeneic stem cell transplant at some point, patient and sibling HLA typing should be carried out shortly after diagnosis.

## TREATMENT STRATEGIES

### INTRODUCTION

Historically, the treatment of newly diagnosed AML is divided into phases. Induction therapy is given to patients to reduce the tumor burden at diagnosis, presumed to be $10^{12}$ cells (1 kg), by approximately three orders of magnitude down to a level at which leukemic cells are no longer detectable in the blood or bone marrow. Although the definition of complete remission[8] has undergone some degree of evolution, in general, the reduction in leukemic cells should occur concomitantly with the resumption of normal hematopoiesis and reasonably normal blood counts. Induction chemotherapy usually is given over approximately 1 week. During that time, patients are monitored carefully for signs of tumor lysis syndrome,[9] in which a rapid release of intracellular contents including potassium and phosphate may cause hyperkalemia, hyperphosphatemia, and secondary hypocalcemia. Secondly, the large load of purine metabolites can lead to high uric acid levels, with the development of renal failure on the basis of urate nephropathy.[9] Tumor lysis syndrome is much less common in AML than in the somewhat more chemotherapy-sensitive lymphoproliferative leukemias, but it is generally accepted that AML patients should receive IV fluids and allopurinol to help prevent this complication. Alkalinization of the urine with the administration of intravenous sodium bicarbonate to maintain uric acid in its more soluble urate form is generally not necessary or advisable. The lysis of leukemic cells can result in exposure to tissue factor and other procoagulants, causing disseminated intravascular coagulopathy (especially in APL),[10] with associated bleeding and/or thrombosis.

Certain patients with AML, particularly those with monocytic subtypes (whose blasts tend to be "sticky"), who present with an absolute blast count of 75,000/uL or greater can experience life-threatening problems with leukostasis. Such complications could include cerebral or pulmonary dysfunction due to plugging of small capillaries in these organs. Treatment for this actual or impending condition is aggressive use of intravenous hydration and cytoreductive measures: usually hydroxyurea[11] and occasionally leukopheresis.

Complete remission is usually achieved 4–6 weeks after beginning induction chemotherapy. At that time, patients generally have recovered from the nonhematologic toxicities of induction chemotherapy, including gastrointestinal and integumentary disruption. After a 1–3-week rest, postremission chemotherapy should be administered to reduce the residual undetectable leukemic burden down to a level compatible with cure. The optimal strategy to achieve such a reduction in residual leukemic cells is controversial; the three major options being several cycles of intensive postremission chemotherapy, high-dose chemotherapy with autologous stem cell rescue (sometimes termed "autotransplant"[12]), and allogeneic transplant from a histocompatible sibling or unrelated donor. While perhaps not completely proven by prospective clinical trials, the choice amongst these options is generally based, at least in part, on the cytogenetic findings at diagnosis.[3] The overall goal of induction and postremission therapy is to prevent leukemic relapse. Just as in the case with failure to achieve remission with standard chemotherapy, a relapse generally signifies a chemotherapy-resistant leukemic cell. Patients may achieve a second complete remission after reinduction chemotherapy (more likely if the initial disease-free interval is greater than 1 year).[13,14] Consolidation of such second remissions should include a high-dose approach (either an autologous or allogeneic transplant )[15,16] if there is to be any possibility of long-term disease-free survival.

### INDUCTION CHEMOTHERAPY

A disappointing fact concerning the treatment of younger adults with AML is that the agents used for induction therapy now are much the same as three decades ago. Three days of an anthracycline (generally, daunorubicin or idarubicin) in conjunction with 7 days of continuous infusional cytarabine (100–200 mg/m$^2$ per day)[17] remains the standard approach. It has been the practice in the Cancer and Leukemia Group B (CALGB) and other cooperative groups to perform a bone marrow examination approximately 2 weeks after the start of induction chemotherapy.[1] If a sufficient degree of myeloblast reduction is not achieved, then 2 days of the same anthracycline and 5 days of cytarabine are administered as a reinduction cycle. Occasionally, serial bone marrows are necessary to clarify whether or not a reinduction cycle should be administered. Approximately 30% of younger adults with AML will require a second course (so-called "2 + 5" reinduction).[1] Although not certain, the requirement for such a reinduction may indicate a worse long-term prognosis.[13] In contrast to a 20–25% death rate in older adults, the mortality associated with induction therapy in younger adults is generally under 10%.[1]

Many attempts to modify or augment standard induction chemotherapy have been made without any clear improvements. Whether one anthracycline is better than another remains controversial. A trial comparing doxorubicin to daunorubicin during induction indicated that doxorubicin was associated with an increase in gastrointestinal complications, without an improvement in response.[17] Several trials conducted in the 1980s[18,19,20] reported a benefit to an idarubicin-based induction compared to daunorubicin; the improved results may have been due to a nonequivalence of the myelosuppresive dose of idarubicin. Although 6-thioguanine is widely used in the United Kingdom and throughout Europe,[2,21] randomized trials comparing 3 + 7 with or without the addition of this agent have not shown a clear-cut benefit with the three-drug versus the two-drug approach.[21] Given the success of high-dose cytarabine (at least 1–1.5 g/m[22] per dose) in the relapse[22] and postremission settings,[1] investigators have tried to either substitute high-dose cytarabine for standard doses[23] or add high-dose cytarabine onto 3 + 7[24] during induction. Although a single institution trial demonstrated a 90% complete remission rate and a 50–60% long-term survival benefit with high-dose cytarabine added on to standard 3 + 7,[24] a cooperative group trial failed to show a benefit for the more aggressive induction.[25] The substitution of high-dose cytarabine for standard-dose cytarabine has also been attempted; although an improved disease-free survival was noted in certain subgroups, there was no clear overall survival benefit.[23] The addition of etoposide, tested by the Australian Leukemic Study Group, was also associated with an improved disease-free, but not an overall, survival advantage.[26] It is not clear whether induction therapies that are associated with a disease-free survival benefit, but not an overall survival benefit, are advantageous.

## POSTREMISSION THERAPY

There is an absolute need to administer postremission chemotherapy in order to yield any chance for the patient to experience long-term disease-free survival. This fact was originally recognized after two trials in the 1970s showed that some chemotherapy led to at least a small long-term survival rate compared to no postremission chemotherapy in which virtually 100% of the patients succumbed to their disease.[27,28] Given our understanding that remission is achieved at a relatively high leukemic burden, this is not surprising. Several studies in the 1980s solidified the concept that intensive chemotherapy represented the standard of care in postremission chemotherapy. High-dose cytarabine was recognized as being biochemically distinct from standard doses of cytarabine; patients resistant to standard-dose cytarabine could enter a remission when doses of 1.5 g/m[2] or greater were administered.[22] A phase II study documented a 40% likelihood of long-term disease-free survival in

patients achieving remission who received high-dose cytarabine.[29] Two cooperative groups in the United States performed randomized trials in the 1980s, comparing standard doses of cytarabine to high-dose ara-C in the postremission setting.[1,30] The Eastern Cooperative Oncology Group compared standard-dose ara-C to one cycle of high-dose ara-C and showed a superior disease-free survival in patients receiving the more intensive arm.[30] CACGB study 8525 probably represents the most important turning point in the chemotherapy-based approach to AML in the last 40 years.[1] In this trial, newly diagnosed patients with AML (adults of all ages) were enrolled and given standard 3 + 7 induction chemotherapy, with daunorubicin and cytarabine. Patients achieving remission were randomized to four cycles of either (a) ara-C at 100 mg/m[2] by continuous infusion for 5 days or (b) cytarabine at 400 mg/m[2] per day by continuous infusion for 5 days, or (c) high-dose cytarabine at 3g/m[2] over 3 h given q 12 h on days 1, 3, and 5 (total six doses). All patients then received an additional four cycles of outpatient daunorubicin for 1 day and low-dose cytarabine for 5 days at 100 mg/m[2] daily. In adults under the age of 60, the best results (superior disease-free and overall survival) were seen in those who were randomized to the high-dose cytarabine. The 45% long-term disease-free survival in such patients achieving remission was comparable to that observed with allogeneic stem cell transplant, and established high-dose cytarabine as the treatment of choice in the postremission setting.

Subsequent trials and practices have deviated from the precise schedule of postremission therapy in CALGB 8525. First, Bloomfield and colleagues showed that not all types of AML benefited equally from the intensive arm.[31] Specifically, most of the benefits of high-dose cytarabine were noted in patients with inversion of chromosome 16 or t(8;21). Both of these abnormalities were recognized to confer a favorable prognosis[3] and also to represent abnormalities of the core-binding factor heterodimer transcription factor.[32] The precise reason why such patients' leukemic cells are so sensitive to intensive chemotherapy remains unknown, but the relatively good prognosis characteristic of these cytogenetic abnormalities has been documented in studies worldwide. Subsequent studies have shown that inversion 16 patients actually do somewhat better than those with t(8;21).[33] Also, clear from reanalysis of CALGB 8525[1,31] and data from other sources[3] is that a subgroup of patients (about 15% of the total) with complex abnormalities or deletion of all or part of chromosomes 5 and/or 7 has a poor prognosis even when intensive postremission chemotherapy is applied. In part because of the difficulty of administering four cycles of postremission intensive chemotherapy followed by four cycles of maintenance chemotherapy, subsequent studies conducted by the CALGB have employed three cycles of high-dose ara-C. It does seem clear that at least three cycles of high-dose ara-C are required to obtain benefit in patients with good prognosis chromosomal abnormalities.[34]

A subsequent CALGB trial randomized patients in remission to receive three cycles of high-dose ara-C or three cycles of a so-called noncross-resistant combination of chemotherapy regimens that included one cycle of etoposide/cyclophosphamide and one cycle of diaziquone (AZQ)/mitoxantrone. No relapse-free or overall survival differences in the randomized arms were seen.[35] While relatively long-term low-dose chemotherapy (maintenance chemotherapy) is routinely employed in the management of patients with acute lymphoblastic leukemia, its use in AML remains controversial. Whereas older studies failed to show benefit for patients receiving maintenance chemotherapy,[36] the good results seen in CALGB 8525 (in which patients received four cycles of a maintenance-type chemotherapy regimen) and recent results from the German Leukemia Cooperative Group[37] have suggested that reexploration of the role of maintenance chemotherapy in AML is appropriate.

Given the adoption of high-dose ara-C or similarly intense regimens as the standard of care for adults with AML, studies have attempted to understand the risk factors for high-dose ara-C-induced cerebellar toxicity[38,39] and to define the role of stem cell transplantation compared to such intense therapy. Even though high-dose ara-C is useful and is associated with a much lower mortality rate than allogeneic stem cell transplantion, the associated neurotoxicity can be devastating, especially if irreversible, as is the case about 50% of the time. The incidence of high-dose ara-C-associated cerebellar toxicity can be lowered if older patients (who do not seem to benefit from this approach)[1,40] and/or those with elevated serum creatinine or impaired liver function are given alternative postremission therapy.

### ROLE OF HEMATOPOIETIC STEM CELL TRANPLANTATION

Improvements in supportive care, as well as the use of high-dose chemotherapy, have made intensive postremission chemotherapy a more attractive option as primary postremission management for most adults with AML in first remission. Similarly, improvements in management of patients after allogeneic stem cell transplantation, including improved graft-versus-host disease prophylaxis, and more recently, the ability to perform molecular histocompatability typing, have resulted in steadily improving the outcome for patients undergoing allogeneic stem cell transplantation. Furthermore, high-dose chemotherapy with autologous peripheral stem cell transplantation is yet another feasible option that can be employed in the postremission management of the younger adult with AML. Four important prospective randomized controlled trials have attempted to define the optimum postremission management of patients with AML, under the age of 50–60, who are in first remission. The trials were all conducted in the 1980s and 1990s, both during the time when intensive high-dose ara-C based chemotherapy was coming into frequent use and when the aforementioned improvements in allogeneic transplantation were being seen. The trial design in each case was similar in that the patients were enrolled at diagnosis; those in remission deemed to be candidates for further aggressive therapy were allocated to allogeneic stem cell transplantation if a sibling donor was identified; and other patients were randomly allocated to chemotherapy or autologous stem cell transplantation. In the case of the trial performed by the Medical Research Council (MRC) in the United Kingdom,[41] patients in each randomized group received the same postremission standard chemotherapy, but those randomized to autologous transplant received this at the conclusion of all therapy. Unfortunately, even after over 2000 patients were enrolled in these trials, the answer remains unclear. In the first published trial,[42] those allocated to allogeneic transplant or randomized to autologous transplant enjoyed a superior relapse-free survival than those randomized to chemotherapy; however, there was no statistically significant improvement in overall survival in those groups, possibly due to salvage of patients in the chemotherapy group, who later relapsed, with an eventual stem cell transplant. The MRC trial[41] did show a relapse-free survival benefit for those randomized to autologous transplant, but again there was no overall survival benefit; this was really a comparison of autologous transplant to no further therapy, in any event. It might have been a "more fair" trial if those randomized to chemotherapy received another cycle of chemotherapy in comparison to the high-dose approach. A French trial showed absolutely no difference in relapse-free survival or long-term survival in the three groups.[43] The United States Intergroup trial[44] actually showed a statistically superior survival for those randomized to chemotherapy, presumably due to unforeseen excess toxicity in the groups that were either allocated to the allogeneic transplant or randomized to high-dose therapy with autologous stem cell rescue.

Given our increased understanding of the heterogeneity of AML based on the chromosome findings at diagnosis,[3] it is not surprising that several of the aforementioned studies comparing chemotherapy to transplantation were reanalyzed based on the impact of each of the potential treatment strategies on patients with various karyotypic risk groups. Unfortunately, none of these studies were prospectively powered to answer questions regarding the advisability of any given treatment based on a certain cytogenetic risk group. Not surprisingly, those patients who present with a favorable chromosomal abnormality at diagnosis (abnormalities of core-binding factor, either inversion of chromosome 16 or t(8;21)) fare well with any of the therapies.[45]

Consequently, most authorities recommend that high-dose ara-C-based chemotherapy be the primary postremission strategy applied to this favorable group of patients, thereby reducing their risk of toxicity. Patients with unfavorable chromosomal abnormalities, such as monosomy 7 or the loss of chromosome 5, should have an allogeneic transplant in first remission.

Given the contemporary favorable results with matched unrelated donor transplants, for the selected young adult who presents with poor chromosomal features at diagnosis, an unrelated matched transplant in first remission could be considered. However, for the 70% of patients who have normal or so-called intermediate chromosomal abnormalities, the benefit of a transplant in terms of reducing the leukemia relapse rate is offset almost exactly by the toxicity of the transplant. Therefore, it is difficult to recommend an optimal strategy for this relatively large group of patients. Patients who have intermediate prognosis chromosomal abnormalities and a sibling donor require a frank discussion of the risks and benefits of each of the approaches. In general, it might be appropriate to delay allogeneic transplant until relapse or second remission, although patients must understand that such delay could compromise their chances for being able to have the transplant if not doing well in the long term. Moreover, children seem to have a more clear-cut benefit from allogeneic transplant as postremission therapy.[46] The younger the adult patient, the more such a strategy makes sense.

## TREATMENT OF APL

The therapeutic approach to patients with APL differs from that in the other histologic subtypes of AML. This topic is discussed briefly here, while more comprehensive discussion appears in Chapter 6.

The use of chemotherapy in conjunction with all-*trans*-retinoic acid (ATRA) is now the most widely accepted standard approach for the induction management of patients with APL. Many questions remain about optimal chemotherapy. Nonetheless, once a diagnosis of APL is established, patients should begin therapy with ATRA because this strategy rapidly ameliorates the disseminated intravascular coagulopathy which can be life threatening. An anthracycline should be started within a few days of beginning ATRA. Studies have conclusively shown that concomitant use of chemotherapy plus ATRA is superior to chemotherapy alone or ATRA followed by chemotherapy.[47,48] Whether or not cytarabine should be included routinely in the induction management of APL is controversial. The Spanish PETHEMA group has had excellent results without the use of this drug.[49] After the chemotherapy is completed, ATRA should be maintained until remission is achieved, an event that may occur at a later time after the initial initiation of induction chemotherapy compared with other subtypes of AML. Once remission has been documented, at least two cycles of an anthracycline-based consolidation regimen are appropriate.[48,49] The need for ara-C in the postremission setting remains controversial. APL is the only type of AML for which maintenance therapy has a clear-cut and widely accepted role.[48,50] Maintenance chemotherapy with ATRA is indicated; the addition of oral antimetabolite therapy, in a manner analogous to that done in pediatric acute lymphoblastic leukemia, will further decrease the relapse rate.[48]

For APL in relapse, arsenic trioxide should be administered. This drug yields a complete remission rate of 85%, even in highly pretreated relapse patients; 85% of those achieving remission do so at a level below the detectability rate for the polymerase chain reaction (PCR)-amplified PML-RARA and fusion transcript.[51] Patients in second remission can be maintained with ATRA or arsenic trioxide; or, if the leukemia is undetectable by PCR analysis, patients should undergo stem cell harvest followed by high-dose chemotherapy with autologous peripheral cell rescue.[52] Given the highly successful and responsive nature of this disease, clinical research is under way, in which patients receive limited amounts of chemotherapy. Investigators of MD Anderson have treated patients with ATRA and gemtuzumab ozogamicin with good initial results.[53]

## TREATMENT OF RELAPSED DISEASE

Patients with relapsed AML cannot be cured with standard chemotherapy. On the other hand, relapsed leukemia is generally treated with reinduction therapy for two reasons. First, this is an important part of the effort to get a patient in second remission, which may have palliative benefit. Most importantly, once the disease is under control, high-dose chemotherapy with hematopoietic stem cell transplant is possible. Second, patients in second remission can be salvaged with high-dose chemotherapy and autologous peripheral stem cell rescue (so-called autologous transplant) with the likelihood of disease-free survival in a second remission being about 30%.[54] In most cases, if an allogeneic donor is available, then it is preferable to consider an allogeneic stem cell transplant. With improved molecular HLA typing, in the absence of a sibling donor, an unrelated molecularly matched donor is an acceptable alternative. Allogeneic transplant can be used in situations where the remission is incomplete; however, this procedure is more likely to be successful if the patient is in fact in a second remission. This topic is covered in greater detail in Chapter 9.

The optimal therapy to use to induce a second remission is not clear. Although in this era most patients under the age of 60 with AML have received a high-dose ara-C-based consolidation regimen during first remission, the same regimen can be used for reinduction. If the first remission duration, the most important prognostic factor for success with reinduction,[55] is greater than 1 year, then standard reinduction therapy can be given with a good chance of success. Otherwise, high-dose ara-C or a combination of high-dose ara-C plus mitoxantrone and etoposide[56] can be employed. Patients with a relatively short first complete remission (CR) duration are reasonable candidates to be enrolled on clinical trials involving novel chemotherapeutic agents and/or targeted agents.

### NOVEL THERAPIES

The burgeoning understanding of the pathophysiology of AML has spurred the development of a host of investigational therapies. Table 4.1 lists a categorization of these therapies and classifies them into therapies that inhibit proliferation, promote apoptosis, improve chemotherapeutic effect, or work by immunotherapeutic means. Because AML is a rare disease that is already associated with fairly effective therapy, the challenge of bringing any of these therapies to improve the natural history of patients with AML is daunting indeed. Nonetheless, there have been two agents relatively recently approved for use in AML.

| Table 4.1  Categories of novel therapies for AML |
| --- |
| Drug-resistance modifiers |
|   Cyclosporine A |
|   Quinine |
|   PSC-833 |
| Proteosome inhibitors (e.g., bortezomib) |
| Proapoptotic approaches (e.g., oblimersen and 18-mer anti-bcl-2) |
| Signal transduction inhibitors |
|   "RAS"—targeted (e.g., farnesyl transferase inhibitors, such as tipifarnib and lonafarnib) |
|   Tyrosine kinase targeted |
|     FLT3 (e.g., PKC 412, CEP 701, and MLN 518) |
|     c-kit (e.g., imatinib) |
| Downstream signal inhibitors |
| Novel cytotoxic chemotherapy |
|   Nucleoside analogs (e.g., troxacitabine and clofarabine) |
|   Alkylating agents (e.g., amonafide) |
| Immunotherapeutic approaches |
|   Antigens known |
|     anti-CD33 (e.g. gemtuzumab ozogamicin) |
|     anti-GM-CSF receptor |
|   Antigens unknown |
|     stimulate immune system (IL-2 and GM-CSF) |
|     present tumor antigens effectively |
|       dendritic cell fusion |
|       transfer hematopoietic growth factor genes |

Just as ATRA was first shown to be effective by investigators in the People's Republic of China,[57] the first reports of the efficacy of arsenic trioxide[58] also emanated from that country. Studies done at Memorial Sloan Kettering Cancer Center[59] and at other US centers[51] demonstrated that intravenously administered arsenic trioxide led to remission in 85% of patients with a relapsed APL. The biological effect of arsenic trioxide occurs via both a promotion of differentiation and an enhancement of apoptosis, but the precise biochemical mechanism remains elusive. The optimal setting for the use of arsenic trioxide in the initial management of AML is being studied as both an alternative to chemotherapy, when used with ATRA,[60] and an early postremission consolidation. Toxicities of arsenic trioxide include prolongation of the QT interval, mandating the close monitoring of electrolytes and electrocardiograms.[61]

Approximately 90% of patients with AML have blasts that express the CD33 antigen on the cell surface[8]; consequently, the humanized monoclonal antibody toxin conjugate gemtuzumab ozogamicin binds to AML cells in 90% of cases. After binding to the cell surface and subsequent internalization, the acidic microenvironment results in release of the calicheamicin toxin, which binds to double-stranded DNA, thereby promoting cell death. A phase I trial demonstrated the feasibility of the intravenous administration of gemtuzumab ozogamicin and was associated with some remissions in relapsed patients.[62] The subsequent phase II trial involving 142 patients yielded a complete remission rate of 30% (half of whom had relatively low platelet count at the time of remission).[63] The phase II trial resulted in the approval of this agent for the treatment of older adults with relapsed AML not deemed to be chemotherapy candidates. As a single agent, significant activity seems to be limited to those with relapsed disease after an initial disease-free interval of at least 3–6 months. The role of gemtuzumab ozogamicin as an adjunct to chemotherapy or in minimal disease settings is being explored.

One of the most important strategies is harnessing our understanding of leukemic pathophysiology to design drugs which will inhibit signaling pathways promoting neoplastic cell growth and survival. Mutations in the FLT3 transmembrane tyrosine kinase occur in 30% of patients with AML. Such mutations are either a 3-33 amino acid repeat in the juxtamembrane region (internal tandem duplication; ITD) which occurs in about 25%, or a point mutation in the so-called activation loop which resides in the cytoplasmic tail (which has a 5% incidence).[64] ITD mutations, particularly if they occur in a homozygous fashion,[65] are associated with an adverse prognosis and may account for a subgroup of patients with normal karyotype, who fare relatively poorly.[66] FLT3 mutations have been preclinically shown to confer growth factor independence in leukemic cell lines and to produce a fatal myeloproliferative syndrome in murine models.[64] Small molecules that inhibit FLT3 have been shown to kill such activated cell lines and model leukemias in mice. Early clinical trials with several FLT3 inhibitors have shown biological activity.[67,68] Farnesyl transferase inhibitors, such as tipifarnib (originally thought to target a posttranslational modification of the *ras* proto-oncogene), also produce remissions in advanced[69] and untreated older patients[70] with AML.

There are several new chemotherapeutic agents, most notably the developmental novel nucleoside analogs troxacitabine[71] and clofarabine,[72] which have produced remissions in patients with relapsed and/or refractory AML. Certain agents such as oblimersen,[73] an 18-mer nucleotide that inhibits the translation of the antiapoptotic bc1-2 protein, are being developed, not as a single agent, but to enhance chemotherapeutic efficacy. One of the reasons for intrinsic disease resistance in certain AML patients, particularly those who are above 60, is the relatively high expression of proteins, such as MDR1, which confer drug resistance.[74] Several clinical trials have attempted to determine whether so-called drug-resistance reversal agents can enhance chemotherapeutic efficacy. Although one randomized trial in relapsed AML showed a survival benefit when cyclosporine A was added to a salvage regimen containing ara-C and daunorubicin,[75] other studies[76] have been less promising.

Immunotherapeutic approaches remain a mainstay of therapy in AML, through the mechanism of graft versus leukemia noted following allogeneic stem cell transplantation.[77] Allogeneic stem cell transplantation, discussed elsewhere, offers, albeit at a significant risk of treatment-related toxicity, an effective antileukemic approach. Whether such a "graft-versus-leukemia" effect can be harnessed without needing to employ high-dose chemotherapy or chemoradiation therapy and receipt of allogeneic stem cells is a subject of active research. Leukemia vaccines have been created, in some cases using leukemia-specific peptides which, presented in the context of an HLA molecule, could engender an immune response.[78] Alternatively, manipulating tumor cells to allow more effective antigen presentation by either dendritic cell fusion[79] or transfection with a gene encoding a relevant cytokine[80] may augment antitumor immunity. Generalized stimulation of the immune system with BCG was ineffective[81]; however, two major randomized trials conducted by the CALGB are determining whether interleukin-2,[82] employed at the conclusion of all-planned postremission therapy, might decrease the relapse rate.

## REFERENCES

1. Mayer RJ, Davis RB, Schiffer CA, et al.: Intensive postremission chemotherapy in adults with acute myeloid leukemia. *N Engl J Med* 331:896–903, 1994.
2. Lowenberg B, Downing JR, Burnett A: Medical progress acute myeloid leukemia. *N Engl J Med* 341:1051, 1999.
3. Grimwade D, Walker H, Oliver F, et al.: The importance of diagnostic cytogenetics on outcome in AML: analysis of 1,612 patients entered into the MRC AML 10 trial. The Medical Research Council Adult and Children's Leukemia Working Parties. *Blood* 92:2322–2333, 1998.
4. Kelly LM, Gilliland DG: Genetics of myeloid leukemics. *Annu Rev Genomics Hum Genet* 3:179–198, 2002.
5. Bennett JM, Catovsky D, Daniel MT, et al.: Proposed revised criteria for the classification of acute myeloid leukemia: a report of the French—American—British Cooperative Group. *Ann Intern Med* 103:620, 1985.
6. Vardiman JW, Harris NL, Brunning RD: The World Health Organization (WHO) classification of the myeloid neoplasms. *Blood* 100:2292–2302, 2002.
7. Fenaux P, Chomienne C, Degos L: Acute promyelocytic leukemia: biology and treatment. *Semin Oncol* 24:92, 1997.
8. Cheson BD, Bennett JM, Kopecky KJ, et al.: International Working Group for diagnosis, standardization of response criteria, treatment outcomes, and reporting standards for therapeutic trials in acute myeloid leukemia. Revised recommendations of the International Working Group for diagnosis, standardization of response criteria, treatment outcomes, and reporting standards for therapeutic trials in acute myeloid leukemia. *J Clin Oncol* 21:4642–4649, 2003.
9. Mitchell C, Bishop M: Tumour lysis syndrome: new therapeutic strategies and classification. *Br J Haematol* 127:3–11, 2004.
10. Gralnick HR, Sultan C: Acute promyelocytic leukemia. Haemorrhagic manifestation and morphologic criteria. *Br J Haematol* 29:373–376, 1975.
11. Grund FM, Armitage JO, Burns CP: Hydroxyurea in the prevention of the effects of leukostasis in acute leukemia. *Arch Intern Med* 137:1246–1247, 1987.
12. Gorin NC: Autologous stem cell transplantation in acute myelocytic leukemia. *Blood* 92:1073–1090, 1998.
13. Estey EH, Shen Y, Thall PF: Effect of time to complete remission on subsequent survival and disease-free survival in AML, RAEB-t and RAEB. *Blood* 95:72–77, 2000.
14. Kantarjian HM, Keating MJ, Walters RS, et al.: The characteristics and outcome of patients with late relapse acute myelogeneous leukemia. *J Clin Oncol* 6:232–238, 1988.
15. Yeager AM, Kaizer H, Santos GW, et al.: Autologous bone marrow transplantation in patients with acute nonlymphocytic leukemia, using ex vivo marrow treated with 4-hydroperoxy-cyclophosphamide. *N Engl J Med* 315:141–147, 1986.
16. Clift RA, Buckner CD, Appelbaum FR, et al.: Allogeneic marrow transplantation during untreated first relapse of acute myeloid leukemia. *J Clin Oncol* 10:1723–1729, 1992.

17. Preisler H, Davis RB, Krishner J, et al.: Comparison of three remission induction regimens and two postinduction strategies for the treatment of acute nonlymphocytic leukemia: a Cancer and Leukemia Group B study. *Blood* 69:1441–1449, 1992.

18. Wiernik PH, Banks PLC, Case DC Jr, et al.: Cytarabine plus idarubicin or daunorubicin as induction and consolidation therapy for previously untreated adult patients with acute myeloid leukemia. *Blood* 79:313, 1992.

19. Berman E, Heller G, Santorsa J, et al.: Results of a randomized trial comparing idarubicin and cytosine arabinoside with daunorubicin and cytosine arabinoside in adult patients with newly diagnosed acute nonlymphocytic leukemia. *Blood* 77:1666, 1991.

20. Vogler WR, Velez-Garcia E, Weiner RS, et al.: A phase three trial comparing idarubicin and daunorubicin in combination with cytarabine in acute myelogenous leukemia. A Southeastern Cancer Group study. *J Clin Oncol* 10:1103, 1992.

21. Hann IM, Stevens RF, Goldstone AH, et al.: Randomized comparison of DAT versus ADE as induction chemotherapy in children and younger adults with acute myeloid leukemia. Results of the Medical Research Council's 10th AML trial (MRC AML10). Adult and Childhood Leukemia Working Parties of the Medical Research Council. *Blood* 89:2311–2318, 1997.

22. Hines JD, Oken MM, Mazza JJ, et al.: High dose cytosine arabinoside and m-AMSA is effective therapy in relapsed acute non-lymphocytic leukemia. *J Clin Oncol* 2:545, 1984.

23. Weick JK, Kopecky KJ, Appelbaum FR, et al.: A randomized investigation of high-dose versus standard-dose cytosine arabinoside with daunorubicin in patients with previously untreated acute myeloid leukemia: a Southwest Oncology Group study. *Blood* 88:2841–2851, 1996.

24. Mitus AJ, Miller KB, Schenkein DP, et al.: Improved survival for patients with acute myelogenous leukemia. *J Clin Oncol* 13:560–569, 1995.

25. Petersdorf S, Rankin C, Terebolo H, et al.: A phase II study of standard dose daunomycin and cytosine arabinoside (ARA-C) with high dose ara-C induction therapy followed by sequential high dose ara-C consolidation for adults with previously untreated acute myelogenous leukemia: a Southwest Oncology Group study (SWOG 9500). *Proc ASCO* 17:55a, 1998.

26. Bishop JF, Mattews JP, Young GA, et al.: Intensified induction chemotherapy with high dose cytarabine and etoposide for acute myeloid leukemia: a review and updated results of the Australian Leukemia Study Group. *Leuk Lymphoma* 28:315–327, 1998.

27. Cassileth PA, Begg CB, Bennett JM, et al.: A randomized study of the efficacy of consolidation therapy in adult acute nonlymphocytic leukemia. *Blood* 63:843–847, 1998.

28. Bloomfield CD: Postremission therapy in acute myeloid leukemia. *J Clin Oncol* 3:1570–1572, 1998.

29. Wolff SN, Herzig RH, Fay JW, et al.: High-dose cytarabine and daunorubicin as consolidation therapy for acute myeloid leukemia in first remission: long-term follow-up and results. *J Clin Oncol* 7:1260, 1989.

30. Cassileth PA, Lynch E, Hines JD, et al.: Varying intensity of postremission therapy in acute myeloid leukemia. *Blood* 79:1924, 1992.

31. Bloomfield CD, Lawrence D, Byrd JC, et al.: Frequency of prolonged remission duration after high-dose cytarabine intensification in acute myeloid leukemia varies by cytogenetic subtype. *Cancer Res* 58:4173–4179, 1998.

32. Strout MP, Marcucci G, Caligiuri MA, Bloomfield CD: Core-binding factor (CBF) and MLL-associated primary acute myeloid leukemia: biology and clinical implications. *Ann Hematol* 78:251–264, 1999.

33. Byrd JC, Mrózek K, Dodge RK, et al.: Pretreatment cytogenetic abnormalities are predictive of induction success, cumulative incidence of relapse, and overall survival in adult patients with de novo acute myeloid leukemia: results from Cancer and Leukemia Group B (CALGB 8461). *Blood* 100:4325–4336, 2002.

34. Byrd JC, Dodge RK, Carroll A, et al.: Patients with t(8;21)(q22;q22) and acute myeloid leukemia have superior failure-free and overall survival when repetitive cycles of high-dose cytarabine are administered. *J Clin Oncol* 17:3767–3775, 1999.

35. Moore JO, Powell B, Velez-Garcia E, et al.: A comparison of sequential non-cross-resistant therapy or ara-C consolidation following complete remission in adult patients below 60 years with acute myeloid leukemia: CALGB 922 (Meeting abstract). *Proc ASCO* 16:50a, 1997.

36. Rai K, Holland JF, Glidewell OS, et al.: Treatment of acute myelocytic leukemia: a study by the Cancer and Leukemia Group B. *Blood* 58:1203–1212, 1981.

37. Bucher T, Hiddemann W, Berdel WE, et al.: German AML Cooperative Group. 6-Thioguanine, cytarabine, and daunorubicin (TAD) and high-dose cytarabine and mitoxantrone (HAM) for induction, TAD for consolidation, and ither prolonged maintenance by reduced monthly TAD or TAD-HAM-TAD and noe course of intensive consolidation by sequential HAM in adult patients at all ages with de novo acute myeloid leukemia (AML): a randomized trial of the German AML Cooperative Group. *J Clin Oncol* 21:4496–4504, 2003.

38. Rubin EH, Andersen JW, Berg DT, et al.: Risk factors for high-dose cytosine arabinoside neurotoxicity: analysis of a CALGB trial of post-remission cytosine arabinoside in patients with acute myeloid leukemia. *J Clin Oncol* 10:948–953, 1992.

39. Smith GA, Damon LE, Rugo HS, Ries CA, Linker CA: High-dose cytarabine dose modification reduces the incidence of neurotoxicity in patients with renal insufficiency. *J Clin Oncol* 15:833–839, 1997.

40. Stone RM, Berg DT, George SL, et al.: Postremission therapy in older patients with de novo acute myeloid leukemia: a randomized trial comparing mitoxantrone and intermediate-dose cytarabine with standard-dose cytarabine. *Blood* 98:548–553, 2001.

41. Burnett A, Goldstone AH, Stevens RM, et al.: Randomized comparison of addition of autologous bone-marrow transplantation to intensive chemotherapy for acute myeloid leukaemia in first remission: results of MRC AML 10 trial. UK Medical Research Council Adult and Children's Leukemia Working Parties. *Lancet* 351:700–708, 1998.

42. Zittoun RA, Mandelli F, Willemze R, et al.: Autologous or allogeneic bone marrow transplantation compared with intensive chemotherapy in acute myelogenous leukemia. *N Engl J Med* 332:217–223, 1995.

43. Harousseau JL, Cahn JY, Pignon B, et al.: Comparison of autologous bone marrow transplantation and intensive chemotherapy as postremission therapy in adult acute myeloid leukemia. The Goupe Ouest Leucemies Aigues Myeloblastiques (GOELAM). *Blood* 90:2978–2986, 1997.

44. Cassileth PA, Harrington DP, Appelbaum FR, et al.: Chemotherapy compared with autologous or allogeneic bone marrow transplantation in the management of acute myeloid leukemia in first remission. *N Engl J Med* 339:1649–1656, 1998.

45. Slovak ML, Kopecky KJ, Cassileth PA, et al.: Karyotypic analysis predicts outcome of preremission and postremission therapy in adult acute myeloid leukemia: a Southwest Oncology Group/Eastern Cooperative Oncology Group study. *Blood* 96:4075–4083, 2000.

46. Woods WG, Neudorf S, Gold S, et al.: A comparison of allogeneic bone marrow transplantation, autologous bone marrow transplantation, and aggressive chemotherapy in children with acute myeloid leukemia in remission: a report from the Children's Cancer Group. *Blood* 97:56–62, 2001.

47. Tallman MS, Andersen JW, Schiffer CA, et al.: All-trans-retinoic acid in acute promyelocytic leukemia. *N Engl J Med* 337:1021–1028, 1997.

48. Fenaux P, Chastang C, Chevret S, et al.: A randomized comparison of all transretinoic acid (ATRA) followed by chemotherapy and ATRA plus chemotherapy and role of maintenance therapy in newly diagnosed acute promyelocytic leukemia. *Blood* 94:1192–1200, 1999.

49. Sanz MA, Martin G, Gonzalez M, Leon A, Rayon C: Risk-adapted treatment of acute promyelocytic leukemia with all-trans-retinoic acid and anthracycline mono-chemotherapy: a multicenter study by the PETHEMA Group. *Blood* 103:1237–1243, 2004.

50. Tallman MS, Andersen JW, Schiffer CA, et al.: All-trans retinoic acid in acute promyelocytic leukemia: long-term outcome and prognostic factor analysis from the North American Intergroup protocol. *Blood* 100:4298–4302, 2002.

51. Soignet SL, Frankel SR, Douer D, et al.: United States multicenter study of arsenic trioxide in relapsed acute promyelocytic leukemia. *J Clin Oncol* 19:3852–3860, 2001.

52. Tallman MS, Nabhan C, Feusner JH, et al.: Acute promyelocytic leukemia: evolving therapeutic strategies. *Blood* 99:759–767, 2002.

53. Estey EH, Giles FJ, Beran M, et al.: Experience with gemtuzumab ozogamicin ("Mylotarg") and all-trans retinoic acid in untreated acute promyelocytic leukemia. *Blood* 99(11):4222–4224, 2002 Jun 1.

54. Yeager AM, Kaizer H, Santos GW, et al.: Autologous bone marrow transplantation in patients with acute nonlymphocytic leukemia, using ex vivo marrow treated with 4-hydroperoxy-cyclophosphamide. *N Engl J Med* 315:141, 1986.

55. Rees JKH, Swirsky D, Gray RG, Hayhoe FGJ: Principal results of the Medical Research Councils 8th acute myeloid leukaemia trail. *Lancet* 2:1236, 1986.

56. Amadori S, Arcese W, Isacchi G, et al.: Mitoxantrone, etoposide, and intermediate-dose cytarabine: an effective and tolerable regimen for the treatment of refractory acute myeloid leukemia. *J Clin Oncol* 9:1210–1214, 1991.

57. Meng-er H, Yu-chen Y, Shu-rong C, et al.: Use of all-trans retinoic acid in the treatment of acute promyelocytic leukemia. *Blood* 72:567, 1988.

58. Shen ZX, Chen GQ, Ni JH, et al.: Use of arsenic trioxide (As203) in the treatment of acute promyelocytic leukemia (APL). II: Clinical efficacy and pharmacokinetics in relapsed patients. *Blood* 89:3354–3360, 1997.

59. Soignet SL, Maslak P, Wang ZG, et al.: Complete remission after treatment of acute promyelocytic leukemia with arsenic trioxide. *N Engl J Med* 339:1341–1348, 1998.

60. Estey EH, Guillermo GM, Ferrajoli A, et al.: Use of all-transretinoic acid (ATRA) + arsenic trioxide (ATO) to eliminate or minimize use of chemotherapy (CT) in untreated acute promyelocytic leukemia (APL). *Blood* 104:abstract 394, 2004.

61. Unnikrishnan D, Dutcher JP, Varshneya N, et al.: Torsades de pointes in 3 patients with leukemia treated with arsenic trioxide. *Blood* 97:1514–1516, 2001.

62. Sievers EL, Applebaum FR, Spielberger RT, et al.: Selective ablation of acute myeloid leukemia using antibody-targeted chemotherapy: a phase I study of an anti-CD33 calicheamicin immunoconjugate. *Blood* 99:3678–3684, 1999.

63. Sievers EL, Larson RA, Stadtmauer EA, et al.: Mylotarg Study Group. Efficacy and safety of gemtuzumab ozogamicin in patients with CD33-positive acute myeloid leukemia in the first relapse. *J Clin Oncol* 19:3244–3254, 2001.

64. Gilliland DG, Griffin JD: The roles of FLT3 in hematopoiesis and leukemia. *Blood* 100:1532–1542, 2002.

65. Whitman SP, Archer KJ, Feng L, et al.: Absence of the wild-type allele predicts poor prognosis in adult de novo acute myeloid leukemia with normal cytogenetics and the internal tandem duplication of FLT3: a Cancer and Leukemia Group B study. *Cancer Res* 61:7233–7239, 2001.

66. Kottaridis PD, Gale RE, Frew ME, et al.: The presence of a FLT3 internal tandem duplication in patients with acute myeloid leukemia (AML) adds important prognostic information to cytogenetic risk group and response to the first cycle of chemotherapy: analysis of 854 patients from the United Kingdom Medical Research Council AML 10 and 12 trials. *Blood* 98:1752–1759, 2001.

67. Smith BD, Lewis M, Beran M, et al.: Single-agent CEP-701, a novel FLT3 inhibitor shows biologic and clinical activity in patients with relapsed or refractory acute myeloid leukemia. *Blood* 103:3669–3676, 2004.

68. Stone RM, DeAngelo DJ, Klimek V, et al.: Patients with acute myeloid leukemia and an activating mutation in FLT3 respond to a small-molecule FLT3 tyrosine kinase inhibitor, PKC412. *Blood* 105:54–60, 2005.

69. Karp J, Lancet JE, Kaufman SH, et al.: Clinical and biological activity of the farnesyl transferase inhibitor R115777 in adults with refractory and relapsed acute leukemias: a phase 1 clinical laboratory correlative trial. *Blood* 2001:97:3361–3369.

70. Lancet JE, Gotlib J, Gojo I, et al.: Tipifarnib (ZARNESTRA™) in previously untreated poor-risk AML of the elderly: updated results of a multicenter phase 2 trial. *Blood* 104:abstract 874, 2004.

71. Giles FJ, Feldman J, Roboz GJ, et al.: Phase II study of troxacitabine, a novel dioxolane nucleoside analog, in patients with untreated or imatinib mesylate-resistant

chronic myelogenous leukemia in blastic phase. *Leuk Res* 27:1091–1096, 2003.

72. Kantarjian H, Gandhi V, Cortes J, et al.: Phase 2 clinical and pharmacologic study of clofarabine in patients with refractory or relapsed acute leukemia. *Blood* 102: 2379–2386, 2003.

73. Marcucci G, Stock W, Dai G, et al.: G3139, a BCL-2 antisense oligo-nucleotide, in AML. *Ann Hematol* 83(suppl 1): S93–S94, 2004.

74. Leith C, Kopecky K, Godwin J, et al.: Acute myeloid leukemia in the elderly: assessment of multidrug resistance (MDR1) and cytogenetics distinguishes biologic subgroups with remarkably distinct responses to standard chemotherapy. A Southwest Oncology Group study. *Blood* 89:3323–3329, 1997.

75. List AF, Kopecky KJ, Willman CL, et al.: Benefit of cyclosporine modulation of drug resistance in patients with poor-risk acute myeloid leukemia: a Southwest Oncology Group study. *Blood* 98:3212–3220, 2001.

76. Greenberg PL, Lee SJ, Advani R, et al.: Mitoxantrone, etoposide, and cytarabine with our without valspodar in patients with relapsed or refractory acute myeloid leukemia and high-risk myelodysplastic syndrome: a phase III trial (E2995). *J Clin Oncol* 22:1078–1086, 2003.

77. Riddell SR, Berger C, Murata M, Randolph S, Warren EH: The graft versus leukemia response after allogeneic hematopoietic stem cell transplantation. *Blood Rev* 17:153–162, 2003.

78. Lu S, Wieder E, Komanduri K, Ma Q, Molldrem JJ: Vaccines in leukemia. *Adv Pharmacol* 51:255–270, 2004.

79. Gong J, Koido S, Kato Y, et al.: Induction of anti-leukemic cytotoxic T lymphocytes by fusion of patient-derived dendritic cells with autologous myeloblasts. *Leuk Res* 28:1302–1312, 2004.

80. Dunussi-Joannopoulos K, Dranoff G, Weinstein HJ, et al.: Gene immunotherapy in murine acute myeloid leukemia: granulocyte-macrophage colony-stimulating factor tumor cell vaccines elicit more potent antitumor immunity compared with B7 family and other cytokine vaccines. *Blood* 91:222, 1998.

81. Omura GA, Vogler R, LeFante J, et al.: Treatment of myelogenous leukemia: influence of three induction regimens and maintenance with chemotherapy or BCG immunotherapy. *Cancer* 49:1530–1536, 1982.

82. Meloni G, Foa R, Vignetti M, et al.: Interleukin-2 may induce prolonged remissions in advanced acute myelogenous leukemia. *Blood* 84:2158, 1994.

## Chapter 5

# TREATMENT APPROACH TO ACUTE MYELOID LEUKEMIA IN OLDER ADULTS

*Mikkael A. Sekeres*

Statistically, it is probably no accident that the first reported case of leukemia (by Velpeau in 1827[1]) occurred in a 63-year old. Acute myeloid leukemia (AML) is a disease of older adults. In the United States, the median age is 68 years and the age-adjusted population incidence is 17.6 per 100,000 for people 65 years of age or older.[2] Compare this to an incidence of 1.8 per 100,000 for people under the age of 65 years.[2] Therefore, of the estimated 11,900 new AML diagnoses in the United States in 2004, over half will affect patients 60 years of age or older,[3] a population considered "elderly" in the leukemia literature.[4–11]

Older adults with AML, when compared to younger patients with the same disease, have a poor prognosis and represent a discrete population in terms of disease features (including the biology of the disease and the incidence of secondary leukemia), treatment-related complications, and overall outcome (Table 5.1). As a result, older patients require distinctive management approaches to determine whether standard treatment, investigational treatment, or low-dose therapy or palliative care is most appropriate.

## DISEASE FEATURES

### CYTOGENETICS

Older adults with AML have a lower incidence of favorable chromosomal abnormalities and a higher incidence of unfavorable abnormalities compared to younger adults with AML.[12–14] In an analysis of outcome of 1213 adult patients with de novo AML assigned varying doses of postremission therapy, only 2% of older patients ($\geq$60 years) had the favorable t(8;21), compared to 9.4% of younger patients (<60 years). Similarly, 3.4% of older patients had inv(16) or t(16;16) compared to 10.4% of younger patients.[15] At the opposite end of the spectrum, with respect to unfavorable cytogenetics, 9.1% of older adults had the $-7$ abnormality compared to 3.2% of younger adults; 6.2%

of older adults had the $+8$ abnormality compared to 4% of younger adults; and 18.3% of older AML patients had complex cytogenetics (defined as three or more cytogenetic abnormalities, not including core-binding factor cytogenetics) compared to only 7.1% of younger patients. Looking specifically within a population of older adults with AML, an analysis of 1065 older patients with de novo and secondary AML enrolled in the Medical Research Council (MRC) AML 11 trial (in which patients were randomized to one of three remission induction regimens and further randomized to postremission therapy) found that 4% of patients had a t(15;17), 2% had a t(8;21), and only 1% had inv(16). Patients fortunate enough to have one of these abnormalities had a survival advantage over other patients. Poor-risk cytogenetics included a complex karyotype (defined here as five or more abnormalities), which was found in 14% of patients, a $+8$ abnormality in 10% of patients, a $-7$ abnormality in 8%, a del(5q) in 8%, and $-5$ abnormality in 5% of older AML patients.[13]

### BONE MARROW BIOLOGY

In older adults, AML is more likely to arise from a proximal bone marrow stem cell disorder,[16] such as myelodysplastic syndrome (MDS),[17] and with leukemia-specific abnormalities in more than one hematopoietic cell lineage.[18] This may explain the different disease behavior in this group, as well as prolonged neutropenia following chemotherapy.[6] Older adults with AML also are more likely to have reduced proliferative capacities in normal hematopoietic stem cells,[19] which also may affect blood count recovery following intensive chemotherapy.

### DRUG-RESISTANCE GENES

The expression of genes that mediate drug resistance occurs with increased frequency in this age cohort.[20] MDR1, the so-called p-glycoprotein (gp170) chemotherapy efflux pump, was found in 71% of leukemic blasts in subjects in a Southwest Oncology Group study

| Table 5.1 Comparison of older and younger adults with AML | | |
|---|---|---|
| Characteristic | Older AML patients[a] | Younger AML patients[a] |
| **Population incidence[b]** | 17.2 | 1.8 |
| **Favorable cytogenetics** | | |
| t(8;21) | 2.0% | 9.4% |
| inv 16 or t(16;16) | 3.4% | 10.4% |
| t(15;17) | 4.0% | 6–12% |
| **Unfavorable cytogenetics** | | |
| –7 | 9.1% | 3.2% |
| +8 | 6.2% | 4.0% |
| Complex | 18.3% | 7.1% |
| **MDR1 expression** | 71% | 35% |
| **Secondary AML** | 24–56% | 8% |
| **Treatment-related mortality[c]** | 25–30% | 5–10% |
| **Complete remission[c]** | 39–61% | 65–73% |
| **Long-term disease-free survival[c]** | 5–15% | 30% |

[a] In general, older AML patients are defined as 60 years of age or older and younger AML patients as below 60 years of age.
[b] New diagnoses, per 100,000 US citizens per year. Older/younger division occurs at 65 years.
[c] Rates following remission induction therapy with an anthracycline- or anthracenedione-based regimen.

Reprinted from Stone RM, O'Donnell MR, Sekeres MA: Acute myeloid leukemia. *Hematology Am Soc Hematol Educ Program* 98–117, 2004, copyright American Society of Hematology, U.S.A.

of AML patients over the age of 55 years. Compare this to an incidence of 35% in younger AML patients.[21,22] MDR1/p-glycoprotein expression is associated with lower complete remission (CR) rates and more chemoresistant disease. In addition, defects in the MSH2 protein involved in DNA mismatch repair and genome protection are expressed with greater frequency in this population.[20] Abnormalities of DNA mismatch repair due to defective MSH2 expression could play a key role in leukemogenesis, in particular in AML arising in older patients or secondary to previous chemotherapy.

### *PRIOR STEM CELL INSULT*

Older adults with AML are more likely to have a secondary leukemia arising from an antecedent MDS or from prior therapy with chemotherapy or radiation therapy for another cancer.[23,24] Patients with this type of AML are predisposed to having abnormalities in chromosome 5 and/or 7.[12,14] Secondary AML (AML that arose after MDS, myeloproliferative disorders, and therapies or other malignancies) comprises 24–56% of AML diagnoses in older patients.[8,22,25] Compare this to the prevalence of approximately 8% in younger AML patients in the MRC AML 10 trial.[12] AML arising from prior bone marrow stem cell disorders, particularly when the process is greater than 10 months in duration

prior to the development of AML, is less responsive to chemotherapy, resulting in shorter event-free survival, a lower CR rate, and conferring a worse prognosis.[26]

## RESPONSE TO THERAPY

Compared to younger patients under the age of 60 years with AML, older adults are not as tolerant of or responsive to remission induction and consolidation chemotherapy. Treatment-related mortality following remission induction therapy, accounting for 5–10% of deaths in younger patients, may be as high as 25–30% in older adults.[7,27–29] These estimates can be considered low, as they derive from clinical trials requiring minimal performance statuses and often excluding patients with certain comorbidities or known secondary AML. High mortality rates likely result from inherent disease biology, an increased prevalence of comorbid disease, and a differential metabolism of induction regimen drugs, particularly cytarabine, resulting in supratherapeutic drug levels.[7,30,31] Concern over potential treatment-related toxicities may result in undertreatment of disease. Paradoxically, administration of full-dose daunorubicin, for example, may result in a reduction in early deaths by effecting a more rapid CR.[18]

The outcome of older adults with AML is worse than that of similarly treated younger patients with the same disease. Adults under the age of 60 years treated with an induction regimen consisting of an anthracycline combined with cytarabine have a 65–73% chance of attaining a CR, while those over 60 years of age have a 39–61% chance of a CR.[6,7,27,28,32–35] Moreover, long-term disease-free survival occurs in approximately 30% of younger adults (or, 45% of those entering a CR), compared to only 5–15% long-term disease-free survival in adults over the age of 60 years.[6,7,28,35–39] The disease features of older adults with AML already elucidated provide the likely explanation for this dismal survival. Again, these numbers represent an optimistic prediction of this population's overall outcome. Thus, approximately 10 patients need to be treated with intensive induction chemotherapy to effect long-term disease-free survival in one. One out of four of those treated patients will not leave their remission induction hospitalization alive.

## INDICATIONS FOR TREATMENT

For 85–95% of older AML patients, any therapy ultimately will be purely palliative. Treatment options range from supportive care (blood and platelet transfusions when needed, antibiotics to treat infections, and growth factor support) to low-dose chemotherapy (e.g., hydroxyurea or low-dose cytarabine arabinoside) or investigational agents, and high-dose chemotherapy (anthracycline- or anthracenedione-based remission induction therapy). The decision of whether or not to offer remission induction therapy (on the part of physicians) or to receive it (on the part of patients) therefore is not straightforward.

Only two clinical trials have compared immediate aggressive induction chemotherapy with an anthracycline-based regimen to an alternative approach in older adults with leukemia. One trial, conducted by the European Organization for Research and Treatment of Cancer Leukemia Group, randomized 60 patients to receive either an anthracycline-based intensive induction regimen or a "wait-and-see" approach followed by mild chemotherapy for palliation of leukemia-related symptoms, begun a median of 9 days after diagnosis.[40] Patients randomized to the intensive therapy group survived a median of 10 weeks longer than those randomized to the "wait-and-see" approach (21 weeks vs 11 weeks, $P = 0.015$)—for a survival time only 16 days longer than the amount of time they spent hospitalized to receive therapy.

The other multi-institutional study randomized 87 patients over the age of 65 years to receive either an anthracycline-based induction regimen or low-dose cytarabine therapy.[41] Fifty-two percent of patients receiving intensive therapy achieved a CR, while only 32% of those receiving low-dose cytarabine entered a CR. On the other hand, the frequency of early deaths was higher in the intensive chemotherapy group (31% vs 10%). Although the CR rates and early death rates were statistically significantly different between the groups, the overall survival (OS) (12.8 months in the intensive therapy group and 8.8 months in the low-dose cytarabine group) was not. In addition, for both studies, the cost in early deaths, length of hospital stay, and transfusion support was substantial.

Given these equivocal results, algorithms of how to approach older AML patients have been proposed.[9,10,18] These suggest that, in the absence of adverse prognostic factors (such as poor-risk cytogenetics, poor performance status, significant comorbidities, or age 80 years or above), patients be offered intensive therapy, including enrollment in clinical trials that use intensive therapy. Alternatively, patients should be given the opportunity to participate in a clinical trial using less intensive therapy, or they should be offered nonintensive therapy or best supportive care.

Our policy is to base treatment decisions on individual patient preference after an *informed* discussion has taken place that incorporates *modified* risk estimates and *functional* patient age (Figure 5.1), without using absolute cutoffs for prognostic factors or chronologic age.

Patients overestimate their chance for cure and 1-year survival, and underestimate the potential for treatment-related mortality. One single-center study found that 74% of patients estimated their chance to be cured by remission induction therapy to be greater than or equal to 50%, and almost 90% estimated their chance of being alive in 1 year to be greater than or equal to 50%. Almost two-thirds of patients reported that they were not offered treatment options other than the one they chose, despite physician documentation of alternatives in all cases.[42] As a communication gap exists between the extent to which physicians believe they are informing patients and what patients report their understanding to be, an informed discussion of treatment options should include multiple explanations by different health care personnel, the use of educational materials, and testing patient understanding.

Outcome and treatment-related mortality estimates should be modified to reflect baseline prognostic factors. For example, patients who fall into the "very elderly"[10] category (80 years or older) can attain a CR with intensive therapy, but their chance of doing so is 30%, and only 7% of treated patients are alive at 1 year.[43] Patients with more than one poor prognostic factor also have diminished CR rates. Taking into account cytogenetics, secondary AML, and MDR1 expression, older AML patients with one of these prognostic factors had CR rates of 44%, compared to CR rates of 24% when patients had two factors and 12% when they had three.[9,22] Conversely, older patients with de novo AML, no MDR1 expression, and intermediate or favorable cytogenetics have CR rates of 72–81% and the potential for a 34% 5-year OS rate.[13,22]

Functional patient age refers to patients who function at an age much younger than their chronologic age might suggest, and thus may derive more benefit from therapy.[44] Formal instruments used to evaluate functional status include The Older American Resources and Services Questionnaire, the Medical Outcomes Study Short Form 36, the Functional Assessment of Cancer Therapy scale, the Charlson Comorbidity Index, and the Karnofsky Performance Status scale, among others.[45–50] An 80-year-old patient scoring well on a functional status evaluation may be a more appropriate candidate for remission induction therapy than a 70-year-old scoring poorly.

## TREATMENT OPTIONS

### REMISSION INDUCTION THERAPY

The backbone of remission induction therapy in AML patients consists of an anthracycline (daunorubicin or idarubicin) or anthracenedione (mitoxantrone) and cytosine arabinoside (ara-C),[6–8,23,32,33,51–58] a regimen that has not changed in over two decades. Typically, daunorubicin is given at a dose of 45 mg/m$^2$/day for 3 days, or idarubicin is given at a dose of 12 mg/m$^2$/day for 3 days, or mitoxantrone is given at a dose of 12 mg/m$^2$/day for 3 days, in combination with ara-C, which is administered as a continuous infusion at 100 or 200 mg/m$^2$/day for 7 days. (*Frequently referred to as 7 + 3 chemotherapy.*) In general, studies have compared different anthracyclines and anthracenediones, varied doses and schedules, and added additional agents with some improvement in CR rates, but without any effect on OS rates (Table 5.2). It is reasonable to tailor the aggressiveness of daunorubicin and ara-C administration

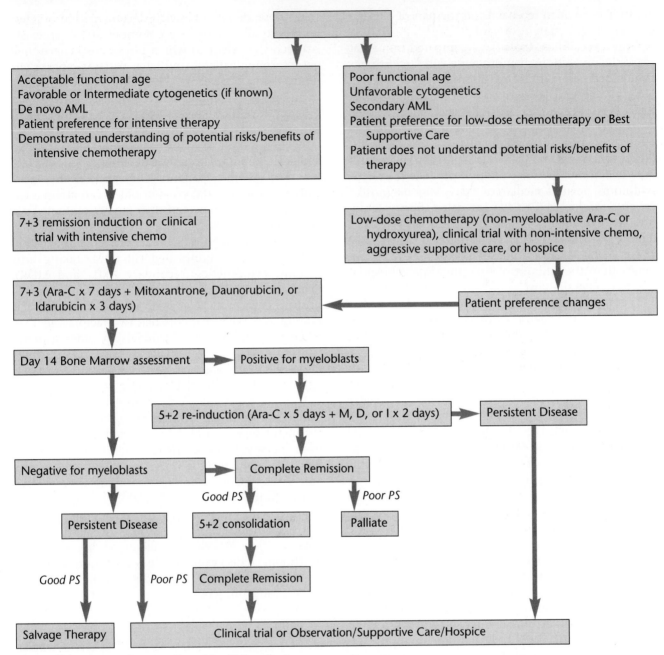

**Figure 5.1**  *Approach to treating older AML patients*

to the functional age of the older AML patient, with the understanding that, theoretically, some degree of efficacy may be compromised.

**Comparing anthracyclines and anthracenediones**

A phase III trial of 489 patients over 60 years of age compared an induction regimen consisting of mitox-antrone and ara-C to the standard of daunorubicin and ara-C.[4] A CR was achieved by 47% of patients treated with mitoxantrone, compared to 38% of patients treated with daunorubicin, a difference that did not achieve statistical significance. Early and postinduction death rates were similar, as were toxicities, with the exception that those treated with mitox-antrone had a significantly higher rate of severe

infections and a trend toward a longer duration of aplasia. OS was similar for both groups.

In older adults with AML, idarubicin may have advantages over daunorubicin that include reduced cardiac toxicity, circumvention of multidrug resistance (MDR), and oral administration.[59] A number of trials have compared the two induction regimens,[60–63] with the majority demonstrating a CR advantage in the idarubicin arm for younger adults, but no reproducible survival advantage. An overview of trials comparing idarubicin to daunorubicin for induction therapy showed similar overall induction failures in patients over 60 years of age receiving either of the two treat-ment arms; an improved CR rate in the idarubicin arm when compared to daunorubicin (50.5% vs 46.1%);

**Table 5.2**    Randomized studies defining remission induction therapy in older adults

| Goal | Remission induction agents | Complete remission | Overall survival | Comments | Reference |
|---|---|---|---|---|---|
| Compare anthracyclines and anthracenediones | M (8 mg/m²/day) + A (100 mg/m²/day) vs D (30 mg/m²/day) + A (100 mg/m²/day) | 47% vs 38% P = 0.07 | 39 weeks (median) 9% (5 years) vs 36 weeks (median) 6% (5 years) P = 0.23 | Early and postinduction death rates were similar for both arms. Patients receiving mitoxantrone had a significantly higher rate of severe infections (25.1% vs 18.6%) and a trend toward a longer duration of aplasia (22 vs 19 days) | 4 |
| | I (8–20 mg/m²/day) + A (100–200 mg/m²/day) vs D (45–50 mg/m²/day) + A (100–200 mg/m²/day) | 51% vs 46% P = ND | 33.6 weeks (median) vs 29.9 weeks (median) P = 0.58 | Early induction failure tended to be higher with idarubicin, while late induction failure was lower. Myelosuppression was greater in patients receiving idarubicin | 64 |
| | I (8 mg/m²/day) + A (100 mg/m²/day) + E (100 mg/m²/day) vs M (7 mg/m²/day) + A (100–200 mg/m²/day) + E (100 mg/m²/day) | 45% vs 50% P = 0.52 | 7 months (median) 21% (2 years) vs 7 months (median) 21% (2 years) P = ND | No difference between groups in degree of myelosuppression or in early death rates | 65 |
| Vary 7 + 3 dose | D (60 mg/m²/day) + A (100 mg/m²/day) vs D (30 mg/m²/day) + A (100 mg/m²/day) | 54% vs 42% P = 0.038 | 16% (5 years) vs 10% (5 years) P = 0.11 | The 30 mg daunorubicin arm was closed prematurely due to higher response rates in the 60 mg arm, resulting in 42 patients receiving lower dose daunorubicin, and 130 patients receiving the higher dose | 34 |
| | D (45 mg/m²/day) + A (100 mg/m²/day) vs D (45 mg/m²/day) + A (200 mg/m²/day) | 44% vs 38% P = 0.68 | 11.0 weeks (median) vs 9.6 weeks (median) P = 0.23 | This study has been criticized for short overall survival times | 27 |
| Add agents | D (50 mg/m²/day) + A (100 mg/m² q 12 h) + T (100 mg/m² q 12 h) vs D (50 mg/m²/day) + A (100 mg/m² q 12 h) + E (100 mg/m²/day) vs M (12 mg/m²/day) + A (100 mg/m²/day) | 62% vs 50% P = 0.002ᵃ vs 55% P = 0.04ᵇ | 12% (5 years) vs 8% (5 years) P = 0.02ᵃ vs 10% (5 years) P = 0.1ᵇ, 0.2ᶜ | There were no significant differences in myelosuppression or other toxicities, though neutrophils were slower to recover in the mitoxantrone arm. Patients receiving ADE had higher rates of induction death (26%, compared to 16% for DAT and 17% for MAC) | 29 |
| | D (60 mg/m²/day) + A (100 mg/m²/day) + E (100 mg/m²/day) vs D (40 mg/m²/day) + A (100 mg/m²/day) + E (60 mg/m²/day) + P (10 mg/kg/day) | 46% vs 39% P = 0.008 | 7 months (median) vs 2 months (median) P = 0.48 | Because of concern about excessive mortality on the ADEP arm (25 deaths vs 12 on the ADE arm), it was closed early to further accrual | 11 |
| Use hematopoietic growth factors | D (45 mg/m²/day) + A (200 mg/m²/day) vs D (45 mg/m²/day) + A (200 mg/m²/day) + GM-CSF (5 µg/kg/day) | 54% vs 51% P = 0.61 | 10.8 months (median) vs 8.4 months (median) P = 0.10 | Median duration of neutropenia was 15 days in the GM-CSF arm and 17 days in the placebo arm (P = 0.02). The duration of hospitalization did not differ between the arms; nor did the rates of life-threatening infection, or persistent leukemia | 6 |

*table continues*

| Table 5.2    continued | | | | | |
| --- | --- | --- | --- | --- | --- |
| Goal | Remission induction agents | Complete remission | Overall survival | Comments | Reference |
| | D (45 mg/m$^2$/day) + A (200 mg/m$^2$/day) | 50% | 9 months (median) | The duration of neutropenia was 15% shorter in the G-CSF arm compared to the placebo arm ($P = 0.14$). The duration of hospitalization did not differ between the arms; nor did the rates of life-threatening infection, or persistent leukemia. | 38 |
| | vs | vs | vs | | |
| | D (45 mg/m$^2$/day) + A (200 mg/m$^2$/day) + | 41% | 6 months (median) | | |
| | G-CSF (400 μg/m$^2$/day) | $P = 0.89$ | $P = 0.71$ | | |

M, mitoxantrone; A, ara-C; D, daunorubicin; I, idarubicin; E, etoposide; T, thioguanine; P, PSC-833; GM-CSF, granulocyte-macrophage colony-stimulating factor; G-CSF, granulocyte-colony-stimulating factor; ND, not done.

[a] For comparison of DAT to ADE.
[b] For comparison of DAT to MAC.
[c] For comparison of ADE to MAC.

Reprinted from Stone RM, O'Donnell MR, Sekeres MA: Acute myeloid leukemia. *Hematology Am Soc Hematol Educ Program* 98–117, 2004, copyright American Society of Hematology, U.S.A.

and no difference in OS in this population.[64] Another study compared an induction regimen consisting of idarubicin, ara-C, and etoposide to mitoxantrone, ara-C, and etoposide in 160 patients over the age of 60 years.[65] There was no statistically significant difference between the two therapy arms in terms of CR rates, neutrophil and platelet recovery (approximately 25 days in both arms), median disease-free survival, 2-year survival, and in treatment-related toxicities.

An Eastern Cooperative Oncology Group (ECOG) study randomized 349 newly diagnosed AML patients older than 55 years to receive ara-C with either daunorubicin, idarubicin, or mitoxantrone as remission induction therapy.[66] Two hundred thirty-six patients underwent subsequent randomization to priming with granulocyte-macrophage colony-stimulating factor (GM-CSF) versus placebo. The overall CR rate was 42%, the median disease-free survival was 7 months and OS was 14 months, and therapy-related toxicity was 16%, with no statistically significant differences among the induction regimens. Interestingly, the CR rate and OS were greater for the first 113 patients who did not have a delay in receiving their induction regimen due to priming regimen versus placebo randomization.

Although some debate exists regarding the equivalency of anthracycline and anthracenedione dosing in comparative trials, given the lack of survival benefit of one agent over another, we consider the three to have equivalent efficacy in the population of older patients with AML, and thus to be interchangeable.

## Varying 7 + 3 doses

There is evidence that higher doses of anthacyclines may affect higher CR rates.[67,68] A direct comparison was conducted by the German AML Cooperative Group. In their study, daunorubicin at a dose of 60 mg/m$^2$/day was compared to daunorubicin at a dose of 30 mg/m$^2$/day in combination with ara-C and 6-thioguanine. The higher dose of daunorubicin resulted in a significantly higher CR rate compared to the lower dose,[69,70] but there was no difference in OS. There has never been a prospective comparison of daunorubicin at doses of 45 mg/m$^2$/day versus 60 mg/m$^2$/day in older adults, and thus we cannot recommend the higher dose.

Similarly, there does not seem to be a benefit to higher doses of ara-C in remission induction therapy. One study randomized 326 patients to receive ara-C at 100 mg/m$^2$/day or ara-C at 200 mg/m$^2$/day combined with daunorubicin.[27] For patients of age 60 years or older, CR rates were actually lower in the higher dose arm, though not significantly, and median OS was similar for both groups, though this study has been criticized for short survival times.[18]

## Additional remission induction agents (7 + 3 + ···)

Another approach is to take advantage of the biological characteristics relatively specific to AML in older adults and add experimental agents to standard anthracycline- or anthracenedione-based therapy. A phase I study of 31 patients of 56 years of age or older with AML involved remission induction therapy which consisted of mitoxantrone, etoposide, and PSC 833, a cyclosporine analog capable of inhibiting the p-glycoprotein efflux pump.[71] The median age of enrolled patients was 71 years, and 70% expressed p-glycoprotein, as would be expected in this population.[22] The overall CR was 50% after a single induction attempt, and the overall median survival was approximately 9 months at the study's termination. A phase III study comparing daunorubicin, ara-C, etoposide, and PSC 833 to daunorubicin, ara-C, and etoposide, on the other hand, had to close accrual to the PSC 833 arm after the first 120 patients were enrolled when an interim analysis revealed an increased early mortality rate compared to the standard arm.[8] Cyclosporine A works in similar ways to overcome the p-glycoprotein pump, thus increasing intracellular anthracycline levels, and is still being evaluated in studies.[72–74]

In direct or historical comparisons, no survival advantage has been found in older AML patients, with the addition to standard 7 + 3 therapy of etoposide or thioguanine.[8,51,65,75] The MRC AML 11 trial randomized 1314 older patients to receive DAT (daunorubicin, ara-C, and thioguanine), ADE (daunorubicin, ara-C, and etoposide), or MAC (mitoxantrone and ara-C).[29] Patients randomized to the DAT arm had significantly higher CR rates, whereas those randomized to the ADE arm had higher rates of induction death, and those receiving MAC had higher rates of resistant disease. There were no substantial differences in long-term survival among the three remission induction arms.

### Gemtuzumab ozogamicin

While standard induction regimens affect the replication of all bone marrow stem cells, antibody-targeted therapy has the potential of selectively ablating malignant myeloid cells while sparing normal stem cells. Gemtuzumab ozogamicin (GO, CMA-676, or Mylotarg) is a humanized monoclonal antibody that targets the CD33 antigen, expressed in 90% of patients with AML.[76–78] It is conjugated to the toxin calicheamycin. GO was approved by the Food and Drug Administration for the treatment of older AML patients with relapsed or refractory AML who are not candidates for other cytotoxic chemotherapy and whose myeloblasts express CD33. This was based on phase 2 data showing overall response rates of 26% and a median relapse-free survival of 6.8 months.[79,80] GO is now being used as single-agent up-front therapy or in combination with 7 + 3 in older AML patients. It will be discussed in more detail in the relapsed or refractory AML setting in Chapter 9.

### Hematopoietic growth factors

In the majority of AML patients, death results from bleeding or infectious complications.[81] This is particularly true in older adults with AML. The utility of hematopoietic growth factors (HGF), including granulocyte colony-stimulating factor (G-CSF) and GM-CSF, for ameliorating the myelosuppressive complications of AML therapy in older adults has been studied extensively.[6,35,36,38,39,67,82,83] These prospective, randomized trials were also designed to determine whether or not HGF had detrimental effects in the inappropriate stimulation of leukemic cell proliferation and thus resistance, or whether they had beneficial effects in "priming" leukemic cells to proliferate prior to the administration of S-phase specific chemotherapy agents such as ara-C.[10,84] With the exception of one ECOG study that demonstrated a CR rate and OS benefit in patients randomized to the GM-CSF arm (compared to patients receiving no growth factor support),[67] these trials found that while HGF are safe, reduce the duration of neutropenia (by a range of 2–6 days), and do not support leukemia cell proliferation,

they also do not reliably improve the CR rate, the length of hospitalization, the induction death rate, or prolong survival.

### POSTREMISSION THERAPY

No randomized trial has ever demonstrated that *any* amount of postremission therapy in older AML patients provides better outcomes than does *no* postremission therapy. That being said, the only studies demonstrating that long-term disease-free remission is possible in older AML patients have included remission induction and postremission therapy.[4,5,7,27–29,32,35,69,83] Standard postremission therapy consists of a repeat of remission induction therapy, single-agent ara-C, or 2 days of an anthracycline or anthracenedione (the same type of drug given at the same doses as with remission induction therapy) combined with 5 days of ara-C, again given at the same dose as with remission induction therapy (*frequently referred to as 5 + 2 postremission therapy*), for one to two cycles.[85]

### Intensive postremission chemotherapy

Younger adults with AML benefit from intensified doses of ara-C therapy in the postremission setting, while older adults, particularly those with liver or kidney abnormalities, do not (Table 5.3).[5,7,30] The Cancer and Leukemia Group B (CALGB) studied 1088 patients with de novo AML who were randomized in first CR (following daunorubicin/ara-C remission induction therapy) to receive one of three postremission therapies: four courses of ara-C at 100 mg/m$^2$/day for 5 days as a continuous intravenous infusion, at 400 mg/m$^2$/ day for 5 days as a continuous intravenous infusion, and at 3 g/m$^2$ in a 3-h infusion every 12 h on days 1, 3, and 5.[7] Three hundred forty-six patients were over 60 years of age. Only 29% of older patients were able to tolerate all four courses of ara-C at 3 g/m$^2$. Neurotoxicity occurred in 32% of older patients in the high-dose arm. Despite the higher rate of toxicity in older adults, disease-free and OS rates in this age group did not differ among the three postremission therapy arms.

A subsequent CALGB study randomized older AML patients in CR following remission induction therapy to one of two postremission regimens: ara-C at 100 mg/m$^2$/day by continuous intravenous infusion over 5 days for four monthly courses, or ara-C at 500 mg/m$^2$ every 12 h in combination with mitoxantrone for six doses, over four monthly courses.[5] Although similar numbers of patients in each arm were able to complete all four postremission courses, survival was again similar at a cost of more toxicity in the higher dose ara-C arm. In another study, the mortality rate among older patients receiving high-dose postremission therapy was 57%, compared to a rate of 13% among younger patients.[37] Given the toxicity of intensive postremission chemotherapy without a gain in survival, it is difficult to justify such treatment in older AML populations.

**Table 5.3    Randomized studies defining postremission therapy in older adults**

| Goal | Postremission agents | Completion of all post-remission cycles | Survival | Comments | Reference |
|---|---|---|---|---|---|
| **Establish therapy intensity** | A (100 mg/m²/day × 5 days) vs A (400 mg/m²/day × 5 days) vs A (3 g/m² q 12 h days 1, 3, 5) | 71% vs 66% vs 29% $P$ = ND | ≤16% (DFS, 4 years) vs ≤16% (DFS, 4 years) vs ≤16% (DFS, 4 years) $P$ = 0.19 | Remission induction with daunorubicin + ara-C. Because of concerns about excessive neuro-toxicity in older patients receiving ara-C at 3 G/m² (32% of 31 patients), it was closed early to further accrual. Overall survival at 4 years in older patients regardless of postremission therapy was 9% | 7 |
| | A (100 mg/m²/day × 5 days) × 4 cycles vs M (5 mg/m² q 12 h days 1–3) + A (400 mg/m² q 12 h days 1–3) × 2 cycles | 71% vs 78% $P$ = ND | 11 months (DFS, median) vs 10 months (DFS, median) $P$ = 0.67 | Remission induction with daunorubicin + ara-C. Higher toxicities, including hemorrhage, infection, dysrhythmias, and malaise, were experienced in the mitoxantrone/ara-C arm. Median overall survival times were 1.6 years in the ara-C arm and 1.3 years in the mitoxantrone/Ara-C arm | 5 |
| **Establish therapy duration** | D (50 mg/m²/day × 2 days) + A (100 mg/m²/day × 7 days) + T (100 mg/m² q 12 h × 7 days) × 1 cycle vs D (50 mg/m²/day × 2 days) + A (100 mg/m²/day × 7 days) + T (100 mg/m² q 12 h × 7 days) × 1 cycle; D (50 mg/m²/day × 2 days) + A (100 mg/m²/day × 5 days) + T (100 mg/m² q 12 h × 5 days) × 1 cycle; C (600 mg/m² × 1 day) + O (1.5 mg/m² × 1 day) + A (100 mg/m²/day × 5 days + Pred (60 mg/m² × 5 days) × 2 cycles | 100% vs 61% $P$ = ND | 23% (OS, 5 years) vs 22% (OS, 5 years) $P$ = NS | Patients randomized to prolonged postremission therapy had a higher 5-year disease-free survival (23% vs 16% for the DAT arm) and lower relapse risk at 5 years (73% vs 81% for the DAT arm), but also more deaths in first complete remission (8% vs 3% in the DAT arm). Differences were not significant | 29 |
| | M (8 mg/m²/day × 1 day) + A (100 mg/m²/day × 7 days) or D (30 mg/m²/day × 1 day) + A (100 mg/m²/day × 7 days) × 1 cycle vs M (8 mg/m²/day × 1 day) + A (100 mg/m²/day × 7 days) or D (30 mg/m²/day × 1 day) + A (100 mg/m²/day × 7 days) × 1 cycle + maintenance with A [10 mg/m² q 12 h × 12 days (q 42 day)] × 8 cycles | ND $P$ = 0.29 | 15% (OS, 5 years) vs 13% (OS, 5 years) | Disease-free survival favored the maintenance therapy arm (at 5 years, 13% vs 7%, $P$ = 0.006). No information is available regarding treatment compliance or toxicity | 4 |

M, mitoxantrone; A, ara-C; DFS, disease-free survival; D, daunorubicin; I, idarubicin; E, etoposide; T, thioguanine; O, vincristine; Pred, prednisone; GM-CSF, granulocyte-macrophage colony-stimulating factor; G-CSF, granulocute colony-stimulating factor; ND, not done; NS, not significant (though actual value not reported).

Reprinted from Stone RM, O'Donnell MR, Sekeres MA: Acute myeloid leukemia. *Hematology AM Soc Hematol Educ Program* 98–117, 2004, copyright American Society of Hematology, U.S.A.

## Protracted postremission chemotherapy

There does not appear to be any additional survival benefit attained from administering one to two cycles of postremission therapy, or in treating older AML patients with maintenance therapy. In the MRC AML 11 trial, 371 patients who entered a CR following anthracycline- or anthracenedione-based remission induction therapy were randomized to receive either one cycle of DAT consolidation therapy or DAT along with three additional cycles of ara-C-based consolidation therapy (for a total of four cycles of postremission therapy).[29] Of patients randomized to the long consolidation course, 61% were able to complete all four cycles. Survival was similar at 5 years for patients randomized to the short and long consolidation arms.

In the phase III trial performed by the Leukemia Cooperative Group of the European Organization for the Research and Treatment of Cancer and the Dutch–Belgian Hemato-oncology Cooperative Hovon Group, patients over 60 years of age were randomized to remission induction regimens consisting of mitoxantrone and ara-C versus daunorubicin and ara-C.[4] Following one cycle of consolidation therapy, 151 patients in CR were further randomized to receive low-dose ara-C maintenance therapy, or to no further treatment. Actuarial disease-free survival was longer for those receiving low-dose postremission therapy compared to those not receiving therapy, with 5-year DFS being 13 and 7% respectively. OS, though, was similar.

## Postremission stem cell transplantation

An even more aggressive approach than induction therapy followed by consolidation or intensification for older adults with AML consists of stem cell transplantation. This topic will be covered in greater detail in Chapter 100. Nonmyeloablative allogeneic stem cell transplants take advantage of a graft-versus-leukemia effect using a less intensive preparative regimen with lower up-front mortality. The reduced treatment-related mortality and ability to perform these transplants in the outpatient setting make them an appealing option for the older AML patient with few comorbidities and an adequate performance status. Preliminary studies that include older AML patients have demonstrated that durable CRs are attainable with this treatment,[86,87] though follow up is still less than 3 years.

### CLINICAL TRIALS

Remission induction therapy for older adults with AML is no panacea, with 5-year survival rates resembling those of patients with advanced lung cancer.[2] It is thus reasonable to consider investigational agents for older AML patients up front, particularly as these patients have a disease that resembles the advanced MDS or secondary AML.[22,88] Potential targets for antileukemia therapy are explained in more detail in Chapter 9. They include specific signaling molecules required for the maintenance of the leukemic state, such as tyrosine kinases; over expression of *bcl-2*, an antiapoptosis signal; DNA methylation, associated with suppression of regulatory genes and with disease progression; indirect pathways that maintain leukemogenesis, including angiogenesis and drug resistance; and investigational agents with mechanisms of action that differ from anthracyclines, anthracenediones, and ara-C, such as nucleoside analogs, farnesyl transferase inhibitors, and MDR modulators.[89–95]

### LOW-DOSE CHEMOTHERAPY/SUPPORTIVE CARE

In the setting of a poor functional age, serious comorbid medical conditions, and particularly patient preference, less intensive chemotherapy or aggressive supportive care may be more appropriate treatment options. Drugs such as hydroxyurea (generally given in doses of 500–3000 mg/day, adjusted to the degree of leukocytosis and/or treatment-related thrombocytopenia) and low-dose ara-C (at a dose of 10 mg/m$^2$) are well tolerated and will reduce leukocytosis for a period of time, though neither will impact survival.[96] We use the phrase *aggressive supportive care* to emphasize that symptoms will be treated vigorously and to distinguish this modality from hospice. Blood and platelet transfusions should be administered to alleviate symptoms stemming from anemia and thrombocytopenia, and antibiotics initiated when appropriate. In addition, integrative therapies such as Reike, therapeutic touch, and herbal medicines may be used by the willing patient. These latter interventions often can be facilitated with involvement of a multidisciplinary team of physicians, nurses, case managers, social workers, therapists, and clergy. Hospice services should be instituted within 6 months of anticipated demise, though some hospice organizations prohibit blood product transfusions, which we consider to be palliative in this population and which may result in improved quality of life in terminal cancer patient populations.[97]

## SUMMARY

Managing AML in older adults can be challenging on a number of levels. While the majority of this population will not enjoy long-term disease-free survival because of disease features and treatment-related complications, a small subset will derive a survival benefit from aggressive chemotherapy approaches. Factors such as functional age can be used to assess which patients might benefit from remission induction and postremission therapy, and which would be done a disservice with such treatment. Studies are needed to assess the trade-off between the slim chance of long-term survival that might be attained with chemotherapy and the quality-of-life issues of low-dose or aggressive supportive therapy.

## REFERENCES

1. Virchow R: Weisses Blut und Milztumoren. *Med Z* 16:9, 1847.
2. Ries L: *SEER Cancer Statistics Review, 1975–2001*. Bethesda, MD: National Cancer Institute, 2004. Available at: http://seer.cancer.gov/csr/1975_2001/.
3. Jemal A: Cancer Statistics, 2004. *CA Cancer J Clin* 54:8, 2004.
4. Lowenberg B: Mitoxantrone versus daunorubicin in induction-consolidation chemotherapy—the value of low-dose cytarabine for maintenance of remission, and an assessment of prognostic factors in acute myeloid leukemia in the elderly: final report. European Organization for the Research and Treatment of Cancer and the Dutch–Belgian Hemato-Oncology Cooperative Hovon Group. *J Clin Oncol* 16:872, 1998.
5. Stone RM: Postremission therapy in older patients with de novo acute myeloid leukemia: a randomized trial comparing mitoxantrone and intermediate-dose cytarabine with standard-dose cytarabine. *Blood* 98:548, 2001.
6. Stone RM: Granulocyte-macrophage colony-stimulating factor after initial chemotherapy for elderly patients with primary acute myelogenous leukemia. Cancer and Leukemia Group B. *N Engl J Med* 332:1671, 1995.
7. Mayer RJ: Intensive postremission chemotherapy in adults with acute myeloid leukemia. Cancer and Leukemia Group B. *N Engl J Med* 331:896, 1994.
8. Baer MR: Phase III study of the multidrug resistance (MDR) modulator PSC-833 in previously untreated acute myeloid leukemia (AML) patients 60 years old: correlation of outcome with functional MDR (CALGB studies 9720 and 9760). *Blood* 98:461a, 2001.
9. Estey EH: How I treat older patients with AML. *Blood* 96:1670, 2000 Sep 1.
10. Stone RM: The difficult problem of acute myeloid leukemia in the older adult. *CA Cancer J Clin* 52:363, 2002.
11. Baer MR: Phase 3 study of the multidrug resistance modulator PSC-833 in previously untreated patients 60 years of age and older with acute myeloid leukemia: Cancer and Leukemia Group B Study 9720. *Blood* 100:1224, 2002.
12. Grimwade D: The importance of diagnostic cytogenetics on outcome in AML: analysis of 1,612 patients entered into the MRC AML 10 trial. The Medical Research Council Adult and Children's Leukaemia Working Parties. *Blood* 92:2322, 1998.
13. Grimwade D: The predictive value of hierarchical cytogenetic classification in older adults with acute myeloid leukemia (AML): analysis of 1065 patients entered into the United Kingdom Medical Research Council AML11 trial. *Blood* 98:1312, 2001.
14. Bloomfield CD: Frequency of prolonged remission duration after high-dose cytarabine intensification in acute myeloid leukemia varies by cytogenetic subtype. *Cancer Res* 58:4173, 1998.
15. Byrd JC: Pretreatment cytogenetic abnormalities are predictive of induction success, cumulative incidence of relapse and overall survival in adult patients with de novo acute myeloid leukemia: results from CALGB 8461. *Blood* 100:4325, 2002.
16. Head DR: Revised classification of acute myeloid leukemia. *Leukemia* 10:1826, 1996.
17. Nagura E: Acute myeloid leukemia in the elderly: 159 Nagoya case studies—Nagoya Cooperative Study Group for elderly leukemia. *Nagoya J Med Sci* 62:135, 1999.
18. Hiddemann W: Management of acute myeloid eukemia in elderly patients. *J Clin Oncol* 17:3569, 1999.
19. Keating S: Prognostic factors of patients with acute myeloid leukemia (AML) allografted in first complete remission: an analysis of the EORTC-GIMEMA AML 8A trial. The European Organization for Research and Treatment of Cancer (EORTC) and the Gruppo Italiano Malattie Ematologiche Maligne dell' Adulto (GIMEMA) Leukemia Cooperative Groups. *Bone Marrow Transplant* 17:993, 1996.
20. Zhu YM: Microsatellite instability and p53 mutations are associated with abnormal expression of the MSH2 gene in adult acute leukemia. *Blood* 94:733, 1999.
21. Leith CP: Frequency and clinical significance of the expression of the multidrug resistance proteins MDR1/P-glycoprotein, MRP1, and LRP in acute myeloid leukemia: a Southwest Oncology Group study. *Blood* 94:1086, 1999.
22. Leith CP: Acute myeloid leukemia in the elderly: assessment of multidrug resistance (MDR1) and cytogenetics distinguishes biologic subgroups with remarkably distinct responses to standard chemotherapy. A Southwest Oncology Group study. *Blood* 89: 3323, 1997.
23. Burnett A: Tailoring the treatment of acute myeloid leukemia. *Curr Opin Oncol* 11:14, 1999.
24. Hoyle CF: AML associated with previous cytotoxic therapy, MDS or myeloproliferative disorders: results from the MRC's 9th AML trial. *Br J Haematol* 72:45, 1989.
25. Bauduer F: De novo and secondary acute myeloid leukemia in patients over the age of 65: a review of fifty-six successive and unselected cases from a general hospital. *Leuk Lymphoma* 35:289, 1999.
26. Estey E: Effect of diagnosis (refractory anemia with excess blasts, refractory anemia with excess blasts in transformation, or acute myeloid leukemia [AML]) on outcome of AML-type chemotherapy. *Blood* 90:2969, 1997.
27. Dillman RO: A comparative study of two different doses of cytarabine for acute myeloid leukemia: a phase III trial of Cancer and Leukemia Group B. *Blood* 78: 2520, 1991.
28. Rees JK: Principal results of the Medical Research Council's 8th acute myeloid leukaemia trial. *Lancet* 2:1236, 1986.
29. Goldstone AH: Attempts to improve treatment outcomes in acute myeloid leukemia (AML) in older patients: the results of the United Kingdom Medical Research Council AML11 trial. *Blood* 98:1302, 2001.
30. Rubin EH: Risk factors for high-dose cytarabine neurotoxicity: an analysis of a Cancer and Leukemia Group B trial in patients with acute myeloid leukemia. *J Clin Oncol* 10:948, 1992.
31. Smith GA: High-dose cytarabine dose modification reduces the incidence of neurotoxicity in patients with renal insufficiency. *J Clin Oncol* 15:833, 1997.
32. Preisler H: Comparison of three remission induction regimens and two postinduction strategies for the

treatment of acute nonlymphocytic leukemia: a Cancer and Leukemia Group B study. *Blood* 69:1441, 1987.

33. Rees JK: Dose intensification in acute myeloid leukaemia: greater effectiveness at lower cost. Principal report of the Medical Research Council's AML9 study. MRC Leukaemia in Adults Working Party. *Br J Haematol* 94:89, 1996.

34. Buchner T: Intensified induction and consolidation with or without maintenance chemotherapy for acute myeloid leukemia (AML): two multicenter studies of the German AML Cooperative Group. *J Clin Oncol* 3:1583, 1985.

35. Witz F: A placebo-controlled study of recombinant human granulocyte-macrophage colony-stimulating factor administered during and after induction treatment for de novo acute myelogenous leukemia in elderly patients. Groupe Ouest Est Leucemies Aigues Myeloblastiques (GOELAM). *Blood* 91:2722, 1998.

36. Heil G: A randomized, double-blind, placebo-controlled, phase III study of filgrastim in remission induction and consolidation therapy for adults with de novo acute myeloid leukemia. The International Acute Myeloid Leukemia Study Group. *Blood* 90:4710, 1997.

37. Cassileth PA: Varying intensity of postremission therapy in acute myeloid leukemia. *Blood* 79:1924, 1992.

38. Godwin JE: A double-blind placebo-controlled trial of granulocyte colony-stimulating factor in elderly patients with previously untreated acute myeloid leukemia: a Southwest Oncology Group study (9031). *Blood* 91:3607, 1998.

39. Lowenberg B: Use of recombinant GM-CSF during and after remission induction chemotherapy in patients aged 61 years and older with acute myeloid leukemia: final report of AML-11, a phase III randomized study of the Leukemia Cooperative Group of European Organisation for the Research and Treatment of Cancer and the Dutch Belgian Hemato-Oncology Cooperative Group. *Blood* 90:2952, 1997.

40. Lowenberg B: On the value of intensive remission-induction chemotherapy in elderly patients of 65+ years with acute myeloid leukemia: a randomized phase III study of the European Organization for Research and Treatment of Cancer Leukemia Group. *J Clin Oncol* 7:1268, 1989.

41. Tilly H: Low-dose cytarabine versus intensive chemotherapy in the treatment of acute nonlymphocytic leukemia in the elderly. *J Clin Oncol* 8:272, 1990.

42. Sekeres MA: Decision-making and quality of life in older adults with acute myeloid leukemia or advanced myelodysplastic syndrome. *Leukemia* 18:809, 2004.

43. DeLima M: Treatment of newly-diagnosed acute myelogenous leukaemia in patients aged 80 years and above. *Br J Haematol* 93:89, 1996.

44. Hurria A: Factors influencing treatment patterns of breast cancer patients age 75 and older. *Crit Rev Oncol Hematol* 46:121, 2003.

45. Karnofsky D: The use of the nitrogen mustards in the palliative treatment of carcinoma. *Cancer* 1:634, 1948.

46. Fillenbaum GG: Screening the elderly. A brief instrumental activities of daily living measure. *J Am Geriatr Soc* 33:698, 1985.

47. George LK: OARS methodology. A decade of experience in geriatric assessment. *J Am Geriatr Soc* 33:607, 1985.

48. Cella DF: The functional assessment of cancer therapy scale: development and validation of the general measure. *J Clin Oncol* 11:570, 1993.

49. Charlson ME: A new method of classifying prognostic comorbidity in longitudinal studies: development and validation. *J Chronic Dis* 40:373, 1987.

50. Ware JE Jr: The MOS 36-item short-form health survey (SF-36). I: Conceptual framework and item selection. *Med Care* 30:473, 1992.

51. Bishop JF: Etoposide in acute nonlymphocytic leukemia. Australian Leukemia Study Group. *Blood* 75:27, 1990.

52. Bishop JF: A randomized study of high-dose cytarabine in induction in acute myeloid leukemia. *Blood* 87:1710, 1996.

53. Weick JK: A randomized investigation of high-dose versus standard-dose cytosine arabinoside with daunorubicin in patients with previously untreated acute myeloid leukemia: a Southwest Oncology Group study. *Blood* 88:2841, 1996.

54. Rai KR: Treatment of acute myelocytic leukemia: a study by Cancer and Leukemia Group B. *Blood* 58:1203, 1981.

55. Preisler HD: Treatment of acute nonlymphocytic leukemia: use of anthracycline-cytosine arabinoside induction therapy and comparison of two maintenance regimens. *Blood* 53:455, 1979.

56. Omura GA: Treatment of acute myelogenous leukemia: influence of three induction regimens and maintenance with chemotherapy or BCG immunotherapy. *Cancer* 49:1530, 1982.

57. Kahn SB: Full dose versus attenuated dose daunorubicin, cytosine arabinoside, and 6-thioguanine in the treatment of acute nonlymphocytic leukemia in the elderly. *J Clin Oncol* 2:865, 1984.

58. Yates J: Cytosine arabinoside with daunorubicin or adriamycin for therapy of acute myelocytic leukemia: a CALGB study. *Blood* 60:454, 1982.

59. Leone G: Idarubicin including regimens in acute myelogenous leukemia in elderly patients. *Crit Rev Oncol Hematol* 32:59, 1999.

60. Vogler WR: A phase III trial comparing idarubicin and daunorubicin in combination with cytarabine in acute myelogenous leukemia: a Southeastern Cancer Study Group study. *J Clin Oncol* 10:1103, 1992.

61. Wiernik PH: Cytarabine plus idarubicin or daunorubicin as induction and consolidation therapy for previously untreated adult patients with acute myeloid leukemia. *Blood* 79:313, 1992.

62. Reiffers J: A prospective randomized trial of idarubicin vs daunorubicin in combination chemotherapy for acute myelogenous leukemia of the age group 55 to 75. *Leukemia* 10:389, 1996.

63. Pignon B: Treatment of acute myelogenous leukaemia in patients aged 50–65: idarubicin is more effective than zorubicin for remission induction and prolonged disease-free survival can be obtained using a unique consolidation course. The Goelam Group. *Br J Haematol* 94:333, 1996.

64. A systematic collaborative overview of randomized trials comparing idarubicin with daunorubicin (or other anthracyclines) as induction therapy for acute myeloid leukaemia. AML Collaborative Group. *Br J Haematol* 103:100, 1998.

65. Archimbaud E: Multicenter randomized phase II trial of idarubicin vs mitoxantrone, combined with VP-16 and cytarabine for induction/consolidation therapy, followed by a feasibility study of autologous peripheral blood stem cell transplantation in elderly patients with acute myeloid leukemia. *Leukemia* 13:843, 1999.

66. Rowe J: A Phase III study of daunorubicin vs idarubicin vs mitoxantrone for older adult patients (>55 years) with acute myelogenous leukemia (AML): A study of the Eastern Cooperative Oncology Group (E3993). *Blood* 92:1284a, 1998.

67. Rowe JM: A randomized placebo-controlled phase III study of granulocyte-macrophage colony-stimulating factor in adult patients (>55 to 70 years of age) with acute myelogenous leukemia: a study of the Eastern Cooperative Oncology Group (E1490). *Blood* 86:457, 1995.

68. Rowe JM: Treatment of acute myelogenous leukemia in older adults. *Leukemia* 14:480, 2000.

69. Buchner T: Daunorubicin 60 instead of 30 mg/sqm improves response and survival in elderly patients with AML. *Blood* 90:583a, 1997.

70. Buchner T: Acute myeloid leukemia: treatment over 60. *Rev Clin Exp Hematol* 6:46, 2002.

71. Chauncey TR: A phase I study of induction chemotherapy for older patients with newly diagnosed acute myeloid leukemia (AML) using mitoxantrone, etoposide, and the MDR modulator PSC 833: a Southwest Oncology Group study 9617. *Leuk Res* 24:567, 2000 Jul.

72. Liu Yin JA: Comparison of "sequential" versus "standard" chemotherapy as re-induction treatment, with or without cyclosporine, in refractory/relapsed acute myeloid leukaemia (AML): results of the UK Medical Research Council AML-R trial. *Br J Haematol* 113:713, 2001.

73. Pea F: Multidrug resistance modulation in vivo: the effect of cyclosporin A alone or with dexverapamil on idarubicin pharmacokinetics in acute leukemia. *Eur J Clin Pharmacol* 55:361, 1999.

74. List AF: Benefit of cyclosporine modulation of drug resistance in patients with poor-risk acute myeloid leukemia: a Southwest Oncology Group study. *Blood* 98:3212, 2001.

75. Bishop JF: Etoposide in the management of leukemia: a review. *Semin Oncol* 18:62, 1991.

76. Appelbaum FR: Antibody-targeted therapy for myeloid leukemia. *Semin Hematol* 36:2, 1999.

77. Sievers EL: Selective ablation of acute myeloid leukemia using antibody-targeted chemotherapy: a phase I study of an anti-CD33 calicheamicin immunoconjugate. *Blood* 93:3678, 1999.

78. Bernstein ID: Monoclonal antibodies to the myeloid stem cells: therapeutic implications of CMA-676, a humanized anti-CD33 antibody calicheamicin conjugate. *Leukemia* 14:474, 2000.

79. Radich J: New developments in the treatment of acute myeloid leukemia. *Oncology (Huntingt)* 14:125, 2000.

80. Sievers EL: Efficacy and safety of Mylotarg (gemtuzumab ozogamicin) in patients with CD33-positive acute myeloid leukemia in first relapse. *J Clin Oncol* 19:3244, 2001.

81. Estey EH: Causes of initial remission induction failure in acute myelogenous leukemia. *Blood* 60:309, 1982.

82. Bolam S: Colony-stimulating factors in the treatment of older patients with acute myelogenous leukaemia. *Drugs Aging* 15:451, 1999.

83. Dombret H: A controlled study of recombinant human granulocyte colony-stimulating factor in elderly patients after treatment for acute myelogenous leukemia. AML Cooperative Study Group. *N Engl J Med* 332:1678, 1995.

84. Rowe J: A Phase III study of priming with yeast-derived granulocyte-macrophage colony-stimulating-factor (rhuGM-CSF) for older adult patients >55 yrs with acute myelogenous leukemia: a study of the Eastern Cooperative Oncology Group. *Blood* 92:2799a, 1998.

85. Vogler WR: A randomized comparison of postremission therapy in acute myelogenous leukemia: a Southeastern Cancer Study Group trial. *Blood* 63:1039, 1984.

86. Bertz H: Allogeneic stem-cell transplantation from related and unrelated donors in older patients with myeloid leukemia. *J Clin Oncol* 21:1480, 2003.

87. McSweeney PA: Hematopoietic cell transplantation in older patients with hematologic malignancies: replacing high-dose cytotoxic therapy with graft-versus-tumor effects. *Blood* 97:3390, 2001.

88. Rossi G: Cytogenetic analogy between myelodysplastic syndrome and acute myeloid leukemia of elderly patients. *Leukemia* 14:636, 2000 Apr.

89. Stone R: PKC412, an Oral FLT3 inhibitor, has activity in mutant FLT3 acute myeloid leukemia (AML): a phase II clinical trial. *Blood* 100:316a, 2002.

90. Giles FJ: New drugs in acute myeloid leukemia. *Curr Oncol Rep* 4:369, 2002.

91. Giles FJ: Acute myeloid leukemia. *Hematology Am Soc Hematol Educ Program* 73, 2002.

92. Karp JE: Clinical and biologic activity of the farnesyl transferase inhibitor R115777 in adults with refractory and relapsed acute leukemias: a phase 1 clinical-laboratory correlative trial. *Blood* 97:3361, 2001.

93. Giles FJ: The emerging role of angiogenesis inhibitors in hematologic malignancies. *Oncology (Huntingt)* 16:23, 2002.

94. Silverman LR: Randomized controlled trial of azacitidine in patients with the myelodysplastic syndrome: a study of the Cancer and Leukemia Group B. *J Clin Oncol* 20:2429, 2002.

95. Giles FJ: SU5416, a small molecule tyrosine kinase receptor inhibitor, has biologic activity in patients with refractory acute myeloid leukemia or myelodysplastic syndromes. *Blood* 20:20, 2003.

96. Robles C: Low-dose cytarabine maintenance therapy vs observation after remission induction in advanced acute myeloid leukemia: an Eastern Cooperative Oncology Group trial (E5483). *Leukemia* 14:1349, 2000 Aug.

97. Sciortino AD: The efficacy of administering blood transfusions at home to terminally ill cancer patients. *J Palliat Care* 9:14, 1993.

Chapter **6**

# TREATMENT APPROACH TO ACUTE PROMYELOCYTIC LEUKEMIA

*James L. Slack*

## INTRODUCTION

Acute promyelocytic leukemia (APL) is a clinically and genetically distinct subtype of AML caused by fusion of the promyelocytic leukemia (*PML*) gene, on chromosome 15, with the retinoic acid receptor α (*RARA*) gene, on chromosome 17. The fusion of PML (or one of the rare variant partner genes) with RARA results in a hybrid protein (PML-RARA) that interferes with function of both the wild-type *PML* and *RARA* genes. The end result is a block in myeloid differentiation, disruption of cellular growth control, and development of clinical APL. The disease was first described clinically in 1957,[1] and the classic reciprocal chromosomal translocation [t(15;17)(q22;q21)] that characterizes APL was identified by Rowley et al. in 1977.[2] Almost three decades later, the molecular pathogenesis of APL is reasonably well understood,[3] and modern treatment regimens have been developed that lead to the cure of more than 70% patients. From a clinical perspective, the challenge is to further increase this cure rate, while reducing (or eliminating) side effects and long-term toxicities associated with intensive chemotherapy. Well-designed clinical trials continue to be the best option for most patients with APL, for it is only in the context of such trials that clinicians can learn how to safely de-escalate therapy in low-risk patients while maintaining excellent outcomes in patients who present with higher risk disease.

## APPROACH TO THE PATIENT WITH APL

### PROGNOSTIC FACTORS

While the presence of the t(15;17) or PML-RARA fusion confers an overall "good" prognosis to APL patients, there nevertheless exists a subset of APL patients who are at high risk of relapse or death despite best available therapy. In 2000, Spanish (PETHEMA: Programa de Estudio y Tratamien to de las Hemopatias Malignas) and Italian (GIMEMA: Gruppo Italiano Malattie Emato logiche dell' adulto) APL investigators defined low-, intermediate-, and high-risk subgroups of APL patients based on presenting white blood cell (WBC) and platelet counts (low risk: WBC count <10,000/μL and platelet count >40,000/μL; intermediate risk: WBC count <10,000/μL and platelet count <40,000/μL; high risk: WBC count >10,000/μL).[4] Based on the above analysis, as well as on data from numerous other groups, it is now well known and accepted that APL patients who present with WBC counts of more than 10,000/μL have a high risk of treatment failure, due both to an increased incidence of deaths during induction and to a higher risk of relapse. Specific genetic findings, such as the bcr-3 PML breakpoint[5] and internal tandem duplication (ITD) of the *FLT3* gene,[6-9] as well as microgranular morphology, are associated with high WBC count, but have not, in general, been found to have independent prognostic significance in patients treated with modern all-*trans*-retinoic acid (ATRA)-based regimens. Also, there is no independent prognostic significance of chromosomal abnormalities in addition to the t(15;17) in patients treated with ATRA-containing regimens.[10,11] Certain immunophenotypic findings seem to be associated with poor prognosis, specifically expression of CD2, CD34, and CD56, but only CD56 expression has been shown to have independent prognostic significance.[12,13]

### THERAPEUTIC MONITORING

APL patients who enter morphologic complete remission (CR) after a single round of induction therapy will often be reverse transcriptase polymerase chain reaction (RT-PCR) positive, and a small minority will have low numbers of residual abnormal promyelocytes. In general, neither finding indicates failure of induction therapy, and such patients should proceed promptly to consolidation. However, a positive RT-PCR result at the end of consolidation, at least in patients treated according to the Italian consolidation regimen, seems to indicate treatment failure.[14] In the Italian study, among 23 patients (out of 683) who were RT-PCR positive at the end of consolidation, 7 were treated "preemptively" with salvage therapy and stem cell transplant, while treatment was delayed in the remaining 16 until development of hematologic relapse. All seven patients treated early (i.e., with persistent molecular disease) were alive, compared to only 2 of the 16 patients treated at the time of hematologic relapse.[14] After consolidation, APL patients who are RT-PCR negative should undergo routine molecular monitoring (e.g., every 2–4 months for at least 2 years) to detect incipient relapse.[15,16] As is discussed below in depth, two successive positive RT-PCR assays (at a sensitivity of 1 in 10$^4$) are highly predictive of subsequent hematologic relapse and cannot be ignored. It is currently not known if blood can substitute for bone marrow for the RT-PCR assays; therefore, bone marrow is the preferred source for collection of cells and isolation of mRNA. A single negative RT-PCR assay has little clinical significance in APL, even at the end of consolidation, and serial monitoring is key to early detection of relapse. Finally, while quantitative RT-PCR assays have been developed and are undergoing clinical testing,[17,18] qualitative RT-PCR assays at a sensitivity of 1 in 10$^4$ remain the "gold standard" for detection of minimal residual disease, and clinicians caring for APL patients need access to a reliable laboratory that can provide this type of serial molecular monitoring.

## TREATMENT OF NEWLY DIAGNOSED APL

### OVERVIEW OF TREATMENT RESULTS IN THE "ATRA ERA"

Table 6.1 presents the results of treatment of over 3000 APL patients from four continents and eight major leukemia cooperative groups since the advent of ATRA-based therapy in approximately 1990. In virtually all of these patients, the diagnosis of APL was confirmed by modern molecular or cytogenetic techniques, and all received ATRA during induction therapy, either alone or in combination with chemotherapy. While it is beyond the scope of this chapter to discuss each trial in detail, careful analysis of the aggregate results illuminates many of the successes (and some of the failures) of treatment of APL over the last 15 years. The most obvious success is the long-term survival rate of approximately 80%, which compares to a rate of 30–40% in the pre-ATRA era.[33] Although 80% is a spectacular number, 5–10% of APL patients die early during induction, another 10% die of refractory disease, and 10% are successfully treated for relapsed APL (but are subjected to the side effects and long-term toxicities of salvage therapies). Furthermore, with the exception of one study,[20] the event-free survival (EFS) of patients with high-risk disease is relatively poor, generally around 50–60%. Thus, as we enter the era of

"third-generation" ATRA-based protocols, exemplified by the APL2000[20] and AIDA2000[26] studies, our challenge is to better manage patients during the initial induction period (particularly those who present with high WBC counts), and to choose appropriate therapies based on accurate risk-group assessment. Questions remain, and newer approaches are under study,[34] but curative, safe treatments for virtually all patients with APL are now available, and it is fair to say that survival free of disease should be attainable for up to 95% of APL patients who survive induction therapy. Assuming a 5% rate of early death, and a small number of relapses and deaths in CR, the EFS target for all future trials of APL should be 85–90%, and anything below this number should be considered unacceptable.

### INDUCTION THERAPY

All of the trials given in Table 6.1 incorporated ATRA into induction therapy and, with few exceptions, reported CR rates are greater than or equal to 90%. What, then, is the best strategy for induction therapy of APL? While the choice of "best" induction therapy may differ for specific subsets of patients, for most patients the weight of evidence supports the use of ATRA, 45 mg/m$^2$/day in divided doses until CR, plus anthracycline-based chemotherapy started on day 2 or 3 (to allow partial improvement of the coagulopathy by ATRA). The choice of anthracycline (daunorubicin vs idarubicin), and the dose, vary by center and group, but excellent results have been achieved using 12 mg/m$^2$ of idarubicin on days 2, 4, 6, and 8,[35] as well as 60 mg/m$^2$ of daunorubicin on days 3–5.[20] This type of combined strategy minimizes the incidence of APL differentiation syndrome, results in disease control in virtually all patients and, in experienced hands, leads to CR rates of more than 95%. Satisfactory rates of CR can also be achieved using ATRA alone for induction, but long-term disease control may be inferior.[21]

### COMPLICATIONS OF INDUCTION THERAPY

The vast majority of APL patients who fail induction do so not because of resistant disease, but because of fatal hemorrhage [usually central nervous system (CNS)], retinoic acid (RA) syndrome (also called "APL differentiation syndrome"), or infection. Rates of early death are, at least historically, much higher in patients with high WBC counts,[29,32,36] as high as 24% in some studies. The Spanish Group has reported an early death rate of 8.4% in 642 patients treated with simultaneous ATRA and idarubicin (AIDA) between 1996 and 2003 in two successive studies[36]; 58% of the early deaths were due to hemorrhage, 31% due to infection, and 10% due to RA syndrome.[36] The rate of early death did not decrease in the more recent LPA99 study, despite the prophylactic use of prednisone (to prevent RA syndrome) and tranexamic acid (to improve the coagulopathy). Renal dysfunction (creatinine >1.4 mg/dL) and high WBC count (>10,000) were the only independent predictors of early death. It is

**Table 6.1** Outcomes of therapy for APL in the "ATRA era"

| Group | Study | Years | N | CR (%) | ED (%) | EFS (%) | OS (%) | RR (%) | HR EFS (%) |
|---|---|---|---|---|---|---|---|---|---|
| ALLG[a] | APML3 | NR | 101 | 90 | 8 | NR | 88 | NR | NR |
| European APL[b] | APL91 | 1991–1992 | 101 | 91 | 9 | 63 | 76 | 31 | 50 |
| European APL[b] | APL93 | 1993–1998 | 404 | 95 | 5 | 66 | 78 | 23 | NR |
| European APL[b] | APL2000 | 2000–2004 | 300 | 96 | 3 | 94 | 97 | 6.6 | 88.4 |
| German AMLCG[c] | TAD/HAM | 1994– | 133 | 89 | 10 | 75 | 80 | 9 | 68 |
| GIMEMA[d] | AIDA93 | 1993–2000 | 807 | 94 | 5.5 | 70 | NR | NR | NR |
| GIMEMA[d] | AIDA0493 | 1997–2000 | 346 | 96 | 4 | 80 | NR | 14 | NR |
| GIMEMA[d] | AIDA2000 | 2000–2003 | 298 | 94 | 6 | 84 | NR | 5 | NR |
| JALSG[e] | JALSG92 | 1992–1997 | 369 | 90 | 8 | 52 | 65 | NR | 38 |
| JALSG[e] | JALSG97 | 1997–2002 | 256 | 95 | 5 | 67 | 84 | NR | 53 |
| MRC (UK)[f] | | 1993–1997 | 120 | 87 | 8 | 64 | 71 | 20 | 29 |
| NA Intergroup[g] | INT0129 | 1992–1995 | 174 | 73 | 11 | 58 | 69 | 29 | NR |
| PETHEMA[h] | LPA96 | 1996–1999 | 175 | 90 | 9.6 | 71 | 78 | 17 | 56 |
| PETHEMA[h] | LPA99 | 1999–2002 | 227 | 90 | 11 | 79 | 85 | 7.5 | 66 |

N, number of enrolled patients; NR, not reported; ED, early death (i.e., death during induction); CR, complete remission; EFS, event-free survival (any event, i.e., death or relapse, after enrollment on study); OS, overall survival; RR, relapse rate; HR EFS, event-free survival in patients with high WBC at diagnosis (>10,000/μL unless otherwise specified).

[a] Data from the Australasian Leukemia and Lymphoma Group.[19]
[b] Data from the European APL Group.[20–23] Results for the APL91 study are from the ATRA arm of that study; EFS and OS are reported at 4 years for the APL91 and APL 93 studies. Data for the APL93 study reported here are for 18–60-year-old adults. EFS, OS, and RR reported for the APL2000 study are at 2 years, and are from the group of patients of age below 60, with WBC count of less than 10,000/μL, who were treated on the ara-C arm of that study (see text for details). EFS, OS, and RR for similar patients treated without ara-C are 83, 90, and 12%.[20]
[c] Results from the German AML Cooperative Group.[24,25] EFS and OS are reported at 4 years; high-risk EFS refers to patients with initial WBC count of more than 5000/μL.
[d] Data from the Italian GIMEMA Cooperative Group.[26,27] For the AIDA93 trial, EFS is reported as of June 2003, while OS is reported at 5.7 years, with median follow up of surviving patients 2.3 years. The data reported for AIDA0493 are from reference [26], and include patients treated on the "AIDA" trial after 1997 (all of whom received 2 years of ATRA-based maintenance). Median follow up in this trial was 4.5 years. Median follow up for the AIDA2000 trial was 2 years. EFS in both studies is reported at 2 years and was calculated by subtracting the ED rate in each group from the reported DFS. Although no EFS was reported for high-risk patients, the cumulative incidence of relapse (CIR) for high-risk patients in the AIDA0493 trial was 29%, versus 2% for high-risk patients in the AIDA2000 trial (see text for details).
[e] Results from the Japanese Acute Leukemia Study Group.[28] EFS and OS are reported at 6 years for the JALSG92 study and at 5 years for the JALSG97 study.
[f] Results from the Medical Research Council (United Kingdom) Adult Leukemia Working Party.[29] Outcome data are at 4 years. The EFS for high-risk patients (WBC count >10,000/μL) was calculated by subtracting the ED rate in this group (24%) from the reported DFS (53%).
[g] Results from the North American Intergroup protocol 0129.[30,31] All data relate to patients on the ATRA arm of this study. EFS and OS are reported at 5 years.[30]
[h] Data from the Spanish cooperative group PETHEMA.[32] EFS in both the LPA96 and LPA99 trials was calculated by subtracting the ED rate in each study from the reported DFS (71 and 79%, respectively for the entire study group, and 66 and 77%, respectively, for the high-risk group). Both EFS and OS are reported at 3 years. The median follow up was 48 months for LPA96 study and 21 months for LPA99 study. The CIR at 3 years for high-risk patients in the LPA96 study was 34.2%, and 21% in the LPA99 study (see text).

also notable that older adults (≥60 years) were more likely to die of infection (56%) than hemorrhage (37.5%).[36]

As the incidence of resistant disease is exceedingly small (less than 1% in most series), strategies to improve CR rates in APL have focused on prevention and/or effective treatment of bleeding and RA syndrome. Although both ATRA and chemotherapy improve the coagulopathy in APL,[37,38] ATRA acts more rapidly, and its use is associated with a more controlled improvement in bleeding and in parameters of disseminated intravascular coagulation and fibrinolysis.[39] Because of this, all patients with a morphologically confirmed (or strongly suspected) diagnosis of APL, particularly those with evidence of significant coagulopathy (or frank bleeding), should be started on ATRA immediately. All patients with APL should receive

aggressive blood product support, including platelet transfusions, in an attempt to maintain a platelet count of 50,000/μL or above, and fresh plasma or cryoprecipitate to maintain fibrinogen levels of 100 mg/dL or higher. This platelet threshold can be adjusted downward as the coagulopathy improves, but 50,000/μL should be the initial target for all patients, particularly around the time of initiation of chemotherapy. The role of heparin therapy in patients who receive ATRA-based induction continues to be controversial.[38,40] As noted above,[36] and although the issue remains unsettled,[41] antifibrinolytic agents such as tranexamic acid and ε-aminocaproic acid do not appear to be effective, and may in fact be detrimental, by increasing the incidence of thrombosis.[42–44] In the recently reported APL2000 trial,[20] the rate of early death was 3% or less in all groups of patients except those of age 60 or above with WBC count of more than 10,000/μL, suggesting that clinicians experience with ATRA, and use of aggressive supportive care measures, may finally be improving the obstinate 8–10% induction death rate that has plagued almost all APL trials.

### APL DIFFERENTIATION SYNDROME

The pathophysiology and treatment of RA syndrome or "APL differentiation syndrome" have recently been reviewed,[45,46] and knowledge of the manifestations of this potentially fatal complication of induction therapy is essential to all clinicians who treat APL. The most common presenting symptoms[47–49] are respiratory distress, fever, pulmonary infiltrates, weight gain, and pleural/pericardial effusions. Less common signs and symptoms include renal failure, cardiac failure, hypotension, and bone pain. These symptoms can develop at virtually any time after presentation (and may be present *before* any therapy), but the median time to development is between weeks 1 and 2 after the start of induction.[47–49] The differential diagnosis includes sepsis/acute respiratory distress syndrome, as well as pulmonary hemorrhage, and the outcome can be fatal if the disorder is not recognized, diagnosed correctly, and properly treated. Treatment of RA syndrome is with corticosteroids (given at the earliest time possible), generally dexamethasone 10 mg q 12 h, and temporary discontinuation of ATRA, at least in severe cases. ATRA can (and should) be safely restarted after the syndrome resolves, and RA syndrome is exceedingly rare in patients who receive ATRA during consolidation or maintenance phases of their treatment. Thus, there should be no hesitation in subsequent use of ATRA in patients who may have developed RA syndrome during induction. The incidence of RA syndrome seems to be lower in patients who receive combined ATRA/chemotherapy induction,[47] and it may be lower in patients who receive prophylactic steroids, but it is clearly not "a problem of the past" and remains a significant clinical issue in the treatment of APL.[46] Finally, note that APL differentiation syndrome also occurs in patients treated with arsenic trioxide for newly diagnosed or relapsed APL,[50] and approximately 50% of such patients develop leukocytosis, which can be marked. In general, the leukocytosis is self-limiting and does not require therapy, but patients with leukocytosis who develop symptoms or signs of coexistent APL differentiation syndrome require treatment with corticosteroids.[50]

### CONSOLIDATION THERAPY

The choice of appropriate postremission therapy will depend on the patient's risk of relapse, which can be estimated based on presenting WBC and platelet counts.[4] APL patients in low- and intermediate-risk groups can generally be successfully consolidated with anthracyclines alone. In recent trials published by the PETHEMA and GIMEMA groups, relapse rates of patients in low and intermediate risk groups were less than 10%, following consolidation with anthracyclines plus ATRA or anthracycline alone (patients generally received induction with idarubicin and ATRA, and 2 years of ATRA-based maintenance).[26,32] However, in the PETHEMA LPA99 trial,[32] patients with high WBC counts continued to have a high risk of relapse (21%), despite addition of ATRA during each course of consolidation, and increased intensity (by approximately twofold) of anthracyclines. High-risk patients appear to be faring somewhat better in the recent AIDA2000 trial,[26] with a relapse rate (at 2 years) of only 2%. Consolidation therapy in this patient group was intensified by addition of ara-C during cycle 1, VP-16 during cycle 2, and ara-C and 6-TG during cycle 3. (All patients also received 15 days of ATRA with each course.) High-risk patients in the APL2000 trial, all of whom received ara-C during consolidation, also have excellent early outcomes, with rates of relapse below 5%.[20] To summarize, consolidation therapy in APL should include, at a minimum, two cycles of ATRA plus anthracyclines; however, APL patients who present with WBC counts of more than 10,000/μL, and perhaps APL patients who express CD56, require additional, or alternative, therapy in addition to standard ATRA and anthracyclines. While further dose escalation of anthracyclines may be possible, current evidence suggests that a significant percentage of high-risk patients may be cured by incorporating ara-C into the induction and/or consolidation regimens. Whether other agents (e.g., arsenic trioxide and gemtuzumab ozogamicin) could substitute for ara-C in this role is not yet known, but this question, at least for arsenic trioxide, is being addressed in the current North American Intergroup trial.

### MAINTENANCE THERAPY

Data from two trials published in the mid-1990s suggested that maintenance therapy with ATRA and/or chemotherapy, generally 6-mercaptopurine (6-MP) plus methotrexate (MTX), was beneficial in increasing the cure rate of APL. For example, in the APL93 study, the 5-year risk of relapse was 39, 29, 24, and 13% in patients who received, respectively, no maintenance, ATRA alone, 6-MP/MTX alone, or combined ATRA/6-MP/MTX.[51] In the group of patients with high WBC count (more than 5000/μL in this study), the relapse risk was 47% without maintenance, but only 8% if patients received ATRA/6-MP/MTX.[51] In the North American Intergroup 0129 study,[30] 5-year disease-free survival was 74% in patients who received ATRA during both induction and maintenance, compared to 55% for patients who received ATRA only during induction. In contrast to the above results, GIMEMA investigators[27] found no differences in molecular disease-free survival according to any of the four maintenance arms (ATRA/6-MP/MTX, ATRA alone, 6-MP/MTX alone, or no maintenance). The ultimate role of maintenance therapy in APL may be difficult to precisely define, as its usefulness may depend on both patient-specific (i.e., risk category) and treatment-specific (i.e., intensity of induction and consolidation therapy) factors. However, currently, ATRA- or arsenic-trioxide-based maintenance therapy is strongly recommended for all patients, and it should be considered mandatory in high-risk patients. Commonly used regimens include 45 mg/m$^2$/day of ATRA every other week, or ATRA at the same dose for 15 days out of each 3-month period. Standard maintenance doses of 6-MP and MTX are 60 mg/m$^2$/day and 20 mg/m$^2$/week, respectively. Treatment should be continued for at least 1 year, but 2 years may be preferable.[51] Maintenance therapy is generally well tolerated, but serious complications can occur, particularly in patients receiving 6-MP and MTX (±ATRA), and include abnormal liver function tests, cytopenias with potentially serious infections, and opportunistic infections such as *Pneumocystis carinii* pneumonia.[51]

## SPECIAL TOPICS IN APL MANAGEMENT

### NOVEL TREATMENT APPROACHES

Investigators from Shanghai[52,53] have recently reported results in 61 newly diagnosed APL patients who received induction therapy with combined ATRA (25 mg/m$^2$/day) plus arsenic trioxide (0.16 mg/kg/day). All patients subsequently received three courses of consolidation chemotherapy, and five cycles of maintenance with sequential ATRA, arsenic, and 6-MP and MTX. Among the 61 patients, 58 (95.1%) entered CR at a median of 26 days and, with a follow up of 20–39 months, all of them were relapse free.[52] Similar results, at least for induction, have been reported by Wang et al.,[54] with a CR rate in 80 newly diagnosed patients treated with low-dose ATRA plus arsenic of 92.5%; there were two early deaths (2.5%), and four cases of resistant leukemia, but no data were presented on long-term outcomes. Estey et al.[34] have treated 44 newly diagnosed APL patients with ATRA (45 mg/m$^2$/ day) plus arsenic trioxide (0.15 mg/kg/day) added at day 10 (with addition of one dose of gemtuzumab ozogamicin if the presenting WBC count was above 10,000/μL or if disease persistence was documented by RT-PCR); treatment with ATRA/arsenic trioxide was continued for 6 months from CR. The rate of CR was 89%, there were four early deaths (9.14%), and 36 of 39 patients were alive in CR at early follow up. Finally, investigators from Iran[55] and India[56] have separately reported results with arsenic trioxide alone as the sole treatment of APL. Rates of CR, were 85.6 and 86% respectively, for the two studies and, relapse rates were approximately 25%.[56,56] In patients with a WBC count lower than 5000 μL, and a platelet count higher than 20,000 μL at dignosis, the EFS was 100%.

Studies such as these must be viewed in context of the data summarized in Table 6.1, particularly the more recent trials. While results with arsenic trioxide alone and ATRA plus arsenic trioxide are encouraging, the number of patients treated to date is relatively small, follow up is short, and extensive experience with these agents is limited to selected centers and countries. In addition, the toxicities of arsenic trioxide and ATRA are not trivial, and there is, as yet, no standardized strategy for postremission therapy in patients who receive this type of induction. Despite these caveats, treatment with arsenic trioxide alone, or arsenic trioxide combined with ATRA, may well be suitable for selected patients with low-risk APL, or for patients who are not candidates for, or who refuse, cytotoxic chemotherapy.

### THE ROLE OF ARA-C

While ara-C has historically been relegated to a minor role in the treatment of APL,[57] more recent data suggest that certain patients, particularly those with high-risk APL, may derive considerable benefit from the addition of ara-C to their treatment. The German AML Co-operative Group,[24,25] which uses high-dose ara-C during induction, is one of the only groups to report essentially equivalent outcomes in patients with high and low WBC counts, suggesting that high-dose ara-C overcomes the negative prognostic impact of high WBC count. In the recently reported AIDA 2000 trial,[26] intensification of consolidation therapy with ATRA and ara-C in high-risk patients led to a cumulative incidence of relapse of 2%, well below the 29% relapse rate seen in the earlier AIDA 0493 trial, and significantly below the 9% relapse rate noted in "intermediate-risk" patients consolidated with anthracyclines and ATRA alone. Finally, the European APL Group[20] has reported preliminary results of a randomized trial in which low-risk patients (below the age of 60 and with WBC counts of less than 10,000/μL) were randomized to receive (group A) or not receive (group B) ara-C during induction and consolidation. All high-risk patients (WBC count >10,000) received standard-dose ara-C during induction and high-dose ara-C (1 or 2 g/m$^2$ every 12 h for eight doses) during consolidation. The preliminary results demonstrate significantly improved EFS (93.6% vs 83.4%) and decrease in relapse rate (3.8% vs 11.9%) in low-risk patients randomized to receive ara-C. Perhaps even more striking, in the nonrandomized high-risk patients (groups C and E, WBC counts >10,000/μL), the relapse rates were 2.6 and 0% respectively, and EFS was extremely impressive, at 88.4% (group C, age <60) and 78.3% (group E, age >60). As reported by the Italian[26] and Spanish groups,[32] cure rates with ATRA- and anthracycline-based therapies are excellent in low-risk patients (WBC count <10,000/μL and platelet count >40,000/μL) and are generally acceptable in intermediate-risk patients (WBC count <10,000/μL and platelet count <40,000/μL), so the need for ara-C in these "low-risk" subgroups remains unclear. However, if longer follow up validates the data from the randomized portion of the APL2000 trial, incorporation of ara-C into the treatment regimen of even low-risk patients may need to be seriously reconsidered. In summary, while the role of ara-C in the treatment of APL remains far from settled, an argument can be made that this agent, particularly at high or intermediate dose, benefits patients with high-risk APL, and as such it should be seriously considered for inclusion into the treatment of all such patients.

### TREATMENT OF APL IN ADULTS OF AGE 60 OR ABOVE

The outcome of treatment of APL in older adults (defined as age 60 or above) remains suboptimal, with rates of EFS and OS of only 55–60% in most studies (Table 6.2). Recently reported results from several large European studies[22,25,58,59] highlight the issues involved in treating this patient population and offer insight into how treatment might be improved. As noted in Table 6.2, CR rates in older adults are approximately 85%, which is marginally, but significantly, lower than the 90–95% rate of CR reported for younger adults treated in the same trials. In the Italian, Spanish, and German AMLCG trials, patients received induction with concurrent ATRA and chemotherapy, while most patients in the European APL93 trial (those above 65 years) were induced with ATRA alone. The comparatively low CR rate seen in all four studies (regardless of induction strategy) was due to a higher rate of deaths during induction, around 15%, which is approximately double of that seen in younger adults. Most of this excess in early deaths is due to infection, as rates of resistant disease, and deaths due to RA syndrome and hemorrhage, are generally similar between older and younger adults.[22,25,58,59] Induction strategies that avoid cytotoxic chemotherapy (with its attendant neutropenia) may be preferable in older adults, particularly those above the age of 70, or with compromised performance status. An appropriate choice for such patients might be ATRA alone, arsenic trioxide alone, or combined ATRA/arsenic trioxide.

The inferior EFS and OS in older adults also relates to a comparatively high rate of deaths during consolidation and maintenance (deaths in CR), again largely due to neutropenia-related infections. This rate of 10–20% could presumably also be improved by decreasing the intensity of the consolidation and/or maintenance therapies. Indeed, a subset of patients in both the APL93 and GIMEMA studies summarized in Table 6.2 received attenuated consolidation (those above 65 years in the APL93 study, and most patients treated after 1997 in the GIMEMA study). In the latter study,[59] the 3-year disease-free and OSs were not different among patients who received three or one cycle of anthracycline-based consolidation (all patients received 2 years of ATRA-based maintenance), suggesting no loss of efficacy with decreasing intensity of therapy. However, the PETHEMA Group[58] has reported the lowest rates of relapse (8.5%) and deaths in CR (9.2%) in adults of age 60 or above, and no planned dose attenuation for older adults was used in that study. The relapse rates in each of the four studies given in Table 6.2 are comparable to relapse rates seen in adults of age below 60, suggesting that, as opposed to most other subtypes of AML, there is no inherent difference in disease biology between APL arising in older versus younger adults. There is a suggestion, however, particularly from the PETHEMA study, that a lower percentage of adults of age 60 or above present with high WBC counts, suggesting that older adults may have an inherently *better* prognosis, at least in terms of disease-related prognostic factors.

Treatment strategies in older adults should thus focus on reducing doses or cycles of chemotherapy, or perhaps omitting chemotherapy altogether. Careful molecular monitoring is mandatory to safely apply this approach, and a certain degree of flexibility is needed to tailor the wide range of therapies available to each patient's clinical course. As with younger patients, risk-adapted strategies[32] should be used, with more intensive regimens reserved for patients who present with

**Table 6.2** Outcomes of therapy for APL in adults of age 60 or above

| Study | N | CR (%) | ED (%) | EFS (%) | OS (%) | RR (%) | Deaths in CR (%) |
|---|---|---|---|---|---|---|---|
| APL93[a] | 129 | 86 | 14 | 53 | 58 | 16 | 18.6 |
| APL2000–Low WBC[b] | 47 | 98 | 2 | 79 | 90 | 11 | NR |
| APL2000–High WBC[b] | 16 | 87 | 13 | 78 | 78 | 0 | NR |
| LPA96/LPA99[c] | 104 | 84 | 15 | 64 | NR | 8.5 | 9.2 |
| AIDA93 and aAIDA97[d] | 134 | 86 | 12 | 47 | 56 | 20 | 12.1 |
| German AMLCG[e] | 32 | 78 | 19 | 54 | 57 | 17 | NR |

N, number of patients enrolled; NR, not reported; ED, early death (death during induction); CR, complete response; EFS, event-free survival (any event, i.e., death or relapse, after enrollment on study); OS, overall survival; RR, relapse rate.

[a] Results from the European APL Group.[22] EFS, OS, and RR are reported at 4 years.

[b] Data are from the European APL Group[20]; EFS, OS, and RR are reported at 2 years. The high WBC count group received intensified induction and consolidation with ara-C.

[c] Results from the PETHEMA Group.[58] Median follow up was 36 months; EFS, OS, and RR were reported at 6 years.

[d] Results from the GIMEMA Group (AIDA93 and amended AIDA97 studies).[59] OS was reported at 6 years. For ease of comparison, the EFS was estimated from the reported DFS (59%) and subtraction of the early death rate (12%).

[e] Data are from the German AML Cooperative Group.[25] EFS, OS, and RR reported at 4 years.

high-risk features, mainly WBC count of more than 10,000/μL. Given that the disease biology is, if anything, more favorable in older adults, there is no reason to believe that, given proper treatment and supportive care, such individuals should not have a cure rate at least equal to younger adults.

## TREATMENT OF RELAPSED APL

Despite the tremendous advances in the treatment of APL discussed above, a small, but significant, percentage of patients will relapse. In the long-term follow up of the APL93 trial,[51] which enrolled 576 patients between 1993 and 1998, 134 (23.3%) patients eventually relapsed (out of 533 who achieved CR). Although most of these relapses occurred within 2.5 years of achieving CR, a substantial percentage (29%) occurred after 2.5 years, with one relapse occurring over 8 years from CR. In the North American Intergroup trial,[30] late relapses were also seen, although by far the highest risk period was the first 2 years after CR. Patients with APL, particularly those who present with high WBC counts, are at risk for relapse in the CNS and other extramedullary sites, including skin and ear.[60–64] Whether this risk has increased in the "ATRA era" is unclear,[62] but of the 22 clinical relapses noted in the PETHEMA LPA96 and LPA99 trials,[32] 6 (27%) occurred in the CNS. Most patients with extramedullary relapse will be found to have occult (i.e., molecular) or overt leukemia in the marrow, and treatment should be directed not only at the site of extramedullary involvement but also at clearance of systemic disease. The high rate of CNS relapse among APL patients with a WBC count of more than 10,000/μL may warrant routine intrathecal prophylaxis in this group of patients, and such a strategy has been adopted by the European APL Group in their APL2000 trial.[20]

As modern management of APL patients includes serial monitoring for residual disease using RT-PCR, many patients are identified with so-called molecular relapse, generally defined as two successive positive PML-RARA RT-PCR assays performed 2–4 weeks apart. Assuming an assay sensitivity of 1 in $10^4$, such a finding is highly predictive of subsequent clinical relapse. While there is little doubt that molecular relapses are a harbinger of hematologic relapse, and thus require treatment, there is very little agreement about what constitutes appropriate therapy in this increasingly common clinical situation. There is no formal proof that treatment of molecular relapse leads to better outcomes compared to treatment at the time of hematologic relapse, but Lo Coco et al.[65] have presented compelling evidence in support of "preemptive" therapy, i.e., at the time of molecular relapse. In that study, among 12 patients with molecular relapse who achieved second molecular CR following salvage with ATRA, ara-C, and mitoxantrone, 10 were alive in sustained

molecular remission at the time of the report, for a 2-year survival of 92%. This compared to a 2-year survival estimate of 44% in a previous series of 37 patients treated by the same investigators with identical therapy, but at the time of hematologic relapse.

While clinicians may be reluctant to subject patients with positive RT-PCR results to intensive chemotherapy (±stem cell transplant), some type of treatment needs to be offered. Options include (1) gemtuzumab ozogamicin[66], (2) arsenic trioxide, (3) ATRA (in patients who have not received ATRA within 6 months), (4) standard anthracycline- or ara-C-based chemotherapy, or (5) some combination of the above. Most of the listed agents should convert patients to molecular negativity, but there is no consensus regarding which agent is most effective in this setting, nor is there consensus regarding the duration of therapy, or the type of further intensification (e.g., stem cell transplant) to offer (if any) after achievement of second molecular remission.

Treatment of frank hematologic relapse requires a more aggressive approach, generally incorporating autologous or allogeneic stem cell transplant in second CR. The best option for initial salvage therapy is probably arsenic trioxide, which has been shown to lead to CR rates of 85–95% in relapsed APL.[67–71] However, the quality of CRs induced by arsenic trioxide is unclear,[72,73] and most clinicians view arsenic trioxide as a "bridge" to stem cell transplant. The goal of salvage therapy, whatever the agent, is attainment of second molecular CR, which is a mandatory prerequisite prior to proceeding to stem cell harvest and possible autologous stem cell transplant. The role of autologous and allogeneic stem cell transplant in the treatment of relapsed APL has received considerable recent attention.[74–80] Initial data from Meloni et al.,[79] and more recent results from the European APL Group,[75] suggest that autologous stem cell transplant may cure as many as 75% of patients who are in molecular remission at the time of stem cell harvest and transplant. Investigators from the Cancer and Leukemia Group B, using a high-dose ara-C/etoposide consolidation/mobilization regimen, have reported an EFS of 74% in APL patients transplanted in second CR.[77] Given the good results with polymerase-chain-reaction-negative autografts in relapsed APL, allogeneic transplant is generally recommended only for those patients who are persistently molecularly positive, or who may have failed previous autologous transplant.[75,78] The role of stem cell transplant in the treatment of relapsed APL has recently been challenged by Au et al.,[67] who treated 42 patients with relapsed APL with a regimen of arsenic trioxide (intravenous or oral), followed by idarubicin consolidation and, in most patients, maintenance with oral arsenic trioxide. With short follow up, 38 of the 42 patients were in hematologic and molecular remission, some of them after subsequent retreatment with arsenic trioxide plus ATRA. If results such as these hold up, the role of stem cell transplant in APL will need to be reexamined; however, at present, autologous or allogeneic transplant offers the best hope for long-term survival for the majority of patients with relapsed APL.

## SUMMARY

The majority of APL patients are now cured with ATRA- or arsenic-trioxide-based regimens combined with anthracycline chemotherapy, but a small percentage of patients fail such therapy and require special attention. In particular, a better understanding of the APL-associated coagulopathy is needed, so that effective therapies can be designed to decrease (or eliminate) early deaths secondary to bleeding. Further exploration of non-myelosuppressive treatments is warranted, especially in low-risk patients or patients with comorbidities that preclude use of aggressive chemotherapy. Finally, patients with high-risk APL require intensified therapy, e.g., with high-dose ara-C or perhaps arsenic trioxide. The goal for the next decade of APL clinical research will be to maintain cure rates for all APL patients while reducing side effects and long-term toxicities of treatment. Patients and physicians alike will continue to benefit from enrollment of patients in carefully designed clinical trials that ask critical questions and provide a framework for rational incorporation of alternative, less-toxic therapies for some or all APL patients. In this way, cure rates will be maintained, the field will move forward, and the ultimate goal of cure of all patients with APL may one day be realized.

## REFERENCES

1. Hillestad LK: Acute promyelocytic leukemia. *Acta Med Scand* 159:189, 1957.
2. Rowley JD, Golomb HM, Vardiman J, et al.: Further evidence for a non-random chromosomal abnormality in acute promyelocytic leukemia. *Int J Cancer* 20:869, 1977.
3. Sirulnik A, Melnick A, Zelent A, et al.: Molecular pathogenesis of acute promyelocytic leukaemia and APL variants. *Best Pract Res Clin Haematol* 16:387, 2003.
4. Sanz MA, Lo Coco F, Martin G, et al.: Definition of relapse risk and role of nonanthracycline drugs for consolidation in patients with acute promyelocytic leukemia: a joint study of the PETHEMA and GIMEMA cooperative groups. *Blood* 96:1247, 2000.
5. Gallagher RE, Willman CL, Slack JL, et al.: Association of PML-RAR alpha fusion mRNA type with pretreatment hematologic characteristics but not treatment outcome in acute promyelocytic leukemia: an intergroup molecular study. *Blood* 90:1656, 1997.
6. Au WY, Fung A, Chim CS, et al.: FLT-3 aberrations in acute promyelocytic leukaemia: clinicopathological associations and prognostic impact. *Br J Haematol* 125:463, 2004.
7. Grimwade D, Gale R, Hills R, et al.: The relationship between FLT3 mutation status, biological characteristics, and outcome in patients with acute promyelocytic leukemia. *Blood* 102:Abstract 334, 2003.
8. Noguera NI, Breccia M, Divona M, et al.: Alterations of the FLT3 gene in acute promyelocytic leukemia: association with diagnostic characteristics and analysis of clinical outcome in patients treated with the Italian AIDA protocol. *Leukemia* 16:2185, 2002.
9. Shih LY, Kuo MC, Liang DC, et al.: Internal tandem duplication and Asp835 mutations of the FMS-like tyrosine kinase 3 (FLT3) gene in acute promyelocytic leukemia. *Cancer* 98:1206, 2003.
10. De Botton S, Chevret S, Sanz M, et al.: Additional chromosomal abnormalities in patients with acute promyelocytic leukaemia (APL) do not confer poor prognosis: results of APL 93 trial. *Br J Haematol* 111:801, 2000.
11. Hernandez JM, Martin G, Gutierrez NC, et al.: Additional cytogenetic changes do not influence the outcome of patients with newly diagnosed acute promyelocytic leukemia treated with an ATRA plus anthracycline based protocol. A report of the Spanish group PETHEMA. *Haematologica* 86:807, 2001.
12. Di Bona E, Sartori R, Zambello R, et al.: Prognostic significance of CD56 antigen expression in acute myeloid leukemia. *Haematologica* 87:250, 2002.
13. Ferrara F, Morabito F, Martino B, et al.: CD56 expression is an indicator of poor clinical outcome in patients with acute promyelocytic leukemia treated with simultaneous all-trans-retinoic acid and chemotherapy. *J Clin Oncol* 18:1295, 2000.
14. Breccia M, Diverio D, Noguera NI, et al.: Clinico-biological features and outcome of acute promyelocytic leukemia patients with persistent polymerase chain reaction-detectable disease after the AIDA front-line induction and consolidation therapy. *Haematologica* 89:29, 2004.
15. Grimwade D: The significance of minimal residual disease in patients with t(15;17). *Best Pract Res Clin Haematol* 15:137, 2002.
16. Lo-Coco F, Breccia M, Diverio D: The importance of molecular monitoring in acute promyelocytic leukaemia. *Best Pract Res Clin Haematol* 16:503, 2003.
17. Gabert J, Beillard E, van der Velden VH, et al.: Standardization and quality control studies of "real-time" quantitative reverse transcriptase polymerase chain reaction of fusion gene transcripts for residual disease detection in leukemia—a Europe Against Cancer program. *Leukemia* 17:2318, 2003.
18. Gallagher RE, Yeap BY, Bi W, et al.: Quantitative real-time RT-PCR analysis of PML-RAR alpha mRNA in acute promyelocytic leukemia: assessment of prognostic significance in adult patients from intergroup protocol 0129. *Blood* 101:2521, 2003.
19. Iland H, Bradstock K, Chong L, et al.: Results of the APML3 trial of ATRA, intensive idarubicin, and triple maintenance combined with molecular monitoring in acute promyelocytic leukemia (APL): a study by the Australasian Leukaemia and Lymphoma Group (ALLG). *Blood* 102:Abstract 484, 2003.
20. Ades L, Raffoux E, Chevret S, et al.: Is ara-C required in the treatment of newly diagnosed APL? Results of a randomized trial (APL2000). *Blood* 104:Abstract 391, 2004.

21. Fenaux P, Chastang C, Chevret S, et al.: A randomized comparison of all transretinoic acid (ATRA) followed by chemotherapy and ATRA plus chemotherapy and the role of maintenance therapy in newly diagnosed acute promyelocytic leukemia. The European APL Group. *Blood* 94:1192, 1999.

22. Ades L, Chevret S, De Botton S, et al.: Outcome of acute promyelocytic leukemia treated with all trans retinoic acid and chemotherapy in elderly patients: the European group experience. *Leukemia* 19:230, 2005.

23. Fenaux P, Chevret S, Guerci A, et al.: Long-term follow-up confirms the benefit of all-trans retinoic acid in acute promyelocytic leukemia. European APL Group. *Leukemia* 14:1371, 2000.

24. Lengfelder E, Reichert A, Schoch C, et al.: Double induction strategy including high dose cytarabine in combination with all-trans retinoic acid: effects in patients with newly diagnosed acute promyelocytic leukemia. German AML Cooperative Group. *Leukemia* 14:1362, 2000.

25. Lengfelder E, Saussele S, Haferlach T, et al.: Treatment of newly diagnosed acute promyelocytic leukemia: the impact of high dose ara-C. *Blood* 102:Abstract 448, 2003.

26. Lo-Coco F, Avvisati G, Vignetti M, et al.: Front-line treatment of acute promyelocytic leukemia with AIDA induction followed by risk-adapted consolidation: Results of the AIDA-2000 trial of the Italian GIMEMA Group. *Blood* 104:Abstract 392, 2004.

27. Avvisati G, Petti MC, Lo Coco F, et al.: The Italian way of treating acute promyelocytic leukemia (APL), final act. *Blood* 102:Abstract 487, 2003.

28. Ohno R, Asou N: The recent JALSG study for newly diagnosed patients with acute promyelocytic leukemia (APL). *Ann Hematol* 83(suppl 1):S77, 2004.

29. Burnett AK, Grimwade D, Solomon E, et al.: Presenting white blood cell count and kinetics of molecular remission predict prognosis in acute promyelocytic leukemia treated with all-trans retinoic acid: result of the randomized MRC trial. *Blood* 93:4131, 1999.

30. Tallman MS, Andersen JW, Schiffer CA, et al.: All-trans retinoic acid in acute promyelocytic leukemia: long-term outcome and prognostic factor analysis from the North American Intergroup protocol. *Blood* 100:4298, 2002.

31. Tallman MS, Andersen JW, Schiffer CA, et al.: All-trans-retinoic acid in acute promyelocytic leukemia. *N Engl J Med* 337:1021, 1997.

32. Sanz MA, Martin G, Gonzalez M, et al.: Risk-adapted treatment of acute promyelocytic leukemia with all-trans-retinoic acid and anthracycline monochemotherapy: a multicenter study by the PETHEMA Group. *Blood* 103:1237, 2004.

33. Tallman MS, Kim HT, Andersen JW, et al.: Outcome of patients with acute promyelocytic leukemia (APL) in the pre-ATRA era: An analysis from the Eastern Cooperative Group (ECOG). *Blood* 102:Abstract 3030, 2002.

34. Estey EH, Garcia-Manero G, Ferrajoli A, et al.: Use of all-trans retinoic acid plus arsenic trioxide as an alternative to chemotherapy in untreated acute promyelocytic leukemia. *Blood* 107:3469, 2006.

35. Mandelli F, Diverio D, Avvisati G, et al.: Molecular remission in PML/RAR alpha-positive acute promyelocytic leukemia by combined all-trans retinoic acid and idarubicin (AIDA) therapy. Gruppo Italiano-Malattie Ematologiche Maligne dell'Adulto and Associazione Italiana di Ematologia ed Oncologia Pediatrica Cooperative Groups. *Blood* 90:1014, 1997.

36. de la Serna J, Martin G, Vellenga E, et al.: Causes of induction failure in newly diagnosed acute promyelocytic leukemia patients treated with simultaneous ATRA and idarubicin (AIDA). *Blood* 104:Abstract 887, 2004.

37. Tallman MS, Lefebvre P, Baine RM, et al.: Effects of all-trans retinoic acid or chemotherapy on the molecular regulation of systemic blood coagulation and fibrinolysis in patients with acute promyelocytic leukemia. *J Thromb Haemost* 2:1341, 2004.

38. Falanga A, Rickles FR: Pathogenesis and management of the bleeding diathesis in acute promyelocytic leukaemia. *Best Pract Res Clin Haematol* 16:463, 2003.

39. Kawai Y, Watanabe K, Kizaki M, et al.: Rapid improvement of coagulopathy by all-trans retinoic acid in acute promyelocytic leukemia. *Am J Hematol* 46:184, 1994.

40. Rodeghiero F, Avvisati G, Castaman G, et al.: Early deaths and anti-hemorrhagic treatments in acute promyelocytic leukemia. A GIMEMA retrospective study in 268 consecutive patients. *Blood* 75:2112, 1990.

41. Black JM, Williams EC, Schwartz BS, et al.: Long term experience using heparin and epsilon-aminocaproic acid for the coagulopathy associated with acute promyelocytic leukemia. *Blood* 100:Abstract 4544, 2002.

42. Escudier SM, Kantarjian HM, Estey EH: Thrombosis in patients with acute promyelocytic leukemia treated with and without all-trans retinoic acid. *Leuk Lymphoma* 20:435, 1996.

43. Hashimoto S, Koike T, Tatewaki W, et al.: Fatal thromboembolism in acute promyelocytic leukemia during all-trans retinoic acid therapy combined with antifibrinolytic therapy for prophylaxis of hemorrhage. *Leukemia* 8:1113, 1994.

44. Mahendra P, Keeling DM, Hood IM, et al.: Fatal thromboembolism in acute promyelocytic leukaemia treated with a combination of all-trans retinoic acid and aprotonin. *Clin Lab Haematol* 18:51, 1996.

45. Larson RS, Tallman MS: Retinoic acid syndrome: manifestations, pathogenesis, and treatment. *Best Pract Res Clin Haematol* 16:453, 2003.

46. Tallman MS: Retinoic acid syndrome: a problem of the past? *Leukemia* 16:160, 2002.

47. de Botton S, Chevret S, Coiteux V, et al.: Early onset of chemotherapy can reduce the incidence of ATRA syndrome in newly diagnosed acute promyelocytic leukemia (APL) with low white blood cell counts: results from APL 93 trial. *Leukemia* 17:339, 2003.

48. de Botton S, Dombret H, Sanz M, et al.: Incidence, clinical features, and outcome of all trans-retinoic acid syndrome in 413 cases of newly diagnosed acute promyelocytic leukemia. The European APL Group. *Blood* 92:2712, 1998.

49. Tallman MS, Andersen JW, Schiffer CA, et al.: Clinical description of 44 patients with acute promyelocytic leukemia who developed the retinoic acid syndrome. *Blood* 95:90, 2000.

50. Camacho LH, Soignet SL, Chanel S, et al.: Leukocytosis and the retinoic acid syndrome in patients with acute promyelocytic leukemia treated with arsenic trioxide. *J Clin Oncol* 18:2620, 2000.

51. Bourgeois E, Chevret S, Sanz M, et al.: Long term follow up of APL treated with ATRA and chemotherapy (CT) including incidence of late relapses and overall toxicity. *Blood* 102:Abstract 483, 2003.

52. Liu YF, Shen ZX, Hu J, et al.: Clinical observation of the efficacy of all-trans retinoic acid (ATRA) combined with arsenic trioxide (As2O3) in newly diagnosed acute promyelocytic leukemia (APL). *Blood* 104:Abstract 888, 2004.

53. Shen ZX, Shi ZZ, Fang J, et al.: All-trans retinoic acid/As2O3 combination yields a high quality remission and survival in newly diagnosed acute promyelocytic leukemia. *Proc Natl Acad Sci U S A* 101:5328, 2004.

54. Wang G, Li W, Cui J, et al.: An efficient therapeutic approach to patients with acute promyelocytic leukemia using a combination of arsenic trioxide with low-dose all-trans retinoic acid. *Hematol Oncol* 22:63, 2004.

55. Ghavamzadeh A, Alimoghaddam K, Ghaffari H, et al.: Treatment of acute promyelocytic leukemia with arsenic trioxide without a TRA and/or chemotherapy. *Ann Oncol* 17:131, 2006.

56. Mathews V, George B, Lakshmi KM, et al.: Single agent arsenic trioxide in the treatment of newly diagnosed acute promyelocytic leukemia: durable remissions with minimal toxicity. *Blood* 107:2627, 2006.

57. Head D, Kopecky KJ, Weick J, et al.: Effect of aggressive daunomycin therapy on survival in acute promyelocytic leukemia. *Blood* 86:1717, 1995.

58. Sanz MA, Vellenga E, Rayon C, et al.: All-trans retinoic acid and anthracycline monochemotherapy for the treatment of elderly patients with acute promyelocytic leukemia. *Blood* 104:3490, 2004.

59. Mandelli F, Latagliata R, Avvisati G, et al.: Treatment of elderly patients (> or = 60 years) with newly diagnosed acute promyelocytic leukemia. Results of the Italian multicenter group GIMEMA with ATRA and idarubicin (AIDA) protocols. *Leukemia* 17:1085, 2003.

60. Breccia M, Petti MC, Testi AM, et al.: Ear involvement in acute promyelocytic leukemia at relapse: a disease-associated "sanctuary?" *Leukemia* 16:1127, 2002.

61. Burry LD, Seki JT: CNS relapses of acute promyelocytic leukemia after all-trans retinoic acid. *Ann Pharmacother* 36:1900, 2002.

62. Specchia G, Lo Coco F, Vignetti M, et al.: Extramedullary involvement at relapse in acute promyelocytic leukemia patients treated or not with all-trans retinoic acid: a report by the Gruppo Italiano Malattie Ematologiche dell'Adulto. *J Clin Oncol* 19:4023, 2001.

63. Sanz MA, Larrea L, Sanz G, et al.: Cutaneous promyelocytic sarcoma at sites of vascular access and marrow aspiration. A characteristic localization of chloromas in acute promyelocytic leukemia? *Haematologica* 85:758, 2000.

64. Breccia M, Carmosino I, Diverio D, et al.: Early detection of meningeal localization in acute promyelocytic leukaemia patients with high presenting leucocyte count. *Br J Haematol* 120:266, 2003.

65. Lo Coco F, Diverio D, Avvisati G, et al.: Therapy of molecular relapse in acute promyelocytic leukemia. *Blood* 94:2225, 1999.

66. Lo Coco F, Cimino G, Breccia M, et al.: Gemtuzumab ozogamicin (Mylotarg) as a single agent for molecularly relapsed acute promyelocytic leukemia. *Blood* 104:1995, 2004.

67. Au WY, Chim CS, Lie AK, et al.: Treatment of relapsed acute promyelocytic leukemia by arsenic-based strategies without hematopoietic stem cell transplantation in Hong Kong: a seven-year experience. *Blood* 104:Abstract 395, 2004.

68. Au WY, Kumana CR, Kou M, et al.: Oral arsenic trioxide in the treatment of relapsed acute promyelocytic leukemia. *Blood* 102:407, 2003.

69. Lazo G, Kantarjian H, Estey E, et al.: Use of arsenic trioxide (As2O3) in the treatment of patients with acute promyelocytic leukemia: the M. D. Anderson experience. *Cancer* 97:2218, 2003.

70. Niu C, Yan H, Yu T, et al.: Studies on treatment of acute promyelocytic leukemia with arsenic trioxide: remission induction, follow-up, and molecular monitoring in 11 newly diagnosed and 47 relapsed acute promyelocytic leukemia patients. *Blood* 94:3315, 1999.

71. Soignet SL, Frankel SR, Douer D, et al.: United States multicenter study of arsenic trioxide in relapsed acute promyelocytic leukemia. *J Clin Oncol* 19:3852, 2001.

72. Carmosino I, Latagliata R, Avvisati G, et al.: Arsenic trioxide in the treatment of advanced acute promyelocytic leukemia. *Haematologica* 89:615, 2004.

73. Raffoux E, Rousselot P, Poupon J, et al.: Combined treatment with arsenic trioxide and all-trans-retinoic acid in patients with relapsed acute promyelocytic leukemia. *J Clin Oncol* 21:2326, 2003.

74. Capria S, Diverio D, Ribersani M, et al.: Autologous stem cell transplantation following BAVC regimen can be a curative approach for APL patients in second molecular remission. *Blood* 102:Abstract 2730, 2003.

75. de Botton S, Fawaz A, Chevret S, et al.: Autologous and allogeneic stem-cell transplantation as salvage treatment of acute promyelocytic leukemia initially treated with all-trans-retinoic acid: a retrospective analysis of the European Acute Promyelocytic Leukemia Group. *J Clin Oncol* 23:120, 2005.

76. Leoni F, Gianfaldoni G, Annunziata M, et al.: Arsenic trioxide therapy for relapsed acute promyelocytic leukemia: a bridge to transplantation. *Haematologica* 87:485, 2002.

77. Linker CA: Autologous stem cell transplantation for acute myeloid leukemia. *Bone Marrow Transplant* 31:731, 2003.

78. Lo-Coco F, Romano A, Mengarelli A, et al.: Allogeneic stem cell transplantation for advanced acute promyelocytic leukemia: results in patients treated in second molecular remission or with molecularly persistent disease. *Leukemia* 17:1930, 2003.

79. Meloni G, Diverio D, Vignetti M, et al.: Autologous bone marrow transplantation for acute promyelocytic leukemia in second remission: prognostic relevance of pretransplant minimal residual disease assessment by reverse-transcription polymerase chain reaction of the PML/RAR alpha fusion gene. *Blood* 90:1321, 1997.

80. Thomas X, Dombret H, Cordonnier C, et al.: Treatment of relapsing acute promyelocytic leukemia by all-trans retinoic acid therapy followed by timed sequential chemotherapy and stem cell transplantation. APL Study Group: Acute promyelocytic leukemia. *Leukemia* 14:1006, 2000.

# Chapter 7

# APPROACHES TO TREATMENT OF SECONDARY ACUTE MYELOID LEUKEMIA AND ADVANCED MYELODYSPLASIA

*Elihu Estey*

## GENERAL ISSUES

Within this chapter, secondary acute myeloid leukemia (AML) and secondary "advanced myelodysplasia (MDS)" (International Prognostic Scoring System categories intermediate-2 and high) are combined based on the likelihood that these illnesses have similar natural histories[1,2]; the somewhat arbitrary criteria used to distinguish them[3]; and, after account is made for other covariates such as cytogenetics and age, their similar response to therapy.[4]

Secondary AML/MDS can mean disease that is diagnosed only after a period of abnormal blood counts (antecedent hematologic disorder, or AHD) or that has arisen following cytotoxic therapy for another illness. In the vast majority of cases, these illnesses are other malignancies, although cases developing after treatment of a "nonmalignant" disease (such as rheumatoid arthritis) with drugs such as methotrexate would also qualify. Using the above definition and using more than one month as the criterion for an AHD, one-half of the 1990 patients treated at M.D. Anderson Hospital from 1991 to present for AML/advanced MDS were secondary cases. Of these cases, 708 had an AHD but no prior chemotherapy (PCH), 108 had PCH without an AHD, and 162 had both an AHD and a PCH. The great majority of these patients received ara-C at $1–2 \text{ g/m}^2$ either daily for 4 or 5 days or $1.5 \text{ g/m}^2$ daily by continuous infusion for 3–4 days combined with idarubicin, fludarabine, topotecan, or troxacitabine. The differences among these regimens are medically insignificant,[5,6] and they are considered together as "standard chemotherapy" (SCH).

Table 7.1 depicts results of SCH in the aforementioned M.D. Anderson patients. Note that the difference in compete remission (CR) rate between de novo patients (66%) and the highest CR rate in the three groups of secondary patients (47%) is greater than the difference between the highest (47%) and lowest CR (40%) rates in the three secondary groups. In general, the same is true when considering probabilities of relapse-free survival (RFS) or survival (Table 7.1, Figure 7.1). These observations provide a rationale for considering patients with a history of PCH or an AHD as secondary AML, to be contrasted with de novo cases (Figure 7.2).

Whether the poor results in secondary AML/MDS are due to some inherent, not currently identified, characteristic of this type of AML/MDS or rather to the presence of other covariates is unclear. The principal predictors of outcome with SCH in AML/MDS are performance status, age, and cytogenetics; the former two are associated with treatment-related mortality (TRM) and the latter with resistance to therapy. Of note, each of these is unevenly distributed between de novo and secondary cases (Table 7.2). Patients with de novo disease are on average 10 years younger, but are twice as likely to have a poor performance status (Zubrod 3 or 4). The association between de novo AML/MDS and poor performance status likely reflects the higher white blood cell count and the correspondingly greater risk for organ infiltration in de novo disease. The tendency of secondary cases to have a relatively high proportion of prognostically unfavorable cytogenetic abnormalities (−5/−7) and a relatively low proportion of better prognosis abnormalities [inv(16), t(8;21)] is well known.[7] In light of these inequalities, it is reasonable to compare outcome in de novo and secondary patients who share a given karyotype, age range, and performance status. Tables 7.3 and 7.4 do so for

| Table 7.1 | Outcome in de novo and secondary AML/MDS | | | | | | | | |
|-----------|-----------|----------|-----------|--------------|------|------|--------------------|------|------|
| | | | CR rate | Probability RFS | | | Probability survival | | |
| AHD | PCH | Patients | (%) | 0.5 y | 1 y | 2 y | 0.5 y | 1 y | 2 y |
| No | No | 998 | 66 | 0.72 | 0.50 | 0.33 | 0.68 | 0.50 | 0.35 |
| Yes | No | 708 | 45 | 0.65 | 0.35 | 0.20 | 0.58 | 0.38 | 0.20 |
| No | Yes | 108 | 47 | 0.51 | 0.32 | 0.18 | 0.46 | 0.32 | 0.14 |
| Yes | Yes | 162 | 40 | 0.59 | 0.39 | 0.26 | 0.49 | 0.24 | 0.16 |

patients under the age of 60 years and 60 or above, respectively. These tables indicate that for every cytogenetic group, with the exception of inv(16)/t(8;21), and in both younger and older patients, the de novo patients have both higher CR rates and longer RFS. Figures 7.3 to 7.5 depict the effect of the de novo/secondary distinction on survival. Goldstone et al. have also noted that secondary disease (an AHD or PCH) remains associated with a worse outcome after accounting for age and cytogenetics.[8]

There are three broad options for treatment of secondary AML/MDS: palliative care only, SCH, or investigational therapy, preferably in the context of a clinical trial. As relapse rates begin to decline sharply once 2–3 years have elapsed from the CR date, patients alive in CR at these times can be considered "potentially cured."[9] Multiplying CR rate by RFS probability indicates that only 10% of secondary cases are predicted to be alive in first CR at 2 years from treatment date if given SCH (Table 7.1). Under these circumstances, investigational therapy may be necessary at some point in the majority of patients with secondary AML/MDS.

It is critical to ask whether there are groups of patients with secondary AML/MDS who should, or plausibly might, receive SCH, which in any event is intuitively preferred by patients and physicians, given the fewer number of unknowns involved. Tables 7.3 and 7.4 indicate that both older and younger patients with inv(16) or t(8;21) should receive SCH. As made clear by Beaumont et al.,[10] standard treatment should also be recommended for patients with secondary acute promyelocytic leukemia (APL). Younger patients with secondary AML and a normal karyotype have a 20% likelihood of remaining alive in first CR at 2 years (a CR rate of 0.69 × an RFS of 0.29; Table 7.3). Whether this result is sufficiently high to justify the use of SCH, given that it is distinctly possible that investigational therapy could be considerably worse, is a subjective decision, except in cases where an internal tandem duplication or mutation of *FLT3*[11] is present and tips the scales to a recommendation for investigational therapy. In the other groups depicted in Tables 7.3 and 7.4, the results with SCH are so poor (less than or equal to 10% probability of potential cure) that investigational therapy is preferred, given that even if it proves worse than SCH, it cannot be much worse. The recommendation that all patients with secondary AML with the exception of those with inv(16) or t(8;21) and, quite plausibly, those under age 60 with good performance status and a normal karyotype are candidates for investigational therapy is, in general, in accord with the recommendation of the National Comprehensive Cancer Network,[12] a consortium of academic medical centers. In those older patients in whom this recommendation cannot be carried out, the option of

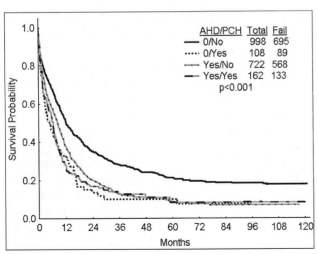

**Figure 7.1** *Survival probabilities of M.D. Anderson patients according to AHD and PCH status*

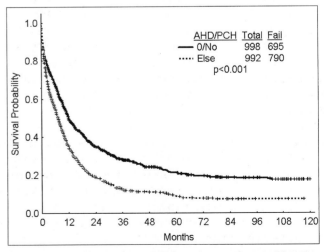

**Figure 7.2** *Survival probabilities when patients with PCH or AHD are considered as one group (secondary AML/MDS) and compared to de novo patients (neither AHD nor PCH)*

| Table 7.2 | Associations with other covariates | |
|---|---|---|
| Predictors | De novo cases | Secondary cases |
| Median age | 55 | 66 |
| Performance status | 126 (13%) | 69 (7%) |
| Zubrod 3 or 4 | | |
| −5/−7 | 180 (18%) | 335 (33%) |
| Inv(16) or t(8;21) | 128 (12%) | 22 (2%) |
| Normal | 932 (39%) | 337 (33%) |
| Other | 265 (26%) | 294 (29%) |
| Insufficient | 47 (5%) | 32 (3%) |

palliative care should be strongly considered given that the 20–30% risk of TRM rate with SCH is not commensurate with the benefits offered by this type of therapy.

Before proceeding to a discussion of investigational therapy, the role of allogeneic stem cell transplant should be discussed. In patients in first CR, "standard" transplant, i.e., using cyclophosphamide and total body irradiation or oral busulfan and cells from an HLA-identical or 1-antigen mismatched sibling donor, is distinguished from "investigational" transplant. The largest trials comparing SCH with standard transplant (allogeneic stem cell transplantation or allo SCT) in first CR minimize selection biases by including patients in the transplant group if they had a donor regardless of whether they had a transplant. These indicate that, on average, patients in the no donor group and donor groups have similar survival.[13,14] No trials address this issue in a similar fashion, restricting attention to patients with secondary AML/MDS. However, there are studies that examine the effect of having a donor in subgroups defined by other prognostic factors. The largest study to examine the effect of cytogenetics[15] found a trend for patients with inv(16) or t(8;21) to live longer if assigned to chemotherapy rather than allo SCT, while patients with prognostically intermediate karyotypes [any but inv(16), t(8;21), −5, −7, 5q−, 7q−, or more than three abnormalities] lived longer with allo SCT, but only if patients were younger than 35. Most importantly, outcome was similarly poor in the adverse karyotype group (−5, −7, 5q−, 7q−, or more than three abnormalities) regardless of whether patients were assigned to

allo SCT or chemotherapy. Similarly, autologous SCT does not affect prognosis in these patients.[16] Both the Medical Research Council (MRC) AML 10 and AML 12 trials[15,17] and a previous MRC study[18] make clear that the principal determinant of outcome remains the prognostic group regardless of patients' donor status. Further suggestion that similar prognostic factors are operative for allo SCT and chemotherapy are data indicating that (1) in patients transplanted in second CR, RFS is influenced by length of the first chemotherapy-maintained CR, as is the case when patients receive chemotherapy to maintain a second CR,[19] and (2) allo SCT does not appear to alter the poor prognosis of patients with FLT3 mutations.[20] Furthermore, although approximately 90% of allo SCT survivors are in good health years after the procedure,[21] they are clearly at increased risk for subsequent development of solid cancers[22,23]; a similar risk is not apparent in long-term survivors of chemotherapy.[9] Thus, unless secondary AML is thought to represent a unique prognostic group, there is no compelling evidence to recommend that patients with secondary AML in first CR receive conventional SCT. If, however, a decision is made to proceed to allo SCT once first CR is observed, administration of consolidation therapy prior to transplantation appears to be of no value.[24]

## INVESTIGATIONAL APPROACHES

As noted above, it is unlikely that secondary AML/MDS possesses unique therapeutic targets. Indeed, because the chromosomal abnormalities characteristic of secondary AML/MDS more frequently occur in older than in younger patients with de novo AML, many of the former may really have "secondary" AML, consequent to prolonged exposure to toxins. Similarly, many patients considered to have de novo AML would be classified as having secondary AML had they happened to visit a physician and have an AHD detected in the months before they were found to have AML. Given these facts, a discussion of investigational approaches to secondary AML is in reality a general discussion of such approaches in worse prognosis AML/MDS. As the ability of the patient to withstand therapy is an important consideration and is often a

| Table 7.3 | Outcome in patients under age 60 with performance status 0–2 by cytogenetics and de novo versus secondary distinction | | | | |
|---|---|---|---|---|---|
| | De novo cases | | | Secondary cases | |
| Cytogenetics | CR rate | RFS at 2 years | | CR rate | RFS at 2 years |
| Intermediate prognosis | 264/352 (75%) | 0.36 | | 120/196 (61%) | 0.27 |
| Normal | 157/206 (76%) | 0.40 | | 69/100 (69%) | 0.29 |
| −5 and/or −7 | 41/63 (65%) | 0.20 | | 43/123 (35%) | 0.08 |
| Inv(16) or t(8;21) | 92/96 (96%) | 0.53 | | 11/11 | 0.54 |

**Table 7.4** Outcome in patients of age 60 and above with performance status 0–2 by cytogenetics and de novo versus secondary distinction

| Cytogenetics | De novo cases | | Secondary cases | |
| --- | --- | --- | --- | --- |
| | CR rate | RFS at 2 years | CR rate | RFS at 2 years |
| Intermediate prognosis | 140/233 (60%) | 0.30 | 183/399 (46%) | 0.23 |
| Normal | 101/151 (67%) | 0.30 | 111/220 (50%) | 0.22 |
| −5 and/or −7 | 36/85 (42%) | 0.11 | 58/181 (32%) | 0.05 |
| Inv(16) or t(8;21) | 11/11 (96%) | 0.14 | 9/11 (81%) | 0.52 |

function of age, older and younger patients will be discussed separately. In each, general issues and strategies will be the focus, rather than a comprehensive list of all new agents in testing.

### OLDER PATIENTS

Detailed studies of the effect of age on outcome in AML suggest that, all else being equal, each additional year increases the risk of death by approximately the same amount.[25] Older patients with AML/MDS are commonly defined as those of age 60 years and above. Given that CR rates in older patients with secondary AML/MDS following SCH are less than 50% (Table 7.4), investigational approaches should be employed at diagnosis. There are three general types of investigational therapies that might be offered to these patients: high-intensity (HI) regimens, low-intensity regimens (LI), and nonablative allogeneic transplant. HI regimens [e.g., clofarabine plus ara-C[26,27] or triapene plus ara-C] are those that produce not only several weeks of severe myelosuppression, but also cause damage to organs, such as the gut or lung. This damage contributes to the 20–30% rate of TRM characteristic of previous HI. This rate, as well as advances in molecular biology, have sparked interest in the development of LI. Examples are the farnesyl transferase

inhibitor R115777[28,29]; the FLT3 inhibitors PKC412 and CEP701[30,31]; other tyrosine kinase inhibitors such as PTK787 and SU5416[32,33]; histone deacetylase (HDAC) inhibitors such as SAHA; and hypomethylating agents such as decitabine[34,35] and 5-azacytidine.[36]

Single-agent studies in high-risk MDS/AML suggest that, in addition to being more "rational" than chemotherapy (CT), LI may have beneficial effects.[28–36] First, they appear to produce less TRM and morbidity than CT. Second, they can produce so-called minor responses (MRs). An example is of "marrow CR" in which, although blood counts remain low, blasts are reduced to "normal" levels in the marrow (<5%) and blood. However, these studies also suggest that CR rates may be considerably lower with HI than with LI, with CR defined as a marrow CR plus "normal" blood counts.[28–36] Thus, most likely, LIs will need to be combined either with each other or with HIs. However, if LI is to be combined with HI in older patients, the HI should presumably be of a type not associated with high rates of TRM. Such combinations, e.g., of LI with low-dose ara-C, can thus be operationally considered "LI" despite the use of chemotherapy. The observations of low CR rates have also prompted an

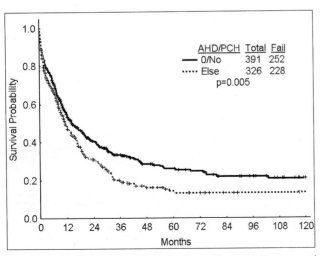

**Figure 7.3** *Survival probabilities in patients with a normal karyotype according to de novo versus secondary distinction*

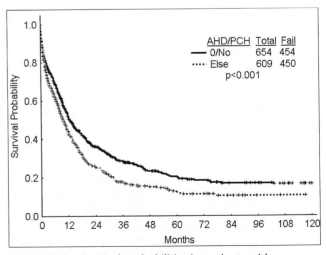

**Figure 7.4** *Survival probabilities in patients with intermediate-risk cytogenetics [normal , +8, del11q, and miscellaneous abnormalities not including −5/−7, inv(16), or t(8;21)] according to de novo versus secondary distinction*

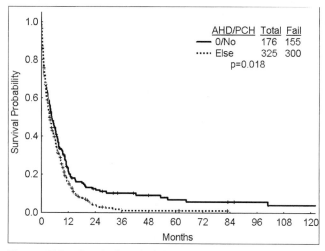

**Figure 7.5** *Survival probabilities in patients with chromosome 5 and/or 7 abnormalities according to de novo versus secondary distinction*

International Working Group (IWG) sponsored by the National Cancer Institute (NCI) to publish criteria for response in MDS, intended with trials of LI in mind, which recognize various categories of MR.[37] Such MRs are also being noted in studies of LI in AML.[28–31] However, as noted by the authors of the IWG report, "it will be important to apply these guidelines prospectively and to critically assess their validity and usefulness."

This statement assumes particular significance given our comparison of the effects on survival of achieving CR versus achieving MR with HI.[38] At M.D. Anderson, we stratified 314 patients with high-risk MDS or AML who survived HI but failed to achieve CR according to whether they exhibited MR on the date they were removed from study. We considered MRs as marrow CR, or as CR with incomplete platelet recovery ($CR_p$) (with less than 5% marrow blasts, normal neutrophil count, and platelet transfusion independence). We then compared survival time in patients according to whether they achieved (1) marrow CR, (2) $CR_p$, (3) CR as usually defined ($CR_p$ and a platelet count >100,000), or (4) none of the above. Survival was dated from date of CR or from date the patient was removed from study. Results are shown in Figure 7.6. Although patients who achieved an MR (marrow CR, $CR_p$) may have done better than patients who did not, the most striking difference was between patients who achieved CR and those who did not.

Findings were similar in patients with high-risk MDS and in those with AML. The results did not reflect differences in time to CR versus time to resistance date or between the times to resistance date in the various subsets of resistant patients. Thus, the observations suggest that only CR potentially lengthens survival in these diseases after administration of HI. This observation is perhaps not surprising. In particular, if many CRs are transient and thus contribute little to an increase in survival time, it may be unrealistic to

expect responses, such as MRs, which are qualitatively inferior to CR, to be associated with a survival benefit. Whether MR will have less effect than that of CR in increasing survival when patients are given LI rather than HI is unknown. However, the data in Figure 7.6 have two consequences. First, they provide an ethical basis for administering either *HI* or *LI* as the initial investigational therapy to older patients with secondary AML/MDS. Specifically, the figure suggests that if the beneficial effect of LIs on TRM is accompanied by a lower CR rate, LI and HI may have equivalent effects on survival. Second, the data emphasize the importance of assessing the relationship between survival and the various categories of MR. Such assessment is facilitated by the short survival of patients of age 60 and above with secondary AML/MDS.

The discussion to date has focused on survival as the principal outcome of interest. However, although they may not improve survival time in older patients with secondary AML/MDS, a major advantage of LIs is the possibility that they will provide better "quality of life" (QOL) than do HIs. Thus, unlike HIs, LIs are often administered by mouth and, in principle, require less time in hospital.[39] However, if HI is more likely to produce a CR than LI, and if achievement of CR is necessary to lower the risk of infection and hemorrhage that are frequent contributors to morbidity in older patients with AML/MDS, HI may be more likely to improve QOL than LI. The above discussion stresses the need for reproducible QOL measurements in patients receiving investigational HI or LI.

A third type of investigational approach in older patients with secondary AML/MDS involves nonablative allogeneic transplant (minitransplant). Minitransplantation relies essentially entirely on a graft-versus-leukemia effect; the purpose of the attenuated doses of chemotherapy used as the preparative regimen is to allow the donor cells to engraft. The source of stem cells is often the blood rather than the bone marrow.[40–42]

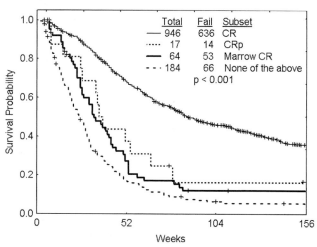

**Figure 7.6** *Subsequent survival in chemotherapy patients according to initial response (see text for details)*

While it is clear that minitransplant produces TRM rates to "only" 20% in patients up to age 75, the potential benefit is less clear. Part of the difficulty in assessing the effectiveness of minitransplant, as well as of various HIs or LIs, is the selection bias that accompanies the initial investigations of these agents. Other avenues of active investigation within transplantation include use of intravenous, rather than oral, busulfan to overcome the erratic pharmacology of the latter,[43] anti-CD45 radiolabeled antibodies as a component of the pretransplant "preparative regimen,"[44] and use of alternative donors (e.g., unrelated, umbilical cord blood).[45] While use of such donors should expand the impact of allo SCT, it is unclear whether donors can be identified within a relevant time frame, particularly if use of donor cells is envisioned during induction. However, it may be possible to wait longer before beginning treatment than is commonly appreciated.[46] This may be particularly true in patients with secondary AML/MDS, who usually present with lower circulating blast counts, than in de novo patients.

### YOUNGER PATIENTS

TRM rates are usually less than 10% in patients under the age of 60. Partly as a consequence of lower TRM rates and again in contrast to older patients, younger patients with secondary AML/MDS generally have CR rates of more than 50% (Tables 7.3 and 7.4). As a result, a case could be made for beginning investigational therapy only once CR has occurred. This approach avoids the ethical issue that might arise consequent to giving investigational therapies to patients with such CR rates, which may be worse than SCH. On the other hand, there is evidence that an induction regimen can influence CR duration.[47] As a practical issue, patients in CR are often ineligible for trials of new agents; this is unfortunate given the short remissions seen in many such patients. Under these circumstances, it is reasonable to administer investigational regimens to younger patients undergoing remission induction for secondary AML/MDS, provided appropriate statistical designs are used (see next section). In younger patients with secondary AML/MDS and abnormalities of chromosomes 5 and/or 7, new regimens should be used at the time of diagnosis since the CR rate in such patients with SCH is less than 40% (Table 7.3). Because younger patients have relatively low TRM rates, reasons to avoid HIs in these patients are less compelling than in older patients, particularly in combination with LIs such as PKC412 or R115777; indeed, trials combining these and similar agents with HI (such as 3 + 7 or even high-dose ara-C) have been proposed or are in progress. Investigational treatments in younger patients thus include both the agents discussed in the section on older patients and exploration of further dose intensification. As an example of the latter, the Cancer and Leukemia Group B (CALGB) has reported that patients under age 60 tolerate daily daunorubicin

doses of 90 mg/m$^2$ in combination with ara-C at 100 mg/m$^2$ given daily for 7 days and etoposide 100 mg/m$^2$ daily.[48] Heretofore, daunorubicin doses rarely exceeded 60 mg/m$^2$ daily. The CALGB is now comparing the 90- and 60-mg/m$^2$ doses.

As noted above, patients with a normal karyotype or abnormalities other than −5/−7 can plausibly begin investigational therapy once CR has occurred. While pharmaceutical companies have provided only a limited number of agents intended for use in patients in remission, commercially available agents can be used for investigational purposes in this setting. For example, 5-azacytidine and decitabine have been approved for use in MDS.[36] The drugs' effectiveness may reflect their ability to demethylate inappropriately hypermethylated genes,[36] thus inducing reexpression of these genes, which might include various "tumor suppressors." There are reasons to think that combinations of demethylating agents and HDAC inhibitors might be particularly effective in this regard. Valproic acid, a pediatric anticonvulsant, is an HDAC inhibitor, although a less potent one than SAHA or depsipeptide. Thus, a combination of 5-azacytidine and valproic acid could be investigated, for example, in patients in remission. Analogous trials could be formulated using commercially available drugs or focusing on the investigational approaches to transplantation, which are described at the conclusion of the section on older patients.

## NEW METHODS FOR CLINICAL TRIALS OF INVESTIGATIONAL AGENTS

The likelihood that many combinations and permutations of LIs, with each other and with HIs, will be investigated in the future leads to consideration of desirable elements to incorporate in the relevant statistical designs. These elements include the need to (1) randomize early in the investigative process; (2) formally monitor multiple outcomes; (3) account for the possibility that the effects of a given treatment may depend on the treatments given before or after; and (4) develop strategy that views drug development as a process rather than as a series of unconnected trials. Topics (2) to (4) are examples of the general problem of "multiplicities." Most statistical designs underlying LI protocols have not focused on these issues.

### NEED FOR EARLY COMPARISON/RANDOMIZATION

The great majority of LIs are tested in single-agent phase II trials. This practice reflects the conventional phase II → phase III paradigm. Specifically, phase II trials are "exploratory," designed to establish activity, with the idea that comparative trials (phase III) should be conducted only after activity has been observed. A fundamental problem with this formulation is that phase II trials are inherently comparative. In particular, patients are vitally interested in whether a particular therapy is superior to another. The comparative nature of phase II trials is implicit in the designs governing their conduct, as these designs specify minimally acceptable response rates,[49] derived via comparison with other available therapies.

Although phase II trials are thus inherently comparative, the current emphasis on single-arm, nonrandomized phase II trials provides an unreliable basis for treatment comparison because of treatment-trial confounding.[50] Indeed, it is logically inconsistent that the need to avoid confounding trial and treatment effects is addressed by randomizing in phase III, yet is ignored in the evaluation of phase II data that determines whether the phase III trial will be conducted in the first place. These considerations emphasize the desirability of randomization among various treatments and strategies in the early stages of their development. Designs for this purpose have been described.[50] In general, these designs call for randomization of a relatively small number of patients among a relatively large number of therapies. Enrolling fewer patients on each trial permits a larger number of treatments to be investigated. This ability is useful because preclinical rationale is an imperfect predictor of clinical success. Thus, although interferon is the only drug currently known to prolong survival in chronic myeloid leukemia (CML), its mechanism of action remains unknown. The development of all-*trans*-retinoic acid (ATRA) for APL is now cited as an exemplar of the "bench-to-bedside" paradigm. However, it is important to remember that the initial Chinese reports of high CR rates were greeted with skepticism in the West; presumably, there would have been less skepticism if a bench-based rationale were readily apparent. Indeed, with the exception of imatinib, most of the drugs that have improved outcome for patients with leukemia (2-chlorodeoxyadenosine in hairy cell leukemia, interferon in CML, ATRA and arsenic trioxide in APL) are examples of "bedside-to-bench" development. If preclinical rationale cannot yet replace empiricism, we should examine a larger number of therapies. Thus, rather than randomizing 240 patients between a standard and an investigational induction regimen, we might be better served by randomizing the same 240 patients among a standard and three investigational induction regimens. It is true that such trials will be nominally "underpowered." However, this argument ignores the false negative rate inherent in the selection of which investigational regimen to study. For example, if there are three potential regimens that could be investigated and if preclinical rationale is, as argued above, a poor predictor of clinical results, then limiting ourselves to one regimen in effect potentially entails a false negative rate of 67%. Simply put, the most egregious false negative results when a treatment is not studied at all.

## NEED TO MONITOR MULTIPLE OUTCOMES

It is commonly accepted that adaptive monitoring (interim analyses) of clinical trials can lower the risk that future patients will receive a therapy already shown to be ineffective/toxic in earlier patients. Adaptive monitoring of most LI trials is limited to interim analyses of response rate, with response defined so as to include MR, which typically is observed much more commonly than is CR.[28-36] The presence of MR indicates that the LI has activity and thus might be worthy of further investigation. However, as emphasized above, the relationship between MR and survival or QOL generally is unknown. Thus, making response the sole focus of interim analyses overlooks the reality that patients are likely to be concerned with response only to the extent that it is known to lead to longer survival and/or a better QOL. This is particularly true in secondary AML/MDS given the short life expectancy of patients with this condition. Indeed, because formal "stopping rules" in trials of LIs are based on response and not on survival, a scenario in which all patients on a trial "respond" but nonetheless die sooner than might be expected if standard HI could, in principle, lead to erroneous continuation of the trial. Because death rates in LI trials are typically monitored informally and on an ad hoc basis, such trials often have very undesirable "operating characteristics" (OCs). OCs include quantities such as the probability of early termination if a treatment arm is truly associated with a higher mortality rate, or the probability of selecting a given treatment if it is truly superior to others, as well as expected sample size.[50]

Survival time usually cannot be fully assessed until several months after entry onto such a trial, while response (MR or CR) can. Because, however, appreciable numbers of secondary AML/MDS patients die within a few months of presentation (e.g., 20–30% at 2 months if given HI), some information about survival is available early on. It follows that both response and survival should be formally monitored several months after beginning a given therapy. Accrual into a treatment arm would stop if either the death rate was too high or the response rate too low. It is possible that a high early death rate might transform into a low later death rate. Similarly, a low response rate might have no effect on survival. However, it is unlikely that patients would accept such possibilities, which should be assessed retrospectively.

Another example is of the use of investigational therapy during remission induction in younger secondary AML/MDS patients in whom SCH produces CR rates in excess of 60% (Table 7.3). The primary goal of using investigational therapy during induction is to improve RFS. Obviously then, this outcome must be monitored. However, because the investigational therapy might reduce a relatively high existing CR rate, it is also important to monitor CR rate. Trade-offs between

CR and RFS can be specified. For example, a high probability that there will be a 5% absolute decrease in CR rate might not cause early stopping, provided there is an equally high probability of a 20% improvement in RFS. These considerations underscore the desirability of including mechanisms for multiple-outcome monitoring in trials in secondary AML/MDS.[51,52]

### NEED TO CONSIDER STRATEGIES AS WELL AS TREATMENTS

Monitoring multiple outcomes simultaneously, ideally based on desirable trade-offs among these outcomes, is an example of a "multiplicity." A second type of multiplicity arises because a given patient with secondary AML/MDS (or cancer) typically receives multiple treatment regimens. Administration of one therapy may affect outcome with a subsequent therapy. For example, because "targeted therapies" may affect multiple targets, a therapy directed at target "X" may also "down (or up) regulate" target "Y," thereby influencing response to a future therapy aimed at Y. It is possible that patients of age 60 and above with high-risk MDS or secondary AML/MDS might have less TRM if given LI first, and HI only should LI fail. However the reverse approach might be preferable if HI's antileukemia effect is significantly greater than that of LI, outweighing any reduction in TRM with the LI first strategy. Thus, the issue is evaluation of a multicourse treatment strategy, rather than a particular treatment, with a goal of assessing which is the preferable sequence of treatments. Conventional statistical designs for LI trials regard each therapy as a distinct entity, thus paying little formal attention to the issue of the sequence in which two or more therapies are administered. It follows that new designs should address this issue.[53]

### NEED TO VIEW DEVELOPMENT OF SECONDARY AML/MDS THERAPY AS A PROCESS

It might be useful to consider drug development as a "process" rather than, as it is currently thought of as, a series of unconnected trials. In this process, referred to as "continuous phase II,"[54] patients are randomized among a number of treatments or strategies. Arms that perform better get used more often. Arms that perform relatively poorly are dropped. An arm that does well enough is recommended for inclusion in a larger cooperative group trial. As more treatments become available, patients are, "seamlessly," randomized among them, without suspending accrual between trials. Application of the continuous phase II processes speeds up drug development. We believe this paradigm is realistic because new statistical designs, based on Bayesian approaches, provide the requisite flexibility and versatility,[50-54] while the recent emergence of powerful computational technology has made the Bayesian paradigm a practical reality. In particular, the OCs of Bayesian designs can now be readily assessed, and conduct of trials monitoring multiple outcomes can be based on a relatively simple user interface.[55]

### REFERENCES

1. Estey EH, Keating MJ, Dixon DO, Trujillo JM, McCredie KB, Freireich EJ: Karyotype is prognostically more important than the FAB system's distinction between myelodysplastic syndrome and acute myelogenous leukemia. *Hemat Path* 1:203–208, 1987.
2. Greenberg P, Cox C, LeBeau MM, et al.: International scoring system for evaluating prognosis in myelodysplastic syndromes. *Blood* 89:2079–2088, 1997.
3. Albitar M, Manshouri T, Shen Y, et al.: Myelodysplastic syndrome is not merely "preleukemia." *Blood* 100:791–798, 2002.
4. Estey E, Thall P, Beran M, Kantarjian H, Pierce S, Keating M: Effect of diagnosis (refractory anemia with excess blasts, refractory anemia with excess blasts in transformation, or acute myeloid leukemia [AML]) on outcome of AML-type chemotherapy. *Blood* 90:2969–2977, 1997.
5. Estey E, Thall P, Cortes J, et al.: Comparison of idarubicin + ara-C-, fludarabine + ara-C-, and topotecan + ara-C-based regimens in treatment of newly diagnosed acute myeloid leukemia, refractory anemia with excess blasts in transformation, or refractory anemia with excess blasts. *Blood* 98:3575–3583, 2001.
6. Giles FJ, Kantarjian HM, Cortes JE, et al.: Adaptive randomized study of idarubicin and cytarabine versus troxacitabine and cytarabine versus troxacitabine and idarubicin in untreated patients 50 years or older with adverse karyotype acute myeloid leukemia. *J Clin Oncol* 21:1722–1727, 2003.
7. Kantarjian H, Keating M, Walters R, et al.: Therapy-related leukemia and myelodysplastic syndromes: clinical, cytogenetic, and prognostic features. *J Clin Oncol* 4:148–1757, 1986.
8. Goldstone AH, Burnett AK, Avivi I, et al.: Secondary AML has a worse outcome than de novo AML even taking into account cytogenetics and age. AML 10,11,12 MRC trials [abstract]. *Blood* 100(11):88a, 2002.
9. De Lima M, Strom SS, Keating M, et al.: Implications of potential cure in acute myelogenous leukemia: development of subsequent cancer and return to work. *Blood* 90:4719–4724, 1997.
10. Beaumont M, Sanz M, Carli P, et al.: Therapy-related acute promyelocytic leukemia. *J Clin Oncol* 21:2123–2137, 2003.
11. Schnittger S, Schoch C, Dugas M, et al.: Analysis of FLT 3 length mutations in 1003 patients with AML: correlation to cytogenetics, FAB subtype, and prognosis in the AMLCG study and usefulness as a maker for detection of minimal residual disease. *Blood* 101:59–66, 2002.
12. National Comprehensive Cancer Network: *NCCN Clinical Practice Guidelines in Oncology* [available on CD-ROM]. 2004 Mar.
13. Zittoun RA, Mandelli F, Willemze R, et al.: Auto or allo bone marrow transplantation compared with intensive chemotherapy in AML. *N Engl J Med* 332:217, 1995.
14. Cassileth PA, Harrington DP, Appelbaum FR, et al.: Chemotherapy compared with auto or allo bone

marrow transplantation in the management of AML in first remission. *N Engl J Med* 339:1649–1656, 1998.

15. Burnett AK, Wheatley K, Stevens R, et al.: Further data to question the use of allo bone marrow transplant in AML 1st remission in addition to intensive chemotherapy: the MRC experience in 715 patients under age 44 years with donors available [abstract]. *Blood* 100(11):74a, 2002.

16. Burnett AK, Goldstone AH, Stevens RMF, et al.: Randomised comparison of addition of auto bone-marrow transplantation to intensive chemotherapy for acute myeloid leukaemia in first remission: results of MRS AML 10 trial. *Lancet* 351:700–708, 1998.

17. Burnett AK, Wheatley K, Goldstone AH, et al.: The value of allo bone marrow transplant in patients with acute myeloid leukaemia at differing risk of relapse: results of the UK MRC AML 10 trial. *Br J Haematol* 118:385–400, 2002.

18. Burnett AK, Goldstone AH, Stevens R, et al.: Biologic characteristics determine the outcome of allo or auto BMT in AML CR1 [abstract]. *Blood* 86(10):614a, 1995.

19. Gale R, Horowitz MM, Rees JKH, et al.: Chemotherapy vs transplants for AML in second remission. *Leukemia* 10:13–19, 1996.

20. Kottaridis PD, Gale RE, Holt M, et al.: Consolidation of AML therapy with autograft and allograft procedures does not negate the poor prognostic impact of FLT3 internal tandem duplications—results from the UK MRC 10 and 12 trials [abstract]. *Blood* 100(11):75a, 2002.

21. Duell T, van Lint MT, Ljungman P, et al.: Health and functional status of long-term survivors of bone marrow transplantation. *Ann Intern Med* 126:184, 1997.

22. Duell T, van Lint MT, Ljungman P, et al.: Health and functional status of long-term survivors of bone marrow transplantation. *Ann Intern Med* 126:184, 1997.

23. Bhatia S, Ramsay NKC, Steinbuch M, et al.: Malignant neoplasms following bone marrow transplantation. *Blood* 87:3633, 1996.

24. Tallman MS, Rowlings PA, Milone G, et al.: Effect of postremission chemotherapy before human leukocyte antigen-identical sibling transplantation for AML in first complete remission. *Blood* 96:1254–1258, 2000.

25. Thall P, Estey E: Graphical methods for evaluating covariate effects in the Cox model. In: Crowley J (ed.) *Handbook of Statistics in Clinical Oncology*. New York: Marcel-Dekker; 2001:411–433.

26. Cortes J, Gandhi V, Plunkett W, et al.: Clofarabine [2-chloro-9- deoxy-2 fluoro-b-D-arabinofuranosyladenine] is active for patients with refractory or relapsed acute leukemias, myelodysplastic syndromes (MDS) and chronic myeloid leukemia in blast phase (CML-BP) [abstract]. *Blood* 100(739):197a, 2002.

27. Faderl S, Gandhi V, Garcia-Manero G, et al.: Clofarabine is active in combination with cytarabine (ara-C) in adult patients (pts) in first relapsed and primary refractory acute leukemia and high-risk myelodysplastic syndrome (MDS) [abstract]. *Blood* 102(11):615a, 2003.

28. Karp JE, Lancet JE, Kaufmann SH, et al.: Clinical and biologic activity of the farnesyltransferase inhibitor R115777 in adults with refractory and relapsed acute leukemias: a phase 1 clinical-laboratory correlative trial. *Blood* 97:3361–3369, 2001.

29. Lancet J, Karp J, Gotlib J, et al.: Zarnestra (R1157777) in previously untreated poor-risk AML and MDS: prelimi-

nary results of a phase II trial [abstract]. *Blood* 100:560a, 2002.

30. Estey E, Fischer T, Giles F, et al.: A randomized phase II trial of the tyrosine kinase inhibitor PKC412 in patients with acute myeloid leukemia (AML)/high-risk myelodysplastic syndromes (MDS) characterized by wild-type (WT) or mutated FLT3 [abstract]. *Blood* 102(11):614a, 2003.

31. Smith BD, Levis M, Beran M, et al.: Single-agent CEP-701, a novel FLT3 inhibitor, shows biologic and clinical activity in patients with relapsed or refractory acute myeloid leukemia. *Blood* 103:3669–3676, 2004.

32. Roboz G, List A, Giles F, et al.: Phase I trial of PTK787/ZK 222584, an inhibitor of vascular growth factor receptor tyrosine kinases, in acute myeloid leukemia and myelodysplastic syndrome [abstract]. *Blood* 100:337a, 2002.

33. Giles FJ, Stopeck AT, Silverman LR, et al.: SU5416, a small molecule tyrosine kinase receptor inhibitor, has biologic activity in patients with refractory acute myeloid leukemia or myelodysplastic syndromes. *Blood* 102:795–801, 2003.

34. Kantarjian HM, O'Brien S, Cortes J, et al.: Results of decitabine (5-aza-2'deoxycytidine) therapy in 130 patients with chronic myelogenous leukemia. *Cancer* 98:522–528, 2003.

35. Issa J-P, Garcia-Manero G, Giles F, et al.: Phase 1 study of low-dose prolonged exposure schedules of the hypomethylating agent 5-aza-2'-deoxycytidine (decitabine) in hematopoietic malignancies. *Blood* 103:1635–1640, 2004.

36. Silverman L, Demakos E , Peterson BL, et al.: Randomized controlled trial of azacytidine in patients with the myelodysplastic syndrome: a study of the Cancer and Leukemia Group B. *J Clin Oncol* 20:2429–2440, 2002.

37. Cheson BD, Bennett JM, Kantarjian H, et al.: Report of an international working group to standardize response criteria for myelodysplastic syndromes. *Blood* 96:3671–3674, 2000.

38. Lopez G, Giles F, Cortes J, et al.: Sub-types of resistant disease in patients with AML, RAEB-t, or RAEB who fail initial induction chemotherapy [abstract]. *Blood* 98:329a, 2001.

39. Pitako J, Haas P, van den Bosch J, Mueller-Berndorf H, Wijermans PW, Lubbert M: Low-dose decitabine (DAC) in elderly MDS patients: quantification of hospitalization vs outpatient management and survival [abstract]. *Blood* 100:793a, 2002.

40. Giralt S, Estey E, Albitar M, et al.: Engraftment of allo hematopoietic progenitor cells with purine analog-containing chemotherapy: harnessing graft-versus-leukemia without myeloablative therapy. *Blood* 89:4531, 1997.

41. Slavin S, Nagler A, Naparstek E, et al.: Non-myeloablative transplant and cell therapy as an alternative to conventional bone marrow transplantation with lethal cytoreduction for the treatment of malignant and non-malignant hematologic diseases. *Blood* 91:756–763, 1998.

42. McSweeny PA, Niederweiser D, Shizuru JA, et al.: Hematopoietic cell transplantation in older patients with hematologic malignancies: replacing high-dose cytotoxic therapy with graft-vs-tumor effect. *Blood* 97:3390–3400, 2001.

43. Andersson BS, Kashyap A, Couriel D, et al.: Intravenous busulfan in pretransplant chemotherapy: bioavailability and patient benefit. *Biol Blood Marrow Transplant* 9(11):722–724, 2003.

44. Pagel JM, Matthews DC, Appelbaum FR, et al.: The use of radioimmunoconjugates in stem cell transplantation. *Bone Marrow Transplant* 29:807–816, 2002.

45. Appelbaum F: The current status of hematopoietic stem cell transplantation. *Annu Rev Med* 54:491–512, 2003.

46. Estey E, Wang X-M, Thall P, et al.: Plausibility of delaying induction therapy in untreated AML. *Blood* 104:879a, Abstract, 2004.

47. Bishop JF, Matthews JP, Young GA, et al.: Intensified induction chemotherapy with high dose cytarabine and etoposide for acute myeloid leukemia: a review and updated results of the Australian Leukemia Study Group. *Leuk Lymphoma* 28:315–327, 1998.

48. Kolitz J, George S, Dodge R, et al.: Dose escalation studies of daunorubicin, ara-C, and etoposide with and without multidrug resistance modulation with PSC 833 in untreated adults with AML <60 years [abstract]. *Blood* 98(11):175a, 2001.

49. Simon R: Optimal two-stage designs for phase II clinical trials. *Control Clin Trials* 10:1–10, 1989.

50. Estey EH, Thall PF: New designs for phase 2 clinical trials. *Blood* 102:442–448, 2003.

51. Thall PF, Simon RM, Estey EH: Bayesian sequential monitoring designs for single-arm clinical trials with multiple outcomes. *Stat Med* 14:357–379, 1995.

52. Thall PF, Simon RM, Estey EH: New statistical strategy for monitoring safety and efficacy in single-arm clinical trials. *J Clin Oncol* 14:296–303, 1996.

53. Thall PF, Sung H-G, Estey EH: Selecting therapeutic strategies based on efficacy and death in multicourse clinical trials. *J Am Stat Assoc* 97:29–39, 2002.

54. Inoue LY, Thall PF, Berry DA: Seamlessly expanding a randomized phase II trial to phase III. *Biometrics* 58:823–831, 2002.

55. Berry DA: Statistical innovations in cancer research. In: Holland J, Frei T, et al. (eds.) *Cancer Medicine*. 6th ed. London: BC Decker; 2003:chap 33, 465–478.

Chapter **8**

# DEFINITION OF REMISSION, PROGNOSIS, AND FOLLOW-UP

## Mikkael A. Sekeres and Matt E. Kalaycio

## INTRODUCTION

The previous chapters in this book have taken us through the epidemiology of acute myeloid leukemia (AML); its pathology and molecular biology; and the nuances of making the diagnosis, treatment options for both younger and older adults, and for special populations of AML patients [such as those with acute promyelocytic leukemia (APL) and secondary AML]. This chapter will address the next step in the thought process about AML, defining remission, predicting which patients are more or less likely to enter a remission and enjoy long-term disease-free survival, and it will provide guidelines for following AML patients once they have achieved a remission.

## DEFINITION OF REMISSION

In broad terms, a complete remission (CR) in AML is defined as the inability to detect leukemia, using standard tests (i.e., peripheral blood smears, bone marrow biopsy and aspirate, and flow cytometry) to the greatest extent possible. It does not indicate or imply cure, though patients may mistake the two and assume that CR and cure are equivalent.[1] Another way of approaching this concept is to consider the following thought experiment. When a patient presents with AML, he or she presumably has $10^{12}$ leukemia cells, which would be approximately the same number of cancer cells present in 1 $cm^3$ of tissue in a solid malignancy [and that would be considered a pathologic enlargement on computed tomographic scan].[2] Standard remission induction therapy usually reduces this number by three or four logs, to $10^9$ or $10^8$ myeloblasts (the amount required to decrease the number of blasts in the bone marrow to less than 5%, in the setting of recovered peripheral blood cell counts).[3] In other words, in the setting of a CR, a patient may still have

between 100 million and 1 billion leukemia cells, necessitating further cycles of chemotherapy to promote further log reductions in blasts, with an ultimate goal of reducing blasts to a finite number, at which point it is hypothesized that the patient's immune system can eliminate the residual leukemia. Only at this point can a patient be said to be cured. In AML, remission status is assessed after a patient's peripheral blood values have recovered, usually between 4 and 6 weeks after the start of remission induction therapy.

The first widely accepted definition of remission in AML was published in 1990 by a National Cancer Institute-sponsored workshop that took place in 1988 on definitions of diagnosis and response in AML.[4,5] This definition was developed for use in clinical trials, though it has been widely applied outside of the trial setting. A CR was defined as a bone marrow biopsy and aspirate, demonstrating normal cellularity with normal erythropoiesis, granulopoiesis, and megakaryopoiesis (typically defined in the context of a bone marrow cellularity of 20%), and containing no more than 5% blasts. In addition, the peripheral blood had to contain at least 1500 granulocytes/$mm^3$ and 100,000 platelets/$mm^3$ for at least 4 weeks in the absence of intervening chemotherapy. The authors went on to comment that CRs were the only responses worth reporting in phase III trials, as lesser responses [e.g., partial responses (PRs)] do not have an impact on survival (the leukemia equivalent of being "a little bit pregnant"). The goal of these definitions was to make clinical trials comparable and interpretable, though the authors concede the lack of evidence supporting portions of their recommendations.

Over the subsequent decade, improvements in diagnostic criteria for AML[6] and insights into the biology and genetics of the disease[7–10] necessitated revisions of these guidelines. An international group of investigators met in Madrid, Spain, in 2001 to develop revised recommendations that incorporated these new insights

| **Table 8.1**   Criteria for a morphologic CR in AML |
| --- |
| Morphologic leukemia-free state |
|   <5% blasts in a bone marrow aspirate |
|   No blasts with Auer rods or persistence of extramedullary disease |
|   Absence of a unique phenotype by flow cytometry identical to what appeared in the initial specimen |
| Absolute neutrophil count <1000 granulocytes/mm³ |
| Platelet count >100,000/mm³ |

and novel therapeutics, and the results of their efforts were published in late 2003.[11]

The authors report different definitions for CR. The first, and most commonly used, is a morphologic CR (Table 8.1). This definition requires that a patient enter a morphologic leukemia-free state, defined as fewer than 5% blasts in a bone marrow aspirate; no blasts with Auer rods or persistence of extramedullary disease; and absence of a unique phenotype by flow cytometry identical to what appeared in the initial specimen (i.e., no persistence of aberrant markers, such as CD7). In the setting of a morphologic leukemia-free state, the patient must demonstrate an absolute neutrophil count of at least 1000 granulocytes/mm³ (the old criteria required 1500) and 100,000 platelets/mm³. Absent are requirements for minimal bone marrow cellularity, minimal hemoglobin values (though patients should be transfusion free), and duration of response, as it was recognized that the 4-week requirement of maintenance of normal blood counts was often impossible in patients undergoing postremission therapy (which often occurs within 4 weeks). The authors also acknowledge that the bone marrow blasts percentage cutoff of 5% is entirely arbitrary.

Subcategories of patients who fulfill the definition of morphologic CR include the following:

1. Those who enter a cytogenetic CR. Patients in this category revert to a normal karyotype at CR from an abnormal one. This category is recommended for use primarily in clinical studies.
2. Those who enter a molecular CR (CRm). Reverse transcriptase polymerase chain reaction (RT-PCR) techniques are sensitive in detecting residual leukemia in AML typified by a specific genetic defect, including the PML/RARA in t(15;17), or the AML1/ETO fusion in t(8;21). The sensitivity of RT-PCR falls in the range of detecting one positive cell in 1000–10,000 cells. The prognostic implication of CRm is well established in monitoring APL[12] and chronic myelogenous leukemia (CML),[13–15] and will become more so in other types of leukemia.
3. Those who enter a morphologic CR with incomplete blood recovery (CRi). In the past, this has been referred to as a CR with the exception of recovery of platelet counts, and was used first on a broad scale

in studies that led to the eventual approval by the Food and Drug Administration for gemtuzumab ozogamicin.[16,17] This category was developed for patients who fulfilled the requirements of a morphologic CR, but with residual neutropenia or thrombocytopenia. These patients do not seem to enjoy the same survival as those who enter a full morphologic CR.

A partial remission is defined as restoration of peripheral blood counts to similar values as in a CR, and a decrease in bone marrow blast percentage by 50% or above, to a total of no more than 25% (but more than 5%, unless Auer rods are present, in which case 5% or less is acceptable to meet the PR definition). Partial remissions are to be used only in the setting of phase I or II trials, in which a signal of activity (in the setting of acceptable safety) may be needed to expand drug testing in a subgroup of patients.

## PROGNOSIS IN AML

Although many clinical and pathologic features of AML have prognostic relevance, only a few prognostic factors are universally agreed upon, validated, and impact clinical practice. Nonetheless, newer biologic markers of prognosis are likely to supplant older clinical markers in the near future.

### Age

As discussed further, and in greater detail in Chapter 5, age greater than 60 years invokes many adverse features that make separation of age from other poor prognostic markers difficult. Nonetheless, the prognosis gets progressively worse for patients with AML and age greater than 60 years, with each incremental decade of age above 60 years. For patients less than age 60, however, age has proven more difficult to prove as an adverse risk factor, suggesting that biologic features of the leukemia, rather than age alone, are most important in predicting outcome.

In the large trial of cytarabine dose-intensification reported by Mayer et al., the remission rate was 75% in patients of age below 40 years and 68% in those of age 40–60 years, but 4-year disease-free survival was 32 and 29%, respectively.[18] Similarly, Zittoun et al. failed to find an adverse impact of increasing age between 10 and 59 years on disease-free survival in a large trial testing the value of stem cell transplant.[19] In contrast, both the Medical Research Council (MRC) and the Southwest Oncology Group and Eastern Cooperative Oncology Group (SWOG/ECOG) intergroup trials found worse survival with age increasing from 18 to 55 years.[20,21] Thus, the impact of age on prognosis in patients less than 60 years of age is uncertain.

APL has an incidence that is similar among all age groups, including the group greater than 60 years of age. There is no evidence that the biology of APL is different in older versus younger patients. Yet, the survival for older patients with APL is significantly worse than it is for younger patients, and it cannot be explained by an inability to tolerate treatment, since remission rates are similar. The experience of APL supports the contention that age is an independent adverse prognostic factor in AML.

## Antecedent hematologic disorders

Some hematologic disorders, such as advanced myelodysplastic syndrome (MDS) and CML, invariably result in transformation to acute leukemia. Others, such as myelofibrosis with myeloid metaplasia, polycythemia rubra vera, and aplastic anemia, do not always terminate in acute leukemia. However, all hematologic disorders that do transform to acute leukemia share an equally poor prognosis with available therapies. In fact, many clinical trials of treatment for acute leukemia exclude patients with antecedent hematologic disorders (AHD) for this very reason. The influential Cancer and Leukemia Group B (CALGB) study that found higher doses of cytarabine after remission improve survival compared to lower doses excluded patients with AHD.[18] Other studies group patients with AHD with those previously exposed to cytotoxic treatments, such as chemotherapy, making distinctions with regard to one group or another difficult.

However, some studies included patients with AHD and analyzed them separately from those with treatment-related AML. One study retrospectively compared 44 patients with an AHD to 152 patients without such a history. The remission rate was lower in patients with an AHD (41% vs 73%), and was only 23% in AHD patients older than 64 years.[22] For patients with AHD who achieved remission, disease-free survival was 17% at 3 years versus 29% ($P = 0.02$) in patients without AHD. Others have reported similar results, but the confounding variables of age and cytogenetics cloud the potential independent adverse prognostic impact of an AHD.

Some patients with AML present with no history of AHD, but have dysplastic changes in their marrow at diagnosis. These patients also have a worse prognosis compared to patients without such morphologic abnormalities.[23,24]

Although some patients who transform from a myeloproliferative disorder into AML achieve remission with standard induction chemotherapy, the duration of response is brief.[25] In a study of 91 cases of myelofibrosis that transformed into AML, 24 patients were treated with standard induction chemotherapy.[26] Of these, none achieved a CR. Although 10 patients reverted to chronic phase disease, their median survival was only 6 months. Importantly, the treatment-related mortality rate was 33% and the median survival of patients treated with chemotherapy (3.9 months) was not significantly different than that achieved without intensive chemotherapy (2.1 months).

## Prior cytotoxic therapy

Patients treated with cytotoxic chemotherapy or radiotherapy for both malignant and nonmalignant conditions are at risk for subsequent, or secondary, AML. Patients with secondary leukemia have an extremely poor prognosis with standard treatments. Secondary leukemias are frequently characterized by clonal cytogenetic abnormalities that by themselves connote a worse prognosis (see below). In one series, only 29% of patients with secondary AML or MDS achieved remission with standard induction chemotherapy, and only 13% of patients survived 2 years.[27] Other recent series confirm these dismal results.[28,29]

However, some secondary leukemias have a more favorable prognosis and should be recognized. Patients with secondary AML characterized by favorable cytogenetics, such as t(8;21) and inv(16), have a worse prognosis compared to patients with favorable cytogenetics and de novo AML, but have a significantly better prognosis than other patients with secondary AML and should be treated with curative intent.[30,31] Rarely, APL is induced by exposure to chemotherapy.[32] When this happens, remission rates and survival are similar to those achieved in the setting of de novo APL.[33]

## Other clinical factors

Some studies suggest that higher white blood cell counts correlate with a worse prognosis,[34] but other studies refute this assertion.[35] In a large study of over 1000 patients, no clinical factor was found to significantly influence survival when cytogenetics and response to treatment were factored in.[21] A recent study suggests that race may be an important, and heretofore unrecognized, prognostic factor. African-American men with AML have a significantly worse remission rate and survival compared to other patients with AML, including African-American women.[36]

We have reviewed our own experience in older patients with AML treated with a uniform induction chemotherapy regimen.[37] Patients who present with a high lactate dehydrogenase level or significant anemia have a survival of less than 5 months.[38] Consistent with reports from larger trials, we found that a delay from diagnosis to the institution of therapy adversely impacts survival.[39,40] In aggregate, these observations suggest that those patients may be identified at diagnosis who will not benefit from standard induction chemotherapy. Furthermore, a leukocyte nadir count of less than 0.04/μL correlates with a poorer prognosis.[41]

## Biologic factors

Evidence is quickly accumulating that biologic factors intrinsic to the leukemic clone have as much, if not more, prognostic significance as do more traditional clinical factors. Cytogenetic analysis has become critical to the management of AML. Further details as to the molecular aberrations induced by cytogenetic

**Table 8.2** Pretreatment cytogenetic risk groups for overall survival in AML

| | SWOG/ECOG[43] | MRC[44] | CALGB[45] |
|---|---|---|---|
| Number of patients | 584 | 1612 | 1213 |
| Favorable risk | Inv(16), t(16;16) | Inv(16), t(16;16) | Inv(16), t(16;16) |
| | del(16q) | del(16q) | t(8;21) |
| | t(8;21) lacking | t(8;21) | del(9q) only if treated |
| | del(9q) or complex | t(15;17) | by stem cell transplant |
| | karyotypes | | [t(15;17) excluded] |
| | t(15;17) | | |
| Intermediate risk | Normal karyotype | Normal karyotype | Normal karyotype |
| | −Y | 11q23 abnormalities | −Y |
| | +8 | +8 | del(5q) |
| | +6 | del(9q) | loss of 7q |
| | del(12p) | del(7q) | t(9;11) |
| | | +21 | +11 |
| | | +22 | del(11q) |
| | | All others | abn(12p) |
| | | | +13 |
| | | | del(20q) |
| | | | +21 |
| Poor risk | Complex karyotype | Complex karyotype | Complex karyotype |
| | 3q abnormalities | 3q abnormalities | Inv(3), t(3;3) |
| | t(6;9) | t(6;9) | t(6;9) |
| | −5, del(5q) | −5, del(5q) | t(6;11) |
| | −7, del(7q) | −7 | −7 |
| | t(9;22) | t(9;22) | +8 |
| | 9q abnormalities | | t(11;19(q23;p13.1) |
| | 11q abnormalities | | |
| | 20q abnormalities | | |
| | 21q abnormalities | | |
| | 17p abnormalities | | |
| Unknown risk | All others | NA | NA |

abnormalities in AML are discussed in Chapter 2. Whether functionally relevant to leukemic pathogenesis or not, the presence or absence of cytogenetic abnormalities provides important prognostic information that is relevant to both younger and older adults with AML.[42]

Three large, multi-institutional efforts have explored the prognostic significance of cytogenetics in detail. As displayed in Table 8.2, there is general agreement as to the prognostic significance of many, but not all, abnormalities.[43–45] Some of the discrepancy may lie in the patient population analyzed. For example, the CALGB study included all patients up to age 86 years, while the other two studies limited their analysis to patients less than 56 years of age. The CALGB study also excluded patients with the t(15;17). The MRC study included children. The SWOG/ECOG and MRC studies each analyzed the results of one study, while the CALGB study compiled data from several clinical trials (as shown in Figure 8.1).

Another complicating factor with regard to the prognostic role of cytogenetics is that all three studies analyzed patients treated differently from the patients in other studies. For example, the CALGB has argued that patients with favorable risk cytogenetics should be treated with multiple cycles of high-dose cytarabine.[46,47] However, other studies, such as the one analyzed by the MRC, show similar survival rates without such therapy.[44,48]

Allogeneic stem cell transplant is often recommended for patients with poor-risk cytogenetics and an available HLA-matched donor. In the SWOG/ECOG study, this approach led to a 5-year overall survival of 44%, compared to 13–15%, in patients treated with chemotherapy alone or autologous stem cell transplant.[43] In contrast, the MRC study showed no benefit to allogeneic transplant for patients with poor-risk cytogenetics in first CR.[49] Nonetheless, the poor results of chemotherapy in all studies, and the relatively better results with allogeneic transplant in most studies, suggest that transplant remains the treatment of choice for patients with poor-risk cytogenetics in first CR.[50,51]

The study of clonal cytogenetic abnormalities has led to the discovery of abnormal and dysregulated genes that result in specific AML phenotypes. Gene expression profiles by microarray analysis confirm the prognostic relevance of cytogenetic risk groups and suggest that other risk groups may yet be identified.[52,53] For example, patients with normal cytogenetics have a

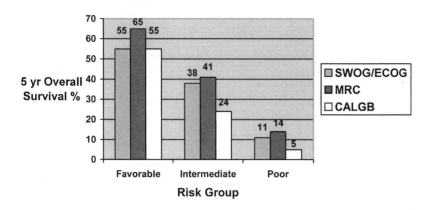

**Figure 8.1**   *Five-year overall survival in AML varies by cytogenetic risk group. SWOG/ ECOG, Southwest Oncology Group/Eastern Cooperative Oncology Group[43]; MRC, Medical Research Council of Great Britain[44]; CALGB, Cancer and Leukemia Group B[45]*

poor prognosis when FLT3 mutations are identified.[54–59] Conversely, the presence of CCAAT/enhancer binding protein-alpha (CEBP-α) mutations[60] and the presence of cytoplasmic nucleophosmin due to translocations involving the *NPM* gene seem to result in a more favorable prognosis.[61] The identification of prognostically relevant molecular pathways should allow for the development of small molecules capable of targeting these pathways and improving survival.

### Follow up

Recommendations for follow up of patients diagnosed with AML who undergo remission induction and postremission therapy and who attain a CR are somewhat arbitrary. While they are based on the recommendations of leukemia experts, they are not grounded in any evidence-based literature that the degree and frequency of surveillance translates to earlier detection of recurrent leukemia, or that this would result in improved survival.

The National Comprehensive Cancer Network has published guidelines on surveillance of AML patients who have attained a remission.[62] This group recom-

mends routinely following patients with complete blood cell counts every 2–3 months for the first 2 years following attainment of remission, and then every 4–6 months for 3 more years, for a total of 5 years of follow up. Bone marrow biopsies should be obtained only in the setting of worrisome peripheral blood counts, and not otherwise regularly, unless a patient is enrolled in a clinical trial that calls for this surveillance.

We recommend obtaining a bone marrow biopsy and aspirate at the conclusion of postremission therapy to document a CR. As is shown in Figure 8.2, we then follow patients with complete blood cell counts every month for 1 year after the postremission therapy CR, and then every 2 months for 1 year. For the third year, we follow patients every 3–4 months for 1 year, and then for years 4–5, every 4–6 months for 2 years, for a total of 5 years of follow up. We further recommend obtaining bone marrow biopsies only in the setting of worrisome blood counts, and urge assessment of cytogenetics at those times to document persistent disease on a molecular level or cytogenetic evolution, which could indicate disease progression and/or treatment-related bone marrow disorders. During the

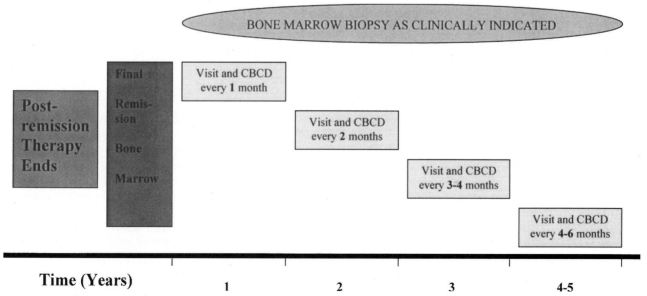

**Figure 8.2**   *Routine follow up of AML patients. CBCD, complete blood cell count with differential*

follow-up period, patients should also resume contact and routine checkups with their primary care physicians.

## SUMMARY

Established criteria should be used to establish whether or not AML patients have entered a remission following standard chemotherapy regimens. Prognostic factors, particularly cytogenetics, are useful in determining the most appropriate risk-adapted approach to postremission therapy, which may include bone marrow transplantation for those in high-risk AML groups. Patients should be followed for 5 years after postremission therapy with routine blood tests, with bone marrow examinations reserved only for suspicion of relapsed disease.

## REFERENCES

1. Sekeres MA, Stone RM, Zahrieh D, et al.: Decision-making and quality of life in older adults with acute myeloid leukemia or advanced myelodysplastic syndrome. *Leukemia* 18(4):809–816, 2004.
2. Pui CH, Ribeiro RC, Hancock ML, et al.: Acute myeloid leukemia in children treated with epipodophyllotoxins for acute lymphoblastic leukemia. *N Engl J Med* 325(24):1682–1687, 1991.
3. Stone RM: The difficult problem of acute myeloid leukemia in the older adult. *CA Cancer J Clin* 52(6):363–371, 2002 .
4. Cheson BD, Cassileth PA, Head DR, et al.: Report of the National Cancer Institute—sponsored workshop on definitions of diagnosis and response in acute myeloid leukemia. *J Clin Oncol* 8(5):813–819, 1990.
5. Vardiman JW, Harris NL, Brunning RD: The World Health Organization (WHO) classification of the myeloid neoplasms. *Blood* 100(7):2292–2302, 2002.
6. Harris NL, Jaffe ES, Diebold J, et al.: The World Health Organization classification of neoplastic diseases of the hematopoietic and lymphoid tissues. Report of the Clinical Advisory Committee meeting, Airlie House, Virginia, November, 1997. *Ann Oncol* 10(12):1419–1432, 1999.
7. Grimwade D, Walker H, Oliver F, et al.: The importance of diagnostic cytogenetics on outcome in AML: analysis of 1,612 patients entered into the MRC AML 10 trial. The Medical Research Council Adult and Children's Leukaemia Working Parties. *Blood* 92(7):2322–2333, 1998.
8. Bloomfield CD, Lawrence D, Byrd JC, et al.: Frequency of prolonged remission duration after high-dose cytarabine intensification in acute myeloid leukemia varies by cytogenetic subtype. *Cancer Res* 58(18):4173–4179, 1998.
9. Leith CP, Kopecky KJ, Chen IM, et al.: Frequency and clinical significance of the expression of the multidrug resistance proteins MDR1/P-glycoprotein, MRP1, and LRP in acute myeloid leukemia: a Southwest Oncology Group study. *Blood* 94(3):1086–1099, 1999.
10. Leith CP, Kopecky KJ, Godwin J, et al.: Acute myeloid leukemia in the elderly: assessment of multidrug resistance (MDR1) and cytogenetics distinguishes biologic subgroups with remarkably distinct responses to standard chemotherapy. A Southwest Oncology Group study. *Blood* 89(9):3323–3329, 1997.
11. Cheson BD, Bennett JM, Kopecky KJ, et al.: Revised recommendations of the International Working Group for Diagnosis, Standardization of Response Criteria, Treatment Outcomes, and Reporting Standards for Therapeutic Trials in Acute Myeloid Leukemia. *J Clin Oncol* 21(24):4642–4649, 2003.
12. Jurcic JG, Nimer SD, Scheinberg DA, DeBlasio T, Warrell RP Jr, Miller WH Jr: Prognostic significance of minimal residual disease detection and PML/RAR-alpha isoform type: long-term follow-up in acute promyelocytic leukemia. *Blood* 98(9):2651–2656, 2001.
13. Branford S, Hughes TP, Rudzki Z, et al.: Monitoring chronic myeloid leukaemia therapy by real-time quantitative PCR in blood is a reliable alternative to bone marrow cytogenetics. Monitoring of BCR-ABL expression using real-time RT-PCR in CML after bone marrow or peripheral blood stem cell transplantation. *Br J Haematol* 107(3):587–599, 1999.
14. Eder M, Battmer K, Kafert S, Stucki A, Ganser A, Hertenstein B: Monitoring of BCR-ABL expression using real-time RT-PCR in CML after bone marrow or peripheral blood stem cell transplantation. *Leukemia* 13(9):1383–1389, 1999.
15. Marin D, Kaeda J, Szydlo R, et al.: Monitoring patients in complete cytogenetic remission after treatment of CML in chronic phase with imatinib: patterns of residual leukaemia and prognostic factors for cytogenetic relapse. *Leukemia* 19(4):507–512, 2005.
16. Sievers EL, Larson RA, Stadtmauer EA, et al.: Efficacy and safety of Mylotarg (gemtuzumab ozogamicin) in patients with CD33-positive acute myeloid leukemia in first relapse. *J Clin Oncol* 19:3244–3254, 2001.
17. Sievers E, Larson R, Estey E, et al.: Comparison of the efficacy and safety of gemtuzumab ozogamicin (CMA-676) in patients <60 and >60 years of age with AML in first relapse. *Proc Am Soc Clin Oncol* 19:8a, 2000.
18. Mayer RJ, Davis RB, Schiffer CA, et al.: Intensive postremission chemotherapy in adults with acute myeloid leukemia. *N Engl J Med* 331:896–903, 1994.
19. Zittoun RA, Mandelli F, Willemze R, et al.: Autologous or allogeneic bone marrow transplantation compared with intensive chemotherapy in acute myelogenous leukemia. European Organization for Research and Treatment of Cancer (EORTC) and the Gruppo Italiano Malattie Ematologiche Maligne dell'Adulto (GIMEMA) Leukemia Cooperative Groups [see comments]. *N Engl J Med* 332(4):217–223, 1995.
20. Cassileth PA, Harrington DP, Appelbaum FR, et al.: Chemotherapy compared with autologous or allogeneic bone marrow transplantation in the management of acute myeloid leukemia in first remission. *N Engl J Med* 339(23):1649–1656, 1998.

21. Wheatley K, Burnett AK, Goldstone AH, et al.: A simple, robust, validated and highly predictive index for the determination of risk-directed therapy in acute myeloid leukaemia derived from the MRC AML 10 trial. *Br J Haematol* 107:69–79, 1999.

22. Gajewski JL, Ho WG, Nimer SD, et al.: Efficacy of intensive chemotherapy for acute myelogenous leukemia associated with a preleukemic syndrome. *J Clin Oncol* 7(11):1637–1645, 1989.

23. Goasguen JE, Matsuo T, Cox C, Bennett JM : Evaluation of the dysmyelopoiesis in 336 patients with de novo acute myeloid leukemia: major importance of dysgranulopoiesis for remission and survival. *Leukemia* 6:520–525, 1992.

24. Brito-Babapulle F, Catovsky D, Galton DA: Myelodysplastic relapse of de novo acute myeloid leukemia with trilineage myelodysplasia: a previously unrecognized correlation. *Br J Haematol* 68:411–415, 1988.

25. Hoyle CF, De Bastios M, Wheatley K, et al.: AML associated with previous cytotoxic therapy, MDS, or myeloproliferative disorders: results from the MRC's 9th AML trial. *Br J Haematol* 72:45–53, 1989.

26. Mesa RA, Li C-Y, Ketterling RP, Schroeder GS, Knudson RA, Tefferi A: Leukemic transformation in myelofibrosis with myeloid metaplasia: a single-institution experience with 91 cases. *Blood* 105(3):973–977, 2005.

27. Kantarjian HM, Estey EH, Keating MJ: Treatment of therapy-related leukemia and myelodysplastic syndrome. *Hematol Oncol Clin North Am* 7(1):81–108, 1993.

28. Josting A, Wiedenmann S, Franklin J, et al.: Secondary myeloid leukemia and myelodysplastic syndromes in patients treated for hodgkin's disease: a report from the German Hodgkin's Lymphoma Study Group. *J Clin Oncol* 21(18):3440–3446, 2003.

29. Smith SM, Le Beau MM, Huo D, et al.: Clinical-cytogenetic associations in 306 patients with therapy-related myelodysplasia and myeloid leukemia: the University of Chicago series. *Blood* 102(1):43–52, 2003.

30. Schoch C, Kern W, Schnittger S, Hiddemann W, Haferlach T: Karyotype is an independent prognostic parameter in therapy-related acute myeloid leukemia (t-AML): an analysis of 93 patients with t-AML in comparison to 1091 patients with de novo AML. *Leukemia* 18:120–125, 2004.

31. Fenaux P, Lucidarme D, Lai JL, Bauters F: Favorable cytogenetic abnormalities in secondary leukemia. *Cancer* 63:2505–2508, 1989.

32. Mistry AR, Felix CA, Whitmarsh RJ, et al.: DNA topoisomerase II in therapy-related acute promyelocytic leukemia. *N Engl J Med* 352(15):1529–1538, 2005.

33. Beaumont M, Sanz M, Carli PM, et al.: Therapy-related acute promyelocytic leukemia. *J Clin Oncol* 21(11):2123–2137, 2003.

34. Preisler H, Davis RB, Kirshner J, et al.: Comparison of three remission induction regimens and two postinduction strategies for the treatment of acute nonlymphocytic leukemia: a Cancer and Leukemia Group B study. *Blood* 69(5):1441–1449, 1987.

35. Swirsky DM, De Bastios M, Parish SE, Rees JKH, Hayhoe FGJ: Features affecting outcome during remission induction of acute myeloid leukaemia in 619 adult patients. *Br J Haematol* 64:435–453, 1986.

36. Sekeres MA, Peterson B, Dodge RK, et al.: Differences in prognostic factors and outcomes in African Americans and whites with acute myeloid leukemia. *Blood* 103(11):4036–4042, 2004.

37. Kalaycio M, Pohlman B, Elson P, et al.: Chemotherapy for acute myelogenous leukemia in the elderly with cytarabine, mitoxantrone, and granulocyte-macrophage colony stimulating factor. *Am J Clin Oncol* 24:58–63, 2001.

38. Abou-Jawde R, Sobecks RM, Pohlman B, Rybicki L, Kalaycio M: Lactate dehydrogenase level is an adverse risk factor for survival in elderly patients with acute myelogenous leukemia. *Blood* 102:Abstract 4594, 2003.

39. Rowe JM, Neuberg D, Friedenberg W, et al.: A phase 3 study of three induction regimens and of priming with GM-CSF in older adults with acute myeloid leukemia: a trial by the Eastern Cooperative Oncology Group. *Blood* 103(2):479–485, 2004.

40. Sekeres MA, Rybicki L, Sobecks RM, et al.: The time interval from diagnosis of acute myeloid leukemia in older adults to start of remission induction therapy predicts survival. *Blood* 102:Abstract 3257, 2003.

41. Han HS, Rybicki L, Kalaycio M, et al.: The Nadir peripheral white blood cell count following remission induction therapy in older adults with acute myeloid leukemia predicts survival. *Blood* 102:Abstract 4679, 2003.

42. Grimwade D, Walker H, Harrison G, et al. The predictive value of hierarchical cytogenetic classification in older adults with acute myeloid leukemia (AML): analysis of 1065 patients entered into the United Kingdom Medical Research Council AML11 trial. *Blood* 98(5):1312–1320, 2001.

43. Slovak ML, Kopecky KJ, Cassileth PA, et al.: Karyotypic analysis predicts outcome of preremission and postremission therapy in adult acute myeloid leukemia: a Southwest Oncology Group/Eastern Cooperative Oncology Group study. *Blood* 96(13):4075–4083, 2000.

44. Grimwade D, Walker H, Oliver F, et al.: The importance of diagnostic cytogenetics on outcome in AML: analysis of 1,612 patients entered into the MRC AML 10 trial. *Blood* 92(7):2322–2333, 1998.

45. Byrd JC, Mrozek K, Dodge RK, et al.: Pretreatment cytogenetic abnormalities are predictive of induction success, cumulative incidence of relapse, and overall survival in adult patients with de novo acute myeloid leukemia: results from Cancer and Leukemia Group B (CALGB 8461). *Blood* 100(13):4325–4336, 2002.

46. Byrd JC, Ruppert AS, Krzysztof M, et al.: Repetitive cycles of high-dose cytarabine benefit patients with acute myeloid leukemia and inv(16)(p13q22) or t(16;16) (p13;q22): results from CALGB 8461. *J Clin Oncol* 22:1087–1094, 2004.

47. Byrd JC, Dodge RK, Carroll A, et al.: Patients with t(8;21)(q22;q22) and acute myeloid leukemia have superior failure-free and overall survival when repetitive cycles of high-dose cytarabine are administered. *J Clin Oncol* 17:3767–3775, 1999.

48. Bradstock KF, Matthews JP, Lowenthal RM, et al.: A randomized trial of high-versus conventional-dose cytarabine in consolidation chemotherapy for adult de novo acute myeloid leukemia in first remission after induction therapy containing high-dose cytarabine. *Blood* 105(2):481–488, 2005.

49. Burnett AK, Wheatley K, Goldstone AH, et al.: The value of allogeneic bone marrow transplant in patients with acute myeloid leukaemia at differing risk of relapse: results of the UK MRC AML 10 trial. *Br J Haematol* 118(2):385–400, 2002.

50. Drobyski W: The role of allogeneic transplantation in high-risk acute myelogenous leukemia. *Leukemia* 18:1565–1568, 2004.

51. Yanada M, Matsuo K, Emi N, Naoe T: Efficacy of allogeneic hematopoietic stem cell transplantation depends on cytogenetic risk for acute myeloid leukemia in first disease remission. *Cancer* 103:1652–1658, 2005.

52. Valk PJM, Verhaak RGW, Beijen MA, et al.: Prognostically useful gene-expression profiles in acute myeloid leukemia. *N Engl J Med* 350(16):1617–1628, 2004.

53. Bullinger L, Dohner K, Bair E, et al.: Use of gene-expression profiling to identify prognostic subclasses in adult acute myeloid leukemia. *N Engl J Med* 350(16):1605–1616, 2004.

54. Frohling S, Schlenk RF, Breitruck J, et al.: Prognostic significance of activating FLT3 mutations in younger adults (16 to 60 years) with acute myeloid leukemia and normal cytogenetics: a study of the AML Study Group Ulm. *Blood* 100(13):4372–4380, 2002.

55. Kiyoi H, Naoe T, Nakano Y, et al.: Prognostic implication of FLT3 and N-RAS gene mutations in acute myeloid leukemia. *Blood* 93(9):3074–3080, 1999.

56. Kottaridis PD, Gale RE, Frew ME, et al.: The presence of a FLT3 internal tandem duplication in patients with acute myeloid leukemia (AML) adds important prognostic information to cytogenetic risk group and response to the first cycle of chemotherapy: analysis of 854 patients from the United Kingdom Medical Research Council AML 10 and 12 trials. *Blood* 98(6):1752–1759, 2001.

57. Ozeki K, Kiyoi H, Hirose Y, et al.: Biologic and clinical significance of the FLT3 transcript level in acute myeloid leukemia. *Blood* 103(5):1901–1908, 2004.

58. Schnittger S, Schoch C, Dugas M, et al.: Analysis of FLT3 length mutations in 1003 patients with acute myeloid leukemia: correlation to cytogenetics, FAB subtype, and prognosis in the AMLCG study and usefulness as a marker for the detection of minimal residual disease. *Blood* 100(1):59–66, 2002.

59. Thiede C, Steudel C, Mohr B, et al.: Analysis of FLT3-activating mutations in 979 patients with acute myelogenous leukemia: association with FAB subtypes and identification of subgroups with poor prognosis. *Blood* 99(12):4326–4335, 2002.

60. Frohling S, Schlenk RF, Stolze I, et al.: CEBPA Mutations in younger adults with acute myeloid leukemia and normal cytogenetics: prognostic relevance and analysis of cooperating mutations. *J Clin Oncol* 22:624–633, 2004.

61. Falini B, Mecucci C, Tiacci E, et al.: Cytoplasmic nucleophosmin in acute myelogenous leukemia with a normal karyotype. *N Engl J Med* 2005;352(3):254–266.

62. NCCN Practice Guidelines in Oncology v.2.2005—Acute Myeloid Leukemia. 2005. Available at: http://www.nccn.org/professionals/physician_gls/PDF/aml.pdf. Accessed June 6, 2005.

# Chapter 9

# TREATMENT OF RELAPSED OR REFRACTORY ACUTE MYELOID LEUKEMIA AND NEW FRONTIERS IN ACUTE MYELOID LEUKEMIA THERAPY

*Frederick R. Appelbaum*

## INTRODUCTION

While there are few easy problems in medical oncology, caring for the patient with relapsed or refractory acute myeloid leukemia (AML) is among the most challenging. Patients and their families are understandably disappointed, frightened, and desperate upon learning that initial therapy did not provide the hoped for results. And their concerns are justified, as treatment for recurrent leukemia is generally far less effective than initial therapy. Further, the physician has only a limited amount of information to help in the selection of therapy since, while there are a large number of studies and review articles dealing with initial therapy of AML, far less is written about recurrent disease. There is also much greater heterogeneity among patients by the time they relapse than at initial diagnosis. Despite, or better, because of the challenges posed by recurrent AML, there are many good reasons to focus on the topic. Given our current abilities and success rates in treating de novo AML, the majority of patients with AML will eventually fall into this category. Further, although outcomes are not outstanding, many patients who have relapsed can still be cured. And finally, this is where research is most needed.

## DEFINITIONS

Although the terms "primary induction failure," "relapsed," and "refractory" are often used, consistent definitions are lacking. "Primary induction failure" is generally used to describe those patients who fail to respond to an initial induction attempt. What constitutes an "induction attempt" is less certain. If induction is taken to mean a single cycle of standard-dose cytarabine plus daunomycin, at least 40% of failing patients will achieve a complete remission (CR) with a second cycle of treatment.[1,2] Although failure to achieve a CR with one cycle of therapy ultimately indicates a poor prognosis, because almost half of patients who fail a single cycle will still achieve a CR with a second cycle of the same therapy, the term primary induction failure should be reserved for patients who fail two cycles of standard-dose therapy. Less is known about patients who fail a single-induction cycle containing high-dose cytarabine. The term "refractory AML" has been used to describe a subset of relapsed AML that is unlikely to respond to further salvage chemotherapy. Hiddemann et al. were among the first to provide a system of definitions and, based on a study of 180 patients, defined "refractory" as patients who had failed initial induction therapy, those who relapsed within 6–12 months of first CR, and those in second or subsequent relapse.[3] Estey et al. performed a retrospective study of 206 patients treated with chemotherapy for recurrent AML at the MD Anderson Cancer Center and were able to identify four groups, based principally on the duration of first CR.[4] Patients with an initial CR in excess of 2 years had a 73% likelihood of obtaining a second CR. Those with an initial CR duration of 1–2 years had a 47% CR rate. Patients with an initial CR lasting less than 1 year or with no initial CR receiving their first salvage attempt had a subsequent

| Table 9.1 | Categories of previously treated active leukemia |
|---|---|
| Category | Comment |
| Primary induction failure | Following two cycles of conventional dose therapy |
| Refractory | First relapse after initial remission of <6 months duration, or second or subsequent relapse |
| Relapse, poor risk | First relapse after initial remission of 6–24 months |
| Relapse, good risk | First relapse after initial remission of >24 months |
| Posttransplant relapse | |

CR rate of 14%. And those receiving a second or subsequent salvage attempt had a 0% CR rate. Both Hiddemann's and Estey's definitions focused on the likelihood of obtaining a second CR. In a subsequent publication, Estey et al. also considered the likelihood of obtaining long-term survival without transplantation and reported that the only group of nontransplanted relapsed patients with survival above 10% 2 years after salvage therapy was the group with an initial CR duration of greater than 2 years.[5] The studies described so far were limited to patients who received aggressive chemotherapy as their initial treatment. Few studies describe the course of patients with AML who relapse after receiving hematopoietic cell transplantation (HCT) as first-line therapy, where it has been examined that the time from marrow transplantation to relapse was the most important predictor of response to reinduction therapy.[6] Thus, at present, as shown in Table 9.1, at least five categories of patients can be defined based on the therapeutic options available to them, their likelihood of obtaining a subsequent remission, and the probability of remaining in remission: primary induction failure, refractory AML, relapsed poor prognosis AML, relapsed favorable prognosis AML, and posttransplant relapse.

There are data to suggest that patient's age, performance status, and cytogenetics also predict the likelihood of obtaining a second CR with salvage chemotherapy. For example, in a review of 254 patients undergoing reinduction therapy, Kern et al. reported that early death during reinduction most closely correlated with patient age, while unfavorable chromosomal abnormalities were associated with a lower CR rate.[7] However, in a multivariate analysis, the only factor associated with time to treatment failure was the duration of first remission. Thus, at present, few data suggest that there are factors independent of the ability to obtain a first CR and its duration to predict response rates or duration following salvage chemotherapy.

There are several categories of patients excluded from the above definition system. Patients with acute promyelocytic leukemia are not included, as their therapy is now so distinct from that used for the majority of AML patients. Also not included are the very elderly or infirm who were not initially treated with aggressive chemotherapy, or who at relapse are not considered to be candidates for such treatment.

## COMBINATION CHEMOTHERAPY FOR PATIENTS IN FIRST RELAPSE

### RETROSPECTIVE STUDIES

A number of retrospective studies have described the outcome of combination chemotherapy for patients with AML in first relapse. At least five have included more than 100 patients (see Table 9.2).[3,8–11] Most of these reports were summaries of multiple regimens and included a fairly wide range of categories of patients. In these five studies, the early death rate ranged from 8 to 32% and the CR rate varied from 30 to 51%. The duration of CR2 was in the range of 5–7.5 months, and the median survival in these trials was 4–10 months. While it is difficult to extract principles of treatment from these retrospective studies, they do provide a realistic sense of what can be expected with fairly standard chemotherapy. They also help confirm the influence of duration of CR on subsequent outcome and the influence of age. For example, in the study reported by Keating et al., the CR rate was 62% in those with a first CR of longer than 12 months versus 19% in those with a shorter first remission, and the CR rates were 36% in those younger than 60 versus 14% in those older than 60 years.[9] While a number of other smaller retrospective studies have reported somewhat more encouraging results, the potential impact of patient selection and the biases imposed by the choice to report and publish these series is substantial, arguing that such studies should be interpreted with considerable caution.

### PROSPECTIVE PHASE II TRIALS

A number of prospective phase II trials exploring various regimens as treatment for AML in first relapse have been published and are included in the excellent summary by Leopold and willemze (see Table 9.3).[12–27] These have generally included a fairly limited number

| Table 9.2 | | Large retrospective reports of treatment of AML in first relapse | |
|---|---|---|---|
| Author | N | CR2 (%) | CR2 median duration (months) | 3-Year survival (%) |
| Rees et al.[8] | 485 | 30 | NA[1] | NA |
| Keating et al.[9] | 187 | 33 | 6 | 8 |
| Thalhammer et al.[10] | 168 | 39 | 7.5 | 19 |
| Hiddemann et al.[3] | 136 | 51 | 5 | <10 |
| Davis et al.[11] | 126 | 40 | 7 | 18 |

N, number; CR2, second complete remission; NA, not available.

**Table 9.3** Selected prospective phase ii studies of chemotherapy for AML in first relapse

| Author et al. | Regimen[a] | N | CR2 (%) | CR2 duration (months) | 3-Year survival (%) |
|---|---|---|---|---|---|
| Archimbaud et al.[12] | MEC | 63 | 76 | 8 | 11 |
| Vignetti et al.[13] | MEC | 50 | 68 | 4 | 29 |
| Carella et al.[14] | ICE | 50 | 50 | 4 | NA |
| Sternberg et al.[15] | IDAC+Mito | 47 | 62 | NA | NA |
| Harousseau et al.[16] | IDAC+IdA | 35 | 60 | 4.5 | NA |
| Peters et al.[17] | IDAC+mAMSA | 27 | 56 | NA | NA |
| Brito-Babapulle et al.[18] | IDAC+Mito | 26 | 58 | 8 | NA |
| Ferrara et al.[19] | FLAG | 26 | 50 | 13 | NA |
| Estey et al.[20] | FA | 25 | 40 | 10 | NA |
| Saito et al.[21] | IDAC+Acl+G | 23 | 87 | NA | 20 |
| Jehn and Heinemann et al.[22] | IDAC+mAMSA | 23 | 78 | 3.3 | 10 |
| Pavlovsky et al.[23] | Ara-c+Rub | 22 | 54 | 4 | NA |
| Kornblau et al.[24] | CECA | 22 | 14 | NA | NA |
| Harousseau et al.[25] | IDAC+Mito | 20 | 60 | NA | NA |
| Ho et al.[26] | Mito+E | 20 | 45 | 5 | NA |

[a]MEC, mitoxantrone, etoposide, cytarabine; ICE, idarubicin, cytarabine, etoposide; IDAC, intermediate-dose cytarabine; Mito, mitoxantrone; IdA, idarubicin; FLAG, fludarabine, cytarabine, granulocyte colony-stimulating factor; FA, fludarabine, cytarabine; Acl, aclarubicin; Rub, rubidizone; CECA, cyclophosphamide, etoposide, carboplatin, cytarabine; E, etoposide; NA, not available.

of patients (from 20 to 63) and have reported CR rates ranging from 40 to 68%. Given the relatively small size of these studies and the potential powerful influence of patient selection on outcome, it is difficult to evaluate the relative merits of these regimens based on these reports. Nonetheless, several of the regimens described in these papers have found their way into common usage. For example, combinations of mitoxantrone, etoposide, and cytarabine (MEC) produced response rates of 60–68% as described by Archimbaud et al. and Vignetti et al. and are now commonly used.[12,13] The

FLAG regimen combining fludarabine, cytarabine, and granulocyte colony-stimulating factor (G-CSF) provided a 50% response rate and is likewise commonly prescribed.[19] These regimens have not been compared in any systematic manner to other regimens.

### PROSPECTIVE RANDOMIZED PHASE III TRIALS
A limited number of phase III randomized trials focusing on the treatment of recurrent AML have been published (see Table 9.4). In a study addressing the question of cytarabine dosing, Kern et al. compared high-dose

**Table 9.4** Randomized trials of AML in first relapse

| Author | Regimen[a] | N | CR2 (%) | CR2 duration (months) | 3-Year survival (%) |
|---|---|---|---|---|---|
| Kern et al.[28] | HiDAC+Mito | 73 | 52 | 5 | NA |
| | IDAC+Mito | 113 | 44 | 3 | NA |
| Vogler et al.[29] | HiDAC | 47 | 40 | 12 | 8 |
| | HiDAC+E | 44 | 45 | 25 | 12 |
| Karanes et al.[b30] | HiDAC | 81 | 32 | 9 | 8 |
| | HiDAC+Mito | 81 | 44 | 5 | 13 |
| Thomas et al.[31] | MEC | 36 | 81 | 4 | 18 |
| | MEC+GM | 36 | 89 | 5 | 18 |
| Ohno et al.[32] | MEC | 26 | 42 | 14 | NA |
| | MEC+G | 24 | 54 | 12 | NA |
| List et al.[c33] | IDAC+D | 107 | 33 | 6 | 9 |
| | IDAC+D+CSP | 119 | 39 | 9 | 20 |

[a]HiDAC, high-dose cytarabine; Mito, mitoxantrone; IDAC, intermediate-dose cytarabine; E, etoposide; MEC, mitoxantrone, etoposide, cytarabine; GM, granulocyte macrophage colony-stimulating factor; G, granulocyte colony-stimulating factor; D, daunomycin; CSP, cyclosporine; NA, not available.
[b]Karanes study included patients with primary refractory disease and first relapse.
[c]List study included patients with primary refractory disease and first relapse (N=177) and patients with AML evolving from MDS (N=49).

versus intermediate-dose cytarabine when combined with mitoxantrone.[28] They reported a trend toward a higher CR rate (52% vs 44%) and a slightly longer duration of second remission (median of 5 vs 3 months) with the higher dose regimen. However, because of a greater early death rate with the higher dose regimen, no benefit in overall survival was seen.

Several studies have addressed the impact of adding other drugs to high-dose cytarabine. Vogler et al. asked whether there was any benefit from adding etoposide to high-dose cytarabine, and reported that CR rates were similar (40% with cytarabine alone vs 45% with cytarabine and etoposide).[29] They also did not see a difference in remission duration in the two arms of the study. Karanes et al. asked whether there was any benefit from adding mitoxantrone to high-dose cytarabine.[30] They reported a significantly higher CR rate with the addition, but no improvement in overall survival.

A third group of studies has attempted to evaluate the impact of the addition of hematopoietic growth factors to chemotherapy for recurrent AML. Thomas et al. asked whether the addition of granulocyte-macrophage colony-stimulating factor (GM-CSF) to the MEC combination improved outcome. In this study, GM-CSF was given during chemotherapy in an effort to recruit cells into cycle, thereby sensitizing them to GM-chemotherapy. The CR rates in both arms of the study were remarkably high (81% without GM-CSF vs 89% with CSF), but not different from each other.[31] The median survival was somewhat better than seen in other studies (8.5 vs 10 months, respectively). Ohno et al. studied the addition of G-CSF to the MEC combination and reported CR rates of 54% with G-CSF versus 42% without G-CSF.[32]

A final group of studies addressed whether inhibition of the multidrug-resistance pump using cyclosporine might benefit patients. In a randomized trial, List et al. found that adding cyclosporine to a combination of high-dose cytarabine and daunomycin led to significantly less treatment failure due to drug resistance, and improved both disease-free survival and overall survival.[33] However, a smaller study from the Dutch group, which tested the addition of cyclosporine to the combination of mitoxantrone and etoposide, found that although the CR rate was higher with cyclosporine (53% vs 43%), there was no improvement in overall survival, possible due to inadequate postinduction therapy as a result of the toxicities of the reinduction treatment.[34]

The experience of the Dutch group is typical. All of these aggressive reinduction regimens are accompanied by significant toxicities, including the risks of significant organ damage and the acquisition of infections, which may make further therapy, including HCT, difficult or impossible. Thus, the search for effective, less toxic therapies continues.

### SINGLE-AGENT THERAPY

Gemtuzumab ozogamicin consists of a humanized anti-CD33 antibody conjugated to a potent chemotherapeutic, calicheamicin. The drug was developed based on the observation that most AML blasts express CD33, while normal stem cells and nonhematopoietic tissue do not. By targeting CD33, an effective, less toxic therapeutic might result. A large trial in patients with AML in first relapse showed that gemtuzumab ozogamicin used as a single agent resulted in complete responses in 26% of patients (approximately half of whom attained a CR with the exception of platelet recovery, or a $CR_p$), and with less toxicity than might be expected with high-dose chemotherapy.[35] Based on these results, the drug was approved by the Food and Drug Administration for the treatment of older patients with recurrent AML in which blasts express CD33. Subsequent studies have shown that, in some combinations, gemtuzumab ozogamicin may contribute to the development of veno-occlusive disease of the liver, so that care should be taken in combining this agent.

## HEMATOPOIETIC CELL TRANSPLANTATION

### PRIMARY INDUCTION FAILURE

Several studies have shown that some patients who fail primary induction therapy can still be cured if treated with allogeneic transplantation. For example, the European Bone Marrow Transplant Group reported long-term survival in 20% of such patients treated with matched sibling transplantation.[36] These results emphasize the importance of HLA-typing patients and family members at the time of diagnosis so that valuable time will not be lost should induction therapy fail. This is particularly important if the patient does not have a matched sibling and an alternative source of stem cells, such as a matched unrelated donor or unrelated cord blood, must be identified.

### TRANSPLANTATION AS SALVAGE THERAPY FOR PATIENTS WITH MATCHED SIBLINGS

Although there are no randomized trials to prove the point, retrospective comparisons suggest that HCT should be considered for almost all patients of age 55 or less with matched siblings who relapse after an initial remission. There are occasional patients with long first remissions (greater than 2 years according to the MD Anderson data) who may do as well with chemotherapy, reserving transplantation for a subsequent relapse, but such patients are uncommon.[37]

Whether patients with AML in first relapse should undergo reinduction therapy before proceeding to transplant from a matched sibling is an unresolved question. A study from Seattle of 126 patients transplanted in untreated first relapse reported a 28% 5-year disease-free survival.[38] This result is only slightly less than what might be expected for matched sibling transplants for AML in second remission. For example, the European Transplant Group reported a 35% 3-year disease-free survival rate among 459 patients transplanted in second remission from matched siblings.[39] However, on an average only approximately 50% of patients in first relapse will be successfully reinduced, 10–15% may die during the reinduction attempt, and others may develop complications that would preclude subsequent transplantation. The results of transplantation in first relapse appear best in those without substantial numbers of circulating blasts. Thus, for those patients with matched siblings where relapse is found early, proceeding straight to allogeneic transplant can be recommended. However, for those with substantial numbers of circulating blasts or those for whom considerable time is required to identify the donor or arrange the logistics for transplantation, reinduction will be necessary.

Discussions of the separate elements of the transplant procedure are included in Chapter 92. However, there have been no randomized trials, addressing the best preparative regimen, source of stem cells, or form of graft-versus-host disease (GvHD) prophylaxis specifically focused on the treatment of AML in first relapse or second remission.

Because of the acute toxicities associated with the high-dose preparative regimens commonly used in the treatment of AML, as well as an increased incidence of GvHD in older patients, allogeneic transplantation in the past was generally restricted to younger patients, generally those less than age 55–60 years. It has long been appreciated that much of the antileukemic effects of allogeneic HCT came from the graft-versus-tumor (GvT) effect. Thus, in an effort to bring the benefits of allogeneic transplantation to an older population of patients, investigators have begun devising strategies to insure allogeneic engraftment without the use of high-dose therapy. A number of reduced-intensity regimens have been developed and used in the treatment of relapsed acute leukemia. These have varied in intensity from low-dose regimens, such as the Seattle regimen consisting of fludarabine 30 mg/kg for 3 days plus 200 cGy total body irradiation (TBI) with posttransplant mycophenolate mofetil and cyclosporine, to regimens of somewhat greater intensity, such as the busulfan 8 mg/kg, fludarabine, and antithymocyte globulin regimen.[40] The Seattle regimen is able to insure engraftment in the large majority of patients and, in patients ranging in age from 50 to greater than 70 years, has been associated with a 100-day nonrelapse mortality of 5–8% and an overall non-relapse mortality of less than 20%.[41] These reduced- intensity regimens have not been, in general, effective for patients in frank relapse, but results in second- remission patients are encouraging. The Seattle group recently reported on a group of 39 patients with AML in second remission who were not

candidates for ablative transplants and recorded the disease-free survival at 3 years as slightly in excess of 40%.[42]

### TRANSPLANTATION AS SALVAGE THERAPY FOR PATIENTS WITHOUT MATCHED SIBLINGS

Patients with AML in second remission but lacking matched family member donors are candidates for either autologous or matched unrelated HCT. Randomized trials comparing the two have not been reported. Relatively small individual trials of autologous transplantation in second remission report 3-year disease-free survival rates ranging from 21 to 52%, with registry data settling at about 30% disease-free survival.[43] Better results can be expected in patients with longer first remissions. A retrospective matched pair analysis of the outcome of 340 patients with AML in second remission treated with either autologous or matched sibling transplantation reported lower relapse rates and somewhat better survival with allogeneic transplantation (39% vs 30% at 4 years).[44] Less data are available about the use of matched unrelated donor transplants for AML in second remission. The 5-year survival rate reported by the National Marrow Donor Program in 473 patients was 31%.[45] Similar results have been published from single institutions.[46] A case-controlled study was conducted by the European Bone Marrow Transplant Group in which the outcome of 46 recipients of unrelated donor transplants for AML in second remission was compared with twice that many autologous recipients.[47] Long-term outcomes, as measured by overall survival, were similar between the groups. While this study has many shortcomings, including its retrospective nature and small sample size, without further data for direction, autologous transplantation might be considered as the best option for older patients and those with more favorable disease characteristics, such as longer first remission, while matched unrelated donor transplantation might be more appropriate for younger patients and those with more unfavorable disease.

Although the amount of data are much more limited, other sources of stem cells are being explored for patients without matched siblings or matched unrelated donors, including the use of haplomismatched donors and the use of cord blood transplants. Both of these approaches are discussed more fully in Chapters 36 and 97.

### TREATMENT OF POSTTRANSPLANT RELAPSE

Patients who relapse following hematopoietic cell transplant present a unique set of problems and, in some cases, opportunities for further therapy. Patients who relapse following an autologous transplant performed for AML in first CR often will respond to further chemotherapy, and the likelihood of response correlates with the length of first CR posttransplant. The results of second allogeneic transplants after failure of first autologous transplants have been reported.[48] Among 24 such patients, the 2-year disease-free survival was surprisingly high, at 46%. The majority of survivors were younger than 17 years and had failed a chemotherapy-only autologous transplant, so that a TBI-containing preparative regimen could be used for the subsequent allogeneic transplant. Such favorable results cannot be expected for older adults who fail a TBI-containing autologous transplant; a strategy of chemotherapy to induce a second remission followed by reduced-intensity allogeneic transplant is probably more appropriate.

Different options are available to the patient who relapses following an allogeneic transplant. Donor lymphocyte infusions (DLI) can, by themselves, induce CRS in 20–30% of patients.[49] Although experience is still limited, most data would suggest that long-term survival after DLI is more likely if patients are first treated back into CR with chemotherapy before receiving DLI. Significant toxicities can follow DLI, including transient marrow hypoplasia, and more importantly, significant GvHD. The extent of GvHD is related to both the total number of T- cells infused and the schedule, with less GVHD being associated with a fractionated infusion schedule. If patients have significant GVHD at the time of relapse, the risks of further DLI outweigh the possible gain, and for such patients options are generally limited to further chemotherapy or palliative care.

## SUMMARY OF TREATMENT OPTIONS FOR RELAPSED AND REFRACTORY AML

Enrolment of patients onto well-designed clinical trials should always be at or near the top of therapeutic options. However, if an appropriate clinical trial is not available or if patients decline participation, the following represents a brief summary of therapeutic options for patients with primary induction failure or recurrent AML.

The only curative approach for patients with AML who fail primary induction is allogeneic HCT, so every effort should be made to identify a donor and proceed to transplant if the patient is a suitable candidate. If no donor is available, investigational or palliative therapy should be considered.

In considering therapeutic approaches for patients with AML who achieve a CR and then relapse, the first question to address is whether the individual patient is a possible candidate for an ablative transplant approach. If so, and if the patient is in early relapse and is known to have a matched sibling, proceeding directly to an allogeneic transplant is recommended. An autologous transplant in untreated first relapse can also be considered if stem cells were stored in first remission and the first remission was of reasonable length. If the patient is a candidate for an ablative

transplant but a donor has not been identified, no stem cells were stored, or there are substantial numbers of circulating blasts at the time relapse, then reinduction therapy is needed. Although the published literature does not permit the identification of a single regimen as the best, based on randomized trials regimens combining high-dose cytarabine with a second agent seem justified, and in at least one randomized trial the use of a multidrug-resistance inhibitor seemed to further improve outcome.[33]

If patients are not transplantation candidates because of age or comorbidities, the wisdom of using aggressive chemotherapy with their accompanying toxicities should be questioned, and consideration for the use of less aggressive therapy, such as single-agent gemtuzumab ozogamicin, might be considered.

## NEW FRONTIERS IN AML THERAPY

### IMPROVED DIAGNOSTICS

In a relatively short time, the application of cytogenetics to clinical decision making in AML has become almost second nature—patients with t(15;17) require all-*trans*-retinoic acid, those with t(8;21) or inv(16) can be successfully managed with chemotherapy alone, while those with monosomy 7 or complex abnormalities may benefit from allogeneic transplant. Given recent advances in gene expression array analyses and, perhaps, proteomics as well, there is every reason to think that many more markers predictive of outcome should be forthcoming.[50,51] In addition to the increased information to be gained at diagnosis, it is almost certain that we should be able to develop tests that will be capable of assaying the results of initial therapy and thus guide further treatment. Quantitative polymerase chain reaction (PCR) assays with considerable predictive power are already being applied to the treatment of accute promyelocytic leukemia and chronic myeloid leukemia (CML).[52,53] The lack of consistent translocations makes it more difficult to develop PCR-based tests widely applicable to all AMLs, but encouraging data with multicolor flow cytometry are emerging.[54] Even without the development of any new therapies, the ability to predict those patients unlikely to be cured with chemotherapy alone and to be able to offer them a bone marrow transplant in first remission, and at the same time spare those likely cured with chemotherapy unnecessary transplant, should improve substantially the overall therapy of AML.

### EMERGING THERAPIES
#### New therapies targeting mutational events
Mutations in receptor tyrosine kinases can be found in a substantial proportion of AML cases. The most commonly affected enzyme is FLT3, which is mutated in approximately 30–35% of cases.[55,56] The majority of

these mutations are internal tandem repeats in the juxtamembrane domain, while a lesser number are point mutations in the activation loop of FLT3. Both types of mutations lead to constitutive activation of the tyrosine kinase and stimulation of growth-related signaling. Retroviral transduction of the activated enzyme into mice results in a myeloproliferative syndrome, but further mutations are required for the development of full-blown leukemia.[57] FLT3 mutations are more commonly seen in t(15;17) and t(6;9) AMLs, but only rarely seen with −7, −5, t(8;21), inv(16), or with mutated RAS.[58] The presence of FLT3 is correlated with a higher white count at diagnosis and a poorer overall outcome of treatment.[59,60] Given the prominent role of FLT3 mutations in AML, efforts have been made to identify and develop compounds capable of inhibiting this tyrosine kinase. At least four compounds have entered clinical trials (reviewed in Ref. 61). CEP-701 (Cephelon, Inc, West Chester, PA) is an indolocarbazole derivative that has entered phase II clinical trials. CT53518 is a piperazinyl quinazoline and is in phase I studies. PKC412 (Novartis Pharmaceuticals, Bazel, Switzerland) is a benzolystaurosporine and has been examined in phase II trials. SU11248 (Sugen, San Francisco, CA) has been examined in a phase I study. While it is too early to reach definitive conclusions, the results of early studies to date show biologic activity of all of these compounds with lowering of blast counts in peripheral blood and marrow.[61] However, sustained complete remissions have not been seen with any frequency, suggesting that, unlike the situation with the tyrosine kinase inhibitor imatinib in CML, it will be necessary to combine kinase inhibitors with other drugs to get any substantial clinical benefits.

c-KIT and FMS are other receptor tyrosine kinases sometimes mutated or overexpressed in AML.[62,63] In a study of SU5416, an inhibitor of c-KIT, only 1 of 38 c-KIT-positive AML patients had a complete response, but 7 had substantial reduction in AML blast counts.[64]

RAS proteins are a group of signaling molecules downstream of many tyrosine kinase receptors which, following receipt of a signal, activate a broad range of proteins involved in cell proliferation and survival including the MAP/ERK kinase involved in cell proliferation, Rac and Rho, which affect cytoskeletal organization, and PI-3 kinase, which opposes apoptosis. Mutations in RAS are found in 15–20% of AML cases, most commonly in N-RAS.[65] RAS proteins are internally synthesized as cytosol precursors and require the addition of a farnesyl group to attach to the cell membrane and transmit signals. Therefore, there was a great interest in exploring farnesyltransferase inhibitors in AML, particularly in those cases with RAS mutations. The most encouraging data to date have been with R115777. In an initial dose-escalation study, central nervous system toxicity was found to be dose limiting at 1200 mg b.i.d. Two complete responses and eight partial responses were seen among 35 patients with recurrent myeloid malig-

nancies.[66] Recent data suggest a higher degree of activity when used in previously untreated patients. Several other farnesyltransferase inhibitors are under study.

Histones are proteins closely associated with chromatin which, in the unacetylated state, anchor the associated chromatin and repress local transcription but, when acetylated, become less anchored to chromatin allowing the structure to relax, unwind, and permit transcription. In certain AMLs, including t(8;21) and t(15;17), the abnormal fusion product resulting from the translocation is thought to bind to its normal promoter target, but also bind the transcriptional repressor complex that includes a histone deacetylase, resulting in deacetylation of the region and thus repression of gene transcription.[67] The repression of these genes may inhibit cell maturation, differentiation, and apoptosis and thus may be important in the leukemic process. On this basis, molecules that inhibit histone deacetylases are being studied as antileukemic agents, including phenylbutyrate, trichostatin, trapoxin, and depsipeptide.[68]

### New therapies targeting adaptive responses

The mutational events that give rise to AML may require the cell to make other adaptive changes in order to survive, particularly when stressed. Since these adaptive changes are not required of normal cells, inhibiting them may result in specific damage or death to AML cells and may specifically sensitize leukemic cells to conventional chemotherapy. One example of such an adaptive change is *Bcl-2*, the antiapoptotic gene that is overexpressed in almost all AML samples, and whose expression is further increased following exposure to chemotherapy.[69,70] An antisense Bcl-2 compound can sensitize AML cells to cytarabine in vitro, providing a strong rationale for ongoing clinical trials combining Bcl-2 antisense with chemotherapy in patients with recurrent AML.[71]

Following exposure to cell-damaging agents, AML blasts markedly increase their cholesterol content, and do so to a much greater degree than do normal bone marrow progenitors. Blocking cholesterol synthesis using mevastatin or zaragozic acid specifically sensitizes most AML cell lines and patient AML samples without a discernible effect on normal hematopoietic progenitors.[72] Dimitroulakos et al. and Wong et al. showed that lovastatin, another inhibitor of de novo cholesterol synthesis, killed six of seven AML cell lines and 13 of 22 primary AML cell cultures.[73,74] Based on these results, current trials are under way, testing combinations of standard chemotherapy combined with increasing doses of statins.

### New immunotherapeutic approaches

Both antibody- and cell-based immunotherapeutic approaches are being explored in AML. As noted earlier, gemtuzumab ozogamicin, an anti-CD33 antibody calicheamicin conjugate, has been approved for treatment of older patients with recurrent AML. Phase II trials of gemtuzumab plus standard chemotherapy for initial treatment of AML have yielded encouraging results, with CR rates in excess of 80%.[75,76] Based on these results, randomized trials are under way, evaluating this approach as initial AML treatment.

Antibodies have also been employed to target radionuclides to the marrow and other sites of disease as part of a transplant preparative regimen. The hypothesis being tested is that by targeting higher doses of radiation to these sites and avoiding normal organs, it should be possible to provide greater antileukemic effects with less toxicity than achievable with TBI. Phase II trials using anti-CD45 monoclonal antibody labeled with [131]I have yielded encouraging results, as have studies of an anti-CD66 antibody labeled with [88]Re.[77,78] A particularly attractive approach under study is the development of an allogeneic transplant regimen combining high-dose targeted radiotherapy for tumor ablation with low-dose fludarabine/TBI to ensure engraftment.

The markedly reduced relapse rates seen with the development of GVHD following allogeneic transplantation coupled with the dramatic tumor responses sometimes seen with DI have fueled interest in the further development of cell-based therapies for AML. The central scientific challenge has been to discover methods to segregate the potentially potent GVT effects from GVHD. Several broad groups of antigens are under study as possible targets capable of this distinction. One set of targets is polymorphic minor histocompatibility antigens, with expression largely limited to hematopoietic tissues. In the setting of allogeneic transplantation, such antigens could serve as targets for donor-derived T-cell clones capable of destroying all normal and malignant host hematopoietic tissue without contributing to GVHD. A number of polymorphic minor histocompatability antigens with expression limited to hematopoietic tissue have been identified by the groups in Seattle and Leiden, and clinical studies involving the use of T-cell clones targeting these antigens are under way.[79,80]

While elegant, the use of T-cell clones targeting minor histocompatability antigens is necessarily restricted to the allogeneic transplant setting. Several classes of nonallogeneic antigens also have the potential capacity to serve as effective targets for T-cell therapy. Mutational antigens, such as the fusion product proteins found in leukemias with t(9;22), t(15;17), or t(6;9), could theoretically serve as specific targets for a cellular immune response. Attempts are being made to elicit antitumor responses to several of these antigens by immunizing patients with vaccines based on these mutant peptides.[81] Perhaps the greatest potential for cell-based therapies comes from the observation that several nonmutated proteins are highly overexpressed in AML cells, including PR3 and WT1.[82,83] Despite that these are self-antigens, because they are normally expressed at such low levels, patients are capable of generating a T-cell response to these proteins. Encouragingly, T cells with specificity to these antigens are able to selectively lyse leukemic blasts without damaging normal CD34-positive hematopoietic cells. Based on these observations, clinical trials involving the adoptive transfer of T cells specific for these antigens are under way, as are trials using these antigens as the basis for AML vaccines.

## SUMMARY

Treatment of the patient with relapsed or refractory AML continues to be a difficult challenge. At the same time, the enormous increase in our understanding of the molecular and immunologic nature of leukemia is beginning to pay dividends in the recent availability of a large number of novel therapies with clear activity in AML. It is now our responsibility as scientists and clinicians to learn how to best use these therapies to benefit our patients.

## REFERENCES

1. Liso V, Iacopino P, Avvisati G, et al.: Outcome of patients with acute myeloid leukemia who failed to respond to a single course of first-line induction therapy: a GIMEMA study of 218 unselected consecutive patients. *Leukemia* 10:1443–1452, 1996.
2. Jourdan E, Reiffers J, Stoppa AM, et al.: Outcome of adult patients with acute myeloid leukemia who failed to achieve complete remission after one course of induction chemotherapy: a report from the BGMT Study Group. *Leuk Lymphoma* 42:57–65, 2001.
3. Hiddemann W, Martin WR, Sauerland CM, et al.: Definition of refractoriness against conventional chemotherapy in acute myeloid leukemia: a proposal based on the results of retreatment by thioguanine, cytosine arabinoside, and daunorubicin (TAD 9) in 150 patients with relapse after standardized first line therapy. *Leukemia* 4:184–188, 1990.
4. Estey E, Kornblau S, Pierce S, et al.: A stratification system for evaluating and selecting therapies in patients with relapsed or primary refractory acute myelogenous leukemia (Letter). *Blood* 88:756, 1996.
5. Estey E: Treatment of refractory AML (Review). *Leukemia* 10:932–936, 1996.
6. Mortimer J, Blinder MA, Schulman S, et al.: Relapse of acute leukemia after marrow transplantation: natural history and results of subsequent therapy. *J Clin Oncol* 7:50–57, 1989.
7. Kern W, Schoch C, Haferlach T, et al.: Multivariate analysis of prognostic factors in patients with refractory and relapsed acute myeloid leukemia undergoing

sequential high-dose cytosine arabinoside and mitox-antrone (S-HAM) salvage therapy: relevance of cytogenetic abnormalities. *Leukemia* 14:226–231, 2000.

8. Rees JK, Gray RG, Swirsky D, et al.: Principal results of the Medical Research Council's 8th acute myeloid leukaemia trial. *Lancet* 2:1236–1241, 1986.

9. Keating MJ, Kantarjian H, Smith TL, et al.: Response to salvage therapy and survival after relapse in acute myelogenous leukemia. *J Clin Oncol* 7:1071–1080, 1989.

10. Thalhammer F, Geissler K, Jager U, et al.: Duration of second complete remission in patients with acute myeloid leukemia treated with chemotherapy: a retrospective single-center study. *Ann Hematol* 72:216–222, 1996.

11. Davis CL, Rohatiner AZ, Lim J, et al.: The management of recurrent acute myelogenous leukaemia at a single centre over a fifteen-year period. *Br J Haematol* 83:404–411, 1993.

12. Archimbaud E, Thomas X, Leblond V, et al.: Timed sequential chemotherapy for previously treated patients with acute myeloid leukemia: long-term follow-up of the etoposide, mitoxantrone, and cytarabine-86 trial. *J Clin Oncol* 13:11–18, 1995.

13. Vignetti M, Orsini E, Petti MC, et al.: Probability of long-term disease-free survival for acute myeloid leukemia patients after first relapse: a single-centre experience. *Ann Oncol* 7:933–938, 1996.

14. Carella AM, Carlier P, Pungolino E, et al.: Idarubicin in combination with intermediate-dose cytarabine and VP-16 in the treatment of refractory or rapidly relapsed patients with acute myeloid leukemia. The GIMEMA Cooperative Group. *Leukemia* 7:196–199, 1993.

15. Sternberg DW, Aird W, Neuberg D, et al.: Treatment of patients with recurrent and primary refractory acute myelogenous leukemia using mitoxantrone and intermediate-dose cytarabine: a pharmacologically based regimen. *Cancer* 88:2037–2041, 2000.

16. Harousseau JL, Reiffers J, Hurteloup P, et al.: Treatment of relapsed acute myeloid leukemia with idarubicin and intermediate-dose cytarabine. *J Clin Oncol* 7:45–49, 1989.

17. Peters WG, Willemze R, Colly LP: Results of induction and consolidation treatment with intermediate and high-dose cytosine arabinoside and m-Amsa of patients with poor-risk acute myelogenous leukaemia. *Eur J Haematol* 40:198–204, 1988.

18. Brito-Babapulle F, Catovsky D, Newland AC, et al.: Treatment of acute myeloid leukemia with intermediate-dose cytosine arabinoside and mitoxantrone. *Semin Oncol* 14:51–52, 1987.

19. Ferrara F, Melillo L, Montillo M, et al.: Fludarabine, cytarabine, and G-CSF (FLAG) for the treatment of acute myeloid leukemia relapsing after autologous stem cell transplantation. *Ann Hematol* 78:380–384, 1999.

20. Estey E, Plunkett W, Gandhi V, et al.: Fludarabine and arabinosylcytosine therapy of refractory and relapsed acute myelogenous leukemia. *Leuk Lymphoma* 9:343–350, 1993.

21. Saito K, Nakamura Y, Aoyagi M, et al.: Low-dose cytarabine and aclarubicin in combination with granulocyte colony-stimulating factor (CAG regimen) for previously treated patients with relapsed or primary resistant acute myelogenous leukemia (AML) and previously untreated elderly patients with AML, secondary AML, and refrac-tory anemia with excess blasts in transformation. *Int J Hematol* 71:238–244, 2000.

22. Jehn U, Heinemann V: Intermediate-dose ara-C/m-AMSA for remission induction and high-dose ara-C/m-AMSA for intensive consolidation in relapsed and refractory adult acute myelogeneous leukemia. *Haematol Blood Transfus* 33:333–338, 1990.

23. Pavlovsky S, Fernandez I, Palau V, et al.: Combination of rubidazone and cytosine arabinoside in the treatment of first relapse in acute myelocytic leukemia. *Ann Oncol* 2:441–442, 1991.

24. Kornblau SM, Kantarjian H, O'Brien S, et al.: CECA-cyclophosphamide, etoposide, carboplatin and cytosine arabinoside—a new salvage regimen for relapsed or refractory acute myelogenous leukemia. *Leuk Lymphoma* 28:371–375, 1998.

25. Harousseau JL, Milpied N, Briere J, et al.: Mitoxantrone and intermediate-dose cytarabine in relapsed or refractory acute myeloblastic leukemia. *Nouv Rev Fr Hematol* 32:227–230, 1990.

26. Ho AD, Lipp T, Ehninger G, et al.: Combination of mitoxantrone and etoposide in refractory acute myelogenous leukemia—an active and well-tolerated regimen. *J Clin Oncol* 6:213–217, 1988.

27. Leopold LH, Willemze R: The treatment of acute myeloid leukemia in first relapse: a comprehensive review of the literature (Review). *Leuk Lymphoma* 43:1715–1727, 2002.

28. Kern W, Aul C, Maschmeyer G, et al.: Superiority of high-dose over intermediate-dose cytosine arabinoside in the treatment of patients with high-risk acute myeloid leukemia: results of an age-adjusted prospective randomized comparison. *Leukemia* 12:1049–1055, 1998.

29. Vogler WR, McCarley DL, Stagg M, et al.: A phase III trial of high-dose cytosine arabinoside with or without etoposide in relapsed and refractory acute myelogenous leukemia. A Southeastern Cancer Study Group trial. *Leukemia* 8:1847–1853, 1994.

30. Karanes C, Kopecky KJ, Grever MR, et al.: A phase III comparison of high dose ARA-C (HIDAC) versus HIDAC plus mitoxantrone in the treatment of first relapsed or refractory acute myeloid leukemia. Southwest Oncology Group study. *Leuk Res* 23:787–794, 1999.

31. Thomas X, Fenaux P, Dombret H, et al.: Granulocyte-macrophage colony-stimulating factor (GM-CSF) to increase efficacy of intensive sequential chemotherapy with etoposide, mitoxantrone and cytarabine (EMA) in previously treated acute myeloid leukemia: a multicenter randomized placebo-controlled trial (EMA91 trial). *Leukemia* 13:1214–1220, 1999.

32. Ohno R, Naoe T, Kanamaru A, et al.: A double-blind controlled study of granulocyte colony-stimulating factor started two days before induction chemotherapy in refractory acute myeloid leukemia. *Blood* 83:2086–2092, 1994.

33. List AF, Kopecky KJ, Willman CL, et al.: Benefit of cyclosporine modulation of drug resistance in patients with poor-risk acute myeloid leukemia: a Southwest Oncology Group study. *Blood* 98:3212–3220, 2001.

34. Daenen S, van der Holt B, Verhoef GE, et al.: Addition of cyclosporin A to the combination of mitoxantrone and etoposide to overcome resistance to chemotherapy in refractory or relapsing acute myeloid leukaemia: a

randomised phase II trial from HOVON, the Dutch–Belgian Haemato-Oncology Working Group for adults. *Leuk Res* 28:1057–1067, 2004.

35. Sievers EL, Larson RA, Stadmauer EA, et al.: Efficacy and safety of gemtuzumab ozogamicin in patients with CD33-positive acute myeloid leukemia in first relapse. *J Clin Oncol* 19:3244–3254, 2001.

36. Biggs JC, Horowitz MM, Gale RP, et al.: Bone marrow transplants may cure patients with acute leukemia never achieving remission with chemotherapy. *Blood* 80(4):1090–1093, 1992.

37. Gale RP, Horowitz MM, Rees JK, et al.: Chemotherapy versus transplants for acute myelogenous leukemia in second remission. *Leukemia* 10:13–19, 1996.

38. Clift RA, Buckner CD, Appelbaum FR, et al.: Allogeneic marrow transplantation during untreated first relapse of acute myeloid leukemia. *J Clin Oncol* 10:1723–1729, 1992.

39. Reiffers J: HLA-identical sibling hematopoietic stem cell transplantation for acute myeloid leukemia. In: Atkinson K (ed.) *Clinical Bone Marrow and Blood Stem Cell Transplantation*. 2nd ed. Cambridge, UK: Cambridge University Press; 2000:433–445.

40. Slavin S, Nagler A, Naparstek E, et al.: Nonmyeloablative stem cell transplantation and cell therapy as an alternative to conventional bone marrow transplantation with lethal cytoreduction for the treatment of malignant and nonmalignant hematologic diseases. *Blood* 91:756–763, 1998.

41. McSweeney PA, Niederwieser D, Shizuru JA, et al.: Hematopoietic cell transplantation in older patients with hematologic malignancies: replacing high-dose cytotoxic therapy with graft-versus-tumor effects. *Blood* 97:3390–3400, 2001.

42. Hegenbart U, Niederwieser D, Sandmaier BM, et al.: Treatment for acute myelogenous leukemia by low-dose, total-body, irradiation-based conditioning and hematopoietic cell transplantation from related and unrelated donors. *J Clin Oncol* 24(3):444–453, 2006.

43. Gorin NC: Autologous stem cell transplantation in acute myelocytic leukemia (Review). *Blood* 92:1073–1090, 1998.

44. Gorin NC, Labopin M, Fouillard L, et al.: Retrospective evaluation of autologous bone marrow transplantation vs allogeneic bone marrow transplantation from an HLA identical related donor in acute myelocytic leukemia. *Bone Marrow Transplant* 18:111–117, 1996.

45. National Marrow Donor Program, Year 2000 Report.

46. Sierra J, Storer B, Hansen JA, et al.: Unrelated donor marrow transplantation for acute myeloid leukemia: an update of the Seattle experience. *Bone Marrow Transplant* 26:397–404, 2000.

47. Ringden O, Labopin M, Gluckman E, et al.: Donor search or autografting in patients with acute leukaemia who lack an HLA-identical sibling? A matched-pair analysis. *Bone Marrow Transplant* 19:963–968, 1997.

48. Radich JP, Gooley T, Sanders JE, et al.: Second allogeneic transplantation after failure of first autologous transplantation. *Biol Blood Marrow Transplant* 6:272–279, 2000.

49. Kolb HJ, Schattenberg A, Goldman JM, et al.: Graft-versus-leukemia effect of donor lymphocyte transfusions in marrow grafted patients. European Group for Blood and Marrow Transplantation Working Party Chronic Leukemia. *Blood* 86:2041–2050, 1995.

50. Bullinger L, Dohner K, Bair E, et al.: Use of gene-expression profiling to identify prognostic subclasses in adult acute myeloid leukemia. *N Engl J Med* 350:1605–1616, 2004.

51. Valk PJ, Verhaak RG, Beijen MA, et al.: Prognostically useful gene-expression profiles in acute myeloid leukemia [see comment]. *N Engl J Med* 350:1617–1628, 2004.

52. Gallagher RE, Yeap BY, Bi W, et al.: Quantitative real-time RT-PCR analysis of PML-RARα mRNA levels in acute promyelocytic leukemia: assessment of prognostic significance in adult patients from intergroup protocol 0129. *Blood* 101:2521–2528, 2003.

53. Hughes TP, Kaeda J, Branford S, et al.: Frequency of major molecular responses to imatinib or interferon alfa plus cytarabine in newly diagnosed chronic myeloid leukemia. *N Engl J Med* 349:1423–1432, 2003.

54. San Miguel JF, Vidriales MB, Lopez-Berges C, et al.: Early immunophenotypical evaluation of minimal residual disease in acute myeloid leukemia identifies different patient risk groups and may contribute to postinduction treatment stratification. *Blood* 98:1746–1751, 2001.

55. Nakao M, Yokota S, Iwai T, et al.: Internal tandem duplication of the flt3 gene found in acute myeloid leukemia. *Leukemia* 10:1911–1918, 1996.

56. Yokota S, Kiyoi H, Nakao M, et al.: Internal tandem duplication of the FLT3 gene is preferentially seen in acute myeloid leukemia and myelodysplastic syndrome among various hematological malignancies. A study on a large series of patients and cell lines. *Leukemia* 11:1605–1609, 1997.

57. Deguchi K, Gilliland DG: Cooperativity between mutations in tyrosine kinases and in hematopoietic transcription factors in AML. *Leukemia* 16:740–744, 2002.

58. Stirewalt DL, Kopecky KJ, Meshinchi S, et al.: *FLT3*, *RAS*, and *TP53* mutations in elderly patients with acute myeloid leukemia. *Blood* 97:3589–3595, 2001.

59. Meshinchi S, Woods WG, Stirewalt DL, et al.: Prevalence and prognostic significance of Flt3 internal tandem duplication in pediatric acute myeloid leukemia. *Blood* 97:89–94, 2001.

60. Thiede C, Steudel C, Mohr B, et al.: Analysis of FLT3-activating mutations in 979 patients with acute myelogenous leukemia: association with FAB subtypes and identification of subgroups with poor prognosis. *Blood* 99:4326–4335, 2002.

61. Tallman MS: New strategies for the treatment of acute myeloid leukemia including antibodies and other novel agents. In: *Hematology*. Washington, DC: American Society of Hematology Education Program Book; 2005:143–150.

62. Ridge SA, Worwood M, Oscier D, et al.: FMS mutations in myelodysplastic leukemic, and normal subjects. *Proc Natl Acad Sci U S A* 87:1377–1380, 1990.

63. Gari M, Goodeve A, Wilson G, et al.: c-kit proto-oncogene exon 8 in-frame deletion plus insertion mutations in acute myeloid leukaemia. *Br J Haematol* 105:894–900, 1999.

64. Fiedler W, Mesters R, Staib P, et al.: SU5416, a novel receptor tyrosine kinase inhibitor, in the treatment of patients with refractory, C-kit positive, acute myeloid leukemia. *Blood* 98(pt 1):124a, Abstract 521, 2001.

65. Radich JP, Kopecky KJ, Willman CL, et al.: N-*ras* mutations in adult de novo acute myelogenous leukemia: prevalence and clinical significance. Blood 76:801–807, 1990.

66. Karp JE, Lancet JE, Kaufmann SH, et al.: Clinical and biologic activity of the farnesyltransferase inhibitor R115777 in adults with refractory and relapsed acute leukemias: a phase 1 clinical-laboratory correlative trial. *Blood* 97:3361–3369, 2001.

67. Wu WS, Vallian S, Seto E, et al.: The growth suppressor PML represses transcription by functionally and physically interacting with histone deacetylases. *Mol Cell Biol* 21:2259–2268, 2001.

68. Ferrara FF, Fazi F, Bianchini A, et al.: Histone deacetylase-targeted treatment restores retinoic acid signaling and differentiation in acute myeloid leukemia. *Cancer Res* 61:2–7, 2001.

69. Campos L, Rouault J-P, Sabido O, et al.: High expression of bcl-2 protein in acute myeloid leukemia cells is associated with poor response to chemotherapy. *Blood* 81:3091–3096, 1993.

70. Banker DE, Groudine M, Norwood T, et al.: Measurement of spontaneous and therapeutic agent-induced apoptosis with BCL-2 protein expression in acute myeloid leukemia. *Blood* 89:243–255, 1997.

71. Konopleva M, Tari AM, Estrov Z, et al.: Liposomal Bcl-2 antisense oligonucleotides enhance proliferation, sensitize acute myeloid leukemia to cytosine-arabinoside, and induce apoptosis independent of other antiapoptotic proteins. *Blood* 95:3929–3938, 2000.

72. Stirewalt DL, Appelbaum FR, Willman CL, et al.: Mevastatin can increase toxicity in primary AMLs exposed to standard therapeutic agents, but statin efficacy is not simply associated with *ras* hotspot mutations or overexpression. *Leuk Res* 27:133–145, 2003.

73. Dimitroulakos J, Nohynek D, Backway KL, et al.: Increased sensitivity of acute myeloid leukemias to lovastatin-induced apoptosis: a potential therapeutic approach. *Blood* 93:1308–1318, 1999.

74. Wong WW, Dimitroulakos J, Minden MD, et al.: HMG-CoA reductase inhibitors and the malignant cell: the statin family of drugs as triggers of tumor-specific apoptosis (Review). *Leukemia* 16:508–519, 2002.

75. Kell WJ, Burnett AK, Chopra R, et al.: A feasibility study of simultaneous administration of gemtuzumab ozogamicin with intensive chemotherapy in induction and consolidation in younger patients with acute myeloid leukemia. *Blood* 102:4277–4283, 2003.

76. De Angelo DJ, Stone RM, Durrant S, et al.: Gemtuzumab ozogamicin (Mylotarg®) in combination with induction chemotherapy for the treatment of patients with de novo acute myeloid leukemia: two age-specific phase 2 trials. *Blood* 102(pt 1):100a, Abstract 341, 2003.

77. Matthews DC, Appelbaum FR: Radioimmunotherapy and hematopoietic cell transplantation. In: Blume KG, Forman SJ, Appelbaum FR (eds.) *Thomas' Hematopoietic Cell Transplantation*. 3rd ed. Oxford, UK: Blackwell Publishing Ltd; 2004:198–208.

78. Bunjes DW, Buchmann I, Duncker C, et al.: Using radio-labeled monoclonal antibodies to intensify the conditioning regimen for patients with high-risk AML and MDS: a single centre experience of 36 transplants. *Blood* 96(pt 1):386a, Abstract 1667, 2000.

79. Warren EH, Greenberg PD, Riddell SR: Cytotoxic T-lymphocyte-defined human minor histocompatibility antigens with a restricted tissue distribution. *Blood* 91:2197–2207, 1998.

80. Mutis T, Verdijk R, Schrama E, et al.: Feasibility of immunotherapy of relapsed leukemia with ex vivo-generated cytotoxic T lymphocytes specific for hematopoietic system-restricted minor histocompatibility antigens. *Blood* 93:2336–2341, 1999.

81. Pinilla-Ibarz J, Cathcart K, Korontsvit T, et al.: Vaccination of patients with chronic myelogenous leukemia with bcr-abl oncogene breakpoint fusion peptides generates specific immune responses. *Blood* 95:1781–1787, 2000.

82. Molldrem JJ, Lee PP, Wang C, et al.: Evidence that specific T lymphocytes may participate in the elimination of chronic myelogenous leukemia. *Nat Med* 6:1018–1023, 2000.

83. Gao L, Bellantuono I, Elsässer A, et al.: Selective elimination of leukemic CD34+ progenitor cells by cytotoxic T lymphocytes specific for WT1. *Blood* 95:2198–2203, 2000.

# Section 2
# ACUTE LYMPHOBLASTIC LEUKEMIA

# Chapter 10
# EPIDEMIOLOGY, RISK FACTORS, AND CLASSIFICATION

*Joseph O. Moore*

## INTRODUCTION

Acute lymphoblastic leukemia (ALL) is a complex and potentially curable hematopoietic cancer that has provided numerous significant firsts in the treatment of malignant disease for children and adults alike. Historically, ALL in children was the first tumor whose treatment attained complete remission in the majority of patients, leading to long-term disease-free survival and cure with combination chemotherapy. In childhood, modern combined modality treatment produces complete response rates of up to 95% and cure rates of up to 64%. In contrast, adults have fared less well, with comparable remission rates up to 93%, but cure rates of 30% or lower in most reported series.[1-4] Reasons for this disparity are likely multifactorial and have been thought to include physician experience and expertise, more rigid adherence to protocols by pediatric oncologists, and different biology of the leukemia in children and adults. Other differences may occur in the presentation of disease, both physically and symptomatically, and in patients' tolerance to aggressive protocol-based treatment, with children more able than adults to follow and remain on an appropriately aggressive protocol. As described below, perhaps more importance lies in more favorable genomic abnormalities in childhood, while in adults very poor prognostic groups, including those expressing the t(9;22) Philadelphia chromosome, occur in almost half of patients.[2]

ALL treatment has influenced all aspects of cancer care. Current success has evolved incrementally, from single-agent chemotherapy to multiple drug combinations and the addition of biologic agents into complex, combined modality therapy. More recently, specific chromosome abnormalities and their associated oncogenes, proto-oncogenes, and signaling pathways have assumed enhanced importance in understanding the biology and treatment of ALL. For example, recognition of the t(9;22) and its balanced exchange of genetic material between bcr (the breakpoint combining region) and the Abelson oncogene (*c-abl*) leads to constitutive activation of the associated tyrosine kinase, producing unregulated cell proliferation. This highlights the interaction of genomics and biology, as well as introduces targeted therapy, with the introduction of the specific bcr/abl kinase inhibitor imatinib mesylate.[5] Additionally, abnormalities of the *MLL* gene and its associated t(4;11) chromosome abnormalities are a predictor of short-duration or low-frequency complete remissions, early relapse, and poor disease-free survival. Documentation of poor overall prognosis has led to a change in therapy for these patients and their early allocation to more aggressive treatment with stem cell transplantation,[3] rather than continuing with more conventional ALL therapy even if complete remission is initially accomplished.[4]

The essential need to identify specific chromosome translocations has also enhanced the importance of

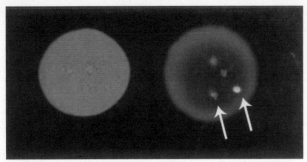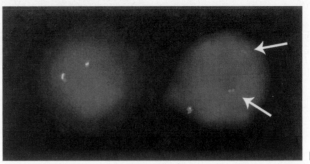

a                                                                                      b

**Figure 10.1**    *FISH techniques: (a) A BCR/ABL dual fusion probe set applied to interphase nuclei. Nucleus at left shows two normal signals for the BCR locus at 22q11.2 (green) and two normal signals for the ABL locus at 9q34 (red). Nucleus at right shows one normal BCR locus (green), one normal ABL locus (red), and two fusion signals (arrows) with juxtaposition of red and green signals, reflecting the rearranged chromosomes 9 and 22. (b) It shows an MLL break apart probe set applied to interphase nuclei. In this probe set, the 5' region flanking MLL is labeled in green and the 3' region flanking MLL is labeled in red. Nucleus at left shows two fusion signals, reflecting the normal (unrearranged) MLL loci at 11q23. Nucleus at right shows one normal (unrearranged) MLL locus. The separation of the green (5' MLL) and red (3' MLL) signals (arrows) shows that rearrangement of this locus has occurred*

diagnostic tools for the identification of these abnormalities rapid and reliable. These include standard cytogenetics, the more targeted fluorescent in situ hybridization (FISH) techniques [Figure 10.1(a) and 10.1(b)], and reverse transcription polymerase chain reaction (RT-PCR), each of which may identify specific chromosome abnormalities, and aid in diagnosis, monitoring of therapeutic response, and identification of minimal residual disease, as further discussed in Chapter 14.[6–9] With both FISH and RT-PCR, it is of critical importance to identify the specific chromosome abnormality or translocation to assure specificity and accuracy of diagnosis and accurate quantitation of the proportion of cells affected.

Current treatment strategies for ALL illustrate progressive and incremental protocol development from single institutions and cooperative group programs, resulting in improved complete response and survival. Numerous groups have contributed, including the Pediatric Oncology Group,[10] the French Cooperative Group,[11] the Cancer and Acute Leukemia Group B,[12–15] the Berlin–Frankfurt–Munster Group,[16–19] the Italian Gruppo Italiano Malaittie Ematologiche Maligne dell'Adulto,[20] the French Leucemie Aigues Lymphoblastique de l'Adulte Group, individual institutions such as St Jude's Children's Hospital,[10] Memorial Sloan-Kettering Cancer Center,[21,22] and MD Anderson Cancer Center,[23] and other more individualized programs,[24] to name but a few. These protocols are described in greater detail in Chapter 13.

Current strategies also illustrate the conceptual importance of sanctuary sites of disease, areas where ALL cells may be protected from destruction by systemic chemotherapy and that require specialized prophylactic treatment targeted to the central nervous system, such as intrathecal chemotherapy delivered by lumbar puncture or an indwelling cerebrospinal access device, or radiation therapy, as might be applied to

other sanctuaries in the testicle and the mediastinum. Preventive treatment of these sanctuaries has had a major positive effect on cure and long-term survival in both children and adults.[4,16,25]

## EPIDEMIOLOGY

The specific cause of ALL is unknown in most patients, and specific epidemiologic associations can be identified in no more than 10% of childhood ALL and in a much lower proportion of adults.[26,27] An extensive review of ALL in children by Buffler et al. details potential occupational exposures in parents of patients, and exposures to aromatic hydrocarbons and household chemicals and pesticides, ionizing radiation, low-frequency magnetic fields, diet, infections, and genetic polymorphisms.[26] Numerous potential predisposing features studied or established include positive associations with the specific genetic syndromes noted below, high birth weight,[28] ethnicity,[29] and a paradoxically negative relation with maternal smoking.[30] While extensively investigated, none of these factors offer potent predictive value for improved diagnosis and increased survival other than the increased risk of leukemia in some hereditary and genetic syndromes (see below). In adults, even fewer associations are apparent; genetic features play a negligible role in disease behavior and in defining and predicting prognosis. The following includes some genomic and other associations in children and adults.

## GENETIC MUTATION

Genetic mutation plays a pivotal role in the etiology of ALL in children born with Down syndrome with the associated trisomy 21 chromosome abnormality.

Alteration and activation of the GATA-1 hematopoietic transcription factor increases the risk for development of ALL and increases the incidence of acute megakaryocytic leukemia as well.[31–35] That hematologic malignancies representing different cell lines may become malignant suggests that multiple signaling pathways may be affected by this and other chromosome abnormalities.[36] Of interest, the more detrimental chromosome abnormalities, t(9;22) and t(4;11), occur infrequently in Down syndrome.[33–35] Favorable abnormalities of the TEL/AML1 fusion, denoted by the t(12;21) translocation, are also less frequent in Down syndrome.

ALL may also arise in the setting of the Li–Fraumeni syndrome, with associated abnormalities of p53, Bloom syndrome, and others predisposing to ALL and to multiple other cancers.[36]

### IN UTERO EVENTS

Toxic exposure in utero to maternal Epstein–Barr virus (EBV) reactivation or other viral entities such as cytomegalovirus and herpes simplex virus has been proposed as a causative factor in some infants and children with ALL.[37] These mutations are not believed to lead directly to ALL, but their effect in delaying cell maturation may allow more genetic abnormalities to occur.[10]

Monozygotic twins carry a small but definite increased risk of concordant ALL. The potential for in utero events leading to postpartum ALL was highlighted in a report of two year-old monozygotic twins, both with ALL, in whom one had two rearranged T-cell receptor δ alleles that were proposed to have occurred in utero, with the transmission of a single allele to the other twin, resulting in ALL.[38] Though these changes were considered critical, other abnormalities or mutations are thought to be necessary to produce ALL in vivo. This suggests that mutations produced in utero may combine with other mutations, leading to leukemia.[32]

### RADIATION EXPOSURE

ALLs occur less frequently following radiation exposure than do acute myeloid leukemias (AML), chronic myeloid leukemia (CML), or myelodysplastic syndromes. The incidence of ALL is modestly increased in populations exposed to ionizing radiation from an atomic bomb,[26,39] and cases are most prevalent among younger survivors.[40] As a general rule, most other forms of radiation may produce an excess of leukemia, again mostly of myeloid origin rather than lymphoid. No study has documented an increase in ALL associated with radiation from diagnostic radiographic procedures.[26]

### TOXIC EXPOSURE

ALL is not increased by exposure to alkylating agents and epipodophyllotoxins,[41] and is not usually considered to be a "secondary" leukemia.

### GENE THERAPY

Gene therapy for X-linked severe combined immunodeficiency syndrome (X-SCID) has led to activation of the LMO2 gene.[42,43] Two of ten patients who received retrovirus vector-mediated gene transfer for X-SCID developed T-cell ALL. This was caused by insertion of the retroviral vector with LMO2 gene activation, leading to leukemic transformation. In normal hematopoiesis, CD34-positive cells may develop into all hematopoietic cell lines. In the lymphoid series, these may differentiate into either B cells or T cells. Ex vivo infection of hematopoietic stem cells by the retrovirus encoding IL2 R gamma c is followed by reinfusion, and it results in activated chromosome translocations with LMO2, including t(ll;14)(p13;q11), or t(7;11)(q35;p13). This represents a classic activation of signaling pathways by the retrovirus-transformed cells leading to T-cell ALL.[42–44]

In adults with ALL, abnormalities of cell cycle regulatory genes are frequently present and may be determinants in leukemogenesis. These include the retinoblastoma gene (Rb), p53, p15 (INK4B), and p16 (INK4A).[45] Pui has detailed and elucidated the initial abnormalities, chromosome aberrations, and their cell signaling consequences in a comprehensive review of ALL, with detailed genomic pathways.[10,33]

## RISK FACTORS

Risk factors, further detailed in subsequent chapters, are a part of the epidemiology of ALL, both with regard to initial factors leading to ALL and factors associated with success or failure of treatment. ALL may occur at any age, but is most frequent in childhood (before age 15), with a consistent incidence in the third to eighth decades of life.[46] In adults, family history and a history of immunologic abnormalities are usually not present. Family history of lymphoma may be present without a definite association being drawn.[27,40]

Risk factors for ALL include Caucasian race as compared to African-American or other ethnic groups in the United States. Rates of ALL are also higher in Northern and Western Europe, North America, and Oceania versus in Asian and black populations.[40] In Israel, Jews have a higher incidence of leukemias, but paradoxically lower rates of ALL.[46]

Exposure to human T-cell leukemia virus 1 may produce a T-cell leukemia presenting with hypercalcemia, bone or skin lesions, lymph node enlargement, which occur in several ethnic populations, such as Japanese from the island of Kyushu and U.S. immigrants from the Caribbean. An initial, more indolent T-cell leukemia may evolve to a very aggressive T-ALL that is treated with great difficulty and responds poorly, with little chance of survival.[44] ALL can also occur as a blastic transformation of CML, and in this setting it is always associated with a t(9;22).

## CLASSIFICATION

The classification of ALL has followed the historical evolution of technology, with cellular morphology by microscopic appearance, immunophenotyping of cell surface markers, lymphocyte subset analysis, and more recently, chromosome evaluation and genomic identification.

Leukemia was first identified and described by Virchow as *weisses blut* (white blood) due to hyper-leukocytosis (elevated white blood cell count), and was further categorized initially using supravital stains of peripheral blood.[47] Subsequent identification of leukemias by cell origin, required separation into groups of myeloid and lymphoid leukemias. Additionally, the identification of acute and chronic varieties of each required more sophisticated techniques of special enzymatic stains, leading to the evolution of our current skills in morphology, cell surface identifications, genomics, and biology as incorporated in the current World Health Organization (WHO) classification.[48]

### MORPHOLOGIC CLASSIFICATION

The French–American–British (FAB) classification system separated AML and ALL based on the visual microscopic appearance of blast forms in peripheral blood and bone marrow, as well as on the activity of selected special enzymatic stains, such as peroxidase, specific and nonspecific esterase, and periodic acid–Schiff for glycogen.[49] Morphologic classification with the FAB system separates three forms of ALL. ALL includes[50]:

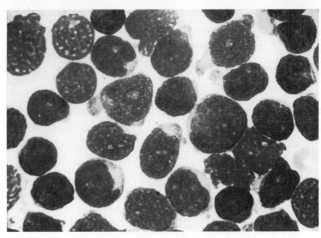

**Figure 10.3**    *L2—variable-sized peripheral blood lymphoblasts with variable chromatin pattern and more frequent nucleoli*

L1—Small lymphocytic variant with uniform small cells having a more "mature" appearance (Figure 10.2).

L2—Variable cell size with large and small cells in the same sample (Figure 10.3). In adults, this variant has a poorer prognosis compared with L1 ALL based on the more frequent presence of the Philadelphia chromosome p190 variant (rather than p210, as with CML), with similar response rates but more rapid relapse and diminished long-term survival.[18,33,48]

L3—Burkitt lymphoma/leukemia, with small uniform lymphoid blasts characterized by vacuolated cytoplasm containing glycogen, and frequent mitotic figures denoting rapid growth (Figure 10.4).

Although classified as a form of ALL, the L3 (Burkitt) variant differs in many respects from other forms of ALL. L3 ALL presents in developed countries as an aggressive disease, often with intra-abdominal lymph

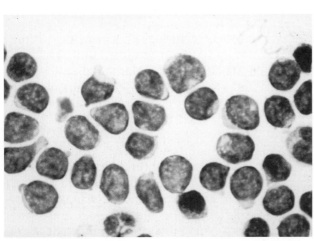

**Figure 10.2**    *L1—uniform small peripheral lymphoid blasts with minimal to moderate cytoplasm, effaced chromatin, and occasional to more numerous nucleoli*

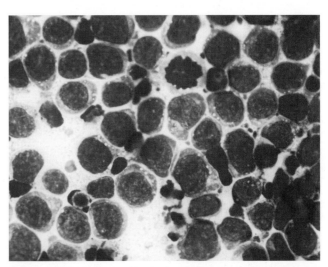

**Figure 10.4**    *L3—Burkitt leukemia in bone marrow with uniform blast forms, cytoplasmic vacuoles, and increased mitoses*

**Table 10.1**    Estimated frequency of specific genotypes of ALL in children and adults

| ALL genotype | Children (%) | Adults (%) |
|---|---|---|
| Hyperdiploidy >50 chromosomes | 25 | 7 |
| TEL/AML1 t(12;21) | 22 | 2 |
| MLL rearrangements [e.g., t(4;11), t(11;19), t(9:11)] | 8 | 10 |
| TAL1 lp32 | 7 | 12 |
| E2A/PBX1 t(1;19) | 5 | 3 |
| BCR/ABL t(9;22) | 3 | 25 |
| HOX11L2 5q35 | 2.5 | 1 |
| MYC t(8;14), t(2;8), t(8,22) | 2 | 4 |
| LYL1 19p13 | 1.5 | 2.5 |
| Hypodiploidy <45 chromosomes | 1 | 2 |
| HOX11 10q24 | 0.7 | 8 |
| MLL/ENL | 0.3 | 0.5 |
| Others | 22 | 23 |

Genetic lesions that are exclusively seen in cases of T-cell lineage leukemias are shaded in gray. All other genetic subtypes are either exclusively or primarily seen in cases of B-cell lineage ALL.

Adapted from data presented in Pui CH, Relling MV, Downing JR: Acute lymphoblastic leukemia. *N Engl J Med* 350:1535–1548, 2004.

**Table 10.2**    Proposed WHO classification of lymphoid neoplasms

B-cell neoplasms
  Precursor B-cell neoplasm
    **Precursor B-lymphoblastic leukemia/lymphoma (precursor B-cell acute lymphoblastic leukemia)**

  Mature (peripheral) B-cell neoplasms[a]
    B-cell chronic lymphocytic leukemia/small lymphocytic lymphoma
    B-cell prolymphocytic leukemia
    Lymphoplasmacytic lymphoma
    Splenic marginal zone B-cell lymphoma (+/− villous lymphocytes)
    Hairy cell leukemia
    Plasma cell myeloma/plasmacytoma
    Extranodal marginal zone B-cell lymphoma of MALT type
    Nodal marginal zone B-cell lymphoma (+/− monocytoid B cells)
    Follicular lymphoma
    Mantle-cell lymphoma
    Diffuse large B-cell lymphoma
    Mediastinal large B-cell lymphoma
    Primary effusion lymphoma
    **Burkitt lymphoma/Burkitt-cell leukemia**

T-cell and NK-cell neoplasms
  Precursor T-cell neoplasm
    **Precursor T-lymphoblastic lymphoma/leukemia (precursor T-cell ALL)**

  Mature (peripheral) T-cell neoplasms[a]
    T-cell prolymphocytic leukemia
    T-cell granular lymphocytic leukemia
    Aggressive NK-cell leukemia
    Adult T-cell lymphoma/leukemia (HTLV1+)
    Extranodal NK/T-cell lymphoma, nasal type
    Enteropathy-type T-cell lymphoma
    Hepatosplenic gamma-delta T-cell lymphoma
    Subcutaneous panniculitis-like T-cell lymphoma
    Mycosis fungoides/Sezary syndrome
    Anaplastic large-cell lymphoma, T/null cell, primary cutaneous type
    Peripheral T-cell lymphoma, not otherwise characterized
    Angioimmunoblastic T-cell lymphoma
    Anaplastic large-cell lymphoma, T/null cell, primary systemic type

HTLV1+, human T-cell leukemia virus; MALT, mucosa-associated lymphoid tissue; NK, natural killer.

[a]B- and T-/NK-cell neoplasms are grouped according to major clinical presentations (predominantly disseminated/leukemic, primary extranodal, and predominantly nodal).

Adapted from Harris NL, Jaffe ES, Diebold J, et al.: World Health Organization classification of neoplastic diseases of the hematopoietic and lymphoid tissues: report of the Clinical Advisory Committee Meeting–Airlie House, Virginia, November 1997. *J Clin Oncol* 17:3835–3849, 1999.

node enlargement and a high growth fraction, in contrast to its African variant, which is associated with EBV and usually presents in a more indolent manner, often as a jaw mass (lumpy jaw), and responds to more modest treatment.[51] The non-African variant is treated with hyperfractionated alkylating agents and cycle-active treatment rather than with conventional ALL protocols, which produce inferior results.[23,52] Several unique chromosome translocations include the typical t(8;14) involving the immunoglobulin gene *IgH* (on chromosome 14, a site frequently involved with a variety of malignant lymphomas and leukemias of lymphoid origin) and the *c-myc* proto-oncogene. Less usual variant translocations t(2;8) and t(8;12) are also seen in morphologically typical Burkitt-type leukemia.[53]

Demonstration of these abnormalities may not be readily apparent by conventional cytogenetics, FISH or even RT-PCR may be required to identify the exact chromosome abnormality and establish cellular origin when morphology suggests Burkitt leukemia or another abnormality, but is not demonstrated by initial chromosome analysis.[6–10]

## B- AND T-CELL LINEAGE

More recently, classification of ALL has been based on B- and T-cell lineage.[54] More than 80% of cases of ALL in adults are of B-cell lineage, with 10–15% arising from T cells.[18,54,55] While protocol chemotherapy and overall treatment usually follow similar pathways, prognosis may be dictated by these subsets and their individual responses to treatment or propensity for relapse.[10,33]

As the B- and T-cell classifications have evolved, these classifications have now been subdivided into diagnostic groups based on immunophenotypic groups extended to specific genetic mutations, and genomics. Treatment planning follows subset or subgroup analysis, including T-cell and mature B-cell ALL, pre-B ALL, and ALL with associated bcr/abl translocation t(9;22), or other detrimental abnormalities demonstrated. These differences in intensity of treatment and various versions of protocols will be considered in Chapter 13.[4,10] Prognosis can now be related to specific subsets based on chromosome mutation and cell signaling pathways; the best examples of these cases, once again, are t(9;22) and t(4;11) as unfavorable predictors, while others may predict a more favorable response and prognosis.[10]

### MORPHOLOGY, IMMUNOPHENOTYPE, AND CYTOGENETICS

Classifications based on morphology, immunophenotype, and cytogenetics (MIC) have further defined subsets of disease based on these parameters for ALL (MIC) and AML (MIC-M), and employ defined subsets of antibodies to delineate diagnostic groups.[56–58] Differences in B- and T-cell incidence in children and adults respectively are detailed in an elegant manner by Pui (Table 10.1). These also relate B- and T-cell lineage to specific subsets of chromosome abnormalities and their incidence by comparison in children and adults.

### WHO CLASSIFICATION

The WHO classification melds morphologic, immunophenotypic, genetic, and clinical characteristics to form a coherent and current classification separating Hodgkin's disease from the non-Hodgkin's lymphomas and differentiating B-cell neoplasms from those of T- and NK (natural killer)-cell origin (Table 10.2). Precursor B- and precursor T-cell leukemias encompass the multiple subsets of ALLs, considered in more detail in the subsequent chapters.[59] An obvious short coming of the WHO system is that its classification does not speak to individual subsets, which may and should require individualization of treatment. Ongoing studies detailing the diagnostic groups above, and studies in animal models such as the zebra fish, will likely supplant current classification systems by defining causative signaling pathways and subsets of disease. These will enhance current prospects for genome-based targeted therapy, such as with the addition of imatinib mesylate to the treatment of bcr/abl-positive ALL, and will lead to more targeted and effective therapy for individual disease subsets in the future.

### SUMMARY

ALL was the first acute leukemia to achieve complete remission, leading to cure in a large proportion of patients, initially in childhood and more recently extending to all age groups. All aspects of leukemia epidemiology, classification, and biology, and more recently, understanding of genomic abnormalities and mechanisms of leukemogenesis, have been advanced by work with ALL and extended to other malignant tumors.

### REFERENCES

1. Laport GF, Larson RA: Treatment of adult acute lymphoblastic leukemia. *Semin Oncol* 24:70–82, 1997.
2. Schiffer CA: Differences in outcome in adolescents with acute lymphoblastic leukemia: a consequence of better regimens? Better doctors? Both? *J Clin Oncol* 21:760–761, 2003.
3. Hoelzer D, Gokbuget N, Digel W, et al.: Outcome of adult patients with T-lymphoblastic lymphoma treated according to protocols for acute lymphoblastic leukemia. *Blood* 99:4379–4385, 2002.
4. Hoelzer D, Gokbuget N: New approaches to acute lymphoblastic leukemia in adults: where do we go? *Semin Oncol* 27:540–559, 2000.
5. Deininger M, Buchdunger E, Druker BJ: The development of imatinib as a therapeutic agent for chronic myeloid leukemia. *Blood* 105:2640–2653, 2005.
6. Cortes J, Giles F, O'Brien S, et al.: Result of high-dose imatinib mesylate in patients with Philadelphia chromosome-positive chronic myeloid leukemia after failure of interferon-alpha. *Blood* 102:83–86, 2003.
7. Radich J, Gathmann I, Kaeda J, et al.: Molecular responses to imatinib and interferon+ ara-C in newly diagnosed CML. *Blood* 102(II):Abstract 635, 2003.
8. Cortes J, O'Brien S, Talpaz M, et al.: Clinical significance of molecular response in chronic myeloid leukemia after imatinib (Gleevec) therapy: low levels of residual disease predict for response duration. *Blood* 102(II):Abstract 1513, 2003.
9. Lowenberg B: Minimal residual disease in chronic myeloid leukemia. *N Engl J Med* 349:1399–1401, 2003.
10. Pui C-H, Relling MV, Downing JR: Acute lymphoblastic leukemia. *N Engl J Med* 350:1535–1548, 2004.
11. Thomas X, Boiron JM, Huguet F, et al.: Outcome of treatment in adults with acute lymphoblastic leukemia: analysis of the LALA-94 trial. *J Clin Oncol* 22:4075–4086, 2004.
12. Cuttner J, Mick R, Budman DR, et al.: Phase III trial of brief intensive treatment of adult acute lymphocytic leukemia comparing daunorubicin and mitoxantrone: a CALGB study. *Leukemia* 5:425–431, 1991.
13. Ellison RR, Mick R, Cuttner J, et al.: The effects of postinduction intensification treatment with cytarabine and daunorubicin in adult acute lymphocytic leukemia: a prospective randomized clinical trial by CALGB. *J Clin Oncol* 9:2002–2015, 1991.
14. Larson RA, Dodge RK, Burns CP, et al.: A five-drug remission induction regimen with intensive consolidation for

adults with acute lymphoblastic leukemia: CALGB study 8811. *Blood* 85:2025–2037, 1995.

15. Szatrowski TP, Dodge RK, Reynolds C, et al.: Lineage specific treatment of adult patients with acute lymphoblastic leukemia in first remission with anti-B4-blocked ricin or high-dose cytarabine: CALGB study 9311. *Cancer* 97:1471–1480, 2003.

16. Schrappe M, Reiter A, Ludwig WD, et al.: Improved outcome in childhood acute lymphoblastic leukemia despite reduced use of anthracyclines and cranial radiotherapy: results of trial ALL-BFM 90. *Blood* 95:3310–3322, 2000.

17. Reiter A, Schrappe M, Ludwig W, et al.: Favorable outcome of B-cell acute lymphoblastic leukemia in childhood: a report of three consecutive studies of the BFM group. *Blood* 20:2471–2478, 1992.

18. Hoelzer D, Thiel E, Loffler H, et al.: Prognostic factors in a multicenter study for treatment of acute lymphoblastic leukemia in adults. *Blood* 71:123–131, 1988.

19. Hoelzer D, Gokbuget N, Digel W, et al.: Outcome of adult patients with T-lymphoblastic lymphoma treated according to protocols for acute lymphoblastic leukemia. *Blood* 99:4379–4385, 2002.

20. Annino L, Vegna ML, Camera A, et al.: Treatment of adult acute lymphoblastic leukemia (ALL): long-term follow-up of the GIMEMA ALL 0288 randomized study. *Blood* 99:863–871, 2002.

21. Reiter A, Schrappe M, Ludwig W, et al.: Favorable outcome of B-cell acute lymphoblastic leukemia in childhood: a report of three consecutive studies of the BFM group. *Blood* 20:2471–2478, 1992.

22. Hussein KK, Dahlberg S, Head D, et al.: Treatment of acute lymphoblastic leukemia in adults with intensive induction, consolidation, and maintenance chemotherapy. *Blood* 73:57–63, 1989.

23. Kantarjian HM, O'Brien S, Smith TL, et al.: Results of treatment with hyper-CVAD, a dose-intensive regimen, in adult acute lymphocytic leukemia. *J Clin Oncol* 18:547–561, 2000.

24. Linker C, Damon L, Ries C, Navarro W: Intensified and shortened cyclical chemotherapy for adult acute lymphoblastic leukemia. *J Clin Oncol* 20:2464–2471, 2002.

25. Surapeneni UR, Cortes JE, Thomas D, et al.: Central nervous system relapse in adults with acute lymphoblastic leukemia. *Cancer* 94:773, 2002.

26. Buffler PA, Kwan ML, Reynolds P, Urayama KY: Environmental and genetic risk factors for childhood leukemia: appraising the evidence. *Cancer Invest* 23:60–75, 2005.

27. Henderson ES, McArthur J: Diagnosis, classification, and assessment of response to treatment. In: Henderson ES, Lister TA (eds.) *Leukemia*. 5th ed. Philadelphia: WB Saunders Co; 1990:733–768.

28. Hjalgrim LL, Rostgaard K, Hjalgrim H, et al.: Birth weight and risk for childhood leukemia in Denmark, Sweden, Norway, and Iceland. *J Natl Cancer Inst* 20:549–556, 2004.

29. Ducore JM, Parikh-Patel A, Gold EB: Cancer occurrence in Southeast Asian children in California. *Pediatr Hematol Oncol* 10:613–618, 2004.

30. Mucci LA, Granath F, Cnattingus S: Maternal smoking and childhood leukemia and lymphoma risk among 1,440,542 Swedish children. *Cancer Epidemiol Biomarkers Prev* 13:1528–1533, 2004.

31. Hitzler JK, Zipursky A: Origins of leukaemia in children with Down syndrome. *Nat Rev Cancer* 5:11–20, 2005.

32. Lange B: The management of neoplastic disorders of haematopoiesis in children with Down's syndrome. *Br J Haematol* 110:512–524, 2000.

33. Pui CH, Raimondi SC, Borowitz MJ, et al.: Immunophenotypes and karyotypes of leukemic cells in children with Down syndrome and acute lymphoblastic leukemia. *J Clin Oncol* 11:1361–1367, 1993.

34. Dordelmann M, Schrappe M, Reiter A, et al.: Down's syndrome in childhood acute lymphoblastic leukemia: clinical characteristics and treatment outcome in four consecutive BFM trials. *Leukemia* 12:645–651, 1998.

35. Chessells JM, Harrison G, Richards SM, et al.: Down's syndrome and acute lymphoblastic leukaemia: clinical features and response to treatment. *Arch Dis Child* 85:321–325, 2001.

36. Vogelstein B, Kinzler KW: Cancer genes and the pathways they control. *Nat Med* 10:789–799, 2004.

37. Pendergrass TW: Epidemiology of acute lymphoblastic leukemia. *Semin Oncol* 12:80–91, 1985.

38. Maia AT, van der velden VH, Harrison CJ: Prenatal origin of hyperdiploid acute lymphoblastic leukemia in identical twins. *Leukemia* 17:2202, 2003.

39. Preston DL, Kusumi S, Tomonaga M, et al.: Cancer incidence in atomic bomb survivors. Part III: Leukemia, lymphoma and multiple myeloma, 1950–1987. *Radiat Res* 137(suppl 9):S68–S97, 1994.

40. Boice JD Jr: Radiation-induced leukemia. In: Henderson ES, Lister TA (eds.) *Leukemia*. 5th ed. Philadelphia: WB Saunders Co; 1990:733–768.

41. Leone G, Mele L, Pulsoni A, Equitani F, Pagano L: The incidence of secondary leukemia. *Haematologica* 84:937–945, 1999.

42. Anson DS: The use of retroviral vectors for gene therapy—what are the risks? A review of retroviral pathogenesis and its relevance to retroviral vector-mediated gene delivery. *Genet Vaccines Ther* 2:9, 2004.

43. Hacein-Bey-Abina S, Von Calle C, Schmidt M, et al.: *LMO2*-associated clonal T cell proliferation in two patients after gene therapy for SCID-X1. *Science* 302:415–419, 2003.

44. Blattner WA: Human retroviruses: their role in cancer. *Proc Assoc Am Physicians* 111:563–572, 1999.

45. Stock W, Tsai T, Golden C, et al.: Cell cycle regulatory gene abnormalities are important determinants of leukemogenesis and disease biology in adult acute lymphoblastic leukemia. *Blood* 95:2364–2371, 2000.

46. Ries LAG, Kosary CL, Hankey BF, Miller BA, Clegg LX, Edwards BK (eds.): *SEER Cancer Statistics Review, 1973–1996*. Bethesda, MD: National Cancer Institute; 1999. NIH publication 99-2789.

47. Virchow RLK: Weisses blut. *N Notiz Geb Natur u Heilk* 36:151, 1845.

48. Gaynor J, Chapman D, Little C, et al.: A cause-specific hazard rate analysis of prognostic factors among 199 adults with acute lymphoblastic leukemia: the Memorial Hospital experience since 1969. *J Clin Oncol* 6:1014–1030, 1988.

49. Bennet JM, Catovsky D, Daniel MT, et al.: Proposals for the classification of the acute leukaemias. French–American–British (FAB) Co-Operative Group. *Br J Hematol* 33:451–458, 1976.

50. Brearley RL, Johnson SA, Lister TA: Acute lymphoblastic leukaemia in adults: clinicopathological correlations with the French–American–British (FAB) Co-Operative group classification. *Eur J Cancer* 15:909–914, 1979.

51. Magrath IT: Small noncleaved cell lymphomas (Burkitt's and Burkitt-like lymphomas. In: Magrath I (ed.) *The Non-Hodgkin's Lymphomas*. 2nd ed. London: Arnold; 1997:781–811.

52. Lee EJ, Petroni GR, Freter CR, et al.: Brief duration high intensity chemotherapy for patients with small non-cleaved cell lymphoma or FAB L3 acute lymphocytic leukemia: results of CALGB 9251. *J Clin Oncol* 19:4014–4022, 2001.

53. Wetzler M, Dodge RK, Mrózek K, et al.: Prospective karyotype analysis in adult acute lymphoblastic leukemia: the Cancer and Leukemia Group B experience. *Blood* 93:3983–3993, 1999.

54. Sobol RE, Royston I, LeBien TW, et al.: Adult acute lymphoblastic leukemia phenotypes defined by monoclonal antibodies. *Blood* 65:730–735, 1985.

55. Foon KA, Billing RJ, Terasaki PI, et al.: Immunologic classification of acute lymphoblastic leukemia. Implications for normal lymphoid differentiation. *Blood* 56:1120–1126, 1980.

56. First MIC Cooperative Study Group: Morphologic, immunologic and cytogenetic (MIC) working classification of acute lymphoblastic leukemia. *Cancer* Genet Cytogenet 23:189–197, 1986.

57. Second MIC Cooperative Study Group: Morphologic, inmunologic and cytogenetic (MIC) working classification of the acute myeloid leukaemias. *Br J Haemat* 68:487–494, 1988.

58. Bene MC, Castoldi G, Knapp W, et al.: Proposals for the immunological classification of acute leukemias. *Leukemia* 9:1783–1786, 1995.

59. Harris NL, Jaffe ES, Diebold J, et al.: World Health Organization classification of neoplastic diseases of the hematopoietic and lymphoid tissues: report of the Clinical Advisory Committee Meeting—Airlie House, Virginia, November 1997. *J Clin Oncol* 17:3835–3849, 1999.

# Chapter 11

# MOLECULAR BIOLOGY, PATHOLOGY, AND CYTOGENETICS OF ACUTE LYMPHOBLASTIC LEUKEMIA

*Meir Wetzler, Krzysztof Mrózek, and Clara D. Bloomfield*

## INTRODUCTION

Acute lymphoblastic leukemia (ALL) is characterized by distinctive morphologic, immunophenotypic, cytogenetic, and molecular genetic features, some of which have important clinical implications for both diagnosis and predicting response to specific treatment regimens, while the role of others is yet to be defined. This chapter focuses on the cytogenetic and molecular aberrations in ALL. Pathologic and immunophenotypic information is provided where it is clearly associated with the cytogenetic and/or molecular aberration.

## MORPHOLOGY

Until recently, ALL was classified based on morphology and cytochemistry according to the French–American–British (FAB) schema, which includes three major subtypes: L1, L2, and L3.[1] However, recent studies have failed to show prognostic significance of the L1 and L2 categories, and their designation has not had a high reproducibility rate among morphologists. Based on these findings, and as a result of improved understanding of the biology of these disorders, the 2001 World Health Organization (WHO) classification considers ALL as a form of lymphoma with a distinctive presentation. Initial classification is based on immunophenotype, and according to FAB, cases considered L1 and L2 are classified under precursor B- and T-cell neoplasms as precursor B-lymphoblastic leukemia/lymphoma and precursor T-lymphoblastic leukemia/lymphoma.[2] In addition to immunophenotype, the WHO classification incorporates molecular, cytogenetic, morphologic, and clinical features in defining disease entities, as described by the WHO Advisory Committee.[2] Table 11.1 shows a comparison between the two classifications.

In the WHO classification, FAB L3 is classified as one of the mature B-cell neoplasms and is designated Burkitt lymphoma/leukemia. It remains a separate entity char-acterized by its morphologic, immunophenotypic, cytogenetic, molecular, and clinical features. The blasts are characteristically medium in size, with dispersed chromatin, multiple nucleoli, and a moderate amount of deep blue cytoplasm with vacuoles. The classic "starry sky" description is derived from the presence of light-colored macrophages (stars) interspersed among sheets of dark blue blasts (sky). Oil red staining can be used to highlight the vacuoles in Burkitt-cell leukemia blasts.

## CYTOGENETIC ABERRATIONS

Cytogenetic aberrations can be structural, e.g., reciprocal and unbalanced translocations, deletions, dicentric chromosomes or inversions, or numerical, e.g., gain of

**Table 11.1** Comparison of the FAB and WHO classifications of ALL

| FAB classification | WHO classification[a] |
|---|---|
| ≥30% blasts | ≥20% blasts[b] |
| L1/L2 (morphology subgroups) | Precursor B-cell ALL (cytogenetic subgroups) |
| | t(9;22)(q34;q11.2) *BCR/ABL* <br> t(V;11)(V;q23) *MLL* rearranged[c] <br> t(1;19)(q23;p13.3) *E2A/PBX1* <br> t(12;21)(p13;q22) *ETV6/RUNX1 (TEL/AML1)* <br> Hypodiploid <br> Hyperdiploid >50 chromosomes <br> Precursor T-cell ALL (cytogenetic subgroups) <br> t(V;14)(V;q11-13) |
| L3 | Burkitt-cell leukemia |

[a]In the WHO classification, ALL and lymphoblastic lymphoma are regarded as a single entity with different clinical presentations.

[b]A disease with less than 20% blasts is defined as lymphoblastic lymphoma.

[c]"V" denotes various partner chromosomes and breakpoints.

a whole chromosome (trisomy) or loss of a whole chromosome (monosomy). In many instances, molecular dissection of structural chromosomal abnormalities, especially reciprocal translocations, has identified specific genes associated with leukemogenesis. The most common structural cytogenetic aberrations and their affected genes in adult ALL are shown in Table 11.2 arranged according to their frequency.

### STRUCTURAL ABERRATIONS
#### t(9;22)(q34;q11.2)

The t(9;22)(q34;q11.2) is the single most frequent chromosomal abnormality in adult ALL, being detected in 11–34% of patients, and is associated with an unfavorable prognosis.[3–11] It rarely occurs in therapy-related ALL.[12] The reciprocal translocation between chromosomes 9 and 22 results in the head-to-tail fusion of variable numbers of 5′ breakpoint cluster region (*BCR*) exons on chromosome band 22q11.2 with the exon 2 of the *ABL* gene (named after the Abelson murine leukemia virus), located on chromosome band 9q34.[13] The protein product of the fusion gene resulting from the t(9;22) plays a central role in the development of this form of ALL. Two main types of fusion proteins, p190$^{BCR/ABL}$ and p210$^{BCR/ABL}$, each containing NH$_2$-terminal domains of BCR and COOH-terminal domains of ABL, are produced, depending on the location of the breakpoint within the *BCR* gene. The p190$^{BCR/ABL}$ product contains the first exon of *BCR* and occurs in 50–78% of the ALL cases with t(9;22).[14–17] The p210$^{BCR/ABL}$ product contains either exon 13 or exon 14 of *BCR* and is less frequent in ALL. However, p190$^{BCR/ABL}$ transcripts are frequently detected at a low level in p210$^{BCR/ABL}$-positive ALL.[18] Clinically, there is no clear distinction between the two molecular variants of the disease,[19–21] except for one report showing that the p210$^{BCR/ABL}$ product is associated with older age patient[22] and another report demonstrating a higher risk of relapse in p190$^{BCR/ABL}$ ALL following allogeneic transplantation.[23] Of interest, imatinib-containing treatment has not revealed any outcome difference between the two disease types.

Secondary chromosomal aberrations accompanying t(9;22) occur in 41–86% of adult ALL patients.[20,21,24–27] The most common additional aberrations in a Cancer and Leukemia Group B series[27] were, in order of decreasing frequency, +der(22)t(9;22), 9p rearrangements, high hyperdiploidy (>50 chromosomes), +8, and −7. In this study, the presence of +der(22)t(9;22) was associated with a higher cumulative incidence of relapse, while the presence of −7 as a sole secondary abnormality was associated with a lower complete remission rate.[27]

At the molecular level, *BCR/ABL* has recently been shown to activate the Src kinases Lyn, Hck, and Fgr in ALL cells.[28] These kinases are less frequently activated in CML, suggesting a unique downstream signaling pathway in *BCR/ABL*-positive ALL. Further, application of DNA microarray gene expression profiling has revealed that *BCR/ABL*-positive pediatric ALL is characterized by gene expression profiles distinct from other prognostically relevant leukemia subtypes. These results were recently partially confirmed and validated in samples from adult ALL patients. Finally, mutations at the ABL kinase domain are frequent and are associated with resistance to imatinib.[29]

The cells of almost all newly diagnosed patients with t(9;22) have a pre-B-cell immunophenotype[4,6,14]; additionally, expression of CD10[14,29] and of myeloid markers[14] is more prevalent in patients with this translocation than in other adult ALL patients. There is some preponderance of FAB L1 over L2 morphology.[6]

#### dic(9;12), dic(9;20), and del(9p)

Structural aberrations involving the short arm of chromosome 9 occur in 5–15% of adult ALL patients.[6,7,9,10] They include dicentric chromosomes: dic(9;12)(p11-13;p11-13) and dic(9;20)(p11;q11), as well as deletions of 9p. Both dicentric chromosomes are associated with a favorable clinical outcome.

**Table 11.2** Most frequent cytogenetic aberrations in adult ALL and their corresponding genes

| Cytogenetic aberration | Genes involved[a] | Frequency (%) |
|---|---|---|
| t(9;22)(q34;q11.2) | *BCR/ABL* | 11–34 |
| del(9p) | *CDKN2A* and *CDKN2B* | 5–15 |
| t(4;11)(q21;q23) | *MLL/AF4* | 3–7 |
| del(12p) or t(12p) | *ETV6* | 4–5 |
| t(14;V)(q11;V)[b] | *TCRA* and *TCRD* | 4–6 |
| t(14;V)(q32;V)[b] | *IGH, BCL11A, TCL-1B,* and *CL11B* | 5 |
| del(6q) | ? | 2–6 |
| t(1;19)(q23;p13.3) | *E2A/PBX1* | 3 |
| t(8;14)(q24;q32) | *MYC/IGH* | 1–2 |
| t(2;8)(p12;q24) | *MYC/IGK* | |
| t(8;22)(q24;q11) | *MYC/IGL* | |

[a]Please refer to text for abbreviations and references for the percentages.
[b]"V" denotes various partner chromosomes and breakpoints.

Other anomalies of 9p, mainly del(9p), are most often associated with the presence of additional clonal aberrations (in up to 90% of patients); in almost one-third of the cases, the additional abnormalities include t(9;22).[10] These data suggest that del(9p) likely represents a secondary cytogenetic abnormality.

### 11q23 aberrations

Chromosome band 11q23 harbors the mixed lineage leukemia gene (*MLL*, also known as *ALL-1*, *HTRX*, or *HRX*),[30] which encodes a putative transcriptional regulator. *MLL* is involved in reciprocal translocations with many partner genes, localized on different chromosomes, both in ALL and in acute myeloid leukemia (AML).[31] While the *MLL* gene can be amplified in a subset of AML patients, its amplification is rare in ALL.[32] The distribution of 11q23/*MLL* translocation partners differs between ALL and AML, with t(4;11)(q21;q23) being by far the most frequent 11q23 translocation in ALL (see below). The partial tandem duplication of *MLL*, described in AML,[33] has not been detected in ALL. 11q23/*MLL* translocations have been described in both de novo and therapy-related disease.[34]

ALL with *MLL* rearrangements also has a unique gene expression profile.[35] Specifically, some *HOX* (homeobox) genes are expressed at higher levels in *MLL*-positive ALL than in *MLL*-negative ALL.[36] Furthermore, gene expression profiles predictive of relapse were recently identified in pediatric *MLL*-positive ALL in one study,[37] although they did not reach statistical significance in another. Further work in this area is on going.

*t(4;11)(q21;q23)* The t(4;11)(q21;q23) is the most frequent chromosomal rearrangement involving the *MLL* gene in adult ALL, being detected in 3–7% of ALL patients, and is associated with an unfavorable outcome.[3–7,9,10] It results in two reciprocal fusion products coding for chimeric proteins derived from *MLL* and from a serine/proline-rich protein encoded by the *AF4* (*ALL1* fused gene from chromosome 4) gene.[38]

Griesinger et al. have demonstrated the presence of *MLL/AF4* fusion gene in adult ALL patients without cytogenetically detectable t(4;11). Another study analyzed the clinical significance of the *MLL/AF4* fusion gene detected molecularly in the absence of karyotypic evidence of t(4;11), and established that patients whose blasts were *MLL/AF4* positive and lacked a t(4;11) had outcomes similar to patients without *MLL/AF4*. This study suggests that additional treatment is not needed for patients whose blasts are *MLL/AF4* positive but t(4;11) negative.

Secondary cytogenetic aberrations in addition to t(4;11) are found in approximately 40% of patients.[6,39,40] The most common additional changes were i(7)(q10) and +6 in one series[39] and +X, i(7)(q10), and +8 in another.[40] With treatment carried out according to risk-adapted therapy, no difference in outcome was observed between patients with and without clonal chromosomal aberrations in addition to t(4;11) at diagnosis,[40] although this series was relatively small.

*Other balanced translocations involving 11q23* Other recurrent, albeit rare in ALL, translocations involving *MLL* include t(6;11)(q27;q23), t(9;11) (p22;q23), t(10;11)(p12;q23), and t(11;19) (q23;p13.3).[41] The respective fusion partners of the *MLL* gene are *AF6*, *AF9*, *AF10*, and *ENL* (eleven-nineteen leukemia). Other less common *MLL* partners have also been described.[42]

Almost all patients with 11q23 translocations have a CD10-negative and CD19-positive B-cell precursor ALL (pre-pre-B ALL).[43] Coexpression of myeloid antigens is well recognized. In one series, 21 of 24 patients with CD10−/CD19+/CD15+ immunophenotype had t(4;11).[20] FAB L2 morphology has been described in up to 44% of patients.[6] Patients with 11q23 aberrations have an unfavorable outcome.[3–10]

### del(12p) or t(12p)

Abnormalities of the short arm of chromosome 12 have been described in 4–5% of adult ALL patients.[6,7,9,10] In one series, 20 of 23 (87%) cases with abnormal 12p had net loss of 12p material: 8 caused by deletions and 12 by unbalanced translocations.[6] It is believed that a putative tumor suppressor gene is located in chromosome band 12p12.3.[44,45] The outcome of patients with abnormalities of 12p, who did not have t(9;22), was favorable in two adult ALL series.[7,10]

A cryptic t(12;21)(p13;q22), commonly found in pediatric ALL and also associated with a favorable outcome, is rare in adult ALL.[46–48] The genes involved in this translocation are *ETV6*[49] and *RUNX1* (runt-related transcription factor 1, also known as *AML1* and *CBFA2*).[50] An intriguing explanation for the favorable outcome of pediatric patients with t(12;21) may lie in the finding that the ETV6/RUNX1 protein can overcome drug resistance through transcriptional repression of multidrug resistance-1 gene expression.[51] Furthermore, t(12;21) ALL is associated with a lower expression of genes involved in purine metabolism and lower de novo purine synthesis.[52] Taken together, these data may explain the favorable outcome of childhood ALL with t(12;21).

### t(14q11-13)

Abnormalities of the proximal part of the long arm of chromosome 14 have been described in 4–6% of adult ALL patients and are associated with the WHO precursor T-lymphoblastic leukemia/lymphoma designation.[6,10] The genes involved in t(14q11-13) are T-cell receptor α (*TCRA*) and δ (*TCRD*).[6]

### Translocations involving band 14q32, other than t(8;14)(q24;q32)

Abnormalities of the distal part of the long arm of chromosome 14 have been described in approximately 5% of adult ALL patients.[10] The genes involved in t(14q32) are the immunoglobulin heavy chain locus (*IGH*)[53] and the Krüeppel zinc-finger gene (*BCL11A*)[54] on chromosome 14q32.3, both in B-lineage ALL; the *TCL1* (T-cell leukemia) gene on chromosome 14q32.1[55] and the distal region of a Krüeppel-like zinc-finger transcription factor *BCL11B* (also called *CTIP2*) on chromosome 14q32.2,[56,57] both in T-lineage ALL.

### del(6q)

Deletions of the long arm of chromosome 6 have been reported in 2–6% of adult ALL patients.[3,6–9,58] In one large series, most deletions encompassed band 6q21 (in 20 of 23 patients), with del(6)(q12q16) being present in 3 remaining patients.[6] In most patients, del(6q) is found together with additional chromosomal abnormalities.[10] It is unclear whether del(6q) represents a primary or secondary cytogenetic abnormality. The outcome of patients with del(6q) was somewhat better than that of patients with a normal karyotype in one large study,[6] but this finding requires confirmation.

### t(1;19)(q23;p13.3)

This aberration is significantly less common in adult than in pediatric ALL. It was recognized as a separate entity in adult ALL in only one series, where it was found in 3% of the patients.[6] There are two cytogenetic variants of the (1;19) translocation: a less common balanced t(1;19)(q23;p13.3) and a predominant unbalanced der(19)t(1;19)(q23;p13.3), which is almost always accompanied by two intact chromosomes 1. The genes involved in this translocation are *E2A* (early region of adenovirus type 2 encoding helix-loop-helix proteins E12/E47) on chromosome band 19p13.3[59,60] and *PBX1* (pre-B-cell leukemia transcription factor 1) on chromosome band 1q23.[61,62] Rare ALL cases with t(1;19) lack the *E2A/PBX1* fusion gene.[63]

The t(1;19) is associated with L1 morphology and CD10 and CD19 positivity in almost all cases.[6,63] Interestingly, up to 25% of cases have been described to have Burkitt-like morphology, even though the immunophenotype was not always of the mature (positive surface immunoglobulin expression) type.[6,63]

### t(8;14)(q24;q32)

This aberration and its variants, t(2;8)(p12;q24) and t(8;22)(q24;q11), are the hallmark of Burkitt lymphoma/leukemia. As a result of t(8;14), the *MYC* gene, located at 8q24, is juxtaposed to the enhancer elements of the *IGH* gene at 14q32. In the case of variant translocations, one of the immunoglobulin light chain genes, mapped to bands 2p12 (*IGK*) and 22q12 (*IGL*), is translocated to a telomeric region of the *MYC* gene at 8q24.[64–67] Consequently, *MYC* is activated and expressed at high levels. Because the product of the *MYC* gene, a DNA-binding protein, is implicated in the regulation of a number of other critical genes, its constitutive production results in uncontrolled proliferation of cells

with one of the translocations. In approximately 45% of ALL L3 cases, one of the primary translocations, t(8;14), t(2;8), or t(8;22), is the sole chromosomal abnormality.[42] The most frequent secondary aberrations include unbalanced structural anomalies of chromosome 1 that lead to gain of material from its long arm, i.e., duplications of 1q, isochromosomes of 1q, and unbalanced translocations involving 1q, and trisomies of chromosomes 7 and 8.[42]

The disease has two major clinical presentations: sporadic/immunodeficiency Burkitt lymphoma/leukemia seen in the Western world, and endemic Burkitt lymphoma/leukemia found in equatorial Africa and almost always associated with Epstein–Barr virus (EBV) infection. They differ not only in regard to clinical manifestations, but also at the molecular level.[68–71]

Burkitt lymphoma/leukemia is associated with mature B-cell immunophenotype with surface IgM, Bcl-6, CD19, CD20, CD22, CD10, and CD79a, and is TdT, CD5, and CD23 negative.

### NUMERICAL ABERRATIONS
### Hyperdiploidy

A high hyperdiploid karyotype, defined by the presence of more than 50 chromosomes, is detected in 2–9% of adult ALL patients.[3,4,6–10] The most common extra chromosomes in 30 adult patients with high hyperdiploidy (range, 51–65 chromosomes) were (in decreasing order) 21, 4, 6, 14, 8, 10, and 17.[6] In pediatric ALL, gain of the X chromosome appears to be the most common chromosomal abnormality, being detected in nearly all children with a high hyperdiploid karyotype and in up to one-third of the patients with low hyperdiploid karyotype (i.e., 47–50 chromosomes).[72] Interestingly, chromosomes 6, 8, and 10 were also the most common chromosomes lost in the hypodiploid group, along with chromosome 21. The reason for the involvement of these specific chromosomes in both types of aberrant karyotypes is unclear. Translocation (9;22) is a common structural aberration in patients with high hyperdiploidy; it was present in 11 of 30 (37%) patients in one series[6] and 7 of 11 (64%) in another.[26] Patients with hyperdiploidy and t(9;22) were older and had shorter disease-free survival (DFS) than those without t(9;22).[6]

The mechanism leading to hyperdiploidy is unknown. Several possibilities have been suggested, including polyploidization with subsequent losses of chromosomes, successive gains of individual chromosomes in consecutive cell divisions, and a simultaneous occurrence of several trisomies in a single abnormal mitosis.[73]

The clinical outcome of adult patients with hyperdiploid karyotypes varies in different series. In two studies, the outcome of patients with hyperdiploid karyotypes was better than that of other adult ALL patients,[3,7,9] while other studies[4,6,10,26] showed poor outcome for these patients except for those with near tetraploidy.[6] The reason for this discrepancy is unclear. In two studies,[7,10] the analysis was restricted to patients with hyperdiploidy without structural abnormalities. The other studies[3,4,6,9,26] did not provide information regarding structural abnormalities. A study of a larger cohort of adult ALL patients analyzing whether hyperdiploid karyotype without structural abnormalities constitutes an independent prognostic factor is warranted.

Almost all cases with high hyperdiploidy have precursor B-lineage ALL.[6,74]

### Hypodiploidy

Hypodiploidy is defined by the presence of less than 46 chromosomes. This karyotype is found in 4–9% of adult ALL patients.[3,6,7,9,75] Patients with hypodiploid karyotypes tend to be somewhat younger than patients with a normal karyotype.[6,7] A recent analysis grouped patients with hypodiploidy into those with near-haploidy (23–29 chromosomes), low hypodiploidy (33–39 chromosomes), and high hypodiploidy (42–45 chromosomes).[75] There were only six adult patients in this series, five of them in the low-hypodiploidy group and one in the high-hypodiploidy group. The most common losses in seven patients with hypodiploidy ranging from 30 to 39 chromosomes involved chromosomes 1, 5, 6, 8, 10, 11, 15, 18, 19, 21, 22, and the sex chromosomes.[6] Only one study reported specifically on hypodiploidy without structural abnormalities.[7] Patients with hypodiploidy have a DFS between 2 and 4 months, and therefore the abnormality is classified as unfavorable.[7]

Most of the patients with hypodiploidy have a B-lineage immunophenotype,[6,7,75] although one report[74] described up to 20% of patients with T-lineage ALL.

### Trisomy 8

Trisomy 8 in ALL is most often associated with other karyotypic abnormalities; it is rare as a sole abnormality.[76] Twelve of 23 (52%) patients with trisomy 8 also had t(9;22). However, patients with trisomy 8 without t(9;22) but with miscellaneous other abnormalities fared as poorly as those with trisomy 8 and t(9;22).[10] It is unclear whether the adverse outcome is due to the other primary abnormalities or associated with the presence of trisomy 8 per se.

### Monosomy 7

As with trisomy 8, monosomy 7 is most often associated with other karyotypic abnormalities; monosomy 7 as a sole abnormality is rare in ALL. Only one adult[10] and one pediatric[77] series defined patients with monosomy 7 as a separate group. In the adult series, 9 of 14 (64%) patients with monosomy 7 had t(9;22). Patients with monosomy 7 without t(9;22) but with miscellaneous other abnormalities fared as poorly as those with monosomy 7 and t(9;22).[10] It is unclear whether the adverse outcome is due to the other primary abnormalities or is associated with the presence of monosomy 7.

## MOLECULAR ABERRATIONS

Molecular aberrations are divided into those that emerge from specific aberrations, gene profiling, and polymorphisms.

### SPECIFIC ABERRATIONS

#### Extrachromosomal amplification of the *NUP214/ABL* fusion gene in T-cell ALL

Two recent studies revealed a novel genetic phenomenon in T-cell ALL: namely cryptic extrachromosomal amplification of a segment from chromosome 9 containing the *ABL* gene. Barber et al. were the first to report that amplification involving the *ABL* gene occurred in 5 of 210 (2.3%) children and 3 of 70 (4.3%) adults with T-cell ALL, even though there was no cytogenetic evidence of amplification, such as double minutes or homogeneously staining regions. The authors suggested that amplified *ABL* sequences were located on submicroscopic circular extrachromosomal DNA molecules called episomes.

### SMAD3

SMAD3 [Sma and Mad (mothers against decapentaplegic) 3] is involved in signal transduction from the transforming growth factor β(TGF-β) superfamily of receptors to the nucleus.[78] SMAD3 protein was recently shown to be absent in T-cell ALL, but present in B-cell ALL and AML. The *SMAD3* transcript was intact in all leukemia subtypes. These data suggest that *SMAD3* is functioning as a tumor suppressor gene in T-cell ALL.

### FLT3

*FLT3* activating mutations are in general rare in ALL, but have been detected in approximately 20% of ALL specimens, with rearrangement of the *MLL* gene,[37,79,80] 25% of hyperdiploid ALL,[80,81] and in the rare subset of CD117/KIT-positive, CD3-positive ALL.[82] Interestingly, the internal tandem duplication of the *FLT3* gene, commonly detected in AML, has thus far not been seen in ALL. FLT3 inhibitors (e.g., PKC412 and CEP-701) can suppress *FLT3*-positive ALL cells in vitro and therefore warrant clinical trials.[79,83]

### TLX1

Gene expression profiles in T cell ALL identified five different signature patterns involving different oncogenes: *TLX1 (HOX11)*, *TLX3 (HOX11L2)*, *TAL1* plus *LMO1/2*, *LYL1* plus *LMO2* and *MLL-ENL*.[85] Only the *TLX1*-expressing samples were associated with a favorable outlook in children[86,87] and adults[88] with T cell ALL.

### Cryptic t(5;14)(q35;q32) and the overexpression of the *TLX3* gene

*TLX3* gene expression represents one of the five oncogenes involved in T-cell ALL. This gene is located on chromosome 5q35 and was found to be transcriptionally activated as a result of a translocation between chromosomes 5 and 14, t(5;14)(q35;q32).[84] A study of samples from 23 childhood T-cell ALL patients revealed that this translocation was cryptic in five of them,[84] which was corroborated by larger studies.[85,86] Overexpression of *TLX3* was reported by one group[87] to bestow poor prognosis but this has not been substantiated by other, larger studies.[85,86]

### NOTCH1

*NOTCH1* point mutations, insertions, and deletions producing aberrant increases in NOTCH1 signaling are frequently present in T-cell ALL.[88–90] Further, NOTCH1 signaling was shown to be required for sustained growth and, in a subset of cell lines, for survival. Finally, experiments with small-molecule inhibitors of γ-secretase, a protease required for normal NOTCH signal transduction and the activity of the mutated forms of NOTCH1, showed inhibitory activity in T-cell ALL with NOTCH1 mutations. These results provide a rationale for clinical trials with NOTCH1 inhibitors, such as γ-secretase antagonists.[89,90]

### GENE PROFILING

#### Relapse-classifying gene sets

Several groups have identified distinctive gene sets in diagnostic samples from patients whose disease subsequently recurred.[91,92] In spite of the different age groups studied (pediatric[91] vs adult[92]), assortment of array platforms, and diverse treatment protocols, all Affymetrix ALL array data and two sets of cDNA arrays validated the predictability of these gene sets to delineate the following cytogenetic prognostic groups: hyperdiploidy, T-lineage ALL, t(12;21), t(4;11), and t(1;19).[93]

#### Resistance-classifying gene sets

A different gene profile was identified when leukemia cells were tested for in vitro sensitivity to the four most commonly used drugs in ALL, i.e., prednisolone, vincristine, asparaginase, and daunorubicin.[94] Interestingly, only three genes for which results were significant in these analyses, *RPL6*, *ARHA*, and *SLC2A14*, have previously been associated with resistance to doxorubicin. Two gene expression profiles that differed according to sensitivity or resistance to the four drugs were compared with treatment outcome. These two gene sets were significantly and independently predictive of outcome. They are now being analyzed in prospective studies to tailor treatment according to patterns of resistance.

## POLYMORPHISMS

Pharmacogenetics is the study of genetic variations in drug-processing genes and individual responses to drugs.[95] It enables the improved identification of patients at higher risk for either disease relapse or chemotherapy-associated side effects.

More than 20 years ago, it was recognized that the activity of thiopurine-*S*-methyltransferase (TPMT), the enzyme involved in the metabolism of 6-mercaptopurine and 6-thioguanine, differs among patients and that approximately 1 in 300 individuals demonstrates reduced enzymatic activity.[96–100] Molecular testing to identify this polymorphism was developed shortly thereafter[101,102] and showed good correlation with the enzymatic activity. Based on molecular testing, it has become clear that homozygous carriers for one of the three *TPMT* mutant alleles experience severe myelotoxicity and increased risk of relapse due to treatment delays.[103,104] Interestingly, patients with the mutated *TPMT* alleles have a significantly higher risk of developing secondary brain tumors if treated with whole-brain radiation.[105] Similarly, there was a trend toward increased risk of secondary AML in patients with decreased enzymatic activity.[106]

Similarly, single-nucleotide polymorphisms involving four of the enzymes involved in methotrexate metabolism have been implicated in increased relapse risk or toxicity in pediatric ALL patients: methylenetetrahydrofolate reductase,[107–111] reduced folate carrier,[112–114] thymidylate synthetase,[115,116] and methylenetetrahydrofolate dehydrogenase.[111]

## FUTURE DIRECTIONS

We believe that progress in cytogenetic and genetic dissection of ALL will lead to risk-adapted treatment in adult ALL, as is already being accomplished for pediatric ALL. Currently, allogeneic transplantation in first remission is offered to adults with unfavorable karyotypes. The future promises more refined approaches, based on the information from genetic analyses, which will hopefully lead to improved outcome in adult ALL.

## ACKNOWLEDGMENTS

This work was supported in part by grant P30CA16058 from the National Cancer Institute, Bethesda, MD, and the Coleman Leukemia Research Fund.

## REFERENCES

1. Bennett JM, Catovsky D, Daniel MT, et al.: The morphological classification of acute lymphoblastic leukaemia: concordance among observers and clinical correlations. *Br J Haematol* 47:553, 1981.
2. Harris NL, Jaffe ES, Diebold J, et al.: World Health Organization classification of neoplastic diseases of the hematopoietic and lymphoid tissues: report of the

Clinical Advisory Committee meeting–Airlie House, Virginia, November 1997. *J Clin Oncol* 17:3835, 1999.

3. Bloomfield CD, Secker-Walker LM, Goldman AI, et al.: Six-year follow-up of the clinical significance of karyotype in acute lymphoblastic leukemia. *Cancer Genet Cytogenet* 40:171, 1989.

4. Fenaux P, Lai JL, Morel P, et al.: Cytogenetics and their prognostic value in childhood and adult acute lymphoblastic leukemia (ALL) excluding L3. *Hematol Oncol* 7:307, 1989.

5. Walters R, Kantarjian HM, Keating MJ, et al.: The importance of cytogenetic studies in adult acute lymphocytic leukemia. *Am J Med* 89:579, 1990.

6. Groupe Français de Cytogénétique Hématologique: Cytogenetic abnormalities in adult acute lymphoblastic leukemia: correlations with hematologic findings outcome. A Collaborative Study of the Groupe Français de Cytogénétique Hématologique. *Blood* 88:3135, 1996.

7. Secker-Walker LM, Prentice HG, Durrant J, et al.: Cytogenetics adds independent prognostic information in adults with acute lymphoblastic leukaemia on MRC trial UKALL XA. *Br J Haematol* 96:601, 1997.

8. Faderl S, Kantarjian HM, Talpaz M, et al.: Clinical significance of cytogenetic abnormalities in adult acute lymphoblastic leukemia. *Blood* 91:3995, 1998.

9. Chessells JM, Hall E, Prentice HG, et al.: The impact of age on outcome in lymphoblastic leukaemia; MRC UKALL X and XA compared: a report from the MRC Paediatric and Adult Working Parties. *Leukemia* 12:463, 1998.

10. Wetzler M, Dodge RK, Mrózek K, et al.: Prospective karyotype analysis in adult acute lymphoblastic leukemia: the Cancer and Leukemia Group B experience. *Blood* 93:3983, 1999.

11. Gleissner B, Rieder H, Thiel E, et al.: Prospective BCR-ABL analysis by polymerase chain reaction (RT-PCR) in adult acute B-lineage lymphoblastic leukemia: reliability of RT-nested-PCR and comparison to cytogenetic data. *Leukemia* 15:1834, 2001.

12. Block AW, Carroll AJ, Hagemeijer A, et al.: Rare recurring balanced chromosome abnormalities in therapy-related myelodysplastic syndromes and acute leukemia: report from an international workshop. *Genes Chromosomes Cancer* 33:401, 2002.

13. Faderl S, Talpaz M, Estrov Z, et al.: The biology of chronic myeloid leukemia. *N Engl J Med* 341:164, 1999.

14. Kantarjian HM, Talpaz M, Dhingra K, et al.: Significance of the P210 versus P190 molecular abnormalities in adults with Philadelphia chromosome-positive acute leukemia. *Blood* 78:2411, 1991.

15. Westbrook CA, Hooberman AL, Spino C, et al.: Clinical significance of the BCR-ABL fusion gene in adult acute lymphoblastic leukemia: a Cancer and Leukemia Group B study (8762). *Blood* 80:2983, 1992.

16. Melo JV, Gordon DE, Tuszynski A, et al.: Expression of the ABL-BCR fusion gene in Philadelphia-positive acute lymphoblastic leukemia. *Blood* 81:2488, 1993.

17. Lim LC, Heng KK, Vellupillai M, et al.: Molecular and phenotypic spectrum of de novo Philadelphia positive acute leukemia. *Int J Mol Med* 4:665, 1999.

18. van Rhee F, Hochhaus A, Lin F, et al.: P190 BCR-ABL mRNA is expressed at low levels in p210-positive chronic myeloid and acute lymphoblastic leukemias. *Blood* 87:5213, 1996.

19. Secker-Walker LM, Craig JM, Hawkins JM, et al.: Philadelphia positive acute lymphoblastic leukemia in adults: age distribution, BCR breakpoint and prognostic significance. *Leukemia* 5:196, 1991.

20. Rieder H, Ludwig WD, Gassmann W, et al.: Prognostic significance of additional chromosome abnormalities in adult patients with Philadelphia chromosome positive acute lymphoblastic leukaemia. *Br J Haematol* 95:678, 1996.

21. Ko BS, Tang JL, Lee FY, et al.: Additional chromosomal abnormalities and variability of BCR breakpoints in Philadelphia chromosome/BCR-ABL-positive acute lymphoblastic leukemia in Taiwan. *Am J Hematol* 71:291, 2002.

22. Gleißner B, Gökbuget N, Bartram CR, et al.: Leading prognostic relevance of the BCR-ABL translocation in adult acute B-lineage lymphoblastic leukemia: a prospective study of the German Multicenter Trial Group and confirmed polymerase chain reaction analysis. *Blood* 99:1536, 2002.

23. Radich J, Gehly G, Lee A, et al.: Detection of BCR-ABL transcripts in Philadelphia chromosome-positive acute lymphoblastic leukemia after marrow transplantation. *Blood* 89:2602, 1997.

24. Preti HA, O'Brien S, Giralt S, et al.: Philadelphia-chromosome-positive adult acute lymphocytic leukemia: characteristics, treatment results, and prognosis in 41 patients. *Am J Med* 97:60–65, 1994.

25. Thomas X, Thiebaut A, Olteanu N, et al.: Philadelphia chromosome positive adult acute lymphoblastic leukemia: characteristics, prognostic factors and treatment outcome. *Hematol Cell Ther* 40:119, 1998.

26. Faderl S, Kantarjian HM, Thomas DA, et al.: Outcome of Philadelphia chromosome-positive adult acute lymphoblastic leukemia. *Leuk Lymphoma* 36:263, 2000.

27. Wetzler M, Dodge RK, Mrózek K, et al.: Additional cytogenetic abnormalities in adults with Philadelphia chromosome-positive acute lymphoblastic leukaemia: a study of the Cancer and Leukaemia Group B. *Br J Haematol* 124:275, 2004.

28. Hu Y, Liu Y, Pelletier S, et al.: Requirement of Src kinases Lyn, Hck and Fgr for BCR-ABL1-induced B-lymphoblastic leukemia but not chronic myeloid leukemia. *Nat Genet* 36:453, 2004.

29. Hofmann WK, Komor M, Hoelzer D, Ottmann OG: Mechanisms of resistance to STI571 (Imatinib) in Philadelphia-chromosome positive acute lymphoblastic leukemia. *Leuk Lymphoma* 45:655, 2004.

30. Specchia G, Mininni D, Guerrasio A, et al.: Ph positive acute lymphoblastic leukemia in adults: molecular and clinical studies. *Leuk Lymphoma* 18(suppl 1):37, 1995.

31. Tkachuk DC, Kohler S, Cleary ML: Involvement of a homolog of *Drosophila* trithorax by 11q23 chromosomal translocations in acute leukemias. *Cell* 71:691, 1992.

32. Harrison CJ, Cuneo A, Clark R, et al.: Ten novel 11q23 chromosomal partner sites. *Leukemia* 12:811, 1998.

33. Cuthbert G, Thompson K, McCullough S, et al.: MLL amplification in acute leukaemia: a United Kingdom Cancer Cytogenetics Group (UKCCG) study. *Leukemia* 14:1885, 2000.

34. Strout MP, Marcucci G, Caligiuri MA, et al.: Core-binding factor (CBF) and MLL-associated primary acute myeloid leukemia: biology and clinical implications. *Ann Hematol* 78:251, 1999.

35. Bloomfield CD, Archer KJ, Mrózek K, et al.: 11q23 balanced chromosome aberrations in treatment-related myelodysplastic syndromes and acute leukemia: report from an international workshop. *Genes Chromosomes Cancer* 33:362, 2002.

36. Rozovskaia T, Ravid-Amir O, Tillib S, et al.: Expression profiles of acute lymphoblastic and myeloblastic leukemias with ALL-1 rearrangements. *Proc Natl Acad Sci USA* 100:7853, 2003.

37. Armstrong SA, Staunton JE, Silverman LB, et al.: MLL translocations specify a distinct gene expression profile that distinguishes a unique leukemia. *Nat Genet* 30:41, 2002.

38. Tsutsumi S, Taketani T, Nishimura K, et al.: Two distinct gene expression signatures in pediatric acute lymphoblastic leukemia with MLL rearrangements. *Cancer Res* 63:4882, 2003.

39. Gu Y, Nakamura T, Alder H, et al.: The t(4;11) chromosome translocation of human acute leukemias fuses the *ALL-1* gene, related to Drosophila *trithorax*, to the *AF-4* gene. *Cell* 71:701, 1992.

40. Pui CH: Acute leukemias with the t(4;11)(q21;q23). *Leuk Lymphoma* 7:173, 1992.

41. Schoch C, Rieder H, Freund M, et al.: Twenty-three cases of acute lymphoblastic leukemia with translocation t(4;11)(q21;q23): the implication of additional chromosomal aberrations. *Ann Hematol* 70:195, 1995.

42. Secker-Walker LM: General report on the European Union Concerted Action Workshop on 11q23, London, UK, May 1997. *Leukemia* 12:776, 1998.

43. Mitelman F, Johansson B, Mertens F (eds.): Mitelman database of chromosome aberrations in cancer. Available at: http://cgap.nci.nih.gov/Chromosomes/Mitelman, 2005.

44. First MIC Cooperative Study Group: Morphologic, immunologic, and cytogenetic (MIC) working classification of acute lymphoblastic leukemias. *Cancer Genet Cytogenet* 23:189, 1986.

45. Aissani B, Bonan C, Baccichet A, et al.: Childhood acute lymphoblastic leukemia: is there a tumor suppressor gene in chromosome 12p12.3? *Leuk Lymphoma* 34:231, 1999.

46. Montpetit A, Larose J, Boily G, et al.: Mutational and expression analysis of the chromosome 12p candidate tumor suppressor genes in pre-B acute lymphoblastic leukemia. *Leukemia* 18:1499, 2004.

47. Aguiar RC, Sohal J, van Rhee F, et al.: TEL-AML1 fusion in acute lymphoblastic leukaemia of adults. *Br J Haematol* 95:673, 1996.

48. Raynaud S, Mauvieux L, Cayuela JM, et al.: TEL/AML1 fusion gene is a rare event in adult acute lymphoblastic leukemia. *Leukemia* 10:1529, 1996.

49. Kwong YL, Wong KF: Low frequency of TEL/AML1 in adult acute lymphoblastic leukemia. *Cancer Genet Cytogenet* 98:137, 1997.

50. Golub TR, Barker GF, Lovett M, et al.: Fusion of PDGF receptor beta to a novel ets-like gene, *tel*, in chronic myelomonocytic leukemia with t(5;12) chromosomal translocation. *Cell* 77:307, 1994.

51. Romana SP, Le Coniat M, Berger R: t(12;21): a new recurrent translocation in acute lymphoblastic leukemia. *Genes Chromosomes Cancer* 9:186, 1994.

52. Asakura K, Uchida H, Miyachi H, et al.: TEL/AML1 overcomes drug resistance through transcriptional repression of multidrug resistance-1 gene expression. *Mol Cancer Res* 2:339, 2004.

53. Zaza G, Yang W, Kager L, et al.: Acute lymphoblastic leukemia with TEL-AML1 fusion has lower expression of genes involved in purine metabolism and lower de novo purine synthesis. *Blood* 104:1435, 2004.

54. Willis TG, Dyer MJ: The role of immunoglobulin translocations in the pathogenesis of B-cell malignancies. *Blood* 96:808, 2000.

55. Satterwhite E, Sonoki T, Willis TG, et al.: The BCL11 gene family: involvement of BCL11A in lymphoid malignancies. *Blood* 98:3413, 2001.

56. Fu TB, Virgilio L, Narducci MG, et al.: Characterization and localization of the TCL-1 oncogene product. *Cancer Res* 54:6297, 1994.

57. MacLeod RAF, Nagel S, Kaufmann M, et al.: Activation of *HOX11L2* by juxtaposition with 3'-*BCL11B* in an acute lymphoblastic leukemia cell line (HPB-ALL) with t(5;14)(q35;q32.2). *Genes Chromosomes Cancer* 37:84, 2003.

58. Bernard OA, Busson-LeConiat M, Ballerini P, et al.: A new recurrent and specific cryptic translocation, t(5;14)(q35;q32), is associated with expression of the Hox11L2 gene in T acute lymphoblastic leukemia. *Leukemia* 15:1495, 2001.

59. Mancini M, Vegna ML, Castoldi GL, et al.: Partial deletions of long arm of chromosome 6: biologic and clinical implications in adult acute lymphoblastic leukemia. *Leukemia* 16:2055, 2002.

60. Mellentin JD, Murre C, Donlon TA, et al.: The gene for enhancer binding proteins E12/E47 lies at the t(1;19) breakpoint in acute leukemias. *Science* 246:379, 1989.

61. Murre C, McCaw PS, Baltimore D: A new DNA binding and dimerization motif in immunoglobulin enhancer binding, daughterless, MyoD, and myc proteins. *Cell* 56:777, 1989.

62. Nourse J, Mellentin JD, Galili N, et al.: Chromosomal translocation t(1;19) results in synthesis of a homeobox fusion mRNA that codes for a potential chimeric transcription factor. *Cell* 60:535, 1990.

63. Kamps MP, Murre C, Sun XH, et al.: A new homeobox gene contributes the DNA binding domain of the t(1;19) translocation protein in pre-B ALL. *Cell* 60:547, 1990.

64. Troussard X, Rimokh R, Valensi F, et al.: Heterogeneity of t(1;19)(q23;p13) acute leukaemias. *Br J Haematol* 89:516, 1995.

65. Neri A, Barriga F, Knowles DM, et al.: Different regions of the immunoglobulin heavy-chain locus are involved in chromosomal translocations in distinct pathogenetic forms of Burkitt lymphoma. *Proc Natl Acad Sci USA* 85:2748, 1988.

66. Gerbitz A, Mautner J, Geltinger C, et al.: Deregulation of the proto-oncogene c-myc through t(8;22) translocation in Burkitt's lymphoma. *Oncogene* 18:1745, 1999.

67. Hecht JL, Aster JC: Molecular biology of Burkitt's lymphoma. *J Clin Oncol* 18:3707, 2000.

68. Boxer LM, Dang CV: Translocations involving c-myc and c-myc function. *Oncogene* 20:5595, 2001.

69. Shiramizu B, Barriga F, Neequaye J, et al.: Patterns of chromosomal breakpoint locations in Burkitt's lymphoma: relevance to geography and Epstein–Barr virus association. *Blood* 77:1516, 1991.

70. Gutierrez MI, Bhatia K, Barriga F, et al.: Molecular epidemiology of Burkitt's lymphoma from South America: differences in breakpoint location and Epstein–Barr virus association from tumors in other world regions. *Blood* 79:3261, 1992.

71. Bhatia K, Spangler G, Gaidano G, et al.: Mutations in the coding region of c-myc occur frequently in acquired immunodeficiency syndrome-associated lymphomas. *Blood* 84:883, 1994.

72. Lieberson R, Ong J, Shi X, et al.: Immunoglobulin gene transcription ceases upon deletion of a distant enhancer. *EMBO J* 14:6229, 1995.

73. Heinonen K, Mahlamaki E, Riikonen P, et al.: Acquired X-chromosome aneuploidy in children with acute lymphoblastic leukemia. *Med Pediatr Oncol* 32:360, 1999.

74. Onodera N, McCabe NR, Rubin CM: Formation of a hyperdiploid karyotype in childhood acute lymphoblastic leukemia. *Blood* 80:203, 1992.

75. Third International Workshop on Chromosomes in Leukemia: Chromosomal abnormalities and their clinical significance in acute lymphoblastic leukemia. *Cancer Res* 43:868, 1983.

76. Harrison CJ, Moorman AV, Broadfield ZJ, et al.: Three distinct subgroups of hypodiploidy in acute lymphoblastic leukaemia. *Br J Haematol* 125:552, 2004.

77. Garipidou V, Yamada T, Prentice HG, et al.: Trisomy 8 in acute lymphoblastic leukemia (ALL): a case report and update of the literature. *Leukemia* 4:717, 1990.

78. Heerema NA, Nachman JB, Sather HN, et al.: Deletion of 7p or monosomy 7 in pediatric acute lymphoblastic leukemia is an adverse prognostic factor: a report from the Children's Cancer Group. *Leukemia* 18:939, 2004.

79. Derynck R, Zhang YE: Smad-dependent and Smad-independent pathways in TGF-β family signalling. *Nature* 425:577, 2003.

80. Armstrong SA, Kung AL, Mabon ME, et al.: Inhibition of FLT3 in MLL. Validation of a therapeutic target identified by gene expression based classification. *Cancer Cell* 3:173, 2003.

81. Taketani T, Taki T, Sugita K, et al.: *FLT3* mutations in the activation loop of tyrosine kinase domain are frequently found in infant ALL with *MLL* rearrangements and pediatric ALL with hyperdiploidy. *Blood* 103:1085, 2004.

82. Armstrong SA, Mabon ME, Silverman LB, et al.: FLT3 mutations in childhood acute lymphoblastic leukemia. *Blood* 103:3544, 2004.

83. Paietta E, Ferrando AA, Neuberg D, et al.: Activating FLT3 mutations in CD117/KIT(+) T-cell acute lymphoblastic leukemias. *Blood* 104:558, 2004.

84. Brown P, Levis M, Shurtleff S, et al.: FLT3 inhibition selectively kills childhood acute lymphoblastic leukemia cells with high levels of FLT3 expression. *Blood* 105:812, 2005.

85. Ferrando AA, Look AT: Gene expression profiling in T-cell acute lymphoblastic leukemia. *Semin Hematol* 40:274, 2003.

86. Ferrando AA, Neuberg DS, Staunton J, et al.: Gene expression signatures define novel oncogenic pathways in T cell acute lymphoblastic leukemia. *Cancer Cell* 1:75, 2002.

87. Cave H, Suciu S, Preudhomme C, et al.: Clinical significance of HOX11L2 expression linked to t(5;14)(q35;q32), of HOX11 expression, and of SIL-TAL fusion in childhood T-cell malignancies: results of EORTC studies 58881 and 58951. *Blood* 103:442, 2004.

88. Ferrando AA, Neuberg DS, Dodge RK, et al.: Prognostic importance of TLX1 (HOX11) oncogene expression in adults with T-cell acute lymphoblastic leukaemia. *Lancet* 363:535, 2004.

89. Bernard OA, Busson-LeConiat M, Ballerini P, et al.: A new recurrent and specific cryptic translocation, t(5;14)(q35;q32), is associated with expression of the Hox11L2 gene in T acute lymphoblastic leukemia. *Leukemia* 15:1495, 2001.

90. Berger R, Dastugue N, Busson M, et al.: t(5;14)/HOX11L2-positive T-cell acute lymphoblastic leukemia. A collaborative study of the Groupe Français de Cytogénétique Hématologique (GFCH). *Leukemia* 17:1851, 2003.

91. Cave H, Suciu S, Preudhomme C, et al.: Clinical significance of HOX11L2 expression linked to t(5;14)(q35;q32), of HOX11 expression, and of SIL-TAL fusion in childhood T-cell malignances: results of EORTC studies 58881 and 58951. *Blood* 103:442, 2004.

92. Ballerini P, Blaise A, Busson-Le Coniat M, et al.: HOX11L2 expression defines a clinical subtype of pediatric T-ALL associated with poor prognosis. *Blood* 100:991, 2002.

93. Weng AP, Ferrando AA, Lee W, et al.: Activating mutations of NOTCH1 in human T cell acute lymphoblastic leukemia. *Science* 306:269, 2004.

94. Pear WS, Aster JC: T cell acute lymphoblastic leukemia/lymphoma: a human cancer commonly associated with aberrant NOTCH1 signaling. *Curr Opin Hematol* 11:426, 2004.

95. Beverly LJ, Capobianco AJ: Targeting promiscuous signaling pathways in cancer: another Notch in the bedpost. *Trends Mol Med* 10:591, 2004.

96. Willenbrock H, Juncker AS, Schmiegelow K, et al.: Prediction of immunophenotype, treatment response, and relapse in childhood acute lymphoblastic leukemia using DNA microarrays. *Leukemia* 18:1270, 2004.

97. Tsukasaki K, Tanosaki S, DeVos S, et al.: Identifying progression-associated genes in adult T-cell leukemia/lymphoma by using oligonucleotide microarrays. *Int J Cancer* 109:875, 2004.

98. Mitchell SA, Brown KM, Henry MM, et al.: Inter-platform comparability of microarrays in acute lymphoblastic leukemia. *BMC Genomics* 5:71, 2004.

99. Holleman A, Cheok MH, den Boer ML, et al.: Gene-expression patterns in drug-resistant acute lymphoblastic leukemia cells and response to treatment. *N Engl J Med* 351:533, 2004.

100. Aplenc R, Lange B: Pharmacogenetic determinants of outcome in acute lymphoblastic leukaemia. *Br J Haematol* 125:421, 2004.

101. Weinshilboum RM, Sladek SL: Mercaptopurine pharmacogenetics: monogenic inheritance of erythrocyte thiopurine methyltransferase activity. *Am J Hum Genet* 32:651, 1980.

102. Lennard L, Lilleyman JS: Are children with lymphoblastic leukaemia given enough 6-mercaptopurine? *Lancet* 2:785, 1987.

103. Lennard L, Van Loon JA, Lilleyman JS, et al.: Thiopurine pharmacogenetics in leukemia: correlation of erythrocyte thiopurine methyltransferase activity and 6-thioguanine nucleotide concentrations. *Clin Pharmacol Ther* 41:18, 1987.

104. Koren G, Ferrazini G, Sulh H, et al.: Systemic exposure to mercaptopurine as a prognostic factor in acute lymphocytic leukemia in children. *N Engl J Med* 323:17, 1990.

105. Schmiegelow K, Schrøder H, Gustafsson G, et al.: Risk of relapse in childhood acute lymphoblastic leukemia is related to RBC methotrexate and mercaptopurine metabolites during maintenance chemotherapy. *J Clin Oncol* 13:345, 1995.

106. Krynetski EY, Schuetz JD, Galpin AJ, et al.: A single point mutation leading to loss of catalytic activity in human thiopurine S-methyltransferase. *Proc Natl Acad Sci USA* 92:949, 1995.

107. Yates CR, Krynetski EY, Loennechen T, et al.: Molecular diagnosis of thiopurine S-methyltransferase deficiency: genetic basis for azathioprine and mercaptopurine intolerance. *Ann Intern Med* 126:608, 1997.

108. McLeod HL, Krynetski EY, Relling MV, et al.: Genetic polymorphism of thiopurine methyltransferase and its clinical relevance for childhood acute lymphoblastic leukemia. *Leukemia* 14:567, 2000.

109. Relling MV, Hancock ML, Boyett JM, et al.: Prognostic importance of 6-mercaptopurine dose intensity in acute lymphoblastic leukemia. *Blood* 93:2817, 1999.

110. Relling MV, Rubnitz JE, Rivera GK, et al.: High incidence of secondary brain tumours after radiotherapy and antimetabolites. *Lancet* 354:34, 1999.

111. Relling MV, Yanishevski Y, Nemec J, et al.: Etoposide and antimetabolite pharmacology in patients who develop secondary acute myeloid leukemia. *Leukemia* 12:346, 1998.

112. Chiusolo P, Reddiconto G, Casorelli I, et al.: Preponderance of methylenetetrahydrofolate reductase C677T homozygosity among leukemia patients intolerant to methotrexate. *Ann Oncol* 13:1915, 2002.

113. Taub JW, Matherly LH, Ravindranath Y, et al.: Polymorphisms in methylenetetrahydrofolate reductase and methotrexate sensitivity in childhood acute lymphoblastic leukemia. *Leukemia* 16:764, 2002.

114. Bernbeck B, Mauz-Korholz C, Zotz RB, et al.: Methylenetetrahydrofolate reductase gene polymorphism and glucocorticoid intake in children with ALL and aseptic osteonecrosis. *Klin Padiatr* 215:327, 2003.

115. Kishi S, Griener J, Cheng C, et al.: Homocysteine, pharmacogenetics, and neurotoxicity in children with leukemia. *J Clin Oncol* 21:3084, 2003.

116. Krajinovic M, Lemieux-Blanchard E, Chiasson S, et al.: Role of polymorphisms in MTHFR and MTHFD1 genes in the outcome of childhood acute lymphoblastic leukemia. *Pharmacogenomics J* 4:66, 2004.

117. Gorlick R, Cole P, Banerjee D, et al.: Mechanisms of methotrexate resistance in acute leukemia. Decreased transport and polyglutamylation. *Adv Exp Med Biol* 457:543, 1999.

118. Belkov VM, Krynetski EY, Schuetz JD, et al.: Reduced folate carrier expression in acute lymphoblastic leukemia: a mechanism for ploidy but not lineage differences in methotrexate accumulation. *Blood* 93:1643, 1999.

119. Laverdiere C, Chiasson S, Costea I, et al.: Polymorphism G80A in the reduced folate carrier gene and its relationship to methotrexate plasma levels and outcome of childhood acute lymphoblastic leukemia. *Blood* 100:3832, 2002.

120. Krajinovic M, Costea I, Chiasson S: Polymorphism of the thymidylate synthase gene and outcome of acute lymphoblastic leukaemia. *Lancet* 359:1033, 2002.

121. Lauten M, Matthias T, Stanulla M, et al.: Association of initial response to prednisone treatment in childhood acute lymphoblastic leukaemia and polymorphisms within the tumour necrosis factor and the interleukin-10 genes. *Leukemia* 16:1437, 2002.

# Chapter 12

# CLINICAL FEATURES AND MAKING THE DIAGNOSIS

*Ronald M. Sobecks*

## CLINICAL FEATURES

### DISEASE PRESENTATION–

Patients with acute lymphoblastic leukemia (ALL) present with signs and symptoms related to impaired hematopoiesis from progressively worsening bone marrow involvement. Anemia may result in fatigue, light-headedness, dyspnea, and pallor. Patients with thrombocytopenia may develop petechiae, purpura, and hemorrhage. Fevers and infections also commonly occur due to neutropenia. Approximately one-third of patients have been reported to have infections, hemorrhage, or constitutional symptoms at the time of diagnosis.[1–3] Clinical characteristics for patients presenting with ALL are given in Table 12.1.

Leukocytosis is often observed at the time of initial disease presentation, and the German Multicenter Trial GMALL 03/87 and 04/89 reported that 51% of their adult patients had a white blood cell (WBC) count of more than $30 \times 10^9$/L.[1] Investigators at MD Anderson Cancer Center noted that 26% of their adult ALL patients had a WBC count of more than $30 \times 10^9$/L and 39% had a WBC count between 5 and $30 \times 10^9$/L.[12] The French Group on Therapy for Adult ALL LALA 87 Trial observed that 31% of adult B-cell ALL patients and 55% of T-cell ALL patients had an initial WBC count of $30 \times 10^9$/L or above.[4] The GIMEMA 0496 study found that 32% of their adult pro-B-cell ALL patients had an initial WBC count of more than $50 \times 10^9$/L.[13] Patients with T-cell ALL have been reported to have a WBC count greater than $100 \times 10^9$/L in 25% of adult patients and in 50–77% of children.[5–7] In addition, 40–50% of children with B-cell ALL have been noted to have an initial WBC count of more than $20–25 \times 10^9$/L.[8,14]

Anemia occurs frequently when patients present with ALL. A hemoglobin of less than or equal to 8 g/dL has been noted in about 30% of adult pro-B-cell ALL patients,[1] while a hemoglobin of less than 12 g/dL has been observed in 85% of B-cell ALL and 65% of T-cell ALL patients.[4] Investigators at MD Anderson Cancer Center found that 69% of their adult ALL patients had an initial hemoglobin of less than 10 g/dL.[12] Fifty-five percent of children with T-cell ALL treated at St Jude Children's Research Hospital were noted to have an initial hemoglobin of less than 11 g/dL.[7] French investigators observed that 42% of their children and 60% of infants with ALL had presenting hemoglobin levels of less than 8 g/dL.[9] More than 80% of children on Children's Cancer Group (CCG) trials were also found to be anemic at diagnosis, with a hemoglobin level of less than or equal to 10 g/dL.[8]

Thrombocytopenia is also commonly observed at the time of diagnosis. Kantarjian et al. noted that 74%

| Table 12.1 | Signs and symptoms at the time of ALL diagnosis | |
|---|---|
| | Reported (%)[a] |
| Hemorrhage | 35–38 |
| Infection | 12–38 |
| B symptoms | 27–33 |
| Lymphadenopathy | |
| B cell | 21–46 (adult), 17–60 (child) |
| T cell | 67–71 (adult), 79 (child) |
| Hepatomegaly | |
| B cell | 13–50 (adult), 3–50 (child) |
| T cell | 34 (adult), 41–72 (child) |
| Splenomegaly | |
| B cell | 30–49 (adult), 5–80 (child) |
| T cell | 52 (adult), 54–84 (child) |
| CNS involvement | |
| B cell | 5–9 (adult), 2–5 (child) |
| T cell | 9–11 (adult), 8–17 (child) |
| Mediastinal mass | |
| B cell | 2–6 (adult), 0.2–11 (child) |
| T cell | 40–91 (adult), 39–54 (child) |
| Pleura involvement | 9–40 (adult), 5–7 (child) |
| Testis involvement | 2–4 (adult), 2 (child) |
| Skin involvement | 2 |
| Kidney involvement | 2 |

[a]Incidences were obtained from Refs. 1–11.

of their adult ALL patients had a presenting platelet count of less than $100 \times 10^9$/L.[12] French investigators similarly reported that approximately 70% of both their B- and T-cell ALL patients had platelet counts of less than or equal to $100 \times 10^9$/L at the time of presentation.[4] The Cancer and Leukemia Group B Study 8364 had found that the initial median platelet counts for B- and T-lineage disease were 47 and $61 \times 10^9$/L, respectively.[10] Of approximately 3700 cases of childhood ALL enrolled on CCG trials, 35–50% had initial platelet counts of less than $50 \times 10^9$/L, 31–36% had platelet counts between 50 and $150 \times 10^9$/L, and 19–29% had platelet counts of more than $150 \times 10^9$/L.[8]

Patients with mature B-cell ALL (Burkitt-type) commonly present with bulky disease from rapid proliferation of the neoplastic cells. Hyperuricemia and a high serum lactate dehydrogenase (LDH) are often observed. Investigators at MD Anderson Cancer Center have reported that 42% of such patients had an initial LDH of 620–4999 U/L, 27% had a level of 5000–10,000 U/L, and 31% had a level of more than 10,000 U/L.[15] They also noted that hepatomegaly, splenomegaly, and lymphadenopathy occurred in 31, 23, and 19% of these patients, respectively. At presentation, 27% of these patients had an initial WBC count of $10 \times 10^9$/L or above, 65% were anemic with a hemoglobin level of less than 10 g/dL, and 77% had a platelet count of less than $100 \times 10^9$/L. As patients with mature B-cell ALL are treated, they also frequently develop tumor lysis syndrome that may further worsen hyperuricemia, which may in turn lead to renal insufficiency. There may also be hyperkalemia, hyperphosphatemia, and a resultant hypocalcemia (see Chapter 107).

### EXTRAMEDULLARY DISEASE
#### Central nervous system disease
Central nervous system (CNS) ALL has been defined as more than five WBCs per microliter of cerebrospinal fluid (CSF) with leukemic lymphoblasts identified after cytocentrifugation.[16,17] There has been some controversy as to whether the presence of blasts in the CSF predicts for more CNS relapses or inferior CNS leukemia-free survival in childhood ALL when the total CSF WBC count is less than 5/μL.[18,19] This is also unknown for adult ALL patients.

At the time of diagnosis, fewer than 5% of children and fewer than 10% of adult ALL patients present with CNS disease.[20] The leukemic cells may traverse superficial cerebral veins into the arachnoid circulation, which then may result in impaired cerebral perfusion. These neoplastic cells can then enter the CSF, resulting in morning headache, emesis, papilledema, signs of meningeal irritation, and impaired cerebral function.[21] In addition, compromise of cranial nerve circulation from leukemia can lead to neuropathies, such as optic neuritis.[22] Endocrinopathies may also

develop from hypothalamic or pituitary involvement.[23] Leukemic infiltration of the leptomeninges may lead to other neurologic symptoms, such as paraparesis.

Adolescent patients, children, and infants have a higher risk of CNS disease than do adults.[24] Approximately 10–40% of patients with mature B-cell ALL (Burkitt-type) develop CNS disease.[15,25,26] This increased incidence is most notable in older ALL patients. Prior to the use of modern ALL treatment regimens, patients with T-cell disease were also more likely than those with B-cell phenotypes to develop CNS disease.[24] In addition, a high leukocyte count, a high serum LDH, and extramedullary disease have been associated with an increased risk of CNS leukemia.[27,28]

Patients with ALL who develop CNS recurrences have a worse prognosis and are at increased risk for systemic relapses. With the use of standard therapies for CNS prophylaxis, the risk of CNS relapses has decreased for both children and adults from approximately 40–50% to 10% or below.[29–31] Of 439 adult ALL patients treated at MD Anderson Cancer Center who achieved a complete remission, 32 (7%) developed a CNS disease relapse.[32] However, when these investigators compared initial characteristics for patients with or without a CNS recurrence, they found no significant differences between the groups with respect to age, WBC count, platelet count, percentage of bone marrow or peripheral blood blasts, bone marrow cellularity, serum LDH, immunophenotype, French–American–British (FAB) classification, or Philadelphia chromosome status.

#### Testicular disease
Patients who develop testicular disease may present with increased testicular size and firmness, as well as nodular lesions in one or both testes that may be painless. The majority of leukemic infiltration involves the interstitium of the testis on the endothelial side.[33] It has been suggested that in children a risk factor for testicular involvement is age older than 10 years during the onset of puberty.[34]

Using autopsy series, ALL involving the testes has been reported to occur in approximately 30–90% of cases.[35] With the use of more effective modern treatment regimens, this incidence may now be considerably lower.[36]

Testicular disease is rare at the time ALL is initially diagnosed. However, testicular involvement is more commonly observed at the time of a disease recurrence, which usually antedates a systemic relapse within months.[37] The Children's Cancer Group reported that, among 3712 childhood ALL cases, there were 113 (8.3%) isolated testicular relapses, 38 (2.8%) concurrent marrow and testicular relapses, 4 (0.3%) concurrent marrow, testicular, and CNS relapses, and 4 (0.3%) concurrent testicular and CNS relapses.[38]

## Lymphatic

Lymphadenopathy is frequently observed and is somewhat more common in T-cell ALL than in B-cell ALL.[1–3,5,9,11] Hepatomegaly and splenomegaly are also commonly identified at the time of disease presentation, and these are also found more often among T-cell phenotypes.[1,2,5,7,9,11] Furthermore, lymphadenopathy and hepatosplenomegaly occur more commonly in children than in adults with T-cell ALL.[5] Although mediastinal masses have been reported in approximately 40–90% of patients at the time of diagnosis of T-cell ALL,[3–7,10] they have also been identified in B-cell ALL patients, but at a much lower frequency.[1,4,9–11]

## MAKING THE DIAGNOSIS

The diagnosis of ALL is usually established by a bone marrow examination from which morphologic assessment, as well as immunophenotypic, cytogenetic, and molecular analyses, may be obtained. Patients presenting with circulating lymphoblasts may also have the diagnosis established by performing these analyses on a peripheral blood sample. ALL and lymphoblastic lymphoma are considered to be the same disease biologically. When patients present with extensive blood and bone marrow involvement with more than 25% blasts, the disease is categorized as ALL. For patients having disease confined to mass lesions and having less than or equal to 25% blasts in the bone marrow, the diagnosis of lymphoblastic lymphoma is used.[39] For patients with lymphoblastic lymphoma, the diagnosis may be established by a biopsy of an involved lymph node(s) or mass lesion(s). An adequate amount of tissue should be obtained to perform the appropriate immunophenotypic, cytogenetic, and molecular analyses.

CNS disease may be detected by a lumbar puncture for CSF cytologic and flow cytometric analyses. Usually, this procedure is not performed initially when there are circulating lymphoblasts in the peripheral blood, as this may theoretically introduce disease into the CSF. Alternatively, a traumatic lumbar puncture may contaminate the CSF specimen with blood containing leukemic lymphoblasts, which could then result in a false positive test for CNS leukemia.

### MORPHOLOGIC ASSESSMENT

A detailed discussion of the pathology of ALL is presented in Chapter 11. The initial morphologic classification for ALL was formulated by the FAB Cooperative Group,[40] which proposed three morphologic subtypes (L1, L2, and L3). The L1 subtype is composed of small cells with a homogeneous nuclear chromatin pattern, regular nuclear shape, and scant cytoplasm that is only slightly to moderately basophilic. The L2 subtype contains cells of more heterogeneous size and are larger than those of the L1 subtype. These blasts also have a more heterogeneous nuclear chromatin pattern, a cytoplasm of variable amount and degree of basophilia, an irregular nuclear shape, and they may have nucleoli that are detected more readily compared to L1 blasts. The L3 subtype consists of blasts of large, uniform size with finely stippled chromatin and regular nuclear shape. Prominent nucleoli are commonly observed, and there are moderate amounts of cytoplasm with deep basophilia and lipid vacuoles. A "starry sky" appearance is often observed, which results from the ingestion of apoptotic neoplastic cells by histiocytes.[41] Although many mitotic figures may be observed, the amount may be greater for T- compared to B-cell phenotypes.

Cytochemistry assessment demonstrates that the lymphoblasts in ALL are negative for myeloperoxidase and Sudan black B stains. Periodic acid–Schiff reaction and nonspecific esterase may be positive.[42] Terminal deoxynucleotidyl transferase (TdT) is also positive in most cases of ALL.

### IMMUNOPHENOTYPIC ASSESSMENT

Specific ALL phenotypes, such as T- or B-cell-lineage disease, cannot be distinguished by morphologic assessment. Immunophenotyping by flow cytometric analysis provides a rapid and accurate method to characterize distinct ALL subtypes. As distinguished in the World Health Organization Scheme, these consist of early precursor B-cell ALL, common B-cell ALL, precursor B-cell ALL, mature B-cell (Burkitt-type) ALL, precursor T-cell ALL, and T-cell ALL.[41–43] Table 12.2 shows the specific lymphoid markers that are expressed with the various ALL subtypes. Further discussion of immunophenotyping for ALL is found in Chapter 11.

### MOLECULAR GENETIC ANALYSIS

Genetic alterations in ALL may be detected by cytogenetic, fluorescent in situ hybridization (FISH), and reverse transcriptase polymerase chain reaction (RT-PCR)

| Table 12.2 | Immunophenotypes of ALL subtypes |
|---|---|
| | Surface markers |
| *B lineages* | |
| Early precursor B cell | TdT+, CD19+, HLA-DR+, cCD79a+, cCD22+ |
| Common B cell | TdT+, CD19+, HLA-DR+, CD10+ |
| Precursor B cell | TdT+, CD19+, HLA-DR+, CD10+, cIg+ |
| Mature B cell | CD19+, CD20+, HLA-DR+, CD10+, CD22+, CD79a, sIg+ |
| *T lineages* | |
| Precursor T cell | TdT+, CD2+, CD7+, cCD3+ |
| T cell | TdT+, CD1a+, CD2+, CD5+, CD7+, sCD3+ |

TdT, terminal deoxynucleotidyl transferase; c, cytoplasmic; s, surface; Ig, immunoglobulin.

| Table 12.3   Genotypes in adult and childhood ALL[41,42,44] | | | |
|---|---|---|---|
| Cytogenetic abnormality | Genetic alteration | Childhood frequency (%) | Adult frequency (%) |
| t(9;22) | BCR/ABL | 3–4 | 25–29 |
| t(12;21) | TEL/AML1 | 22–29 | 2 |
| t(4;11), t(11;19), t(9;11) | MLL | 8 | 10 |
| t(1;19) | PBX/E2A | 5–6[a] | 3 |
| t(8;14), t(8;22), t(2;8) | MYC | 2 | 4 |
| 5q35 | HOX11L2 | 3 | 1 |
| 19p13 | LYL1 | 2 | 3 |
| 10q24 | HOX11 | 1 | 8 |
| 1p32 | TAL1 | 7 | 12 |
| Hyperdiploid (>50) | | 25 | 7 |
| Hypodiploid (<45) | | 1–5 | 2 |

[a]The frequency is approximately 25% for childhood precursor B-cell ALL.

analyses. These diagnostic techniques allow for precise determination of specific ALL genotypes that provide important prognostic information. Molecular genetic alterations in ALL are given in Table 12.3. DNA microarray analysis may also provide unique gene expression profiles which will continue to refine the classification of ALL subtypes.[45,46] Chapter 11 also specifically reviews the molecular biology of ALL. As FISH and RT-PCR are more sensitive techniques at detecting prognostically important cytogenetic abnormalities than is traditional karyotyping, we recommend use of one of these modalities to determine the presence of t(9;22) or t(4;11).

### DIFFERENTIAL DIAGNOSIS
The differential diagnosis for ALL includes acute myeloid leukemia, aplastic anemia, chronic myeloid leukemia in lymphoid blast crisis, a minimally differentiated and reactive bone marrow with increased hematogones, bilineal acute leukemia in which two distinct leukemic populations coexist, and biphenotypic acute leukemia in which a single leukemic population coexpresses a sufficient amount of both myeloid and lymphoid markers. Although chronic lymphoid leukemia and other lymphoid malignancies with circulating lymphoma cells may initially be considered in the differential diagnosis of ALL based upon an initial complete blood count and differential, ALL is usually easily distinguished from these diseases by morphologic review and immunophenotyping.

Lymphoblastic lymphoma and Burkitt lymphoma are biologically the same disease as their leukemic counterparts. However, their differential diagnosis also includes other aggressive lymphomas, thymoma, and other solid tumors from the respective anatomic locations in which they are found. An adequate biopsy specimen from which appropriate morphologic, immunophenotypic (e.g., TdT), and molecular studies (e.g., BCR/ABL) can be performed usually allows the diagnosis to be definitively established.

### REFERENCES

1. Ludwig W-D: Immunophenotypic and genotypic features, clinical characteristics, and treatment outcome of adult pro-B acute lymphoblastic leukemia: results of the German Multicenter Trials GMALL 03/87 and 04/89. *Blood* 92:1898, 1998.
2. Thomas X: Philadelphia chromosome positive adult acute lymphoblastic leukemia: characteristics, prognostic factors and treatment outcome. *Hematol Cell Ther* 40:119, 1998.
3. Hoelzer D: Outcome of adult patients with T-lymphoblastic lymphoma treated according to protocols for acute lymphoblastic leukemia. *Blood* 99:4379, 2002.
4. Boucheix C: Immunophenotype of adult acute lymphoblastic leukemia, clinical parameters, and outcome: an analysis of a prospective trial including 562 tested patients (LALA87). *Blood* 84:1603, 1994.
5. Garand R: Comparison of outcome, clinical, laboratory, and immunological features in 164 children and adults with T-ALL. *Leukemia* 4:739, 1990.
6. Goldberg JM: Childhood T-cell acute lymphoblastic leukemia: the Dana-Farber Cancer Institute Acute Lymphoblastic Leukemia Consortium experience. *J Clin Oncol* 21:3616, 2003.
7. Pui C-H: Heterogeneity of presenting features and their relation to treatment outcome in 120 children with T-cell acute lymphoblastic leukemia. *Blood* 75:174, 1990.
8. Steinherz PG: Treatment of patients with acute lymphoblastic leukemia with bulky extramedullary disease and T-cell phenotype or other poor prognostic features. Randomized controlled trial from the Children's Cancer Group. *Cancer* 82:600, 1998.
9. Lenormand B: PreB1 (CD10-) acute lymphoblastic leukemia: immunophenotypic and genomic

characteristics, clinical features and outcome in 38 adults and 26 children. *Leuk and Lymphoma* 28:329, 1998.

10. Czuczman MS: Value of immunophenotype in intensively treated adult acute lymphoblastic leukemia: Cancer and Leukemia Group B study 8364. *Blood* 93:3931, 1999.

11. Ng SM: Age, sex, haemoglobin level, and white cell count at diagnosis are important prognostic factors in children with acute lymphoblastic leukemia treated with BFM-type protocol. *J Trop Pediatr* 46:338, 2000.

12. Kantarjian HM: Results of treatment with hyper-CVAD, a dose-intensive regimen, in adult acute lymphocytic leukemia. *J Clin Oncol* 18:547, 2000.

13. Cimino G: Clinico-biologic features and treatment outcome of adult pro-B-ALL patients enrolled in the GIMEMA 0496 study: absence of the ALL1/AF4 and of the BCR/ABL fusion genes correlates with a significantly better clinical outcome. *Blood* 102:2014, 2003.

14. Pui C-H: Clinical significance of CD10 expression in childhood acute lymphoblastic leukemia. *Leukemia* 7:35, 1993.

15. Thomas DA: Hyper-CVAD program in Burkitt's-type adult acute lymphoblastic leukemia. *J Clin Oncol* 17:2461, 1999.

16. Tubergen DG: Blasts in CSF with a normal cell count do not justify alteration of therapy for acute lymphoblastic leukemia in remission: a Children's Cancer Group study. *J Clin Oncol* 12:273, 1994.

17. Mastrangelo R: Report and recommendations of the Rome workshop concerning poor-prognosis acute lymphoblastic leukemia in children: biologic basis for staging, stratification, and treatment. *Med Pediatr Oncol* 14:191, 1986.

18. Mahmoud HH: Low leukocyte counts with blast cells in cerebrospinal fluid of children with newly diagnosed acute lymphoblastic leukemia. *N Engl J Med* 329:314, 1993.

19. Gilchrist GS: Low numbers of CSF blasts at diagnosis do not predict for the development of CNS leukemia in children with intermediate-risk acute lymphoblastic leukemia: a Children's Cancer Group report. *J Clin Oncol* 12:2594, 1994.

20. Cortes J: Central nervous system involvement in adult acute lymphocytic leukemia. *Hematol Oncol Clin North Am* 15:145, 2001.

21. Pochedly C: Neurologic manifestations of leukemia. I: Symptoms due to increased CSF pressure and hemorrhage. II: Involvement of the cranial nerves, hypothalamus, spinal cord, and peripheral neuropathy. In: Pochedly C (ed.) *Leukemia and Lymphoma in the Central Nervous System*. Springfield, IL: Charles C. Thomas; 1977:3.

22. Ingram LC: Cranial nerve palsy in childhood acute lymphoblastic leukemia and non-Hodgkin's lymphoma. *Cancer* 67:2262, 1991.

23. Pinkel D: Prevention and treatment of meningeal leukemia in children. *Blood* 84:355, 1994.

24. Pavlovsky S: Factors that influence the appearance of central nervous system leukemia. *Blood* 42:935, 1973.

25. Gururangan S: Outcome of CNS disease at diagnosis in disseminated small noncleaved-cell lymphoma and B-cell leukemia. A Children's Cancer Group study. *J Clin Oncol* 18:2017, 2000.

26. Todeschini G: Eighty-one percent event-free survival in advanced Burkitt's lymphoma/leukemia: no difference in outcome between pediatric and adult patients treated with the same intensive pediatric protocol. *Ann Oncol* 8:77, 1997.

27. Kantarjian HM: Identification of risk groups for development of central nervous system leukemia in adults with acute lymphocytic leukemia. *Blood* 72:1784, 1988.

28. Stewart DJ: Natural history of central nervous system acute leukemia in adults. *Cancer* 47:184, 1981.

29. Pui CH: Acute lymphoblastic leukemia in children. *Curr Opin Oncol* 12:3, 2000.

30. Omura GA: Combination chemotherapy of adult acute lymphoblastic leukemia with randomized central nervous system prophylaxis. *Blood* 55:199, 1980.

31. Cortes J: The value of high-dose systemic chemotherapy and intrathecal therapy for central nervous system prophylaxis in different risk groups of adult acute lymphoblastic leukemia. *Blood* 86:2091, 1995.

32. Surapaneni UR: Central nervous system relapse in adults with acute lymphoblastic leukemia. *Cancer* 94:773, 2002.

33. Kay HEM: Testicular infiltration in acute lymphoblastic leukemia. *Br J Haematol* 53:537, 1983.

34. Ritzén EM: Testicular relapse of acute lymphoblastic leukemia (ALL). *J Reprod Immunol* 18:117, 1990.

35. Hustu HO: Extramedullary leukaemia. *Clin Haematol* 7:313, 1978.

36. Brecher ML: Intermediate dose methotrexate in childhood acute lymphoblastic leukemia resulting in decreased incidence of testicular relapse. *Cancer* 58:1024, 1986.

37. Sullivan MP: Radiotherapy (2500 rad) for testicular leukemia: local control and subsequent clinical events: a Southwest Oncology Group study. *Cancer* 46:508, 1980.

38. Gaynon PS: Survival after relapse in childhood acute lymphoblastic leukemia. Impact of site and time to first relapse--the Children's Cancer Group experience. *Cancer* 82:1387, 1998.

39. Murphy SB: Childhood non-Hodgkin's lymphoma. *N Engl J Med* 299:1446, 1978.

40. Bennett JM: Proposals for the classification of the acute leukaemias. French–American–British (FAB) Co-Operative Group. *Br J Haematol* 33:451, 1976.

41. Diebold J, Jaffe ES, Raphael M, et al.: Burkitt lymphoma. In: Jaffe ES, Harris NL, Stein H, Vardiman JW (eds.) *World Health Organization Classification of Tumours: Tumours of Haematopoietic and Lymphoid Tissues*. Lyon, France: IARC Press; 2001:181.

42. Brunning RD, Borowitz M, Matutes E, et al.: Precursor B lymphoblastic leukaemia/lymphoblastic lymphoma (Precursor B-cell acute lymphoblastic leukaemia). In: Jaffe ES, Harris NL, Stein H, Vardiman JW (eds.) *World Health Organization Classification of Tumours: Tumours of Haematopoietic and Lymphoid Tissues*. Lyon, France: IARC Press; 2001:111.

43. van't Veer MB: Acute lymphoblastic leukaemia in adults: immunological subtypes and clinical features at presentation. *Ann Hematol* 66:277, 1993.

44. Pui CH: Mechanisms of disease—acute lymphoblastic leukemia. *N Engl J Med* 350:1535, 2004.

45. Yeoh EJ: Classification, subtype discovery, and prediction of outcome in pediatric acute lymphoblastic leukemia by gene expression profiling. *Cancer Cell* 1:133, 2002.

46. Armstrong SA: Inhibition of FLT3 in MLL: validation of a therapeutic target identified by gene expression based classification. *Cancer Cell* 3:173, 2003.

# Chapter 13

# TREATMENT APPROACH TO ADULT ACUTE LYMPHOBLASTIC LEUKEMIA

## Elizabeth S. Rich, Cara A. Rosenbaum, and Wendy Stock

In acute lymphoblastic leukemia (ALL), normal hematopoiesis is suppressed by accumulation in the bone marrow of clonal, malignant lymphoblasts. Arrested at various stages of development, different subtypes of ALL are characterized by distinct immunophenotypic, cytogenetic, and molecular features. In contrast to pediatric ALL, where cure rates approach 80%, only one-third of adult patients with ALL achieve long-term disease-free survival (DFS). To improve the outcome of patients with adult ALL, insight gained from the characterization of ALL has led to a risk-adapted approach to therapy.[1] Further understanding of the biology of this disease will refine this risk-adapted approach, with the ultimate goal of improving the cure rates of adult patients with ALL.

## BACKGROUND

ALL is a relatively rare disease in adults, representing approximately 20% of adult acute leukemias. The estimated number of new cases of ALL in the year 2003 in the United States was 3600. The age-adjusted incidence is 1.6 per 100,000 in adults.[2] There is a bimodal distribution to the incidence of the disease, with an initial peak in early childhood and a second smaller peak in patients older than 50 years.[3] Secondary acute leukemias can occur following chemotherapy or radiation treatment for other malignancies. Although most of these leukemias are myeloid, an increasing number of ALL cases are being reported following exposure to chemotherapy with topoisomerase II inhibitors. These therapy-related ALL cases have been associated with chromosomal rearrangements involving the *MLL* gene and typically occur within 2 years of initial exposure to the chemotherapeutic agent(s).[4] A longer time to development of leukemia has been observed following exposure to alkylating agents and the development of therapy-related leukemias.

## PROGNOSTIC FACTORS AND RISK STRATIFICATION

Recognized prognostic factors in adult ALL that impact on treatment allocation are discussed below (Table 13.1).

### AGE AT DIAGNOSIS

Most clinical trials[5–9] have noted a marked difference in both complete remission (CR) rate and DFS in ALL patients, depending on patient age. Both comorbid medical conditions resulting in increased toxicity of induction and postremission therapy and the presence of higher risk biologic features contribute to the adverse prognosis of older adults with ALL. DFS is consistently less than 20% in patients older than 60 years. Shorter remission duration in older adults is also a consequence of the higher frequency of adverse cytogenetic features, including the t(9;22)(q34;q11), or Philadelphia chromosome, which may occur in as many as 40% of adults older than 50 years.[10,11]

### LEUKOCYTE COUNT AT PRESENTATION

The majority of clinical studies have identified a high presenting white blood cell (WBC) count as an adverse prognostic factor that influences both CR rate and duration.[5,12–14] Despite intensification of recent regimens, lower remission durations in this subset of patients persist, particularly in those with precursor B ALL and WBC counts of higher than 100,000/μL.[15] The same degree of hyperleukocytosis has not been as clearly associated with an adverse prognosis in precursor T ALL, in which patients routinely present with higher WBC counts.

### FAILURE TO ATTAIN A CR IN LESS THAN 4–5 WEEKS

Several clinical studies have identified the importance of time required to attain first remission as a significant prognostic factor in adult ALL.[8,16]

**Table 13.1** Prognostic factors in adult ALL identifying risk groups for treatment—stratification

| Prognostic factor | Ref | Good risk | Standard risk | Poor risk |
|---|---|---|---|---|
| Clinical age<br>Presenting WBC<br>Time to CR | 5, 6–16 | <30 years<br><30,000/uL<br><2–4 weeks | 30–60 years old<br><30,000/uL<br>2–4 weeks | 60 years<br>>30,000/uL (precursor B)<br>>2–4 weeks |
| Immunophenotype | 17–19 | Mature<br>B-Burkitt type<br>Precursor T | Precursor B | Pro-B<br>early T (only 1–3 T-cell markers) |
| Molecular/cytogenetics | 20 | High hyperdiploid<br>t(8;14), t(2;8), or<br>t(8;22) | Normal karyotype | t(9;22)/BCR-ABL<br>t(4;11)/MLL-AF4<br>+(8)<br>del(7) |
| MRD[a] | 21–28 | $<10^{-4}$ after induction<br>$<10^{-4}$ or negative<br>during first years | | $>10^{-3}$ after induction<br>$>10^{-4}$ or increasing during first year<br>of therapy |

[a]Remains to be validated in a large, prospective series.

## CYTOGENETICS/MOLECULAR GENETICS

Cytogenetic abnormalities occur in about 60–70% of adults with ALL and are among the most important prognostic factors; therefore, cytogenetic analysis is a critical component of the diagnostic workup.[14,21] The Cancer and Leukemia Group B (CALGB) stratified patients into three prognostic groups based on cytogenetics: poor [including t(9;22), t(4;11), −7, and +8]; normal diploid; and miscellaneous (all other structural aberrations), with DFS rates of 11, 38, and 52%, respectively.[29] In this series, a higher frequency (35%) of patients with precursor T ALL had a normal karyotype. In particular, all larger series have identified that the presence of the Philadelphia chromosome, t(9;22) (q34;q11), and translocations involving the *MLL* gene on chromosome 11q23—the most common of which is the t(4;11)(q21;q23)—are independently associated with short CR duration and survival.[20,21,30] The Philadelphia chromosome is the most common recurring abnormality (overall 25–30%) in adult ALL, and it increases in frequency with age. Allogeneic stem cell transplantation (allo SCT) in first remission is advocated for these high-risk patients and is discussed below. In contrast, patients with precursor T ALL and the t(10;14) appear to have durable remissions.[5]

## MINIMAL RESIDUAL DISEASE STUDIES

Polymerase chain reaction (PCR) and flow cytometry have been used to monitor the persistence of the leukemic clone during treatment in an attempt to identify patients in morphologic and cytogenetic remission, but in whom there is persistence of subclinical or minimal residual disease (MRD), which may increase the risk of relapse. These sensitive techniques rely on the ability to identify a unique marker of the leukemia cells. For example, PCR techniques monitor a recurring fusion gene (e.g., *BCR-ABL*) or a clone-specific rearrangement of the immunoglobulin heavy chain or T-cell receptor gene.[19] MRD monitoring by flow cytometry of an aberrant immunophenotype of the leukemic blasts (e.g., presence of myeloid antigens on a lymphoid progenitor cell) can be identified at diagnosis and used for MRD monitoring. These molecular techniques have far greater sensitivity than standard cytogenetic analysis and may detect anywhere from one leukemia cell in a background of 10,000 to 1 million normal cells. Using both semiquantitative and more precise quantitative techniques, a number of studies in both pediatric and adult ALL have now provided preliminary evidence that MRD detection at specific time points following achievement of remission is an independent prognostic factor that may predict early relapse.[22–26]

## RISK-ADAPTED THERAPY

The factors described above can be used to provide a general risk assessment for prognosis and treatment planning. As many as 75% of adults with ALL can be considered relatively "high risk," with an expected DFS of 25–35%. Only approximately 25% of patients can be considered "standard risk," with anticipated survival rates of more than 50%. Nevertheless, until recently, most adults with ALL have been treated similarly regardless of patient-specific clinical and biologic risk features. To date, "risk-adapted" therapy in adult ALL has focused primarily on two disease subsets: patients with mature B-cell (Burkitt-type) ALL and those with Philadelphia-chromosome-positive (Ph+) ALL. These two groups are considered separately in the "Treatment" section that follows. The role of dose intensification with SCT in first remission and age-adapted therapeutic strategies will also be reviewed.

## TREATMENT STRATEGIES IN ADULT ALL

Treatment programs in adult ALL have evolved from the successful strategies employed in pediatric ALL and incorporate multiple active agents into complex regimen-specific sequential therapies. The goal of these dose-intensive regimens is rapid cytoreduction with restoration of normal hematopoiesis; prevention of the emergence of drug-resistant subclones; prophylaxis of sanctuary sites such as the central nervous system (CNS); and eradication of persistent MRD with prolonged maintenance chemotherapy. Therapy is generally divided into several phases: induction, postremission consolidation or intensification, CNS prophylaxis, and maintenance therapy.

### REMISSION INDUCTION THERAPY

Prednisone, vincristine, and L-asparaginase, based on pediatric regimens, formed the backbone of early trials in adult ALL. CR rates were 40–65%, with remission duration of only 3–7 months. However, the addition of an anthracycline (daunorubicin or doxorubicin) increased the CR rate to between 72 and 92%, and increased the median remission duration to approximately 18 months.[6,31–34] CR rates were similar when different anthracyclines (daunorubicin and mitoxantrone) were compared during induction therapy in a CALGB trial.[35] Intensification of the daunorubicin dose during induction has been reported to improve CR rates and DFS,[36,37] and was the focus of a recently completed trial in the CALGB.[38]

From several pediatric ALL clinical trials, it appears that dexamethasone provides better antileukemic activity than prednisone; in part, this may be because of its ability to achieve higher drug levels in the CNS.[39–41] The MD Anderson adult ALL trials have used dexamethasone during induction and postremission therapy as part of their "hyper-CVAD" regimen.[42] The CALGB is exploring the substitution of dexamethasone for prednisone during induction and postremission therapy.

L-Asparaginase has resulted in significant toxicities, including hepatotoxicity, neurotoxicity, pancreatitis, and coagulopathy in older adults with ALL, and its importance in adult ALL regimens remains somewhat controversial. A retrospective analysis performed by the CALGB demonstrated a marginal benefit in DFS for adults who received all prescribed doses of L-asparaginase in comparison to those who failed to receive all recommended doses.[43] Currently, the optimization of L-asparaginase pharmacokinetics utilizing the polyethylene glycol conjugate of this agent is being studied in both pediatric and adult regimens.

The usual four-drug induction regimen (anthracycline, glucocorticoid, vincristine, and L-asparaginase) yields CR rates of up to 75–95% (see Table 13.2), and it has been difficult to demonstrate further improvement with additional drugs. The German Multicenter ALL Cooperative Group (GMALL) has also used a 5–7-day "prophase" with prednisone and cyclophosphamide given prior to standard induction therapy for cytoreduction in an effort to minimize the risk of tumor lysis and its complications.[50] Randomized studies have not demonstrated a benefit to the addition of agents such as cyclophosphamide or cytarabine,[49,51] although the addition of these agents to specific subsets of ALL may improve outcome.

To avoid exposure to the toxicities of L-asparaginase, steroids, and vincristine, investigators at Memorial Sloan Kettering Cancer Center have studied an alternative induction regimen for adults with ALL. This effective approach employs high-dose cytarabine and mitoxantrone and has resulted in a CR rate of 84%.[52] L-Asparaginase has been omitted from the hyper-CVAD regimen at MD Anderson.[42] The key components of hyper-CVAD consist of alternating cycles of fractionated doses of cyclophosphamide, high-dose methotrexate (MTX), and cytarabine with intensive CNS prophylaxis, followed by 2 years of maintenance with 6-mercaptopurine (6-MP), MTX, vincristine, and prednisone (POMP). In a long-term follow-up of results for this hyper-CVAD regimen in ALL, the overall CR rate was 92%. With a median follow-up of 63 months, the 5-year survival and CR duration rates were 38%.[53]

### CONSOLIDATION/INTENSIFICATION

Although induction CR rates are 90% in many series of adult ALL, the long-term DFS over the last decade remains 25–50%, despite attempts to modify and improve postremission therapy through schedules with a variety of drugs that are active in ALL. These agents include oral and higher doses of intravenous MTX, antimetabolites such as 6-MP and 6-thioguanine, low- and high-dose cytarabine, and etoposide. In addition, many of the drugs that are used during induction therapy (anthracyclines, glucocorticoids, vincristine, and L-asparaginase) have also been reintroduced during postremission therapy. The value of postremission dose intensity has been addressed in several large prospective clinical trials with promising results. In a large phase II study from the CALGB, patients received both early and late intensification courses of treatment with eight drugs followed by maintenance chemotherapy for 2 years after diagnosis.[44] Compared to previous CALGB trials where less intensive postremission therapy was administered, the median remission duration and survival improved to 29 and 36 months, respectively. Investigators at MD Anderson center have also explored dose intensification in their hyper-CVAD regimen. As mentioned above, the median survival for 288 patients treated between 1992 and 2000 was 32 months, with a 5-year survival of 38%.[53]

Successive German multicenter trials have evaluated the impact of subset-specific dose intensification during postremission therapy.[54] Recently, patients

**Table 13.2    Results of recent chemotherapy studies in adult ALL**

| Trial | Ref | Year | Number of patients | Randomized | Intervention /Design | CR rate (%) | PFS% (years) | Comments |
|---|---|---|---|---|---|---|---|---|
| CALGB 9111 | 44 | 1998 | 198 | Yes | Benefit of G-CSF and consolidation | 82 | 23 months[a] | G-CSF improved CR rates, decreased induction deaths, but did not improve DFS or OS |
| PETHEMA ALL-89 | 45 | 1998 | 108 | Yes | Benefit of delayed intensification | 86 | 41% (5 years) | No benefit to intensification |
| MDACC | 42 | 2000 | 203 | No | "Hyper-CVAD" alternating cycles of intensive therapy | 91 | 39% (5 years) | No L-asparaginase/no cranial RT is administered in this regimen |
| MRC UKALL XA | 46 | 1993 | 618 | Yes | Benefit of early or late intensification | 88 | 28% (5 years) | No clear benefit to intensification, but decrease relapses in patients with early intensification |
| University of California (San Francisco) #8707 | 47 | 2002 | 84 | No | Intensified/cyclical but shortened postremission therapy | 93 | 52% (5 years) | Approach may be effective for standard-risk ALL |
| GMALL 05/93 | 48 | 2001 | 1200 | Yes | (a) Intensification by risk group (b) Intensification of maintenance therapy | 86 | 47% (5 years) | Long-term follow up ongoing |
| GIMEMA ALL 0288 | 49 | 2002 | 794 | Yes | (a) Addition of cyclophosphamide to induction (b) Benefit of early intensification | 82 | 2 years[a] | Neither induction nor postremission intensification improved CR or DFS |

[a]Median survival.

with standard-risk B-lineage ALL received high-dose MTX, while T-ALL patients received postremission cyclophosphamide and cytarabine, and high-risk B-lineage patients received both high-dose MTX and high-dose cytarabine.[48] The median remission duration was 57 months for standard-risk patients, with a 5-year survival of 55%. However, this approach did not appear to improve the outcome of high-risk patients except for those with pro-B ALL who achieved a continuous CR rate of 41%, in contrast to only 19% for other high-risk patients. The outcome for high-risk patients, with SCT in CR1, has been explored by other groups and is discussed below.

### NEWER "TARGETED" AGENTS
Recently, monoclonal antibodies targeted to epitopes present on lymphoblasts have also been evaluated. Rituximab, a chimeric humanized mouse antibody directed against CD20, which is expressed in approximately 20% of ALL cases, is being explored as an adjunct to standard chemotherapy in frontline and salvage therapy. Initial reports suggest that its addition may improve response rates, but with short-term follow-up[55]; longer follow-up will be needed to determine its potential to improve DFS. Campath-1H is a monoclonal humanized form of a rat antibody active against CD52, an antigen on nearly all normal B and T lymphocytes that may be present on the surface of most cases of ALL.[56,57] Although the experience with this antibody in relapsed, refractory ALL has been limited, Campath-1H has been shown to clear blasts from the peripheral blood after failure of traditional chemotherapy.[57,58] The CALGB has recently begun testing the feasibility of incorporating Campath-1H into the initial treatment of adult ALL in an attempt to eradicate MRD in early CR1 (CALGB 10102).

Other novel agents are being considered for addition to frontline therapy for this disease subset. For example, clofarabine, a purine analog, was recently approved for refractory or relapsed pediatric ALL.[59] Nelarabine (GW506U78), a prodrug of guanosine arabinoside, has been shown to have activity in relapsed precursor T ALL.[60–62]

### CNS PROPHYLAXIS
Although only 2–10% of adults with ALL present with CNS involvement at diagnosis,[63] 50–75% of patients will relapse in the CNS at 1 year in the absence of CNS-directed therapy.[64,65] The diagnosis of CNS leukemia requires the presence of more than five leukocytes per microliter in the cerebrospinal fluid (CSF) and the identification of lymphoblasts in the CSF differential.[66] Patients with CSF involvement may be asymptomatic, or can present with headache, meningismus, malaise, fever, or cranial nerve palsies. False-negative CSF results may occur in patients with predominantly cranial nerve involvement. Mature B-cell ALL, high serum lactate dehydrogenase (LDH) levels, and high proliferative index (more than 14% of lymphoblasts in the G2M/S phase of the cell cycle at diagnosis) have been associated with a higher risk of CNS disease in adult ALL.[63]

There is no consensus regarding the best approach for CNS prophylaxis in adult ALL. Concomitant use of cranial irradiation and IT therapy is often toxic and may result in delays in delivery of postremission intensification therapy. Alternative strategies have included triple IT therapy with MTX, cytarabine, and a corticosteroid without cranial irradiation,[67] or IT therapy combined with high-dose systemic therapy with CSF-penetrating drugs, including MTX, cytarabine, L-asparaginase, and corticosteroids. Systemic administration of dexamethasone achieves higher CSF levels than of prednisone and has a longer half-life in the CSF than prednisone.[68] As discussed previously, in a randomized pediatric trial, dexamethasone resulted in a lower incidence of CNS relapse compared to prednisone.[39] Although some studies suggest that CNS relapse rates of less than 5% can be achieved in adults with ALL using combination IT and high-dose systemic chemotherapy without cranial irradiation,[42,63,69] in the GMALL studies, attempts to omit or postpone CNS irradiation led to higher CNS relapse rates.[70] The omission of CNS irradiation may be of particular concern for patients with precursor T ALL; the pediatric oncology groups in the United States have generally continued to use prophylactic irradiation for high-risk patients with T-lineage disease. Future trials may explore a risk-oriented approach to CNS prophylaxis, with the goals of minimizing toxicity and optimizing efficacy.

### MAINTENANCE CHEMOTHERAPY
Long-term maintenance therapy typically consists of 6-MP given daily and MTX weekly for 18–36 months, often with the addition of periodic "pulses" of vincristine and prednisone or dexamethasone. Maintenance therapy is based on the theory of using prolonged exposure to antimetabolites to kill slowly dividing, potentially drug-resistant subclones remaining after induction and consolidation therapy, and has been demonstrated to reduce relapse rates in randomized trials in pediatric ALL. Although there have been no randomized studies justifying the use of maintenance therapy in adult ALL, attempts at omitting maintenance therapy in several different adult ALL studies have yielded unchanged or inferior results.[35,71,72] Importantly, there appears to be no benefit to prolonged maintenance therapy for patients with mature B-cell ALL who respond well to short-term dose-intensive regimens, as described below, and rarely relapse beyond the first year of treatment.

### STEM CELL TRANSPLANTATION
#### Allo SCT in first remission
The overall role of allo SCT in CR1 remains controversial; however, for ALL patients with adverse cytogenetics, including the t(9;22) and t(4;11), allo SCT in CR1 is the treatment of choice.

Survival for adult ALL patients following matched sibling allo SCT in first remission is approximately 50% (range, 20–80%).[73] The International Bone Marrow Transplant Registry (IBMTR) compared 251 patients who received intensive postremission chemotherapy with 484 patients who received matched sibling allo SCT.[74] Although 9-year DFS rates were similar—32% for chemotherapy and 34% for allo SCT—a higher recurrence rate of 66% was observed for chemotherapy patients versus 30% for those receiving allo SCT, with treatment-related mortality being the main cause of failure in patients who received allo SCT.

Allo SCT and autologous stem cell transplantation (auto SCT) in first remission were compared in a large French multicenter trial (LALA 87).[75] Based on an intent-to-treat analysis, survival at 10 years was 46% for those receiving allo SCT compared to 31% for those receiving consolidation chemotherapy alone ($p = 0.04$). The value of allo SCT was even more apparent after patients were classified into standard-risk and high-risk groups. High -risk was defined as having one more of the following factors: presence of the Philadelphia chromosome (Ph+), null ALL, age above 35 years, WBC count more than $30 \times 10^9$/L, and time to CR more than 4 weeks. In the high-risk group, the overall survival (OS) at 10 years was 44%, versus only 11% for the control arm ($p = 0.009$). In the standard-risk group, there did not appear to be a distinct survival advantage for allo SCT over chemotherapy. These results support the value of allo SCT in first CR for high-risk patients.

Based on the results above, the LALA-94 trial evaluated the benefit of a risk-adapted postremission approach in ALL and concluded, in a recently published paper, that allo SCT improved DFS in high-risk ALL in first CR.[76] Auto SCT did not confer a significant benefit over chemotherapy for high-risk ALL.

The Medical Research Council (MRC) UKALL12/ ECOG 2993 study is the largest prospective randomized trial designed to evaluate the role of allo SCT as postremission therapy in adult ALL, and accrual is ongoing.[77] All patients receive two phases of induction therapy and are assigned in first remission to receive allo SCT if they have a histocompatible sibling donor, while those without a related donor are randomized to auto SCT versus consolidation and maintenance chemotherapy. More than 1300 patients have been recruited, and the results reported so far have focused on the Ph+ patients ($n = 875$). An intention to treat analysis showed a significantly reduced relapse rate of 24% in Ph− patients assigned to allograft ($n = 190$) in comparison to 60% for those randomized to auto SCT or chemotherapy ($p = 0.0001$). There was an improved 5-year event-free survival (EFS) of 52% in patients assigned to allo SCT versus 36% for the randomized group ($p = 0.05$) that was most noticeable for patients classified as standard risk (5-year EFS of 64% for allo SCT vs 46%, $p = 0.05$). In contrast to the LALA study,

these data suggest that allo SCT may be beneficial for all younger adult ALL patients (of age below 50) in first remission, regardless of risk group; however, the trial is ongoing and definitive conclusions cannot yet be made.

Recently, the French Cooperative Group (GOE-LAMS) published its results of 198 patients with precursor B ALL who were randomized to early allo SCT in CR1 (if HLA-matched sibling donor available) or to consolidation/intensification therapy followed by auto SCT in CR1.[78] These investigators found a significant benefit to allo SCT in CR1. Using an intent to treat analysis, OS at 6 years was 75% for ALL patients younger than 50 years who received allo SCT, compared to 40% for those receiving auto SCT.

## Autologous Stem Cell Transplantation

The prospective, randomized studies described above in adult ALL demonstrate that relapse-free survival is inferior for auto SCT when compared to allo SCT. Moreover, no advantage in survival has been demonstrated with auto SCT compared with continued postremission chemotherapy alone.[79] DFS at 3 years following auto SCT in first remission in two of the largest trials reported was only 28–39%,[80–82] which is not better than survival rates reported in recent chemotherapy trials of adult ALL. Therefore, auto SCT does not currently have a role in the treatment of ALL, outside of the setting of a clinical trial.

## RISK-ADAPTED THERAPY

### MATURE B-CELL ALL

Clearly, a separate disease from the precursor cell acute leukemias, mature B-cell (Burkitt-type) ALL, is the least common subtype of ALL, comprising fewer than 5% of adult ALL cases. Patients with mature B-cell ALL must be identified at diagnosis, as specific therapeutic strategies have been shown to improve outcome dramatically for this disease subset.

Although the peak incidence is seen in children and young adults, patients older than 60 years make up one-third of adult cases.[83] The distinction between mature B-cell ALL and Burkitt lymphoma with marrow involvement is arbitrary; absence of extramedullary disease would favor the former.[84] Lymphoblasts of the FAB-L3 subtype express monoclonal surface immunoglobulin (sIg) along with B-cell-associated antigens CD19, CD20, and CD22. Certain characteristic cytogenetic abnormalities define the disease: The t(8;14), t(2;8), or t(8;22) represent variant translocations of the *c-myc* proto-oncogene at band 8q24 to the immunoglobulin gene at either the heavy chain or light chain locus, respectively.

The recent improvements in outcome for adults with mature B-cell ALL have resulted from adaptation of successful pediatric regimens. The French were the first to apply pediatric protocols to the therapy of adults with mature B-cell ALL, and were able to provide a CR rate of 79%, with a 3-year OS of 57%.[85] In what remains as the largest published series of adults to date with this disorder, Hoelzer et al. reported CR rates of 63 and 74%, and 4–8-year OS rates of 49–51%, respectively, in 59 adults treated with the pediatric Berlin-Frankfurt-Münster (BFM) protocols B-NHL 83 and B-NHL 86.[86] These protocols shared several important components: a cytoreductive prephase with low-dose cyclophosphamide and prednisone given 1 week before the start of intensive therapy, intermediate- to high-dose cytarabine, podophyllotoxins, doxorubicin, vincristine, high-dose MTX, fractionated high-dose cyclophosphamide/ifosfamide, aggressive IT chemotherapy, and tailored cranial radiotherapy for patients with CNS disease, all given in repeated cycles of short duration over a 4–6-month period. Relapse rarely occurred after the first year; thus, prolonged maintenance was not necessary.

An alternative successful approach using similar principles is the hyper-CVAD regimen developed at the MD Anderson Cancer Center.[87] Twenty-six patients with B-cell ALL and a median age of 58 years were treated with eight cycles of hyperfractionated cyclophosphamide, vincristine, doxorubicin, and dexamethasone, alternating with courses of high-dose intravenous MTX and cytarabine, with prophylactic CNS therapy consisting of MTX and cytarabine. A CR rate of 81% was attained, with a 3-year OS of 49% and a 3-year DFS of 61%. Overall, the hyper-CVAD regimen produced favorable results for all patient subsets, except for those presenting with very high LDH, CNS disease, and age over 60 years.

To improve response rates, the CALGB has also recently studied two separate cohorts of patients with advanced Burkitt lymphoma and mature B-cell ALL treated with intensive, pediatric-derived protocols, with the two cohorts differing in degrees of CNS-directed therapy given.[88,89] The first cohort was treated with a modified GMALL BFM protocol consisting of a pretreatment phase, fractionated ifosfamide and cyclophosphamide, high-dose MTX, vincristine, dexamethasone, and doxorubicin, alternating with etoposide and cytarabine by continuous infusion. Triple IT CNS therapy and prophylactic cranial irradiation were given to all patients. For the 24 B-cell ALL patients, CR rates of 75% were attained, with 3-year leukemia-free survival (LFS) and OS of 61 and 46%, respectively. Significant and often irreversible neurologic toxicity was noted with this intensive CNS-directed therapy; it was thus amended to reduce the number of IT injections, and cranial irradiation was omitted except for those with overt CNS or high-risk disease. A second cohort with this modified approach resulted in CR, 3-year LFS, and OS rates of 68, 67, and 50%, respectively, and CNS failure rates were not increased. Most importantly, severe neurologic toxicity was dramatically reduced from 60 to 23%. The authors concluded that high-dose antimetabolites and IT chemotherapy alone can prevent CNS failure, and cranial radiotherapy may be omitted in the absence of proven CNS involvement. The results of these and several other treatment programs that have been developed for Burkitt lymphoma and mature B-cell ALL are summarized in Table 13.3.

Recently, the therapeutic focus for mature B-cell ALL has turned to the addition of the monoclonal antibody, rituximab, for these strongly CD20+ leukemias. Preliminary results of the MD Anderson group, in which combining rituximab was combined with the hyper-CVAD regimen, demonstrated a CR rate of 93% and 1-year DFS of 86%.[94] Their preliminary data suggest a particular advantage for older adults treated with this approach. The CALGB also has a phase II study under way, in which patients with Burkitt lymphoma and leukemia are treated with rituximab and a high-intensity chemotherapy regimen. The GMALL study group has a similar prospective trial underway, with rituximab for the treatment of B-cell ALL and Burkitt lymphoma.

For treatment of advanced Burkitt lymphoma and mature B-cell ALL, both allo SCT and auto SCT are generally reserved for salvage therapy in relapsed or refractory disease. The general consensus has been that there is no role for this therapy in first CR in the standard-risk patient, as intensive high-dose chemotherapeutic regimens now yield such high CR rates and few long-term relapses. However, allogeneic stem cell transplant may be considered for patients with high-risk presenting features or for those failing to attain a CR within 4 weeks of initiation of therapy.

### PHILADELPHIA-CHROMOSOME-POSITIVE ALL

The t(9;22) occurs in 20–30% of patients with adult ALL. Although the remission rate is approximately 60–80% with intensive induction therapy, Ph+ ALL is not considered curable with standard chemotherapy, with long-term survival rates of less than 10%.[29,95] To improve outcome in Ph+ ALL, efforts have focused on dose intensification with allo SCT in first remission, which is currently the recommended treatment. In a preliminary report from the MRC UKALL X11/ECOG E2993 study, the EFS was 38% at 3 years for 35 patients with Ph+ ALL who received postremission allo SCT in CR1, compared to only 5% for those who received postremission chemotherapy or auto SCT in CR1.[96] Although difficult to compare because of variability in patient characteristics and treatment regimen, other small series report survival rates between 30 and 60%,[97–102] and all share the conclusions that Ph+ ALL patients appear to do best when an allo SCT is performed in first remission. For Ph+ ALL patients without HLA-matched sibling donors, the efficacy of matched unrelated donor (MUD) transplants has also been evaluated. In one small series of 18 young patients (median age was only 25 years) with Ph+ ALL

**Table 13.3**  Adult mature B-cell ALL studies[a]

| Author/protocol | Number of Patients | Age range | Elderly patients (%) | Median age | M/F ratio | CR (%) | DFS (% years) | OS (% years) | Induction mortality (%) |
|---|---|---|---|---|---|---|---|---|---|
| Fenaux[84]/ Protocol 3 LMB-86 | 7 | 17–66 | NA | 32 | 7 | 87 | 57   7mos (plateau) | 50   1 | 12 |
| Soussain[85]/ LMB-84/86 | 28 | 17–65 | 25 | 29.5 | 1.6 | 79 | 57   3 | 57   3 | 11 |
| Hoelzer[86]/ B-NHL 83 B-NHL 86 | 24 / 35 | 15–58 / 18–65 | 28 | 33 / 36 | 3.8 / 3.4 | 63 / 74 | 50  8 / 71  4 | 49  8 / 51  4 | 8 / 9 |
| Todeschini[90]/ POG 8617 | 7 | 19–64 | NA | 35 | 3 | 100 | NR | EFS 75 / Mean f/u 28months | 0 |
| Thomas[87]/ Hyper-CVAD | 26 | 17–79 | 46 / 58 | 58 | 4.2 | 81 | 61   3 | 49   3 | 19 |
| Magrath[91]/ 77-04 NCI 89-C-41 | 11 / 3 | 18–56 / 18–59 | NA | 24 / 25 | 3.3 / 4 | NR / 100 | NR / 100  2 | EFS 19  2 / 100  2 | NR / 0 |
| Mead[92]/ CODOX-M/IVAC | All stages 39 / Stage IV only 26 | 16–60 | NA | NR | NR | 74 | NR | 70   2 | NR |
| Lee[88]/ CALGB 9251 | Stage IV/L3 43 / L3 only 24 | 18–72 / 20–72 | 19 / 35 | 44 / 45 | 1.8 / 5 | All stages 80 / L3 only 75 | All stages 65  3 / L3 only 61  3 | All stages 52  3 / L3 only 46  3 | 4 / 4 |
| Rizzieri[89]/ CALGB 9251 (Cohort#2) | All stages 40 / Stage IV only 34 | 17–78 | 23 | 50 | 4 | 68 | 67   3 | 50   3 | 12 |
| Oriol[93]/ PETHEMA- LAL3/97 | All stages 39 / L3 only 25 | 15–74 | 17 | 35 | 1.8 | L3 only 68 | All stages 60   2 | L3 only 39   2 | All stages 18 |
| Thomas[94] Rituximab and Hyper-CVAD | All stages 15 | 27–72 | N/A | 50 | 5.3 | 93 | 86   1 | NR | NR |

CR, complete remission; LFS, leukemia-free survival; OS, overall survival; EFS, event-free survival; NR, not recorded; L3, mature B-cell ALL.
[a]Only data for intensive, high-dose chemotherapy protocols included; includes patients with mature B-cell ALL or stage IV Burkitt lymphoma unless specified, some data extrapolated.

who underwent a MUD allo SCT, the DFS at 2 years was 49% in this selected group, which is similar to the rates reported for HLA-matched sibling transplants.[101] With improvements in graft-versus-host disease prophylaxis, MUD transplants are also being explored in older patients with Ph+ ALL in CR1.

Imatinib mesylate (STI571, Gleevec; Novartis, East Hanover, NJ), a selective inhibitor of the BCR-ABL tyrosine kinase,[102] has shown promise in the treatment of Ph+ ALL. A CR rate of 29% was achieved in a group of 56 recurrent and refractory Ph+ ALL patients who received imatinib at 400 mg or 600 mg daily,[103] although only 6% of patients sustained a response of at least 4 weeks. Because of these promising results in highly refractory patients, imatinib is being tested by a number of groups for its ability to reduce disease burden prior to and following allo SCT or auto SCT (for patients without an HLA-matched sibling donor) for Ph+ ALL in CR1.[104–107] Preliminary results from these studies are encouraging, with high CR rates (79–100%) when imatinib was combined with induction chemotherapy. The majority of these patients were eligible for an allo SCT in early CR1. With limited follow-up, DFS rates of 78–90% are reported in these studies.

Combining imatinib with nontransplant chemotherapy may be a particularly promising approach for older Ph+ patients for whom allo SCT may not be feasible. The GMALL has initiated a randomized multicenter phase II study to determine the safety and efficacy of imatinib in Ph+ ALL patients greater than 55 years of age as first-line single-agent induction therapy, with administration of postremission consolidative chemotherapy for a duration of up to 1 year. Preliminary results suggest that combination treatment is tolerable, and early response rates appear favorable, with a CR rate of 93% for older Ph+ patients (median age of 67). This impressive CR rate compares favorably to a historical control CR rate of only 44% for a similar older high-risk group of patients.[108] Second-generation-targeted tyrosine kinase inhibitors (nilotinib, Novartis, Hanover, NJ, and dasatinib, Bristol-Myers Squibb, NY) that overcome imatinib resistance are now being tested in patients with relapsed Ph+ ALL. Thus, it appears that the principles that have resulted in the spectacular success of molecular targeted therapy using imatinib in patients with CML may now be applied to improve outcome for this most challenging subset of ALL.

### ALL WITH 11q23 (MLL) ABNORMALITIES

The t(4;11)(q21;q23) is the most common recurring abnormality involving the *MLL* gene on chromosome 11q23, and it occurs in 5–10% of adult ALL cases.[109–111] Patients often present with high leukocyte counts, hepatosplenomegaly, and CNS involvement. Survival for these patients is poor with chemotherapy alone, with DFS less than 15% at 5 years.[29] In contrast, when an allo SCT is performed in CR1, the GMALL reported more than 50% of patients with the t(4;11) achieving long-term DFS.[112] These investigators attributed their good results to the combination of high-dose cytarabine and mitoxantrone intensification followed by allo SCT. Based on these data, the current recommendation is to identify a donor for allo SCT early in CR1 for patients with the *MLL* gene rearrangements. In addition, they may benefit from intensive cytoreduction with a high-dose cytarabine-based regimen that may be given as early consolidative therapy while a suitable donor is being identified.

## AGE-STRATIFIED THERAPY

A series of systematic clinical trials in children with ALL has resulted in such high cure rates for the majority of patients (EFS of more than 75% for most patients) that current risk-adapted clinical trials in the pediatric cooperative groups are beginning to explore less intensive therapy for very good risk patients, with the goal of achieving similar results with fewer long-term side effects. In contrast, as discussed in detail above, the outcome for ALL in adults is considerably less favorable, with overall cure rates of less than 30%. Factors contributing to this marked difference include significant differences in the molecular genetics of adult ALL, with a higher incidence (30% in adults and 5% in children) of the unfavorable (9;22) Philadelphia chromosome translocation in adults and a virtual absence of the favorable *TEL-AML1* fusion gene resulting from a cryptic translocation, the t(12;21).[113–115] In addition, other negative risk factors include comorbid medical conditions in the aging population and poorer tolerance of chemotherapy, particularly of intensive treatment with L-asparaginase and higher dose MTX, drugs that have been used with great success in the pediatric population.[116]

### ADOLESCENT ALL

From subset analyses of both pediatric and adult ALL clinical trials, the adolescent and young adult (AYA) population has a distinctive outcome. In pediatric studies, adolescents are considered a high-risk group, receiving more intensive treatment with the intent of improving outcome to achieve the successes noted in good-risk children of age 2–10.[117,118] In the adult cooperative groups, AYA have traditionally received similar treatment to older adults and have been viewed as a relatively good risk group.[5] Several retrospective analyses have recently unveiled some striking differences in the outcome of AYA patients, depending upon "the door" they enter at the time of their diagnosis in determining enrollment on pediatric versus adult clinical trials.[119–121] Retrospective comparisons of pediatric versus adult clinical trials for ALL in North America, France, and the Netherlands all reached similar conclusions: AYA patients fared significantly better when

**Table 13.4**    Outcome comparison of adolescent/young adults with ALL on pediatric versus adult clinical trials

| Cooperative group | Study period/ number of patients | Age (years) | CR (%) | EFS (%) |
|---|---|---|---|---|
| North America[119] | 1988–1998 | 16–21 | | |
| CCG 1882 (pediatrics) | 196 patients | | 96 | 64 |
| CALGB 8811–9511 (adults) | 103 patients | | 93 | 38 |
| French[120] | 1993–1994 | 15–20 | | |
| FRALLE-93 (pediatrics) | 77 patients | | 94 | 67 |
| LALA-94   (adults) | 100 patients | | 83 | 41 |
| Dutch[121] | 1985–1999 | 15–21 | | |
| SKION ALL 6–9 (pediatrics) | 47 patients | | 98 | 69 |
| HOVON 5 and 18 (adults) | 73 patients | | 91 | 31 |
| | | | | 46 |

they were treated on pediatric protocols, despite that CR rates for AYA patients were generally comparable between adult and pediatric trials (Table 13.4).

### Factors Affecting Treatment Outcome: Drug Dosage, Schedule, the Doctors, and the Patients

All of these studies have engendered vigorous debate about whether the disparity in outcome for AYAs on pediatric versus adult trials can be accounted for primarily by differences in the drug regimens and planned dose intensity, or whether the precision with which actual dose was delivered might have a significant role in patient outcome. In general, the pediatric regimens contained significantly higher cumulative doses of nonmyelosuppressive drugs, including glucocorticoids, vincristine, and L-asparaginase. In addition, more frequent IT therapy was administered in the pediatric regimens, and maintenance therapy was generally administered for longer periods of time. As these are retrospective studies, dose delivery has been difficult to examine and may be influenced significantly by differences in adult versus pediatric physician attitude and experience with treatment of ALL. In addition, the attitudes, family support, and compliance of AYAs treated by adult versus pediatric oncologists may be different and relevant.

### OLDER ADULTS WITH ALL

A review of the annual age-specific leukemia incidence in the United States underscores the observation that ALL is relatively uncommon in the middle adult years, but increases rapidly in incidence over the age of 60. These patients have only rarely been included in clinical trials, and as yet, there are no optimal treatment programs available.

In a recent report from the northern counties of England, approximately one-third of ALL cases in adults occurred in patients older than 60 years.[122] Various treatment approaches have been taken in this older group of patients, but the outcomes are uniformly poor (Table 13.4). Investigators at the MD

Anderson Hospital have reported on 52 patients treated with infusional vincristine, adriamycin, and dexamethasone (VAD). This regimen produced a high CR rate with relatively low toxicity in older patients.[6] In the most recent CALGB trials, a CR rate of 65% was observed in older patients (60–80 years old, with a median age of 65).[5,44] Nevertheless, the 3-year survival in all three of these reports remains poor. The low tolerance of elderly patients for intensive chemotherapy remains one of the obstacles to increasing the overall cure rate in adults.[123] It is now estimated that as many as 40–50% of patients older than 60 years are Ph+; therefore, the focus on novel nonmyelosuppressive molecular targeted treatment strategies, as discussed above, is particularly needed for this very high risk group of patients. As previously discussed, the promising early results of combination chemotherapy with imatinib in older patients with Ph+ ALL are an example of the potential to significantly improve CR rates and, perhaps, OS in elderly patients with ALL.

## SUPPORTIVE CARE

Infectious disease complications secondary to neutropenia are the primary cause of treatment-related morbidity and mortality in acute leukemia, and the risks seem to be especially high in older patients.[44] Several studies have focused on preventing prolonged neutropenia in adults with ALL, with prophylactic use of granulocyte-stimulating growth factors.[44,124] Two sequential studies of granulocyte colony-stimulating factor (G-CSF) use during induction therapy performed by the GMALL demonstrated a reduction in the duration of neutropenia, a reduction in the number of nonviral infections, and less frequent interruptions in chemotherapy schedules. These benefits, however, did not translate into improved DFS or OS.[125]

In 1998, the CALGB published results of its large, prospective, randomized trial of G-CSF given during induction and consolidation chemotherapy.[44] Subjects who received G-CSF required fewer days to neutrophil recovery following induction chemotherapy for ALL. Subjects in the G-CSF group also had a shorter hospitalization time, a higher CR rate (87% vs 77%), and fewer induction deaths (5% vs 11%). However, G-CSF did not allow for a compressed course of chemotherapy or shorten the overall time required to undergo induction and consolidation. Nevertheless, in patients older than 60 years, the CR rate for patients receiving G-CSF was 81%, compared with 55% in the placebo arm. Despite the improvement in CR rates in older adults, however, none of the studies has demonstrated improvement in DFS or OS when hematopoietic growth factors were added to standard therapies.[126]

## TREATMENT ALGORITHM

Our current approach to treatment of adult ALL is beginning to incorporate these principles of risk adapted therapy. We advocate strongly the participation in clinical trials for adults with ALL. For younger patients, we have turned our focus to trying to achieve the same improvements in outcome noted by the pediatric cooperative groups for high-risk adolescents, where DFS is now routinely over 70%. To this end, an intergroup trial (CALGB and SWOG) will treat patients younger than 30 years with a regimen that is currently being used in the Children's Oncology Group (COG) for all adolescents and other high-risk children with ALL. The ECOG continues to explore the benefit of allo SCT in first remission for suitable younger patients, and their preliminary results also appear encouraging.

Current clinical trial efforts for adults with precursor B and T ALL have been directed toward the addition of novel targeted agents to reduce MRD and prolong DFS. Based on preliminary results from the GMALL and MD Anderson Cancer Center, the incorporation of rituximab into front-line therapy for CD20+ precursor B ALL appears promising. The ongoing CALGB study, as noted above, explores the substitution of dexamethasone for prednisone during induction and postremission therapy, and incorporates an alternative monoclonal antibody, Campath-1H, during postremission therapy for CD52+ precursor B and T ALL.

For suitable patients with a t(9;22), t(4;11), or other high-risk ALL, an allo SCT in first remission remains our treatment of choice. For the t(9;22) patients, the addition of imatinib to frontline therapy may improve outcome. We are participating in a US intergroup trial that explores the addition of imatinib pre- and post-stem cell transplant. Based on the exciting preliminary results described above in the section on Ph+ ALL, the incorporation of imatinib into standard induction and postremission therapy for older patients with ALL is rational, appears to be well tolerated, and significantly increases CR rates, with further follow up needed to validate the improvement noted in DFS and OS.

Finally, the outcome for patients with mature B-cell ALL has steadily improved, using short course-intensive therapy with fractionated alkylating agents, high-dose MTX and cytarabine, and intensive CNS prophylaxis. The addition of rituximab for these strongly CD20+ patients may further improve response rates and has been incorporated into frontline therapies for mature B-cell ALL in both North American and European cooperative group trials.

## REFERENCES

1. Stock W: Treatment of adult acute lymphoblastic leukemia: risk-adapted strategies. *Hematology 1999.* Washington, DC: American Society of Hematology Education Program Book; 1999:87.
2. Jemal A, Murray T, Samuels A, et al.: Cancer statistics, 2003. *CA Cancer J Clin* 53:5, 2003.
3. Ries L, Smith MA, Gurney JG: *Cancer Incidence and Survival among Children and Adolescents: United States SEER Program 1975–1995.* Bethesda: National Cancer Institute, 1999.
4. Andersen MK, Christiansen DH, Jensen BA, et al.: Therapy-related acute lymphoblastic leukaemia with MLL rearrangements following DNA topoisomerase II inhibitors, an increasing problem: report on two new cases and review of the literature since 1992. *Br J Haematol* 114:539, 2001.
5. Larson RA, Dodge RK, Burns CP, et al.: A five-drug remission induction regimen with intensive consolidation for adults with acute lymphoblastic leukemia: Cancer and Leukemia Group B study 8811. *Blood* 85:2025, 1995.
6. Kantarjian HM, Walters RS, Keating MJ, et al.: Results of the vincristine, doxorubicin, and dexamethasone regimen in adults with standard- and high-risk acute lymphocytic leukemia. *J Clin Oncol* 8:994, 1990.
7. Lazzarino M, Morra E, Alessandrino EP, et al.: Adult acute lymphoblastic leukemia. Response to therapy according to presenting features in 62 patients. *Eur J Cancer Clin Oncol* 18:813, 1982.
8. Hoelzer D, Thiel E, Loffler H, et al.: Prognostic factors in a multicenter study for treatment of acute lymphoblastic leukemia in adults. *Blood* 71:123, 1988.
9. Chessells JM, Hall E, Prentice HG, et al.: The impact of age on outcome in lymphoblastic leukaemia; MRC UKALL X and XA compared: a report from the MRC Paediatric and Adult Working Parties. *Leukemia* 12:463, 1998.
10. Secker-Walker LM, Craig JM, Hawkins JM, et al.: Philadelphia positive acute lymphoblastic leukemia in adults: age distribution, BCR breakpoint and prognostic significance. *Leukemia* 5:196, 1991.
11. Secker-Walker LM: Distribution of Philadelphia positive acute lymphoblastic leukemia: geographical heterogeneity or age related incidence? *Genes Chromosomes Cancer* 3:320, 1991.

12. Linker CA, Levitt LJ, O'Donnell M, et al.: Treatment of adult acute lymphoblastic leukemia with intensive cyclical chemotherapy: a follow-up report. *Blood* 78:2814, 1991.

13. Hoelzer D, Thiel E, Ludwig WD, et al.: The German multicentre trials for treatment of acute lymphoblastic leukemia in adults. The German Adult ALL Study Group. *Leukemia* 6(suppl 2):175, 1992.

14. Faderl S, Albitar M: Insights into the biologic and molecular abnormalities in adult acute lymphocytic leukemia. *Hematol Oncol Clin North Am* 14:1267, 2000.

15. Mandelli F, Annino L, Rotoli B: The GIMEMA ALL 0183 trial: analysis of 10-year follow-up. GIMEMA Cooperative Group, Italy. *Br J Haematol* 92:665, 1996.

16. Gaynor J, Chapman D, Little C, et al.: A cause-specific hazard rate analysis of prognostic factors among 199 adults with acute lymphoblastic leukemia: the Memorial Hospital experience since 1969. *J Clin Oncol* 6:1014, 1988.

17. Brunning RD, Borowitz M, Matutes E, et al.: *World Health Organization Classification of Tumours: Pathology and Genetics of Haematopoietic and Lymphoid Tissues.* Lyon, France: IARC Press, 2001.

18. Baer MR: Assessment of minimal residual disease in patients with acute leukemia. *Curr Opin Oncol* 10:17, 1998.

19. Stock W, Estrov Z: Studies of minimal residual disease in acute lymphocytic leukemia. *Hematol Oncol Clin North Am* 14:1289, 2000.

20. Faderl S, Kantarjian HM, Talpaz M, et al.: Clinical significance of cytogenetic abnormalities in adult acute lymphoblastic leukemia. *Blood* 91:3995, 1998.

21. Groupe Francais de Cytogenetic abnormalities in adult acute lymphoblastic leukemia: correlations with hematologic findings outcome. A Collaborative Study of the Group Francais de Cytogenetique Hematologique. *Blood* 87:3135, 1996.

22. Cave H, van der Werff ten Bosch J, Suciu S, et al.: Clinical significance of minimal residual disease in childhood acute lymphoblastic leukemia. European Organization for Research and Treatment of Cancer–Childhood Leukemia Cooperative Group. *N Engl J Med* 339:591, 1998.

23. van Dongen JJ, Seriu T, Panzer-Grumayer ER, et al.: Prognostic value of minimal residual disease in acute lymphoblastic leukaemia in childhood. *Lancet* 352:1731, 1998.

24. Foroni L, Coyle LA, Papaioannou M, et al.: Molecular detection of minimal residual disease in adult and childhood acute lymphoblastic leukaemia reveals differences in treatment response. *Leukemia* 11:1732, 1997.

25. Mortuza FY, Papaioannou M, Moreira IM, et al.: Minimal residual disease tests provide an independent predictor of clinical outcome in adult acute lymphoblastic leukemia. *J Clin Oncol* 20:1094, 2002.

26. Sher D, Dodge R, Bloomfield CD, et al.: Clone-specific quantitative real-time PCR of IgH or TCR gene rearrangements in adult ALL following induction chemotherapy identifies patients with a poor prognosis: pilot study from the Cancer and Leukemia Group B (CALGB 20101). *Blood* 100:153a, 2002.

27. Schrappe M, Flohr T, Beier R, et al.: Risk stratification in childhood acute lymphoblastic leukemias based on clone-specific detection of minimal residual disease (MRD) with molecular genetics: performance in German trial ALL-BFM 2000. *Hematol J* 1:695a, 2001.

28. Hoelzer D, Gokbuget N, Bruggemann M: Clinical impact of minimal residual disease in trial design for adult ALL. *Blood* 98:584, 2001.

29. Wetzler M, Dodge RK, Mrozek K, et al.: Prospective karyotype analysis in adult acute lymphoblastic leukemia: the Cancer and Leukemia Group B experience. *Blood* 93:3983, 1999.

30. Secker-Walker LM, Prentice HG, Durrant J, et al.: Cytogenetics adds independent prognostic information in adults with acute lymphoblastic leukaemia on MRC trial UKALL XA. MRC Adult Leukaemia Working Party. *Br J Haematol* 96:601, 1997.

31. Hussein KK, Dahlberg S, Head D, et al.: Treatment of acute lymphoblastic leukemia in adults with intensive induction, consolidation, and maintenance chemotherapy. *Blood* 73:57, 1989.

32. Schauer P, Arlin ZA, Mertelsmann R, et al.: Treatment of acute lymphoblastic leukemia in adults: results of the L-10 and L-10M protocols. *J Clin Oncol* 1:462, 1983.

33. Gottlieb AJ, Weinberg V, Ellison RR, et al.: Efficacy of daunorubicin in the therapy of adult acute lymphocytic leukemia: a prospective randomized trial by Cancer and Leukemia Group B. *Blood* 64:267, 1984.

34. Radford JE Jr, Burns CP, Jones MP, et al.: Adult acute lymphoblastic leukemia: results of the Iowa HOP-L protocol. *J Clin Oncol* 7:58, 1989.

35. Cuttner J, Mick R, Budman DR, et al.: Phase III trial of brief intensive treatment of adult acute lymphocytic leukemia comparing daunorubicin and mitoxantrone: a CALGB study. *Leukemia* 5:425, 1991.

36. Todeschini G, Tecchio C, Meneghini V, et al.: Estimated 6-year event-free survival of 55% in 60 consecutive adult acute lymphoblastic leukemia patients treated with an intensive phase II protocol based on high induction dose of daunorubicin. *Leukemia* 12:144, 1998.

37. Linker C, Damon L, Ries C, et al.: Intensified and shortened cyclical chemotherapy for adult acute lymphoblastic leukemia. *J Clin Oncol* 20:2464, 2002.

38. Stock W, Yu D, Johnson J, et al.: Intensified daunorubicin during induction and post-remission therapy of adult acute lymphoblastic leukemia (ALL): results of CALGB 19802. *Blood* 102:379a, 2003.

39. Jones B, Freeman AI, Shuster JJ, et al.: Lower incidence of meningeal leukemia when prednisone is replaced by dexamethasone in the treatment of acute lymphocytic leukemia. *Med Pediatr Oncol* 19:269, 1991.

40. Hurwitz CA, Silverman LB, Schorin MA, et al.: Substituting dexamethasone for prednisone complicates remission induction in children with acute lymphoblastic leukemia. *Cancer* 88:1964, 2000.

41. Bostrom BC, Sensel MR, Sather HN, et al.: Dexamethasone versus prednisone and daily oral versus weekly intravenous mercaptopurine for patients with standard-risk acute lymphoblastic leukemia: a report from the Children's Cancer Group. *Blood* 101:3809, 2003.

42. Kantarjian HM, O'Brien S, Smith TL, et al.: Results of treatment with hyper-CVAD, a dose-intensive regimen, in adult acute lymphocytic leukemia. *J Clin Oncol* 18:54, 2000.

43. Larson RA, Fretzin MH, Dodge RK, et al.: Hypersensitivity reactions to L-asparaginase do not impact on the remission duration of adults with acute lymphoblastic leukemia. *Leukemia* 12:660, 1998.

44. Larson RA, Dodge RK, Linker CA, et al.: A randomized controlled trial of filgrastim during remission induction and consolidation chemotherapy for adults with acute lymphoblastic leukemia: CALGB study 9111. *Blood* 92:1556, 1998.

45. Ribera JM, Ortega JJ, Oriol A, et al.: Late intensification chemotherapy has not improved the results of intensive chemotherapy in adult acute lymphoblastic leukemia. Results of a prospective multicenter randomized trial (PETHEMA ALL-89). Spanish Society of Hematology. *Haematologica* 83:222, 1998.

46. Durrant IJ, Richards SM: Results of Medical Research Council trial UKALL IX in acute lymphoblastic leukaemia in adults: report from the Medical Research Council Working Party on adult leukaemia. *Br J Haematol* 85:84, 1993.

47. Linker C, Damon L, Ries C, et al.: Intensified and shortened cyclical chemotherapy for adult acute lymphoblastic leukemia. *J Clin Oncol* 20:2464, 2002.

48. Gokbuget N, Arnold R, Buechner T, et al.: Intensification of induction and consolidation improves only subgroups of adult ALL: analysis of 1200 patients in GMALL study 05/93. *Blood* 98:802a, 2001.

49. Annino L, Vegna ML, Camera A, et al.: Treatment of adult acute lymphoblastic leukemia (ALL): long-term follow-up of the GIMEMA ALL 0288 randomized study. *Blood* 99:863, 2002.

50. Gokbuget N, Hoelzer D, Arnold R, et al.: Treatment of adult ALL according to protocols of the German Multicenter Study Group for Adult ALL (GMALL). *Hematol Oncol Clin North Am* 14:1307, 2000.

51. Rohatiner AZ, Bassan R, Battista R, et al.: High dose cytosine arabinoside in the initial treatment of adults with acute lymphoblastic leukaemia. *Br J Cancer* 62:454, 1990.

52. Weiss M, Maslak P, Feldman E, et al.: Cytarabine with high-dose mitoxantrone induces rapid complete remissions in adult acute lymphoblastic leukemia without the use of vincristine or prednisone. *J Clin Oncol* 14:2480, 1996.

53. Kantarjian H, Thomas D, O'Brien S, et al.: Long-term follow-up results of hyperfractionated cyclophosphamide, vincristine, doxorubicin, and dexamethasone (hyper-CVAD), a dose-intensive regimen, in adult acute lymphocytic leukemia. *Cancer* 101:2788, 2004.

54. Hoelzer D, Thiel E, Ludwig WD, et al.: Follow-up of the first two successive German multicentre trials for adult ALL (01/81 and 02/84). German Adult ALL Study Group. *Leukemia* 7(suppl 2):S130, 1993.

55. Thomas D, Cortes J, Giles F: The modified hyper-CVAD regimen in newly diagnosed adult acute lymphoblastic leukemia. *Blood* 98:590a, 2001.

56. Hale G, Swirsky D, Waldmann H, et al.: Reactivity of rat monoclonal antibody CAMPATH-1 with human leukaemia cells and its possible application for autologous bone marrow transplantation. *Br J Haematol* 60:41, 1985.

57. Dyer MJ, Hale G, Hayhoe FG, et al.: Effects of CAMPATH-1 antibodies in vivo in patients with lymphoid malignancies: influence of antibody isotype. *Blood* 73:1431, 1989.

58. Kolitz JE, O'Mara V, Willemze R: Treatment of acute lymphoblastic leukemia with campath. *Blood* 84:301a, 1994.

59. Faderl S, Gandhi V, Kozuch P, et al.: Clofarabine is active in combination with cytarabine in adult patients in first relapsed and primary refractory acute leukemia and high-risk myelodysplastic syndrome. *Blood* 102:615a, 2003.

60. Gandhi V, Plunkett W, Rodriguez CO Jr, et al.: Compound GW506U78 in refractory hematologic malignancies: relationship between cellular pharmacokinetics and clinical response. *J Clin Oncol* 16:3607, 1998.

61. Kisor DF, Plunkett W, Kurtzberg J, et al.: Pharmacokinetics of nelarabine and 9-beta-D-arabinofuranosyl guanine in pediatric and adult patients during a phase I study of nelarabine for the treatment of refractory hematologic malignancies. *J Clin Oncol* 18:995, 2000.

62. De Angelo DJ, Yu D, Richards SM: A phase II study of 2-amino-9-alpha-D-arabinosyl-6-methoxy-9H-purine (506U78) in patients with relapsed or refractory T-lineage acute lymphoblastic leukemia (ALL) or lymphoblastic lymphoma (LBL): CALGB study 19801. *Blood* 100:198a, 2002.

63. Kantarjian HM, Walters RS, Smith TL, et al.: Identification of risk groups for development of central nervous system leukemia in adults with acute lymphocytic leukemia. *Blood* 72:1784, 1988.

64. Law IP, Blom J: Adult acute leukemia: frequency of central system involvement in long term survivors. *Cancer* 40:1304, 1977.

65. Cortes J, O'Brien SM, Pierce S, et al.: The value of high-dose systemic chemotherapy and intrathecal therapy for central nervous system prophylaxis in different risk groups of adult acute lymphoblastic leukemia. *Blood* 86:2091, 1995.

66. Mastrangelo R: The problem of "staging" in childhood acute lymphoblastic leukemia: a review. *Med Pediatr Oncol* 14:121, 1986.

67. Pullen J, Boyett J, Shuster J, et al.: Extended triple intrathecal chemotherapy trial for prevention of CNS relapse in good-risk and poor-risk patients with B-progenitor acute lymphoblastic leukemia: a Pediatric Oncology Group study. *J Clin Oncol* 11:839, 1993.

68. Balis FM, Lester CM, Chrousos GP, et al.: Differences in cerebrospinal fluid penetration of corticosteroids: possible relationship to the prevention of meningeal leukemia. *J Clin Oncol* 5:202, 1987.

69. Mandelli F, Annino L, Vegna ML, et al.: GIMEMA ALL 0288: a multicentric study on adult acute lymphoblastic leukemia. Preliminary results. *Leukemia* 6(suppl 2):182, 1992.

70. Gokbuget N, Auion-Freire E, Diedrich H, et al.: Characteristics and outcome of CNS relapse in patients with adult acute lymphoblastic leukemia. *Blood* 94:288a, 1999.

71. Cassileth PA, Andersen JW, Bennett JM, et al.: Adult acute lymphocytic leukemia: the Eastern Cooperative Oncology Group experience. *Leukemia* 6(suppl 2):178, 1992.

72. Dekker AW, van't Veer MB, Sizoo W, et al.: Intensive postremission chemotherapy without maintenance therapy in adults with acute lymphoblastic leukemia. Dutch Hemato-Oncology Research Group. *J Clin Oncol* 15:476, 1997.

73. De Witte T, Awwad B, Boezeman J, et al.: Role of allogeneic bone marrow transplantation in adolescent or adult patients with acute lymphoblastic leukaemia or lymphoblastic lymphoma in first remission. *Bone Marrow Transplant* 14:767, 1994.

74. Horowitz MM, Messerer D, Hoelzer D, et al.: Chemotherapy compared with bone marrow transplantation for adults with acute lymphoblastic leukemia in first remission. *Ann Intern Med* 115:13, 1991.

75. Sebban C, Lepage E, Vernant JP, et al.: Allogeneic bone marrow transplantation in adult acute lymphoblastic leukemia in first complete remission: a comparative study. French Group of Therapy of Adult Acute Lymphoblastic Leukemia. *J Clin Oncol* 12:2580, 1994.

76. Thomas X, Boiron J-M, Huguet F, et al.: Outcome of treatment in adults with acute lymphoblastic leukemia: analysis of the LALA-94 trial. *J Clin Oncol* 22:1, 2004.

77. Avivi I, Rowe JM, Goldstone AH: Stem cell transplantation in adult ALL patients. *Best Pract Res Clin Haematol* 15:653, 2002.

78. Hunault M, Harousseau J-L, Delain M: Better outcome of adult acute lymphoblastic leukemia after early genoidentical allogeneic bone marrow transplant (BMT) than after late high-dose therapy and autologous BMT: a GOELAMS trial. *Blood* 104:3028, 2004.

79. Vey N, Blaise D, Stoppa AM, et al.: Bone marrow transplantation in 63 adult patients with acute lymphoblastic leukemia in first complete remission. *Bone Marrow Transplant* 14:383, 1994.

80. Thiebaut A, Vernant JP, Degos L, et al.: Adult acute lymphocytic leukemia study testing chemotherapy and autologous and allogeneic transplantation. A follow-up report of the French protocol LALA 87. *Hematol Oncol Clin North Am* 14:1353, 2000.

81. Attal M, Blaise D, Marit G, et al.: Consolidation treatment of adult acute lymphoblastic leukemia: a prospective, randomized trial comparing allogeneic versus autologous bone marrow transplantation and testing the impact of recombinant interleukin-2 after autologous bone marrow transplantation. BGMT Group. *Blood* 86:1619, 1995.

82. Fiere D, Lepage E, Sebban C, et al.: Adult acute lymphoblastic leukemia: a multicentric randomized trial testing bone marrow transplantation as postremission therapy. The French Group on Therapy for Adult Acute Lymphoblastic Leukemia. *J Clin Oncol* 11:1990, 1993.

83. Taylor PR, Reid MM, Bown N, et al.: Acute lymphoblastic leukemia in patients aged 60 years and over: a population-based study of incidence and outcome. *Blood* 80:1813, 1992.

84. Fenaux P, Bourhis JH, Ribrag V: Burkitt's acute lymphocytic leukemia (L3ALL) in adults. *Hematol Oncol Clin North Am* 15:37, 2001.

85. Soussain C, Patte C, Ostronoff M, et al.: Small noncleaved cell lymphoma and leukemia in aduts. A retrospective study of 65 adults treated with the LMB pediatric protocols. *Blood* 85:664, 1995.

86. Hoelzer D, Ludwig WD, Thiel E, et al.: Improved outcome in adult B-cell adult lymphoblastic leukemia. *Blood* 87:495, 1996.

87. Thomas DA, Cortes J, O'Brien S: Hyper-CVAD program in burkitt's-type acute lymphoblastic leukemia. *J Clin Oncol* 17:2461, 1999.

88. Lee EJ, Petroni GR, Schiffer CA: Brief-duration high-intensity chemotherapy for patients with small non-cleaved-cell lymphoma or FAB L3 acute lymphocytic leukemia: results of Cancer and Leukemia Group B study 9251. *J Clin Oncol* 19:4014, 2001.

89. Rizzieri DA, Johnson JL, Niedzwiecki D, et al.: Intensive chemotherapy with and without cranial radiation for Burkitt leukemia and lymphoma: final results of Cancer and Leukemia Group B study 9251. *Cancer* 100:1438, 2004.

90. Todeschini G, Tecchio C, Degani D, et al.: Eighty-one percent event-free survival in advanced Burkitt's lymphoma/leukemia: no differences in outcome between pediatric and adult patients treated with the same intensive pediatric protocol. *Ann Oncol* 8(suppl 1):77, 1997.

91. Magrath I, Adde M, Shad A, et al.: Adults and children with small non-cleaved-cell lymphoma have a similar excellent outcome when treated with the same chemotherapy regimen. *J Clin Oncol* 14:925, 1996.

92. Mead GM, Sydes MR, Salewski J, et al.: An international evaluation of CODOX-M and CODOX-M alternating with IVAC in adult Burkitt's lymphoma: results of United Kingdom Lymphoma Group LY06 study. *Ann Oncol* 13:1264, 2002.

93. Oriol A, Ribera JM, Esteve J, et al.: Lack of influence of human immunodeficiency virus infection status in the response to therapy and survival of adult patients with mature B-cell lymphoma or leukemia. Results of the PETHEMA-LAL3/97 study. *Haematologica* 88:445, 2003.

94. Thomas DA, Cortes J, Faderl S: Outcome of the hyper-CVAD and rituximab regimen in Burkitt (BL) and Burkitt-like (BLL) leukemia/lymphoma. *Blood* 104:901a, 2004.

95. Faderl S, Garcia-Manero G, Thomas DA, et al.: Philadelphia chromosome-positive acute lymphoblastic leukemia–current concepts and future perspectives. *Rev Clin Exp Hematol* 6:142, 2002; discussion: 200.

96. Rowe JM, Richards SM, Burnett AK, et al.: Favorable results of allogeneic bone marrow transplantation (BMT) for adults with Philadelphia (Ph)-chromosome-negative acute lymphoblastic leukemia (ALL) in first complete remission (CR): results from the international ALL trial (MRC UKALL XII/ECOG E2993). *Blood* 98:481a, 2001.

97. Dunlop LC, Powles R, Singhal S, et al.: Bone marrow transplantation for Philadelphia chromosome-positive acute lymphoblastic leukemia. *Bone Marrow Transplant* 17:365, 1996.

98. Stockschlader M, Hegewisch-Becker S, Kruger W, et al.: Bone marrow transplantation for Philadelphia-chromosome-positive acute lymphoblastic leukemia. *Bone Marrow Transplant* 16:663, 1995.

99. DeaneM, Koh M, Foroni L, et al.: FLAG-idarubicin and allogeneic stem cell transplantation for Ph-positive ALL beyond first remission. *Bone Marrow Transplant* 22:1137, 1998.

100. Snyder DS, Nademanee AP, O'Donnell MR, et al.: Long-term follow-up of 23 patients with Philadelphia chromosome-positive acute lymphoblastic leukemia treated with allogeneic bone marrow transplant in first complete remission. *Leukemia* 13:2053, 1999.

101. Sierra J, Radich J, Hansen JA, et al.: Marrow transplants from unrelated donors for treatment of Philadelphia chromosome-positive acute lymphoblastic leukemia. *Blood* 90:1410, 1997.

102. Druker BJ, Tamura S, Buchdunger E, et al.: Effects of a selective inhibitor of the Abl tyrosine kinase on the growth of Bcr-Abl positive cells. *Nat Med* 2:561, 1996.

103. Ottmann OG, Druker BJ, Sawyers CL, et al.: A phase 2 study of imatinib in patients with relapsed or refractory Philadelphia chromosome-positive acute lymphoid leukemias. *Blood* 100:1965, 2002.

104. Thomas D, Cortes J, Giles FJ: Combination of hyper-CVAD and imatinib mesylate (STI571) for Philadelphia positive adult lymphoblastic leukemia or chronic myelogenous leukemia in lymphoid blast phase. *Blood* 98:803a, 2001.

105. Thomas DA, Faderl S, Cortes J: Treatment of Philadelphia chromosome-positive acute lymphocytic leukemia with hyper-CVAD and imatinib mesylate. *Blood* 103:4396, 2004.

106. Towatari M, Yanada M, Usui N: Combination of intensive chemotherapy and imatinib can rapidly induce high-quality complete remission for a majority of patients with newly diagnosed BCR-ABL-positive acute lymphoblastic leukemia. *Blood* 104:3507, 2004.

107. Lee S, Kim Y-J, Min C-K: The effect of first-line imatinib interim therapy on the outcome of allogeneic stem cell transplantation in adults with newly diagnosed philadelphia chromosome-positive acute lymphoblastic leukemia. *Blood* 105:3449, 2005.

108. Wassmann B, Gokbuget N, Scheuring UJ, et al.: A randomized multicenter open label phase II study to determine the safety and efficacy of induction therapy with imatinib (Glivec, formerly STI571) in comparison with standard induction chemotherapy in elderly (>55 years) patients with Philadelphia chromosome-positive (Ph+/BCR-ABL+) acute lymphoblastic leukemia (ALL) (CSTI571ADE 10). *Ann Hematol* 82:716, 2003.

109. Thirman MJ, Gill HJ, Burnett RC, et al.: Rearrangement of the MLL gene in acute lymphoblastic and acute myeloid leukemias with 11q23 chromosomal translocations. *N Engl J Med* 329:909, 1993.

110. Pui CH, Frankel LS, Carroll AJ, et al.: Clinical characteristics and treatment outcome of childhood acute lymphoblastic leukemia with the t(4;11)(q21;q23): a collaborative study of 40 cases. *Blood* 77:440, 1991.

111. Reiter A, Schrappe M, Ludwig WD, et al.: Chemotherapy in 998 unselected childhood acute lymphoblastic leukemia patients. Results and conclusions of the multicenter trial ALL-BFM 86. *Blood* 84:3122, 1994.

112. Ludwig WD, Rieder H, Bartram CR, et al.: Immunophenotypic and genotypic features, clinical characteristics, and treatment outcome of adult pro-B acute lymphoblastic leukemia: results of the German multicenter trials GMALL 03/87 and 04/89. *Blood* 92: 1898, 1998.

113. Faderl S, Kantarjian HM, Talpaz M, et al.: Clinical significance of cytogenetic abnormalities in adult acute lymphoblastic leukemia. *Blood* 91:3995, 1998.

114. Secker-Walker LM, Craig JM, Hawkins JM, et al.: Philadelphia chromosome positive acute lymphoblastic leukemia in adults: age distribution, BCR breakpoint and prognostic significance. *Leukemia* 5:196, 1991.

115. Rubnitz JE, Downing JR, Pui CH, et al.: TEL gene rearrangement in acute lymphoblastic leukemia: a new genetic marker with prognostic significance. *J Clin Oncol* 15:1150, 1997.

116. Silverman LB, Gelber RD, Delton VK, et al.: Improved outcome for children with acute lymphoblastic leukemia: results of Dana-Farber consortium protocol 91–01. *Blood* 97:1211, 2001.

117. Schrappe M, Reiter A, Ludwig WD, et al.: Improved outcome in childhood acute lymphoblastic leukemia despite reduced use of anthracyclines and cranial radiotherapy: results of trial ALL-BFM 90, German–Austrian–Swiss ALL-BFM Study Group. *Blood* 95:3310, 2000.

118. Nachman JB, Sather HN, Sesel MG, et al.: Augmented post-induction therapy for children with high-risk acute lymphoblastic leukemia and a slow response to initial therapy. *N Eng J Med* 338:1663, 1998.

119. Stock W, Sather H, Dodge RK, et al.: Outcome of adolescents and young adults with ALL: a comparison of Children's Cancer Group (CCG) and Cancer and Leukemia Group B (CALGB) regimens. *Blood* 96:467a, 2000.

120. Boissel N, Auclerc M-F, Lheritier V, et al.: Should adolescents with acute lymphoblastic leukemia be treated as old children or young adults? Comparison of the French FRALLE-93 and LALA-94 trials. *J Clin Oncol* 21:774, 2003.

121. de Bont JM, ver der Holt B, Dekker AW, et al.: Significant difference in outcome for adolescents with acute lymphoblastic leukemia (ALL) treated on pediatric versus adult ALL protocols. *Leukemia* 18:2032–2035, 2004.

122. Taylor PR, Reid MM, Proctor SJ: Acute lymphoblastic leukaemia in the elderly. *Leuk Lymphoma* 13: 373, 1994.

123. Thomas X, Olteanu N, Charrin C, et al.: Acute lymphoblastic leukemia in the elderly: the Edouard Herriot Hospital experience. *Am J Hematol* 67:73, 2001.

124. Ottmann OG, Hoelzer D: Growth factors in the treatment of acute lymphoblastic leukemia. *Leuk Res* 22:1171, 1998.

125. Geissler K, Koller E, Hubmann E, et al.: Granulocyte colony-stimulating factor as an adjunct to induction chemotherapy for adult acute lymphoblastic leukemia– a randomized phase-III study. *Blood* 90:590, 1997.

126. Ozer H, Armitage JO, Bennett CL, et al.: 2000 update of recommendations for the use of hematopoietic colony-stimulating factors: evidence-based, clinical practice guidelines. American Society of Clinical Oncology Growth Factors Expert Panel. *J Clin Oncol* 18:3558, 2000.

# Chapter 14

# DEFINITION OF REMISSION, PROGNOSIS, AND FOLLOW-UP

*Meir Wetzler*

## INTRODUCTION

This chapter will define remission, prognosis, and follow-up criteria for acute lymphoblastic leukemia (ALL). As opposed to acute myeloid leukemia (AML), where the International Working Group has established the definitions[1] [see Chapter 8], no such project was undertaken in ALL.

## DEFINITION OF REMISSION

The importance in achieving a consensus on the definition of remission is to allow comparison of results from an assortment of studies and different institutions to provide the basis on which to make decisions about the care of patients. Consensus, as such, is required, but its achievement is compounded by the quality of the bone marrow specimen and the experience of the pathologist evaluating it. A morphologic complete remission (CR) is defined as having a neutrophil count $\geq 1.0 \times 10^9$/L, platelet count $\geq 100 \times 10^9$/L, normal bone marrow cellularity with trilineage hematopoiesis, with <5% blasts and resolution of all extramedullary disease.[1] Note that hemoglobin concentration or hematocrit are not included when evaluating remission status, but the patient has to be transfusion independent. Partial remission (PR) is not used for studies in which the objective is cure, but is used for phase I and II studies, conducted in patients with refractory or relapsed disease. In such cases, the aim is to record any significant activity. PR is then defined as $\geq 5$% but <20% blasts.

### HEMATOGONES

Occasionally it is difficult to distinguish between persistent disease and the presence of hematogones.[2–4] Hematogones are nonmalignant lymphoid progenitor cells found in the bone marrow, and are similar to lymphoblasts. Hematogones are usually heterogenous in size and are nonclonal. If the ALL blasts express myeloid markers, the hematogones, by definition, are devoid of these and therefore can be distinguished from leukemia blasts. If the hematogones do not express myeloid markers, it is difficult to distinguish them from leukemia blasts. Most experts would recommend repeating marrow examinations, weekly or every other week, until either the disappearance of the hematogones or emergence of the leukemic clone.

### MORPHOLOGIC CR

Morphologic CR without complete recovery of platelet count is not considered a category of CR in AML patients.[1] The same is true for ALL patients. Time to platelet recovery seems to predict outcome of patients with de novo ALL who have achieved CR.[5] In one study, patients who did not achieve platelet recovery by day 48 had a significantly worse outcome than those who achieved platelet recovery by day 12. Therefore, in ALL, morphologic CR without platelet count recovery ($\geq 100 \times 10^9$/L) should not be regarded as CR.

Finally, the definition of CR in AML was previously associated with a requirement for a 4-week duration of persistent remission to qualify as a CR. However, in ALL, postremission therapy is administered without any delays, and therefore the definition of CR should not be time dependent; retrospective designation of CR based on subsequent clinical course is not recommended. This correlates with the recently revised definition of CR in AML.[1]

### IMMUNOPHENOTYPIC CR

Patients who achieve morphologic CR can be further categorized based on additional and more sensitive methods. Flow cytometry identifies leukemia-associated marker patterns on the surface of, or inside, the blasts. These patterns include over-expression (e.g., for B lineage: CD10, CD19, CD20) as well as under-expression (e.g., CD45) of markers compared with their expression on normal lymphoid cells. Overall, persistence of a unique phenotype determined by flow cytometry, e.g., CD10 and CD20 coexpression, has been associated with worse outcome and should be viewed as

**Table 14.1**    Sensitivity of minimal residual disease detection by flow cytometry

| Disease | Sensitivity[a] | References |
|---|---|---|
| Adult T ALL | $1:1 \times 10^4$ | 13 |
| ALL (age ≥14 years old) | $1:2 \times 10^3$ | 14 |
| Adult and childhood ALL | TdT $<100 \times 10^3$, CD10 $>50 \times 10^3$, CD19 $>11 \times 10^{3b}$ | 10 |
| Childhood ALL | $1:1 \times 10^4$ | 11 |
| Childhood ALL | $1:1 \times 10^4$ | 12 |
| Childhood ALL | 1 blast/$\mu$L | 15 |
| Pre-B cell line | $1:1 \times 10^6$ | 6 |
| Breast cancer | $1:1 \times 10^7$ | 7 |
| Breast cancer | $1:1 \times 10^7$ | 8 |

[a]Ratio of malignant cell and normal nonmalignant cells.
[b]Molecules per cell.

residual disease.[6–15] However, the sensitivity and reliability of these tests depend on the number of cells to be analyzed (Table 14.1). Flow cytometry allows detection of one abnormal cell in $10^6$ cells, if at least $10^7$ cells are analyzed. Such large numbers are rarely available during remission, and therefore a more realistic sensitivity to detect minimal residual disease would be one abnormal cell in $10^4$–$10^5$ cells.[16] This level of sensitivity is achievable only if the antibodies can clearly distinguish the leukemic blasts from normal cells. In addition, antibodies with nonspecific light scattering will lower the sensitivity of the test. It is therefore recommended to use serially diluted leukemic blasts with normal cells to confirm the level of sensitivity. Finally,

clonal evolution may cause disappearance of one or more antigens detected at diagnosis.[17–23] Therefore, after taking into consideration all the caveats mentioned above, lack of minimal residual disease by quantitative flow cytometry at the end of remission induction therapy was associated with better clinical outcome in some studies of adult ALL patients.[10,13–15] However, because of a multitude of methods and lack of consensus, it is still not possible to make a clear recommendation of how to use flow cytometry to detect minimal residual disease.

### CYTOGENETIC CR

There are no prospective studies to evaluate the role of complete cytogenetic remission in ALL. Cytogenetic analysis, based on at least 20 metaphases, can detect one residual metaphase, resulting in a sensitivity of 5%. As was described earlier, flow cytometry and molecular testing (see below) can detect one abnormal cell in $10^3$–$10^4$ normal cells. Minimal residual disease, detected by either of these two methods, was proven to be an independent prognostic factor in ALL (see above for flow cytometry and below for molecular target). Therefore, complete cytogenetic remission should be evaluated prospectively in ALL clinical trials to determine its significance for the prediction of outcome.

### MOLECULAR CR

Molecular CR has been associated with clinical outcome in ALL[12,24–40] (Table 14.2). However, the degree of sensitivity may have an impact on the correlation with clinical outcome. For example, Roberts and colleagues[41] detected one abnormal cell in $10^5$ or more normal cells, and concluded that their finding did not predict relapse because the test either detected preleukemic or nondividing cells. Detecting one abnormal cell in $10^4$ or fewer

**Table 14.2**    Sensitivity of minimal residual disease detection by molecular analyses

| Disease | Molecular target | Sensitivity | References |
|---|---|---|---|
| ALL (age ≥15 years old) | IgH | $1-5:10^2-10^3$ | 29 |
| ALL (age ≥15 years old) | TCRD, TCRG | $1:10^3-10^5$ | 31 |
| Adult and childhood ALL | IgH | $1:5 \times 10^3$ | 24 |
| Adult and childhood ALL | IgH, IgK, TCRD, TCRG | $1:10^4$ to $1:10^6$ | 27 |
| Adult and childhood ALL | IgH, IgK, TCRD, TCRG | $1:10^3$ to $1:10^6$ | 12 |
| Adult and childhood ALL | TCRD, TCRG, TAL-1 | NOS | 32 |
| Adult and childhood ALL | TCRB | $1:5 \times 10^4$ | 39 |
| Adult ALL | IgH, IgK, TCRB, TCRD | $1:10^4$ to $1:10^5$ | 38 |
| Childhood ALL | IgH, TCRD, TCRG | $1:10^6$ | 34 |
| Childhood ALL | IgK-Kde, TCRD, TCRG, TAL-1 | $1:10^3-10^6$ | 25 |
| Childhood ALL | IgH, TCRD, TCRG | $1:10^5$ | 26 |
| ALL (NOS) | WT1 | $1:10^6$ | 30 |
| ALL (NOS) | WT1 | $10^0$ copies/100-ng cDNA | 28 |
| Adult ALL | WT1 | 1 copy:$10^5$ ABL copies | 35 |
| BCR/ABL-ALL (NOS) | BCR/ABL | $1:10^5$ | 36,37 |
| MLL/AF4-childhood ALL | MLL/AF4 | $1:10^3$ | 40 |
| Childhood ALL[a] | HOX11L2 | Normalized to ABL | 33 |

NOS: not otherwise specified.
[a]Only 2 patients were followed for MRD.

normal cells has been shown to predict outcome,[24,26,28,29,31–35,39,40] while others were able to demonstrate prediction of outcome with more sensitive tests.[12,25,27,30,34,36] These tests varied in their techniques, studying either tumor-specific DNA to detect residual malignant B cells by immunoglobulin gene rearrangement or residual malignant T cells by T-cell receptor genes,[12,24–27,29,31,32,38,39] or tumor-specific RNA to detect fusion gene transcripts (e.g., *BCR/ABL*, *TEL/AML1*, *MLL/AF4*)[36,40,42,43] or aberrantly expressed genes [e.g., *FLT3*,[33,44] *WT1*,[28,30,35] *HOX11*[33]]. The tests also differed in the time points to analyze minimal residual disease, e.g., day 11 versus end of induction. Therefore, a molecular CR must incorporate the sensitivity of the test and timing, and also the gene analyzed to allow comparisons among different studies. Because of these issues, it is not possible to make a clear recommendation of how to use molecular testing to detect minimal residual disease outside of a correlative study to a clinical trial.

### TREATMENT FAILURE

Treatment failure has not been defined specifically for ALL, and therefore the revised criteria set forth recently for AML should be used,[1] with some modifications. Treatment failure includes all patients who did not achieve a CR, or in phase I or II trials, a PR, and should be subclassified into several categories. "Treatment failure due to refractory disease" should be defined differently than it is in AML[1] because the induction treatment in ALL spreads over at least 3 weeks. One could define treatment failure as patients who have persistent peripheral blood blasts 7 days from initiation of induction treatment,[45,46] or persistent bone marrow blasts (>5%) 14 days from initiation of induction treatment.[45,46] Table 14.3 demonstrates the number of patients analyzed for each recommendation. "Treatment failure due to complications from aplasia" was described in AML[1] but, to the best of our knowledge, was not described in ALL. "Finally, treatment failure of indeterminate cause" should be defined for ALL. It can include two categories as described for AML[1] with modifications due to different treatment regimens. One category should include those patients who die less than 7 days after initiation of treatment and the other category should include those patients who survive seven or more days after the initiation of treat-

ment, whose most recent peripheral blood smear does not show persistent leukemia, and who did not have a bone marrow examination subsequent to therapy.

### RELAPSE

Relapse is defined as in AML[1]: that is, morphologic relapse, after achievement of CR, is the reappearance of leukemic blasts in the peripheral blood or ≥5% blasts in the bone marrow, or the reappearance of cytologically proven extramedullary disease. Genetic or molecular relapse is defined by reappearance of a cytogenetic or molecular abnormality.

## PROGNOSTIC FACTORS

Prognostic factors in adult ALL represent an evolving concept and depend on the advent of new research findings. Independent prognostic factors that were established by more than one group are summarized in Table 14.4. Other prognostic factors that emerged in small studies asking a particular question about one or another factor are beyond the scope of this Chapter.

## FOLLOW-UP

The follow-up of ALL patients is intended to measure the duration of survival or remission. As in AML,[1] four different categories are used: overall survival, relapse-free survival, event-free survival, and remission duration. The main reason to have an assortment of definitions is to handle the possibility of competing events. For example, there can be two competing events for survival: relapsed disease or massive myocardial infarction. Even though both are fatal, only one counts toward ALL treatment outcome.[80,81] In another manner, the massive myocardial infarction may have precluded ALL relapse from occurring.

### OVERALL SURVIVAL

Overall survival is measured from the time of diagnosis to the time of death from any cause. If the patient is not known to be deceased, overall survival is censored on the date the patient was last known to be alive. Overall survival is usually not subject to competing risks. However, if overall survival following regimen A is sought, and the patient is then undergoing an allogeneic transplantation and dies from transplant-related complications, death from transplantation becomes a competing risk for regimen A.

### RELAPSE-FREE SURVIVAL

Relapse-free survival is used only for patients who achieve CR and is calculated from the date CR was attained to the time of relapse or death, whichever occurs first. As described above, if the patient is not

| Table 14.3 | Number of patients analyzed for persistence of peripheral blood and bone marrow blasts during remission induction | |
|---|---|---|
| | Number of patients | Reference |
| Day 7 | 255 | 45 |
| Day 7 | 79 | 46 |
| Day 14 | 299 | 45 |
| Day 15 | 437 | 47 |

**Table 14.4  Prognostic factors in adult ALL**

| Risk factor | Note |
|---|---|
| Age | Age at diagnosis is one of the most important pretreatment risk factors, with advancing age being associated with a worse prognosis. Chronic and intercurrent diseases impair tolerance to aggressive therapy; acute medical problems at diagnosis may reduce the likelihood of survival.[48–58]<br>■ High risk: age >60 years |
| Performance status | Performance status, independent of age, also influences the ability to survive induction therapy, and thus respond to treatment.[54,57]<br>■ High risk: poor performance status. |
| Leukocyte count | A high presenting leukocyte count is an independent prognostic factor; duration of CR is inversely related to the presenting leukocyte count.[48–50,53,55,58–61]<br>■ High risk: leukocyte count >30,000/µL in B-lineage disease and >100,000/µL in T-lineage disease |
| Immunophenotype | Immunophenotype at diagnosis is an independent prognostic factor. In brief, T-lineage immunophenotype confers better outcome than B lineage and the presence of 6 or more T-cell markers is associated with favorable prognosis.[48,54,61–63]<br>■ High risk: B-lineage disease. |
| Karyotype | Chromosome findings at diagnosis are an independent prognostic factor. In brief, t(9;22), +8, t(4;11), −7, and hypodiploid karyotypes are associated with unfavorable outcome; normal karyotype, +21, and del(9p) or t(9p) confer an intermediate outcome; and del(12p) or t(12p) and t(14q11-q13) may be associated with favorable outcome.[48,54,55,61,64–70]<br>■ High risk: t(9;22), +8, t(4;11), −7, and hypodiploid karyotypes |
| HOX11 oncogene[a] | The expression of HOX11 oncogene has a favorable outcome in adult T-lineage ALL.[71]<br>■ High risk: lack of HOX11 gene expression |
| Multidrug resistance | The expression of multidrug resistance proteins is associated with an unfavorable outcome in adult ALL.[72–77]<br>■ High risk: expression of multidrug resistance proteins |
| Bone marrow biopsy morphology | Persistence of normal residual hematopoiesis and intense leukemic cells mitotic activity are associated with favorable outcome.[78] |
| Lactic dehydrogenase (LDH) level | High LDH level is associated with poor outcome[54] and with CNS disease in some studies.[54,79]<br>■ High risk: elevated LDH |
| Cytoreduction | Eradication of the leukemic blasts from the peripheral blood or bone marrow at day 7 or day 14 was shown to be associated with a favorable outcome.[45–47,53]<br>■ High risk: lack of cytoreduction |
| Achievement of CR | In addition to pretreatment variables, achievement of CR correlates with prognosis in ALL.[58,61]<br>■ High risk: lack of achievement of CR with the first cycle of chemotherapy |

[a]Even though this factor was described only once in adult ALL, several studies described its significance in pediatric ALL and therefore this factor is mentioned herein.

known to have relapsed, or deceased, relapse-free survival is censored on the date the patient was last seen. Relapse-free survival is not subject to competing risks.

### EVENT-FREE SURVIVAL

Event-free survival is measured from the date of diagnosis until treatment failure, defined as either resistant disease, disease relapse, or death from any cause, whichever occurs first. If none of these events occur, the event-free survival is censored at the date the patient was last seen. Event-free survival, for patients who do not achieve a CR, is defined as the time to progression, or death, whichever occurs first. As with overall survival and relapse-free survival, event-free survival is not subject to competing risks.

### REMISSION DURATION

Remission duration, as the name suggests, is reserved only for patients who achieve CR, and is calculated from the date CR was attained to the date of relapse. For patients who die without a report of relapse, remission duration is censored at the date of death, regardless of the cause. Finally, for patients whose disease does not relapse, remission duration is defined until the day the patient was last seen. This is the only measure, of the above four, as defined by Cheson and colleagues,[1] subject to competing risks (e.g., death without relapse).

**Table 14.5  Proposed follow-up for adult ALL patients**

| Category | How? | How often? |
|---|---|---|
| Remission status | Ask about constitutional symptoms and symptoms of anemia, thrombocytopenia, and granulocytopenia | Every month during the first year, every 3 months for the second and third years posttherapy, and then at least every 6 months for 3 years |
| Remission status | Look for pallor, petechiae, lymphadenopathy | Every month for 1 year posttherapy, and then every 3 months for 2 more years, and at least every 6 months for 3 years |
| Remission status | Complete blood count with differential | Every month for 1 year posttherapy, and then every 3 months for 2 more years, and at least every 6 months for 3 years |
| Remission status | Bone marrow aspiration and biopsy for morphology and cytogenetics | Once, 3 months post completion of chemotherapy, and then no specific guidelines, unless on clinical trial |
| Remission status | PCR for specific chromosomal aberrations | No specific guidelines |
| Remission status | PCR with patient-specific junctional regions of rearranged immunoglobulin or T-cell receptor genes | No specific guidelines |
| Remission status | Flow cytometry to detect specific phenotypes | No specific guidelines |
| Avascular necrosis | Ask about pain in hips while walking | With each history taking as mentioned above |
| Heart failure | Ask about swollen ankles, shortness of breath, etc. | With each history taking as mentioned above |
| Sterility | Ask about pregnancies | With each history taking as mentioned above |
| Hypothyroidism | Ask about cold intolerance, fatigue, somnolence | With each history taking as mentioned above |

PCR, polymerase chain reaction.

Other definitions of outcomes have been used in clinical trials.[1] For example, when postremission therapy was studied, all patients had to be in a CR at the time of enrollment, and therefore time until relapse or death should be measured from the date of study entry following CR.

## LONG-TERM FOLLOW-UP

Follow-up plans for patients on a clinical trial should adhere to the scheme described in the study. There is no consensus for the follow-up of patients not enrolled on clinical trials. A general recommendation (Table 14.5) would be to follow the patients monthly during the first year, every 2 to 3 months during the second and third years, and then at least every 6 months during the next 3 years. At 6 years and thereafter, patients can be monitored annually with history and physical examination, complete blood count with differential, and careful attention for second malignancies, heart failure, sterility, avascular necrosis, and hypothyroidism—all potential sequelae of therapy. Assessment of minimal residual disease should preferably be associated with clinical trials.

## REFERENCES

1. Cheson BD, Bennett JM, Kopecky KJ, et al.: Revised recommendations of the International Working Group for Diagnosis, Standardization of Response Criteria, Treatment Outcomes, and Reporting Standards for Therapeutic Trials in Acute Myeloid Leukemia. *J Clin Oncol* 21:4642, 2003.
2. Lai R, Hirsch-Ginsberg CF, Bueso-Ramos C: Pathologic diagnosis of acute lymphocytic leukemia. *Hematol Oncol Clin North Am* 14:1209, 2000.
3. Rimsza LM, Larson RS, Winter SS, et al.: Benign hematogone-rich lymphoid proliferations can be distinguished from B-lineage acute lymphoblastic leukemia by integration of morphology, immunophenotype, adhesion molecule expression, and architectural features. *Am J Clin Pathol* 114:66, 2000.
4. Kroft SH, Asplund SL, McKenna RW, et al.: Haematogones in the peripheral blood of adults: a four-colour flow cytometry study of 102 patients. *Br J Haematol* 126:209, 2004.
5. Faderl S, Thall PF, Kantarjian HM, et al.: Time to platelet recovery predicts outcome of patients with de novo acute lymphoblastic leukaemia who have achieved a complete remission. *Br J Haematol* 117:869, 2002.
6. Gross HJ, Verwer B, Houck D, et al.: Detection of rare cells at a frequency of one per million by flow cytometry. *Cytometry* 14:519, 1993.
7. Gross HJ, Verwer B, Houck D, et al.: Model study detecting breast cancer cells in peripheral blood mononuclear cells at frequencies as low as 10(–7). *Proc Natl Acad Sci USA* 92:537, 1995.

8. Rehse MA, Corpuz S, Heimfeld S, et al.: Use of fluorescence threshold triggering and high-speed flow cytometry for rare event detection. *Cytometry* 22:317, 1995.

9. Rosenblatt JI, Hokanson JA, McLaughlin SR, et al.: Theoretical basis for sampling statistics useful for detecting and isolating rare cells using flow cytometry and cell sorting. *Cytometry* 27:233, 1997.

10. Farahat N, Morilla A, Owusu-Ankomah K, et al.: Detection of minimal residual disease in B-lineage acute lymphoblastic leukaemia by quantitative flow cytometry. *Br J Haematol* 101:158, 1998.

11. Coustan-Smith E, Behm FG, Sanchez J, et al.: Immunological detection of minimal residual disease in children with acute lymphoblastic leukaemia. *Lancet* 351:550, 1998.

12. Malec M, Bjorklund E, Soderhall S, et al.: Flow cytometry and allele-specific oligonucleotide PCR are equally effective in detection of minimal residual disease in ALL. *Leukemia* 15:716, 2001.

13. Krampera M, Vitale A, Vincenzi C, et al.: Outcome prediction by immunophenotypic minimal residual disease detection in adult T-cell acute lymphoblastic leukaemia. *Br J Haematol* 120:74, 2003.

14. Vidriales MB, Perez JJ, Lopez-Berges MC, et al.: Minimal residual disease in adolescent (older than 14 years) and adult acute lymphoblastic leukemias: early immunophenotypic evaluation has high clinical value. *Blood* 101:4695, 2003.

15. Dworzak MN, Panzer-Grumayer ER: Flow cytometric detection of minimal residual disease in acute lymphoblastic leukemia. *Leuk Lymphoma* 44:1445, 2003.

16. Campana D, Coustan-Smith E: Detection of minimal residual disease in acute leukemia by flow cytometry. *Cytometry* 38:139, 1999.

17. Borella L, Casper JT, Lauer SJ: Shifts in expression of cell membrane phenotypes in childhood lymphoid malignancies at relapse. *Blood* 54:64, 1979.

18. Greaves M, Paxton A, Janossy G, et al.: Acute lymphoblastic leukaemia associated antigen. III Alterations in expression during treatment and in relapse. *Leuk Res* 4:1, 1980.

19. Lauer S, Piaskowski V, Camitta B, et al.: Bone marrow and extramedullary variations of cell membrane antigen expression in childhood lymphoid neoplasias at relapse. *Leuk Res* 6:769, 1982.

20. Raghavachar A, Thiel E, Bartram CR: Analyses of phenotype and genotype in acute lymphoblastic leukemias at first presentation and in relapse. *Blood* 70:1079, 1987.

21. Pui CH, Raimondi SC, Head DR, et al.: Characterization of childhood acute leukemia with multiple myeloid and lymphoid markers at diagnosis and at relapse. *Blood* 78:1327, 1991.

22. Abshire TC, Buchanan GR, Jackson JF, et al.: Morphologic, immunologic and cytogenetic studies in children with acute lymphoblastic leukemia at diagnosis and relapse: a Pediatric Oncology Group study. *Leukemia* 6:357, 1992.

23. van Wering ER, Beishuizen A, Roeffen ET, et al.: Immunophenotypic changes between diagnosis and relapse in childhood acute lymphoblastic leukemia. *Leukemia* 9:1523, 1995.

24. Foroni L, Coyle LA, Papaioannou M, et al.: Molecular detection of minimal residual disease in adult and childhood acute lymphoblastic leukaemia reveals differences in treatment response. *Leukemia* 11:1732, 1997.

25. van Dongen JJ, Seriu T, Panzer-Grumayer ER, et al.: Prognostic value of minimal residual disease in acute lymphoblastic leukaemia in childhood. *Lancet* 352:1731, 1998.

26. Cavé H, van der Werff ten Bosch J, Suciu S, et al.: Clinical significance of minimal residual disease in childhood acute lymphoblastic leukemia. European Organization for Research and Treatment of Cancer—Childhood Leukemia Cooperative Group. *N Engl J Med* 339:591, 1998.

27. Nakao M, Janssen JW, Flohr T, et al.: Rapid and reliable quantification of minimal residual disease in acute lymphoblastic leukemia using rearranged immunoglobulin and T-cell receptor loci by LightCycler technology. *Cancer Res* 60:3281, 2000.

28. Kreuzer KA, Saborowski A, Lupberger J, et al.: Fluorescent 5'-exonuclease assay for the absolute quantification of Wilms' tumour gene (WT1) mRNA: implications for monitoring human leukaemias. *Br J Haematol* 114:313, 2001.

29. Mortuza FY, Papaioannou M, Moreira IM, et al.: Minimal residual disease tests provide an independent predictor of clinical outcome in adult acute lymphoblastic leukemia. *J Clin Oncol* 20:1094, 2002.

30. Cilloni D, Gottardi E, De Micheli D, et al.: Quantitative assessment of WT1 expression by real time quantitative PCR may be a useful tool for monitoring minimal residual disease in acute leukemia patients. *Leukemia* 16:2115, 2002.

31. Gameiro P, Mortuza FY, Hoffbrand AV, et al.: Minimal residual disease monitoring in adult T-cell acute lymphoblastic leukemia: a molecular based approach using T-cell receptor G and D gene rearrangements. *Haematologica* 87:1126, 2002.

32. Nirmala K, Rajalekshmy KR, Raman SG, et al.: PCR-heteroduplex analysis of TCR gamma, delta and TAL-1 deletions in T-acute lymphoblastic leukemias: implications in the detection of minimal residual disease. *Leuk Res* 26:335, 2002.

33. Ballerini P, Blaise A, Busson-Le Coniat M, et al.: HOX11L2 expression defines a clinical subtype of pediatric T-ALL associated with poor prognosis. *Blood* 100:991, 2002.

34. Nyvold C, Madsen HO, Ryder LP, et al.: Precise quantification of minimal residual disease at day 29 allows identification of children with acute lymphoblastic leukemia and an excellent outcome. *Blood* 99:1253, 2002.

35. Garg M, Moore H, Tobal K, et al.: Prognostic significance of quantitative analysis of WT1 gene transcripts by competitive reverse transcription polymerase chain reaction in acute leukaemia. *Br J Haematol* 123:49, 2003.

36. Scheuring UJ, Pfeifer H, Wassmann B, et al.: Serial minimal residual disease (MRD) analysis as a predictor of response duration in Philadelphia-positive acute lymphoblastic leukemia (Ph+ALL) during imatinib treatment. *Leukemia* 17:1700, 2003.

37. Hughes T, Deininger M, Hochhaus A, et al.: Monitoring CML patients responding to treatment with tyrosine kinase inhibitors: review and recommendations for harmonizing current methodology for detecting BCR-ABL transcripts and kinase domain mutations and for expressing results. *Blood* 108:28, 2006.

38. Bruggemann M, Raff T, Flohr T, et al.: Clinical significance or minimal residual disease quantification in adult

patients with standard-risk acute lymphoblastic leukemia. *Blood* 107:1116, 2006.

39. Bruggemann M, van der Velden VH, Raff T, et al.: Rearranged T-cell receptor beta genes represent powerful targets for quantification of minimal residual disease in childhood and adult T-cell acute lymphoblastic leukemia. *Leukemia* 18:709, 2004.

40. Metzler M, Brehm U, Langer T, et al.: Asymmetric multiplex-polymerase chain reaction—a high through-put method for detection and sequencing genomic fusion sites in t(4;11). *Br J Haematol* 124:47, 2004.

41. Roberts WM, Estrov Z, Ouspenskaia MV, et al.: Measurement of residual leukemia during remission in childhood acute lymphoblastic leukemia. *N Engl J Med* 336:317, 1997.

42. van der Velden VH, Hochhaus A, Cazzaniga G, et al.: Detection of minimal residual disease in hematologic malignancies by real-time quantitative PCR: principles, approaches, and laboratory aspects. *Leukemia* 17:1013, 2003.

43. Endo C, Oda M, Nishiuchi R, et al.: Persistence of TEL-AML1 transcript in acute lymphoblastic leukemia in long-term remission. *Pediatr Int* 45:275, 2003.

44. Nakao M, Janssen JW, Erz D, et al.: Tandem duplication of the FLT3 gene in acute lymphoblastic leukemia: a marker for the monitoring of minimal residual disease. *Leukemia* 14:522, 2000.

45. Cortes J, Fayad L, O'Brien S, et al.: Persistence of peripheral blood and bone marrow blasts during remission induction in adult acute lymphoblastic leukemia confers a poor prognosis depending on treatment intensity. *Clin Cancer Res* 5:2491, 1999.

46. Legrand O, Marie JP, Cadiou M, et al.: Early cytoreduction: a major prognostic factor in adult acute lymphoblastic leukemia. *Leuk Lymphoma* 15:433, 1994.

47. Sebban C, Browman GP, Lepage E, et al.: Prognostic value of early response to chemotherapy assessed by the day 15 bone marrow aspiration in adult acute lymphoblastic leukemia: a prospective analysis of 437 cases and its application for designing induction chemotherapy trials. *Leuk Res* 19:861, 1995.

48. Larson RA, Dodge RK, Burns CP, et al.: A five-drug remission induction regimen with intensive consolidation for adults with acute lymphoblastic leukemia: cancer and leukemia group B study 8811. *Blood* 85:2025, 1995.

49. Group. FL: Long-term survival in acute lymphoblastic leukaemia in adults: a prospective study of 51 patients. Finnish Leukaemia Group. *Eur J Haematol* 48:75, 1992.

50. Hoelzer D, Ludwig WD, Thiel E, et al.: Improved outcome in adult B-cell acute lymphoblastic leukemia. *Blood* 87:495, 1996.

51. Legrand O, Marie JP, Marjanovic Z, et al.: Prognostic factors in elderly acute lymphoblastic leukaemia. *Br J Haematol* 97:596, 1997.

52. Chessells JM, Hall E, Prentice HG, et al.: The impact of age on outcome in lymphoblastic leukaemia; MRC UKALL X and XA compared: a report from the MRC Paediatric and Adult Working Parties. *Leukemia* 12:463, 1998.

53. Ueda T, Miyawaki S, Asou N, et al.: Response-oriented individualized induction therapy with six drugs followed by four courses of intensive consolidation, 1 year maintenance and intensification therapy: the ALL90 study of the Japan Adult Leukemia Study Group. *Int J Hematol* 68:279, 1998.

54. Thomas X, Danaila C, Le QH, et al.: Long-term follow-up of patients with newly diagnosed adult acute lymphoblastic leukemia: a single institution experience of 378 consecutive patients over a 21-year period. *Leukemia* 15:1811, 2001.

55. Takeuchi J, Kyo T, Naito K, et al.: Induction therapy by frequent administration of doxorubicin with four other drugs, followed by intensive consolidation and maintenance therapy for adult acute lymphoblastic leukemia: the JALSG-ALL93 study. *Leukemia* 16:1259, 2002.

56. Hallbook H, Simonsson B, Ahlgren T, et al.: High-dose cytarabine in upfront therapy for adult patients with acute lymphoblastic leukaemia. *Br J Haematol* 118:748, 2002.

57. Kantarjian H, Thomas D, O'Brien S, et al.: Long-term follow-up results of hyperfractionated cyclophosphamide, vincristine, doxorubicin, and dexamethasone (Hyper-CVAD), a dose-intensive regimen, in adult acute lymphocytic leukemia. *Cancer* 101:2788, 2004.

58. Robak T, Szmigielska-Kaplon A, Wrzesien-Kus A, et al.: Acute lymphoblastic leukemia in elderly: the Polish Adult Leukemia Group (PALG) experience. *Ann Hematol* 83:225, 2004.

59. Campos L, Sabido O, Sebban C, et al.: Expression of BCL-2 proto-oncogene in adult acute lymphoblastic leukemia. *Leukemia* 10:434, 1996.

60. Daenen S, van Imhoff GW, van den Berg E, et al.: Improved outcome of adult acute lymphoblastic leukaemia by moderately intensified chemotherapy which includes a 'pre-induction' course for rapid tumour reduction: preliminary results on 66 patients. *Br J Haematol* 100:273, 1998.

61. Linker C, Damon L, Ries C, et al.. Intensified and shortened cyclical chemotherapy for adult acute lymphoblastic leukemia. *J Clin Oncol* 20:2464, 2002.

62. Boucheix C, David B, Sebban C, et al.: Immunophenotype of adult acute lymphoblastic leukemia, clinical parameters, and outcome: an analysis of a prospective trial including 562 tested patients (LALA87). French Group on Therapy for Adult Acute Lymphoblastic Leukemia. *Blood* 84:1603, 1994.

63. Czuczman MS, Dodge RK, Stewart CC, et al.: Value of immunophenotype in intensively treated adult acute lymphoblastic leukemia: cancer and leukemia Group B study 8364. *Blood* 93:3931, 1999.

64. Bloomfield CD, Secker-Walker LM, Goldman AI, et al.: Six-year follow-up of the clinical significance of karyotype in acute lymphoblastic leukemia. *Cancer Genet Cytogenet* 40:171, 1989.

65. Fenaux P, Lai JL, Morel P, et al.: Cytogenetics and their prognostic value in childhood and adult acute lymphoblastic leukemia (ALL) excluding L3. *Hematol Oncol* 7:307, 1989.

66. Walters R, Kantarjian HM, Keating MJ, et al.: The importance of cytogenetic studies in adult acute lymphocytic leukemia. *Am J Med* 89:579, 1990.

67. Groupe Français de Cytogénétique Hématologique: Cytogenetic abnormalities in adult acute lymphoblastic leukemia: correlations with hematologic findings outcome. A collaborative study of the Groupe Français de Cytogénétique Hématologique. *Blood* 88:3135, 1996.

68. Secker-Walker LM, Prentice HG, Durrant J, et al.: Cytogenetics adds independent prognostic information in adults with acute lymphoblastic leukaemia on MRC trial UKALL XA. MRC Adult Leukaemia Working Party. *Br J Haematol* 96:601, 1997.

69. Wetzler M, Dodge RK, Mrozek K, et al.: Prospective karyotype analysis in adult acute lymphoblastic leukemia: the cancer and leukemia Group B experience. *Blood* 93:3983, 1999.

70. Ribera JM, Ortega JJ, Oriol A, et al.: Prognostic value of karyotypic analysis in children and adults with high-risk acute lymphoblastic leukemia included in the PETHEMA ALL-93 trial. *Haematologica* 87:154, 2002.

71. Ferrando AA, Neuberg DS, Dodge RK, et al.: Prognostic importance of TLX1 (HOX11) oncogene expression in adults with T-cell acute lymphoblastic leukaemia. *Lancet* 363:535, 2004.

72. Goasguen JE, Dossot JM, Fardel O, et al.: Expression of the multidrug resistance-associated P-glycoprotein (P-170) in 59 cases of de novo acute lymphoblastic leukemia: prognostic implications. *Blood* 81:2394, 1993.

73. Ohno N, Tani A, Chen ZS, et al.: Prognostic significance of multidrug resistance protein in adult T-cell leukemia. *Clin Cancer Res* 7:3120, 2001.

74. Damiani D, Michelutti A, Michieli M, et al.: P-glycoprotein, lung resistance-related protein and multidrug resistance-associated protein in de novo adult acute lymphoblastic leukaemia. *Br J Haematol* 116:519, 2002.

75. Tafuri A, Gregorj C, Petrucci MT, et al.: MDR1 protein expression is an independent predictor of complete remission in newly diagnosed adult acute lymphoblastic leukemia. *Blood* 100:974, 2002.

76. Plasschaert SL, Vellenga E, de Bont ES, et al.: High functional P-glycoprotein activity is more often present in T-cell acute lymphoblastic leukaemic cells in adults than in children. *Leuk Lymphoma* 44:85, 2003.

77. Suvannasankha A, Minderman H, O'Loughlin KL, et al.: Breast cancer resistance protein (BCRP/MXR/ABCG2) in adult acute lymphoblastic leukaemia: frequent expression and possible correlation with shorter disease-free survival. *Br J Haematol* 127:392, 2004.

78. Thomas X, Le QH, Danaila C, et al.: Bone marrow biopsy in adult acute lymphoblastic leukaemia: morphological characteristics and contribution to the study of prognostic factors. *Leuk Res* 26:909, 2002.

79. Kantarjian HM, Walters RS, Smith TL, et al.: Identification of risk groups for development of central nervous system leukemia in adults with acute lymphocytic leukemia. *Blood* 72:1784, 1988.

80. Shen Y, Thall PF: Parametric likelihoods for multiple non-fatal competing risks and death. *Stat Med* 17:999, 1998.

81. Gooley TA, Leisenring W, Crowley J, et al.: Why Kaplan-Meier fails and cumulative incidence succeeds when estimating failure probabilities in the presence of competing risks. In: Crowley L, ed. *Handbook of Statistics in Clinical Oncology*. New York: Marcel Dekker, 2001:513.

# Chapter 15

# TREATMENT OF RELAPSED OR REFRACTORY ACUTE LYMPHOBLASTIC LEUKEMIA AND NEW FRONTIERS IN THERAPY

*Nicole Lamanna and Mark A. Weiss*

## INTRODUCTION

One of the great success stories of medical oncology has been the treatment of acute lymphoblastic leukemia (ALL) in children. Through a strong cooperative group effort, the recruitment of a high proportion of afflicted patients, and the conduct of multiple randomized trials, there have been successive improvements in treating childhood ALL, so that now 60–75% of the children with ALL can achieve long-term disease-free survival.[1] Unfortunately, adults with ALL do not fare as well. Despite complete remissions (CRs) in 60–90% , long-term disease-free survival still remains at 20–40%.[2,3] In addition to deaths (5–10%) during remission induction, approximately 10–25% of patients have resistant disease. Even for patients who achieve a CR, 60–70% will relapse, often within 2 years of achieving the remission (a time when most patients are still receiving maintenance therapy). Management of both primary refractory and relapsed patients poses a great challenge to clinicians; it occurs commonly, and long-term survival in these patients is typically poor. Newer treatment strategies and novel agents are urgently needed to improve the prognosis for these patients. This chapter will review some of the prognostic features that influence the likelihood of failing to achieve a CR, chemotherapy strategies often employed in the salvage setting, stem cell transplantation, and special cases, including patients with Philadelphia (Ph)-chromosome disease, patients with central nervous system (CNS) relapse, and the use of newer agents.

## PROGNOSTIC FEATURES

While several analyses of prognostic features in ALL have been performed, two classic multivariate analyses, one by the German multicenter group and another by the Memorial Sloan-Kettering Cancer Center (MSKCC) group, were reported in 1988. These and other studies indicate the importance of five prognostic features: white blood cell (WBC) count at diagnosis, age, leukemic cell immunophenotype, cytogenetics (particularly Philadelphia-chromosome-positive disease), and the time to achieve CR.[4,5]

An elevated WBC count at the time of diagnosis is associated with a poor prognosis. The multivariate analyses indicate that there is both a reduced likelihood of achieving a CR, as well as a shorter duration of remission, and ultimately worse overall survival. In part, the poor prognosis associated with an elevated WBC reflects an increased disease burden, but it is also related to the propensity of poor cytogenetic subtypes (i.e., t(4:11) and t(9:22)) to present with hyperleukocytosis. Different studies have used different WBC levels as their cutoff for an adverse feature. In the MSKCC study, WBC counts greater than 10,000/μL were associated with a lower frequency of achieving a CR, and counts greater than 20,000/μL were associated with a shorter duration of CR. In the German study, WBC counts greater than 30,000/μL carried an adverse prognosis.

Older age in adult ALL patients is also associated with a worse prognosis, and similar to an elevated WBC count, age is probably a continuous variable (i.e., the older the patient, the worse the prognosis). Different studies have defined different ages as having a poor prognosis; the German group identified age 35, while the MSKCC study identified age 60.

The immunophenotype of the leukemic cell also has prognostic significance.[4-6] Traditionally, T-cell disease has had a favorable prognosis, pre-B-cell (common) ALL an intermediate prognosis, and mature B-cell disease was associated with a poorer prognosis (using conventional treatments). Recently, however, modern intensive treatment regimens designed specifically for this rare subtype have improved the prognosis for patients with mature B-cell (Burkitt's type) lymphoblastic disease, and it is no longer considered to have a comparatively poor prognosis.[7,8]

Cytogenetic abnormalities, specifically t(9;22) (Philadelphia-chromosome-positive disease) and t(4;11), portend poor prognoses. These patients are essentially never cured by chemotherapeutic regimens, with 5-year disease-free survival rates of 0–15%, using conventional therapy. A minority may be cured with an allogeneic transplant in first CR.[9a-c] Also unclear is the impact that therapy with the tyrosine kinase inhibitor imatinib mesylate will have on Philadelphia-chromosome-positive disease. Another karyotype, t(8;14), involving the c-myc locus, has traditionally carried an unfavorable prognosis, though again, this may change with current intensive therapy.

Many studies have shown that the time to achieve a CR during remission induction therapy carries significant prognostic implications. The likelihood of being cured diminishes with the greater amount of time it takes the patient to achieve a CR. Notably, time to CR greater than 4 or 5 weeks substantially diminishes the likelihood of cure.[5] However, it is uncertain whether a shorter duration in achieving a CR reflects an innate sensitivity of the disease to the chemotherapeutic agents used, or whether the rapid cytoreduction of the leukemic cell mass minimizes the development of drug resistance and thus ultimately allows for the cure of the patient.

Note however the above-listed prognostic features relate primarily to initial therapy. At relapse, the prognosis is poor, with only a small fraction of patients salvaged. In this setting, long duration of first remission and isolated sanctuary site relapse are the two most important favorable prognostic factors.

## CHEMOTHERAPY STRATEGIES

Several common treatment strategies have been used in patients who have refractory or resistant ALL. One option is to administer a regimen that is similar to the original remission induction therapy, particularly if there has been a long duration of remission prior to their eventual relapse (>1–2 years). However, this strategy is likely to be ineffective in patients with primary refractory disease. Variations on traditional induction therapy, usually including vincristine, prednisone, and an anthracycline intensified with cyclophosphamide and/or L-asparaginase, are frequently used in the salvage setting. A second CR can occasionally be achieved in the subset of patients who had a long first remission or who developed recurrent disease after completing maintenance chemotherapy.[10] Even one of the most favorable reports, however, achieved a CR in only 44% of the patients.[11] Furthermore, the median survival for these patients was only 8 months, and 3-year survival was only 10%.

As many patients develop recurrent disease within the first 2 years of achieving their first remission, the likelihood of achieving a second CR with regimens similar to the remission induction therapy is low.[12-15] Likewise, for those patients whose disease is primarily refractory to standard remission induction therapy, simply repeating the same induction treatments is usually futile. Thus, another option is to use other agents that are relatively distinct from the agents used in the traditional induction treatment programs. One of the most commonly used agents in this setting is cytarabine arabinoside (ara-C) administered at a high dose. As a single agent, high-dose cytarabine (given at doses of, for example, $2–3\ G/m^2$ every 12 h for 6–12 doses) may induce a CR in approximately 30% of patients with relapsed or refractory ALL.[15] In combination with other agents, such as L-asparaginase,[16-18] doxorubicin,[19] idarubicin,[20-22] or mitoxantrone[23-26], higher response rates can be achieved, with CRs as high as 72% reported. An example of such a regimen is the combination of high-dose cytarabine with a single high-dose of idarubicin, which was reported by the MSKCC group as producing a CR in 44–58% of the patients.[27,28] Of course, a direct comparison of these regimens is impossible given the differences in patient characteristics, the number of prior regimens and doses and schedules of the agents used, as well as the variable use of subsequent autologous or allogeneic stem cell transplantation and noncomparative trials.

Unfortunately, for many patients, even if a second CR is achieved, it is notoriously difficult to maintain, and each subsequent response is of a shorter duration than the prior one. Thus, in general, patients with a suitable allogeneic transplant option that is not precluded by age, performance status, or other concurrent illness should be referred for such a transplant in second CR.

## STEM CELL TRANSPLANTATION

### ALLOGENEIC TRANSPLANTATION

Allogeneic transplantation with an HLA-matched identical sibling has been performed in adults with ALL in a number of settings. In a small subset of patients, this dose-intense treatment has the ability to eradicate residual leukemia in patients whose disease is refractory to conventional chemotherapy. However, there are three main prerequisites that should be met prior to a patient undergoing this intense procedure. First, it is imperative that the patient be in an acceptable physical condition to withstand the demands and complications of the transplant. Secondly, it is preferable that the patient be in CR or in a minimal disease state to decrease the likelihood of relapse after transplant. Finally, a suitable donor must be identified and available. It is generally recommended that at the time of initial diagnosis the patient and immediate family members have HLA typing performed, as the process can be time consuming and, if done at the time of relapse, can cause unwanted delays. If no immediate family member is identified as a match, we recommend no additional testing until a transplant is needed (at the time of relapse). At such a time, a more extended family search can be performed along with a preliminary search of unrelated donors. The initial search through the National Marrow Donor Program (NMDP) registry is performed free of charge and is a one-time search used to identify potential candidates. An international search can also be initiated depending on the patient's racial and ethnic background, and depending on whether or not a match is found using the NMDP. Unfortunately, the lack of availability of human leukocyte antigen (HLA)-matched donors often limits the utility of this approach. In one study by Davies et al., the outcome of 115 consecutive patients with recurrent ALL were examined over a 2-year period.[29] A matched related donor was identified in 35%. Of the 75 patients without a related donor, 58 patients had an unrelated donor search initiated. Only 37% of these patients had an unrelated donor identified. Finding a matched unrelated donor is even more complicated if the patient has a diverse ethnic or racial background.

Even if a suitable donor is identified, allogeneic transplant is not a panacea for treating relapsed ALL. Limitations of transplant in patients with ALL are highlighted by reviewing patterns of failure. Patients with ALL who undergo allogeneic transplantation suffer from both treatment-related mortality as well as a significant rate of relapse. This differs from patients with acute myeloid leukemia (AML), who fail allogeneic transplantation primarily because of treatment-related mortality. This appears to be due to the "graft-versus-leukemia" effect in which the transplanted (donor) immune system eliminates residual leukemic cells being less effective in ALL than in AML or chronic myeloid leukemia (CML). Supporting this concept is data from the International Bone Marrow Transplant Registry, which compared identical twin (syngeneic) transplants to HLA-identical sibling (allogeneic) transplants.[30] As with graft-versus-host disease, the graft-versus-leukemia is more pronounced in the allogeneic transplants as compared with syngeneic transplants. The results of the IBMTR study demonstrated a significantly higher rate of relapse in the syngeneic transplants for patients with AML or CML, but not for those patients with ALL, implying that graft-versus-leukemia is less potent in ALL compared to its effect in CML or AML. Another example supporting the concept that graft-versus-leukemia is less active in ALL comes from an analysis of studies of donor T-cell infusions used to treat relapsed leukemia after allogeneic stem cell transplant. In the "classic" study, donor lymphocyte infusions produced complete responses in 73% of patients with CML, 29% of patients with AML, and 0% of patients with ALL.[31]

The use and timing of allogeneic transplantation in adult patients with ALL is another dilemma. At the Fred Hutchinson Cancer Center, in 192 adults with ALL transplanted in second CR or beyond, the 5-year disease-free survival was only 15%.[32] Another more recent study demonstrated a similar outcome for transplants performed beyond first CR, and included a treatment-related mortality rate of 43%.[33] There have been two large comparative studies of allogeneic transplant versus standard chemotherapy for patients in first CR. Neither study was able to demonstrate improved survival for the transplant arm and therefore with the exception of patients with t(9;22) and t(4;11) allogeneic transplant in first remission cannot be routinely recommended.[34,35]

### AUTOLOGOUS TRANSPLANTATION

Autologous transplantation for adult ALL is even less successful than allogeneic transplantation.[36] In part, this is likely related to the amount of disease burden prior to autologous transplantation and whether the residual leukemia cells were sufficiently eradicated prior to reinfusion. Many investigators have attempted to purge residual disease ex vivo by using different chemotherapeutic agents or monoclonal antibodies.[37-41] Not only are results of autologous transplantation disappointing in second CR, but even in first CR this modality has a limited applicability. Both a non-randomized and a randomized trial in patients in first CR have shown no benefit to autologous transplantation compared with maintenance chemotherapy.[42,43] Therefore, autologous transplantation in patients with relapsed ALL should still be considered investigational and not routinely recommended to patients in first CR outside of a clinical trial.

## PHILADELPHIA-CHROMOSOME-POSITIVE DISEASE

Patients with Ph-chromosome-positive ALL (Ph+ ALL) have a poor prognosis even with modern treatment regimens. Thus, it is generally recommended that these patients undergo allogeneic transplantation in first CR, as this strategy is curative in a minority of patients.[44,45] The development of imatinib, a tyrosine kinase inhibitor with relative specificity for bcr-abl, has dramatically altered the natural history and treatment of patients with CML.[46] Imatinib also has some activity in Ph+ ALL, although less so than in patients with CML, with only 29% of relapsed or refractory patients achieving a CR.[47] In addition, the median time to progression for responding patients is only 2.2 months, illustrating the development of resistance to imatinib in this patient group.[48,49] A recent study investigated prognostic factors for response to imatinib mesylatetherapy in patients with ALL.[50] Prior CR <6 months, WBC count >$10 \times 10^9$/L, circulating peripheral blood blasts at diagnosis, additional Ph chromosomes, and at least 2 bcr-abl fusion signals were all associated with a significantly inferior frequency of response and response duration to imatinib mesylate. Given the disappointing responses seen in patients with Ph+ ALL compared with patients with CML treated with imatinib mesylate, many investigators are evaluating the role of imatinib mesylate combination chemotherapy in both the initial treatment setting[51] as well as in the relapsed setting.[52]

## CNS RELAPSE

Approximately 10% of patients who have received appropriate CNS prophylaxis will develop relapse in the CNS. Systemic relapse can often be identified simultaneously or shortly after CNS relapse is documented. Therefore, it is generally recommended that in addition to the treatment for CNS disease, patients should receive systemic reinduction chemotherapy. Treatment of established CNS disease often requires a combination of radiotherapy and intrathecal chemotherapy. The radiotherapy should be administered to the whole brain, consisting of 1800–2400 cGy (in 150- to 200-cGy fractions). Higher doses should be avoided due to both the risk of late toxicity (such as cognitive deficits or necrosis) as well as the potential later requirement of total body irradiation as part of the conditioning regimen for an allogeneic transplant. In addition, despite encouraging results in children, spinal radiotherapy should be avoided in adults, as the dose of radiotherapy to marrow-bearing areas subsequently limits the ability to administer necessary systemic chemotherapy. Furthermore, although this approach can help control the CNS disease, it does not prolong survival, as these patients typically succumb to relapsed system disease.[53] Intrathecal or intraventricular therapy for patients with established CNS disease should include methotrexate (12–15 mg) or ara-C, preferably administered intraventricularly via an Ommaya reservoir. It should be administered as often as two to three times per week with at least 1 day off between doses until the cerebrospinal fluid (CSF) is cleared of leukemic blasts, then twice a week for 2–3 weeks, and then twice a month for 2 or 3 additional months (total of 8–12 doses). Patients who develop CNS disease despite prophylaxis with intrathe-

cal methotrexate, and those patients who do not clear the blasts promptly from the CSF (within two treatments), should receive intraventricular therapy with ara-C at a dose of 60 mg.

## NEW THERAPIES

As the overall survival for adult patients with relapsed or refractory ALL remains poor, newer therapies are needed. In addition to different combination chemotherapy strategies with traditional agents, investigators are examining the role of newer, investigational agents in the treatment of these patients.

*Clofarabine.* Clofarabine is a nucleoside analog that is a hybrid of fludarabine and cladribine. In a small phase II study of refractory or relapsed patients with ALL ($n = 12$), there was one CR (8%) that lasted 4 months.[54a] Clofarabine has recently been approved by the FDA for use in pediatric ALL.[54b]

*Nelarabine.* Nelarabine is a prodrug of ara-G. Evaluation of this arabinosyl analog of deoxyguanosine has shown some promising activity.[55,56] In a phase I study of 26 patients, there were 10 responses (five CRs); 7/8 patients with T-cell ALL, 1 with T-lymphoid blast crises of CML, 1 with T-cell lymphoma, and 1 with B-cell CLL.[55] Interestingly, responses were not observed in patients with B-lineage ALL, and some investigators believe that one mechanism of T-cell selective cytotoxicity may result from high ara-GTP accumulation in T cells resulting in an S-phase dependent apoptosis, which may lead to a T-cell specific signal for the induction and liberation of soluble Fas ligand, thereby inducing an apoptotic response in neighboring non-S-phase cells.[57]

*Alemtuzumab.* Alemtuzumab is a monoclonal antibody that binds to CD52, an antigen present on nearly all normal B and T lymphocytes. It has been approved by the Food and Drug Administration for use in patients with chronic lymphocytic leukemia (CLL) who are refractory to fludarabine, and it has been studied extensively in patients with CLL.[58–60] The experience of alemtuzumab in patients with refractory or relapsed ALL is limited.[61] It has been incorporated into purging techniques for autologous transplant, in conditioning regimens for allogeneic transplant, and used as an immunosuppressant for graft-versus-host disease.[62–64]

## CONCLUSION

Unfortunately, the treatment of patients with relapsed or refractory ALL remains a daunting challenge to investigators and treating physicians. Hopefully, as we gain more insight into the biology of this disease, we can improve not only upon the treatment of patients who have relapsed, but also on initial treatment strategies, thereby minimizing those who require treatment in the relapsed setting. In addition, as we develop better techniques to assess for minimal residual disease, perhaps allowing for earlier intervention before overt clinical relapse, we may improve the outcome of these patients. Currently, the best chance for patients with relapsed disease is to induce a second CR (for suitable patients we favor high-dose cytarabine with high-dose anthracycline) followed by an allogeneic transplant.

## ACKNOWLEDGMENT

This study was supported in part by the Lymphoma Foundation and Victoria's Smile Foundation.

## REFERENCES

1. Pui CH, Evans WE: Acute lymphoblastic leukemia. *N Engl J Med* 339:605, 1998.
2. Copelan EA, McGuire EA: The biology and treatment of acute lymphoblastic leukemia in adults. *Blood* 85:1151, 1995.
3. Lamanna N, Weiss M: Treatment options for newly diagnosed patients with adult acute lymphoblastic leukemia. *Curr Hematol Rep* 3(1):40–46, 2004.
4. Hoelzer D, Thiel E, Loffler H, et al.: Prognostic factors in a multicenter study for treatment of acute lymphoblastic leukemia in adults. *Blood* 71:123, 1988.
5. Gaynor J, Chapman D, Little C, et al.: A cause-specific hazard rate analysis of prognostic factors among 199 adults with acute lymphoblastic leukemia: the Memorial Hospital experience since 1969. *J Clin Oncol* 6:1014, 1988.
6. Boucheix C, David B, Sebban C, et al.: Immunophenotype of adult acute lymphoblastic leukemia, clinical parameters and outcome: an analysis of a prospective trial including 562 tested patients (LALA87). *Blood* 84:1603, 1994.
7. Hoelzer D, Ludwig WD, Thiel E, et al.: Improved outcome in adult B-cell acute lymphoblastic leukemia. *Blood* 87:495, 1996.
8. Thomas DA, Cortes J, O'Brien S, et al.: Hyper-CVAD program in Burkitt's type adult lymphoblastic leukemia. *J Clin Oncol* 17:2461, 1999.
9a. Barrett AJ, Horowitz MM, Ash RC, et al.: Bone marrow transplantation for Philadelphia chromosome-positive acute lymphoblastic leukemia. *Blood* 79:3067, 1992.
9b. Wetzler M, Dodge RK, Mrozek K, et al.: Prospective karyotype analysis in adult acute lymphoblastic leukemia: The Cancer and Leukemia Group B Experience. *Blood* 93(11):3983, 1999.
9c. Secker-Walker LM, Prentice HG, Durrant J, et al.: On behalf of the MRC Adult Leukemia Working Party: Cytogenetics adds independent prognostic information in adults with acute lymphoblastic leukemia on MRC trial UKALLXA. *Br J Haematol* 96:601, 1997.
10. Woodruff R, Lister T, Paxton A, et al.: Combination chemotherapy for hematologic relapse in adult acute lymphoblastic leukemia (ALL). *Am J Hematol* 4:173–177, 1978.
11. Capizzi RI, Poole M, Cooper MR, et al.: Treatment of poor risk acute leukemia with sequential high-dose Ara-C and asparaginase. *Blood* 63:694, 1984.
12. Amadori S, Papa F, Avvisati G, et al.: Sequential combination high-dose Ara-C and asparaginase for the treatment of advanced acute leukemia and lymphoma. *Leuk Res* 8:729, 1984.
13. Wells RJ, Feusner J, Devney R, et al.: Sequential high-dose cytosine arabinoside-asparaginase treatment in advance childhood leukemia. *J Clin Oncol* 3:998, 1985.
14. Ishii E, Mara T, Ohkubo K, et al.: Treatment of childhood acute lymphoblastic leukemia with intermediate-dose cytosine arabinoside and adriamycin. *Med Pediatr Oncol* 14:73, 1986.
15. Kantarjian HM, Estey EH, Plunkett W, et al.: Phase I–II clinical and pharmacologic studies of high-dose cytosine arabinoside in refractory leukemia. *Am J Med* 81:387, 1986.
16. Capizzi RI, Poole M, Cooper MR, et al.: Treatment of poor risk acute leukemia with sequential high-dose Ara-C and asparaginase. *Blood* 63:694, 1984.
17. Amadori S, Papa F, Avvisati G, et al.: Sequential combination high-dose Ara-C and asparaginase for the treatment of advanced acute leukemia and lymphoma. *Leuk Res* 8:729, 1984.
18. Wells RJ, Feusner J, Devney R, et al.: Sequential high-dose cytosine arabinoside-asparaginase treatment in advance childhood leukemia. *J Clin Oncol* 3:998, 1985.
19. Ishii E, Mara T, Ohkubo K, et al.: Treatment of childhood acute lymphoblastic leukemia with intermediate-dose cytosine arabinoside and adriamycin. *Med Pediatr Oncol* 14:73, 1986.
20. Giona F, Testi A, Amadori G, et al.: Idarubicin and high-dose cytarabine in the treatment of refractory and relapsed acute lymphoblastic leukemia. *Ann Oncol* 1:51, 1990.
21. Tan C, Steinherz P, Meyer P: Idarubicin in combination with high-dose cytosine arabinoside in patients with acute leukemia in relapse [abstract]. *Proc Annu Meet Am Assoc Cancer Res* 31:A1133, 1990.
22. Camera A, Annino L, Chiurazzi F, et al.: GIMEMA ALL – Rescue 97: a salvage strategy for primary refractory or relapsed adult acute lymphoblastic leukemia. *Haematologica* 89:145–153, 2004.
23. Hiddemann W, Kreutzman H, Straif K, et al.: High-dose cytosine arabinoside in combination with mitoxantrone for the treatment of refractory acute myeloid and lymphoblastic leukemia. *Semin Oncol* 14:73, 1987.
24. Leclerc J, Rivard G, Blanch M, et al.: The association of once a day high-dose Ara-C followed by mitoxantrone for three days induces a high rate of complete remission in children with poor prognosis acute leukemia [abstract]. *Blood* 72(suppl):210, 1988.
25. Kantarjian H, Walters R, Keating M, et al.: Mitoxantrone and high-dose cytosine arabinoside for the treatment of refractory acute lymphocytic leukemia. *Cancer* 65:5, 1990.
26. Feldman EJ, Alberts DS, Arlin Z, et al.: Phase I clinical and pharmacokinetic evaluation of high-dose mitoxantrone in combination with cytarabine in patients with acute leukemia. *J Clin Oncol* 11:2002, 1993.

27. Weiss MA, Drullinsky P, Maslak P, et al.: A phase I trial of a single high dose of idarubicin combined with high-dose cytarabine as induction therapy in relapsed or refractory adult patients with acute lymphoblastic leukemia. *Leukemia* 12(6):865–868, 1998.

28. Weiss MA, Aliff TB, Tallman MS, et al.: A single, high dose of idarubicin combined with cytarabine as induction therapy for adult patients with recurrent or refractory acute lymphoblastic leukemia. *Cancer* 95(3):581–587, 2002.

29. Davies SM, Ramsay NK, Weisdorf DJ: Feasibility and timing of unrelated donor identification for patients with ALL. *Bone Marrow Transplant* 17:737–740, 1996.

30. Gale RP, Horowitz MM, Ash RC, et al.: Identical-twin bone marrow transplants for leukemia. *Ann Intern Med* 120:646, 1994.

31. Kolb H-J, Scattenberg A, Goldman JM, et al.: Graft-versus-leukemia effect of donor lymphocyte transfusions in marrow grafted patients. *Blood* 86:2041, 1995.

32. Doney K, Fisher LD, Appelbaum FR, et al.: Treatment of adult acute lymphoblastic leukemia with allogeneic bone marrow transplantation. Multivariate analysis of factors affecting acute graft-versus-host disease, relapse, and relapse-free survival. *Bone Marrow Transplant* 7:453, 1991.

33. Annaloro C, Curioni ACE, Molteni M, et al.: Hematopoietic stem cell transplantation in adult acute lymphoblastic leukemia: a single-centre analysis. *Leuk Lymph* 45:1175, 2004.

34. Sebban C, Lepage E, Vernant J-P, et al.: Allogeneic bone marrow transplantation for acute lymphoblastic leukemia in first complete remission: a comparative study. *J Clin Oncol* 12:2580, 1994.

35. Zhang M-J, Hoelzer D, Horowitz MM, et al.: Long-term follow-up of adults with acute lymphoblastic leukemia in first remission treated with chemotherapy or bone marrow transplantation. *Ann Intern Med* 123:428, 1995.

36. Attal M, Blaise D, Marit G, et al.: Consolidation treatment of adult acute lymphoblastic leukemia: a prospective, randomized trial comparing allogeneic versus autologous bone marrow transplantation and testing the impact of recombinant interleukin-2 after autologous bone marrow transplant. *Blood* 86:1619, 1995.

37. Capizzi RL, Keeser LW, Sartorelli AC: Combination chemotherapy: theory and practice. *Semin Oncol* 4:227, 1977.

38. Beatty PG, Hansen JA, Longton GM, et al.: Marrow transplantation from HLA-matched unrelated donors for treatment of hematologic malignancies. *Transplantation* 51:443, 1991.

39. Gunther R, Chelstrom LM, Finnegan D, et al.: In vivo anti-leukemic efficacy of anti-CD7-pokeweed antiviral protein immunotoxin against human T-lineage acute lymphoblastic leukemia/lymphoma in mice with severe combined immunodeficiency. *Leukemia* 7:298, 1993.

40. Mehta J, Powles R, Treleaven J, et al.: Autologous transplantation with CD52 monoclonal antibody-purged marrow for acute lymphoblastic leukemia: Long-term follow-up. *Leuk Lymphoma* 25:479, 1997.

41. Maldonado MS, Diaz-Heredia C, Badell I, et al.: Autologous bone marrow transplantation with mono-clonal antibody purged marrow for children with acute lymphoblastic leukemia in second remission—Spanish Working Party for BMT in Children. *Bone Marrow Transplant* 22:1043, 1998.

42. Thiebaut A, Vernant JP, Degos L, et al.: Adult acute lymphocytic leukemia study testing chemotherapy and autologous and allogeneic transplantation. A follow-up report of the French protocol LALA 87 (Review). *Hematol Oncol Clin N Amer* 14:1353–1366, 2000.

43. Fiere D, Lepage E, Sebban C, et al.: Adult acute lymphoblastic leukemia: a multicentric randomized trial testing bone marrow transplantation as postremission therapy. *J Clin Oncol* 11:1990, 1993.

44. Barrett AJ, Horowitz, MM, Ash RC, et al.: Bone marrow transplantation for Philadelphia chromosome-positive acute lymphoblastic leukemia. *Blood* 79:3067–3070, 1992.

45. Dombret H, Gabert J, Boiron JM, et al.: Outcome of treatment in adults with Philadelphia chromosome-positive acute lymphoblastic leukemia: results of the prospective multicenter LALA-94 trial. *Blood* 100:2357–2366, 2002.

46. Druker BJ, Talpaz M, Resta DJ, et al.: Efficacy and safety of a specific inhibitor of the BCR-ABL tyrosine kinase in chronic myeloid leukemia. *N Engl J Med* 344:1031–1037, 2001.

47. Ottmann OG, Druker BJ, Sawyers CL, et al.: A phase 2 study of imatinib in patients with relapsed or refractory Philadelphia chromosome-positive acute lymphoid leukemias. *Blood* 100:1965–1971, 2002.

48. Hoffman WK, Jones JC, Lemp NA, et al.: Ph+ acute lymphoblastic leukemia resistant to the tyrosine kinase inhibitor STI571 has a unique BCR-ABL gene mutation. *Blood* 99:1860–1862, 2002.

49. Hoffman WK, Komor M, Wassman B, et al.: Presence of the BCR-ABL mutation Glu255Lys prior to STI571 (imatinib) treatment in patients with Ph+ acute lymphoblastic leukemia. *Blood* 102:659–661, 2003.

50. Wassman B, Pfeifer H, Scheuring UJ, et al.: Early prediction of response in patients with relapsed or refractory Philadelphia chromosome-positive acute lymphoblastic leukemia (Ph+ ALL) treated with imatinib. *Blood* 103:1495–1498, 2004.

51. Thomas DA, Faderl S, Cortes J, et al.: Treatment of Philadelphia chromosome-positive acute lymphocytic leukemia with hyper-CVAD and imatinib mesylate. *Blood* 103(12):4396–4407, 2004.

52. Wassmann B, Scheuring U, Pfeifer H, et al.: Efficacy and safety of imatinib mesylate (Glivec) in combination with interferon-alpha (IFN-alpha) in Philadelphia chromosome-positive acute lymphoblastic leukemia (Ph+ ALL). *Leukemia* 17:1919–1924, 2003.

53. Sanders KE, Ha CS, Cortes-Franco JE, et al.: The role of craniospinal irradiation in adults with a central nervous system recurrence of leukemia. *Cancer* 100:216–2180, 2004.

54a. Kantarjian H, Gandhi V, Cortes J, et al.: Phase 2 clinical and pharmacologic study of clofarabine in patients with refractory or relapsed acute leukemia. *Blood* 102:2379, 2003.

54b. Jeha S, Gaynon PS, Razzouk BI, et al.: Phase II study of clofarabine in pediatric patients with refractory or relapsed acute lymphoblastic leukemia. *J Clin Oncol* 24(12):1917, 2006.

55. Gandhi V, Plunkett W, Rodriguez CO Jr, et al.: Compound GW506U78 in refractory hematologic

malignancies: relationship between cellular pharmaco-kinetics and clinical response. *J Clin Oncol* 16: 3607–3615, 1998.

56. Gandhi V, Plunkett W, Weller S, et al.: Evaluation of the combination of nelarabine and fludarabine in leukemias: clinical response, pharmacokinetics, and pharmacodynamics in leukemia cells. *J Clin Oncol* 19(8):2142–2152, 2001.

57. Rodriguez CO Jr, Stellrecht CM, Gandhi V: Mechanisms of T-cell selective cytotoxicity of arabinosylguanine. *Blood* 102(5):1842–1848, 2003.

58. Keating MJ, Byrd J, Rai K, et al.: Campath-1H Collaborative Study Group: Multicenter study of Campath-1H in patients with chronic lymphocytic leukemia (B-CLL) refractory to fludarabine [abstract]. *Blood* 94(suppl 1):705a, 1999. Abstract 3118.

59. Osterborg A, Dyer MJ, Bunjes D, et al.: Phase II multi-center study of human CD52 antibody in previously treated chronic lymphocytic leukemia, European Study Group of Campath-1H Treatment in Chronic Lymphocytic Leukemia. *J Clin Oncol* 15:1567, 1997.

60. Rai KR, Freter CE, Mercier RJ, et al.: Alemtuzumab in previously treated chronic lymphocytic leukemia patients who also had received fludarabine. *J Clin Oncol* 20:3891–3897, 2002.

61. Dyer MJS, Hale G, Hayhoe FGJ, et al.: Effects of Campath-1H antibodies in vivo in patients with lym-phoid malignancies: influence of antibody isotype. *Blood* 73:1431, 1989.

62. Mehta J, Powles R, Treleaven J, et al.: Autologous trans-plantation with CD52 monoclonal antibody-purged marrow for acute lymphoblastic leukemia: long-term follow-up. *Leuk Lymphoma* 25:479–486, 1997.

63. Piccaluga PP, Martineli G, Malagola M, et al.: Anti-leukemic and anti-GVHD effects of campath-1H in acute lymphoblastic leukemia relapsed after stem-cell transplantation. *Leuk Lymphoma* 45:731–733, 2004.

64. Novitzy N, Thomas V, Hale G, Waldmann H: Ex vivo depletion of T cells from bone marrow grafts with Campath-1H in acute leukemia: graft-versus-host disease and graft-versus-leukemia effect. *Transplantation* 67:620–626, 1999.

# Section 3
# CHRONIC MYELOGENOUS LEUKEMIA

## Chapter 16
## EPIDEMIOLOGY, RISK FACTORS, AND CLASSIFICATION OF CHRONIC MYELOID LEUKEMIA

*Tariq I. Mughal and John M. Goldman*

## INTRODUCTION

Chronic myeloid leukemia (CML), historically also known as chronic myelogenous leukemia, chronic myelocytic leukemia, and chronic granulocytic leukemia, is a form of chronic myeloproliferative disease (CMPD) with a well-defined genetic defect known as the Philadelphia (Ph) chromosome.[1,2] The Ph chromosome is associated with a *BCR-ABL* fusion gene expressed as an oncoprotein, p210BCR-ABL, which is generally considered as the initiating event for the chronic phase of CML. All CMPDs are clonal hematopoietic stem cell disorders characterized by proliferation in the bone marrow of one or more of the myeloid cell lineages that gradually displaces normal haematopoiesis (Table 16.1). The remaining forms of CMPD do not have a specific genetic defect and the diagnosis, for the most part, relies upon clinical and hematologic features. The recent observations supporting the notion of JAK2 as a candidate gene involved in the molecular pathogenesis of some of the CMPD, specifically polycythemia vera, essential thrombocythemia and primary myelofibrosis, should herald an enhanced understanding of these disorders and might lead to a new classification of these disorders and, perhaps, novel treatments.[3–5] In this chapter, we review the epidemiology, risk factors, and classification of CML.

CML originates in an abnormal hematopoietic stem cell, which acquires a Ph chromosome, and the *BCR-ABL* fusion gene, which is considered to be the principal pathogenetic event[6,7] (Figure 16.1). The Ph chromosome and the *BCR-ABL* gene are found in all myeloid lineage cells and some, but not all, B and T lymphocytes. Clinically, CML is a biphasic or triphasic disease that is usually diagnosed in the initial "chronic" phase and then spontaneously evolves after a median time of 4–5 years into an "advanced" phase, which resembles an acute leukemia. The transformation into an advanced phase (called blast crisis) can occur abruptly or via a period of acceleration (called accelerated phase).

| Table 16.1 WHO classification of CMPD |
| --- |
| Chronic myeloid leukemia (also referred to as chronic myelogenous leukemia) |
| Chronic neutrophilic leukemia |
| Chronic eosinophilic leukemia (and the hypereosinophilic syndrome) |
| Polycythemia vera |
| Chronic idiopathic myelofibrosis (with extramedullary hemopoiesis) |
| Essential thrombocythemia |
| Chronic myeloproliferative disease, unclassifiable |

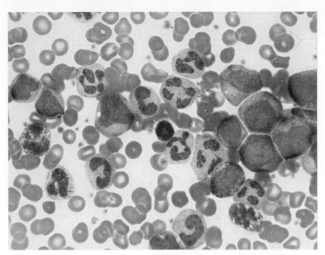

**Figure 16.1** *A peripheral blood film of a patient with classical CML*

## EPIDEMIOLOGY

CML is the most common of the CMPDs. It accounts for about 15–20% of all cases of adult leukemias, but less than 5% of all childhood leukemias. It is slightly more common in males than in females and occurs exceedingly rarely during the first decade of life. It has a median age of onset of about 50 years. The incidence of CML is about 1–1.5 per 100,000 persons per annum.[8] There appears to be no association with social class or ethnicity, and its incidence appears to be remarkably constant worldwide.[9] Some reports suggest a slightly higher prevalence in some parts of India and China, in particular Hong Kong, but these remain unconfirmed.

## RISK FACTORS

Almost all cases of CML have no identifiable predisposing factors, and even when there might be a plausible causal link, it is extremely difficult to incriminate any factor in individual patients. Exposure to ionizing radiation is the only known etiological factor; the incidence of CML was increased to a minor but significant degree in patients treated with radiation therapy for ankylosing spondylitis or metropathia hemorrhagica.[10,11] The most compelling link between radiation exposure and CML comes from a [Life Span] study of survivors of the atomic bomb explosions in Hiroshima and Nagasaki (Japan) in 1945.[12,13] There was an increased risk of CML among the survivors. An increased risk of leukemia, but not of CML, has also been reported in an area immediately surrounding the British nuclear fuel facility at Calder Hall in Cumbria, U.K. (although a government commission of enquiry was unable to confirm this).

There are no firm associations of exposure to toxic chemicals or any infectious agent and CML.

Chemicals that damage the bone marrow, in particular aromatic hydrocarbons and benzene, appear to predispose to acute myeloid leukemia (AML), but it is impossible to be certain that leukemia would not have developed in a particular patient in the absence of exposure to the suspect substance. Recently, it has been shown that benzene activates an oncogene that causes AML.

Though a small number of families with a high incidence of CML have been reported, there is no confirmed familial predisposition and no definite association with human leukocyte antigen (HLA) genotypes and CML.[14] Interestingly, two HLA types are associated with a decreased incidence of CML.[15] Relapse of CML originating in donor cells following related allogeneic stem cell transplantation has been recorded.[16] It is also noteworthy that only rarely does the identical twin brother or sister of a person with CML also develop leukemia. In a study of 40 pairs of identical twins in which one twin had CML, there was no instance in which the other twin developed CML.

Unlike the case in certain common epithelial cancers, there are no known dietary or social habits that increase the risk of acquiring CML. Smoking cigarettes has been weakly implicated. This link is dependent on the duration of exposure and the age of starting to smoke.

## CLASSIFICATION

The classification of CML, though not entirely straightforward, has recently been the subject of much revision by the World Health Organization (WHO).[17] Patients with classical CML have a well-defined disease characterized by splenomegaly, leukocytosis, and the finding of a *BCR-ABL* fusion gene in all leukemic cells. The classical Ph chromosome is easily identifiable in 80% of CML patients; in a further 10% of patients, variant translocations may be "simple," involving chromosome 22 and a chromosome other than chromosome 9, or "complex," in which chromosome 9, 22, and additional chromosomes are involved. About 8% of patients with classical clinical and hematologic features of CML lack the Ph chromosome and are referred to as the cases of "Ph-negative CML." About half such patients have a *BCR-ABL* gene and are referred to as Ph-negative, BCR-ABL-positive cases. The remainder, perhaps less than 5% of patients with hematologically "acceptable" CML, are BCR-ABL negative, and some of these have mutations in the *ras* gene. These patients are usually classified as having Ph-negative, BCR-ABL-negative CML or atypical CML (sometimes also referred to as subacute myeloid leukemia), chronic myelomonocytic leukemia (CMML) or chronic neutrophilic (CNL) (Table 16.2). Children may have a disease previously referred to as juvenile CML, and now juvenile myelomonocytic leukemia (JMML). Importantly, in none of these variants is there a Ph

| Table 16.2    Classification of CML and its variants |
|---|
| Classical Ph-positive CML |
| Ph-negative, bcr/abl-positive hematologically typical CML |
| Ph-negative, bcr/abl-negative hematologically atypical CML |
| Juvenile myelomonocytic leukemia |
| Chronic myelomonocytic leukemia |
| Chronic neutrophilic leukemias |

| Table 16.3    WHO classification of myelodysplastic/myeloproliferative diseases |
|---|
| Chronic myelomonocytic leukemia |
| Atypical chronic myeloid leukemia |
| Juvenile myelomonocytic leukemia |
| Myelodysplastic/myeloproliferative disease, unclassifiable |

chromosome. Patients with atypical CML, CMML, and JMML usually have clinical and hematological features that suggest an overlap between CMPD and myelodysplastic syndrome (MDS), and the contemporary classification of myelodysplastic/myeloproliferative diseases is appropriate (Table 16.3).

CNL is a rare disease, which is of considerable academic interest since it is sometimes associated with a Ph chromosome and a BCR-ABL related oncoprotein, the p230[18]; currently fewer than 100 patients with Ph-positive CNL have been reported worldwide. CNL affects older adults, compared to CML. It is of considerable interest that in about 20% of the reported cases, there was an associated malignancy, typically multiple myeloma, but none of these patients exhibited clonality in their myeloid cells. Distinctions among chronic phase, accelerated phase, and blast crisis CML are discussed in Chapter 17.

## REFERENCES

1. Nowell PC, Hungerford DA: A minute chromosome in human chronic granulocytic leukemia. *Science* 132:1497, 1960.
2. Deininger M, Goldman JM, Melo JV: The molecular biology of chronic myeloid leukemia. *Blood* 96:3343–3356, 2000.
3. Kralovics R, Passamonti F, Buser AS, et al.: A gain-of-function mutation of JAK2 myeloproliferative disorders. *N Engl J Med* 352:1779–1790, 2005.
4. Baxter EJ, Scott LM, Campbell PJ, et al.: Acquired mutation of the tyrosine kinase JAK2 in human myeloproliferative disorders. *Lancet* 365:1054–1061, 2005.
5. Levine RL, Wadleigh M, Cools J, et al.: Activating mutation in the tyrosine kinase JAK2 in polycythemia, essential thrombocythemia, and myeloid metaplasia with myelofibrosis. *Cancer Cell* 7:387–397, 2005.
6. Groffen J, Heisterkamp, N. The chimeric BCR-ABL gene. *Baillière's Clin Hematol* 10:187, 1997.
7. Mughal TI, Goldman JM: Chronic myeloid leukemia: current status and controversies. *Oncology* 18:837–854, 2004.
8. Morrison VA: Chronic leukemias. *Cancer J Clin* 44:353, 1994.
9. Muir CS, Waterhouse J, Mack T, Powell J, Whelan S: *Cancer incidence in 5 continents, vol 5*. IARC Scientific Publication no. 88. Lyon: International Agency for Research on Cancer, 1987.
10. Court Brown W, Abbatt J: Mortality from cancer causes after radiotherapy for ankylosing spondylitis. *Br Med J* 2:1327–1329, 1965.
11. Doll R, Smith PG: The long term effects of X-irradiation in patients treated for metropathia haemorrhagica. *Br J Radiol* 41:362–368, 1968.
12. Heyssel R, Brill B, Woodbury L: Leukemia in Hiroshima atomic bomb survivors. *Blood* 15:313–331, 1960.
13. Kato H, Schull WJ: Studies on the mortality of A-bomb survivors 1950–1971. *Radiat Res* 90:395, 1982.
14. Eglin RP, Swann RA, Isaacs D, Moon ER: Chronic leukaemia in siblings. *Lancet* 2:984, 1984.
15. Posthuma EFM, Falkenburg JHF, Apperley JF, et al.: On behalf of the Chronic Leukemia Working Party of the EBMT. HLA-B8 and the HLA-A3 co expressed with HLA-B8 are associated with a reduced risk of the development of chronic myeloid leukemia. *Blood* 93:3863–3865, 1999.
16. Marmont A, et al.: Recurrence of Ph[1]–leukemia in donor cells after marrow transplantation for chronic granulocytic leukemia. *N Engl J Med* 31:990, 1988.
17. Jaffe ES, Harris NL, Stein H, Vardiman JW (eds.): *World Health Organization Classification of Tumours. Pathology and Genetics of Tumours of Haematopoietic and Lymphoid Tissues*. Lyon, France: IARC Press; 2001, pp. 15–60.
18. Melo JV: The diversity of the BCR-ABL fusion proteins and their relationship to leukemia phenotype. *Blood* 96: 3343–3356, 2000.

# Chapter 17
# MOLECULAR BIOLOGY, PATHOLOGY, AND CYTOGENETICS

## Michael Deininger

Chronic myeloid leukemia (CML) is probably the most extensively studied malignancy and has served as a pacemaker for the development of new concepts and strategies in oncology. It was the description of the first CML cases, independently by Bennet[1] and Virchow,[2] which led to the term "leukemia," Greek for "white blood." CML was the first human cancer consistently associated with a chromosomal abnormality, the Philadelphia (Ph) chromosome.[3] It was also the first malignancy that was faithfully reproduced in an animal model based on precise knowledge of the causal molecular lesion.[4] Lastly, CML was the first malignant condition, where the identification of the causal abnormality led to a specific therapy.[5] Despite intensive efforts, important aspects of CML pathogenesis are not well understood, such as the mechanisms underlying the progression to blast crisis. This chapter reviews the pathogenesis of CML, with a slight emphasis on clinical applications. Due to the wealth of data, this review cannot be comprehensive, and many important aspects had to be omitted because of space constraints.

## MORPHOLOGY

### CHRONIC PHASE

Approximately 85% of patients with CML are diagnosed in the chronic phase.[6] A presumptive diagnosis can be established based on a Giemsa-stained peripheral blood or bone marrow aspirate. The peripheral blood demonstrates variable degrees of leukocytosis with a striking left shift in the white blood cell differential, basophilia, and less frequently, eosinophilia. Thrombocytosis is also common as is a moderate degree of anemia (Table 17.1).[7] The morphology of the peripheral blood cells is normal; dysplasia is not a typical feature of CML and points to alternative diagnoses (see below). In the bone marrow, cellularity is increased with a predominance of granulopoiesis over erythropoiesis. Basophils and eosinophils may be increased, usually in proportion to their numbers in the peripheral blood. Megakaryocytes are frequently increased in numbers, tend to be small and hypolobulated (micromegakaryocytes), and form clusters or sheets. Other findings include pseudo-Gaucher cells or sea-blue histiocytes, both representing macrophages that are unable to metabolize the increased glucocerebroside load associated with the high cell turnover. Bone marrow histology yields additional information and is mandatory in the case of a "dry tap," as it may reveal increased blasts that are not apparent on the blood smear. Various degrees of reticulin fibrosis are a common finding, particularly in patients with more advanced disease.[8] Angiogenesis is also increased but vessel density is not part of standard histologic reports, since it requires special stains.[9] Overall, the morphologic findings allow establishing the diagnosis of a myeloproliferative syndrome, consistent with CML. However, a definitive diagnosis of CML should be made only after the presence of the Ph chromosome, or the *BCR-ABL* translocation has been documented by cytogenetic or molecular techniques (see below).

### ACCELERATED PHASE

The diagnostic criteria for accelerated phase have been a matter of debate and the issue has not been resolved

| Table 17.1 Blood white cell differential count at diagnosis ($n = 90$) | |
|---|---|
| | Percent of total leukocytes |
| Myeloblasts | 3 |
| Promyelocytes | 4 |
| Myelocytes | 12 |
| Metamyelocytes | 7 |
| Band forms | 14 |
| Segmented forms | 38 |
| Basophils | 3 |
| Eosinophils | 2 |
| Nucleated red cells | 0.5 |
| Monocytes | 8 |
| Lymphocytes | 8 |

**Table 17.2**   Diagnostic criteria for accelerated phase

Blasts 15–29%[a]
Blasts plus promyelocytes >30% (with blasts alone <30%)[a]
Basophils >20%[a]
Platelets <100 × 109/L, unrelated to therapy

[a]Refers to peripheral blood or bone marrow.

completely. The most widely accepted criteria are given in Table 17.2.[10] Percentages of blasts, promyelocytes, and basophils, as well as thrombocytopenia that is not related to therapy, were all demonstrated to be independent adverse prognostic indicators in multivariate analysis, and these parameters were used to define accelerated phase in the recent large trials of imatinib in advanced CML.[11] It is controversial whether clonal evolution (CE), i.e., the presence of cytogenetic abnormalities in addition to the Ph chromosome, is indicative of accelerated phase at diagnosis in the absence of any of the other criteria. However, there is consensus that CE in a patient undergoing therapy indicates disease progression. In addition to the criteria in Table 17.2, a number of "soft" parameters are used clinically, such as decreased responsiveness to drug therapy, increasing splenomegaly, or pronounced B symptoms. Although features like this are clearly suggestive of disease progression, they are difficult to cast into an unambiguous definition and therefore should not be used in isolation to establish a diagnosis of accelerated phase.

## BLASTIC PHASE (BLAST CRISIS)

A diagnosis of blastic phase is made when more than or equal to 30% blasts are present in the blood or bone marrow. Immunophenotyping is mandatory to determine whether the blasts have myeloid (60–70% of cases) or lymphoid differentiation (20–30% of cases), since this has major implications for optimal management. In the case of myeloid blast crisis, the blasts may fulfill the diagnostic criteria for any of the French–American–British (FAB) subgroups, but myelomonocytic differentiation is most frequent. Immunophenotypic analysis reveals positivity for myeloperoxidase and myeloid markers (CD13, CD14, and CD33). Lymphoid blast crisis usually has a pre-B-cell phenotype, with positivity for B-cell markers (CD19 and CD20), CD10, and TdT.[12,13] T-lymphoid blast crisis is extremely rare. Approximately 10% of cases are undifferentiated or biphenotypic. Regardless of the phenotype, the blasts almost invariably express the CD34 antigen. A diagnosis of blastic phase is also established in the case of extramedullary disease, with the exception of liver or spleen involvement.

## CYTOGENETICS

### CONVENTIONAL G BANDING AND R BANDING

The cytogenetic hallmark of CML is the Ph chromosome, which is demonstrable in approximately 90%

of patients with a diagnosis of CML based on clinical and morphologic criteria. The Ph chromosome, originally thought to be a shortened chromosome 22 and thus referred to as 22[−3] is the result of a reciprocal translocation between the long arms of chromosomes 9 and 22 [t(9;22)(q34;q11)].[14] As a consequence, genetic sequences from the *BCR* gene on 22q34 are fused 5′ of the *ABL** gene on 9q11, and vice versa, generating a *BCR-ABL* fusion gene on the derivative chromosome 22 and an *ABL-BCR* fusion gene on the derivative chromosome 9 [Figure 17.1(a) and 17.1(b)].[15,16] Approximately 10% of patients with typical CML are negative for the t(9;22)(q34;q11) by conventional G- or R-banding techniques. In approximately half of these patients, the *BCR-ABL* translocation is detectable by fluorescence in situ hybridization (FISH) or reverse transcription polymerase chain reaction (RT-PCR), a situation referred to as cryptic or silent Ph translocation. The clinical course of these individuals is not different from classical Ph-chromosome-positive CML, while the remaining 5% of patients have truly *BCR-ABL*-negative disease. According to the World Health Organization, CML is defined by presence of the *BCR-ABL* translocation, and thus the term Ph-negative or *BCR-ABL*-negative CML should not be used any longer. Depending on specific features, it may be possible to classify such patients as having chronic myelomonocytic leukemia if there is persistent monocytosis of more than 10[9]/L, or atypical CML if there is prominent dysgranulopoiesis. Otherwise, the disease should be referred to as chronic myeloproliferative disease, unclassifiable. The exclusive definition of CML as the *BCR-ABL*-positive disease has become even more important with the advent of imatinib as a specific targeted therapy for this disorder.[17]

### FLUORESCENCE IN SITU HYBRIDIZATION

Fluorescent probes to detect the *BCR-ABL* translocation have become widely available and are equally suitable for analysis of metaphases and interphases [Figure 17.1(c)]. Using FISH on metaphase spreads allows for analysis of several hundred cells, which increases the sensitivity for detection of residual disease by one order of magnitude.[18] Analysis of interphase nuclei permits making a diagnosis of CML in cases that fail to grow metaphases. FISH on interphase nuclei from the peripheral blood correlates with bone marrow cytogenetics.[19] However, the fact that the Ph status of B cells is unpredictable can lead to over- or underestimation, when unselected peripheral blood white cells are analyzed.[20] For diagnostic purposes, it

---

* The correct designation of ABL is ABL-1, as there is the ABL-related gene (ARG) that is referred to as ABL-2. However, as "ABL" is still much more commonly used in the medical literature than ABL-1, ABL will be used throughout this chapter.

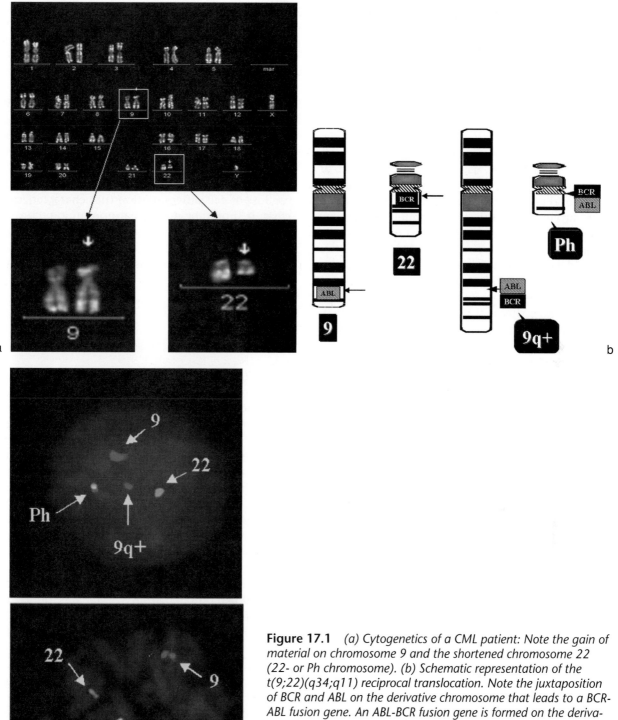

**Figure 17.1** *(a) Cytogenetics of a CML patient: Note the gain of material on chromosome 9 and the shortened chromosome 22 (22- or Ph chromosome). (b) Schematic representation of the t(9;22)(q34;q11) reciprocal translocation. Note the juxtaposition of BCR and ABL on the derivative chromosome that leads to a BCR-ABL fusion gene. An ABL-BCR fusion gene is formed on the derivative chromosome 9 but does not appear to play a role in the pathogenesis of CML. (c) Fluorescence in situ hybridization (FISH): The upper panel shows an interphase nucleus, and the lower panel a metaphase. FISH was done with the LSI bcr/abl ES probe (Vysis, Downer's Grove, IL) that detects the BCR-ABL fusion as well as the (red) signal on the derivative chromosome 9. (Courtesy of Christel Mueller, Department of Hematology, University of Leipzig, Germany)*

is crucial to establish the false-positive and false-negative rates of the probe set used, which vary significantly between different commercially available kits.[21] The obvious disadvantage of FISH is that it screens only for the presence of the *BCR-ABL* translocation, and does not detect other cytogenetic abnormalities.

### DELETIONS FLANKING THE BCR-ABL BREAKPOINT

It was recently observed that 10–15% of CML patients harbor large deletions, flanking the breakpoint on chromosome 9 and, less frequently, chromosome 22, or both.[22,23] Patients with such deletions have a much shorter survival with interferon-alpha-based therapy and appear to have a shorter time to progression on imatinib.[24] These observations led to the speculation that the deleted region may contain a tumor suppressor gene. One candidate on chromosome 9q is PRDM12, a zinc-finger protein, which may function as a negative transcriptional regulator.[25,26] Deletions on the derivative chromosome 9 are detectable with most commercially available FISH probes.[27] In addition, patients with loss of genetic material on either side of the breakpoint are negative for *ABL-BCR* mRNA.[28] This however does not fully account for the fact that about one-third of CML patients fail to express this reciprocal fusion mRNA.[29] Although the prognostic significance of deletions flanking the *BCR-ABL* breakpoint awaits evaluation in a prospective fashion, "deletion status" should become part of diagnostic reports.[30] It has recently been shown that the frequency of deletions is much higher in patients with so-called variant Ph translocations that involve one or two chromosomes in addition to chromosomes 9 and 22. These variants may be generated at the time of the initial translocation event or, less frequently, may be acquired during disease progression, where they represent an unusual form of clonal cytogenetic evolution (see below).[31] The inferior survival of patients with variant Ph translocations could be convincingly attributed to high frequency of derivative chromosome 9 deletions, as elimination of this group of patients eliminated the difference.[31]

### CYTOGENETIC CLONAL EVOLUTION (CE)

The acquisition of nonrandom karyotypic abnormalities in addition to the Ph chromosome is referred to as CE. CE is strongly associated with disease progression, occurring in more than 50% of patients with blastic transformation.[32] Although many different chromosomal abnormalities have been reported, there are a few specific changes that account for the majority of cases.[33] Hyperdiploid karyotypes predominate, most commonly trisomy 8, 19, 21, or a second Ph chromosome. Another frequent finding is isochromosome 17, while monosomy 7, loss of the Y chromosome, and reciprocal translocations, such as t(3;21)(q21;q26), are relatively rare. Progressively more abnormalities are

often acquired during further disease progression. Intriguingly, the sequence of acquisition of these additional changes is apparently nonrandom, following certain "routes" of CE,[33] and there are geographical and ethnic differences, whose etiology is not understood.[34] Events like t(3;21)(q21;q26) that involves the *EVI-1* gene, a transcription factor, may conceivably dysregulate myeloid cell differentiation, a key feature of blastic transformation, and thus explain the phenotype of blast crisis compared to chronic phase. However, in most instances, it is not known how the recurrent chromosomal changes may contribute to the loss of cell differentiation that characterizes blast crisis. It should be noted that nonrandom chromosomal abnormalities have been detected in the Ph-chromosome-negative cells of some patients, with a complete cytogenetic response to imatinib.[35] This yet unexplained phenomenon should not be referred to as CE.

## MOLECULAR PATHOGENESIS

### MOLECULAR ANATOMY OF THE BCR-ABL FUSION

The breakpoints in ABL are spread over a large genomic region and may occur 5' of ABL exon Ib, between ABL exons Ia and II or, most frequently, between the two alternative first ABL exons (Figure 17.2) (reviewed in Ref. 36). Despite this variation, the ABL portion in the fusion mRNA and protein is usually constant, encompassing ABL exons 2–11. This is thought to be the result of posttranscriptional processing of the primary transcript. In contrast, the breakpoints in BCR localize to three distinct breakpoint cluster regions (*bcr*),[16] which are associated with the three major types of Bcr-Abl fusion proteins. Breaks in the minor *bcr* (m-*bcr*) give rise to an e1a2 fusion mRNA and a 190-kd protein (p190$^{BCR-ABL}$) that is found in two-third of patients with Ph-chromosome-positive acute lymphoblastic leukemia (ALL) and in rare patients with CML. Unlike typical CML, these patients are characterized by monocytosis.[37] Breaks in the major *bcr* (M-*bcr*) result in e13a2 or e14a2 fusion mRNAs (previously referred to as b2a2 and b3a2, according to the original numbering of exons within the major breakpoint cluster region) and a 210-kd protein (p210$^{BCR-ABL}$). p210$^{BCR-ABL}$ is typical of CML but also occurs in one-third of patients with Ph-chromosome-positive ALL.[36] Many efforts were made toward identifying consistent differences between patients expressing e13a2 (b2a3) or b14a2 (b3a2). However, the only association that seems to stand the test of time is the notion of slightly higher platelet counts in patients with e14a2 transcripts.[38] The third recognized cluster, termed micro-*bcr* (μ-*bcr*), is localized in BCR intron 19 and generates a 230-kd protein (p230$^{BCR-ABL}$) that is associated with the rare and relatively benign condition of chronic neutrophilic leukemia.[39] The fact that the Abl portion

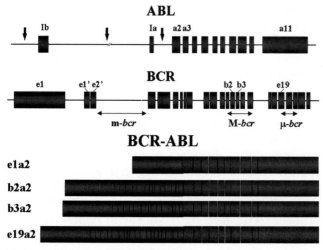

**Figure 17.2** *Location of the breakpoints in BCR and ABL and structure of the various BCR-ABL mRNAs. Breakpoints in ABL are spread over a large genomic region and may occur upstream of exon Ib, between exons Ia and II, or between exons Ib and Ia. In contrast, breakpoints in the BCR cluster in defined breakpoint cluster regions (bcr), a fact that led to the gene's naming. ABL exons 2–11 are contained in the BCR-ABL mRNA, regardless of the breakpoint location, as a result of splicing. In contrast, different types of fusion mRNA and protein are generated from the different breakpoint cluster regions in BCR. (Reproduced from Deininger et al.: Blood 96:3343, 2000; with permission)*

in the different fusion proteins is constant while the Bcr portion is variable provides circumstantial evidence that the transforming principle is likely to reside in Abl, while the Bcr part appears to modify the disease phenotype, with retention of a larger BCR portion rendering the disease less aggressive. Although the three major types of *BCR-ABL* fusion mRNA account for more than 99% of cases of Bcr-Abl-positive leukemia, many more *BCR-ABL* variants have been seen in anecdotal cases or small series of patients.[38] Most of these variants have atypical breakpoints in BCR, generating fusion mRNAs, such as e6a2[40] or e8-insert-a2, where the open reading frame is retained by interposition of intronic sequences. However, fusions between BCR exon 1 and ABL exon 3 have also been described in CML patients.[41] Due to the small numbers of reported cases, it has been difficult to convincingly ascribe a particular clinical phenotype to any of these rare *BCR-ABL* variants; however, the general theme seems to be that the retention of more BCR sequences within the fusion protein attenuates the disease, consistent with the observations in the major types of Bcr-Abl fusion proteins.

### HEMATOPOIETIC LINEAGE INVOLVEMENT

CML is frequently referred to as a stem cell disease, since all three myeloid lineages (granulopoiesis, megakaryopoiesis, and erythropoiesis) carry the Ph chromosome. Data regarding the lymphoid cell compartment have been more conflicting, and there is

apparently variation between different patients. In most patients, at least a proportion of the peripheral blood B cells are Ph positive.[42] Mature T cells are usually Ph negative,[43] while T-cell precursors were found to be positive in one study.[44] The existence of myeloid and B-lymphoid (and in rare instances T-lymphoid) blastic transformation (see below), as well as the observation that endothelial cells may be Ph positive,[45] is further support for the involvement of an early progenitor cell. There is still controversy as to whether Ph-positive ALL with a p210$^{BCR-ABL}$ fusion and lymphoid blast crisis are different entities or not.[46] The fact that the hematopoiesis that recovers after intensive chemotherapy is usually Ph negative in the case of ALL but Ph positive in the case of lymphoid blast crisis argues for two distinct entities. The ability of interferon alpha,[47] autologous stem cell transplantation,[48] and, more impressively, imatinib[5] to restore Ph-negative hematopoiesis in many patients indicates that normal hematopoietic progenitor cells survive in the presence of the CML cell clone. Remarkably, the most primitive stem cell compartment appears to be predominantly Ph negative in early phases of the disease, despite the fact that the peripheral myeloid cells are almost exclusively Ph positive.[49,50] This has led to the notion that Bcr-Abl initially favors the expansion of committed progenitor cells (such as colony-forming units granulocyte-macrophage), while the stem cell compartment may be more resistant. Clearly, the question how the Bcr-Abl-positive cell clone outcompetes normal hematopoiesis is at the very heart of CML pathogenesis and is discussed in more detail further below.

### MULTISTEP VERSUS SINGLE-STEP PATHOGENESIS

It is generally thought that Bcr-Abl alone is necessary and sufficient to induce the chronic phase of CML. This notion is supported by murine disease models (see below), the ability of certain therapies to restore Ph-negative polyclonal hematopoiesis,[35,51,52] and the lack of detectable genetic abnormalities in addition to the Ph chromosome in newly diagnosed patients. However, there are some arguments against this view. Mathematical modeling suggested that the epidemiology of chronic phase CML is more compatible with two or three genetic events than with one.[53] X-chromosome-based clonality studies in Ph-negative Epstein–Barr-virus-transformed B-cell lines from CML patients showed evidence for "skewing" toward the genotype of the leukemia clone in a subset of patients, consistent with a clonal abnormality that predated the acquisition of the Ph chromosome.[54] Lastly, *BCR-ABL* mRNA is detectable at very low levels in the blood of many healthy individuals, suggesting that Bcr-Abl alone may not be sufficient to induce the CML phenotype.[55,56] Another observation pointing to the possibility of a pathological "pre-Philadelphia" state is the observation of cytogenetic abnormalities in the

Ph-negative cells of some patients, with a cytogenetic response to imatinib.[35,57,58] Although in the vast majority of cases the respective abnormalities, many of them typical of myelodysplastic syndromes, are not present in Bcr-Abl-positive cells, arguing against the acquisition of Ph as a secondary event, it remains possible that the Ph-negative hematopoiesis as a whole is abnormal. In this scenario, different abnormal clones would emerge, including the Bcr-Abl-positive clone that has the greatest proliferation capacity and leads to clinical CML.

## THE PHYSIOLOGICAL FUNCTION OF THE TRANSLOCATION PARTNERS

Abl is a 145-kd nonreceptor tyrosine kinase with multiple and complex functions. Two isoforms (Abl-A and Abl-B) exist that differ in their N-terminal regions, depending on the usage of exon Ia or exon Ib (Figure 17.3). Only Abl-B, which is 19 amino acids longer than Abl-A, is myristoylated at the N-terminus,[59] a feature that has recently been linked to autoinhibition of kinase activity.[60,61] Further toward the C-terminus, there is a Src homology (SH) 3 domain that interacts with proline-rich domains of other proteins, an SH2 domain capable of binding to phosphorylated tyrosine residues of interacting proteins, and an SH1 domain, which carries tyrosine kinase activity.[36] While the N-terminus exhibits a high degree of homology to other nonreceptor tyrosine kinases, such as Src, the C-terminus is unique to Abl. Three DNA-binding domains, a nuclear localization signal, nuclear export signal, a proline-rich region, and an actin-binding domain can be defined within the C-terminus. Under physiological circumstances, Abl is nuclear, and its tyrosine kinase activity is tightly regulated.

The function of Abl has been studied extensively, and a very complex picture has emerged (for reviews, see Refs. 62 and 63). There is evidence for an inhibitory role of Abl in cell cycle regulation, which led to the notion that it may be considered a tumor suppressor.[64] A number of studies have implicated Abl tyrosine kinase in the regulation of the cellular response to DNA damage, by interaction with several proteins involved in DNA repair or response to genotoxic stress.[65–70] Yet other data suggest a role in the signal transduction from and to integrin receptors on the cell surface,[71,72] and there is evidence for activation of Abl kinase upon ligand binding to the platelet-derived growth factor receptor.[73] Mice with homologous disruption of the ABL locus suffer from high perinatal mortality and have multiple defects, including defective immune function and skeletal abnormalities, and suffer from a poorly characterized wasting syndrome.[74,75] However, there is no indication that the rate of spontaneous tumors is increased in these mice, arguing against a tumor suppressor function of Abl. Importantly, simultaneous disruption of the ABL-related gene, ARG, also referred to as ABL-2, is embryonically lethal, due to a failure of neuronal development, which argues that the ARG may partially compensate for the loss of Abl function in the ABL knockout mice.[76] The mechanism underlying the tight regulation of Abl kinase activity in physiological conditions has recently been clarified, at least for the Abl-B isoform, by a combination of mutational structure function analysis and crystallography.[60,61] These studies revealed a critical role for the N-terminal cap region of the protein, which inhibits the kinase by an intramolecular interaction. This does not exclude that other mechanisms, such as transacting molecules, may also be involved in regulating the kinase.[77]

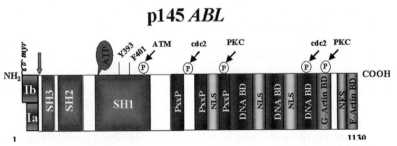

**p145 ABL**

**Figure 17.3** *Structure of the Abl protein. The type Ia isoform is slightly shorter than type Ib, which contains a myristoylation (myr) site for attachment to the plasma membrane. Note the three SrC-homology (SH) domains situated toward the NH$_2$-terminus. Y393 is the major site of autophosphorylation within the kinase domain, while phenylalanine 401 (F401) is highly conserved in PTKs containing SH3 domains. The middle of the protein is dominated by proline-rich regions (PxxP) capable of binding to SH3 domains and also harbors one of three nuclear localization signals (NLS). The carboxy-terminus contains DNA as well as G- and F-actin-binding domains. Phosphorylation sites by Atm, cdc2, and PKC are shown. The arrowhead indicates the position of the breakpoint in the Bcr-Abl fusion protein. (Blood 96:3343, 2000; with permission)*

# p160 BCR

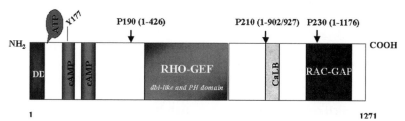

**Figure 17.4** *Structure of the Bcr protein. Note the dimerization domain (DD) and the two cAMP kinase homologous domains at the N-terminus. Y177 is the autophosphorylation site crucial for binding to Grb-2. The center of the molecule contains a region homologous to Rho guanidine nucleotide exchange factors (Rho-GEF) as well as dbl-like and pleckstrin homology (PH) domains. Toward the C-terminus a putative site for calcium-dependent lipid binding (CaLB) and a domain with activating function for Rac-GTPase (Rac-GAP) are found. Arrowheads indicate the position of the breakpoints in the Bcr-Abl fusion proteins. (Blood 96:3343, 2000; with permission)*

The function of BCR (Figure 17.4) is even less well understood than that of Abl. The N-terminus contains a dimerization domain as well as a serine/threonine kinase activity. The center of the molecule is dominated by dbl-like and pleckstrin homology (PH-) domains that have guanidine nucleotide exchange function for small G proteins, including RhoA, Rac, and Cdc42. The C-terminus has GTPase-activating function for Rac (reviewed in Ref. 36). In contrast to ABL knockout mice, BCR knockout mice are practically normal, and an increased oxidative burst of their neutrophils is the only recognized anomaly.[78]

## ESSENTIAL FEATURES OF THE BCR-ABL PROTEIN

Mutational analysis of Bcr-Abl identified several domains and amino acid residues that are crucial to the molecule's capacity to transform hematopoietic cells. Most importantly, deletion of the tyrosine kinase function abrogates transformation and leukemogenicity,[79] although more recent data suggest that even the kinase-dead protein may modify certain cellular functions, such as adhesion and migration.[80] A second critical structural motif is the N-terminus of BCR that contains the dimerization domain.[81] This domain can be replaced by other sequences that allow dimerization; for example, ETV-6 in the Etv-6-Abl fusion protein that has sporadically been found in patients with ALL.[82] Since the N-terminus of Abl is crucial to the autoregulation of the kinase, it is conceivable that the principal consequence of dimerization is the abrogation of autoinhibition.[60,61] Many other motifs within Bcr-Abl have important functions but are not essential to leukemogenesis. Rather than that, they modulate the aggressiveness of the disease or influence its phenotype in murine models of Bcr-Abl-positive leukemia. For example, tyrosine 177 of BCR is crucial to the induction of myeloid but not lymphoid leukemia,[83] and deletion of the Abl SH3 domain attenuates the disease.[84]

## ACTIVATION OF SIGNALING PATHWAYS

As a result of the constitutive tyrosine kinase activity, multiple substrates are tyrosine phosphorylated in Bcr-Abl-positive cells, including the oncoprotein itself. As mentioned above, Bcr-Abl has several functional domains that are capable of binding other proteins in tyrosine-dependent and -independent manners. Additional binding sites are generated by autophosphorylation. The net result is a multiprotein complex held together by multiple protein–protein interactions.[85,86] In addition, Bcr-Abl phosphorylates a host of substrates that are not directly bound to the protein but impact on crucial cellular functions. Examples include adhesion protein like paxillin and tensin or the focal adhesion kinase (reviewed in Ref. 36).

Research over the past two decades has revealed that multiple signaling pathways are activated in Bcr-Abl-transformed cells. This includes the Ras/Raf/mitogen-activated kinase pathway,[87] phosphatidyl inositol 3 kinase (PI3 kinase),[88] STAT5,[89] Myc[90], and many others (reviewed in Refs. 36,91). Overall, there is extensive redundancy. For example, Ras may be activated in two different ways. One possibility is binding of the adapter protein Grb-2 to phosphorylated tyrosine 177 that subsequently binds and activates the GTP exchange factor Sos, which in turn stabilizes Ras in the active GTP-bound form.[92] The second option is activation via the adapter protein Shc, which requires the Abl SH2 domain but not tyrosine 177.[93] Studies in cell lines frequently indicated important or even essential functions for individual pathways, suggesting that the respective pathways may be attractive therapeutic targets. However, data obtained in murine models of Bcr-Abl-positive leukemia that employed knockout animals to test for the requirement of certain signaling components in vivo were usually less convincing. For example, the induction of a myeloproliferative syndrome in mice is not impaired in animals with a homozygous deletion of the *STAT5A* and *STAT5B* genes[94] or the inter leukin 3 (IL-3) and granulocyte-macrophage colony-stimulating factor genes.[95] Although the rather aggressive phenotype of the murine CML models raises the question whether more subtle effects would be detectable with a model that is closer to the clinical disease, these observations support the view that the redundancy within the signaling network of Bcr-Abl-transformed cells may compensate for the loss of individual components.

## BIOLOGICAL PROPERTIES OF CML CELLS

Compared to their normal counterparts, CML progenitor cells are able to enter the cell cycle in the absence of growth factors,[96] although they are not cytokine-independent.[97] Nonetheless, the reduced requirement for external stimuli may lend a growth advantage to CML cells that is sufficient to outcompete normal hematopoiesis over time. There is evidence that autocrine production of IL-3 and granulocyte colony-stimulating factor by CML progenitor cells may be the underlying mechanism.[98] In addition to inducing proliferation, Bcr-Abl has been shown to inhibit apoptosis by multiple mechanisms, including upregulation of the antiapoptotic protein Bcl-X$_L$ and downregulation of proapoptotic Bim.[99–103] A third biological feature that characterizes Bcr-Abl-positive cells is a perturbation of their adhesion to stroma[104] and migration in response to chemokines such as SDF-1,[105] which may explain extramedullary hematopoiesis. It has been difficult to link certain biological properties to the activation of specific signaling pathways that are activated by Bcr-Abl, and the issue is complicated by the fact that much of the data are derived from studies in cell lines rather than primary CML cells. Proliferation and inhibition of apoptosis are strictly dependent on Bcr-Abl kinase activity, whereas the defects in adhesion and migration are not completely reversible upon inhibition of Bcr-Abl.[106] If this is clinically significant in the setting of targeted therapy of CML with imatinib remains to be seen.

## MECHANISMS OF DISEASE PROGRESSION

One could argue that CML would not pose a clinical problem if the disease remained in the chronic phase. Clinical observation holds that the time-to-disease progression is extremely variable from patient to patient, with some individuals progressing to blast crisis within weeks from what seemed a diagnosis of standard chronic phase disease, and others remaining stable for many years, even with conventional hydroxyurea-based therapy. The mechanisms underlying disease progression are not well understood. Studies from a number of laboratories have suggested that the expression of Bcr-Abl may adversely affect several DNA repair pathways.[107–111] It is thought that over time this favors the accumulation of additional genetic abnormalities, such as the inactivation of tumor suppressor genes. Another possibility is that accelerated

loss of telomere length predisposes the CML cells to the acquisition of additional chromosomal abnormalities. In fact reduced telomere length correlated with an adverse prognosis.[112] However, no consistent genetic abnormalities have been associated with disease progression. Deletions of the INK4A locus, resulting in inactivation of the p16 cyclin-dependent kinase inhibitor and—presumable—p14$^{ARF}$, occur in approximately 50% of patients with lymphoid blast crisis, without impacting prognosis.[113,114] Deletion of p53 has been observed in another subset of patients[115] and deletion of the retinoblastoma susceptibility gene in isolated cases.[116] All these abnormalities fail to explain the most striking feature that distinguishes blastic from chronic phase CML, namely the block of differentiation. In acute myeloid leukemia (AML), the concept that two types of mutations are required to induce the disease phenotype has recently received much attention.[117] According to this model, a type I mutation, such as an activating mutation of Ras or a tyrosine kinase, leads to increased proliferation and reduced apoptosis, while differentiation is maintained. A second, type II mutation, such as the AML1-ETO fusion, affects a transcription factor that is crucial for myeloid cell differentiation. The result is a differentiation block that leads to the full AML phenotype. Experimental evidence in support of this concept has accumulated from murine leukemia models. For example, transplantation of murine bone marrow cells expressing constitutively active Flt3 into syngeneic recipients induces a myeloproliferative syndrome, but coexpression of Aml1-Eto induces acute leukemia. Similarly, transplantation of bone marrow cells expressing both Bcr-Abl and a NUP98-HOXA9 fusion protein induces AML.[118] In contrast to AML, translocations involving the core-binding factors CBFβ and AML1 have only occasionally been observed in blast crisis, and there is little evidence for point mutations in these key regulators of myeloid differentiation. A more attractive candidate is EVI-1/MDS-1, a transcription factor that is affected by several chromosomal aberrations, such as t(3;21)(q26;q22), inv(3)(q21q26), or t(3;3)(q21q26), that belong to the recurrent nonrandom abnormalities in patients with transition to blast crisis.[33] In addition, increased expression of EVI-1 mRNA has been observed in patients with blast crisis.[119] Mice transplanted with bone marrow cells expressing both Bcr-Abl and Aml1-Evi-1 develop AML, and both components of the chimeric protein are required for induction of this phenotype.[120,121] Very recently, an AML1-EVI-1 fusion protein has been shown to suppress the transcription factor CEBPA in AML.[122] CEBPA has also been implicated by a study that showed that CEBPA expression is inhibited in blast crisis cells as a result of posttranscriptional modification by the poly (rC) binding protein hnRNP E2.[123] Another transcription factor implicated in blast crisis is Wnt, whose activation in progenitor cells may endow them with increased self-renewal capacity,[124] which however does not readily explain their failure to differentiate. Lastly, it should be mentioned that increased expression of Bcr-Abl protein[125] and methylation of the ABL promoter[126] have also been linked to disease progression.

### MURINE MODELS OF Bcr-Abl-POSITIVE LEUKEMIA

In a seminal study Daley and colleagues showed that transplantation of murine bone marrow infected with a Bcr-Abl retrovirus into lethally irradiated syngeneic recipients induced a myeloproliferative syndrome that resembled human CML.[4] This study provided strong evidence that Bcr-Abl is the causative agent responsible for CML and suggested that no additional abnormalities are required for leukemogenicity. However, disease penetrance with the model was relatively low. In addition, a proportion of mice developed atypical Bcr-Abl-positive tumors, such as macrophage tumors. Subsequent studies showed that the conditions used for retroviral infection of murine bone marrow greatly impact the phenotype of the disease.[127] For example, mice transplanted with marrow harvested from donor mice not treated with 5-fluorouracil almost invariably develop B-cell ALL, not a myeloproliferative syndrome. Another important variable is the promoter used to drive the expression of Bcr-Abl. Thus, a more recently developed model uses the promoter of the murine stem cell leukemia and employs high viral titers for transduction.[128] With this approach, 100% of animals develop a myeloproliferative syndrome resembling CML with a latency of approximately 25 days. Although the refinements to the murine disease model have greatly increased its usefulness, one remaining concern is that the Bcr-Abl-positive myeloproliferative syndrome, though phenotypically resembling chronic phase CML, is in reality a very aggressive and rapidly lethal leukemia, in contrast to the chronic phase of human CML. This may be due the fact that levels of Bcr-Abl protein are much higher than in human CML cells.

Transgenic approaches placing Bcr-Abl under the control of the Bcr promoter were initially not successful, due to embryonic lethality.[129] However, with the use of a tetracycline-repressible system and enhancer elements of the SCL locus, it has recently been possible to generate transgenic mice that develop a myeloproliferative syndrome that reproduces some of the features of chronic phase CML and is reversible on re-exposure to tetracyclin.[130]

## SUMMARY

CML is defined by the presence of a *BCR-ABL* fusion gene that gives rise to a cognate chimerical protein with constitutive tyrosine kinase activity. Cytogenetically, the *BCR-ABL* translocation is evident as a Ph chromosome, but some 5% of patients have a cryptic translocation that is detectable only by FISH or RT-PCR. It is thought that the *BCR-ABL* translocation occurs in a pluripotent hematopoietic stem cell and is the only event required for the induction of chronic phase CML, although this has been questioned. Bcr-Abl tyrosine kinase activity maintains a complicated and redundant network of signaling pathways, individual components of which are frequently dispensable for malignant transformation. The biological hallmarks of CML cells, increased proliferation, reduced apoptosis, and perturbed adhesion to extracellular matrix, are almost exclusively dependent on Bcr-Abl's tyrosine kinase activity, indicating that the latter is an ideal therapeutic target. The mechanisms underlying disease progression are not well understood. Analogy to AML suggests that the function of a transcription factor may be disrupted that is essential for coordinated myeloid cell differentiation.

### REFERENCES

1. Bennett JH: Case of hypertrophy of the spleen and liver in which death took place from suppuration of the blood. *Edinb Med Surg J* 64:413, 1845.
2. Virchow R: Weisses Blut. *Frorieps Notizen* 36:151, 1845.
3. Nowell P, Hungerford D: A minute chromosome in human chronic granulocytic leukemia. *Science* 132: 1497, 1960.
4. Daley GQ, Van Etten RA, Baltimore D: Induction of chronic myelogenous leukemia in mice by the P210bcr/abl gene of the Philadelphia chromosome. *Science* 247:824, 1990.
5. Druker BJ, Talpaz M, Resta DJ, et al.: Efficacy and safety of a specific inhibitor of the *BCR-ABL* tyrosine kinase in chronic myeloid leukemia. *N Engl J Med* 344:1031, 2001.
6. Cervantes F, Hernandez-Boluda JC, Ferrer A, et al.: The changing profile of Ph-positive chronic myeloid leukemia at presentation: possible impact of earlier diagnosis on survival. *Haematologica* 84:324, 1999.
7. Lichtman, MA: Chronic myelogenous leukemia and related disorders. In Williams WJ, Beutler E, Erslev A, Lichtman MA (eds.) *Hematology*, 4th ed. New York: McGraw-Hill; 1991:202.
8. Buesche G, Georgii A, Duensing A, et al.: Evaluating the volume ratio of bone marrow affected by fibrosis: a parameter crucial for the prognostic significance of marrow fibrosis in chronic myeloid leukemia. *Hum Pathol* 34:391,2003.
9. Aguayo A, Kantarjian H, Manshouri T, et al.: Angiogenesis in acute and chronic leukemias and myelodysplastic syndromes. *Blood* 96:2240, 2000.
10. Kantarjian HM, Talpaz M: Definition of the accelerated phase of chronic myelogenous leukemia. *J Clin Oncol* 6:180, 1988.
11. Talpaz M, Silver RT, Druker BJ, et al.: Imatinib induces durable hematologic and cytogenetic responses in patients with accelerated phase chronic myeloid

leukemia: results of a phase 2 study. *Blood* 99:1928, 2002.

12. Favre G, Passweg J, Hoffmann T, et al.: Immunophenotype of blast crisis in chronic myeloid leukemia. *Schweiz Med Wochenschr* 128:1624, 1998.

13. Cervantes F, Villamor N, Esteve J, et al.: "Lymphoid" blast crisis of chronic myeloid leukaemia is associated with distinct clinicohaematological features. *Br J Haematol* 100:123, 1998.

14. Rowley JD: A new consistent chromosomal abnormality in chronic myelogenous leukaemia identified by quinacrine fluorescence and Giemsa staining. *Nature* 243:290, 1973.

15. Bartram CR, de Klein A, Hagemeijer A, et al.: Translocation of c-abl oncogene correlates with the presence of a Philadelphia chromosome in chronic myelocytic leukaemia. *Nature* 306:277, 1983.

16. Groffen J, Stephenson JR, Heisterkamp N, et al.: Philadelphia chromosomal breakpoints are clustered within a limited region, bcr, on chromosome 22. *Cell* 36:93, 1984.

17. Vardiman JW, Pierre R, Thiele J, et al.: Chronic myeloproliferative diseases. In: Jaffe ES, Harris NL, Stein H, Vardiman JW (eds.) *Tumors of Haematopoietic and Lymphoid Tissues*. Lyon, France: IARC Press; 2001:15.

18. Schoch C, Schnittger S, Bursch S, et al.: Comparison of chromosome banding analysis, interphase- and hyper-metaphase-FISH, qualitative and quantitative PCR for diagnosis and for follow-up in chronic myeloid leukemia: a study on 350 cases. *Leukemia* 16:53, 2002.

19. Le Gouill S, Talmant P, Milpied N, et al.: Fluorescence in situ hybridization on peripheral-blood specimens is a reliable method to evaluate cytogenetic response in chronic myeloid leukemia. *J Clin Oncol* 18:1533, 2000.

20. Reinhold U, Hennig E, Leiblein S, et al.: FISH for *BCR-ABL* on interphases of peripheral blood neutrophils but not of unselected white cells correlates with bone marrow cytogenetics in CML patients treated with imatinib. *Leukemia* 17:1925, 2003.

21. Chase A, Grand F, Zhang JG, et al.: Factors influencing the false positive and negative rates of *BCR-ABL* fluorescence in situ hybridization. *Genes Chromosomes Cancer* 18:246, 1997.

22. Huntly BJ, Reid AG, Bench AJ, et al.: Deletions of the derivative chromosome 9 occur at the time of the Philadelphia translocation and provide a powerful and independent prognostic indicator in chronic myeloid leukemia. *Blood* 98:1732, 2001.

23. Sinclair PB, Nacheva EP, Leversha M, et al.: Large deletions at the t(9;22) breakpoint are common and may identify a poor-prognosis subgroup of patients with chronic myeloid leukemia. *Blood* 95:738, 2000.

24. Huntly BJ, Guilhot F, Reid AG, et al.: Imatinib improves but may not fully reverse the poor prognosis of patients with CML with derivative chromosome 9 deletions. *Blood* 102:2205, 2003.

25. Kolomietz E, Marrano P, Yee K, et al.: Quantitative PCR identifies a minimal deleted region of 120 kb extending from the Philadelphia chromosome ABL translocation breakpoint in chronic myeloid leukemia with poor outcome. *Leukemia* 17:1313, 2003.

26. Reid AG, Nacheva EP: A potential role for PRDM12 in the pathogenesis of chronic myeloid leukemia with derivative chromosome 9 deletion. *Leukemia* 18:178, 2004.

27. Muller C, Hennig E, Franke C, et al.: The BCR/ABL-extra signal fluorescence in situ hybridization system reliably detects deletions upstream of the ABL locus: implications for reporting of results and followup of chronic myelogenous leukemia patients. *Cancer Genet Cytogenet* 136:149, 2002.

28. Huntly BJ, Bench AJ, Delabesse E, et al.: Derivative chromosome 9 deletions in chronic myeloid leukemia: poor prognosis is not associated with loss of ABL-BCR expression, elevated *BCR-ABL* levels, or karyotypic instability. *Blood* 99:4547, 2002.

29. Melo JV, Gordon DE, Cross NC, et al.: The ABL-BCR fusion gene is expressed in chronic myeloid leukemia. *Blood* 81:158, 1993.

30. Huntly BJP, Bench A, Green AR: Double jeopardy from a single translocation: deletions of the derivative chromosome 9 in chronic myeloid leukemia. *Blood* 102:1160, 2003.

31. Reid AG, Huntly BJ, Grace C, et al.: Survival implications of molecular heterogeneity in variant Philadelphia-positive chronic myeloid leukaemia. *Br J Haematol* 121:419, 2003.

32. Mitelman F: The cytogenetic scenario of chronic myeloid leukemia. *Leuk Lymphoma* 11(suppl 1):11, 1993.

33. Johansson B, Fioretos T, Mitelman F: Cytogenetic and molecular genetic evolution of chronic myeloid leukemia. *Acta Haematol* 107:76, 2002.

34. Johansson B, Mertens F, Mitelman F: Geographic heterogeneity of neoplasia-associated chromosome aberrations. *Genes Chromosomes Cancer* 3:1, 1991.

35. Bumm T, Muller C, Al Ali HK, et al.: Emergence of clonal cytogenetic abnormalities in Ph− cells in some CML patients in cytogenetic remission to imatinib but restoration of polyclonal hematopoiesis in the majority. *Blood* 101:1941, 2003.

36. Deininger MW, Goldman JM, Melo JV: The molecular biology of chronic myeloid leukemia. *Blood* 96:3343, 2000.

37. Melo JV, Myint H, Galton DA, et al.: P190 *BCR-ABL* chronic myeloid leukaemia: the missing link with chronic myelomonocytic leukaemia? *Leukemia* 8:208, 1994.

38. Melo JV: The diversity of *BCR-ABL* fusion proteins and their relationship to leukemia phenotype. *Blood* 88:2375, 1996.

39. Pane F, Frigeri F, Sindona M, et al.: Neutrophilic chronic myeloid leukemia: a distinct disease with a specific molecular marker (BCR/ABL with C3/A2 junction). *Blood* 88:2410, 1996.

40. Hochhaus A, Reiter A, Skladny H, et al.: A novel *BCR-ABL* fusion gene (e6a2) in a patient with Philadelphia chromosome-negative chronic myelogenous leukemia. *Blood* 88:2236, 1996.

41. Al Ali HK, Leiblein S, Kovacs I, et al.: CML with an e1a3 *BCR-ABL* fusion: rare, benign, and a potential diagnostic pitfall. *Blood* 100:1092, 2002.

42. Reinhold U, Hennig E, Leiblein S, et al.: FISH for *BCR-ABL* on interphases of peripheral blood neutrophils but not of unselected white cells correlates with bone marrow cytogenetics in CML patients treated with imatinib. *Leukemia* 17:1925, 2003.

43. Garicochea B, Chase A, Lazaridou A, et al.: T lymphocytes in chronic myelogenous leukaemia (CML): no evidence of the BCR/ABL fusion gene detected by fluorescence in situ hybridization in 14 patients. *Leukemia* 8:1197, 1994.

44. Takahashi N, Miura I, Saitoh K, et al.: Lineage involvement of stem cells bearing the Philadelphia chromosome in chronic myeloid leukemia in the chronic phase as shown by a combination of fluorescence-activated cell sorting and fluorescence in situ hybridization. *Blood* 92:4758, 1998.

45. Gunsilius E, Duba HC, Petzer AL, et al.: Evidence from a leukaemia model for maintenance of vascular endothelium by bone-marrow-derived endothelial cells. *Lancet* 355:1688, 2000.

46. Deininger M: Src kinases in Ph+ lymphoblastic leukemia. *Nat Genet* 36:440, 2004.

47. Talpaz M, Kantarjian H, Kurzrock R, et al.: Interferon-alpha produces sustained cytogenetic responses in chronic myelogenous leukemia. Philadelphia chromosome-positive patients. *Ann Intern Med* 114:532, 1991.

48. McGlave PB, De Fabritiis P, Deisseroth A, et al.: Autologous transplants for chronic myelogenous leukaemia: results from eight transplant groups. *Lancet* 343:1486,1994.

49. Petzer AL, Eaves CJ, Barnett MJ, et al.: Selective expansion of primitive normal hematopoietic cells in cytokine-supplemented cultures of purified cells from patients with chronic myeloid leukemia. *Blood* 90:64, 1997.

50. Petzer AL, Eaves CJ, Lansdorp PM, et al.: Characterization of primitive subpopulation of normal and leukemic cells present in the blood of patients with newly diagnosed as well as established chronic myeloid leukemia. *Blood* 88:2162, 1996.

51. Bergamaschi G, Podesta M, Frassoni F, et al.: Restoration of normal polyclonal haemopoiesis in patients with chronic myeloid leukaemia autografted with Ph-negative peripheral stem cells. *Br J Haematol* 87:867, 1994.

52. Carella A, Lerma E, Corsetti MT, et al.: Autografting with Philadelphia chromosome-negative mobilized hematopoietic progenitor cells in chronic myelogenous leukemia. *Blood* 93:1534, 1999.

53. Vickers M: Estimation of the number of mutations necessary to cause chronic myeloid leukaemia from epidemiological data. *Br J Haematol* 94:1, 1996.

54. Raskind WH, Ferraris AM, Najfeld V, et al.: Further evidence for the existence of a clonal Ph-negative stage in some cases of Ph-positive chronic myelocytic leukemia. *Leukemia* 7:1163, 1993.

55. Biernaux C, Loos M, Sels A, et al.: Detection of major bcr-abl gene expression at a very low level in blood cells of some healthy individuals. *Blood* 86:3118, 1995.

56. Bose S, Deininger M, Gora-Tybor J, et al.: The presence of *BCR-ABL* fusion genes in leukocytes of normal individuals: implications for the assessment of minimal residual disease. *Blood* 92:3362, 1998.

57. O'Dwyer ME, Gatter KM, Loriaux M, et al.: Demonstration of Philadelphia chromosome negative abnormal clones in patients with chronic myelogenous leukemia during major cytogenetic responses induced by imatinib mesylate. *Leukemia* 17:481, 2003.

58. Terre C, Eclache V, Rousselot P, et al.: Report of 34 patients with clonal chromosomal abnormalities in Philadelphia-negative cells during imatinib treatment of Philadelphia-positive chronic myeloid leukemia. *Leukemia* 18:1340, 2004.

59. Daley GQ, Van Etten RA, Jackson PK, et al.: Nonmyristoylated Abl proteins transform a factor-dependent hematopoietic cell line. *Mol Cell Biol* 12:1864, 1992.

60. Hantschel O, Nagar B, Guettler S, et al.: A myristoyl/phosphotyrosine switch regulates c-Abl. *Cell* 112:845, 2003.

61. Nagar B, Hantschel O, Young MA, et al.: Structural basis for the autoinhibition of c-Abl tyrosine kinase. *Cell* 112:859, 2003.

62. Pendergast AM: The Abl family kinases: mechanisms of regulation and signaling. *Adv Cancer Res* 85:51, 2002.

63. Van Etten RA: Cycling, stressed-out and nervous: cellular functions of c-Abl. *Trends Cell Biol* 9:179, 1999.

64. Sawyers CL, McLaughlin J, Goga A, et al.: The nuclear tyrosine kinase c-Abl negatively regulates cell growth. *Cell* 77:121, 1994.

65. Gong JG, Costanzo A, Yang HQ, et al.: The tyrosine kinase c-Abl regulates p73 in apoptotic response to cisplatin-induced DNA damage. *Nature* 399:806, 1999.

66. Kharbanda S, Ren R, Pandey P, et al.: Activation of the c-Abl tyrosine kinase in the stress response to DNA-damaging agents. *Nature* 376:785, 1995.

67. Shafman T, Khanna KK, Kedar P, et al.: Interaction between ATM protein and c-Abl in response to DNA damage. *Nature* 387:520, 1997.

68. Yuan ZM, Huang Y, Ishiko T, et al.: Regulation of Rad51 function by c-Abl in response to DNA damage. *J Biol Chem* 273:3799, 1998.

69. Yuan ZM, Huang Y, Whang Y, et al.: Role for c-Abl tyrosine kinase in growth arrest response to DNA damage. *Nature* 382:272, 1996.

70. Yuan ZM, Shioya H, Ishiko T, et al.: p73 is regulated by tyrosine kinase c-Abl in the apoptotic response to DNA damage. *Nature* 399:814, 1999.

71. Lewis JM, Baskaran R, Taagepera S, et al.: Integrin regulation of c-Abl tyrosine kinase activity and cytoplasmic-nuclear transport. *Proc Natl Acad Sci U S A* 93:15174, 1996.

72. Lewis JM, Schwartz MA: Integrins regulate the association and phosphorylation of paxillin by c-Abl. *J Biol Chem* 273:14225, 1998.

73. Plattner R, Irvin BJ, Guo S, et al.: A new link between the c-Abl tyrosine kinase and phosphoinositide signalling through PLC-gamma1. *Nat Cell Biol* 5:309, 2003.

74. Schwartzberg PL, Stall AM, Hardin JD, et al.: Mice homozygous for the ablm1 mutation show poor viability and depletion of selected B and T cell populations. *Cell* 65:1165, 1991.

75. Tybulewicz VL, Crawford CE, Jackson PK, et al.: Neonatal lethality and lymphopenia in mice with a homozygous disruption of the c-abl proto-oncogene. *Cell* 65:1153, 1991.

76. Koleske AJ, Gifford AM, Scott ML, et al.: Essential roles for the Abl and Arg tyrosine kinases in neurulation. *Neuron* 21:1259, 1998.

77. Wen ST, Van ER: The PAG gene product, a stress-induced protein with antioxidant properties, is an Abl

SH3-binding protein and a physiological inhibitor of c-Abl tyrosine kinase activity. *Genes Dev* 11:2456, 1997.

78. Voncken JW, van Schaick H, Kaartinen V, et al.: Increased neutrophil respiratory burst in bcr-null mutants. *Cell* 80:719, 1995.

79. Lugo TG, Pendergast AM, Muller AJ, et al.: Tyrosine kinase activity and transformation potency of bcr-abl oncogene products. *Science* 247:1079, 1990.

80. Wertheim JA, Forsythe K, Druker BJ, et al.: BCR-ABL-induced adhesion defects are tyrosine kinase-independent. *Blood* 99:4122, 2002.

81. McWhirter JR, Galasso DL, Wang JY: A coiled-coil oligomerization domain of Bcr is essential for the transforming function of Bcr-Abl oncoproteins. *Mol Cell Biol* 13:7587, 1993.

82. Papadopoulos P, Ridge SA, Boucher CA, et al.: The novel activation of ABL by fusion to an ets-related gene, TEL. *Cancer Res* 55:34, 1995.

83. He Y, Wertheim JA, Xu L, et al.: The coiled-coil domain and Tyr177 of bcr are required to induce a murine chronic myelogenous leukemia-like disease by bcr/abl. *Blood* 99:2957, 2002.

84. Skorski T, Nieborowska-Skorska M, Wlodarski P, et al.: The SH3 domain contributes to BCR/ABL-dependent leukemogenesis in vivo: role in adhesion, invasion, and homing. *Blood* 91:406, 1998.

85. Gaston I, Johnson KJ, Oda T, et al.: Coexistence of phosphotyrosine-dependent and -independent interactions between Cbl and Bcr-Abl. *Exp Hematol* 32:113, 2004.

86. Salgia R, Sattler M, Pisick E, et al.: p210BCR/ABL induces formation of complexes containing focal adhesion proteins and the protooncogene product p120c-Cbl. *Exp Hematol* 24:310, 1996.

87. Cortez D, Reuther GW, Pendergast AM: The *BCR-ABL* tyrosine kinase activates mitotic signaling pathways and stimulates G1-to-S phase transition in hematopoietic cells. *Oncogene* 15:2333, 1997.

88. Skorski T, Kanakaraj P, Nieborowska Skorska M, et al.: Phosphatidylinositol-3 kinase activity is regulated by BCR/ABL and is required for the growth of Philadelphia chromosome-positive cells. *Blood* 86:726, 1995.

89. Sillaber C, Gesbert F, Frank DA, et al.: STAT5 activation contributes to growth and viability in Bcr/Abl-transformed cells. *Blood* 95:2118, 2000.

90. Sawyers CL, Callahan W, Witte ON: Dominant negative MYC blocks transformation by ABL oncogenes. *Cell* 70:901, 1992.

91. Melo JV, Deininger MW: Biology of chronic myelogenous leukemia–signaling pathways of initiation and transformation. *Hematol Oncol Clin North Am* 18:545–viii, 2004.

92. Pendergast AM, Quilliam LA, Cripe LD, et al.: BCR-ABL-induced oncogenesis is mediated by direct interaction with the SH2 domain of the GRB-2 adaptor protein. *Cell* 75:175, 1993.

93. Goga A, McLaughlin J, Afar DE, et al.: Alternative signals to RAS for hematopoietic transformation by the *BCR-ABL* oncogene. *Cell* 82:981, 1995.

94. Sexl V, Piekorz R, Moriggl R, et al.: Stat5a/b contribute to interleukin 7-induced B-cell precursor expansion, but abl- and bcr/abl-induced transformation are independent of stat5. *Blood* 96:2277, 2000.

95. Li S, Gillessen S, Tomasson MH, et al.: Interleukin 3 and granulocyte-macrophage colony-stimulating factor are not required for induction of chronic myeloid leukemia-like myeloproliferative disease in mice by BCR/ABL. *Blood* 97:1442, 2001.

96. Jonuleit T, Peschel C, Schwab R, et al.: Bcr-Abl kinase promotes cell cycle entry of primary myeloid CML cells in the absence of growth factors. *Br J Haematol* 100:295, 1998.

97. Amos TA, Lewis JL, Grand FH, et al.: Apoptosis in chronic myeloid leukaemia: normal responses by progenitor cells to growth factor deprivation, X-irradiation and glucocorticoids. *Br J Haematol* 91:387, 1995.

98. Jiang X, Lopez A, Holyoake T, et al.: Autocrine production and action of IL-3 and granulocyte colony-stimulating factor in chronic myeloid leukemia. *Proc Natl Acad Sci U S A* 96:12804, 1999.

99. Amarante Mendes GP, McGahon AJ, Nishioka WK et al.: Bcl-2-independent Bcr-Abl-mediated resistance to apoptosis: protection is correlated with up regulation of Bcl-xL. *Oncogene* 16:1383, 1998.

100. Amarante Mendes GP, Naekyung Kim C, Liu L, et al.: Bcr-Abl exerts its antiapoptotic effect against diverse apoptotic stimuli through blockage of mitochondrial release of cytochrome C and activation of caspase-3. *Blood* 91:1700, 1998.

101. Bedi A, Barber JP, Bedi GC, et al.: *BCR-ABL*-mediated inhibition of apoptosis with delay of G2/M transition after DNA damage: a mechanism of resistance to multiple anticancer agents. *Blood* 86:1148, 1995.

102. Cortez D, Kadlec L, Pendergast AM: Structural and signaling requirements for *BCR-ABL*-mediated transformation and inhibition of apoptosis. *Mol Cell Biol* 15:5531, 1995.

103. Kuribara R, Honda H, Matsui H, et al.: Roles of Bim in apoptosis of normal and Bcr-Abl-expressing hematopoietic progenitors. *Mol Cell Biol* 24:6172, 2004.

104. Gordon MY, Dowding CR, Riley GP, et al.: Altered adhesive interactions with marrow stroma of haematopoietic progenitor cells in chronic myeloid leukaemia. *Nature* 328:342, 1987.

105. Salgia R, Quackenbush E, Lin J, et al.: The BCR/ABL oncogene alters the chemotactic response to stromal-derived factor-1alpha. *Blood* 94:4233, 1999.

106. Ramaraj P, Singh H, Niu N, et al.: Effect of mutational inactivation of tyrosine kinase activity on BCR/ABL-induced abnormalities in cell growth and adhesion in human hematopoietic progenitors. *Cancer Res* 64:5322, 2004.

107. Canitrot Y, Falinski R, Louat T, et al.: p210 BCR/ABL kinase regulates nucleotide excision repair (NER) and resistance to UV radiation. *Blood* 102:2632, 2003.

108. Canitrot Y, Lautier D, Laurent G, et al.: Mutator phenotype of BCR—ABL transfected Ba/F3 cell lines and its association with enhanced expression of DNA polymerase beta. *Oncogene* 18:2676, 1999.

109. Deutsch E, Dugray A, Abdul Karim B, et al.: *BCR-ABL* down-regulates the DNA repair protein DNA-PKcs. *Blood* 97:2084, 2001.

110. Dierov J, Dierova R, Carroll M: BCR/ABL translocates to the nucleus and disrupts an ATR-dependent intra-S phase checkpoint. *Cancer Cell* 5:275, 2004.

111. Takedam N, Shibuya M, Maru Y: The *BCR-ABL* onco-protein potentially interacts with the xeroderma pigmentosum group B protein. *Proc Natl Acad Sci U S A* 96:203, 1999.

112. Brummendorf TH, Holyoake TL, Rufer N, et al.: Prognostic implications of differences in telomere length between normal and malignant cells from patients with chronic myeloid leukemia measured by flow cytometry. *Blood* 95:1883, 2000.

113. Hernandez-Boluda JC, Cervantes F, Colomer D, et al.: Genomic p16 abnormalities in the progression of chronic myeloid leukemia into blast crisis: a sequential study in 42 patients. *Exp Hematol* 31:204, 2003.

114. Sill H, Goldman JM, Cross NC: Homozygous deletions of the p16 tumor-suppressor gene are associated with lymphoid transformation of chronic myeloid leukemia. *Blood* 85:2013, 1995.

115. Feinstein E, Cimino G, Gale RP, et al.: p53 in chronic myelogenous leukemia in acute phase. *Proc Natl Acad Sci U S A* 88:6293, 1991.

116. Towatari M, Adachi K, Kato H, et al.: Absence of the human retinoblastoma gene product in the megakaryoblastic crisis of chronic myelogenous leukemia. *Blood* 78:2178, 1991.

117. Deguchi K, Gilliland DG: Cooperativity between mutations in tyrosine kinases and in hematopoietic transcription factors in AML. *Leukemia* 16:740, 2002.

118. Dash AB, Williams IR, Kutok JL, et al.: A murine model of CML blast crisis induced by cooperation between BCR/ABL and NUP98/HOXA9. *Proc Natl Acad Sci U S A* 99:7622, 2002.

119. Carapeti M, Goldman JM, Cross NC: Overexpression of EVI-1 in blast crisis of chronic myeloid leukemia. *Leukemia* 10:1561, 1996.

120. Cuenco GM, Ren R: Cooperation of *BCR-ABL* and AML1/MDS1/EVI1 in blocking myeloid differentiation and rapid induction of an acute myelogenous leukemia. *Oncogene* 20:8236, 2001.

121. Cuenco GM, Ren R: Both AML1 and EVI1 oncogenic components are required for the cooperation of AML1/MDS1/EVI1 with BCR/ABL in the induction of acute myelogenous leukemia in mice. *Oncogene* 23:569, 2004.

122. Helbling D, Mueller BU, Timchenko NA, et al.: The leukemic fusion gene AML1-MDS1-EVI1 suppresses CEBPA in acute myeloid leukemia by activation of Calreticulin. *Proc Natl Acad Sci U S A* 101:13312, 2004.

123. Perrotti D, Cesi V, Trotta R, et al.: *BCR-ABL* suppresses C/EBPalpha expression through inhibitory action of hnRNP E2. *Nat Genet* 30:48, 2002.

124. Jamieson CH, Ailles LE, Dylla SJ, et al.: Granulocyte-macrophage progenitors as candidate leukemic stem cells in blast-crisis CML. *N Engl J Med* 351:657, 2004.

125. Gaiger A, Henn T, Hoerth E, et al.: Increase of *BCR-ABL* chimeric mRNA expression in tumor cells of patients with chronic myeloid leukemia precedes disease progression. *Blood* 86:2371, 1995.

126. Asimakopoulos FA, Shteper PJ, Krichevsky S, et al.: ABL1 methylation is a distinct molecular event associated with clonal evolution of chronic myeloid leukemia. *Blood* 94:2452, 1999.

127. Elefanty AG, Cory S: Hematologic disease induced in BALB/c mice by a bcr-abl retrovirus is influenced by the infection conditions. *Mol Cell Biol* 12:1755, 1992.

128. Pear WS, Miller JP, Xu L, et al.: Efficient and rapid induction of a chronic myelogenous leukemia-like myeloproliferative disease in mice receiving P210 bcr/abl-transduced bone marrow. *Blood* 92:3780, 1998.

129. Heisterkamp N, Jenster G, Kioussis D, et al.: Human bcr-abl gene has a lethal effect on embryogenesis. *Transgenic Res* 1:45, 1991.

130. Koschmieder S, Goettgens B, Zhang P, et al.: Inducible chronic phase of myeloid leukemia with expansion of hematopoietic stem cells in a transgenic model of *BCR-ABL* leukemogenesis. *Blood* 105:324, 2005.

# Chapter 18

# TREATMENT APPROACH TO CHRONIC-PHASE CHRONIC MYELOGENOUS LEUKEMIA

*Jorge E. Cortes*

The treatment of chronic myelogenous leukemia (CML) has been characterized in recent years by some of the most remarkable achievements in the treatment of cancer.[1] Some of the best results obtained with allogeneic stem cell transplantation (SCT) have been reported in CML, and some of the leading observations that triggered our current knowledge about graft-versus-leukemia effect and the immunology of transplant were pioneered in CML. CML was probably also one of the first malignancies in which a biologic agent, interferon alpha (IFN-α), was able to eliminate the disease, substantiated by the achievement of a complete cytogenetic remission in a fraction of all patients treated. Most recently, the introduction of imatinib mesylate represents one of the best examples of a target-specific therapy that has resulted in complete responses for the majority of patients with this disease. The availability of several treatment modalities that may improve the survival of patients with any malignancy is welcome. The current challenge, however, is to learn to integrate these strategies in a way that will result in the greatest probability of long-term survival for most patients diagnosed with CML. It is no longer a matter of treatment options, but of treatment strategies. In this chapter, we will discuss the current treatment alternatives for patients with CML in chronic phase. This is an evolving field not free of controversy, and the major elements of this controversy will be discussed here. Although IFN-α has been largely replaced by imatinib as the centerpiece of the management of patients with chronic-phase CML, the lessons learned from IFN-α are important and will therefore be discussed first.

## IFN-α

Treatment with IFN-α resulted in a complete cytogenetic remission (i.e., 0% Philadelphia-chromosome (Ph)-positive metaphases) in 5–25% of the patients treated. A partial cytogenetic response (i.e., 1–34% Ph-positive metaphases) was achieved in 10–15% of the patients treated, for a major cytogenetic remission rate (i.e., 0–34% Ph-positive) of 30–35%.[2] With the addition of other agents, particularly cytarabine, a complete cytogenetic response was achieved in up to 35% of patients and a major remission in up to 50%.[3-7] Achieving a complete cytogenetic remission was associated with an improved survival: 78% of the patients who achieved a complete response are alive at 10 years.[8] Patients with a partial cytogenetic remission have a survival advantage (39% at 10 years) over those with a minor cytogenetic response (i.e., 35–95% Ph-positive) or no cytogenetic response (25% at 10 years), although survival is not as favorable as that for patients achieving a complete remission. Thus, the goal of therapy in the IFN-α era became achievement of a complete cytogenetic remission, in contrast to the hematologic response, which was the goal of therapy in the hydroxyurea/busulfan era.

Among patients who achieve a complete cytogenetic remission, there is a significant variability in terms of their molecular response. Patients who retain high levels of minimal residual disease by quantitative polymerase chain reaction (Q-PCR) have a high probability of relapse, whereas 80% of those with levels <0.045% remained in remission after 3 years.[9] Furthermore, approximately 30% of patients who achieve a complete cytogenetic remission have undetectable disease by PCR (i.e., achieve complete molecular remission). These patients are cured from CML, with none having relapsed after a median follow-up of 10 years.[8] Among those with residual disease by PCR, 40–60% have remained in cytogenetic remission after 10 years in what has been called "functional cure." Although this finding emphasizes the significance of achieving a molecular remission, it also points to the fact that some patients might live with low levels of minimal residual disease with no clinical evidence of CML. This has been attributed to immune mechanisms stimulated by IFN-α. In fact, cytotoxic T lymphocytes specific for PR1, a peptide derived from proteinase 3, which is overexpressed in CML, are found in patients in complete remission after IFN-α therapy (or SCT) but not in those without complete cytogenetic remission or those treated with chemotherapy.[10] These lymphocytes may be responsible for the elimination or control of the residual leukemic cells.

## STEM CELL TRANSPLATATION (SCT)

The results, techniques, and practical aspects of SCT will be described in detail in Chapter 37. However, some important aspects of SCT in CML and its integration with other treatment options are discussed here. First, SCT may be curative for a significant fraction of eligible patients who receive a transplant from a human leukocyte antigen (HLA)-identical sibling. Unfortunately, because of the requirements for age, adequate organ function and performance status, and availability of donor, only a fraction of patients are eligible for this procedure. The expected proportion of all patients with CML that may be eligible for a stem cell transplant is unknown, but considering that the median age is 66 years,[11] it is probably a small percentage.

The expected results with this procedure can be exemplified by a recent series from Seattle.[12] This study used targeted busulfan plus cyclophosphamide as the conditioning regimen for 131 patients in early chronic phase with a median age of 43 years (range, 14–66 years). At 3 years, the projected nonrelapse mortality rate was 14%, and 78% were projected to be alive and free of disease. Among survivors, 60% had extensive chronic graft-versus-host disease (GVHD) 1 year after transplantation, but only 10% had a Karnofsky score less than 80%. Interestingly, 11% of patients had minimal residual disease documented by PCR, but had not relapsed at the time of the report, suggesting that a mechanism such as immune surveillance could prevent relapse of the disease.[12] This phenomenon would be similar to the "functional cure" described with IFN-α. Occasionally, patients may relapse many years after SCT. Few series have analyzed the very long-term results of SCT, and thus the magnitude of this problem is difficult to measure. A recent series analyzed the very long-term follow-up of 89 patients transplanted at a single institution.[13] Twenty-eight (32%) were alive 10 or more years after their transplant. The mean time to hematologic or cytogenetic relapse was 7.7 years, with five patients relapsing more than 10 years after transplantation.

Results with SCT for patients transplanted in more advanced stages of the disease (accelerated or blast phase) are worse, with 5-year survival probabilities of 40–60% for patients in accelerated phase and 10–20% for those in blast phase. Patients in blast phase who are transplanted in second chronic phase may have long-term outcomes similar to those of patients in accelerated phase. For patients who do not have a sibling donor, transplantation from a matched unrelated donor (MUD) is an option. The results with MUD transplants have been inferior, mostly because of the increased risk of GVHD. The long-term disease-free survival rate after MUD transplant for young patients transplanted within 1 year from diagnosis is 57% compared to 67% for those receiving transplants from matched siblings.[14] The results with MUD are, however, improving in recent years with decreasing rates of GVHD and improving probability of long-term survival with the use of molecularly matched donors, although this may further limit the availability of donors. In an attempt to make the SCT option available to more patients, nonmyeloablative transplants have been used for those of older age or with other health considerations that would otherwise prevent them from receiving a SCT. Long-term results are not yet available with these techniques, but early results in small series report disease-free survival rates as high as 85% at 70 months.[15] If these results hold in larger series with long-term follow-up, stem cell transplant would be applicable for the more typical patients (i.e., median age 66 years) who have matched sibling donors. The use of alternative donors, such as cord blood or haploidentical donors, is still in early investigational stages and has not demonstrated any advantage over nontransplant investigational options.

One important aspect to consider in the setting of other effective treatment options is the timing of SCT. Earlier results from the IBMTR suggested that SCT performed after 12 months from the time of diagnosis had a significantly inferior outcome. Recently, it has been suggested that transplant within the first 24 months,[16] and in some series within 36 months,[17] have similar outcomes to those performed within the first 12 months. Thus, decisions regarding SCT must be made early and reevaluated at early time points in patients who are treated with imatinib but are transplant candidates. These considerations will be further discussed later in the chapter.

Another important consideration is the possible effect that prior therapy with other agents may have on the results expected with stem cell transplant. Some studies had suggested that prior therapy with IFN-α adversely affected the outcome after transplantation.[18] However, several subsequent trials demonstrated that no such adverse effect exists.[19–22] Some early observations suggest that prior therapy with imatinib has no adverse impact on the outcome after SCT.[23,24] Although these observations are still limited and have short follow-up, there is little reason to believe that a significant effect may be observed.

## IMATINIB MESYLATE

The first clinical use of imatinib mesylate (imatinib) in CML was among patients who had failed prior therapy with IFN-α-based therapy or who could not tolerate this therapy. In a dose-finding study, using daily doses of 25–1000 mg daily, few responses were observed at doses of up to 250 mg daily.[25] However, 98% of patients receiving a dose of at least 300 mg daily achieved a complete hematologic response (CHR), and 54% achieved a cytogenetic response. In addition, imatinib proved to be well tolerated at doses up to 1000 mg, with no dose limiting toxicity identified, and a maximum tolerated dose was not reached.[25] A dose of 400 mg daily was selected for a subsequent study including 454 patients in late chronic phase who had failed or were intolerant to IFN-α therapy.[26] At the most recent update, a CHR was achieved in 95% and a major cytogenetic response in 60 % (complete in 48%). After a median follow-up of 18 months, the progression-free survival rate was 89%, and 95% of the patients were alive.[26] Similar results have been reported in more recent, smaller series.[9,10] The use of imatinib in this setting is now over 5-years old, and longer-term follow-up has been reported in a cohort of 261 patients treated at a single institution.[27] A major cytogenetic response has been achieved in 73% of patients, including a complete response in 61%. Responses have been durable, with over 90% of patients who achieved a complete cytogenetic response maintaining a major response. With a median follow-up of nearly 4 years, 80% of patients were alive and free of progression and 86% are alive. More importantly, the molecular responses to imatinib have continued to improve, with 31% of patients with a BCR-ABL/ABL ratio of <0.05% and 15% with undetectable BCR-ABL transcripts by nested PCR. These results show that the favorable response to imatinib is durable after 4 years for the majority of patients; these results may continue to improve with continuation of therapy.[27]

These favorable results have been confirmed with imatinib in early chronic-phase CML when used as first-line therapy. A multicenter randomized trial compared imatinib with IFN-α and low-dose ara-C in patients with previously untreated, early chronic-phase CML (IRIS trial).[28] After a median follow-up of 18 months, the estimated rate of a major cytogenetic response was 87% in the imatinib group and 35% in the IFN-α plus ara-C group (p <0.001). The estimated rates of complete cytogenetic response were 76% and 15%, respectively (p <0.001). At 18 months, the estimated rate of freedom from progression to accelerated or blastic phase was 97% in the imatinib group and 92% in the IFN-α group (p <0.001). The toxicity profile and quality of life were significantly better for patients treated with imatinib.[29] However, a survival advantage could not be demonstrated in this study for patients treated with imatinib, mostly due to early crossover from IFN-α to imatinib (by protocol design or by patient's choice) in over 85% of the patients randomized to IFN-α. An analysis of imatinib-treated patients compared to a historical control treated with IFN-α-based therapy shows the significant survival advantage that would be expected with the higher rate of cytogenetic and molecular responses seen with imatinib.[30] A recent update of the IRIS trial reported a rate of complete cytogenetic response of 86%. These responses have been durable, with 93% of patients who achieved a complete cytogenetic response still having this response after 60 months. The estimated survival free of transformation at 5 years is 93% and the overall survival is 89% (95% if only CML-related deaths are considered). Another independent series of 50 similar patients treated with the standard dose (400 mg) of imatinib reported similar results: a major cytogenetic response in 90% and a complete cytogenetic response in 72%.[31] Thus, imatinib has become the standard initial therapy for patients with CML. A discussion regarding the decision between transplant and imatinib and treatment algorithms will be presented at the end of this chapter.

### DOSE

The standard imatinib dose for patients treated in chronic phase is 400 mg daily. The selection of this dose after the dose-finding phase I study was somewhat arbitrary, as no dose limiting toxicity was identified at doses of up to 1000 mg daily.[25] It also provided some suggestion of improved responses with higher doses, as few responses were observed at the lowest doses, and 53% of those treated with 140–250 mg daily had a hematologic response (11% had a cytogenetic response). Nearly all patients treated at doses of 300 mg or higher had a hematologic response and 54% achieved a cytogenetic response.[25] Thus, current recommendations are to avoid treating patients with less than 300 mg of imatinib daily. Furthermore, there is a growing evidence that higher doses of imatinib (600–800 mg daily) may result in significantly higher response rates (and faster responses) compared to the standard dose. One study used 800 mg daily for patients who had failed prior IFN-α-based therapy but had never received imatinib.[32] A complete cytogenetic response was achieved in 90% of the patients, compared to the historical 48% with standard dose in a similar population. More importantly, 50% of the patients had undetectable levels of BCR-ABL with nested PCR.[32] A subsequent study used the same approach for untreated patients with CML in early chronic phase. Among 114 such patients treated with 800 mg of imatinib daily (in two divided doses of 400 mg), a complete cytogenetic response was achieved in 90%, most within 6 months of the start of therapy. After 18 months of therapy, 28% of the patients had undetectable BCR-ABL by nested PCR, compared to 4–10% with standard dose imatinib.[32] A third study, from a different group, used 600 mg of imatinib and previously untreated patients with early chronic-phase CML, increasing the dose to 800 mg if responses were not progressing according to predetermined desired endpoints. After 6 months of therapy, 79% of patients had achieved a complete cytogenetic response. Patients who received the target dose with no dose reductions had a significantly better molecular response than those receiving lower average doses, even if higher than the standard, suggesting improved molecular responses with increasing doses.[33] Thus, although today the standard dose of imatinib for chronic-phase CML is still 400 mg daily, the data summarized above suggest that this may be changing in the near future.

### MONITORING

For many years, hematologic response was the goal of therapy with agents such as hydroxyurea and busulfan. The most important legacy of the IFN-α era was to demonstrate that achieving a cytogenetic response would prolong the survival of patients with CML.[8,34] The goal of therapy became achieving a major, and particularly a complete cytogenetic response. With most patients achieving a complete cytogenetic response on imatinib, the goal of therapy is shifting again now toward achieving a molecular response. Eliminating all evidence of minimal residual disease (at least according to currently available techniques) is associated with improved probability of long-term remissions in many tumors. This is clearly true also in CML.

The clinical significance of molecular monitoring in CML is best documented in patients treated with an SCT. Patients who have BCR-ABL detectable by PCR, particularly if later than 6 months after transplant, have a significantly higher probability of relapse.[35,36] Furthermore, Q-PCR has become an important tool to determine the risk of relapse. Patients with the highest levels of BCR-ABL transcripts have the highest risk of relapse.[35,36] Molecular monitoring with Q-PCR is thus routine after SCT. Indeed, early intervention (e.g., donor lymphocyte infusion) is frequently indicated based on increasing levels of BCR-ABL transcripts, with the best results obtained when intervention occurs at the first evidence of relapse. Among patients treated with IFN-α, there is a considerable heterogeneity in the levels of BCR-ABL transcripts detectable among those who achieve a complete cytogenetic response. However, the risk of relapse is minimal for patients with levels below the median, while most of those with higher levels lose their response.[9] Indeed, approximately one-third of patients who achieve a complete cytogenetic response have undetectable BCR-ABL transcripts by nested PCR, and none of these patients has lost this response after 10 years.[8]

Despite the relatively brief follow-up available for patients treated with imatinib, there is mounting evidence that molecular monitoring has important clinical implications. The IRIS trial demonstrated a significantly improved molecular response with imatinib compared to IFN-α at each time point from the achievement of complete cytogenetic response.[37] Overall, after a median follow-up of 18 months, nearly 40% of the patients treated with imatinib had a 3-log reduction of BCR-ABL transcripts, and 4–10% had undetectable BCR-ABL levels. This magnitude of response was rare among patients treated with IFN-α. This may have been due, in fact, to the short follow-up for patients treated with IFN-α, as over 80% of patients crossed over to the imatinib arm after a short period of time. Still, with the significantly higher rate of complete cytogenetic responses achieved with imatinib, it is likely that a significant difference would have been observed even if patients had continued IFN-α therapy. Furthermore, obtaining a molecular response earlier has important clinical implications. Among patients who achieved a complete cytogenetic response with imatinib, those who had at least a 3-log reduction in BCR-ABL transcripts at 12 months from the start of therapy had a significantly better probability of progression-free survival compared to those who had a less pronounced reduction.[37] In another study of patients in chronic phase, who had achieved a complete cytogenetic response after imatinib therapy, those who achieved levels of BCR-ABL/ABL ratio of <0.05% (i.e., major molecular response) had a significantly lower probability of losing their cytogenetic response compared to those who did not reach these levels.[38] The difference was even more significant when considering only patients who achieved a complete molecular response (i.e., undetectable BCR-ABL). Similarly, those who had achieved a major molecular response after 12 months of therapy had a significantly better predicted probability of a sustained complete cytogenetic remission.[38] A third study with a relatively smaller cohort of patients confirmed a longer duration of complete cytogenetic response for patients who had a maximum reduction of BCR-ABL transcripts of at least 2 logs.[39] It has also been suggested that patients who have lower levels of transcripts detectable after the first few months of therapy with imatinib have a significantly lower probability of developing point mutations conferring resistance to imatinib. Thus, it is evident from these studies that the objective of therapy in the imatinib era should be to achieve at least a major molecular response, and that achieving this response early increases the probability of a long-term durable response.

A recommended algorithm for monitoring patients receiving therapy with imatinib is presented in Table 18.1. At the time of diagnosis, it is recommended that all patients have a regular karyotype as well as Q-PCR

**Table 18.1** Recommendations for monitoring of patients treated with imatinib

| Timing | Recommended tests and frequency |
|---|---|
| At diagnosis | • Cytogenetics, Q-PCR, ?FISH |
| First year | • Cytogenetics every 3–6 months |
| | • Q-PCR every 3–6 months |
| After first year | • Cytogenetics every 6–12 months |
| | • Q-PCR every 3–6 months |

Q-PCR = quantitative polymerase chain reaction; FISH = fluorescent in situ hybridization.

(real-time PCR) done. As will be discussed later in this chapter, the first 12 months of therapy may be the most critical to establish the long-term prognosis of the patient, and therefore to make treatment decisions. Thus, during these first months, repeat monitoring is recommended every 3–6 months. This should include Q-PCR and cytogenetics. The major inconvenience of monitoring with cytogenetics is the need for a bone marrow aspiration. However, this is the only test to date that gives reliable information regarding other chromosomal abnormalities. The presence of additional chromosomal abnormalities may reduce the probability of response to imatinib and the overall survival.[40–42] In addition, 6–8% of patients who respond to imatinib may develop chromosomal abnormalities in the Ph-negative metaphases.[42–44] Although the long-term implications of these abnormalities are still uncertain, it is important to recognize and follow this phenomenon. After the first 12 months of therapy, Q-PCR should be performed at least every 6–12 months and a routine cytogenetic analysis every 12 months. Fluorescent in situ hybridization can be used to monitor the cytogenetic response between cytogenetic analysis, as it can be done in peripheral blood. However, even with the newest probes, there is a small percentage of false positivity. For the determination of molecular response, a Q-PCR (i.e., real-time PCR) is needed. Unfortunately, this test is not widely available. Furthermore, there is considerable heterogeneity between the reports from different laboratories, and the results from many laboratories that offer this test have not been clinically validated. In addition, the analysis of the results from the IRIS trial, the largest to date to report on molecular monitoring, initiated molecular monitoring only after the patients achieved complete cytogenetic response. To determine the log reduction at different time points, a baseline was derived from results obtained from 30 patients. Thus, a 3-log reduction in fact corresponds to levels of <0.036%, which is a 3-log reduction from the standardized base line of 36% for the sample cohort. Using each patient's individual baseline value to determine the 3-log reduction has not been validated as an important endpoint.

## CONTINUATION OF THERAPY

Once a patient starts therapy with imatinib, early endpoints are predictive of longer-term response and should be followed carefully. The initial report on patients in chronic phase treated with imatinib after IFN-α failure showed that patients who have no cytogenetic response after 3 months of therapy have only a 12% probability of later achieving a complete cytogenetic response with continuation of therapy. In contrast, patients who have achieved at least a minor cytogenetic response after 3–12 months of therapy have a 35–50% probability of later achieving a complete response.[45] A similar analysis of patients with previously untreated chronic-phase CML derived from the IRIS population has recently been presented.[46] Patients with no or minor cytogenetic response after 3 months of therapy have a 50% probability of achieving a complete cytogenetic response at 2 years. However, patients with no cytogenetic response after 6 months of therapy have only approximately a 10% probability of achieving a complete cytogenetic response at 2 years, compared with 50% for those with at least a minor response. After 12 months of therapy, only those patients who have achieved a partial cytogenetic response have a reasonable probability of achieving a complete response with continuation of therapy.[46] These observations have been incorporated into the treatment algorithm proposed in Figure 18.1.

## DISCONTINUATION OF THERAPY

An important consideration is whether imatinib therapy can be safely discontinued for patients who have an adequate response (e.g., complete cytogenetic or molecular response) and if so when to do it. There is only limited published information in this regard, including case reports or small series.[47–49] Two patients have been reported to have a sustained response after discontinuation of therapy. However, one series of three patients and one patient from another series have all lost their response after discontinuation of therapy following a complete molecular response. Interestingly, the responses were lost rapidly (i.e., within 3–6 months) after discontinuation of therapy, uncovering more rapid kinetics of the disease than are traditionally recognized. In at least two patients where imatinib was reinitiated, patients again rapidly responded, suggesting that resistance to imatinib had not evolved, but rather that continuation of therapy was required. It has been suggested that the earliest, probably quiescent, progenitor cells in CML are insensitive to imatinib in vitro.[50] It is conceivable that these progenitors might trigger proliferation of leukemia once the inhibitory pressure of imatinib is eliminated. In view of these observations, even when limited, the current recommendation is to continue therapy with imatinib indefinitely.

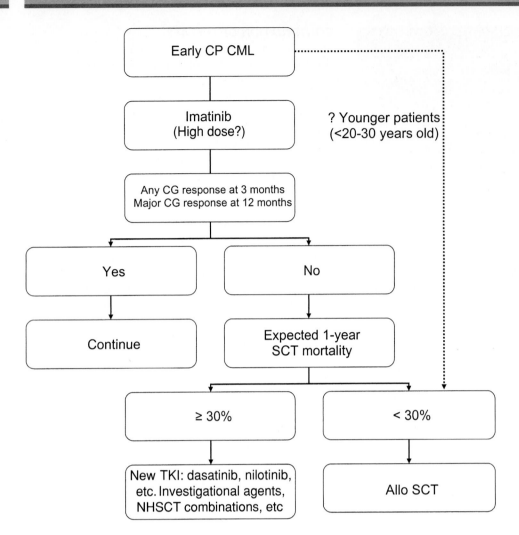

**Figure 18.1** *Proposed treatment algorithm for patients with CML in early chronic phase. TKI, tyrosine kinase inhibitors)*

### MANAGEMENT OF MYELOSUPPRESSION

Overall, imatinib is well tolerated. Probably the most common adverse event with imatinib is myelosuppression. Grade 3 or higher neutropenia (i.e., neutrophils $<1 \times 10^9/L$) occurs in up to 35–45% of patients, and thrombocytopenia in 20–25%.[26,28,32,51,52] Severe anemia is less common, occurring in 5–10% of the patients. All of these are more common in patients who have failed prior therapies (e.g., IFN-α), and are dose-related, occurring more frequently among patients treated with higher doses. Patients who develop grade 3 or higher neutropenia or thrombocytopenia may have a lower probability of achieving a cytogenetic response. The adverse prognosis is particularly noticeable among patients whose myelosuppression lasts longer than 2 weeks.[51,53] This has been attributed to a decreased dose intensity, as the current recommendation is to interrupt therapy in patients who develop this degree of myelosuppression and reduce the doses for those who take more than 2 weeks to recover.[54] To try to overcome these events, hematopoietic growth factors have been used. Most patients who develop neutropenia respond rapidly to the use of filgrastim (G-CSF)[55–57],

allowing for more continued therapy with imatinib and improved response in many instances. A similar effect has been reported with oprelvekin (interleukin-11) for patients with thrombocytopenia.[58] Patients with anemia do not carry an inferior prognosis.[59] This is probably due to the fact that most patients have only grade 1 or 2 anemia, and it is not currently recommended to interrupt therapy for anemia grade 3 or higher. There have been reports about the effective use of erythropoietin[59,60] and darbepoetin[61] for these patients. Although these short series suggest that the use of these growth factors is safe in these settings, their use is not currently standard or approved and should be considered with caution. In addition, most patients who develop myelosuppression will not need hematopoietic growth support. This adverse event is more frequently seen during the first few months of therapy. Treatment interruption is frequently all that is needed for recovery, and most patients will not even require dose reductions. Myelosuppression after the first 3 months of therapy is less common and it is in this setting that it may represent a more significant management problem, particularly when prolonged or recurrent.

**Table 18.2** Management of adverse events associated with imatinib therapy

*Myelosuppression*

Monitor CBC weekly for 2–3 months, then every 4–6 weeks

Hold therapy for grade ≥3 neutropenia or thrombocytopenia:
- ANC $<1 \times 10^9$/L
- Platelets $<50 \times 10^9$/L

Do not hold for anemia

Monitor CBC at least weekly after holding

Restart when ANC $\geq 1 \times 10^9$/L, platelets $\geq 50 \times 10^9$/L
- If recovery occurs within 2 weeks, restart at the same dose
- If recovery takes longer than 2 weeks, decrease the dose (not less than 300 mg/d)

Consider use of growth factors (G-CSF, IL-11, EPO) for patients with recurrent myelosuppression

*Nonhematologic toxicity*

Manage grade ≤2 toxicity early. Some suggestions include

| Adverse event | Management |
| --- | --- |
| Nausea | Antiemetics (Compazine, |
| Diarrhea | Zofran, etc) |
| Skin rash | Antiadiarrhea (Imodium, |
| Peripheral edema | Lomotil, etc) |
| Periorbital edema | Topical and/or systemic |
| Muscle cramps | steroids, antihistamines |
| Bone aches | Diuretics |
| Liver dysfunction | Preparation H |
| | Tonic water, quinine, calcium supplements |
| | Nonsteroidal anti-inflammatory agents |
| | Monitor frequently |

Hold therapy for grade ≥3 toxicity or persistent grade 2 toxicity not responding to optimal management

Restart therapy at a lower dose when toxicity resolves to grade ≤1

CBC, complete blood count; ANC, absolute neutrophil count.

### *MANAGEMENT OF OTHER TOXICITIES*

Although nonhematologic adverse events are relatively common with imatinib, these are frequently mild, and can be managed easily. Grade 3 or higher adverse events are seen seldomly, and only 2–3% of the patients require permanent discontinuation of therapy because of toxicity. A guideline for the management of the most common adverse events is presented in Table 18.2. Early intervention is important to help avoid more significant problems and unnecessary treatment interruptions and dose reductions. There has been some concern regarding the possibility of late adverse events with prolonged therapy with imatinib in view of its inhibition of c-kit and platelet derived growth factor receptor (PDGFR). However, to date, there is no evidence of any unexpected late complications.

## TREATMENT RECOMMENDATIONS

The most complex and controversial aspect of therapy is the treatment algorithm for a patient with previously untreated CML in early chronic phase. The results with imatinib, particularly with higher doses, are excellent. The one major drawback of imatinib treatment is the relatively short follow-up, as this modality has been used for patients with previously untreated chronic-phase CML for only approximately 6 years and as a first line of therapy for approximately 5 years. As the results continue to improve, imatinib would become the preferred therapy for all patients, as it is associated with minimal toxicity and with no treatment-related mortality. If an extrapolation can be made from the IFN-α data, it is reasonable to expect that a significant proportion of patients may be cured with imatinib. Seventy-eight percent of patients who achieve a complete cytogenetic response with IFN-α are alive after 10 years, but only 25–35% of patients achieve this response with IFN-α-based therapy. With imatinib, 80–90% of patients achieve this response. Responses also occur earlier with imatinib, and early responses are associated with an improved long-term outcome. More importantly, the rate of molecular responses is significantly higher with imatinib, suggesting that there are not only more, but better responses with this agent compared to IFN-α. However, the immune modulation that is associated with IFN-α therapy is lacking with imatinib. Immune phenomena are thought to be responsible for the long-term durable cytogenetic and hematologic responses after IFN-α therapy, even in the setting of minimal residual disease (i.e., "functional cures" or dormant state).[10,62] Allogeneic SCT can be curative in a significant proportion of patients eligible to receive this approach. Besides availability of a donor and age, the major consideration of whether or not to pursue this therapy is the risk of early mortality and the long-term complications. Early mortality is usually lowest among younger patients, particularly those younger than age 20–30 years. Most studies of SCT emphasize the results in the first few years, but late relapses and complications should also be taken into consideration. Extensive chronic GVHD can be seen in as many as 60% of the patients treated,[12] and late relapses can occur in some patients.[13] All of these issues need to be evaluated when deciding on SCT, and the local experience at the site where the transplant is to be performed needs to be taken into account. When alternative transplant options are being sought, the increased risks and lack of long-term data should be recognized. Matched unrelated transplants may be associated with increased mortality and GVHD, although molecular matching has decreased these risks considerably. Thus, if the local experience is favorable, these transplants could be considered for younger patients.

Nonmyeloablative conditioning regimens have allowed offering transplantation to patients in older age groups or with comorbid conditions. The early mortality is decreased with these transplants, though late complications may be similar to full ablative regimens. These are still relatively new options and there is little long-term data on efficacy and late complications. As longer-term follow-up becomes available regarding the incidence of late relapses and complications, these options may become more standard. Transplantations with alternative donors, such as mismatched and haploidentical donors and umbilical cords, should be considered investigational and considered only when other options have failed.

For a patient who has no option for a stem cell transplant, the decision regarding frontline therapy is simple and the treatment of choice is undoubtedly imatinib. More controversial at this time is the proper dose at which treatment should be initiated. The standard dose is 400 mg daily. However, as mentioned earlier, results with higher doses have strongly suggested that these doses are more effective and well tolerated for the majority of patients. Ideally, all patients should be included in clinical trials looking at either high-dose imatinib or imatinib-based combinations. Several trials of this nature are currently being performed around the world. For the patient who will not be entered in a clinical trial, although higher doses may be preferred, they may not be practical for financial or other considerations. In such instances, the standard dose can be initiated. Close monitoring is of the outmost importance in such cases, and increasing the dose when response goals are not being met at the desired times should be encouraged.

The decision regarding therapy is more complicated and controversial for young patients who have a fully matched sibling. Results with transplant are best among those younger than age 25–30 years, and SCT should be given consideration. As a patient's age increases, the risks involved with transplantation also increase. For most patients, an initial trial with imatinib is probably adequate. However, if the decision is made to start therapy with imatinib, it is important, particularly in the case of the younger patients with an adequate sibling donor, to monitor the patient closely with cytogenetic and molecular monitoring to be certain that the response is progressing as desired.

The proposed ideal goals for patients being treated with imatinib are presented in Table 18.3. For a patient who has not achieved a hematologic response by 3 months, or a minor cytogenetic response by 6 months or partial by 12 months, changing therapies should be strongly considered. What the alternative therapy should be in these cases varies from patient to patient. Increasing the dose of imatinib to 800 mg daily would be the first choice for patients who are being treated with standard dose of imatinib and have had no significant nonhematologic toxicity. If the patient has had hematologic toxicity at the lower doses, the use of hematopoietic growth factors can be considered. For patients who have already been taking higher dose imatinib, and who have the option of an allogeneic stem cell transplant, this option should be considered if the expected 1-year mortality is <40%.

Some scenarios are controversial, and sufficient information may be lacking to make strong recommendations. Patients who achieve a complete cytogenetic remission but have less than a 3-log reduction in transcript levels have a worse prognosis than those who have at least a 3-log reduction. However, the progression-free survival at 3 years is still 92% and it probably does not justify a change in therapy, particularly when there is a significant risk of mortality or other serious complications. Patients who show an increase in transcript levels after reaching a nadir also pose a dilemma. It has been suggested that a twofold increase may herald the appearance of mutations,[63] but this data has not been confirmed by other studies. Also, the short survival proposed for patients with P-loop mutations has not been confirmed in other studies. Thus, at this time, strong recommendations cannot be made based on molecular monitoring alone, particularly when the risks involved with the proposed new therapy are high. The same can be said about the appearance of chromosomal abnormalities in Ph-negative metaphases that occurs in up to 16% of patients. The few instances in which such patients have been diagnosed with myelodysplastic syndromes have been based on soft criteria. Indeed, in many instances these abnormalities may spontaneously disappear. Thus, in the absence of clear data suggesting that these changes affect the long-term outcome of patients, they deserve no more than careful monitoring.

**Table 18.3**  Recommendations regarding continuation of therapy with imatinib by response at various times after initiation of imatinib therapy

| Response | Months of treatment | | | |
| --- | --- | --- | --- | --- |
| | 3 | 6 | 9 | 12 |
| No CHR | Change | Change | Change | Change |
| CHR, >95% Ph-positive | Continue | Change | Change | Change |
| CHR, 35–95% Ph-positive | Continue | Continue | Continue | Change |
| CHR, 1–35% Ph-positive | Continue | Continue | Continue | Change |

CHR, complete hematologic response.

## CONCLUSION

The introduction of imatinib has changed our considerations for treatment for patients with CML in chronic phase. For most patients, imatinib should be the standard and therapy should be optimized with the intention to achieve a molecular remission as early as possible. Controversy exists regarding the ideal strategy for young patients with the option of an allogeneic stem cell transplant, and probably either option is appropriate as a first-line therapy. Adequate management is particularly important in these patients if one is to optimize the probability of achieving long-term durable remissions and minimize the risks for the majority of patients with CML.

## *REFERENCES*

1. Faderl S, Talpaz M, Estrov Z, Kantarjian HM: Chronic myelogenous leukemia: biology and therapy. *Ann Intern Med* 131:207–219, 1999.
2. Kantarjian HM, Smith T, O'Brien S, et al.: Prolonged survival in chronic myelogenous leukemia after cytogenetic response to interferon-therapy. *Ann Intern Med* 122:254–261, 1995.
3. O'Brien S, Kantarjian H, Koller C, et al.: Sequential homoharringtonine and interferon-alpha in the treatment of early chronic phase chronic myelogenous leukemia. *Blood* 93:4149–4153, 1999.
4. O'Brien S, Talpaz M, Cortes J, et al.: Simultaneous homoharringtonine and interferon-alpha in the treatment of patients with chronic-phase chronic myelogenous leukemia. *Cancer* 94:2024–2032, 2002.
5. Baccarani M, Rosti G, de Vivo A, et al.: A randomized study of interferon-alpha versus interferon-alpha and low-dose arabinosyl cytosine in chronic myeloid leukemia. *Blood* 99:1527–1535, 2002.
6. Kantarjian HM, O'Brien S, Smith TL, et al.: Treatment of Philadelphia chromosome-positive early chronic phase chronic myelogenous leukemia with daily doses of interferon alpha and low-dose cytarabine. *J Clin Oncol* 17:284–292, 1999.
7. Guilhot F, Chastang C, Michallet M, et al.: Interferon alfa-2b combined with cytarabine versus interferon alone in chronic myelogenous leukemia. French Chronic Myeloid Leukemia Study Group [see comments]. *N Engl J Med* 337:223–229, 1997.
8. Kantarjian HM, O'Brien S, Cortes JE, et al.: Complete cytogenetic and molecular responses to interferon-alpha-based therapy for chronic myelogenous leukemia are associated with excellent long-term prognosis. *Cancer* 97:1033–1041, 2003.
9. Hochhaus A, Reiter A, Saussele S, et al.: Molecular heterogeneity in complete cytogenetic responders after interferon-alpha therapy for chronic myelogenous leukemia: low levels of minimal residual disease are associated with continuing remission. German CML Study Group and the UK MRC CML Study Group. *Blood* 95:62–66, 2000.
10. Molldrem JJ, Lee PP, Wang C, et al.: Evidence that specific T lymphocytes may participate in the elimination of chronic myelogenous leukemia. *Nat Med* 6:1018–1023, 2000.
11. Ries LAG, Eisner MP, Kosary CL, et al.: *SEER Cancer Statistics Review, 1975–2001, Vol. 2004.* Bethesda, MD: National Cancer Institute; 2004. Available at: http://seer.cancer.gov/csr/1975α2001/

12. Radich JP, Gooley T, Bensinger W, et al.: HLA-matched related hematopoietic cell transplantation for chronic-phase CML using a targeted busulfan and cyclophosphamide preparative regimen. *Blood* 102:31–35, 2003.
13. Kiss TL, Abdolell M, Jamal N, Minden MD, Lipton JH, Messner HA: Long-term medical outcomes and quality-of-life assessment of patients with chronic myeloid leukemia followed at least 10 years after allogeneic bone marrow transplantation. *J Clin Oncol* 20:2334–2343, 2002.
14. Weisdorf DJ, Anasetti C, Antin JH, et al.: Allogeneic bone marrow transplantation for chronic myelogenous leukemia: comparative analysis of unrelated versus matched sibling donor transplantation. *Blood* 99:1971–1977, 2002.
15. Or R, Shapira MY, Resnick I, et al.: Nonmyeloablative allogeneic stem cell transplantation for the treatment of chronic myeloid leukemia in first chronic phase. *Blood* 101:441–445, 2003.
16. Clift RA, Buckner CD, Thomas ED, et al.: Marrow transplantation for patients in accelerated phase of chronic myeloid leukemia. *Blood* 84:4368–4373, 1994.
17. Gratwohl A, Hermans J, Niederwieser D, et al.: Bone marrow transplantation for chronic myeloid leukemia: long-term results. Chronic Leukemia Working Party of the European Group for Bone Marrow Transplantation. *Bone Marrow Transplant* 12:509–516, 1993.
18. Morton AJ, Gooley T, Hansen JA, et al.: Association between pretransplant interferon-alpha and outcome after unrelated donor marrow transplantation for chronic myelogenous leukemia in chronic phase. *Blood* 92:394–401, 1998.
19. Giralt SA, Kantarjian HM, Talpaz M, et al.: Effect of prior interferon alfa therapy on the outcome of allogeneic bone marrow transplantation for chronic myelogenous leukemia. *J Clin Oncol* 11:1055–1061, 1993.
20. Giralt S, Szydlo R, Goldman JM, et al.: Effect of short-term interferon therapy on the outcome of subsequent HLA-identical sibling bone marrow transplantation for chronic myelogenous leukemia: an analysis from the international bone marrow transplant registry. *Blood* 95:410–415, 2000.
21. Hehlmann R, Hochhaus A, Kolb HJ, et al.: Interferon-alpha before allogeneic bone marrow transplantation in chronic myelogenous leukemia does not affect outcome adversely, provided it is discontinued at least 90 days before the procedure. *Blood* 94:3668–3677, 1999.
22. Lee SJ, Klein JP, Anasetti C, et al.: The effect of pretransplant interferon therapy on the outcome of unrelated

donor hematopoietic stem cell transplantation for patients with chronic myelogenous leukemia in first chronic phase. *Blood* 98:3205–3211, 2001.

23. Holowiecki J, Kruzel T, Wojnar J, et al.: Allogeneic stem cell transplantation from unrelated and related donors is effective in CML Ph+ and ALL Ph+ patients pretreated with imatinib [abstract]. *Blood* 102:436b, 2003. Abstract #5473.

24. Prejzner W, Zaucha JM, Szatkowski D, et al.: Imatinib therapy prior to myeloablative allogeneic stem cell transplantation does not increase acute transplant related toxicity [abstract]. *Blood* 102:911a, 2003. Abstract #3389.

25. Druker BJ, Talpaz M, Resta DJ, et al.: Efficacy and safety of a specific inhibitor of the BCR-ABL tyrosine kinase in chronic myeloid leukemia. *N Engl J Med* 344:1031–1037, 2001.

26. Kantarjian H, Sawyers C, Hochhaus A, et al.: Hematologic and cytogenetic responses to imatinib mesylate in chronic myelogenous leukemia. *N Engl J Med* 346:645–652, 2002.

27. Kantarjian HM, Cortes JE, O'Brien S, et al.: Long-term survival benefit and improved complete cytogenetic and molecular response rates with imatinib mesylate in Philadelphia chromosome-positive chronic-phase chronic myeloid leukemia after failure of interferon-alpha. *Blood* 104:1979–1988, 2004.

28. O'Brien SG, Guilhot F, Larson RA, et al.: Imatinib compared with interferon and low-dose cytarabine for newly diagnosed chronic-phase chronic myeloid leukemia. *N Engl J Med* 348:994–1004, 2003.

29. Hahn EA, Glendenning GA, Sorensen MV, et al.: Quality of life in patients with newly diagnosed chronic phase chronic myeloid leukemia on imatinib versus interferon alfa plus low-dose cytarabine: results from the IRIS Study. *J Clin Oncol* 21:2138–2146, 2003.

30. Kantarjian H, O'Brien S, Cortes J, et al.: Analysis of the impact of imatinib mesylate therapy on the prognosis of patients with Philadelphia chromosome-positive chronic myelogenous leukemia treated with interferon-alpha regimens for early chronic phase. *Cancer* 98:1430–1437, 2003.

31. Kantarjian HM, Cortes JE, O'Brien S, et al.: Imatinib mesylate therapy in newly diagnosed patients with Philadelphia chromosome-positive chronic myelogenous leukemia: high incidence of early complete and major cytogenetic responses. *Blood* 101:97–100, 2003.

32. Cortes J, Giles F, O'Brien S, et al.: Result of high-dose imatinib mesylate in patients with Philadelphia chromosome-positive chronic myeloid leukemia after failure of interferon-alpha. *Blood* 102:83–86, 2003.

33. Hughes T, Branford S, Matthews J, et al.: Trial of higher dose imatinib with selective intensification in newly diagnosed CML patients in the chronic phase [abstract]. *Blood* 102:31a, 2003. Abstract #95.

34. Talpaz M, Kantarjian H, Kurzrock R, Trujillo JM, Gutterman JU: Interferon-alpha produces sustained cytogenetic responses in chronic myelogenous leukemia. Philadelphia chromosome-positive patients. *Ann Intern Med* 114:532–538, 1991.

35. Radich JP, Gehly G, Gooley T, et al.: Polymerase chain reaction detection of the BCR-ABL fusion transcript after allogeneic marrow transplantation for chronic myeloid leukemia: results and implications in 346 patients. *Blood* 85:2632–2638, 1995.

36. Radich JP, Gooley T, Bryant E, et al.: The significance of bcr-abl molecular detection in chronic myeloid leukemia patients "late," 18 months or more after transplantation. *Blood* 98:1701–1707, 2001.

37. Hughes TP, Kaeda J, Branford S, et al.: Molecular responses to Imatinib (STI571) or Interferon + Ara-C as initial therapy for CML; results of the IRIS Study [abstract]. *Blood* 100:93a, 2002. Abstract #345.

38. Cortes J, O'Brien S, Talpaz M, et al.: Clinical significance of molecular response in chronic myeloid leukemia after imatinib (Gleevec) therapy: low levels of residual disease predict for response duration [abstract]. *Blood* 102:416a, 2003. Abstract #1513.

39. Rosti G, Martinelli G, Bassi S, et al.: Molecular response to imatinib in late chronic-phase chronic myeloid leukemia. *Blood* 103:2284–2290, 2004.

40. O'Dwyer ME, Mauro MJ, Blasdel C, et al.: Clonal evolution and lack of cytogenetic response are adverse prognostic factors for hematologic relapse of chronic phase CML patients treated with imatinib mesylate. *Blood* 103:451–455, 2004.

41. Cortes JE, Talpaz M, Giles F, et al.: Prognostic significance of cytogenetic clonal evolution in patients with chronic myelogenous leukemia on imatinib mesylate therapy. *Blood* 101:3794–3800, 2003.

42. Cortes J, O'Dwyer ME: Clonal evolution in chronic myelogenous leukemia. *Hematol Oncol Clin North Am* 18:671–684, 2004.

43. Medina J, Kantarjian H, Talpaz M, et al. Chromosomal abnormalities in Philadelphia chromosome-negative metaphases appearing during imatinib mesylate therapy in patients with Philadelphia chromosome-positive chronic myelogenous leukemia in chronic phase. *Cancer* 98:1905–1911, 2003.

44. Bumm T, Muller C, Al-Ali HK, et al.: Emergence of clonal cytogenetic abnormalities in Ph-cells in some CML patients in cytogenetic remission to imatinib but restoration of polyclonal hematopoiesis in the majority. *Blood* 101:1941–1949, 2003.

45. Kantarjian H, Talpaz M, O'Brien S, et al.: Prediction of initial cytogenetic response for subsequent major and complete cytogenetic response to imatinib mesylate therapy in patients with Philadelphia chromosome-positive chronic myelogenous leukemia. *Cancer* 97:2225–2228, 2003.

46. Druker BJ, Gathmann I, Bolton AE, Larson RA, IRIS: Probability and impact of obtaining a cytogenetic response to imatinib as initial therapy for chronic myeloid leukemia (CML) in chronic phase [abstract]. *Blood* 102:182a, 2003. Abstract #634.

47. Cortes J, O'Brien S, Kantarjian H: Discontinuation of imatinib therapy after achieving a molecular response. *Blood* 104:2204–2205, 2004.

48. Mauro MJ, Druker BJ, Maziarz RT: Divergent clinical outcome in two CML patients who discontinued imatinib therapy after achieving a molecular remission. *Leuk Res* 28:71–73, 2004.

49. Ghanima W, Kahrs J, Dahl TG, III, Tjonnfjord GE: Sustained cytogenetic response after discontinuation of imatinib mesylate in a patient with chronic myeloid leukaemia. *Eur J Haematol* 72:441–443, 2004.

50. Graham SM, Jorgensen HG, Allan E, et al.: Primitive, quiescent, Philadelphia-positive stem cells from patients with chronic myeloid leukemia are insensitive to STI571 in vitro. *Blood* 99:319–325, 2002.

51. Sneed TB, Kantarjian HM, Talpaz M, et al.: The significance of myelosuppression during therapy with imatinib mesylate in patients with chronic myelogenous leukemia in chronic phase. *Cancer* 100:116–121, 2004.

52. Kantarjian H, Talpaz M, O'Brien S, et al.: High-dose imatinib mesylate therapy in newly diagnosed Philadelphia chromosome-positive chronic phase chronic myeloid leukemia. *Blood* 103:2873–2878, 2004.

53. Cashen A, DiPersio JF, Khoury H: Does early imatinib-induced myelosuppression predict hematologic responses in patients with advanced-phase chronic myeloid leukemia? *J Clin Oncol* 21:4255–4256, 2003.

54. Deininger MW, O'Brien SG, Ford JM, Druker BJ: Practical management of patients with chronic myeloid leukemia receiving imatinib. *J Clin Oncol* 21:1637–1647, 2003.

55. Quintas-Cardama A, Kantarjian H, O'Brien S, et al.: Granulocyte-colony-stimulating factor (filgrastim) may overcome imatinib-induced neutropenia in patients with chronic-phase chronic myelogenous leukemia. *Cancer* 100:2592–2597, 2004.

56. Mauro MJ, Kurilik G, Balleisen S, O'Dwyer ME, Reese SF, Druker B: Myeloid growth factors for neutropenia during iamtinib mesylate (STI571) therapy for CML: preliminary evidence of safety and efficacy. *Blood* 98:139a, 2001.

57. Marin D, Marktel S, Foot N, et al.: G-CSF reverses cytopenia and may increase cytogenetic responses in patients with CML treated with imatinib mesylate [abstract]. *Blood* 100:782a, 2002. Abstract #3091.

58. Ault P, Kantarjian H, Welch MA, Giles F, Rios MB, Cortes J: Interleukin 11 may improve thrombocytopenia associated with imatinib mesylate therapy in chronic myelogenous leukemia. *Leuk Res* 28:613–618, 2004.

59. Cortes J, O'Brien S, Quintas A, et al.: Erythropoietin is effective in improving the anemia induced by imatinib mesylate therapy in patients with chronic myeloid leukemia in chronic phase. *Cancer* 100:2396–2402, 2004.

60. Mauro MJ, Blasdel C, O'Dwyer ME, Kurilik G, Capdeville R, Druker B: Erythropoietin for anemia during imatinib mesylate (STI571) therapy for CML: preliminary evidence of safety and efficacy [abstract]. *Proc ASCO* 21:27a, 2002. Abstract #106.

61. Ault P, Kantarjian H, O'Brien S, Garcia-Manero G, Rios MB, Cortes J: Use of darbopoietin alfa for the treatment of anemia occuring during imatinib therapy for CML: preliminary evidence of safety and efficacy [abstract]. *Proc ASCO* 22:613, 2003. Abstract #2467.

62. Talpaz M, Estrov Z, Kantarjian H, Ku S, Foteh A, Kurzrock R: Persistence of dormant leukemic progenitors during interferon-induced remission in chronic myelogenous leukemia. Analysis by polymerase chain reaction of individual colonies. *J Clin Invest* 94:1383–1389, 1994.

63. Branford S, Rudzki Z, Parkinson I, et al.: Real-time quantitative PCR analysis can be used as a primary screen to identify imatinib-treated patients with CML who have BCR-ABL kinase domain mutations. *Blood* 104:2926–2932, 2004.

Chapter **19**

# TREATMENT APPROACH TO ACCELERATED-PHASE OR BLAST-CRISIS CHRONIC MYELOGENOUS LEUKEMIA

*Eric J. Feldman*

## INTRODUCTION

Until recently, the progression to blast phase was considered inevitable for almost all patients with chronic myelogenous leukemia (CML).[1] Except for a minority of patients able to tolerate interferon and achieve a complete cytogenetic response, or for those with an HLA-matched sibling and young enough to survive a bone marrow transplant, most patients entered the blastic phase of CML and died within 6 months to a year.[2] Fortunately, advances in both transplantation and nontransplantation therapy have improved the outlook for patients with chronic-phase CML, and by extension, have changed the way in which patients entering the blast phase present and are approached therapeutically.

Imatinib mesylate, widely available by the year 2000, is currently the initial treatment of choice for the majority of patients with CML. Although follow-up is short, preliminary results have demonstrated that close to 80% are achieving complete remissions and less than 10% of the patients have progressed to blast phase by 4 years.[3] Concurrently, the development of large marrow donor registries, coupled with improved transplantation techniques for older patients and for those undergoing unrelated donor transplants, have led to an increased use of transplantation for patients unresponsive to imatinib, who in the past would have been deemed ineligible for this procedure.[4]

Although the duration of response to imatinib is still unknown, and concerns over drug resistance have emerged, several situations seem probable: (1) a significant percentage of patients treated with imatinib will be long-term survivors and will not enter the blast phase; (2) patients entering the blast phase of disease will have already been treated with imatinib, which may influence their ability to respond to subsequent therapy; and (3) an increasingly higher percentage of chronic-phase CML patients will undergo hematopoietic stem cell transplantation at the development of clinical or laboratory evidence of imatinib failure with an expanding pool of "acceptable" donors. It is with this background we can examine the treatment options available to patients in the advanced phases of CML.

## IMATINIB MESLATE IN ACCELERATED- AND BLAST-PHASE CML

Although it is unlikely that patients, nowadays, will enter blastic or accelerated phase without having received prior treatment with imatinib, it is worthwhile to review the results of imatinib therapy in imatinib-naive patients for historical interest, as well as to gain some understanding of the role of bcr/abl in the growth and proliferation of CML cells during transformation to the blast phase.

The clinical development of imatinib mesylate followed the traditional development of cytotoxic agents in leukemia with the finding of the maximally tolerated dose in a phase I study[5] and then subsequent phase II evaluations in subsets of CML patients. Two separate trials evaluated the efficacy of imatinib in CML patients in accelerated phase and in blastic phase, with further subset analysis of patients in either myeloid or lymphoid blast transformation.[6–10]

The accelerated-phase study, reported by Talpaz et al.,[6] included 181 confirmed patients with accelerated phase as defined by a set of criteria that had been demonstrated retrospectively to correlate with survival rates compared to chronic-phase patients, and that were different than that of blastic-phase patients. These criteria included the presence of 15–30% blasts, or 30% blasts and promyelocytes, or 20% basophils in the blood or marrow, or a platelet count less than $100 \times 10^3$ /L unrelated to anticancer therapy. Patients were treated with 400 or 600 mg of imatinib daily. Overall, 69% of the patients achieved a sustained hematologic response, 34% complete, and the rest either achieved a blast percentage in the marrow under 5% with incomplete peripheral blood recovery (marrow response) or a return to a second chronic phase (no criteria for accelerated disease as defined above). The rate of complete cytogenetic response was 17%, and the 1-year progression-free and overall survival was 59 and 74%, respectively. Patients treated with 600 mg compared to 400 mg realized greater benefit with a higher overall cytogenetic responses (28% vs 16%) and better progression-free and overall 1-year survival rates (67 and 78% vs 44 and 65%), with no significant increases in toxicity.

Although the definition of accelerated phase of CML by hematologic criteria, as outlined above, was used in the initial studies of imatinib, subsequent patients have been labeled accelerated phase purely on the basis of clonal evolution, i.e, the development of chromosomal abnormalities in addition to a single t(9;22). In an analysis by O'Dwyer et al., the results of treatment with imatinib at a dose of 600 mg was evaluated based on the criteria used for defining accelerated phase.[11] Patients with accelerated disease based on hematologic criteria without clonal evolution had a significantly worse response rate and time to treatment failure compared to patients with clonal evolution as the sole criterion for defining accelerated disease. Patients with clonal evolution alone had a major cytogenetic response rate of 73% and a treatment failure rate at 1 year of 0% compared to a major cytogenetic response rate of 31% and a 1-year treatment failure rate of 28% in patients with hematologic criteria alone for accelerated disease. Patients with both hematologic and clonal evidence of accelerated disease did the worst of all three groups, with cytogenetic response rates of 12.5%, a 1-year treatment failure rate of 67%, and a median time to treatment failure of 8 months. This experience suggests that patients with clonal evolution alone, without other evidence of accelerated disease, have a similar response rate to that of patients with chronic-phase disease, provided they receive doses of 600 mg or higher of imatinib.

The myeloid blast-phase study reported by Sawyers et al.[9] included 229 evaluable patients with more than 30% blasts in the blood or marrow, with a myeloid phenotype demonstrated by immunophenotypic and cytochemical evaluation. As in the accelerated-phase study, patients were treated with either 400 or 600 mg of imatinib. Overall, 31% of the patients achieved a sustained hematologic response. Hematologic responses were complete in only 8% of the patients, with the majority being classified as a return to chronic phase. Major and complete cytogenetic responses were observed in 16 and 7%, respectively. Patients previously untreated for the blast phase of disease fared better, experiencing an overall and complete hematologic response (CHR) rate of 36 and 9%, compared to 21 and 6%, respectively, for patients who had received prior induction chemotherapy for blast-phase disease. Major cytogenetic responses were observed in 16% of the patients, in whom 7% were complete. The median survival for all patients was 6.9 months, with 32% of the patients still alive at 1 year. The impact of the dose of imatinib was significant, with overall hematologic responses of 34% for patients treated with 600 mg compared to 9% for patients receiving 400 mg of imatinib. Cytogenetic responses were also significantly better with the higher doses of imatinib (18% vs 6%).

Transformation of CML to a lymphoid blast phase is less common than myeloid transformation, and patients in this category treated with imatinib have been grouped together with patients with Ph+ acute lymphoblastic leukemia. In both phase I and phase II studies, imatinib demonstrated efficacy in lymphoid blast-phase patients similar to responses seen in patients with myeloid blast phase.[10] Overall, 25% of the patients in lymphoid blast phase achieved a sustained hematologic response to imatinib, but responses were generally of short duration, with a median time to progression of 2.2 months. Similar to patients with Ph+ ALL, imatinib alone has limited efficacy in lymphoid blast phase, and further development is based on the incorporation of imatinib into chemotherapy-based regimens.[12]

In addition to the inability of imatinib alone to control established lymphoid blast disease, imatinib has been shown, in some instances, to fail to prevent the onset of lymphoid transformation in patients in chronic phase. Sudden onset of blast-phase disease, especially lymphoid transformation, has been observed in patients prior to the development of imatinib, including patients who had a complete cytogenetic response on treatment with interferon alpha or postallogeneic transplantation.[13] Recent observations have demonstrated a similar phenomenon in patients in cytogenetic remission on imatinib.[14] In addition, complete response to imatinib does not protect against the development of meningeal involvement by lymphoid blast cells. In several patients, meningeal relapse occurred despite control of marrow disease.[15] Imatinib levels in these patients were demonstrated to be approximately 2 logs lower in the cerebrospinal fluid compared to plasma.[16]

The results of these trials in patients with advanced phases of CML have demonstrated that imatinib, a relatively specific tyrosine kinase inhibitor of bcr/abl, was effective in inducing sustained responses, which compared favorably to results with more intensive chemotherapy-based regimens. Importantly, imatinib's biologic activity in these patients with advanced disease demonstrated that signal transduction mediated by the BCR/ABL protein was still a relevant target for therapeutic inhibition, but that mechanisms of resistance, genetic reexpression or mutation of BCR/ABL, and/or clonal evolution, leads to eventual loss of clinical activity and progression of disease.[17,18] Efforts to overcome resistance have included dose escalation of imatinib[19] and the addition of other chemotherapeutic or molecularly directed agents to imatinib.[20,21] Other efforts currently underway are the development of newer tyrosine kinase inhibitors with activity in the mutated forms of BCR/ABL.[22]

## CHEMOTHERAPY FOR ACCELERATED- AND BLAST-PHASE CML

Prior to the development of imatinib, the outlook for patients entering the advanced phases of CML was dismal. Chemotherapy was the mainstay for these patients, and the choice of chemotherapeutic agents generally followed the treatment plans for acute myeloid and lymphoblastic leukemia: patients with accelerated or myeloid blast phase received cytarabine/anthracycline-based regimens, while patients with lymphoid transformation received standard vincristine/prednisone-based protocols. Although imatinib may now be considered the treatment of choice for patients with CML entering the accelerated or blast phase, most patients in the future will have already received imatinib as part of treatment for chronic-phase disease, and thus chemotherapy must still be considered as an important part of therapy. What has changed, however, is that patients entering advanced phases will have been treated with imatinib, and whether this changes the efficacy of chemotherapy is yet to be determined.

Several experiences using acute myeloid leukemia AML-type chemotherapy for patients with advanced-phase CML have been published. Problems arise in the interpretation of the outcomes of these studies. First, institutional differences exist in the response criteria used, which makes the comparison of results often suboptimal. Most investigators agree on the definition of a CHR, which has been defined using acute leukemia criteria with the necessity of achieving <5% blasts in the bone marrow and recovery of neutrophil and platelet counts. Partial or incomplete responses, however, are frequently included in the overall response rates, and the definitions of responses that are not complete are inconsistent. Patients achieving all criteria for CHR, but with incomplete platelet recovery, have been designated "hematologic improvement" (HI) or complete remission with incomplete platelet recovery (CRp). Other response criteria have included the term "return to chronic phase," which has been defined differently in some series. By some criteria, this category of response requires the disappearance of blast-phase features, defined as peripheral or marrow blast percentage under 15%, basophils under 20%, blasts plus promyelocytes under 30%, and return of platelet counts to >100,000/L. Other criteria for return to a second

chronic phase have called for a blast percentage in the blood of 5% and less than 10% in the marrow, with no defined criteria for recovery of neutrophils or platelets.

In addition to problems associated with nonstandardized response criteria, differences in criteria that distinguish accelerated from blast phase have been used (discussed earlier), making comparisons between treatment outcomes unclear. An important by-product of the development of imatinib, and the international collaborations required for its rapid development, was the adoption of more universally accepted definitions of disease stage, as well as a greater standardization of response criteria. Undoubtedly, in the future this will lead to easier interpretations of clinical studies in patients with CML; however, most chemotherapy-based regimens for advanced-phase CML were evaluated prior to imatinib; therefore, making direct comparisons between studies harder.

## CYTARABINE-BASED COMBINATION REGIMENS

The largest series incorporating AML-type chemotherapy in patients with myeloid blast phase (blast count > 30%) involved 162 patients treated at MD Anderson Cancer Center over an 11-year period from 1986 to 1997.[23] Ninety patients received intensive combination chemotherapy, largely high-dose cytarabine-based. Overall, 28% of the patients responded to treatment, with CHR in 8% of the patients, and an additional 7% achieving all criteria for CHR, but with incomplete platelet count recovery. In addition, 11% of the patients achieved a return to chronic phase, and 2% of the patients were termed a partial response. The duration of response was approximately 4 months, which corresponded with survival as well. In a series of patients treated at the Karolinska Hospital in Sweden,[24] 47% of 83 patients with accelerated or myeloid blast-phase disease, treated with an anthracycline/cytarabine-based regimen, achieved a return to chronic phase, the definition of which was less stringent than the MD Anderson data. Overall survival was similar, however, in the 4–6 month range. In this series, patients with accelerated-phase disease had similar responses to those of blast-phase, although they demonstrated a slight, but statistically insignificant, improvement in survival. These studies, as well as numerous other smaller experiences,[25–29] have demonstrated that standard AML-type regimens have limited efficacy in advanced-phase patients and, despite widespread application, it is not clear that higher-doses of ara-C are better than standard doses in this setting.

## SINGLE-AGENT THERAPY

A number of novel chemotherapeutic agents have been studied as single agents in advanced-phase disease. To date, the most promising agents have been the hypomethylating agents, decitabine (5-aza 2'deoxycytidine) and azacytidine (5-azacytidine). These agents act in part by reversing the methylation, or silencing, of numerous tumor suppressive genes that exert antiproliferative effects, thus potentially reversing or slowing the progression of CML. Decitabine has been the most extensively studied hypomethylating agent in CML, whereas azacitidine has been used more commonly in patients with myelodysplastic syndrome.[30] In a study conducted at MD Anderson Cancer Center, 64 myeloid blast-phase and 51 accelerated-phase Ph+ CML patients were treated with repetitive monthly cycles of decitabine. In blast-phase patients, 28% achieved a response, which included a CHR in approximately 9%. In accelerated patients, a 55% overall response rate, with an approximate 23% CHR rate, was observed.[31] Response durations and survival rates were quite poor in blastic phase patients, with a 3-year survival rate of only 5%. Accelerated-phase patients had significantly better outcomes, with 3-year survival rates of 27%, again pointing out the importance of distinguishing between these stages of CML. Despite the myelosuppressive properties of decitabine, only 3% of all patients treated died of complications of cytopenias. These results suggested that single-agent decitabine, although still relatively ineffective, resulted in equivalent outcomes to that of the high-dose cytarabine-based regimens with less toxicity.

Several other agents have been tried alone or in combination with cytarabine in patients with advanced-phase CML. These have included topotecan, carboplatin, homoharringtonine, amsacrine, and mithramycin.[32–36] None have demonstrated enhanced activity compared to standard antileukemia agents. Most recently, troxacitabine, a novel nucleoside analog, has been evaluated both in AML and in myeloid blast-phase CML.[37] Of particular interest is that this agent has been tested in patients either previously treated with imatinib or in imatinib-naive patients. In an initial phase II evaluation in myeloid blast phase, 6 of 16 (37%) of patients responded to troxacitabine in a cohort in which only 3 patients had received prior treatment with imatinib.[38] In a subsequent larger trial, a 13% response rate was seen in 51 myeloid blast-phase patients in whom 93% had progressed on treatment with imatinib.[39] Although no specific data have been reported for response rates for cytarabine-based regimens or hypomethylating agents comparing outcomes by prior exposure to imatinib, the results with troxacitabine suggest that patients progressing on treatment with imatinib may be particularly resistant.

## LYMPHOID BLAST PHASE

Approximately one-fourth of patients entering blast phase will have a lymphoid phenotype compared to the more common presentation of a myeloid or undifferentiated blastic phase. Patients entering lymphoid phase are often younger and less often have a prior accelerated phase documented compared to patients entering myeloid blast phase. A sudden onset of blast phase is more common in patients entering lymphoid blast phase, and in fact can occur in patients seemingly in stable chronic phase responding to therapy with interferon and/or imatinib.[40] There appears to be no evidence that prior treatment with interferon selects for patients entering the lymphoid blast phase, however.

Therapy for patients in lymphoid blast phase is generally more successful than for patients with myeloid transformation, as more patients enter a second chronic phase, which is durable enough to consider a hematopoietic stem cell transplant (see below). In a review published by the MD Anderson Cancer Center, overall, 49% of patients responded to therapy.[41] In this series, patients given traditional drugs used to treat acute lymphoblastic leukemia (vincristine, prednisone, cyclophosphamide, adriamycin) had a higher rate of return to a chronic phase compared to patients treated with high-dose ara-C or methotrexate combined with L-asparaginase (61% vs 33% and 25%, respectively). Other series, however, have demonstrated high response rates (50% +) using high-dose cytarabine/anthracycline-based regimens.[42] Median survival rates for lymphoid blast-phase patients are approximately 9 months, compared to the median 3-4 months observed in patients with myeloid blast-phase disease. As with patients with myeloid blast phase, the impact of prior treatment with imatinib on the effectiveness of subsequent chemotherapy for lymphoid blast phase is, at present, unknown.

## ALLOGENEIC HEMATOPOIETIC STEM CELL TRANSPLANTATION THERAPY

Most patients with an HLA-compatible donor, sibling or otherwise, will preferentially undergo transplantation therapy while still in chronic phase.[43] This will occur either as initial treatment or in patients not responding to interferon or imatinib therapy. The results of transplantation therapy for patients in blast phase are poor, and many institutions are reluctant to perform this procedure unless the patient is able to achieve a second chronic phase with chemotherapy or imatinib prior to transplantation. The decision not to offer transplantation to patients with advanced-phase CML has been based on results from cooperative groups and/or large single institutions that have reported long-term survival for transplantation in blast phase of 0–14% and survival rates for accelerated-phase patients of 15–20%.[44,45] On the other hand, since no other therapies exist for these patients that are associated with long-term survival, many patients are transplanted in advanced phases of disease for want of better treatment.

To better identify patients likely to survive transplantation, despite entering the advanced phases of disease, several groups have employed prognostic scoring systems generated from multivariate analyses of transplantation outcomes in relatively large numbers of patients. One of these scoring systems, the Gratwohl Score, based on results of transplantation in patients reported by the European Blood and Marrow Transplantation Group, has been widely used.[46] In this scoring system, a higher score (associated with a worse survival) is given based on several pre-transplantation variables predictive for poor outcome, including increasing patient age, advanced stage of disease, incompatibility of donor and recipient, prolonged time from diagnosis to transplant, and donor –recipient sex mismatch. Thus, a young patient (age, 20–40) with an HLA-identical sibling match, transplanted within 12 months of diagnosis may still be a suitable candidate for transplantation, even in the accelerated or blast phase of disease, whereas a patient above the age of 40 in blast phase undergoing a matched unrelated transplantation would have a small chance for long-term survival. Although improvement continues in the supportive care and treatment of graft-versus host disease for patients undergoing allogeneic hematopoietic stem cell transplantation, transplantation of CML in the advanced stages should be avoided with every effort being made to identify those patients unlikely to be long-term survivors with nontransplantation therapy and plan transplantation prior to disease progression to accelerated and blast phase.

## FUTURE DIRECTIONS IN THERAPY FOR ADVANCED-PHASE CML

The success of imatinib will clearly result in fewer patients with CML progressing to the advanced phases. Is blastic phase CML a disease of the past? Further observational time will let us know what percent of patients with CML will be cured with imatinib. Although leukemia cells resistant to imatinib have been detected in patients with CML, this has mostly occurred in advanced-phase patients who received imatinib for the first time, having received prior treatment with other agents.[47] The incidence of imatinib resistance so far in newly diagnosed chronic-phase patients is still quite low. However, if imatinib resistance is observed, these patients will be at risk for progression to blast-phase disease, and thus future development of therapies in CML will clearly be aimed at preventing the emergence of imatinib-resistant subclones with therapies that may enhance the activity of imatinib[48] and/or the use of newer inhibitors with effectiveness in mutated forms of bcr/abl. Initial clinical investigation of these new agents are planned for advanced-phase patients progressing on treatment with imatinib.

## REFERENCES

1. Kantarjian H: Chronic myelogenous leukemia: a concise update. *Blood* 82:691–703, 1993.
2. Faderl S: Chronic myelogenous leukemia: biology and therapy. *Ann Intern Med* 131:207–219, 1996.
3. O'Brien SG: Imatinib compared with interferon and low-dose cytarabine for newly diagnosed chronic phase chronic myeleid leukemia. *N Engl J Med* 348(11):994–1004, 2003.
4. McGlave PB: Unrelated donor marrow transplantation for chronic myelogenous leukemia: 9 years experience of the National Marrow Donor Program. *Blood* 95(7):2219–2225, 2000.
5. Druker BJ: Activity of a specific inhibitor of the Bcr-Abl tyrosine kinase in the blast crisis of chronic myeloid leukemia and acute lymphoblastic leukemia with the Philadelphia chromosome. *N Engl J Med* 344(14):1038–1042, 2001.
6. Talpaz M: Imatinib induces durable hematologic and cytogenetic responses in patients with accelerated phase chronic myeloid leukemia: results of a phase 2 study. *Blood* 99(6):1928–1937, 2002.
7. Kantarjian HM: Treatment of Philadelphia chromosome-positive, accelerated-phase chronic myelogenous leukemia with imatinib mesylate. *Clin Cancer Res* 8(7):2167–2176, 2002.
8. Kantarjian HM: Imatinib mesylate (STI571) therapy for Philadelphia chromosome-positive chronic myelogenous leukemia in blast phase. *Blood* 99(10):3547–3553, 2002.
9. Sawyers CL: Imatinib induces hematologic and cytogenetic responses in patients with chronic myelogenous leukemia in myeloid blast crisis: results of a phase II study. *Blood* 99(10):3530–3539, 2002.
10. Ottmann OG: A phase 2 study of imatinib in patients with relapsed or refractory Philadelphia chromosome-positive acute lymphoid leukemias. *Blood* 100(6):1965–1971, 2002.
11. O'Dwyer ME: The impact of clonal evolution on response to imatinib mesylate (STI571) in accelerated phase CML. *Blood* 100(5):1628–1633, 2002.
12 Thomas DA: Treatment of Philadelphia chromosome-positive acute lymphocytic leukemia with hyper-CVAD and imatinib mesylate. *Blood* 103(12):4396–4407, 2004.
13. Kantarjian H: Sudden onset of the blastic phase of chronic myelogenous leukemia: patterns and implications. *Cancer* 98(1):81–85, 2003.
14. Avery S: Lymphoid transformation in a CML patient in complete cytogenetic remission following treatment with imatinib. *Leuk Res* 28(suppl 1):S75–S77, 2004.
15. Bujassoum S: Isolated central nervous system relapse in lymphoid blast crisis chronic myeloid leukemia and acute lymphoblastic leukemia in patients on imatinib therapy. *Leuk Lymphoma* 45(2):401–403, 2004.

16. Leis JF: Central nervous system failure in patients with chronic myelogenous leukemia lymphoid blast crisis and Philadelphia chromosome positive acute lymphoblastic leukemia treated with imatinib (STI-571). *Leuk Lymphoma* 45(4):695–698, 2004.

17. Mahon FX: Selection and characterization of BCR-ABL positive cell lines with differential sensitivity to the tyrosine kinase inhibitor STI571: diverse mechanisms of resistance. *Blood* 96(3):1070–1079, 2000.

18. Weisberg E: Mechanisms of resistance to the ABL tyrosine kinase inhibitor STI571 in BCR/ABL-transformed hematopoietic cell lines. *Blood* 95:3498–3505, 2000.

19. Zonder JA: The effect of dose increase of imatinib mesylate in patients with chronic or accelerated phase chronic myelogenous leukemia with inadequate hematologic or cytogenetic response to initial treatment. *Clin Cancer Res* 9(6):2092–2097, 2003.

20. Gardembas M: Results of a prospective phase 2 study combining imatinib mesylate and cytarabine for the treatment of Philadelphia-positive patients with chronic myelogenous leukemia in chronic phase. *Blood* 102(13):4298–4305, 2003 Dec 15.

21. Nakajima A: Efficacy of SCH66336, a farnesyl transferase inhibitor, in conjunction with imatinib against BCR-ABL-positive cells. *Mol Cancer Ther* 2(3):219–224, 2003 Mar.

22. Tipping AJ: Efficacy of dual-specific Bcr-Abl and Src-family kinase inhibitors in cells sensitive and resistant to imatinib mesylate. *Leukemia* 18(8):1352–1356, 2004 Aug.

23. Sacchi S: Chronic myelogenous leukemia in nonlymphoid blastic phase: analysis of the results of first salvage therapy with three different treatment approaches for 162 patients. *Cancer* 86(12):2632–2641, 1999.

24. Axdorph U: Intensive chemotherapy in patients with chronic myelogenous leukaemia (CML) in accelerated or blastic phase—a report from the Swedish CML Group. *Br J Haematol* 118(4):1048–1054, 2002.

25. Bauduer F: Treatment of chronic myelogenous leukemia in blast crisis and in accelerated phase with high- or intermediate-dose cytosine arabinoside and amsacrine. *Leuk Lymphoma* 10(3):195–200, 1993.

26. Seiter K: Phase I clinical and laboratory evaluation of topotecan and cytarabine in patients with acute leukemia. *J Clin Oncol* 15(1):44–51, 1997.

27. Koller CA: A phase I-II trial of escalating doses of mitoxantrone with fixed doses of cytarabine plus fludarabine as salvage therapy for patients with acute leukemia and the blastic phase of chronic myelogenous leukemia. *Cancer* 86(11):2246–2251, 1999.

28. Kantarjian HM: Treatment of the blastic phase of chronic myelogenous leukemia with mitoxantrone and high-dose cytosine arabinoside. *Cancer* 62(4):672–676, 1988.

29. Dutcher JP: Phase II study of mitoxantrone and 5-azacytidine for accelerated and blast crisis of chronic myelogenous leukemia: a study of the Eastern Cooperative Oncology Group. *Leukemia* 6(8):770–775, 1992.

30. Silverman LR: Randomized controlled trial of azacitidine in patients with the myelodysplastic syndrome: a study of the Cancer and Leukemia Group B. *J Clin Oncol* 20(10):2429–2440, 2002.

31. Kantarjian HM: Results of decitabine (5-aza-2'deoxycytidine) therapy in 130 patients with chronic myelogenous leukemia. *Cancer* 98(3):522–528, 2003.

32. Park SJ: Topotecan-based combination chemotherapy in patients with transformed chronic myelogenous leukemia and advanced myelodysplastic syndrome. *Korean J Intern Med* 15(2):122–126, 2000.

33. Dutcher JP: Phase II study of carboplatin in blast crisis of chronic myeloid leukemia: Eastern Cooperative Oncology Group study E1992. *Leukemia* 12(7):1037–1040, 1998.

34. O'Brien S: Homoharringtonine therapy induces responses in patients with chronic myelogenous leukemia in late chronic phase. *Blood* 86(9):3322–3326, 1995 Nov 1.

35. Arlin ZA: Philadelphia chromosome (Ph1)-positive acute lymphoblastic leukemia (ALL) is resistant to effective therapy for Ph1-negative ALL. *Acta Haematol* 81(4):217–8, 1989.

36. Koller CA: Preliminary observations on the therapy of the myeloid blast phase of chronic granulocytic leukemia with plicamycin and hydroxyurea. *N Engl J Med* 315(23):1433–1438, 1986 Dec 4.

37. Giles F: Troxacitabine, a novel dioxolane nucleoside analog, has activity in patients with advanced leukemia. *J Clin Oncol* 19(3):762–771, 2001.

38. Giles FJ: Phase II study of troxacitabine, a novel dioxolane nucleoside analog, in patients with refractory leukemia. *J Clin Oncol* 20(3):656–664, 2002 Feb 1.

39. Giles FJ: Phase II study of troxacitabine, a novel dioxolane nucleoside analog, in patients with untreated or imatinib mesylate-resistant chronic myelogenous leukemia in blastic phase. *Leuk Res* 27(12):1091–1096, 2003.

40. Kantarjian HM: Sudden onset of the blastic phase of chronic myelogenous leukemia: patterns and implications. *Cancer* 98(1):81–85, 2003.

41. Derderian PM: Chronic myelogenous leukemia in the lymphoid blastic phase: characteristics, treatment response, and prognosis. *Am J Med* 94(1):69–74, 1993.

42. Feldman EJ: Phase I clinical and pharmacokinetic evaluation of high-dose mitoxantrone in combination with cytarabine in patients with acute leukemia. *J Clin Oncol* 11(10):2002–2009, 1993.

43. Thomas ED: Marrow transplantation for the treatment of chronic myelogenous leukemia. *Ann Intern Med* 104(2):155–163, 1986.

44. Clift RA: Marrow transplantation for patients in accelerated phase of chronic myeloid leukemia. *Blood* 84(12):4368–4373, 1994.

45. Martin PJ: HLA-identical marrow transplantation during accelerated-phase chronic myelogenous leukemia: analysis of survival and remission duration. *Blood* 72(6):1978–1984, 1988.

46. Gratwohl A: Allogeneic bone marrow transplantation for chronic myeloid leukemia. Working Party Chronic Leukemia of the European Group for Blood and Marrow Transplansplantation (EBMT). *Bone Marrow Transplant* (suppl 3):S7–S9, 1996.

47. Hochaus A: Molecular and chromosomal mechanisms of resistance to imatinib (STI571). *Leukemia* 16:2190–2196, 2002.

48. Nimmanapalli R: Cotreatment with the histone deacetylase inhibitor suberoylanilide hydroxamic acid (SAHA) enhances imatinib-induced apoptosis of Bcr-Abl-positive human acute leukemia cells. *Blood* 101(8):3236–3239, 2003.

# Chapter 20

# DEFINITION OF REMISSION, PROGNOSIS, AND FOLLOW-UP

*Matt E. Kalaycio and Ilka Warshawsky*

## DEFINITION OF REMISSION

As the therapy of chronic myelogenous leukemia (CML) has improved over the years, the definitions of response have changed. Before the recognition that allogeneic hematopoietic stem cell transplant (HSCT) could cure CML, the treatment of CML was palliative. Thus, remission meant that the blood counts were normalized and symptoms were controlled. This definition is inadequate today.

Table 20.1 lists the three categories of remission in CML, namely hematologic, cytogenetic, and molecular, as well as their most common definitions.

### HEMATOLOGIC REMISSION

Hematologic remission is the goal of purely palliative therapy. Hematologic remission does not impact the natural history of CML to a significant degree. In the Italian CML Study Group trial comparing palliative hydroxyurea or busulfan with interferon α, complete hematologic remission was obtained in 68–87% of patients after 8 months of any therapy.[1] Those patients treated without interferon had a median survival of 52 months and only 29% were alive at 6 years. These results are comparable to what one might expect in the absence of any therapy.[2,3] In contrast, patients treated with either interferon or imatinib enjoy both increased hematologic remission rates and improved survival compared to hydroxyurea or busulfan. The improved survival rates achieved by interferon and imatinib stem directly from their ability to induce cytogenetic remission, a characteristic both hydroxyurea and busulfan lack.

### CYTOGENETIC REMISSION

Cytogenetic remission is defined as a reduction in the number of identifiable Philadelphia (Ph+) chromosomes by standard metaphase karyotypic analysis. The degree of reduction determines the completeness of remission, and this degree of reduction has prognostic significance with regard to survival. The importance of achieving a major or complete cytogenetic remission (CCR) is highlighted by the results of several randomized clinical trials comparing interferon-α to chemotherapy such as hydroxyurea. In these studies, the only patients achieving a significant cytogenetic remission were those treated with interferon.[1,4,5] For patients achieving CCR on interferon, the 10-year overall survival rate was 72%.[6]

With interferon alone, however, only a minority of patients actually achieved a CCR. In a randomized trial of interferon alone versus the combination of interferon plus low-dose cytarabine in chronic-phase CML patients, the combination treatment arm induced more major cytogenetic remissions than did the interferon alone arm (35% vs 21%; $P = 0.001$).[7] This difference translated into a 5-year overall survival advantage for the combination arm of 70% versus 62% ($P = 0.02$). Thus, cytogenetic remission, and in particular CCR, is an important endpoint not only to determine efficacy, but also to maximize the chances for long-term disease-free survival.

Cytogenetic analysis is the gold standard method for predicting clinical outcomes in CML and is typically performed on bone marrow samples. However, there are many practical disadvantages to monitoring CML therapy by bone marrow cytogenetics, including the requirement for proliferating cells and the poor sensitivity (typically 5%) for detecting low-level minimal residual disease. Fluorescent in situ hybridization (FISH) allows for detection of the *bcr/abl* translocation in either metaphase or interphase cells. Because interphase cells are suitable, FISH can be performed on blood leukocytes. Moreover, large numbers of cells can be examined, which increases the sensitivity over that of metaphase cytogenetics. A negative FISH result correlates very well with CCR.[8,9]

### MOLECULAR REMISSION

Reverse transcriptase-polymerase chain reaction (RT-PCR) is the most sensitive method for detecting the *bcr/abl* transcript. A complete molecular remission means that the *bcr/abl* transcript cannot be detected by

**Table 20.1    Definitions of remission in CML**

| Remission | | Definition | 5-Years survival with interferon |
|---|---|---|---|
| **Hematologic** | | | |
| | Complete | Normal WBC and PLT<br>Normal WBC differential<br>No palpable splenomegaly<br>No symptoms referable to CML | 30–40% |
| | Partial | Decrease of WBC to <50% of the pretreatment level and <20,000/μL<br>Or<br>Normal WBC, but persistent splenomegaly or abnormal WBC differential | |
| **Cytogenetic** | | | |
| | Complete | 0% Ph+ metaphases<br>Or<br>Absence of FISH signal | 86% |
| | Major | 1–34% Ph+ metaphases | 80% |
| | Minor | 35–90% Ph+ metaphases | 60% |
| | None | 91–100% Ph+ metaphases | 20% |
| **Molecular** | | | |
| | Complete | No detectable bcr/abl transcripts | NA |
| | Major | >3-log reduction in bcr/abl transcripts | |

RT-PCR.[10] Before the advent of imatinib for the treatment of CML, the only therapeutic modality capable of inducing a complete molecular remission was allogeneic HSCT. In fact, molecular relapse or failure to induce molecular remission after HSCT predicts hematologic relapse and is an indication for salvage therapy including donor lymphocyte infusions.[11] Thus, a complete molecular remission is tantamount to cure after HSCT and is the ultimate goal of non-HSCT therapies if they aspire to cure CML.

Imatinib can induce molecular remission, though not as uniformly or as quickly as with an allogeneic HSCT. At a dose of 400 mg daily in untreated patients with chronic-phase CML, imatinib induces a complete molecular remission in fewer than 5% of patients.[12] Although higher doses of imatinib may induce a higher rate of complete molecular remission, most patients in CCR still have detectable bcr/abl transcripts.[13] For these patients in CCR who still have detectable bcr/abl transcripts, a reduction in the number of these transcripts may be just as important as complete molecular remission.

A note of caution must be inserted when considering the definition of a complete molecular response as determined by RT-PCR analysis. RT-PCR techniques may fail to detect extremely low levels of bcr/abl, and lab-to-lab differences in methodology preclude the practical comparison of results generated between laboratories. To account for variations in methodology and RT-PCR sensitivity, optimal post-therapy monitoring of disease is better accomplished using quantitative rather than qualitative RT-PCR assays. The log reduction in bcr/abl transcripts compared to a baseline level obtained at the time CCR was achieved has been introduced as a method to standardize the reporting of molecular responses after treatment for CML.[12] In general, a 3-log reduction in the number of detectable bcr/abl transcripts constitutes a major molecular remission.

## PROGNOSIS

CML has a variable prognosis largely determined by clinical features present at diagnosis. Clearly, patients in chronic phase have a better prognosis than those in either accelerated or blast phase (see Chapters 19 and 20). However, patients in chronic phase may also be risk stratified according to what treatment they receive.

### CML TREATED WITH HYDROXYUREA (OR BUSULFAN)

A large study of patients treated mostly with hydroxyurea was the basis for the first widely recognized prognostic scoring system. Sokal et al. performed a multiple regression analysis of 625 chronic-phase patients aged 5–45 years and identified age, spleen size, hematocrit, platelet count, and the percentage of circulating blast cells as significant prognostic factors.[14] The "Sokal" scoring system devised by this analysis classifies patients into risk categories that predict survival in patients treated with hydroxyurea.

### CML TREATED WITH INTERFERON

As interferon became the treatment of choice, the validity of the Sokal system came into question. To address the question of prognostic factors in patients treated with interferon, Hasford et al. analyzed data on 1303 patients aged 10–85 years and treated with interferon.[15] This analysis identified age, spleen size, percentages of circulating blasts, basophils, and eosinophils, as well as platelet counts as significant prognostic factors. The resulting "Hasford" score was then validated on 322 different patients. This scoring system categorizes patients treated with interferon into low, intermediate, and high risk for survival, and does so more effectively than the Sokal score.[16]

Many, if not most, patients initially treated with interferon are now taking imatinib. Whether the Sokal and/or Hasford scoring systems are appropriate for prognostic determination in patients treated with imatinib is uncertain. In fact, in a study of 351 patients treated with imatinib after failure of interferon, age did not appear to be a significant prognostic indicator as it was in both the Sokal and Hasford scoring systems.[17]

Marin et al. studied 145 patients treated with imatinib after failure of interferon in chronic-phase CML.[18] The analysis identified two independent predictors of progression-free survival after 3 months of therapy. Both a neutrophil count $<1 \times 10^9/L$ and $\geq 65\%$ Ph+ metaphases predicted poor survival. Patients who had neither risk factor had an 18-month survival of 100% compared to a survival of 33% if they had both. The investigators concluded that myelosuppression from imatinib and failure to achieve cytogenetic remission after 3 months predicts poor survival in patients treated with imatinib. Sneed et al. confirmed this observation in a study of 143 patients treated with imatinib after failure with interferon.[19] In this study, drug-induced grade III myelosuppression reduced the CCR rate from 63–36% ($P = 0.001$).

### CML TREATED WITH IMATINIB

Imatinib has not been available for a long enough period of time to make firm conclusions with regard to long-term prognosis using the Sokal and Hasford scoring systems. Data are becoming available, however, with regard to the ability of imatinib to induce cytogenetic and molecular remissions that perhaps can be used as surrogate markers of long-term prognosis.

In the International Randomized Study of Interferon and STI-571 (IRIS) trial, patients with chronic-phase CML were randomized to treatment with either the combination of interferon and cytarabine or imatinib at a dose of 400 mg/day. The IRIS investigators attempted to calculate Sokal and Hasford scores at the time of enrollment into the trial. Unfortunately, 30% of patients lacked the necessary values to calculate the prognostic score. However, for those patients with a high-risk Sokal or Hasford score, the rates of CCR at 18 months were 56% and 66%, respectively, for patients treated with imatinib.[20] At the time the study was published, the duration of follow-up was too short to determine with confidence the applicability of either scoring system to survival in patients treated with imatinib. In contrast, a study of 77 patients treated with imatinib 400 mg daily in combination with interferon showed that both the Sokal and Hasford systems were useful in predicting major cytogenetic remission rates.[21] In this study, only 23% and 17% patients with high-risk scores by Sokal and Hasford criteria, respectively, achieved a major cytogenetic remission. Thus, firm conclusions about the applicability of these scoring systems to patients treated with imatinib await further analysis. Given the uncertainty surrounding the applicability of the Sokal and Hasford scoring systems, these scoring systems should not be routinely applied to patients treated with imatinib.

The prognostic scoring systems applied to patients with CML may be supplanted by newer, biologically-based, prognostic factors. Derivative chromosome 9 deletions are found in 10–15% of patients with chronic-phase CML at diagnosis.[22,23] The presence of these deletions clearly portends a worse prognosis in patients treated with either hydroxyurea or interferon and does so independently of either the Sokal or Hasford scores.[24] Patients harboring derivative chromosome 9 deletions have a better prognosis when treated with imatinib, but may not have as favorable a prognosis as those patients treated with imatinib in the absence of deletions.[25] In addition, the prognosis of patients with derivative chromosome 9 deletions treated with allogeneic HSCT may be poorer compared to those patients without deletions.[26]

Additional analysis of the IRIS trial has provided insight into other potential markers of prognosis in patients treated with imatinib for chronic-phase CML. Approximately 25% of patients fail to achieve CCR with imatinib 400 mg daily. These patients have a median progression-free survival of 85% at 24 months of follow-up. In contrast, patients achieving a CCR with imatinib have a 95–100% 24-month progression-free survival ($P = <0.001$) depending on the degree of molecular remission.[12,20] Therefore, the features of patients that predict for failure to achieve CCR with imatinib are also likely to portend poor survival and these patients might be suitable candidates for allogeneic HSCT as an initial treatment strategy.

Another strategy to predict outcome in patients treated with imatinib may be to monitor the quantitative reduction in *bcr/abl* transcript levels. In one study of 106 patients treated with imatinib and monitored by quantitative RT-PCR, the probability of a major cytogenetic response was significantly higher in patients with a *bcr-abl/bcr* ratio <20% after 2 months of imatinib therapy.[27]

Some patients have CML that is intrinsically resistant to imatinib at diagnosis. As many as 23% of untreated CML patients fail to achieve major cytogenetic remission after 6 months of imatinib dosed at 400 mg daily.[20] These patients generally acquire resistance to imatinib, although imatinib resistant mutations in *bcr/abl* have been reported before the treatment begins.[28,29] Acquired mutations that confer resistance are not useful as a prognostic tool at diagnosis. However, once recognized, some acquired mutations are associated with a worse prognosis than others.[30] There is no consensus as to how the detection of such mutations should guide therapy and whether or not allogeneic HSCT can impact on an otherwise poor prognosis.

### CML TREATED WITH ALLOGENEIC HSCT

The prognosis for patients initially treated with HSCT is generally favorable (see Chapter 37). However, certain clinical features do predict for improved survival after HSCT. The European Group for Blood and Marrow Transplantation (EGBMT) registry analyzed data in 3142 patients treated for CML between 1989 and 1997.[31] They developed a prognostic risk score based on known risk factors for outcome after HSCT such as age, donor/recipient gender, donor/recipient histocompatibility, stage of disease, and time from diagnosis to transplant. The scoring system that came of this analysis is given in Table 20.2. The total score derived from this system not only predicts transplant-related mortality, but also 5-year leukemia-free survival as depicted in Table 20.3.

Stem cell transplantation, however, is not a static field. Techniques are continually improving, as are reported results. Indeed, in a recent report of a single-institution experience of HLA identical sibling allogeneic HSCT, the reported 3-year disease-free survival

**Table 20.3**  The EGBMT scoring system predicts treatment-related mortality and leukemia-free survival

| Score | Treatment-related mortality (%) | 5-year leukemia-free survival (%) |
|---|---|---|
| 0 | 20 | 62 |
| 1 | 23 | 61 |
| 2 | 31 | 44 |
| 3 | 46 | 34 |
| 4 | 51 | 28 |
| 5 | 71 | 37 |
| 6 | 73 | 15 |
| 7 (only 4 patients) | NA | NA |

was 78% in 131 patients treated for chronic-phase CML.[32] Thus, the prognostic scoring systems of the past may not apply to the modern HSCT techniques available today.

The prognostic information available to the newly diagnosed patient with CML is both a blessing and a curse. While the patient may take comfort in knowing that cure is possible (and likely) with allogeneic HSCT, the relative safety, but lack of long-term prognostic information, of imatinib clouds decision making with regard to optimal treatment approaches. Clearly, patients with accelerated- or blast-phase CML should proceed as soon as possible to HSCT. For patients in chronic-phase CML, the issues are more controversial.

To sort through these issues, an expert panel was convened to provide treatment recommendations. They recommend that all patients be initiated on treatment with imatinib at diagnosis.[33] "Selected" patients may be considered for HSCT prior to a full therapeutic trial of imatinib. Although the panel does not elaborate on the definition of "selected," one could imagine that a young patient with high-risk features, such as anemia, splenomegaly, and thrombocytosis, would be a good candidate for an initial transplant approach. Failure to achieve CCR on imatinib, or failure to tolerate imatinib, is also an indication for HSCT.[33] The National Comprehensive Cancer Network (NCCN) has offered similar and more comprehensive guidelines.[34]

**Table 20.2**  The EGBMT prognostic scoring system for patients with CML treated with HSCT

| Risk factor | | Score |
|---|---|---|
| Donor | HLA identical sibling | 0 |
| | Matched unrelated donor | 1 |
| Disease stage | First chronic phase | 0 |
| | Accelerated phase | 1 |
| | Blast crisis of higher chronic phase | 2 |
| Age of recipient | <20 years | 0 |
| | 20–40 years | 1 |
| | >40 years | 2 |
| Gender combination | Other | 0 |
| | Male recipient female donor | 1 |
| Times from diagnosis to HSCT | ≤12 months | 0 |
| | >12 months | 1 |

## FOLLOW-UP

### CHRONIC PHASE

The patient with chronic-phase CML treated with imatinib requires close monitoring to determine response and to adjust therapy accordingly. Complete blood counts should be monitored weekly for at least 1

**Table 20.4**  Recommended follow-up evaluations for patients with CML in chronic phase being treated with imatinib

| | First year | | Subsequent years | | |
| --- | --- | --- | --- | --- | --- |
| | Every 3 months | Every 6 months | Every 3 months | Every 6 months | Every 12 months |
| *Blood sample* | | | | | |
| CBC and diff | X | | X | | |
| FISH analysis | X | | | | |
| QT-PCR | | X* | | X* | |
| *Bone marrow* | | | | | |
| Histology | | X | | | X |
| Cytogenetics | | X | | | X |

*Only if negative for bcr/abl by FISH.

month following the initiation of therapy. In the absence of significant myelosuppression, the monitoring interval may be successively increased up to about every 3 months.[33,35] A recommended approach to *bcr/abl* monitoring is provided in Table 20.4.

An assessment of treatment response should be made at 3-month intervals in the first year of therapy. Failure to tolerate imatinib or to achieve hematologic remission by 3 months is an indication for either increasing the dose of imatinib or proceeding to HSCT in appropriate patients.[33,36] More than half of patients will have achieved a major cytogenetic remission with imatinib at 3 months of follow-up.[20]

However, a bone marrow exam should be performed annually to include standard karyotype analysis even in the setting of a CCR. The development of additional cytogenetic abnormalities to the Ph+ clone predicts for relapse and progression to accelerated-phase disease after a response to imatinib.[37] Emerging results of treatment with imatinib have revealed another disturbing finding. Some patients develop clonal cytogenetic abnormalities in Philadelphia-chromosome-negative (Ph−) hematopoietic progenitors.[38] Although fewer than 10% of treated patients have been identified with Ph− clonal evolution,[39] the appearance of trisomy 8 and monosomy 7 among the reported abnormalities is a cause for concern. Indeed, several case reports of myelodysplasia, but not acute leukemia, have been reported in this setting.[38,40,41] Clonal evolution in a patient with chronic-phase CML should prompt a discussion of allogeneic HSCT as a viable treatment alternative.

If a patient achieves a CCR after 6–12 months of imatinib therapy, most investigators recommend imatinib be continued indefinitely. These patients are likely to have a relatively favorable prognosis although cure is by no means assured. The prognosis is particularly favorable if while in CCR, the level of *bcr/abl* transcripts becomes either undetectable or reduced more than 3-logs as determined by RT-PCR. These patients in molecular remission enjoy 100%

progression-free survival after 24 months of imatinib therapy.[12]

As previously discussed, patients who fail to achieve cytogenetic remission within 6 months of treatment with imatinib have a poorer prognosis, and one mechanism of imatinib resistance is mutations in *bcr/abl*. A second mechanism for imatinib resistance is up-regulation of *bcr/abl* by gene amplification, and these patients are candidates for either dose-escalation of imatinib or allogeneic HSCT.[29,42–46] Indeed, accelerated-phase CML with *bcr/abl* gene amplification responds better to a daily dose of 600 mg of imatinib than to a daily dose of 400 mg. Patients with chronic-phase CML resistant to 400 mg of imatinib may also achieve responses with higher doses.[36] However, these responses tend not to be durable, and alternative treatments, such as HSCT, have been recommended.[47] Similarly, patients who fail to achieve a major molecular remission, or have increasing titers of *bcr/abl*, after 9–12 months of imatinib therapy are candidates for alternative treatments including HSCT.

With regard to mechanisms of imatinib resistance, unfortunately, there is no practical widely available test that reliably distinguishes mechanisms of resistance to imatinib.

### ACCELERATED- AND BLAST-PHASE CML

The follow-up of patients with advanced CML depends largely on whether or not they are HSCT candidates. Although some patients with accelerated-phase CML can achieve relatively durable remissions (see Chapter 19), cure is unlikely, and progression is often rapid. Thus, patients with advanced CML should be considered for HSCT even if they respond favorably to imatinib therapy.

Not all patients are transplant candidates, however, and these patients will need to be monitored for evidence of progressive disease. Dose escalation of imatinib is a viable treatment option for patients progressing on standard doses. Whether combinations of imatinib with other active agents will prove beneficial is uncertain, but participation in clinical trials is recommended.

## REFERENCES

1. The Italian Cooperative Study Group on Chronic Myeloid Leukemia: Interferon alfa-2a as compared with conventional chemotherapy for the treatment of chronic myeloid leukemia. *N Engl J Med* 330(12):820–825, 1994.

2. Silver RT: Chronic myeloid leukemia: a perspective of the clinical and biologic issues of the chronic phase. *Hematol Oncol Clin North Am* 4(2):319–335, 1990.

3. Cervantes F, Rozman C: A multivariate analysis of prognostic factors in chronic myeloid leukemia. *Blood* 60(6):1298–1304, 1982.

4. Allan NC, Richards SM, Shepherd PCA, et al.: UK Medical Research Council randomised, multicentre trial of interferon-an1 for chronic myeloid leukaemia: improved survival irrespective of cytogenetic response. *Lancet* 345:1392–1397, 1995.

5. Hehlmann R, Berger U, Pfirrmann M, et al.: Randomized comparison of interferon alpha and hydroxyurea with hydroxyurea monotherapy in chronic myeloid leukemia (CML-study II): prolongation of survival by the combination of interferon alpha and hydroxyurea. *Leukemia* 17(8):1529–1537, 2003.

6. Bonifazi F, de Vivo A, Rosti G, et al.: Chronic myeloid leukemia and interferon-a: a study of complete cytogenetic responders. *Blood* 98(10):3074–3081, 2001.

7. Guilhot F, Chastang C, Michallet M, et al.: Interferon alfa-2b combined with cytarabine versus interferon alone in chronic myelogenous leukemia. *N Engl J Med* 337(4):223–229, 1997.

8. Le Gouill S, Talmant P, Milpied N, et al.: Fluorescence in situ hybridization on peripheral-blood specimens is a reliable method to evaluate cytogenetic response in chronic myeloid leukemia. *J Clin Oncol* 18:1533–1538, 2000.

9. Reinhold U, Hennig E, Leiblein S, et al.: FISH for BCR-ABL on interphases of peripheral blood neutrophils but not of unselected white cells correlates with bone marrow cytogenetics in CML patients treated with imatinib. *Leukemia* 17(10):1925–1929, 2003.

10. Kim YJ, Kim DW, Lee S, et al.: Comprehensive comparison of FISH, RT-PCR, and RQ-PCR for monitoring the BCR-ABL gene after hematopoietic stem cell transplantation in CML. *Eur J Haematol* 68(5):272–280, 2002.

11. Radich JP, Gooley T, Bryant E, et al.: The significance of bcr-abl molecular detection in chronic myeloid leukemia patients "late," 18 months or more after transplantation. *Blood* 98(6):1701–1707, 2001.

12. Hughes TP, Kaeda J, Branford S, et al.: Frequency of major molecular responses to imatinib or interferon alfa plus cytarabine in newly diagnosed chronic myeloid leukemia [see comment]. *N Engl J Med* 349(15):1423–1432, 2003.

13. Cortes J, Giles F, O'Brien S, et al.: Result of high-dose imatinib mesylate in patients with Philadelphia chromosome-positive chronic myeloid leukemia after failure of interferon-alpha. *Blood* 102(1):83–86, 2003.

14. Sokal JE, Cox EB, Baccarani M, et al.: Prognostic discrimination in "good-risk" chronic granulocytic leukemia. *Blood* 63:789–799, 1984.

15. Hasford J, Pfirrmann M, Hehlmann R, et al.: A new prognostic score for survival of patients with chronic myeloid leukemia treated with interferon-alfa. *J Natl Cancer Inst* 90:850–858, 1998.

16. Hasford J, Pfirrmann M, Hehlmann R, et al.: Prognosis and prognostic factors for patients with chronic myeloid leukemia: nontransplant therapy. *Semin Hematol* 40(1):4–12, 2003.

17. Cortes J, Talpaz M, O'Brien S, et al.: Effects of age on prognosis with imatinib mesylate therapy for patients with Philadelphia chromosome-positive chronic myelogenous leukemia. *Cancer* 98(6):1105–1113, 2003.

18. Marin D, Marktel S, Bua M, et al.: Prognostic factors for patients with chronic myeloid leukaemia in chronic phase treated with imatinib mesylate after failure of interferon alfa. *Leukemia* 17(8):1448–1453, 2003.

19. Sneed TB, Kantarjian HM, Talpaz M, et al.: The significance of myelosuppression during therapy with imatinib mesylate in patients with chronic myelogenous leukemia in chronic phase. *Cancer* 100(1):116–121, 2004.

20. O'Brien SG, Guilhot F, Larson RA, et al.: Imatinib compared with interferon and low-dose cytarabine for newly diagnosed chronic-phase chronic myeloid leukemia. *N Engl J Med* 348(11):994–1004, 2003.

21. Rosti G, Trabacchi E, Bassi S, et al.: Risk and early cytogenetic response to imatinib and interferon in chronic myeloid leukemia. *Haematologica* 88(3):256–259, 2003.

22. Herens C, Tassin F, Lemaire V, et al.: Deletion of the 5'-ABL region: a recurrent anomaly detected by fluorescence in situ hybridization in about 10% of Philadelphia-positive chronic myeloid leukaemia patients. *Br J Haematol* 110(1):214–216, 2000.

23. Sinclair PB, Nacheva EP, Leversha M, et al.: Large deletions at the t(9;22) breakpoint are common and may identify a poor-prognosis subgroup of patients with chronic myeloid leukemia. *Blood* 95(3):738–743, 2000.

24. Huntly BJ, Bench A, Green AR: Double jeopardy from a single translocation: deletions of the derivative chromosome 9 in chronic myeloid leukemia. *Blood* 102(4):1160–1168, 2003.

25. Huntly BJ, Guilhot F, Reid AG, et al.: Imatinib improves but may not fully reverse the poor prognosis of patients with CML with derivative chromosome 9 deletions. *Blood* 102(6):2205–2212, 2003.

26. Kolomietz E, Al-Maghrabi J, Brennan S, et al.: Primary chromosomal rearrangements of leukemia are frequently accompanied by extensive submicroscopic deletions and may lead to altered prognosis. *Blood* 97(11):3581–3588, 2001.

27. Merx K, Muller MC, Kreil S, et al.: Early reduction of BCR-ABL mRNA transcript levels predicts cytogenetic response in chronic phase CML patients treated with imatinib after failure of interferon alpha. *Leukemia* 16(9):1579–1583, 2002.

28. Roche-Lestienne C, Lai JL, Darre S, et al.: A mutation conferring resistance to imatinib at the time of diagnosis of chronic myelogenous leukemia. *N Engl J Med* 348(22):2265–2266, 2003.

29. Kreuzer KA, Le Coutre P, Landt O, et al.: Preexistence and evolution of imatinib mesylate-resistant clones in chronic myelogenous leukemia detected by a PNA-based PCR clamping technique. *Ann Hematol* 82(5):284–289, 2003.

30. Branford S, Rudzki Z, Walsh S, et al.: Detection of BCR-ABL mutations in patients with CML treated with imatinib is

virtually always accompanied by clinical resistance, and mutations in the ATP phosphate-binding loop (P-loop) are associated with a poor prognosis. *Blood* 102(1): 276–283, 2003.

31. Gratwohl A, Hermans J, Goldman JM, et al.: Risk assessment for patients with chronic myeloid leukaemia before allogeneic blood or marrow transplantation. *Lancet* 352:1087–1092, 1998.

32. Radich JP, Gooley T, Bensinger W, et al.: HLA-matched related hematopoietic cell transplantation for chronic-phase CML using a targeted busulfan and cyclophosphamide preparative regimen. *Blood* 102(1):31–35, 2003.

33. Nimer SD, DiPersio JF, Kantarjian H, et al.: Practical Management Guidelines in CML: a consensus report. In: Nimer SD (ed.) The Philadelphia Consortium Roundtable; 2002 March, 2003; Philadelphia, PA: AOI Communications; 2002.

34. Network NCC: Chronic myelogenous leukemia: clinical practice guidelines in oncology. *J Natl Compr Cancer Netw* 1(1 suppl):S14–S40, 2003.

35. Deininger MW, O'Brien SG, Ford JM, Druker BJ: Practical management of patients with chronic myeloid leukemia receiving imatinib. *J Clin Oncol* 21(8):1637–1647, 2003.

36. Kantarjian HM, Talpaz M, O'Brien S, et al.: Dose escalation of imatinib mesylate can overcome resistance to standard-dose therapy in patients with chronic myelogenous leukemia. *Blood* 101(2):473–475, 2003.

37. O'Dwyer ME, Mauro MJ, Blasdel C, et al.: Clonal evolution and lack of cytogenetic response are adverse prognostic factors for hematologic relapse of chronic phase CML patients treated with imatinib mesylate. *Blood* 103(2):451–455, 2004.

38. O'Dwyer ME, Gatter KM, Loriaux M, et al.: Demonstration of Philadelphia chromosome negative abnormal clones in patients with chronic myelogenous leukemia during major cytogenetic responses induced by imatinib mesylate. *Leukemia* 17(3):481–487, 2003.

39. Medina J, Kantarjian H, Talpaz M, et al.: Chromosomal abnormalities in Philadelphia chromosome-negative metaphases appearing during imatinib mesylate therapy in patients with Philadelphia chromosome-positive chronic myelogenous leukemia in chronic phase. *Cancer* 98(9):1905–1911, 2003.

40. Bumm T, Muller C, Al-Ali H-K, et al.: Emergence of clonal cytogenetic abnormalities in Ph- cells in some CML patients in cytogenetic remission to imatinib but restoration of polyclonal hematopoiesis in the majority. *Blood* 101(5):1941–1949, 2003.

41. Andersen MK, Pedersen-Bjergaard J, Kjeldsen L, et al.: Clonal Ph-negative hematopoiesis in CML after therapy with imatinib mesylate is frequently characterized by trisomy 8. *Leukemia* 16(7):1390–1393, 2002.

42. Azam M, Latek RR, Daley GQ: Mechanisms of autoinhibition and STI-571/imatinib resistance revealed by mutagenesis of BCR-ABL. *Cell* 112(6):831–843, 2003.

43. Hochhaus A, Kreil S, Corbin AS, et al.: Molecular and chromosomal mechanisms of resistance to imatinib (STI571) therapy. *Leukemia* 16(11):2190–2196, 2002.

44. Weisberg E, Griffin JD: Mechanism of resistance to the ABL tyrosine kinase inhibitor STI571 in BCR/ABL-transformed hematopoietic cell lines. *Blood* 95(11): 3498–3505, 2000.

45. Mahon FX, Deininger MWN, Schultheis B, et al.: Selection and characterization of BCR-ABL positive cell lines with differential sensitivity to the tyrosine kinase inhibitor STI571: diverse mechanisms of resistance. *Blood* 96(3):1070–1079, 2000.

46. le Coutre P, Tassi E, Varella-Garcia M, et al.: Induction of resistance to the Abelson inhibitor STI571 in human leukemic cells through gene amplification. *Blood* 95(5): 1758–1766, 2000.

47. Zonder JA, Pemberton P, Brandt H, et al.: The effect of dose increase of imatinib mesylate in patients with chronic or accelerated phase chronic myelogenous leukemia with inadequate hematologic or cytogenetic response to initial treatment. *Clin Cancer Res* 9(6): 2092–2097, 2003.

# Chapter 21

# NEW FRONTIERS IN THE TREATMENT OF RELAPSED OR REFRACTORY CHRONIC MYELOGENOUS LEUKEMIA

*Seema Gupta, Javier Pinilla-Ibarz, Peter Maslak, and David Scheinberg*

## INTRODUCTION

The introduction of imatinib mesylate to the therapy of chronic myeloid leukemia (CML) radically changed the clinical management of patients with this disorder and ushered in the era of effective targeted therapy for this disease. The results from the initial clinical studies have established imatinib as the standard for newly diagnosed therapy of chronic phase CML. As an increasing number of patients are treated with imatinib and as the long-term follow-up data on the durability of responses to imatinib continue to evolve, attention has focused on both the development of resistance to this therapy and the potential clinical implications such resistance has on the management of this disease.

Questions regarding the ultimate efficacy of imatinib have been framed in the context of whether this agent can eliminate the clonogenic BCR/ABL-positive leukemia cell. While most patients who successfully undergo allogeneic stem cell transplantation are rendered BCR/ABL negative via reverse transcriptase polymerase chain reaction (RT-PCR), this is generally not the case with imatinib. Instead, data suggest that quantitative PCR and the ability to induce a 3-log reduction below the baseline BCR/ABL transcript is predictive of long-term response. The results from a large randomized international study demonstrated that patients who were able to achieve a ≥3-log reduction (major molecular response or MMR) in BCR/ABL by RT-PCR had a better prognosis than those who were unable to do so.[1] In this trial, 58% of patients who were in complete cytogenetic remission (CCR) at the 12-month mark did not progress over the next 12 months.[1] Patients who were in a CCR and who did not achieve a ≥3-log reduction had a 5% chance of disease progression. In this study, however, an MMR was achieved in 39% of the patients who were randomized to imatinib therapy but only 2% of patients randomized to the IFN-α plus ara-C arm. In addition, early and prompt reduction in the BCR/ABL transcript level has been shown to be predictive of CCR.[2,3] In another study, 106 patient samples were analyzed and the level of BCR/ABL transcript at 2 months predicted for major cytogenetic response (MCR) at 6 months. Both of these studies raise the issue of the clinical relevancy of current available surrogate endpoints and whether qualitative or quantitative measurements should be used to gauge the efficacy of therapy. While complete eradication of the leukemic clone to a level undetectable by the most sensitive method available could be the ultimate goal of therapy, the ability to achieve long-term survival may also correlate with a decrease in the amount of minimal residual disease below a "critical" level. In this scenario, trace amounts of the disease may be present, but not clinically relevant as a patient continues in complete clinical remission.

## IMATINIB RESISTANCE—EVOLUTION OF THE TARGET

Published criteria defines primary resistance to imatinib mesylate as the inability to reach complete hematologic remission (CHR) by 3 months, MCR (defined as (≤35% of cells positive for the BCR/ABL transcript) by 6 months, or CCR by 12 months of therapy. Approximately 20–30% of newly diagnosed patients are resistant to imatinib using such criteria.[1,2] MD Anderson Cancer Center (MDACC) has reported that primary resistance can be reduced to about 10% by increasing the standard administered dose of imatinib to 800 mg/day.[3] Acquired resistance to imatinib may, however, develop as the neoplastic cells exhibit alternative mechanisms to maintain sufficient amounts of active BCR/ABL signal to maintain growth. Clinically, acquired resistance is defined as the loss of an established hematologic, cytogenetic, or molecular response or the progression of disease to an accelerated or blastic phase. In the large randomized imatinib study discussed above, approximately 8% of patients had an acquired resistance to imatinib by 18 months on treatment.[1]

Clinical resistance may develop by several mechanisms, including BCR/ABL gene amplification, incomplete inhibition of BCR/ABL cells with the subsequent selection of resistant cells, BCR/ABL gene mutations, and possibly, increased expression of the *MDR-1* gene encoded P-glycoprotein. Increased expression of BCR/ABL by chromosome or gene amplification appears to be the most common mechanism of acquired resistance in vitro.[4,5] In the clinical setting, however, several studies have shown that another common cause of acquired resistance is the development of mutations in the kinase domain of BCR/ABL.[6–8] Several groups have reported at least 20 different point mutations from the leukemic cells of patients resistant to imatinib. The two most common kinase domain mutations, T315I and E255K, change the conformation of the protein and prevent the binding of imatinib to the BCR/ABL protein.[6,9,10] Although these mutations were not identified in patient samples taken prior to initiation of therapy with imatinib, they were most likely present in undetectable quantities at the time of diagnosis. This has been shown in patients with Ph-positive ALL prior to therapy with imatinib.[11]

Under the selective pressure of imatinib treatment, these resistant molecules emerge, giving rise to progressive disease. When patients are identified as becoming imatinib resistant, direct sequencing of BCR/ABL can be employed to define the possible mechanism of resistance. Such a strategy may, in the future, help guide treatment decisions as alternative targets and agents become available. Table 21.1 summarizes some novel therapies for treatment of imatinib-resistant CML.

## STRATEGIES FOR OVERCOMING IMATINIB RESISTANCE

### DOSE ESCALATION OF IMATINIB

If clinical resistance is modulated by an increase in the amount of BCR/ABL, it might be possible to overcome the resistance by increasing either the dose of imatinib or the ability of imatinib to bind to its target. Mutations such as T315I and E255K confer steric changes that are difficult to overcome even with higher doses of imatinib. Other mutations, such as M244V, F311L, and M351T, however, may be overcome by escalating the dose of imatinib.[7] Certain other mutations, namely those in the ATP phosphate-binding loop (P loop), such as E255K, may confer a poor prognosis. In one Australian study, 12/13 patients with mutations in the P loop had a median survival of only 4.5 months.[7] Mutations in the activation loop (A loop), downstream from the A loop, and in the imatinib-binding regions of the kinase may be at least partially sensitive to higher doses of imatinib. As these different mutations retain varying sensitivities to imatinib, it is rational to attempt dose escalation in such patients.

| Table 21.1 | Novel therapies to treat imatinib-resistant CML | |
|---|---|---|
| Therapy | Mechanism | Developmental status |
| Transplantation (auto or allo) | GvL | Established therapy |
| Dose escalation of imatinib (600–800 mg) | Inhibition of partially resistant bcr/abl mutants | Phase II/III trials ongoing |
| Geldanamycin, 17-AAG, ATO, siRNA, ribozymes | Downregulation of intracellular BCR/ABL levels | Preclinical/phase I/II |
| PD173955, PD166326, AP23464, BMS354825 | Second-generation tyrosine kinase inhibitors | Preclinical/phase I/II/III |
| FTIs (tipifarnib), zolendronate | Inhibition of downstream Ras signaling pathway | Phase I |
| Rapamycin, CCI-779 | Inhibitor of downstream effector m-tor in PI-3 kinase pathway | Phase I |
| Leptomycin B | Nuclear entrapment of bcr/abl preventing its antiapoptotic effect | Preclinical |
| PSC833, verapamil | P-glycoprotein inhibitors | Preclinical |
| HHT | Plant alkaloid, unknown | Phase I/II |
| Bortezimib | Proteosome inhibition | Phase I/II |

Alternatively, the upregulation of the BCR/ABL signal through mechanisms of gene amplification may also be amenable to dose escalation. In this scenario, the intrinsic sensitivity of the cell is retained, and the desired clinical effect is a function of the dose-response curve. Critical levels of imatinib are needed to inhibit BCR/ABL function and may be achieved by increasing the doses of the agent. The experience reported by MDACC demonstrates better responses when higher doses of imatinib are used as initial therapy, and has laid the groundwork for this strategy.

## DOWNREGULATION OF INTRACELLULAR BCR/ABL LEVELS

Noxious stimuli to cells activate the synthesis of some proteins while inhibiting the synthesis of others. The heat-shock proteins are molecular chaperones that stabilize the tertiary conformation of key cellular proteins, including proteins involved in signal transduction. Misfolding of proteins can produce inactive aggregated forms. Heat-shock protein 90 (hsp90) is a specific molecular chaperone that affects the stability and function of multiple oncogenic proteins, including BCR/ABL.[12,13] Geldanamycin is a benzoquinone ansamycin antibiotic that inhibits hsp90 by competitively binding to an ATP-binding pocket in the amino terminus of the hsp90 molecule.[12–14] Inactivation of hsp90 causes dysfunction and rapid degradation of their "client proteins" (including Raf-1, v-Src, p185[c-erbB-2], and BCR/ABL)[13,15,16] via the proteosome pathway. A less toxic analog of geldanamycin, 17-AAG, has been shown in preclinical studies to down regulate BCR/ABL in Ph-positive cell lines K562 and transfected HL60.[13] When the hsp90 protein is inhibited, BCR/ABL is rendered sensitive to cellular physiologic mechanisms and can be degraded by the ubiquitin-proteosome pathway -3 activating the intrinsic apoptotic pathway.[13] This appears to be the mechanism of action of this class of drugs. Preclinical laboratory studies have shown that BCR/ABL point mutations isolated from imatinib-resistant CML are degraded in vitro by both geldanamycin and 17-AAG. This effect has been demonstrated in both the T3151 and E255K cell lines.[17] In both cell lines, the BCR/ABL protein was depleted at a low concentration of geldanamycin (30 nm).[12] Leukemic blasts taken from three patients with CML blast crisis, who progressed while on imatinib, have been shown in vitro to be susceptible to 17-AAG-induced apoptosis.[18] These laboratory observations have raised the possibility of combining other therapeutic agents with 17-AAG in an effort to reverse the drug-resistant phenotype in patients with advanced stage disease.

Arsenic trioxide (ATO) represents a novel agent that has shown preclinical activity in the treatment of imatinib-resistant CML by inducing alteration of mitochondrial inner transmembrane potential, leading to the release of cytochrome c with subsequent caspase activation and apoptosis.[19] Recently, ATO has also been shown to interfere with the translation of BCR/ABL by inhibition of ribosomal p70S6 kinase activity.[20,21] Based on this rationale, the ATO and imatinib combination has been studied in numerous Ph-positive cell lines. Studies using the K562 and HL60/BCR/ABL cell lines have shown that the proapoptotic activity of imatinib is enhanced in the presence of ATO.[21] Cotreatment of K562 and transfected MO7p210 cells with approximately equipotent doses of ATO and imatinib additively inhibited growth proliferation.[22] In colony-forming assays using CML patient samples, the combination of ATO and imatinib showed increased antiproliferative activity compared to imatinib alone.[22] The additive effect of the ATO in combination with imatinib has initiated several phase I and II clinical trials examining the combination.

Interruption of the messenger RNA (mRNA) of mutant BCR/ABL may also be a target for therapeutic intervention. Antisense oligonucleotides could be designed that are complementary to the sequences on mutant BCR/ABL fusion transcripts. These small molecules would interfere with translation by physically blocking ribosome access to mRNA of the aberrant CML cells without affecting normal cells. Other mechanisms may potentially play a role in the antisense effects on BCR/ABL. DNA—RNA hybrids are more susceptible to RNAse activity, and several studies have shown that this strategy is feasible in CML cells in vitro.[23–26] However, these agents have been difficult to study and implement in humans, even though they can be delivered relatively safely. This difficulty may, in part, be due to the long half-life of the BCR/ABL protein in vivo and the inability to deliver the drug in a manner that will allow it to be present in the cell for longer periods of time (i.e., 24–48 h). In addition, poor uptake of these antisense oligonucleotides into cells may prohibit their clinical usefulness. A similar strategy is based on RNA interference (RNAi). Several groups have reported in vitro BCR/ABL inhibitory effects, using small interfering RNA oligonucleotides (siRNA) in CML cell lines.[27–29] Ribozymes (RNA) and DNAzymes (DNA) are designed to hybridize to specific RNA molecules and initiate hydrolysis of phosphodiester bonds in the target RNA. These strategies have all shown promise in the preclinical setting, but the clinical feasibility in imatinib-resistant patients has not yet to be established.

## SECOND-GENERATION TYROSINE KINASE INHIBITORS

Agents that have a different conformational binding to BCR/ABL than imatinib provide another potential approach to imatinib-resistant CML. Such compounds may be particularly useful in patients who have developed point mutations in the ABL domain and are no longer able to bind imatinib in the kinase pocket and inhibit ATP binding. Second-generation tyrosine kinase inhibitors may still be able to bind the appropriate binding site and block ATP from binding. Several of these agents are currently being developed in both the laboratory and the clinic. PD173955 (Pfizer) is a more potent inhibitor of BCR/ABL than is imatinib. Unlike imatinib, this small molecule has been shown to bind Abl independent of its phosphorylation state.[30] Hence, more potent tyrosine kinase inhibitors may be able to maintain activity against mutated clones. PD166326 (Pfizer), a novel compound in the pyridopyrimidine class of tyrosine kinase inhibitors, has been shown to be a potent inhibitor of BCR/ABL tyrosine kinase activity and BCR/ABL-dependent proliferation.[31] The activity of PD166326 against BCR/ABL-induced leukemia in an in vivo mouse model has recently been reported (N Wolff, ASH 2003). PD166326- and imatinib-treated mice had improved survival, lower white blood cell (WBC) count, and less splenomegaly than placebo-treated mice, suggesting that PD166326 was superior to imatinib in decreasing the overall leukemic burden. Thus, in this CML animal model, the novel tyrosine kinase inhibitor PD166326 exhibited greater antileukemic activity than imatinib, suggesting that further development of this or a related compound may lead to even more potent drugs for the treatment of human CML. The investigators have postulated that, similar to the experience with combination chemotherapy, combinations of different kinase inhibitors at the initiation of therapy may suppress the emergence of resistant clones and improve therapeutic outcomes.

In vitro data on the novel dual selective SRC/ABL inhibitor, AP23464 (ARIAD pharmaceuticals, Cambridge, MA), has shown that this drug inhibits in vitro growth of cells that express either wild-type BCR/ABL or the most prevalent mutations induced by imatinib in BCR/ABL: Q252H, Y253F, E255K, M351T, or H396P.[32] AP23464 was approximately eightfold more potent than imatinib in inhibiting the growth of Ba/F3 cells expressing wild-type BCR/ABL. Also, AP23464 inhibited the growth of Ba/F3 cells expressing all mutant forms of BCR/ABL except for T315I at the same nanomolar concentrations as the wild type.[32] Studies to assess the in vivo activity of AP23464 and key analogs are currently in progress.

Another second-generation tyrosine kinase inhibitor that is currently in clinical trials is BMS-354825. The studies are being conducted in patients with chronic phase CML who are resistant to imatinib.[33]

### INHIBITORS OF THE DOWNSTREAM PATHWAYS
### Ras signaling

Activation of the Ras signaling pathway is essential for BCR/ABL function. After BCR/ABL has activated Ras, Ras requires several additional posttranslational modifications, including prenylation. Prenylation involves adding a lipid anchor to the target protein, which facilitates binding of this protein to cellular membranes, allowing them to function as intermediates in the process(es) of signal transduction. In the Ras pathway, prenylation is catalyzed by farnesyl protein transferase; the farnesyl transferase inhibitors (FTIs) interfere with this step by inhibiting this enzyme. Given the central role that the *ras* oncogene plays in controlling cellular metabolism, multiple FTI compounds are currently being developed and tested across a wide range of hematologic malignancies. A phase I/II study of tipifarnib, an FTI, in patients with a spectrum of myeloproliferative disorders reported preliminary results in 23 patients.[34] Tipifarnib was administered at a dose of 300 mg p.o. b.i.d. for 21 days every 4 weeks. Clinical WBC responses [normalization of WBC, complete remission (CR); or >50% WBC count reduction, partial remission] were seen in 5 of 21 (24%) evaluable patients. No cytogenetic responses were seen in six evaluable patients. Grade 2 anemia and greater than grade 3 thrombocytopenia were the most common hematologic toxicities.[34] Two other phase I studies of tipifarnib in combination with imatinib for the treatment of CML have also been reported. Cortes et al. conducted a phase I study of the combination of tipifarnib with imatinib in patients with CML in chronic phase who had failed imatinib therapy.[35] Doses of tipifarnib of 300 mg p.o. b.i.d. for the first 14 days of each 21-day cycle were administered with imatinib 300 mg daily. Subsequent doses of 300 and 400 mg, and 400 and 400 mg, respectively, in the same schedule were also administered. Nine patients were treated; three at each dose level. Hematologic responses were seen in patients with abnormal blood counts but none of the patients achieved a cytogenetic response.[35] A second phase I trial also combined tipifarnib with imatinib, but in patients with accelerated (AP) or blastic phase (BP) of CML with hematologic relapse or cytogenetic resistance to imatinib. Imatinib was given at 600 mg p.o. daily and combined with escalating doses of tipifarnib (200–600 mg p.o. b.i.d.). The combination therapy was administered for 21 days. Of the six evaluable patients, in the first cohort, three patients reached a complete hematologic response. No cytogenetic responses were seen.[36]

Zolendronate, a bisphosphonate, has been shown to inhibit downstream signaling of Ras in vitro. Additional in vitro and murine model studies have shown synergy between imatinib and zolendronate, providing a rationale for examining this combination in the clinical setting.[37]

### PI-3K/AKT pathway

PI-3 kinase activation is essential for the BCR/ABL-mediated transformation of cells. PI-3 kinase is a heterodimer consisting of catalytic (p110) and regulatory (p85) segments. BCR/ABL interacts with the p85 subunit. Two PI-3 kinase inhibitors are currently in clinical development. Wortmannin and LY294002 are active compounds and synergize with imatinib in vitro.[38,39] Wortmannin is a naturally occurring compound and is highly unstable in solution, making it a challenging compound to develop clinically.

Several downstream effectors in this PI-3 kinase pathway have been identified. One is m-TOR, which is involved in the phosphorylation of several signaling proteins, including the S6 ribosomal protein, an important target of BCR/ABL.[40] Inhibitors of m-TOR, such as rapamycin, have been attractive as possible therapeutic agents in CML. These agents have already undergone phase I/II clinical testing in a variety of other tumors and are currently beginning clinical trials in CML.[41]

### OTHER NOVEL APPROACHES TO THERAPY OF RELAPSED CML

Imatinib-resistant cell lines have been shown to overexpress the multidrug-resistance drug transport protein P-glycoprotein. Sensitivity to imatinib could be partially restored in vitro when the cells were exposed to verapamil or PSC833, both P-glycoprotein inhibitors.[42]

Leptomycin B is a novel therapeutic responsible for nuclear entrapment of BCR/ABL. BCR/ABL exerts an antiapoptotic effect in the cytoplasm of cells. Leptomycin B is an inhibitor of the nuclear export of BCR/ABL, preventing it from reaching the cytoplasm, thus abrogating its antiapoptotic effect on cells. It has also been shown that nuclear BCR/ABL induces apoptosis of cells in vitro.[43] Nuclear entrapment is thus another potential therapeutic strategy for imatinib-resistant disease.

Homoharringtonine (HHT) is a plant alkaloid derived from the *Cephalotaxus fortuneii* tree, known to have antileukemia activity when first used by the Chinese in the treatment of both acute myeloid leukemia (AML) and CML in the late 1970s.[44,45] MDACC has performed several studies in the pre-imatinib era using HHT alone and in combination with IFN-α in chronic phase CML, and has demonstrated the ability of this drug to induce CR. Seventy-two percent of 58 patients in late chronic phase were able to achieve a CHR with HHT alone. However, only 31% of patients had a cytogenetic response. In vitro data suggests that there is a synergistic effect of HHT in combination with imatinib in vitro, providing a potential rationale for combination therapy in resistant patients.[46]

The ubiquitin-proteasome pathway is the primary intracellular pathway responsible for the degradation of proteins. Proteasome inhibitors are being investigated as potential therapies in a wide variety of hematologic malignancies. Inactivation of NF-κB appears to be crucial in the activity of proteosome inhibitors. NF-κB is inhibited in the cytoplasm through binding to IκB, a substrate for proteasomes.[47] In CML, BCR/ABL activates NF-κB-dependent transcription, and NF-κB is necessary for BCR/ABL-mediated cell proliferation.[48–50] PS-341 is a potent and selective inhibitor of the proteosome that has shown significant clinical activity in multiple myeloma. In vitro, PS-341 induced significant growth inhibition and apoptosis in several BCR/ABL-positive cell lines, including both imatinib-sensitive and -resistant cell lines.[51] Clinical studies in imatinib-resistant patients are ongoing.

## IMMUNOTHERAPY

### ROLE OF ALLOGENEIC TRANSPLANTATION

Since the first demonstration of its curative potential, allogeneic stem cell transplantation has played an important role in the management of CML. The results for a wide range of these clinical studies are reviewed in Chapter 37. The ability of both interferon and imatinib to affect the natural history of the disease has altered the initial treatment paradigms, and some debate has surrounded both the institution and the timing of stem cell transplantation in the course of therapy. Such treatment decisions are tempered by consideration of the risk/benefit ratio particularly, as it pertains to specific groups of patients.

Despite the current controversy surrounding the most appropriate time to proceed with allogeneic stem cell transplantation in CML, the experience with this modality has proven valuable as proof of concept regarding the clinical efficacy of immunotherapy. The model of the "graft-versus-leukemia" (GvL) effect has been further refined and, in turn, has given rise to immunology-based therapeutic strategies, such as donor leukocyte infusions (DLI) and reduced intensity, nonmyeloblative transplantation ("mini-transplants"). Such approaches have been pioneered in CML and applied, with varying degrees of success, in other forms of human leukemia.

### SPECIFIC IMMUNOTHERAPY WITH BCR/ABL-DERIVED PEPTIDE VACCINES

As discussed above, many clinicians still consider allogeneic stem cell transplantation to be the "gold standard" for curative therapy in CML by virtue of the long-term survival achieved and the ability of this modality to render the patient BCR/ABL negative using PCR-based assays. The importance of the immunologic properties of the graft has received a great amount of attention, with attempts to recapitulate a GvL effect while separating it from the side effects of conventional transplantation regimens undertaken by a number of investigators. The potential to induce and then employ specific antileukemic immune effectors is attractive and has seen realization in the formulation of a vaccine strategy for this disease.

The unique amino acid sequences encompassing the b3a2, b2a2, or e1a2 in BCR/ABL breakpoints can be considered truly tumor-specific antigens because they contain sequences that are not expressed in any normal cellular protein. Despite the intracellular location of these proteins, short peptides produced by cellular processing of the fusion protein products can be presented on the cell surface within the cleft of HLA molecules, and in this form, they can be recognized by T cells.[52–54] Several investigators have demonstrated the immunogenicity from fusion-region-derived peptides of p210-b3a2 in the context of MHC class I and class II. By screening large numbers of fusion peptides from the junctional sequences of CML, several peptides have been derived from the b3a2 CML breakpoint that bind with high, intermediate, or low affinity to HLA-A0201, A3, A11, and B8.[53,55–58] Recent mass spectrometry studies have further demonstrated the presence of cell-surface HLA-associated BCR/ABL peptides previously described as binders of HLA-A0301 in primary CML cells from HLA-A3-positive patients.[59] This is the first direct evidence of naturally processed and expressed endogenous BCR/ABL peptides on the surface of CML cells. Support for the immunogenicity of synthetic BCR/ABL fusion peptides capable of interacting with class II MHC molecules has been accumulating as well. Peptides corresponding to the b3a2 fusion sequences have been shown to bind DR3 (DRB1*0301), DR4 (DRB1*0402), and DR11 (DRB1*1101), and b3a2 peptides have been shown to induce HLA-DR1 (DRB1*0101), DR2 (DRB1*1501), DR4 (DRB1*0401), DR9 (DRB1*0901), and DR11 (DRB1*1101) restricted proliferative responses of CD4-positive T lymphocytes and cytotoxic cell responses associated with DRB1*0901.[55,60–64] Indirect evidence for processing and recognition of p210-b3a2 class II has been described.[60,64,65] Evidence for immunogenicity on class I and class II b2a2 and e1a2 peptides-derived breakpoint translocations have also been reported.

Based on the immunogenic evidence of b3a2 peptides-derived translocation, the Memorial Sloan-Kettering Cancer Center (MSKCC) Group initiated studies to evaluate the safety and immunogenicity of a multidose, multivalent BCR/ABL breakpoint peptide vaccine in CML patients, with a b3a2 breakpoint.

Based on these results, a phase II trial in adult CML patients with any HLA type and a b3a2 breakpoint was undertaken. Patients were vaccinated five times over a 10-week period using a preparation of six peptides (100 μg each) and the immunologic adjuvant QS-21 (100 μg). Immunologically responding patients received three additional monthly vaccinations, and those with continued response received another three bimonthly vaccinations. Immune and clinical responses were measured. All 14 patients developed delayed-type hypersensitivity (DTH) and/or CD4 proliferative responses, and 11 of 14 patients showed IFN-γ release by CD4 ELISPOT. A peptide-specific CD8-positive IFN-γ ELISPOT was found in four patients; two of them had received an allogeneic stem cell transplantation prior to relapse. Four patients in hematologic remission had a decrease in Ph percentage (three concurrently receiving IFN-α and one on imatinib), and three patients in molecular relapse after allogeneic transplant became transiently PCR negative after vaccination. Two of these patients received DLI after the first vaccination in an attempt to vaccinate the naive donor leukocytes within the recipient (vaccination by proxy). All five patients on IFN ultimately reached a complete cytogenetic remission. These results suggested that a tumor-specific BCR/ABL breakpoint peptide-derived vaccine could be safely administered to patients and that such a vaccine could elicit measurable peptide-specific CD4 immune responses in all treated patients, including patients post stem cell transplantation, on interferon, or on imatinib. A causal relationship between clinical response and vaccination, however, remains unclear and requires further study in the context of well-designed clinical trials.

Recently, an Italian group has reported results using the same BCR/ABL vaccine. In this study, 16 evaluable patients with CML in chronic phase with at least one of a group of designated specific HLA subtypes (HLA A3, A11, B8, DR11, DR1, or DR4) were treated. Patients with a b3a2, BCR/ABL breakpoint were vaccinated subcutaneously six times over a 12-week period (every 2 weeks) using a preparation of five peptides mixed with QS-21 and granulocyte-macrophage colony-stimulating factor (GM-CSF) the day before and the day of vaccination. Patients who responded immunologically received two booster vaccinations at 4- and 8-month interval from the date of the last vaccination. As in the prior study, no significant toxic effects were observed. Thirteen of 16 patients developed CD4 proliferative responses and 9 of 16 DTH. In 10 patients treated with imatinib, 5 of 9 patients became CCR after three to six vaccinations.[66] Three of the five CCR patients were also able to achieve a molecular response. In six patients treated with IFN-α, two had a CCR. These results supported the findings from the MSKCC Group regarding the safety and measurable peptide-specific CD4 immune responses in all treated patients, and provide a rationale for future clinical trials in the context of minimal residual disease induced by imatinib.[66]

### SELF-ANTIGENS FOR IMMUNOTHERAPY OF CML

Proteinase 3, a serine protease stored in azurophilic granules, is a differentiation antigen associated with myeloid granule formation and is overexpressed in a variety of myeloid leukemia types, including CML cells. Therefore, it has been considered a possible target antigen for specific active immunotherapy. CTLs specific for an HLA-A2.1-restricted nonpolymorphic peptide (PR1) derived from proteinase 3 have shown HLA-restricted cytotoxicity, and selectively inhibit CML progenitors over normal marrow cells.[67,68] PR1-specific T cells have been identified by HLA-A2-PR1 peptide HLA tetramers in a majority of CML patients who responded to either IFN-α or allogeneic stem cell transplantation.[69] PR1-specific CTLs isolated from these patients were capable of lysing fresh leukemia cells. Follow-up studies in patients with relapsed CML revealed a selective loss of the high-avidity PR1-CTL population by tetramer determination. A functional PR1-specific CTL immune response was also lost prior to CML relapse, suggesting a possible therapeutic role for "add back" of high-affinity PR1-CTL.

The results of a phase I vaccine trial using a PR1 peptide in patients with HLA A0201 have been reported. This trial included a total of 15 patients: 6 with CML (interferon resistant or relapsed after stem cell transplantation), 8 with AML (smoldering relapse or ≥second CR), and 1 with MDS with no detectable antibodies to proteinase 3 (antineutrophil cytoplasmic autoantibody negative). Patients were treated with three dose levels of PR1 peptide in incomplete Freud's adjuvant (Montanide ISA-51) and 70 µg of GM-CSF every 3 weeks for three injections. Eight of 15 patients (53%) had some evidence of immune response to the peptide vaccine as assessed by tetramer staining and flow cytometric detection of intracellular IFN-γ. In this group, five patients experienced a clinical response, including three patients with a molecular response and one with a cytogenetic response. In one patient, tetramer sort-purified PR1-CTL obtained after vaccination showed PR1 specificity against peptide-pulsed T2 cells, as well as significant lysis of BM cell at diagnosis but not at remission. This study provided evidence that peptide vaccination against PR1 of leukemia patients can elicit highly active specific cellular immunity against leukemia.

## CONCLUSION

The introduction of imatinib therapy has altered the paradigm for the clinical management of patients with CML. Despite the overwhelmingly positive results with this agent, a potential flaw with a targeted therapy like imatinib is that the target needs to be present in a form or amount that is sensitive to this specific modality in every clonogenic cell. The inherent genetic instability of CML poses both a theoretical and practical problem for single-agent therapy. Patients who have primary resistance to imatinib or who develop resistance following therapy require alternative approaches to control and ultimately cure the disease. As new targets are identified, agents can be introduced to complement imatinib and administer as part of combination therapy. Alternatively, immunologic approaches will continue to be used for patients who fail first line therapy as the models of active specific immunity are refined and the adoptive cellular therapies receive more widespread application.

## REFERENCES

1. Hughes TP, Kaeda J, Branford S, et al.: Frequency of major molecular responses to imatinib or interferon alfa plus cytarabine in newly diagnosed chronic myeloid leukemia. *N Engl J Med* 349(15):1423–1432, 2003.

2. O'Brien SG, Guilhot F, Larson RA, et al.: Imatinib compared with interferon and low-dose cytarabine for newly diagnosed chronic-phase chronic myeloid leukemia. *N Engl J Med* 348(11):994–1004, 2003.

3. Kantarjian H, Talpaz M, O'Brien S, et al.: High-dose imatinib mesylate therapy in newly diagnosed Philadelphia chromosome-positive chronic phase chronic myeloid leukemia. *Blood* 103(8):2873–2878, 2004.

4. Mahon FX, Deininger MW, Schultheis B, et al.: Selection and characterization of BCR-ABL positive cell lines with differential sensitivity to the tyrosine kinase inhibitor STI571: diverse mechanisms of resistance. *Blood* 96(3):1070–1079, 2000.

5. le Coutre P, Tassi E, Varella-Garcia M, et al.: Induction of resistance to the Abelson inhibitor STI571 in human leukemic cells through gene amplification. *Blood* 95(5):1758–1766, 2000.

6. Branford S, Rudzki Z, Walsh S, et al.: High frequency of point mutations clustered within the adenosine triphosphate-binding region of BCR/ABL in patients with chronic myeloid leukemia or Ph-positive acute lymphoblastic leukemia who develop imatinib (STI571) resistance. *Blood* 99(9):3472–3475, 2002.

7. Branford S, Rudzki Z, Walsh S, et al.: Detection of BCR-ABL mutations in patients with CML treated with imatinib is virtually always accompanied by clinical resistance, and mutations in the ATP phosphate-binding loop (P-loop) are associated with a poor prognosis. *Blood* 102(1):276–283, 2003.

8. Shah NP, Nicoll JM, Nagar B, et al.: Multiple BCR-ABL kinase domain mutations confer polyclonal resistance to the tyrosine kinase inhibitor imatinib (STI571) in chronic phase and blast crisis chronic myeloid leukemia. *Cancer Cell* 2(2):117–125, 2002.

9. Gorre ME, Mohammed M, Ellwood K, et al.: Clinical resistance to STI-571 cancer therapy caused by BCR-ABL gene mutation or amplification. *Science* 293(5531):876–880, 2001.

10. von Bubnoff N, Schneller F, Peschel C, Duyster J: BCR-ABL gene mutations in relation to clinical resistance of Philadelphia-chromosome-positive leukaemia to STI571: a prospective study. *Lancet* 359(9305):487–491, 2002.

11. Hofmann WK, Komor M, Wassmann B, et al.: Presence of the BCR-ABL mutation Glu255Lys prior to STI571 (imatinib) treatment in patients with Ph+ acute lymphoblastic leukemia. *Blood* 102(2):659–661, 2003.

12. Blagosklonny MV, Fojo T, Bhalla KN, et al.: The Hsp90 inhibitor geldanamycin selectively sensitizes Bcr-Abl-expressing leukemia cells to cytotoxic chemotherapy. *Leukemia* 15(10):1537–1543, 2001.

13. Nimmanapalli R, O'Bryan E, Bhalla K: Geldanamycin and its analogue 17-allylamino-17-demethoxygeldanamycin lowers Bcr-Abl levels and induces apoptosis and

differentiation of Bcr-Abl-positive human leukemic blasts. *Cancer Res* 61(5):1799–1804, 2001.

14. An WG, Schulte TW, Neckers LM: The heat shock protein 90 antagonist geldanamycin alters chaperone association with p210bcr-abl and v-src proteins before their degradation by the proteasome. *Cell Growth Differ* 11(7):355–360, 2000.

15. Blagosklonny MV, Toretsky J, Neckers L: Geldanamycin selectively destabilizes and conformationally alters mutated p53. *Oncogene* 11(5):933–939, 1995.

16. Xu Y, Lindquist S: Heat-shock protein hsp90 governs the activity of pp60v-src kinase. *Proc Natl Acad Sci U S A* 90(15):7074–7078, 1993.

17. Gorre ME, Ellwood-Yen K, Chiosis G, Rosen N, Sawyers CL: BCR-ABL point mutants isolated from patients with imatinib mesylate-resistant chronic myeloid leukemia remain sensitive to inhibitors of the BCR-ABL chaperone heat shock protein 90. *Blood* 100(8):3041–3044, 2002.

18. Nimmanapalli R, Bhalla K: Novel targeted therapies for Bcr-Abl positive acute leukemias: beyond STI571. *Oncogene* 21(56):8584–8590, 2002.

19. Zhu XH, Shen YL, Jing YK, et al.: Apoptosis and growth inhibition in malignant lymphocytes after treatment with arsenic trioxide at clinically achievable concentrations. *J Natl Cancer Inst* 91(9):772–778, 1999.

20. Nimmanapalli R, Bali P, O'Bryan E, et al.: Arsenic trioxide inhibits translation of mRNA of bcr-abl, resulting in attenuation of Bcr-Abl levels and apoptosis of human leukemia cells. *Cancer Res* 63(22):7950–7958, 2003.

21. Porosnicu M, Nimmanapalli R, Nguyen D, Worthington E, Perkins C, Bhalla KN: Co-treatment with As2O3 enhances selective cytotoxic effects of STI-571 against Brc-Abl-positive acute leukemia cells. *Leukemia* 15(5):772–778, 2001.

22. La Rosee P, Johnson K, O'Dwyer ME, Druker BJ: In vitro studies of the combination of imatinib mesylate (Gleevec) and arsenic trioxide (Trisenox) in chronic myelogenous leukemia. *Exp Hematol* 30(7):729–737, 2002.

23. Wu Y, Yu L, McMahon R, Rossi JJ, Forman SJ, Snyder DS: Inhibition of bcr-abl oncogene expression by novel deoxyribozymes (DNAzymes). *Hum Gene Ther* 10(17):2847–2857, 1999.

24. de Fabritis P, Amadori S, Petti MC, et al.: In vitro purging with BCR-ABL antisense oligodeoxynucleotides does not prevent haematologic reconstitution after autologous bone marrow transplantation. *Leukemia* 9(4):662–664, 1995.

25. Skorski T, Szczylik C, Malaguarnera L, Calabretta B: Gene-targeted specific inhibition of chronic myeloid leukemia cell growth by BCR-ABL antisense oligodeoxynucleotides. *Folia Histochem Cytobiol* 29(3):85–89, 1991.

26. Szczylik C, Skorski T, Nicolaides NC, et al.: Selective inhibition of leukemia cell proliferation by BCR-ABL antisense oligodeoxynucleotides. *Science* 253(5019):562–565, 1991.

27. Wilda M, Fuchs U, Wossmann W, Borkhardt A: Killing of leukemic cells with a BCR/ABL fusion gene by RNA interference (RNAi). *Oncogene* 21(37):5716–5724, 2002.

28. Scherr M, Battmer K, Winkler T, Heidenreich O, Ganser A, Eder M: Specific inhibition of bcr-abl gene expression by small interfering RNA. *Blood* 101(4):1566–1569, 2003.

29. Wohlbold L, van der Kuip H, Miething C, et al.: Inhibition of bcr-abl gene expression by small interfering RNA sensitizes for imatinib mesylate (STI571). *Blood* 102(6):2236–2239, 2003.

30. Nagar B, Bornmann WG, Pellicena P, et al.: Crystal structures of the kinase domain of c-Abl in complex with the small molecule inhibitors PD173955 and imatinib (STI-571). *Cancer Res* 62(15):4236–4243, 2002.

31. von Bubnoff N, Veach DR, Miller WT, et al.: Inhibition of wild-type and mutant Bcr-Abl by pyrido-pyrimidine-type small molecule kinase inhibitors. *Cancer Res* 63(19):6395–6404, 2003.

32. O'Hare T, Pollock R, Stoffregen EP, et al.: Inhibition of wild-type and mutant Bcr-Abl by AP23464, a potent ATP-based oncogenic protein kinase inhibitor: implications for CML. *Blood* 104(8):2532–2539, 2004.

33. Shah NP, Tran C, Lee FY, Chen P, Norris D, Sawyers CL: Overriding imatinib resistance with a novel ABL kinase inhibitor. *Science* 305(5682):399–401,2004.

34. Lancet J, Gojo I, Gotlib J: Tipifarnib in previously untreated poor-risk AML and MDS: interim results of a phase 2 trial. *Blood* 102(11):Abstract 613, 2003.

35. Cortes J, Albitar M, Thomas D, et al.: Efficacy of the farnesyl transferase inhibitor R115777 in chronic myeloid leukemia and other hematologic malignancies. *Blood* 101(5):1692–1697, 2003.

36. Gotlib J, Mauro MJ, O'Dwyer M, et al.: Tipifarnib (Zarnestra) and imatinib (Gleevec) combination therapy in patients with advanced chronic myelogenous leukemia (CML); preliminary results of a phase I study. *Blood* 102(11): Abstract 3384, 2003.

37. Kuroda J, Kimura S, Segawa H, et al.: The third-generation bisphosphonate zoledronate synergistically augments the anti-Ph+ leukemia activity of imatinib mesylate. *Blood* 102(6):2229–2235, 2003.

38. Klejman A, Rushen L, Morrione A, Slupianek A, Skorski T: Phosphatidylinositol-3 kinase inhibitors enhance the anti-leukemia effect of STI571. *Oncogene* 21(38):5868–5876, 2002.

39. Skorski T, Kanakaraj P, Nieborowska-Skorska M, et al.: Phosphatidylinositol-3 kinase activity is regulated by BCR/ABL and is required for the growth of Philadelphia chromosome-positive cells. *Blood* 86(2):726–736, 1995.

40. Edinger AL, Linardic CM, Chiang GG, Thompson CB, Abraham RT: Differential effects of rapamycin on mammalian target of rapamycin signaling functions in mammalian cells. *Cancer Res* 63(23):8451–8460, 2003.

41. Ly C, Arechiga AF, Melo JV, Walsh CM, Ong ST: Bcr-Abl kinase modulates the translation regulators ribosomal protein S6 and 4E-BP1 in chronic myelogenous leukemia cells via the mammalian target of rapamycin. *Cancer Res* 63(18):5716–5722, 2003.

42. Mahon FX, Belloc F, Lagarde V, et al.: MDR1 gene overexpression confers resistance to imatinib mesylate in leukemia cell line models. *Blood* 101(6):2368–2373, 2003.

43. Vigneri P, Wang JY: Induction of apoptosis in chronic myelogenous leukemia cells through nuclear entrapment of BCR-ABL tyrosine kinase. *Nat Med* 7(2):228–234, 2001.

44. Chinese People's Liberation Army 187th Hospital: Harringtonine in acute leukemias. Clinical analysis of 31 cases. *Chin Med J (Engl)* 3(5):319–324, 1977.

45. Yongji Z, Hui Y, Xueying L, et al.: Experimental studies on the toxicity of harringtonine and homoharringtonine. *Chin Med J (Engl)* 92(3):175–180, 1979.

46. Scappini B, Onida F, Kantarjian HM, et al.: In vitro effects of STI 571-containing drug combinations on the growth of Philadelphia-positive chronic myelogenous leukemia cells. *Cancer* 94(10):2653–2662, 2002.

47. Adams J, Palombella VJ, Sausville EA, et al.: Proteasome inhibitors: a novel class of potent and effective antitumor agents. *Cancer Res* 59(11):2615–2622, 1999.

48. Reuther JY, Reuther GW, Cortez D, Pendergast AM, Baldwin AS Jr: A requirement for NF-kappaB activation in Bcr-Abl-mediated transformation. *Genes Dev* 12(7):968–981, 1998.

49. Hamdane M, David-Cordonnier MH, D'Halluin JC: Activation of p65 NF-kappaB protein by p210BCR-ABL in a myeloid cell line (P210BCR-ABL activates p65 NF-kappaB). *Oncogene* 15(19):2267–2275, 1997.

50. Dou QP, McGuire TF, Peng Y, An B: Proteasome inhibition leads to significant reduction of Bcr-Abl expression and subsequent induction of apoptosis in K562 human chronic myelogenous leukemia cells. *J Pharmacol Exp Ther* 289(2):781–790, 1999.

51. Gatto S, Scappini B, Pham L, et al.: The proteasome inhibitor PS-341 inhibits growth and induces apoptosis in Bcr/Abl-positive cell lines sensitive and resistant to imatinib mesylate. *Haematologica* 88(8):853–863, 2003.

52. Nieda M, Nicol A, Kikuchi A, et al.: Dendritic cells stimulate the expansion of bcr-abl specific CD8+ T cells with cytotoxic activity against leukemic cells from patients with chronic myeloid leukemia. *Blood* 91(3):977–983, 1998.

53. Yotnda P, Firat H, Garcia-Pons F, et al.: Cytotoxic T cell response against the chimeric p210 BCR-ABL protein in patients with chronic myelogenous leukemia. *J Clin Invest* 101(10):2290–2296, 1998.

54. ten Bosch GJ, Kessler JH, Joosten AM, et al.: A BCR-ABL oncoprotein p210b2a2 fusion region sequence is recognized by HLA-DR2a restricted cytotoxic T lymphocytes and presented by HLA-DR matched cells transfected with an Ii(b2a2) construct. *Blood* 94(3):1038–1045, 1999.

55. Bocchia M, Korontsvit T, Xu Q, et al.: Specific human cellular immunity to bcr-abl oncogene-derived peptides. *Blood* 87(9):3587–3592, 1996.

56. Bocchia M, Wentworth PA, Southwood S, et al.: Specific binding of leukemia oncogene fusion protein peptides to HLA class I molecules. *Blood* 85(10):2680–2684, 1995.

57. Greco G, Fruci D, Accapezzato D, et al.: Two brc-abl junction peptides bind HLA-A3 molecules and allow specific induction of human cytotoxic T lymphocytes. *Leukemia* 10(4):693–699,1996.

58. Buzyn A, Ostankovitch M, Zerbib A, et al.: Peptides derived from the whole sequence of BCR-ABL bind to several class I molecules allowing specific induction of human cytotoxic T lymphocytes. *Eur J Immunol* 27(8):2066–2072, 1997.

59. Clark RE, Dodi IA, Hill SC, et al.: Direct evidence that leukemic cells present HLA-associated immunogenic peptides derived from the BCR-ABL b3a2 fusion protein. *Blood* 98(10):2887–2893, 2001.

60. Mannering SI, McKenzie JL, Fearnley DB, Hart DN: HLA-DR1-restricted bcr-abl (b3a2)-specific CD4+ T lymphocytes respond to dendritic cells pulsed with b3a2 peptide and antigen-presenting cells exposed to b3a2 containing cell lysates. *Blood* 90(1):290–297, 1997.

61. Pawelec G, Max H, Halder T, et al.: BCR/ABL leukemia oncogene fusion peptides selectively bind to certain HLA-DR alleles and can be recognized by T cells found at low frequency in the repertoire of normal donors. *Blood* 88(6):2118–2124, 1996.

62. Bosch GJ, Joosten AM, Kessler JH, Melief CJ, Leeksma OC: Recognition of BCR-ABL positive leukemic blasts by human CD4+ T cells elicited by primary in vitro immunization with a BCR-ABL breakpoint peptide. *Blood* 88(9):3522–3527, 1996.

63. Tsuboi A, Oka Y, Ogawa H, et al.: Cytotoxic T-lymphocyte responses elicited to Wilms' tumor gene WT1 product by DNA vaccination. *J Clin Immunol* 20(3):195–202, 2000.

64. Yasukawa M, Ohminami H, Kaneko S, et al.: CD4(+) cytotoxic T-cell clones specific for bcr-abl b3a2 fusion peptide augment colony formation by chronic myelogenous leukemia cells in a b3a2-specific and HLA-DR-restricted manner. *Blood* 92(9):3355–3361, 1998.

65. Chen W, Peace DJ, Rovira DK, You SG, Cheever MA: T-cell immunity to the joining region of p210BCR-ABL protein. *Proc Natl Acad Sci U S A* 89(4):1468–1472, 1992.

66. Bocchia M, Gentili S, Abruzzese E, et al.: Imatinib plus CMLVAX100 (p210-derived peptide vaccine): induction of Comlete molecular responses in patients with CML showing persistent residual disease during treatment with imatinib mesylate. *Blood* 102(11):Abstract 93, 2003.

67. Molldrem J, Dermime S, Parker K, et al.: Targeted T-cell therapy for human leukemia: cytotoxic T lymphocytes specific for a peptide derived from proteinase 3 preferentially lyse human myeloid leukemia cells. *Blood* 88(7):2450–2457, 1996.

68. Molldrem JJ, Clave E, Jiang YZ, et al.: Cytotoxic T lymphocytes specific for a nonpolymorphic proteinase 3 peptide preferentially inhibit chronic myeloid leukemia colony-forming units. *Blood* 90(7):2529–2534, 1997.

69. Molldrem JJ, Lee PP, Wang C, et al.: Evidence that specific T lymphocytes may participate in the elimination of chronic myelogenous leukemia. *Nat Med* 6(9):1018–1023, 2000.

# Section 4
# CHRONIC LYMPHOCYTIC LEUKEMIA

## Chapter 22
## MOLECULAR BIOLOGY, PATHOLOGY, AND CYTOGENETICS OF CHRONIC LYMPHOCYTIC LEUKEMIA

*Martin J.S. Dyer and Randy D. Gascoyne*

## INTRODUCTION

CLL is a disease of a subtype of mature B cells characterized by expression of a specific combination of cell surface molecules: CD5[+], CD19[+], CD23[+]; surface immunoglobulin (sIg) and CD20 are expressed at only low levels. Histologically, the disease is rather bland, and usually, should present little problem in diagnosing. However, despite the morphological homogeneity, the disease varies enormously in prognosis, with some patients requiring no treatment for many years, if ever, while others die rapidly with chemotherapy-resistant disease.

In the basic biology of CLL, considerable progress has been made. The paradigm of CLL we have lived with for the past 40 years, that CLL is a disease of immunologically inert mature B cells, arising due to suppressed apoptosis, is being increasingly challenged. In the peripheral blood, viability of CLL cells appears to be dependent on intercellular contact with specialized subsets of dendritic or "nurse-like" cells, while other cell types may fulfil comparable roles in other sites.[1,2] In vivo metabolic labeling with heavy water suggests an unexpectedly high turnover of cells[3] (see also www.kinemed.com). Studies on the sequences of the expressed immunoglobulin (*IG*) variable region (*IGHV*) gene sequences are shedding new light on the possible pathogenesis of this disease. Furthermore, a subclinical expansion of CLL cells has been described, which appears to be the equivalent of monoclonal gammopathy of undetermined significance (MGUS).[4]

Within molecular cytogenetics analysis, progress has been hampered by the lack of a consistent cytogenetic lesion. The most common abnormality, involving deletion of a small region of chromosome 13q14, may involve loss of expression of micro RNA gene expression.[5] Clinically, molecular genetic analysis of the tumor cells, not only by molecular cytogenetics but also by mutational analysis of *IGHV* sequences, are now mandatory components for diagnosis in CLL and will eventually predict therapy.[6] Notably, patients with mutated *IGHV* have a much better prognosis than those with germline segments.[7] Similarly, patients with deletions and mutations involving either the p53 gene on chromosome 17p13.3 or the *ATM* gene on 11q23.1 fare badly.[8] Determining the nature of the molecular events associated with these different subgroups is now a major challenge.

## FAMILIAL CLL

It is apparent from several studies that there is a familial clustering of cases of CLL, perhaps in as many as 5% of cases.[8,9] The pedigrees are not normally large, usually affecting only two generations. The genetic defect(s) underlying the familial form of the disease remain unknown but are now the subject of a number of epidemiologic and molecular studies. A number of "candidate genes" have been investigated, but none has shown involvement. Application of whole genomic techniques to these cases may allow identification of the key gene(s). Conventional comparative genomic hybridization has been used in order to identify regions of recurrent genomic loss in DNA from patients with familial CLL; four areas of loss were identified, including Xp11.2-p21, Xq21-qter, 2p12-p14, and 4q11-q21.[10] Use of bacterial artificial chromosomes (BAC) arrays would greatly enhance the resolution of this analysis.[11]

Cases may show anticipation, with both generations often presenting concurrently; whether this reflects trinucleotide expansion, as seen in neurological disorders that exhibit this phenomenon (increasing expansion being associated with an earlier age of onset of disease), is not yet clear. However, anticipation is not a feature of all series and may reflect ascertainment bias.

Please see http://www.icr.ac.uk for further information and how to enter families into an international collaborative study.

## CD5+ B CELLS AND THE POSSIBLE ROLE OF CLONAL LYMPHOCYTES OF UNKNOWN SIGNIFICANCE IN CLL

CLL is a disease of CD5+ B cells. CD5 is a highly conserved single-chain 67-kDa transmembrane glycoprotein containing three scavenger receptor cysteine-rich (SRCR) domains. CD5 expression is found on all human T cells, but only on a subset of B cells. Despite its sequence conservation, CD5 expression in T cells and B cells varies widely from species to species; in some, all B cells are CD5 positive. Studies on CD5-deficient mice have shown that CD5 functions as a negative regulator of B-cell receptor-mediated signaling. Murine CD5+ (B1) B cells may represent a distinct lineage of B-cell development, arising early and self-renewing, producing low affinity, polyreactive antibodies that may contribute to the development of autoimmune diseases.[12] Whether CD5 expression in human B cells marks a functionally distinct lineage, or whether it reflects its function as an activation antigen, is unclear.

Both CD5+ and CD5− B cells may be found in the peripheral blood of normal individuals. It seems likely that CLL arises from the former. The evidence for this comes from an intriguing recent finding of clonal CD5+ B cells with the composite immunophenotype typical of CLL (namely CD19+/CD5+/ with low CD20 and CD79b) in the peripheral blood of 3.5% of normal individuals older than 40 years.[4] These cells, detected by four-color flow cytometry, were present at low levels (median, 0.013; range, 0.002–1.458 × 10$^9$ cells/L), and in most cases, represented only a minority of B cells (median, 11%; range, 3–95%). Clonality was demonstrated using *IGH* PCR, and sequence analysis showed the presence of mutated *IGHV* sequences. Moreover, these cells are markedly increased in frequency in first-degree relatives of patients with the familial form of CLL.[13]

The precise significance of these cells is not clear; in analogy with the situation in myeloma, they have been termed *clonal lymphocytes of uncertain significance* or "CLUS." Long-term follow-up will be necessary to determine whether the relationship between the low-level "CLL" cells and clinical disease is similar to that seen in MGUS and myeloma. More recently, another study has not only confirmed these findings of low-level CLL-like cells in the peripheral blood of normal individuals, but has also shown the presence of clonal B cells with different immunophenotypes.[14] In both studies, the frequency of clonal cells increased with age.

Further study of these populations should allow insights into the pathogenesis of both familial and sporadic forms of CLL.

## CYTOLOGY/HISTOPATHOLOGY

The key diagnostic feature of CLL relies on a careful examination of the peripheral blood smear. In a typical case, there is a lymphocytosis of small, round, mature-appearing lymphocytes with scant amounts of cytoplasm and mature chromatin. Typically, the chromatin has a characteristic clumped appearance with absent nucleoli. Disrupted lymphocytes, known as smudge cells, are a common finding in CLL (Figure 22.1). A lymphocytosis of 5 × 10$^9$ lymphocytes/L has been a mandatory part of the diagnostic criteria (see Chapter 23), although this will have to be reviewed in light of the description of CLUS.

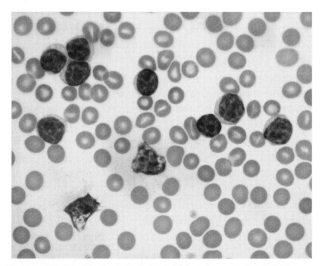

**Figure 22.1** *Typical peripheral blood smear in CLL showing small cells with clumped nuclear chromatin and occasional smudge cells*

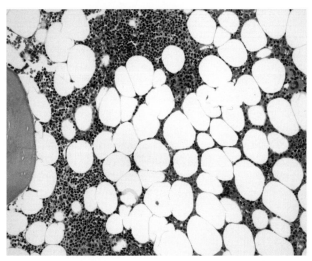

**Figure 22.2** *Bone marrow showing minimal nodular pattern of involvement*

A small number of larger cells resembling prolymphocytes may be seen at diagnosis. Characteristically, these account for <10% of the WBC differential. In time the prolymphocytes can increase, leading to a variant form of CLL referred to as CLL/PL. This represents a type of progression of CLL. In most cases, prolymphocytes account for <55% of the total WBC. The morphology in these cases is characteristically dimorphic, a finding that is particularly helpful for diagnosis. An uncommon form of CLL may occur and is referred to as CLL of mixed cell type. Such cases demonstrate a spectrum of morphologies and thus differ from the typical dimorphic appearance of CLL with scattered prolymphocytes.

The bone marrow in CLL is virtually always involved, but a number of differing presentations may be encountered. These include a nodular pattern,/—interstitial, mixed, and diffuse (Figures 22.2 and 22.3).

Some data suggest that these histologic patterns may have independent prognostic relevance in CLL. Occasionally, bone marrow biopsies may reveal the presence of growth centers, a characteristic histologic finding in the lymph nodes of patients with CLL. These represent scattered pale-staining areas where focal collections of prolymphocytes and so-called paraimmunoblasts reside. As the name indicates, this is where tumor growth is thought to occur and where one would typically encounter the otherwise uncommon mitotic figures.

A predominantly lymph-node-based form of the disease can occur, and is referred to as small lymphocytic lymphoma (SLL). The lymph node histology, immunophenotype, and cytogenetic/molecular alterations are identical to classic CLL. Although this represents an uncommon diagnosis, some cases of SLL may never develop an absolute lymphocytosis. This fact alone lends credence to the suggestion that CLL and SLL are related, but unknown factors that distinguish a predominantly leukemic disease from a tissue-based illness are poorly understood. As noted above, the histology of CLL and SLL are identical. The infiltrates are diffuse, but the presence of growth centers imparts a pseudofollicular architecture that is diagnostic. This finding is the result of scattered growth centers that produce an alternating dark and light staining pattern (Figures 22.4 and 22.5). The lightly staining areas harbor prolymphocytes and paraimmunoblasts, larger cells with more vesicular chromatin and prominent nucleoli. Occasional cases may lack prominent growth centers and typically these same cells are scattered diffusely throughout the lymph node. This can lead to problems with the diagnosis if the typical cytological appearance of the CLL/SLL cells is not appreciated. In some cases, growth centers may begin to sheet-out, suggesting histologic transformation. Importantly, this finding is not tantamount to the so-called Richter's syndrome, but rather represents a form of disease progression. Immunohistochemical staining of

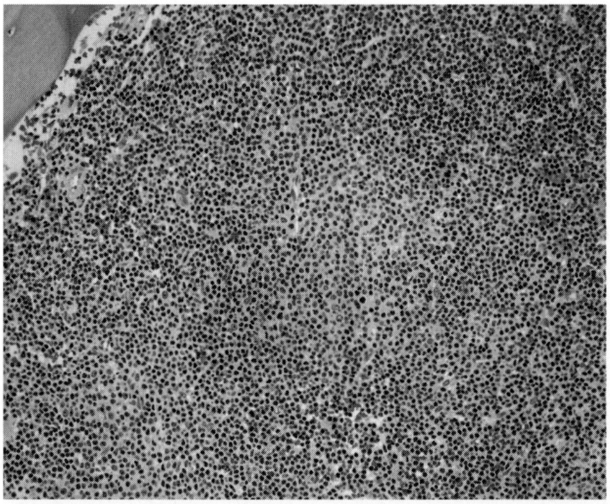

**Figure 22.3** *Heavy, diffuse bone marrow involvement in CLL. A growth center can be identified in the biopsy*

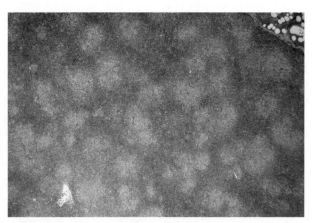

**Figure 22.4** *Low magnification image of a lymph node in CLL with "pseudo-follicular" pattern*

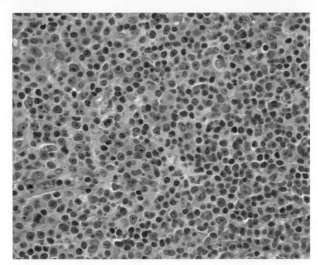

**Figure 22.5** *Higher magnification of the same lymph node showing growth centers with increased prolymphocytes and paraimmunoblasts*

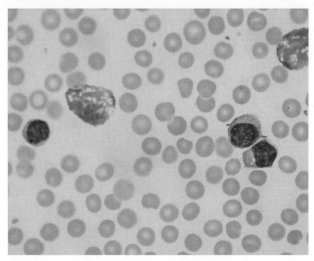

**Figure 22.6** *Peripheral blood smear with "atypical" CLL. Cells have slightly less clumped chromatin and more flowing cytoplasm*

sections of lymph nodes involved by CLL/SLL demonstrate weak expression of CD20 (stronger within the growth centers), expression of CD79a, coexpression of CD5 and CD23, and absence of cyclin D1.

CLL in most cases is easily diagnosed based on a combination of morphology and immunophenotypic findings. Rarely, cases are encountered where the distinction from other lymphoid leukemias or lymphomas is difficult, requiring ancillary studies such as cytogenetics, fluorescent in situ hybridization (FISH), and molecular genetics. In particular, the differential diagnosis of CLL includes a small group of other lymphoid malignancies with B cells coexpressing CD5. This list includes mantle cell lymphoma (MCL) and uncommon cases of marginal zone lymphoma (MZL) that may show CD5 expression. MCL typically has a distinct morphology, characterized by a cytologic spectrum rather than the typical dimorphic appearance of CLL. The peripheral blood may be involved at diagnosis in as many as one-third of cases. MCL in most cases reveals a small number of circulating blast cells, a feature that is never seen in CLL. However, rare cases exist that appear to overlap these two diseases, making accurate subclassification difficult. For these uncommon cases, other strategies can then be used to help distinguish between CLL and MCL. The immunophenotype of MCL is different from CLL in the majority of cases. The expression of CD20 is typically brighter than CLL, the cells express more sIg, they fail to express CD23, and virtually always express FMC7, an unusual epitope associated with the CD20 molecule. When a combination of morphology and immunophenotype do not allow a distinction between CLL and MCL, then FISH and/or standard cytogenetic studies are useful. MCL always shows the presence of a disease-defining translocation t(11;14)(q13;q32) involving *CCND1* (cyclin D1) on chromosome 11. This translocation is never seen in CLL/SLL.

Lastly, infrequent cases of CLL are characterized by an atypical morphology (Figure 22.6). Such cases often show unusual morphologic features such as nuclear irregularity and more abundant, flowing cytoplasm. The cells may coexpress CD11c, a variable finding in typical CLL. These cases contain the subset of CLL in which the t(14;19)(q32;q13) involving *BCL3* on chromosome 19q13 appears to be more common and tends to be associated with more aggressive clinical behavior. Chronic B-cell leukemias in which the cells lack CD5 coexpression should not be designated as CLL. Such cases frequently represent splenic MZL and may be associated with a slightly different morphology and the presence of some cells showing villous cytoplasmic projections. In the absence of other evidence to support a diagnosis of splenic MZL, based solely on the peripheral blood examination, such cases should be labeled as chronic B-cell leukemia, not otherwise specified.

## IMMUNOPHENOTYPE

The immunophenotype of most cases of CLL allows ready distinction from other malignancies of mature B cells using only a limited panel of antibodies. The coexpression of CD5 and CD23 in the presence of low-level expression of CD20 and sIg is diagnostic (Table 22.1). CD23-negative CLL is rare and has been associated with a poor prognosis; whether it harbours specific genetic abnormalities is not yet known.

A more comprehensive analysis of the CLL cell surface has been performed assessing expression of a variety of other cell surface molecules in order to differentiate possible prognostic subgroups.[18] All B-CLLs express the phenotype of activated B cells with overexpression of the activation markers CD23, CD25, CD69,

**Table 22.1**  The immunophenotype and functions of some of the molecules associated with CLL

| CD antigen | Expression in lymphoid cells | Functions and comments |
|---|---|---|
| CD5 | All T cells<br>B-cell subset<br><br>CD5+ DLBCL<br>Mantle cell lymphoma<br>Most (All) CLL | 1. Negative regulator of B-cell receptor (BCR) signalling.<br>2. Stimulates autocrine IL10 production inhibiting apoptosis. |
| CD23/ FCεR2 | Activated B cells<br><br>Rare in DLBCL<br>MCL usually negative.<br><br>Most CLL | 1. A key molecule for B-cell activation and growth.<br>2. Low-affinity IgE receptor.<br>3. Soluble forms (released by catalytic activity of ADAM 8/15/28) have potent mitogenic activity. Levels correlate with disease activity.<br>4. Upregulated by IL4. |
| CD79b | B-cells—component with CD79a of the BCR<br><br>LOW expression in CLL. | CD79a/b heterodimer is critical for BCR signaling and regulates allelic exclusion, proliferation, differentiation, anergy, and apoptosis in mature B cells. ΔCD79b, an alternative splice transcript, is expressed preferentially in CLL. |
| CD20 FMC7 | Broad expression in B-cell malignancies<br><br>LOW expression in CLL. | Tetraspan family member. Only 47 amino acids in one loop potentially exposed at the cell surface. Mediates store-operated cation entry. Localized to microvilli.[15]<br><br>FMC7 is a CD20 epitope. |
| CD38 | Broad hemopoietic expression.<br>High-level expression on plasma cells.<br>High expression in poor prognosis CLL. | CD38 is a cyclic ADP-ribose hydrolase. |
| ZAP70 | Normal T cells<br>Various B-cell and T-cell malignancies<br>Low-level expression in CLL with unmutated *IGHV* gene segments. | Intracellular kinase that transduces signals from the T-cell antigen receptor involved in BCR signaling in CLL.[16]<br>May also be involved in CXCR4/SDF1 signaling<br>Predominantly nuclear expression in CLL[17] |

and CD71, whereas, conversely, all exhibit down-regulation of CD22, FcγRIIb, CD79b, and IgD, molecules known to be down-regulated by cell triggering and activation. This composite phenotype is typical of memory B cells and is consistent with the gene expression profile of CLL.

The immunophenotype of CLL proliferation centers, however, differs significantly from that of cells in the peripheral blood.[2,16] Such cells express Ki67, high-levels of CD20 and CD23, and unlike cells in the peripheral blood survivin. Whether cells in the proliferation centers preferentially express activation-induced cytidine deaminase (AID), an enzyme necessary for somatic hypermutation (SHM), class-switching of the *IGH* genes, and expressed in only a subclone in CLL, is not yet known.[19] These and other data discussed below indicate that the proliferating cells in CLL may have a different phenotype and behavior from the bulk of cells in the peripheral blood.

The best molecule for prognostic evaluation is the intracellular tyrosine kinase, ZAP70.[20] This molecule was found to be expressed in CLL from gene expression profiling (GEP) experiments. This was an unanticipated finding, as until then ZAP70 had been described as a T-cell specific molecule involved in signal transduction from the T-cell receptor for antigen. ZAP70 expression has since been described in a variety of B-cell malignancies, where its expression is unexpectedly within the nucleus rather than the cytoplasm (Table 22.1). Its functions in B-cell malignancies are unknown, although it has been suggested that, as in T-cells, it may be involved in signal transduction from the B-cell receptor (BCR) for antigen(reviewed in Ref. 16). The major clinical interest in ZAP70 in CLL is that expression correlates strongly with absence of mutations within the *IGHV* region gene segments (qv), and may substitute for *IGHV* mutational analysis. ZAP70 expression may be detected by flow cytometry, although problems with using this method include expression in residual T-cells and the low-level expression of the molecule in CLL.[21] High ZAP70 expression correlates with a more aggressive clinical course.

## CYTOGENETICS AND MOLECULAR CYTOGENETICS

Regular cytogenetic analysis of CLL is confounded by the low proliferative rate of the bulk of the cells and the presence of residual normal T cells. Comprehensive analysis has been performed by a number of dedicated centers worldwide, where conditions for CLL cytogenetics have been optimized. From these studies it is clear that, unlike the related diseases of mature B cells, such as follicular lymphoma or MCL, there is no obvious consistent cytogenetic lesion in CLL.

A number of recurrent abnormalities have been identified, although the molecular consequences of some remain to be unequivocally identified. Practically, these lesions can be readily detected using interphase FISH methods, either using individual BAC clones or using CLL specific BAC arrays.[22] However, interphase methods will miss many of the complex cytogenetic events that may occur in CLL.[23] A further problem is that many of these events, including both 11q and 17p13 deletions, are secondary and thus only present in a fraction of cells at diagnosis; this may limit the clinical use of BAC arrays, whose sensitivity is not presently adequate to detect such minor changes.

As with acute lymphoblastic leukemia (ALL), detection of these genomic abnormalities is associated with specific prognostic groups and will form the basis for stratified therapy in future clinical trials.[24]

**Del(13)(q14)**: Loss of a region of 13q14 is the commonest lesion seen in CLL, one allele being lost in about 40% of the cases and both alleles in about 10–20% by interphase FISH analysis. Some of these deletions may be extremely small and may therefore be missed by interphase FISH. Deletions of this region in the absence of other abnormalities are associated with good prognosis disease in CLL. More recently, it has become apparent that deletions of this region may be seen not only in several other B-cell malignancies including MCL, diffuse large B-cell non-Hodgkin's lymphoma (DLBCL), and myeloma, but in solid tumors as well.

These data strongly suggest the presence of a tumor suppressor gene (TSG) within this region. However, despite characterization of many transcripts within the deleted region, the nature of the involved gene remains obscure (see for example Ref. 25 and references therein). According to Knudson's hypothesis for "classical" TSGs, deletion of one allele should be associated with mutation of the other; no mutations have been found in any of the candidate genes.

Similarly, no hypermethylation of the promoter regions, which would also result in reduced expression, has been observed in CLL. Haploinsufficiency, where loss of one allele alone results in a phenotype, may be the answer to this conundrum, but validation will require careful in vivo modeling.[26]

Another possibility is that the 13q14 deletion may involve micro-RNAs (miRNAs), 19–22 nucleotide long genes that regulate key processes including apoptosis and proliferation.[27] Some miRNAs are developmentally regulated and some are B-cell specific; some are directly involved in chromosomal translocations, indicating a direct role in the pathogenesis of neoplasia.[28] It has been suggested that the target genes in CLL may be two adjacent miRNAs, miRNA15 and 16, clustered together on chromosome 13q14 within the final intron of the *DLEU2* gene[5] (see also http://www.sanger.ac.uk/Software/Rfam/mirna/index.shtml). Furthermore, the same group has used an miRNA array to demonstrate that specific subgroups of CLL may be associated with specific miRNA "signatures."[29,30] However, these data are controversial and need to be confirmed. The possible role of many of the other 206 miRNAs so far identified in the pathogenesis of B-cell malignancies remains to be investigated; it is of some considerable interest that many map to the sites of recurrent DNA damage in malignancy.

**Del(11)(q22.3-q23.1)**: Deletions of this region are observed in about 12–15% of the cases. These deletions are molecularly variable and often secondary, but tend to be associated with progressive disease occurring in younger men with bulky lymph node disease. The association with poor prognosis may not be present in elderly patients with deletions of this region, about 50% of which appear to involve the gene that causes ataxia-telangectasia, the *ATM* gene. This gene comprises 63 exons and encodes a huge protein of 3056 amino acids; consequently, mutational analysis is technically difficult. Mutations of *ATM* are seen in all cases of T-cell prolymphocytic leukemia and may also be found in 50% of CLL patients with 11q deletions. However, some of these "mutations" may in fact represent rare germline polymorphisms.

The ATM protein is an important cell cycle checkpoint kinase that functions as an activator/regulator of a wide variety of downstream proteins, including p53, checkpoint proteins RAD17 and RAD9A, and DNA repair proteins. Loss of ATM functions results in loss of responses to DNA damage, and consequently genomic instability.[31]

**Del(17)(p13)**: deletion of the short arm of chromosome 17 is seen in about 5–7% of cases of CLL at diagnosis. This is often a secondary abnormality and therefore may be seen in only a fraction of the neoplastic cells. The target gene of this deletion is cases *TP53*, although deletion of one allele with no *TP53* mutations in the remaining allele may occur, suggesting the presence of another, more telomeric TSG on chromosome 17p.

Abnormalities within the *TP53/ATM* axis have a profound impact on the biological behavior of CLL; patients with either abnormality, but particularly those with *TP53* mutations, fare badly with conventional chemotherapy. Their detection may be an indication for early therapy with agents such as CAMPATH-1H (alemtuzumab), where elimination of the neoplastic cells does not depend on p53 function. Given the importance of changes in *TP53* and *ATM* to eventual clinical outcome, and the difficulties in assessing both genes, a simple functional assay may be of value. The response to ionizing irradiation in terms of increased p21 expression allows a direct assessment of both p53 and ATM functions.[32]

Although the consequences of *ATM* and *TP53* inactivation are similar, they are by no means identical. Genome-wide expression experiments have indicated that the worse response of patients with *TP53* mutations may reflect the loss of p53-dependent apoptotic pathways.[33]

**Trisomy 12**: This abnormality occurs in about 15% of CLL patients and again is usually only seen in a fraction of the cells. The percentage of cells with trisomy 12 often does not increase with transformation. The specific molecular consequences of this abnormality, which again is not specific for CLL, are not clear.

## IG TRANSLOCATIONS IN CLL

Although *IG* translocations are rare in CLL[34] and probably comprise no more than 5% of cases, they have allowed the identification of a number of genes of interest. They appear to be associated with aggressive disease. The presence of a t(11;14)(q13;q32) in a mature B-cell malignancy precludes the diagnosis of CLL; MCL in leukemic phase, a specific subtype of MCL, is most likely. Detection of *IGH* translocations is now performed by interphase FISH, but these methods have not been used to detect *IG* light chain translocations in any large series of CLL patients.

*BCL2*: All cases of CLL express high levels of *BCL2* RNA and protein. It has been suggested that this high-level expression is due to hypomethylation of the *BCL2* promoter. Chromosomal translocations involving *BCL2* are rare and probably occur in no more than 2% of the cases. *BCL2* translocations may be secondary events in CLL. The prognostic implication of *BCL2* translocations in CLL is uncertain, as the levels of protein expression are very high in cases lacking the translocation.

The nature of *BCL2* translocations in CLL suggests a pathogenetic mechanism distinct from that seen in follicular non-Hodgkin's lymphoma. Unlike *BCL2* translocations in follicular lymphoma, in CLL, most involve the *IG* light chain gene segments. The breakpoints within *BCL2* are also different; most breakpoints in CLL involve the 5′ region of the gene within the variant cluster region.

*BCL3*: Originally identified by its involvement in t(14:19)(q32;q13), *BCL3* is a member of the IkB family of proteins, which mediates transcriptional up-regulation of NFκB target genes through interaction with p50/p52 homodimers. The translocation is not specific for CLL and occurs in several B-cell malignancies.

*BCL11A*: This gene, which encodes a Krüppel zinc finger protein, was cloned from its direct involvement in t(2;14)(p13;q32) in cases of aggressive CLL. How BCL11A transforms B cells remains unknown. It is a transcriptional repressor that binds directly to BCL6; however, BCL6 is not usually expressed at high levels, if at all, in CLL. *BCL11A* translocations are rare in CLL. All cases to date have retained germline *IGHV* segments, despite having undergone class switch recombination.

## IGHV AND BCL6 MUTATIONAL ANALYSIS IN CLL

SHM of the *IGHV* gene segments is an essential component in the generation of high affinity antibodies during the immune response. This process introduces targeted mutations primarily into the complementarity determining regions (CDRs) of productively rearranged *IGHV* segments at extremely high rates. *IGHV* mutational analysis should reflect the history of a B cell: mutations indicate encounter with antigen in the germinal center, while unmutated *IGHV* sequences indicate antigen naïve B cells. SHM is potentially a dangerous, mutagenic process, and errors in SHM have been implicated in the pathogenesis of B-cell lymphomas through the generation of *IG* chromosomal translocations. SHM may also act on other non-*IG* genes in both normal and malignant B cells.

Mutational analysis of *IGHV* gene segments in CLL has been and continues to shed significant light on the pathogenesis of the disease (reviewed in Refs. 16 and 35). In 1999, two groups independently showed that the presence or absence of *IGHV* mutations defined prognostically important subgroups of CLL; patients lacking *IGHV* mutations fared worse than patients with mutated sequences. One simple interpretation of these data is that the unmutated CLL represents malignant transformation of antigen naïve B cells. However, these data are not consistent with either the activated B-cell phenotype of CLL, or the gene expression profile, both of which are most similar to memory B cells with continued environmental stimulation.

Mature B cells depend on maintained stimulation via the BCR for antigen, and loss of this complex results in rapid B-cell death by apoptosis.[36] One possible explanation for the presence of unmutated *IGHV* in CLL might be the strength of antigenic stimulation with persistent environmental or autoantigenic stimulation driving at least the early phases of development of the neoplastic clone. Such cells might persist and be antigenically challenged without negotiating a classical germinal center reaction. If persistent exogenous antigenic stimulation were confirmed, it would be analogous to the development of extranodal mucosa-associated lymphoid tissue lymphomas, which have been shown to be dependent on chronic antigenic stimulation of an increasing number of microbial antigens.[37]

Consistent with this hypothesis of recurrent antigenic stimulation is the restricted IGHV and IG light chain (IGL) repertoires in at least some cases of CLL.[35,38,39] Individual IGHV segments tend either to be mutated or unmutated and to have similar if not identical CDRs. For instance, in one study of class-switched non-IgM producing CLL, five cases of sIgG+ CLL were found to share CDR motifs not only in the heavy chain but also in the light chain. Three-dimensional modeling indicated that these antibodies could bind the same antigenic epitope. On the basis of the restricted antibody responses to carbohydrate antigens, it was suggested that this epitope might be a carbohydrate determinant.[38] In a study of 1220 CLL patients, 164 (13.8%) had VH1-69 and of these 163 were in germline configuration[39]; moreover, there appeared to be marked restriction in the CDR3 region in at least 15 of these patients, who also had the same light chain gene. These data suggest that there is either a strong antigenic selection process, or that B cells bearing this particular combination of IG recombination events are somehow more sensitive to transformation. The presence of such restricted antibody specificities allows new experimental approaches into the pathogenesis of CLL.

However, not all mutated CLL behave "well." It is apparent from several series that patients with mutations in the IGHV3-21 segment have progressive disease.[40] In at least some cases this would appear to be due to an association with the TP53 mutation.[41]

BCL6 mutations, clustering within the region subject to chromosomal translocations in follicular and DLBCL and presumably arising due to the actions of SHM, have been reported in CLL.[34] In two reports there was concordance between presence of IGHV mutations, but not in the third. This controversy remains to be resolved. In contrast to DLBCL, where SHM-induced mutations may commonly occur in other proto-oncogenes, such mutations appear to be rare in CLL.

## GENOME-WIDE GEP

GEP experiments using either the Lymphochip or Affymetrix arrays have shown that all CLL samples have a remarkably consistent profile, independent of IGHV mutational status, consistent with their origination from memory B cells. In this regard, CLL differs from other B-cell diseases such as DLBCL, where the profile differs markedly from case to case. CLL expresses genes not expressed in normal memory B cells, including ROR1 receptor tyrosine kinase and CD200, and conversely, lacks expression of other genes normally expressed in normal memory cells, such as histone H2AX and RAD9. The biological relevance of these observations remains to be determined; some of these may be of direct pathological significance in the development of CLL.

Despite the relative constancy of the CLL gene signature, a number of genes were identified whose expression segregated with the presence or absence of mutations. As mentioned earlier, ZAP70 expression correlated most strongly with the unmutated IGHV subset of CLL. Other genes differentially expressed between the two subsets of disease included BCL7A, FGFR1, and PAK1. Many of the genes that were more highly expressed in unmutated CLL were induced during activation of blood B cells.

More recent GEP experiments have focussed on responses of CLL to irradiation-induced DNA damage and defining pathways that mediate resistance.[33,42]

## BIOLOGY OF CLL

An observation made years ago is that CLL B cells isolated from the peripheral blood undergo rapid apoptosis in vitro. The rate of apoptosis varies substantially, but there appears to be no simple correlation between rates of apoptosis in vitro and clinical outcome. A similar rapid rate of in vitro apoptosis is also observed in B cells derived from involved lymph nodes in patients with follicular lymphoma. As both populations express large amounts of BCL2 protein, these data may indicate that BCL2 alone is insufficient to suppress "spontaneous" apoptosis.

CLL cells in vivo do not appear to undergo such rapid apoptosis; work has been done to elucidate signaling pathways that maintain the viability in vitro, as definition of these pathways might define new therapeutic targets. A number of signaling pathways have been implicated, including IL4, IL7, CXCR4/SDF1, BAFF, and integrin signaling; the possible clinical relevance of these remains to be determined. Comparison of experiments is difficult because of differing culture conditions used. Serum-free conditions for the maintenance of CLL cells in vitro have been defined, but have not been widely used.[43] Also, in most cases adequate definition of the CLL cells used in the experiments, in terms of both IGHV mutational and molecular cytogenetic analysis, has not been performed.

Spontaneous apoptosis may be suppressed simply by either

a) *culturing at high density,*[44] most in vitro experiments use much lower concentrations of cells ($10^6$ cells/mL) than those actually seen in a patient, or
b) *culturing in the presence of albumin.*[45]

Culturing CLL in the presence of adherent cells from a wide variety of sources, including marrow mesenchymal cells, may also prevent apoptosis.[46,47] The presence in the peripheral blood, specialized dendritic or "nurse" cells may maintain the viability of CLL for prolonged periods.[1]

Prevention of proteolytic degradation of the anti-apoptotic molecule MCL1 appears to be a key event in most of these experiments[48]; the rapid turnover of this protein may make it a target for a variety of therapeutic approaches. However, all of the above techniques do not result in proliferation of CLL cells, but rather in maintained viability. CLL cells in the blood are in the $G_0$ phase of the cell cycle. As with spontaneous apoptosis, a large number of simple manoeuvres, such as CpG dinucleotide stimulation along with IL2, or TNFα and IL6, can result in proliferation.[49]

However, the physiological and biological relevance of all of the above observations is not clear. Nor is it certain that cells derived from the peripheral blood are the correct population to be studied. Few studies have been done on either bone marrow or lymph node CLL cells, which may differ considerably from cells within the blood.

Moreover, a number of interesting studies in vivo suggest that CLL, rather than being a disease of suppressed apoptosis with only gradual accumulation of cells, may in fact, like other malignancies, be a disease of proliferation. First, there is evidence using metabolic labeling with $D_2O$ or heavy water and mass spectrometry that patients with clinical stage A disease with stable peripheral blood lymphocytes may nevertheless turnover the entire clone in a matter of months 3. Secondly, and less directly, B-CLL cells have been shown to have significantly shorter telomeres than those in autologous neutrophils and B cells from healthy age-matched subjects; patients with unmutated IGHV genes had significantly shorter telomeres than those in mutated IGHV genes.[50,51] These data suggest that a considerable number of cell divisions must have occurred in the leukemic cells after their genesis.

Taken together, these results indicate that CLL may be rapidly turning over in vivo and that several cell–cell interactions are required in order to maintain the viability of CLL cells. The necessity for persistent signaling suggests new therapeutic approaches.

There are also profound immunological defects in CLL whose biology remains poorly understood. Suppression of residual normal B cells as detected by low serum immunoglobulin levels is a feature, and worsens with disease progression. One explanation might be the release of immunosuppressive cytokines, such as IL10 or TGFβ, from CLL B cells. However, there are also marked abnormalities of the T-cell populations in CLL. Somewhat surprisingly, their numbers are usually increased in CLL and their persistence may be essential for progression of CLL (reviewed in Ref. 16).

## CONCLUSIONS

Historically, CLL has lagged behind the other B-cell malignancies in terms of molecular and biological analysis. This situation is now changing rapidly. We are beginning to make progress in our understanding of the basic biology of CLL. The paradigm of gradual accumulation of apoptotis defective mature B cells is now being replaced by a much more complex and dynamic picture of proliferating CLL stem cells[52] continued superantigen drive, and persistent stimulation by a variety of different stromal and perhaps T cells, with constant turnover of cells in the periphery. The nature of the CLL stem cell and the nature of the initiating genetic events in this cell population are key aims; identification of both would hopefully allow the development of more effective and targeted therapies, along the lines of the paradigm established in chronic myeloid leukemia and imatinib.

## REFERENCES

In the interest of space not all pertinent references have been cited here; we apologise to our colleagues for glaring omissions. A more comprehensive list may be obtained on request to the authors.

1. Tsukada N, Burger JA, Zvaifler NJ, Kipps TJ: Distinctive features of "nurselike" cells that differentiate in the context of chronic lymphocytic leukemia. *Blood* 99:1030, 2002.
2. Caligaris-Cappio F: Role of the microenvironment in chronic lymphocytic leukaemia. *Br J Haematol* 123:380, 2003.
3. Messmer BT, Messmer D, Allen SL, et al.: In vivo measurements document the dynamic cellular kinetics of chronic lymphocytic leukemia B cells. *J Clin Invest* 115(3):755, 2005.
4. Rawstron AC, Green MJ, Kuzmicki A, et al.: Monoclonal B lymphocytes with the characteristics of "indolent" chronic lymphocytic leukemia are present in 3.5% of adults with normal blood counts. *Blood* 100:635, 2002.
5. Calin GA, Dumitru CD, Shimizu M, et al.: Frequent deletions and down-regulation of micro- RNA genes miR15 and miR16 at in chronic lymphocytic leukemia. *Proc Natl Acad Sci USA* 99:15524, 2002.
6. Shanafelt TD, Geyer SM, Kay NE: Prognosis at diagnosis: integrating molecular biologic insights into clinical practice for patients with CLL. *Blood* 103:1202, 2004.
7. Ries LAG, Eisner MP, Kosary, CL, et al. (eds.): *SEER Cancer Statistics Review, 1975-2000.* Bethesda, MD: National Cancer Institute; 2003. Available at: http://seer.cancer.gov/csr/1975_2000
8. Houlston RS, Sellick G, Yuille M, Matutes E, Catovsky D: Causation of chronic lymphocytic leukemia–insights from familial disease. *Leuk Res* 27:871, 2003.

9. Caporaso N, Marti GE, Goldin L: Perspectives on familial chronic lymphocytic leukemia: genes and the environment. *Semin Hematol* 41:201, 2004.

10. Summersgill B, Thornton P, S. Atkinson S, et al.: Chromosomal imbalances in familial chronic lymphocytic leukaemia: a comparative genomic hybridisation analysis. *Leukemia* 16;1229, 2002.

11. Ishkanian AS, Malloff CA, Watson SK, et al.: A tiling resolution DNA microarray with complete coverage of the human genome. *Nat Genet* 36:299, 2004.

12. Carsetti R, Rosado MM, Wardmann H: Peripheral development of B cells in mouse and man. *Immunol Rev* 197:179, 2004.

13. Rawstron AC, Yuille MR, Fuller J, et al.: Inherited predisposition to CLL is detectable as subclinical monoclonal B-lymphocyte expansion. *Blood* 100:2289, 2002.

14. Ghia P, Prato G, Scielzo C, et al.: Monoclonal CD5+ and CD5- B-lymphocyte expansions are frequent in the peripheral blood of the elderly. *Blood* 103:2337, 2004.

15. Li H, Ayer LM, Polyak MJ, Mutch CM, et al.: The CD20 calcium channel is localized to microvilli and constitutively associated with membrane rafts: antibody binding increases the affinity of the association through an epitope-dependent cross-linking-independent mechanism. *J Biol Chem* 279:19893, 2004.

16. Stevenson FK, Caligaris-Cappio F: Chronic lymphocytic leukemia: revelations from the B-cell receptor. *Blood* 103:4389, 2004.

17. Admirand JH, Rassidakis GZ, Abruzzo LV, et al.: Immunohistochemical detection of ZAP-70 in 341 cases of non-Hodgkin and Hodgkin lymphoma. *Mod Pathol* 17:954, 2004.

18. Damle RN, Ghiotto F, Valetto A, et al.: B-cell chronic lymphocytic leukemia cells express a surface membrane phenotype of activated, antigen-experienced B lymphocytes. *Blood* 99: 4087, 2002.

19. Albesiano E, Messmer BT, Damle RN, et al.: Activation-induced cytidine deaminase in chronic lymphocytic leukemia B cells: expression as multiple forms in a dynamic, variably sized fraction of the clone. *Blood,* 102:3333, 2003.

20. Wiestner A, Rosenwald A, Barry TS, et al.: ZAP-70 expression identifies a chronic lymphocytic leukemia subtype with unmutated immunoglobulin genes, inferior clinical outcome, and distinct gene expression profile. *Blood* 101:4944, 2003.

21. Orchard JA, Ibbotson RE, Davis Z, et al.: ZAP-70 expression and prognosis in chronic lymphocytic leukaemia. *Lancet* 363:105, 2004.

22. Schwaenen C, Nessling M, Wessendorf S, et al.: Automated array-based genomic profiling in chronic lymphocytic leukemia: development of a clinical tool and discovery of recurrent genomic alterations. *Proc Natl Acad Sci USA* 101:1039, 2004.

23. Gardiner AC, Corcoran MM, Oscier DG: Cytogenetic, fluorescence in situ hybridisation, and clinical evaluation of translocations with concomitant deletion at 13q14 in chronic lymphocytic leukaemia. *Genes Chromosomes Cancer* 20:73, 1997.

24. Stilgenbauer S, Bullinger L, Lichter P, Dohner H:. Genetics of chronic lymphocytic leukemia: genomic aberrations and V$_H$ gene mutation status in pathogenesis and clinical course. *Leukemia* 16:993, 2002.

25. Corcoran MM, Hammarsund M, Zhu C, et al.: *DLEU2* encodes an antisense RNA for the putative bicistronic *RFP2/LEU5* gene in humans and mouse. *Genes Chromosomes Cancer* 40:285, 2004.

26. Santarosa M, Ashworth A: Haploinsufficiency for tumour suppressor genes: when you don't need to go all the way. *Biochim Biophys Acta* 1654: 105, 2004.

27. Bartel DP: MicroRNAs: genomics, biogenesis, mechanism, and function. *Cell* 116: 281, 2004.

28. Chen CZ, Li L, Lodish HF, Bartel DP: MicroRNAs modulate hematopoietic lineage differentiation. *Science* 303:83, 2004.

29. Liu CG, Calin GA, Meloon B, et al.: An oligonucleotide microchip for genome-wide microRNA profiling in human and mouse tissues. *Proc Natl Acad Sci USA* 101:9740, 2004.

30. Calin GA, Liu CG, Sevignani C, et al.: MicroRNA profiling reveals distinct signatures in B cell chronic lymphocytic leukemias. *Proc Natl Acad Sci USA* 101(32):11755, 2004.

31. Stankovic T, Stewart GS, Fegan C, et al.: Ataxia telangiectasia mutated-deficient B-cell chronic lymphocytic leukemia occurs in pregerminal center cells and results in defective damage response and unrepaired chromosome damage. *Blood* 99:300, 2002.

32. Pettitt AR, Sherrington PD, Stewart G, et al.: p53 dysfunction in B-cell chronic lymphocytic leukemia: inactivation of *ATM* as an alternative to *TP53* mutation. *Blood* 98:814, 2001.

33. Stankovic T, Hubank M, Cronin D, et al.: Microarray analysis reveals that TP53- and ATM-mutant B-CLLs share a defect in activating proapoptotic responses after DNA damage but are distinguished by major differences in activating prosurvival responses. *Blood* 103:291, 2004.

34. Dyer MJS, Oscier DG: The configuration of the immunoglobulin genes in B cell chronic lymphocytic leukemia. *Leukemia* 16:973, 2002.

35. Chiorazzi N, Ferrarini M: B cell chronic lymphocytic leukemia: lessons learned from studies of the B cell antigen receptor. *Annu Rev Immunol* 21:841, 2003.

36. Kraus M, Alimzhanov MB, Rajewsky N, Rajewsky K: Survival of resting mature B lymphocytes depends on BCR signaling via the Igalpha/beta heterodimer. *Cell* 117:787, 2004.

37. Isaacson PG, Du MQ: Timeline: MALT lymphoma: from morphology to molecules. *Nat Rev Cancer* 4:644, 2004.

38. Ghiotto F, Fais F, Valetto A, et al.: Remarkably similar antigen receptors among a subset of patients with chronic lymphocytic leukemia. *J Clin Invest* 113:1008, 2004.

39. Widhopf GF, II, Rassenti LZ, Toy TL, et al.: Chronic lymphocytic leukemia B cells of more than one percent of patients express virtually identical immunoglobulins. *Blood* 104(8):2499, 2004.

40. Tobin G, Thunberg U, Johnson A, et al.: Somatically mutated Ig V$_H$3-21 genes characterize a new subset of chronic lymphocytic leukemia. *Blood* 99:2262, 2002.

41. Lin K, Manocha S, Harris RJ, et al.: High frequency of p53 dysfunction and low level of V$_H$ mutation in chronic lymphocytic leukemia patients using the V$_H$3-21 gene segment. *Blood* 102:1145, 2003.

42. Vallat L, Magdelenat H, Merle-Beral H, et al.: The resistance of B-CLL cells to DNA damage-induced apoptosis defined by DNA microarrays. *Blood* 101:4598, 2003.

43. Levesque MC, O'Loughlin CW, Weinberg JB: Use of serum-free media to minimize apoptosis of chronic lymphocytic leukemia cells during *in vitro* culture. *Leukemia* 20:1305, 2001.

44. Pettitt AR, Moran EC, Cawley JC: Homotypic interactions protect chronic lymphocytic leukaemia cells from spontaneous death *in vitro*. *Leuk Res* 25:1003, 2001.

45. Jones DT, Ganeshaguru K, Anderson RJ, et al.: Albumin activates the AKT signaling pathway and protects B-chronic lymphocytic leukemia cells from chlorambucil- and radiation-induced apoptosis. *Blood* 101:3174, 2003.

46. Ghia P, Caligaris-Cappio F: The indispensable role of microenvironment in the natural history of low-grade B-cell neoplasms. *Adv Cancer Res* 79:157, 2000.

47. Cuni S, Perez-Aciego P, Perez-Chacon G, et al.: A sustained activation of PI3K/NF-κB pathway is critical for the survival of chronic lymphocytic leukemia B cells. *Leukemia* 18:1391, 2004.

48. Opferman JT, Letai A, Beard C, et al.: Development and maintenance of B and T lymphocytes requires antiapoptotic MCL-1. *Nature* 426:671, 2003.

49. Bogner C, Schneller F, Hipp S, et al.: Cycling B-CLL cells are highly susceptible to inhibition of the proteasome: involvement of p27, early D-type cyclins, Bax, and caspase-dependent and -independent pathways. *Exp Hematol* 31:218, 2003.

50. Hultdin M, Rosenquist R, Thunberg U, et al.: Association between telomere length and $V_H$ gene mutation status in chronic lymphocytic leukaemia: clinical and biological implications. *Br J Cancer* 88:593, 2003.

51. Damle RN, Batliwalla FM, Ghiotto F, et al.: Telomere length and telomerase activity delineate distinctive replicative features of the B-CLL subgroups defined by immunoglobulin V gene mutations. *Blood* 103:375, 2004.

52. Scadden DT: Cancer stem cells refined. *Nat Immunol* 5:701, 2004.

# Chapter 23

# CLINICAL FEATURES AND MAKING THE DIAGNOSIS

## William G. Wierda, Joan H. Admirand, and Susan M. O'Brien

## INTRODUCTION

Chronic lymphocytic leukemia (CLL) is characterized by accumulation of monoclonal malignant B cells in blood, lymph nodes, liver, spleen, and bone marrow. These cells have a unique immunophenotype and biology. With time, patients may develop progressive lymphocytosis, lymphadenopathy, hepatosplenomegaly, anemia, and thrombocytopenia. Prior to the availability of flow cytometry, cytogenetic, and molecular analyses, the diagnosis was made based on an elevated white blood cell count with morphologic examination of the blood smear demonstrating characteristically small, well-differentiated lymphocytes. Some patients also presented with lymphadenopathy and/or hepatosplenomegaly. Flow cytometry has made evaluation and characterization of B-cell lymphoproliferative diseases more precise and has enabled identification of subgroups of patients with clinically distinct diagnoses. Karyotypic analyses, including standard metaphase chromosome analysis and fluorescence in situ hybridization (FISH), have also been key in identifying subgroups of patients with B-cell lymphoproliferative diseases. Still, CLL remains a diagnosis for which diverse clinical courses are observed and are dictated by characteristics of the individual patients' leukemic clone. Continued work to identify important and significant prognostic factors will enable identification of clinical entities that represent distinct diseases within the group of patients currently diagnosed with CLL. In this chapter, we will review diagnostic criteria and clinical characteristics of patients with CLL.

## EPIDEMIOLOGY

CLL is the most common adult form of leukemia in Western society. According to a recent analysis of the Surveillance Epidemiology and End Results database,[1] the annual overall age-adjusted incidence in the United States between 1997 and 2001 was 3.5/100,000 people: 5.0/100,000 for males and 2.5/100,000 for females. This is a disease of older adults with distinct and unique clinical characteristics and concerns. The majority of individuals are diagnosed when over 65 years of age, and the incidence increases with increasing age. The incidence for individuals over age 70 years is 50/100,000. The median age at diagnosis between 1997 and 2001 was 72 years: for males 70 years and 74 years of age for females. This median has risen over the past 10–15 years, likely due to aging of the U.S. population. The 5-year survival (1995–2000) was 73% overall: 71% for males and 76% for females. The median age at death was 78 years: 76 for males and 81 years for females.

In the United States, CLL is most common in the Caucasian population and less common in African-Americans and individuals from the Far East. The age-adjusted annual incidence between 1975 and 2001 for Caucasians was 3.9/100,000 and for African-Americans 2.8/100,000.[1] CLL is rare in individuals of Japanese ancestry.

Ghia et al. screened blood from 500 unselected healthy individuals over age 65 and identified a population of monoclonal (by light-chain analysis) $CD5^+/19^+/23^+$ B cells in 3.8% of these individuals.[2] These asymptomatic individuals did not have lymphocytosis or clinical evidence of disease, and did not fulfill diagnostic criteria for CLL. Whether or not some or all of these individuals will progress to fulfill diagnostic criteria or develop symptomatic disease is unclear. Nevertheless, this indicates that the incidence of a monoclonal lymphoproliferative process is potentially much more common in the elderly population than has been previously appreciated.

The demographics of newly diagnosed patients are different today than 20 years ago. Due to the widespread availability of routine automated blood counts, a large proportion of patients is diagnosed based on incidental finding of lymphocytosis in the absence of any significant symptoms. These patients are therefore being diagnosed at an earlier stage. The overwhelming majority of patients present to private practice physicians and are followed and treated in this setting. Patients followed and treated at tertiary referral centers tend to be younger and more heavily pretreated. The median age for both previously untreated and previously treated patients on clinical trials at such institutions is roughly 60 years of age.

## CLINICAL PRESENTATION

The clinical presentation of CLL patients is diverse, with variability in presenting symptoms, physical examination findings, and laboratory test results. As noted above, patients often present without any symptoms, and the diagnosis is made on the basis of an elevated absolute lymphocyte count found on routine complete blood count (CBC). Less commonly, patients present with nontender lymphadenopathy, and are noted to have an elevated blood lymphocyte count on further evaluation. Some patients present with concomitant illnesses such as infection or chronic rhinitis, or less commonly, autoimmune phenomena such as autoimmune hemolytic anemia (AIHA) or immune thrombocytopenia purpura (ITP).

## CRITERIA FOR DIAGNOSIS

The National Cancer Institute (NCI) sponsored a working group in 1988 that developed criteria and guidelines for clinical protocols, as well as general-practice recommendations for patients with CLL.[3] In 1996, the criteria and guidelines were revised to those in current use.[4] These guidelines importantly include indications for treatment and criteria for evaluating response to treatment. The diagnosis of CLL requires a sustained absolute lymphocytosis of greater than 5000 lymphocytes/μL. This value is also important for making the academic distinction between CLL and small lymphocytic lymphoma (SLL), in which the absolute lymphocyte count is less than 5000 lymphocytes/μL. Patients with greater than 55% prolymphocytes on differential or greater than 15,000 prolymphocytes/μL meet the diagnostic criteria for prolymphocytic leukemia (PLL). Morphologic assessment and flow cytometry immunophenotyping are critical to confirming the diagnosis of CLL and will be discussed subsequently in this chapter.

Although a bone marrow aspirate and biopsy are not required for making the diagnosis of CLL, if performed, the aspirate smear should show greater than 30% of nucleated cells to be lymphocytes according to the NCI criteria.[4] Evaluation of the sectioned bone marrow core biopsy will identify the pattern of involvement, which has prognostic value. As the bone marrow is always involved and is the last to be cleared with standard chemotherapy, a bone marrow examination is most helpful in evaluating response to treatment and is required to confirm complete remission. A bone marrow aspirate and biopsy are also useful in evaluating patients with thrombocytopenia to differentiate between an autoimmune process and lack of platelet production due to CLL marrow infiltration.

## DIFFERENTIAL DIAGNOSIS

A malignant lymphoproliferative disorder should be suspected when the absolute lymphocyte count is greater than 5000 lymphocytes/μL. The differential diagnosis for patients with lymphocytosis, lymphadenopathy, and/or organomegaly includes numerous malignant lymphoproliferative disorders (Table 23.1). These include CLL, PLL, adult peripheral T-cell lymphoma, natural killer cell leukemia, mantle cell lymphoma, marginal zone lymphoma (nodal, extranodal, or splenic), hairy cell leukemia, SLL, lymphoplasmacytic leukemia, and follicular center lymphoma in a leukemic phase. Distinguishing CLL from other lymphoproliferative disorders is based on morphology and, more importantly, on immunophenotype (Figure 23.1).

Lymphocytosis may be reactive and therefore polyclonal and benign (Table 23.2). This must be distinguished from the malignant monoclonal lymphoproliferative disorders. Reactive lymphocytosis may be due to viral or bacterial infections. In addition, individuals may have elevated lymphocyte counts following splenectomy. For B-cell lymphoproliferative diseases, monoclonality is usually established by immunoglobulin (Ig) light-chain restriction.[5]

| Table 23.1 Differential diagnosis for monoclonal B-cell lymphoproliferative disorders | |
|---|---|
| Clonal lymphocyte population | Disease |
| B Cell | Chronic lymphocytic leukemia |
| | Mantle cell lymphoma |
| | Follicular lymphoma |
| | Hairy cell leukemia |
| | Splenic marginal zone lymphoma |
| | Splenic lymphoma with villious lymphocytes |
| | Lymphoplasmacytoid lymphoma |
| | B-cell prolymphocytic leukemia |
| T Cell | Sezary syndrome |
| | Large granular lymphocyte leukemia |
| | Adult T-cell leukemia/lymphoma |
| | HTLV-1+ T-cell leukemia |
| | T-cell prolymphocytic leukemia |

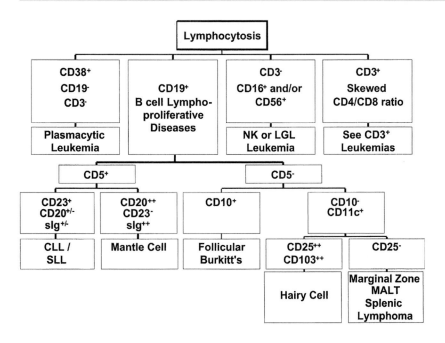

**Figure 23.1** *Characterization of malignant lymphocytosis by flow cytometry. Lymphoproliferative disorders are characterized by flow cytometry based on T- and B-cell markers. This figure further classifies CD19+ lymphoproliferative diseases based on B-cell markers*

## SYMPTOMS

Many patients are asymptomatic at diagnosis, particularly patients with early stage disease. Symptoms may include weakness, malaise, fatigue, night sweats, and low-grade fever without evidence of infection. Unintentional weight loss is not common but if it reaches or exceeds 10% body weight in a 6-month period, it is an indication for treatment. Classical B symptoms are uncommon in patients with CLL, and if present in those with long-standing disease may indicate transformation to large-cell lymphoma (Richter transformation). Less commonly, patients may complain of rheumatology-type symptoms, such as arthralgias and myalgias. These rheumatologic symptoms may be associated with rheumatoid factor.[6] It is uncommon for progressive adenopathy to produce pain, airway or vascular compromise, or obstruction of the gastrointestinal tract. Organomegaly, particularly splenomegaly, also occurs with progressive disease. Splenomegaly is usually painless, but may cause early satiety and bloating. Patients with CLL can have exaggerated reactions to mosquito or other insect bites.[7–9] The pathophysiology for this hyperresponsiveness is unknown.

## PHYSICAL FINDINGS

The most common finding on physical examination is adenopathy, which is most easily appreciated in the cervical, axillary, and inguinal regions. Adenopathy is typically symmetric, but may be more prominent in a particular region of the body, such as the neck. If adenopathy is asymmetric, or there is rapid increase in a localized nodal group, suspicion should be raised for Richter transformation. Organomegaly typically involves the spleen; hepatomegaly due to leukemic infiltration is less comman. Although extranodal involvement is rare, patients may develop leukemic infiltrates in the skin,[10,11] mucosa-associated lymphoid tissue,[12,13] or lungs.[14–16] Central nervous system involvement with leukemia is rare, but can cause headache, meningitis, cranial nerve palsy, mental status changes, or coma.[17] The kidneys or collecting system may be involved with leukemia.[18–21] This is rare and difficult to document by histology. When present, it may be characterized by a progressive rise in creatinine that improves following treatment. Overall, patients with extranodal involvement tend to have more aggressive disease and a worse prognosis.

| Table 23.2 Benign lymphocytosis | |
|---|---|
| Lymphocyte population | Etiology |
| B Cell | Postsplenectomy<br>Persistent polyclonal<br>B-cell lymphocytosis |
| T Cell | Viral infection (EBV, CMV, influenza, hepatitis, HTLV)<br>Bordetella pertussis<br>Syphilis<br>Mycobacterium tuberculosis<br>Serum sickness<br>Thyrotoxicosis<br>Addison disease<br>Postsplenectomy |

EBV, Epstein–Barr virus; CMV, cytomegalovirus; HTLV, human T-lymphotrophic virus.

## LABORATORY FINDINGS

### BLOOD FINDINGS

In previously untreated patients, lymphocytosis must be present. Lymphocytosis may be affected by treatment, and some patients may have prominent adenopathy with minimal lymphocytosis following treatment. The leukemic cells of patients with CLL are typically small-to-medium size, well differentiated, and have a thin rim of cytoplasm and a dense, homogenous, round nucleus that is slightly eccentrically located [Figure 23.2(a)].[22] The chromatin is clumped and nucleoli are usually not prominent. Prolymphocytes are larger with dispersed chromatin, a single nucleolus, and more abundant cytoplasm [Figure 23.2(b)]. For typical CLL, there should be fewer than 10% prolymphocytes.[23] CLL with increased prolymphocytes (CLL/PL) is defined by more than 10% but fewer than 55% prolymphocytes. Patients with greater than 55% prolymphocytes or greater than 15,000 prolymphocytes/μL meet the diagnostic criteria for PLL. Smudge cells may be present on the peripheral blood smear of patients with CLL [Figure 23.2(c)].[24] These are leukemia cell artifacts that result from rupture of fragile lymphocytes with processing and preparation of the blood smear. Patients with CLL almost never experience leukostasis syndrome. With a rising absolute lymphocyte count, there is a relative reduction in the number of neutrophils; previously untreated patients may develop neutropenia (≤500 neutrophils/μL). This may be a dilution effect, but may also be due to reduced production as a result of CLL bone marrow infiltration.

## STAGING

Stage has prognostic importance for patients with CLL. It is also used as a guide to initiate treatment. Staging is most useful at diagnosis, prior to administration of any treatment. There are two major staging systems:

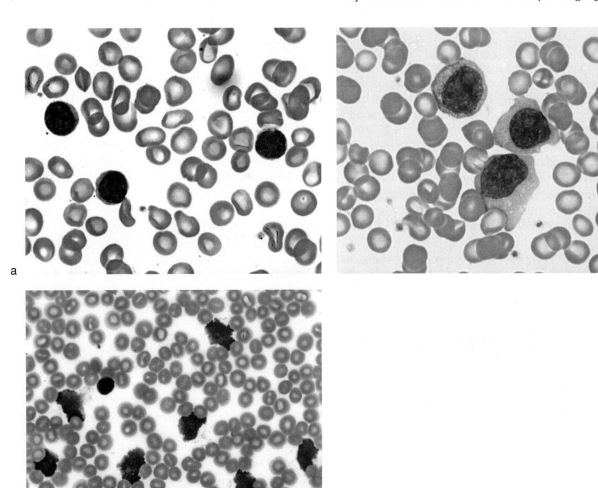

**Figure 23.2** *Morphology and histology of CLL in peripheral blood and lymph node. (a) Peripheral blood smear of a patient with CLL (1000 × magnification). Typical CLL lymphocytes are small and well differentiated, with round nuclei and clumped chromatin. (b) Peripheral blood smear of a patient with PLL. Prolymphocytes comprise greater than 55% of cells and are larger with dispersed chromatin, prominent, single nucleoli, and abundant cytoplasm (1000 × magnification). (c) Peripheral blood smear of a patient with CLL, illustrating "smudge cells" (500 × magnification)*

the Rai staging system,[25,26] used in the United States, and the Binet staging system,[27] used more commonly in Europe (Table 23.3). The Rai staging system was initially proposed as a five-stage system, with stage 0 characterized by lymphocytosis, stage I by adenopathy, stage II by organomegaly, stage III by anemia, and stage IV by thrombocytopenia.[25] This five-stage system was simplified into three stages, consisting of low risk (stage 0), intermediate risk (stages I and II), and high risk (stages III and IV).[26] The estimated median survival for patients with low-risk disease was >10 years, for intermediate-risk disease 7 years, and for high-risk disease 1.5–4 years. The Binet system is a three-stage system and is based on the number of lymph node sites involved and the presence or absence of cytopenias. Generally, patients progress through the stages with progression of their disease, in the absence of treatment.

The prognostic significance of stage is more obvious for patients with advanced-stage disease. However, the majority of patients are diagnosed with early stage disease, of whom about half will have an indolent clinical course and the other half will have a more progressive course. Therefore, significant effort has gone into identifying prognostic factors for patients with early stage disease that predict for rapidly progressive disease. Recently identified important prognostic factors that have been identified include immunoglobulin heavy-chain variable ($IgV_H$) gene mutational status,[28,29] expression of surface CD38,[29,30] and ZAP-70 expression.[31–34] These prognostic factors are most useful for counseling patients with early stage disease, as approximately half of these patients will be nonprogressors with an indolent clinical course and half will have progressive disease, requiring treatment in a short period.

## EVALUATION OF PATIENTS WITH CLL

Initial evaluation (Table 23.4) of patients suspected of having CLL should begin with a complete history and physical examination. There are no known associations between CLL and environmental exposures; therefore, exposure history is usually noncontributory. There is a strong association between genetics and risk for CLL,[35–37] making family history an important part of the evaluation. Physical examination should concentrate on evaluation for adenopathy and hepatosplenomegaly. CBC with differential and morphologic examination of the blood smear provides both diagnostic and staging information. Immunophenotype analysis of blood or bone marrow is also required. Phenotypic markers for a complete workup should include Ig light chains (κ and λ), CD5, CD19, CD23, CD20, CD79b, FMC7, CD11c, CD22, CD25, CD10, and CD38 (prognostic). Karyotype analysis by FISH for 13q deletion, 17p deletion, 11q deletion, and trisomy 12 yields useful prognostic information for counseling patients; standard metaphase karyotype is of lower yield and will often miss 13q deletion. Serum chemistries should be performed, including serum creatinine, especially if it is likely that treatment will be initiated. Measure of serum β-2-microglobulin

| Table 23.3 | Staging systems for CLL | | |
|---|---|---|---|
| Staging system | Simplified three-stage system | Clinical features at diagnosis | Estimated median survival (years) |
| **Rai stage** | | | |
| 0 | Low risk | Lymphocytosis in blood and marrow only | >10 |
| I | Intermediate risk | Lymphocytosis and lymphadenopathy | 7 |
| II | | Lymphocytosis and splenomegaly and/or hepatomegaly | |
| III | High risk | Lymphocytosis and anemia (Hgb <11 g/dL) | 1.5–4 |
| IV | | Lymphocytosis and thrombocytopenia (PLT <100,000/μL) | |
| **Binet stage** | | | |
| A | | Blood and marrow lymphocytosis and <3 areas of palpable node/organ enlargement (cervical, axillary, or inguinal; liver or spleen) | >7 |
| B | | Blood and marrow lymphocytosis and ≥3 areas of palpable node/organ enlargement (cervical, axillary, or inguinal; liver or spleen) | <5 |
| C | | Same as B with anemia (Hgb <11 g/dL for men and <10 g/dL for women) or thrombocytopenia (PLT <100,000/μL) | <2 |

Hgb, hemoglobin; PLT, platelets.

**Table 23.4    Evaluation of newly diagnosed patients with CLL**

Essential studies
  History and physical examination
  CBC and differential
  Morphologic examination of peripheral blood smear
  Immunophenotype of blood or bone marrow aspiration
  Markers include surface Ig (IgM, IgD, and IgG), Ig light chains (κ and λ), CD5, CD19, CD20, CD23, CD79b, CD11c, CD22, CD38, CD10, and FMC7
  Cytogenetic analysis with FISH for 13q deletion, 11q deletion, trisomy 12, and 17p deletion
  Serum chemistries including creatinine, β-2-microglobulin, quantitative Ig
  Serial CBC to determine lymphocyte doubling time

Optional studies
  Bone marrow aspirate and core biopsy
  Leukemia cell ZAP-70 expression
  $IgV_H$ gene sequence

provides prognostic information.[38,39] Quantitative immunoglobulin levels should be obtained to assess for hypogammaglobulinemia. Occasionally, IgG or IgM will be elevated, in which case serum protein electrophoresis with immunofixation can be obtained to evaluate for the presence of a monoclonal paraprotein.[40,41] If available, ZAP-70 expression should be measured as a prognostic marker. Further evaluation should be directed by clinical judgment. If AIHA is suspected, then reticulocyte count, direct and indirect Coomb test, haptoglobin level, lactate dehydrogenase, and fractionated bilirubin should be evaluated. Radiographic studies are not required for staging; however, they should be obtained when clinically indicated.

## IMMUNE DEFECTS

The immune system is composed of unique and diverse effector cells and soluble factors (proteins) that must be carefully orchestrated in order to carry out innate and adaptive protective functions. CLL B cells disrupt the immune function of patients with CLL (Table 23.5). The most evident manifestation of immune dysfunction is the increased risk and frequency of infection. Many patients with CLL succumb to infection or ineffectively treated autoimmunity.[42–44] The treatments used for CLL, such as purine analogs, further immunosuppress patients and put them at increased risk for opportunistic infections and may exacerbate or unmask autoimmunity.[45–47]

### HUMORAL DEFECTS
#### Immunoglobulin
Hypogammaglobulinemia is a common and progressive immune defect in patients with CLL and is another factor that increases the risk of infection.[44,48] Furthermore, dysregulated humoral immunity is associated with ineffective production of antigen-specific antibodies.[49]

Hypogammaglobulinemia is not always present at diagnosis, but frequently develops as the disease progresses. It follows that the incidence increases with duration of disease and with advancing stage.[50–52] It is progressive and tends to be irreversible; immunoglobulin levels rarely return to normal even in those patients achieving complete remission with treatment. This refractoriness to recovery may be related to prolonged lymphopenia induced by purine analogs.

**Table 23.5    Immune defects in patients with CLL**

| Defect | Characteristic |
|---|---|
| T cell | Inverted blood CD4/CD8 ratio<br>Poor T-cell response to mitogens<br>Defective expression of function-associated surface molecules<br>Increased CD8$^+$ suppressor cell function<br>Anergy/hyporesponsive skin testing |
| B cell | Reduced number in blood<br>Reduced immunoglobulin production |
| Neutrophil | Quantitative decrease in neutrophils<br>Functional defects—chemotaxis, phagocytosis, and chemiluminescence |
| Hypogammaglobulinemia | Overall decreased serum immunoglobulin levels<br>Decreased serum IgG3, IgG4, and IgA<br>Decreased mucosal IgA and IgM |
| Complement Deficiency | Decreased C1 and C4<br><br>C1 esterase inhibitor deficiency |

Hypogammaglobulinemia is directly related to morbidity and mortality in patients with CLL since it increases the risk for infection with encapsulated bacteria, and infection is the cause of death in 30–50% of patients with CLL.[52–55] Also, reduced mucosal IgA and IgM are risk factors for developing respiratory tract infections, such as pneumonia. The risk of morbidity and mortality appears to increase when IgG levels fall below 700 mg/dL; reduced serum IgA levels are also correlated with shorter survival.[56] It is intriguing that certain isotypes and subclasses tend to be more commonly affected, particularly IgG3 and IgG4.[55,57] Some patients have marked hypogammaglobulinemia but do not develop infections, leading to speculation that certain Ig subclasses may be more critical for protection than currently appreciated.

### AUTOIMMUNITY

Although CLL is characterized by progressive hypogammaglobulinemia and defective T-cell immunity, a paradoxical event is the development of autoimmunity in some patients with this disease. The autoimmune targets are predominately hematopoietic cells, specifically mature red blood cells, platelets, or red blood cell precursors. AIHA is the most common feature and together with ITP may occur in as many as 35% of patients.[58,59] Much less commonly, patients may develop a lupus-like condition[60] or rheumatoid arthritis.[6] The mechanism by which patients develop this autoimmunity is unclear. Occasionally, such events can be severe, refractory to treatment, and lead to significant morbidity and mortality.

Autoantibodies are more common in the elderly population,[61] nearly as frequent as seen with individuals with CLL; however, the incidence of AIHA is higher in patients with CLL than normal age-matched individuals. CLL is the most common cause of secondary AIHA.[62] AIHA in CLL is characterized by production of polyclonal antibodies against mature red blood cells. These are "warm antibodies" and are demonstrated with the Coomb test. The autoantibodies are typically IgG isotype, indicating participation of activated T cells and memory cells. The prevalence of AIHA increases with advanced stage and progression of the disease.[63] CLL B cells have been shown to produce Ig with low-level autoreactivity, but there is no evidence that the leukemia cells produce the autoantibodies responsible for AIHA or ITP. A significant proportion of patients (over 20%) with CLL have positive direct Coomb tests; however, not all of these patients will develop clinically significant AIHA. In addition, not all patients with active hemolysis will have a positive direct or indirect Coombs tests.

Treatment, particularly with the purine analog fludarabine, has been associated with development of AIHA.[64,65] However, randomized trials comparing fludarabine to alkylating-agent-based therapy have not shown a significantly higher incidence of AIHA in patients receiving fludarabine. The mechanism for treatment-induced autoimmunity is likely unmasking of autoimmunity after alteration of T-lymphocyte populations.

ITP occurs in 2–5% of patients with CLL.[58,63,66] ITP is more difficult to diagnose than is AIHA due to a lack of reliable diagnostic laboratory tests. Antiplatelet antibody studies are unreliable. In addition, there are other causes for thrombocytopenia patients with CLL. Specifically, thrombocytopenia may be caused by progressive bone marrow infiltration by leukemia cells with disease progression. In addition, splenomegaly that develops with disease progression may contribute to thrombocytopenia through sequestration. Despite this, it is unusual for marrow infiltration or splenomegaly to result in a platelet count less than 10,000/μL. If patients develop thrombocytopenia to this degree in the absence of cytotoxic chemotherapy, then ITP is high on the differential diagnosis.

Similarly to AIHA, ITP results from production of polyclonal antibodies of IgG isotype. Production of such antibodies implies the participation of activated T cells in this reaction and production of memory cells. Cytotoxic chemotherapy has also been reported to trigger ITP in patients with CLL. Notably, approximately one-third of patients with ITP associated with CLL also have a positive direct Coomb test.[67]

## CONCLUSIONS

Great progress has been made over the past 10–20 years in characterizing B-cell lymphoproliferative diseases, particularly CLL. Immunophenotypic analysis, as well as molecular genetics, has significantly contributed to this characterization. However, significant heterogeneity still exists in the clinical courses of patients diagnosed with this disease. Further progress in defining subsets of patients with a more homogenous prognosis will likely be aided by further identification of molecular aberrations in this disease.

### REFERENCES

1. National Cancer Institute: SEER Cancer Statistics Review 1975–2001. Available at: http://seer.cancer.gov/csr/1975_2001/.

2. Ghia P, Prato G, Scielzo C, et al.: Monoclonal CD5+ and CD5- B-lymphocyte expansions are frequent in the peripheral blood of the elderly. *Blood* 103:2337, 2004.

3. Cheson BD, Bennett JM, Rai KR, et al.: Guidelines for clinical protocols for chronic lymphocytic leukemia: recommendations of the National Cancer Institute-sponsored working group. *Am J Hematol* 29:152, 1988.

4. Cheson BD, Bennett JM, Grever M, et al.: National Cancer Institute-sponsored working group guidelines for chronic lymphocytic leukemia: revised guidelines for diagnosis and treatment. *Blood* 87:4990, 1996.

5. Batata A, Shen B: Diagnostic value of clonality of surface immunoglobulin light and heavy chains in malignant lymphoproliferative disorders. *Am J Hematol* 43:265, 1993.

6. Taylor HG, Nixon N, Sheeran TP, et al.: Rheumatoid arthritis and chronic lymphatic leukaemia. *Clin Exp Rheumatol* 7:529, 1989.

7. Weed RI: Exaggerated delayed hypersensitivity to mosquito bites in chronic lymphocytic leukemia. *Blood* 26:257, 1965.

8. Kolbusz RV, Micetich K, Armin AR, et al.: Exaggerated response to insect bites. An unusual cutaneous manifestation of chronic lymphocytic leukemia. *Int J Dermatol* 28:186, 1989.

9. Barzilai A, Shpiro D, Goldberg I, et al.: Insect bite-like reaction in patients with hematologic malignant neoplasms. *Arch Dermatol* 135:1503, 1999.

10. Cerroni L, Zenahlik P, Hofler G, et al.: Specific cutaneous infiltrates of B-cell chronic lymphocytic leukemia: a clinicopathologic and prognostic study of 42 patients. *Am J Surg Pathol* 20:1000, 1996.

11. Kaddu S, Smolle J, Cerroni L, et al.: Prognostic evaluation of specific cutaneous infiltrates in B-chronic lymphocytic leukemia. *J Cutan Pathol* 23:487, 1996.

12. Kuse R, Lueb H: Gastrointestinal involvement in patients with chronic lymphocytic leukemia. *Leukemia* 11(suppl 2):S50, 1997.

13. Johnston R, Altman KW, Gartenhaus RB: Chronic lymphocytic leukemia manifesting in the paranasal sinuses. *Otolaryngol Head Neck Surg* 127:582, 2002.

14. Berkman N, Polliack A, Breuer R, et al.: Pulmonary involvement as the major manifestation of chronic lymphocytic leukemia. *Leuk Lymphoma* 8:495, 1992.

15. Dear AE, Goldstein D, Hayman JA: Malignant pulmonary lymphoid disease: case reports illustrating anatomical pattern of disease as a prognostic marker. *Pathology* 28:20, 1996.

16. Ahmed S, Siddiqui AK, Rossoff L, et al.: Pulmonary complications in chronic lymphocytic leukemia. *Cancer* 98:1912, 2003.

17. Elliott MA, Letendre L, Li CY, et al.: Chronic lymphocytic leukaemia with symptomatic diffuse central nervous system infiltration responding to therapy with systemic fludarabine. *Br JHaematol* 104:689, 1999.

18. Pangalis GA, Boussiotis VA, Kittas C: B-chronic lymphocytic leukemia. Disease progression in 150 untreated stage A and B patients as predicted by bone marrow pattern. *Nouv Rev Fr Hematol* 30:373, 1988.

19. Haraldsdottir V, Haanen C, Jordans JG: Chronic lymphocytic leukaemia presenting as renal failure with lymphocytic infiltration of the kidneys. *Neth J Med* 41:64, 1992.

20. Phillips JK, Bass PS, Majumdar G, et al.: Renal failure caused by leukaemic infiltration in chronic lymphocytic leukaemia. *J Clin Pathol* 46:1131, 1993.

21. Comerma-Coma MI, Sans-Boix A, Tuset-Andujar E, et al.: Reversible renal failure due to specific infiltration of the kidney in chronic lymphocytic leukaemia. *Nephrol Dial Transplant* 13:1550, 1998.

22. Bennett JM, Catovsky D, Daniel MT, et al.: Proposals for the classification of chronic (mature) B and T lymphoid leukaemias. French–American–British (FAB) Cooperative Group. *J Clin Pathol* 42:567, 1989.

23. Matutes E, Oscier D, Garcia-Marco J, et al.: Trisomy 12 defines a group of CLL with atypical morphology: correlation between cytogenetic, clinical and laboratory features in 544 patients. *Br J Haematol* 92:382, 1996.

24. Macdonald D, Richardson H, Raby A: Practice guidelines on the reporting of smudge cells in the white blood cell differential count. *Arch Pathol Lab Med* 127:105, 2003.

25. Rai KR, Sawitsky A, Cronkite EP, et al.: Clinical staging of chronic lymphocytic leukemia. *Blood* 46:219, 1975.

26. Rai KR: A critical analysis of staging in CLL. In: Gale RP, Rai KR (eds.) *Chronic Lymphocytic Leukemia: Recent Progress, Future Direction.* New York: Liss; 1987:253.

27. Binet JL, Auquier A, Dighiero G, et al.: A new prognostic classification of chronic lymphocytic leukemia derived from a multivariate survival analysis. *Cancer* 48:198, 1981.

28. Hamblin TJ, Davis Z, Gardiner A, et al.: Unmutated Ig V(H) genes are associated with a more aggressive form of chronic lymphocytic leukemia. *Blood* 94:1848, 1999.

29. Damle RN, Wasil T, Fais F, et al.: Ig V gene mutation status and CD38 expression as novel prognostic indicators in chronic lymphocytic leukemia. *Blood* 94:1840, 1999.

30. Ibrahim S, Keating M, Do KA, et al.: CD38 expression as an important prognostic factor in B-cell chronic lymphocytic leukemia. *Blood* 98:181, 2001.

31. Wiestner A, Rosenwald A, Barry TS, et al.: ZAP-70 expression identifies a chronic lymphocytic leukemia subtype with unmutated immunoglobulin genes, inferior clinical outcome, and distinct gene expression profile. *Blood* 101:4944, 2003.

32. Crespo M, Bosch F, Villamor N, et al.: ZAP-70 expression as a surrogate for immunoglobulin-variable-region mutations in chronic lymphocytic leukemia. *N Engl J Med* 348:1764, 2003.

33. Orchard JA, Ibbotson RE, Davis Z, et al.: ZAP-70 expression and prognosis in chronic lymphocytic leukaemia. *Lancet* 363:105, 2004.

34. Rassenti LZ, Huynh L, Toy TL, et al.: ZAP-70 compared with immunoglobulin heavy-chain gene mutation status as a predictor of disease progression in chronic lymphocytic leukemia. *N Engl J Med* 351:893, 2004.

35. Gunz FW: The epidemiology and genetics of the chronic leukaemias. *Clin Haematol* 6:3, 1977.

36. Cartwright RA, Bernard SM, Bird CC, et al.: Chronic lymphocytic leukaemia: case control epidemiological study in Yorkshire. *Br J Cancer* 56:79, 1987.

37. Goldgar DE, Easton DF, Cannon-Albright LA, et al.: Systematic population-based assessment of cancer risk in first-degree relatives of cancer probands. *J Natl Cancer Inst* 86:1600, 1994.

38. Hallek M, Wanders L, Ostwald M, et al.: Serum beta(2)-microglobulin and serum thymidine kinase are independent predictors of progression-free survival in chronic lymphocytic leukemia and immunocytoma. *Leuk Lymphoma* 22:439, 1996.

39. Molica S, Levato D, Cascavilla N, et al.: Clinico-prognostic implications of simultaneous increased serum levels of

soluble CD23 and beta2-microglobulin in B-cell chronic lymphocytic leukemia. *Eur J Haematol* 62:117, 1999.

40. Deegan MJ, Abraham JP, Sawdyk M, et al.: High incidence of monoclonal proteins in the serum and urine of chronic lymphocytic leukemia patients. *Blood* 64:1207, 1984.

41. Pangalis GA, Moutsopoulos HM, Papadopoulos NM, et al.: Monoclonal and oligoclonal immunoglobulins in the serum of patients with B-chronic lymphocytic leukemia. *Acta Haematol* 80:23, 1988.

42. Hamblin TJ, Oscier DG, Young BJ: Autoimmunity in chronic lymphocytic leukaemia. *J Clin Pathol* 39:713, 1986.

43. Morra E, Nosari A, Montillo M: Infectious complications in chronic lymphocytic leukaemia. *Hematol Cell Ther* 41:145, 1999.

44. Tsiodras S, Samonis G, Keating MJ, et al.: Infection and immunity in chronic lymphocytic leukemia. *Mayo Clin Proc* 75:1039, 2000.

45. Wijermans PW, Gerrits WB, Haak HL: Severe immunodeficiency in patients treated with fludarabine monophosphate. *Eur J Haematol* 50:292, 1993.

46. Anaissie EJ, Kontoyiannis DP, O'Brien S, et al.: Infections in patients with chronic lymphocytic leukemia treated with fludarabine. *Ann Intern Med* 129:559, 1998.

47. Keating MJ, O'Brien S, Lerner S, et al.: Long-term follow-up of patients with chronic lymphocytic leukemia (CLL) receiving fludarabine regimens as initial therapy. *Blood* 92:1165, 1998.

48. Ultmann JE, Fish W, Osserman E, et al.: The clinical implications of hypogammaglobulinemia in patients with chronic lymphocytic leukemia and lymphocytic lymphosarcoma. *Ann Intern Med* 51:501, 1959.

49. Shaw R, Szwed C, Boggs D, et al.: Infection and immunity in chronic lymphocytic leukemia. *Arch Intern Med* 106:467, 1960.

50. Davey FR, Kurec AS, Tomar RH, et al.: Serum immunoglobulins and lymphocyte subsets in chronic lymphocytic leukemia. *Am J Clin Pathol* 87:60, 1987.

51. Orfao A, Gonzalez M, San Miguel JF, et al.: Surface phenotype and immunoglobulin levels in B-cell chronic lymphocytic leukaemia. *Haematologia* 23:49, 1990.

52. Itala M, Helenius H, Nikoskelainen J, et al.: Infections and serum IgG levels in patients with chronic lymphocytic leukemia. *Eur J Haematol* 48:266, 1992.

53. Griffiths H, Lea J, Bunch C, et al.: Predictors of infection in chronic lymphocytic leukaemia (CLL). *Clin Exp Immunol* 89:374, 1992.

54. Molica S, Levato D, Levato L: Infections in chronic lymphocytic leukemia. Analysis of incidence as a function of length of follow-up. *Haematologica* 78:374, 1993.

55. Aittoniemi J, Miettinen A, Laine S, et al.: Opsonising immunoglobulins and mannan-binding lectin in chronic lymphocytic leukemia. *Leuk Lymphoma* 34:381, 1999.

56. Rozman C, Montserrat E, Vinolas N: Serum immunoglobulins in B-chronic lymphocytic leukemia. Natural history and prognostic significance. *Cancer* 61:279, 1988.

57. Copson ER, Ellis BA, Westwood NB, et al.: IgG subclass levels in patients with B cell chronic lymphocytic leukaemia. *Leuk Lymphoma* 14:471, 1994.

58. Ebbe S, Wittels B, Dameshek W: Autoimmune thrombocytopenic purpura (ITP type) with chronic lymphocytic leukemia. *Blood* 19:23, 1962.

59. Bergsagel DE: The chronic leukemias: a review of disease manifestations and the aims of therapy. *Can Med Assoc J* 96:1615, 1967.

60. Lugassy G, Lishner M, Polliack A: Systemic lupus erythematosus and chronic lymphocytic leukemia: rare coexistence in three patients, with comments on pathogenesis. *Leuk Lymphoma* 8:243, 1992.

61. Ramos-Casals M, Garcia-Carrasco M, Brito MP, et al.: Autoimmunity and geriatrics: clinical significance of autoimmune manifestations in the elderly. *Lupus* 12:341, 2003.

62. Engelfriet CP, Overbeeke MA, von dem Borne AE: Autoimmune hemolytic anemia. *Semin Hematol* 29:3, 1992.

63. Hamblin TJ, Oscier DG, Young BJ: Autoimmunity in chronic lymphocytic leukaemia. *J Clin Pathol* 39:713, 1986.

64. Tertian G, Cartron J, Bayle C, et al.: Fatal intravascular autoimmune hemolytic anemia after fludarabine treatment for chronic lymphocytic leukemia. *Hematol Cell Ther* 38:359, 1996.

65. Gonzalez H, Leblond V, Azar N, et al.: Severe autoimmune hemolytic anemia in eight patients treated with fludarabine. *Hematol Cell Ther* 40:113, 1998.

66. Duhrsen U, Augener W, Zwingers T, et al.: Spectrum and frequency of autoimmune derangements in lymphoproliferative disorders: analysis of 637 cases and comparison with myeloproliferative diseases. *Br J Haematol* 67:235, 1987.

67. Diehl LF, Ketchum LH: Autoimmune disease and chronic lymphocytic leukemia: autoimmune hemolytic anemia, pure red cell aplasia, and autoimmune thrombocytopenia. *Semin Oncol* 25:80, 1998.

# Chapter 24

# INDICATIONS FOR TREATMENT AND TREATMENT APPROACH FOR CHRONIC LYMPHOCYTIC LEUKEMIA

## *Kanti R. Rai and Bhoomi Mehrotra*

The answer to the question of when to initiate cytotoxic therapy in a patient with chronic lymphocytic leukemia (CLL) has been modified and refined in the past 5 years, and to some extent that process of "refinement" is, perhaps, still an ongoing one.[1]

## "WAIT & WATCH" POLICY INITIALLY UPON DIAGNOSIS

CLL is one of the few hematologic malignancies in which it is advisable not to start treatment merely because a patient has just been diagnosed with this disease. Except for circumstances when, at the time of diagnosis, certain unusual clinical findings are present (discussed below), patients with CLL are initially followed on a "wait and watch" basis.[2]

A newly diagnosed patient without symptoms, and in whom the disease was discovered because of a routine (or yearly) medical checkup, or accidentally in the process of investigations of unrelated problems, is kept under observation, and is asked to return to the clinic at 3-month intervals for re-evaluation.[2]

## WHEN TO INITIATE CYTOTOXIC THERAPY

The method we have used in our clinic for deciding to institute therapy in a CLL patient who has been under observation since the initial diagnosis is based on any of the following features:

1. Development of symptoms attributable to CLL.
2. Evidence of progressive increase in the extent of disease.
3. Development of disease-related complications.

### "USUAL" SYMPTOMS ATTRIBUTABLE TO CLL
In CLL, the usual disease-related symptoms are the same as "B" symptoms found in lymphomas[2]: profound night-sweats; weight loss (10% or more from usual weight over 6–12 month period) without trying; fever without overt infections and extreme fatigue. Emergence of any of these symptoms in a previously asymptomatic patient is an indication for therapy.

### ASSESSMENT OF EXTENT OF DISEASE
Clinical staging continues to remain a readily available method of assessing the extent of disease in a patient with CLL. The five-part Rai system, or its three-part modification (Table 24.1), and the Binet system (Table 24.2) are being used both in the clinic as well as in clinical investigations.[3]

In the Binet system, there are five areas of lymphoid enlargement identified in a focused physical examination: (1) cervical; (2) axillary; (3) inguino-femoral (whether unilateral or bilateral on each site is counted as one site); (4) spleen; and (5) liver. In both systems, no additional weight is given to large, bulky tumor sizes of the palpable organs. However, the disease is considered to be active and progressive if the size of any palpable mass rapidly increases, and that becomes an appropriate reason to consider initiating cytotoxic therapy. Worsening of clinical stage, from the low-risk to the intermediate- or high-risk category is evidence, also, of disease progression and initiation of therapy.

Both the Binet and Rai staging systems were formulated before computerized axial tomography (CAT) scanning had become routine, and when enlargement of lymph nodes, spleen, or liver were recognized, they became clinically palpable.[1] To this day, for assignment of stage of a disease, only findings upon a physical

**Table 24.1    Rai Staging System in CLL**

| Risk-Category (Modified Rai) | Clinical Stage | Criteria | Median Survival (Months) |
|---|---|---|---|
| Low Risk | 0 | Lymphocytosis only | 120+ |
| Intermediate Risk | 1 | Lymphocytosis + Palpably enlarged Lymph nodes | 95 |
| | II | Lymphocytosis + Palpably enlarged Spleen and/or liver | 72 |
| High-Risk | III | Lymphocytosis + Anemia (hemoglobin <11 gm%) | 30 |
| | IV | Lymphocytosis + Thrombocytopenia (platelets < 100,000/mm³) | 30 |

examination are taken into account, for it is recognized that if CAT scans are made the basis for staging, few patients would fall into stage 0 (low-risk category), because it is likely that CAT scan would reveal an enlarged node in the chest, abdomen, or pelvis. Similarly, many of Binet's stage A patients might become stage B, and their respective prognostic and clinical implications would become unclear. In view of both systems of staging having certain weaknesses, and that their true value is to provide some direction for decision making for therapeutic intervention and assessment of success or failure of any therapy, clinical staging in CLL should continue to be based only on findings following physical examination.

In addition to clinical staging, certain other features also have been recognized as helpful in decision-making of whether initiation of treatment is indicated.

**Table 24.2    Binet Staging System in CLL**

| Clinical Stage | Criteria | Median Survival (months) |
|---|---|---|
| A | Two or fewer sites of palpably enlarged lymph nodes, spleen or liver | 120+ |
| B | Three or more sites of palpable enlarged lymph nodes, spleen or liver | 61 |
| C | Anemia (hemoglobin < 10gm%) and/or thrombocytopenia (platelet <100,000/mm³) | 32 |

**Rate of increase in absolute lymphocyte count**

In an untreated patient, if the absolute lymphocyte count (ALC) is increasing at a rapid rate, doubling in a short period, usually considered to be less than 6 months, (although some observers consider doubling in less than 12 months as rapid rate), the disease is progressing rapidly, and therapy should be started. It is our opinion that this feature of rapid lymphocyte doubling time should not be enough if it exists as a sole feature, i.e., in absence of "B" symptoms or worsening of clinical stage, etc. Also, the height of the ALC should also be taken into account; for example, ALC doubling from a relatively low number, e.g., 6000 to 12,000/mm³ in 6–12 months in an asymptomatic patient carries less weight than a high baseline, e.g., 100,000/mm³ ALC projected to be doubling in the same period of 6–12 months. Similarly, hyperlymphocytosis, for example, an ALC of 250,000/mm³ or higher, might cause hyperviscosity of circulating blood, and thus pose an increased risk of thromboembolic events in the microcirculation in an organ, with potentially catastrophic results. Thus, hyperlymphocytosis by itself in some circumstances should become a trigger to initiate therapy.

Is histopathologic pattern of lymphoid infiltration in the biopsy specimens of bone marrow by itself a factor in decision making? In our opinion, although a diffuse infiltration pattern is generally associated with a worse prognosis than nodular or interstitial (nondiffuse) patterns, this feature is not powerful enough to deserve to be factored in making this decision.

Other clinical characteristics that have been reported to be helpful in determining whether CLL is active or progressing are elevated serum levels of β2-microglobulin, thymidine kinase, and soluble CD23.[1] Although each one of these tests has some validity as a prognostic marker in CLL, none of them has been tested and proven to be powerful in prospectively conducted studies; nor have they been consistently used by all clinicians. Therefore, we have not integrated any of these in our decision-making algorithm in this disease.

### ROLE OF OTHER DISEASE-RELATED COMPLICATIONS

CLL patients are known to be at an increased risk of developing autoimmune hematologic complications. The most frequent among these is Coombs positivity with or without resulting autoimmune hemolytic anemia (AIHA) and immune thrombocytopenia (ITP). Pure red cell aplasia (PRCA) is a relatively rare complication, while immune neutropenia is extremely rare in CLL. When AIHA, ITP, or PRCA occur even in a patient who has not received any prior cytotoxic therapy, we consider these complications indications for instituting therapy.

Finally, a small minority of CLL patients develop Richter's transformation in the form of diffuse large cell lymphoma or prolymphocytic leukemia. Both of these conditions might have developed from the original CLL clone or from a new clone as a separate, new malignancy. Both of these conditions have been known to occur in patients who had received prior chemotherapy regimens for CLL, and also in previously untreated patients. These complications have been treated with a wide range of chemotherapy agents, but unfortunately none has been found to be consistently and reproducibly effective.

### IMPACT OF RECENTLY IDENTIFIED BIOLOGIC AND CYTOGENETIC PROGNOSTIC MARKERS ON TREATMENT DECISIONS

Considerable degrees of excitement and hopes for improving the treatment of CLL have recently been generated following the discovery of four prognostic features.

### MUTATION STATUS OF IgVH GENES

Leukemic lymphocytes of nearly 50% of the CLL patients have somatic mutations in *IgVH* genes, and the remaining 50% have unmutated *VH* genes.[4,5] There is a strong correlation between longer survival and overall better clinical course among patients with mutated *VH* genes compared to their unmutated counterparts. Thus, it is reasonable to consider the unmutated *VH* gene patients for early therapeutic intervention. This, we believe, will happen in the foreseeable future, but at this moment, the testing for the mutation is neither generally available (it is labor intensive and costly), nor has its methodology been standardized. Also, there is a lack of consensus among experts as to how to define "mutated." Does it require 2% mutations, or 2.5%, or 3%? This is not a trivial issue,

because the counterparts of each of these ratios will thus be called unmutated, and whether those patients labeled "unmutated" will have to have more than 98% homology, more than 97.5%, or more than 97% homology is a matter which is yet to be resolved. Once this is resolved, it is possible that a symptom-free, early stage CLL patient who might otherwise be followed on wait-and-watch basis would become a candidate for immediate chemotherapeutic intervention if that patient has unmutated *VH* genes. However, at this time we include this parameter only in research-based investigational therapeutic trials.

### COEXPRESSION OF CD38 ON LEUKEMIC B LYMPHOCYTES

It has been observed that CLL patients whose leukemic lymphocytes do not coexpress CD38 have a better prognosis than those who are CD38 positive.[4] Thus, it would seem logical to include CD38 positive patients (similar to VH-unmutated patients) among those in whom early intervention will be appropriate. This recommendation also appears reasonable, but there is a lack of agreement as to whether 30% or greater positivity should be considered CD38 positive, or the threshold should be set at 13%. As in the case of VH mutations, we believe that defining when CD38 is called positive will be resolved soon, but until that happens, in our clinical practice, we do not make therapeutic decisions on that basis alone.

### ZAP-70 EXPRESSION IN CLL B LYMPHOCYTES

CLL patients whose leukemic lymphocytes do not have ZAP-70 positivity have been reported to have strong correlation with mutated VH status.[6,7] However, we have not yet allowed introduction of ZAP-70 in clinical practice, and in decision-making for initiation of therapy, because other laboratories have found testing for ZAP-70 difficult to reproduce from one time to the next. Until the issues of correct methodology and predictable reproducibility of results have been resolved, we consider it premature to incorporate this test for making a decision if therapeutic intervention is appropriate.

### FISH CYTOGENETICS IN CLL

It has previously been shown that conventional cytogenetics, using banding techniques, provide inconsistently reliable results in CLL because leukemic lymphocytes in this disease do not readily yield readable metaphases.[8] The development of fluorescence in situ hybridization (FISH) techniques and the availability of DNA probes for all chromosomes of interest in CLL have made it possible to study chromosomal abnormalities in this disease. Using FISH, we now can divide CLL patients into distinct prognostic categories based on chromosomal abnormalities.[8] Patients with 13q deletions as a single abnormality have the best survival. High-risk abnormalities and the shortest survival were observed with 11q del and 17p del, while trisomy 12 (12+) and no chromosomal abnormality patients form the intermediate survival group.[8] As FISH methodology has become standardized, we believe that low-risk or intermediate-risk (by clinical staging) group patients who are free of symptoms but have 17p del or 11q del could be considered for early intervention, especially when they participate in a prospectively randomized study with one arm consisting of wait and watch (currently the standard of practice for patients in these clinical stages), and the other arm consisting of some regimen of effective chemotherapy.

## TREATMENT APPROACH FOR PATIENTS WITH CLL

Once we have made an assessment that a patient with CLL, who has been on a "wait and watch" method of follow-up, should start cytotoxic therapy, we first try to determine what our therapeutic endpoint should be. This assessment is made on a case-by-case basis and, therefore, is highly individualized. For example, for a relatively young patient with no other major comorbid conditions, we would take an aggressive approach with an intent to achieve a complete remission or a good quality partial remission, and then, as the next step, depending upon the ability of the patient to actively participate in the decision-making process, we would engage the patient in a discussion of whether he/she would be willing to enter any prospectively conducted clinical trials aimed at elimination of minimal residual disease with targeted monoclonal antibody therapy in an adjuvant setting, or with hematopoietic stem cell transplantation following a nonmyeloablative conditioning regimen. The latter courses are still unproven for their ability to achieve a cure or even to improve the duration of remission and survival time, but are accompanied by a higher likelihood of treatment-related morbidity and mortality.

If, on the other hand, we are dealing with an older patient whose actuarial life expectancy is considered to be about 10 years, aggressive and curative therapeutic approaches would be inappropriate, because of a treatment-associated significant incidence of morbidity and mortality. In those cases, a palliative approach is indicated, with the objective of relief of symptoms and reduction of body burden of overall tumor mass, while, to a certain extent, preserving the quality of life. Additionally, if these patients have other major comorbid conditions, our treatment objective would be rather conservative, and palliative therapy aimed at relief of symptoms but with less potential toxicity would be the recommended method of management.

## REFERENCES

1. IWCLL-Initiated Working Group on Prognostic and diagnostic parameters in CLL: Perspectives on the use of new diagnostic tools in the treatment of chronic lymphocytic leukemia. *Blood* 107:859–61, 2006.
2. Cheson BD, Bennett JM, Grever M, et al.: National Cancer Institute-Sponsored Working Group Guidelines for CLL: revised guidelines for diagnosis and treatment. *Blood* 87:4990–4997, 1996.
3. Chronic lymphocytic leukemia: recommendations for diagnosis, staging and response criteria. International Workshop on CLL. *Ann Intern Med* 110: 236–238, 1989.
4. Damle RN, Wasil T, Fais F, et al.: IgV gene mutation status and CD38 expression as novel prognostic indicators in CLL. *Blood* 94:1840–1847, 1999.
5. Hamblin TJ, Davis Z, Gardiner A, Oscier DG, Stevenson FK: Unmutated IgV(H) genes are associated with a more aggressive form of CLL. *Blood* 94:1848–1854, 1999.
6. Crespo M, Bosch F, Villamor N, et al.: ZAP-70 expression as a surrogate for immunoglobulin-variable region mutations in CLL. *N Engl J Med* 348: 1764–1775, 2003.
7. Rassenti LZ, Huynh L, Toy TL, et al.: ZAP-70 compared with immunoglobulin heavy chain gene mutation status as a predictor of disease progression in CLL. *N Engl J Med* 351:893–901, 2004.
8. Dohner H, Stilgenbauer S, Benner A, et al.: Genomic aberrations and survival in patients with CLL. *N Engl J Med* 343:1910–1916, 2000.

# Chapter 25

# RESPONSE CRITERIA, PROGNOSIS, AND FOLLOW-UP IN CHRONIC LYMPHOCYTIC LEUKEMIA

*Emili Montserrat*

## RESPONSE CRITERIA

The *National Cancer Institute–Working Group* (NCI-WG) and the *International Workshop on Chronic Lymphocytic Leukemia* (IWCLL) independently proposed criteria for assessing response in patients with chronic lymphocytic leukemia (CLL) (Table 25.1), the NCI proposal having gained wider acceptance and being the one usually employed.[1,2]

These criteria have proved to be extremely useful to conduct and compare trials, thereby contributing to progress in CLL therapy. Nevertheless, these proposals were elaborated in an era in which no effective therapy for CLL existed. Today, treatment of CLL is based on purine analogs, particularly fludarabine, along with other agents. This results not only in a high complete remission (CR) rate but also in the disappearance, in many instances, of minimal residual disease (MRD)—a situation difficult to envisage when NCI-WG and IWCLL criteria were proposed.

Because of this, classical response criteria are now somewhat obsolete. For example, according to such criteria, patients with less than 30% lymphocytes in a bone marrow aspirate may be classified as complete responders, provided clinical and laboratory findings return to normal. In addition, patients with lymphoid aggregates in bone marrow biopsy are considered to be in nodular partial response, yet these nodules may

| Table 25.1 | Chronic lymphocytic leukemia: Response criteria | |
|---|---|---|
| Response | IWCLL criteria | NCI-WG criteria |
| CR | No evidence of disease | Absence of lymphadenopathy, hepatomegaly, splenomegaly or constitutional symptoms. Normal blood count: neutrophils $> 1.5 \times 10^9$/L, platelets $> 100 \times 10^9$/L, Hb $> 11$ g/dL, lymphocytes $< 4.0 \times 10^9$/L, BM biopsy with normal cellularity and lymphocytes $< 30\%$. |
| nPR | | CR criteria with presence of lymphoid aggregates in bone marrow biopsy |
| PR | Change from stage C to stage A or B; from stage B to A | 50% reduction in blood lymphocytes and 50% reduction in lymphadenopathy and/or 50% reduction in splenomegaly and/or hepatomegaly. Neutrophils $> 1.5 \times 10^9$/L or 50% improvement over baseline; platelets $> 100 \times 10^9$/L or 50% improvement over baseline; Hb $> 11.0$ g/dL (not supported by transfusion) or 50% improvement over baseline. |
| SD | No change in the stage of the disease | No CR, PR, or PD. |
| PD | Change from stage A disease to stage B or C, or from stage B to C | At least one of the following: $> 50\%$ increase in the size of at least two lymph nodes or new palpable lymph nodes; $\geq 50\%$ increase of splenomegaly or hepatomegaly or appearance if there was no transformation to a more aggressive histology, Richter or prolymphocytic leukemia; $> 50\%$ increase in the absolute number or circulating lymphocytes. |

CR = complete response; nPR = same as CR with presence of lymphoid aggregates in bone marrow biopsy; PR = partial response; SD = stable disease; PD = progressive disease.

represent either leukemic or nonneoplastic T cells. In other words, some patients considered to be in CR by current criteria can still harbor leukemic cells, whereas others who are deemed to be in partial remission (PR) may have achieved CR.

A step forward in evaluating the response in CLL has been the assessment of MRD by either allele-specific polymerase chain reaction (PCR) or four-color cytofluorometry, classical combinations being CD19/CD5/CD79b/CD20 or CD19/CD5/CD43/C20.[3–5] However, these combinations are less effective in situations where leukemia cells lack CD20, e.g., in patients treated with combinations including rituximab. Antigenic combinations that circumvent that problem include CD79b/CD43/CD19/CD5; CD81/CD22/CD19/CD5; and CD20/CD38/CD19/CD5.[6] Although PCR has a slightly higher sensitivity than four-color cytofluorometry, both methods are similarly useful from the clinical point of view, and four-color cytofluorometry is cheaper and more widely applicable.

Analyzing MRD may be useful for assessing and monitoring the response to therapy. There is already proof that eradicating MRD results not only in longer freedom-from-progression but also longer survival,[3,7–9] making the MRD eradication a desirable goal in CLL therapy.

Note that some patients considered in NCI-WG PR because of treatment-related cytopenias (normalization of peripheral blood cell counts is a requisite for CR in classical response criteria) may have achieved an MRD-negative status, and these patients have a better prognosis than those in CR by NCI-WG criteria but with persistent MRD.[9] This indicates that MRD status may be more important than NCI-WG criteria to predict outcome after therapy.

A practical point is, therefore, that with the newer, more effective, but also more myelotoxic treatments, a time window of 2–3 months that would allow patients to recover from treatment-related cytopenias should be required before evaluating response and that treatment-related cytopenias should not necessarily disqualify for CR. Also, and more importantly, MRD-negative CR should be incorporated as a new response category in the assessment of CLL therapy.

Another criticism to current response criteria is that the disappearance of immunologic abnormalities that may be present before treatment (e.g., hypogammaglobulinemia, autoimmune hemolytic anemia (AIHA), positive Coombs test) is not considered as a criterion for CR. This is not an easy issue since current therapies cause a profound immunosuppression and may trigger autoimmune phenomena.[10] However, whether the outcome of patients in whom the immunologic abnormalities are corrected upon treatment is better than those in whom such abnormalities persist should be investigated.

Finally, the assessment of lymphadenopathy, splenomegaly, and hepatomegaly is made clinically both when assessing clinical stage and when evaluating response to therapy. The role of imaging studies (e.g., CT scans) in staging and response to therapy evaluation should be evaluated.

## PROGNOSIS

The median survival of patients with CLL is about 10 years. Some patients have a survival not different from that of the general population, but there are others who have a rapidly fatal course. Clinical stages have been the most useful prognostic parameters in CLL[11,12] (Table 25.2; Figure 25.1). They, however, have some limitations. For example, an important condition of all prognostic parameters is that they identify a *substantial* proportion of patients with different outcome. Since the majority of patients with CLL are diagnosed on the occasion of routine medical examinations, when still asymptomatic, most patients (70–80%) are in early clinical stage at diagnosis, thus limiting the prognostic value of clinical stages.[13,14] Moreover, progressive and indolent forms of the disease are not identified. In addition, the mechanisms accounting for cytopenias are not taken into consideration, yet there is some indication that patients with cytopenias of immune origin may have a better outcome than those in whom the cytopenia is caused by a massive infiltration of the bone marrow by neoplastic cells.[15,16]

Because of the limitations discussed above, other prognostic factors able to increase the prognostic power of clinical stages have been proposed. In addition to clinical stages, other widely used prognostic factors include the degree of bone marrow infiltration, blood lymphocyte levels, lymphocyte doubling time, and lymphocyte morphology. A number of serum markers, including lactate dehydrogenase (LDH), thymidine kinase, B2-microglobulin, CD23, CD25, and CD20 serum levels have also been found to be good indicators of survival(reviewed in Refs. 17,18).

Differences in the natural history of CLL and its prognosis reflect the biological heterogeneity of the disease, which is rapidly unfolding. Thus, in up to 90% of the patients it is possible to detect cytogenetic abnormalities by fluorescent in situ hybridization studies. Although nonspecific, there are interesting correlates between some cytogenetic aberrations and clinical features and prognosis. For example, patients with del(13q) as a single anomaly have an excellent prognosis whereas those with del(11q) or del(17p) do not respond to chemotherapy and tend to have a rapidly evolving disease. Moreover, trisomy 12 is associated with atypical morphology and immunophenotype of the leukemic cells, and del(6q) is more frequently observed in patients whose lymphocytes display plasmacytoid features and intermediate prognosis.[19–21] Also, overexpression of *MDR-1* and *MDR-3* genes and P-glycoprotein detection on neoplastic cells has been correlated in some studies with resistance to therapy and poor prognosis.[22,23]

| Table 25.2 | Staging systems for chronic lymphocytic leukemia | | |
| --- | --- | --- | --- |
| *Staging system* | *Stage* | *Clinical features* | *Median survival (yrs)* |
| **Rai** | | | |
| Low-risk | 0 | Lymphocytosis alone | 14.5 |
| Intermediate-risk | I | Lymphocytosis Lymphadenopathy | 7.5 |
| | II | Lymphocytosis Spleen or liver enlargement | |
| High-risk | III | Lymphocytosis Hemoglobin < 11 g/dL | 2.5 |
| | IV | Lymphocytosis Platelets < 100,000/microliter | |
| **Binet** | | | |
| Low-risk | A | No anemia, no thrombocytopenia < 3 lymphoid areas* enlarged | 15.5 |
| Intermediate-risk | B | No anemia, no thrombocytopenia ≥ 3 lymphoid areas enlarged | 5.5 |
| High-risk | C | Hemoglobin < 10 g/dL or Platelets < 100,000/microliter | 3 |

*The Binet staging system takes into consideration the following lymphoid areas: lymph nodes (whether unilateral or bilateral) in the head and neck, axillae, and groin; spleen, and liver.

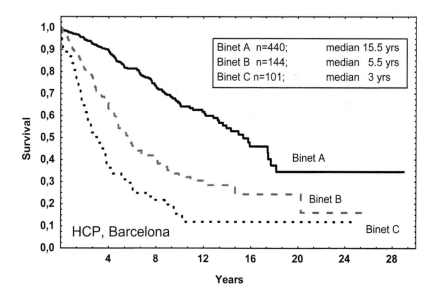

Binet A  n=440;     median 15.5 yrs
Binet B  n=144;     median 5.5 yrs
Binet C  n=101;     median 3 yrs

**Figure 25.1** *Chronic lymphocytic leukemia. Survival of a large series of patients from the Hospital Clínic, Barcelona, according to Binet's clinical stages*

The mutational status of *IgVH* genes separates CLL into two forms with distinct presenting features and outcome. Thus, as compared to those with IgVH mutations, patients with unmutated IgVH genes have a more malignant disease, including evidence of advanced, progressive disease, atypical cell morphology, adverse cytogenetic features, and resistance to therapy.[24–26] The prognostic significance of IgVH mutations is independent from that of clinical stages and cytogenetic abnormalities. Unfortunately, studying IgVH mutations is not yet possible on a routine basis, hence the interest in finding a surrogate for IgVH mutations easily applicable in clinical practice. CD38 expression on leukemic lymphocytes correlates, although not absolutely, with IgVH mutations; moreover, CD38 expression may vary over time.[27] Recently, it has been demonstrated that ZAP-70 expression on leukemic cells, as evaluated by cytofluorometry or PCR, strongly correlates with IgVH mutations and has important prognostic significance by itself. The expression of ZAP-70 in more than 20% of neoplastic lymphocytes correlates with unmutated IgVH genes and conveys a poor prognosis.[28–31] It has also been shown that high expression of activation-induced cytidine deaminase mRNA is associated with unmutated *IgVH* gene status and unfavorable cytogenetic aberrations in CLL[32]; however, the clinical applicability of this test has not yet been established.

Besides findings at diagnosis, evolutive features are also important in prognosis. In about 3–10% of patients, the disease undergoes transformation into a more aggressive type, most commonly large-cell lymphoma (Richter syndrome), which is usually revealed by fever, weight loss, night sweats, enlarged lymphadenopathy, and increased LDH serum levels.[33–35] The prognosis of such an event is poor, with a median survival of less than 6 months.

Patients with CLL may also experience transformation into prolymphocytoid leukemia (PL), in which larger lymphocytes (prolymphocytes) coexist with small, typical CLL cells; the prognosis of the so-called CLL/PL is poorer than that of the typical CLL.[36]

In addition, the outcome of patients with CLL can be blurred by the appearance of second malignancies to which patients with CLL are prone.[37,38] Risk assessment, however, is not easy because of the variability in the criteria used to evaluate it. In a study based on data from population-based cancer registries, the observed/expected ratio was 1.20, with an increased risk for Kaposi sarcoma, malignant melanoma, larynx cancers, lung cancer, and also bladder and gastric cancer in men. No relationship was found between the characteristics of the disease and its treatment with the incidence of second cancers.[37] Recently, cases of myelodysplasia/acute leukemia have been reported in patients treated with chlorambucil and fludarabine[39]; because of the increasing use of purine analogs in combination with other agents in CLL therapy, physicians should be alert to this possible complication.

Hypogammaglobulinemia may be observed in up to 60% of the patients with advanced disease, and contributes to the increased risk for infections, occasionally opportunistic, that patients with CLL may present and that are the most important cause of death.[40,41]

Patients with CLL may also develop AIHA, which can be triggered by treatment; although it usually responds to corticosteroids, some fatal cases of AIHA have been reported.[42]

As previously discussed, response to therapy is an important prognostic parameter in itself,[7–9,43–45] the higher the degree of response the better the outcome. Thus, the patients who achieve MRD-negative status have a better prognosis than those with inferior response to therapy, including those in CR by classical criteria but with persistence of MRD.[9] In addition, the detection of MRD predicts clinical relapse with the exception of patients submitted to allogeneic transplantation, thus reflecting the importance of a graft-versus-leukemia effect in such a context.[46,47]

## FOLLOW-UP

There is no consensus on how to follow patients with CLL and, in fact, no specific recommendations have been made by the NCI-WG,[1] the IWCLL,[2] or in some more recent guidelines.[41,42] Follow-up must be individualized on the basis of the characteristics of the patient and the disease. Patients with low-risk disease do not need to be monitored as frequently as those with poor prognostic features. Thus, patients with low-risk, stable disease may be evaluated every 6–12 months, whereas those with high-risk disease need to be seen at shorter intervals, e.g., every 3 months. Attention must be paid to the appearance of signs of disease progression or complications such as those discussed above, including disease transformation, second neoplasias, autoimmune phenomena, hypogammaglobulinemia, or infections.

## REFERENCES

1. International Workshop on CLL: Chronic lymphocytic leukemia: recommendations for diagnosis, staging, and response criteria. International Workshop on Chronic Lymphocytic Leukemia. *Ann Intern Med* 110:236–238, 1989.
2. Cheson BD, Bennett JM, Grever M, et al.: National Cancer Institute-sponsored working group guidelines for chronic lymphocytic leukemia: revised guidelines for diagnosis and treatment. *Blood* 87:4990–4997, 1996.
3. van Dongen JJM, Langerak AW, Brüggemann M, et al.: Design and standardization of PCR primers and protocols for detection of clonal immunoglobulin and T cell receptor gene recombinations in suspect lymphoproliferations: report of the BIOMED-2 Concerted Action BMH4-CT98-3936. *Leukemia* 17:2257–2317, 2003.
4. Rawstron AC, Kennedy B, Evans PA, et al.: Quantitation of minimal disease levels in chronic lymphocytic leukemia using a sensitive flow cytometric assay improves the prediction of outcome and can be used to optimize therapy. *Blood* 98:29–35, 2001.
5. Böttcher S, Ritgen M, Pott C, et al.: Comparative analysis of minimal residual disease detection using four-color flow cytometry, consensus IgH-PCR, and quantitative IgH PCR in CLL after allogeneic and autologous stem cell transplantation. *Leukemia* 18:1637–1645, 2004.
6. Rawstron AC, Villamor N, Zehnder JL, et al.: International standardized approach to molecular and flow cytometric disease monitoring in CLL [abstract]. *Blood* 104:15, 2004.
7. Provan D, Bartlett-Pandite L, Zwicky C, et al.: Eradication of polymerase chain reaction-detectable chronic lymphocytic leukemia cells is associated with improved outcome after bone marrow transplantation. *Blood* 88:2228–2235, 1996.
8. Bosch F, Ferrer A, López-Guillermo A, et al.: Fludarabine, cyclophosphamide and mitoxantrone in the treatment

of resistant or relapsed chronic lymphocytic leukaemia. *Br J Haematol* 119:976–984, 2002.

9. Moreton P, Kennedy B, Lucas G, et al.: Eradication of minimal residual disease (MRD) in B-cell chronic lymphocytic leukemia after alemtuzumab therapy is associated with prolonged survival. *J Clin Oncol* 23:2971–2979, 2005.

10. Cheson BD: Infectious and immunosuppresive complications of purine analog therapy. *J Clin Oncol* 13:2431–2448, 1995.

11. Rai KR, Sawitsky A, Cronkite EP, et al.: Clinical staging of chronic lymphocytic leukemia. *Blood* 46:219–234, 1975.

12. Binet JL, Auquier A, Dighiero G, et al.: A new prognostic classification of chronic lymphocytic leukemia derived from a multivariate survival analysis. *Cancer* 48:198–206, 1981.

13. Rozman C, Bosch F, Montserrat E: Chronic lymphocytic leukemia: a changing natural history? *Leukemia* 11:775–778, 1997.

14. Molica S, Levato D: GAT is changing in the natural history of chronic lymphocytic leukemia? *Haematologica* 86:8–12, 2001.

15. Mauro FR, Foa R, Cerretti R, et al.: Autoimmune hemolytic anemia in chronic lymphocytic leukemia: clincial, therapeutic, and prognostic features. *Blood* 95:2788–2792, 2000.

16. Kyasa MJ, Parrish RS, Schichman SA, Zent CS: Autoimmune cytopenia does not predict poor prognosis in chronic lymphocytic leukemia/small lymphocytic lymphoma. *Am J Hematol* 74:1–8, 2003.

17. Montserrat E: Assessing prognosis in patients with chronic lymphocytic leukemia a quarter of century after Rai and Binet staging systems. *Ann Oncol* 15:450–451, 2004.

18. Zent CS, Kay NE: Advances in the understanding of biology and prognosis in chronic lymphocytic leukemia. *Curr Oncol Rep* 5:348–354, 2004.

19. Döhner H, Stilgenbauer S, Benner A, et al.: Genomic aberrations and survival in chronic lymphocytic leukemia. *N Engl J Med* 343:1910–1916, 2000.

20. Döhner H, Stilgenbauer S, Döhner K, Bentz M, Lichter P: Chromosome aberrations in B-cell chronic lymphocytic leukemia: reassessment based on molecular cytogenetic analysis. *J Mol Med* 77:266–281, 1999.

21. Cuneo A, Rigolin GM, Bigoni R, et al.: Chronic lymphocytic leukemia with 6q- shows distinct haematological features and intermediate prognosis. *Leukemia* 18:476–483, 2004.

22. Friedenberg WR, Spencer SK, Musser C, et al.: Multi-drug resistance in chronic lymphocytic leukemia. *Leuk Lymphoma* 34:171–178, 1999.

23. Pepper C, Thomas A, Hidalgo de Quintana J, Davies S, Hoy Y, Bentley P: Pleiotropic drug resistance in B-cell chronic lymphocytic leukaemia-the role of Bcl-2 family disregulation. *Leuk Res* 1007–1014, 1999.

24. Hamblin TJ, Davis Z, Gardiner A, Oscier DG, Stevenson FK: Unmutated Ig V(H) genes are associated with a more aggressive form of chronic lymphocytic leukemia. *Blood* 94:1848–1854, 1999.

25. Damle RN, Wasil T, Fais F, et al.: Ig V gene mutation status and CD38 expression as novel prognostic indicators in chronic lymphocytic leukemia. *Blood* 94:1840–1847, 1999.

26. Krober A, Seiler T, Benner A, et al.: V(H) mutation status, CD38 expression level, genomic aberrations, and prognosis in chronic lymphocytic leukemia. *Blood* 100:1410–1416, 2002.

27. Hamblin TJ, Orchad JA, Ibbotson RE, et al.: CD38 expression and immunoglobulin variable region mutations are independent prognostic variables in chronic lymphocytic leukemia, but CD38 expression may vary during the course of the disease. *Blood* 99:1023–1029, 2002.

28. Crespo M, Bosch F, Villamor N, et al.: ZAP-70 expression as a surrogate for immunoglobulin-variable-region mutations in chronic lymphocytic leukemia. *N Engl J Med* 348:1764–1775, 2003.

29. Wiestner A, Rosenwald A, Barry TS, et al.: ZAP-70 expression identifies a chronic lymphocytic leukemia subtype with unmutated immunoglobulin genes, inferior clinical outcome, and distinct gene expression profile. *Blood* 101:4944–4951, 2003.

30. Orchad JA, Ibbotson RW, Davis Z, et al.: ZAP-70 expression and prognosis in chronic lymphocytic leukemia. *Lancet* 363:105–111, 2004.

31. Rassenti LZ, Huynh L, Toy TL, et al.: ZAP-70 compared with immunoglobulin heavy-chain gene mutation status as predictor of disease progression in chronic lymphocytic leukemia. *N Engl J Med* 351:893–901, 2004.

32. Heintel D, Kroemer E, Kienle D, et al.: High expression of activation-induced cytidine deaminase (AID) mRNA is associated with unmutated IgVH gene status and unfavorable cytogenetic aberrations in patients with chronic lymphocytic leukemia. *Leukemia* 4:756–762, 2004.

33. Richter MN: Generalized reticular cell sarcoma of lymph nodes associated with lymphatic leukemia. *Am J Pathol* 4:285–292, 1928.

34. Robertson LE, Pugh W, O'Brien S, et al.: Richter's syndrome: a report on 39 patients. *J Clin Oncol* 11:1985–1989, 1993.

35. Giles FJ, O'Brien SM, Keating MJ: Chronic lymphocytic leukemia in (Richter's) transformation. *Semin Oncol* 25:117–125, 1998.

36. Enno A, Catovsky D, O'Brien M, et al.: 'Prolymphocytoid' transformation of chronic lymphocytic leukemia. *Br J Haematol* 41:9–18, 1979.

37. Greene MH, Hoover RN, Fraumeni JF: Subsequent cancer in patients with chronic lymphocytic leukemia. A possible immunologic mechanism. *J Natl Cancer Inst* 61:337–340, 1978.

38. Hisada M, Biggar RJ, Greene MH, et al.: Solid tumors after chronic lymphocytic leukemia. *Blood* 98:1979–1981, 2001.

39. Morrison VA, Rai KR, Peterson BL, et al.: Therapy-related myeloid leukemias are observed in patients with chronic lymphocytic leukemia after treatment with fludarabine and chlorambucil: results of an intergroup study, Cancer and Leukemia Group B. *J Clin Oncol* 20:3878–3884, 2002.

40. Rozman C, Montserrat E, Viñolas N: Serum immunoglobulins in B-chronic lymphocytic leukaemia. Natural history and prognostic significance. *Cancer* 61:279–283, 1988.

41. Molica S: Infections in chronic lymphocytic leukemia: Risk factors, an impact on survival, and treatment. *Leuk Lymphoma* 13:203–214, 1994.

42. Weiss RB, Freiman J, Kweder SL, Diehl LF, Byrd JC: Hemolytic anemia after fludarabine therapy for chronic lymphocytic leukemia. *J Clin Oncol* 16:1885–1889, 1998.

43. Montserrat E, Alcala A, Parody R, et al.: A randomized trial comparing chlorambucil plus prednisone versus cyclophosphamide, vincristine, and prednisone. *Cancer* 56:2369–2375, 1985.

44. Catovsky D, Fooks I, Richards S: Prognostic factors in chronic lymphocytic leukaemia: the importance of age, sex, and response to treatment in survival. A report from the MRC CLL 1 trial. *Br J Haematol* 72:141–149, 1989.

45. Keating MI, O'Brien S, Kantarjian H, et al.: Long-term follow-up of patients with chronic lymphocytic leukemia treated with fludarabine as a single agent. *Blood* 81: 2878–2884, 1993.

46. Esteve J, Villamor N, Colomer D, Montserrat E: Different clinical value of minimal residual disease after autolo-gous and allogeneic stem cell transplantation for chronic lymphocytic leukemia. *Blood* 99:1873–1874, 2002.

47. Mattson J, Uzuel M, Remberger M, et al.: Minimal resid-ual disease is common after allogeneic stem cell trans-plantation in patients with B cell chronic lymphocytic leukemia and may be controlled by graft-versus-host dis-ease. *Leukemia* 14:247–254, 2000.

48. Hallek M, Bergmann M, Emmerich B (for the German CLL Study Group). Chronic lymphocytic leukemia: up-dated recommendations on diagnosis and treatment. *Onkologie* 27:97–104, 2004.

49. Anonymous: Guidelines on the diagnosis and manage-ment of chronic lymphocytic leukaemia. *Br J Haematol* 15:294–317, 2004.

# Chapter 26

# TREATMENT OF CHRONIC LYMPHOCYTIC LEUKEMIA

*Matt E. Kalaycio*

## INTRODUCTION

Once the diagnosis of chronic lymphocytic leukemia (CLL) is made (Chapter 23) and there is an indication to begin therapy (Chapter 24), treatment should then begin without delay. The initial treatment has traditionally been palliative, as no treatment to date has demonstrably prolonged overall survival. However, new paradigms are emerging that promise to increase complete remission (CR) rates and eliminate minimal residual disease (MRD). These innovative strategies (Table 26.1) may yet prove to prolong survival and are the subject of intense investigation.

## INITIAL TREATMENT WITH CHEMOTHERAPY

### CHLORAMBUCIL VERSUS FLUDARABINE

Introduced into clinical practice in the early 1960s, chlorambucil (CLB) is an orally administered alkylating agent with significant activity against CLL. In two prospectives, randomized trials of CLB versus observation in patients with asymptomatic, low-risk disease, the overall response (OR) rates to CLB 0.1 mg/kg daily or 0.3 mg/kg for 5 days monthly were 76% and 69%, respectively.[1] More recently, a randomized trial of CLB 20 mg/m$^2$ every 28 days versus fludarabine (FLU) 25 mg/m$^2$ daily for 5 days monthly for 6 months in patients with symptomatic CLL showed an advantage for FLU versus CLB in response rate and progression-free survival (PFS).[2] The results of this study largely relegated CLB to the treatment of older and more infirm patients who were felt to be unable to tolerate FLU.

### FLUDARABINE VERSUS FLUDARABINE PLUS CYCLOPHOSPHAMIDE

The observation of higher than expected response rates with the combination of FLU with cyclophosphamide (CTX)[3] prompted prospective, randomized trials of the combination compared to FLU alone. These studies consistently demonstrated improved response rates and longer PFS for the combination treatment.[4] Although toxicities were increased and there was no improvement in overall survival with the combination, the improved response rates and prolonged PFS strongly suggest that in patients able to tolerate intensive therapy, the combination of FLU plus CTX is preferred to FLU alone.

## INITIAL TREATMENT WITH MONOCLONAL ANTIBODIES

### RITUXIMAB

As CLL cells express CD20, there is a rationale to treat the disease with the anti-CD20 monoclonal antibody rituximab. In one study, 44 untreated but symptomatic patients were treated with rituximab 375 mg/m$^2$ weekly for 4 weeks. The response rate was 51%, but only 4% of patients achieved a CR after the first course.[5] With additional courses administered every 6 months, the remission rate improved to 59%, but with only a 9% CR rate. The median PFS was 18.6 months.

### ALEMTUZUMAB

CD52 is expressed on all hematopoietic cells, including CLL. Alemtuzumab is an anti-CD52 monoclonal antibody that is effective against advanced lymphoid malignancies. In a study of 41 patients treated with alemtuzumab, given at a dose of 30 mg subcutaneously three times per week for 18 weeks, the OR rate was 87%, with a CR rate of 19%.[6] A randomized comparison of alemtuzumab versus CLB untreated but symptomatic patients with CLL is being completed.

## INITIAL TREATMENT WITH CHEMOTHERAPY PLUS MONOCLONAL ANTIBODIES

### FLUDARABINE PLUS RITUXIMAB

The combination of FLU and rituximab was studied in a randomized, Phase II trial of concurrent therapy

**Table 26.1**    Common treatment regimens for chronic lymphocytic leukemia

| Agent | Dose | Method | Frequency | Duration |
|---|---|---|---|---|
| Chlorambucil | 20–40 mg/m² | Oral | Once monthly | 6 months |
| Fludarabine | 25 mg/m² | IV | Daily for 5 days every 28 days | 6 months |
| Fludarabine | 25 mg/m² | IV | Daily for 5 days | |
| Cyclophosphamide | 250 mg/m² | IV | Daily for 3 days every 28 days | 6 months |
| Fludarabine | 25 mg/m² | IV | Daily for 5 days | |
| Cyclophosphamide | 250 mg/m² | IV | Daily for 3 days | |
| Rituximab | 375 mg/m² | IV | First cycle | |
| | 500 mg/m² | IV | Monthly every 28 days | 6 months |
| Pentostatin | 4 mg/m² | IV | Every 28 days | 6 months |
| Cyclophosphamide | 600 mg/m² | IV | | |
| Rituximab | 375 mg/m² | IV | (with second cycle) | |
| Alemtuzumab | 1 mg | IV | Day 1 | 12 weeks |
| | 10 mg | IV | Day 2 | |
| | 30 mg | IV | Day 3, then thrice weekly | |
| Or | | | | |
| Alemtuzumab | 30 mg | SQ | Thrice weekly | 12 weeks |

versus sequential therapy in untreated, but symptomatic, patients with CLL. One hundred and four patients were randomized to either FLU 25 mg/m² daily for 5 days monthly for 6 months, or FLU at the same dose and schedule plus rituximab 375 mg/m² on day 1 and 4 of the first cycle, then on day 1 of the subsequent 5 cycles. All patients were then treated with rituximab 375 mg/m² weekly for 4 weeks as consolidation therapy. The remission rate for patients enrolled on the concurrent arm was 90%, while the remission rate was 77% for patients on the sequential arm; there was no difference in either PFS or overall survival.[7] Furthermore, patients receiving the concurrent regimen experienced more grade 3 or 4 neutropenia compared to those on the sequential arm (74% vs 41%, respectively) and grade 3 or 4 infusion-related toxicity (20% vs 0%, respectively).

### FLUDARABINE PLUS RITUXIMAB PLUS CYCLOPHOSPHAMIDE

After finding the combination of FLU, CTX, and rituximab (FCR) to be active in relapsed and refractory CLL, investigators at the MD Anderson Cancer Center tested FCR in untreated, but symptomatic patients. They treated 224 patients with FLU 25 mg/m² and CTX 250 mg/m² for 3 days every 28 days, for six courses. In addition, rituximab 375 mg/m² was given the day prior to the first dose of FLU, and then 500 mg/m² was given on the first day of the subsequent five courses. The OR rate was 95%, and an impressive 70% achieved a CR.[8] The median PFS at the time the study was published had not been reached, with a median of 48 months of follow-up. Toxicity was significant, but manageable, with myelosuppression and infections relatively frequent. This combination is

being compared to other regimens in randomized clinical trials, but given the extraordinary results FCR is a standard first-line therapeutic option.

## CONSOLIDATION THERAPY TO ELIMINATE MINIMAL RESIDUAL DISEASE

A CR by current criteria (see Chapter 25) goes beyond the former definition of the absence of detectable disease by histologic review of a bone marrow sample. Modern flow cytometric techniques are capable of detecting CLL clones well below our ability to see them histologically. The presence of residual disease that eludes our ability to detect it histologically is known as mininal residual disease (MRD). Nearly every study that has explored the clinical importance of MRD has concluded that patients with MRD following a course of cytotoxic treatment have a worse prognosis than do those who have no detectable MRD.[8,9] Other studies suggest that treatment of MRD improves survival in those who have it successfully eradicated.[10–12] However, it is not proven that the elimination of MRD in those patients who have it will improve their otherwise poor survival. The treatment of MRD remains an area of active investigation, but cannot yet be considered standard therapy.

## RELAPSED OR REFRACTORY CLL

### MONOCLONAL ANTIBODIES

CD20 is only dimly expressed on CLL cells. In advanced CLL, treatment with rituximab at standard doses results in only a 15% response rate.[13] Higher doses can achieve higher response rates, but PFS is generally short.[14,15] Furthermore, the use of rituximab earlier in treatment is likely to result in rituximab resistance. Thus, as a single agent, rituximab has a limited role in the treatment of advanced CLL.

Alemtuzumab has been explored as a treatment for relapsed or refractory CLL in several clinical trials. A consistent response rate of 30–40%, and PFS of approximately 1 year in responders, is reported by these studies when the drug is administered at 30 mg as an IV infusion three times a week for 3–4 months.[16–20] Alemtuzumab is particularly useful in the treatment of CLL characterized by 17p deletions that are known to be chemotherapy resistant.[21] The drug is associated with significant and sometimes severe infusion reactions, however. These reactions are muted, with no apparent loss of efficacy, when alemtuzumab is administered subcutaneously, though this administration route in no way abrogates its immunosuppressive side effects.[22,23] Patients treated with alemtuzumab require antimicrobial prophylaxis against bacteria, *Pneumocystis jeroveci*, and H*erpes* viruses.[24] In addition, there is a substantial risk of cytomegalovirus reactivation and infection that requires a high level of suspicion for fevers of undetermined origin at a minimum, and possibly oral prophylaxis.[25–27]

### CHEMOTHERAPY PLUS MONOCLONAL ANTIBODIES

The limited single-agent activity of the monoclonal antibodies has led to combination treatment strategies. The FCR regimen has been shown to have superior activity to other FLU-based regimens.[28] In a study of 177 relapsed or refractory patients treated with FCR, the overall remission rate was 73%.[29] The median time to progression was 28 months, but 39 months for those patients who achieved a CR.

Another regimen combines the purine analog pentostatin 4 mg/m$^2$ with CTX 600 mg/m$^2$ IV on 1 day every month for 6 months. Rituximab 375 mg/m$^2$ is added with the second cycle. This regimen results in an OR rate of 75%, but unlike the FCR regimen, was given with prophylactic antibiotics and routine hematopoietic growth factor support.[30]

Patients previously treated with purine analogs such as FLU usually remain responsive to purine analogs as long as their disease does not progress or relapse within 6 months of treatment. Those who do progress or relapse with 6 months are considered "FLU refractory" and respond poorly to purine analog-based treatment. These patients are candidates for alemtuzumab or investigational approaches.

### FUTURE DIRECTIONS

As long as CLL remains incurable, multiple new avenues of research will be explored for patients with CLL. Newer approaches target antigenic determinants,

enhance apoptotic pathways, improve allogeneic stem cell transplantation, and explore vaccination strategies. Some of these exciting approaches are nearing use in the clinic.

### FLAVOPIRIDOL

Flavopiridol inhibits cyclin-dependent kinases that may induce apoptosis. With a pharmacokinetically guided dose schedule of a 30-mg IV bolus, followed by a 30–50-mg 4 -hour infusion, 45% of patients with advanced CLL achieved a remission that lasted approximately 1 year.[31] This regimen, however, is associated with significant toxicity, including a severe tumor lysis syndrome that excludes patients with a white blood cell count greater than 200/μL and mandates hospitalization for aggressive hydration and prophylactic rasburicase. The drug is also myelosuppressive, with 100% grade 3–4 neutropenia.

### LENALIDOMIDE

Lenalidomide is an immunomodulatory agent with an uncertain mechanism of action in CLL. In one trial of 45 patients treated orally with 25 mg daily for 21 days of a 28-day cycle, 47% of patients achieved a remission.[32] Treatment was complicated by a "flare reaction" characterized by a transient worsening of disease in the setting of fevers and sweats. This reaction could be prevented or treated by corticosteroids and dose-

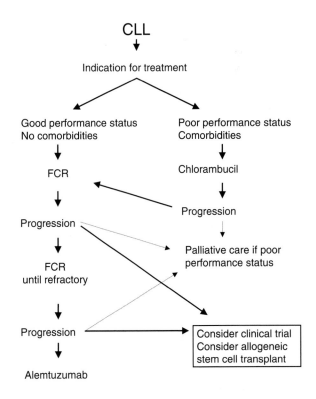

(Consider clinical trial at all decision points)

**Figure 26.1** *Treatment approach to chronic lymphocytic leukemia*

escalation rather than by initiating therapy at 25 mg per day. Myelosuppression was also commonly experienced.

### OBLIMERSEN

As a single agent, the anti-BCL2 antisense oligonucleotide, oblimersen, induced remission in less than 10% of patients and was complicated by a cytokine release syndrome characterized by fever, hypotension, and back-pain.[33] However, in a randomized study of FLU and CTX administered either with or without an infusion of oblimersen, a higher response rate was induced in the treatment arm that included oblimersen.

### BENDAMUSTINE

Bendamustine is a bifunctional alkylating agent that induced remission in 75% of patients with relapsed or refractory CLL in one study.[34] In another study, a remission rate of 56% was achieved in a similar population of patients.[35] The toxicity of bendamustine is largely limited to myelosuppression, infections, and allergic skin reactions.

## SUMMARY

The treatment of CLL is evolving as investigators test new treatments and new combinations. The optimal approach has yet to be defined. In Figure 1, the approach taken by the group at the Cleveland Clinic Taussig Cancer Center is outlined. Treatment is delayed until the onset of symptomatic progression, at which time the most effective therapy, FCR, is administered in the hope that a higher CR rate will translate into longer remission and improved overall survival. Post-remission treatment is investigational. Treatment with FCR is continued until the patient becomes FLU refractory. If no clinical trial is available, alemtuzumab is given.

The approach outlined in Figure 26.1 largely assumes that all patients have the same disease. As discussed in Chapter 25, this assumption is false. Unfortunately, we are currently unable to offer patients with adverse risk factors, such as ZAP-70 expression, treatment options that are known to improve their prognosis. Risk-adapted approaches to CLL are as desperately needed as are new drugs and methods, which advocate for accrual to innovative clinical trials.

## REFERENCES

1. Dighiero G, Maloum K, Desablens B, et al.: Chlorambucil in indolent chronic lymphocytic leukemia. French Cooperative Group on Chronic Lymphocytic Leukemia. *N Engl J Med* 338(21):1506–1514, 1998.
2. Rai KR, Peterson BL, Appelbaum FR, et al.: Fludarabine compared with chlorambucil as primary therapy for chronic lymphocytic leukemia. *N Engl J Med* 343(24):1750–1757, 2000.
3. Flinn IW, Byrd JC, Morrison C, et al.: Fludarabine and cyclophosphamide with filgrastim support in patients with previously untreated indolent lymphoid malignancies. *Blood* 96(1):71–75, 2000.
4. Eichhorst BF, Busch R, Hopfinger G, et al.: Fludarabine plus cyclophosphamide versus fludarabine alone in first-line therapy of younger patients with chronic lymphocytic leukemia. *Blood* 107(3):885–891, 2006.
5. Hainsworth JD, Litchy S, Barton JH, et al.: Single-agent rituximab as first-line and maintenance treatment for patients with chronic lymphocytic leukemia or small lymphocytic lymphoma: a phase II trial of the Minnie Pearl Cancer Research Network. *J Clin Oncol* 21(9):1746–1751, 2003.
6. Lundin J, Kimby E, Bjorkholm M, et al.: Phase II trial of subcutaneous anti-CD52 monoclonal antibody alemtuzumab (Campath-1H) as first-line treatment for patients with B-cell chronic lymphocytic leukemia (B-CLL). *Blood* 100(3):768–773, 2002.
7. Byrd JC, Peterson BL, Morrison VA, et al.: Randomized phase 2 study of fludarabine with concurrent versus sequential treatment with rituximab in symptomatic, untreated patients with B-cell chronic lymphocytic leukemia: results from Cancer and Leukemia Group B 9712 (CALGB 9712). *Blood* 101(1):6–14, 2003.
8. Keating MJ, O'Brien S, Albitar M, et al.: Early results of a chemoimmunotherapy regimen of fludarabine, cyclophosphamide, and rituximab as initial therapy for chronic lymphocytic leukemia. *J Clin Oncol* 23(18):4079–4088, 2005.
9. Rawstron AC, Kennedy B, Evans PA, et al.: Quantitation of minimal disease levels in chronic lymphocytic leukemia using a sensitive flow cytometric assay improves the prediction of outcome and can be used to optimize therapy. *Blood* 98(1):29–35, 2001.
10. Montillo M, Tedeschi A, Miqueleiz S, et al.: Alemtuzumab as consolidation after a response to fludarabine is effective in purging residual disease in patients with chronic lymphocytic leukemia. *J Clin Oncol* 24(15):2337–2342, 2006.
11. Moreton P, Kennedy B, Lucas G, et al.: Eradication of minimal residual disease in B-cell chronic lymphocytic leukemia after alemtuzumab therapy is associated with prolonged survival. *J Clin Oncol* 23(13):2971–2979, 2005.
12. Wendtner CM, Ritgen M, Schweighofer CD, et al.: Consolidation with alemtuzumab in patients with chronic lymphocytic leukemia (CLL) in first remission—experience on safety and efficacy within a randomized multicenter phase III trial of the German CLL Study Group (GCLLSG). *Leukemia* 18(6):1093–1101, 2004.
13. Huhn D, von Schilling C, Wilhelm M, et al.: Rituximab therapy of patients with B-cell chronic lymphocytic leukemia. *Blood* 98(5):1326–1331, 2001.

14. O'Brien SM, Kantarjian H, Thomas DA, et al.: Rituximab dose-escalation trial in chronic lymphocytic leukemia. *J Clin Oncol* 19(8):2165–2170, 2001.
15. Byrd JC, Murphy T, Howard RS, et al.: Rituximab using a thrice weekly dosing schedule in B-cell chronic lymphocytic leukemia and small lymphocytic lymphoma demonstrates clinical activity and acceptable toxicity. *J Clin Oncol* 19(8):2153–2164, 2001.
16. Fiegl M, Falkner A, Hopfinger G, et al.: Routine clinical use of alemtuzumab in patients with heavily pretreated B-cell chronic lymphocytic leukemia: a nation-wide retrospective study in Austria. *Cancer* 107(10):2408–2416, 2006.
17. Keating MJ, Flinn I, Jain V, et al.: Therapeutic role of alemtuzumab (Campath-1H) in patients who have failed fludarabine: results of a large international study. *Blood* 99(10):3554–3561, 2002.
18. Knauf W, Rieger K, Blau W, et al.: Remission induction using alemtuzumab can permit chemotherapy-refractory chronic lymphocytic leukemia (CLL) patients to undergo allogeneic stem cell transplantation. *Leuk Lymphoma* 45(12):2455–2458, 2004.
19. McCune SL, Gockerman JP, Moore JO, et al.: Alemtuzumab in relapsed or refractory chronic lymphocytic leukemia and prolymphocytic leukemia. *Leuk Lymphoma* 43(5):1007–1011, 2002.
20. Osterborg A, Dyer MJ, Bunjes D, et al.: Phase II multicenter study of human CD52 antibody in previously treated chronic lymphocytic leukemia. European Study Group of CAMPATH-1H Treatment in Chronic Lymphocytic Leukemia. *J Clin Oncol* 15(4):1567–1574, 1997.
21. Lozanski G, Heerema NA, Flinn IW, et al.: Alemtuzumab is an effective therapy for chronic lymphocytic leukemia with p53 mutations and deletions. *Blood* 103(9):3278–3281, 2004.
22. Bowen AL, Zomas A, Emmett E, Matutes E, Dyer MJ, Catovsky D: Subcutaneous CAMPATH-1H in fludarabine-resistant/relapsed chronic lymphocytic and B-prolymphocytic leukaemia. *Br J Haematol* 96(3):617–619, 1997.
23. Cortelezzi A, Pasquini MC, Sarina B, et al.: A pilot study of low-dose subcutaneous alemtuzumab therapy for patients with hemotherapy-refractory chronic lymphocytic leukemia. *Haematologica* 90(3):410–412, 2005.
24. Martin SI, Marty FM, Fiumara K, Treon SP, Gribben JG, Baden LR: Infectious complications associated with alemtuzumab use for lymphoproliferative disorders. *Clin Infect Dis* 43(1):16–24, 2006.
25. O'Brien SM, Keating MJ, Mocarski ES: Updated guidelines on the management of cytomegalovirus reactivation in patients with chronic lymphocytic leukemia treated with alemtuzumab. *Clin Lymphoma Myeloma* 7(2):125–130, 2006.
26. Laurenti L, Piccioni P, Cattani P, et al.: Cytomegalovirus reactivation during alemtuzumab therapy for chronic lymphocytic leukemia: incidence and treatment with oral ganciclovir. *Haematologica* 89(10):1248–1252, 2004.
27. Nguyen DD, Cao TM, Dugan K, Starcher SA, Fechter RL, Coutre SE: Cytomegalovirus viremia during Campath-1H therapy for relapsed and refractory chronic lymphocytic leukemia and prolymphocytic leukemia. *Clin Lymphoma* 3(2):105–110, 2002.
28. Wierda W, O'brien S, Faderl S, et al.: A retrospective comparison of three sequential groups of patients with Recurrent/Refractory chronic lymphocytic leukemia treated with fludarabine-based regimens. *Cancer* 106(2):337–345, 2006.
29. Wierda W, O'Brien S, Wen S, et al.: Chemoimmunotherapy with fludarabine, cyclophosphamide, and rituximab for relapsed and refractory chronic lymphocytic leukemia. *J Clin Oncol* 23(18):4070–4078, 2005.
30. Lamanna N, Kalaycio M, Maslak P, et al.: Pentostatin, cyclophosphamide, and rituximab is an active, well-tolerated regimen for patients with previously treated chronic lymphocytic leukemia. *J Clin Oncol* 24(10):1575–1581, 2006.
31. Byrd JC, Lin TS, Dalton JT, et al.: Flavopiridol administered using a pharmacologically derived schedule is associated with marked clinical efficacy in refractory, genetically high-risk chronic lymphocytic leukemia. *Blood* 109(2):399–404, 2007.
32. Chanan-Khan A, Miller KC, Musial L, et al.: Clinical efficacy of lenalidomide in patients with relapsed or refractory chronic lymphocytic leukemia: results of a phase II study. *J Clin Oncol* 24(34):5343–5349, 2006.
33. O'Brien SM, Cunningham CC, Golenkov AK, Turkina AG, Novick SC, Rai KR: Phase I to II multicenter study of oblimersen sodium, a Bcl-2 antisense oligonucleotide, in patients with advanced chronic lymphocytic leukemia. *J Clin Oncol* 23(30):7697–7702, 2005.
34. Kath R, Blumenstengel K, Fricke HJ, Hoffken K: Bendamustine monotherapy in advanced and refractory chronic lymphocytic leukemia. *J Cancer Res Clin Oncol* 127(1):48–54, 2001.
35. Bergmann MA, Goebeler ME, Herold M, et al.: Efficacy of bendamustine in patients with relapsed or refractory chronic lymphocytic leukemia: results of a phase I/II study of the German CLL Study Group. *Haematologica* 90(10):1357–1364, 2005.

# Chapter **27**

# AGGRESSIVE TRANSFORMATION AND PARANEOPLASTIC COMPLICATIONS OF CHRONIC LYMPHOCYTIC LEUKEMIA

*Terry J. Hamblin*

## AGGRESSIVE TRANSFORMATION

There is much confusion about aggressive transformation in chronic lymphocytic leukemia (CLL). Unlike chronic myeloid leukemia where such a transformation is the rule, in CLL it is rare. Moreover, transformation to acute lymphoblastic leukemia (ALL), although reported in the literature,[1] is a myth based on a misunderstanding of the nature of CLL. We can, however, recognize different ways in which CLL can transform (Table 27.1).

### *RICHTER'S SYNDROME*
### Incidence
In 1928, Maurice Richter described an aggressive lymphoma occurring in a patient with CLL.[2] Richter's syndrome is now recognized as a rare but regular culmination of CLL. In the largest series of cases, Robertson et al.[3] reported 39 patients with Richter's syndrome among 1374 with CLL (2.8%). The accuracy of this estimate of prevalence is not clear. Patients with CLL are often elderly when diagnosed, and elderly patients dying of disseminated cancer may never have the type of cancer elucidated. This point was emphasized by a series of 1011 patients from Rome.[4] There were 12 cases of Richter's syndrome among the 207 aged under 55 years (5.9%), but only 10 among the 807 cases over 55 (1.2%). As the authors stated, "the rate of lymphomas in the old age group is possibly underestimated, because very old patients with advanced and unresponsive disease are not always submitted, for ethical reasons, to surgical biopsies." On the other hand, both the MD Anderson Cancer Center and the University "La Sapienza" in Rome are special places that attract the most difficult cases. It is probable that nonprogressive, uncomplicated cases of CLL not requiring treatment are underrepresented in both series and that Richter's syndrome is even rarer than has been reported.

### Definition
It has been accepted that any type of aggressive lymphoma occurring in a patient with CLL may be called Richter's syndrome. Thus, cases of diffuse large B-cell lymphoma, Hodgkin's disease,[5] and even high-grade T-cell lymphoma[6] have received that appellation.

### Clinical features
Richter's transformation is often characterized by sudden clinical deterioration and development of systemic symptoms of fever and weight loss.[3] There is usually a rapid enlargement of lymph node masses, especially of retroperitoneal lymph nodes. Hepatomegaly and splenomegaly are common, and extranodal disease is often seen. A rise in serum lactate dehydrogenase is usual, and in nearly half the patients, a monoclonal immunoglobulin can be detected. Hypercalcemia may be seen and this may or may not be accompanied by lytic bone lesions.

### Pathogenesis
It is clear that there are at least two separate phenomena involved: the first is a true transformation to a clonally related, aggressive lymphoma, and the second is the occurrence of a clonally unrelated, new tumor, perhaps because of diminished immune surveillance.

*Clonally related tumors* The relationship between CLL and aggressive lymphoma was originally tested by examining the light-chain type of the surface immunoglobulin,[7] but this is not sufficient to either confirm or refute an origin from a single clone, and subsequent studies have used a combination of immunophenotyping,[8] karyotyping,[9] fluorescent in situ hybridization,[10] restriction fragment length polymorphism analysis,[11] reaction with anti-idiotypic antibody,[12] and immunoglobulin variable

| Table 27.1 | Transformation of CLL |
|---|---|

Richter's syndrome
  Clonally related
    Diffuse large cell lymphoma—B cell
    Hodgkin's disease
  Clonally unrelated
    EBV related
      Hodgkin's disease
      Diffuse large-cell lymphoma—B cell
      Diffuse large-cell lymphoma—T cell
    EBV status unknown

Prolymphocytoid transformation
  Transient
  Stable
  Progressive

Acute lymphoblastic leukemia
  Blastic mantle cell lymphoma
  Mythologic

region heavy-chain (*IgVH*) gene sequencing.[13] The conclusion of these studies is that sometimes the two tumors are clonally related and sometimes they are not. An interesting study using *IgVH* gene sequencing showed that in five out of six patients whose CLL used unmutated *IgVH* genes, the diffuse large-cell lymphoma (DLCL) clone evolved from the CLL clone, whereas in the two CLL patients whose disease used mutated *IgVH* genes, the DLCL clone was unrelated to the CLL clone.[13]

With the recognition that Hodgkin's disease is a tumor of B cells, it is perhaps less surprising than would have been thought a decade ago that Reed–Sternberg cells should have an identical IgH CDRIII sequence to that of the CLL cells in two out of three cases of Hodgkin's disease supervening in CLL.[14] A remarkable case was investigated by van den Berg et al.[15] in which histology demonstrated a composite lymphoma consisting in part of small-cell lymphoma, in part Hodgkin's disease, and in part anaplastic large-cell lymphoma. All three tumors were clonally related. The CLL component was CD5 negative.

***Clonally unrelated tumors*** If the second lymphoid tumor is not clonally related, is it any more than part of the spectrum of second cancers long been believed to occur in patients with CLL?[16] Among more recent studies, Davis[17] found a relative risk for second lymphoid tumors of 4.5 and for nonlymphoid tumors of 2.3 among 419 patients with CLL in Washington. Travis[18] analyzed data for 9456 patients with CLL from the National Cancer Institute's Surveillance, Epidemiology, and End results (SEER) program. The observed over expected (O/E) ratio for second malignancies was 1.28 (confidence intervals [CI] 1.19–1.37). Significant excesses were found for cancers of the lung and brain, melanoma (including intraocular melanoma), and

Hodgkin's disease. A Danish study of 7391 patients again found standardized incidence ratios of 2.0 for men and 1.2 for women for second malignancies.[19] Increased risks were found for carcinoma of the kidney, nonmelanomatous skin cancer and sarcoma for both sexes, and lung and prostate cancer for men. A more recent evaluation of the SEER program,[20] now totaling 16,367 patients, found a standardized incidence ratio for second malignancies of 1.2 (CI 1.15–1.26), with significant excesses for Kaposi's sarcoma (O/E 5.09) and melanoma (O/E 3.18) and cancers of the larynx (O/E 1.72) and lung (O/E 1.66). In men, brain cancers were more common (O/E 1.91), and in women cancers of the stomach (O/E 1.76) and bladder (O/E 1.52) were commoner.

These figures need to be interpreted with caution. In many series, cancers diagnosed concurrently with or before the CLL are included. Since CLL is diagnosed as an incidental finding in 75% of cases and is clinically silent in a large proportion of patients, there is an inbuilt bias in favor of diagnosing CLL in cancer patients who have more blood tests than the general population. Patients with cancer are often nonspecifically unwell before the diagnosis of cancer is made and will have blood tests to investigate this, with the result that the inconsequential CLL is diagnosed before the cancer reveals itself. In addition, patients with CLL are seen more frequently by doctors than members of the general population, and other cancers are more readily detected.

It is also possible that treatment of CLL, particularly with alkylating agents, predisposes the patient to the development of a second malignancy. This may account for the higher incidence of bladder cancer among women in the latest SEER analysis. Some excesses in specific tumors may be the consequence of data dredging, especially if the tumor excess is confined to one sex.

One important question is whether the immunodeficiency of CLL is what that leads to second malignancies. Kaposi's sarcoma is a disease of impaired immunity, and both melanomas and renal cell cancers are tumors known to be influenced by the immune system. It is also likely that the excess of lymphomas is mediated by the immune deficiency. However, apart from these, any increase in second cancers may be more apparent than real.

The suspicion that clonally unrelated lymphomas occurring in CLL might be virally induced was raised by Momose et al.[21] Occasionally, apparent Reed–Sternberg cells can be found scattered among the small lymphocytes in the lymph node histology of CLL. Among 13 cases where these were found, Momose et al. detected Epstein–Barr virus (EBV) RNA in 12 by in situ hybridization. Three of these cases later developed disseminated Hodgkin's disease. Rubin et al.[22] studied two cases of Richter's syndrome with Hodgkin's disease characteristics in which they found EBV DNA in the lymph nodes using the polymerase chain reaction (PCR) and EBV latent membrane protein (LMP) in the Reed–Sternberg cells by immunohistochemistry.

Matolcsy et al.[23] found EBV genome integration in the DLCL component but not the CLL component of a case of Richter's syndrome where the clones were unrelated. Petrella et al.[24] reported two further cases where EBV could be detected in Reed–Sternberg cells by in situ hybridization. A Japanese case was reported by Otsuka et al.[25] in which EBV nuclear antigen and LMP could be detected in the DLCL cells and in situ hybridization revealed the presence of EBV-encoded small RNA. Ansell et al. studied 25 patients with Richter's syndrome presenting to the Mayo Clinic.[26] Four showed evidence of EBV in the DLCL cells: three with a B-cell phenotype were positive for LMP, and EBV DNA and RNA, and one with a T-cell phenotype was positive for EBV RNA. Six further cases (four from Italy and two from Belgium) of Hodgkin's disease supervening on CLL all support the hypothesis that this is often an EBV-driven event.[27,28] In a delicate study using single-cell PCR, Kanzler et al.[29] enunciated the principle that Hodgkin's disease may be clonally unrelated to the CLL, in which case it is driven by EBV, but in rare cases it is clonally related to the CLL and in these cases EBV cannot be detected. The same may be said for DLCL, though cases with a T-cell immunophenotype are presumably always clonally unrelated. The evidence for EBV involvement in Richter's syndrome is very sparse except in the case of Hodgkin's disease, and for the vast majority of cases of DLCL occurring in patients with CLL, there is no information as to pathogenesis.

That lymphomas may arise from EBV-driven clones in CLL questions the wisdom of treating CLL with agents that reinforce the already-present immunodeficiency, especially in patients without poor prognostic factors. Agents such as fludarabine and alemtuzumab are potent immunosuppressants and their use may lead to EBV reactivation.[30]

### Treatment

Richter's syndrome has a poor prognosis. A study of 25 patients from France in 1981[5] reported a median survival of 4 months and a complete remission rate following intensive chemotherapy of 24%. Seventeen years later a survey of the experience of the MD Anderson Cancer Center in Houston[31] found a median survival of 6 months. There have been no large-scale studies of treatment of Richter's syndrome, but the MD Anderson reported two phase II studies of combination chemotherapy regimens. The first[32] described the use of hyper-CVXD (fractionated cyclophosphamide, vincristine, DaunoXome, and dexamethasone) in 29 patients. Although there were 11 complete responses, they were mostly short lived. There was a treatment-related mortality of 20% during the first course of therapy, and the median survival was only 10 months. The second trial[33] was of the combination of fludarabine, cytarabine, cyclophosphamide, cisplatin, and granulocyte-macrophage colony-stimulating factor in 15 patients with Richter's syndrome together with a small number of other patients with refractory low-grade lymphomas. Only one patient achieved a complete remission, and there was considerable toxicity.

Despite these dismal results, there have been anecdotal reports of good responses to conventional chemotherapy for both the Hodgkin's and non-Hodgkin's varieties of Richter's syndrome.[34–36] Allogeneic stem cell transplantation has been reported in eight patients, three of whom were alive at 14, 47, and 67 months.[37] An interesting patient was reported by Espanol et al.[38] Richter's syndrome developed in a patient 4 months after an allogeneic stem cell transplant for CLL. Complete remission and full donor chimerism was obtained by withdrawal of immunosuppression and donor lymphocyte infusions.

### PROLYMPHOCYTOID TRANSFORMATION
### Definition

Prolymphocytes are large lymphocytes, some 10–15 μm in diameter compared to 7–10 μm for CLL cells. They have round or indented nuclei with chromatin that is less dense than that of CLL cells, but more dense than that of lymphoblasts. They possess a single prominent nucleolus. The cytoplasm is more abundant than that of a typical CLL cell, and in Romanowsky-stained specimens it is pale blue and agranular. Although small numbers of prolymphocytes are usually found in CLL, there is a distinct B-cell prolymphocytic leukemia (PLL) that is completely unrelated to CLL. Clinically, splenomegaly without lymphadenopathy is the rule, but it is defined by the presence of >55% circulating prolymphocytes.[39] It is immunophenotypically distinct, with strong positivity for surface immunoglobulin, CD20, CD22, CD79b, and FMC7, while it is negative for CD23 and mouse rosettes. The reaction with CD5 is controversial. Most cases are CD5 negative, but perhaps 20% are CD5 positive. This may be explained by the discovery of a splenomegalic form of mantle cell lymphoma with t(11;14) that morphologically resembles PLL.[40,41]

Prolymphocytoid transformation of CLL was first reported by David Galton's group at the Royal Postgraduate Medical School in London.[42] It was specifically noted that the cells retained the immunophenotype of CLL cells. In a series of papers,[43–46] the Galton Group defined typical CLL as having <10% prolymphocytes and CLL/PLL as those cases with between 10 and 55% prolymphocytes. Although as a group patients with CLL/PLL had more surface immunoglobulin than those with typical CLL, there was no sudden transition from a lower density at an earlier stage of the disease, and the immunophenotype of small and large cells was indistinguishable.

Contrary to the common perception, in a study of 55 cases of CLL/PLL,[44] half showed a stable picture without a progressive increase in prolymphocytes. The prognosis of this group was similar to that of stable CLL without prolymphocytes. In one-third of cases, the increase in prolymphocytes was unsustained, and in only 18% was there a definite progression toward a more malignant phase of the disease. In a multivariate analysis of prognostic factors in CLL/PLL, only an absolute number of prolymphocytes and spleen size were of independent prognostic significance. The median survival for patients with prolymphocytes $>15 \times 10^9$/L was 3 years.[39]

### Karyotype

Cellular morphology seems to be closely related to karyotype. In a study of 544 patients, Matutes et al.[47] found trisomy 12 in 18%. Thirty-one percent of these had CLL/PLL compared to 10% of the whole series. Subsequent studies have shown that such atypical morphology is also associated with a deletion at 6q21[48] and t(14;19) translocations,[49] both of which are associated with an adverse prognosis. Even more significantly, 80% of patients with p53 abnormalities have CLL/PLL morphology.[50]

Oscier et al. found evidence of karyotypic evolution in 16% of 112 patients with CLL studied by sequential cytogenetic studies.[51] Finn et al. found a higher incidence of 43% in 51 patients.[52] The most common extra abnormality was a structural abnormality of 6q21. Bea et al. found sequential increases in chromosomal abnormalities in six out of ten patients with Richter's transformation or other types of clinical progression.[53]

Treatment may induce evolution. It may be thought of as a selective pressure-inducing change. Just as antibiotics can select for drug-resistant bacteria, similarly chemotherapy may kill only the susceptible cells, allowing drug-resistant cells to regrow. These may be morphologically more extreme, karyotypically different, and may express greater amounts of CD38.[54]

### Implications for management

Merely finding increased numbers of prolymphocytes in the blood is not necessarily an indication of transformation of CLL. The increase may be transient, indicative of a recent infection or other unknown event. Some karyotypic abnormalities (such as trisomy 12) are associated with >15% circulating prolymphocytes; yet these patients may remain stable for many years. Increasing numbers of prolymphocytes and karyotypic evolution usually have a poor prognosis. Most authors have been unable to attach an independent prognostic effect to deletions at 6q21, but acquisition of p53 abnormalities at 17p13 carries the worse possible prognosis.[55–57] This is often associated with morphologic change (prolymphocytoid transformation[50] or Richter's syndrome[53]) and drug resistance.[58]

The indications for treatment in CLL/PLL are the same as those for CLL itself: systemic symptoms and bone marrow failure. The presence of prolymphocytes should raise the possibility of abnormalities of the p53 pathway, indicating potential drug resistance and a call for nonstandard therapy, such as alemtuzumab or high-dose methylprednisolone.

### TRANSFORMATION TO ACUTE LEUKEMIA

Transformation of CLL to ALL used to be regularly reported. The first report mentioned blast cells with surface immunoglobulin, which would be uncharacteristic for classical ALL.[59] One of the two cases in this study had surface IgMκ, with rheumatoid factor activity on both lymphocytes and lymphoblasts, and it now seems more likely that this and subsequent cases represent either a Richter-like transformation of CLL with peripheral blood spillover of the high-grade lymphoma cells, or a similar high-grade transformation of a different B-cell lymphoma with a superficial resemblance to CLL.

In at least one of the reported cases, the CD5 antigen was retained during the blastic phase,[60] which raises the possibility of a blastic version of mantle cell lymphoma occurring in a patient with the type of mantle cell lymphoma that closely resembles CLL,[41] and this seems certainly to be the explanation for the most recent case report where both the small-cell version and the blastic version had the t(11;14) translocation.[61] However, in another case the blasts were shown to be terminal deoxynucleotidyl transferase positive,[62] and in this and other cases the blast cells had the characteristics of ALL.[63] In such cases, however, it has not been established that the ALL belongs to the same clone as the CLL.

There is no convincing evidence that CLL ever transforms into ALL.

## PARANEOPLASTIC COMPLICATIONS

Although there are a few paraneoplastic complications of CLL of uncertain origin, the majority are caused by altered immunity (Table 27.2). For unknown reasons, CLL has a profound effect on the normal immune system, although it has been suggested that CLL is a tumor of regulatory B cells, and exerts its effect in this way.[64] The altered immunity manifests itself as immune deficiency, which will not be considered in this chapter, and autoimmunity.

### AUTOIMMUNITY

The association of autoimmune disease and CLL is well known but misunderstood. There is no general tendency for patients with CLL to develop autoimmune disease. The only autoimmune conditions seen in CLL with any frequency are autoimmune hemolytic anemia (AIHA) and immune thrombocytopenia (ITP). A few other rare conditions occur in CLL more commonly than would be expected, but the common autoimmune diseases, such as rheumatoid arthritis,

| Table 27.2   Paraneoplastic complications of CLL |
| --- |
| **Autoimmune** |
|   Antibody produced by tumor |
|     Cold agglutination syndrome |
|     Acquired angioedema |
|     Some cases of glomerulonephritis or nephrotic syndrome |
|   Antibody produced by residual lymphoid tissue |
|     Autoimmune hemolytic anemia |
|     Immune thrombocytopenia |
|     Immune neutropenia |
|     Pure red cell aplasia |
|     Paraneoplastic pemphigus |
|     Some cases of glomerulonephritis or nephrotic syndrome |
| **Nonimmune** |
|   Hypercalcemia |
|   Severe reactions to insect bites |
| **Obscure and uncertain** |
|   Bell's palsy |
|   Peripheral neuritis |
|   Parkinson's disease |
|   RS3PE |

thyroid disease, pernicious anemia, and systemic lupus erythematosus (SLE) are no commoner in CLL than in age-matched controls.[65]

## Autoimmune hemolytic anemia

Using the technique of differential agglutination, Berlin was the first to show shortened red cell survival in nine patients with CLL.[66] Later, Wasserman et al.[67] found hemolytic anemia in 9 of 58 consecutive patients with CLL, with 5 out of 7 testing positive in the direct antiglobulin test. Following this, a series of studies suggested that AIHA occurs at some time in the course of CLL in 10–26% of cases.[68]

AIHA is commoner in CLL than in the general population. The reported prevalence varies from 1.8 to 35%.[69,70] The disparity is because prevalence is closely related to stage and progression. In stable stage A disease, Hamblin et al.[65] found a prevalence of 2.9%, compared to 10.5% in stage B and C disease and 18.2% in progressive stage A disease.

From a different point of view, CLL is the commonest known cause. In a large series of patients with AIHA, Engelfriet et al.[71] found that 14% were associated with CLL, compared to 7% for SLE, the next most common cause. However, in about half the cases of AIHA no cause is found. AIHA occurs about eight times more commonly in CLL than in other forms of non-Hodgkin's lymphoma, and about two and a half times more commonly than in Hodgkin's disease.

## Immune thrombocytopenia

Minot and Buckman[72] reported that half their patients with CLL had thrombocytopenia at presentation. Once an immune cause for thrombocytopenia had been recognized, Harrington and Arimura[73] reported seven cases of ITP occurring in CLL. Ebbe et al.[74] reported five more cases and suggested that the prevalence of ITP in CLL was 2%, and this was confirmed by Hamblin et al.[65] and Dührsen et al.[75] However, the numbers were small in all three series and the reliability of the diagnoses suspect. The diagnosis of ITP in CLL depends on the presence of isolated thrombocytopenia, and normal or increased bone marrow megakaryocytes with an excess of early forms. More sophisticated, though not entirely reliable, tests are increased mean platelet volume and platelet distribution width, and detection of platelet antibodies in the serum or on the platelet membrane.

The diagnosis of ITP is difficult. Bone marrows heavily infiltrated with CLL cells make megakaryocytic numbers difficult to assess. Tests for platelet antibodies are still unsatisfactory. Increased levels of platelet-associated IgG was found in 30% of thrombocytopenic patients with CLL and 10% of nonthrombocytopenic patients.[76] Even higher rates were found in non-Hodgkin's lymphomas. This test is known to have a high false-positive rate. The diagnosis is often made by exclusion and confirmed by response to therapy. About one-third of patients with ITP secondary to CLL also have a positive direct antiglobulin test (Evans' syndrome), a much higher rate than for primary ITP.[77]

## Autoimmune neutropenia

When a CLL patient becomes neutropenic, it is usually because of marrow infiltration or treatment. Early reports of immune neutropenia in CLL[78] probably referred to the well-recognized syndrome of large granular lymphocytic (LGL) leukemia with neutropenia.[79] A study from Crete[80] reported higher numbers of CD3[+], CD8[+], and CD57[+] cells in neutropenic patients with CLL and demonstrated that CD8[+] cells from neutropenic patients exerted a greater suppressive effect on colony-forming unit–granulocyte-macrophage colony growth than that of similar cells from nonneutropenic patients. More recently, it has been suggested that the secretion of high levels of Fas ligand is the cause of the neutropenia that is sometimes seen in B CLL.[81] Antineutrophil antibodies seem to be involved only rarely, if at all.

## Pure red cell aplasia

Although well recognized in CLL,[82] pure red cell aplasia (PRCA) is also a frequent complication of LGL leukemia; indeed, this is probably its commonest cause.[83] Nevertheless, Chikkappa et al.[84] recognized PRCA in 23 cases of B CLL, and subsequently it has been reported on at least five occasions.[77] From their own cases, Chikkappa et al.[84] estimated the prevalence at 6%, but this seems an exaggeration. In our series, about 1% of our 800 unselected patients with CLL have developed PRCA. The recent spate of cases of PRCA following treatment with erythropoietin has provided an easy assay for determining the autoimmune nature of PRCA.[85]

### Other types of autoimmune disease

The idea that CLL was regularly associated with all types of autoimmune disease was reinforced by reviews by Miller[86] and Dameshek.[87] However, in an elderly population, autoantibodies are recognized quite commonly. Hamblin et al.[65] found that 21.5% of a control population of individuals over 60 years of age had tissue-specific autoantibodies detected by immunofluorescence. In an age-matched series of 195 patients with CLL, the prevalence of autoantibodies was exactly the same. Dührsen et al.[75] confirmed this. However, there are three conditions that should be looked at more closely.

*Nephrotic syndrome and glomerulonephritis* Nephrotic syndrome occurs more commonly in CLL than would be expected by chance. In 1974, Dathan et al.[88] reported two patients with CLL who developed nephrotic syndrome caused by an immune complex glomerulonephritis. Almost immediately, Cameron and Ogg[89] reported another three cases, but subsequent letters to the same journal were rejected because there were so many. This complication is therefore much commoner than the 50 cases, mostly in the form of single case reports, uncovered by a PubMed search. Either membranous glomerulonephritis or membranoproliferative glomerulonephritis may be seen on renal histology. There have been two reports of antineutrophil cytoplasmic antibodies, one of which followed treatment with fludarabine.[90,91]

*Acquired angioedema* As with hereditary angioedema, the acquired form is characterized by recurrent bouts of angioedema and abdominal pain. It is caused by a deficiency of the inhibitor of the first component of complement (C1-INH). It differs from the hereditary form in that there is no family history, and the onset is not until the fifth decade of life. Type I is associated with lymphoproliferative diseases, including CLL, and type II with autoantibodies. The normal C1-INH molecule has a molecular weight (MW) of 105 kd, with a binding site for the serine protease C1s. The autoantibodies recognize two synthetic peptides (peptides 2 and 3) that span the reactive site of the molecule.

A study of six cases of acquired angioedema (AAE) demonstrated that the autoantibodies were monoclonal whether or not they were associated with a lymphoproliferative disease[92]; and the distinction may well be an artificial one, depending on how hard a lymphoproliferative disease is to find. In both types of AAE, a nonfunctional C1-INH molecule of MW 95 kd is found in the serum. The mechanism of action of the antibody is to cause or allow the cleavage of the C1-INH molecule, rendering it inactive.[93]

*Blistering skin diseases* The first report of a patient with CLL and a pemphigoidlike skin disease was by Oppenheim in 1910,[94] although the two patients reported by Sachs in 1921[95] had a more secure diagnosis of CLL. In 1974, Cuni et al. described a single case of bullous pemphigoid, established by the presence of antibasement membrane antibody.[96] In their review of the literature, they discovered 16 other cases of CLL with either bullous or vesicular skin lesions. Goodnough and Muir[97] reported the next case 6 years later, but in the same year Laskaris et al.[98] reported two cases of CLL associated with oral pemphigus.

The confusion over pemphigus and pemphigoid was resolved when Anhalt et al.[99] described paraneoplastic pemphigus. The clinical features are of painful erosions of the oropharynx, and vermilion borders of the lips that are resistant to conventional treatment. There is severe pseudomembranous conjunctivitis. There are several types of itchy cutaneous lesions including confluent erythema with skin denudation, and papules on the trunk and extremities forming target lesions, with central blistering. Anhalt reported that patients with this condition had often been previously misdiagnosed as pemphigus vulgaris or erythema multiforme. Histologically, he observed three elements: suprabasilar intraepithelial acantholysis, necrosis of individual keratinocytes, and vacuolar interface change. Immunofluorescence studies revealed the presence in the serum of antibodies that reacted with the intracellular spaces, such as is seen in pemphigus vulgaris or foliaceus. However, direct immunofluorescence studies of the skin also demonstrated complement deposition along the basement membrane typical of bullous pemphigoid.

Investigation of patients' sera showed immunoprecipitation of a complex of four polypeptides from keratinocyte extracts with MWs of 250, 230, 210, and 190 kd, respectively. Subsequently, several groups confirmed this pattern of autoantibodies,[100–102] but two groups also found an antibody against a 130-kd component.[103,104] These antigenic components have subsequently been identified. The 130-kd glycoprotein is characteristically involved in pemphigus vulgaris. It has been cloned and sequenced[105] and termed desmoglein 3. It belongs to the cadherin family of cell adhesion molecules. Antibodies to the 230-kd polypeptide are characteristically found in the sera of patients with bullous pemphigoid. The protein is known as BPAG2,[100] is intracellular, and localizes to the hemidesmosomal plaque. The 250-kd protein is desmoplakin I,[100] the 210-kd protein is envoplakin,[106] and the 190-kd protein is periplakin.[107]

Although it is rare, paraneoplastic pemphigus is a discrete autoimmune blistering skin disease with characteristic clinical features, a pathognomonic pattern of antibody specificity, and an association with lymphoid tumors. It may occur in an array of lymphoid tumors, and especially in Castleman's disease, but about 30% of cases occur in CLL.[108]

## Mechanisms of autoimmunity in CLL

*Secretion of autoantibody by tumor cells* Perhaps the simplest explanation for autoimmune disease in CLL would be that the autoantibodies were the product of the tumor. Using a sensitive immunoblotting technique, Beaume et al.[109] found monoclonal immunoglobulin in the sera of 80% of CLL patients. However, the light-chain type was the same as that of the surface immunoglobulin in only half the cases. In CLL, serum monoclonal immunoglobulins cannot be assumed to have been produced by the tumor.

There is some evidence that CLL lymphocytes may be induced to produce autoantibodies. When stimulated with phorbol ester cells, 12 of 14 patients with CLL secreted IgM that reacted with a variety of autoantigens.[110] Similar polyreactive antibodies have been described by Sthoeger et al.[111] The antibodies were of the same light-chain types as the surface Ig of the CLL cells, and therefore not the product of contaminating normal B cells. These findings give weight to the hypothesis that CLL is derived from a B cell of separate lineage akin to the Ly-1 (CD5) B cell of mice, although this hypothesis is in increasing disrepute.[68]

Sthoeger et al.[112] reported two cases of CLL with AIHA where immunoglobulin eluted from direct antiglobulin positive red cells reacted with anti-κ, but not anti-λ antibodies. In addition, the CLL cells produced in culture a monoclonal IgM that reacted with red cells, though more strongly at 4°C than at 37°C. Most agree that the antibody in AIHA is polyclonal and the product of the residual lymphoid tissue, and not of the tumor cells. A study by Sikora et al.[113] demonstrated that the monoclonal Ig rescued from CLL cells was not responsible for a concurrent warm antibody AIHA.

On the other hand, in cold agglutination syndrome, most cases seem to be caused by a monoclonal IgM. The molecular basis for this reaction is now understood. A rat monoclonal antibody, 9G4, raised against the surface IgM of a B-cell lymphoma recognized a shared idiotypic determinant on all anti-I or anti-i cold agglutinins.[114] B cells from patients with cold agglutination syndrome were immortalized with EBV. The 9G4-positive lines were investigated for the use of immunoglobulin $V_H$ genes and found exclusively to use the $V_{4-34}$ gene.[115,116] This specificity was retained whether the $V_H$ gene was in germline configuration or showed evidence of somatic mutation. The detailed biochemistry of both the reaction with red cells and with the 9G4 monoclonal has been elucidated.[117]

However, cold agglutination syndrome is rare in CLL. CLL cells do not usually secrete enough immunoglobulin for it to be detected by conventional methods. Thus although 6 of 78 patients with persistent cold agglutinins had CLL,[118] the definition then in use for CLL would not have excluded diseases like splenic marginal zone lymphoma, which has a greater propensity for secreting large amounts of monoclonal immunoglobulin. The same is true of the single case report from Feizi et al.[119] and the single case of CLL with cold agglutination syndrome reported by Hamblin et al.[65] which, in retrospect, had a spillover lymphoma. A more recent case was also CD5 negative,[112] an almost certain indication that this also was a different type of lymphoma. In this case, the heavy-chain gene used by the surface immunoglobulin was $DP54$ and not $V_{4-34}$, an indication that the cold agglutinin was not the product of the tumor. In the last 5 years, we have seen a single patient with long-standing cold agglutination syndrome who developed definite CLL during his last illness. Both his anti-I antibody and the surface immunoglobulin used the $V_{H4-34}$ gene; the same is true for the case reported recently by Ruzickova et al.[120]

As far as other autoimmune syndromes are concerned, there is little evidence that the autoantibodies are the product of the CLL cell. It is believed that CLL-associated angioedema,[92] and possibly CLL-associated glomerulonephritis,[121] may be caused in this way. On the other hand, a recent publication suggests that the anti-230-kd autoantibody associated with paraneoplastic pemphigus is not synthesized by CLL cells.[122]

*Autoimmunity triggered by treatment* Although the suggestion that autoimmunity might be triggered by treatment in CLL was made nearly 40 years ago,[123] there were few corroborating reports[124–126] until the association with fludarabine was realized. The first report of two cases appeared as a letter,[127] though in only one of the cases was the association with treatment secure. A contrary view was reported by investigators from the MD Anderson Cancer Center, who argued that the cases represented the natural prevalence of AIHA in CLL.[128] Five out of 112 patients treated with fludarabine developed hemolysis after between 1 and 6 courses of therapy, and a further four patients with preexisting AIHA deteriorated after fludarabine treatment, though four further patients with preexisting AIHA received fludarabine safely.

Two years later, Myint et al.[129] reported that of 52 heavily pretreated patients, 12 developed AIHA after between 2 and 6 courses of fludarabine. Since then, many reports involving well over 100 patients have confirmed the association. The frequency of hemolysis depends on how much previous treatment the patient has received. Only about 2% of patients treated for the first time develop AIHA, compared with about 5% of patients who have received some previous treatment, and over 20% of heavily pretreated patients.

Among 1203 patients studied at University "La Sapienza" in Rome,[130] 52 cases of AIHA were observed (4.3%). In 19 patients, the AIHA was present at the time of diagnosis of the CLL, and a further 20 developed AIHA while still untreated. Ten developed AIHA while on therapy, seven on low-dose chlorambucil (1.8% of those so treated) and three on fludarabine (2.5% of those so treated). Current thinking is that AIHA triggered by treatment has been underreported in the past, and is probably as common after chlorambucil treatment as after fludarabine, but after fludarabine it is more severe and difficult to treat. Early suggestions are that the risk is less with the fludarabine/cyclophosphamide combination.

Autoimmune thrombocytopenia may also be triggered by fludarabine. Montillo et al.[131] first reported relapse of CLL-associated ITP after exposure to fludarabine. Over 30 cases of fludarabine-related ITP have now been reported.[68] Only one possible case of immune neutropenia[132] and three cases of PRCA have been reported.[68] Paraneoplastic pemphigus has been reported in five cases.[68] There have been two cases of postfludarabine glomerulonephritis.[68]

The other purine analogs, cladribine and pentostatin, are also capable of triggering autoimmune complications.[68] As the best known toxicity of the purine analogs is their profound T-cell suppression, it is interesting to note that treatment with Campath-1H can also trigger autoimmunity in CLL.[68] Interestingly, paraneoplastic pemphigus may also be triggered by radiotherapy.[68]

From these observations some general conclusions can be drawn. Most cases of postfludarabine autoimmunity have occurred in heavily pretreated patients. Usually, patients have previously received an alkylating agent. The complication is severe and often difficult to treat. In many cases it has been fatal. If control is achieved, then reexposure to any of the purine analogs retriggers the complication. Even alkylating agents may retrigger it. The recurrence is likely to be even more virulent. Although commonest in CLL, autoimmunity may also be induced in other low-grade lymphoproliferative diseases.

### Synthesis: why is CLL complicated by autoimmunity?

The cause of the autoimmune complications of CLL is unknown. Although they are a feature of all low-grade B-cell lymphomas, they are worse in CLL, just as the immunodeficiency is worse. Both the immunodeficiency and the autoimmunity are made worse by treatment. They are probably related. Noting the almost AIDS-like, CD4 T-cell suppression that occurs after treatment with fludarabine, Hamblin[68] suggested that autoimmunity in CLL is caused by loss of T-cell regulatory control of autoreactive T cells.

In most cases of AIHA, the autoantibody preferentially reacts with components of the Rh antigen. A recent study has demonstrated that CLL cells act as the most potent antigen presenting cells for purified Rh antigen.[133]

### Treatment of autoimmune complications

*Acquired angioedema* Treatment of AAE has been recently reviewed by Markovic et al.[134] They recommend treatment of the CLL as the most important element of the management. The androgens, stanozolol and danazol, have been widely used for both the hereditary and acquired form of the disease and are generally successful. They act by increasing the production of C1 esterase inhibitor by the liver. For those who are unhappy taking androgenic steroids, tranexamic acid (0.5 g three times daily) is as successful in the acquired form as in the in the hereditary form.

*Autoimmune hemolytic anemia* There are no controlled trials of treatment of AIHA secondary to CLL, and treatment does not differ from AIHA in other circumstances. Prednisolone 1 mg/kg for 10–14 days has been the standard treatment for acute hemolysis for 50 years.[135] As most cases occur in progressive CLL, it would be usual to also treat the CLL, with either chlorambucil or fludarabine, but this carries a risk. For patients in whom the AIHA has been triggered by fludarabine, further exposure to purine analogs or even to any other cytotoxic drug may be hazardous. Patients failing to respond to prednisolone, or relapsing when the dose is reduced, are offered azathioprine or cyclophosphamide.

There are few data on the value of splenectomy in this condition. In a series of 113 splenectomies for AIHA, only 4 were for hemolysis secondary to CLL.[136] The hazards of splenectomy are well known, and are certainly increased in frail, elderly, immunodeficient patients. Nevertheless, it may be lifesaving.

Among 73 cases of AIHA treated with intravenous immunoglobin (IVIG) detailed in the literature,[137] 40% responded. Doses of 0.4 g/kg/day for 5 days were effective. Only 18 of the 73 cases also had CLL. Response was transient, lasting only 3–4 weeks, but retreatment was effective.[77]

Cyclosporine is used in AIHA when other modalities have failed.[138] The dose is 5–8 mg/kg/day, tapering to a maintenance dose of about 3 mg/kg/day. We aim to keep the blood level at about 100 μg/L.

The severity of hemolysis following fludarabine is often extreme, and several reports detail fatalities. Patients who develop these complications are often immunosuppressed and prone to infection. Further immunosuppressive treatment will intensify this risk. Anticipating that the complication will be difficult to control, we move rapidly to secondary treatments. Where steroids have failed, we have found success with IVIG and splenectomy, but many of our patients have required cyclosporine and, because responses are often delayed, we move rapidly to prescribing it.[68]

A special risk is the retriggering of autoimmunity by reexposure to fludarabine, cladribine, or pentostatin.[68] Even chlorambucil may retrigger the complication.[68] The current Medical Research Council trial suggests that there is no extra hazard in treating a patient with a positive direct antiglobulin test (DAT), but there is if the patients has preexisting AIHA.

Rituximab infusion is rapidly gaining favor for the treatment of autoimmune complications of CLL, especially those occurring after exposure to fludarabine. Zaja et al. reported remarkable responses in cases of AIHA, ITP, cold agglutination syndrome, and axonal degenerating neuropathy.[139]

***Autoimmune thrombocytopenia*** This complication is so rarely diagnosed that there is next to no guidance in the literature on treatment. It therefore seems wise to follow the Clinical Guidelines of the American Society of Hematology[140] for the treatment of idiopathic thrombocytopenic purpura, and to treat the CLL independently as required. Thus, asymptomatic thrombocytopenia should only be treated when the platelet count is $<30 \times 10^9$/L. Hospitalization should be confined to patients with mucous membrane or other severe bleeding. Conventional dose oral prednisolone is the treatment of choice for those who need any treatment (those with severe bleeding or a platelet count $<30 \times 10^9$/L).

Prednisolone is given in the same dose as for AIHA. Patients failing to respond are treated with IVIG 0.4 g/kg/day for 5 days. The response rate is higher than that for AIHA. Splenectomy is also more effective than in AIHA, with response rates of over 70% in patients unresponsive to steroids.[141] Other treatments found to be successful in AIHA may also be tried. Unique to autoimmune thrombocytopenia is treatment with vinca alkaloids. Vincristine 1 mg i.v. weekly $\times$ 6 is often effective, but vinblastine has also been used. The drugs may be given as boluses or by slow infusion.[68]

ITP complicating CLL may be severe, causing intractable bleeding. Special measures may need to be taken to control the bleeding, including IVIG followed immediately by platelet transfusion. Alternatively, methylprednisolone 1 g/day i.v. $\times$ 3 followed by platelet transfusion may be effective. Tranexamic acid is worth trying, as is recombinant factor VIIa.[142]

***Pure red cell aplasia*** Treatment for this complication has been reviewed by Diehl and Ketchum.[77] On the basis of literature reports of 41 treatments in 33 patients, they recommend instituting treatment to control the CLL, as this will be necessary to achieve long-term remission of the PRCA. At the same time, the PRCA is treated with prednisolone 1 mg/kg/day. If there is no response, then cyclosporine is added. The

reticulocyte count should increase within 2–3 weeks, and the hemoglobin normalize in 1–2 months. At this point, the steroid dose can be reduced and stopped. Cyclosporine should be continued for 6–7 months and then gradually withdrawn.

***Paraneoplastic pemphigus*** This syndrome is frequently fatal[68]; four of the original five patients died, and two patients who developed it following fludarabine also succumbed. One patient has survived post-fludarabine paraneoplastic pemphigus after having been treated with prednisolone 500 mg/day, cyclophosphamide 100 mg/day for several weeks, together with IVIG 120 mg over the first 3 days. Other patients with a similar syndrome, unrelated to malignancy, have responded to IVIG. Three British patients responded to the combination of high-dose steroids and cyclosporine or cyclophosphamide, although one later died from sepsis.

***Rapidly progressive glomerulonephritis*** Treatment for glomerulonephritis involves intense immunosuppression with high-dose intravenous methylprednisolone and cyclophosphamide.[68] Plasma exchange has a role in those cases that present with renal failure requiring dialysis. Aggressive immunosuppression has the added benefit of suppressing the CLL. It is moot whether control of the CLL or control of the autoimmune process is responsible for the beneficial effect of such treatment.

## NONIMMUNE COMPLICATIONS
### Hypercalcemia
Hypercalcemia is a rare complication of CLL.[143] The cause is obscure. Rossi et al.[144] have suggested that cases of CLL might have abnormal osteoclast differentiation, leading to increased bone resorption.

### Abnormal reactions to insect bites
There has long been a story that patients with CLL respond abnormally to insect bites. Two recent studies have entered the literature.[145,146] Histology showed T- and B-cell infiltrates with prominent eosinophil infiltration and eosinophil granule deposition. One patient developed bullous lesions.

### Neurologic complications
Hamblin[147] reported patients with various neurologic complications, including Bell's palsy, Parkinson's disease, and peripheral neuropathy. It is difficult to know whether such complications are neoplastic, paraneoplastic, or incidental. Creange et al.[148] reported seven cases of inflammatory neuromuscular disorders in which there was clear evidence of infiltration with CLL cells. Bell's palsy is now thought to be a complication of Herpes simplex infections in most cases, and Hamblin[147] reported a temporal relationship of Parkinson's disease to severe Herpes zoster infections.

## RS3PE

Recurrent symmetrical seronegative synovitis with pitting edema (RS3PE) is a strange condition of old men who are HLA-B7 positive. It is associated with hematologic disorders in 30% of cases, most commonly CLL and the myelodysplastic syndromes.[149]

### REFERENCES

1. Zarrabi MH, Grunwald HW, Rosner F: Chronic lymphocytic leukemia terminating in acute leukemia. *Arch Intern Med* 137:1059, 1977.
2. Richter M: Generalised reticular sarcoma of lymph nodes associated with lymphatic leukemia. *Am J Pathol* 4:285, 1928.
3. Robertson LE, Pugh W, O'Brien S, et al.: Richter's syndrome: a report on 39 cases. *J Clin Oncol* 11:1985, 1993.
4. Mauro FR, Foa R, Giannarelli D, et al.: Clinical characteristics and outcome of young chronic lymphocytic leukemia patients: a single institution study of 204 cases. *Blood* 94:448, 1999.
5. Harousseau JL, Flandrin G, Tricot G, et al.: Malignant lymphoma supervening in chronic lymphocytic leukemia and related disorders. Richter's syndrome: a study of 25 cases. *Cancer* 48:1302, 1981.
6. Lee A, Skelly ME, Kingma DW, et al.: B-cell chronic lymphocytic leukemia followed by high grade T-cell lymphoma. An unusual variant of Richter's syndrome. *Am J Clin Pathol* 103:348, 1995.
7. McDonnell JM, Beshorner WE, Staal SP, et al.: Richter's syndrome with two different B-cell clones. *Cancer* 58:2031, 1986.
8. Miyamura K, Osada H, Yamauchi T, et al.: Single clonal origin of neoplastic B-cells with different immunoglobulin lightchains in a patient with Richter's syndrome. *Cancer* 66:140, 1990.
9. Koduru PR: Serial phenotypic, cytogenetic and molecular genetic studies in Richter's syndrome: demonstration of lymphoma development from chronic lymphocytic leukemia cells. *Br J Haematol* 85:613, 1993.
10. Kruger A: Use of a retinoblastoma gene probe to investigate clonality in Richter's syndrome. *Leukemia* 7:1891, 1993.
11. Michiels JJ, van Dongen JJ, Hagemeijer A, et al.: Richter's syndrome with identical immunoglobulin gene rearrangements in the chronic lymphocytic leukemia and the supervening non-Hodgkin lymphoma. *Leukemia* 3:819, 1989.
12. Bertoli LF, Kubagawa H, Borzillo GV, et al.: Analysis with antiidiotype antibody of a patient with chronic lymphocytic leukemia and a large cell lymphoma (Richter's syndrome). *Blood* 70:45, 1987.
13. Cherepakhin V: Common clonal origin of chronic lymphocytic leukemia and high grade lymphomas of Richter's syndrome. *Blood* 82:3141, 1993.
14. Ohno T, Smir BN, Weisenburger DD, et al.: Origin of the Hodgkin/Reed–Sternberg cells in chronic lymphocytic leukemia with "Hodgkin's transformation." *Blood* 91:1757, 1998.
15. van den Berg A, Maggio E, Rust R, et al.: Clonal relation in a case of CLL, ALCL, and Hodgkin composite lymphoma. *Blood* 100:1425, 2002.
16. Beresford OD: Chronic lymphatic leukaemia associated with malignant disease. *Br J Cancer* 6:339, 1952.
17. Davis JW: Second cancers in patients with chronic lymphocytic leukemia. *J Natl Cancer Inst* 78:91, 1987.
18. Travis LB: Second cancers in patients with chronic lymphocytic leukemia. *J Natl Cancer Inst* 84:1422, 1992.
19. Mellemgaard A, Geisler CH, Storm HH: Risk of kidney cancer and other second solid malignancies in patients with chronic lymphocytic leukemia. *Eur J Haematol* 53:218, 1994.
20. Hisada M, Biggar RJ, Greene MH, et al.: Solid tumors after chronic lymphocytic leukemia. *Blood* 98:1979, 2001.
21. Momose H, Jaffe ES, Shin SS, et al.: Chronic lymphocytic leukemia/small lymphocytic lymphoma with Reed–Sternberg-like cells and possible transformation to Hodgkin's disease. Mediation by Epstein–Barr virus. *Am J Surg Pathol* 16:859, 1992.
22. Rubin D, Hudnall SD, Aisenberg A, et al.: Richter's transformation of chronic lymphocytic leukemia with Hodgkin's-like cells associated with Epstein–Barr virus infection. *Mol Pathol* 7:91, 1994.
23. Matolcsy A, Unghirami G, Knowles DM: Molecular genetic demonstration of the diverse evolution of Richter's syndrome (chronic lymphocytic leukemia and subsequent large cell lymphoma). *Blood* 83:1363, 1994.
24. Petrella T, Yaziji N, Collin F, et al.: implication of the Epstein–Barr virus in the progression of chronic lymphocytic leukemia/small lymphocytic lymphoma to Hodgkin-like lymphoma. *Anticancer Res* 17:3907, 1997.
25. Otsuka E, Miyazaki Y, Moriyama K, et al.: Epstein–Barr virus associated Richter's syndrome accompanied by interstitial pneumonia. *Rinsho Ketsueki* 40:402, 1999.
26. Ansell SM, Li CY, Lloyd RV, et al.: Epstein–Barr virus in Richter's transformation. *Am J Hematol* 60:99, 1999.
27. Pescarmona E, Pignoloni P, Mauro FR, et al.: Hodgkin/Reed–Sternberg cells and Hodgkin's disease in patients with B-cell chronic lymphocytic leukaemia: an immunohistological, molecular and clinical study of four cases suggesting a heterogeneous pathogenetic background. *Virchows Arch* 437:128, 2000.
28. de Leval L, Vivario M, De Prijck B, et al.: Distinct clonal origin in two cases of Hodgkin's lymphoma variant of Richter's syndrome associated with EBV infection. *Am J Surg Pathol* 28:679, 2004.
29. Kanzler H, Kuppers R, Helmes S, et al.: Hodgkin and Reed–Sternberg-like cells in B-cell chronic lymphocytic leukemia represent the outgrowth of single germinal-center B-cell derived clones: potential precursors of Hodgkin and Reed–Sternberg cells in Hodgkin's disease. *Blood* 95:1023, 2000.
30. Lazzarino M, Orlandi E, Baldanti F, et al.: The immunosuppression and potential for EBV reactivation of fludarabine combined with cyclophosphamide and dexamethasone in patients with lymphoproliferative disorders. *Br J Haematol* 107:877, 1999.
31. Giles FJ, O'Brien SM, Keating MJ. Chronic lymphocytic leukemia in (Richter's) transformation. *Semin Oncol* 25:117, 1998.

32. Dabaja BS, O'Brien SM, Kantarjian HM, et al.: Fractionated cyclophosphamide, vincristine, liposomal daunorubicin (daunoXome), and dexamethasone (hyperCVXD) regimen in Richter's syndrome. *Leuk Lymphoma* 42:329, 2001.

33. Tsimberidou AM, O'Brien SM, Cortes JE, et al.: Phase II study of fludarabine, cytarabine (ara-C), cyclophosphamide, cisplatin and GM-CSF (FACPGM) in patients with Richter's syndrome or refractory lymphoproliferative disorders. *Leuk Lymphoma* 43:767, 2002.

34. Robak T, Kasznicki M, Bartkowiak J, et al.: Richter's syndrome following cladribine therapy for chronic lymphocytic leukemia first manifested as pathologic fracture of the femur. *Leuk Lymphoma* 42:789, 2001.

35. Jelic S, Jovanovic V, Milanovic N, et al.: Richter syndrome with emphasis on large-cell non-Hodgkin lymphoma in previously unrecognized subclinical chronic lymphocytic leukemia. *Neoplasma* 44:63, 1997.

36. Alliot C, Tabuteau S, Desablens B: Hodgkin's disease variant of Richter's syndrome: complete remission of the both malignancies after 14 years. *Hematology* 8:229, 2003.

37. Rodriguez J, Keating MJ, O'Brien S, et al. Allogeneic haematopoietic transplantation for Richter's syndrome. *Br J Haematol* 110:897, 2000.

38. Espanol I, Buchler T, Ferra C, et al.: Richter's syndrome after allogeneic stem cell transplantation for chronic lymphocytic leukaemia successfully treated by withdrawal of immunosuppression, and donor lymphocyte infusion. *Bone Marrow Transplant* 31:215, 2003.

39. Melo JV, Catovsky D, Galton DA: Chronic lymphocytic leukemia and prolymphocytic leukemia: a clinico-pathological reappraisal. *Blood Cells* 12:339, 1987.

40. Ruchlemer R, Parry-Jones N, Brito-Babapulle V, et al.: B-prolymphocytic leukaemia with t(11;14) revisited: a splenomegalic form of mantle cell lymphoma evolving with leukaemia. *Br J Haematol* 125:330, 2004.

41. Orchard J, Garand R, Davis Z, et al.: A subset of t(11;14) lymphoma with mantle cell features displays mutated IgVH genes and includes patients with good prognosis, non-nodal disease. *Blood* 101:4975, 2003.

42. Enno A, Catovsky D, O'Brien M, et al.: "Prolymphocytoid" transformation of chronic lymphocytic leukaemia. *Br J Haematol* 41:9, 1979.

43. Melo JV, Catovsky D, Galton DA: The relationship between chronic lymphocytic leukaemia and prolymphocytic leukaemia. I: Clinical and laboratory features of 300 patients and characterization of an intermediate group. *Br J Haematol* 63:377, 1986.

44. Melo JV, Catovsky D, Galton DA: The relationship between chronic lymphocytic leukaemia and prolymphocytic leukaemia. II: Patterns of evolution of "prolymphocytoid" transformation. *Br J Haematol* 64:77, 1986.

45. Melo JV, Wardle J, Chetty M, et al.: The relationship between chronic lymphocytic leukaemia and prolymphocytic leukaemia. III: Evaluation of cell size by morphology and volume measurements. *Br J Haematol* 64:469, 1986.

46. Melo JV, Catovsky D, Gregory WM, et al.: The relationship between chronic lymphocytic leukaemia and prolymphocytic leukaemia. IV: Analysis of survival and prognostic features. *Br J Haematol* 65:23, 1987.

47. Matutes E, Oscier D, Garcia-Marco J, et al.: Trisomy 12 defines a group of CLL with atypical morphology: correlation between cytogenetic, clinical and laboratory features in 544 patients. *Br J Haematol* 92:382, 1996

48. Cuneo A, Rigolin GM, Bigoni R, et al.: Chronic lymphocytic leukemia with 6q- shows distinct hematological features and intermediate prognosis. *Leukemia* 18:476, 2004.

49. Michaux L, Dierlamm J, Wlodarska I, et al.: t(14;19)/BCL3 rearrangements in lymphoproliferative disorders: a review of 23 cases. *Cancer Genet Cytogenet* 94:36, 1997.

50. Lens D, Dyer MJ, Garcia-Marco JM, et al.: p53 abnormalities in CLL are associated with excess of prolymphocytes and poor prognosis. *Br J Haematol* 99:848, 1997.

51. Oscier D, Fitchett M, Herbert T, et al.: Karyotypic evolution in B-cell chronic lymphocytic leukaemia. *Genes Chromosomes Cancer* 3:16, 1991.

52. Finn WG, Kay NE, Kroft SH, et al.: Secondary abnormalities of chromosome 6q in B-cell chronic lymphocytic leukemia: a sequential study of karyotypic instability in 51 patients. *Am J Hematol* 59:223, 1998.

53. Bea S, Lopez-Guillermo A, Ribas M, et al.: Genetic imbalances in progressed B-cell chronic lymphocytic leukemia and transformed large-cell lymphoma (Richter's syndrome). *Am J Pathol* 161:957, 2002.

54. Hamblin TJ, Orchard JA, Ibbotson RE, et al.: CD38 expression and immunoglobulin variable region mutations are independent prognostic variables in chronic lymphocytic leukemia, but CD38 expression may vary during the course of the disease. *Blood* 99:1023, 2002.

55. Oscier DG, Gardiner AC, Mould SJ, et al.: Multivariate analysis of prognostic factors in CLL: clinical stage, $V_H$ gene mutational status, and loss or mutation of the *p53* gene are independent prognostic factors. *Blood* 100:1177, 2002.

56. Lin K, Sherrington PD, Dennis M, et al.: Relationship between p53 dysfunction, CD38 expression, and IgV(H) mutation in chronic lymphocytic leukemia. *Blood* 100:1404, 2002.

57. Krober A, Seiler T, Benner A, et al.: V(H) mutation status, CD38 expression level, genomic aberrations, and survival in chronic lymphocytic leukemia. *Blood* 100:1410, 2002.

58. Cano I, Martinez J, Quevedo E, et al.: Trisomy 12 and p53 deletion in chronic lymphocytic leukemia detected by fluorescence in situ hybridization: association with morphology and resistance to conventional chemotherapy. *Cancer Genet Cytogenet* 90:118, 1996.

59. Brouet JC, Preud'homme JL, Seligman M, et al.: Blast cells with surface immunoglobulin in two cases of acute blast crisis supervening on chronic lymphocytic leukaemia. *Br Med J* 4:23, 1973.

60. Miller ALC, Habershaw JA, Dhaliwhal HS, et al.: Chronic lymphocytic leukaemia presenting as a blast cell crisis. *Leuk Res* 8:905, 1984.

61. Mohamed AN, Compean R, Dan ME, et al.: A clonal evolution of chronic lymphocytic leukemia to acute lymphoblastic leukemia. *Cancer Genet Cytogenet* 86:143, 1996.

62. Januszewicz E, Cooper IA, Pilkington G, et al.: Blastic transformation of chronic lymphocytic leukemia. *Am J Hematol* 15: 399, 1983.

63. Frenkel EP, Ligler FS, Graham MS, et al.: Acute lymphocytic leukemia transformation of chronic lymphatic leukemia: substantiation by flow cytometry. *Am J Hematol* 10:391, 1981.

64. Stevenson FK, Caligaris-Cappio F: Chronic lymphocytic leukemia: revelations from the B-cell receptor. *Blood* 103:4389, 2004.

65. Hamblin TJ, Oscier DG, Young BJ: Autoimmunity in chronic lymphocytic leukaemia. *J Clin Pathol* 39:713, 1986.

66. Berlin R: Red cell survival studies in normal and leukaemic subjects; latent hemolytic syndrome in leukaemia with splenomegaly–nature of anemia in leukaemia–effect of splenomegaly. *Acta Med Scand* 139(suppl 252):1, 1951.

67. Wasserman LR, Stats D, Schwartz L, et al.: Symptomatic and hemopathic hemolytic anemia. *Am J Med* 18:961, 1955.

68. Hamblin TJ: Autoimmune disease and its management in chronic lymphocytic leukemia. In: Cheson BD (ed.) *Chronic Lymphocytic Leukemia: Scientific Advances and Clinical Developments*. 2nd ed. New York: Marcel Dekker; 2001:435.

69. Bergsagel DE: The chronic leukemias: a review of disease manifestations and the aims of therapy. *Can Med Assoc J* 96:1615, 1967.

70. Dighiero G. Hypogammaglobulinemia and disordered immunity in CLL. In: Cheson BD (ed.) *Chronic Lymphocytic Leukemia: Scientific Advances and Clinical Developments*. New York: Marcel Dekker; 1993:167.

71. Engelfriet CP, Overbeeke MAM, von dem Borne AEGK: AIHA. *Semin Hematol* 29:3, 1992.

72. Minot GR, Buckman TE: The blood platelets in the leukemias. *Am J Med Sci* 169:477, 1925.

73. Harrington WJ, Arimura G: Immune reactions of platelets. In: Johnson SA, Monto RW, Rebuck JW, Horn RC (eds.) *Blood Platelets*. Boston, MA: Little Brown; 1961:117.

74. Ebbe S, Wittels B, Dameshek W: Autoimmune thrombocytopenic purpura ("ITP type") with chronic lymphocytic leukemia. *Blood* 19:23, 1962.

75. Dührsen U, Augener W, Zwingers T, et al.: Spectrum and frequency of autoimmune derangements in lymphoproliferative disorders: analysis of 637 cases and comparison with myeloproliferative diseases. *Br J Haematol* 67:235, 1987.

76. Hegde UM, Williams K, Devereux S, et al.: Platelet associated IgG and immune thrombocytopenia in lymphoproliferative and autoimmune disorders. *Clin Lab Haematol* 5:9, 1983.

77. Diehl LF, Ketchum LH: Autoimmune disease and chronic lymphocytic leukemia: AIHA, pure red cell aplasia and autoimmune thrombocytopenia. *Semin Hematol* 25:80, 1998.

78. Killman S-Å: Auto-aggressive leukocyte agglutinins in leukaemia and chronic leukopenia. *Acta Med Scand* 163:207, 1959.

79. Loughran TP, Kardin ME, Starkebaum G, et al.: Leukemia of large granular lymphocytes: association with clonal chromosomal abnormalities and autoimmune neutropenia, thrombocytopenia, and hemolytic anemia. *Ann Intern Med* 102:169, 1985.

80. Katrinakis G, Kyriakou D, Alexandrakis M, et al.: Evidence for involvement of activated CD8+/HLA-DR+ cells in the pathogenesis of neutropenia in patients with B-cell chronic lymphocytic leukaemia. *Eur J Haematol* 55:33, 1995.

81. Lamy T, Loughran TP: Current concepts: large granular lymphocyte leukaemia. *Blood Rev* 13:230, 1999.

82. Abeloff MD, Waterbury MD: Pure red cell aplasia and chronic lymphocytic leukemia. *Arch Intern Med* 134:721, 1974.

83. Lacy MQ, Kurtin PJ, Tefferi A: Pure red cell aplasia: association with large granular lymphocytic leukemia and the prognostic value of cytogenetic abnormalities. *Blood* 87:3000, 1996.

84. Chikkappa G, Zarrabi MH, Tsan MF: Pure red cell aplasia in patients with chronic lymphocytic leukemia. *Medicine (Baltimore)* 65:339–351, 1986.

85. Casadevall N, Nataf J, Viron B, et al.: Pure red-cell aplasia and anti-erythropoietin antibodies in patients treated with recombinant erythropoietin. *N Engl J Med* 346:469, 2002.

86. Miller DG: Patterns of immunological deficiency in lymphomas and leukemias. *Ann Intern Med* 57:703–715, 1962.

87. Dameshek W: Chronic lymphocytic leukemia–an accumulative disease of immunologically incompetent lymphocytes. *Blood* 24:566–584, 1967.

88. Dathan JRE, Heyworth MF, MacIver AG: Nephrotic syndrome in chronic lymphocytic leukaemia. *Br Med J* 3:655, 1974.

89. Cameron S, Ogg CS: Nephrotic syndrome in chronic lymphocytic leukaemia. *Br Med J* 3:164, 1974.

90. Tisler A, Pierratos A, Lipton JH: Crescentic glomerulonephritis associated with p-ANCA positivity in fludarabine-treated chronic lymphocytic leukaemia. *Nephrol Dial Transplant* 11:2306, 1996.

91. Dussol B, Brunet P, Vacher-Coponat H, et al.: Crescentic glomerulonephritis with antineutrophil cytoplasmic antibodies associated with chronic lymphocytic leukaemia. *Nephrol Dial Transplant* 12:785, 1997.

92. He S, Tsang S, North J, et al.: Epitope mapping of C1 inhibitor autoantibodies from patients with acquired C1 inhibitor deficiency. *J Immunol* 156:2009, 1996.

93. Chevailler A, Arlaud G, Ponard D, et al.: C-1-inhibitor binding monoclonal immunoglobulins in three patients with acquired angioneurotic edema. *J Allergy Clin Immunol* 97:998, 1996.

94. Oppenheim M: Verhandlungen der Weiner dermatologischen Gesellschaft. *Arch Belg Dermatol Syphiligr* 101:379, 1910.

95. Sachs O: Ueber Pemphigoide Hauteruption in Einem Falle von Lymphatischer Leukaemie. *Wien Klin Wochenschr* 34:317, 1921.

96. Cuni LJ, Grünwald H, Rosner F: Bullous pemphigoid in chronic lymphocytic leukemia with the demonstration of anti-basement membrane antibodies. *Am J Med* 57:987, 1974.

97. Goodnough LT, Muir A: Bullous pemphigoid as a manifestation of chronic lymphocytic leukemia. *Arch Intern Med* 140:1526, 1980.

98. Laskaris GC, Papavasilou SS, Bovopoulou OD, et al.: Association of oral pemphigus with chronic lymphocytic leukemia. *Oral Surg Oral Med Oral Pathol* 50:244, 1980.

99. Anhalt GJ, Kim SC, Stanley JR, et al.: Paraneoplastic pemphigus. An autoimmune mucocutaneous disease associated with neoplasia. *N Engl J Med* 323:1729, 1990.

100. Camisa C, Helm TN, Liu YC, et al.: Paraneoplastic pemphigus: a report of three cases including one long term survivor. *J Am Acad Dermatol* 27:547, 1992.

101. Su WP, Oursler JR, Muller SA: Paraneoplastic pemphigus: a case with high titer of circulating anti-basement membrane zone antibodies. *J Am Acad Dermatol* 30:841, 1994.

102. Rodot S, Botcazou V, Lacour JP, et al.: Paraneoplastic pemphigus: review of the literature, apropos of a case associated with chronic lymphocytic leukemia. *Rev Med Interne* 16:938, 1995.

103. Joly P, Thomine E, Gilbert D, et al.: Overlapping distribution of autoantibody specificities in paraneoplastic pemphigus and pemphigus vulgaris. *J Invest Dermatol* 103:65, 1994.

104. Hashimoto T, Amagai M, Ning W, et al.: Novel non-radioisotope immunoprecipitation studies indicate involvement of pemphigus vulgaris antigen in paraneoplastic pemphigus. *J Dermatol Sci* 17:132, 1998.

105. Amagai M, Klaus-Kovtun V, Stanley JR: Autoantibodies against a novel cadherin in pemphigus vulgaris, a disease of call adhesion. *Cell* 67:869, 1991.

106. Kim SC, Kwon YD, Lee IJ, et al.: cDNA cloning of the 210-kDa paraneoplastic pemphigus antigen reveals that envoplakin is a component of the antigen complex. *J Invest Dermatol* 109:365, 1997.

107. Ruhrberg C, Hajibagheri MA, Parry DA, et al.: Periplakin, a novel component of cornified envelopes and desmosomes that belongs to the plakin family and forms complexes with envoplakin. *J Cell Biol* 39:1835, 1997.

108. Anhalt GJ, Nousari HC: Paraneoplastic autoimmune syndromes. In: Rose NR, Mackay IR (eds.) *The Autoimmune Diseases*. 3rd ed. San Diego, CA: Academic; 1998:795.

109. Beaume A, Brizard A, Dreyfus B, et al.: High incidence of serum monoclonal Igs detected by a sensitive immunoblotting technique in B-cell chronic lymphocytic leukemia. *Blood* 84:1216, 1994.

110. Broker BM, Klajman A, Youinou P, et al.: Chronic lymphocytic leukemias (CLL) cells secrete multispecific autoantibodies. *J Autoimmun* 1:469, 1988.

111. Sthoeger ZM, Wakai M, Tse DB, et al.: Production of autoantibodies by CD5-expressing B lymphocytes from patients with chronic lymphocytic leukemia. *J Exp Med* 169:255, 1989.

112. Sthoeger ZM, Stoeger D, Shtalrid M, et al.: Mechanism of AIHA in chronic lymphocytic leukemia. *Am J Hematol* 43:259, 1993.

113. Sikora K, Kirkorian J, Levy R: Monoclonal immunoglobulin rescued from a patient with chronic lymphocytic leukemia and AIHA. *Blood* 54:513, 1979.

114. Stevenson FK, Wrightham M, Glennie MJ, et al.: Antibodies to shared idiotypes as agents for analysis and therapy for human B cell tumours. *Blood* 68:430, 1986.

115. Pascual V, Victor K, Lelsz D, et al.: Nucleotide sequence analysis of the V regions of two IgM cold agglutinins. Evidence that the $V_H4$-21 gene segment is responsible for the major cross-reactive idiotype. *J Immunol* 146:4385, 1991.

116. Pascual V, Victor K, Spellerberg M, et al.: VH restriction among human cold agglutinins: the VH4-21 gene segment is required to encode anti-I and anti-i specificities. *J Immunol* 149:2337, 1992.

117. Potter KN, Li Y, Pascuel V, et al.: Molecular characterization of a cross-reactive idiotope on human immunoglobulins utilizing the $V_H4$-21 gene segment. *J Exp Med* 178:1419, 1993.

118. Crisp D, Pruzanski W: B-cell neoplasms with homogeneous cold-reacting antibodies (cold agglutinins). *Am J Med* 72:915, 1982.

119. Feizi T, Wernet P, Kunkel HG, et al.: Lymphocytes forming red cell rosettes in the cold in patients with chronic cold agglutinin disease. *Blood* 42:753, 1973.

120. Ruzickova S, Pruss A, Odendahl M, et al.: Chronic lymphocytic leukemia preceded by cold agglutinin disease: intraclonal immunoglobulin light-chain diversity in V(H)4-34 expressing single leukemic B cells. *Blood* 100:3419, 2002.

121. Gouet D, Marechaud R, Touchard G, et al.: Nephrotic syndrome associated with chronic lymphocytic leukaemia. *Nouv Presse Med* 11:3047, 1982.

122. Lisery L, Cambazard F, Rimokh R, et al.: Bullous pemphigoid associated with chronic B-cell lymphatic leukemia: the anti-230-kDa autoantibody is not synthesized by leukemic cells. *Br J Dermatol* 141:155, 1999.

123. Lewis FB, Schwarz RS, Damashek W: X-irradiation and alkylating agents as possible trigger mechanisms in autoimmune complications of malignant lymphoproliferative diseases. *Clin Exp Immunol* 1:3, 1966.

124. Hansen MM: Chronic lymphocytic leukaemia: clinical studies based on 189 cases followed for a long time. *Scand J Haematol* 18(suppl 1):1, 1973.

125. Catovsky D, Foa R: B-cell chronic lymphocytic leukaemia. In: Catovsky D, Foa R (eds.) *The Lymphoid Leukaemias*. London: Butterworths; 1990:73.

126. Thompson-Moya L, Martin T, Heuft HG, et al.: Allergic reaction with immune hemolytic anemia arising from chlorambucil. *Am J Hematol* 32:230, 1989.

127. Bastion Y, Coiffier B, Dumontet C, et al.: Severe autoimmune hemolytic anemia in two patients treated with fludarabine for chronic lymphocytic leukemia. *Ann Oncol* 3:171, 1992.

128. Di Raimondo F, Guistolisi R, Cacciola E, et al.: Autoimmune hemolytic anemia in chronic lymphocytic leukemia patients treated with fludarabine. *Leuk Lymphoma* 11:63, 1993.

129. Myint H, Copplestone JA, Orchard J, et al.: Fludarabine-related autoimmune haemolytic anaemia in patients with chronic lymphocytic leukaemia. *Br J Haematol* 91:341, 1995.

130. Mauro FR, Foa R, Cerretti R, et al.: Autoimmune hemolytic anemia in chronic lymphocytic leukemia: clinical, therapeutic, and prognostic features. *Blood* 95:2786, 2000.

131. Montillo M, Tedeschi A, Leoni P: Recurrence of autoimmune thrombocytopenia after treatment with

fludarabine in a patient with chronic lymphocytic leukemia. *Leuk Lymphoma* 15:187, 1994.

132. Stern SC, Shah S, Costello C: Probable autoimmune neutropenia induced by fludarabine treatment for chronic lymphocytic leukaemia. *Br J Haematol* 106:836, 1999.

133. Hall AM, Vickers MA, McLeod E, et al.: Rh Autoantigen presentation to helper T cells in chronic lymphocytic leukemia by malignant B-cells. *Blood* 105:2175, 2005.

134. Markovic SN, Inwards DJ, Frigas EA, et al.: Acquired C1 esterase inhibitor deficiency. *Ann Intern Med* 132: 144, 2000.

135. Dameshek W, Komninos ZP: The present status of treatment of autoimmune hemolytic anemia with ACTH and cortisone. *Blood* 11:648, 1956.

136. Coon WW: Splenectomy in the treatment of hemolytic anemia. *Arch Surg* 120:625, 1985.

137. Flores G, Cunningham-Rundles C, Newland AC, et al.: Efficacy of intravenous immunoglobulin in the treatment of autoimmune hemolytic anemia: results in 73 patients. *Am J Hematol* 44:237, 1993.

138. Ruess-Borst MA, Waller HD, Muller CA: Successful treatment of steroid resistant hemolysis in chronic lymphocytic leukemia with cyclosporine A. *Am J Hematol* 9:357, 1994.

139. Zaja F, Vianelli N, Sperotto A, et al.: Anti-CD20 therapy for chronic lymphocytic leukemia-associated autoimmune diseases. *Leuk Lymphoma* 44:1951, 2003.

140. The American Society of Hematology ITP Practice Guideline Panel: Diagnosis and treatment of idiopathic thrombocytopenic purpura: recommendations of the American Society of Hematology. *Ann Intern Med* 126:319, 1997.

141. McMillan R: Therapy for adults with refractory chronic immune thrombocytopenic purpura. *Ann Intern Med* 126:307, 1997.

142. Culic S: Recombinant factor VIIa for refractive haemorrhage in autoimmune idiopathic thrombocytopenic purpura. *Br J Haematol* 120:909, 2003.

143. Laughen RH, Carey RM, Wills MR, et al.: Hypercalcemia associated with chronic lymphocytic leukemia. *Arch Intern Med* 139:1307, 1979.

144. Rossi JF, Cappard D, Marcelli C, et al.: Micro-osteoclast resorption as a characteristic feature of B-cell malignancies other than multiple myeloma. *Br J Haematol* 76:469, 1990.

145. Davis MD, Perniciaro C, Dahl PR, et al.: Exaggerated arthropod-bite lesions in patients with chronic lymphocytic leukemia: a clinical, histopathologic, and immunopathologic study of eight patients. *J Am Acad Dermatol* 39:27, 1998.

146. Blum RR, Phelps RG, Wei H: Arthropod bites manifesting as recurrent bullae in a patient with chronic lymphocytic leukemia. *J Cutan Med Surg* 5:312, 2001.

147. Hamblin TJ: Chronic lymphocytic leukaemia. *Baillieres Clin Haematol* 1:449, 1987.

148. Creange A, Theodorou I, Sabourin J-C, et al.: Inflammatory neuromuscular disorders associated with chronic lymphoid leukemia: evidence for clonal B cells within muscle and nerve. *J Neurol Sci* 137:35, 1996.

149. Cobeta-Garcia JC, Domingo-Morera JA, Martinez-Burgui J: RS3PE syndrome and chronic lymphocytic leukemia. *Intern Med* 34:15, 1995.

# Section 5
# HAIRY CELL LEUKEMIA

## Chapter 28

# EPIDEMIOLOGY, RISK FACTORS, AND CLASSIFICATION OF HAIRY CELL LEUKEMIA

*Diane M. BuchBarker*

## EPIDEMIOLOGY

Hairy cell leukemia (HCL) is one of the B-cell lymphoproliferative disorders and is quite rare.

There is little known about epidemiologic factors of importance in patients with HCL.

### INCIDENCE

Hairy cell leukemia is an uncommon malignancy, encompassing only 1–2% of all leukemias in the United States. It is slightly lower at 1.12% of all leukemias in Mexico.[1] Incidence is reported as 2.9 per million persons per year for men and 0.6 per million persons per year for women, and is similar to that reported in England and Wales.[2] The incidence in Hong Kong is much lower, at only 0.0035 per million persons per year.[3] The highest documented incidence is derived from nationwide information from Iceland—at 4.7 per million persons per year.[4] Generally, the disease is indolent with a prolonged clinical course.

Patients presenting with HCL are usually in their middle ages, with the median age of 52 years at diagnosis. There is a striking male predominance, with a male/female ratio of 4:1. This male predominance holds true throughout all countries.

There is also ratio discordance with race. Caucasians have a higher frequency of HCL than other races. Jewish males have a higher risk than Jewish females or those of other religion groups.[5]

### GENETIC PREDISPOSITION

There is no proven genetic predisposition to the development of HCL, although approximately 15 cases of what appears to be familial HCL have been reported over the past 20 years. They have all shared the HLA haplotype A2, Bw4, and Bw6 suggesting that these haplotypes may play a role in genetic predisposition.[6,7]

### MORTALITY DATA

In untreated patients, the rate of survival at 5 and 10 years was 34.4% and 29.6%, respectively. For splenectomized patients the 5-year survival was approximately 60% and for those receiving pentostatin, the 5-year survival was 90%.[8]

## RISK FACTORS

The interest in identifying risk factors for all cancers is rising with the increasing incidences of cancer. Most likely because of the rarity of this disease, there is little information on risk factors for HCL. Studies have identified a number of potential risk factors for HCL, including occupational hazards, chemical exposure, and infectious predispositions.

### CHEMICAL EXPOSURE AND HAIRY CELL LEUKEMIA

Several studies have hinted at chemical exposure as a risk factor, consistent with data seen in other hematologic malignancies. The tendency of HCL to occur in men at a 4:1 ratio suggests that there may be occupational risk factors as well. Summaries of these studies are as follows: Hardel et al. reported on a population-based cancer registry analysis of 515 cases and 1141 controls. They identified increased risks for subjects exposed to herbicides, insecticides, fungicides, and impregnating agents.[9] A significant association was found between HCL and insecticides, fungicides, and herbicides, with an overall odds ratio ranging from 1.5 to 2.4 in a study of 226 men with HCL reported by Clavel.[10] Nordstrom et al., in the *British Journal of Cancer*, published a study that also identified exposure to the above mentioned same agents as risk factors.[11]

### OCCUPATIONAL HAZARDS AND HAIRY CELL LEUKEMIA

In the study by Nordstrom et al. data supported agriculture-related exposures as an increased risk for HCL. There was also an overall elevated odds ratio for exposure to farm animals, specifically cattle, horses, hogs, poultry, and sheep. There is, however, a question of recall bias affecting these results.[11] Ruiz-Arguelles reported on 27 patients with HCL in Mexico and found that the proportion of patients with leukemia to be higher in the northern region of the country where farming and agriculture is more prevalent.[1] Clavel reports on 225 men with HCL and 425 matched controls, and found that 20.8% of the cases were farmers.[10]

Organic solvents have been implicated in the etiology of HCL in several series.[12–14] One of the larger case-control studies of 291 cases with HCL and 541 matched controls was published in the *British Journal of Hematology*[15] and did not find an association with jobs involving exposure to solvents. The study admittedly lacked the power to investigate higher odds ratio for some jobs, such as spray painters. Previous studies have suggested an association with organic solvents.

### INFECTIOUS EXPOSURES AND HAIRY CELL LEUKEMIA

The contribution of infectious pathogens to the etiology of cancer is being investigated for a multitude of cancers. Because of the association of Non-Hodgkin's lymphoma with Epstein-Barr virus (EB), Nordstrom reported on the correlation of exposure to Epstein-Barr virus and exposure to organochlorines as risk factors for HCL. High titres of antibodies to EB early antigen IgG, along with higher blood concentrations of chlordanes, and hexachlorobenzene were correlated with an increased risk for HCL.[16]

A population-based case control study performed in Sweden through a mailed questionnaire to investigate the possible role of previous medical history and medications as risk factors for HCL was conducted by Nordstrom et al. Elevated odds ratio was found in those with a history of appendicitis and pneumonia, NSAID use, as well as a history of malignancy.[17] There

was no association found between cigarette smoking, alcohol, or coffee consumption and HCL.[11,15]

### RISK OF SECOND MALIGNANCIES

In an epidemiological study of HCL in Los Angeles County in 1990, it was noted that patients with a history of HCL were more than twice as likely as other cancer patients to have multiple cancer diagnoses.[5] Since that time, multiple studies have confirmed that HCL patients have an increased risk for secondary malignancies. The rationale for this observation is probably dual. The primary treatment of HCL involves the use of nucleoside analogs, which lead to prolonged immunosuppression, with lower than normal numbers of CD4+ cells for more than 3.5 years.[18,19] This prolonged immunosuppression leads to an increase in second malignancies.[19] Cheson et al. looked at patients with either chronic lymphocytic leukemia (CLL) or HCL who had undergone treatment with Nucleoside Analogs and found a total of 150 secondary cancers in 146 patients. Most of these cases were solid tumors, with a higher than expected frequency of prostate cancer.[20] In a study from British Columbia, Au et al. reported that of 117 patients with HCL diagnosed between 1976 and 1996, 30.7% had at least one additional malignancy. Twenty percent were diagnosed either at the same time or within a few years of the diagnosis of HCL, with a peak incidence at 2 years afterwards. All secondary malignancies were solid tumors.[21]

Interestingly, previous studies of other immunocompromised populations found an increased incidence of hematologic malignancies, yet more solid tumors were found in patients with HCL. They were detected prior to or concomitant with the diagnosis of HCL. There is one case report of a patient with a myeloproliferative disorder (essential thrombocythemia) treated with hydroxyurea who later developed HCL.[22] There have been two reports of pre-existing polycythemia vera followed by a diagnosis of HCL.[23]

Interferon alpha is an effective treatment for HCL. This suggests that the immune system may help modulate disease progression.[24,25] Multiple tumors were found in some studies either prior to or concomitant with the diagnosis of HCL, raising the suspicion that there may be an underlying impaired immune response in patients with HCL.[26]

Not all studies support the theory that patients with HCL are at an increased risk for second malignancies. The following reported that the incidence of second malignancies was not significantly higher than expected. Fifty-four of 1,022 patients in the Italian Cooperative Group for the Study of HCL developed second cancers; this was not significantly higher than the expected rate, although the incidence of lymphoid neoplasms was significantly higher.[27] Data on 350 patients with HCL obtained from the M.D. Anderson Cancer Center Cancer Registry found that, although there was an increase in the number of second malignancies, statistical significance was not achieved, and the excess malignancies were not thought to be associated with therapy.[28]

## CLASSIFICATION

Hairy cell leukemia is a rare chronic monoclonal B-cell neoplasm. There is no internationally recognized classification system for HCL. In fact, the World Health Organization classification of hematopoietic and lymphoid malignancy represents the first worldwide consensus document on the classification of lymphoma/leukemia.

Classically, three immunophenotypic variants are described. All hairy cells express the pan-B-cell antigens CD19 and CD20. They are negative for CD5, CD10, and CD23. The classic variant coexpresses CD11c, CD25, and CD103. The variant group accounts for 10% of hairy cell cases and expresses CD11c, but not CD25. Expression of CD103 is variable. The survival of the variant form seems to be inferior to the classic type, most likely due to chemoresistance. The Japanese variant is CD11c positive, and occasionally CD103 positive, but CD25 negative.[29–32]

## REFERENCES

1. Ruiz-Arguelles GJ, Cantu-Rodriquez OG, Gomez-Almaguer F, et al.: Hairy cell leukemia is infrequent in Mexico and has a geographic distribution. *Am J Hematol* 52(4):316–318, 1995 Aug.
2. Staines A, Cartwright RA: Hairy cell leukemia: Descriptive epidemiology and a case study. *Br J Hematol* 85(4):714–717, 1993 Dec.
3. Au WY, Kwong YL, Ma SK, et al.: Hairy cell leukemia in Hong Kong Chinese: a 12-year retrospective survey. *Hematol Oncol* 18(4):155–159, 2000 Dec.
4. Kristinsson Sy, Vidarsson B, Agnarsson BA, et al.: Epidemiology of hairy cell leukemia in Iceland. *Hematol J* 3(3):145–147, 2002.
5. Bernstein L, Newton P, Ross RK: Epidemiology of hairy cell leukemia in Los Angeles County. *Cancer Res* 50(12):3605–3609, 1990 June 15.
6. Gramatovici M, Bennett JM, Hiscock JG, Grewal KS: Three cases of familial hairy cell leukemia. *Am J Hematol* 42(4):337–339, April 1993.
7. Cetiner M, Adiguzel C, Argon D, et al.: Hairy cell leukemia in father and son. *Med Oncol* 20(4):375–378, 2003 Jan.
8. Flinn IW, Kopecky Kj, Foucar MK, et al.: Long-term follow-up of remission duration, mortality, and second malignancies in hairy cell leukemia patients treated with pentostatin. *Blood* 96(9):2981–2986, 2000 Nov.
9. Hardell L, Eriksson M, Nordstrom M: Exposure to pesticides as risk factor for Non-Hodgkin's lymphoma and hairy cell leukemia: Pooled analysis of two Swedish case-control studies. *Leukemia Lymphoma* 43(5):1043–1049, 2002 May.
10. Clavel J, Hemon D, Mandereau L, et al.: Farming, pesticide use and hairy-cell leukemia. *Scand J Work Environ Health* 22(4):285–293, 1996 Aug.
11. Nordstrom M, Hardell L, Magnuson A, et al.: Occupational exposures, animal exposure and smoking as risk factors for hairy cell leukaemia evaluated in a case-control study. *Br J Cancer* 77(11):2048–2052, 1998 June.
12. Flandrin G, Collado S: Is male predominance in hairy cell leukaemia related to occupational exposure to ionizing radiation, benzene and other solvents? *Br J Haematol* 67:119–120, 1987.
13. Oleske D, Golomb HM, Farber MD,et al.:A case-control inquiry into the etiology of hairy cell leukemia. *Am J Epidemiol* 121:675–683, 1985.
14. Staines A, Cartwright RA: Hairy cell leukaemia: descriptive epidemiology and a case-control study. *Br J Haematol* 85:714–717, 1993.
15. Clavel J, Mandereau L, Cordier S, et al.: Hairy cell leukaemia, occupation, and smoking. *Br J Haematol* 91(1):154–161, 1995 Sept.
16. Nordstrom M, Hardell L, Lindstrom G, et al.: Concentrations of organochlorines related to titers to Epstein-Barr virus early antigen IgG as risk factors for hairy cell leukemia. *Environ Health Perspec* 108(5):441–415, 2000 May.
17. Nordstrom M, Hardell L, Fredrikson M: Previous medical history and medications as risk factors for hairy cell leukaemia. *Oncol Rep* 6(2):415–419, 1999 Mar-Apr.
18. Seymour JF, Talpaz M, Kurzrock R: Response duration and recovery of CD4+ lymphocytes following deoxycoformycin I interferon-alpha-resistant hairy cell leukemia; 7-year followup. *Leukemia* 11:42–47, 1997.
19. Seymour JF, Kurzrock R, Freireich EJ, et al.: 2-Chlorodeoxyadenosine induces durable remissions and prolonged suppression of CD4+ lymphocyte counts in patients with hairy cell leukemia. *Blood* 83:2906–2911, 1994.
20. Cheson B, Vena DA, Barrett J, Freidlin B: Second malignancies as a consequence of Nucleoside Analog therapy for chronic lymphoid leukemias. *J Clin Oncol* 17(8):2454–2460, 1999 Aug.
21. Au WY, Klasa RJ, Gallagher R, et al.: Second malignancies in patients with hairy cell leukemia in British Columbia; a 20-year experience. *Blood* 92(4):1160–1164, 1998 Aug.
22. Azagury M: Development of hairy cell leukemia in a patient treated with cytoreductive agents for essential thrombocythemia. *Leukemia Lymphoma* 44(6):1067–1069, 2003 June.
23. Kelly NP: Hairy cell leukemia variant developing in a background of polycythemia vera. *Archives Pathol Lab Med* 127(4):209–211, 2003 Apr.
24. Zhang HG: Aging, immunity, and tumor susceptibility. *Immunol Allergy Clin North Am* 23(1):83–102, 2003 Feb.
25. Seymour JF, Estey EH, Keating MJ, et al.: Response to interferon-alpha in patients with hairy cell leukemia relapsing after treatment with 2-chlorodeoxyadenosine. *Leukemia* 9:929–932, 1995 May.
26. Saven A, Burian C, Koziol J, Piro L: Long-term follow-up of patients with hairy cell leukemia after cladribine treatment. *Blood* 92(6):1918–1926, 1998 Sept.

27. Federico M:Risk of second cancer in patients with hairy cell leukemia: long-term follow-up. *J Clin Oncol* 20(3):638–646,2002 Feb.

28. Kurzrock R: Second cancer risk in hairy cell leukemia: analysis of 350 patients. *J Clin Oncol* 15(5):1803–1819, 1997 May.

29. Wu Ml, Kwaan HCl, Goolsby Cl: Atypical hairy cell leukemia. *Arch Pathol Lab Med* 124(11):1710–1713, 2000 Nov.

30. Katayama I, Hirashima K, Maruyama K, et al.: Hairy cell leukemia in Japanese patients: a study with molecular antibodies. *Leukemia* 1(4):301–305, 1987 Apr.

31. Machii T, Tokumine Y, Inoue R, Kitani T.: Predominance of a distinct subtype of hairy cell leukemia in Japan. *Leukemia* 7(2):181–186, 1993 Feb.

32. Matutes E: The variant form of hairy-cell leukaemia. *Best Prac Res Clin Hematol* 16(1):41–56, 2003 Mar.

# Chapter 29

# MOLECULAR BIOLOGY, PATHOLOGY, AND CYTOGENETICS IN HAIRY CELL LEUKEMIA

## *Mirko Zuzel and John C. Cawley*

## INTRODUCTION

Hairy cell leukemia (HCL) is a clonal expansion of abnormal memory-type B cells with specific features of activation, including the distinctive "hairy" morphology of the malignant cells that give the disease its name. The malignant hairy cells (HCs) display specific patterns of activated signaling components, express a spectrum of activation antigens and activated adhesion receptors, and spontaneously secrete a number of autocrine cytokines. Many recent studies clearly indicate that the pathology of HCL is, to a large extent, a direct reflection of this activated phenotype of the malignant cells.

Although HCL is a largely homogenous disease with respect to its cell-biological and clinicopathological features, no consistent abnormal cytogenetic profile has yet been demonstrated, and the nature of the oncogenic transformation of HCs remains unclear.

Here we first describe the specific cell-biological and molecular characteristics of HCs and discuss their importance for the distinctive clinicopathological features and therapy of HCL. We also present the currently known cytogenetics of this disease.

## CELL AND MOLECULAR BIOLOGY

### HAIRY CELLS AS MEMORY B CELLS

It is well established that HCs are mature clonal B cells that express a range of B-cell markers (e.g., CD19, CD20, CD22) together with surface immunoglobulin which has often undergone class-switch recombination and relatively low levels of somatic hypermutation (Table 29.1). Moreover, individual HCs can express multiple heavy chain isotypes that are generated by splicing of long RNA transcripts.[1] Studies of a limited number of cases failed to show clear evidence of biased $V_H$ gene segment usage or cell selection by antigen(s).[2]

| Table 29.1 HCs as mature B cells |
| --- |
| • Express strong surface immunoglobulin |
| • All heavy-chain isotypes except IgE potentially expressed; IgG3 predominant |
| • Coexpression of multiple isotypes the result of RNA splicing |
| • Often VH mutated without further clonal evolution |
| • No clear biased usage of VH gene segments |
| • Lack naïve (e.g., CD23) and germinal centre antigens (e.g., CD10, BCL-6) |
| • Do not express plasma-cell markers (MUM-1, CD138, BLIMP 1) |

Although HCs express the plasma-cell antigen PCA1,[3] and the CD85 expressed by plasma cells and other mature B cells, they have little or no propensity to differentiate into antibody-secreting cells. Recent gene expression profiling clearly places HCs, along with chronic lymphocytic leukemia (CLL) cells, at the memory stage of B-cell development.[4] Reactivity with a phage-derived antibody known as phab V-3 and high levels of CD11c expression indicate that HCs may originate from a subpopulation of normal CD11c-positive memory B cells with similar phab V-3 reactivity.[5] This subpopulation is VH-mutated and possesses the memory-cell marker CD27 that has also been reported to be present on HCs.[4]

### ACTIVATION FEATURES OF HAIRY CELLS

Long before the advent of CD antibodies, the distinctive morphology of HCs was highly suggestive of the activated nature of the malignant cells. Subsequent studies have indeed shown the HCs express a number of antigens (e.g., FMC7, CD22, CD25, CD72, CD40L) associated with the activation of B cells and other cell types (Table 29.2),[6] but lack CD23, which is expressed by CLL cells and upregulated during normal B-cell activation.[6] Moreover, certain HC-"restricted" antigens,

| Table 29.2 Activation features |
|---|
| Upregulated activation antigens<br>(e.g., FMC-7, CD22, CD25, CD72, CD40L) |
| Downregulation of antigens often reduced during<br>activation of other cells types (e.g., CD21 and CD24) |
| HC-"restricted" antigens probably indicative of activation<br>(e.g., CD11c, CD68, CD103, HC-2, cyclin D1 and TRAP[a]) |
| Surface microvilli and ruffles, relatively abundant<br>basophilic cytoplasm, open nuclear chromatin |

[a]TRAP = tartrate-resistant acid phosphatase.

such as CD11c, CD68c, CD103, HC-2, cyclin D1, and TRAP, have also been associated with the activation of certain lymphoid and non-lymphoid cell types.[7] Interestingly, both the CD21 and CD24 markers, normally lost after B-cell activation, are expressed by HCs only at low levels.[6]

### OTHER DISTINCTIVE PHENOTYPIC FEATURES

In addition to the HC-"restricted" activation antigens alluded to above, global gene-expression analysis has identified a large number of new genes differentially expressed by HCs as compared to normal memory B cells and a range of normal and malignant B-cell-types.[4] Genes of particular potential importance identified by this technology include those related to HC morphology, to the long-known "monocytic" features of HCs, to the adhesion and homing of the malignant cells, and to their propensity to alter the extracellular matrix of bone marrow and hepatic portal tracts. These phenotypic features are listed in Table 29.3 and will be

| Table 29.3 Newly identified differentially expressed genes of potential pathogenetic importance |
|---|
| Morphology related<br>pp52 (LSP-1), β-actin, Gas 7 and EPB4.IL-2 |
| '"Monocytic" features<br>annexin 1, CD63, CPVL, CD68, c-Maf |
| Unusual tissue distribution<br>CCR7 and CXCR5 chemokine receptors downregulated<br>TIMP-1, TIMP-4 and RECK matrix metalloproteinase<br>inhibitors upregulated |
| Matrix remodeling<br>Overexpression of FGF-2 and FGFR1 confirm previous<br>evidence for involvement of this autocrine loop in the<br>stimulation of the production of HC-derived fibronectin<br>responsible for the bone marrow fibrosis of HCL |

considered further in the section dealing with the pathology of the disease.

### ACTIVATED SIGNALLING COMPONENTS

A number of signaling components are now known to be activated in HCs. The so-far identified activation signals and their likely mutual relationships are summarized in Table 29.4. Some of these signals are transient and clearly originate from cell stimulation by components of the in vivo microenvironment, but some persist in vitro, suggesting that they are truly constitutive. It is, however, not yet clear which of these constitutive signals is a direct consequence of the still unknown oncogenic event(s), and which are attributable to autocrine cytokine production. The pathogenetic role

| Table 29.4 Activation signals in HCs | | |
|---|---|---|
| Signal | Possible origin | Functional relevance |
| Elevated intracellular $[Ca^{2+}]$ | Release from intracellular stores in response to autocrine cytokine.<br>Influx via highly expressed and phosphorylated CD20 | Activation messenger |
| Increased protein tyrosine phosphorylation | Constitutively activated Src | Downsteam activation of Rho GTPases, PKCs and MAP kinases |
| Active Rac and Cdc42 | Src-activated GEF(s) | Formation of surface ruffles and microvilli and downstream activation of MAP kinases |
| Activated PKCs | Upstream activators include high $[Ca^{2+}]$,PLC-generated DAG and Src | Rgulation of MAP kinases and NFκB involved in cell survival and proliferation |
| Activated MAP kinases | ERK activation constitutive and PKC dependent<br>p38 and JNK induced by external signals (e.g., TNF) and suppressed by active PKCα | ERK provides a pro-survival signal<br>p38 is pro-apoptotic<br>JNK stimulates CD11c expression via AP-1 complex formation |
| Activated NFκB | Autocrine TNF and integrin signaling | Stimulates IAP production.<br>Suppression of IAPs involved in the αIFN-induced sensitivity of HCs to TNF killing |

of these signals will be considered in the section dealing with the pathology of the disease.

The first demonstration of a messenger that could be responsible for the activated state of HCs was provided by Genot et al., who showed elevated $[Ca^{2+}]$ in HCs and identified phosphorylated CD20 as an influx channel involved in this $Ca^{2+}$ elevation.[8,9] $Ca^{2+}$ / calmodulin-dependent protein kinase II may be responsible for the CD20 phosphorylation and for the maintenance of $Ca^{2+}$ influx.[9] Interestingly, HC treatment with α interferon reduced CD20 phosphorylation and the cytosolic $Ca^{2+}$ level,[10] and the authors suggested that this might be a part of the mechanism of the therapeutic action of this agent in HCL.

Increased expression of Src and high protein tyrosine kinase activity in HCs have also been recognized for some time.[11] More recently, it was demonstrated that Src-dependent tyrosine phosphorylation is responsible for downstream activation of many other signaling components, including Rho GTPases,[12] PKCs, and MAP kinases.[13] Rac and Cdc42, the two constitutively active Rho GTPases in HCs, are responsible for the distinctive morphological features of these malignant cells,[12] as well as for their adhesive and motile behavior on different substrates.[14] In addition to regulating cytoskeletal dynamics, Rac and Cdc42 are also likely to be involved in the activation of MAPKs.[15]

PKC(s) involvement in activation of HCs has long been suspected, as other B cells treated with phorbol esters acquire HC-like morphology and TRAP expression. More recent work has revealed the presence in HCs of at least six PKC isoforms, of which only PKCα was consistently found to be strongly constitutively active.[13] Furthermore, PKCs were found to be crucially involved in the regulation of MAPKs in HCs. Thus, HC incubation with PKC inhibitors caused a rapid four-fold increase in p38 MAP kinase activation and an equally rapid downregulation of constitutive ERK activity.[13] This was followed by pronounced shortening of cell survival, a finding in accordance with the proposed central role of the balance between activations of cytoprotective ERK and pro-apoptotic p38/JNK in the regulation of cell survival.[16]

HCs produce large amount of TNF and possess both TNFR1 and TNFR2.[17,18] Autocrine TNFα increases cell survival,[19] but in the presence of αIFN this pro-survival effect is converted to a pro-apoptotic one.[20] This cell killing is brought about by IFN-induced suppression of IAP (inhibitors of apoptosis) production regulated by the NFκB-dependent arm of TNF signaling. HC adhesion to vitronectin and fibronectin stimulates IAP production that is not inhibited by αIFN, and can therefore provide relative protection of HCs from this IFN-induced, TNF-mediated killing.[20]

Thus, intrinsic activation of malignant HCs is highly relevant for both pathogenesis and therapy of HCL. Therefore, studies of the signaling pathways involved may suggest new therapies, and may give some insight into the elusive nature of the primary oncogenic event(s) responsible for the intrinsic activation and developmental arrest of HCs.

### ADHESION RECEPTORS

HCs are highly adherent and, on some substrates, spontaneously motile cells. This indicates that receptors involved in the adhesion and motility of these cells are constitutively activated. This conclusion is supported by the demonstration that HCs readily interact

| Table 29.5 | Expression and function of HC adhesion receptors | |
| --- | --- | --- |
| Integrins | (CD) | Possible functions |
| **Adhesion receptors** | | |
| $\alpha_4\beta_1$ | (49d/29) | Involved in binding to matrix (fibronectin, FN) and accessory cells via CD106 (VCAM) |
| $\alpha_5\beta_1$ | (49e/29) | Involved, together with $\alpha_4\beta_1$ in binding to, and assembly of, FN matrix |
| $\alpha_M\beta_2$ | (11b/18) | Weakly expressed. Constitutes a monocytic feature of HCs and may be involved in endocytosis |
| $\alpha_x\beta_2$ | (11c/18) | Diagnostically important. Receptor for a number of ligands, including ICAM-1 (CD54), but function in HCs unclear |
| $\alpha_v\beta_3$ | (51/61) | Receptor for vitronectin (VN) and PECAM-1 (CD31). Important in HC motility |
| $\alpha_E\beta_7$ | (103/b$_7$) | Diagnostically important. Receptor for E cadherin, but function in HCL unclear |
| **Other adhesion receptors** | | |
| CD44 | | Highly expressed. HC receptor for hyaluronan. Several isoforms expressed (VH3, V3, V6). CD44H signals for FGF-2 (bFGF) production; V3 (heparan sulphate-containing isoform) acts as a co-receptor with FGFR-1 for stimulation of HC FN production by FGF-2 |
| L-selectin | (62L) | Little or no expression. Shed on cell activation |

**Table 29.6    Cytokines produced by HCs**

| Cytokine | Receptors on HCs | Comment |
|---|---|---|
| TNF-α | TNFRI and RII present | Involved in HC survival and response to IFN therapy |
| IL-6 | Present | Production may be induced by TNF. May participate in the proliferative effects of TNF |
| IL-10 | Not studied | Suppresses TH1 cytokine production |
| GM-CSF | Receptor present | Prolongs the survival of HCs and inhibits their motility |
| M-CSF | Receptor present | Stimulates chemokinesis and chemotaxis of HCs |
| bFGF | Both FGFR1 and CD44v3 co-receptor present | Involved in FN production by HA-adherent HCs. May stimulate increased angiogenesis in HCL bone marrow |
| TGFβ | Not studied | Elevated in HCL serum and BM. May be involved in suppression of the production and function of normal hematological cells, and stimulates BM fibroblasts to produce the collagen component of reticulin fibrosis |
| IFNα | Receptor present | Induces HC apoptosis in the absence of cell adhesion and may induce autocrine production of TNF |

with a number of extracellular matrix (ECM) components including fibronectin (FN), vitronectin (VN), and hyaluronan (HA) (see Table 29.5). On FN, HCs firmly adhere and assume a spread morphology, whereas on VN and HA they display polarized morphology and pronounced motility.[14,21] This spectrum of behavior is likely to reflect both differences in the interaction of various adhesion receptors with the activated cortical cytoskeleton, as well as differences in signals generated by these receptors upon ligand binding. With regard to their interaction with FN, HCs are unique among B cells because of their ability to synthesize this protein and also to assemble it into matrix,[22] in a process that requires FN binding to activated $\alpha_5\beta_1$ integrin.[23,24]

### AUTOCRINE CYTOKINES

Pathogenetically relevant cytokines produced by HCs and their autocrine and paracrine effects are summarized in Table 29.6. Among these, TNF, IL-6 and GM-CSF have been reported to promote HC survival/proliferation,[25–27] while GM- and M-CSF affect malignant-cell adhesion / motility.[28,29] HCs also produce bFGF, TGFβ, and IL-10, which are involved in processes by which HCs modify extracellular and cellular components of their microenvironment. Thus, bFGF and TGFβ are respectively involved in the stimulation of FN production by HCs and of collagen by fibroblasts.[30,31] Moreover, TGFβ can inhibit normal hematopoiesis and also, together with IL-10, suppress the immune functions of T cells and monocytes.[32,33]

In addition to responding to autocrine cytokines, HCs possess a number of receptors for cytokines produced by other cells. Thus, IL-1 is known to upregulate the surface expression of Ig and PCA-1 antigen by HCs,[34] while IL-4 and IL-15, alone or in synergy with other growth factors, stimulate the cells to synthesize DNA.[35] HCs also possess IL-2 and IL-3 receptors;

expression of the IL-2 receptor (CD25) is of diagnostic importance, but no functional effects of either IL-2 or IL-3 have so far been demonstrated.

In summary, cytokines play a part in most, if not all, pathogenetically important reactions of HCs, including their clonal expansion, their distinctive tissue homing and their influence on both cellular and extracellular components of the invaded tissues. This ultimately results in the suppression of both normal hematopoiesis and immunity—the two most damaging aspects of the disease.

## PATHOLOGY

The principal distinctive pathological features of HCL (Table 29.7) have been known for more than 20 years, but their pathogenesis has only recently started to be defined. Thus, the cell-signaling and gene-expression studies described above have now largely elucidated the causes of the unusual morphology of HCs. Also, investigations of the expression and function of adhesion receptors, together with the identification of pathogenetically important cytokines, have provided data that could explain the predilection of HCs for homing

**Table 29.7    Key pathological feature of HCL**

- Pathognomonic HC
- TRAP expression by HCs
- BM infiltration and fibrosis
- Invasion of splenic red pulp and pseudosinus formation
- Hepatic infiltration with sinusoidal and portal tract involvement
- Lymph nodes relatively spared
- Cytopenias (especially monocytopenia), T-cell dysfunction and immune defect

to bone marrow, spleen and liver, while largely sparing other lymphoreticular sites.

## CYTOLOGY AND (IMMUNO)CYTOCHEMISTRY OF HAIRY CELLS

In stained films of blood and bone marrow, HCs appear as distinctive large cells (15–30 μm in diameter) with abundant light-blue cytoplasm and peripheral hair-like protrusions. The nucleus is usually eccentric and has relatively open chromatin with inconspicuous nucleoli. HCs are unique among hemic cells in displaying strong cytoplasmic staining for tartrate-resistant acid phosphatase. Both the surface appearance and TRAP positivity of HCs are the result of the intrinsic activation described earlier.

As at the level of the light microscope, the ultrastructure of HCs corresponds to that of highly metabolically active cells. Thus, HCs display only modest peripheral nuclear chromatin condensation and possess abundant cytoplasm with plentiful mitochondria and frequent ribosomes. A relatively specific ultrastructural feature is the presence of ribosome–lamellar complexes in a variable proportion of cells (Fig. 29.1). Although these structures were described many years ago,[36] their nature and functions are still unclear. HCs contain a large amount of F-actin, which supports the prominent surface ruffles and microvilli best seen by scanning electron microscopy (Fig. 29.2).

Recent studies have identified a number of molecules which, by interacting with F-actin, may be involved in the generation of the hairy appearance of the malignant cells. These include pp52 (LSP-1), Gas-7, and EPB4.1L2—recently found by gene microarray analysis to be overexpressed in HCs (Table 29.3).[4] pp52 has been previously found to be abundant in the F-actin-rich protrusions of HCs,[37] while, by interacting

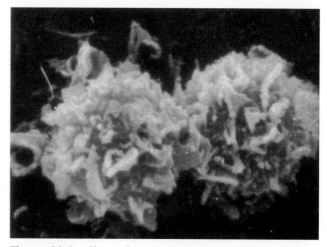

**Figure 29.2** *The surface structure of HCs. This scanning electron micrograph shows the surface of two adjacent HCs. Note the distinctive mixture of surface ruffles and microvilli*

with F-actin, ectopically expressed Gas 7 induces excessive surface projections and dramatic changes in cell shape.[38] EPB4.1L2 is also involved in the regulation of cell shape through interaction with β-actin underneath the plasma membrane.[4]

In addition to possessing a unique morphology, HCs are unusual among lymphoid cells in displaying a spectrum of features normally associated with monocytes and macrophages. HCs are able to phagocytose a range of particles and microorganisms,[39] a property that has recently been linked to the specific upregulation of annexin A1, CD68, and a novel serine carboxypeptidase CPVL which was first identified in macrophages.[40] Although the expression of CD11c is possibly an activation feature of HCs and is also found on certain other lymphoid cell types, this integrin α chain, together with CD63, is commonly regarded as a macrophage marker. In addition, HCs have been shown to overexpress c-Maf, a transcription factor linked to macrophage differentiation.[41] Finally, overexpression or underexpression by HCs of a number of genes outlined in Table 29.3 could be relevant for the unusual tissue distribution of HCs and for the matrix remodeling by the malignant cells that are such distinctive features of HCL.

### BONE MARROW

The bone marrow (BM) is variably infiltrated by widely spaced HCs surrounded by clear areas, which impart a halo appearance. This loose packing probably reflects cell spreading on the altered ECM and has been likened to a fried-egg appearance.[42] This appearance is also seen when HCs adhere to FN-coated surfaces in vitro.[43]

In the BM microenvironment, the FN component of the distinctive reticulin fibrosis is largely, if not exclusively, synthesized by HCs themselves.[22,30] As mentioned above, adhesion receptors, together with autocrine bFGF, play a key role in this matrix remodeling. It has been demonstrated that in BM and hepatic

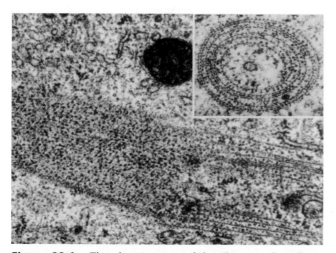

**Figure 29.1** *The ultrastructure of the ribosome–lamellar complex. In the lower right part of this electron micrograph, the R–L complex is sectioned longitudinally, while on the left the complex is cut obliquely. The inset shows the complex in transverse section. In three dimensions, the R–L complex probably resembles a coiled roll of chicken wire*

portal tracts adhesion to hyaluronan via the standard hematopoietic form of CD44 stimulates HCs to secrete bFGF.[30] This bFGF binds to both FGFR1 and CD44v3 on HCs and stimulates them to produce FN.[30] Secreted FN is then assembled into a matrix by a process involving $\alpha_5\beta_1$ FN receptors on the malignant cells.[22] The importance of HA for the initiation of this process is indicated by the absence of fibrosis in the infiltrated red pulp of the spleen, which does not contain HA.

### SPLEEN

The spleen is usually the major site of HC infiltration. The malignant cells accumulate in the red pulp, while the white pulp of the enlarged spleen is greatly reduced. Within the sinuses of the red pulp, the HCs have a propensity to replace the endothelium and to remodel the sinuses so that they enlarge, forming the vascular lakes or pseudosinuses pathognomonic of the disease.[42] The mechanism of splenic homing is likely to involve HC interaction with endothelium and also, via $\alpha_V\beta_3$ integrin, with VN present in the spleen.[43] The candidate chemoattractant to the red pulp is M-CSF produced by macrophages,[29] while the likely first step in vascular remodeling is HC interaction with endothelial cells via $\alpha_4\beta_1$-to-VCAM binding.[44] This is followed by replacement of endothelial linings by HCs in a process that may involve $\alpha_V\beta_3$-mediated movement of HCs in between and underneath endothelium. The likely binding partners of $\alpha_V\beta_3$ during this process could be PECAM on endothelial cells and VN on basement membranes. The tendency of HCs to remain confined to the vascular spaces of the red pulp could possibly be explained by the reduced or absent expression of the chemokine receptors CCR5 and CXCR4, and by upregulation of the metalloproteinase inhibitors TIMP-1, TIMP-4 and RECK (Table 29.3).[4] This could severely limit or abolish the ability of HCs to receive stimuli for exit from the red pulp and to employ metalloproteinases to traverse basement membranes and invade other compartments of the spleen.

### LIVER

Hepatic infiltration by HCs is a constant feature of HCL, but the organ is usually not markedly enlarged, and its general architecture remains intact. Both sinusoids and portal tracts are involved. In the sinusoids, the HCs may lie free within the lumen or be closely associated with the endothelium and adjacent hepatocytes.[6] In the portal tracts, the infiltrate is associated with marked fibrosis. This fibrosis is likely to involve the same mechanisms as described for BM.[30]

### LYMPH NODES

Although clinical lymphadenopathy is uncommon in HCL, at postmortem some lymph node involvement is usually found. The infiltration is paracortical and at least some follicles are usually preserved.[42] This relative sparing of lymph nodes may be the result of low or absent L-selectin (CD62L)[7] and CCR7.[4]

In advanced disease, prominent upper abdominal lymphadenopathy may occur. The infiltrating HCs are larger and of more immature appearance than typical HCs, suggesting that such node enlargement is a consequence of disease transformation.[45]

### OTHER BLOOD CELLS

At presentation, most patients have evidence of suppressed hematopoiesis. Abnormalities of monocytes, T cells, NK cells, dendritic cells, platelets, and neutrophils have all been described in HCL.[6,46] Among these, the monocytopenia of the disease and altered T-cell function have attracted particular attention because of their potential contribution to the marked immune deficiency present in active disease.

The cause of the almost complete absence of circulating monocytes remains unclear. It has been proposed that reduction in antigen presentation, as a result of monocytopenia and reduced numbers of dentritic cells, is partly responsible for the defective immune responses in HCL. However, since tissue macrophages are plentiful,[6] abnormalities of T cells and of their interactions with antigen-presenting cells seem to be of a greater importance. T-cell abnormalities include both quantitative and qualitative defects. Overall T-cell numbers are often reduced, the CD4[+] / CD8[+] cell ratio is reversed, and the percentage of $\gamma\delta$ T cells is frequently increased.[47–49] Moreover, the response of T cells to alloantigens in mixed lymphocyte cultures is grossly abnormal.[48,49] This abnormality has been attributed to reduced or absent CD28 expression on a large proportion of CD4[+], as well as CD8[+] cells.[49] Among CD4[+] T cells, CD45RO[+] memory cells are grossly reduced.[50]

Studies of the T-cell receptor (TCR) in HCL have demonstrated oligoclonality in most patients, with a markedly skewed repertoire of TCRβV genes.[51] Moreover, some gene segments of the normal repertoire were absent from the T cells of HCL.[49,52] Interestingly, αIFN treatment leads to both the disappearance of the selected clones and to a gradual full restoration of the normal TCR repertoire,[52] suggesting a direct influence of the malignant cells on T-cell development in HCL. Some of the apparently expanded clones are found to recognize antigens overexpressed by (but not necessarily specific to) HCs, as is the case with overexpressed synaptojanin 2.[53] However, T cells that were found to be clonally expanded in HCL seem to have no cytotoxic effect on the malignant cells,[54] and therefore are unlikely to have a beneficial effect on disease progression.

Thus, although abnormalities of the immune system in HCL have over the years received considerable attention, many questions regarding the immunobiology of the disease remain to be answered. It should be pointed out, however, that the clinical importance of the immune system dysfunction in HCL has been significantly reduced by the current successful early therapy of the disease.

## CYTOGENETICS

The most important aspects of the cytogenetics of HCL are given in Table 29.8. Although many karyotypic abnormalities have been described,[55] none are specific and none are consistently found in all HCL patients. Therefore, karyotypic analysis has not yet given any insight into the primary oncogenic event(s) responsible for the disease.

As pointed out by Basso et al.,[4] HCs and CLL cells, unlike other malignant B cells, typically lack reciprocal balanced chromosomal translocations. Since these translocations are generated during Ig VDJ recombination, class switching and somatic hypermutation, their absence supports the proposition that both HCL and CLL are malignancies of mature memory B cells in which these processes are switched off.

HCL was the first hematological malignancy analyzed by comparative expressed sequence hybridization (CESH) to chromosomes.[56] This showed a consistent expression profile of different chromosome regions that carry a "splenic signature," along with HC-specific under-or overexpressed regions.[56] Moreover, these regions contained many genes which had also been found to be differentially expressed by gene-array analysis,[4] and which encode proteins of potential pathogenetic importance (Tables 29.2 and 29.3). However, neither cytogenetics nor gene-expression analysis have yet identified abnormalities common to all HCL cases that could explain the remarkable homogeneity of the disease, and at the same time provide clues concerning the events responsible for malignant transformation and maturational arrest of HCs.

| Table 29.8 Cytogenetics of HCL |
|---|
| • No consistent or specific cytogenetic abnormality |
| • Absence of translocations suggests malignant transformation of post-GC-type cells |
| • Most frequent recurrent abnormalities involve chromosomes 5(trisomy 5, 5q13 aberrations) and 14 (add (14)q(32) and del(14)(q) |
| • A range of other structural and numerical abnormalities of a number of chromosomes reported |
| • CESH profiling showed a uniform pattern of over- and underexpression of chromosome regions consistent with gene expression profiles established by DNA microarray analysis |
| • Uniform clinicopathological, DNA microarray and CESH profiles suggest that none of the described cytogenetic abnormalities play a primary pathogenetic role |

## REFERENCES

1. Forconi F, Sahota SS, Raspadori D, et al.: Tumor cells of hairy cell leukemia express multiple clonally related immunoglobulin isotypes via RNA splicing. *Blood* 98:1174, 2001.

2. Maloum K, Magnac C, Azgui Z, et al.: VH gene expression in hairy cell leukaemia. *Br J Haematol* 101:171, 1998.

3. Anderson KC, Boyd AW, Fisher DC, et al.: Hairy cell leukemia: a tumor of pre-plasma cells. *Blood* 65:620, 1985.

4. Basso K, Liso A, Tiacci E, et al.: Gene expression profiling of hairy cell leukemia reveals a phenotype related to memory B cells with altered expression of chemokine and adhesion receptors. *J Exp Med* 199:59, 2004.

5. van Der Vuurst De Vries AR, Logtenberg T: A phage antibody identifying an 80-kDa membrane glycoprotein exclusively expressed on a subpopulation of activated B cells and hairy cell leukemia B cells. *Eur J Immunol* 29:3898, 1999.

6. Burthem J, Cawley JC: *Hairy-Cell Leukaemia*. Berlin: Springer-Verlag; 1996.

7. Zuzel M, Cawley JC: The biology of hairy cells. *Best Pract Res Clin Haematol* Mar, 16:1, 2003.

8. Genot E, Bismuth G, Degos L, et al.: Interferon-alpha downregulates the abnormal intracytoplasmic free calcium concentration of tumor cells in hairy cell leukemia. *Blood* 80:2060, 1992.

9. Genot EM, Meier KE, Licciardi KA, et al.: Phosphorylation of CD20 in cells from a hairy cell leukemia cell line. Evidence for involvement of calcium/calmodulin-dependent protein kinase II. *J Immunol* 151:71, 1993.

10. Genot E: Interferon alpha and intracytoplasmic free calcium in hairy cell leukemia cells. *Leuk Lymphoma* 12:373, 1994.

11. Lynch SA, Bvrugge JS, Fromowitz F, et al.: Increased expression of the src proto-onocgene in hairy cell leukemia and a subgroup of B-cell lymphomas. *Leukemia* 7:1416, 1993.

12. Zhang X, Machii T, Matsumura I, et al.: Constitutively activated Rho guanosine triphosphatases regulate the growth and morphology of hairy cell leukemia cells. *Int J Hematol* 77:263, 2003.

13. Kamiguti AS, Harris RJ, Slupsky JR, et al.: Regulation of hairy-cell survival through constitutive activation of mitogen-activated protein kinase pathways. *Oncogene* 22:2272, 2003.

14. Burthem J, Baker PK, Hunt JA, et al.: Hairy cell interactions with extracellular matrix: expression of specific integrin receptors and their role in the cell's response to specific adhesive proteins. *Blood* 84:873, 1994.

15. Lim L, Manser E, Leung T, et al.: Regulation of phosphorylation pathways by p21 GTPases. The p21 Ras-related Rho subfamily and its role in phosphorylation signalling pathways. *Eur J Biochem* 242:171, 1996.

16. Xia Z, Dickens M, Raingeaud J, et al.: Opposing effects of ERK and JNK-p38 MAP kinases on apoptosis. *Science* 270:1326, 1995.

17. Foa R, Guarini A, Francia di Celle P, et al.: Constitutive production of tumor necrosis factor-alpha in hairy cell leukemia: possible role in the pathogenesis of the cytopenia(s) and effect of treatment with interferon-alpha. *J Clin Oncol* 10:954, 1992.

18. Trentin L, Zambello R, Agostini C, et al.: Expression and functional role of tumor necrosis factor receptors on leukemic cells from patients with type B chronic lymphoproliferative disorders. *Blood* 81:752, 1993.

19. Schmid M, Porzsolt F: Autocrine and paracrine regulation of neoplastic cell growth in hairy cell leukemia. *Leuk Lymphoma* 17:401, 1995.

20. Baker PK, Pettitt AR, Slupsky JR, et al.: Response of hairy cells to IFN-alpha involves induction of apoptosis through autocrine TNF-alpha and protection by adhesion. *Blood* 100:647, 2002.

21. Aziz KA, Till KJ, Zuzel M, et al.: Involvement of CD44-hyaluronan interaction in malignant cell homing and fibronectin synthesis in hairy cell leukemia. *Blood* 96:3161, 2000.

22. Burthem J, Cawley JC: The bone marrow fibrosis of hairy-cell leukemia is caused by the synthesis and assembly of a fibronectin matrix by the hairy cells. *Blood* 83:497, 1994.

23. Wu C, Keivens VM, O'Toole TE, et al.: Integrin activation and cytoskeletal interaction are essential for the assembly of a fibronectin matrix. *Cell* 83:715, 1995.

24. Pankov R, Cukierman E, Katz BZ, et al.: Integrin dynamics and matrix assembly: tensin-dependent translocation of alpha(5) beta (1) integrins promotes early fibronectin fibrillogenesis. *J Cell Biol* 148:1075, 2000.

25. Schiller JH, Bittner G, Spriggs DR: Tumor necrosis factor, but not other hematopoietic growth factors, prolongs the survival of hairy cell leukemia cells. *Leuk Res* 16:337, 1992.

26. Barut B, Chauhan D, Uchiyama H, et al.: Interleukin-6 functions as an intracellular growth factor in hairy cell leukemia in vitro. *J Clin Invest* 92:2346, 1993.

27. Harris RJ, Pettitt AR, Schmutz C, et al.: Granulocyte-macrophage colony-stimulating factor as an autocrine survival factor for mature normal and malignant B lymphocytes. *J Immunol* 164:3887, 2000.

28. Till KJ, Burthem J, Lopez A, et al.: Granulocyte-macrophage colony-stimulating factor receptor: stage-specific expression and function on late B cells. *Blood* 88:479, 1996.

29. Burthem J, Baker PK, Hunt JA, et al.: The function of c-fms in hairy-cell leukemia: macrophage colony-stimulating factor stimulates hairy-cell movement. *Blood* 83:1381, 1994.

30. Aziz KA, Till KJ, Chen H, et al.: The role of autocrine FGF-2 in the distinctive bone marrow fibrosis of hairy-cell leukaemia (HCL). *Blood* 102:1051, 2003.

31. Shehata M, Schwarzmeier JD, Hilgarth M, et al.: TGF-beta 1 induces bone marrow reticulin fibrosis in hairy cell leukemia. *J Clin Invest* 113:676, 2004.

32. Beck C, Schreiber H, Rowley D: Role of TGF-beta in immune-evasion of cancer. *Microsc Res Tech* 52:387, 2001.

33. Prud'homme GJ, Piccirillo CA: The inhibitory effects of transforming growth factor-beta-1 (TGF-beta 1) in autoimmune diseases. *J Autoimmun* 14:23, 2000.

34. Takeuchi H, Katayama I: Interleukin 1 (IL-1 alpha and IL-1 beta) induces differentiation/activation of B cell chronic lymphoid leukemia cells. *Cytokine* 6:243, 1994.

35. Barut BA, Cochran MK, O'Hara C, et al.: Response patterns of hairy cell leukemia to B-cell mitogens and growth factors. *Blood* 76:2091, 1990.

36. Katayama I, Nagy GK, Balogh K Jr: Light microscopic identification of the ribosome-lamella complex in "hairy cells" of leukemic reticuloendotheliosis. *Cancer* 32:843, 1973.

37. Miyoshi EK, Stewart PL, Kincade PW, et al.: Aberrant expression and localisation of the cytoskeleton-binding pp52 (LSP1) protein in hairy cell leukemia. *Leuk Res* 25:57, 2001.

38. She BR, Liou GG, Lin-Chao S: Association of the growth-arrest-specific protein Gas7 with F-actin induces reorganisation of microfilaments and promotes membrane outgrowth. *Exp Cell Res* 273:34, 2002.

39. Rosner MC, Golomb HM: Phagocytic capacity of hairy cells from seventeen patients. *Virchows Arch B Cell Pathol Incl Mol Pathol* 40:327, 1982.

40. Mahoney JA, Ntolosi B, DaSilva RP, et al.: Cloning and characterisation of CPVL, a novel serine carboxypeptidase, from human macrophages. *Genomics* 72:243, 2001.

41. Hegde SP, Zhao J, Ashmun RA, et al.: c-Maf induces monocytic differentiation and apoptosis in bipotent myeloid progenitors. *Blood* 94:1578, 1999.

42. Bethel KJ, Sharpe RW: Pathology of hairy-cell leukaemia. *Best Pract Res Clin Haematol* 16:15, 2003.

43. Burthem J, Vincent A, Cawley JC: Integrin receptors and hairy cell leukaemia. *Leuk Lymphoma* 21:211, 1996.

44. Vincent AM, Burthem J, Brew R, et al.: Endothelial interactions of hairy cells: the importance of alpha 4 beta 1 in the unusual tissue distribution of the disorder. *Blood* 88:3945, 1996.

45. Mercieca J, Matutes E, Moskovic E, et al.: Massive abdominal lymphadenopathy in hairy cell leukaemia: a report of 12 cases. *Br J Haematol* 82:547, 1992.

46. Kraut EH: Clinical manifestations and infectious complications of hairy-cell leukaemia. *Best Pract Res Clin Haematol* 16:33, 2003.

47. Kluin-Nelemans JC, Kester MG Oving I, et al.: Abnormally activated T lymphocytes in the spleen of patients with hairy-cell leukemia. *Leukemia* 8:2095, 1994.

48. Van De Corput L, Falkenburg JH, Kluin-Nelemans JC: T-cell dysfunction in hairy cell leukemia: an updated review. *Leuk Lymphoma* 30:31, 1998.

49. Van de Corput L, Falkenburg JH, Kester MG, et al.: Impaired expression of CD28 on T cells in hairy cell leukemia. *Clin Immunol* 93:256, 1999.

50. Van der Horst FA, van der Marel A, den Ottolander GJ, et al.: Decrease of memory T helper cells (CD4+ CD45R0+) in hairy cell leukemia. *Leukemia* 7:46, 1993.

51. Kluin-Nelemans JC, Kester MG, Melenhorst JJ, et al.: Persistent clonal excess and skewed T-cell repertoire in T cells from patients with hairy cell leukemia. *Blood* 87:3795, 1996.

52. Kluin-Nelemans HC, Kester MG, van de Corput L, et al.: Correction of abnormal T-cell receptor repertoire during interferon-alpha therapy in patients with hairy cell leukemia. *Blood* 91:4224, 1998.

53. Spaenij-Dekking EH, Van Delft J, Van Der Meijden E, et al.: Synaptojanin 2 is recognised by HLA class II-restricted hairy cell leukemia-specific T cells. *Leukemia* 17:2467, 2003.

54. Spaenij-Dekking EH, Van der Meiijden ED, Falkenburg JH, et al.: Clonally expanded T cells in hairy cell leukemia patients are not leukemia specific. *Leukemia* 18:176, 2004.

55. Sambani C, Trafalis DT, Mitsoulis-Mentzikoff C, et al.: Clonal chromosome rearrangements in hairy cell leukemia: personal experience and review of literature. *Cancer Genet Cytogenet* 129:138, 2001.

56. Vanhentenrijk V, De Wolf-Peeters C, Wlodarska I: Comparative expressed sequence hybridization studies of hairy cell leukemia show uniform expression profile and imprint of spleen signature. *Blood* 104:250, 2004.

# Chapter 30

# CLINICAL FEATURES AND MAKING THE DIAGNOSIS OF HCL

## Olga Frankfurt, Martin S. Tallman, and LoAnn C. Peterson

## CLINICAL PRESENTATION

Hairy cell leukemia (HCL) is a rare chronic lymphoproliferative disorder, characterized by circulating B lymphocytes displaying prominent cytoplasmic projections and infiltrating the bone marrow and the spleen. The disease was first described as a distinct clinicopathologic entity in 1958 by Bourouncle et al., who referred to the disorder as "leukemic reticuloendotheliosis".[1] The descriptive term "hairy cell leukemia" was suggested by Schrek and Donnely in 1966.[2]

The typical patient is a Caucasian middle-aged man, presenting with splenomegaly, pancytopenia, and occasionally recurrent infections. Circulating hairy cells are usually present in the peripheral blood.[3]

### LABORATORY FINDINGS

Although the majority of patients are generally well at the time of diagnosis, some present with symptoms related to anemia, neutropenia, or thrombocytopenia (Table 30.1). Pancytopenia is present in approximately half of the patients, and the remaining half usually exhibit a combination of cytopenias. In a series of 102 patients with HCL, 86 had anemia, 84 had thrombocytopenia, and 78 were neutropenic at the time of diagnosis.[4] Approximately 25% of patients report weakness and fatigue, 25% suffer from opportunistic infections in the setting of neutropenia, and another quarter have easy bruising from thrombocytopenia. About 25% of patients are incidentally discovered to have splenomegaly or an abnormal peripheral blood count, at the time of evaluation for an unrelated condition.[5]

Coagulopathy, manifested by TTP and anti-factor VIII antibodies and paraproteinemia have been reported in patients with HCL.[6,7]

### PHYSICAL FINDINGS

Splenomegaly is present in 80–90% of patients with HCL. The spleen is frequently massive, and palpable at

| Table 30.1 | Clinical features of hairy-cell leukemia |
|---|---|
| *Clinical symptoms* | |
| Fatigue | 25% |
| Repeated infections | 25% |
| *Abnormal findings on physical examination* | |
| Splenomegaly | 80–90% |
| Hepatomegaly | 20–35% |
| Lymphadenopathy | 25% |
| *Laboratory abnormalities* | |
| Circulating hairy cells | 90% |
| Pancytopenia | 70% |
| Anemia | 80% |
| Thrombocytopenia | 70–80% |
| Neutropenia | 80% |
| Leukemic phase | 20% |
| Liver function abnormalities | 20% |
| Azotemia | 27% |
| Hypergammaglobulinemia | 18% |
| *Other findings* | |
| Osteolytic bone lesions | 3% |
| Autoimmune diseases | rare |

least 5 cm below the left costal margin in approximately 60% of patients.[8] Early satiety or abdominal fullness caused by splenomegaly is present is 25% of patients at diagnosis.[5]

Hepatomegaly, rarely a significant finding, is present in 20% of patients. Unlike many other lymphoproliferative disorders, peripheral adenopathy is uncommon at diagnosis, with fewer than 10% of patients having lymph nodes larger than 2 cm. However, with the advent of computed tomography and other diagnostic imaging modalities, significant internal adenopathy can be demonstrated in about 30% of patients. Although not common at diagnosis, internal lymphadenopathy may develop after a prolonged disease course[9] and is present in 75% of patients at autopsy.[10] Such characteristic localization of HCL is likely due to the expression of the integrin receptor, α4β1, by the hairy cells and its interaction with the vascular adhesion molecule-1 (VCAM-1) found on splenic and hepatic endothelia, bone marrow, and splenic stroma.[11]

Spontaneous splenic rupture, spinal cord compression with paralysis due to neuronal infiltration by leukemic cells, protein-losing enteropathy from bowel infiltration by leukemic cells, esophageal perforation, uveitis, serous and chylous ascites, and pleural and pericardial effusion have been described in patients with HCL.[12–14]

### INFECTIOUS COMPLICATIONS

Significant neutropenia and monocytopenia predispose patients with HCL to infections from a wide variety of typical and opportunistic organisms.[15] Infections with *Mycobacterium kansasii*, *Pneumocystis carinii*, aspergillus, histoplasma, cryptococcus, *Listeria monocytogene*, and *Toxoplasma gondii* have been described.[15–17] In addition to neutropenia and monocytopenia, the milieu making patients susceptible to infections includes T-cell dysfunction, decreased numbers of dendritic and antigen-presenting cells, as well as impaired interferon production by mononuclear cells.[18–21]

### ASSOCIATION WITH AUTOIMMUNE PHENOMENA

The association between HCL and autoimmune disorders such as scleroderma, polymyositis, Raynaud's phenomenon, and various vasculitis, has been described.[22,23] Among the vasculopathic syndromes polyarteritis nodosa represents the most frequently associated disorder, with 18 cases reported so far. It has been suggested that a common membrane antigen expressed in leukemia cells and vascular endothelium may lead to a vasculitis by generating cross-reacting antibody.[24] Four cases of scleroderma in the setting of HCL have been reported.[25–27] It has been postulated that sarcoidosis may be induced directly through hairy cell antigen-mediated activation of T cells or indirectly through promotion of the nonspecific inflamatory response.[27] The presence of cutaneous lesions, such as erythematous maculopapules and pyoderma gangrenosum, have been noted in patients with HCL.[28–30]

### BONE LESIONS

About 3% of patients with HCL present with painful bony lesions, most commonly involving the proximal femur. Diffuse osteoporosis, focal and diffuse osteosclerosis, as well as lytic lesions of the skeleton have been described in patients with HCL. Patients who suffer from such skeletal complications tend to have higher tumor burden, with the marrow being diffusely infiltrated by hairy cells.[31–33]

## DIAGNOSIS

The initial evaluation of a patient with HCL includes a history and physical examination, a complete blood count with differential count, review of the peripheral blood smear, routine serum electrolytes, blood urea nitrogen and creatinine, hepatic transaminases, a bone marrow aspirate and core biopsy, and immunophenotyping by flow cytometry of peripheral blood or bone marrow aspirate.

### HISTOPATHOLOGY
#### Peripheral blood and bone marrow
Hairy cells can be identified in Wright's-stained blood smears from almost all patients with HCL, although the number of circulating hairy cells is usually low. The bone marrow is often inaspirable, resulting in a "dry tap". However, when aspiration is successful, hairy cells are morphologically similar to those in the blood.

The morphologic features of hairy cells are distinctive, Figure 30.1(a). They are approximately one to two

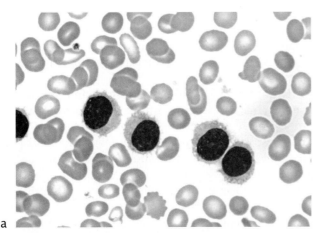
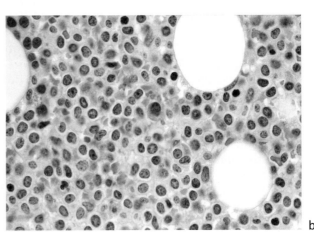

a                                                                          b

**Figure 30.1** *(a) Peripheral smear of a patient with hairy-cell leukemia, demonstrating classic feature of the hairy cells, including bean-shaped nucleus, homogenous, ground-glass chromatin, and abundant pale blue cytoplasm with "hairy" projections. Presence of leukocytosis is atypical for HCL. (b) Bone marrow trephine biopsy of a patient with hairy-cell leukemia, showing diffuse infiltration of hairy cells with abundant pale cytoplasm*

times the size of a small lymphocyte, with nuclei that appear round, oval, indented, monocytoid, and occasionally convoluted.[34] The chromatin pattern is net-like in appearance and nucleoli are indistinct or absent. The amount of cytoplasm varies from scant to abundant and is pale blue-gray in color. The cytoplasmic borders are irregular and exhibit fine, hair-like projections or irregular borders. Occasionally, cytoplasmic granules are present. Examination of the bone marrow biopsy is important in the diagnosis of HCL because of its characteristic histopathology.[35–38] In most patients, the bone marrow is hypercellular, although the cellularity may be normal or decreased, Figure 30.1(b). Hairy cell infiltration is diffuse, patchy, or interstitial, or a combination of these patterns. In patients with diffuse involvement, large areas of the bone marrow are replaced by hairy cells, with complete effacement of marrow in some patients. With patchy infiltration, subtle, small clusters of hairy cells are present focally or scattered throughout the bone marrow. Unlike most lymphomas, the hairy cells do not form well-defined, discrete aggregates; instead, they merge subtly with the surrounding residual hematopoietic tissue. In the interstitial pattern of involvement, variable numbers of hairy cells infiltrate between normal hematopoietic cells and fat, leaving the overall bone marrow architecture preserved. Hairy-cell nuclei in sections are round, oval, or indented and typically are widely separated from each other by abundant, clear, or lightly eosinophilic cytoplasm; rarely, the cells are convoluted or spindle shaped, Figure 30.2(a). The nuclear chromatin is lightly condensed, nucleoli are inconspicuous, and mitotic figures are rare or absent. Extravasated red blood cells are often observed. Reticulin stains of the bone marrow trephine biopsy in HCL show a moderate to marked increase in reticulin fibers, Figure 30.2(b). Normal hematopoietic cells are usually decreased in HCL, with granulocytes being typically more severely reduced than erythroid precursors and megakary-

ocytes. In about 10–20% of patients with HCL, the bone marrow is hypocellular. The hypocellularity may be severe and may strongly resemble aplastic anemia.[39]

### Spleen and other sites

The spleen in patients with HCL is usually enlarged, with a median weight of 1300 g.[40] Splenic involvement in HCL is characterized by diffuse infiltration of the red pulp cords and sinuses, with atrophy or replacement of the white pulp. Blood-filled sinuses, referred to as "pseudosinuses", lined by hairy cells, are often present, but are not pathognomonic of HCL.[41] The liver shows both sinusoidal and portal infiltration by hairy cells. Involved lymph nodes commonly exhibit partial effacement, with hairy cells infiltrating the paracortex and medulla in a leukemic pattern. The hairy cells often surround residual lymphoid follicles and extend through the capsule.

### *CYTOCHEMISTRY*

Cytochemical studies demonstrating tartrate-resistant acid phosphatase (TRAP) activity, traditionally have been used to confirm the diagnosis of HCL, although the routine use of immunophenotyping for the diagnosis of chronic lymphoproliferative disorders has diminished reliance on the TRAP stain. Immunohistochemical stains for TRAP are also available and can be used in paraffin-embedded sections to demonstrate the activity of this enzyme. Similar to cytochemistry, a positive immunohistochemical stain is not pathognomonic for HCL; positivity has been reported in systemic mastocytosis and Gaucher's disease.[42] However, the presence of cells positive for both CD20 and TRAP activity confirm the diagnosis of HCL.

### *IMMUNOPHENOTYPIC PROFILE*

Flow cytometric immunophenotyping is a critical part of the diagnostic evaluation of HCL, and helps to distinguish it from other lymphoproliferative disorders.

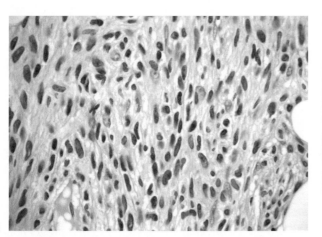
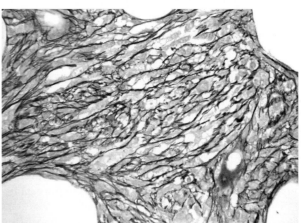

a                                                                                                 b

**Figure 30.2** *(a) Bone marrow trephine biopsy showing hairy cells with spindle shape nuclei. (b) Bone marrow trephine biopsy stained for reticulin, demonstrating extensive fibrosis surrounding the individual hairy cells, typical for HCL*

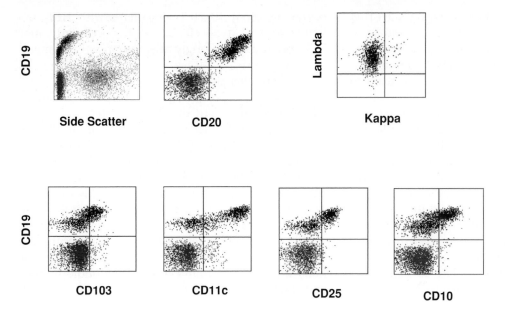

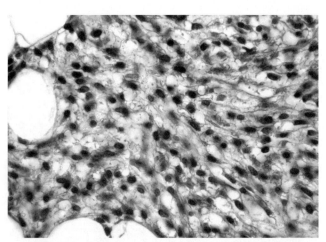

**Figure 30.3** *Flow immunocytometry of a patient with HCL. Hairy cells (red) express B-cell antigens CD19/CD20, λ light-chain restriction and are positive for CD11c and CD25. CD10 positivity is noted in the minority of patients with HCL*

As hairy cells exhibit distinctive light scatter characteristics and immunophenotype Figure 30.3, they are identified by peripheral blood flow cytometry in most of the patients with HCL, even when the HC represent less than 1% of lymphocytes.[43] This observation is useful at the time of diagnosis and after therapy to assess residual disease.[44,45]

Hairy cells show bright CD45 expression with increased forward and side scatter, resembling that of large lymphocytes or monocytes. They express one or more heavy chains and monotypic light chains. The number of cases expressing either kappa or lambda light chains is approximately equal.[43,46]

Hairy cells strongly express the pan B-cell antigens CD19, CD20, CD22, and CD79b.[47] They also express high levels of CD11c, CD25, FMC7, and CD103 surface antigens.[43,48] The CD11c antigen, the 150-kD α chain of the 150/95 $\beta_2$-integrin normally expressed on neutrophils and monocytes, is expressed at levels 30-fold higher than those in chronic lymphocytic leukemia.[49,50] CD25, the α chain of interleukin-2 (IL-2) receptor, is expressed in HCL, while the β-chain of IL-2 receptor is expressed in variant HCL.[51] Serum levels of soluble IL-2 receptor can be monitored in HCL patients and correlates with disease activity following treatment.[52]

CD103 has the greatest sensitivity and specificity for HCL. CD103 is a $\alpha^E$ subunit of the $\alpha^E\beta_7$-integrin, also known as human mucosal lymphocyte 1 (HML-1) antigen due to its primary expression by intraepithelial T lymphocytes. This integrin is believed to be involved in the process of lymphocytes homing and adhesion.[53]

CD123, a monoclonal antibody that identifies α chain of human interleukin-3 receptor, is expressed in HCL cells as well as in other acute leukemias and a variety of normal hematopoietic cells. Recently, CD123 was determined to be a useful marker for distinguishing HCL from hairy-cell leukemia variant and marginal zone splenic lymphoma, with 91–96% sensitivity and 97–100% specificity.[54]

In a small study of nine patients with HCL, CD52 was expressed in most leukemic cells in all the patients. Specifically, greater than 92% of HC stained positive in all nine cases, while 99% positivity was observed in six. The presence of CD52 on HC provides a theoretical basis for use of targeted therapy, such as the monoclonal antibody alemtuzumab, for the treatment of HCL.[55] CD10 (CALLA antigen) and CD5 are weakly expressed in 26% and 5% of patients with HCL, respectively.

### IMMUNOHISTOCHEMISTRY

Several B-cell associated antibodies, including CD20, CD79a, and DBA.44, can be used in routinely processed paraffin tissue sections of the bone marrow to detect hairy cells, Figure 30.4. Although these antibodies are not specific for HCL, they can be used to document the

**Figure 30.4** *Immunohistochemistry stain (MB2) of bone marrow trephine biopsy indicating that hairy cells are of B-cell origin*

B-cell nature of the infiltrate and highlight the extent of bone marrow infiltration at the time of diagnosis and following therapy.[56,57] Immunohistochemical techniques can also be used to evaluate bone marrow sections for TRAP.[42]

### GENE PROFILE

Genetic and molecular events leading to the development of HCL are not well established. Cytogenetic data confirmed by comparative genomic hybridization studies show that the majority of HCL cases have a normal, or at least balanced karyotype.[58–60] Abnormalities involving chromosomes 1, 2, 3, 4, 5, 6, 11, 13, 14, 15, 17, 19, and 20 have been reported. Among a few recurrent aberrations, are abnormalities of chromosome 5 (trisomy 5, 5q13) and chromosome 14 (add (14)(q32) and del (14)(q)).[61–63] Overexpression of cyclin D1, found in about 50–75% of HCL cases, is not associated with genomic rearrangement of 11q13/BCL1.[64]

Mutated $V_H$ gene status in HCL cells suggests that HCL originates from an antigen-experienced memory B-cell subset. The mutation pattern and gene usage resemble that for reactive marginal zone (MZ) B cells, particularly their mutated subset, and MALT-type MZL.[60,65]

### ELECTRON MICROSCOPY

By electron microscopy inspection, hairy cells have circumferential cytoplasmic projections and a few blunt microvilli.[66] Ribosomal lamella complexes, cylindrical cytoplasmic inclusions composed of a central hollow space surrounded by the multiple parallel lamellae with ribosomal-like granules in the inter-lamellar space, are discovered in 50% of patients with HCL by electron microscopy.[67] However, such complexes are not pathognomonic for HCL, and have been described in other lymphoproliferative disorders.[68]

## DIFFERENTIAL DIAGNOSIS

The differential diagnosis of HCL includes other B-cell lymphoproliferative disorders, and systemic mastocytosis (SM) (see Table 30.2 and 30.3).

### HAIRY CELL LEUKEMIA VARIANT

HCLv is a rare clinicopathologic entity first described in 1980. Most patients with HCL reported from Japan also exhibit features similar to those of the HCLv.[69,70] Unlike HCL, HCLv is associated with prominent leukocytosis,

| Table 30.2 | Differential diagnosis of hairy-cell leukemia |
|---|---|

Hairy cell leukemia variant (HCLv)
Polyclonal hairy B-cell lymphoproliferative disorder (HBLD)
Splenic marginal zone lymphoma (SMZL)
Systemic mastocytosis (SM)
Chronic lymphocytic leukemia (B-CLL)

| Table 30.3 | Differential diagnosis of hairy-cell leukemia |
|---|---|

Immunophenotype of B-cell chronic lymphoid leukemias

| Antigen | CLL | B-PLL | HCL | SMZL | HCL-v |
|---|---|---|---|---|---|
| SIg | + (dim) | + | + | + | + |
| CD19 | + | + | + | + | + |
| CD20 | + (dim) | + | + | + | + |
| CD22 | +/− | + | + | + | + |
| FMC7 | − | + | + | + | |
| CD79b | − | + | − | + | + |
| CD5 | + | +/− | − | − | − |
| CD23 | + | +/− | − | − | |
| CD25 | +/− | − | + | − | + |
| CD11c | +/− | − | + | +/− | +/− |
| CD103 | − | − | + | − | +/− |
| CD10 | − | − | − | − | − |

+ = most cases are positive for the antigen; − = most cases are negative; +/− = cases are variably positive; CLL = chronic lymphocytic leukemia; PLL = prolymphocytic leukemia; HCL = hairy cell leukemia; sIg = surface immunoglobulin.

lack of male preponderance, aspirable bone marrow with lack of fibrosis, and absence of monocytopenia. The neoplastic cells express surface immunoglobulins with Ig light-chain restriction as well as pan-B cell antigens CD19/20. They are negative for CD5, CD10, and CD25 antigens, while CD103 and CD11c may be positive. The bone marrow typically shows an interstitial infiltrate accompanied by an intrasinusoidal component. Similar to HCL, HCLv cells have a villous cytoplasm; however, they generally exhibit a more condensed chromatin, higher nuclear-to-cytoplasm ratio, and more pronounced central nucleoli than do the cells in patients with HCL Figure 30.5.[71] TRAP staining of HCLv cells is negative.[54] The biologic relationship between HCLv and HCL remains unknown.

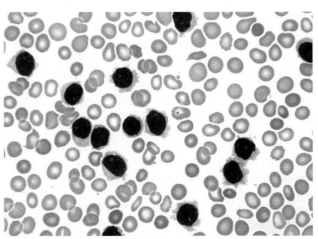

**Figure 30.5** *Peripheral smear of a patient with hairy-cell variant, demonstrating abundant cytoplasm with irregular borders and visible nucleoli (in contrast to HCL)*

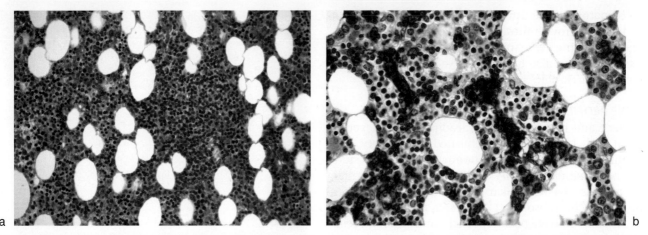

a                                                                              b

**Figure 30.6**    *Bone marrow trephine biopsy of a patient with splenic marginal zone lymphoma showing (a) focal lymphoid aggregates and (b) immunostaining for CD20 delineates intrasinusoidal and interstitial infiltration by lymphocytes*

## POLYCLONAL B-CELL LYMPHOPROLIFERATIVE DISORDER

An entity called polyclonal hairy B-cell lymphoproliferative disorder (HBLD) has been described in Japan.[72,73] All of the patients were females, had splenomegaly and minimal or no lymphadenopathy; persistent lymphocytosis was noted in all the patients, some having anemia and thrombocytopenia. Abnormal lymphocytes present in the peripheral blood and bone marrow had round nuclei and abundant pale cytoplasm with long microvilli and prominent membranous ruffles. They expressed CD5– CD10– CD11c+ CD19+ CD20+ CD23– by flow cytometry studies. Although these findings were similar to those of HCL, the surface marker of the kappa and lambda chains was unbiased and studies of immunoglobulin gene rearrangements and expressions showed a polyclonal proliferation of B cells.[73]

## SPLENIC MARGINAL ZONE LYMPHOMA

The clinical presentation of patients with splenic marginal zone lymphoma (SMZL) may resemble that of HCL, including massive splenomegaly and absence of lymphadenopathy. However, unlike HCL, lymphocytosis is common, the lymphocytes exhibit more basophilic cytoplasm, and the cytoplasmic projections are subtle or absent; TRAP staining is usually negative or only weakly positive.[34,74] Both HCL and SMZL cells are of B-cell lineage and are CD19 and CD20 positive, with Ig light-chain restriction, as well as CD10 and CD5 negative. However, the SMZL cells are usually CD103 and CD123 negative.[54,75–77] The bone marrow infiltrates are sharply demarcated from the surrounding normal tissue, and intrasinusoidal infiltration is often prominent, Figures 30.6(a) and (b). In addition, sections of spleen show predominantly white pulp involvement resembling that of low-grade lymphoma.[74]

## SYSTEMIC MASTOCYTOSIS

Infiltrates of systemic mastocytosis in the bone marrow may closely resemble that of HCL. However, immunohistochemical studies show that the mast cells, unlike hairy cells, are negative for B-cell antigens, but react with mast cell tryptase.[78]

## CHRONIC LYMPHOCYTIC LEUKEMIA

Finally, aged blood from patients with B-cell chronic lymphocytic leukemia (B-CLL) may demonstrate artifactual cytoplasmic projections due to cytoplasmic distortion. Leukocytosis in CLL is usually more pronounced than in HCL, and monocytopenia is typically absent. In addition, CLL has a distinct phenotypic profile differentiating it from HCL, including CD5 positivity.[79]

## REFERENCES

1. Bouroncle BA, Wiseman BK, Doan CA: Leukemic reticuloendotheliosis. *Blood* 13(7):609–630, 1958.
2. Schrek R, Donnelly WJ: "Hairy" cells in blood in lymphoreticular neoplastic disease and "flagellated" cells of normal lymph nodes. *Blood* 27(2):199–211, 1966.
3. Polliack A: Hairy cell leukemia and allied chronic lymphoid leukemias: current knowledge and new therapeutic options. *Leuk Lymphoma* 26 (Suppl) 1:41–51, 1997.
4. Turner A, Kjeldsberg CR: Hairy cell leukemia: a review. *Medicine* (Baltimore);57(6):477–499, 1978.
5. Flandrin G, Sigaux F, Sebahoun G, Bouffette P: Hairy cell leukemia: clinical presentation and follow-up of 211 patients. *Semin Oncol* 11(4 Suppl 2):458–471, 1984.
6. Moses J, Lichtman SM, Brody J, Wisch N, Moake J: Hairy cell leukemia in association with thrombotic thrombocytopenic purpura and factor VIII antibodies. *Leuk Lymphoma* 22(3–4):351–354, 1996.
7. Golomb HM: Hairy cell leukemia: the importance of accurate diagnosis and sequential management. *Adv Intern Med* 29:245–269, 1984.
8. Golomb HM, Catovsky D, Golde DW: Hairy cell leukemia: a clinical review based on 71 cases. *Ann Intern Med* 89(5 Pt 1):677–683,1978.
9. Mercieca J, Matutes E, Moskovic E, et al.: Massive abdominal lymphadenopathy in hairy cell leukaemia: a report of 12 cases. *Br J Haematol* 82(3):547–554, 1992.

10. Vardiman JW, Golomb HM: Autopsy findings in hairy cell leukemia. *Semin Oncol* 11(4):370–380,1984.

11. Vincent AM, Burthem J, Brew R, Cawley JC: Endothelial interactions of hairy cells: the importance of alpha 4 beta 1 in the unusual tissue distribution of the disorder. *Blood* 88(10):3945–3952, 1996.

12. Bouroncle BA: Unusual presentations and complications of hairy cell leukemia. *Leukemia* 1(4):288–293, 1987.

13. Davies GE, Wiernik PH: Hairy cell leukemia with chylous ascites. *Jama* 238(14):1541–1542, 1977.

14. Robinson A, Eting E, Zeidman A, Djaldetti M, Mittelman M, Savir H: Ocular manifestation of hairy cell leukemia with dramatic response to 2-chloro-deoxy-adenosine. *Am J Ophthalmol* 121(1):97–99, 1996.

15. Bouza E, Burgaleta C, Golde DW: Infections in hairy-cell leukemia. *Blood* 51(5):851–859, 1978.

16. Knecht H, Rhyner K, Streuli RA: Toxoplasmosis in hairy-cell leukaemia. *Br J Haematol* 62(1):65–73, 1986.

17. Guerin JM, Meyer P, Habib Y: Listeria monocytogenes infection and hairy cell leukemia. *Am J Med* 83(1):188, 1987.

18. Siegal FP, Shodell M, Shah K, et al.: Impaired interferon alpha response in hairy cell leukemia is corrected by therapy with 2-chloro-2'-deoxyadenosine: implications for susceptibility to opportunistic infections. *Leukemia* 8(9):1474–1479, 1994.

19. Yam LT, Chaudhry AA, Janckila AJ: Impaired marrow granulocyte reserve and leukocyte mobilization in leukemic reticuloendotheliosis. *Ann Intern Med* 87(4):444–446, 1977.

20. Van De Corput L, Falkenburg JH, Kluin-Nelemans JC: T-cell dysfunction in hairy cell leukemia: an updated review. *Leuk Lymphoma* 30(1–2):31–39, 1998.

21. Bourguin-Plonquet A, Rouard H, Roudot-Thoraval F, et al.: Severe decrease in peripheral blood dendritic cells in hairy cell leukemia. *Br J Haematol* 116(3):595–597, 2002.

22. Blanche P, Bachmeyer C, Mikdame M, Dreyfus F, Sicard D: Scleroderma, polymyositis, and hairy cell leukemia. *J Rheumatol* 22(7):1384–1385, 1995.

23. Dorsey JK, Penick GD: The association of hairy cell leukemia with unusual immunologic disorders. *Arch Intern Med* 142(5):902–903, 1982.

24. Carpenter MT, West SG: Polyarteritis nodosa in hairy cell leukemia: treatment with interferon-alpha. *J Rheumatol* 21(6):1150–1152, 1994.

25. Berthiot G: Hairy cell leukemia and sarcoidosis. *Eur J Med* 2(1):61, 1993.

26. Myers TJ, Granville NB, Witter BA: Hairy cell leukemia and sarcoid. *Cancer* 43(5):1777–1781, 1979.

27. Schiller G, Said J, Pal S: Hairy cell leukemia and sarcoidosis: a case report and review of the literature. *Leukemia* 17(10):2057–2059, 2003.

28. Lawrence DM, Sun NC, Mena R, Moss R: Cutaneous lesions in hairy-cell leukemia. case report and review of the literature. *Arch Dermatol* 119(4):322–325, 1983.

29. Kaplan RP, Newman G, Saperia D: Pyoderma gangrenosum and hairy cell leukemia. *J Dermatol Surg Oncol* 13(9):1029–1031, 1987.

30. Cartwright PH, Rowell NR: Hairy-cell leukaemia presenting with pyoderma gangrenosum. *Clin Exp Dermatol* 12(6):451–452, 1987.

31. Lal A, Tallman MS, Soble MB, Golubovich I, Peterson L: Hairy cell leukemia presenting as localized skeletal involvement. *Leuk Lymphoma* 43(11):2207–2211, 2002.

32. Quesada JR, Keating MJ, Libshitz HI, Llamas L: Bone involvement in hairy cell leukemia. *Am J Med* 74(2):228–231, 1983.

33. Lembersky BC, Ratain MJ, Golomb HM: Skeletal complications in hairy cell leukemia: diagnosis and therapy. *J Clin Oncol* 6(8):1280–1284, 1988.

34. Hanson CA, Ward PC, Schnitzer B: A multilobular variant of hairy cell leukemia with morphologic similarities to T-cell lymphoma. *Am J Surg Pathol* 13(8):671–679, 1989.

35. Burke JS: The value of the bone-marrow biopsy in the diagnosis of hairy cell leukemia. *Am J Clin Pathol* 70(6):876–884, 1978.

36. Bartl R, Frisch B, Hill W, Burkhardt R, Sommerfeld W, Sund M: Bone marrow histology in hairy cell leukemia. Identification of subtypes and their prognostic significance. *Am J Clin Pathol* 79(5):531–545, 1983.

37. Burke JS, Rappaport H: The diagnosis and differential diagnosis of hairy cell leukemia in bone marrow and spleen. *Semin Oncol* 11(4):334–346, 1984.

38. Katayama I: Bone marrow in hairy cell leukemia. *Hematol Oncol Clin North Am* 2(4):585–602, 1988.

39. Lee WM, Beckstead JH: Hairy cell leukemia with bone marrow hypoplasia. *Cancer* 50(10):2207–2210, 1982.

40. Golomb HM, Vardiman JW: Response to splenectomy in 65 patients with hairy cell leukemia: an evaluation of spleen weight and bone marrow involvement. *Blood* 61(2):349–352, 1983.

41. Nanba K, Soban EJ, Bowling MC, Berard CW: Splenic pseudosinuses and hepatic angiomatous lesions: distinctive features of hairy cell leukemia. *Am J Clin Pathol* 67(5):415–426, 1977.

42. Hoyer JD, Li CY, Yam LT, Hanson CA, Kurtin PJ: Immunohistochemical demonstration of acid phosphatase isoenzyme 5 (tartrate-resistant) in paraffin sections of hairy cell leukemia and other hematologic disorders. *Am J Clin Pathol* 108(3):308–315, 1997.

43. Robbins BA, Ellison DJ, Spinosa JC, et al.: Diagnostic application of two-color flow cytometry in 161 cases of hairy cell leukemia. *Blood* 82(4):1277–1287, 1993.3

44. Sausville JE, Salloum RG, Sorbara L, et al.: Minimal residual disease detection in hairy cell leukemia. Comparison of flow cytometric immunophenotyping with clonal analysis using consensus primer polymerase chain reaction for the heavy chain gene. *Am J Clin Pathol* 119(2):213–217, 2003.

45. Babusikova O, Tomova A: Hairy cell leukemia: early immunophenotypical detection and quantitative analysis by flow cytometry. *Neoplasma* 50(5):350–356, 2003.

46. Cornfield DB, Mitchell Nelson DM, Rimsza LM, Moller-Patti D, Braylan RC: The diagnosis of hairy cell leukemia can be established by flow cytometric analysis of peripheral blood, even in patients with low levels of circulating malignant cells. *Am J Hematol* 67(4): 223–226, 2001.

47. Falini B, Schwarting R, Erber W, et al.: The differential diagnosis of hairy cell leukemia with a panel of monoclonal antibodies. *Am J Clin Pathol* 83(3):289–300, 1985.

48. Visser L, Shaw A, Slupsky J, Vos H, Poppema S: Monoclonal antibodies reactive with hairy cell leukemia. *Blood* 74(1):320–325, 1989.

49. Schwarting R, Stein H, Wang CY: The monoclonal antibodies alpha S-HCL 1 (alpha Leu-14) and alpha S-HCL 3

(alpha Leu-M5) allow the diagnosis of hairy cell leukemia. *Blood* 65(4):974–983, 1985.

50. Hanson CA, Gribbin TE, Schnitzer B, Schlegelmilch JA, Mitchell BS, Stoolman LM: CD11c (LEU-M5) expression characterizes a B-cell chronic lymphoproliferative disorder with features of both chronic lymphocytic leukemia and hairy cell leukemia. *Blood* 76(11):2360–2367, 1990.

51. de Totero D, Tazzari PL, Lauria F, et al.: Phenotypic analysis of hairy cell leukemia: "variant" cases express the interleukin-2 receptor beta chain, but not the alpha chain (CD25). *Blood* 82(2):528–535, 1993.

52. Steis RG, Marcon L, Clark J, et al.: Serum soluble IL-2 receptor as a tumor marker in patients with hairy cell leukemia. *Blood* 71(5):1304–1309, 1988.

53. Micklem KJ, Dong Y, Willis A, et al.: HML-1 antigen on mucosa-associated T cells, activated cells, and hairy leukemic cells is a new integrin containing the beta 7 subunit. *Am J Pathol* 139(6):1297–1301, 1991.

54. Del Giudice I, Matutes E, Morilla R, et al.: The diagnostic value of CD123 in B-cell disorders with hairy or villous lymphocytes. *Haematologica* 89(3):303–308, 2004.

55. Quigley MM, Bethel KJ, Sharpe RW, Saven A: CD52 expression in hairy cell leukemia. *Am J Hematol* 74(4):227–230, 2003.

56. Hounieu H, Chittal SM, al Saati T, et al.: Hairy cell leukemia. Diagnosis of bone marrow involvement in paraffin-embedded sections with monoclonal antibody DBA.44. *Am J Clin Pathol* 98(1):26–33, 1992.

57. Hakimian D, Tallman MS, Kiley C, Peterson L: Detection of minimal residual disease by immunostaining of bone marrow biopsies after 2-chlorodeoxyadenosine for hairy cell leukemia. *Blood* 82(6):1798–1802, 1993.

58. Dierlamm J, Stefanova M, Wlodarska I, et al.: Chromosomal gains and losses are uncommon in hairy cell leukemia: a study based on comparative genomic hybridization and interphase fluorescence in situ hybridization. *Cancer Genet Cytogenet* 128(2):164–167, 2001.

59. Nessling M, Solinas-Toldo S, Lichter P, et al.: Genomic imbalances are rare in hairy cell leukemia. Genes Chromosomes *Cancer* 26(2):182–183, 1999.

60. Vanhentenrijk V, De Wolf-Peeters C, Wlodarska I: Comparative expressed sequence hybridization studies of hairy cell leukemia show uniform expression profile and imprint of spleen signature. *Blood* 104(1):250–255, 2004.

61. Haglund U, Juliusson G, Stellan B, Gahrton G: Hairy cell leukemia is characterized by clonal chromosome abnormalities clustered to specific regions. *Blood* 83(9): 2637–2645, 1994.

62. Kluin-Nelemans HC, Beverstock GC, Mollevanger P, et al.: Proliferation and cytogenetic analysis of hairy cell leukemia upon stimulation via the CD40 antigen. *Blood* 84(9):3134–3141, 1994.

63. Sambani C, Trafalis DT, Mitsoulis-Mentzikoff C, et al.: Clonal chromosome rearrangements in hairy cell leukemia: personal experience and review of literature. *Cancer Genet Cytogenet* 129(2):138–144, 2001.

64. Bosch F, Campo E, Jares P, et al.: Increased expression of the PRAD-1/CCND1 gene in hairy cell leukaemia. *Br J Haematol* 91(4):1025–1030, 1995.

65. Vanhentenrijk V, Tierens A, Wlodarska I, Verhoef G, Wolf-Peeters CD: V(H) gene analysis of hairy cell leukemia reveals a homogeneous mutation status and suggests its marginal zone B-cell origin. *Leukemia* 18(10):1729–1732, 2004.

66. Katayama I, Li CY, Yam LT: Ultrastructural characteristics of the "hairy cells" of leukemic reticuloendotheliosis. *Am J Pathol* 67(2):361–370, 1972.

67. Rosner MC, Golomb HM: Ribosome-lamella complex in hairy cell leukemia. Ultrastructure and distribution. *Lab Invest* 42(2):236–247, 1980.

68. Brunning RD, Parkin J: Ribosome-lamella complexes in neoplastic hematopoietic cells. *Am J* Pathol 79(3):565–578, 1975.

69. Machii T, Tokumine Y, Inoue R, Kitani T: Predominance of a distinct subtype of hairy cell leukemia in *Japan Leukemia* 7(2):181–186, 1993.

70. Miyazaki M, Taguchi A, Sakuragi S, Mitani N, Matsuda K, Shinohara K: Hairy cell leukemia, Japanese variant, successfully treated with cladribine. *Rinsho Ketsueki* 45(5):405–407, 2004.

71. Cawley JC, Burns GF, Hayhoe FG: A chronic lymphoproliferative disorder with distinctive features: a distinct variant of hairy-cell leukaemia. *Leuk Res* 4(6):547–559, 1980.

72. Machii T, Yamaguchi M, Inoue R, et al.: Polyclonal B-cell lymphocytosis with features resembling hairy cell leukemia-Japanese variant. *Blood* 89(6):2008–2014, 1997.

73. Yagi Y, Sakabe H, Kakinoki R, et al.: A hairy B cell lymphoproliferative disorder resembling hairy cell leukemia. *Rinsho Ketsueki* 45(4):312–315, 2004.

74. Sun T, Susin M, Brody J, et al.: Splenic lymphoma with circulating villous lymphocytes: report of seven cases and review of the literature. *Am J Hematol* 45(1):39–50, 1994.

75. Matutes E, Morilla R, Owusu-Ankomah K, Houlihan A, Catovsky D: The immunophenotype of splenic lymphoma with villous lymphocytes and its relevance to the differential diagnosis with other B-cell disorders. *Blood* 83(6):1558–1562, 1994.

76. Matutes E, Morilla R, Owusu-Ankomah K, Houliham A, Meeus P, Catovsky D: The immunophenotype of hairy cell leukemia (HCL). Proposal for a scoring system to distinguish HCL from B-cell disorders with hairy or villous lymphocytes. *Leuk Lymphoma* 14 Suppl 1:57–61, 1994.

77. Troussard X, Valensi F, Duchayne E, et al.: Splenic lymphoma with villous lymphocytes: clinical presentation, biology and prognostic factors in a series of 100 patients. Groupe Francais d'Hematologie Cellulaire (GFHC). *Br J Haematol* 93(3):731–736, 1996.

78. Ruck P, Horny HP, Kaiserling E: Immunoreactivity of human tissue mast cells. *Acta Pathol Jpn* 42(3):227–228, 1992.

79. Keating MJ: Chronic lymphoproliferative disorders: chronic lymphocytic leukemia and hairy-cell leukemia. *Curr Opin Oncol* 5(1):35–41, 1993.

# Chapter 31

# INDICATIONS FOR TREATMENT AND INITIAL TREATMENT APPROACH TO HAIRY CELL LEUKEMIA

*Alan Saven, Andrew P. Hampshire and Lyudmila Bazhenova*

## INDICATIONS FOR TREATMENT

Hairy cell leukemia is an indolent lymphoproliferative disorder, which, prior to the advent of successful systemic therapy, had a median survival of 53 months. Approximately 10% of the patients diagnosed with this disorder never require therapy. This population is characterized by older age, smaller spleen size, and minimal circulating hairy cells.[1] The following criteria, though not validated, are commonly accepted as appropriate indications for therapy: neutropenia characterized by an absolute neutrophil count (ANC) $<1 \times 10^9$/L, anemia with a hemoglobin $<10$ g/dL, or thrombocytopenia $<(50-100) \times 10^9$/L, recurrent serious infections, or symptomatic splenomegaly. Much less commonly, bulky or painful lymphadenopathy, constitutional symptoms including fevers, chills, sweats, or weight loss, vasculitis, bone involvement, or leukocytosis with a high proportion of circulating hairy cells (white cell count $>20 \times 10^9$/L) are also indications for treatment. Bone marrow involvement, no matter what the degree, is not an indication for therapy in the absence of peripheral blood cytopenias. The early initiation of therapy results in neither a survival nor a response benefit. Therefore, a strategy of careful observation is appropriate in patients who do not meet these criteria for the initiation of therapy.

## INITIAL TREATMENT APPROACH

In the past, treatment decisions regarding the initial therapy for hairy cell leukemia evaluated the merit of a 12-month course of interferon-α versus that of splenectomy. However, the success of 2-chlorodeoxyadenosine (2-CdA; cladribine) and 2′-deoxycoformycin (DCF; pentostatin) has relegated both interferon and splenectomy to be used only in certain uncommon clinical situations.

### 2-CHLORODEOXYADENOSINE
#### Mechanism of action
Lymphocytes possess high levels of deoxycytidine kinase. Cells low in adenosine deaminase activity accumulate deoxypurine nucleotides, and cell death ensues. This is similar to the situation in severe combined immunodeficiency syndrome, in which one-third of children exhibit an adenosine deaminase deficiency. These observations led to the development of cladribine, or 2-CdA, by Professor Dennis Carson in 1980.[2] Cladribine is a purine nucleoside characterized by the substitution of chlorine for hydrogen at position 2 of the purine ring. This substitution confers resistance to cladribine from the action of adenosine deaminase. The high activity of deoxycytidine kinase in lymphocytes, in combination with the resistance to adenosine deaminase, drives the conversion and intracellular accumulation of 2-CdA triphosphate and its subsequent incorporation into the lymphocyte's DNA (see Figure 31.1). Once these nucleotides become incorporated into DNA, strand breakage ensues, leading to cell death. Cladribine is toxic to both resting and dividing lymphocytes, making it a therapeutically attractive candidate in low-grade lymphoproliferative disorders.

#### Treatment results
The first use of cladribine in the treatment of hairy cell leukemia was published in 1987 by Carrera et al.[3] In 1990, investigators at Scripps Clinic in La Jolla reported on 12 patients with hairy cell leukemia treated with a single 7-day course of 2-CdA at a dose of 0.1 mg/kg daily by continuous intravenous infusion; 11 of the 12 patients achieved a complete response (CR), and the remaining patient had a partial response

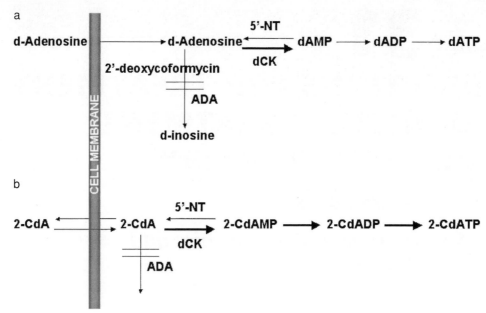

**Figure 31.1** *(a) Normal pathway for deoxynucleotide metabolism and the mechanism of action of 2'-deoxycoformycin (pentostatin). Deoxyadenosine is normally converted to deoxyinosine through the action of adenosine deaminase. In the congenital absence of adenosine deaminase (such as in severe combined immunodeficiency), or in the presence of DCF, a potent direct inhibitor of adenosine deaminase, deoxyadenosine triphosphate accumulates because of the high ratio of deoxycytidine kinase (dCK) relative to 5'-nucleotidase (5'-NT). This accumulation of deoxyadenosine triphosphate results in cell death. (b) Mechanism of action of 2-chlorodeoxyadenosine (cladribine). 2-CdA enters the cell through an efficient transport system. It is resistant to the action of adenosine deaminase. Because of the high ratio of deoxycytidine kinase to 5'-nucleotidase in lymphocytes, 2-chlorodeoxyadenosine triphosphate accumulates and results in DNA strand breaks, leading to cell death*

(PR); on follow-up, none of the patients had relapsed, with a 15.5-month median remission duration.[4]

These encouraging results led to further investigations, and in 1998, Saven et al. published the long-term follow-up of 358 patients treated with a single course of continuous intravenous infusion of 2-CdA for 7 days.[5] Ninety-one percent of their 349 evaluable patients achieved a CR, with resolution of peripheral cytopenias (i.e., ANC $>1.5\times10^9$/L, hemoglobin $\geq12$ g/dL, and platelets $>100\times10^9$/L), no evidence of hairy cells morphologically in the bone marrow, and resolution of all adenopathy and splenomegaly. Seven percent of the patients achieved a PR, for an overall response rate (ORR) of 98%. Twenty-six percent of these patients relapsed at a median of 29 months from therapy. An additional CR was achieved in 62% of the relapsed patients who were treated with a second course of 2-CdA; 26% of these retreated patients achieved a PR. The treatment failure rate at 48 months was 18.7% with a 96% overall survival at 48 months.

Goodman et al. reported in 2003 on the extended follow-up of these patients treated at Scripps Clinic.[6] Of the 209 patients treated at that institution with at least 7 years of follow-up, there was a 95% CR rate and a 5% PR rate. The median response duration was 98 months.

Of the 37% experiencing a relapse, the median time to relapse was 42 months. Of these relapsed patients treated with a second course of 2-CdA, 75% achieved a CR and 17% a PR. The overall survival at 108 months was 97%.

These excellent response rates and response durations with the use of a single infusion of cladribine have been confirmed in other single-institution series (see Table 31.1). In 1992, Estey et al. reported on 46 patients with hairy cell leukemia treated at MD Anderson Cancer Center, Houston, TX.[7] They delivered the 2-CdA by continuous intravenous infusion at a dose of 40 mg/m² per day for 7 days; the CR rate was 78% and the PR rate was 11%. Only one patient relapse was observed in the group of responding patients, but follow-up was limited at 37 weeks.

In 1996, Tallman et al. described the experience at Northwestern University in 52 consecutive patients with a 2-CdA treatment protocol of 0.1 mg/kg per day, by continuous intravenous infusion for 7 days.[8] They observed an 80% CR rate with an 18% PR rate. Fourteen percent of the patients relapsed at a median of 24 months. Of five patients retreated with a second course of 2-CdA, two patients achieved a CR and three a PR. The overall survival at 4 years was 86%. Hoffman

**Table 31.1**    Trial results of 2-CdA in hairy cell leukemia

| Author | Institution | Year | N | CR | PR | ORR | Relapse[b] | F/U |
|---|---|---|---|---|---|---|---|---|
| Carrera[3] | Scripps Clinic | 1990 | 12 | 92% | 8% | 100% | 0 | 16 months |
| Saven[5] | Scripps Clinic | 1998 | 349 | 91% | 7% | 98% | 18.7% | 48 months |
| Goodman[a,6] | Scripps Clinic | 2003 | 207 | 95% | 5% | 100% | 37% | >84 months |
| Estey[7] | MDACC[c] | 1992 | 46 | 78% | 11% | 89% | 2.4% | 37 weeks |
| Tallman[8] | Northwestern | 1996 | 52 | 80% | 18% | 98% | 28% | 48 months |
| Hoffman[9] | LI Jewish[d] | 1997 | 49 | 76% | 24% | 100% | 20% | 55 months |
| Cheson[10] | NCI[e] | 1998 | 861 | 50% | 37% | 87% | 12% | 52 months |
| Dearden[11] | Royal Marsden[f] | 1999 | 45 | 84% | 16% | 100% | 29% | 45 months |

[a] Study reports on the subset of patients previously reported by Saven et al.[5] with more than 7 years of follow-up.
[b] Relapse is reported within the follow-up period listed.
[c] MD Anderson Cancer Center, Houston, TX.
[d] Long Island Jewish, New York.
[e] National Cancer Institute.
[f] Royal Marsden Hospital, London, England

et al. reported in 1997 on 49 patients with hairy cell leukemia treated at Long Island Jewish Medical Center, with a single 7-day continuous infusion of 2-CdA.[9] They reported a 76% CR rate and a 24% PR rate. At 55-months median follow-up, there was an 80% relapse-free survival rate and a 95% overall survival rate.

In the largest study on the use of 2-CdA to treat hairy cell leukemia, Cheson et al. reported in 1998 on 979 patients treated through the Group C protocol mechanism at the National Cancer Institute.[10] Of 861 evaluable patients, a CR was obtained in 50% and a PR in 37%. The relapse rate at a median follow-up of 52 months was 12%. Although the CR in this study, which the authors felt approximated general clinical practice to a greater degree than single-institution studies, was lower, this may have been related to the lack of central pathology review.

Finally, in a British study published in 1999, Dearden et al. from the Royal Marsden Hospital in London described their long-term results with both pentostatin and cladribine in patients with hairy cell leukemia.[11] Forty-five patients were treated with cladribine, with 84% achieving a CR, and a 16% PR rate was observed. At 45 months, the relapse rate was 29%.

Despite the durability of the responses generated by cladribine, it is clear that a proportion of patients in apparent CR without morphologic evidence of residual disease in the bone marrow actually have demonstrable disease when more sensitive tests to detect minimal residual disease are used. In a study reported by Hakimian et al. from Northwestern University, 5 of their 24 patients in apparent CR 3 months after treatment with 2-CdA had residual disease when paraffin blocks of their bone marrows were stained with anti-CD20 and anti-CD45Ro antibodies.[12] In a separate investigation, 154 complete remission bone marrow biopsies from HCL patients treated with 2-CdA at Scripps Clinic were analyzed with anti-CD20 and DBA.44 immunostains.[13] Overall, 50% of the biopsies exhibited staining with anti-CD20 and/or DBA.44 in hairy cells, indicating residual disease. However, in those patients with immunophenotypic minimal residual disease and normal peripheral blood counts, there was no documented increase in the number of marrow hairy cells on serial bone marrow evaluation. So, although it is clear that a significant proportion of patients in morphologic CR actually harbor minimal residual disease, the clinical significance of this finding remains unclear.

In summary, a single course of cladribine given as a 7-day continuous intravenous infusion induces a complete remission in a high proportion of patients who meet the indications for therapy. The ORR approaches 100%. With extended follow-up, the responses achieved are durable, and the majority of patients with relapsed disease achieve further responses with retreatment. However, even with extended follow-up, there is no clear plateau on the time to treatment failure curve, and it remains to be seen to what extent 2-CdA represents curative therapy.

### Alternate methods of administration

A variety of different 2-CdA routes and schedules of administration have been investigated in an attempt to reproduce the high response rates seen with the 7-day continuous infusion schedule while also decreasing the associated myelosuppression and improving convenience of administration. On the basis of their earlier pharmacokinetic studies revealing a terminal half-life of 7–10 h for 2-CdA, Juliusson et al. reported in 1995 on their experience in hairy cell leukemia with daily subcutaneous injections of 2-CdA for seven consecutive days.[14] They documented a CR rate of 81% in their 73 patients, similar to the excellent rates achieved with continuous intravenous infusion. In addition, they did not observe significant injection site reactions.

Lauria et al. treated 25 hairy cell leukemia patients who had severe cytopenias (ANC $<1.0 \times 10^9$/L prior to therapy) with a regimen of weekly 2-CdA, dosed at 0.15 mg/kg intravenously for 6 weeks.[15] They observed a CR in 76% of their patients, a PR in 24%, and only a 16% incidence of severe neutropenia (ANC $<0.5 \times 10^9$/L). The median duration of response in these 19 patients, however, was only 15 months. Liliemark et al. studied the feasibility of delivering 2-CdA by the oral route.[16] In 13 patients with B-cell chronic lymphocytic leukemia (CLL) and low-grade non-Hodgkin's lymphoma (NHL), they delivered intravenous, subcutaneous, and oral preparations of 2-CdA (either in liquid or capsule form) in an alternating fashion. On the basis of pharmacokinetic data, they concluded that an AUC resembling that of a 2-h intravenous infusion could be obtained with an oral preparation at double the dose.

There have been additional investigations using 2-CdA delivered as a 2-h intravenous infusion in other low-grade lymphoproliferative disorders, including CLL, NHL, and lymphoplasmacytic lymphoma. These investigations have all documented equivalent feasibility and tolerability. However, there have not been any comparative studies of 2-CdA demonstrating a superiority of any alternate mode of delivery over the traditional 7-day continuous intravenous infusion in hairy cell leukemia. Because of the excellent long-term efficacy and safety data using this route and schedule, 0.1 mg/kg of 2-CdA delivered by continuous intravenous infusion daily for 7 days remains the regimen of choice.

## Acute toxicity

The major acute toxicity of 2-CdA is myelosuppression. In their long-term follow-up study, investigators at Scripps Clinic noted a 16% incidence of Grade 3 and a 71% incidence of Grade 4 neutropenia in the first 135 consecutive treated patients.[5] Ten percent had Grade 3 and 10% had Grade 4 thrombocytopenia. Grade 3 anemia occurred in 20% and Grade 4 in 2%. Forty-two percent developed neutropenic fever, though in only 13%, was an infection documented. Of these, the most common infecting organism was *Staphylococcus*, usually associated with the indwelling intravenous catheter. Although there were several oral herpetic infections and acute dermatomal herpes reactivations, no fungal infections were found. This high rate of neutropenia with culture negative neutropenic fever was also noted at similar rates in other single-institution series with 2-CdA. Despite the frequency of myelosuppression, additional acute toxicities were uncommon. There were no significant rates of nausea, vomiting, alopecia, myalgias, neuropathy, or allergic reactions.

Given the high rate of febrile neutropenia following cladribine therapy for hairy cell leukemia, Saven et al. studied the efficacy of filgrastim priming, followed sequentially by 2-CdA and later by daily filgrastim at 5 µg/kg until an ANC of $>2 \times 10^9$/L for two consecutive days was achieved.[17] Even though the median nadir ANC increased significantly over historical controls, and the median number of neutropenic days was 9 (compared to 22 among historical controls), no significant improvement in the percentage of febrile patients, number of febrile days, or hospitalization rates for febrile neutropenia was observed.

## Delayed toxicity

The delayed toxicity profile of 2-CdA in hairy cell leukemia is dominated by its immunosuppressive effects. CD4[+] lymphocyte counts become suppressed, and remain so for prolonged periods, after a single 7-day continuous course. The most common late infection in all series was recurrent dermatomal herpes zoster. The severity, duration, and clinical sequelae of this CD4[+] lymphocyte depletion was characterized by Seymour et al. in a cohort of 40 patients with hairy cell leukemia treated with continuous infusion 2-CdA at MD Anderson Cancer Center.[18] Prior to therapy, 18 patients had lymphocyte subsets analyzed and the median CD4[+] count was 743/µL (range, 58–2201/µL) with a median CD8[+] count of 238/µL (range, 75–2342/µL). Within 4 months of treatment, 25 patients had nadir lymphocyte subsets analyzed with the median CD4[+] count suppressed to 139/µL (range, 25–580/µL), and CD8[+] to 92/µL (range, 26–879/µL). This suppression was prolonged, with a median time of 40 months until CD4[+] counts returned to the normal range. CD8[+] counts returned to normal levels sooner, with a median recovery time of 23 months. The clinical implication of this profound and prolonged lymphopenia is uncertain; however, given that in this small series only one opportunistic infection, dermatomal herpes zoster, was documented. Nonetheless, the delayed toxicity profile of 2-CdA is characterized by late infections, primarily dermatomal herpes zoster. In the long-term follow-up of 358 patients at Scripps Clinic, seven (2%) suffered dermatomal herpes zoster activation within a range of 10–69 months following therapy.

In the same group of patients, with extended follow-up, Goodman and colleagues recorded 58 second malignancies among 47 patients (22% of their cohort) with an observed to expected ratio of second malignancies, compared with NCI SEER data, of 2.03 (95% confidence intervals (CI) 1.49–2.71).[6] Debate continues regarding the degree and the nature of the risk of second malignancies in patients with hairy cell leukemia treated with cladribine or other purine analogs. It remains unclear whether any significant increased risk exists, and if so, whether this is secondary to the underlying disease or to the corresponding therapy. A retrospective review of 350 hairy cell patients treated at MD Anderson Cancer Center and followed for 6 years, reported by Kurzrock et al., reported 26 patients with a second malignancy, for an observed-to-expected ratio of 1.34 (p = 0.08).[19] No evidence of a treatment effect for 2-CdA, interferon-α, or DCF was observed.

The Italian Cooperative Group for the study of hairy cell leukemia reviewed 1022 patients and documented 54 malignancies, with a standardized incidence ratio (SIR) of 1.01.[20] Although no overall increased risk was observed, an increased risk specifically of NHL was noted (SIR = 5.3; CI, 1.9–11.5). Of the 979 patients with hairy cell leukemia treated with 2-CdA at the National Cancer Institute and described by Cheson et al., the relative risk of developing a second malignancy at a median of 3.4 years was 1.71 (CI, 1.24–2.30).[21] Of the 117 patients with hairy cell leukemia diagnosed over a 20-year period in British Columbia, Canada, Au et al. reported 44 additional tumors in 36 patients (30.7%), with 25 of these diagnosed after the occurrence of their leukemia.[22] Of these 25, 20% were nonmelanoma skin cancer. An increased rate of second malignancies was calculated compared with age- and sex-matched controls, and peaked at 2 years after treatment. There was no significant treatment effect on the risk of second malignancy, with the exception of a small group of patients initially treated with interferon-α followed by a purine analog, who had a relative risk that ranged from 1.60 to 4.31.

## 2'-DEOXYCOFORMYCIN
### Mechanism of action
2'-Deoxycoformycin directly mimics the metabolic consequences of congenital adenosine deaminase defi-ciency. A product of *Streptomyces antibioticus*, DCF is a tight inhibitor of adenosine deaminase that results in lymphocyte depletion (see Figure 31.1). It was first shown to have therapeutic activity in hairy cell leukemia in 1983.[23]

### Treatment results
Cassileth et al. reported on 50 patients with hairy cell leukemia treated with DCF and followed for a median of 39 months.[24] After treatment for a median of 3 months, patients achieved a 64% CR and a 20% PR rate, with relapses in 6 of the 42 responders (14%) (see Table 31.2). In another early trial through the National Cancer Institute–Canadian Clinical Trials Group, Johnston et al. documented a CR in 25 of 28 (89%) evaluable patients with all remaining patients achieving a PR (11%).[25] Patients were treated with 4 mg/m² intravenously weekly for three consecutive weeks, repeated every 8 weeks, and continued for two additional cycles beyond CR. Overall toxicity included a 48% incidence of fever and infection, a 62% incidence of lethargy, and a 76% incidence of nausea and vomiting. Additional side effects included anorexia, dry skin, altered taste, and paresthesias.

Early results from the Eastern Cooperative Oncology Group, reported by Spiers et al., used a regimen of 5 mg/m² given on two consecutive days every 2 weeks until a CR was attained.[26] In 34 patients treated with this approach, 53% achieved a CR and 38% a PR. Treatment with DCF was associated with a 96% incidence of Grade 3/4 myelosuppression, a 19% incidence of serious infection, and two treatment related fatalities. With a median follow-up of 82 months, Kraut et al. described their experience in a group of 24 patients with HCL treated with DCF delivered every other week at a

| Table 31.2 | Trial results of DCF in hairy cell leukemia | | | | | | | |
|---|---|---|---|---|---|---|---|---|
| Author | Institution | Year | N | Treatment | CR | PR | Relapse | F/U |
| Cassileth[24] | Univ. of Penn. | 1991 | 50 | 5 mg/m² × 2d q.2 weeks | 64% | 20% | 14% | 39 months |
| Johnston[25] | NCI-CCTG[a] | 1988 | 28 | 4 mg/m², IV, per week ×3, q.8 weeks | 89% | 11% | NR | 429 days |
| Spiers[26] | ECOG[b] | 1987 | 34 | 5 mg/m² × 2d q.2 weeks | | 53% | 38% | NR NR |
| Kraut[27] | The Ohio State Univ. | 1994 | 24 | 4 mg/m², IV q.2 weeks | N/A[c] | N/A[c] | 48% | 82 months |
| Ribeiro[28] | Centre Hospitalier Lyon-Sud, France | 1999 | 50 | 4 mg/m², IV q.2 weeks | 44% | (36/16)%[d] | 10% | 33 months |
| Grever[29] | Intergroup[e] | 1995 | 154 | 4 mg/m², IV q.2 weeks | 76% | 3% | 9% | 57 months |
| Flinn[30] | Intergroup[e,f] | 2000 | 241 | 4 mg/m², IV q.2 weeks | N/A[f] | N/A | 18%[f] | 9.3 years |

[a] National Cancer Institute – Canadian Clinical Trials Group.
[b] Eastern Cooperative Oncology Group.
[c] All patients in the study had attained a CR, and were followed for relapse, survival, and long-term toxicity.
[d] 38% good PR (bone marrow involvement <5%), 19% PR.
[e] Southwest Oncology Group, Eastern Cooperative Oncology Group, Cancer and Leukemia Group B, National Cancer Institute- Canadian Clinical Trials Group.
[f] Long-term follow-up of the randomized Intergroup study, which included all patients treated with DCF initially or on crossover from interferon. The 5- and 10-year relapse-free survival were 85% and 67%, respectively.

dose of 4 mg/m$^2$, again until a CR was attained.[27] Only 1 of the patients died, but 11 of the remaining 23 patients had relapsed at a median time of 30 months from therapy. There were no serious infectious complications, nor was there a dramatic increase in second malignancies, with the exception of epithelial skin cancers.

Similar results were observed in 50 patients treated with an identical regimen of every-other-week DCF in a French study reported by Ribeiro et al.[28] With a median follow-up of 33 months, responses were documented in 96% of the patients, including 44% of those who achieved a CR, 36% with a "good" PR (bone marrow involvement of <5%), and 16% with a PR. There were two deaths. The toxicity included Grade 3/4 neutropenia in 13 of the patients (26%), fever with infection in 13 patients (26%), nausea and vomiting despite the prophylactic use of antiemetics in 14 (28%), and rash in 9 patients. Second malignancies were observed in 10% of the patients.

In an Intergroup study, the response and duration of relapse-free survival in patients with hairy cell leukemia treated with interferon-α or DCF were compared and their toxicities described.[29] Three hundred and thirteen eligible patients were randomized to either interferon α-2a, 3 million units subcutaneously three times per week for 6 months (prolonged to a full year for an objective response) versus DCF at 4 mg/m$^2$ administered intravenously every other week (given two doses past a CR, continued to 12 months if a PR was achieved, and stopped at 6 months in the absence of a response). Crossover was allowed. While only 11% of the interferon-α treated patients achieved a CR and 27% a PR with no early deaths, 76% of the DCF patients achieved a CR and 3% a PR, with three early deaths. Grade 4 myelosuppression was significantly greater with DCF than with interferon-α, as was the incidence of suspected infections in the DCF group (53% vs 35%, respectively). The median relapse-free survival of the 134 patients who achieved a CR was significantly longer in the DCF treated group (and had not yet been reached) than the 20-month relapse-free survival calculated in the interferon-α group, after a median follow-up of 57 months. Once a median follow-up of 9.3 years had been reached, the updated relapse, toxicity, and survival data of the 154 patients initially treated with DCF, and the 87 patients treated upon crossover from interferon-α failure, was reported by Flinn et al.[30] The 5- and 10-year survival of 90% and 81% was no different from that calculated from an age and sex matched control population. The 5- and 10-year relapse-free survival were 85% and 67%, respectively, based on the 173 patients who achieved a CR. After lymphoid, hematologic, and epithelial skin cancers were excluded, the 25 diagnoses of solid tumors recorded was not any greater than that expected in the general population.

In summary, complete remission can be achieved in a high percentage of patients with hairy cell leukemia treated with DCF at the standard dose of 4 mg/m$^2$ intravenously given every other week until the attainment of remission. It appears that these remissions are durable despite a lack of clear evidence that the therapy is, in fact, curative.

**Toxicity**

The major toxicity of DCF is related to profound immunosuppression with significant granulocytopenia, as well as CD4$^+$ lymphopenia. Rates of severe neutropenia vary with the regimen used, but range from 26% up to 96%. Associated rates of infection range from 26% up to 53%. Although uncommon, treatment-related deaths have been reported in many of the published series. Additional common toxicities include dermatitis, nausea, and vomiting, and less common toxicities include lethargy, altered taste, paresthesias, and conjunctivitis. Although the immunosuppression appears prolonged, there is no evidence that this results in an increase in serious delayed infections or second malignancies.

## SPLENECTOMY

Splenomegaly is present in the majority of patients with hairy cell leukemia, with leukemic infiltration primarily within the red pulp.[31,32] Therefore, removal of the spleen eradicates one of the major sites of disease accumulation.

Splenectomy was the treatment of choice for hairy cell leukemia before the introduction of effective cytotoxic therapies. In the majority of cases, the peripheral blood counts responded favorably and patients survived for years after the operation, often without additional therapy. Splenectomy removes splenic sequestration of blood elements, thereby alleviating pancytopenia. However, in situations in which pancytopenia is secondary to bone marrow infiltration by hairy cells, splenectomy is less beneficial. CR, defined as hemoglobin greater than 11.0 g/dL, granulocyte count greater than 1000/mm$^3$, and a platelet count greater than 100,000/mm$^3$ (Catovsky criteria), has been reported in 40–67% of patients (see Table 31.3). Improvement in at least one cytopenia is seen in up to 90% of patients. The most common hematologic parameter to improve postsplenectomy is the platelet count, often seen within days of the surgery. Patients who achieve a CR have improved survival compared to partial responders.[33,35,37,41] However, an overall survival benefit from splenectomy has not been consistently demonstrated.[34,36,39,42] Before the introduction of effective systemic therapies, patients who did not respond to splenectomy had a poor prognosis. Both the probability of response as well as the duration of response inversely correlates with the degree of bone marrow involvement. The duration of response to splenectomy has been evaluated extensively (see Table 31.3).

| Table 31.3 Splenectomy in the treatment of hairy cell leukemia | | | | |
|---|---|---|---|---|
| Author | Number of subjects | CR (%) | PR (%) | Response duration (months) |
| Catovsky[33] | 28 | 61 | 39 | 2.5-16 |
| Golomb[34] | 71 | NR | 91 | NR |
| Mintz and Golomb[35] | 26 | 42 | 58 | NR |
| Jansen[36] | 225 | 40 | 39 | NR |
| Ingoldby[37] | 21 | 62 | 24 | 4-31 |
| Golomb[38] | 65 | 42 | 58 | NR |
| Flandrin[39] | 85 | 61 | 73 | NR |
| Magee[40] | 26 | 77 | 11 | 4-20 |
| Van Norman[41] | 42 | 67 | 19 | NR |

CR: complete response; PR: partial response; NR: not reported.

Despite a concern about an increased incidence of infections following splenectomy, Golomb found no change in infectious complications in postsplenectomy patients.[34,43] Nevertheless, vaccinations against encapsulated organisms are recommended prior to splenectomy.

With the advent of new, more effective treatment modalities, splenectomy has fallen out of favor. It is now considered a temporizing measure, with a median time to treatment failure of 8.3 months (range, 1–22 months). Even prior to the adoption of modern surgical techniques, including laparoscopic splenectomy, surgical mortality was low, estimated at 2% in some reports.[41] Splenectomy has been safely performed at the twenty-fourth week of gestation in a pregnant patient with hairy cell leukemia.[44]

Current indications for splenectomy as an initial treatment approach to hairy cell leukemia include active or uncontrolled infections in the setting of severe and refractory neutropenia secondary to hairy cell leukemia, thrombocytopenic bleeding, massive, painful, or ruptured splenomegaly, or contraindications to chemotherapy (e.g., pregnancy or medical comorbidities).

### INTERFERON

When splenectomy was used commonly as a first-line treatment approach to HCL, one of every two to three patients relapsed following the procedure. Other chemotherapeutic agents were tried with limited success.[45–47] The demonstration of activity of interferon-α against hairy cell leukemia was viewed as a significant advance, as it was the first agent that could partially eradicate the hairy cell population from the bone marrow, thus eventually changing the response criteria. However, much like splenectomy, interferon-α is only rarely indicated in the current approach to initial management, and only under certain clinical circumstances.

The first experience with interferon in hairy cell leukemia was reported in 1984 by Quesada et al.[48] They treated seven patients with partially purified human interferon and showed a dramatic improvement in all blood counts within a 2- to 3-month period. Once recombinant interferon became available, Golomb et al. treated 69 patients with interferon α-2b at $2 \times 10^6$ U/m$^2$ subcutaneously three times weekly for a year.[49–51] Interferon-α demonstrated an ORR of 91% with 13% of the patients achieving a CR, defined as <5% of hairy cells in the bone marrow and normalization of peripheral blood counts. Relapses were uncommon during therapy and for the first 6–9 months thereafter. Median actuarial failure-free survival was 25.4 months.

Interferon α-2a (Roferon-A, Roche, Nutley, NJ) has also been studied in hairy cell leukemia. Quesada et al.[52] treated 25 patients with $3 \times 10^6$ U/m$^2$ of interferon α-2a daily for 4–6 months, followed by three times a week for a year. They documented a response rate of 87%, with 30% of the patients exhibiting a CR. Median time to remission was 3.5 months. Discontinuation of the treatment resulted in clinical relapse in 33% of the patients.

Numerous other trials have shown comparable results (see Table 31.4). Response rates range from 43% to 100%, the majority of which are partial. Hematologic changes follow a well-described pattern. Platelet counts increase first, often as early as 2 weeks into therapy, reaching a normal value by approximately 1.5–2 months. During the first 2 months of treatment there is a notable decrease in the white count and hemoglobin.[53] Full granulocytic response is usually delayed until 3–5 months. Hemoglobin response lags behind, with responses still seen as far as 9 months into the therapy.[58,59] In general, treatment naive patients exhibit higher response rates. In addition to improving peripheral blood counts, interferon-α also reduces splenomegaly size. Interferon-α is effective in patients with an intact spleen as well as in splenectomized patients.

Neither the optimal dose nor the optimal duration of interferon therapy has been clearly established. Standard regimens include either interferon α-2b (Intron A) $2 \times 10^6$ U/m$^2$ subcutaneously three times per week for a year or interferon α-2a (Roferon-A) $3 \times 10^6$ U/m$^2$ daily for 4–6 months, followed by three times a week a for a year.

Despite impressive ORRs, between 33% and 86% patients relapse at a median of 6–30 months (see Table 31.3).[51,56,60,62–64]

With long-term follow-up, an increased incidence of second malignancies has been noted following interferon-α treatment.[65] After a median follow-up of 91 months, 13 patients (19%) developed a second malignancy. Six were hematopoietic and seven adenocarcinomas. The excess frequency was 4.33 compared

**Table 31.4** Results of interferon therapy in patients with hairy cell leukemia

| Author | Type of interferon | Dose and schedule | Number of subjects | CR (%) | PR (%) | Duration (month) of response |
|---|---|---|---|---|---|---|
| Quesada[48] | Interferon alpha-N1 | $3 \times 10^6$ U daily | 7 | 42 | 57 | 6–10 |
| Jacobs[53] | Interferon alpha-2b | $2 \times 10^6$ U/m$^2$, three times weekly | 22 | 0 | 43 | NR |
| Quesada[52] | Interferon alpha-2a | $3 \times 10^6$ U daily for 4–6 months, followed by three times weekly for 1 year | 30 | 30 | 57 | 10+ |
| Castaigne[54] | Interferon alpha-2° Interferon alpha-2b Interferon alpha-N1 | $3 \times 10^6$ U daily $2 \times 10^6$ U/m$^2$, three times weekly $3 \times 10^6$ U daily | 27 | 7 | 29 | NR |
| Thompson[55] | Interferon alpha-2b | $2 \times 10^6$ U/m$^2$ three times weekly for 1 year | 212 | 4 | 74 | NR |
| Berman[56] | Interferon alpha-2a | $3 \times 10^6$ U daily for 4–6 months, followed by three times weekly for 18 months | 35 | 0 | 69 | 25 |
| Smith[57] | Interferon alpha-2a | $3 \times 10^6$ U daily for 4–6 months, followed by three times weekly for 1 year | 53 | 2 | 74 | NR |
| Golomb[51] | Interferon alpha-2b | $2 \times 10^6$ U/m$^2$, three times weekly | 69 | 13 | 62 | 25.4 |
| Smalley[58] | Interferon alpha-N1 | $2 \times 10^6$ U/m$^2$, daily for 28 days followed by three times weekly for 22 weeks | 10 | 2 | 60 | NR |
| Grever[29] | Interferon alpha-2a | $3 \times 10^6$ U 3 times per week | 159 | 11 | 38 | 9–27 |
| Rai[59] | Interferon alpha-2b | $2 \times 10^6$ U/m$^2$ three times weekly for 1 year | 64 | 24 | 49 | 18 |
| Zinzani[60] | Interferon alpha-2a | $3 \times 10^6$ U daily | 44 | 18 | 64 | 14 |
| Damasio[61] | Interferon alpha-2a | $3 \times 10^6$ U 3 times per week | 64 | 0 | 90 | NR |

CR: complete response; PR: partial response; NR: not reported.

to the general population, and for patients with hematologic neoplasms, it was 40 times the expected frequency. However, other single institution series indicate a risk equal to the general population, but with an increase in lymphoid neoplasms.[20]

The toxicity profile of interferon includes a mild influenza-like syndrome. This syndrome occurs in 95% of patients and is characterized by fevers, myalgias, and fatigue; it improves after 2–4 weeks despite the continuation of therapy and responds well to acetaminophen. Cutaneous side effects, including both generalized rash as well as injection site reactions, are noted in approximately 50% of the patients. Central nervous system side effects include depression and somnolence. Although transient myelosuppression is observed during the first 2 months of therapy, patients treated with interferon have fewer incidences of infections compared to an untreated cohort.[52] Reversible liver enzyme abnormalities are observed in 20–30% of the patients.

In summary, interferon-α remains a palliative treatment strategy without observed complete eradication of the disease. Compared to nucleoside analogs, the response is usually slower and only rarely complete. It is now rarely the initial treatment of choice, but can be considered for hairy cell leukemia patients with active uncontrolled infection, for a disease which has relapsed or is refractory to first-line therapy, or in those with an unacceptably high risk for febrile neutropenia. This may include elderly patients with medical comorbidities, which preclude the use of purine analogs, or those with significant renal insufficiency. In addition, although experience with interferon-α in pregnant patients with hairy cell leukemia is limited, safety has been demonstrated when used in similar patients with chronic myelogenous leukemia.

## SUMMARY

Hairy cell leukemia is an uncommon, low-grade lymphoproliferative disorder. Although the mere documentation of the presence of this leukemia is not itself an indication for therapy, the majority of patients will eventually require treatment for their disease. Although, historically, the initial treatment approach has evolved from splenectomy to interferon-α, contemporary treatment options include either a single-week-long course of 2-CdA, traditionally delivered by continuous intravenous infusion, or 4–6 months of DCF, given as a short infusion every other week. Although there have been no randomized trials comparing these two approaches, both therapies result in prolonged, unmaintained remissions in the vast majority of patients. In addition, both therapies are associated with profound and prolonged immunosuppression, although the subsequent infectious complication rates are low.

## REFERENCES

1. Golomb HM, Catovsky D, Golde DW: Hairy cell leukemia. A clinical review based on 71 cases. *Ann Intern Med* 89(Part 1):677, 1978.
2. Carson DA, Wasson DB, Beutler E: Antileukemia and immunosuppressive activity of 2-chloro-2′-deoxyadenosine. *Proc Natl Acad Sci U S A* 81:2232, 1981.
3. Carrera CJ, Piro LD, Miller WE, et al.: Remission induction in hairy cell leukemia by treatment with 2-chlorodeoxyadenosine: Role of DNA strand breaks and NAD depletion [abstract]. *Clin Res* 35:597A, 1987.
4. Piro LD, Carrera CJ, Carson DA, et al.: Lasting remissions in hairy cell leukemia induced by a single infusion of 2-chlorodeoxyadenosine. *N Engl J Med* 322:1117, 1990.
5. Saven A, Burian C, Koziol JA, et al.: Long-term follow-up of patients with hairy cell leukemia after cladribine treatment. *Blood* 92:1918, 1998.
6. Goodman GR, Burian C, Koziol JA, et al.: Extended follow-up of patients with hairy cell leukemia after treatment with cladribine. *J Clin Oncol* 21:891, 2003.
7. Estey EM, Kurzrock R, Kantarjian HM, et al.: Treatment of hairy cell leukemia with 2-chlorodeoxyadenosine (2-CdA). *Blood* 79:882, 1992.
8. Tallman MS, Hakimian D, Rademaker AW, et al.: Relapse of hairy cell leukemia after 2-chlorodeoxyadenosine: Long-term follow-up of the Northwestern University experience. *Blood* 88:1954, 1996.
9. Hoffman MA, Janson D, Rose E, et al.: Treatment of hairy cell leukemia with cladribine: response, toxicity and long-term follow-up. *J Clin Oncol* 15:1138, 1997.
10. Cheson BD, Vena DA, Montello MJ, et al.: Treatment of hairy cell leukemia with 2-chlorodeoxyadenosine via the Group C Protocol Mechanism of the National Cancer Institute: a report of 979 patients. *J Clin Oncol* 16:3007, 1998.
11. Dearden CE, Matutes E, Hilditch BL, Swansbury GJ, Catovsky D: Long-term follow-up of patients with hairy cell leukaemia with pentostatin or cladribine. *Br J Haematol* 106:515, 1999.
12. Hakimian D, Tallman MS, Kiley C, et al.: Detection of minimal residual disease by immunostaining of bone marrow biopsies after 2-chlorodeoxyadenosine for hairy cell leukemia. *Blood* 82:1798, 1993.
13. Ellison DJ, Sharpe RW, Robbins BA, et al.: Immunomorphologic analysis of bone marrow biopsies after treatment with 2-chlorodeoxyadenosine for hairy cell leukemia. *Blood* 84:4310, 1994.
14. Juliusson G, Heldal D, Hippe E, et al.: Subcutaneous injections of 2-chlorodeoxyadenosine for symptomatic hairy cell leukemia. *J Clin Oncol* 13:989, 1995.
15. Lauria F, Bocchia M, Marotta G, et al.: Weekly administration of 2-chlorodeoxyadenosine in patients with hairy cell leukemia: a new treatment schedule effective and safer in preventing infectious complications (Letter). *Blood* 89:1838, 1998.
16. Liliemark J, Albertioni F, Hassan M, et al.: On the bioavailability of oral and subcutaneous 2-chloro-2′-deoxyadenosine in humans: alternative routes of administration. *J Clin Oncol* 10:1514, 1992.
17. Saven A, Burian C, Adusumalli J, et al.: Filgrastim for cladribine-induced neutropenic fever in patients with hairy cell leukemia. *Blood* 93:2471, 1999.
18. Seymour J, Kurzrock R, Freireich EJ, et al.: 2-Chlorodeoxyadenosine induces durable remissions and prolonged suppression of CD4+ lymphocyte counts in patients with hairy cell leukemia. *Blood* 83:2906, 1994.
19. Kurzrock R, Strom SS, Estey E, et al.: Second cancer risk in hairy cell leukemia: analysis of 350 patients. *J Clin Oncol* 15:1803, 1997.
20. Federico M, Zinzani PL, Frassoldati A, et al.: Risk of second cancer in patients with hairy cell leukemia: long-term follow-up. *J Clin Oncol* 20:638, 2002.
21. Cheson BD, Vena DA, Barrett J, et al.: Second malignancies as a consequence of nucleoside analog therapy for chronic lymphoid leukemias. *J Clin Oncol* 17:2454, 1999.
22. Au WY, Klasa RJ, Gallagher R, et al.: Second malignancies in patients with hairy cell leukemia in British Columbia: a 20-year experience. *Blood* 92:1160, 1998.
23. Spiers ASD, Parekh SJ: Pentostatin (2′-deoxycoformycin, DCF) is active in hairy cell leukemia (HCL) [abstract]. *Blood* 62:208a, 1983.
24. Cassileth PA, Cheuvant B, Spiers ASD, et al.: Pentostatin induces durable remissions in hairy cell leukemia. *J Clin Oncol* 9:243, 1991.
25. Johnston JB, Glazer RI, Pugh L, et al.: The treatment of hairy cell leukemia with 2′-deoxycoformycin. *Br J Haematol* 63:525, 1986.
26. Spiers ASD, Moore D, Cassileth PA, et al.: Remissions in hairy cell leukemia with pentostatin (2′-deoxycoformycin). *N Engl J Med* 316:825, 1987.
27. Kraut EH, Grever MR, Bouroncle BA: Long-term follow-up of patients with hairy cell leukemia after treatment with 2′-deoxycoformycin. *Blood* 84:4061, 1994.
28. Ribeiro P, Bouaffia F, et al.: Long term outcome of patients with hairy cell leukemia treated with pentostatin. *Cancer* 84:65, 1999.
29. Grever M, Kopecky K, Foucar MK, et al.: Randomized comparison of pentostatin versus interferon alfa-2a in previously untreated patients with hairy cell leukemia: an intergroup study. *J Clin Oncol* 13:974, 1995.
30. Flinn IW, Kopecky KJ, Foucar MK, et al.: Long-term follow-up of remission duration, mortality, and second malignancies in hairy cell leukemia patients treated with pentostatin. *Blood* 96:2981, 2000.

31. Golomb HM: Hairy cell leukemia. An unusual lympho-proliferative disease: a study of 24 patients. *Cancer* 42:946, 1978.

32. Katayama I, Finkel HE: Leukemic reticuloendotheliosis. A clinicopathologic study with review of the literature. *Am J Med* 57:115, 1974.

33. Catovsky D: Hairy cell leukemia and prolymphocytic leukemia. *Clin Haematol* 6:245, 1977.

34. Golomb HM, Catovsky D, Golde DW: Hairy cell leukemia: a five-year update on seventy-one patients. *Ann Intern Med* 99:485, 1983.

35. Mintz U, Golomb HM: Splenectomy as initial therapy in twenty-six patients with leukemic reticuloendotheliosis (hairy cell leukemia). *Cancer Res* 39:2366, 1979.

36. Jansen J, Hermans J: Splenectomy in hairy cell leukemia: a retrospective multicenter analysis. *Cancer* 47:2066, 1981.

37. Ingoldby CJ, Ackroyd N, Catovsky D, et al.: Splenectomy for hairy cell leukaemia. *Clin Oncol* 7:325, 1981.

38. Golomb HM, Vardiman JW: Response to splenectomy in 65 patients with hairy cell leukemia: an evaluation of spleen weight and bone marrow involvement. *Blood* 61:349, 1983.

39. Flandrin G, Sigaux F, Sebahoun G, et al.: Hairy cell leukemia: clinical presentation and follow-up of 211 patients. *Semin Oncol* 11:458, 1984.

40. Magee MJ, McKenzie S, Filippa DA, et al.: Hairy cell leukemia: durability of response to splenectomy in 26 patients and treatment of relapse with androgens in six patients. *Cancer* 56:2557, 1985.

41. Van Norman AS, Nagorney DM, Martin JK, et al.: Splenectomy for hairy cell leukemia: a clinical review of 63 patients. *Cancer* 57:644, 1986.

42. Bouroncle BA: The history of hairy cell leukemia: characteristics of long-term survivors. *Semin Oncol* 11:479, 1984.

43. Golomb HM, Hadad LJ: Infectious complications in 127 patients with hairy cell leukemia. *Am J Hematol* 16:393, 1984.

44. Stiles GM, Stanco LM, Saven A, et al.: Splenectomy for hairy cell leukemia in pregnancy. *J Perinatol* 18:200, 1998.

45. Golomb HM: Progress report on chlorambucil therapy in postsplenectomy patients with progressive hairy cell leukemia. *Blood* 57:464, 1981.

46. Stewart DJ, Benjamin RS, McCredie KB, et al.: The effectiveness of rubidazone in hairy cell leukemia (leukemic reticuloendotheliosis). *Blood* 54:298, 1979.

47. Calvo F, Castaigne S, Sigaux F, et al.: Intensive chemotherapy of hairy cell leukemia in patients with aggressive disease. *Blood* 65:115, 1985.

48. Quesada JR, Reuben J, Manning JT, et al.: Alpha-interferon for induction of remission in hairy cell leukemia. *N Engl J Med* 310:15, 1984.

49. Ratain MJ, Golomb HM, Vardiman JW, et al.: Treatment of hairy cell leukemia with recombinant alpha-2 interferon. *Blood* 65:644, 1985.

50. Golomb HM, Jacobs A, Fefer A, et al.: Alpha-2 interferon therapy of hairy cell leukemia: a multicenter study of 64 patients. *J Clin Oncol* 4:900, 1986.

51. Golomb HM, Ratain MJ, Mick R, et al.: Interferon treatment for hairy cell leukemia: An update on a cohort of 69 patients treated from 1983–1986. *Leukemia* 6:1177, 1992.

52. Quesada JR, Hersh EM, Manning J, et al.: Treatment of hairy cell leukemia with recombinant alpha-interferon. *Blood* 68:493, 1986.

53. Jacobs AD, Champlin RE, Golde DW: Recombinant alpha-2 interferon for hairy cell leukemia. *Blood* 65:1017, 1985.

54. Castaigne S, Sigaux F, Cantell K: Interferon alpha in the treatment of hairy cell leukemia. *Cancer* 57(8):1681, 1986.

55. Thompson JA, Fefer A: Interferon in the treatment of hairy cell leukemia. *Cancer* 59:605, 1987.

56. Berman E, Heller G, Kempin S, et al.: Incidence of response and long-term follow-up in patients with hairy cell leukemia with recombinant alpha-2a. *Blood* 75:839, 1990.

57. Smith JW, II, Longo DL, Urba WJ, et al.: Prolonged, continuous treatment of hairy cell leukemia patients with recombinant interferon-alpha 2a. *Blood* 78:1664, 1991.

58. Smalley RV, Connors J, Tuttle RL, et al.: Splenectomy vs. alpha interferon: a randomized study in patients with previously untreated hairy cell leukemia. *Am J Hematol* 41:13, 1992.

59. Rai KR, Davey F, Peterson B, et al.: Recombinant alpha-2b-interferon in therapy of previously untreated hairy cell leukemia: long-term follow-up results of study by Cancer and Leukemia Group B. *Leukemia* 9:1116, 1995.

60. Zinzani PL, Lauria F, Raspadori D, et al.: Comparison of low-dose versus standard-dose alpha-interferon regimen in the hairy cell leukemia treatment. *Acta Haematol* 85:16, 1991.

61. Damasio EE, Clavio M, Masoudi B, et al.: Alpha-interferon as induction and maintenance therapy in hairy cell leukemia: a long term follow-up analysis. *Eur J Haematol* 64:47, 2000.

62. Golomb HM, Ratain MJ, Fefer A, et al.: Randomized study of the duration of treatment with interferon alfa-2b in patients with hairy cell leukemia. *J Natl Cancer Inst* 80:369, 1988.

63. Ratain MJ, Golomb HM, Bardawil RG: Durability of responses to interferon alfa-2b in advanced hairy cell leukemia. *Blood* 69:872, 1987.

64. Ratain MJ, Golomb HM, Vardiman JW, et al.: Relapse after interferon alpha-2b therapy for hairy cell leukemia: analysis of diagnostic variables. *J Clin Oncol* 6:1714, 1988.

65. Kampmeier P, Spielberger R, Dickstein J, et al.: Increased incidence of second neoplasms in patients treated with interferon α-2b for hairy cell leukemia: a clinicopathologic assessment. *Blood* 83:2931, 1994.

# Chapter 32

# DEFINITION OF REMISSION, PROGNOSIS, AND FOLLOW-UP IN HAIRY CELL LEUKEMIA

*Eric H. Kraut*

## TREATMENT AND REMISSION DEFINITION

### NATURAL HISTORY

Hairy Cell Leukemia (HCL) is a chronic lymphoproliferative disorder usually presenting with pancytopenia, recurrent systemic infections, and splenomegaly.[1] The major cause of death in untreated patients is infection, usually due to an immune deficiency state related to neutropenia, monocytopenia, natural killer cell deficiency, and dendritic cell deficiency.[2,3] Therapy prior to 1980 temporarily improved blood counts, but had no dramatic effect on the immune deficiency or overall survival, with patients dying as a result of their disease within 5 years of diagnosis.[4] The dramatic change in survival as a result of the treatments outlined in Chapter 31 has transformed HCL from a fatal disorder to a chronic one, with some patients cured of their disease.

### SPLENECTOMY

The definition of remission in a malignancy is established in order to distinguish the effectiveness of different treatment options and determine whether treatment has an impact on survival and quality of life. The development of these definitions for HCL has paralleled the improved management of this disease.

For many years, the major treatment for patients with HCL was splenectomy.[5] Splenectomy was undertaken either due to pain and discomfort secondary to an enlarged spleen or for the cytopenias seen in this disease. Responses to splenectomy were classified according to those established by Catovsky[6] (Table 32.1). A complete response (CR) was defined as an increase in hemoglobin level above 11 g/dL, neutrophils above $1 \times 10^9$/L, and platelets above $100 \times 10^9$/L. A partial response (PR) was the same degree of improvement in one or two of the blood elements or improvement in all three, but below the values for CR. These criteria took into account that splenectomy did

improve cytopenias in 60–100% of the patients, but did not significantly affect the bone marrow infiltration or circulating hairy cells.[5,7] In fact, the degree of bone marrow involvement prior to splenectomy appeared to predict the degree of success with this procedure, and thus patients with marked infiltration of the marrow with hairy cells were less likely to respond.[7]

### INTERFERON

In 1984, a major advance in the treatment of HCL was achieved with the evidence that alpha interferon was cytotoxic to hairy cells and could induce complete remissions in some patients.[9] The ability to eradicate the hairy cell population from the bone marrow led to more stringent criteria for response, culminating in the consensus resolution for the response published in 1987[8] (Table 32.1). A CR now required a hemoglobin level ≥12 g/dL, a neutrophil count ≥1500/μL, and

| Table 32.1 Criteria for response assessment in hairy cell leukemia[8] | |
|---|---|
| Complete response | Partial response* |
| Neutrophils ≥1500μL[a] | Reduction in organomegaly >50% |
| Platelets ≥100,000/μL | <5% circulating hairy cells |
| Hemoglobin ≥12 g/dL[a] | Decrease by 50% hairy cells in |
| No hairy cells in bone marrow by H&E[a] | bone marrow |
| Regression of spleen to normal by physical exam[a] | Hemoglobin ≥12 g/dL |
| No circulating hairy cells[a] | Neutrophils ≥ 1500/μL |
| | Platelets ≥ 100,000/μL |

[a]Catovsky[6] definition allowed 1000 neutrophils and hemoglobin of 11 for complete remission and does not include clearance of marrow or peripheral blood for hairy cells. Partial remission just required improvement of two of three blood valus to the CR definition or improvement in all three values.

clearance of hairy cells from blood and bone marrow, with resolution of organomegaly on physical exam. A PR required a 50% decrease in organomegaly and less than 5% circulating hairy cells, with normalization of the blood counts as described for a CR.

Despite its obvious activity, interferon rarely completely eliminated the hairy cells from the bone marrow, and the majority of patients were left with significant bone marrow infiltration.[10,11] The amount of remaining hairy cell involvement in the marrow after treatment had prognostic significance, with early relapse occurring in patients with greater than 30% hairy cell infiltration.

### PURINE NUCLEOSIDES

The introduction of the purine nucleosides pentostatin (2-deoxycoformycin) and 2-chlorodeoxyadenosine (2-CdA) revolutionized the management of HCL and raised the possibility of cure. Both of these drugs induce a high percentage of true complete remissions, which are durable in a significant number of patients.[12–14] Using the stringent guidelines outlined in the consensus resolution, over 90% of the patients had responses, and those with responses experienced marked improvement in survival. However, using more sophisticated techniques such as flow cytometry and immunohistochemistry, up to 50% of the patients in complete remission by standard criteria have minimal residual disease remaining in their bone marrow.[15,16] The impact of this observation on the outcome of patients is unclear.

Several investigators have examined the remission duration and survival in patients who have negative bone marrows by morphology, but positive bone marrows by immunohistochemistry and flow cytometry.[16–18] Tallman et al.[16] evaluated 66 patients treated with either pentostatin or 2-CdA, and in complete remission by clinical and morphologic criteria. The estimated 4-year relapse-free survival was 55% in the patients with minimal residual disease by immunohistochemistry and 88% in the patients without minimal residual disease. Matutes et al.[17] evaluated 23 patients after treatment with 2-deoxycoformycin and in complete remission by standard criteria. He reported no difference in relapse rates in the patients with or without minimal residual disease by immunophenotyping of bone marrow or peripheral blood.

For future clinical trials in HCL, it is reasonable to incorporate immunohistochemistry and flow data on the patient's bone marrow, and add a category of complete remission with minimal residual disease by special studies. This will provide us with information on how necessary it is to completely eradicate the hairy cell population, and give us better methods to compare new therapies.

## PROGNOSIS

The change in the prognosis of patients with HCL is best demonstrated by comparing data from patients followed and treated prior to 1985, largely with splenectomy, to patients followed after treatment with interferon and the purine nucleosides (Table 32.2).

| Table 32.2 | Remission duration and survival | | | |
|---|---|---|---|---|
| Author | N | Treatment | Median PFS | Median survival |
| Bouroncle[19] | 105 | +/− Spelnectomy | | 5.8 years |
| Golomb and Golde[4] | 71 | +/− Splenectomy | | 5.8 years |
| Jansen and Hermans[20] | 391 | +/− Splenectomy | | 4 years |
| Ratain et al.[11] | 69 | Interferonα | 25.4 months | not reached 91%/4years |
| Federico et al.[21] | 166 | Interferonα | | not reached 96%/5years |
| Grever et al.[13] | 17 | Interferonα | 20 months | not reached At 57 months |
| Goodman et al.[14] | 209 | Cladribine | 99 months | not reached 97%/9 years |
| Tallman[22] | 52 | Cladrbine | 72%/48 months | 96%/4 years |
| Flinn et al.[23] | 241 | Pentostatin | 85% at 60 months 67% at 120 months | not reached 90%/10 years |
| Kraut et at.[24] | 24 | Pentostatin | | not reached 96%/6.8 years |

PFS, pregression-free survival.

## SPLENECTOMY AND NATURAL HISTORY

Bouroncle[19] reported on 105 patients followed with or without splenectomy, and noted a median survival of 5.8 years. Golomb et al.[4] gave an update on 71 patients with a median survival, measured starting at the development of symptoms (not from diagnosis), of 70 months. Jansen and Hermans[20] analyzed 391 patients from multiple institutions to evaluate the effectiveness of splenectomy, and noted an overall median survival of 48 months. Patients in this series, who underwent a splenectomy, had a survival benefit. The other observation from these reports was that several parameters had prognostic importance, including the degree of cytopenias and a history of infections.

## INTERFERON

Although interferon was the first drug with significant activity in HCL patients, long-term studies are limited because of the subsequent introduction of the purine nucleoosides. Ratain et al.[11] reported on 69 patients who received alpha interferon, and noted a 91% survival at 4 years. However, the median time for a patient requiring treatment (usually due to cytopenia) was 25.4 months. Federico et al.[21] followed 166 patients who received interferon therapy, and reported a 96% survival at 5 years, with most patients progressing by 4 years. Grever described that 12 of 17 patients who were in complete remission after interferon therapy relapsed with a median time of 20 months. Median survival had not been reached at a median follow-up of 57 months. Thus, although the disease is not eradicated, survival appears improved over splenectomy.

## PURINE NUCLEOSIDES

Patients treated with either cladribine or pentostatin have a disease course that resembles patients with indolent lymphoma, with prolonged responses to therapy and overall survival longer than relapse-free survival.[22] Goodman et al.[14] reported on 209 patients treated with cladribine and followed them for at least 7 years. Of the 207 patients evaluated, 95% had a CR and 5% a PR. The median duration of a CR was 99 months (range, 8–172 months) and that of a PR was 37 months (range, 10–116 months). Seventy six patients (37%) relapsed after the first course of treatment, with a median time to relapse of 42 months (range, 8–118 months). The risk of relapse was increased with short disease duration prior to therapy, lower hemoglobin levels, and higher white blood counts at baseline. Sixty patients in first relapse after cladribine were retreated, with a CR rate of 75% in the 59 evaluable patients and a median duration of second remission of 35 months (range, 4–92 months). Second relapses were seen in 20 patients, with 6 of 10 patients treated again achieving CR. When survival was evaluated for all patients, only six patients (3%), all complete responders, had died. However, only one of these patients died from causes related to disease. The overall survival rate in this series was 97% at 108 months.

Flinn et al.[23] reported a 9-year follow-up of a large intergroup study of HCL patients treated with pentostatin. A total of 241 patients were treated with pentostatin initially or after interferon failure. There were 40 deaths, with only 2 deaths due to HCL. And 201 patients were followed for a median of 9.3 years, with a Kaplan-Meier estimate of survival of 90% at 5 years and 81% at ten years. The 173 patients (71%) who achieved a confirmed CR had an overall relapse-free survival of 85% at 5 years and 67% at 10 years. There was no comment on retreatment after relapse.

Kraut et al.[24] reported 24 patients followed after pentostatin therapy for a median of 82 months (range, 54–104 months). Out of 24 patients 23 were alive, with one dying of refractory/recurrent disease. Twelve patients remained in remission and 11 patients relapsed. Seven patients were retreated, with 5 achieving a second complete remission. The overall survival from treatment initiation of this group was 93 months (range, 63–116 months). There have been only two documented deaths in this group, and neither related to disease.

In summary, patients treated with purine nucleosides have a dramatic increase in their survival, and few responding patients have died due to their disease. The development of other therapies for resistant disease, such as rituximab[25] or anti-CD-22 recombinant immunotoxin (BL 22),[26] and the potential benefit of splenectomy or interferon in treatment failures, may further extend survival.

## LONG-TERM COMPLICATIONS

The initial concern for patients treated with the purine nucleosides was for an increased risk of infection and the development of second malignancies due to the profound long-term suppression of CD4 and CD8 lymphocytes.[27,28] However, a significant increase in infections is not seen in patients who have responded to treatment and have normal neutrophil counts. In our series, during the 7-year median follow-up, only herpes zoster was seen in remission patients.[24]

A variety of second malignancies have been reported in patients with HCL both prior to and following diagnosis and treatment. They include both solid tumors and malignancies of the lymphoid and hematopoietic system.[3] These have been reported in the pre-chemotherapy era, as well as in long-term follow-up after treatment with interferon and purine antimetabolites. Several papers have tried to answer the question of whether the risk of second malignancy is inherently increased in hairy cell patients and/or does treatment increase the risk. In a retrospective review of 117 patients from British Columbia with a median follow-up of 5 years, there were 44 malignancies in 36 patients.[29] This was greater than expected when compared to age-matched controls, but there did not appear to be a relationship to treatment with interferon or purine analogs. In a study from the University of Chicago of HCL patients who received interferon, there were 13 malignancies, including six hematologic, among 69 patients.[30] This was more than the expected three patients, though whether this increase was drug or disease related could not be determined.

In the multicenter study comparing interferon with pentostatin treatment,[23] 241 patients were followed; 39 malignancies developed, including eight hematologic malignancies. This was slightly greater than the 26 expected, but when solid tumors alone were evaluated, there was no difference compared to age-matched controls. In a retrospective review of 725 Italian HCL patients, including patients treated with interferon and chemotherapy, the incidence of second malignancies was only 3.7%, not significantly greater than expected in this older population.[31] It is thus not yet determined whether HCL is associated with second malignancies or the possible role of treatment in their development. Long-term evaluation will be needed to define the true risk, but as of now second malignancies have not impacted survival.

In summary, as the result of effective initial treatment of HCL patients and the ability to retreat when patients relapse, survival was similar to that predicted for the general population. Additionally, long-term complications after treatment are not frequent and do not affect overall survival.

## GUIDELINES FOR FOLLOW-UP AND RETREATMENT

HCL is a low-growth malignancy, and the usual pattern of relapse that we have seen is progressive cytopenia, but only after marked marrow infiltration occurs. Thus, measurement of peripheral blood counts alone may not detect relapsed disease.

### SOLUBLE INTERLEUKIN-2 RECEPTOR
The interleukin-2 (IL-2) receptor is defined by reactivity with CD25 monoclonal antibodies and is expressed on the surface of hairy cells.[32] Soluble forms of the receptor (sIL-2R) are detected in the peripheral blood of hairy cell patients, and can be used as a marker of disease response and relapse.[25,33] We performed serial measurements of sIL-2R levels in patients after pentostatin treatment, and demonstrated that a rising sIL-2R value predicted hematologic relapse (unpublished observations). This is similar to data from other investigators, and is another means of following patients for disease progression. Additionally, it has been used effectively for determining response and predicting resistance.[25,33]

### FOLLOW-UP RECOMMENDATIONS
The efficacy of pentostatin and 2-CDA and the ability to reinduce patients has influenced our approach to follow-up. During our initial trials of pentostatin, patients routinely had repeat bone marrows while in remission, and retreatment was started with marrow repopulation. However, it has been demonstrated that the patients with a marked degree of marrow infiltration still respond to treatment[12,22]; thus early treatment is not required.

We see patients after remission induction every 4–6 months, with blood counts and repeat sIL-2R levels performed prior to bone marrow biopsies if there is a change in blood counts. For patients not on protocol, we only perform bone marrows when treatment is indicated. The criteria for retreatment included persistent granulocytopenia $\leq 500/\mu L$, platelets $\leq 50,000/\mu L$, hemoglobin $\leq 10 g/dL$, painful splenomegaly, and recurrent infections related to immune deficiency. This is more conservative than what is recommended by Goodman et al.,[14] who recommend treatment for neutrophils $\leq 1000/\mu L$ and platelets $\leq 100,000/\mu L$. With our criteria, we have had no difficulties retreating patients, and have had no severe complications in patients, being observed without therapy.

## SUMMARY

For many years, a diagnosis of HCL was to be feared because of a shortened survival with multiple complications from infections, marked splenomegaly, and severe anemia and thrombocytopenia. Moreover, treatment options were limited, and often only supportive measures were available. Now in the twenty-first century we can list it along with the other triumphs in medical oncology, including Hodgkin's disease and testicular carcinoma. The goals of treatment, to extend survival and improve the quality of life, have been reached.

### REFERENCES

1. Bouroncle BA, Wiseman BK, Doan CA: Leukemic reticuloendotheliosis. *Blood* 13:609, 1958.
2. Bourquin-Pionquet A, Rouard H, Roudot-Thoraval F et al.: Severe decrease in peripheral blood dendritic cells in hairy cell leukemia. *Br J Haematol* 116: 595,2002.
3. Kraut E: Clinical manifestations and infectious complications in hairy cell leukemia. *Best Pract Res Clin Haematol* 16:33, 2003.
4. Golomb HM, Catovsky D, Golde D: Hairy cell leukemia: a clinical review based on 71 cases. *Ann Intern Med* 89:677, 1978.

5. Zakarija A, Peterson L, Tallman M: Splenectomy and treatments of historical interest. *Best Pract Res Clin Haematol.* 16:57, 2003.

6. Catovsky D: Hairy cell leukemia and prolymphocytic leukemia. *Clin Haematol* 6:245, 1977.

7. Golomb H, Vardiman J: Response to splenectomy in 65 patients with hairy cell leukemia an evaluation of spleen weight and bone marrow involvement. *Blood* 61:349, 1983.

8. Anonymous: Consensus resolution: proposed criteria for the evaluation of response to treatment in hairy cell leukemia. *Leukemia* 1:405, 1987.

9. Quesada J, Reuben J, Manny J, et al.: Alpha interferon for induction of remission in hairy cell leukemia. *N Engl J Med* 310:15, 1984.

10. Ahmed S, Rai K: Interferon in the treatment of hairy cell leukemia. *Best Pract Res Clin Haematol* 16:61, 2003.

11. Ratain M, Golomb HM, Vardiman J, et al.: Relapse after interferon alpha 2b therapy for hairy cell leukemia analysis of prognostic variables. *J Clin Oncol* 6:1714, 1988.

12. Kraut E: Phase II trials of pentostatin (Nipent) in hairy cell leukemia. *Semin Oncol* 27(suppl 5):27, 2000.

13. Grever M, Kopecky K, Foucar K, et al.: Randomized comparison of pentostatin versus interferon alfa2a in previously treated patients with hairy cell leukemia. *J Clin Oncol* 13:974, 1995.

14. Goodman G, Beutler E, Saven A (eds.): Cladribine in the treatment of hairy cell leukemia. *Best Pract Res Clin Haematol* 16:101, 2003.

15. Bethel C, Sharpe R: Pathology of hairy cell leukemia. *Best Pract Res Clin Haematol* 16:15, 2003.

16. Tallman M, Hakimian D, Kopecky K, et al.: Minimal residual disease in patients with hairy cell leukemia in complete remission treated with 2-chlorodeoxyadenosine or 2'deoxycoformycin and prediction of early relapse. *Clin Cancer Res* 5:1665,1999.

17. Matutes E, Meeus K, McLennen K, Catovsky D: The significance of minimal residual disease in hairy cell leukemia treated with deoxycoformycin: a long term followup study. *Br J Haematol* 98:375, 1998.

18. Bastie J, Cazals-Hatem D, Daniel M, et al.: Five year followup after 2-chlorodeoxyadenosine. *Leuk Lymphoma* 35:555, 1999.

19. Bouroncle B: Thirty five years in the progress of hairy cell leukemia. *Leuk Lymphoma* 14(suppl 1):1, 1994.

20. Jansen J, Hermans J: Splenectomy in hairy cell leukemia. *Cancer* 47:2066, 1981.

21. Federico M, Frassoldati A, Lamparelli, et al.: Long term results of alpha interferon as initial therapy and splenectomy as consolidation therapy in patients with hairy cell leukemia. *Ann Oncol* 5:725,1994.

22. Tallman M: Current treatment strategies for patients with hairy cell leukemia. *Rev Clin Exp Hematol* 64:323, 2002.

23. Flinn I, Kopecky K, Foucar K, et al.: Long term followup of remission duration, mortality, and second malignancies in hairy cell leukemia patients treated with pentostatin. *Blood* 96:2981, 2000.

24. Kraut E, Grever M, Bouroncle B: Long term followup of patients with hairy cell leukemia after treatment with 2'deoxycoformycin. *Blood* 84:4061, 1994.

25. Thomas D, O'Brien S, Bueso-Ramos C: Rituximab in relapsed or refractory hairy cell leukemia. *Blood* 102:3906, 2003.

26. Kreitman R, Wilson W, Bergeron K, et al.: Efficacy of the anti-CD22 recombinant immunotoxin BL22 in chemotherapy-resistant hairy cell leukemia. *N Engl J Med* 345:241, 2001.

27. Kraut E, Neff J, Bouroncle B, Grever M: Immunosuppressive effects of pentostatin. *J Clin Oncol* 8:848, 1990.

28. Seymour J, Kurzrock R, Freireich E, et al.: 2'Chlorodeoxyadenosine induces durable remissions and prolonged suppression of CD41lymphocyte counts in patients with hairy cell leukemia. *Blood* 83:2906, 1994.

29. Au W, Klasa R, Gallagher R, et al.: Second malignancies in patients with hairy cell leukemia in British Columbia: a 20 year experience. *Blood* 92:1160, 1998.

30. Kampmeier P, Spielberger R, Dickstein J, et al.: Increased incidence of second neoplasms in patients treated with interferon 2b for hairy cell leukemia: a clinical pathologic assessment. *Blood* 84:3242, 1994.

31. Frassoldati A, Lamparelli T, Federico M, et al.: Hairy cell leukemia: a clinical review based on 725 cases of the Italian Cooperative Group. *Leuk Lymphoma* 13:307, 1994.

32. Rubin L, Nelson D: The soluble interleukin 2 receptor biology function and clinical application. *Ann Intern Med* 113:619, 1990.

33. Arun B, Curt B, Longo D, et al.: Elevations in serum soluble IL2 receptor levels predict relapse in patients with hairy cell leukemia. *Cancer J Sci Am* 6:21, 2000.

Chapter **33**

# TREATMENT OF RELAPSED OR REFRACTORY HAIRY CELL LEUKEMIA AND NEW FRONTIERS IN HAIRY CELL LEUKEMIA THERAPY

*Robert J. Kreitman*

## INTRODUCTION

As reviewed in Chapter 28, hairy cell leukemia (HCL) is a B-cell malignancy comprising 2% of all leukemias,[1,2] and is highly responsive, but not curable, with known therapy. Patients present with pancytopenia and splenomegaly, and have malignant cells in the blood, bone marrow, and spleen with eccentric kidney-shaped spongiform nuclei and hairlike cytoplasmic projections. The diagnosis was classically made by tartrate-resistant acid phosphatase (TRAP) staining.[3,4] More recently, the diagnosis is most accurately made by fluorescent-activated cell sorting (FACS) analysis (or flow cytometry), which demonstrates HCL cells strongly positive for B-cell antigens CD19, CD20, and CD22, and often other antigens including CD103 (B-ly7) CD11c, CD25, and CD123.[5–7] The differential diagnosis, which is important to consider in relapsed or refractory patients, includes splenic lymphoma with villous lymphocytes (SLVL), which may be distinguished from HCL by polar distribution of villous cytoplasmic projections, lack of pancytopenia, and CD25, CD103, and/or CD123 negativity.[7–9] HCL variant (HCLv) is a disorder comprising about 20% of HCL in which the malignant cells may have bilobed nuclei, prominent nucleoli, and may be clumped in the marrow. The HCLv cells may be CD25, CD103, CD11c, and/or CD123 negative, and patients are primarily refractory to purine analogs and other therapies.[6,7,10–12]

## TREATMENT OF RELAPSED HCL WITH STANDARD THERAPY

### SALVAGE SPLENECTOMY IN HCL

In patients with pancytopenia due to relapsed or refractory HCL with hypersplenism, splenectomy provides an excellent palliative benefit. Thrombocytopenia has been reported to improve in up to 92% of patients.[13] Early nonrandomized studies suggested a survival benefit, particularly in young symptomatic patients with large spleens and pancytopenia.[4,14,15] Nevertheless, it is currently accepted that splenectomy does not affect long-term survival.[16] Splenectomy can be accomplished safely in most patients by laparoscopy,[17,18] which minimizes recovery time. Patients without significant anemia and with a spleen tip less than 4 cm below the left costal margin are unlikely to respond well to splenectomy.[19] Although splenectomy often results in increased hairy cell infiltration into the bone marrow, blood, and abdominal lymph nodes,[20] some HCL patients can benefit early after splenectomy with a systemic reduction in malignant cells; complete pathologic remissions in the blood and marrow are rare. Patients with end-stage refractory HCL with transfusion dependence should not be denied splenectomy, as the procedure may be lifesaving in such patients. Nevertheless, splenectomy may be delayed for most relapsed or refractory patients wishing to try a variety of other salvage therapies.

## INTERFERON IN PURINE ANALOG-RESISTANT HCL

Because interferon was used more often prior to the reported efficacy of purine analogs in HCL, there is only limited data on its efficacy in purine-resistant HCL. In 10 patients from the Intergroup study who crossed over from pentostatin to interferon, there were no responses. Interferon was effective in patients after failure of splenectomy and prior chemotherapy, but it was not clear, and perhaps unlikely, that any of these patients had received prior therapy with purine analogs.[21] Nevertheless, interferon is a treatment recommended for relapsed HCL, particularly when cytopenias are severe and avoidance of myelotoxicity from purine analogs is a goal.[22]

## FLUDARABINE FOR PURINE ANALOG-RESISTANT HCL

Fludarabine is a fluorinated monophosphorylated purine nucleoside analog that resists deamination by adenosine deaminase and is cytotoxic after conversion to the triphosphate form.[23] Known better for its excellent efficacy for CLL, fludarabine is capable of inducing responses in HCL. Of four reported responses of HCL to fludarabine, one partial response (PR) was observed in HCLv, and one of four responses was a marginal response.[24,25] Several of these patients were resistant to purine analogs. Fludarabine can also be used in combination with monoclonal antibody (mAb) therapy, as in CLL.[26]

## THE DECISION FOR NONSTANDARD BIOLOGIC THERAPY VERSUS ADDITIONAL PURINE ANALOG THERAPY

As mentioned above, both purine analogs are quite effective in HCL, even as second or even third courses. In fact, it is often unclear who should receive a repeat course of purine analog and who should receive salvage therapy. This decision depends somewhat on the toxicity of cladribine and pentostatin. Either agent has been reported to deplete resting T cells, particularly CD4+ lymphocytes, for up to 4 years.[27,28] The length of prior response to the last course of purine analog is often used to decide whether to repeat the course. If the last response was brief, a repeat course of purine analog might risk cumulative overlapping damage to CD4+ lymphocyte populations. Furthermore, as both the likelihood and the duration of complete remission (CR) decline with repeated courses of purine analogs, the chance of benefit is lower in patients with short-lived prior response. In general, most physicians will use a repeat course of purine analog if the last response was greater than 2 years, particularly if only one prior course of purine analog was given. Patients with less than 1 year of response to prior cladribine or pentostatin should be offered other therapy. Patients having 1–2-year response to the last course of purine analog may be appropriate for nonstandard therapy, and this may also be the case for patients with a 2–4-year response to a second or later course of purine analog.

## MONOCLONAL ANTIBODY THERAPY OF HCL

### CD20, A TARGET FOR B-CELL MALIGNANCIES INCLUDING HCL

CD20 is a 297-amino-acid glycoprotein that participates in B-cell activity and regulation of B-cell growth.[29] It has two transmembrane domains, so that both the carboxyl and amino termini are present on the cytosolic surface of the membrane. Only a small loop of 44 amino acid residues is extracellular, so CD20 is tightly held by the cell membrane and not shed. CD20 is expressed on >95% of B-cell non Hodgkin's lymphoma (NHL), but not on stem cells or plasma cells.[30] Its expression is lower in CLL, but higher in HCL.[6,31]

### DEVELOPMENT OF RITUXIMAB FOR TARGETING CD20+ CELLS

Rituximab is a chimeric anti-CD20 mAb (Figure 33.1), containing the mouse variable domains of the mAb 2B8 grafted to the human IgG1 constant domains. Rituximab kills CD20+ cells by several mechanisms, including (1) complement-dependent cellular cytotoxicity, (2) antibody-dependent cellular cytotoxicity, and (3) induction of apoptosis.[32] Both early phase II testing and phase II pivotal testing of rituximab at 375 mg/m$^2$ per week × 4 in relapsed low-grade NHL demonstrated overall response rates of up to 48% (6% CR). The majority of toxic events were infusion related (hypotension, bronchospasm, rhinitis, pruritis, rash, urticaria, and tumor pain) and decreased with repeated dosing. Human antimouse antibodies (HAMA) were not observed. This led to Food and Drug Administration's approval of rituximab for indolent NHL. Its effect against indolent NHL was greatly enhanced by combining the drug with chemotherapy, with 95% overall response rates and 55% CR in patients receiving CHOP [cyclophosphamide, hydroxydaunomycin (doxorubicin), Oncovin (vincristine), and prednisone] plus rituximab.[33] Activity with or without chemotherapy was reported in other B-cell malignancies, including aggressive NHL, mantle cell lymphoma, CLL, and Waldenstrom's macroglobulinemia.[34–36]

### CLINICAL TESTING OF RITUXIMAB IN CLINICAL HCL TRIALS

Several case reports treating HCL with rituximab have appeared since 1999.[37–41] Four small studies have been reported in which rituximab was administered to patients with HCL (Table 33.1). Hagberg and Lundholm reported 11 classic HCL patients treated with rituximab at 375/m$^2$/week × 4.[42] Three patients were newly diagnosed and eight were relapsed. All eight relapsed patients had received one to three courses of cladribine, and seven out of eight of these patients also had received one to two courses of interferon. Of the 11 patients, 7 had cytopenias as defined by hemoglobin, granulocytes,

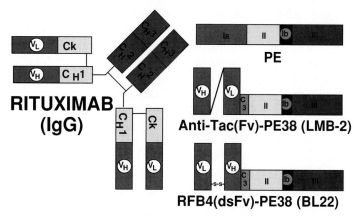

**Figure 33.1** *Structure of biologic salvage therapies in HCL. Rituximab is a chimeric anti-CD20 mAb containing the mouse variable domains ($V_L$ and $V_H$) of the mAb 2B8 grafted to the human IgG1 constant domains (C and $C_H1$-$C_H2$-$C_H3$). Pseudomonas exotoxin (PE) contains 613 amino acids. Domain Ia (amino acids 1–252) is the binding domain, domain II (amino acids 253–364) is responsible for translocating the toxin to the cytosol, and domain III (amino acids 400–613) contains the ADP-ribosylating enzyme which inactivates elongation factor 2 (EF-2) in the cytosol. The function of domain Ib (amino acids 365–399) is unknown. PE38 is a truncated form of PE devoid of domain Ia and amino acids 365–380 of domain Ib. The single-chain recombinant immunotoxin anti-Tac(Fv)-PE38 (LMB-2) contains the variable heavy domain ($V_H$) of the anti-Tac mAb fused via the peptide linker (G4S)3 to the variable light domain ($V_L$), which in turn is fused to PE38. The recombinant immunotoxin RFB4(dsFv)-PE38 (BL22) is composed of the $V_L$ from the mAb RFB4 disulfide bonded to a fusion of $V_H$ with PE38. The disulfide bond connecting $V_H$ and $V_L$ is formed between two cysteine residues replacing Arg44 of $V_H$ and Gly100 of $V_L$*

and platelets not greater than 12 g/dL, 1500/mm³, and 100,000/mm³, respectively. There were six CRs, including one previously reported.[38] One patient had a PR, and four patients had stable disease. At a median follow-up of more than 14 months, the duration of response was 1–33 months, with all responses ongoing. Of the six complete responders, only two had cytopenias. A second study was reported by Lauria et al., in which 10 patients with HCL were treated with rituximab (referred to as Mabthera, Roche, Inc).[43] All of the patients were previously pretreated with purine analogs and interferon, and all had prior cytopenias. Responses included one CR (previously reported[37]), four PRs, and three marginal responses. No patients progressed at 10–24 (median 16) months from finishing therapy. Patients responded quickly, with cytopenias correcting in all responders by 3 months, except in a partial responder who had an improvement in granulocytes from 1000 to 1200/mm³. Cytopenias corrected in some of the marginal responders as well. Splenomegaly

| Number of patients | Prior CdA/DCF T× | Number of doses | Responses | Median F/U duration (range) in months | Relapse from CR + PR | CRs–non–CRs with cytopenias | Reference |
|---|---|---|---|---|---|---|---|
| 11 | CdA 8/11 | 4 | 6 CR, 1 PR | 14 (0–34) | 0 | 2/6 vs 5/5 | Hagberg and Lundholm[42] |
| 10 | CdA DCF 10/10 | 4 | 1 CR, 4 PR | 16 (10–24) | 0 | 1/1 vs 9/9 | Lauria et al.,[43] |
| 24 | CdA 24/24 | 4 | 3 CR, 3 PR | 14.6 | 2 | 3/3 vs ?/21 | Nieva et al.,[44] |
| 15 | CdA/DCF 15/15 | 4–12 | 8 CR, 4 PR | 32 (8-45) | 5 | 5/8 vs 7/7 | Thomas et al.,[45] |

**Table 33.1** Rituximab trials in patients with HCL

Prior CdA/DCF T× indicates the number of patients enrolled who had prior therapy with cladribine (CdA) and/or pentostatin (DCF). Cytopenias are considered present when patients have (1) neutrophil count <1500/mm³, (2) platelets count <100,000/mm³, or (3) Hb <11g/dl.

In Thomas et al., two of the four PRs were reported as CR-RD, meaning 1–5% hairy cells in the marrow but otherwise in CR.

was present in two cases and resolved in both. Circulating hairy cells were eradicated in six of the seven patients. In a phase II trial from the Scripps Clinic, of 24 patients treated with rituximab, there were 3 CRs, 3 PRs, and 2 responders relapsed at a median of 15 months.[44] Higher activity was observed in a trial reported by Thomas et al., in which more than four doses were given.[45] Out of 15 patients, 7 who received eight doses attained a CR, and an additional patient had a CR after 12 doses. Two patients had a PR with 4 and 12 doses, and two patients had a CR with 1–5% residual marrow infiltration after 4 and 8 doses, for an overall response rate of 80%. Preexisting cytopenias were present in five of the eight CRs and in all seven patients not achieving a CR.

### CONCLUSIONS OF RITUXIMAB TREATMENT IN HCL

The case reports and trials clearly show that rituximab has significant activity in HCL, with a total of 18 CRs out of 60 patients (30%) treated on the four small trials. Trials with the highest CR rates (53–55%) were small and included patients without preexisting cytopenias, but it is also possible that 8–12 doses of rituximab were more effective than 4. As rituximab was associated with minimal toxicity in HCL patients, it should be strongly considered in patients who relapse from purine analog therapy. Rituximab has also shown efficacy for treating autoimmune thrombocytopenia,[46] and was reported to effectively treat this condition as a complication from pentostatin therapy.[47]

### TARGETING CD52 ON HCL CELLS WITH ALEMTUZUMAB

CD52 is a 12-amino-acid glycoprotein that is present on lymphocytes at up to 450,000 sites/cell.[48,49] It is also present on monocytes, macrophages, eosinophils, and the male reproductive tract.[50,51] Quigley et al. at the Scripps Clinic recently reported that in nine cases of classic HCL and one of HCLv, all patients expressed CD52 on 92–100% of the HCL cells.[52] Fietz et al. reported recently that a patient with HCL and short-lived or poor responses to cladribine, interferon, splenectomy, and rituximab had hematologic benefit with alemtuzumab.[53] The patient tolerated rituximab more poorly than alemtuzumab because of an allergic reaction to the former. With both mAbs, the patient had an improvement in thrombocytopenia, but failed to reverse blood transfusion dependence.

## LMB-2, TARGETING CD25⁺ HCL

### DEVELOPMENT OF LMB-2 FOR THE TREATMENT OF CD25⁺ MALIGNANCIES

The interleukin 2 receptor (IL-2R) is composed of $\alpha$(CD25), $\beta$(CD122), and $\gamma$(CD132) chains. IL-2 binds with high affinity ($K_d \sim 10^{-11}$ M) to the complex containing all three of them, but with low affinity ($K_d \sim 10^{-8}$ M) to CD25 alone, also called p55 or Tac.[54] In contrast, the mAb anti-Tac binds to CD25 with high affinity ($K_d \sim 10^{-10}$ M).[55] CD25 is overexpressed in a variety of hematologic malignancies, including adult T-cell leukemia (ATL) and HCL, other T- and B-cell leukemias and lymphomas, and Hodgkin's disease.[56–58] CD25 usually far outnumbers other subunits of the IL-2R on cells, and in some tumors is the only IL-2R subunit present. To construct an anti-CD25 recombinant immunotoxin, the variable heavy domain of anti-Tac ($V_H$) was fused to the variable light domain via a 15-amino-acid linker to the variable light domain ($V_L$), which in turn was fused to PE40.[59] Both anti-Tac(Fv)-PE40 and the slightly shorter derivative anti-Tac(Fv)-PE38 (Figure 33.1) bound well to CD25, and were very cytotoxic to CD25⁺ cell lines and activated human T cells, which mediate autoimmune disease.[59,60] LMB-2 induced complete regression of CD25⁺ human xenografts in mice[61,62] and killed fresh leukemic cells from patients with ATL,[60,62] HCL, and other leukemias.[63] In monkeys, LMB-2 caused reversible transaminase elevations, but not death, at dose levels up to 1000 $\mu$g/kg q.o.d. $\times$ 3.[62,64] Large-scale production of LMB-2 was accomplished after expression of a DNA plasmid in *Escherichia coli*.[65–67]

### ELIGIBILITY AND DOSING IN A PHASE I TRIAL OF LMB-2

The phase I trial of LMB-2 began in 1996 and included patients with a histologically confirmed diagnosis of Hodgkin's disease (HD), NHL, or leukemia with evidence of CD25 on malignant cells, except in HD not amenable to biopsy.[58] All patients had prior standard and salvage therapy (see Table 33.2), and those with indolent disease were in need of treatment. For first-time or repeat cycles, patients could not have high levels of neutralizing antibodies. LMB-2 was administered for three doses by 30-min infusion (q.o.d. $\times$ 3). The maximum tolerated dose (MTD) was defined as the highest dose level for which 0–1 out of 6 patients had dose limiting toxicity (DLT). Patients without progressive disease or neutralizing antibodies could be retreated, and could be dose escalated to the dose level below that which new patients were permitted to receive. Plasma levels of LMB-2 were quantitated by a cytotoxicity assay and enzyme-linked immunosorbent assays.

### RESULTS OF PHASE I TESTING OF LMB-2

LMB-2 was administered at 2–63 $\mu$g/kg q.o.d. $\times$ 3 to a total of 35 patients with chemotherapy-resistant hematologic malignancies, including 11 with Hodgkin's disease, 6 with B-cell NHL, 8 with CLL, 4 with HCL, 3 with peripheral T-cell lymphoma (PTCL), 1 with cutaneous T-cell lymphoma (CTCL), and 2 with ATL.[68] DLT was observed at 63 $\mu$g/kg i.v. q.o.d. $\times$3, the dose at which one patient had grade 4 transaminase elevations and another had nausea, vomiting, and diarrhea followed by a transient cardiomyopathy.

**Table 33.2** LMB–2 in patients with HCL

| Patient number | Age/ sex | Prior TX | Spleen/ cytopenias | HCL cells/uL | Dose level (μg/ kg × 3) | Total cycles | DLT | Peak level (ng/mL) | Neut ABs | Response | % Decr HCL |
|---|---|---|---|---|---|---|---|---|---|---|---|
| 15 | 63/M | IFN, CdA | Large/+ | 63,900 | 30 | 1 | – | 219 | – | PR | 99.8 |
| 30 | 47/M | IFN, CdA, | Absent/+ | 478 | 63 | 2 | – | 593 | – | CR | 100 |
| 32 | 60/F | IFN, CdA, DCF | Absent/+ | 350 | 63 | 1 | Heart | 1094 | – | PR | 99 |
| 35 | 35/M | IFN, CdA | Absent/+ | 60,700 | 40 | 2 | – | 487 | + | PR | 98 |

Prior treatments T−X included interferon (IFN), cladribine (CdA), and pentostatin (DCF). Patients with absent spleens had prior splenectomy. The presence absence (+ or −) of cytopenias is also listed to indicate whether patients had ANC <1500/mm$^3$, platelets <100,000/mm$^3$, or Hb <11 g/dL on enrollment. Neutralizing antibodies (Neut ABs) were + if the serum neutralized 1000 ng/mL of the cytotoxic activity of LMB-2 toward CD25+SP2/Tac cells. Peak levels indicate the highest plasma level achieved with any of the doses of LMB-2 administered, as measured by cytotoxicity assay of plasma on SP2/Tac cells using pure LMB-2 for a standard curve. Responses included partial response (PR) or complete remission (CR). The percent decrease in circulating HCL count (% Decr HCL) as a result of LMB-2 treatment is shown.

The most common first-cycle toxicity at the MTD (40 μg/kg q.o.d. × 3) in nine patients was transaminase (aspartate transaminase and alanine transaminase) elevations. Nausea, fever, and weight gain were also common toxicities. Symptomatic pulmonary edema or other features of dose-limiting vascular leak syndrome (VLS) were not seen, although hypoalbuminemia was common. Reversible anaphylaxis to LMB-2 was observed in one patient who had been pretreated with anti-Tac mAb and had developed nonneutralizing anti-idiotype antibody prior to LMB-2 enrollment. The median half-life of LMB-2 was about 4 h at the MTD. After cycle 1, only 6 of 35 patients (17%) made neutralizing antibodies at high enough levels to disqualify them from further treatment. Thus, patients were retreated for a total of two to six cycles. None of eight CLL patients receiving a total of 16 cycles developed any trace of neutralizing antibodies. PRs were observed in one patient with ATL, HD, CTCL, and CLL.

### RESPONSES TO LMB-2 IN HCL PATIENTS

All four patients with HCL, who had failed at least cladribine and interferon, had major responses.[69] Patient 30 [see Figure 33.2(a)] prior to treatment had pancytopenia, with a pretransfusion hemoglobin as low as 8.5 g/dL, a platelet count of 47,000/mm$^3$, an absolute neutrophil count (ANC) of 360/mm$^3$, and an enlarged spleen and precarinal lymph nodes. The pancytopenia resolved with elimination of the tumor cells. The hairy cell count of 478/μL decreased >90% from just one dose of LMB-2, as assessed on day 3. By day 8, the HCL count had decreased by >99%, and was cleared following cycle 2. Flow cytometry is able to quantify HCL cells making up <0.01% of the lymphocytes. The CR in patient 30 was associated with resolution of baseline splenomegaly and precarinal adenopathy, and transfusion independence. Recovery of normal counts is shown in Figure 33.2(a), with the platelet count first to recover, improving from a pretreatment baseline of 53,000–133,000/μL by day 22.

The granulocyte count improved next, from a baseline of 390–1430/μL by 66 days after beginning LMB-2. The hemoglobin improved to normal by 150 days, and has remained above 11 for >6 years without further treatment. Three patients had PR to LMB-2 after one cycle of 30, 63, and 40 μg/kg q.o.d. × 3, with >98–99.8% decreases in circulating HCL cells. CR was not achieved in these patients, probably because they could not be effectively retreated.

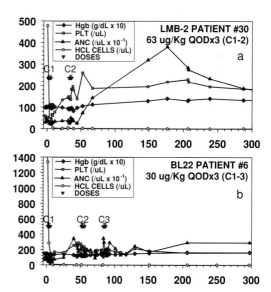

**Figure 33.2** *Complete remission of HCL patients to recombinant immunotoxins. LMB-2 patient 30 (a) received two cycles of LMB-2 at 63 μg/kg q.o.d. × 3. The three doses of each cycle are indicated by a coalescence of three arrows. The hemoglobin (Hb), platelet count (PLT), absolute neutrophil count (ANC), and circulating HCL count (HCL) is shown from several days before to 300 days after the first dose. Similar data are shown for BL22 patient 6 (b) who received three cycles of BL22 at 30 μg/kg q.o.d. × 3*

## BL22, TARGETING CD22⁺ HCL

### RATIONALE FOR TARGETING CD22

In many B-cell lymphomas and leukemias, CD22 is displayed by the malignant cells more often than CD25.[58,70–72] Moreover, CD25⁻ HCL is one of the most common features of HCLv. These patients are overrepresented in the population of HCL patients requiring salvage therapy, because they do not respond well to standard therapy, even if previously untreated.[10,73] CD22 is considered one of the best antigens to target in HCL and is essentially always strongly expressed.[31] Although CD22 is found on normal B cells, it is not expressed on stem cells. As mentioned above, a variety of immunotoxin chemical conjugates have been used to target CD22⁺ leukemias and lymphomas in preclinical and clinical studies, not related to HCL.[74–79]

### PRECLINICAL DEVELOPMENT OF BL22

To produce a stable anti-CD22 recombinant immunotoxin, the variable domains of the anti-CD22 mAb RFB4 were connected by a disulfide bond instead of a peptide linker, and $V_H$ was fused to PE38, resulting in BL22 (see Figure 33.1).[80] The disulfide bond was created by mutating Arg44 of $V_H$ and Gly100 of $V_L$ to cysteines. This technology had been used previously for stabilizing Fvs of a variety of different mAbs, including anti-Tac.[81,82] Chemical reactions are not needed to make the recombinant immunotoxin, since the disulfide bond between $V_L$ and $V_H$-PE38 forms automatically during in vitro renaturation of the two fragments. Complete regressions in mice of human CD22⁺ B-cell lymphoma xenografts were observed at plasma levels which could be tolerated in cynomolgus monkeys.[83] CRs of these xenografts were observed whether BL22 was administered by bolus injection q.o.d. × 3 or by continuous infusion. Leukemic cells freshly obtained from patients with CLL and NHL were incubated ex vivo with BL22.[72] This study, which showed specific killing of such cells, was important for preclinical development because malignant cells freshly obtained from patients typically display far fewer CD22 sites/cell compared to cell lines.

### METHODS AND PATIENTS FOR TESTING BL22 IN HCL

BL22 was administered to 16 patients with HCL as part of a phase I trial in patients with B-cell malignancies.[84] Like LMB-2, patients were dosed by 30-min infusion q.o.d. × 3. Patients without progressive disease or neutralizing antibodies to the toxin could be retreated at 3-week intervals. Disease was staged by blood counts with flow cytometry, bone marrow biopsy with immunohistochemistry, and computerized tomography. Neutralizing antibody and pharmacokinetic assays were performed by cytotoxicity assay as with LMB-2. Of 16 patients,[84] 13 had classic HCL and 3 had HCLv. As shown in Table 33.3, the median age was 54 years and the male-to-female ratio was 3/1, similar to what is reported for HCL.[85,86] All patients were pretreated with cladribine. Patients 5, 8, 9, 11, 13, and 14 were pretreated with one course, patients 4, 6, 10, 12, and 15 with two courses, patients 3, 7, and 16 with three courses, patient 1 with five courses, and patient 2 with six prior courses of cladribine. Patients often had one or several courses of prior interferon, pentostatin, and rituximab as well. About half the patients had prior splenectomy. Circulating HCL counts were typically high in patients after splenectomy but were highest (132,000/μL) in patient 4, who had a large spleen. All three HCLv patients (14, 18, and 26) had high circulating malignant counts. Dose levels included 3, 6, 10, 20, 30, 40, and 50 μg/kg q.o.d. × 3, and patients often were retreated with a variety of different dose levels.

### RESPONSE TO BL22 IN PATIENTS WITH HCL

A total of 87 cycles of BL22 were administered to 16 patients, each patient receiving 1–15 cycles (Table 33.3). A total of 11 out of 16 patients (68%) attained a CR, and 2 patients had a PR (12%). Patients 2 and 5 had marginal responses, with 98 and 99.5% reductions in circulating HCL counts, respectively, but less than 50% decreases in lymph node masses. A CR was attained in all three HCLv patients. Of 11 CRs, 6 (patients 6, 8, 9, 11, 12, and 16) had a CR after cycle 1, and patients 3, 4, 7, 10, and 13 had a CR after cycles 2, 9, 4, 3, and 2, respectively. Only one (patient 12) of the CRs had minimal residual disease in the bone marrow biopsy by immunohistochemistry at the time CR was documented. Complete clearing of circulating HCL cells was documented in 10 out of 11 CRs, and patient 7 had a decrease in HCL count from 32,000 to 1 cell/μL. Cytopenias resolved in all responders. Within the follow-up time of 4–22 (median 12) months, relapse was documented in three patients (patients 4, 7, and 12 after 8, 12, and 7 months, respectively), and all three of them were returned to CR with additional BL22. These relapses were asymptomatic in that they were detected by routine bone marrow biopsies, and the patients had not redeveloped cytopenias.

### BL22 IMMUNOGENICITY, PLASMA LEVELS, AND TOXICITY IN HCL PATIENTS

High levels of neutralizing antibodies were observed in patients 5, 9, and 12 after cycles 1, 1, and 5, respectively. Patient 5 had preexisting low levels of neutralizing antibodies prior to receiving BL22. Patient 2 had low levels of neutralizing antibodies after cycle 5. Plasma levels in patients with high disease burden increased greatly on subsequent cycles after patients responded. Dose-limiting toxicity in patient 5 included a cytokine release syndrome in patient 5 with fever, hypotension, bone pain, and weight gain (VLS) without pulmonary edema, which resolved within 3 days. Patients 8 and 13 had a completely reversible hemolytic uremic syndrome (HUS),

**Table 33.3  BL22 in patients with HCL**

| Patient number | Age/ sex | Prior TX | Spleen/ cytopenias | HCL cells/uL | Dose level (µg/ kg × 3) | Total cycles | DLT | Peak level (ng/mL) | Neut ABs | Response | % Decr HCL |
|---|---|---|---|---|---|---|---|---|---|---|---|
| 1 | 71/F | IFN, CdA, DCF, Ritux | Absent/+ | 88,000 | 3 | 1 | – | 13 | – | PD | – |
| 2 | 54/M | IFN, DCF, CdA, B4bR | Absent/+ | 690 | 6–10 | 5 | – | 115 | – | MR | 98 |
| 3 | 42/F | CdA | Large/+ | 11 | 10–20 | 4 | – | 693 | – | CR | 100 |
| 4 | 46/M | IFN, CdA, DCF, Flud, Ritux | Large/+ | 132,000 | 30–50 | 14 | – | 1033 | – | CR | 100 |
| 5 | 54/M | CdA, IFN | Absent/+ | 180 | 30 | 2 | VLS | 1602 | + | MR | 99.5 |
| 6 | 61/M | CdA, IFN | Large/+ | 1330 | 30 | 3 | – | 1716 | – | CR | 100 |
| 7 | 70/M | CdA, IFN | Large/+ | 32,00 | 30–40 | 9 | – | 1805 | – | CR | 99.997 |
| 8 | 50/M | CdA | Large/+ | 46 | 30 | 2 | HUS | 772 | – | CR | 100 |
| 9 | 45/F | CdA, IFN, DCF | Large/+ | 22 | 30 | 2 | – | 840 | + | CR | 100 |
| 10 | 59/M | IFN, CdA, DCF | Absent/+ | 4700 | 40–50 | 5 | – | 2604 | – | CR | 100 |
| 11 | 56/M | CdA | Acc/– | 44,000 | 40–50 | 3 | – | 2222 | – | CR | 100 |
| 12 | 43/M | CdA, IFN | Large/+ | 9 | 40–50 | 5 | – | 1847 | + | CR | 100 |
| 13 | 57/F | CdA, IFN | Absent/+ | 38 | 50 | 2 | HUS | 1498 | – | CR | 100 |
| 14 | 37/M | CdA, Ritux | Large/+ | 26 | 40 | 15 | – | 1497 | – | PR | 100 |
| 15 | 54/M | CdA | Large/+ | 65 | 40 | 13 | – | 1920 | – | PR | 100 |
| 16 | 55/M | CdA | Absent/– | 6 | 40 | 2 | – | 1652 | – | CR | 100 |

Prior treatments T× included interferon (IFN), cladribine (CdA), pentostatin (DCF), rituximab (Ritux), anti-B4 blocked ricin (B4bR, and fludarabine (Flud). Patients with prior splenectomy are indicated with either absent spleen or as having an accessory (Acc) spleen. The presence or absence (+ or −) of cytopenias is also listed to indicate whether patients had ANC <500/mm³, platelets <100,000/mm³, or Hb <11g/dL on enrollment. Patient 4 had splenectomy after cycle 3 due to an HCL-related bleeding disorder; the bleeding disorder responded but disease progressed in the peripheral blood prior to receiving the remaining 11 cycles of BL22. Dose-limiting toxicity included either vascular leak syndrome (VLS) or hemolytic uremic syndrome (HUS). Peak levels indicate the highest plasma level achieved with any of the doses of BL22 administered, as measured by cytotoxicity assay of plasma on Raji cells using pure BL22 for a standard curve. Neutralizing antibodies (Neut ABs) were + if the serum neutralized 1000 ng/mL of the cytotoxic activity of BL222 toward CD22⁺ Raji cells. Responses included partial response (PR) or complete remission (CR). The percent decrease in circulation HCL count (% Decr HCL) as a result of BL22 treatment is shown.

confirmed by renal biopsy. In each case, HUS presented with hematuria and hemoglobinuria by day 8 of cycle 2. These patients required 6–10 days of plasmapheresis, but not dialysis for complete resolution of renal function and correction of thrombocytopenia and anemia. Both patients achieved a CR, patient 8 prior to HUS and patient 13 afterward, and in both cases all preexisting cytopenias resolved, as well as those related to HUS.

### CONCLUSIONS OF CLINICAL TESTING OF BL22 IN HCL

BL22 is the first agent since purine analogs that can induce a CR in the majority of patients with HCL, and appears at least as active as rituximab for this disease. All patients treated with HCL had prior cladribine and had responded unsatisfactorily to at least the last course, and this includes patients with HCLv. Its success in chemoresistant patients is related to its different mechanism of action compared to purine analogs, and the fact that CD22 is highly conserved at high density on HCL cells despite purine analog resistance. Lack of CR was usually related to easily identifiable factors, including low doses due to the phase I design, and secondary immune response after cycle 1, which prevented effective retreatment. Patient 14 had significant splenomegaly which required several cycles to resolve, but disease in the marrow was still evident after cycle 12. In further follow-up, this patient was actually found to enter CR finally after cycle 14. The cause of HUS in patients receiving BL22 is not known, and since HUS has not been observed in over 100 patients receiving PE38 fused to ligands other than RFB4(dsFv), the mechanism must in part be mediated by CD22.

### SUMMARY

Effective therapeutic options for patients with relapsed or refractory HCL include repeated courses of purine analogs, palliative splenectomy, or interferon, rituximab, and the recombinant immunotoxins BL22 and LMB-2. Data are insufficient to determine whether BL22 is better than LMB-2 for CD25⁺ HCL, but as 20% of HCL patients have CD25⁻ HCL cells, BL22 is the agent that has been developed more for this disease. Additional phase II clinical testing is under way to establish the safety and optimal dosing of BL22 for efficacy, and similar testing is also being done with rituximab.

## REFERENCES

1. Cheson BD, Martin A: Clinical trials in hairy cell leukemia. Current status and future directions [published erratum appears in *Ann Intern Med* 107(4):604, 1987 Oct]. *Ann Intern Med* 106:871–878, 1987.

2. Bouroncle BA, Wiseman BK, Doan CA: Leukemic reticuloendotheliosis. *Blood* 13:609–630, 1958.

3. Katayama I, Li CY, Yam LT: Histochemical study of acid phosphatase isoenzyme in leukemic reticuloendotheliosis. *Cancer* 29:157–164, 1972.

4. Golomb HM, Catovsky D, Golde DW: Hairy cell leukemia: a clinical review based on 71 cases. *Ann Intern Med* 89:677–683, 1978.

5. Hassan IB, Hagberg H, Sundstrom C: Immunophenotype of hairy-cell leukemia. *Eur J Haematol* 45:172–176, 1990.

6. Robbins BA, Ellison DJ, Spinosa JC, et al.: Diagnostic application of two-color flow cytometry in 161 cases of hairy cell leukemia. *Blood* 82:1277–1287, 1993.

7. DelGiudice I, Matutes E, Morilla R, et al.: The diagnostic value of CD123 in B-cell disorders with hairy or villous lymphocytes. *Haematologica* 89:303–308, 2004.

8. Azemar M, Masche A, Schaefer HE, Unger C: Splenic lymphoma with villous lymphocytes—difficulties in differential diagnosis. *Onkologie* 21:235–239, 1998.

9. Treton D, Valensi F, Troussard X, et al.: Cytokine response of B lymphocytes from splenic lymphoma with villous lymphocytes: correlation with TNF-RII (p75) and CD11c expression. *Hematol Cell Ther* 38:345–352, 1996.

10. Blasinska-Morawiec M., Robak T, Krykowski E, Hellmann A, Urbanska-Rys H: Hairy cell leukemia-variant treated with 2-chlorodeoxyadenosine—a report of three cases. *Leuk Lymphoma* 25:381–385, 1997.

11. Dunn P, Shih LY, Ho YS, Tien HF: Hairy cell leukemia variant. *Acta Haematol* 94:105–108, 1995.

12. Wu ML, Kwaan HC, Goolsby CL: Atypical hairy cell leukemia. *Arch Pathol Lab Med* 124:1710–1713, 2000.

13. Van Norman AS, Nagorney DM, Martin JK, Phyliky RL, Ilstrup DM: Splenectomy for hairy cell leukemia. A clinical review of 63 patients. *Cancer* 57:644–648, 1986.

14. Jansen J, Hermans J, Remme J, den Ottolander GJ, Cardozo PL: Hairy cell leukaemia. Clinical features and effect of splenectomy. *Scand J Haematol* 21:60–71, 1978.

15. Jansen J, Hermans J: Splenectomy in hairy cell leukemia: a retrospective multicenter analysis. *Cancer* 47:2066–2076, 1981.

16. Bouroncle BA: The history of hairy cell leukemia: characteristics of long-term survivors. *Semin Oncol* 11:479–485, 1984.

17. Baccarani U, Terrosu G, Donini A, Zaja F, Bresadola F, Baccarani M: Splenectomy in hematology. Current practice and new perspectives. *Haematologica* 84:431–436, 1999.

18. Walsh RM, Heniford BT: Laparoscopic splenectomy for non-Hodgkin lymphoma. *J Surg Oncol* 70:116–121, 1999.

19. Golomb HM, Vardiman JW: Response to splenectomy in 65 patients with hairy cell leukemia: an evaluation of spleen weight and bone marrow involvement. *Blood* 61:349–352, 1983.

20. Mercieca J, Puga M, Matutes E, Moskovic E, Salim S, Catovsky D: Incidence and significance of abdominal lymphadenopathy in hairy cell leukaemia. *Leuk Lymphoma* 14(suppl 1):79–83, 1994.

21. Golomb HM, Jacobs A, Fefer A, et al.: Alpha-2 interferon therapy of hairy-cell leukemia: a multicenter study of 64 patients. *J Clin Oncol* 4:900–905, 1986.

22. Lauria F, Forconi F: Towards the pharmacotherapy of hairy cell leukaemia. *Expert Opin Pharmacother* 5:1523–1533, 2004.

23. Chun HG, Leyland-Jones B, Cheson BD: Fludarabine phosphate: a synthetic purine antimetabolite with significant activity against lymphoid malignancies. *J Clin Oncol* 9:175–188, 1991.

24. Kantarjian HM, Schachner J, Keating MJ: Fludarabine therapy in hairy cell leukemia. *Cancer* 67:1291–1293, 1991.

25. Kraut EH, Chun HG: Fludarabine phosphate in refractory hairy cell leukemia. *Am J Hematol* 37:59–60, 1991.

26. Byrd JC: Concurrent vs sequential rituximab and fludarabine elicits higher complete response in CLL. *Oncol News Int* 11:22, 2002.

27. Seymour JF, Kurzrock R, Freireich E J, Estey EH: 2-chlorodeoxyadenosine induces durable remissions and prolonged suppression of CD4+ lymphocyte counts in patients with hairy cell leukemia. *Blood* 83:2906–2911, 1994.

28. Seymour JF, Talpaz M, Kurzrock R: Response duration and recovery of CD4+ lymphocytes following deoxycoformycin in interferon-alpha-resistant hairy cell leukemia: 7- year follow-up. *Leukemia* 11:42–47, 1997.

29. Riley JK, Sliwkowski MX: CD20: a gene in search of a function. *Semin Oncol* 27:17–24, 2000.

30. Maloney DG, Smith B, Rose A: Rituximab: mechanism of action and resistance. *Semin Oncol* 29:2–9, 2002.

31. Cordone I, Annino L, Masi S, et al.: Diagnostic relevance of peripheral blood immunocytochemistry in hairy cell leukaemia. *J Clin Pathol* 48:955–960, 1995.

32. Taji H, Kagami Y, Okada Y, et al.: Growth inhibition of CD20-positive B lymphoma cell lines by IDEC-C2B8 anti-CD20 monoclonal antibody. *Jpn J Cancer Res* 89:748–756, 1998.

33. Czuczman MS, GrilloLopez AJ, White CA, et al.: Treatment of patients with low-grade B-cell lymphoma with the combination of chimeric anti-CD20 monoclonal antibody and CHOP chemotherapy. *J Clin Oncol* 17:268–276, 1999.

34. Coiffier B: Rituximab in combination with CHOP improves survival in elderly patients with aggressive non-Hodgkin's lymphoma. *Semin Oncol* 29:18–22, 2002.

35. Byrd JC, Murphy T, Howard RS, et al.: Rituximab using a thrice weekly dosing schedule in b-cell chronic lymphocytic leukemia and small lymphocytic lymphoma demonstrates clinical activity and acceptable toxicity. *J Clin Oncol* 19:2153–2164, 2001.

36. Dimopoulos MA, Zervas C, Zomas A, et al.: Treatment of Waldenstrom's macroglobulinemia with rituximab. *J Clin Oncol* 20:2327–2333, 2002.

37. Zinzani PL, Ascani S, Piccaluga PP, Bendandi M, Pileri S, Tura S: Efficacy of rituximab in hairy cell leukemia treatment. *J Clin Oncol* 18:3875–3877, 2000.

38. Hagberg H: Chimeric monoclonal anti-CD20 antibody (rituximab)—an effective treatment for a patient with relapsing hairy cell leukaemia. *Med Oncol* 16:221–222, 1999.

39. Hoffman M, Auerbach L: Bone marrow remission of hairy cell leukaemia induced by rituximab (anti-CD20 monoclonal antibody) in a patient refractory to cladribine. *Br J Haematol* 109:900–901, 2000.

40. Sokol L, Agosti SJ: Simultaneous manifestation of chronic lymphocytic leukemia (CLL) and hairy cell leukemia (HCL). *Am J Hematol* 75:107–109, 2004.

41. Pollio F, Pocali B, Palmieri S, et al.: Rituximab: a useful drug for a repeatedly relapsed hairy cell leukemia patient. *Ann Hematol* 81:736–738, 2002.

42. Hagberg H, Lundholm L: Rituximab, a chimaeric anti-CD20 monoclonal antibody, in the treatment of hairy cell leukaemia. *Br J Haematol* 115:609–611, 2001.

43. Lauria F, Lenoci M, Annino L, et al.: Efficacy of anti-CD20 monoclonal antibodies (Mabthera) in patients with progressed hairy cell leukemia. *Haematologica* 86:1046–1050, 2001.

44. Nieva J, Bethel K, Saven A: Phase 2 study of rituximab in the treatment of cladribine-failed patients with hairy cell leukemia. *Blood* 102:810–813, 2003.

45. Thomas DA, O'Brien S, Bueso-Ramos C, et al.: Rituximab in relapsed or refractory hairy cell leukemia. *Blood* 102:3906–3911, 2003.

46. Cooper N, Stasi R, CunninghamRundles SS, et al.: The efficacy and safety of B-cell depletion with anti-CD20 monoclonal antibody in adults with chronic immune thrombocytopenic purpura. *Br J Haematol* 125:232–239, 2004.

47. Hensel M, Ho AD: Successful treatment of a patient with hairy cell leukemia and pentostatin-induced autoimmune thrombocytopenia with rituximab. *Am J Hematol* 73:37–40, 2003.

48. Hale G: Biology of the CD52 antigen. *CLL Cutting Edge* 6:2, 2001.

49. Hale G: The CD52 antigen and development of the CAMPATH antibodies. *Cytotherapy* 3:137–143, 2001.

50. Elsner J, Hochstetter R, Spiekermann K, Kapp A: Surface and mRNA expression of the CD52 antigen by human eosinophils but not by neutrophils. *Blood* 88:4684–4693, 1996.

51. Hale G, Rye PD, Warford A, Lauder I, Brito-Babapulle A: The glycosylphosphatidylinositol-anchored lymphocyte antigen CDw52 is associated with the epididymal maturation of human spermatozoa. *J Reprod Immunol* 23: 189–205, 1993.

52. Quigley MM, Bethel KJ, Sharpe RW, Saven A: CD52 expression in hairy cell leukemia. *Am J Hematol* 74: 227–230, 2003.

53. Fietz T, Rieger K, Schmittel A, Thiel E, Knauf W: Alemtuzumab (Campath 1H) in hairy cell leukaemia relapsing after rituximab treatment. *Hematol J* 5: 451–452, 2004.

54. Taniguchi T, Minami Y: The IL2/IL-2 receptor system: a current overview. *Cell* 73:5–8, 1993.

55. Uchiyama T, Nelson DL, Fleisher TA, Waldmann TA: A monoclonal antibody (anti-Tac) reactive with activated and functionally mature human T cells. II: Expression of Tac antigen on activated cytotoxic killer T cells, suppressor cells, and on one of two types of helper T cells. *J Immunol* 126:1398–1403, 1981.

56. Kodaka T, Uchiyama T, Ishikawa T, et al.: Interleukin-2 receptor -chain (p70-75) expressed on leukemic cells from adult T cell leukemia patients. *Jpn J Cancer Res* 81:902–908, 1990.

57. Yagura H, Tamaki T, Furitsu T, et al.: Demonstration of high-affinity interleukin-2 receptors on B-chronic lymphocytic leukemia cells: functional and structural characterization. *Blut* 60:181–186, 1990.

58. Sheibani K, Winberg CD, Velde SVD, Blayney DW, Rappaport H: Distribution of lymphocytes with interleukin-2 receptors (TAC antigens) in reactive lymphoproliferative processes, Hodgkin's disease, and non-Hodgkin's lymphomas: an immunohistologic study of 300 cases. *Am J Pathol* 127:27–37, 1987.

59. Chaudhary VK, Queen C, Junghans RP, Waldmann TA, FitzGerald DJ, Pastan I: A recombinant immunotoxin consisting of two antibody variable domains fused to *Pseudomonas* exotoxin. *Nature* 339:394–397, 1989.

60. Kreitman RJ, Chaudhary VK, Waldmann TA, et al.: Cytotoxic activities of recombinant immunotoxins composed of *Pseudomonas* toxin or diphtheria toxin toward lymphocytes from patients with adult T-cell leukemia. *Leukemia* 7:553–562, 1993.

61. Kreitman RJ, Bailon P, Chaudhary VK, FitzGerald DJP, Pastan I: Recombinant immunotoxins containing anti-Tac(Fv) and derivatives of *Pseudomonas* exotoxin produce complete regression in mice of an interleukin-2 receptor-expressing human carcinoma. *Blood* 83:426–434, 1994.

62. Kreitman RJ, Pastan I: Targeting *Pseudomonas* exotoxin to hematologic malignancies. *Semin Cancer Biol* 6:297–306, 1995.

63. Robbins DH, Margulies I, Stetler-Stevenson M, Kreitman RJ: Hairy cell leukemia, a B-cell neoplasm which is particularly sensitive to the cytotoxic effect of anti-Tac(Fv)-PE38 (LMB-2). *Clin Cancer Res* 6:693–700, 2000.

64. Kreitman RJ, Pastan I: Targeted toxin hybrid proteins. In: Oxender D, Post LE (eds.) *Novel Therapeutics from Modern Biotechnology*. Berlin/Germany: Springer-Verlag; 1997:89–110.

65. Buchner J, Pastan I, Brinkmann U: A method for increasing the yield of properly folded recombinant fusion proteins: single-chain immunotoxins from renaturation of bacterial inclusion bodies. *Anal Biochem* 205:263–270, 1992.

66. Kreitman RJ, Pastan I: Purification and characterization of IL6-PE$^{4E}$, a recombinant fusion of interleukin 6 with *Pseudomonas* exotoxin. *Bioconjug Chem* 4:581–585, 1993.

67. Kreitman RJ, Pastan I: Making fusion toxins to target leukemia and lymphoma. In: Francis GE, Delgado C (eds.) *Drug Targeting*. Vol. 25.Riverview, NJ: Humana Press Inc; 2000:215–226.

68. Kreitman RJ, Wilson WH, White JD, et al.: Phase I trial of recombinant immunotoxin anti-Tac(Fv)-PE38 (LMB-2) in patients with hematologic malignancies. *J Clin Oncol* 18:1614–1636, 2000.

69. Kreitman RJ, Wilson WH, Robbins D, et al.: Responses in refractory hairy cell leukemia to a recombinant immunotoxin. *Blood* 94:3340–3348, 1999.

70. Strauchen JA, Breakstone BA: IL-2 receptor expression in human lymphoid lesions. *Am J Pathol* 126:506–512, 1987.

71. Clark EA: CD22, a B cell-specific receptor, mediates adhesion and signal transduction. *J Immunol* 150: 4715–4718, 1993.

72. Kreitman RJ, Margulies I, Stetler-Stevenson M, Wang QC, FitzGerald DJP, Pastan I: Cytotoxic activity of

disulfide-stabilized recombinant immunotoxin RFB4(dsFv)-PE38 (BL22) towards fresh malignant cells from patients with B-cell leukemias. *Clin Cancer Res* 6:1476–1487, 2000.

73. Sainati L, Matutes E, Mulligan S, et al.: A variant form of hairy cell leukemia resistant to alpha-interferon: clinical and phenotypic characteristics of 17 patients. *Blood* 76:157–162, 1990.

74. Ghetie M-A, May RD, Till M, et al.: Evaluation of ricin A chain-containing immunotoxins directed against CD19 and CD22 antigens on normal and malignant human B-Cells as potential reagents for in vivo therapy. *Cancer Res* 48:2610–2617, 1988.

75. Ghetie M-A, Richardson J, Tucker T, Jones D, Uhr JW, Vitetta ES: Antitumor activity of Fab′ and IgG-anti-CD22 immunotoxins in disseminated human B lymphoma grown in mice with severe combined immunodeficiency disease: effect on tumor cells in extranodal sites. *Cancer Res* 51:5876–5880, 1991.

76. Bregni M, Siena S, Formosa A, et al.: B-cell restricted saporin immunotoxins: activity against B-cell lines and chronic lymphocytic leukemia cells. *Blood* 73:753–762, 1989.

77. Senderowicz AM, Vitetta E, Headlee D, et al.: Complete sustained response of a refractory, post-transplantation, large B-cell lymphoma to an anti-CD22 immunotoxin. *Ann Intern Med* 126:882–885, 1997.

78. Kreitman RJ, Hansen HJ, Jones AL, FitzGerald DJP, Goldenberg DM, Pastan I: *Pseudomonas* exotoxin-based immunotoxins containing the antibody LL2 or LL2-Fab′ induce regression of subcutaneous human B-cell lymphoma in mice. *Cancer Res* 53:819–825, 1993.

79. Theuer CP, Kreitman RJ, FitzGerald DJ, Pastan I: Immunotoxins made with a recombinant form of *Pseudomonas* exotoxin A that do not require proteolysis for activity. *Cancer Res* 53:340–347, 1993.

80. Mansfield E, Amlot P, Pastan I, FitzGerald DJ: Recombinant RFB4 immunotoxins exhibit potent cytotoxic activity for CD22-bearing cells and tumors. *Blood* 90:2020–2026, 1997.

81. Reiter Y, Brinkmann U, Kreitman RJ, Jung S-H, Lee B, Pastan I: Stabilization of the Fv fragments in recombinant immunotoxins by disulfide bonds engineered into conserved framework regions. *Biochemistry* 33:5451–5459, 1994.

82. Reiter Y, Kreitman RJ, Brinkmann U, Pastan I: Cytotoxic and antitumor activity of a recombinant immunotoxin composed of disulfide-stablized anti-Tac Fv fragment and truncated *Pseudomonas* exotoxin. *Int J Cancer* 58:142–149, 1994.

83. Kreitman RJ, Wang QC, FitzGerald DJP, Pastan I: Complete regression of human B-cell lymphoma xenografts in mice treated with recombinant anti-CD22 immunotoxin RFB4(dsFv)-PE38 at doses tolerated by cynomolgus monkeys. *Int J Cancer* 81:148–155, 1999.

84. Kreitman RJ, Wilson WH, Bergeron K, et al.: Efficacy of the anti-CD22 recombinant immunotoxin BL22 in chemotherapy-resistant hairy-cell leukemia. *N Engl J Med* 345:241–247, 2001.

85. Flandrin G, Sigaux F, Sebahoun G, Bouffette P: Hairy cell leukemia: clinical presentation and follow-up of 211 patients. *Semin Oncol* 11:458–471, 1984.

86. Frassoldati A, Lamparelli T, Federico M, et al.: Hairy cell leukemia: a clinical review based on 725 cases of the Italian Cooperative Group (ICGHCL). Italian Cooperative Group for Hairy Cell Leukemia. *Leuk Lymphoma* 13:307–316, 1994.

# Section 6
# SPECIAL TOPICS IN LEUKEMIA

## Chapter 34

# MANAGEMENT OF FEVER AND NEUTROPENIA IN LEUKEMIA

*Robin K. Avery*

## OVERVIEW OF FEVER AND NEUTROPENIA

### INTRODUCTION

The febrile neutropenic patient is a central topic in the management of hematologic malignancy. Empiric antimicrobial therapy for fever in the neutropenic patient has been the standard of care for decades, but opinions still vary as to the optimal antibacterial agent or agents, the nature and timing of antifungal therapy, and other issues. This chapter will review basic principles of the physical examination, laboratory studies, radiography, and clinical syndromes. It will also provide updates on the spectrum of infecting organisms, antimicrobial resistance, newer antimicrobial agents, and innovative strategies, such as outpatient and home intravenous (i.v.) therapy. A brief section will summarize highlights of infection control.

The Infectious Disease Society of America (IDSA) has published updated 2002 Guidelines for the Use of Antimicrobial Agents in Neutropenic Patients with Cancer.[1] This comprehensive document features a rating system reflecting the strength of the recommendation (A–E) and the quality of the evidence (I–III), and is highly recommended.

### DEFINITION OF FEVER AND NEUTROPENIA

A commonly accepted definition of fever, used in the IDSA guidelines, is a single oral temperature of 38.3 °C (101 °F) or more, or a temperature of ≥38.0 °C (100.4 °F) for ≥1 h. The route of temperature measurement is important. Although rectal temperatures are more accurate than oral or axillary temperatures, rectal temperatures are usually contraindicated in the neutropenic patient due to the risk of promoting bacteremia from colorectal organisms.

The definition of neutropenia used in the IDSA Guidelines is an absolute neutrophil count (ANC) of <500 cells/mm³, or a count of <1000 cells/mm³ if a decrease to <500 cells/mm³ is expected.

### RISK STRATIFICATION

Both the degree and duration of neutropenia are important in determining the risk for infection. Profoundly neutropenic patients, with an ANC of <100 cells/mm³, are at highest risk for infection. Those with neutrophil counts of <500 mm³ are at higher risk than those with counts of <1000/mm³. A patient who is expected to recover from chemotherapy-induced neutropenia has a different level of risk from a patient in whom neutrophil recovery is not anticipated. Neutropenia of 10 days or more duration confers greater risk. Neutropenia in patients with acute leukemia is generally of longer duration than in patients with solid tumors.

Several models of risk stratification have been developed.[2] Additional risk factors for infection among leukemic patients include mucosal or integumentary breaks such as mucositis, surgical wounds, pressure ulcers, or *C. difficile* colitis; renal or other organ dysfunction; metabolic and nutritional factors; age; comorbidities such as diabetes mellitus; steroids or other immunosuppressive agents; and immune defects such as hypogammaglobulinemia. It is helpful to keep a paradigm of risk stratification in mind in assessing the febrile neutropenic patient.

### HISTORY OF FEVER AND NEUTROPENIA THERAPY

In the 1960s and '70s, it was recognized that the most immediate threat came from Gram-negative infections, particularly *E. coli*, *Klebsiella*, and *Pseudomonas*, which could cause rapid overwhelming sepsis.[3] Thus, empiric therapy regimens have historically been directed at preventing these Gram-negative infections. The combination of an antipseudomonal beta-lactam and an aminoglycoside has been widely used to achieve synergy against such organisms as *Pseudomonas*. Concerns about potential toxicity, and the development of third-generation cephalosporins and carbapenems, have led to a preference for monotherapy at some centers.

As discussed below, there has been a shift in recent years, from predominantly Gram-negative toward Gram-positive organisms. Whether or not to include an agent such as vancomycin in the initial regimen has been vigorously debated. The emergence of resistance factors such as extended-spectrum beta-lactamases has also caused alteration in regimens at some centers. In general, growing antimicrobial resistance should prompt frequent reconsideration of empiric antibiotic regimens.[4]

## MICROBIOLOGY OF INFECTION IN THE NEUTROPENIC PATIENT

### CLASSIC MICROBIOLOGY: GRAM-NEGATIVE ORGANISMS; RECENT EMERGENCE OF GRAM-POSITIVE ORGANISMS

Landmark papers on fever and neutropenia cited organisms such as *E. coli*, *Klebsiella*, and *Pseudomonas* as major pathogens,[2] presumed to originate from the patient's own intestinal flora. However, there has been a shift toward Gram-positive organisms, which now constitute the majority of positive blood culture isolates. Reasons cited for this include use of indwelling i.v. catheters, oral mucositis from current chemotherapy regimens, and use of quinolone prophylaxis.[5] Catheters are most likely to become infected with cutaneous flora; oral mucositis predisposes to viridans streptococcal infection, which can be fulminant.[6] Quinolones are powerful agents against aerobic Gram-negative bacilli, and may lead to overgrowth of organisms such as staphylococci, streptococci, and enterococci.

### ANTIMICROBIAL RESISTANCE PATTERNS

The emergence of extended-spectrum beta-lactamases in *E. coli*, *Klebsiella*, and other organisms has limited the utility of penicillins and traditional cephalosporins at some centers.[7] Although imipenem, meropenem, and cefepime have extremely broad spectrums of activity, organisms resistant to these agents have also been described.[4,5] Methicillin resistance in coagulase-negative *staphylococci* and *Staphylococcus* aureus (MRSA) has become increasingly common, as has vancomycin-resistant *Enterococcus* (VRE).

Organisms such as *Stenotrophomonas*, *Leukonostoc*, and *Corynebacterium jekeium* are now appearing,[5] some of which are not covered by standard antibiotics. For example, *Stenotrophomonas* is often resistant to all but sulfa-based agents.[4,5]

Frequent reconsideration of antibiotic regimens is important. If a patient is deteriorating on therapy, consideration should be given to expanding antibiotic coverage to include the multiresistant bacteria that may be specific to that hospital. Updates from the hospital microbiology laboratory and infection control committee can provide valuable information about changing susceptibility patterns.

### FUNGAL PATHOGENS, INCLUDING EMERGING FUNGI

Fungal infections occur with increasing frequency when neutropenia is prolonged (see below). In the past, most fungal infections were caused by species of *Candida* or *Aspergillus*. *Candida* are frequent colonizers of skin, oropharynx, and the gastrointestinal tract, and may cause localized or disseminated infection. *Aspergillus* spores are widespread in the environment and can also be nosocomial pathogens, particularly in relation to building construction. Sinus or airway colonization may become an invasive infection in the setting of neutropenia. Those with a history of marijuana use, gardening, farming, or construction work are at a higher risk for being colonized.

In recent years, resistance to antifungal agents has increasingly occurred. Fluconazole has been used for therapy or prophylaxis of yeast infections, as it avoids the toxicities of amphotericin B. However, pathogens such as *Candida glabrata* (frequently fluconazole resistant) and *Candida krusei* (always resistant) have emerged in the setting of increasing fluconazole usage. In addition, unusual fungi such as *Fusarium*, *Trichosporon*, *Paecilomyces*, and *Scedosporium* are seen with more frequency. Some of these display resistance to traditional antifungal agents.

## CLINICAL PRESENTATIONS

### HISTORY AND PHYSICAL EXAMINATION

The history should include determination of the underlying cancer, the type and date of most recent chemotherapy, concomitant immunosuppressive medications, and exposures. Symptoms relating to the sinuses, eyes, ears, respiratory and gastrointestinal systems, skin, and catheter sites are of particular importance. The magnitude of the fever and the presence of rigors are also indicators of the severity of illness.

On physical examination, attention should be given to the sinuses, oropharynx, lung and heart exams, catheter site, abdomen, external perianal exam, and skin. Classic signs of inflammation may be absent in the setting of neutropenia. For example, pneumonia is not usually accompanied by lobar consolidation or sputum. Fever, dry cough, and dyspnea might be the only signs of pneumonitis. Peritoneal signs are often absent, and nonspecific abdominal pain might reflect appendicitis, typhlitis, or even perforated viscus. Any proptosis, chemosis, limitation of extraocular motion, or dark nasal or oropharyngeal lesions should prompt emergent surgical consultation for possible invasive fungal infection. Lethargy or focal neurologic signs should prompt emergent imaging of the central nervous system (CNS).

External perianal inspection should be performed, but internal rectal examination should be avoided.

Skin lesions may be the only clues to the etiology of a fever, and biopsy and culture of these lesions can be crucial for diagnosis (see below).

### LABORATORY STUDIES

The degree of neutropenia is important, and a complete blood count with differential is essential. Renal or hepatic dysfunction may reflect acute sepsis or may be preexisting. Acidosis is worrisome for impending sepsis.

Cultures of blood and urine should be obtained, and antibiotics initiated promptly. If an i.v. catheter is present, cultures through each lumen of the catheter should be obtained in addition to a peripheral blood culture. Sputum cultures are low-yield, and bronchoscopy is more useful in the patient with pneumonitis. Lumbar punctures are rarely necessary and may be contraindicated in the thrombocytopenic patient. Stool samples for *C. difficile* and for enteric pathogens and parasites should be obtained in a patient with diarrheal illness. Any drainage from a catheter site or wound should be sent for Gram stain and cultures.

If bronchoscopy or open lung biopsy is performed, a complete panel of stains and cultures should be sent, including Gram stain and bacterial cultures; fungal; *Nocardia*; AFB stains and cultures; *Pneumocystis* stain; Legionella direct fluorescent assay and culture; and cultures for cytomegalovirus (CMV), herpes simplex virus (HSV), and respiratory viruses (influenza, parainfluenza, respiratory syncytial virus (RSV), and adenovirus).

Serologic testing is of limited value in the diagnosis of acute infection in this population. Useful antigen detection tests include cryptococcal antigen in serum or cerebrospinal fluid (CSF), and *Histoplasma* urinary antigen.

### RADIOGRAPHIC STUDIES

The chest X-ray is important, but may provide incomplete information. While patchy interstitial infiltrates or a faint localized haze may reflect pulmonary infection, more sensitive chest CT (computed tomography)

scanning may reveal small nodules, cavities, the halo sign of aspergillosis, and other signs that may not be visualized on chest X-ray. The CT can guide decisions for procedures such as bronchoscopy and lung biopsy, as well as empiric therapy.

The abdominal CT scan is helpful in patients with abdominal pain, as the physical exam may lack classic signs. The CT can reveal abscesses, adenopathy, intestinal wall thickening, or phlegmon suggestive of typhlitis, lesions of hepatosplenic candidiasis, and other conditions.[8]

The brain magnetic resonance imaging (MRI) (or contrast CT if MRI is not rapidly available) is important for evaluation of mental status changes, seizures, or focal neurologic signs. Brain abscesses, septic embolic infarcts, or evidence of rapidly progressive fungal infection may be found on MRI. Additional cuts of the sino-orbital region, mastoid, and ear canal should be obtained in patients with symptoms referable to those areas.

### CLINICAL SYNDROMES

#### Fever without localizing signs

The majority of patients display no obvious source of infection. Bacteremia may be present due to the entry of intestinal or oropharyngeal flora into the bloodstream, or catheter-related infection without external signs. Frequent exams can determine if any new localizing signs are developing. As the leukocyte count rises, previously infected areas often develop more classic signs of inflammation.

#### Abdominal pain and gastrointestinal symptoms

Abdominal pain should always be taken seriously, as peritoneal signs may be absent. Acute appendicitis, cholecystitis, perforated gastric or duodenal ulcers, and diverticulitis can be sources of rapid deterioration. Bacterial infections of the upper urinary tract or biliary system are more likely to be severe in the presence of obstruction due to kidney stones, tumor, or choledocholithiasis.

Neutropenic enterocolitis (typhlitis) is a feared complication involving infection of the intestinal wall. Typhlitis may progress to full-thickness involvement of the right colon, with necrosis and gangrene of the cecum. Though classically associated with *Pseudomonas*, typhlitis may be caused by other Gram-negative bacteria. Surgery may be required, but milder cases may be managed with protracted antibiotic therapy.

*C. difficile* colitis may occur due to use of antibiotics. Wall thickening of the colon on CT scans due to *C. difficile* may be confused with typhlitis. *C. difficile* colitis is more ominous in the setting of ileus and abdominal distention without diarrhea. Repeated plain films of the abdomen can identify colonic dilatation. A stool sample for *C. difficile* toxin assay should be obtained, but occasional false negatives may occur.

#### Pulmonary infiltrates

The lungs are a frequent site of bacterial, fungal, and viral infection.[9] The radiographic pattern on Chest X-ray

(CXR) or CT is helpful. Lobar infiltrates are uncommon, but may reflect postobstructive pneumonia. Bacterial infection more commonly appears as patchy, sometimes multilobar infiltrates. Diffuse infiltrates suggest viral or overwhelming bacterial or fungal pneumonia, or noninfectious etiologies such as pulmonary hemorrhage. Nodular infiltrates are more likely to be fungal, nocardial, or mycobacterial. The presence of cavitary lesions suggests fungi, mycobacteria, bacterial lung abscess, septic pulmonary emboli, or tumor. The "halo sign" is often indicative of aspergillosis.[10] Evidence of old granulomatous disease, such as calcified hilar lymph nodes, suggests dormant fungal or mycobacterial infection that could reactivate in the neutropenic patient.

Patients with pulmonary infiltrates may progress rapidly to respiratory failure and mechanical ventilation. This should prompt broadening of the antibiotic regimen, including systemic antifungal therapy. Patients whose white blood cell counts begin to recover may actually experience a respiratory exacerbation.

Bronchoscopy with bronchoalveolar lavage (BAL) is far more likely than sputum to yield a diagnosis, but BAL cultures may show no growth even in active infection, particularly with prior antibiotic therapy. The BAL is more sensitive for *Pneumocystis* than for fungi, and mycobacteria often require protracted time to grow. CMV in BAL cultures is not necessarily indicative of CMV pneumonitis. Lung biopsy can add considerably to the diagnostic yield of bronchoscopy, but severe thrombocytopenia makes transbronchial biopsy problematic. Open lung biopsy may be warranted in such situations.

Aspiration pneumonia may occur, particularly in elderly patients or those with mental status changes or severe nausea and vomiting. In this situation, bronchoscopy is often nondiagnostic or may grow mixed flora.

Infection control issues are important in patients with pulmonary infiltrates, as devastating outbreaks of respiratory viral infection have occurred (influenza, parainfluenza, RSV, and adenovirus).[11] During influenza season, or any time a community-acquired respiratory virus is suspected, any patient with an unexplained infiltrate should be placed in respiratory isolation initially.

Other causes of pulmonary infiltrates can mimic infection, and should be considered. These include pulmonary hemorrhage, septic pulmonary emboli, congestive heart failure, chemotherapy and radiation toxicity, and adult respiratory distress syndrome from nonpulmonary sepsis.

### Ophthalmologic and otolaryngologic signs

Symptoms referable to the eye, sinuses, orbit, ear, nose, or mastoid should be considered potential emergencies. Fulminant mucormycosis or aspergillosis may progress rapidly to the CNS. Sino-orbital infection (fungal or bacterial) may lead to orbital cellulitis, abscess, meningitis, or cavernous sinus thrombosis. Otologic infection may lead to progression of infection in the mastoid or temporal lobe. Rapid, surgical debridement, combined with high-dose broad-spectrum therapy, represents the best chance for survival.

### Focal neurologic signs and mental status changes

New focal neurologic signs or mental status changes in a neutropenic patient should prompt vigorous evaluation. Focal signs may reflect brain parenchymal abnormalities (intracranial hemorrhage, metastases, cerebral vascular accident, brain abscesses, progressive fungal infection). Antibiotic choice should include agents that cross the blood–brain barrier. Such as third-generation Cephalosporins and Vancomycin.

Seizures may result from focal abnormalities, CNS infections, or medication toxicity. Mental status changes may be a nonspecific presenting sign of sepsis or may reflect drug effect, as well as CNS infection. Among antibiotics, imipenem and ciprofloxacin may contribute to mental status changes in the elderly or in those with renal dysfunction. In addition, antiemetics, pain medications, and sleep medications may cause mental status changes. Meningitis may occur, most commonly due to *Pneumococcus, Listeria, Cryptococcus* (in patients with cellular immune defects), or other fungi, but meningeal signs are uncommon. More indolent mental status changes or focal abnormalities may reflect subacute fungal infection, bacterial brain abscess, toxoplasmosis, or progressive multifocal leukoencephalopathy.

In endemic areas (See the Centers for Disease Control and Prevention Website: www.cdc.gov for maps and more information about areas in which West Nile virus transmission is occurring), West Nile virus encephalitis should be ruled out in any patient with neurologic signs, lethargy, flaccid paralysis, or multiorgan failure. Serology from blood and CSF has been the standard for diagnosis, but molecular testing may improve diagnostic yield.

Prompt radiologic imaging should be performed in cases of suspected CNS infection, as discussed above. Lumbar puncture is problematic in thrombocytopenic patients, but if strongly indicated, can be obtained with platelet transfusion support. Space-occupying lesions and cerebral edema should be ruled out first. Rapid neurologic and neurosurgical consultation should be obtained in patients with progressive symptoms.

### Skin lesions

As disseminated infections with filamentous fungi or mycobacteria are difficult to diagnose in a timely fashion, biopsies and cultures of suspicious skin lesions are often helpful. *Pseudomonas, Candida* spp., and *Fusarium* are particularly likely to be associated with skin lesions. Lesions of ecthyma gangrenosum most often reflect disseminated infection with *Pseudomonas*. Disseminated candidiasis can present with nodular or papular scattered lesions. Dark necrotic-appearing lesions can reflect either bacterial or fungal infection. Peripheral embolic phenomena reflecting endovascular infection may occur in the absence of positive blood cultures.

### Indwelling i.v. catheters
Tunneled catheters are subject to several types of infection: exit site cellulitis, bacteremia with or without external signs, tunnel infection, and septic thrombophlebitis. The most common causative organisms are coagulase-negative staphylococci, but *Staphylococcus aureus*, *Enterococcus*, Gram-negative bacilli, other skin flora, yeast, and occasionally nontuberculous mycobacteria also may be causative organisms. Decisions regarding catheter removal often must be made in the face of fever, neutropenia, and need for multilumen access. In general, tunnel infections require catheter removal regardless of the organism, and pain over the tunnel may be the only sign in a neutropenic patient. In *Candida*, VRE, or *Bacillus* infection, it is particularly important to remove the catheter, and it is often desirable to do so for *Staphylococcus aureus* and Gram-negative bacilli. On the other hand, in the absence of tunnel infection, coagulase-negative staphylococcal infection can often be cleared without catheter removal. If the catheter is to be left in place, repeat blood cultures on therapy should be obtained to document initial clearing, then again after therapy is completed, to document cure. Many clinicians recommend alternating catheter lumens for administration of the i.v. antibiotic.

Persistent positive blood cultures on therapy may reflect septic thrombophlebitis, or less commonly endocarditis, and indicates a need to remove the catheter.

## CHOICE OF EMPIRIC ANTIMICROBIAL THERAPY

### ANTIBACTERIAL THERAPY
#### Beta-lactam plus aminoglycoside therapy
Such combinations have been used for empiric therapy for decades.[1,3] The beta-lactams chosen may be higher-generation penicillins (piperacillin, ticarcillin, mezlocillin, piperacillin-tazobactam, or ticarcillin-clavulanate) or higher-generation cephalosporins (ceftazidime or cefepime) with antipseudomonal activity. Doses should be in the high end of the dosing range. Aminoglycosides include gentamicin, tobramycin, and amikacin, used either with traditional dosing or more recently with single-daily dosing.[12] Advantages to this strategy include synergy against organisms such as *Pseudomonas*, and broad-spectrum activity, especially at centers with marked antimicrobial resistance. Disadvantages include the toxicities of aminoglycosides (nephrotoxicity, ototoxicity, and vestibular toxicity.) Measurement of serum trough levels is important, with dose adjustment whenever renal function changes.

### Monotherapy
Monotherapy is used in a number of centers, and includes agents such as ceftazidime, cefepime, imipenem, or meropenem.[13] Except for ceftazidime, these agents have Gram-positive as well as Gram-negative coverage. Advantages include a simpler regimen and less toxicity. Disadvantages include the risk of missing resistant organisms. Although randomized trials and meta-analyses have documented the efficacy of monotherapy,[14] growing antimicrobial resistance may require reevaluation of this strategy in the future.[13]

### Timing of Gram-positive therapy
There has been considerable debate regarding the inclusion of Gram-positive coverage (particularly vancomycin) in the initial regimen, with studies suggesting that vancomycin can be safely added later.[15] However, some institutions use vancomycin because of the fulminant syndrome that can occur with viridans streptococci, including those with reduced susceptibility to penicillins, and the rise of methicillin-resistant staphylococci in patients with indwelling catheters. Vancomycin may, however, predispose to VRE infection, renal dysfunction, and rash. The Hospital Infection Control Practices Advisory Committee (HICPAC) has issued guidelines, which discourage empiric use of vancomycin except in situations where the risk of omitting it is high.[16] However, the benefits may still outweigh the risks at some centers with a high rate of methicillin resistance.

Some centers choose to add vancomycin secondarily if there is no response to the initial regimen. Another strategy is to include vancomycin initially, then omit it after 48 h if cultures are negative and the catheter site shows no sign of infection. Serum trough levels of vancomycin should be monitored, and adjustments made for changing renal function. Many centers include vancomycin in the initial regimen of a critically ill patient, or when there is an evidence of catheter-related infection.

### Change of therapy
When fever persists for 72 h or longer despite the initial empiric regimen, consideration should be given to changing therapy. A vigorous search for a fever source should be continued, including repeat exams, cultures, chest X-ray, and sometimes CT scans. If positive cultures have been obtained, the regimen can be adjusted accordingly but should retain broad-spectrum coverage, as the patient may still be neutropenic.

Changes in empiric therapy include (1) addition of a second agent to a monotherapy regimen; (2) changing one or more agents in the regimen, such as a carbapenem in place of a beta-lactam; (3) addition of vancomycin; and (4) addition of systemic antifungal therapy (see below).

## Stopping antimicrobial therapy

With positive blood cultures, an appropriate duration of therapy should be administered, which may involve home i.v. antibiotics. For fever with negative cultures, the IDSA Guidelines state that antimicrobial therapy may be discontinued when the ANC is 500 cells/mm³ or greater for two consecutive days, if the patient has become afebrile by day 3 of antibiotics.[1] If the patient became afebrile after day 3 of antibiotic therapy, the guidelines suggest continuing therapy until the ANC has been 500 cells/mm³ or greater for 4–5 days. The more difficult question is what to do if the patient remains neutropenic. The IDSA Guidelines allow for discontinuation of therapy if the patient is afebrile 5–7 days, has defervesced by day 3, is persistently neutropenic by day 7 without positive cultures, and was initially low risk without subsequent complications. However, many centers will elect to trim the antibiotic regimen without complete discontinuation in such cases. In a patient who is at high risk, antibiotics should be continued. If the patient is still febrile on day 3, and later is afebrile but with a neutrophil count which is persistently less than 500 cells/mm³, the recommendation is to reassess and continue antibiotic therapy for two more weeks.[1]

## Oral therapy

As part of the trend toward risk stratification, and to avoid risks and costs of lengthy hospital-based care, there has been an increased interest in early discharge and even initial oral therapy.[17] Randomized trials have demonstrated safety and efficacy of oral therapy in certain *low-risk* groups of patients.[18] The presence of chills, hypotension, dyspnea, radiographic abnormalities, or localizing signs such as abdominal pain, or anything worrisome to the clinician immediately takes the patient out of the "low-risk" group. A multinational scoring system for identifying low-risk patients has been developed, which included the following: absence of symptoms or mild-to-moderate symptoms; absence of hypotension, dehydration, or chronic obstructive pulmonary disease; presence of solid tumor, absence of previous fungal infection in patients with hematologic malignancies, outpatient status, and age less than 60 years.[19] Other factors cited as part of low-risk criteria include cancer in partial or complete remission, temperature less than 39 °C, normal chest X-ray, absence of rigors, respiratory rate 24 breaths/min or less, and absence of diabetes, confusion, mental status changes, or blood loss.

The oral combination most frequently used to treat fever and neutropenia is a combination of ciprofloxacin and amoxicillin–clavulanate.[17,18] This combination is less useful at centers where there is already significant quinolone resistance. With any patient in whom oral therapy is used, the patient should be closely monitored and should be immediately placed on broad-spectrum i.v. antibiotics if fever or any other worrisome clinical change occurs.

## Outpatient and home i.v. antibiotic therapy

Home i.v. antibiotic therapy is useful in the patient with resolved neutropenia who needs to complete a course of therapy for a defined infection. There has also been recent interest in early discharge of the stable neutropenic patient on home i.v. antibiotic therapy or oral therapy after initial i.v. therapy in the hospital.[17,19] Again, this is only appropriate to consider in the patient without signs of severe infection, who is tolerating antibiotic therapy appropriate to initial culture results, and who is reliable and is closely monitored. If the patient is at high risk, continued inpatient treatment is preferred.

### *ANTIFUNGAL THERAPY*
### Timing of antifungal therapy

Early studies have shown that the risk of occult fungal infection increases sharply when the neutropenic patient has been febrile on broad-spectrum antibiotics for 5–7 days or more. Traditionally, i.v. amphotericin B has been added at this time.[1] The patient with pulmonary infiltrates is also more likely to have occult fungal infection.[9] However, toxicities of amphotericin B have been problematic, including renal insufficiency, electrolyte abnormalities, and infusion-related chills and dyspnea. The availability of newer antifungals has expanded the choices available to the clinician. Interpretation of the literature is complicated by the multiplicity of studies and issues in clinical trial design.[20,21]

Lipid formulations of amphotericin, including amphotericin B lipid complex (ABLC) and liposomal amphotericin, are less nephrotoxic than conventional amphotericin, but are costly; infusion-related reactions may still occur (less so with liposomal amphotericin). Fluconazole is primarily useful for prevention of infection with sensitive *Candida* species, and does not have activity against *Aspergillus*. Centers with extensive fluconazole use may see a rise in fluconazole-resistant yeast, including *C. glabrata* and *C. krusei*. Itraconazole has activity against *Aspergillus* and is sometimes used as antifungal prophylaxis. However, oral tolerability is decreased in patients with chemotherapy-induced nausea, and the i.v. formulation cannot be used in patients with renal dysfunction.

Caspofungin and micafungin are echinocandin antifungals with broad activity against yeasts and molds including *Aspergillus* (not *Cryptococcus*). They are generally well tolerated and available only in an i.v. formulation. Liver function tests should be monitored with their use.

Voriconazole is a broad-spectrum antifungal agent with both i.v. and oral formulations. It covers many *Candida* species resistant to other azoles, has excellent activity against *Aspergillus*, and also a number of emerging fungal pathogens, but not mucormycetes. As with itraconazole, the i.v. formulation cannot be used in patients with renal insufficiency. Visual symptoms occur in many patients, especially early in therapy. Patients should be warned in advance that these symptoms may occur.

## Randomized trials and meta-analyses of empiric antifungal therapy

Multiple randomized trials have been performed using different antifungal agents, in patients who either have persistent fever or who require prophylaxis. A randomized trial by Winston et al. compared fluconazole (400 mg) to placebo at initiation of chemotherapy.[22] Fluconazole decreased fungal colonization and superficial fungal infections, but did not clearly decrease invasive fungal infections; aspergillosis was infrequent in both groups.[22] A later randomized trial of 317 patients by Winston et al. compared i.v. fluconazole versus amphotericin B for patients with persistent fever, and found no significant differences, inefficacy, and fewer infusion-related reactions with fluconazole.[23] Similarly, in another randomized trial, Boogaerts et al. found that the efficacy of itraconazole was similar to that of amphotericin B, but itraconazole was associated with fewer side effects.[24]

Antifungal agents may also be used as prophylaxis prior to the onset of fever. The Canadian Fluconazole Prophylaxis Study Group found that fluconazole, compared with placebo, reduced invasive fungal infection and fungal-related mortality.[25] A study by Menichetti et al. of 820 patients receiving prophylaxis with oral fluconazole versus oral amphotericin showed no difference in efficacy, but better tolerability of oral fluconazole.[26] The same group performed a placebo-controlled trial of itraconazole oral solution and found that itraconazole reduced proven and suspected deep fungal infection and candidemia.[27] Concerns have been raised, however, about the increasing incidence of colonization with *C. glabrata* and *C. krusei* in patients receiving fluconazole prophylaxis.[28]

Several trials have assessed lipid formulations of amphotericin B. Prentice et al. conducted two multicenter trials (one in adults and one in children) comparing conventional versus liposomal amphotericin in patients with fever and neutropenia.[29] Liposomal amphotericin was associated with fewer side effects, and defervescence occurred in 64% of those on 3 mg/kg/day liposomal amphotericin as opposed to 49% of those on conventional amphotericin ($p = 0.03$).[29] Mattiuzzi et al. compared liposomal amphotericin B versus the combination of fluconazole and itraconazole prophylaxis.[30] Efficacy was similar, but liposomal amphotericin was associated with more increases in serum creatinine and bilirubin.[30] Wingard et al. compared liposomal amphotericin with ABLC and found similar efficacy, but fewer infusion-related reactions with liposomal amphotericin.[31] Walsh et al. (NIAID Mycoses Study Group) compared liposomal amphotericin B with conventional amphotericin B in a study of 687 patients.[32] Resolution of fever, survival, and rates of discontinuation of the study drug were similar in both groups, but there were fewer proven breakthrough fungal infections in the liposomal amphotericin group as well as less infusion-related toxicity and nephrotoxicity.[32]

Walsh et al. also compared voriconazole with liposomal amphotericin B in a randomized trial of 837 patients with persistent fever and neutropenia.[33] The overall success rate was similar; however, there were fewer breakthrough fungal infections, less nephrotoxicity, and fewer infusion-related reactions with voriconazole.[33]

Given the number of randomized trials comparing antifungal medications, several meta-analyses have been performed. Gotzsche and Johansen in 2002 analyzed 30 trials in which antifungal therapy had been compared with placebo or no treatment.[34] Antifungal treatment with amphotericin B, itraconazole, or fluconazole decreased the incidence of invasive fungal infection. A meta-analysis of 38 trials from 2002 by Bow et al. showed that antifungal prophylaxis reduced the use of parenteral antifungal therapy, and superficial and deep fungal infections. For the overall population, mortality was not reduced, but it was reduced in the subgroups with prolonged neutropenia and who had received hematopoietic stem cell transplantation.[35] Glasmacher et al. analyzed 13 randomized trials of itraconazole prophylaxis and concluded that itraconazole solution (not capsules) reduced the incidence of invasive fungal infections, invasive yeast infections, and mortality from fungal infections but not overall mortality.[36]

There is still no consensus on the optimal antifungal agent to use, or whether to start this agent before fever occurs. The 2002 IDSA guidelines state that amphotericin B has usually been the drug of choice.[1] Lipid formulations of amphotericin B can be used as alternatives, with similar efficacy, less toxicity, and higher cost. Fluconazole is an acceptable alternative at institutions at which invasive mold infections and *C. krusei* infections are uncommon. Voriconazole and caspofungin are increasingly used, and newer antifungal agents are still being developed.

## MANAGEMENT OF ANTIMICROBIAL TOXICITY
### Renal dysfunction

When multiple antimicrobial agents are administered, the risk of drug toxicity increases. Renal dysfunction may result from fluid shifts, hypotension, chemotherapy, other medications, or sepsis. Aminoglycosides and amphotericin B are particularly likely to cause nephrotoxicity. Less commonly, vancomycin, or occasionally beta-lactams (via interstitial nephritis), can be nephrotoxic. When the creatinine rises, there are several possibilities for alteration of the regimen. If an aminoglycoside is being used in combination with a beta-lactam, it may be replaced with a quinolone or aztreonam, unless cultures dictate otherwise. Amphotericin B may be replaced by a lipid formulation of amphotericin. i.v. itraconazole and voriconazole are prepared in a cyclodextrin vehicle, which cannot be used in renal dysfunction, so these may have to be changed to oral therapy or to other antifungals.

## Rash

Drug-associated dermatitis is common in the febrile neutropenic patient, and drug fever may occur with or without rash. Antibiotic-associated rashes are frequently diffuse and maculopapular or confluent, but occasionally appear as palpable purpura, and sometimes progress to desquamation. Consideration should be given to changing antibiotics when a rash occurs, particularly beta-lactams and vancomycin, or less commonly quinolones or azoles. Rashes due to aminoglycosides or amphotericin are uncommon. Drug rashes may progress for several days after discontinuation.

Discontinuation of vancomycin is prudent if the treated patient develops a rash, as some vancomycin reactions can become severe. If needed to treat a methicillin-resistant Gram-positive infection, another agent, such as clindamycin, daptomycin, or quinupristin-dalfopristin may be substituted. If a beta-lactam agent is discontinued due to rash, consideration should be given to avoiding related drugs, such as cephalosporins or carbapenems.

## Clostridium difficile colitis

Diarrhea is common in the neutropenic patient, with common causes including chemotherapy-induced mucositis and antibiotics. Only a fraction of these cases reflect *C. difficile* colitis, but this can be clinically severe, especially when ileus and abdominal distention develop. Bacteremias due to enteric flora are more likely to occur from disruption of colonic mucosa. As febrile neutropenic patients requireongoing antibiotic therapy, treatment of *C. difficile* colitis is challenging. In addition to therapy with oral metronidazole (or oral vancomycin in the patient who has failed metronidazole), it may be helpful to change the antibiotic regimen to omit clindamycin or cephalosporins. If the patient is unable to take oral medication or has severe ileus, i.v. metronidazole is preferred.

### OTHER TOPICS IN ANTIMICROBIAL THERAPY
## Pneumocystis prophylaxis

The use of prophylaxis for *Pneumocystis jiroveci* (formerly *P. carinii*) pneumonia (PCP) has been most extensively studied in children with acute lymphoblastic leukemia, who have an overall 21% risk of PCP without prophylaxis, and in whom risk depends on the intensity of maintenance therapy.[37] PCP occurs in other leukemic patients as well. Prophylaxis with thrice weekly trimethoprim–sulfamethoxazole (TMP–SMX) is highly effective.[37] Whereas the IDSA guidelines do not recommend TMP–SMX prophylaxis for all neutropenic patients, they do recommend such prophylaxis for all patients at high risk for PCP, whether neutropenic or not, including leukemic patients receiving steroid therapy.[1] In addition, any patient with a prior episode of PCP should receive long-term secondary prophylaxis.

## Antiviral therapy

Although CMV infection is a common occurrence in the allogeneic HSCT recipient, it is uncommonly seen in the nontransplanted leukemic patient unless the patient also has some defect in cellular immunity. Therefore, anti-CMV therapy is not generally a part of the empiric regimen in febrile neutropenia. It is, however, appropriate to perform diagnostic tests for CMV in a patient with persistent unexplained fever or pulmonary infiltrates.

HSV reactivation may occur in the setting of chemotherapy and neutropenia, and acyclovir prophylaxis is commonly used to prevent oral mucosal and perineal HSV in that setting.

Respiratory viruses, such as influenza, parainfluenza, RSV, and adenovirus, can be devastating. Where such illness is suspected, rapid isolation of the patient is crucial for prevention of nosocomial transmission. Under certain outbreak circumstances, it may be appropriate for a whole ward to receive antiinfluenza prophylaxis (e.g., with oseltamivir). As immunocompromised patients may have a suboptimal antibody response to yearly influenza vaccination (though they should still receive it), *all* health care workers and family members in contact with neutropenic patients should be strongly advised to be vaccinated against influenza, using the injected vaccine (rather than the inhaled vaccine, which is live).

## Previous infections

When assessing a patient who has had previous significant infections, previous microbiologic data may be helpful. For example, a previous catheter-related bacteremia with a *Pseudomonas* resistant to ceftazidime, even though fully treated, might make the clinician choose something other than ceftazidime monotherapy for this patient's next episode of neutropenic fever.

Similarly, knowing the details of past invasive fungal infections, and verification that these were treated with an appropriate length of therapy and radiographic resolution, is crucial.

## Hypogammaglobulinemia

In addition to the immune defect conferred by neutropenia, certain patients may also have humoral immune defects that contribute to infection risk. Hypogammaglobulinemia is most frequently seen in patients with CLL and in the early phase after allogeneic bone marrow transplant. Low immunoglobulin levels (IgG below 400 mg/dl) predispose to recurrent and severe bacterial infections; immunoglobulin replacement can be helpful.

## INFECTION CONTROL

Space does not permit a detailed discussion of infection control issues, but highlights will be briefly outlined. The reader is referred to monographs from the

Centers for Disease Control and Prevention, Infectious Diseases Society of America, and American Society of Blood and Marrow Transplantation,[38] as well as other reviews,[39] for more details.

### HAND HYGIENE

Although numerous infection control measures have been proposed to protect neutropenic patients, the most universal agreement concerns the importance of hand hygiene. The importance of health care workers' washing their hands thoroughly before and after patient contact cannot be overemphasized, yet compliance is surprisingly incomplete. Recently, antimicrobial hand rubs have been introduced as an alternative to traditional handwashing, and appear to be effective.[39]

### AIR AND VENTILATION MANAGEMENT

Laminar air-flow rooms and/or high-efficiency particulate air (HEPA) filtration have been advocated as measures to reduce the concentration of potential airborne pathogens, particularly fungal spores . The efficacy of such measures is most established for high-risk patients, such as those with prolonged neutropenia and/or HSCT transplantation. The importance of such measures for patients with lower risk, shorter duration neutropenia is less well established.[39]

When hospital construction is taking place, it is prudent to take all preventive measures possible to prevent exposure of vulnerable patients to increased fungal spores. These measures may include masks when patients leave the floor, protective barriers, air surveillance, or even moving an entire ward during phases of construction. When outbreaks of unexpected fungal infection occur, air and ventilation issues in the unit in question should be thoroughly examined.[39]

### RESPIRATORY ISOLATION AND OTHER SPECIAL PRECAUTIONS

As discussed above, patients with suspected respiratory virus should be placed in isolation rooms with negative airflow to reduce the possibility of airborne spread of these viruses to other patients. Visitors with any symptoms of respiratory infection should not be allowed to visit the oncology ward. Mild illness in a visitor could result in devastating infection in one or more patients.

Documented or suspected tuberculosis or primary varicella (chickenpox) also require respiratory isolation. Hospitals vary in their infection control measures for resistant pathogens such as MRSA, VRE, and multiresistant Gram-negative bacteria.

### OTHER POTENTIAL NOSOCOMIAL EXPOSURES

One of the best-known pathogens to be transmitted through hospital water sources is *Legionella*.[40] Hospitals vary in their *Legionella* incidence, and infection control and surveillance measures differ from one institution to another. Copper–silver ionization systems have been described as the most effective way to control potential sources.[40]

Hospital visitors should not be permitted to visit if they have any fever or respiratory illness. Visitors should wash their hands before and after leaving the patient's room. In outbreak settings such as respiratory viruses in the community, it may be prudent to restrict visitation to immediate family members.

## REFERENCES

1. Hughes WT, Armstrong D, Bodey GP et al.: 2002 Guidelines for the use of antimicrobial agents in neutropenic patients with cancer. *Clin Infect Dis* 34:730–751, 2002.
2. Rolston KV: New trends in patient management: risk-based therapy for febrile patients with neutropenia. *Clin Infect Dis* 29:515–521, 1999.
3. Bodey GP: Infections in cancer patients. *Cancer Treat Rev* 2:89–128, 1975.
4. Shlaes DM, Binczewski B, Rice LB: Emerging antimicrobial resistance and the immunocompromised host. *Clin Infect Dis* 17(suppl 2):S527–S536, 1993.
5. Zinner SH: Changing epidemiology of infections in patients with neutropenia and cancer; emphasis on Gram-positive and resistant bacteria. *Clin Infect Dis* 29: 490–494, 1999.
6. Cohen J, Donnelly JP, Worsley AM, et al.: Septicaemia caused by viridans streptococci in neutropenic patients with leukemia. *Lancet* 2(8365–8366): 1452–1454, 1983.
7. Paterson DL, Ko WC, Von Gottberg A, et al.: Antibiotic therapy for *Klebsiella pneumoniae* bacteremia: implications of production of extended-spectrum beta-lactamases. *Clin Infect Dis* 39:31–37, 2004.
8. Kirkpatrick IDC, Greenberg HM: Gastrointestinal complications in the neutropenic patient: characterization and differentiation with abdominal CT. *Radiology* 226:668–674, 2003.
9. Maschmeyer G, Beinert T, Buchheidt D, et al.: Diagnosis and antimicrobial therapy of pulmonary infiltrates in febrile neutropenic patients—guidelines of the Infectious Diseases Working Party (AGIHO) of the German Society of Hematology and Oncology (DGHO). *Ann Hematol* 82(suppl 2):S118–S126, 2003.
10. Kuhlman JE, Fishman EK, Siegelman SS: Invasive pulmonary aspergillosis in acute leukemia: characteristics findings on CT, the CT halo sign, and the role of CT in early diagnosis. *Radiology* 157:611–614, 1985.
11. Raad I, Abbas J, Whimbey E: Infection control of nosocomial respiratory virus disease in the immunocompromised host. *AM J Med* 102(3A):48–52, 1997.
12. Barza M, Iaonnidis JP, Cappelleri JC, Lau J: Single or multiple daily doses of aminoglycosides: a meta-analysis. *BMJ* 312:338–345, 1996.
13. Ramphal R: Is monotherapy for febrile neutropenia still a viable alternative? *Clin Infect Dis* 29:508–514, 1999.

14. Paul M, Soares-Weiser K, Leibovici L: Beta lactam monotherapy versus beta lactam-animoglycoside combination therapy for fever with neutropenia: systematic review and meta-analysis. *BMJ* 326:1111, 2003.
15. Rubin M, Hathorn JW, Marshall D, et al.: Gram-positive infections and the use of vancomycin in 550 episodes of fever and neutropenia. *Ann Intern Med* 108:30–35, 1988.
16. Hospital Infection Control Practices Advisory Committee: Recommendations for preventing the spread of vancomycin resistance. Recommendations of the Hospital Infection Control Practices Advisory Committee (HICPAC). *MMWR Recomm Rep* 44(RR-12):1–13, 1995.
17. Rolston KV: Oral antibiotic administration and early hospital discharge is a safe and effective alternative for treatment of low-risk neutropenic fever. *Cancer Treat Rev* 29:551–554, 2004.
18. Freifeld A, Marchigiani D, Walsh T, et al.: A double-blind comparison of empirical oral and intravenous antibiotic therapy for low-risk febrile patients with neutropenia during cancer chemotherapy. *N Engl J Med* 341:305–311, 1999.
19. Klastersky J, Paesmans M, Rubenstein EB, et al.: The multinational association for supportive care in cancer risk index: a multinational scoring system for identifying low-risk febrile neutropenic cancer patients. *J Clin Oncol* 18:3038–3051, 2000.
20. Bennett JE, Powers J, Walsh T, et al.: Forum report: issues in clinical trials of empirical antifungal therapy in treating febrile neutropenic patients. *Clin Infect Dis* 36(suppl 3): S117–S122, 2003.
21. Marr KA: Antifungal therapy for febrile neutropenia: issues in clinical trial design. *Curr Opin Investig Drugs* 5: 202–207, 2004.
22. Winston DJ, Chandrasekar PH, Lazarus HM, et al.: Fluconazole prophylaxis of fungal infections in patients with acute leukemia. Results of a randomized placebo-controlled, double-blind, multicenter trial. *Ann Intern Med* 118:495–503, 1993.
23. Winston DJ, Hathorn JW, Schuster MG, Schiller GJ, Territo MC: A multicenter, randomized trial of fluconazole versus amphotericin B for empiric antifungal therapy of febrile neutropenic patients with cancer. *Am J Med* 108:282–289, 2000.
24. Boogaerts M, Winston DJ, Bow EJ, et al.: Intravenous and oral itraconazole versus intravenous amphotericin B deoxycholate as empirical antifungal therapy for persistent fever in neutropenic patients with cancer who are receiving broad-spectrum antibacterial therapy. A randomized, controlled trial. *Ann Intern Med* 135: 412–422, 2001.
25. Rotstein C, Bow EJ, Lavardiere M, et al.: Randomized placebo-controlled trial of fluconazole prophylaxis for neutropenic cancer patients: benefit based on purpose and intensity of cytotoxic therapy. The Canadian Fluconazole Prophylaxis Study Group. *Clin Infect Dis* 28: 331–340, 1999.
26. Menichetti F, Del Favero A, Martino P, et al.: Preventing fungal infection in neutropenic patients with acute leukemia: fluconazole compared with oral amphotericin B. The GIMEMA Infection Program. *Ann Intern Med* 120: 913–918, 1994.
27. Menichetti F, Del Favero A, Martino P, et al.: Itraconazole oral solution as prophylaxis for fungal infections in neutropenic patients with hematologic malignancies: a randomized, placebo-controlled, double-blind, multicenter trial. GIMEMA Infection Program. *Clin Infect Dis* 28:250–255, 1999.
28. Wingard JR, Merz WG, Rinaldi MG, et al.: Increase in *Candida krusei* infection among patients with bone marrow transplantation and neutropenia treated prophylactically with fluconazole. *N Engl J Med* 325: 1274–1277, 1991.
29. Prentice HG, Hann IM, Herbrecht R, et al.: A randomized comparison of liposomal versus conventional amphotericin B for the treatment of pyrexia of unknown origin in neutropenic patients. *Br J Haematol* 98:711–718, 1997.
30. Mattiuzzi GN, Estey E, Raad I, et al.: Liposomal amphotericin B versus the combination of fluconazole and itraconazole as prophylaxis for invasive fungal infections during induction chemotherapy for patients with acute myelogenous leukemia and myelodysplastic syndrome. *Cancer* 97:450–456, 2003.
31. Wingard JR, White MH, Anaissie E, et al.: A randomized double-blind comparative trial evaluating the safety of liposomal amphotericin B versus amphotericin B lipid complex in the empirical treatment of febrile neutropenia. *Clin Infect Dis* 31:1155–1163, 2000.
32. Walsh TJ, Finberg RW, Arndt C, et al.: Liposomal amphotericin B for empirical therapy in patients with persistent fever and neutropenia. *N Engl J Med* 340: 764–771, 1999.
33. Walsh TJ, Pappas P, Winston DJ, et al.: Voriconazole compared with liposomal amphotericin B for empirical antifungal therapy in patients with neutropenia and persistent fever. *N Engl J Med* 346:225–234, 2002.
34. Gotzsche PC, Johansen HK: Routine versus selective antifungal administration for control of fungal infections in patients with cancer. *Cochrane Database Syst Rev* CD000026, 2002.
35. Bow EJ, Lavardiere M, Lussier N, et al.: Antifungal prophylaxis for severely neutropenic chemotherapy recipients: a meta-analysis of randomized-controlled clinical trials. *Cancer* 94:3230–3246, 2002.
36. Glasmacher A, Prentice A, Gorschluter M, et al.: Itraconazole prevents invasive fungal infections in neutropenic patients treated for hematologic malignancies: evidence from a meta-analysis of 3,597 patients. *J Clin Oncol* 21:4615–4626, 2003.
37. Hughes WT, Rivera GK, Schell MJ, Thornton D, Lott L: Successful intermittent chemoprophylaxis for *Pneumocystis carinii* pneumonitis. *N Engl J Med* 316: 1627–1632, 1977.
38. Centers for Disease Control and Prevention: Guidelines for preventing opportunistic infections among hematopoietic stem cell transplant recipients. *MMWR Recomm Rep* 49:1–125, 2000.
39. Avery RK, Longworth DL: Infection control issues after hemopoietic stem cell transplantation. In: Bowden RA, Ljungman P, and Paya CV (eds.) *Transplant Infections.* 2nd ed. Philadelphia, PA: Lippincott Williams and Wilkins; 2003:chap 36, 577–588.
40. Sabria M, Yu VL: Hospital-acquired legionellosis: solutions for a preventable infection. *Lancet Infect Dis* 2: 368–373, 2002.

Chapter **35**

# AUTOLOGOUS STEM CELL TRANSPLANTATION FOR LEUKEMIA

## Alexander E. Perl, Selina M. Luger, and Edward A. Stadtmauer

## AUTOLOGOUS STEM CELL TRANSPLANTATION: INTRODUCTION AND HISTORY

### INTRODUCTION

If high-dose therapy (HDT) and autologous stem cell transplant (ASCT) are to be successful as a curative therapy for leukemia, then one or more of the following must be true:

1. HDT overcomes drug resistance, and therefore eliminates minimal and otherwise undetectable leukemic burden in the patient that could potentially lead to relapse.
2. The processing and purging of stem cells eliminates contaminating leukemia cells from the graft, thereby resulting in cure, once HDT has been administered.
3. There is some not-well-understood difference between high-dose chemotherapy (HDCT) and conventional dose therapy that stimulates the host immune system to eradicate minimal residual leukemia cells in a form of adoptive immunotherapy.

Numerous phase III trials have compared standard, dose-intensive chemotherapy for acute leukemia to ASCT. Limitations of the studies' designs and/or execution has, however, left many questions at present unanswered, making the precise utility of ASCT in the treatment of leukemia still a point of great debate.

### HISTORY

The potential for cryopreservation of human cells was first realized in the late 1940s,[1] when viability of spermatocytes following long-term, ultra-low temperature storage in glycerol was initially reported. Approximately one decade later, dimethylsulfoxide (DMSO) was also shown to be an effective cyropreserving agent.[2]

Following successes in the development of myeloablative chemotherapy, attempts to provide the clinical benefits of myeloablative therapy to patients who lacked histocompatible marrow donors were undertaken. The first report of autologous stem cell transplantation for acute myeloid leukemia (AML) was published in the late 1970s by Gorin et al.[3] This patient with AML had had marrow collected and cryopreserved at first remission that was thawed and reinfused following a myeloablative regimen at the time of first relapse. Fefer et al. reported a series of patients with refractory AML who underwent syngeneic donor transplants, and also demonstrated long-term relapse-free survival (RFS).[4] A number of reports followed, utilizing first remission marrow for hematopoetic rescue after HDT for refractory AML, all demonstrating high response rates, but few cures. With these promising reports of activity, the procedure was moved earlier into the course of disease, at first or subsequent remission.

## AUTOLOGOUS STEM CELL TRANSPLANTATION FOR ACUTE MYELOGENOUS LEUKEMIA

### RATIONALE

Increased dose and dose intensity of post-remission therapy have been shown to clearly improve outcome in AML. In 1988, Cassileth et al. demonstrated that low-dose cytosine arabinoside (Ara-C) maintenance CT was superior to no post-remission therapy in first remission AML.[5] Indeed, all patients who did not receive further therapy relapsed, with a median time to progression of only 4 months. Subsequent studies established a dose response effect of post-remission cytarabine among patients under the age of 60, ultimately leading to 4-year continuous complete

**Table 35.1**  Factors that affect relapse risk following autologous transplantation for leukemia

- Age
- Karyotype
- Minimal residual disease status at time of harvest
- Disease status at time of transplant (initial remission, second remission, etc.)
- Time from achievement of remission to transplant
- Post-remission chemotherapy prior to harvest (in AML)
- Presence of FLT3-ITD (in AML)

FLT3-ITD: *fms*-like tyrosine kinase 3-internal tandem duplication mutation.

**Table 35.2**  Risk stratification of acute myeloid leukemia

| *Favorable* |
| --- |
| Age <60 |
| WBC <100,000 |
| De novo leukemia |
| t(15;17); t(8;21); inv16 (or t(16;16)) |
| absence of high risk cytogenetic abnormalities or FLT3-ITD |

| *Unfavorable* |
| --- |
| Age >60 |
| WBC >100,000 |
| Antecedent hematologic condition (e.g., myelodysplasia) or prior chemotherapy/radiation |
| Deletions/monosomies of chromosome 3, 5, 7, or complex karyotype (≥3 per SWOG or ≥5 per MRC), t6;9, 11q23 rearranged |
| FLT3-ITD |

| *Intermediate/indeterminate* |
| --- |
| all others |

SWOG: Southwest Oncology Group; MRC: Medical Research Council (United Kingdom); FLT3-ITD: *fms*-like tyrosine kinase 3-internal tandem duplication mutation.

remissions in more than 40% of patients treated with the most dose-intensive regimens.[6] These data strongly suggested that increasing intensity of post-remission therapy was a critical strategy to achieve cure of AML. SCT was the logical progression of this idea: administering myeloablative doses of CT, hopefully toxic enough to leukemic cells that hematopoietic stem cell (HSC) replacement was necessary for marrow recovery.

### PROGNOSTIC FACTORS

A number of patient characteristics have now been identified as prognostic factors in the treatment of AML (Table 35.1). Interpretation of clinical trial results must take into account these different prognostic subtypes. Factors that have consistently been found to predict poor therapeutic outcome with standard CT include old age, high white blood cell (WBC) count at diagnosis, AML arising from an antecedent stem cell disorder (e.g., myelodysplasia), therapy-related leukemia, extramedullary disease, more than one cycle of induction chemotherapy to achieve complete remission (CR), MDR-1 expression by flow cytometry, poor-risk cytogenetics (including abnormalities of chromosomes 3q, 5q, 7, 11q23, or complex karyotype), internal tandem duplications of the FLT3 receptor tyrosine kinase, or the presence of minimal residual disease at completion of consolidation CT (Table 35.2).[7-11] Favorable prognostic factors include the lack of the above characteristics. In addition, these include cytogenetic abnormalities, such as the 15;17 translocation in acute promyelocytic leukemia, or transcriptional repression of the core binding factor complex associated with 8;21 translocation or inversion of chromosome 16.[9]

In general, patients with secondary or therapy-related AML, myelodysplasia, and residual cytogenetic abnormalities are rarely treated with ASCT. All other subgroups have been considered appropriate for clinical trials.

### METHODS OF SCT
#### Myeloablative regimens

A number of myeloablative regimens have been used for SCT in AML. The two most common were derived by the pioneering work in AML by the Seattle and Johns Hopkins groups. To this day, total body irradiation (TBI) and cyclophosphamide (Cy) or the busulfan (Bu) and Cy, are the most common regimens utilized. Traditional Bu/Cy consists of 1 mg/kg oral Bu given every 6 h for 16 total doses (16 mg/kg), followed by 2–4 days Cy for a total of 120–200 mg/kg. Most centers utilize the Bu/Cy (2) regimen, as comparison between it and Bu/Cy (4) has shown reduced toxicity for BuCy (2) without an impact on efficacy. Recently, Bu dosing has been guided and adjusted pharmacokinetically by measuring area under the curve (AUC) to correct for erratic GI absorption and first-pass hepatic metabolism. Maintenance of steady-state Bu levels within a narrow range seems to reduce toxicity, particularly hepatic veno-occlusive disease. More recently, an intravenous formulation of busulfan has become available, with the benefit of far more predictable pharmacokinetics, minimal patient to patient variability, and potentially less toxicity. The most common radiation-containing preparative regimen for autografting is 120 mg/kg Cy with six fractionated doses of 200 cGy. No definitive data suggest a clear benefit of a radiation-containing regimen over a CT regimen.

### Stem cell source

Pluripotent HSCs can be derived from bone marrow (BM) via numerous percutaneous aspirations or by leukapheresis of cells circulating in the blood following growth factor stimulation or recent chemotherapy, or both. Blood-derived stem cells appear to consistently shorten the time to neutrophil and platelet recovery, compared to BM. Peripheral blood cells have all but replaced bone marrow in general practice due to ease of collection, superior engraftment, and equivalence of relapse risk and survival from comparison studies between the two approaches.[12]

### Stem cell in vitro purging

As stated at the outset of this chapter, due to the nature of harvesting stem cells in a marrow disorder such as leukemia, one can expect tumor contamination of grafts. A number of approaches to reduce tumor burden among harvested grafts have been undertaken to reduce the likelihood of relapse following ASCT. Such relapses can be expected to arise from one of the two sources: harvested cells in the autograft, or unharvested, drug-resistant clones that survive the preparative regimen. A combination of the two etiologies is likely. Studies of relapses after syngeneic transplantation demonstrate relapse rates of more than 50%, demonstrating that the myeloablative regimen itself may be a greater source of therapeutic failure than inability to achieve a tumor-free graft at the time of reinfusion.[13] The corollary to the syngeneic data, however, shows that residual leukemia is frequently present at the time of harvesting. It is therefore not surprising that grafts should have a high risk of tumor contamination, and that—even with improvements in myeloablative regimens—this may contribute to relapse.

Contamination of autografts at the time of harvesting occurs frequently and is readily confirmed by immunophenotype, clonogenic assay, or PCR. Experiments in which harvested marrow was transfected with a retroviral construct containing the neomycin-resistance gene were found to show incorporation of the marker gene in a subset of leukemia cells at the time of relapse. This suggests that a component of the relapse was indeed caused by leukemia cells from the reinfused harvest product.[14] Purging of the graft therefore makes intuitive sense to minimize the risk of reinfusion of clonogenic leukemia cells.

Purging of marrow is accomplished by chemical, immunologic, or physical means. Chemotherapeutic agents such as the prodrugs 4-hydroperoxycyclophosphamide (4-HC) or mafosfamide are particularly toxic to committed progenitors and leukemic blasts, but spare the earliest hematopoietic elements. These stem cells express relatively high levels of the detoxifying enzyme aldehyde dehydroxygenase, decreasing intracellular generation of active metabolites such as phosphoramine mustard and limiting stem cell injury from either agent.[15] Regardless of this fact, purging with cytotoxic agents lowers stem cell dose. In combination with the slow self-renewal rates of early progenitors, it is not surprising that engraftment is typically delayed following purging with cytotoxic agents, and this may be associated with increased bleeding or risk of infection.

Numerous studies have demonstrated that purging can decrease the degree of leukemic burden in the autograft, and that this is associated with a lower relapse rate.[16,17] There are no prospective randomized trials to examine whether purging is associated with improved survival as compared to unmanipulated autografts. The largest study investigating the benefits of purging in AML is a retrospective analysis of nearly 300 autologous transplants from the Autologous Blood and Marrow Registry.[18] In all of these cases, transplantation occurred within 6 months of complete remission, minimizing the bias of delay prior to transplantation that confounds numerous studies of purging. A multivariate analysis of this data showed purging with 4-HC was associated with an improved leukemia-free survival (56% vs 31% in first CR; 29% vs 10% in second CR, respectively) and overall survival (62% vs 40% in first CR; 46% vs 17% in second CR, respectively), with comparable transplant-related morbidity and mortality. Significant differences were noted between the two groups in terms of time to engraftment, with a median time to ANC >500 of 40 days in the purged group and 30 days in those receiving unpurged transplants. Differences in regimen-related toxicities, as well as some disparities in baseline characteristics of the patients receiving each type of transplant may have contributed to the study's findings. However, the overall survival of 46% among purged transplants beyond the first remission deserves note, as this survival is more typical of the survival plateau among historical studies of unpurged transplants in first remission. Indeed, there are few, if any large series of unpurged transplants that significantly exceed this level, regardless of disease status.

A number of monoclonal antibodies have been employed to purge contaminating early hematopoietic cells, such as anti-CD33 and CD14, along with immunomagnetic beads or complement fixation.[19–22] Other methods that have been used include density-gradient centrifugation, elutriation, hyperthermia, and cytokines, such as interleukin-2.[23] Like the effect of chemotherapeutic purging, molecular and immunologic purging of autografts, even when associated with reduction in leukemic burden, lowers stem cell count. Numerous retrospective and phase II studies have shown that graft manipulation delays engraftment. Attempts to use myeloid growth factors, such as granulocyte or granulocyte-monocyte stimulating factors have not been pursued to determine if these agents can minimize some of this toxicity. Alternatively, amifostine has been examined as a cytoprotective agent, to allow for the sparing of normal hematopoietic stem cells in the graft.[24]

Despite a sound rationale and both laboratory and clinical evidence for the feasibility and efficacy of autograft purging, the benefit of purging remains speculative. The labor-intensive procedure adds substantial cost to transplant, as well as the potential for increased transplant-related morbidity from delayed engraftment. This has kept the practice from widespread acceptance. From available literature, patients that seem to benefit the most from the practice are those who are beyond the first remission at the time of transplant. However, this is a heterogeneous group and this complicates analysis of data from various centers and purging agents. It is also unclear if there would be a benefit of purging marrow obtained in second remission above that of using stem cells harvested and stored early in the course of disease (i.e., as soon as feasible once in first remission). In the absence of randomized data, the practice of autograft purging for leukemia remains investigational at present.

### Stem cell in vivo purging

Treatment with chemotherapy, antibodies, or molecularly targeted agents prior to stem cell harvest provides an ability to perform graft purging in vivo. Given that relapse following initial remission is universal among patients with acute leukemia, some form of post-remission therapy appears necessary to ensure a purified stem cell harvest. Chemotherapy purging with high dose cytarabine (HDAC)-containing regimens are most commonly used to this end, an approach pioneered at the City of Hope.[25] The number of post-remission cycles needed for adequate purging is unanswered. Additional cytoreduction from multiple cycles of chemotherapy may produce a "cleaner" harvest, but whatever benefit is achieved is counterbalanced against increased regimen-related toxicity, as well as a decreased ability to adequately collect cells with each cycle delivered. For this reason, most centers harvest cells following 1–2 cycles of HDAC-based chemotherapy. The University of California, San Francisco group developed a feasible, two-step approach to autologous transplant based on this work.[26] This center used a single consolidation cycle of HDAC plus infusional etoposide, followed by peripheral stem cell harvest at GCSF-supported recovery. This approach provided more than $5 \times 10^6$ CD34+ cells/kg at collection for more than 99% of patients so treated. Ninety-one percent of these patients were subsequently able to receive the intended stem cell transplant. With a median follow-up of over 5 years, a disease-free survival of 55% in 133 patients transplanted with unpurged cells was observed, with a DFS of 74% among those with favorable cytogenetics.[27]

In addition to intensive chemotherapy, a newer agent that is potentially suitable for in-vivo purging is gemtuzumab ozogamicin. Gemtuzumab is an antibody directed against CD33 that is linked to an anthracycline-like toxin, calicheamicin. The agent produces complete responses in approximately one-third of patients treated at relapse, and is associated with a favorable toxicity profile compared to reinduction chemotherapy. However, a number of patients reinduced with gemtuzumab developed hepatic veno-occlusive disease during subsequent allogeneic transplant.[28] This has tempered enthusiasm for this agent in relapsed patients who are expected to proceed to transplant once in remission. The drug, however, may not be associated with this toxicity if administered during remission, particularly since lower doses may provide adequate in vivo purging of minimal disease following stem cell harvest. This approach is currently being assessed in cooperative group trials.

### CLINICAL RESULTS OF AUTOLOGOUS TRANSPLANTATION FOR ACUTE MYELOID LEUKEMIA
#### Phase II trials in AML

Numerous phase II trials have demonstrated the efficacy of ASCT as a consolidation therapy for AML in remission. Trials in second and subsequent remission generally demonstrate a 20–30% long-term RFS; studies in first remission show less uniform results, ranging from 34% to 70% long-term RFS. This likely depends largely upon quality of pre-transplant in vivo purging with chemotherapy and pre-treatment cytogenetics. Given that some studies suggest dramatic efficacy (RFS of up to 70%), caution must be used in interpreting these data. Additional factors that might influence how these results are interpreted include the duration between initial remission and transplant, baseline differences among patients likely to enter innovative trials (generally healthier and younger than historical controls), and variations in induction, consolidation, and preparative therapies. Lastly, most relapses following ASCT occur within first two years, and therefore adequate follow up prior to publication is necessary to avoid premature conclusions of efficacy.

#### Phase III trials in AML

There have been four large, prospective, randomized trials comparing the outcome of newly diagnosed patients with AML treated with post-remission intensive consolidation chemotherapy versus autologous versus allogeneic transplant and a fifth comparing auto to allo-BMT (Table 35.3). In all cases, allogeneic transplant was not based upon randomization, but on availability of a human leukocyte antigen (HLA)-matched sibling donor. Randomization of remaining patients to either chemotherapy or autologous transplantation was performed. With the exception of the US intergroup study, the other four studies used unpurged marrows as a stem cell source and none used growth factor support following marrow reinfusion. All studies present their results by intention-to-treat analysis.

The AML-8A EORTC-GIMEMA (European Organization for the Research and Treatment of Cancer-Gruppo Italiano Mallatie Ematologiche Maligne dell'Adulto) trial included 941 eligible and evaluable children and younger adults with newly diagnosed AML.[29] Median age was 33 years (range 11–59). All patients received infusional ara-C at 200 mg/m² for 7 days plus daunorubicin 45 mg/m² by bolus on days 1–3. Those in remission after 1–2 cycles received a single course of intensive consolidation, consisting of intermediate dose cytarabine (500–1000 mg/m² q12h on days 1–4) with amsacrine. Seventeen

**Table 35.3** AML: Phase III trials of autologous transplant versus intensive chemotherapy or allogeneic transplant

| Reference | Treatment | Purging | TRM/deaths in CR (%) | Number tx/intended | LFS (%) | OS (%) |
|---|---|---|---|---|---|---|
| Zittoun et al. (GIMEMA/EORTC AML-8A)[29] | ABMT | No | 12 | 95/128 | 48 | 56 |
| | DA | | 9 | 104/126 | 30 | 46 |
| | AlloBMT | | 29 | 144/168 | 55 | 59 |
| Harousseau et al. (GOELAMS)[31] | ABMT | No | NR[a] | 75/86 | 44 | 50 |
| | IA/RA | | NR[a] | 71/78 | 40 | 54.5 |
| | AlloBMT | | NR[a] | 73/78 | 44 | 52.5 |
| Burnett et al. (MRC AML10)[32] | MidAC/ABMT | No | 12 | 126/190 | 54 | 57 |
| | MiDAC | | 4 | 186/191 | 40 | 45 |
| | AlloBMT | | 19 | 257/419 | 50 | 55 |
| Cassileth et al. (US intergroup)[33] | ABMT | 4-HC | 14 | 63/116 | 37 | 47 |
| | HDAC | | 3 | 99/118 | 35 | 54 |
| | AlloBMT | | 25 | 105/120 | 43 | 46 |
| Suciu et al. (GIMEMA/EORTC AML-10)[30] | ASCT (peripheral blood cells) | No | 4 | 246/441 | 42 | 51 |
| | AlloBMT | | 17 | 202/293 | 52 | 58 |

ABMT: autologous bone marrow transplant; alloBMT: allogeneic bone marrow transplant; DA: daunorubicin, ara-C; IA: idarubicin, ara-C; RA: rubidazone, ara-C; MiDAC: mitoxantrone, intermediate dose ara-C; HDAC: high dose ara-C; ASCT: autologous stem cell transplant.

[a] NR not reported by intention-to-treat. The toxic death rate for patients who actually underwent autologous transplant, intensive chemotherapy, and allogeneic transplant on this study were 6.5%, 3%, and 22%, respectively. Unlike patients assigned allogeneic BMT, patients treated with either intensive chemotherapy or autologous transplant also underwent an additional cycle of intensive chemotherapy, associated with a 2.5% mortality rate.

percent of patients received T-cell depleted grafts using elutriation. Those assigned to autologous transplant received at least $1 \times 10^8$ nucleated cells/kg, without graft manipulation or purging. Patients assigned to intensive consolidation chemotherapy received a second intensive chemotherapy cycle consisting of high dose ara-C (2 gm/m$^2$ q12h on days 1–4) with daunorubicin (45 mg/m$^2$ on days 5–7).

Of the 941 patients enrolled, the complete remission rate was 66% (623 patients). Due to early relapses, toxic death, non-lethal toxicity, or refusal of assigned therapy, 201 patients received no further therapy than induction or the single post-remission course of intensive chemotherapy. Of the 422 patients who completed intensive consolidation and proceeded to further therapy, approximately one-third (168) of these patients were found to be eligible for allo-BMT. The number of patients randomized to autologous transplant was 128 and 126 to intensive chemotherapy. Seventy-nine patients (19%) did not receive the intended post-remission therapy for aforementioned reasons; these patients were roughly equally distributed among the three groups. Ultimately, 144 patients

received an allograft, 95 patients received an autograft, and 104 patients received a second cycle of intensive chemotherapy.

With the obvious exception of age due to the established cutoff in the allo-BMT arm, baseline characteristics were well matched among the treatment arms, including cytogenetic risk groups, FAB classification, number of cycles needed to achieve CR, and initial WBC count at diagnosis. Time to hematopoietic recovery was significantly longer in the autologous group. The time from documented remission to initiation of assigned therapy was significantly longer in the autologous and allogeneic arms (14 and 15 months, respectively) than in the chemotherapy arm (10 months, $p < 0.0001$). This delay may have accounted for the decrease in early relapses in the chemotherapy group (5 vs 12 and 18 in the autologous and allogeneic arms, respectively). This difference in timing of therapy may have selected for high-risk disease among those in the CT group, since patients destined to ultimately relapse may have been more likely to have received their assigned therapy prior to this event due to treatment delay in the other arms. Accordingly, this might underestimate the treatment effect of their post-consolidation therapy.

The 4-year RFS estimates were 55%, 48%, and 30% for allotransplant, autotransplant, and chemotherapy, respectively. These differences in estimated RFS between the two transplant arms were non-significant. However, the survival estimates of either were significantly better than that of CT ($p = 0.05$). Death in first remission was most likely in those treated with allo-BMT. Interestingly, the 4-year OS was not statistically significantly different in any arm, with rates of 59%, 56%, and 46% for allotransplant, autotransplant, and CT, respectively ($p = 0.43$). A high rate of salvage was seen among patients treated with consolidation CT who relapsed. Of these patients, 62% (36/58) achieved a second remission and nearly two-thirds (22/36) of those achieving a second remission were subsequently treated with an autologous transplant. While relapses among those transplanted in first remission were less frequent, the salvage rate in the autologous and allogeneic arms was inferior, at 38% (11/29) and 40% (8/20), although the authors did not report whether this finding was of statistical significance. Second transplants were rarely performed (two in each treatment arm).

Following these results, the EORTC/GIMEMA abandoned the use of intensive post-remission chemotherapy and designed their next study (AML-10) to compare the benefit of autologous BMT/PSCT with that of allo-BMT in younger patients.[30] To minimize bias, this study also attempted to place transplant in as early a point in post-remission therapy as possible and analyzed the data on the basis of allogeneic donor versus no donor. Patients in the age group of 15–45 years with newly diagnosed AML were treated with infusional ara-C (100 mg/m$^2$ d1-7) and three doses of an anthracycline on days 1, 3, and 5. Patients in CR were treated with one cycle of intermediate dose ara-C (500 mg/m$^2$ q12h d1-6) and those without a histocompatible sibling underwent either bone marrow or peripheral blood harvest of stem cells. The intended conditioning regimen for all patients was Bu/Cy (2), although many patients received Cy/TBI. Approximately one quarter of patients assigned to allo-BMT received T-cell depletion. Autologous grafts were unmanipulated.

A total of 1136 patients were eligible for study entry. Of these patients, 822 (74%) entered a CR following induction and 734 received further therapy and were eligible for analysis. Of these, 293 had HLA-matched siblings and were designated "donor" and the remaining 441 were considered to have "no donor". The two groups were well balanced for age, FAB subtype, number of induction cycles. Cytogenetics were unavailable in approximately 40% of patients in each group, but their outcome paralleled the group for which cytogenetics was known. For those with a known karyotype, the two groups were well matched except for highest risk cytogenetics (abnormal 3q, 5, 7, 11q23, t(6;9),

t(9;22), or complex karyotype), which were seen in 14% patients in the no-donor group but 24% in the donor group (no $p$ value provided). 69% of patients who had a donor identified actually received an allogeneic transplant and 56% of those lacking a donor received an autograft. The median follow-up was 4 years; during this time, 293 relapses occurred and 66 patients died in CR1. The 4-year DFS was improved among those patients with a donor versus no donor (52% vs 42%, respectively, $p = 0.044$), although 9 months of follow-up was needed before the survival curves showed this difference. Despite this decrease in relapse risk among those with donors, no statistically significant difference in overall survival was noted (58% vs 51% for donor vs no donor, respectively, $p = 0.18$).

The French Cooperative, Groupes Ouest Est Leucemies Aigues Myeloblastiques (GOELAM), trial[31] was designed to compare the outcome of patients treated with two cycles of intensive post-remission therapy with that of one cycle of intensive chemotherapy followed by autologous transplantation. This study enrolled patients from the age group of 15 to 50 in remission following either rubidazone or idarubicin plus infusional ara-C for 1–2 cycles. Those under 40 years of age with an HLA-identical sibling received an allogeneic transplant. Most of these patients were treated with one cycle of post-remission amsacrine and standard dose ara-C (100 mg/m$^2$ SQ) while awaiting allogeneic transplant. The remaining patients on the study received one cycle of intensive chemotherapy using high dose ara-C (3 gm/m$^2$ q12 h d1-4) and idarubicin or rubidazone. These patients were randomized either to receive a subsequent autologous transplant or a second cycle of intensive chemotherapy using etoposide and amsacrine. Unmanipulated bone marrow was harvested following the first intensive consolidation cycle and contained at least $1 \times 10^8$ nucleated cells/kg. The conditioning regimen for the autologous transplant arm was Bu/Cy (4) in all patients. Those receiving an allogeneic transplant were predominantly conditioned with Cy/TBI, although about one-fourth of patients received Bu/Cy. No T-cell depletion was performed and most patients received cyclosporine plus methotrexate as immunosuppression and GVHD prophylaxis. The median follow-up was 62 months.

The median age of enrolled patients was 36 years. Of the 504 enrolled and evaluable patients, 367 (73%) achieved a CR, with no statistical difference in the success or toxicity of the two induction regimens. Of the patients in CR, 88 were assigned to allo-BMT and 73 actually received the intended therapy. Of the remaining patients eligible for randomization, only 164 were able to be randomized, with 86 assigned auto-SCT and 78 assigned CT. The large patient drop out prior to randomization was due to early relapse, poor hematologic reconstitution, infections, toxic death, patient refusal, or protocol violations. The time from initial remission to intended therapy was shortest in those who received allogeneic transplants (68 days), followed by CT (91 days) and autologous transplant (109 days). Baseline characteristics in terms of cytogenetic groups, FAB classification, presenting WBC, or number of cycles required for initial CR were well matched between groups, with the exception of the cytogenetic risk profile of the group assigned allo-BMT, which had a statistically significant lower percentage of patients with intermediate or unfavorable risk karyotypes (17% vs 47% in CT arm, $p = 0.001$). The 4-year RFS and OS were 44% and 52.5% for allo-BMT, 44% and 55% for ABMT, and 40% and 54.5% for CT, with all comparisons among groups not statistically significant. The time to hematopoietic recovery was similar for the ABMT and CT groups, except for that of time-to-platelet recovery, which was significantly longer in the transplant group (110 vs 19 days), likely again related to the relatively low stem cell dose.

The UK Medical Research Council AML 10 trial[32] asked a very different question from the previously described studies. It examined whether autologous or allogeneic transplant improved outcome in patients who had otherwise completed a full course of intensive post-remission chemotherapy. In this study, newly diagnosed children and young adults (age less than 56 years) were randomly assigned to either daunorubicin, ara-C, and etoposide (ADE) or daunorubicin, ara-C, and thioguanine (DAT) for two cycles, with those in CR proceeding to one cycle of standard-dose ara-C ($200$ mg/m$^2$ CI d1-5) based consolidation. Patients with HLA-identical siblings were eligible to receive an allogeneic BMT following an additional cycle of intermediate dose ara-C ($1$ gm/m$^2$ d1-3) plus mitoxantrone (MiDAC). The remainder underwent bone marrow harvest of at least $1 \times 10^8$ nucleated cells followed by MiDAC consolidation. Following this cycle, patients were randomized to receive either an unpurged autologous transplant or no further therapy. If patients relapsed in the observation group, reinduction was attempted and those salvaged were consolidated with autologous cells from the prior harvest. The myeloablative preparative regimen was Cy/TBI for both allogeneic and autologous transplants and patients received immunosuppression and GVHD prophylaxis based upon institutional preferences.

Of the 1857 patients enrolled on this trial, 81% (1509) entered CR. Number of patients in CR found to have HLA-matched sibling donors was 370, leaving 1131 patients eligible for randomization. However, the majority (620) of these patients were not randomized, with most choosing not to receive treatment after the fourth cycle of chemotherapy (481), and some choosing autologous transplant (79). Only 25% of those initially entering remission (381) were randomized to either autologous BMT ($n = 190$) or no further therapy ($n = 191$) following four cycles of chemotherapy. Of the patients randomized to autologous transplant, 126 received the intended therapy (66%). The median

bone marrow harvest dose was $2.18 \times 10^8$ mononuclear cells/kg. Patients randomized to autologous BMT showed a significant reduction in relapse risk as compared to those assigned no further therapy (37% vs 58%, $p = 0.0007$). There was no evidence for a weighted risk reduction based on age or cytogenetic risk group. Relapse following autologous transplant was associated with a notably poorer risk of achieving a second CR than among patients who had received no further therapy (34% vs 59%). No difference in survival was seen between autologous transplant and those who received no further therapy (57% vs 45%, $p = 0.2$). Most relapses in the auto-BMT group occurred within 2 years, while there was an increase in relapses after 2 years in remission among those who received no further therapy. When survival past 2 years was analyzed separately, a statistically significant benefit for autologous BMT was seen. A subsequent analysis based upon allogeneic donor versus no-donor status showed a statistically significant decrease in relapse risk at 7 years based on the presence of a donor (36% vs 52%, $p = 0.0001$), but only a trend toward improved survival (56% vs 50%, $p = 0.1$) was noted.

In addition to the small number of patients who were eligible for randomization, a criticism of this study is that the total post-remission dose of ara-C is relatively low in comparison to other randomized studies of consolidation therapy. Patients treated with MACE and MiDAC received a total of 4 gm/m$^2$ of ara-C. By contrast, those treated on the EORTC/GIMEMA study received a total of 20 gm/m$^2$, patients on the GOELAM trial received 24 gm/m$^2$, those on the US intergroup study received 36 gm/m$^2$,[33] and, finally, those treated on the initial CALGB study that established the benefits of dose escalating post-remission ara-C received an impressive 72 gm/m$^2$ over their four consolidation cycles.[6] The UK MRC-AML10 is the only study of the four phase III trials comparing intensive chemotherapy with autologous or allogeneic transplant to show a significant survival benefit of autologous transplant compared with intensive chemotherapy. In this context, one must question if the post-remission therapeutic intensity of the chemotherapy arm was adequate to draw any firm conclusions regarding its efficacy.

The Eastern Cooperative Oncology Group-led North American Intergroup trial[33] enrolled patients with newly diagnosed AML between the age groups of 16 and 55. Subjects received induction therapy with 1–2 cycles of idarubicin and infusional ara-C (3+7) followed by intensification with identical agents (2+5). Patients with HLA-compatible siblings were assigned to allo-BMT using Bu/Cy (4) conditioning and all others were randomized to receive either a single cycle of high dose ara-C (3 gm/m$^2$ q12 h d1-6) or ABMT using Bu/Cy (4) conditioning and perfosfamide (4-HC, 4-hydroperoxycyclophosphamide) purging. The CR rate for the 740 evaluable patients enrolled was 70% (518).

Of these enrolled patients 120 were assigned to allo-BMT; 116 and 120 patients were randomized to ABMT and HDAC consolidation, respectively. Ultimately 105, 63, and 99 patients went on to receive their assigned allotransplant, autotransplant, or HDAC consolidation, respectively. With a median follow-up of 4 years, DFS was not significantly different at 43%, 37%, and 35%, respectively. OS was slightly better in the HDAC arm, at 54%, than either tha allo- or auto-BMT arms at 46% and 47%, respectively ($p = 0.05$). The 100-day mortality after post-remission therapy was 3% in the HDAC arm, 14% in the auto-BMT arm, and 21% in the allo-BMT arm. The median time-to-platelet recovery was 64 days in the autoBMT arm versus 24 days in the alloBMT arm. Subsequent studies by the same cooperative group using unpurged peripheral blood stem cells have shown comparable efficacy with transplant-related mortality of 0% ($n = 32$), suggesting that the use of bone marrow source and purging may have accounted for some of the surprisingly high mortality rate in this arm.[34]

### Correlation of cytogenetic risk group with response to autologous transplant in AML

A benefit of the five randomized comparisons of post-remission therapy was the enrollment and categorization of more than 4000 patients with AML in the US, UK, and Western Europe. Several publications have reinforced the concept that pre-treatment karyotype is among the strongest predictors of outcome for newly diagnosed patients. Classifications of favorable, indeterminate/intermediate, and poor-risk (see Methods of SCT) were applied fairly uniformly to the various studies. Regardless of the differences in treatment algorithms on the individual trials, the three risk groups showed remarkably similar long-term outcome from study to study, validating this prognostic model. Subgroup analyses of the various treatment arms ensued to determine if a particular post-remission approach (CT, ABMT, or alloBMT) was best suited to particular risk groups.

The MRC-AML 10, US-intergroup, and EORTC/GIMEMA AML-10 studies all included detailed analyses based upon cytogenetic risk groups.[30–36] In both the US intergroup and EORTC/GIMEMA study, patients with poor-risk cytogenetics had a dismal leukemia-free and overall survival when treated with intensive chemotherapy or autoBMT. When analyzed on a donor versus no-donor basis, the difference in overall survival was improved among those with donors, and this met statistical significance in both studies ($p = 0.043$ and $p = 0.035$, respectively). By contrast, the MRC study showed no statistically significant benefit to any arm. Patients with indeterminate/intermediate cytogenetic risk showed no consistent benefit to any post-remission strategy in any of the studies. The results in the favorable cytogenetics group varied most from study to study. In each study, however, the allograft arm had an inferior overall survival, and this met statistical significance in the MRC

study. In the US intergroup study, autografted patients in the favorable risk cytogenetics group had a superior survival to those treated with chemotherapy or allografting. However, this study had a surprisingly poor outcome of those in the favorable risk category who were treated with high dose ara-C consolidation. Indeed, in comparison to historical controls[9] or even to patients in the study with indeterminate/intermediate risk cytogenetics, the favorable risk group had notably inferior disease free and overall survival.

The benefit of autologous BMT for acute promyelocytic leukemia is well established by several trials. FAB M3 disease was allowed on all of the randomized phase III studies listed above except for the EORTC/GIMEMA AML10, which began accrual following the widespread availability of all-trans retinoic acid in induction regimens. Given the superb results of ATRA-based chemotherapy regimens (OS of approximately 70%), it is felt that historical results of autologous transplant or allogeneic transplant in CR1 do not improve upon this performance. Given the increased toxicity associated with these regimens, transplantation in CR1 is not justified. Most patients with M3 AML do not receive transplantation unless they relapse and subsequently achieve a second remission with reinduction chemotherapy. Several studies have looked at the outcome of transplants for second remission APL, and the outcome of autologous transplant in this setting is excellent. Meloni et al. showed that achieving a molecular remission by RT-PCR for PML-RARa fusion was a strong predictor of survival following unpurged autograft in CR2. Although the group studied was small, the difference in relapse rate among those with RT-PCR negative harvests (1/9) as compared to those with detectable minimal residual disease harvests (7/7) was impressive.[37] A larger, retrospective report of the European Acute Promyelocytic Group[38] documented the outcome of patients with relapsed APL who underwent successful salvage. Patients who subsequently underwent autologous transplant had a superior overall survival compared to those who received an allogeneic transplant or chemotherapy alone (60 vs 52 vs 40%, respectively, $p = 0.04$). A potential limitation of these data is the absence of arsenic for salvage, which is currently considered the standard of care and might obviate the need for subsequent transplantation.

### Autologous BMT for AML: Conclusions

Adult patients with AML in first CR currently have three effective post-remission therapies. Five large, randomized trials have failed to establish clear superiority of one approach over another, although available data suggest that patients with high risk cytogenetics may be best benefited by allografting, when feasible. Autologous transplant for AML in first complete remission seems to provide comparable leukemia-free and overall survival to allogeneic transplant for patients with standard or favorable risk cytogenetics. In comparison to intensive chemotherapy, autologous transplant may provide superior initial antileukemic therapy, particularly among those with favorable cytogenetics, but has not clearly been shown to offer a survival benefit. This is likely due to the high salvage rate among those treated with intensive chemotherapy, many of whom may receive subsequent myeloablative therapy in second remission. Quality of life scores among patients treated with autologous transplant are typically superior to those of patients who underwent allogeneic transplant but inferior to those of patients treated with intensive chemotherapy, particularly regarding impaired fertility and libido.[39] The choice of post-remission therapy remains largely an individual one, based on cytogenetics and other risk stratification, availability of histocompatible sibling donors, as well as physician and patient preference.

The benefits of ABMT for patients with AML in second and subsequent remissions are clear, particularly for those without HLA-compatible donors and patients with acute promyelocytic leukemia, given the low likelihood of conventional chemotherapy to be curative. Because of the efficacy of all-trans retinoic acid plus anthracycline-based chemotherapy at inducing remission and preventing relapse with comparably low toxicity, autologous transplant should no longer be offered to patients with acute promyelocytic leukemia in first CR. However, ABMT in second remission should be considered the standard of care for patients without RT-PCR evidence of PML-RAR fusion. There remains a strong need for innovative phase I and phase II trials to develop novel therapies in AML.

## AUTOLOGOUS STEM CELL TRANSPLANTATION FOR ACUTE LYMPHOBLASTIC LEUKEMIA

### RATIONALE

Acute lymphoblastic leukemia (ALL) is an uncommon disease in adults. It is initially very responsive to chemotherapy and the vast majority enters remission. However, relapse is common and the ultimate long-term survival rate hovers at approximately 20–30%. Poor prognostic factors include very young or old age, high WBC count at diagnosis, the presence of the Philadelphia chromosome (Ph+), and slow initial response to therapy (Table 35.4).[40]

The chance for long-term RFS after relapse without transplant is very limited. It seems paramount to adequately achieve initial leukemic control due to low response rate to salvage and lack of durability of subsequent remissions, regardless of consolidation strategy.

### PURGING

In vitro HSC purging is well studied in ALL, due to the well-known antigens that characterize this disease and the ability to raise monoclonal antibodies (mAbs)

| Table 35.4    Risk stratification of acute lymphoblastic leukemia |
| --- |
| *High risk* |
| Time to CR >4 wks |
| t(9;22) (BCR-ABL) or t(4;11), t(1;19), +8, −7 |
| WBC >100,000 (for precursor-B ALL) |
| Age >30 |
| *Favorable risk* |
| Time to CR <4 weeks |
| No high risk cytogenetics |
| Precursor-T ALL or precursor-B ALL with WBC <30,000 |
| Age <30 |

against these antigens, mAbs against anti-CD 9, 10, 19, 20 have been most commonly used in B-cell ALL[41] and anti-CD5, and anti-CD7 for T-cell ALL.[42] Similar antibodies have been combined with immunotoxins or magnetic beads. 4-HC has also been used as a purging agent. In vitro laboratory studies demonstrate significant reduction in contaminating tumor cells, but, as with other purging techniques, there has not been substantial clinical evidence to demonstrate the efficacy of this procedure. Most recently, CD34 selection columns have been used to positively screen and select pluripotent HSCs and to passively purge pure contaminating leukemia cells. The limited degree of selection of these devices, and the possibility of CD34 expression on leukemic blasts, make this approach less promising. In vivo purging with mobilizing chemotherapy prior to blood stem cell collection is also under investigation in ALL.

The development of imatinib is increasing interest in autografting in Ph+ ALL. The drug is being investigated as an in vivo purging agent, as well as post-autograft maintenance therapy. Already, several groups—notably MD Anderson and the German Multicenter ALL cooperative group—have reported feasibility of incorporating imatinib into standard regimens such as Hyper-CVAD[43] and BFM-style inductions. In the latter group, greater molecular responses at the time of stem cell harvest were noted when imatinib was started within two weeks of initiation of chemotherapy and no planned treatment breaks occur up to the time of stem cell mobilization.[44] The ECOG/MRC ALL study has recently amended its treatment protocol to incorporate 4 weeks of imatinib as in vivo purging prior to stem cell harvest, as well as maintenance post transplant for all Ph+ patients. As is true with the agent in CML, longer follow-up of clinical trials is necessary to see if the often impressive early hematologic and cytogenetic responses to imatinib are paired with clinically meaningful outcomes such as improved LFS and OS.

There are case reports showing successful use of rituximab for CD20+ ALL as in vivo purging but no large series or trials to support its use.[45,46] Unfortunately, the antigen is only rarely expressed among precursor B-ALL, making its use in autologous transplant only suitable to a minority of patients. Due to frequent expression in Burkitt (FAB L3 ALL) leukemia, it may be an attractive choice in the small number of patients with this disease who require autografting.

A final antibody that may ultimately prove relevant as an in vitro purging agent is the anti-CD52 mAb (Campath 1H). CD-52 is expressed in the majority of pre-B ALL, and alemtuzumab is well tolerated as an injectible chemotherapy in the treatment of B-cell malignancies. The drug is already being used as an immunomodulatory agent in allogeneic transplantation due to its in vivo T-cell depletion ability without the typical side effects of reduced stem cell dose from graft manipulation. Whether the drug will develop a role in autologous transplantation remains to be seen, but it has been employed successfully in small series.[22]

### HIGH DOSE REGIMENS

Common regimens for ALL include cytoxan and TBI, with or without the addition of etoposide. Traditionally, the TBI is fractionated, sometimes with an increased dose of 1200–1400 cGy, particularly in the pediatric population. No one regimen has been demonstrated to be superior to another. Rapid engraftment is typically seen.

### CLINICAL RESULTS OF PHASE II TRIALS OF AUTOLOGOUS TRANSPLANTATION FOR ACUTE LYMPHOBLASTIC LEUKEMIA

Numerous small phase II trials have been conducted of ABMT for ALL, in first or second remission, or with refractory disease. OS has generally ranged between 5% and 20% for relapsed leukemia and 2-year DFS was 30–60%, when transplant is conducted in first CR. Interpretation of these trials suffers from the likely selection bias inherent in phase II trials and the varying pre-transplant regimens and prognostic factors for the patients studied.

### CLINICAL RESULTS OF PHASE III TRIALS OF AUTOLOGOUS TRANSPLANTATION FOR ACUTE LYMPHOBLASTIC LEUKEMIA

The Leucemie Aigues Lymphblastiques de l'Adulte (LALA) 94 trial[47] was a follow-up to the LALA 87 trial, which randomized patients with newly diagnosed ALL in remission to standard chemotherapy, autologous transplant, or allogeneic transplant. This study showed no difference in outcome between post-remission therapies in ALL among standard risk disease, but clear superiority of allogeneic transplant among those with high-risk disease.[48] Autologous transplant showed a trend toward improved outcome in comparison to standard chemotherapy, but was inferior to alloBMT among high risk patients. The LALA 94 trial further examined the role of intensified consolidation and risk-directed post-remission therapy in a large

multicenter trial. Following a standard, four-drug induction, patients were stratified into one of four risk categories. Those with standard risk ALL (defined by WBC < 30K, time to CR < 4 weeks, absence of high risk cytogenetics, absence of CNS disease at presentation, and typical immunophenotype with absent myeloid markers) were randomized to either standard or intensive consolidation followed by 2 years of consolidation/maintenance. High risk patients (albeit Ph⁻ and without CNS disease) all received intensive consolidation and those who lacked histocompatible donors were randomized to receive either an autologous transplant or standard consolidation/maintenance. High risk patients with HLA-matched siblings received an allogeneic BMT. All Ph⁺ patients received intensive consolidation and were assigned to allogeneic or autologous transplant, depending on availability of an HLA-matched donor (sibling or unrelated). Lastly, patients with CNS disease received triple intrathecal therapy, whole brain radiation, and intensive consolidation followed by either allogeneic or autologous transplant, depending on donor status. All transplants used Cy/TBI conditioning, except for patients who were Ph⁺, who also received high dose etoposide. Autografts were unpurged except in rare cases.

Over 8 years, the LALA94 study enrolled 1000 patients, of which 922 were evaluable; 771 (84%) achieved CR; 706 received subsequent therapy and were risk-stratified. Of the high risk patients, 82 had a sibling donor and were assigned to transplant. The remaining 129 were randomized to chemotherapy versus autologous transplant. Of those randomized to autograft, 87% actually received the intended therapy. Seventy-eight Ph⁺ patients were assigned to allo-BMT, while 65 had no donor. 18 patients with CNS disease had matched-family donors, while 30 were assigned to autograft. In all three risk groups where autologous transplant and/or standard chemotherapy was compared to allo-BMT there was a statistically superior DFS, 3-year survival, and 5-year survival favoring the allogeneic arm. In the comparison between autologous transplant and standard consolidation among high risk patients, there was a trend among autografted patients toward improved median LFS (15 vs 11 months, $p = 0.08$), 3-year survival (39 vs 24%, no $p$ value given), and 5-year survival (25 vs 15%, no $p$ value given). A notable difference in the two groups was the pattern of relapse, specifically the absence of late relapses among those autografted. By contrast, the chemotherapy-treated group had a continuous pattern of relapse over time.

The largest prospective, randomized trial to assess the utility of post-remission strategies in ALL is the ECOG 2993/MRC UKALL XII study, which randomizes newly diagnosed patients with ALL to either standard chemotherapy or an autologous PSC transplant. Patients under age 55 with an HLA-matched sibling are given an allo-BMT and those with Ph⁺ disease may receive a matched, unrelated donor transplant. The conditioning regimen for all transplants is TBI/VP16. The study uses a two-month, modified BFM induction followed by high dose methotrexate and asparaginase intensification. After intensification, patients receive either a transplant or four cycles of consolidation followed by 18 months of maintenance therapy. Interim results have been presented in an abstract form.[49] To date, over 1500 patients have been enrolled for this study worldwide, including more than 550 patients who received transplants as consolidation therapy. The CR rate is 93% among those with Ph⁻ disease and 84% in the Ph⁺ subgroup. The trial shows substantial improvement in the 5-year OS among those treated with allogeneic transplant as compared to autograft (55% vs 39%, $p < 0.05$). The effect was robust regardless of age, donor source (sibling or unrelated), or cytogenetics. No comparative data among the randomized arms have been disclosed to date as the study continues to accrue patients. The survival of patients after relapse was dismal, with only 13 patients (6%) alive at 5 years after relapse, regardless of subsequent therapy.

## CONCLUSIONS

The results of the ECOG 2993/MRC UKALL XII may ultimately define a role for autologous transplant in the management of adult ALL. At present, there is no clear group for which it should be considered a standard of care. Available data recommend allogeneic transplant in CR1 for all patients with ALL, though the data seem to be more robust among high risk patients. Outside clinical trials, autologous transplantation should be reserved for patients with poor prognostic factors in first remission who are not candidates for allogeneic SCT, or patients in second and subsequent remission.

## AUTOLOGOUS SCT FOR CHRONIC MYELOGENOUS LEUKEMIA

### HISTORY

CML has traditionally been the most common indication for allogeneic transplantation and the curative potential of allo-BMT in this disease is well established. The majority of preparative regimens used for leukemia were developed to treat this disease. It was also the model for adoptive immunotherapy in the form of graft-versus-tumor that established the practice of donor lymphocyte infusion. The development of imatinib has substantially decreased the number of patients who are treated with stem cell transplants, but it remains the standard bearer for patients treated with curative intent.

Autologous transplant plays a less established role in CML management than allogeneic BMT. However, given the lack of potential histocompatible donors for many patients, as well as the tendency for the disease to present after the age of 50 years, autologous transplant has enjoyed a fair amount of interest in terms of offering the potential benefits of myeloablative therapy to more patients with CML. This is particularly true for advanced phase disease, for which there are no effective therapies outside of transplant. The initial reports of autologous transplant in CML used stem cells frozen from chronic phase to rescue patients treated with myeloablaative chemotherapy at a time of blast crisis. A second chronic phase ensued in many patients, but relapses typically occurred in less than 1 year.[50] Due to persistence of leukemia following autologous transplantation, attempts using a number of in vitro purging agents ensued, none of which consistently provided protection against relapse. Ultimately the development of imatinib may have rekindled interest in harvesting of PCR negative stem cells for use in future because of imatinib failure. Given the low toxicity of the drug, however, there is little interest in autologous transplant as initial therapy.

### RATIONALE

CML derives from disordered proliferation of a Ph⁺ clone that arises from an early hematopoietic stem cell. Marrows of patients with CML may contain chimerism between malignant Ph⁺ and non-malignant Ph⁻cells. The results of chemotherapy, interferon, or imatinib to induce cytogenetic responses, as well as the ability to grow CFU of Ph⁻ cells from cultured CML marrow, demonstrates this point. Collecting stem cells purified for Ph⁻ clones has been the elusive goal of studies of autologous transplant for CML. To this end, a number of purging approaches have been investigated. However, data regarding syngeneic transplantation show a high relapse rate and suggest that graft versus leukemia may be equivalent to—if not more important than—myeloablation and infusion of a tumor-free graft.[13]

### PHASE I AND II TRIALS OF ABMT IN CHRONIC MYELOGENOUS LEUKEMIA

Most autologous transplant trials in CML consist of small series of patients at single institutions (Table 35.5).There are no randomized data to compare the merits of autologous transplant against any other therapy for CML. By far, most series instead attempt to define a novel method of isolating Ph⁺ cells for harvest, typically via purging of Ph⁺ clones. Among the agents used in attempts to purge Ph⁻ cells in vitro have been chemicals such as 4-HC,[51] mafosfamide,[52] interferon gamma.[53] Other approaches included differentiation agents, such as GM-CSF[54] or extended culture to purify for Ph⁻ clones. In small series, all of these approaches were seen to have transient significant activity, frequently leading to engraftment with complete cytogenetic responses. However, relapse across these studies, was near universal, typically after only a

**Table 35.5** Selected trials of autologous transplantation for chronic myeloid leukemia

| References | Purging | Number treated | CR | PR | Graft failure |
|---|---|---|---|---|---|
| Carlo-Stella et al.[52] | Mafosfamide | 10 | 6 | 1 | |
| McGlave et al.[53] | IFN-γ | 44 | 10 | 12 | |
| Barnett et al.[32] | Long-term culture | 22 | 13 | 3 | 5 |
| Coutinho et al. (1997) | Long-term culture | 9 | 4 | 3 | 2 |
| DeFabritis et al. (1998) | Bcr-abl antisense | 8 | 2 | 0 | 0 |
| Luger et al.[55] | c-myb antisense | 25 | 2 | 3 | 5 |
| Reiffers et al.[12] | Unpurged | 49 | 10 | 5 | |
| Simonsson et al. (1996) | In vivo | 30 | 13 | 10 | |
| Carella et al. (1996) | In vivo | 30 | 16 | 10 | 0 |
| Verfaillie et al. (1998) | In vivo | 47 | 4 | 9 | 1 |
| Rapoport et al. (2004) | Post-transplant co-stimulated T-cell infusion | 9 | 4 (3 negative BCR-ABL RT-PCR) | 0 | |

few months of remission. It is unclear if survival among treated patients would exceed that expected by the natural history of this chronic disease.

Autografts for CML have been one of the first places that gene-directed therapy with antisense oligodeoxynucleotides (AS-ODN) have been employed. Two pilot studies deserve note. Not surprisingly, AS-ODN directed against BCR-ABL were the first target to be tested in CML. Eight patients in transformation to advanced disease were subjected to autologous transplantation using marrow that had had antisense against BCR-ABL incubating for 24–72 hours prior to cyropreservation. Two patients had a complete cytogenetic response by FISH. The remainder had minimal or no response. Toxicity was negligible. Another oligodeoxynucleotide target protein has been the c-myb proto-oncogene,[55] which is felt to play an essential role in both hematopoiesis and leukemogenesis. Because leukemia cells show enhanced reliance upon myb's ability to transactivate a number of important growth regulatory genes important in CML, myb inhibition is an attractive therapeutic target in this disease. Twenty-four patients underwent bone marrow harvest with incubation of their marrow for either 24 or 72 hours in AS-ODN targeted against c-myb. After conditioning with busulfan with or without cytoxan, the purged marrow cells were reinfused. Myb and RNA transcript numbers decreased appreciably in approximately half of patients. Two patients achieved a complete cytogenetic response and three more had major cytogenetic responses. However, unlike the AS-ODN targeted against BCR-ABL, significant delayed engraftment was seen among all those treated with 72-hour incubation, requiring back up marrow infusion in a number of patients.

Imatinib has been utilized both prior to harvesting and following autologous transplantation.[56,57] Given its impressive success in upfront CML therapy, the number of autologous stem cell transplants that have been performed for this disease has plummeted.

However, imatinib has only transient activity in advanced phase disease.[58] A role for imatinib in combination with autografting may ultimately be established among patients initially presenting with advanced phase disease who are either poor candidates for allogeneic transplant or lack suitable donors. Several groups have shown that Ph⁻ stem cell collection is feasible among patients treated with complete cytogenetic responses to imatinib who are mobilized with GCSF.[59]

Because approximately one quarter of patients treated with imatinib will achieve more than 3 log reduction or even molecular clearance of BCR-ABL, these patients could be considered ideal candidates for harvesting of stem cells, either for immediate use or during disease progression period on imatinib. At present, one remaining question is: for whom would this approach be warranted? Patients with negative quantitative PCR studies for BCR-ABL would initially seem to be attractive candidates, since these patients are most likely to be able to mobilize BCR-ABL negative harvests as measured by PCR. Yet disease progression models consider such patients to be at the lowest risk of progression, with current estimates ranging as low as less than 1% risk of progression/year.[60] Those for whom disease control is suboptimal and progression is probable are unlikely to produce uncontaminated grafts even with imatinib.

### CONCLUSION

Allogeneic transplant remains the only proven cure for CML and should be strongly considered in young, highly motivated patients with HLA-identical siblings. Current disease models also suggest that survival is extended by imatinib, and therefore an initial therapeutic trial of the agent is also reasonable. Autologous BMT is rarely performed for CML due to the predictability of response to imatinib and the low level of toxicity. As data regarding imatinib resistance have come to prominence, novel approaches to treat resistant disease are sought. Here it is possible that autologous transplant may return to prominence as the cohort currently being treated with imatinib ages and resistance becomes more common over time. A growing number of second-generation *abl* kinase inhibitors have been developed to treat this looming threat.

Given the lack of durable responses in most ABMT series, it is unlikely that autologous transplant will gain much prominence in the future of this disease unless more effective purging or adoptive immunotherapy is able to be incorporated into autologous regimens.

## REFERENCES

1. Polge C, Smith AU, Parkes AS: Revival of spermatozoa after vitrification and dehydration at low temperatures. *Nature* 1949(164):666, 1991.
2. Lovelock JE, Bishop MWH: Prevention of freezing damage to living cells by dimethylsulphoxide. *Nature* 1959(183):1394–1395, 1959.
3. Gorin NC, Najman A, et al.: Autologous bone-marrow transplantation in acute myelocytic leukaemia. *Lancet* 1(8020):1050, 1977.
4. Fefer A, Cheever MA, et al.: Bone marrow transplantation for refractory acute leukemia in 34 patients with identical twins. *Blood* 57(3):421–430, 1981.
5. Cassileth PA, Harrington DP, et al.: Maintenance chemotherapy prolongs remission duration in adult acute nonlymphocytic leukemia. *J Clin Oncol* 6(4):583-587, 1988.
6. Mayer RJ, Davis RB, et al.: Intensive postremission chemotherapy in adults with acute myeloid leukemia. Cancer and Leukemia Group B. *N Engl J Med* 331(14):896–903, 1995.
7. Willman CL: The prognostic significance of the expression and function of multidrug resistance transporter proteins in acute myeloid leukemia: studies of the Southwest Oncology Group Leukemia Research Program. *Semin Hematol* 34(4 Suppl 5):25–33, 1997.
8. Byrd JC, Weiss RB, et al.: Extramedullary leukemia adversely affects hematologic complete remission rate and overall survival in patients with t(8;21)(q22;q22): results from Cancer and Leukemia Group B 8461. *J Clin Oncol* 15(2):466–475, 1997.
9. Byrd JC, Mrozek K, et al.: Pretreatment cytogenetic abnormalities are predictive of induction success, cumulative incidence of relapse, and overall survival in adult patients with de novo acute myeloid leukemia: results from Cancer and Leukemia Group B (CALGB 8461). *Blood* 100(13):4325–4336, 2002.
10. Kottaridis PD, Gale RE, et al.: Prognostic implications of the presence of FLT3 mutations in patients with acute myeloid leukemia. *Leuk Lymphoma* 44(6):905–913, 2003.
11. Venditti A, Buccisano F, et al.: Level of minimal residual disease after consolidation therapy predicts outcome in acute myeloid leukemia. *Blood* 96(12):3948–3952, 2000.
12. Reiffers J, Labopin M, et al.: Autologous blood cell vs marrow transplantation for acute myeloid leukemia in complete remission: an EBMT retrospective analysis. *Bone Marrow Transplant* 25(11):1115–1119, 2000.
13. Gale RP, Horowitz MM, et al.: Identical-twin bone marrow transplants for leukemia. *Ann Intern Med* 120(8):646–652, 1994.
14. Brenner MK, Rill DR, et al.: Gene-marking to trace origin of relapse after autologous bone-marrow transplantation. *Lancet* 341(8837):85–86, 1993.
15. Kastan MB, Schlaffer E, et al.: Direct demonstration of elevated aldehyde dehydrogenase in human hematopoietic progenitor cells. *Blood* 75(10):1947–1950, 1990.
16. Miller CB, Zehnbauer BA, et al.: Correlation of occult clonogenic leukemia drug sensitivity with relapse after autologous bone marrow transplantation. *Blood* 78(4):1125–1131, 1991.
17. Gorin NC, Labopin M, et al.: Importance of marrow dose on posttransplant outcome in acute leukemia: models derived from patients autografted with mafosfamide-purged marrow at a single institution. *Exp Hematol* 27(12):1822–1830, 1999.
18. Miller CB, Rowlings PA, et al.: The effect of graft purging with 4-hydroperoxycyclophosphamide in autologous bone marrow transplantation for acute myelogenous leukemia. *Exp Hematol* 29(11):1336–1346, 2001.
19. Lemoli RM, Gasparetto C, et al.: Autologous bone marrow transplantation in acute myelogenous leukemia: in vitro treatment with myeloid-specific monoclonal antibodies and drugs in combination. *Blood* 77(8):1829–1836, 1991.
20. Selvaggi KJ, Wilson JW, et al.: Improved outcome for high-risk acute myeloid leukemia patients using autologous bone marrow transplantation and monoclonal antibody-purged bone marrow. *Blood* 83(6):1698–1705, 1994.
21. De Rosa L, Montuoro A, et al.: Progenitor cells purging: negative selection. *Int J Artif Organs* 16(Suppl 5):102–107, 1993.
22. Mehta J, Powles R, et al.: Autologous transplantation with CD52 monoclonal antibody-purged marrow for acute lymphoblastic leukemia: long-term follow-up. *Leuk Lymphoma* 25(5–6):479–486, 1997.
23. Beaujean F, Bernaudin F, et al.: Successful engraftment after autologous transplantation of 10-day cultured bone marrow activated by interleukin 2 in patients with acute lymphoblastic leukemia. *Bone Marrow Transplant* 15(5):691–696, 1995.
24. Balzarotti M, Grisanti S, et al.: Ex vivo manipulation of hematopoietic stem cells for transplantation: the potential role of amifostine. *Semin Oncol* 26(2 Suppl 7):66–71, 1999.
25. Stein AS, O'Donnell MR, et al.: In vivo purging with high-dose cytarabine followed by high-dose chemoradiotherapy and reinfusion of unpurged bone marrow for adult acute myelogenous leukemia in first complete remission. *J Clin Oncol* 14(8):2206–2216, 1996.
26. Linker CA, Ries CA, et al.: Autologous stem cell transplantation for acute myeloid leukemia in first remission. *Biol Blood Marrow Transplant* 6(1):50–57, 2000.
27. Linker CA: Autologous stem cell transplantation for acute myeloid leukemia. *Bone Marrow Transplant* 31(9):731–738, 2003.

28. Wadleigh M, Richardson PG, et al.: Prior gemtuzumab ozogamicin exposure significantly increases the risk of veno-occlusive disease in patients who undergo myeloablative allogeneic stem cell transplantation. *Blood* 102(5):1578–1582, 2003.

29. Zittoun R, Mandelli, F, et al.: EORTC-GIMEMA AML8 protocol. A phase III study on autologous bone-marrow transplantation in acute myelogenous leukemia (AML). *Leuk Lymphoma* 13(Suppl 1):101, 1994.

30. Suciu S, Mandelli F, et al.: Allogeneic compared with autologous stem cell transplantation in the treatment of patients younger than 46 years with acute myeloid leukemia (AML) in first complete remission (CR1): an intention-to-treat analysis of the EORTC/GIMEMAAML-10 trial. *Blood* 102(4):1232–1240, 2003.

31. Harousseau JL, Cahn JY, et al.: Comparison of autologous bone marrow transplantation and intensive chemotherapy as postremission therapy in adult acute myeloid leukemia. The Groupe Ouest Est Leucemies Aigues Myeloblastiques (GOELAM). *Blood* 90(8): 2978–2986, 1997.

32. Burnett AK, Goldstone AH, et al.: Randomised comparison of addition of autologous bone-marrow transplantation to intensive chemotherapy for acute myeloid leukaemia in first remission: results of MRC AML 10 trial. UK Medical Research Council Adult and Children's Leukaemia Working Parties. *Lancet* 351(9104):700–8, 1998.

33. Cassileth PA, Harrington DP, et al.: Chemotherapy compared with autologous or allogeneic bone marrow transplantation in the management of acute myeloid leukemia in first remission. *N Engl J Med* 339(23): 1649–1656, 1998.

34. Cassileth P, Lee S, et al.: Intensified induction chemotherapy in adult acute myeloid leukemia followed by high-dose chemotherapy and autologous peripheral blood stem cell transplantation: an eastern cooperative oncology group trial (E4995). *Leuk Lymphoma* 46(1): 55–61, 2005.

35. Slovak ML, Kopecky KJ, et al.: Karyotypic analysis predicts outcome of preremission and postremission therapy in adult acute myeloid leukemia: a Southwest Oncology Group/Eastern Cooperative Oncology Group Study. *Blood* 96(13):4075–4083, 2000.

36. Grimwade D, Walker H, et al.: The importance of diagnostic cytogenetics on outcome in AML: analysis of 1,612 patients entered into the MRC AML 10 trial. The Medical Research Council Adult and Children's Leukaemia Working Parties. *Blood* 92(7):2322–2333, 1998.

37. Meloni G, Diverio D, et al.: Autologous bone marrow transplantation for acute promyelocytic leukemia in second remission: prognostic relevance of pretransplant minimal residual disease assessment by reverse-transcription polymerase chain reaction of the PML/RAR alpha fusion gene. *Blood* 90(3):1321–1325, 1997.

38. de Botton S, Fawaz A, et al.: Autologous and allogeneic stem-cell transplantation as salvage treatment of acute promyelocytic leukemia initially treated with all-trans-retinoic acid: a retrospective analysis of the European acute promyelocytic leukemia group. *J Clin Oncol* 23(1):120–126, 2003.

39. Watson M, Wheatley K, et al.: Severe adverse impact on sexual functioning and fertility of bone marrow transplantation, either allogeneic or autologous, compared with consolidation chemotherapy alone: analysis of the MRC AML 10 trial. *Cancer* 86(7):1231–1239, 1999.

40. Hoelzer D: Prognostic factors in acute lymphoblastic leukemia. *Leukemia* 6(Suppl 4):49–51, 1992.

41. Martin H, Atta J, et al.: Purging of peripheral blood stem cells yields BCR-ABL-negative autografts in patients with BCR-ABL-positive acute lymphoblastic leukemia. *Exp Hematol* 23(14):1612–1618, 1995.

42. Uckun FM, Kersey JH, et al.: Autologous bone marrow transplantation in high-risk remission T-lineage acute lymphoblastic leukemia using immunotoxins plus 4-hydroperoxycyclophosphamide for marrow purging. *Blood* 76(9):1723–1733, 1990.

43. Thomas DA, Faderl S, Cortes J, et al.: Update of the hyper-CVAD and imatinib mesylate regimen in Philadelphia (Ph) positive acute lymphocytic leukemia. *Blood*, 104(abstract):11, 2004.

44. Ottman OG, Wassmann B, Pfeifer H, et al.: Imatinib given concurrently with induction chemotherapy is superior to imatinib subsequent to induction and consolidation in newly diagnosed Philadelphia-positive acute lymphoblastic leukemia *Blood*, 104(abstract):11, 2004

45. Jandula BM., Nomdedeu J, et al.: Rituximab can be useful as treatment for minimal residual disease in bcr-abl-positive acute lymphoblastic leukemia. *Bone Marrow Transplant* 27(2):225–227, 2001.

46. Corbacioglu S, Eber S, et al.: Induction of long-term remission of a relapsed childhood B-acute lymphoblastic leukemia with rituximab chimeric anti-CD20 monoclonal antibody and autologous stem cell transplantation. *J Pediatr Hematol Oncol* 25(4):327–329, 2003.

47. Thomas X, Boiron JM, et al.: Outcome of treatment in adults with acute lymphoblastic leukemia: analysis of the LALA-94 trial. *J Clin Oncol* 22(20):4075–4086, 2004.

48. Thiebaut A, Vernant JP, et al.: Adult acute lymphocytic leukemia study testing chemotherapy and autologous and allogeneic transplantation. A follow-up report of the French protocol LALA 87. *Hematol Oncol Clin North Am* 14(6):1353–1366, 2000.

49. Goldstone et al.: The outcome of 551 1st CR transplants in adult ALL from the UKALL XII/ECOG 2993 Study. *Blood*, 104(abstract):11, 2004.

50. Reiffers J, Trouette R, et al.: Autologous blood stem cell transplantation for chronic granulocytic leukaemia in transformation: a report of 47 cases. *Br J Haematol* 77(3):339–345, 1991.

51. Degliantoni G, Mangoni L, et al.: In vitro restoration of polyclonal hematopoiesis in a chronic myelogenous leukemia after in vitro treatment with 4-hydroperoxycyclophosphamide. *Blood* 65(3):753–757, 1985.

52. Carlo-Stella C, Mangoni L, et al.: Autologous transplant for chronic myelogenous leukemia using marrow treated ex vivo with mafosfamide. *Bone Marrow Transplant* 14(3):425–32, 1994.

53. McGlave PB, Arthur D, et al.: Autologous transplantation for CML using marrow treated ex vivo with recombinant human interferon gamma. *Bone Marrow Transplant* 6(2):115–120, 1990.

54. Gladstone DE, Bedi A, et al.: Philadelphia chromosome-negative engraftment after autologous transplantation with granulocyte-macrophage colony-stimulating factor for chronic myeloid leukemia. *Biol Blood Marrow Transplant* 5(6):394–399, 1999.

55. Luger SM, O'Brien SG, et al.: Oligodeoxynucleotide-mediated inhibition of c-myb gene expression in autografted bone marrow: a pilot study. *Blood* 99(4): 1150–1158, 2002.

56. Fischer T, Reifenrath C, et al.: Safety and efficacy of STI-571 (imatinib mesylate) in patients with bcr/abl-positive chronic myelogenous leukemia (CML) after autologous peripheral blood stem cell transplantation (PBSCT). *Leukemia* 16(7):1220–1228, 2002.

57. Kreuzer KA, Kluhs C, et al.: Filgrastim-induced stem cell mobilization in chronic myeloid leukaemia patients during imatinib therapy: safety, feasibility and evidence for an efficient in vivo purging. *Br J Haematol* 124(2): 195–199, 2004.

58. Kantarjian HM, Cortes J, et al.: Imatinib mesylate (STI571) therapy for Philadelphia chromosome-positive chronic myelogenous leukemia in blast phase. *Blood* 99(10):3547–3553, 2002.

59. Hui CH, Goh KY, et al.: Successful peripheral blood stem cell mobilisation with filgrastim in patients with chronic myeloid leukaemia achieving complete cytogenetic response with imatinib, without increasing disease burden as measured by quantitative real-time PCR. *Leukemia* 17(5):821–828, 2003.

60. Hughes TP, Kaeda J, et al.: Frequency of major molecular responses to imatinib or interferon alfa plus cytarabine in newly diagnosed chronic myeloid leukemia. *N Engl J Med* 349(15):1423–1432, 2003.

# Chapter **36**

# ALLOGENEIC HEMATOPOIETIC STEM CELL TRANSPLANTATION FOR THE ACUTE LEUKEMIAS IN ADULTS

*Corey Cutler and Joseph H. Antin*

## INTRODUCTION

Acute lymphoblastic leukemia (ALL) is an uncommon malignancy in adults, with an incidence rate of 0.3–0.8 cases/$10^5$ individuals between the ages of 20 and 50. In comparison, acute myeloid leukemia (AML) occurs in 1.2–2.4/$10^5$ individuals between the ages of 20 and 50.[1] Nevertheless, AML and ALL represent the two most common indications for allogeneic stem cell transplantation worldwide, as reported to the International Bone Marrow Transplant Registry in 2002, accounting for over 7000 reported transplants worldwide.[2]

Modest advances in the therapy for ALL and AML have been made in the last decade; but despite these advances, long-term outcomes for these diseases, particularly in adults, remain poor, as less than half of these patients achieve a durable remission.[3,4] This chapter discusses the established and emerging role of allogeneic stem cell transplantation as therapy for the acute leukemias.

## ALLOGENEIC STEM CELL TRANSPLANTATION FOR ALL

### TRANSPLANTATION IN FIRST COMPLETE REMISSION

ALL has a relatively poor prognosis in adults with long-term survival in only 30–40% of newly diagnosed individuals.[5] Traditional risk factors defining "high-risk" disease include advanced age, very elevated WBC at presentation, immunophenotype (Pro-B cell ALL), the presence of adverse cytogenetic changes (i.e., t(9:22) and t(4:11)), and a delay in the time to achieve a first remission.[5] Newer prognostic factors include the presence of minimal residual disease detected by sensitive molecular techniques and gene-expression profile

hierarchical clustering and expression analysis.[4] As outcome in high-risk disease is significantly worse than for standard risk disease (most notably for adverse cytogenetic changes), many analyses on cohorts of high-risk patients transplanted in first remission have been performed.

Single center data on transplantation for ALL are extremely heterogeneous. One report of an experience treating 39 adults with high-risk features in first remission, with a uniform conditioning regimen of total body irradiation and etoposide, yielded a relapse rate of only 15%, with an event-free survival of 64% at 10 years.[6] However, a review of 99 patients from six trials, all with Ph+ ALL transplanted in first remission using fully matched, sibling or unrelated donors demonstrated disease-free survival of 0–86%.[7] Numerous other single-arm studies have reported similarly heterogeneous outcomes.[8]

True randomized evidence supporting the role of allogeneic transplantation for ALL in first complete remission is lacking. An attempt to address this question has been addressed with studies of biologic assignment, where patients with histocompatible donors are assigned to allogeneic transplantation, while those patients without suitable donors are randomized to autologous transplantation or conventional chemotherapy. Table 36.1 summarizes the results from the published comparative trials. The GOELAM used a biologic assignment strategy and assigned allogeneic transplantation or consolidative chemotherapy followed by autologous transplantation to 156 patients younger than 50 years, all with high-risk ALL. Transplant-related mortality was only 15% and at 6 years, disease-free survival was greater in the allogeneic transplant arm (75 vs 46%, *p* = 0.0027; Figure 36.1).[10] The LALA group used a similar strategy and assigned allogeneic transplant to Ph+ patients with a sibling donor and compared outcomes

**Table 36.1** Trials of biologic randomization in ALL, since 1990

| Trial, (year of publication) | Entry criteria and methodology | Comparison | N | Survival | | Relapse | Survival by risk | Comments |
|---|---|---|---|---|---|---|---|---|
| EORTC ALL-3, (2004)[9] | Age 15–50<br>Standard and high –risk<br>Ph-<br>Biologic randomization<br>2nd randomization for no donor group | AlloBMT vs<br>AutoBMT +<br>chemotherapy | 68<br><br>116 | 6 yr DFS<br>38.2%<br>36.8%<br>p = 0.69 | OS<br>41.2%<br>38.8%<br>p = 0.95 | 38.2%<br>56.3%<br>p = 0.01 | No differences when stratified by risk | Only 69% of AlloBMT group underwent transplantation.<br>AutoBMT and chemotherapy arms analyzed together |
| GOELAL02, (2004)[10] | Age 15–50<br>High -risk<br>Biologic randomization | AlloBMT vs<br>AutoSCT | 41<br>115 | 6 yr DFS<br>75%<br>33%<br>p = 0.0027<br>p < 0.001 | OS<br>75%<br>40% | 12%<br>56%<br>p = 0.0001 | | 9 patients aged 50–59 assigned AutoBMT not included in these data.<br>2nd randomization after AutoBMT to Interferon. |
| Gupta et al. (2004)[11] | Age 16–54<br>Standard and high risk<br>Retrospective review of Biologic randomization | AlloBMT vs<br>chemotherapy | 48<br>39 | 3 yr DFS<br>37%<br>44%<br>p = NS | OS<br>43%<br>60%<br>p = NS | 40%<br>61%<br>p = 0.007 | High risk<br>34 vs. 17%, p = NS<br>(includes Ph+ patients)<br>Standard risk<br>54 vs. 64%, p = NS | Patients not enrolled prospectively<br>Ph+ patients were offered URD transplantation and are not included in this analysis |
| LALA 94, (2002)[12] | Age 15–55<br>Ph+ only<br>Biologic randomization with physician preference | AlloBMT vs URD<br>AlloBMT +<br>AutoPBSCT | 46<br>14<br>43 | 3 yr OS<br>37%<br>12%<br>p = 0.02 | | 50%<br>90%<br>p < 0.01 | | Physician preference influenced whether URD search was performed for patients without sibling donors.<br>Survival predicted by minimal residual disease after intensification chemotherapy. |
| MRC UKALL, XII/ECOG E2993 (2001)[13] | Age 14–60<br>Ph– reported<br>Biologic randomization<br>2nd randomization for no donor group | AlloBMT vs<br>AutoBMT +<br>chemotherapy | 170<br>264 | 5 yr DFS<br>54%<br>34%<br>p = 0.04 | | 23%<br>61%<br>p = 0.001 | High risk<br>44 vs. 26%, p = 0.3<br>Standard risk<br>66 vs. 45%, p = .06 | Abstract publication to date |

| Trial, (year of publication) | Entry criteria and methodology | Comparison | N | Survival | Relapse | Survival by risk | Comments |
|---|---|---|---|---|---|---|---|
| LALA 87, (2000)[14-16] | Age 15–40<br>Standard and high risk<br>Biologic randomization | AlloBMT vs chemotherapy | 116<br>141 | 10 yr OS<br>46%<br>31%<br>p = 0.04 | | High risk<br>44 vs 11%, p = 0.009<br>Standard risk<br>49 vs. 43%, p = NS | Induction chemotherapy less intense than current regimens |
| Suzuki et al. (1997)[17] | Age 15–44<br>Biologic randomization | AlloBMT vs chemotherapy | 13<br>16 | 10 yr DFS<br>52%<br>30%<br>p = NS | | | |
| Attal et al. (1995)[18] | Age 15–55<br>Biologic randomization<br>2nd randomization for no donor group | AlloBMT vs AutoBMT | 43<br>77 | 3 yr DFS<br>68%<br>26%<br>p < 0.001 | 12%<br>62% | | Second randomization to IL-2 after AutoBMT only, which did not alter results |
| Blaise et al. (1990)[19] | Age >15<br>High risk only<br>Comparative cohort analysis, Biologic assignment | AlloBMT vs AutoBMT | 25<br>22 | 3 yr DFS<br>71%<br>40%<br>p = NS    OS<br>71%<br>62%<br>p = NS | 9%<br>57%<br>p < 0.01 | | Purged autologous grafts given and T cell depletion used in some AlloBMT patients |

a

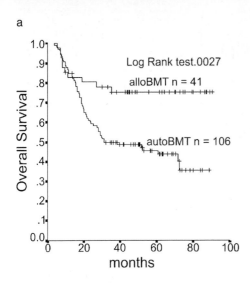

b

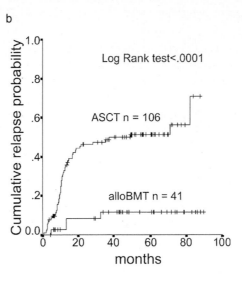

**Figure 36.1** *(a) Overall survival and (b) Relapse from the GOELAL02 trial*

with a group that received autologous and unrelated donor transplantation. Overall survival was 37% in the transplant arm in comparison with 12% in the chemotherapy cohort.[12] The prior LALA randomized trial also demonstrated an advantage to transplant in first remission among high-risk patients.[14] Preliminary results from the MRC UKALL/ECOG co-operative study suggest that even for standard risk ALL, allogeneic transplant in first remission may be beneficial (54 vs 34% 5 year OS, $p = 0.04$).[13] In contrast, recent studies published by the EORTC[9] and Gupta et al.,[11] demonstrated that transplantation in first remission did not increase survival in either high-risk or standard risk cohorts. Interestingly, all of the trials found similar outcomes in patients receiving autologous SCT and chemotherapy, suggesting that autologous transplantation does not improve survival in ALL.

All of the biologic assignment studies have agreed that the relapse rate after allogeneic transplantation is lower than after autologous transplantation or consolidative chemotherapy. However, transplant-related morbidity and mortality offsets survival gains through reduction in relapse rates. Nonetheless, the results of these large studies have made allogeneic transplantation from an HLA-matched sibling the therapy of choice for patients with high-risk ALL in first remission.

There has been reluctance to offer unrelated donor stem cell transplantation in first remission, even to patients with high-risk ALL, because of anticipated higher rates of treatment-related mortality when unrelated donors are used. However, with high resolution HLA typing and improvements in immunosuppression and antibiotic management, morbidity and mortality after unrelated transplantation for ALL is not greatly increased in comparison with related donor transplantation. Therefore there is now interest in offering unrelated donor transplantation in first remission to patients without suitable related donors in whom transplant is indicated. A retrospective review conducted through the National Marrow Donor Program evaluated matched, or

single-antigen mismatched, unrelated transplantation for high-risk ALL in first remission.[20] In this study, overall survival at 4 years was 32%, which is similar to the sibling transplantation results reported above. In another retrospective study comparing outcomes for patients in first remission and beyond who underwent transplantation, no difference in outcome for patients receiving related and unrelated donor transplants was noted (42 vs 45% 5 year DFS).[21] Similarly, a retrospective cohort analysis suggested that outcomes after matched, unrelated transplant in first remission were similar to, or better than, outcomes after autologous transplantation (51 vs 44% 3 year OS).[22]

For patients with standard risk leukemia, the biologic assignment studies do not conclusively support routine transplantation at this time, although the results of the MRC UKALL/ECOG study are promising. While biologic assignment and intention-to-treat analysis are the most appropriate methodology for policy development on the issue of the role of transplant in first remission,[23] for the individual patient, the results of these studies may be inappropriate to help guide therapy. Reported very rarely, as-treated analyses are more helpful in the situation in deciding on the role of transplantation, once a remission has been attained, a suitable donor is identified, and the patient is deemed to be a suitable transplant candidate. Two other factors need to be considered for patients with standard risk ALL. With the widespread use of intensive and continuous chemotherapy regimens as primary therapy for ALL, it is possible that the achievement of second remission after relapse will become less likely, as tumors may develop resistance to chemotherapy. This may actually worsen outcomes for transplantation for relapsed disease[24] and make a strategy of salvage transplant for relapsed disease less likely to be successful. Second, the morbidity and mortality after transplantation while in remission continues to decline. Taken together, a strategy to maximize long-term survival among standard-risk ALL patients may include allogeneic transplantation from an HLA-identical sibling in first remission.

## TRANSPLANTATION FOR ADVANCED ALL

Allogeneic transplantation is the therapy of choice in relapsed ALL, as durable remissions with chemotherapy alone are rare in adults. Transplantation in untreated first relapse and second remission yield roughly equivalent results; however, long-term remission rates are significantly lower when compared to transplantation in first remission. In a retrospective analysis of 182 adults will ALL, 5 year overall survival after transplantation in second or greater remission ($n = 46$) and relapse ($n = 95$) were 23% and 9%, respectively, in comparison with 43% for patients transplanted in first remission.[25] In a retrospective review of 147 patients transplanted for advanced ALL (the majority with matched, related donors), overall survival was less than 10% among 79 patients with a pre-B phenotype.[26]

Only a minority of patients with advanced ALL will have suitable matched, related donors. Since the outcome of relapsed or refractory ALL is so poor with chemotherapy alone, unrelated or alternative donor transplantation is warranted in this setting. In a study of 63 patients in second or greater remission or with refractory ALL, overall survival was 17% for patients in remission and 5% for patients with refractory disease;[20] however, survival for patients in second remission was greater (36% at 5 years) in another study facilitated by the NMDP that included patients of all risk types transplanted in second remission.[27] In this study, unrelated transplantation was not statistically better than autologous transplantation in second remission (36 vs 27%, $p = 0.11$), but a Cox multivariable regression analysis demonstrated an improvement in long-term survival in patients receiving allogeneic transplantation who survived 6 months after transplantation. Again, lower relapse rates after allogeneic transplantation were offset by the mortality of the transplant procedure itself. In a matched-pair analysis of matched, unrelated donor transplantation in comparison with autologous transplantation, the EBMT demonstrated similar survival outcomes (39 vs 31%, $p = 0.19$).[28]

In summary, transplantation for advanced ALL should be performed whenever feasible. Despite trends toward improved outcomes with unrelated donor transplantation over autologous transplantation, no single comparative trial has demonstrated convincing evidence of superiority. Since outcomes after unrelated allogeneic transplantation have been improving as HLA matching techniques improve, it is likely that allogeneic transplantation, rather than autologous transplantation, will become the strategy of choice to reduce relapse with advanced disease.

## ALLOGENEIC TRANSPLANTATION IN COMBINATION WITH IMATINIB

Imatinib mesylate (formerly known as STI-571, Gleevec,™ Novartis AG) is a potent, reversible inhibitor of bcr/abl tyrosine kinase activity.[29] When added to induction chemotherapy, this drug has been shown to increase remission rates among Ph+ ALL patients.[30,31] Similarly, this drug may be effective for relapsed Ph+ ALL.[32] By increasing remission rates among newly diagnosed Ph+ ALL patients, the long-term success of allogeneic transplantation may be improved, as disease status at the time of transplantation is a powerful predictor of long-term survival.[25] Furthermore, imatinib use may increase the window of opportunity for patients with newly diagnosed or relapsed disease to find suitable allogeneic donors by prolonging remission time. Imatinib has been given to newly diagnosed, refractory or relapsed patients prior to allogeneic transplantation.[33–36] At this time, all that can be concluded from this experience is that imatinib therapy prior to transplantation does not impair engraftment of transplanted hematopoietic progenitor cells.[33] Since the number of patients reported at this time is limited, estimates of the long-term impact of imatinib use prior to transplantation are difficult to predict. Whether empiric imatinib after transplantation will be effective as a preventative strategy against relapse is also unpredictable.

## NONMYELOABLATIVE TRANSPLANTATION

Transplantation with nonmyeloablative or reduced-intensity conditioning regimens eliminates much of the morbidity and mortality associated with high-dose transplantation.[37,38] As such, this approach has been used widely in older individuals, in individuals with comorbid illnesses, and in those who have undergone prior high-dose therapy approaches. Without high-dose chemoradiotherapy, this approach to transplantation relies exclusively on the development of a potent graft-versus-leukemia (GVL) reaction. While GVL reactions are prominent in some hematologic malignancies, they may be less pronounced in aggressive lymphoid malignancies, such as ALL. However, after ablative transplantation, the presence of GVHD has been shown to be protective against relapse, invoking the power of a potent GVL response.[26,39–41]

No single study has prospectively accrued sufficient subjects to make reliable conclusions on the role of nonmyeloablative transplant for ALL; however, investigators from four large trials[42–46] have pooled their results and reported outcomes on 27 patients.[47] The median age of the patients was 50 years, and most had advanced disease (only four were in first remission while 12 were chemorefractory or in relapse at the time of transplant) or adverse cytogenetic features (Philadelphia chromosome in 11). In this study, multiple conditioning regimens, GVHD prophylaxis regimens, stem cell donor types, and stem cell sources were used. Despite this, donor-derived hematopoiesis occurred in all patients, with a 63% incidence of Grade II–IV acute GVHD and a 72% rate of chronic GVHD among evaluable patients. Treatment-related mortality was 23%. Eight of 27 patients are alive without disease at a median of

816 days from transplantation (range 381–1375 days), which is considered a promising result, given the otherwise poor prognosis of these patients without transplantation. In this study, a correlation between the incidence of acute GVHD and protection from relapse was noted (hazard rate for relapse prevention 3.3, $p = 0.05$), invoking an active GVL reaction.

A more uniform cohort of 22 high-risk ALL patients enrolled in a multicenter German trial has been reported.[48] The majority of these patients received a fludarabine-busulfan conditioning regimen followed by an infusion of peripheral blood stem cells (PBSC) from matched related (13), unrelated (8), and mismatched related (1) donors. Despite similar rates of acute GVHD as reported in the pooled analysis, the overall survival in this cohort was 18% at a median follow-up of 16.5 months for survivors (range 5–30 months). In summary, at the present time, there remains insufficient data to routinely recommend nonmyeloablative transplant outside of a clinical trial.

### OTHER ISSUES IN TRANSPLANTATION FOR ALL
#### Stem cell source and preparative regimen
There is no preparative regimen that yields superior results when used prior to transplant for ALL. Many centers employ regimens that include etoposide; however, this agent has not been shown to improve transplant outcomes among adults. The IBMTR has analyzed the outcomes in 298 patients who received HLA-matched sibling transplants for ALL in first or second remission. Long-term survival was superior in patients who received ≥ 13 Gy of TBI, but no differences were noted when cyclophosphamide and etoposide use were compared.[49] Regarding stem cell source, no randomized trial has directly compared PBSC with bone marrow for ALL transplantation because of the rarity of this disease and large sample size that a clinical trial would need to demonstrate differences. While superior disease-free survival has been demonstrated with PBSC transplantation over stem cell transplantation using HLA-identical sibling donors, particularly with advanced malignancies, subgroup analyses in ALL are too small to demonstrate differences.[50] A single retrospective analysis of 102 ALL patients who received an unrelated stem cell transplant demonstrated inferior survival among PBSC patients despite no differences in grade II–IV acute GVHD or chronic GVHD incidence.[51] In this study, PBSC patients were less likely to receive TBI as conditioning ($p = 0.06$), which may have influenced outcome.[49] Although used infrequently, umbilical cord transplantation has been attempted in adults with advanced ALL. The advantage of cord blood transplantation is the rapid access to stem cells and the potential for less GVHD than with other unrelated stem cell products. Too few transplants for ALL have been performed to make conclusive comments on the role of cord blood transplanta-

tion; however, the relative lack of GVHD could be associated with a high risk of relapse.

#### Therapy of relapse: DLI and imatinib
ALL in relapse after transplantation is rarely salvaged by donor lymphocyte infusion. This observation is consistent but confusing, since there does appear to be a measurable GVL response in primary transplantation. Less than 20% of patients will achieve a remission to DLI alone[52,53]; however, this number may be increased with concomitant chemotherapy. Despite this, remissions are rarely durable. Imatinib has been used as therapy for relapse after transplantation of ALL[54]; however, the majority of the reported experience in relapsed Ph+ malignancies is in chronic myeloid leukemia (CML)[55,56] or the lymphoblastic phase of CML.[57,58] The combination of imatinib and DLI may prove to an important therapeutic modality for relapsed ALL. Attempts at second transplantation have been made with reasonable success, with long-term survival in up to 30% of patients.[59]

## ALLOGENEIC STEM CELL TRANSPLANTATION FOR AML

### TRANSPLANTATION IN FIRST COMPLETE REMISSION
There have been at least 12 prospective trials that have used a biologic randomization strategy to assign allogeneic stem cell transplant or consolidative chemotherapy (with or without autologous stem cell transplantation) for patients with AML in first remission (Table 36.2). Several recurring themes have emerged as a result of this vast experience involving over 3600 patients. First, it is clear that a profound GVL effect exists, as relapse rates after allogeneic transplantation are uniformly lower after allogeneic transplant in comparison with nonallogeneic postremission strategies. Second, allogeneic transplantation continues to be a risky medical procedure, as mortality while in remission is markedly higher in the allogeneic transplant arms of the prospective trials. Third, the risks of reduced relapse rates but higher treatment-related mortality have led to modest gains in disease-free and overall survival in the more recent comparative trials of allogeneic stem cell transplantation.

The decision to undertake allogeneic stem cell transplantation while in first complete remission is usually based on risk stratification according to cytogenetics.[74] The greatest controversy on the role of transplantation for AML in first complete remission has focused on the group of patients with intermediate risk cytogenetics, where long-term remissions without transplantation occur in less than 40% of affected individuals. The EORTC/GIMEMA AML-10 trial compared 293 patients with AML in first remission with an HLA-identical sibling to 441 patients in whom a suitable HLA-matched family member donor was not available.[62] Subjects

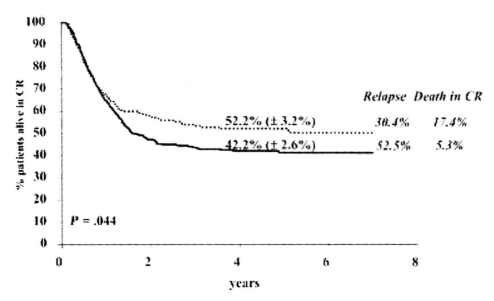

**Figure 36.2** *Disease-free survival from ORTC/GIMEMA AML-10 trial*

without a suitable stem cell donor were assigned to autologous stem cell transplantation, although only 56% of these subjects underwent the procedure. Up to 40% of the patients in both arms had no cytogenetic information available, but approximately 35% of the remaining patients were classified as having intermediate risk cytogenetics. Overall, the 4 year disease-free survival in the transplant group, in an intent-to-treat fashion, was superior to the nontransplant group (52.2 vs 42.2%, $p$ = 0.044; Figure 36.2); however, in subgroup analysis, the intermediate risk group alone did not show a trend toward improved survival. The favorable differences in outcome were more prominent in the younger age groups, suggesting that the combination of a relative decrease in treatment-related mortality associated with young age and the gains in relapse prevention was sufficient to generate a clinical benefit. The prior EORTC/GIMEMA AML 8A trial was unable to demonstrate a difference between allogeneic and autologous transplantation strategies, although in this trial, both forms of transplantation were superior to chemotherapy alone as postremission consolidation therapy.[66]

The MRC AML 10 trial compared the outcomes of 419 patients in remission and assigned to allogeneic transplant on the basis of an available HLA-identical sibling with 868 patients with no sibling donor, all of whom were assigned autologous transplantation.[64] Disease-free survival was prolonged in the transplantation group in comparison with the nontransplant cohort (50 vs 42% at 7 years, $p$ = 0.001; Figure 36.3). Overall survival was marginally, but not statistically, better (56 vs 50%, $p$ = 0.1). Although this trial was designed to decide whether allogeneic transplantation was superior to autologous transplantation, only 23% of the no-donor arm actually underwent autologous transplantation, making the interpretation of these results questionable. Nonetheless, in the intermediate-risk subgroup, allogeneic transplantation was associated with an improvement in disease-free survival (50 vs 39%, $p$ = 0.004; Figure 36.3) and overall survival (54 vs 44%, $p$ = 0.02).[64]

For patients with intermediate cytogenetic risk AML in first complete remission, consolidation with allogeneic transplantation is superior antileukemic therapy in comparison with chemotherapy or autologous transplantation. While no trial has focused uniquely on patients with intermediate risk cytogenetics, this group represented the majority of patients studied in most of the trials, and as such, the best estimate of the effect in this majority subgroup is the overall effect of the trial, as long as significant heterogeneity among the subgroups is absent.[75] The three largest trials demonstrated a reduction in relapse rates after allogeneic transplant of 21–26% and an absolute improvement in disease-free or overall survival of 8–13%.[62,64,66,67] Many other trials have been performed that addressed this question (Table 36.2), and three additional small trials have been able to demonstrate the statistical superiority of allogeneic transplantation over consolidation chemotherapy or autologous transplantation,[70,72,73] while the other trials were too small and underpowered to demonstrate differences,[60,63,71] or no differences were noted.[68,69]

The favorable cytogenetic changes in AML (t(8;21), t(15;17), inv(16), t(16;16), and del(16q)) comprise a distinct minority of favorable-outcome adult AML cases. Only a few trials have accrued sufficient numbers of favorable-risk subjects to properly examine the role of transplantation for AML with favorable cytogenetics. The SWOG/ECOG Intergroup trial included 121 patients with favorable cytogenetics, 84% of whom achieved a complete remission to induction chemotherapy and were subsequently assigned to allogeneic stem cell transplant if an HLA-identical sibling was available ($n$ = 19) or randomized to autologous transplantation ($n$ = 26) or chemotherapy ($n$ = 22).[68,76] Thirty one additional patients were

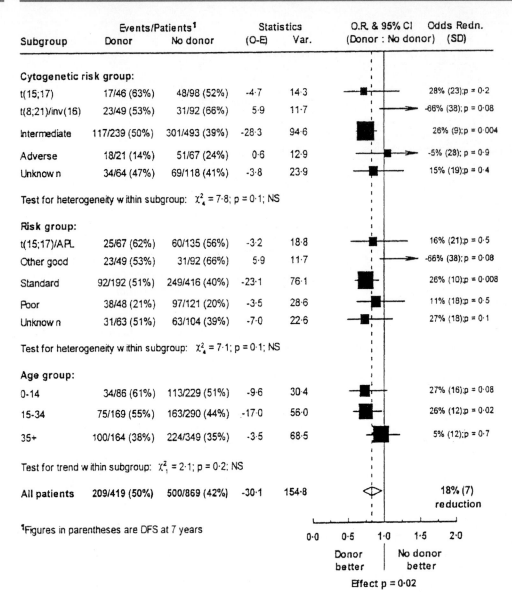

| Subgroup | Events/Patients[1] Donor | No donor | Statistics (O-E) | Var. | O.R. & 95% CI (Donor : No donor) | Odds Redn. (SD) |
|---|---|---|---|---|---|---|
| **Cytogenetic risk group:** | | | | | | |
| t(15;17) | 17/46 (63%) | 48/98 (52%) | -4.7 | 14.3 | | 28% (23);p = 0.2 |
| t(8;21)/inv(16) | 23/49 (53%) | 31/92 (66%) | 5.9 | 11.7 | | -66% (38);p = 0.08 |
| Intermediate | 117/239 (50%) | 301/493 (39%) | -28.3 | 94.6 | | 26% (9);p = 0.004 |
| Adverse | 18/21 (14%) | 51/67 (24%) | 0.6 | 12.9 | | -5% (28); p = 0.9 |
| Unknown | 34/64 (47%) | 69/118 (41%) | -3.8 | 23.9 | | 15% (19);p = 0.4 |

Test for heterogeneity within subgroup: $\chi^2_4 = 7.8$; p = 0.1; NS

| Subgroup | Events/Patients Donor | No donor | Statistics (O-E) | Var. | | Odds Redn. (SD) |
|---|---|---|---|---|---|---|
| **Risk group:** | | | | | | |
| t(15;17)/APL | 25/67 (62%) | 60/135 (56%) | -3.2 | 18.8 | | 16% (21);p = 0.5 |
| Other good | 23/49 (53%) | 31/92 (66%) | 5.9 | 11.7 | | -66% (38);p = 0.08 |
| Standard | 92/192 (51%) | 249/416 (40%) | -23.1 | 76.1 | | 26% (10);p = 0.008 |
| Poor | 38/48 (21%) | 97/121 (20%) | -3.5 | 28.6 | | 11% (18);p = 0.5 |
| Unknown | 31/63 (51%) | 63/104 (39%) | -7.0 | 22.6 | | 27% (18);p = 0.1 |

Test for heterogeneity within subgroup: $\chi^2_4 = 7.1$; p = 0.1; NS

| Subgroup | Events/Patients Donor | No donor | Statistics (O-E) | Var. | | Odds Redn. (SD) |
|---|---|---|---|---|---|---|
| **Age group:** | | | | | | |
| 0-14 | 34/86 (61%) | 113/229 (51%) | -9.6 | 30.4 | | 27% (16);p = 0.08 |
| 15-34 | 75/169 (55%) | 163/290 (44%) | -17.0 | 56.0 | | 26% (12);p = 0.02 |
| 35+ | 100/164 (38%) | 224/349 (35%) | -3.5 | 68.5 | | 5% (12);p = 0.7 |

Test for trend within subgroup: $\chi^2_1 = 2.1$; p = 0.2; NS

| | | | | | | |
|---|---|---|---|---|---|---|
| **All patients** | 209/419 (50%) | 500/869 (42%) | -30.1 | 154.8 | | 18% (7) reduction |

[1]Figures in parentheses are DFS at 7 years

0.0    0.5    1.0    1.5    2.0

Donor better | No donor better

Effect p = 0.02

**Figure 36.3** *Disease-free survival from the MRC AML-10 subgroup analyses*

not treated on study. The outcome of allogeneic transplantation and autologous transplantation (5 year OS 63% and 71%, respectively) was superior to the result for chemotherapy alone (5 year OS 35%), which is significantly lower than in other reported series of favorable risk AML.[74,77,78] The EORTC/GIMEMA trial, which studied 123 patients with favorable risk cytogenetic profiles did not demonstrate a difference in outcomes among patients (68.1 vs 73.9% 4 year DFS)[62] although patients with favorable cytogenetic changes benefited most from transplantation.[76] Nonetheless, consolidative chemotherapy remains the most commonly applied consolidation strategy for favorable-risk patients.

Patients with unfavorable cytogenetics have a very poor prognosis, despite similar rates of remission after induction chemotherapy compared with other AML cytogenetic risk groups. For this reason, transplantation in first remission is widely accepted as standard therapy, wherever a suitable donor is identified. The biologic assignment studies have confirmed that allogeneic transplantation is a superior therapy in comparison with consolidative chemotherapy or autologous transplantation. The EORTC/GIMEMA trial even suggested that with an increasingly unfavorable prognosis prior to transplantation, the greater the benefits that can be achieved with transplant therapy.[62] The prognosis of unfavorable cytogenetic risk AML is poor enough that unrelated allogeneic stem cell transplantation is generally undertaken in first remission, when a suitable HLA-matched sibling donor is unavailable. Since matched, related transplantation is not yet the accepted standard for either intermediate or favorable cytogenetic risk AML in first remission, unrelated donor transplantation cannot be routinely recommended.

### TRANSPLANTATION FOR ADVANCED AML

Once relapsed, AML carries a poor prognosis, with very few long-term remissions induced by chemotherapy

## Table 36.2 Trials of biologic assignment in AML, since 1990

| Trial (year of publication) | Entry criteria and methodology | Comparison | N | Survival | Relapse | Survival by risk | Comments |
|---|---|---|---|---|---|---|---|
| CETLAM (2004)[60] | Age ≤50 Intermediate, adverse cytogenetics Biologic randomization | AlloSCT vs AutoSCT | 28 36 | 4 yr OS 48% 60% $p$ = NS | | | Uniform induction, consolidation chemeotherapy regimen PBSC and BM used, T depleted in majority Multiple GVHD regimens As treated analyses presented |
| Heil et al. (2004)[61] | Age <60 Adverse cytogenetics Biologic randomization | AlloPBSCT vs AutoPBSCT | 25 20 | 5 yr DFS 37% 45% $p$ = NS | | | Intermediate cytogenetic risk patients also included, but outcomes comparing transplant strategies are not reported As treated analysis, nonactuarial statistics |
| EORTC/GIMEMA AML-10 (2003)[62] | Age 15–45 All cytogenetic risk groups Biologic randomization | AlloSCT vs AutoSCT | 293 441 | 4 yr DFS 52.2% 42.2% $p$ = 0.044 | 30.4% 52.5% $p$ < 0.001 | 4 yr OS Favorable: 68.1 vs 73.9% Intermediate: 53.4 vs 54.3% Adverse (pooled) 50.2 vs 29.4% | Unknown cytogenetics unknown in ~40% Only 56% of AutoSCT group and 69% of AlloSCT group underwent transplant after achieving CR Age was predictor of disease-free outcome at 4 years: Age 15–25: 64.0 vs 50.8%, Hazard : 0.65 (0.41–1.04), 26–35: 61.9 vs 49.6% 0.69 (0.46–1.02) 36–45: 53.4 vs 51.6% 0.97 (0.7–1.33) Cox model suggests: Worse prognosis associated with most gain from AlloSCT |
| Hellenic Cooperative Group (2003)[63] | Age <50 All cytogenetic groups Biologic randomization 2nd randomization of no donor group. | AlloSCT vs AutoPBSCT vs chemotherapy | 15 19 15 | 3 yr OS 73% 58 46 $p$ = 0.41 | | | As-treated analysis Favorable risk cytogenetics with no sibling assigned chemo. Chemotherapy group received only 2 cycles of HiDAC Intermediate risk alloSCT group significantly younger than autoPBSCT or chemotherapy group |
| MRC AML 10 (2002)[64,65] | Age ≤55 All cytogenetic groups Biologic randomization | AlloBMT vs AutoBMT | 419 868 | 7 yr DFS OS 50% 56% 42% 50% $p$ = 0.001 $p$ = 0.1 | 36 52% $p$ < 0.001 | 7 yr OS Favorable 63 vs 77% Intermediate 56 vs 45% ($p$ <0.05) Adverse 21 vs 24% | Patient accrual between 1985 and 1995 Cytogenetics unknown in 13% Only 61% of AlloBMT group and 23% of AutoBMT underwent transplant Intermediate risk patients benefited from AlloBMT |
| EORTC/GIMEMA 8A (1998)[66,67] | Age 10–45 All cytogenetic groups Biologic randomization | AlloBMT vs AutoBMT + chemotherapy | 295 | 6 yr DFS OS 46% 51% | 42 | 6 yr OS Favorable: 61 vs 56%, $p$ = NS | Uniform induction and consolidation therapy Randomization after CR1 attained Only 61% of AlloBMT group underwent |

*table continues*

Table 36.2  continued

| Trial, (year of publication) | Entry criteria and methodology | Comparison | N | Survival | Relapse | Survival by risk | Comments |
|---|---|---|---|---|---|---|---|
| | 2nd randomization of no donor group. | | 377 | 33% p = 0.01<br>43% p = 0.24 | 63% p < 0.001 | Intermediate:<br>46 vs 38%, p = NS<br>Adverse<br>28 vs 22%, p = NS | transplant DFS improved, but not OS, even when adjusted in Cox model |
| Intergroup (1998)[68] | Age 16–55<br>All cytogenetic groups<br>Biologic randomization<br>2nd randomization of no donor group | AlloBMT vs<br>AutoBMT vs<br>chemotherapy | 113<br>116<br>117 | 4 yr DFS<br>43%<br>35%<br>35%<br>OS<br>46%<br>43%<br>52% | 29<br>48<br>61 | | Purged autotransplantation performed<br>Only 54% of AutoBMT group underwent transplantation Chemotherapy better than autoBMT (p = 0.05) and AlloBMT (p = 0.04)<br>No difference between AlloBMT and AutoBMT |
| GOELAM (1997)[69] | Age 15–40<br>Biologic randomization (donor vs. no donor)<br>2nd randomization of no donor group.<br>All cytogenetic groups | AlloBMT vs<br>AutoBMT +<br>chemotherapy | 88<br>134 | 4 yr DFS<br>44%<br>38%<br>p = NS<br>OS<br>53%<br>53%<br>p = NS | 37%<br>N/A | 4 yr OS<br>Favorable:<br>71.5 vs 66.5% p = NS<br>Intermediate:<br>40.5 vs 56.5% p = NS<br>Adverse (pooled)<br>41 vs 30%, p = NS | Uniform induction and consolidation therapy<br>AutoBMT and chemotherapy arms analyzed together |
| BGMT 87 (1996)[70] | Age 15–45<br>All cytogenetic groups<br>Biologic randomization<br>2nd randomization of no donor group. | AlloBMT vs<br>AutoBMT +<br>ChemoRx | 36<br>60 | 3 yr DFS<br>66.5%<br>42.4%<br>p < 0.05<br>OS<br>65%<br>50.9%<br>p = NS | 24.1%<br>56%<br>p < 0.009 | | Uniform induction and consolidation therapy.<br>Study performed to confirm BGMT 87 |
| Mitus et al. (1995)[71] | Age <65<br>All cytogenetic groups<br>Biologic randomization | AlloBMT vs<br>AutoBMT | 31<br>53 | 5 yr DFS<br>56%<br>45%<br>p = NS | 20%<br>50% | | Nonuniform treatment, including T cell depletion |
| Ferrant et al. (1991)[72] | Age ≤55<br>All cytogenetic groups<br>Biologic randomization | AlloBMT vs<br>AutoBMT | 24<br>72 | 4 yr DFS<br>53%<br>16%<br>p = 0.003 | 41%<br>78%<br>p = 0.01 | | Uniform induction, consolidation therapy<br>Identical conditioning therapy for AlloBMT and AutoBMT<br>Only 44% assigned AutoBMT underwent transplantation |
| HOVON (1990)[73] | Age 15–60<br>Biologic randomization | AlloBMT vs<br>AutoBMT | 21<br>32 | 3 yr DFS<br>51<br>35<br>p = 0.12<br>OS<br>66%<br>37%<br>p = 0.05 | 34<br>60 p = 0.03 | | Treatment administered between 1984 and 1987<br>T cell depletion used uniformly<br>As treated analysis |

alone.[79] Patients with favorable prognostic features, including a longer duration of first remission[79,80] and favorable cytogenetic features at presentation,[81] have more favorable outcomes. The CALGB tested autologous transplantation in a cohort of 50 individuals with AML in second remission. With a short follow-up, 25% of patients remain in remission.[82] While other small series exist, because of short follow-up, autologous transplantation cannot be routinely recommended for patients in second or subsequent remission. Allogeneic stem cell transplantation is the recommended therapy for second or subsequent remission AML. The French Bone Marrow Transplant Group (SFGM) retrospectively reviewed the outcomes in 310 patients with relapsed AML who underwent transplantation. The 5-year probability of survival was 35% in patients who underwent transplant in second or subsequent complete remission. This was significantly better than the outcomes for patients transplanted in untreated or refractory relapse (14% and 11%, respectively).[83] Overall, patients with sibling donors fared better than patients with unrelated donors ($p = 0.001$), mainly due to differences in transplant-related mortality. While transplantation in untreated relapse is certainly feasible,[84] recent analyses suggest that reinduction chemotherapy may have some value, if only to help determine prognosis with transplantation.

Despite anthracycline-based induction chemotherapy, up to 30% of patients with newly diagnosed AML will not achieve a complete remission. The long-term prognosis for these patients with primary refractory AML is extraordinarily grim, with essentially no long-term survivors in the absence of allogeneic stem cell therapy. Salvage transplantation can result in long-term remissions in approximately 10–30% of individuals when family members or unrelated volunteers are used as donors.[83,85–87] In this setting, the use of unrelated donors and adverse cytogenetics negatively impact long-term survival.[86] The timing and number of chemotherapy cycles prior to transplantation for refractory AML is likely critical, as patients exposed to multiple rounds of chemotherapy and infectious complications of prolonged neutropenia have a higher incidence of transplant-related morbidity and mortality. Achieving a remission after primary induction failure does not appear to influence long-term outcome[86] and so multiple attempts to induce a remission are likely detrimental.

### NONMYELOABLATIVE TRANSPLANTATION

Similar to the situation in ALL, nonmyeloablative transplantation for AML has been shown to reduce transplant-related morbidity and mortality, mainly by reducing the incidence of serious complications in the immediate posttransplant period. Here as well, the GVL reaction is an important component of therapy. The Spanish Group for Hematopoietic Transplantation demonstrated a significant improvement in outcome for patients who developed grade II–IV acute GVHD in comparison with patients who experienced no GVHD after nonmyeloablative transplantation (13 vs 58% disease progression at 1 year, $p = 0.008$).[88]

The use of transplantation for patients with AML in first remission has been demonstrated to be safe. Feinstein *et al.* transplanted 18 patients with AML in first remission and demonstrated that nonrelapse mortality was only 17% at 1 year. The majority of treatment failures in this cohort were related to disease relapse, which was responsible for 70% of the deaths in this trial.[89] Nonmyeloablative transplantation has been used as consolidation therapy for patients in second remission, for relapsed disease after failed autologous transplantation or prior high-dose allogeneic stem cell transplantation and for patients with refractory leukemia. In these settings, the most important predictors of long-term outcome include cytogenetics and remission status at the time of transplantation.

To explore the utility of nonmyeloablative transplantation in a cohort of individuals traditionally considered eligible for ablative transplantation approaches, Ruiz-Arguelles et al. transplanted 24 young patients (median age 35 years) with AML, using nonmyeloablative conditioning.[90] The median survival of this cohort exceeds 7 years and has not been reached and progression-free survival at 2 years is 66%. Transplant-related toxicity was very minor, and the majority of transplants occurred in an outpatient setting. Similarly, Alyea et al. compared the results of ablative and nonmyeloablative conditioning in a cohort of individuals above the age of 50, the majority of whom had AML. No differences in outcome were noted; however, interestingly, it appeared that patients <50 years did better with ablative regimens.[91] While results from larger series need to confirm these findings, the combination of reduced treatment-related morbidity and mortality with an active GVL effect may make nonmyeloablative transplantation the therapy of choice for individuals in first remission with either intermediate or unfavorable cytogenetic risks, but is not recommended routinely at this time.

### THERAPY OF RELAPSE AFTER TRANSPLANTATION

Relapse after allogeneic transplantation for AML is not uncommon and represents a difficult challenge to the clinician. Rates of response to donor lymphocyte infusions (DLI) are roughly the same for AML as for ALL and occur in roughly 15–40% of cases.[52,92,93] Most of these responses are short-lived and are often associated with either acute or chronic GVHD. To be effective most DLI must be performed in remission.

For patients who do not respond to DLI, the option of a second allogeneic transplant exists. Using a second, matched related donor, 3 year leukemia-free survival among 125 patients with relapsed AML after a first matched, related transplant was 27%.[59] The majority of these patients received allografts from the same donor, and the majority had myeloablative conditioning regimens. Factors that predicted survival included the length of remission from initial transplant, remission status at the time of second transplant, and the age of the recipient.[59] Similar findings were reported from three European studies[94–96], although the transplant-related mortality in the French study was 68%.[96] In this study, chronic GVHD was associated with a more favorable outcome (hazard rate 3.2 for overall survival, $p = 0.0005$), suggesting that GVL is required for favorable long-term outcome.[96] These outcomes are only observed if the transplant takes place more than a year after the first transplant. Attempts at transplantation within 1 year are associated with increased transplant-related mortality. The use of unrelated donors to harness more potent GVL effects[97] and the use of nonmyeloablative conditioning to reduce transplant-related mortality have been attempted as well.[98]

## SPECIAL TOPICS IN TRANSPLANTATION FOR AML
### Stem cell source

As in ALL, trials have prospectively enrolled patients to determine if outcomes using PBSC are superior, equivalent, or inferior to stem cell transplantation. The Stem Cell Trialists group demonstrated in an individual-patient meta-analysis that for all hematologic malignancies, disease-free outcomes were slightly superior for PBSC transplantation, although this was not seen in the AML subgroup. In a large retrospective IBMTR review, outcome for patients with AML in first remission was no different for PBSCT in comparison with BMT (1 year DFS 70% vs 61%, $p = 0.25$); however, patients in second remission benefited significantly with PBSCT (1 year DFS 77% vs 57%, $p = 0.003$).[99] This is in contrast to a large EBMT survey where no differences were noted,[100] and a second EBMT survey where CD34+ rich stem cell transplantation was associated with improved outcome for patients with AML in first remission.[101]

The use of umbilical cord transplantation has been explored for patients with AML, and until recently was considered outside a clinical trial only when a sibling or suitable unrelated donor was not available. Two recent trials have recently demonstrated that although there are differences in rates of GVHD and time to engraftment with cord blood transplantation, long-term outcomes are similar to unrelated stem cell transplantation.[102,103] Whether cord blood transplantation is equivalent to unrelated PBSC transplantation is unknown.

### Transplantation for secondary AML

Therapy-related AML or AML arising from a myelodysplastic syndrome (collectively, secondary AML, sAML) is considered incurable with standard chemotherapeutic approaches. Secondary AML is often associated with adverse cytogenetic features including loss of part or all of chromosome 7, loss of chromosome 5q, translocations involving MLL gene at 11q23, or a complex karyotype with multiple cytogenetic aberrations. As in de novo AML, these cytogenetic changes are associated with poor prognosis[104] and wherever possible a suitable allogeneic donor should be identified once secondary AML is diagnosed.[105,106] Since many patients with sAML are of advanced age, the less toxic approaches of autologous and nonmyeloablative stem cell transplantation have been used with varying degrees of success. The EBMT reported outcomes in 173 patients with MDS or secondary AML who underwent autologous transplantation. The risk of relapse was 55%, which was higher than for allogeneic stem cell recipients.[107] There are currently no long-term studies supporting the use of autologous transplantation for sAML. Allogeneic transplantation is the preferred therapeutic modality, leading to long-term remission in approximately 20–30%, when ablative conditioning is utilized.[105,108]

### Acute promyelocytic leukemia

Acute promyelocytic leukemia (APL), associated with the t(15;17) translocation has the most favorable prognosis of the AMLs, with long-term remission rates of approximately 80% with ATRA-based induction strategies.[109] Nonetheless, relapses occur and frequently involve the CNS.[110] Fortunately, reinduction with arsenic-based regimens is often successful at inducing second remissions.[111] As consolidative therapy for APL in second remission, both autologous and allogeneic transplant approaches have been attempted. Meloni et al. demonstrated the value of PCR testing for minimal residual disease in a series of patients who underwent autologous transplantation for APL in second clinical remission. Patients with detectable translocations between the PML and RAR α genes all relapsed, while the in patients without minimal residual disease by PCR relapsed rarely.[112] In a series of patients with APL in second clinical remission who received allogeneic stem cell transplants from HLA-identical siblings, long-term disease-free survival was 46%.[113] Sustained remissions were noted even in patients with persistent minimal residual disease prior to transplantation. This suggests that an active GVL effect can cure APL, when autologous transplantation is not indicated. While autologous or allogeneic transplantation are generally only indicated for patients with APL in first remission when standard therapy cannot be administered, patients in second remission benefit from autologous transplantation, when minimal residual disease is undetectable or allogeneic transplantation when minimal residual disease persists.

# REFERENCES

1. SEER *Cancer Statistics Review*, 1975–2001. Accessed 2004, available at: http://seer.cancer.gov/csr/1975_2001.

2. International Bone Marrow Transplant Registry. *Report on State of the Art in Blood and Marrow Transplantation.* ccessed 2004, available at: http://www ibmtr org/infoserv/infoserv5 html.

3. Giles F, Keating A, Goldstone A, et al.: Acute myeloid leukemia. *Hematology 2002. American Society of Hematology Education Program Book,* 73–110, 2002.

4. Pui CH, Relling MV, Downing JR. Acute lymphoblastic leukemia. *N Engl J Med* 350:1535–1548, 2004.

5. Hoelzer D, Gökbuget N, Ottman O, et al.: Acute lymphoblastic leukemia. *Hematology 2002. American Society of Hematology Education Program Book,* 162–192, 2002.

6. Jamieson CH, Amylon MD, Wong RM, Blume KG: Allogeneic hematopoietic cell transplantation for patients with high-risk acute lymphoblastic leukemia in first or second complete remission using fractionated total-body irradiation and high-dose etoposide: a 15-year experience. *Exp Hematol* 31:981–986, 2003.

7. Snyder DS: Allogeneic stem cell transplantation for Philadelphia chromosome-positive acute lymphoblastic leukemia. *Biol Blood Marrow Transplant* 6:597–603, 2000.

8. Martin TG, Gajewski JL: Allogeneic stem cell transplantation for acute lymphocytic leukemia in adults. *Hematol Oncol Clin North Am* 15:97–120, 2001.

9. Labar B, Suciu S, Zittoun R, et al.: Allogeneic stem cell transplantation in acute lymphoblastic leukemia and non-Hodgkin's lymphoma for patients 50 years old in first complete remission: results of the EORTC ALL-3 trial. *Haematologica* 89:809–817, 2004.

10. Hunault M, Harousseau JL, Delain M, et al.: Better outcome of adult acute lymphoblastic leukemia after early genoidentical allogeneic bone-marrow transplantation (BMT) than after late high-dose therapy and autologous BMT: a GOELAMS trial. *Blood* 104:3028–3037, 2004.

11. Gupta V, Yi QL, Brandwein J, et al.: The role of allogeneic bone marrow transplantation in adult patients below the age of 55 years with acute lymphoblastic leukemia in first complete remission: a donor vs no donor comparison. *Bone Marrow Transplant* 33:397–404, 2004.

12. Dombret H, Gabert J, Boiron JM, et al.: Outcome of treatment in adults with Philadelphia chromosome-positive acute lymphoblastic leukemia—results of the prospective multicenter LALA-94 trial. *Blood* 100:2357–2366, 2002.

13. Rowe K, Richards S, Burnett A, et al.: Favorable results of allogeneic bone marrow transplantation (BMT) for adults with Philadelphia (Ph)-chromosome-negative acute lymphoblastic lymphoma (ALL) in first completeremission (CR): results from the International ALL Trial (MRC UKALL XII/ECOG E2993). *Blood* 98:481a, 2001.

14. Thiebaut A, Vernant JP, Degos L, et al.: Adult acute lymphocytic leukemia study testing chemotherapy and autologous and allogeneic transplantation. A follow-up report of the French protocol LALA 87. *Hematol Oncol Clin North Am* 14:1353–1366, 2000.

15. Sebban C, Lepage E, Vernant JP, et al.: Allogeneic bone marrow transplantation in adult acute lymphoblastic leukemia in first complete remission: a comparative study. French Group of Therapy of Adult Acute Lymphoblastic Leukemia. *J Clin Oncol* 12:2580–2587, 1994.

16. Fiere D, Lepage E, Sebban C, et al.: Adult acute lymphoblastic leukemia: a multicentric randomized trial testing bone marrow transplantation as postremission therapy. The French Group on Therapy for Adult Acute Lymphoblastic Leukemia. *J Clin Oncol* 11:1990–2001, 1993.

17. Suzuki N, Koike T, Furukawa T, et al.: Comparison of long-term survival between bone marrow transplantation and maintenance chemotherapy for adult acute lymphoblastic leukemia in first remission. *Rinsho Ketsueki* 38:95–99, 1997.

18. Attal M, Blaise D, Marit G, et al.: Consolidation treatment of adult acute lymphoblastic leukemia: a prospective, randomized trial comparing allogeneic versus autologous bone marrow transplantation and testing the impact of recombinant interleukin-2 after autologous bone marrow transplantation. BGMT Group. *Blood* 86:1619–1628, 1995.

19. Blaise D, Gaspard MH, Stoppa AM, et al.: Allogeneic or autologous bone marrow transplantation for acute lymphoblastic leukemia in first complete remission. *Bone Marrow Transplant* 5:7–12, 1990.

20. Cornelissen JJ, Carston M, Kollman C, et al.: Unrelated marrow transplantation for adult patients with poor-risk acute lymphoblastic leukemia: strong graft-versus-leukemia effect and risk factors determining outcome. *Blood* 97:1572–1577, 2001.

21. Kiehl MG, Kraut L, Schwerdtfeger R, et al.: Outcome of allogeneic hematopoietic stem-cell transplantation in adult patients with acute lymphoblastic leukemia: no difference in related compared with unrelated transplant in first complete remission. *J Clin Oncol* 22:2816–2825, 2004.

22. Weisdorf D, Bishop M, Dharan B, et al.: Autologous versus allogeneic unrelated donor transplantation for acute lymphoblastic leukemia: comparative toxicity and outcomes. *Biol Blood Marrow Transplant* 8:213–220, 2002.

23. Gray R, Wheatley K: How to avoid bias when comparing bone marrow transplantation with chemotherapy. *Bone Marrow Transplant* 7(Suppl 3):9–12, 1991.

24. Mengarelli A, Iori AP, Cerretti R, et al.: Increasing risk of relapse after allogeneic stem cell transplant for adult acute lymphoblastic leukemia in > or = 2nd complete remission induced by highly intensive chemotherapy. *Haematologica* 87:782–784, 2002.

25. Doney K, Hagglund H, Leisenring W, et al.: Predictive factors for outcome of allogeneic hematopoietic cell transplantation for adult acute lymphoblastic leukemia. *Biol Blood Marrow Transplant* 9:472–481, 2003.

26. Grigg AP, Szer J, Beresford J, et al.: Factors affecting the outcome of allogeneic bone marrow transplantation for adult patients with refractory or relapsed acute leukaemia. *Br J Haematol* 107:409–418, 1999.

27. Weisdorf D, Bishop M, Dharan B, et al.: Autologous versus allogeneic unrelated donor transplantation for acute lymphoblastic leukemia: comparative toxicity and outcomes. *Biol Blood Marrow Transplant* 8:213–220, 2002.

28. Ringden O, Labopin M, Gluckman E, et al.: Donor search or autografting in patients with acute leukaemia who lack an HLA-identical sibling? A matched-pair analysis. Acute Leukaemia Working Party of the European Cooperative Group for Blood and Marrow Transplantation (EBMT) and the International Marrow Unrelated Search and Transplant (IMUST) Study. *Bone Marrow Transplant* 19:963–968, 1997.

29. Druker BJ, Sawyers CL, Kantarjian H, et al.: Activity of a specific inhibitor of the BCR-ABL tyrosine kinase in the blast crisis of chronic myeloid leukemia and acute lymphoblastic leukemia with the Philadelphia chromosome. *N Engl J Med* 344:1038–1042, 2001.

30. Thomas DA, Faderl S, Cortes J, et al.: Treatment of Philadelphia chromosome-positive acute lymphocytic leukemia with hyper-CVAD and imatinib mesylate. *Blood* 103:4396–4407, 2004.

31. Towatari M, Yanada M, Usui N, et al.: Combination of intensive chemotherapy and imatinib can rapidly induce high-quality complete remission for a majority of patients with newly diagnosed BCR-ABL positive acute lymphoblastic leukemia. *Blood* 104(12):3507–3512, 2004.

32. Ottmann OG, Druker BJ, Sawyers CL, et al.: A phase 2 study of imatinib in patients with relapsed or refractory Philadelphia chromosome-positive acute lymphoid leukemias. *Blood* 100:1965–1971, 2002.

33. Shimoni A, Kroger N, Zander AR, et al.: Imatinib mesylate (STI571) in preparation for allogeneic hematopoietic stem cell transplantation and donor lymphocyte infusions in patients with Philadelphia-positive acute leukemias. *Leukemia* 17:290–297, 2003.

34. Yamada M, Miyamura K, Fujiwara T, et al.: Imatinib mesylate in conjunction with allogeneic hematopoietic stem cell transplantation in patients with Philadelphia chromosome positive leukemias: report of 4 cases. *Tohoku J Exp Med.* 204:79–84, 2004.

35. Lee S, Kim DW, Kim YJ, et al.: Minimal residual disease-based role of imatinib as a first-line interim therapy prior to allogeneic stem cell transplantation in Philadelphia chromosome-positive acute lymphoblastic leukemia. *Blood* 102:3068–3070, 2003.

36. Wassmann B, Pfeifer H, Scheuring U, et al.: Therapy with imatinib mesylate (Glivec) preceding allogeneic stem cell transplantation (SCT) in relapsed or refractory Philadelphia-positive acute lymphoblastic leukemia (Ph+ALL). *Leukemia* 16:2358–2365, 2002.

37. Khouri IF, Keating M, Korbling M, et al.: Transplant-lite: induction of graft-versus-malignancy using fludarabine-based nonablative chemotherapy and allogeneic blood progenitor-cell transplantation as treatment for lymphoid malignancies. *J Clin Oncol* 16:2817–2824, 1998.

38. Slavin S, Nagler A, Naparstek E, et al.: Nonmyeloablative stem cell transplantation and cell therapy as an alternative to conventional bone marrow transplantation with lethal cytoreduction for the treatment of malignant and nonmalignant hematologic diseases. *Blood* 91:756–763, 1998.

39. Nordlander A, Mattsson J, Ringden O, et al.: Graft-versus-host disease is associated with a lower relapse incidence after hematopoietic stem cell transplantation in patients with acute lymphoblastic leukemia. *Biol Blood Marrow Transplant* 10:195–203, 2004.

40. Zikos P, Van Lint MT, Lamparelli T, et al.: Allogeneic hemopoietic stem cell transplantation for patients with high risk acute lymphoblastic leukemia: favorable impact of chronic graft-versus-host disease on survival and relapse. *Haematologica* 83:896–903, 1998.

41. Weisdorf DJ, Nesbit ME, Ramsay NK, et al.: Allogeneic bone marrow transplantation for acute lymphoblastic leukemia in remission: prolonged survival associated with acute graft-versus-host disease. *J Clin Oncol* 5:1348–1355, 1987.

42. Kottaridis PD, Milligan DW, Chopra R, et al.: In vivo CAMPATH-1H prevents graft-versus-host disease following nonmyeloablative stem cell transplantation. *Blood* 96:2419–2425, 2000.

43. Chakraverty R, Peggs K, Chopra R, et al.: Limiting transplantation-related mortality following unrelated donor stem cell transplantation by using a nonmyeloablative conditioning regimen. *Blood* 99:1071–1078, 2002.

44. Corradini P, Tarella C, Olivieri A, et al.: Reduced-intensity conditioning followed by allografting of hematopoietic cells can produce clinical and molecular remissions in patients with poor-risk hematologic malignancies. *Blood* 99:75–82, 2002.

45. Martino R, Caballero MD, Canals C, et al.: Allogeneic peripheral blood stem cell transplantation with reduced-intensity conditioning: results of a prospective multicentre study. *Br J Haematol* 115:653–659, 2001.

46. Giralt S, Thall PF, Khouri I, et al.: Melphalan and purine analog-containing preparative regimens: reduced-intensity conditioning for patients with hematologic malignancies undergoing allogeneic progenitor cell transplantation. *Blood* 97:631–637, 2001.

47. Martino R, Giralt S, Caballero MD, et al.: Allogeneic hematopoietic stem cell transplantation with reduced-intensity conditioning in acute lymphoblastic leukemia: a feasibility study. *Haematologica* 88:555–560, 2003.

48. Arnold R, Massenkeil G, Bornhauser M, et al.: Nonmyeloablative stem cell transplantation in adults with high-risk ALL may be effective in early but not in advanced disease. *Leukemia* 16:2423–2428, 2002.

49. Marks D, Forman S, Blume K, et al.: A comparison of cyclophosphamide and total body irradiation with etoposide and total body irradiation as conditioning regimens for patients undergoing sibling allografts for acute lymphoblstic leukemia in first or second complete remission. The improtance of the dse of total body irradiation. *Biol Blood Marrow Transplant* 12(4): 438–453, 2006.

50. Stem Cell Trialists Group. Allogeneic peripheral blood stem cell transplant vs. bone marrow transplant in the management of hematological malignancies: an individual patient data meta-analysis of 9 randomized trials. *J Clin Oncol* 23(22):5074–5087, 2005.

51. Garderet L, Labopin M, Gorin NC, et al.: Patients with acute lymphoblastic leukaemia allografted with a matched unrelated donor may have a lower survival

with a peripheral blood stem cell graft compared to bone marrow. *Bone Marrow Transplant* 31:23–29, 2003.

52. Collins RH, Jr, Shpilberg O, Drobyski WR, et al.: Donor leukocyte infusions in 140 patients with relapsed malignancy after allogeneic bone marrow transplantation. *J Clin Oncol* 15:433–444, 1997.

53. Luznik L, Fuchs EJ: Donor lymphocyte infusions to treat hematologic malignancies in relapse after allogeneic blood or marrow transplantation. *Cancer Control* 9:123–137, 2002.

54. Au WY, Lie AK, Ma SK, et al.: Tyrosine kinase inhibitor STI571 in the treatment of Philadelphia chromosome-positive leukaemia failing myeloablative stem cell transplantation. *Bone Marrow Transplant* 30:453–457, 2002.

55. McCann SR, Gately K, Conneally E, Lawler M: Molecular response to imatinib mesylate following relapse after allogeneic SCT for CML. *Blood* 101:1200–1201, 2003.

56. Olavarria E, Craddock C, Dazzi F, et al.: Imatinib mesylate (STI571) in the treatment of relapse of chronic myeloid leukemia after allogeneic stem cell transplantation. *Blood* 99:3861–3862, 2002.

57. Gopcsa L, Barta A, Banyai A, et al.: Salvage chemotherapy with donor lymphocyte infusion and STI 571 in a patient relapsing with B-lymphoblastic phase chronic myeloid leukemia after allogeneic bone marrow transplantation. *Pathol Oncol Res* 9:131–133, 2003.

58. Wassmann B, Scheuring U, Thiede C, et al.: Stable molecular remission induced by imatinib mesylate (STI571) in a patient with CML lymphoid blast crisis relapsing after allogeneic stem cell transplantation. *Bone Marrow Transplant* 31:611–614, 2003.

59. Eapen M, Giralt SA, Horowitz MM, et al.: Second transplant for acute and chronic leukemia relapsing after first HLA-identical sibling transplant. *Bone Marrow Transplant* 34:721–727, 2004.

60. Brunet S, Esteve J, Berlanga J, et al.: Treatment of primary acute myeloid leukemia: results of a prospective multicenter trial including high-dose cytarabine or stem cell transplantation as post-remission strategy. *Haematologica.* 89:940–949, 2004.

61. Heil G, Krauter J, Raghavachar A, et al.: Risk-adapted induction and consolidation therapy in adults with de novo AML aged </= 60 years: results of a prospective multicenter trial. *Ann Hematol* 83:336–344, 2004.

62. Suciu S, Mandelli F, de Witte T, et al.: Allogeneic compared with autologous stem cell transplantation in the treatment of patients younger than 46 years with acute myeloid leukemia (AML) in first complete remission (CR1): an intention-to-treat analysis of the EORTC/GIMEMAAML-10 trial. *Blood* 102:1232–1240, 2003.

63. Tsimberidou AM, Stavroyianni N, Viniou N, et al.: Comparison of allogeneic stem cell transplantation, high-dose cytarabine, and autologous peripheral stem cell transplantation as postremission treatment in patients with de novo acute myelogenous leukemia. *Cancer* 97:1721–1731, 2003.

64. Burnett AK, Wheatley K, Goldstone AH, et al.: The value of allogeneic bone marrow transplant in patients with acute myeloid leukaemia at differing risk of relapse: results of the UK MRC AML 10 trial. *Br J Haematol* 118:385–400, 2002.

65. Burnett AK, Goldstone AH, Stevens RM, et al.: Randomised comparison of addition of autologous bone-marrow transplantation to intensive chemotherapy for acute myeloid leukaemia in first remission: results of MRC AML 10 trial. UK Medical Research Council Adult and Children's Leukaemia Working Parties. *Lancet* 351:700–708, 1998.

66. Keating S, de Witte T, Suciu S, et al.: The influence of HLA-matched sibling donor availability on treatment outcome for patients with AML: an analysis of the AML 8A study of the EORTC Leukaemia Cooperative Group and GIMEMA. European Organization for Research and Treatment of Cancer. Gruppo Italiano Malattie Ematologiche Maligne dell'Adulto. *Br J Haematol* 102:1344–1353, 1998.

67. Zittoun RA, Mandelli F, Willemze R, et al.: Autologous or allogeneic bone marrow transplantation compared with intensive chemotherapy in acute myelogenous leukemia. European Organization for Research and Treatment of Cancer (EORTC) and the Gruppo Italiano Malattie Ematologiche Maligne dell'Adulto (GIMEMA) Leukemia Cooperative Groups. *N Engl J Med* 332:217–223, 1995.

68. Cassileth PA, Harrington DP, Appelbaum FR, et al.: Chemotherapy compared with autologous or allogeneic bone marrow transplantation in the management of acute myeloid leukemia in first remission. *N Engl J Med* 339:1649–1656, 1998.

69. Harousseau JL, Cahn JY, Pignon B, et al.: Comparison of autologous bone marrow transplantation and intensive chemotherapy as postremission therapy in adult acute myeloid leukemia. The Groupe Ouest Est Leucemies Aigues Myeloblastiques (GOELAM). *Blood* 90:2978–2986, 1997.

70. Reiffers J, Stoppa AM, Attal M, et al.: Allogeneic vs autologous stem cell transplantation vs chemotherapy in patients with acute myeloid leukemia in first remission: the BGMT 87 study. *Leukemia* 10:1874–1882, 1996.

71. Mitus AJ, Miller KB, Schenkein DP, et al.: Improved survival for patients with acute myelogenous leukemia. *J Clin Oncol* 13:560–569, 1995.

72. Ferrant A, Doyen C, Delannoy A, et al.: Allogeneic or autologous bone marrow transplantation for acute non-lymphocytic leukemia in first remission. *Bone Marrow Transplant* 7:303–309, 1991.

73. Lowenberg B, Verdonck LJ, Dekker AW, et al.: Autologous bone marrow transplantation in acute myeloid leukemia in first remission: results of a Dutch prospective study. *J Clin Oncol* 8:287–294, 1990.

74. Grimwade D, Walker H, Oliver F, et al.: The importance of diagnostic cytogenetics on outcome in AML: analysis of 1,612 patients entered into the MRC AML 10 trial. The Medical Research Council Adult and Children's Leukaemia Working Parties. *Blood* 92:2322–2333, 1998.

75. Wheatley K: Current controversies: which patients with acute myeloid leukaemia should receive a bone marrow transplantation?—a statistician's view. *Br J Haematol* 118:351–356, 2002.

76. Slovak ML, Kopecky KJ, Cassileth PA, et al.: Karyotypic analysis predicts outcome of preremission and postremission therapy in adult acute myeloid leukemia: a Southwest Oncology Group/Eastern Cooperative Oncology Group Study. *Blood* 96:4075–4083, 2000.

77. Byrd JC, Mrozek K, Dodge RK, et al.: Pretreatment cytogenetic abnormalities are predictive of induction success, cumulative incidence of relapse, and overall survival in adult patients with de novo acute myeloid leukemia: results from Cancer and Leukemia Group B (CALGB 8461). *Blood* 100:4325–4336, 2002.

78. Grimwade D, Walker H, Harrison G, et al.: The predictive value of hierarchical cytogenetic classification in older adults with acute myeloid leukemia (AML): analysis of 1065 patients entered into the United Kingdom Medical Research Council AML11 trial. *Blood* 98:1312–1320, 2001.

79. Gale RP, Horowitz MM, Rees JK, et al.: Chemotherapy versus transplants for acute myelogenous leukemia in second remission. *Leukemia* 10:13–19, 1996.

80. Ferrara F, Palmieri S, Mele G: Prognostic factors and therapeutic options for relapsed or refractory acute myeloid leukemia. *Haematologica* 89:998–1008, 2004.

81. Kern W, Haferlach T, Schnittger S, et al.: Karyotype instability between diagnosis and relapse in 117 patients with acute myeloid leukemia: implications for resistance against therapy. *Leukemia* 16:2084–2091, 2002.

82. Linker C, George S, Hurd S, Larson R: Autologous stem cell transplantation for acute myeloid leukemia in second remission—CALGB 9620. *Blood* 98:689a, 2001.

83. Michallet M, Thomas X, Vernant JP, et al.: Long-term outcome after allogeneic hematopoietic stem cell transplantation for advanced stage acute myeloblastic leukemia: a retrospective study of 379 patients reported to the Societe Francaise de Greffe de Moelle (SFGM). *Bone Marrow Transplant* 26:1157–1163, 2000.

84. Clift RA, Buckner CD, Appelbaum FR, et al.: Allogeneic marrow transplantation during untreated first relapse of acute myeloid leukemia. *J Clin Oncol.* 10:1723–1729, 1992.

85. Chiang KY, van Rhee F, Godder K, et al.: Allogeneic bone marrow transplantation from partially mismatched related donors as therapy for primary induction failure acute myeloid leukemia. *Bone Marrow Transplant* 27:507–510, 2001.

86. Fung HC, Stein A, Slovak M, et al.: A long-term follow-up report on allogeneic stem cell transplantation for patients with primary refractory acute myelogenous leukemia: impact of cytogenetic characteristics on transplantation outcome. *Biol Blood Marrow Transplant* 9:766–771, 2003.

87. Singhal S, Powles R, Henslee-Downey PJ, et al.: Allogeneic transplantation from HLA-matched sibling or partially HLA-mismatched related donors for primary refractory acute leukemia. *Bone Marrow Transplant* 29:291–295, 2002.

88. Martino R, Caballero MD, Simon JA, et al.: Evidence for a graft-versus-leukemia effect after allogeneic peripheral blood stem cell transplantation with reduced-intensity conditioning in acute myelogenous leukemia and myelodysplastic syndromes. *Blood* 100:2243–2245, 2002.

89. Feinstein LC, Sandmaier BM, Hegenbart U, et al.: Non-myeloablative allografting from human leucocyte antigen-identical sibling donors for treatment of acute myeloid leukaemia in first complete remission. *Br J Haematol* 120:281–288, 2003.

90. Ruiz-Arguelles GJ, Gomez-Almaguer D, David-Gomez-Rangel J, et al.: Allogeneic hematopoietic stem cell transplantation with non-myeloablative conditioning in patients with acute myelogenous leukemia eligible for conventional allografting: a prospective study. *Leuk Lymphoma* 45:1191–1195, 2004.

91. Alyea EP, Kim H, Cutler C, et al.: Similar outcome of non-myeloablative and myeloablative allogeneic hematopoietic cell transplantation for patients greater than fifty years of age. *Blood* 104:300a, 2004 (Abstract).

92. Alyea E: Donor lymphocyte infusions. In: Soiffer R (ed.) *Stem Cell Transplantation for Hematologic Malignancies.* Totowa, NJ: Humana Press; 453–467, 2004.

93. Porter DL, Collins RH, Jr, Hardy C, et al.: Treatment of relapsed leukemia after unrelated donor marrow transplantation with unrelated donor leukocyte infusions. *Blood* 95:1214–1221, 2000.

94. Bosi A, Bacci S, Miniero R, et al.: Second allogeneic bone marrow transplantation in acute leukemia: a multicenter study from the Gruppo Italiano Trapianto Di Midollo Osseo (GITMO). *Leukemia* 11:420–424, 1997.

95. Bosi A, Laszlo D, Labopin M, et al.: Second allogeneic bone marrow transplantation in acute leukemia: results of a survey by the European Cooperative Group for Blood and Marrow Transplantation. *J Clin Oncol* 19:3675–3684, 2001.

96. Michallet M, Tanguy ML, Socie G, et al.: Second allogeneic haematopoietic stem cell transplantation in relapsed acute and chronic leukaemias for patients who underwent a first allogeneic bone marrow transplantation: a survey of the Societe Francaise de Greffe de moelle (SFGM). *Br J Haematol* 108:400–407, 2000.

97. Lipton JH, Messner H: The role of second bone marrow transplant using a different donor for relapsed leukemia or graft failure. *Eur J Haematol* 58:133–136, 1997.

98. Feinstein LC, Sandmaier BM, Maloney DG, et al.: Allografting after nonmyeloablative conditioning as a treatment after a failed conventional hematopoietic cell transplant. *Biol Blood Marrow Transplant* 9:266–272, 2003.

99. Champlin RE, Schmitz N, Horowitz MM, et al.: Blood stem cells compared with bone marrow as a source of hematopoietic cells for allogeneic transplantation. *Blood* 95:3702–3709, 2000.

100. Ringden O, Labopin M, Bacigalupo A, et al.: Transplantation of peripheral blood stem cells as compared with bone marrow from HLA-identical siblings in adult patients with acute myeloid leukemia and acute lymphoblastic leukemia. *J Clin Oncol* 20:4655–4664, . 2002.

101. Gorin NC, Labopin M, Rocha V, et al.: Marrow versus peripheral blood for geno-identical allogeneic stem cell transplantation in acute myelocytic leukemia: influence of dose and stem cell source shows better outcome with rich marrow. *Blood* 102:3043–3051, 2003.

102. Laughlin MJ, Eapen M, Rubinstein P, et al.: Outcomes after transplantation of cord blood or bone marrow from unrelated donors in adults with leukemia. *N Engl J Med* 351:2265–2275, 2004.

103. Rocha V, Labopin M, Sanz G, et al.: Transplants of umbilical-cord blood or bone marrow from unrelated donors in adults with acute leukemia. *N Engl J Med.* 351:2276–2285, 2004.

104. Kern W, Haferlach T, Schnittger S, Hiddemann W, Schoch C: Prognosis in therapy-related acute myeloid leukemia and impact of karyotype. *J Clin Oncol* 22:2510–2511, 2004.

105. Witherspoon RP, Deeg HJ, Storer B, et al.: Hematopoietic stem-cell transplantation for treatment-related leukemia or myelodysplasia. *J Clin Oncol* 19:2134–2141, 2001.

106. Anderson JE, Gooley TA, Schoch G, et al.: Stem cell transplantation for secondary acute myeloid leukemia: evaluation of transplantation as initial therapy or following induction chemotherapy. *Blood* 89:2578–2585, 1997.

107. de Witte T, Hermans J, Vossen J, et al.: Haematopoietic stem cell transplantation for patients with myelodysplastic syndromes and secondary acute myeloid leukaemias: a report on behalf of the Chronic Leukaemia Working Party of the European Group for Blood and Marrow Transplantation (EBMT). *Br J Haematol* 110:620–630, 2000.

108. Yakoub-Agha I, de La SP, Ribaud P, et al.: Allogeneic bone marrow transplantation for therapy-related myelodysplastic syndrome and acute myeloid leukemia: a long-term study of 70 patients-report of the French society of bone marrow transplantation. *J Clin Oncol* 18:963–971, 2000.

109. Tallman MS, Nabhan C, Feusner JH, Rowe JM: Acute promyelocytic leukemia: evolving therapeutic strategies. *Blood* 99:759–767, 2002.

110. Burry LD, Seki JT: CNS relapses of acute promyelocytic leukemia after all-trans retinoic acid. *Ann Pharmacother* 36:1900–1906, 2002.

111. Tallman MS: Arsenic trioxide: its role in acute promyelocytic leukemia and potential in other hematologic malignancies. *Blood Rev* 15:133–142, 2001.

112. Meloni G, Diverio D, Vignetti M, et al.: Autologous bone marrow transplantation for acute promyelocytic leukemia in second remission: prognostic relevance of pretransplant minimal residual disease assessment by reverse-transcription polymerase chain reaction of the PML/RAR alpha fusion gene. *Blood* 90:1321–1325, 1997.

113. Lo Coco F, Romano A, Mengarelli A, et al.: Allogeneic stem cell transplantation for advanced acute promyelocytic leukemia: results in patients treated in second molecular remission or with molecularly persistent disease. *Leukemia* 17:1930–1933, 2003.

# Chapter 37

# TRANSPLANTATION IN CHRONIC LEUKEMIA

## Thomas S. Lin and Edward A. Copelan

## CHRONIC MYELOGENOUS LEUKEMIA

Allogeneic stem cell transplantation is the only proven curative treatment for chronic myelogenous leukemia (CML). More allogeneic transplants have been performed for CML and more cures achieved than for any other disease. Paradoxically, while the results of transplantation in CML appear to be improving over the last several years, the number of allogeneic transplants for CML has decreased over the same period. This decrease has occurred as an increasing proportion of patients are placed on imatinib mesylate (Gleevec) as initial treatment and as a result of the effectiveness of this agent.

Important questions remain regarding the appropriate timing of allogeneic transplantation in the treatment of CML. First, which patients should undergo transplantation shortly after diagnosis? Secondly, when should patients who initially receive treatment with imatinib to be considered for transplantation? Although most clinicians are familiar with recent clinical studies with imatinib, many are less knowledgeable about the results of recent transplant studies. The following section details the current status of transplantation in CML.

## MYELOABLATIVE ALLOGENEIC TRANSPLANTATION IN CML

Texts and review articles commonly provide a wide range of survival and mortality rates in patients with CML who undergo allogeneic transplantation. [1-5] The lower range of survival and higher range of mortality rates generally quoted are derived from studies of patients who underwent transplantation 20 or more years ago. [6-11] Results have improved with time. [6-12]

Allogeneic transplantation using myeloablative regimens works through two different mechanisms. The myeloablative regimen eradicates nearly all malignant cells in most patients. A retrospective analysis of iden-

tical twins with CML demonstrated a 3-year probability of leukemia-free survival of 59%, compared to 61% for HLA-identical sibling transplants. [14] Although the 3-year probability of treatment-related mortality was only 3% for the twins, their risk of relapse was 40% at three years, compared to 7% for a cohort of HLA-identical sibling transplants. The fact that some patients with CML are cured by syngeneic transplants demonstrates that myeloablative therapy alone can eradicate all malignant cells in some patients. The higher relapse rate indicates a role for allogeneic cells in complete eradication of disease. Lower relapse rates in patients who undergo unrelated transplants and in those who develop graft-versus-host disease [15-17] further support the importance of the allogeneic effect. The sustained elimination of Ph+ cells following infusion of donor lymphocytes, in patients who relapse following transplantation, is clear demonstration of the potency of the allogeneic affect. [18-20]

## MATCHED SIBLING TRANSPLANTS

Five-year estimates of leukemia-free survival following myeloablative transplantation using sibling donors do not precisely reflect rates of long-term disease-free survival in chronic phase CML. Extended follow-up demonstrates that deaths from chronic GVHD and relapses occur beyond 5 years. [21,22] However, donor lymphocyte infusion (DLI) results in sustained leukemia-free survival in a substantial proportion of patients who relapse following transplantation, and who would be considered treatment failures by conventional analysis. "Current DFS" [23] more accurately assesses long-term results of allogeneic transplantation by appropriately recognizing patients who achieve sustained remission following DLI. With current approaches, including the use of DLI, approximately two-thirds of patients with chronic phase CML can be cured by myeloablative transplantation. Twenty-five to 30% of patients die from complications of transplantation, and 5% of relapsed disease.

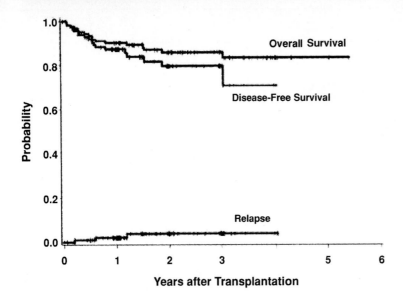

**Figure 37.1** *Outcomes after transplantation using a targeted BU/CY regimen. Estimates of survival, DFS, and relapse at 3 years after transplantation are 86%, 78%, and 8%, respectively*

Along with improvements in supportive care, modifications in preparative regimens may play an important role in improving results. Although busulfan has not been proven statistically superior to total body irradiation (TBI) as preparation for allogeneic transplantation, some studies report lower rates of transplant-related mortality and relapse, and higher rates of leukemia-free survival using busulfan.[24-26] Continued refinement of busulfan-based regimens, including the use of intravenous busulfan[27,28] and/or pharmacological targeting[13] of busulfan, appears to improve results. Radich et al. reported that 78% of patients transplanted in Seattle have sustained leukemia-free survival using dose adjustment of busulfan to ensure "targeted" concentrations[13] (Figure 37.1).

## MYELOABLATIVE TRANSPLANTATION FROM UNRELATED DONORS

The outcomes in patients receiving unrelated transplants have improved more rapidly than have outcomes in patients with sibling donors. More sophisticated techniques for determining HLA compatibility and better understanding of the relative importance of matching of specific HLA antigens are largely responsible. Leukemia-free survival rates with well-matched unrelated donors in patients 40 years and younger, undergoing transplantation within a year of diagnosis, appear to be similar to those obtained with related donors.[29-31] Yet, patients without histocompatible sibling donors are rarely considered for transplantation early in the course of disease. Although identification of donors and procurement of stem cells can not be accomplished as quickly as for sibling donors, preliminary studies can be used to estimate the likelihood of finding a fully matched donor. In most cases, donor stem cells can be obtained expeditiously. Appropriate patients without sibling donors should be offered this potential therapy.

## PROGNOSTIC FACTORS IN ALLOGENEIC TRANSPLANTATION

Identification of significant prognostic factors represents an important advance in transplantation in CML. In some situations, an understanding of these factors, such as the interval between diagnosis and transplantation, provides an opportunity to optimize results. In others it permits a more accurate assessment of outcome. Prognostic factors can also identify patients who would be at high risk for complications of transplantation, and for whom a transplant is not an appropriate therapy.

### AGE

Older age is perceived by many to be among the most important adverse factors in transplantation. For allogeneic transplantation in general, the adverse influence of older age largely results from the favorable outcome of pediatric compared to adult patients.[32,33] Differences between younger and older adults are less dramatic.

Studies using TBI in the preparative regimen for transplantation in CML have demonstrated a significant adverse influence of advancing age.[34,35] The Seattle program described a significant adverse affect of age in CML using TBI, but not in patients who receive busulfan[13,36,37] (Figure 37.2). Others have similarly failed to identify age as a significant independent prognostic factor in patients who receive busulfan.[38,39] Results from Ohio State have demonstrated that the influence of age is attributable to other factors, including interval from diagnosis to transplantation, which is generally longer in older patients.[39]

### INTERVAL FROM DIAGNOSIS TO TRANSPLANTATION
The incidence of transplant-related mortality increases and leukemia-free survival decreases with prolongation of the interval from diagnosis to transplantation.

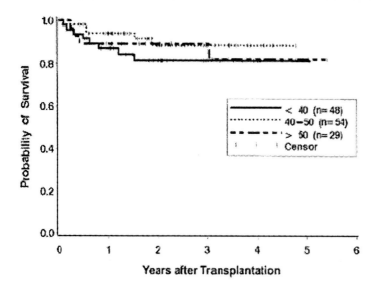

**Figure 37.2** *Effect of age on survival. There are no statistically significant differences in survival of patients aged younger than 40 years, 40 to 50 years, and older than 50 years (p = 0.55)*

Although most studies have suggested a threshold at 1 or 2 years, at which point patients transplanted beyond this cutoff fare significantly worse, analysis of data from Ohio State demonstrates that interval is a continuous variable. Patients undergoing transplantation less than 3 months following diagnosis had 5 years of leukemia-free survival in excess of 90% (Figure 37.3).[39] Data from Seattle indicate favorable outcomes in patients who undergo transplantation fewer than 6 months from diagnosis.[40]

The higher rate of transplant-related mortality associated with prolonged intervals between diagnosis and transplantation likely results from subclinical toxicities due to therapy. Prior busulfan[41] and interferon therapy[42,43] are associated with more regimen-related toxicity than hydroxyurea. The adverse influence of interferon is not seen with short-term treatment (<6 months)[44] or when therapy is discontinued at least 3 months prior to transplantation.[45] Preliminary results of transplantation in patients who took imatinib have not generally indicated an adverse influence, but data suggesting a possible adverse affect have been presented.[46]

### PHASE OF DISEASE

The prior discussion refers to patients with chronic phase disease. Patients with accelerated or blastic phase disease have substantially worse outcomes with allogeneic transplantation. Approximately one in three patients with accelerated phase disease is cured by allogeneic transplantation.[1–6,47] Higher rates of success have been reported in some studies; however, the use of different definitions of accelerated phase disease complicates interpretation of these data. Only one in ten patients with blastic phase disease is cured by transplantation.[1–7,47]

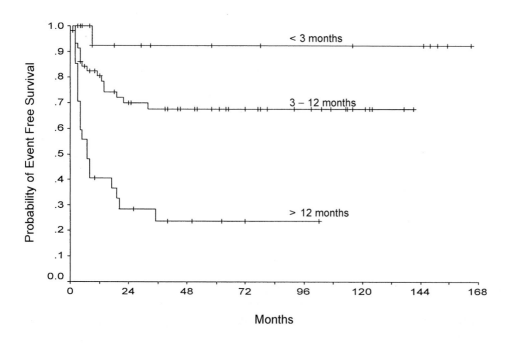

**Figure 37.3** *The probability of event-free survival for patients with chronic phase chronic myelogenous leukemia undergoing allogeneic transplantation less than 3 months, 3 months to a year, or more than a year*

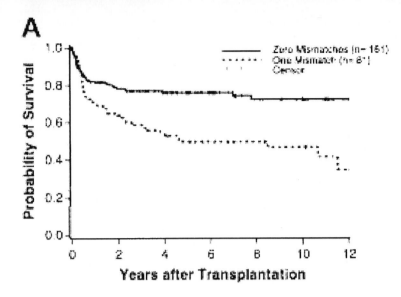

**Figure 37.4** *No deaths occurred beyond 12 years in any group. Among low-risk patients, 12 in the matched group and four in the mismatched group have follow-up beyond 12 years and are indicated as censored observation at 12 years*

## DONOR SOURCE

Unrelated transplantation is perceived by many clinicians to be substantially more dangerous than transplantation using sibling donors. Although overall sustained LFS is roughly 10% lower using unrelated donors, according to international registry data, results in selected patients closely resemble those achievable with siblings. Patients aged 50 years or younger, with well-matched donors, who undergo transplantation within a year of diagnosis, have sustained survival rates of approximately 70%.[29]

The difference in outcome between siblings and matched unrelated donors is closely related to the degree of HLA incompatibility between donor and recipient (Figure 37.4). Patients with chronic phase CML within 2 years of diagnosis, mismatched at a single HLA-A, B, C, DRB1, or DQB1 allele have a significantly worse outcome than their counterparts with no mismatch. A single mismatch of an HLA-C allele or antigen, an occurrence largely unrecognized historically because of the failure to prospectively match donor–recipient pairs at this site, confers a significantly increased risk of mortality.[49]

Multiple mismatches further increase transplant risk. Those involving HLA-DQB increase mortality compared to those not involving HLA-DQB.[49] These findings emphasize the necessity of performance of and appropriate analysis of molecular typing of HLA alleles for donor selection.

## MARROW VERSUS PERIPHERAL BLOOD

The use of peripheral blood cells have been associated with more rapid engraftment and less severe regimen-related toxicities, compared to marrow, in several studies.[50–54] An increased incidence of chronic GVHD with peripheral blood cells has offset this advantage, and most studies indicate similar overall outcomes.

## APPROACH TO PATIENTS

The Gratwohl score estimates transplant outcome using age, disease, stage, interval from diagnosis to transplant, type of donor, and donor–recipient genders.[35] IBMTR data have confirmed the value of this model.[55]

Newly diagnosed patients should be provided with extensive information on imatinib and on transplantation. Most patients who understand well the two approaches will determine their own initial treatment. Physicians must be certain that patients are well informed. Many do not understand the significant influence of treatment delay on transplant outcome, the ease with which the potential for unrelated donor matches can be determined, nor even that molecular evidence of disease is present in patients who respond well to imatinib.

For patients who receive imatinib as initial therapy, response to treatment is predictive of outcome. Patients who achieve a major cytogenetic remission have a prolonged survival. Those who achieve complete cytogenetic remission enjoy the greatest survival advantage.[56,57] Quantitative assays demonstrate that patients who achieve complete cytogenetic remission with imatinib are more than twice as likely as those achieving complete remission with interferon plus cytarabine to have 3 log reductions in Bcr-Abl transcript levels.[58] All patients who achieve this level of reduction are free from progression at 2 years.[58,59] These patients should continue imatinib until they demonstrate progressive disease.

At many centers, patients who fail to achieve substantial reductions in Bcr-Abl positive cells within

3–4 months, or a cytogenetic remission by 6 months, are considered for allogeneic transplantation without further delay. For patients who achieve cytogenetic remission, but later have progressive increase in the proportion of Bcr-Abl positive cells, transplantation is similarly considered without delay.

## MANAGING RELAPSE

Relapse of CML occurs in approximately 10% of patients who undergo myeloablative allogeneic transplantation for chronic phase disease, and in more than 50% of patients with blastic phase disease. Higher relapse rates occur in identical twins and in T-cell depleted transplants, and lower relapse rates occur in patients developing GVHD. These data led to the use of donor lymphocyte infusions to treat patients who relapsed following allogeneic transplantation.[19,20] A majority of patients who recur achieve sustained molecular remissions with appropriately administered DLI. Escalating dose schedules of DLI reduce the frequency of GVHD and marrow aplasia, and improve the effectiveness of this procedure.[20]

Molecular testing for Bcr-Abl transcripts can be used to identify patients who are likely to relapse. Detection of Bcr-Abl transcripts 6 to 12 months following transplantation is highly predictive of subsequent relapse, whereas detection less than 3 months or more than 18 months from transplantation is less predictive.

Quantification of Bcr-Abl offers more reliable prediction of hematologic relapse. Patients with persistently high levels of transcripts or with increasing Bcr-Abl transcripts are highly likely to relapse.

## REDUCED-INTENSITY STEM CELL TRANSPLANTATION

The desire to reduce transplant-related mortality, the effectiveness of donor lymphocyte infusions, and evidence in canine models that low doses of TBI provide sufficient immunosuppression to permit engraftment of histocompatible donor hematopoietic cells[60,61] led to the development and application of reduced intensity regimens in CML.[62–64] Although treatment was initially restricted to patients whose age or co-morbidities placed them at high risk for complications, present studies are designed to evaluate their effectiveness in a broader range of patients.

Reduced-intensity regimens result in less acute toxicity and reduced regimen-related morbidity and mortality.[62–66] However, the incidence of severe GVHD may be similar to that seen with myeloablative regimens.[65–67] Graft rejection[68,69] and relapse occur more frequently,[65,66,68–70] while infectious complications occur at a similar rate.[66,68,71] These regimens permit allogeneic transplantation of individuals who would

not be considered good candidates for myeloablative transplantation. Their widespread application requires further investigation.

## AUTOLOGOUS TRANSPLANTATION

Autografting using Ph-negative stem cells harvested during recovery from induction chemotherapy may result in short-term cytogenetic remission and prolong survival modestly.[72,73] However, Ph-positive hematopoiesis generally recurs quickly.

Several ongoing studies collect mobilized stem cells from patients who are not candidates for allogeneic transplantation and who achieve cytogenetic remissions with imatinib. When patients progress, autotransplantation is carried out. Such studies require sufficient accrual and follow-up to render meaningful results.[74]

## SUMMARY

Multiple areas of controversy surround the appropriate timing of transplantation in individuals with CML. Although the discussion focuses on transplantation as initial therapy, timing of transplantation in patients who first receive imatinib is equally important and more frequently encountered.

Age and the availability of a sibling donor are the two variables most commonly used to determine candidacy for transplantation as initial therapy. Older age does not appear to be a significant adverse factor for allogeneic transplantation when busulfan-based preparative regimens are used. Results with well-matched unrelated donors are similar to those achieved with sibling donors. The ability to assess preliminary results, estimate the probability of finding a suitable donor, and perform allogeneic transplantation quickly, has made early transplantation with unrelated donors a reasonable possibility in a sizable number of patients.

In patients who receive imatinib as initial treatment, monitoring Bcr-Abl transcript levels or, at the least, monitoring of marrow cytogenetics to evaluate initial response and early evidence of progression are vital to provide appropriate care. The effectiveness of reduced-intensity transplants, particularly in patients with progressive disease, has not been firmly established. Reduced-intensity transplantation and autografting should be performed only on appropriate clinical trials.

## CHRONIC LYMPHOCYTIC LEUKEMIA

Chronic lymphocytic leukemia (CLL), the most common leukemia in the Western hemisphere, remains incurable with standard therapies. The increasing use of genetic risk stratification factors, such as cytogenetic abnormalities,[00-00] zeta-associated protein 70 (ZAP-70),[00-00] and immunoglobulin heavy chain variable region (IgVH) mutational status[00-00] allows physicians to identify high-risk patients who likely will fare poorly with standard chemotherapy. CLL patients with unmutated IgVH have a much poorer prognosis than patients with mutated CLL[00-00] and comprise a target population for whom SCT should be considered. However, despite considerable interest in the use of SCT for CLL, the long-term survival benefit of SCT remains unclear in this disease. Autologous SCT has failed to demonstrate a durable long-term survival benefit, whereas myeloablative allogeneic SCT is associated with significant treatment-related mortality (TRM). Non-myeloablative allogeneic SCT has demonstrated promise, but long-term follow-up is lacking. The role of SCT in CLL has been extensively reviewed[00-00]; therefore, this section will focus on selected topics.

## AUTOLOGOUS SCT

Studies of autologous SCT in CLL have produced mixed results, due to patient selection and the variable use of purging techniques. Disease-free survival (DFS) has ranged from 25% to 69%, with similar discrepancies in overall survival (OS).[00-00] Until recently, the best results (63–69% 4-year DFS, 85–94% 4-year OS) were achieved using purged SCT in patients with relatively early disease.[00-00] However, a British MRC study recently reported that autologous SCT using unpurged stem cells achieved 5-year DFS and OS rates of 78% and 52%, respectively, in 65 patients.[00-00] Sixteen of 20 evaluable patients achieved molecular remission by PCR examination of IgVH gene rearrangement. The benefit of stem cell purging has not been demonstrated by randomized studies, and this recent British study showed that excellent results can be obtained without purging.[00-00] Therefore, the use of stem cell purging should remain experimental.

The utility of autologous SCT in high-risk patients with unmutated IgVH has been examined. A retrospective German study of 58 CLL patients (20 mutated, 38 unmutated) showed that unmutated IgVH remained an adverse prognostic factor despite autologous SCT.[00-00] Median time to clinical relapse was 37 months in the unmutated group, whereas only one mutated patient relapsed 4 years post-SCT; the 2-year probability of relapse was 19% and 0%, respectively, for unmutated and mutated patients. Nonetheless, unmutated patients still enjoyed a 2-year OS of 89%. A similar study examined 325 consecutive CLL patients enrolled on clinical studies at the University of Heidelberg.[00-00] Forty-four patients who underwent autologous SCT were matched with 44 similar patients who received chemotherapy without SCT. Unmutated IgVH was

seen in 66% of both cohorts. Median survival from diagnosis for unmutated patients was 139 months for SCT, versus 73 months for chemotherapy, with a hazard ratio (HR) of 0.31 ($p = 0.02$). These studies demonstrate that, while patients with genetic risk factors, such as unmutated IgVH, still do poorly compared to good- or intermediate-risk patients who undergo autologous SCT, autologous SCT still confers benefit onto high-risk CLL patients. Thus, an autologous SCT as part of a clinical trial should be considered for poor-risk CLL patients who are unable to undergo allogeneic SCT.

Despite the promising results of these studies, the utility of autologous SCT in CLL is limited by several factors. Firstly, patients with CLL often have significant marrow and blood involvement that may result in contamination of the stem cell product despite cytoreductive therapy[00-00] Secondly, the predominant chemotherapeutic agent in CLL, fludarabine, is profoundly myelosuppressive and may hamper collection of an adequate number of autologous stem cells. For example, peripheral stem cell mobilization was unsuccessful in 33% of patients in the MRC study.[00-00] Thirdly, the high-dose conditioning regimens used in autologous SCT are associated with a significant risk of secondary myelodysplasia (MDS) or AML; 8% of patients in the MRC study developed MDS/AML.[00-00] Finally, extensive studies in follicle center lymphoma[00-00] and multiple myeloma[00-00] have not demonstrated that autologous SCT is curative in hematologic malignancies that are incurable with standard chemotherapy. In particular, this last factor has dampened enthusiasm for further studies of autologous SCT for CLL, particularly for patients who have an HLA-identical sibling donor. Given the limitations of autologous SCT, the major focus of clinical research in SCT for CLL has shifted to allogeneic SCT.

## MYELOABLATIVE ALLOGENEIC SCT

Allogeneic SCT offers several theoretical advantages over autologous SCT in CLL. First, contamination of the stem cell source and inadequate stem cell collection are not obstacles for allogeneic SCT. Secondly, the use of an allogeneic donor allows for an immunological graft-versus-leukemia (GVL) effect. Although GVL is not as pronounced in allogeneic SCT for CLL as it is for CML, studies have demonstrated that this immunological effect is still important.[00-00] Limited data suggest that TBI-containing conditioning regimens are superior to busulphan and cytotan (BuCy) in CLL. A small study of 25 patients by the Seattle group revealed a 100-day TRM of 57% for BuCy ($n = 7$), compared to 17% for TBI regimens ($n = 18$). Five-year actuarial survival was 56% for 14 patients transplanted with TBI regimens from 1992 to 1999.[00-00] An MD

Anderson study of Cy/TBI in 28 CLL patients observed a 100-day TRM of 11%. Five-year PFS and OS were 78% and 78%, respectively, for chemo-sensitive patients, compared to 26% and 31% for refractory patients.[00-00] Thus, TBI-containing myeloablative regimens offer the potential of long-term survival with acceptable TRM. Although results are superior for chemo-sensitive patients, myeloablative allogeneic SCT benefits a substantial minority of refractory patients.

Although prospective studies of myeloablative allogeneic SCT for CLL have been limited by small sample size and inadequate follow-up, large, retrospective multi-center registry analyses have examined the use of allogeneic SCT in large numbers of CLL patients.[00-00] A retrospective EBMT study of 135 patients showed a 54% 3-year OS and 40% 100-day TRM.[00-00] Similar findings were reported by the IBMTR, with a 45% 3-year OS and 30% 100-day TRM in 242 patients. [00-00] Although patients in these analyses were relatively young (median age 45 and 47), with a median of only two prior therapies, the high TRM may be explained in part by the late stage of the disease in many of these patients. Median time from diagnosis to SCT was 41 and 46 months in the two studies, respectively,[00-00] and 37% of patients in the EBMT study were chemo-refractory entering transplant.[00-00] Although there are no randomized studies, a retrospective comparison showed a 3-year DFS of 57% for allogeneic SCT, versus 24% for purged autologous SCT.[00-00]

Thus, myeloablative allogeneic SCT may offer superior DFS in CLL, compared to autologous SCT. Although 3-year DFS after allogeneic SCT is approximately 50%,[00-00] longer follow-up is needed to determine if this disease remission proves durable over time. However, the advantage in markedly decreased relapse rates with allogeneic SCT is offset by a higher TRM,[00-00] decreasing enthusiasm for this treatment modality in CLL, which is often an indolent disease. Limited data indicate that Bu/Cy may be particularly toxic in this population; in contrast, TBI regimens appear to induce acceptable TRM.[00-00] In order to preserve the immunological GVL effect while reducing TRM, the focus of clinical SCT research in CLL has turned to non-myeloablative allogeneic SCT in recent years (discussed below). However, the ability of myeloablative allogeneic SCT to achieve DFS in a significant minority of chemo-refractory patients indicates that a full allogeneic SCT should be considered for this group of patients. Cy/TBI or a similar TBI regimen should be considered for any CLL patient undergoing full alloegeneic SCT.

## NON-MYELOABLATIVE ALLOGENEIC SCT

The major focus of clinical transplant research in CLL has shifted to non-myeloablative allogeneic SCT. Ideally, the GVL effect of allogeneic SCT can be harnessed, while reducing TRM from acute GVHD, acute infection and organ toxicity associated with myeloablative SCT. Although many reports of non-myeloablative SCT have included CLL with other indolent lymphoproliferative diseases, such as follicle center lymphoma, several studies have specifically examined CLL.[00-00] Fludarabine, busulfan, and ATG were administered to 30 German CLL patients; the stem cell source was a matched related (n = 15) or unrelated (n = 15) donor.[00-00] Grade 2–4 acute GVHD was observed in 56% patients, while 75% developed chronic GVHD.[00-00] Responses were seen in 93% patients, with 40% achieving CR. Of note, it took up to 2 years for patients to achieve CR, suggesting a GVL effect. All patients achieved a molecular CR by PCR, but only six patients were in continued molecular CR after a median follow-up of two years. Two-year TRM, PFS, and OS were 15%, 67%, and 72%, respectively.[00-00]

The EBMT retrospectively examined 77 CLL patients who received a variety of non-myeloablative conditioning regimens, followed by allogeneic SCT. [00-00] Median follow-up was 18 months. Complete chimerism and best response were achieved a median of 3 months post-SCT. One-year TRM was 18%, and the 2-year probability of relapse was 31%. Two-year DFS and OS were 56% and 72%, respectively. Nineteen patients received donor lymphocyte infusion (DLI) for relapse or incomplete donor chimerism, but only seven responded to DLI (37%). Unfortunately, the interpretation of this study was compromised by the heterogeneity of conditioning regimens, and the use of ATG or Campath-1H for T-cell depletion in 40% of patients.

A recent, small German study indicated that non-myeloablative allogeneic SCT may be superior to autologous SCT in obtaining clinical and molecular remissions in high-risk CLL patients with unmutated IgVH, due to a GVL effect. Seven of nine patients (78%) became negative by PCR for allele-specific IgVH after day + 100 post-SCT; attainment of molecular CR occurred after DLI or development of chronic GVHD. In contrast, only six of 26 control CLL patients (23%) achieved a PCR-negative state after autologous SCT.[00-00] Thus, an immunological GVL effect appears to be important in CLL and may confer a long-term survival advantage for allogeneic over autologous SCT, given sufficient time. Finally, the MD Anderson administered fludarabine and cyclophosphamide to 17 patients, 10 of whom also received rituximab, followed by allogeneic SCT. [00-00] Ten patients subsequently received DLI for persistent CLL; 7 achieved a CR, and 2 a PR. Of the 17 patients, 12 achieved a CR and 4 a PR, for an overall response rate of 94%. Interestingly, OS was 100% for patients who received rituximab with conditioning, compared to 14% for patients who did not. Although these results were intriguing, this was a small study, and it is unclear how rituximab may augment or facilitate the GVL effect of allogeneic SCT in CLL.

## SUMMARY

Despite advances in chemotherapy for CLL, this disease remains incurable by standard therapies. Thus, SCT should be considered, especially for younger patients and patients with high-risk genetic features who likely will do poorly with chemotherapy. Non-myeloablative allogeneic SCT is the most promising transplant modality in CLL, and is the focus of most clinical transplant studies in CLL. Short-term DFS of 50–75% has been obtained with acceptable TRM, and molecular responses have been obtained with the onset of GVHD or the therapeutic use of DLI. However, long-term follow-up is lacking, and it is unclear whether the DFS observed during 2 years will prove durable over time. Myeloablative allogeneic SCTs should be considered for patients with bulky or refractory disease; a TBI-containing regimen should be used to reduce TRM. Finally, autologous SCT should be considered for high-risk CLL patients who do not have an allogeneic option. Although autologous SCT has not proven curative in CLL, it still confers a survival advantage on patients with unmutated IgVH. However, it is necessary to limit the number of prior therapies, particularly fludarabine-based regimens, given that insufficient stem cells are collected from a third or more of CLL patients being considered for autologous SCT.

## REFERENCES

1. Rabinowitz I, Larsson R: Chronic myelogenous leukemia: *Wintrobe's Clinical Hematology*. Philadelphia: Lipincott Williams and Wilkins; 2004.
2. Mughal TI, Goldman JM: Chronic myeloid leukemia: *Oxford Textbook of Medicine*. Oxford: Oxford University Press; 2003.
3. Sawyer CL: Chronic myeloid leukemia. *N Eng J Med* 304:1330, 1999.
4. Goldman JM: Chronic myeloid leukemia: current treatment options. *Blood* 98:2039, 2001.
5. Faderal S: Chronic myelogenous leukemia: update on Biology and treatment. *Oncology* 13:169, 1999.
6. Kantarjian HM: Chronic myelogenous leukemia: a multivariate analysis of the association of patient characteristics and therapy with survival. *Blood* 66:1326, 1985.
7. Speck B: Bone marrow transplantation for chronic myeloid leukemia *Semin Hematol* 21:48, 1984.
8. Doney KC: Treatment of chronic granulocytic leukemia by chemotherapy, total body irradiation and allogeneic bone marrow transplantation. *Exp Hematol* 6:738, 1978.
9. Doney KC: Allogeneic bone marrow transplantation for chronic granulocytic leukemia. *Exp Hematol* 9:966, 1981.
10. Clift RA Treatment of chronic granulocytic leukaemia in chronic phase by allogeneic marrow transplantation. *Lancet* 2:621, 1982.
11. Champlin R: Allogeneic bone marrow transplantation for chronic myelogenous leukemia in chronoic or accelerated phase. *Blood* 60:1038, 1982.
12. Thomas ED: Marrow transplantation for the treatment of chronic myelogenous leukemia. *Ann Intern Med* 104:155, 1986.
13. Radich J: HLA-matched related hematopoietic cell transplantation for chronic-phase CML using a targeted busulfan and cycophosphamide preparative regimen. *Blood* 102:31, 2003.
14. Gale RP: Identical-twin bone marrow transplants for leukemia. *Ann Int Med* 120:646, 1994.
15. Horowitz MM: Graft-versus-leukemia reactions after bone marrow transplantation. *Blood* 75:555, 1990.
16. Sullivan KM: Influence of acute and chronic graft-versus-host disease on relapse and survival after one marrow transplantation for HLA-identical siblings as treatment of acute and chronic leukemia. *Blood* 74:1180, 1989.
17. Gratwohl A: Graft-versus-host disease and outcome in HLA-identical sibling transplantation for chronic myeloid leukemia. *Blood* 100:3877, 2002.
18. Glucksberg H: Clinical manifestations of graft-versus-host disease in human recipients of HL-A matched sibling donors. *Transplantation* 18:295, 1974.
19. Levine JE: Prospective trial of chemotherapy and donor leukocyte infusions for relapse of advance myeloid malignancies after allogeneic stem-cell transplantation. *J Clin Oncol* 20:405, 2002.
20. Dazzi F: Comparision of single-dose and escalating-dose regimens of donor lymphocyte infusion for relapse after allografting for chronic myeloid leukemia. *Blood* 95:67, 2000.
21. Daniels EH: Related donor marrow transplant for chronic myeloid leukemia: patient characteristics predicitive of outcome. *Bone Marrow Transplant* 17:537, 1996.
22. van Rhee F: Relapse of chronic myeloid leukemia after allogeneic bone marrow transplants: the case for giving donor leukocyte transfusions before the onset of hematologic relapse. *Blood* 83:3377, 1994.
23. Craddock C: Estimating leukemia-free survival after allografting for chronic myeloid leukemia: a new method that takes into account patients who relapses and are restored to complete remission. *Blood* 96:86, 2000.
24. Clift RA: Marrow transplant for chrionic myeloid leukemia: a randomized study comparing cyclophosphamide and total body irradiation with busulfan and cyclophosphamide. *Blood* 84:2036, 1994.
25. Kroger N: Camparison of total body irradiation vs busulfan in combination with cyclophosphamide as conditioning for unrelated stem cell transplantation in CML patients. *Bone Marrow Transplant* 27:349, 2001.
26. Kim I: Allogeneic bone marrow transplantation for chronic myeloid leukemia: A retrospective study of

busulfan-cytoxan versus total body irradiation-cytoxan as preparative regimen in Koreans. *Clin Transplant* 15:167, 2001.

27. Andersson BS: Conditioning therapy with intravenous busulfan and cyclophosphamide (IV BuCy2) for hematologic malignancies prior to allogeneic stem cell transplantation: a phase II study. *Biol Blood Marrow Transplant* 8:145, 2002.

28. Thall PF.: Comparison of 100-day mortality rates associated with i.v. busulfan and cyclophosphamide vs other preparative regimens in allogeneic bone marrow transplantation for chronic myelogenous leukemia: Bayesian sensitivity analyses of confounded treatment and center effects. *Bone Marrow Transplantation* 33:1191, 2004.

29. Hansen JA: Bone marrow transplants from unrelated donors for patients with chronic myeloid leukemia. *N Engl J Med* 338:962, 1998.

30. Davies SM.: Equivalent outcomes in patients with chronic myelogenous leukemia after early transplantation of phenotypically matched bone marrow from marrow from related or unrelated donors. *Am J Med* 110:339, 2001.

31. Weisdorf DJ: Allogeneic bone marrow transplantation for chronic myelogenous leukemia: comparative analysis of unrelated versus matched sibling donor transplantation. *Blood* 99:1971, 2002.

32. Bolwell BJ: Is bone marrow transplantation appropriate in older patients? In: Bolwell BJ (ed.) *Current Controversies in Bone Marrow Transplantation.* Totowa, NJ: Humana Press; 2000:29:40.

33. Bolwell BJ: Are predictive factors clinically useful in bone marrow transplantation? *Bone Marrow Transplantation* 32:853, 2003.

34. Clift RA: Marrow transplantation for CML: the Seattle experience. *Bone Marrow Transplantation* 17 (Suppl 3): S1, 1996.

35. Gratwohl AH: Risk assessment for patients with chronic myeloid leukaemia before allogeneic blood or marrow transplantation. Chronic Leukemia Working Party of the European Group for Blood and Marrow Transplantation. *Lancet* 352:1087, 1998.

36. Radich JP: The significance of bcr-abl molecular detection in chronic myeloid leukemia patients "late", 18 months or more after transplantation. *Blood* 00098:1701, 2001.

37. Radich JP: Allogeneic hematopoietic stem cell transplantation for chronic myeloid leukemia. *Hematol Oncol Clin N Am* 18:685, 2004.

38. Copelan EA: The influence of early transplantation, age, GVHD prevention regimen, and other factors on outcome of allogeneic transplantation for CML following BuCy. *Bone Marrow Transplantation* 26:1037, 2000.

39. Copelan EA: The influence of early transplantation, age, GVHD prevention regimen, and other factors on outcome of allogeneic transplantation for CML following BuCy. *Bone Marrow Transplantation* 26:1037, 2000.

40. Appelbaum FR: Bone marrow transplantation for chronic myelogenous leukemia. *Semi Oncol* 22:405, 1995.

41. Goldman JM: Choice of pretransplant treatment and timing of transplants for chronic myelogenous leukemia in chronic phase. *Blood* 82:2235, 1993.

42. Beelen DW: Prolonged administration of interferon-alpha in patients with chronic-phase Philadelphia chromosome-positive chronic myelogenous leukemia before allogeneic bone marrow transplantation may adversely affect transplant outcome. *Blood* 85:2981, 1995.

43. Morton AJ: Association between pretransplant interferon-alpha and outcome after unrelated donor marrow transplantation for myelogenous leukemia in chronic phase. *Blood* 92:394, 1998.

44. Gurakt S: Effect of short-term interferon therapy on the outcome of subsequent HLA-identical sibling gone marrow transplantation for chronic myelogenous leukemia: an analysis from the international bone marrow transplant registry. *Blood* 95:410, 2000.

45. Hehlmann, R: Interferon-alpha before allogeneic bone marrow transplantation in chronic myelogenous leukemia does not affect outcome adversely, provided it is discontinued at least 90 days before the procedure. *Blood* 94:3668, 1999.

46. Zander, A: Pre-treatment with glivec increases transplant-related mortality after allogeneic transplant. *Bone Marrow Transplantation* 33:S60, 2004.

47. Horowitz MM: Allogeneic bone marrow transplantation for CML: a report from the International Bone Marrow Transplant Registry. *Bone Marrow Transplantation* 17:S5, 1996.

48. Kernan NA: Analysis of 462 transplantations from unrelated donors facilitated by the National Marrow Donor Program. *N Engl J Med.* 328:593, 1993.

49. Petersdorf EW: Limits of HLA mismatching in unrelated hematopoietic cell transplantation. *Blood* 10B:1182, 2004.

50. Bensinger WI: Transplantation of bone marrow as compared with peripheral-blood cells for HLA-identical relative in patients with hematologic cancers. *N Engl J Med* 344:175, 2001.

51. Blaise D: Randomized trial of bone marrow versus lenograstim primed blood cell allogeneic transplantation in patient with early-stage leukemia: a report from the Societe Francaise de Greffe deMoelle. 18:537, 2000.

52. Heldal D: A randomized study of allogeneic transplantation with stem cells from blood or bone marrow. *Bone Marrow Transplantation* 25:1129, 2000.

53. Morton JH: Granulocyte-colony stimulation factor (G-CSF)-prime allogeneic bone marrow: significantly less graft-versus-host disease and comparable engraftment to G-CSF-mobilized peripheral blood stem cells. *Blood* 98:3186, 2001.

54. Schmitz N: Transplantation of mobilized peripheral blood cells HLA-identical siblings with standard-risk leukemia. *Blood* 100:761, 2002.

55. Passweg J: Validation of the EBMT risk score for recipients of allogeneic hematopoietic stem cell transplants for chronic myelogenous leukemia (CML) (abstract). *Blood.* 2001;98:349a.

56. Marin D: Survival of patients with chronic-phase chronic myeloid leukaemia on imatinib after failure on interferon. *Lancet* 362:617, 2003.

57. Mughal TI: Chronic myeloid leukemia: Current status and controversies. *Oncology* 18:837, 2004.

58. Hughes TP: Frequency of major molecular responses to imatinib or interferon alfa plus cytarabine in newly

diagnosed chronic myeloid leukemia, *N Engl J Med* 349;15 October 2003.

59. Hochhaus A: Imatinib therapy in chronic myelogenous leukemia: strategies to avoid and overcome resistance. *Leukemia* 1:11, 2004.

60. Yu C: DLA-identical bone marrow grafts after low-dose total body irradiation: effects of high-dose corticosteroids and cyclosporine on engraftment. *Blood* 86:4376, 1995.

61. Georges GE: Adoptive immunotherapy in canine mixed chimeras after non-myeloablative hematopoietic cell transplantation. *Blood* 95:3262, 2000.

62. Champlin RE: FLAG-IDA, a non-ablative preparative regimen, with allogeneic PBSC transplantation for CML. *Blood* 96:S1, 2000.

63. Or R: Nonmyeloablative allogeneic stem cell transplantation for the treatment of chronic myeloid leukemia in first chronic phase. *Blood* 101:441, 2003.

64. Bornhauser M: Cooperative German Transplant Study Group. Dose-reduced conditioning for allografting in 44 patients with chronic myeloid leukaemia: a retrospective analysis. *Br J Haematol* 115:119, 2001.

65. Sloand E: The graft-versus-leukemia effect of nonmyeloablative stem cell allografts may not be sufficient to cure chronic myelogenous leukemia. *Bone Marrow Transplantation* 32:897, 2003.

66. Muzaffar H: Nonmyeloablative stem cell transplantation for chroinic myeloid leukemia. *Hematol Oncol Clin North Am* 18:703, 2004.

67. Couriel D: Graft-versus-host disease after nonmyeloablative versus myeloablative conditioning regimens in fully matched sibling donor hematopoietic stem cell transplants. *Blood* 96:408, 2000.

68. Sandmaier BM: Induction of molecular remissions in CML with nonmyeloablative HLA-identical sibling allografts. *Blood* 96:201a, 2000.

69. Giralt S: Nonmyeloablative stem cell transplantation: lessons from the first generation trials. *Leuk Lymphoma Updates* 2:4, 1999.

70. Giralt S: Melphalan and purine analog-containing preparative regimens: reduce-intensity conditioning for patients with hematologic malignancies undergoing allogeneic progenitor cell transplantation. *Blood* 97:631, 2001.

71. Bornhauser M: Cooperative German Transplant Study Group. dose reduced conditioning for allografting in 44 patients with chronic myeloid leukemia: a retrospective analysis. *Br J Haematol* 115(1):119, 2001.

72. Carella AM: Mobilization and transplantation of Philadelphia-negative peripheral blood progenitor cells early in chronic myelogenous leukemia. *J Clin Oncol* 15:1575, 1997.

73. Carella AM: Autografting with Philadelphia chromosome-negative mobilized hematopoietic progenitor cells in chronic myelogenous leukemia. *Blood* 93:1534, 1999.

74. Carella AM.: Autografting in chronic myeloid leukemia. *Semi Hematol*, 40:72, 2003.

75. Lee SJ: Physicians' attitudes about quality of life issues in hematopoietic stem cell transplantation. *Blood* 10:1182, 2004.

76. Caldera H: Stem cell transplantation for multiple myeloma: current status future direction. *Curr Hematol Rep* 3: 249–256, 2004.

77. Crespo M: ZAP-70 expression as a surrogate for immunoglobulin variable region mutations in chronic lymphocytic leukemia. *N Engl J Med* 348:1764–1775, 2003.

78. Damie RN: Ig V gene mutation status and CD38 expression as novel prognostic indicators I chronic lymphocytic leukemia. *Blood* 1840–1847, 1999.

79. Dohner H: Gene deletion predicts for poor survival and non-response to therapy with purine analogs in chronic B-cell leukemias. *Blood* 85:1580–1589, 1995.

80. Dohner H: Genomic aberrations and survival in chronic lymphocytic leukemia. *N Engl J Med* 343: 1910–1916, 2000.

81. Doney KC: Allogeneic related donor hematopoietic stem cell transplantation for treatment of chronic lymphocytic leukemia. *Bone Marrow Transplant* 29:817–823, 2002.

82. Dreger P: Treatment-related mortality and graft-versus-leukemia activity after allogeneic stem transplantation for chronic lymphocytic leukemia using intensity-reduced conditioning. *Leukemia* 17:841–848, 2003.

83. Dreger P: The prognostic impact of autologous stem cell transplantation in patients with chronic lymphocytic leukemia: a risk-matched analysis based on the VH gene mutational status. *Blood* 103:2850–2858, 2004.

84. Dreger P: Prognostic factor for survival after autologous stem cell transplantation for chronic lymphocytic leukemia (CLL): The EBMT experience. 2000.

85. Dreger P: Efficacy and prognostic implications of early autologous stem cell transplantation for poor-risk chronic lymphocytic leukemia (CLL). *Blood* 96:483a, 2000.

86. El Rouby S: p53 gene mutation in B-cell chronic lymphocytic leukemia is associated with drug resistance and is independent of MDR1/MDR3 gene expression. *Blood* 82:3452–3459, 1993.

87. Hamblin TJ: Unmutated Ig VH genes are associated with a more aggressive form of chronic lymphocytic leukemia. *Blood* 94:1848–1854, 1999.

88. Hamblin TJ: Immunoglobulin V genes associated with a more aggressive form of chronic lymphocytic leukemia. *Blood* 95:2455–2457, 2000.

89. Hamblin TJ: CD38 expression and immunoglobulin variable region mutations are independent prognostic variables in chronic lymphocytic leukemia, but CD38 expression may vary during the course of the disease. *Blood* 99:1023–1029, 2002.

90. Horowitz M: Hematopoietic stem cell transplantation (SCT) for chronic lymphocytic leukemia (CLL). *Blood* 96:522a, 2000.

91. Jabbour E: Stem cell transplantation for chronic lymphocytic leukemia: should not more patients get a transplant? *Bone Marrow Transplant* 34:289–297, 2004.

92. Khouri IF: Hematopoietic stem cell transplantation for chronic lymphocytic leukemia. *Curr Opin Hematol* 5:454–459, 1998.

93. Khouri IF: Long-term follow-up of patients with CLL treated with allogeneic hematopoietic transplantation. *Cytotherapy* 4:217–221, 2002.

94. Khouri IF: Nonablative allogeneic stem cell transplantation for chronic lymphocytic leukemia: impact of

rituximab on immunomodulation and survival. *Exp Hematol* 32:28–35, 2004.

95. Lin TS: Augologous stem cell transplantation for non-Hodgkin's lymphoma. *Curr Hematol Rep* 2:310–315, 2003.

96. Michallet MR: Allogeneic hematopoietic stem cell transplantation (HSCT) for chronic lymphocytic leukemia (CLL): results and prognostic factors for survival after transplantation: analysis from EBMT registry. *Blood* 96:205a, 2000.

97. Milligan DW: Autografting for younger patients with chronic lymphocytic leukemia is safe and achieves a high percentage of molecular responses: results of the MRC Pilot Study. *Blood*. In press.

98. Montserrat E: Autologus stem cell transplantation (ASCT) for chronic lymphocytic leukemia (CLL): results in 107 patients. *Blood* 94:396a, 1999.

99. Rabinowe SN: Autologous and allogeneic bone marrow transplantation for poor prognosis patients with B-cell chronic lymphocytic leukemia. *Blood* 82:1366–1376, 1993.

100. Rassenti LZ: ZAP-70 is a more reliable marker of disease progression risk than immunoglobulin mutation status in chronic lymphocytic leukemia. *Blood* 102:34a, 2003.

101. Ritgen M: Unmutated immunoglobulin variable heavy-chain gene status remains an adverse prognostic factor after autologous stem cell transplantation for chronic lymphocytic leukemia. *Blood* 101:2049–2053, 2003.

102. Ritgen M: Graft-versus-leukemia activity may overcome therapeutic resistance of chronic lymphocytic leukemia with unmutated immunoglobulin variable heavy chain gene status: implications of minimal residual disease measurement with quantitative PCR. *Blood*. In press.

103. Schetelig: Reduced non-relapse mortality after reduced intensity conditioning in advance chronic lymphocytic leukemia. *Ann Hematol* 81(Suppl 2):S47–48, 2002.

104. Schetelig J: Evidence of a graft-versus-leukemia effect in chronic lymphocytic leukemia after reduced-intensity conditioning and allogeneic stem-cell transplantation: the Cooperative German Transplant Study Group. *J Clin Oncol* 21: 2747–2753, 2003.

105. Petersdof EW: Limits of HLA mismatching in unrelated hematopoietic cell transplantation. *Blood* 104:9. 2004.

# Section 1
# MYELODYSPLASTIC SYNDROMES

## Chapter 38

# MYELODYSPLASTIC SYNDROMES: MOLECULAR BIOLOGY, PATHOLOGY, AND CYTOGENETICS

*Rami Komrokji and John M Bennett*

## INTRODUCTION

The myelodysplastic syndrome (MDS) is a heterogeneous group of clonal neoplastic stem cell disorders. The disease is characterized clinically by bone marrow failure with peripheral cytopenias and a tendency to progress to acute myeloid leukemia (AML). Pathologically, dysplastic morphologic features in the peripheral blood and bone marrow gives the disease its misnomer as myelodysplastic syndrome, although it is truely neoplastic.[1]

The recognition and classification of MDS have evolved over the years as we learn more about the disease. The description of refractory anemia early in the past century was followed by the observation of progression to leukemia. MDS was then recognized as a primary bone marrow failure disorder. The French-American-British classification (FAB) and its revision addressed the heterogeneity in the subtypes and noted the variability in progression to AML.[2,3] The new World Health Organization (WHO) classification refined the FAB classification in an attempt to better predict outcome by using more homogenous and distinct subgroups.[4]

MDS is predominantly a disease of the older adults, probably reflecting the requirement of multiple and prolonged leukemogens for the disease to develop. MDS may be more common than chronic lymphocytic leukemia (CLL). The estimated incidence is 4/100,000 US citizens per year and it increases with age.[5] Majority of patients will succumb to the disease, more so because of infections and their complications rather than AML evolution.[6] Only one third of patients will eventually progress to AML, a process that may result from accumulating further DNA damage, as well as from clonal evolution.

## PATHOGENESIS MODEL

The occurrence of MDS is best viewed in the framework of a multi-hit theory. Hereditary and multiple environmental factors result in a neoplastic stem cell clone.[7] The MDS clone is characterized by altered gene functions; the gene alterations result either from single-gene mutations, chromosomal abnormalities (mostly deletions), or gene silencing. Many of those altered genes are suppressor genes that function in a recessive manner. Various gene alterations of MDS clone result in an intrinsic increase in the susceptibility of the clone to apoptosis. MDS clone is also recognized by the immune system leading, in some cases, to clonal T-cell proliferation that leads to release of various cytokines, including TNF alpha.[8–10] The cytokines cause the apoptosis of the MDS clone and of normal hematopoietic cells.[11] This intrinsic and immune-mediated susceptibility to apoptosis are the hallmarks of early MDS pathogenesis, explaining the clinical findings of peripheral cytopenias despite a hypercellular bone marrow.[12]

## EVIDENCE OF CLONALITY

The neoplastic MDS clone arises from a pluripotent stem cell. The evidence of clonality was originally demonstrated through G6PD mosaicism.[13] Subsequently, cytogenetic studies revealed two clones with and without trisomy eight in patients with sideroblastic anemia.[14] Clonality is also supported by restriction fragment length polymorphisms (RFLPs) of X-chromosome genes and by the use of fluorescence in-situ hybridization (FISH).[15] The assay is based on differences in X chromosome inactivation patterns between normal and neoplastic tissues of female patients. In a polyclonal cell population, the maternal X chromosome is active in half the cells and inactive in the other half, while in a monoclonal cell population, the maternal X chromosome is either active or inactive in all the cells. This difference in the pattern of X chromosome inactivation between normal and neoplastic cell populations can be demonstrated, in females heterozygous for a particular RFLP, by a Southern blot analysis using X-linked DNA probes with restriction enzymes capable of differentially cleaving the material from the paternal X chromosome on one hand, and the active from the inactive X chromosome on the other. Several studies have also shown evidence of clonality in lymphoid lineages as well, suggesting that the MDS clone arises from early pluripotent stem cells capable of myeloid and lymphoid differentiation.[16,17] Karyotypic evolution and complex karyotypic changes may occur with progression of MDS and transformation to AML.

## GENE ALTERATIONS

Loss or gain of gene function can result from single-gene mutations, chromosomal translocations (unbalanced or balanced), and epigenetic alterations, such as silencing of gene expression by hypermethylation. The net result is either gain of an oncogene function or loss of tumor-suppressor gene function. Tumor-suppressor gene function in a recessive fashion that requires loss of both alleles.[18] Haploinsufficiency (loss of a single gene copy) can result in reduction of the gene products and a predisposition to malignancies.[19]

The RAS gene family is the most studied in MDS. Ten to forty percent of patients with MDS have RAS mutations. The most common mutation is a single base change at codon 12 of the N-RAS family. The resultant mutated N-RAS protein retains an active GTP form, promoting continuous signaling to the nucleus. N-RAS mutations carry a higher risk of AML transformation and portend a worse prognosis.

Other gene mutations described in MDS include P53 tumor suppression gene (5–10% of cases);[20] FLT3 oncogene receptor tyrosine kinase (5% of cases);[21] P15 ink4b, a tumor suppressor gene that is transcriptionally repressed through promoter silencing by hypermethylation (can be present in up to 50% of high-grade MDS).[22] The abnormality is seen with the 7q- syndrome and is associated with shorter survival.[23] Microsatellite instability (MSI) resulting from defective mismatch repair genes (MMR) has been described particularly in therapy related MDS (t-MDS).[24] Table 38.1 lists a few of the described genes that are altered in MDS.

Certain co-existing gene mutations may increase the individual susceptibility to develop MDS; the NQO1 gene mutation increases the risk for t-MDS in both the homozygotic and heterozygotic states. NQO1 is a quinone oxireductase required for detoxifying benzene derivatives.[25,26]

| Table 38.1 | Altered genes in MDS | | |
|---|---|---|---|
| Gene | Abnormality | Significance in MDS | Function |
| BCL-2 | Overexpression | High risk MDS | Anti-apoptosis |
| CSF1R/FMS | Mutation | High risk MDS | Encodes macrophage CSF |
| GCSFR | Mutation | Congenital neutropenia and progression to MDS/AML | Encodes G-CSF receptor |
| FLT 3 | Internal tandem duplication | High risk MDS, progression to AML | Encodes tyrosine kinase receptor |
| MDR1 | Expressed | Drug resistance | Transmembrane efflux pump |
| MPL | Overexpressed | High risk MDS | Encodes thrombopoeitin receptor |
| NF1 | Mutation | Pediatric MDS | Tumor suppressor gene |
| NRAS | Mutation | Early MDS | Cell signaling pahtway |
| P15 ink4b | Hypermethylation | High risk MDS | Cycline-dependent kinase inhibitor |
| P53 | Mutation | Early and high risk MDS, poor prognosis | Arrests cell cycle to allow DNA damage repair |
| Telomerase | Increase activity | High risk MDS | Maintain telomere length |

## MICROARRAY ANALYSIS IN MDS

The introduction of microarray analysis revolutionized the analysis of gene profiles. Not only can thousands of genes be analyzed together, but the technique also identifies gene profiles, "molecular signatures" that can help refine the disease, categorize its subtypes, better predict outcomes, and hopefully tailor therapies.

Microarray analysis studies in MDS identified new important genes, profiles that may help distinguish MDS from AML, as well as low risk from high risk MDS. In one study, investigators were able to discriminate between healthy control bone marrow samples and samples from MDS patients using the expression profile of 11 selected genes representing different gene classes. The gene expression profile was also able to discriminate between low risk and high risk MDS. The retinoic acid induced gene (RAI3), radiation-inducible immediate early response gene (IEX1), and the stress-induced phosphoprotein 1 (STIP1) gene were among the genes down-regulated in low risk MDS reflecting that the CD34 MDS, stem cells may lack the defensive proteins and thus be more susceptible to damage.[27] In another study, researchers were able to distinguish between AML blasts and MDS blasts by using gene profiles. Delta-like gene (Dlk), Tec gene, and inositol 1,4,5-triphosphate receptor type 1 gene were among those highly specific for MDS. The Dlk 1 gene, for example, may be an important gene in cell proliferation and may allow stromal cells to support stem cells.[28] Gene sets identified for early stage MDS included the PIASy gene (PIAS family are a group of signaling proteins), which functions as a tumor-suppressor gene. As MDS progresses and transforms to AML, those gene expressions are decreased.[29]

## CYTOGENETICS

Chromosomal abnormalities are described in 40–70% of all MDS cases.[30] Chromosomal abnormalities usually consist of an unbalanced loss, deletion, or translocation. It may be surprising to find a normal karyotype in 30–60% of a clonal disease; however, this could be explained by technical failures, as well as karyotypic evolution over time. A normal karyotype does, however, carry a better prognosis, similar to the 5q- syndrome, 20q-, or loss of chromosome Y. A complex karyotype is defined as the presence of three or more different cytogenetic abnormalities. It occurs in 10–20% of primary MDS and in up to 90% of therapy-related MDS. Table 38.2 lists the most common chromosomal abnormalities in primary and therapy related MDS.[31] More cytogenetic abnormalities occur in high risk MDS and therapy related MDS. The reported frequency of cytogenetic abnormalities under the new WHO classification are: refractory anemia 25%; refractory anemia with ring sideroblasts 10%; refractory

**Table 38.2** Cytogenetic abnormalities in MDS

| Cytogenetic abnormality | Primary MDS | Therapy-related MDS |
|---|---|---|
| All over | 40–70% | 80–90% |
| −5/ del (5q) | 10–20% | 90% −5 or −7 |
| −7/ del (7q) | 5–10% | |
| +8 | 10% | 10% |
| −Y | 10% | |
| 17 p− | 7% | |
| del(20q) | 5% | |
| t(11q23) | 5–6% | 3% |
| Complex karyotype | 10–20% | 90% |

cytopenia with multi-lineage dysplasia 50%; and refractory anemia with excess blasts type I & II 30–50%.[32] Cytogenentic abnormalities do not correlate with WHO subtypes, except for the 5q- syndrome, which represents a separate entity, and isodicentric X chromosome associated with ring sideroblasts.[31]

### LOSS OF CHROMOSOME 5/del(5q)

Loss of chromosome 5 or interstitial deletion of its long arm is one of the most common chromosomal abnormalities described in primary and therapy-related MDS (see Table 38.2). This abnormality is associated with previous exposure to carcinogens, including benzene, alkylating agents, and radiation.[33] This −5/del(5q) abnormality is distinguished from the 5q-syndrome. The 5q- syndrome is associated with a macrocytic anemia and often thrombocytosis. It occurs more commonly in upper middle age females, and carries the best prognosis of MDS subtypes. The deletion in the 5q- syndrome breakpoint, which involves band 5q33, contains a different myeloid tumor-suppressor gene from the 5q31 band that is commonly involved in -5/del (5q).[31]

### LOSS OF CHROMOSOME 7/Del(7q)

Monosomy 7 or deletion of the long arm of chromosome 7 is well described in therapy-related MDS and primary MDS (see Table 38.2). The breakpoint 7q22 is more commonly associated with MDS cases. A monosomy 7 syndrome entity is described in the pediatric literature, and is common in juvenile myelomonocytic leukemia (JMML). Interestingly, −7/del(7q) is the most common abnormality described in patients with hereditary predispositions to MDS, such as Fanconi anemia.[31,34]

Loss of 7q is associated with AML1 gene mutations. Monosomy 7 or deletion of the long arm of chromosome 7 is associated with a poor outcome in children and adults.

### TRISOMY 8

Trisomy 8 is described in different hematological malignancies including MDS. Its significance is not well understood.[31,34]

### LOSS OF Y CHROMOSOME

Loss of chromsome Y is described in patients with hematological and non-hematological diseases, and by itself does not represent diagnostic evidence of a hematological process.[35] Once present, however, in MDS it may carry a favorable prognosis.

### LOSS OF THE SHORT ARM OF CHROMOSOME 17

17p syndrome is associated morphologically with the classical pseudo-Pelger-Huët hypolobulation. The p53 gene is located on 17p13.1 and is often involved in this syndrome.[31]

### DELETION OF THE LONG ARM OF CHROMOSOME 20

Del (20q) carries a favorable prognosis as an isolated abnormality. It is more often seen in early MDS. Prominent erythrocytic and megakaryocytic dysplasia is often seen. Mature granulocytes from the peripheral blood may lack the abnormality, suggesting an increased propensity for apoptosis in the clone carrying this abnormality.[31,34] Isochromosome 20q with loss of interstitial material i (20q-) was described recently in six MDS patients out of a registry of 998. This was seen more commonly in older patients, whose MDS behaved different clinically from the 20q-syndrome, with its rapid progression and shorter survival. The i (20q-) could represent a further evolution of the 20q karyotype, thus predicting disease progression.[36]

### 11q23 SYNDROME

Translocations involving 11q23 are classically described in therapy-related MDS secondary to topoisomerase II class drugs.[37,38] The MLL (mixed lineage leukemia) gene is located on 11q23, and in acute leukemia usually portends a poor prognosis. The exact involvement of the MLL gene in primary MDS is not well defined.[34]

### OTHER CHROMOSOMAL ABNORMALITIES

t(5;12)(q33;p13) occurs in 2–3% of CMML cases. The translocation results in a fusion oncogene TEL/PDGFßR. TEL is a transcription factor gene located on chromosome 12p13.1. It is involved in angiogenesis and hematopoesis. TEL fuses to the transmembrane and cytoplasmic domains of PDGFR, replacing the ligand-binding site, and leads to autoactivation of the PDGFR.[39,40] CMML patients with this translocation may benefit from therapy with imatinib mesylate as well as other tyrosine kinase inhibitors.[40–42] Other translocations reported in CMML includes: t(5;17)(q33;p13) (Rabaptin-5/PDGFßR),[43] t(5;7)(q33; p11.2) (HIP1/PDGFßR),[44] and t(5;10)(q33;q21) (H4-D10S170/PDGFßR).[43] Cytogenetic abnormalities are seen in 20–30% of CMML cases.[45]

t(3,21) is described in t-MDS/AML. EAP (Epstein-Barr virus small RNAs associated protein) at 3q26 fuses to the RUNX1 gene (AML gene) on 21q22 leading to truncation of RUNX1 and loss of its function. Two other genes described on 3q26 include EVI1 (ecotropic virus infection site) and MDS/EVI1 (MDS associated sequences). The MDS/EVI1 gene fuses to RUNX1, leading to a different EVI1 protein.[31] Patients with MDS who have EVII abnormalities may benefit from therapy with arsenic trioxide.

The Philadelphia chromosome t(9,22) has been described in MDS. Ph+MDS patients had a median survival of 13 months in one review.[46] Translocations seen in AML, such as t(8,21) or inv(16), have also been described in MDS.

### CYTOGENETICS AND PROGNOSIS OVERVIEW

The international prognostic scoring system (IPSS) is one of the best available systems to predict prognosis and AML evolution in MDS. The IPSS was developed by the international MDS risk analysis workshop. Data were pooled from seven previous studies that used independent risk-based prognostic systems. In a multivariate analysis age, gender, cytogenetics, cytopenias, and bone marrow blasts were significant independent prognostic variables.[47]

According to cytogenetics, patients were placed into three categories: a good prognosis group with normal cytogenetics, −Y, del(5q), and del(20q); a poor prognosis group, including patients with three or more cytogenetic anomalies or chromosome 7 anomalies; and other anomalies, classified in the intermediate group. The median survival in years for good, intermediate, and poor prognosis groups were 3.8, 2.4, and 0.8 years, respectively. The time to 25% AML evolution was 5.6, 1.6, and 0.9 years, respectively.[47,48]

## APOPTOSIS IN MDS

Apoptosis may carry the explanation for the paradoxical observation of peripheral cytopenias and a normo- or hypercellular bone marrow in MDS.[49,12] Evidence of apoptosis in MDS is supported by various techniques. Apoptosis was first observed by electron microscopic examination of the bone marrow in MDS patients. Evidence of apoptosis was also shown by biochemical techniques, in situ methods, and flow cytometric studies.[12]

Apoptosis seems to be greater in the early stages of MDS and decreases as MDS progresses and transforms to AML. Flow cytometric studies revealed that the proportion of CD34+ cells in G1-DNA phase is higher in early MDS. Also, the ratio of c-Myc (a pro-apoptotic gene) to BCL 2 (an anti-apoptotic gene) decreases as MDS progresses to AML.[50] It is controversial whether apoptosis is restricted to CD34+ progenitors, or whether it also includes mature cells.[12]

Several mechanisms can explain the observation of excessive apoptosis in MDS. The MDS clone itself may carry an intrinsic liability for apoptosis due to altered gene functions and expression; however, there is a lack of correlation between cytogenetic abnormalities and apoptosis, suggesting that the phenomenon is not only restricted to the MDS clone.[51,52] Increased apoptosis in MDS could also be secondary to inhibitory cytokines (mainly TNF-α) that can induce apoptosis and may affect both the MDS clone and normal cells.[53,54] Increased expression of FAS ligand (CD 95 cell surface protein) in MDS bone marrow cells could also be one of the mechanisms contributing to apoptosis.[55] Other potential mechanisms include cell cycle abnormalities and mithochondrial abnormalities leading to increased apoptosis. Mutations of mitochondrial DNA may also impair iron metabolism, contributing to sideroblastic anemia.[12]

## MICROENVIRONMENT IN MDS

The hematopoietic microenvironment refers to the fibroblasts, adipose cells, macrophages, endothelial cells, and the supportive matrix of the bone marrow.[56] Though still somewhat controversial, there is growing evidence that abnormalities of the supporting stroma affect its ability to effectively support normal hematopoiesis in MDS.[56–59]

Using in vitro studies, abnormalities of the hematopoietic microenvironment in patients with MDS were demonstrated.[60] Adherent cell layers were developed in long-term bone marrow cultures (LTMC) from MDS patients and normal marrows. The adherent cell layer consisted of a mixture of cells, mostly fibroblasts and macrophages. Morphologically, the adherent cell layer appeared to be normal in MDS, however, it produced more IL-6 and TNF compared to normal bone marrow. The adherent cell layers were then separated into macrophage, and fibroblast-enriched cell layers, both of which demonstrated increased apoptosis. The macrophage-enriched cell layer produced significantly higher TNF-α, while the fibroblast-enriched layer produced significantly higher IL-6 than normal marrows. A dysfunctional stroma may also contribute to the pathogenesis of MDS. Reports of donor cell leukemia or MDS after allogeneic stem cell transplant may represent supporting evidence for the role of the microenvironment and stroma in disease pathogenesis.[61]

## PATHOLOGY

Pathological dysplastic features are the hallmark of MDS. The diagnosis of MDS requires careful examination of the peripheral blood, bone marrow aspirate, and core biopsy. MDS is a diagnosis of exclusion, and no single dysplastic or morphological feature is pathognomonic. The pathological examination should provide information regarding the presence of dysplasia, the cell lines involved, the percentage of bone marrow blasts, and the presence and percentage of ring sideroblasts.

The French-American-British (FAB) system served as the gold standard classification for MDS for more than 20 years.[2,3] The new WHO classification was built on the FAB classification system with further attempts to refine the classification.[4] Table (38.3) summarizes the WHO subtypes and the required criteria for the diagnosis of each. Briefly, the major changes in the WHO classification include the introduction of multi-lineage dysplasia (defined as more than 10% dysplastic progeny of two or more cell lines and less than 5% blasts) and preservation of the subtypes refractory anemia and refractory anemia with ring sideroblasts to uni-lineage dysplasia and less than 10% dysplasia in either the myeloid or the megakaryocytic cell lines. Refractory anemia with excess blasts is subdivided into type I (5-9% blasts) and type II (10-19%) blasts. Refractory anemia with excess blasts in transformation is eliminated and the threshold for diagnosis of AML is lowered to 20% blasts instead of 30% blasts. Chronic myelomonocytic leukemia is moved to a separate category (myelodysplastic/myeloproliferative disorders) along with atypical chronic myelogenous leukemia (CML) and JMML. Finally, the 5q- syndrome is recognized as a distinct entity due to its unique clinical presentation and favorable outcome.[32,62,48].

The recommendations for the diagnosis of MDS are the same in the WHO and FAB classifications.[32] Peripheral blood and a bone marrow aspirate and biopsy should be examined. Cytogenetics should be tested when feasible. The standard stains (Romanowsky, hematoxylin and eosin) should be done, in addition to the Prussian blue stain for iron and the reticulin stain for fibrosis. Silver stains may reveal sideroblasts in cases of iron deficiency anemia.[63] To determine the percentage of blasts, a 500-cell differential should be performed on the bone marrow and a 200-cell differentiation on the peripheral blood.

The dysplastic features in the bone marrow and peripheral blood include:

*Dyserythropoietic features*: In the bone marrow these include multinuclearity, nuclear fragments, megaloblastoid changes, cytoplasmic abnormalities, and increased erythroblasts (Figure 38.1(a) and (b)). In the peripheral blood manifestations may include poikilocytosis, anisocytosis, nucleated red blood cells, and basophilic stippling.

*Dysgranulopoietic features*: These include hypolobulation, nuclear sticks, ring-shaped nuclei, and hypogranulation. The classical pseudo-Pelger-Huët neutrophils should be seen in more than 10% of the peripheral neutrophils (Figure 38.1(a)).

*Dysmegakaryocytopoietic features*: These include micromegakaryocytes, large mononuclear forms, and multiple small nuclei (Figure 38,1(c)).

*Abnormal sideroblasts*: These are defined by five or more iron granules. When the granules encircle one third or more of the nucleus in iron stained smears, the term

**Table 38.3**    The WHO classification of MDS and required criteria for diagnosis

| Category | Percentage of MDS cases | Peripheral blood | Bone marrow |
|---|---|---|---|
| Refractory anemia (RA) | 5–10% | Anemia <br> <1% blasts <br> $< 1 \times 10^9$ monocytes | Erythroid dysplasia <br> < 10 % myeloid or megakaryocytic dysplasia <br> < 5% blasts <br> < 15% sideroblasts |
| Refractory anemia with ring sideroblasts (RARS) | 10–15% | Anemia <br> < 1% blasts <br> $< 1 \times 10^9$ monocytes | Erythroid dysplasia <br> < 10 % myeloid or megakaryocytic dysplasia <br> < 5% blasts <br> > 15% sideroblasts |
| Refractory cytopenia with multilineage dysplasia (RCMD) | 24% | Bi-or pancytopenia <br> < 1% blasts <br> $< 1 \times 10^9$ monocytes | Dysplasia in > 10% of the cells in two or more cell lines <br> < 5% blasts in BM <br> < 15% sideroblasts |
| Refractory anemia with multilineage dysplasia and ring sideroblasts (RCMD-RS) | 15% | Bi-or pancytopenia <br> < 1% blasts <br> $< 1 \times 10^9$ monocytes | Dysplasia in > 10% of the cells in two or more cell lines <br> < 5% blasts in BM <br> > 15% sideroblasts |
| Refractory anemia with excess blasts type I and II (RAEB-1 & RAEB II) | 40% | Cytopenia <br> Type I: 1–5% blasts <br> Type II: 6–19% blasts | Uni or multilineage dysplasia <br> Type I 5–9% blasts <br> Type II 10–19% blasts |
| 5q syndrome | ? | Normal or elevated platelets <br> < 5% blasts | Normal or increased megakaryocytes <br> < 5% blasts |
| MDS unclassified ( MDS-U) | ? | Cytopenia <br> < 1% blasts | Unilineage dyplasia of myeloid or megakaryocytic line <br> < 5% blasts |

"ringed sideroblast" is applied (Figure 38.1(d)). Ring sideroblast MDS subtypes have more than 15% ring sideroblasts and less than 5% blasts.

In addition to the aspirate, the bone marrow biopsy may give helpful information. A bone marrow biopsy allows for a better assessment of cellularity. MDS bone marrow is typically normo or hypercellular;[64] however, hypoplastic MDS, an entity that resembles aplastic anemia, could be challenging to differentiate from aplastic anemia or hypocellular AML.[65] A bone marrow biopsy can also help assess the degree of fibrosis, as in 50% of MDS cases some degree of fibrosis may be seen on reticulin stains.[66,67] Dysmegakaryocytes may be easier to identify on a bone marrow biopsy. Finally, identification of abnormal localization of immature precursors (ALIP) may carry a poor prognosis. ALIP are defined as the presence of three or more foci of immature cells—myeloblasts or promyelocytes—displaced from the paratrabecular area to the intertrabecular areas.[68]

Cytochemical and immunocytochemical stains could be an adjunct in the diagnosis of MDS in identifying its subtypes. Peroxidase and Sudan Black stains are helpful in distinguishing the myeloid origin of the blasts, though peroxidase can decrease over the course of MDS.[69] Esterase and double esterase stain can help distinguish dysplastic granulocytes from early monocytes.[70] Staining megakaryocytes for GP IIb/IIIa using alkaline phosphatase anti-alkaline phosphatase (APAAP)

can help distinguish small dysplastic megakaryocytes that could be mistaken for lymphocytes.[71] Flow cytometry can detect immunophenotypic abnormalities in cases when combined morphology and cytogenetics are nondiagnostic.[72] Immunophenotypic myeloid dysplasia features include hypogranular neutrophils based on orthogonal scatter, CD64 negativity, and low CD11b, CD16, and CD13 expression. Erythroid immunophenotypic dysplasia includes decreased CD71 (transferrin receptor) expression on glycophorin A+ precursors. Megakaryocytic lineage dysplasia is, however, difficult to recognize currently immunophenotypically.

## SUMMARY

The myelodysplastic syndromes are heterogeneous clonal stem cell disorders characterized by dysplastic pathological features, clinical peripheral cytopenias, and a tendency to progress to AML.

The pathogenesis of MDS includes clonal gene function alterations due to single-gene alteration, chromosomal abnormalities or epigenetic phenomenon. Apoptosis can explain the paradoxical observation of peripheral cytopenias and normo- or hypercellular bone marrow. Different mechanisms, such as abnormal cytokines production and intrinsic clonal susceptibility lead to excessive apoptosis. Alterations in the

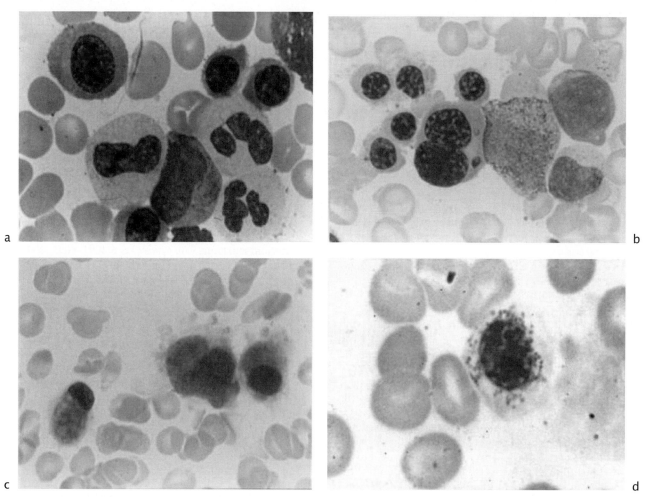

**Figure 38.1** *Bone marrow: (a) megaloblastoid erythroid precursor, pseudo-Pelger-Huët neutrophils (bilobed and hypogranular), and a myeloblast with Auer rods; (b) dysplastic erythroid precursors, bi-nucleated erythroid precursor, and a myeloblast; (c) mononuclear and micromegakaryocytes; (d) Prussian blue stain of the bone marrow showing a ring sideroblast*

immune system and bone marrow microenvironment clearly contribute to the development of MDS.

Pathologically, dysplasia is the hallmark of the disease. A careful pathological exam of the peripheral blood and bone marrow aspirate, and biopsy is necessary for diagnosis and better classification. MDS remains a diagnosis of exclusion. Cytogenetic testing using conventional analysis as well as molecular methods, such as fluorescence in-situ hybridization should be done when feasible. The clinician should use the information from pathologic examination and cytoge-

netic testing to better classify the disease, predict the prognosis, and hopefully tailor the treatment.

In the future, we will continue to explore the molecular biology and different pathogenetic aspects of the disease to develop a better understanding and to translate the basic science findings into targeted therapies. The new WHO classification may allow us to classify the disease into more homogenous classes, to develop treatments for those subtypes, and to continue refining the classification, as we understand the biology and behavior of the disease.

### REFERENCES

1. Bennett JM, Komrokji R, Kouides P: The myelodysplastic syndromes. In: Abeloff Martin D, Armitage James O, Niederhuber John E., et al. (eds.) *Clinical Oncology.* 3rd ed. New York: Churchill Livingstone; 2004.
2. Bennett JM, Catovsky D, Daniel MT, et al.: Proposals for the classification of theacute leukaemias. French-American-British (FAB) Co-operative Group. *Br J Haematol* 33:451–458, 1976.
3. Bennett JM, Catovsky D, Daniel MT, et al.: Proposals for the classification of the myelodysplastic syndromes. *Br J Haematol* 51:189–199, 1982.
4. Harris NL, Jaffe ES, Diebold J, et al.: World Health Organization classification of neoplastic diseases of the hematopoietic and lymphoid tissues: report of the Clinical Advisory Committee meeting—Airlie House, Virginia, November 1997. *J Clin Oncol* 17(12):3835–3849, 1999.
5. Aul C, Gattermann N, Schneider W: Age-related incidence and other epidemiological aspects of myelodysplastic syndromes. *Br J Haematol* 82:358–367, 1992.
6. Pomeroy C, Oken MM, Rydell RE, et al: Infection in the myelodysplastic syndromes. *Am J Med* 90:338–344, 1991.

7. Gallagher A, Darley RL, Padua R: The molecular basis of myelodysplastic syndromes. *Haematologica* 82:191–204, 1997.

8. Smith MA, Smith JG: The occurrence subtype and significance of haemopoietic inhibitory T cells (HIT cells) in myelodysplasia: an in vitro study. *Leuk Res* 15:597–601, 1991.

9. Molldrem JJ, Jiang YZ, Stetler-Stevenson M, et al.: Haematological response of patients with myelodysplastic syndrome to antithymocyte globulin is associated with a loss of lymphocyte-mediated inhibition of CFU-GM and alterations in T-cell receptor Vbeta profiles. *Br J Haematol* 102:1314–1322, 1998.

10. Kitagawa M, Saito I, Kuwata T, et al.: Overexpression of tumor necrosis factor (TNF)-alpha and interferon (IFN)-gamma by bone marrow cells from patients with myelodysplastic syndromes. *Leukemia* 11:2049–2054, 1997.

11. Deeg HJ, Beckham C, Loken MR, et al.: Negative regulators of hemopoiesis and stroma function in patients with myelodysplastic syndrome. *Leuk Lymphoma* 37:405–414, 2000.

12. Yoshida Y: The role of apoptosis in the myelodysplastic syndromes. In: Bennett JM (ed.) *The Myelodysplastic Syndromes:Pathobiology and Clinical Management.* New York: Marcel Dekker;2002:177–201.

13. Prchal JT, Throckmorton DW, Carroll AJ, et al.: A common progenitor for human myeloid and lymphoid cells. *Nature* 274:590–591, 1978.

14. Amenomori T, Tomonaga M, Jinnai I, et al.: Cytogenetic and cytochemical studies on progenitor cells of primary acquired sideroblastic anemia (PASA): involvement of multipotent myeloid stem cells in PASA clone and mosaicism with normal clone. *Blood* 70:1367–1372, 1987.

15. Anastasi J, Feng J, Le Beau MM, et al.: Cytogenetic clonality in myelodysplastic syndromes studied with fluorescence in situ hybridization: lineage, response to growth factor therapy, and clone expansion. *Blood* 81:1580–1585, 1993.

16. Lawrence HJ, Broudy VC, Magenis RE, et al.: Cytogenetic evidence for involvement of B lymphocytes in acquired idiopathic sideroblastic anemias. *Blood* 70:1003–1005, 1987.

17. Janssen JW, Buschle M, Layton M, et al.: Clonal analysis of myelodysplastic syndromes: evidence of multipotent stem cell origin. *Blood* 73:248–254, 1989.

18. Knudson AG Jr: Mutation and cancer: statistical study of retinoblastoma. *Proc Natl Acad Sci US.* 68:820–823, 1971.

19. Song WJ, Sullivan MG, Legare RD, et al.: Haploinsufficiency of CBFA2 causes familial thrombocytopenia with propensity to develop acute myelogenous leukaemia. *Nature Genetics* 23:166–175, 1999.

20. Fenaux P, Morel P, Lai JL: Cytogenetics of myelodysplastic syndromes. *Semin Hematol* 33:127–138, 1996.

21. Nakamura K, Inokuchi K, Dan K: Abnormalities of the p53, N-ras, DCC and FLT-3 genes in myelodysplastic syndromes. *J Nippon Med Sch* 68:143–148, 2001.

22. Quesnel B, Guillerm G, Vereecque R, et al.: Methylation of the p15(INK4b) gene in myelodysplastic syndromes is frequent and acquired during disease progression. *Blood* 91:2985–2990, 1998.

23. Christiansen DH, Andersen MK, Pedersen-Bjergaard J: Methylation of p15INK4B is common, is associated with deletion of genes on chromosome arm 7q and predicts a poor prognosis in therapy-related myelodysplasia and acute myeloid leukemia. *Leukemia* 17:1813–1819, 2003.

24. Sheikhha MH, Tobal K, Liu Yin JA: High level of microsatellite instability but not hypermethylation of mismatch repair genes in therapy-related and secondary acute myeloid leukaemia and myelodysplastic syndrome. *Br J Haematol* 117:359–365, 2002.

25. Larson RA, Wang Y, Banerjee M, et al.: Prevalence of the inactivating 609C–>T polymorphism in the NAD(P)H:quinone oxidoreductase (NQO1) gene in patients with primary and therapy-related myeloid leukemia. *Blood* 94:803–807, 1999.

26. Naoe T, Takeyama K, Yokozawa T, et al.: Analysis of genetic polymorphism in NQO1, GST-M1, GST-T1, and CYP3A4 in 469 Japanese patients with therapy-related leukemia/ myelodysplastic syndrome and de novo acute myeloid leukemia. *Clin Cancer Res* 6:4091–4095, 2000.

27. Hofmann WK, de Vos S, Komor M, et al.: Characterization of gene expression of CD34+ cells from normal and myelodysplastic bone marrow. *Blood* 100:3553–3560, 2002.

28. Miyazato A, Ueno S, Ohmine K, et al.: Identification of myelodysplastic syndrome-specific genes by DNA microarray analysis with purified hematopoietic stem cell fraction. *Blood* 98:422–427, 2001.

29. Ueda M, Ota J, Yamashita Y, et al.: DNA micro array analysis of stage progression mechanism in myelodysplastic syndrome. *Br J Haematol* 123:288–296, 2003.

30. Vallespi T, Imbert M, Mecucci C, et al.: Diagnosis, classification, and cytogenetics of myelodysplastic syndromes. *Haematologica* 83:258–275, 1998.

31. Olney HJ, Le Beau MM: The cytogenetics of myelodysplastic syndromes. *Best Pract Res Clin Haematol* 14:479–495, 2001.

32. Brunning RD BJ, Flandrin G, et al.: Myelodysplastic syndromes. In: Jaffe E Harris N, Stein H (eds.) *Pathology and Genetics of Tumors of Haematopoietic and Lymphoid Tissue. Lyon,* France: IARC Press; 2001:61.

33. West RR, Stafford DA, White AD, et al.: Cytogenetic abnormalities in the myelodysplastic syndromes and occupational or environmental exposure. *Blood* 95:2093–2097, 2000.

34. Mecucci C: Molecular features of primary MDS with cytogenetic changes. *Leuk Res* 22:293–302, 1998.

35. Loss of the Y chromosome from normal and neoplastic bone marrows. United Kingdom Cancer Cytogenetics Group (UKCCG). *Genes Chromosomes Cancer* 5:83–88, 1992.

36. Li T, Xue Y, Wu Y, et al.: Clinical and molecular cytogenetic studies in seven patients with myeloid diseases characterized by i(20q-). *Br J Haematol* 125:337–342, 2004.

37. Pedersen-Bjergaard J, Philip P: Two different classes of therapy-related and de-novo acute myeloid leukemia? *Cancer Genet Cytogenet* 55:119–124, 1991.

38. Pedersen-Bjergaard J, Pedersen M, Roulston D, et al.: Different genetic pathways in leukemogenesis for patients presenting with therapy-related myelodysplasia and therapy-related acute myeloid leukemia. *Blood* 86:3542–3552, 1995.

39. Carroll M, Tomasson MH, Barker GF, et al.: The TEL/platelet-derived growth factor beta receptor (PDGF beta R) fusion in chronic myelomonocytic leukemia is a transforming protein that self-associates and activates PDGF beta R kinase-dependent signaling pathways. *Proc Natl Acad Sci USA* 93:14845–14850, 1996.

40. Sternberg DW, Tomasson MH, Carroll M, et al.: The TEL/PDGFbetaR fusion in chronic myelomonocytic leukemia signals through STAT5-dependent and STAT5-independent pathways. *Blood* 98:3390–3397, 2001.

41. Cain JA, Grisolano JL, Laird AD, et al.: Complete remission of TEL-PDGFRB-induced myeloproliferative disease in mice by receptor tyrosine kinase inhibitor SU11657. *Blood* 2004. [Epub ahead of print.]

42. Magnusson MK, Meade KE, Nakamura R, et al.: Activity of STI571 in chronic myelomonocytic leukemia with a platelet-derived growth factor beta receptor fusion oncogene. *Blood* 100:1088–1091, 2002.

43. Magnusson MK, Meade KE, Brown KE, et al.: Rabaptin-5 is a novel fusion partner to platelet-derived growth factor beta receptor in chronic myelomonocytic leukemia. *Blood* 98:2518–2525, 2001.

44. Ross TS, Bernard OA, Berger R, et al.: Fusion of Huntingtin interacting protein 1 to platelet-derived growth factor beta receptor (PDGFbetaR) in chronic myelomonocytic leukemia with t(5;7)(q33;q11.2). *Blood* 91:4419–4426, 1998.

45. Chronic myelomonocytic leukemia: single entity or heterogeneous disorder? A prospective multicenter study of 100 patients. Groupe Francais de Cytogenetique Hematologique. *Cancer Genet Cytogene* 55:57–65, 1991.

46. Keung YK, Beaty M, Powell BL, et al.: Philadelphia chromosome positive myelodysplastic syndrome and acute myeloid leukemia-retrospective study and review of literature. *Leuk Res* 28:579–586, 2004.

47. Greenberg P, Cox C, LeBeau MM, et al.: International scoring system for evaluating prognosis in myelodysplastic syndromes. *Blood* 89:2079–2088, 1997.

48. Komrokji R, Bennett JM. The myelodysplastic syndromes: classification and prognosis. *Curr Hematol Rep* 2:179–185, 2003.

49. Yoshida Y: Hypothesis: apoptosis may be the mechanism responsible for the premature intramedullary cell death in the myelodysplastic syndrome. *Leukemia* 7:144–146, 1993.

50. Rajapaksa R, Ginzton N, Rott LS, et al.: Altered oncoprotein expression and apoptosis in myelodysplastic syndrome marrow cells. *Blood* 88:4275–4287,1996.

51. Parker JE, Fishlock KL, Mijovic A, et al.: "Low-risk" myelodysplastic syndrome is associated with excessive apoptosis and an increased ratio of pro- versus anti-apoptotic bcl-2-related proteins. *Br J Haematol* 103:1075–1082, 1998.

52. Bogdanovic AD, Trpinac DP, Jankovic GM, et al.: Incidence and role of apoptosis in myelodysplastic syndrome: morphological and ultrastructural assessment. *Leukemia* 11:656–659, 1997.

53. Raza A, Mundle S, Shetty V, et al.: Novel insights into the biology of myelodysplastic syndromes: excessive apoptosis and the role of cytokines. *Int J Hematol* 63:265–278,1996.

54. Allampallam K, Shetty VT, Raza A: Cytokines and MDS. *Cancer Treat Res* 108:93–100, 2001.

55. Bouscary D, De Vos J, Guesnu M, et al.: Fas/Apo-1 (CD95) expression and apoptosis in patients with myelodysplastic syndromes. *Leukemia* 11:839–845, 1997.

56. Deeg HJ: Marrow stroma in MDS: culprit or bystander? *Leuk Res* 26:687–688, 2002.

57. Flores-Figueroa E, Gutierrez-Espindola G, Guerrero-Rivera S, et al.: Hematopoietic progenitor cells from patients with myelodysplastic syndromes: in vitro colony growth and long-term proliferation. *Leuk Res* 23:385–394,1999.

58. Coutinho LH, Geary CG, Chang J, et al.: Functional studies of bone marrow haemopoietic and stromal cells in the myelodysplastic syndrome (MDS). *Br J Haematol* 75:16–25, 1990.

59. Aizawa S, Nakano M, Iwase O, et al.: Bone marrow stroma from refractory anemia of myelodysplastic syndrome is defective in its ability to support normal CD34-positive cell proliferation and differentiation in vitro. *Leuk Res* 23:239–246, 1999.

60. Flores-Figueroa E, Gutierrez-Espindola G, Montesinos JJ, et al.: In vitro characterization of hematopoietic microenvironment cells from patients with myelodysplastic syndrome. *Leuk Res* 26:677–686, 2002.

61. Rami Komrokji, Jainulabdeen J Ifthikharuddin, Raymond E Felgar, et al.: Donor cell myelodysplastic syndrome after allogeneic stem cell transplantation responding to donor lymphocyte infusion: casreport and literature review. *Am J Hematol* 76, 2004 (in press)

62. Bennett JM: World Health Organization classification of the acute leukemias and myelodysplastic syndrome. *Int J Hematol* 72:131–133, 2000.

63. Tham KT CJ, Macon WR: Silver stain for ringed sideroblasts. A sensitive method that differs from Perls' reaction in mechanism and clinical application. *Am J Clin Pathol* 94:73, 1990.

64. Ho PJ GJ, Vincent P, Joshua D: The myelodysplastic syndromes: diagnostic criteria and laboratory evaluation (review). *Pathology* 25:297, 1993.

65. Maschek H, Kaloutsi V, Rodriguez-Kaiser M, et al. Hypoplastic myelodysplastic syndrome: incidence, morphology, cytogenetics, and prognosis. *Ann Hematol* 66:117, 1993.

66. Tricot G, De Wolf-Peeters C, Hendrickx B, et al.: Bone marrow histology in myelodysplastic syndromes. I. Histological findings in myelodysplastic syndromes and comparison with bone marrow smears. *Br J Haematol* 57:423–430,1984.

67. Rios A, Canizo MC, Sanz MA, et al.: Bone marrow biopsy in myelodysplastic syndromes: morphological characteristics and contribution to the study of prognostic factors. *Br J Haematol* 75:26–33, 1990.

68. Tricot G, De Wolf-Peeters C, Vlietinck R, et al.: Bone marrow histology in myelodysplastic syndromes. II. Prognostic value of abnormal localization of immature precursors in MDS. *Br J Haematol* 58:217–225, 1984.

69. Seo IS, Li CY, Yam LT: Myelodysplastic syndrome: diagnostic implications of cytochemical and immunocytochemical studies. *Mayo Clin Proc* 68:47–53,1993.

70. Scott CS, Cahill A, Bynoe AG, et al.: Esterase cytochemistry in primary myelodysplastic syndromes and megaloblastic anaemias: demonstration of abnormal staining patterns associated with dysmyelopoiesis. *Br J Haematol* 55:411–418,1983.

71. Kawaguchi M, Nehashi Y, Aizawa S, et al.: Comparative study of immunocytochemical staining versus Giemsa stain for detecting dysmegakaryopoiesis in myelodysplastic syndromes (MDS). *Eur J Haematol* 44:89–94,1990.

72. Stetler-Stevenson M, Arthur DC, Jabbour N, et al.: Diagnostic utility of flow cytometric immunophenotyping in myelodysplastic syndrome. *Blood* 98:979-987, 2001.

# Chapter 39

# CLINICAL FEATURES AND MAKING THE DIAGNOSIS OF MYELODYSPLASTIC SYNDROMES

## Lewis R. Silverman

## CLINICAL FEATURES

### PHYSICAL: SIGNS, SYMPTOMS, AND EXAM

Although the myelodysplastic syndromes (MDS) have occasionally been described in children and adolescents, they are primarily encountered in adults in their sixth decade or older.[1,2] In most reports, the median age is over 65 and there appears to be a male predominance.[2,3] The clinical and laboratory presentation, although nonspecific in most patients, is dominated by and often reflects the fact that MDS derives from a defect involving a multipotent hematopoietic stem cell affecting one or more cell lineages.

Symptoms relate primarily to the peripheral blood cytopenias, with those attributable to anemia being most common. These may produce signs and symptoms on their own, or exacerbate those attributable to other pre-existing comorbid conditions. Most patients present for medical evaluation because of complaints relating to these symptoms. These include weakness, fatigue, dyspnea, poor exercise tolerance, angina pectoris, pallor, and signs of cardiac failure relating to the degree of anemia. Signs and symptoms in association with neutropenia and thrombocytopenia are encountered less frequently. These include bacterial infections involving the lungs, kidneys, bladder, and skin; easy bruising, ecchymosis, petechiae, epistaxis, gingival bleeding, and hematuria. Patients with severe thrombocytopenia (i.e., platelets $<20 \times 10^9$/L) may manifest life threatening gastrointestinal, pulmonary, gynecologic, or neurologic hemorrhage.

Physical findings are also nonspecific. The exam will often reveal signs relating to the underlying cytopenias. Hepatic and/or splenic enlargement are reported in 10–40% of patients and are most commonly found in chronic myelomonocytic leukemia (CMML). Lymphadenopathy and skin infiltration are uncommon,[4-9] although the appearance of leukemia cutis in patients with MDS may herald the transformation to acute leukemia by weeks or months. Identification of leukemia cutis may also signal the development of a more aggressive clinical course, and in one study appeared to be associated with a poor prognosis.[10] Similar to patients with AML, patients with MDS develop Sweet's syndrome (neutrophilic dermatosis).[11,12] Other skin findings include vasculitis and pyoderma gangrenosum.[12,13]

## LABORATORY

Hematologic laboratory findings demonstrate peripheral blood cytopenias in one or more cell lines associated with dysmorphic features. These reflect dysmaturation of one or one or more of the cell lines and are detailed in Table 39.1. These maturational defects may be identified not only in the lines with diminished production but may also be seen in the lines where bone marrow production is still conserved. The bone marrow is most often hypercellular and features morphologic abnormalities involving one, two, or all of the cell lineages (Table 39.1 and Figures 39.1 and 39.2). The dysmorphic features are critical to establish the diagnosis, and both the French–American–British (FAB) and World Health Organization (WHO) classification systems are based primarily on these findings (see Chapter 38). A diagnosis without maturational abnormalities in at least one cell line would be difficult to support.

Histologic examination of bone marrow trephine biopsies by Tricot and colleagues have pointed to abnormalities of the microenvironment.[14] They noted the presence of clusters of immature precursor cells in the central intertrabecular region of the marrow, rather than along the endosteal surfaces. They cited this as evidence of abnormal localization of immature precursors (ALIP).[14,15] ALIP was detected even before bone marrow smears revealed an excess of blasts. In a series of 40 patients, the presence of ALIP correlated significantly with shortened survival and was associated with an increased risk of transformation to AML. These findings were independent of the FAB subtype and were detected even in patients with refractory

**Table 39.1    Morphologic and functional cellular abnormalities**

*Erythrocytes*
Morphology
  Anisocytosis
  Poilkilocytosis
  Oval macrocytes
  Microcytes
  Basophilic stippling
  Howell–Jolly bodies
  Circulating nucleated red cells
  Ringed sideroblasts
  Increased stainable iron
  Megaloblastoid maturation*
  Multinucleated precursors*
  Nuclear fragmentation*
  Nuclear budding*
  Karryohexis*
  Defective hemoglobinization*
*Leukocytes*
Morphology
  Pseudo Pelger-Huet Cells
  Monocytosis
  Defective granule formation (hypogranulation)
  Megaloblastoid maturation
  Auer rods
  Abnormal chromatin clumping
  Abnormal nuclear bridging
  Increased myeloblasts
*Megakaryocytes*
Morphology
  Circulating megakaryocyte fragments
  Giant platelets
  Micromegakaryocytes*
  Hypolobulated nuclei*
  Hyperlobulated nuclei*
  Large mononulcear forms*
*Erythrocytes*
Function
  Decrease or loss of blood group antigens
  Increased fetal hemoglobin
  Aberrant globin chain synthesis
  Disordered ferrokinetics

Enzymes
  Increased hexokinase
  decreased pyruvate kinase
  decreased 2,3 diphophoglycerate mutase
  decreased phosphofructokinase
  increased adenosine deaminase
  increased pyruvate kinase
*Leukocytes*
Function
  Increased leukocyte alkaline phosphatase
  Decreased myeloperoxidase
  Increased muramidase (CMML)
  Loss of granule membrane glycoproteins
  Inappropriate surface antigens
  Decreased adhesion
  Defective chemotaxis
  Deficient phagocytosis
  Impaired bacteriocidal activity
*Megakaryocytes*
Function
  Defective platelet aggregation
  Deficiency in thromboxane $A_2$
  Bernard–Soulier-like defect
*Immune Deficiencies*
  Decreased T-cell IL-2 receptors
  Decreased IL-2 production
  Decreased NK activity
  Decreased NK response to gamma inteferon
  Decreased gamma interferon production
  Decreased response to mitogens
  Decreased $T_4$ cells
  Immunoglobulin abnormalities
  Autoanibodies
  Autoimmune phenomenon
  Impaired self-recognition

CMML, Chronic myelomonocytic leukemia
*Bone marrow findings

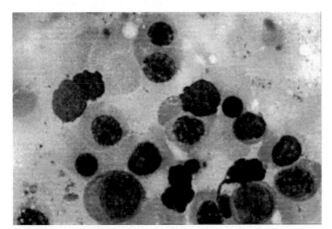

**Figure 39.1**    *Bone marrow smear with marked erythrodyspoiesis and binucleared erythroid progenitors*

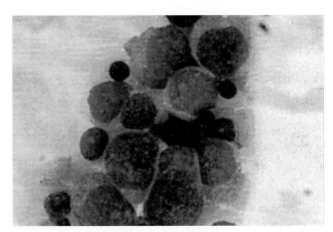

**Figure 39.2**    *Bone marrow smear with increased myeloblasts*

anemia. Care must be applied to differentiate true ALIP from pseudo-ALIP. In the latter case, the clusters of cells are either of erythroid or megakaryocytic origin and do not convey the same prognostic information compared to the former, where the immature cells are of myeloid origin. The determination of the immature precursor phenotype by immunohistochemical methods may be helpful in distinguishing pseudo and true ALIP, and thus permit identification of specific MDS subgroups with a poor prognosis.[16] ALIP is not, however, specific to patients with MDS, and therefore not useful as a diagnostic tool.[16]

Functional abnormalities can occur in all three cell lines and range in severity from minor laboratory defects to those impairments associated with major clinical manifestations. These functional defects may exacerbate underlying existing cytopenias (i.e., anemia, neutropenia, and thrombocytopenia) or may produce a functionally deficient state even when peripheral blood counts remain in the normal range. Thus, patients with normal neutrophil counts may still experience recurrent bacterial infections reflecting functional neutropenia. Erythroid enzyme defects, aberrant expression of red cell surface antigens, and abnormalities of hemoglobin production and iron metabolism have all been described. Some of the changes in enzyme activity, such as those that occur with pyruvate kinase, may affect red cell survival.[17,18] Impaired activity of A and H transferase and galactosyltransferase has resulted in changes in blood types.[19,20] Hemoglobin production is affected with increased fetal hemoglobin, aberrant globin chain synthesis, and disordered ferrokinetics.[21,22] Acquired alpha-thalassemia has been described secondary to a deletion of the alpha-globin chain cluster or an inactivating mutation of the transcriptional factor ATRX, resulting in down-regulation of the alpha-globin chain synthesis.[23]

The myeloid series often reveals leukopenia with immature forms and increased numbers of large unstained cells. Neutropenia is more commonly found in patients with refractory anemia with excess blasts (RAEB) and RAEB-T than in patients with refractory anemia (RA) and refractory anemia with ringed sideroblasts (RARS).[8] Leukocytosis most often accompanies CMML, and by definition requires an absolute monocytosis ($>1 \times 10^9$/L) for diagnosis. Monocytosis may, however, also be present in the other MDS subtypes.[8] Cytoplasmic abnormalities result in cells with hypogranule or defective granule formation, Auer rods, or abnormal azurophilic granules. Histocytochemical studies reveal cells with increased or decreased levels of leukocyte alkaline phosphatase, decreased myeloperoxidase staining, and loss of granule membrane glycoproteins.[24–28] Surface antigen analysis has shown loss of lineage-specific antigens, with persistent or increased expression of inappropriate antigens and lineage infidelity.[29–32] In some instances, the abnormal persistence of antigens or an increased proportion of cells expressing those antigens was associated with an increased risk of leukemic transformation and shortened survival. Abnormal expression of an activated surface phenotype on monocytes has been demonstrated in patients within all FAB subtypes, while expression of activated surface antigens on granulocytes was almost exclusively seen in patients with excess blasts.[33] Impaired granulocyte function includes impaired respiratory burst, deficit in chemotaxis and superoxide release, as well as a defect in neutrophil stimulation signaling.[33,34] Nuclear abnormalities such as pseudo Pelger-Huet cells and functional abnormalities are further outlined in Table 39.1.[35]

Megakaryocytes can be decreased and their morphology is often bizarre (Table 39.1). Patients with RAEB and RAEB-T more commonly have thrombocytopenia, decreased megakaryocytes, and greater degrees of dysmegakaryopoiesis.[8] Megakaryocyte fragments and giant thrombocytes may circulate in the peripheral blood. Hemorrhagic symptoms in these patients may be due to thrombocytopenia and functionally defective platelets. Dysfunction can result from defective platelet aggregation, deficiencies in thromboxane A2 activity, or the development of a Bernard–Soulier-type platelet defect. This latter defect has developed from a deficiency in the membrane glycoprotein GP 1b-IX complex.[36,37]

A small percentage of patients present with hypoplastic bone marrows and cytopenias which morphologically may be difficult to distinguish from aplastic anemia.[38] Cytogenetic analysis with or without interphase FISH may be helpful in establishing a diagnosis.

The relationship of MDS to abnormalities of the immune system is of particular interest given the broad range of abnormalities described. There is a decrease in the number of T-cell interleukin-2 (IL-2) receptors, as well as IL-2 production. The latter is due in part to a failure of immunoregulatory B cells.[39] Natural Killer (NK) cell activity and responsiveness to alpha-interferon is decreased, as is alpha-interferon production, while total numbers of NK cells are variable.[39] There are decreases in the number of T cells, responsiveness to mitogenic stimulation, the total number of cells, and the T4/T8 ratio.[31,40,41] The latter is due predominantly to a decrease in T4 cells. Overexpression of HLA-DR15 may occur in some patients, and may be a useful predictive factor for response to immunotherapeutic interventions.[42]

Immunoglobulin abnormalities manifest as autoantibodies or a positive direct Coombs' test.[43,44] The relationship of the disease to the immune abnormalities is poorly understood. A general dysregulation of the immune system is prevalent in many patients. Many patients will present with evidence of associated autoimmune disorders.[13] This may include polyserositis with frank, nonspecific inflammatory pericarditis and pleuritis with significant effusions,[13] or it may be associated with other autoimmune diseases, such as Crohn's and Behcet's disease.[45,46] Additional autoimmune mediated conditions associated with MDS include relapsing polychondritis, arthritis, polyneuropathy, hemolytic anemia, and immune thrombocytopenia. Recent reports have also described glomerulonephritis and nephrotic syndrome.[47,48] In some cases, increased serum lyzozyme (muramidase) in patients with CMML may be the inciting nephrotoxic agent. Although the pathophysiologic relationship of these autoimmune phenomenas and MDS is uncertain, it appears that the prognostic factors relating to MDS are the primary determinants for outcome, rather than the autoimmune disease.[49] Consistent with this is the finding of altered antibody repertoires of self-reactive IgM and IgG in MDS patients, indicating a disturbance in self-recognition mechanisms.[50] Whether some abnormalities relate in part to the number of red cell transfusions, or whether they are reversible with effective treatment, is unknown. Given the nature of the defect in a multipotent stem cell with the potential to differentiate along multiple pathways,[51] the dysregulation of T and B cells is not surprising. A report of 20 patients with nontherapy-related MDS and concurrent lymphoid or plasmacytic malignant neoplasms provides further evidence to the multipotency of the stem cell affected, and to the derivative generalized immune dysregulation.[8,43]

## ESTABLISHING A DIAGNOSIS

The diagnosis of MDS in most patients is readily established with standardized testing, which should include history and physical examination, complete blood count, and review of the peripheral blood smear. The findings of cytopenias in the absence of explanation from biochemical, vitamin deficiency, hemorrhage, toxin/drug, or infectious etiology should lead to a bone marrow aspirate and biopsy with routine cytogenetic evaluation. The diagnosis of MDS is based primarily on morphologic criteria demonstrating dysmorphic features in the peripheral blood and bone marrow precursors (described above and Table 39.1). Although some of the classification systems include cytogenetic information (IE:WHO), they are based primarily on bone marrow and peripheral blood morphology. A diagnosis of MDS cannot be definitively established without examination of a bone marrow aspirate. Peripheral blood smears may be suggestive, but not conclusive. Some in the hematologic community believe a bone marrow smear alone is adequate for diagnosis. In some instances a smear is sufficient, however, a bone marrow biopsy provides complimentary information on cellularity, infiltrative disease, megakaryocyte morphology, and fibrosis that is often important in completing the evaluation and is informative for thera-

peutic decisions. Analysis of the marrow population, using flow cytometric analysis has become standard for the diagnosis and subtyping in patients with acute leukemia. It is more routinely being applied to establish a diagnosis of MDS, as well. Abnormal populations and skewed antigen expression can be identified.[52–58] However, comparative studies of bone marrow morphology and flow cytometry results have not been conducted, and thus one cannot be certain if used alone whether flow cytometry results can reliably establish a diagnosis and classification of MDS. Accurate classification according to FAB or WHO criteria must be based, at least in part, on bone marrow morphology. Thus, flow cytometry should be viewed as a complementary examination, but not sufficient to establish the diagnosis and classification.

## DIAGNOSTIC DILEMMAS

Certain patients with MDS may present with unusual or uncharacteristic features and represent a diagnostic challenge. These cases usually represent a small but difficult subset of patients in which to confidently establish the diagnosis. Patients may present with isolated thrombocytopenia that may antedate the diagnosis of MDS by months or years.[59] The bone marrow may reveal increased megakaryocytes, and an antiplatelet antibody may be identified in the serum. However, as noted above, this may be seen in conjunction with MDS, and may not represent a true case of immune thrombocytopenic purpura (ITP). Often, treatments typically used for ITP are ineffective. In these patients, careful examination of peripheral blood and bone marrow morphology may reveal the correct diagnosis. As in other patients in whom establishment of a diagnosis may be problematic, cytogenetic analysis may be helpful in leading to the correct diagnosis of MDS. Finding a cytogenetic abnormality frequently associated with MDS can often lead to the appropriate diagnosis. This applies both to these patients and to others described below.

Some patients with MDS present with features also suggestive of a myeloproliferative disorder (MPD), representing an "overlap syndrome."[60,61] In these patients, cytopenias may present simultaneously with elevated white blood cell or platelet counts. In some patients, an increased leukocyte count may be accompanied by a monocytosis. Under current classification systems, some of these patients will be clearly defined as having an MPD, while others are still categorized as having MDS depending on the upper limit of the WBC count permitted in the classification system (see Chapter 38). Others may have myelofibrosis with or without marked splenomegaly and peripheral blood cytopenias,[59,61–63] yet also have dysplastic features suggesting MDS. These patients are more difficult to classify. Those with myelofibrosis with markedly enlarged spleens and a leukoerythroblastic peripheral smear are more likely to have classical myelofibrosis with myeloid metaplasia, while patients without significant splenomegaly and/or the peripheral leukoerythroblastic picture may be considered to have primary MDS with fibrosis.

The hypoplastic MDS variant is often indistinguishable from aplastic anemia, and may have many features in common.[53,64–67] Those patients with increased expression of HLA-DR15 and the paroxysmal nocturnal hemoglobinuria (PNH) phenotype (decreased expression of CD59), whether having MDS or aplastic anemia, may respond to immunomodulatory treatments. Cytogenetic abnormalities, if present, involving chromosomes frequently abnormal in MDS may suggest the diagnosis of MDS, but does not completely exclude aplastic anemia.[68]

Finally, there are patients who present with severe pancytopenia and bone marrow findings that are nondiagnostic (i.e., minimal if any dysmorphic changes, no increase in myeloblasts) and without any cytogenetic abnormalities. Some of these patients may have MDS and only with continued observation and testing will a diagnosis be unequivocally established. Others may have been exposed to a bone marrow insult (toxin, infectious agent, etc.), which may never be identified, but which may permit eventual complete or partial marrow recovery over months or years. In these latter individuals, in the absence of clear diagnostic evidence, patience, continued observation, and supportive care may be the best approach pending a declarative diagnosis. One other consideration for these patients would be an immune-mediated injury to hematopoietic stem cells. The differential in these patients includes large granular lymphocytic leukemia, where T-cell receptor and immunoglobulin gene rearrangement studies may be informative.[69]

Thus, MDS represents a disease with protean clinical and laboratory features. In the majority, with the appropriate evaluation, a diagnosis can be readily established, permitting accurate classification and appropriate therapeutic decisions.

## REFERENCES

1. Creutzig U, Cantu-Rajnoldi A, Ritter J, et al.: Myelodysplastic syndromes in childhood. *Am. J. Ped Hematol/Oncol* 9:324, 1987.
2. Silverman L: The myelodysplastic syndrome. In: Kufe D, Pollack R, Weichselbaum R, et al. eds. *Cancer Medicine.* Hamilton, ON, BC Decker; 2003:2077–2093.
3. Silverman LR, Demakos EP, Peterson BL, et al.: Randomized controlled trial of azacitidine in patients with the myelodysplastic syndrome: a study of the cancer and leukemia group B. *J Clin Oncol* 20:2429–2440, 2002.
4. Foucar K, Langdon RM II, Armitage JO, Olson DB, Carroll TJ Jr: Myelodysplastic syndromes. A clinical and pathologic analysis of 109 cases. *Cancer* 56:553–561, 1985.
5. Mufti GJ, Stevens JR, Oscier DG, Hamblin TJ, Machin D: Myelodysplastic syndromes: a scoring system with prognostic significance. *Br J Haematol* 59:425–432, 1985.
6. Tricot G, Vlietinck R, Boogaerts MA, et al.: prognostic factors in the myelodysplastic syndromes: importance of initial data on peripheral blood counts, bone marrow cytology, trephine biopsy and chromosomal analysis. *Br J Haematol* 60:19–27, 1985.
7. Varela BL, Chuang C, Woll JE, Bennett JM: Modifications in the classification of primary myelodysplastic syndromes: the addition of a scoring system. *Hematol Oncol* 3:55–65, 1985.
8. Vallespi T, Torrabadella M, Julia A, et al.: Myelodysplastic syndromes: a study of 101 cases according to the FAB classification. *Br J Haematol* 61:83–92, 1985.
9. Yunis JJ, Lobell M, Arnesen MA, et al.: Refined chromosome study helps define prognostic subgroups in most patients with primary myelodysplastic syndrome and acute myelogenous leukemia. *Br J Haematol* 68:189, 1988.
10. Paydas S, Zorludemir S: Leukaemia cutis and leukaemic vasculitis. *Br J Dermatol* 143:773–779, 2000.
11. Avivi I, Rosenbaum H, Levy Y, Rowe J: Myelodysplastic syndrome and associated skin lesions: a review of the literature. *Leuk Res* 23:323–330, 1999.
12. Megarbane B, Bodemer C, Valensi F, et al.: Association of acute neutrophilic dermatosis and myelodysplastic syndrome with (6; 9) chromosome translocation: a case report and review of the literature. *Br J Dermatol* 143:1322–1324, 2000.
13. Enright H, Jacob HS, Vercellotti G, Howe R, Belzer M, Miller W: Paraneoplastic autoimmune phenomena in patients with myelodysplastic syndromes: response to immunosuppressive therapy. *Br J Haematol* 91:403–408, 1995.
14. Tricot G, De Wolf-Peeters C, Hendrickx B, Verwilghen RL: Bone marrow histology in myelodysplastic syndromes: histological findings in myelodysplastic syndromes and comparison with bone marrow smears. *Br J Haematol* 57:423, 1984.
15. Tricot G, De Wolf-Peeters C, Vlietinck R, Verwilghen RL: Bone marrow histology in myleodysplastic syndromes: Prognostic value of abnormal localization of immature precursors in MDS. *Br J Haematol* 58:217, 1984.
16. Mangi MH, Salisbury JR, Mufti GJ: Abnormal localization of immature precursors (ALIP) in the bone marrow of myelodysplastic syndromes: current state of knowledge and future directions. *Leuk. Res* 15:627–639, 1991.
17. Tani K, Fujii H, Takahashi K, et al.: Erythrocyte enzyme activities in myelodysplastic syndromes: elevated pyruvate kinase activity. *Am J Hematol* 30:97, 1989.
18. Breton-Gorius J, Houssay D, Dreyfus B: Partial myeloperoxidase deficiency in a case of preleukaemia. I: Studies of fine structure and peroxidase synthesis of promyelocytes. *Br J Haematol* 30:273, 1975.
19. Dreyfus B, Sultan C, Rochant H, et al.: Anomalies of blood group antigens and erythrocyte enzymes in two

types of chronic refractory anaemia. *Br J Haematol* 16:303, 1969.

20. Yoshida A, Kumazaki T, Dave V, Blank J, Dzik WH: Suppressed expression of blood group B antigen and blood group galactosyltransferase in a preluekemic subject. *Blood* 66:990, 1985.

21. Uchida T, Kokubun K, Abe R, et al.: Ferrokinetic evaluation of erythropoiesis in patients with myelodysplastic syndromes. *Acta Haematol* 79:81, 1988.

22. Peters RE, May A, Jacobs A: Increased alpha:non-alpha globin chain synthesis ratios in myelodysplastic syndromes and myeloid leukaemia. *J Clin Pathol* 39:1233, 1986.

23. Steensma DP, Gibbons RJ, Higgs DR: Acquired alpha-thalassemia in association with myelodysplastic syndrome and other hematologic malignancies. *Blood* 105:443–452, 2005.

24. Elghetany M, MacCallum J, Nelson D, et al.: Abnormal granulocytes in myelodysplastic syndromes: A morphologic, cytochemical and immunocytochemical study of 71 patients. *Blood* 76(suppl):267a, 1990.

25. Elghetany MT, Molina CP, Patel J, Martinez J, Schwab H, Velagaleti GV: Expression of CD4 on peripheral blood granulocytes. A novel finding in a case of myelodysplastic syndrome in association with t(5;12). *Cancer Genet Cytogenet* 136:38–42, 2002.

26. Elghetany MT, Peterson B, MacCallum J, et al.: Deficiency of neutrophilic granule membrane glycoproteins in the myelodysplastic syndromes: a common deficiency in 216 patients studied by the cancer and leukemia group B. *Leuk Res* 21:801–806, 1997.

27. Elghetany MT, Peterson B, MacCallum J, et al.: Double esterase staining and other neutrophilic granule abnormalities in 237 patients with the myelodysplastic syndrome studied by the cancer and leukemia group B. *Acta Haematol* 100:13–16, 1998.

28. Breton-Gorius J, Houssay D, Dreyfus B: Partial myeloperoxidase deficiency in a case of preleukaemia. I: Studies of fine structure and peroxidase synthesis of promyelocytes. *Br J Haematol* 30:273, 1975.

29. Baumann MA, Keller RH, McFadden PW, Libnoch JA, Patrick CW: Myeloid cell surface phenotype in myelodysplasia: evidence for abnormal persistence of an early myeloid differentiation antigen. *Am J Hematol* 22:251, 1986.

30. Clark RE, Smith SA, Jacobs A: Myeloid surface antigen abnormalities in myelodysplasia: Relation to prognosis and modification by 13-cis retinoic acid. *J. Clin. Pathol* 40:652, 1987.

31. Hokland P, Kerndrup G, Griffin JD, Ellegaard J: Analysis of leukocyte differentiation antigens in blood and bone marrow from preleukemia (refractory anemia) patients using monoclonal antibodies. *Blood* 67:898, 1986.

32. Silverman LR, Yagi MJ, Holland JF, Bekesi JG: Lineage infidelity with coexpression of myeloid and lymphoid markers and IL-2 receptor are common in myelodysplastic syndromes. *Proc. Am. Assoc. Can. Res.* 33:152, 1992.

33. Felzman T, Gisslinger H, Krieger O, Majdic O, Ludwig H, Köller U: Immunophenotypic characterization of myelomonocytic cells in patients with myelodysplastic syndrome. *Br J Haematol* 84:428–435, 1993.

34. Lowe GM, Dang Y, Watson F, Edwards SW, Galvani DW: Identification of a subgroup of myelodysplastic patients

with a neutrophil stimulation-signalling defect. *Br J Haematol* 86:761–766, 1994.

35. Felman P, Bryon PA, Gentilhomme O, et al.: The syndrome of abnormal chromatin clumping in leucocytes: a myelodysplastic disorder with proliferative features? *Br J Haematol* 70:49–54, 1988.

36. Russell NH, Keenan JP, Bellingham AJ: Thrombocytopathy in preleukaemia: association with a defect of thromboxane A2 activity. *Br J Haematol* 41:417, 1979.

37. Raman KS, Van Slyck EJ, Riddle J, Sawdyk MA, Abraham JP, Saeed SM: Platelet function and structure in myeloproliferative disease, myelodysplastic syndrome, and secondary thrombocytosis. *Am J Clin Pathol* 91:647, 1989.

38. Tuzuner N, Cox C, Rowe J, Watrous D, Bennett J: Hypocellular myelodysplastic syndromes: new proposals. *Br J Haematol* 91:612–617, 1995.

39. Sorskaar D, Forre O, Albrechtsen D, Stavem P: Decreased natural killer cell activity versus normal natural killer cell markers in mononuclear cells from patients with smouldering leukemia. *Scand J Haematol* 37:154, 1986.

40. Merchav S, Nagler A, Silvian I, Carter A, Tatarsky I, Spira G: Immunoglobulin synthesis in myelodysplastic syndromes: normal B-cell and immunoregulatory T-cell functions. *Clin Immunol Immunopathol* 42:195, 1987.

41. Mufti GJ, Figes A, Hamblin TJ, Oscier DG, Copplestone JA: Immunological abnormalities in myelodysplastic syndromes. *Br J Haematol* 63:143, 1986.

42. Saunthararajah Y, Nakamura R, Nam JM, et al.: HLA-DR15 (DR2) is overrepresented in myelodysplastic syndrome and aplastic anemia and predicts a response to immunosuppression in myelodysplastic syndrome. *Blood* 100:1570–1574, 2002.

43. Mufti GJ, Figes A, Hamblin TJ, Oscier DG, Copplestone JA: Immunological abnormalities in myelodysplastic syndromes. *Br J Haematol* 63:143, 1986.

44. Economopoulos T, Economidou J, Giannopoulos G, et al.: Immune abnormalities in myelodysplastic syndromes. *J Clin Pathol* 38:908, 1985.

45. Bosch X, Bernadich O, Vera M: The association between Crohn disease and the myelodysplastic syndromes. Report of 3 cases and review of the literature. *Medicine* (Baltimore) 77:371–377, 1998.

46. Della Rossa A, Tavoni A, Tognetti A, Testi C, Bombardieri S: Behcet's disease with gastrointestinal involvement associated with myelodysplasia in a patient with congenital panhypopituitarism. *Clin Rheumatol* 17:515–517, 1998.

47. Bogdanovic R, Kuzmanovic M, Markovic-Lipkovski J, et al.: Glomerular involvement in myelodysplastic syndromes. *Pediatr Nephrol* 16:1053–1057, 2001.

48. Saitoh T, Murakami H, Uchiumi H, et al.: Myelodysplastic syndromes with nephrotic syndrome. *Am J Hematol* 60:200–204, 1999.

49. Giannouli S, Voulgarelis M, Zintzaras E, Tzioufas AG, Moutsopoulos HM: Autoimmune phenomena in myelodysplastic syndromes: a 4-yr prospective study. *Rheumatology* (Oxford) 43:626–632, 2004.

50. Stahl D, Egerer G, Goldschmidt H, Sibrowski W, Kazatchkine MD, Kaveri SV: Altered self-reactive antibody repertoires are a general feature of patients with myelodysplastic syndrome. *J Autoimmun* 16:77–86, 2001.

51. Prchal JT, Throckmorton DW, Carroll AJ, Fuson EW, Gams RA: A common progenitor for human myeloid and lymphoid cells. *Science* 274:590, 1978.

52. Ogata K, Nakamura K, Yokose N, et al.: Clinical significance of phenotypic features of blasts in patients with myelodysplastic syndrome. *Blood* 100:3887–3896, 2002.

53. Kasahara S, Hara T, Itoh H, et al.: Hypoplastic myelodysplastic syndromes can be distinguished from acquired aplastic anaemia by bone marrow stem cell expression of the tumour necrosis factor receptor. *Br J Haematol* 118:181–188, 2002.

54. Eighetany MT: Diagnostic utility of flow cytometric immunophenotyping in myelodysplastic syndrome. *Blood* 99:391–392, 2002.

55. Stetler-Stevenson M, Arthur DC, Jabbour N, et al.: Diagnostic utility of flow cytometric immunophenotyping in myelodysplastic syndrome. *Blood* 98:979–987, 2001.

56. Miller DT, Stelzer GT: Contributions of flow cytometry to the analysis of the myelodysplastic syndrome. *Clin Lab Med* 21:811–828, 2001.

57. Ito S, Ishida Y, Murai K, Kuriya S: Flow cytometric analysis of aberrant antigen expression of blasts using CD45 blast gating for minimal residual disease in acute leukemia and high-risk myelodysplastic syndrome. *Leuk Res* 25:205–211, 2001.

58. Chang CC, Cleveland RP: Decreased CD10-positive mature granulocytes in bone marrow from patients with myelodysplastic syndrome. *Arch Pathol Lab Med* 124:1152–1156, 2000.

59. Sashida G, Takaku TI, Shoji N, et al.: Clinico-hematologic features of myelodysplastic syndrome presenting as isolated thrombocytopenia: an entity with a relatively favorable prognosis. *Leuk Lymphoma* 44:653–658, 2003.

60. Bain BJ: The relationship between the myelodysplastic syndromes and the myeloproliferative disorders. *Leuk Lymphoma* 34:443–449, 1999.

61. Gupta R, Abdalla SH, Bain BJ: Thrombocytosis with sideroblastic erythropoiesis: a mixed myeloproliferative myelodysplastic syndrome. *Leuk Lymphoma* 34:615–619, 1999.

62. Lambertenghi-Deliliers G, Orazi A, Luksch R, Annaloro C, Soligo D: Myelodysplastic syndrome with increased marrow fibrosis: a distinct clinico-pathological entity. *Br J Haematol* 78:161–166, 1991.

63. Lambertenghi-Deliliers G, Annaloro C, Oriani A, Soligo D: Myelodysplastic syndrome associated with bone marrow fibrosis. *Leuk Lymphoma* 8:51–55, 1992.

64. Maciejewski JP, Follmann D, Nakamura R, et al.: Increased frequency of HLA-DR2 in patients with paroxysmal nocturnal hemoglobinuria and the PNH/aplastic anemia syndrome. *Blood* 98:3513–3519, 2001.

65. Maciejewski JP, Risitano A, Kook H, Zeng W, Chen G, Young NS: Immune pathophysiology of aplastic anemia. *Int J Hematol* 76 (suppl 1):207–214, 2002.

66. Maciejewski JP, Selleri C: Evolution of clonal cytogenetic abnormalities in aplastic anemia. *Leuk Lymphoma* 45:433–440, 2004.

67. Paquette RL: Diagnosis and management of aplastic anemia and myelodysplastic syndrome. *Oncology* (Williston Park) 16:153–161, 2002.

68. Maciejewski JP, Selleri C: Evolution of clonal cytogenetic abnormalities in aplastic anemia. *Leuk Lymphoma* 45:433–440, 2004.

69. Saunthararajah Y, Molldrem JL, Rivera M, et al.: Coincident myelodysplastic syndrome and T-cell large granular lymphocytic disease: clinical and pathophysiological features. *Br J Haematol* 112:195–200, 2001.

# Chapter 40

# TREATMENT APPROACH TO EARLY MYELODYSPLASTIC SYNDROMES

## *Virginia M. Klimek and Stephen D. Nimer*

## INTRODUCTION

Developing a standard treatment algorithm for patients with myelodysplastic syndrome (MDS) is difficult, due to the tremendous heterogeneity of the disease and the limited, variably toxic available therapies. In this chapter, we attempt to place into context the currently available treatment options for patients with MDS, focusing on supportive care and low-intensity therapies. In our summary, we propose a treatment approach to MDS, based on specific clinical presentations.

MDS patients can be classified according to the French–American–British (FAB) classification system,[1] the World Health Organization classification system,[2] and most recently, the International Prognostic Scoring System (IPSS)[3], which integrate a variety of clinical features. These systems do not take into account the biological basis of this set of diseases, which remain ill-defined. The development of targeted therapies for leukemia and related diseases is dependent on identifying genetic lesions that are critical for the growth of the malignant cell or for monoclonal antibody-based therapy, and on identifying cell surface markers that are abundantly expressed on the target cell. No such critical genetic lesions or cell surface markers have been identified for the vast majority of MDS patients; their identification has been hampered by the lack of an animal model of MDS and by difficulties in isolating "MDS-initiating cells" in the laboratory. Thus, other than the use of imatinib for rare chronic myelomonocytic leukemia (CMML) patients with t(5;12), i.e., TEL-PDGFRβ-positive CMML, targeted therapies cannot yet be applied to MDS.

The few recurrent genetic abnormalities identified in MDS patients, such as point mutations in the *AML1* gene, the t(3;5) that generates the NPM-MLF1 fusion protein, or the t(3;21) (which generates an AML1-EVI-1 fusion), are infrequent. While del(5q), del(7q), del (20q), and trisomy 8 are the most frequent cytogenetic abnormalities found in MDS, the gene(s) affected by these abnormalities have still not been determined. Given the absence of identified genetic abnormalities in MDS hematopoietic cells and the heterogeneity of the disease, studies have also focused on defining the bone marrow milieu that supports or sustains the MDS process. Overactive macrophage function (with increased cytokine secretion), changes in microvessel density, and abnormalities in the maintenance of telomeres have been observed in some MDS patients. Immunologic abnormalities have also been identified in patients with MDS, and these abnormalities (especially those also found in aplastic anemia (AA) patients) have provided the rationale for the testing of immunomodulatory treatments.

Recent discoveries, such as the lack of circulating natural killer T cells in these patients, may provide additional therapeutic options in the future, although some cellular abnormalities may simply represent "down-stream" effects of the impaired hematopoiesis found in MDS, and may not provide insight into new therapies. Similarly, the excess production of inhibitory cytokines by macrophages (and other bone marrow cells) that can suppress hematopoiesis has led to testing of a variety of forms of anticytokine therapy. Though thus far largely unsuccessful, such approaches may be used more effectively in the future. A thorough discussion of the novel therapies being applied to subsets of MDS patients will be covered in Chapter X.

## SUPPORTIVE CARE

Many patients with MDS require close monitoring only during the early phase of their disease. However, once patients become symptomatic from cytopenias, the timely use of supportive care measures can impact significantly on their quality of life (QOL). Supportive care measures generally consist of packed red blood cell (PRBC) transfusions to treat or prevent the symptoms and physiologic consequences of anemia, antibiotics to treat or prevent infection, and platelet transfusions to prevent or treat bleeding.

The "optimal" hemoglobin concentration for anemic, transfusion-dependent MDS patients has never been defined. Nonetheless, a commonly used threshold for PRBC transfusions has been a hemoglobin level of less than 8.0 g/dL. This may be too low for many patients, as studies in patients with cancer and chemotherapy-induced anemia suggest that a hemoglobin level of 11.0–12.0 g/dL may provide optimal symptom relief.[4] During the routine care of MDS patients, this level may be difficult to achieve or maintain because of the frequency and amount of blood required and the poorer response of MDS bone marrow to erythropoietic agents. Therefore, the threshold for individual MDS patients will vary depending on the patient's age, conditioning, level of activity, and the presence or absence of cardiopulmonary disease. QOL studies should aid in defining the benefit of maintaining higher hemoglobin levels in MDS patients.

Platelet transfusions are used to prevent or treat bleeding due to severe thrombocytopenia or platelet dysfunction. Assuming normal platelet function, prophylactic transfusions are generally reserved for patients with a platelet count of $<10,000/\mu L$. Patients with evidence of significant platelet dysfunction should be evaluated on a case-by-case basis. Otherwise, thrombocytopenic MDS patients who are not bleeding can be observed if they have no other risk factors for significant bleeding. For patients undergoing active therapy for MDS, it may be desirable to maintain a platelet count of $>20,000/\mu L$ during periods of reversible, treatment-related myelosuppression. A diagnosis of immune-mediated thrombocytopenia (ITP) should be considered in thrombocytopenic patients, as ITP and other autoimmune phenomenas are associated with MDS.[5] Potent thrombopoietic agents, however, are not currently available. Interleukin-11 has been tested in thrombocytopenic MDS patients, but its safety and efficacy has not been established. A variety of thrombopoietin "mimics" are currently being evaluated, with some activity being seen in thrombocytopenic patients.

Supportive care for MDS patients includes managing infectious complications from neutropenia. Fever or signs of infection should be assessed promptly in neutropenic patients and treated with antibiotics. During brief periods of neutropenia, antibiotic prophylaxis may be appropriate. Granulocyte transfusions may improve survival in patients with transient neutropenia and severe bacterial or fungal infections that are not responding to appropriate antibiotics. However, their efficacy in patients with unremitting neutropenia is not established. Other supportive care measures include vaccinating MDS patients (and their close contacts) against influenza, and considering the use of pneumococcal vaccines.

Chronic PRBC transfusion therapy can result in iron overload, and prevention of hemochromatosis should be considered in patients with stable disease. Liver biopsy is the gold standard for assessing iron overload, but it may not be feasible in some patients because of thrombocytopenia or other medical concerns. Superconducting quantum interference device imaging can quantitate hepatic iron deposition, but this technology is available at few sites throughout the world. MRI of the liver or heart can be used to document iron overload,[6] and despite its limitations, serial serum ferritin levels can also be used to estimate systemic iron burden. Patients with chronically elevated ferritin levels (1500–2500 ng/mL or greater), and those who have received 25–50 units of PRBCs, should be considered for iron chelation therapy with subcutaneous desferrioxamine.[7,8] Unfortunately, because of the cost, discomfort, and time involved in its administration, desferrioxamine therapy is frequently refused or administered irregularly by MDS patients. Oral chelating agents are being evaluated in Europe (deferiprone) and in the United States (ICL670), primarily in patients with thalassemia. If shown to be effective and safe in MDS, oral chelating agents may be used with or instead of desferrioxamine in the future.

Other risks of transfusion therapy include acute transfusion reactions, alloimmunization, transfusion-associated graft-versus-host disease, and rarely, the transmission of infectious diseases, such as HIV, hepatitis viruses, or even more rarely West Nile virus.[9,10] These risks, as well as iron overload, can be lessened with the judicious use of transfusions. Irradiated blood products should be used for patients with MDS undergoing intensive therapy or ablative transplant conditioning to prevent transfusion-associated graft-versus-host disease. Furthermore, leukocyte depletion of RBC and platelet transfusions can reduce the incidence of human leukocyte antigen (HLA) alloimmunization, transmission of viral infections, and transfusion reactions.

## LOW-INTENSITY THERAPY

Low-intensity therapies include hematopoietic growth factors (such as recombinant erythropoietin), immunosuppressive therapy (IST), hypomethylating agents (5-azacytadine and decitabine, though only in specific subsets of early MDS patients), and antiangiogenic/immunomodulatory agents (such as thalidomide or lenalidomide). They may be administered as standard care, when appropriate, or in the context of a clinical trial. For patients with IPSS low or intermediate-1 risk disease, these treatments may be used before or concomitant with supportive care measures, or when supportive care measures are no longer effective or interfere significantly with a patient's QOL (e.g., due to frequent transfusions, infections). Low-intensity therapy may also be used for higher risk patients who are elderly or have significant comorbid conditions that prevent them from receiving higher intensity therapies, or at times used in preparation for such high-intensity treatment.

### GROWTH FACTORS

Following the Food and Drug Administration (FDA) approval of recombinant human erythropoietin (rHuEPO) therapy for treating anemia in hemodialysis patients, rHuEPO was given to patients with anemia, including those with MDS, in a variety of clinical trials.

These studies are summarized in Table 40.1. A meta-analysis of 17 early, small studies in anemic MDS patients revealed an overall erythroid response rate of 16%, generally at rHuEPO doses >150 U/kg three times per week.[11] Predictors for a response (a rise in hemoglobin $\geq$2.0 g/dL or becoming PRBC transfusion independent) included a low serum-erythropoietin level, nontransfusion-dependent anemia, and a diagnosis of refractory anemia (RA) or refractory anemia with excess blasts (RAEB). Patients with low erythropoietin levels and few or no transfusion requirements had a response rate >50%. High doses of erythropoietin are

| Table 40.1 | Larger trials of rHuEPO (alone or with rHuG-CSF or rHuGM-CSF) to treat anemia in MDS patients | | | | | |
|---|---|---|---|---|---|---|
| Reference | Trial design | Number of patients | Overall erythroid response rate | Erythroid response | | Response correlates |
| | | | | Major | Minor | |
| 11 | Phase II Meta-analysis EPO | 205 | 16% | ND | ND | EPO <200 U/L; no prior PRBC transfusions |
| (Rose, Abels et al. 1995) | Phase II EPO | 115 (100 evaluable) | 28% | ND | ND | RA; EPO <100 U/L |
| (Terpos, Mougiou et al. 2002) | Phase II EPO | 292 (281 evaluable) | 18% at 12 weeks / 45% at 26 weeks | 8% at 12 weeks / 27% at 26 weeks | 10% at 12 weeks / 18% at 26 weeks | EPO <150 U/L; IPSS good risk cytogenetics |
| 15 | Phase III, EPO vs. Placebo | 87 (75 evaluable -38 on EPO arm) | 37% (vs. 11%, $P = 0.007$) | 13% (vs. 0%) | 24% (vs. 11%) | RA; EPO <200 U/L; no prior PRBC transfusions |
| (Negrin, Stein et al. 1996) | Phase II, EPO + G-CSF | 55 | 48% | 32% | 16% | Low EPO level |
| (Hellstrom-Lindberg, Ahlgren et al. 1998) | Phase II, EPO + G-CSF | 56 (47 evaluable) | 38% | 21% | 17% | EPO level <500 U/LI; $\leq$2 u PRBC/mos. |
| (Remacha, Arrizabalaga et al. 1999) | Phase II, EPO + G-CSF | 32 | 50% | 38% | 13% | Predicitive model (Hellstrom-Lindberg, Negrin et al. 1997) |
| (Mantovani, Lentini et al. 2000) | Phase II, EPO + G-CSF | 33 (28 evaluable at 12 weeks) | 61% at 12 weeks / 80% at 26 weeks | 43% at 12 weeks / −56% at 36 weeks | 18% at 12 weeks / −25% at 36 weeks | Higher pre-tx HGB level |
| (Hellstrom-Lindberg, Gulbrandsen et al. 2003) | Phase II, EPO + G-CSF | 63 (53 evaluable) | 42% | 28% | 13% | Predicitive model (Hellstrom-Lindberg, Negrin et al. 1997) |
| (Casadevall, Durieux et al. 2004) | EPO + G-CSF vs. supp. care | 60 (24 evaluable in treatment arm) | 42% vs. 0% ($p = 0.01$) | 2/24; 8/24 | 8/24; 7/24 | RA and RARS |
| (Thompson, Gilliland et al. 2000) | EPO + GM-CSF | 45 | 9% | ND | ND | EPO <500 U/L |

EPO, recombinant erythropoietin; G-CSF, recombinant granulocyte colony-stimulating factor; GM-CSF, recombinant granulocyte-macrophage colony-stimulating factor; PRBC, packed red blood cell transfusions; RA, refractory anemia; RARS, refractory anemia with ringed sideroblasts; Hgb, hemoglobin (g/DL); ND, not determined.

needed to grow BFU-E and CFU-E from MDS bone marrows,[12] and inappropriately low serum-erythropoietin levels are seen in only approximately one third of patients with MDS[13,14]; perhaps these features account for the low clinical response rates seen. In the only randomized, placebo-controlled, phase III rHuEPO trial, 87 MDS patients with a Hgb <9.0 g/dL were treated with rHuEPO at a dose of 150 U/kg/day for 8 weeks. An overall response rate of 36.8% was detected.[15] Patients with RA or refractory anemia with ringed sideroblasts (RARS) were the most responsive, and nontransfused patients fared better than those that had been transfused. Although rHuEPO can improve hematocrit levels in relatively low-risk patients with low erythropoietin levels and low transfusion requirements, its impact on survival and QOL is not well characterized. Also, most patients in these clinic trials received rHuEPO three or more times per week. This frequent self-injection schedule may be too cumbersome or uncomfortable for most patients, and it is unknown whether similar results can be achieved in a routine outpatient setting.

rHuEPO is well tolerated in patients with anemia, and although some cases of pure red cell aplasia have been associated with rHuEPO, these episodes appeared to be related to packaging and storage problems with a specific rHuEPO formulation (used primarily in Europe) that may have increased the immunogenicity of the drug.[16] As transfusion therapy can be associated with short-term and long-term complications, the use of rHuEPO in responding anemic MDS patients has major advantages over transfusion therapy.

Granulocyte colony-stimulating factor (G-CSF) (and Granulocyte-macrophage colony-stimulating factor (GM-CSF) to a lesser extent) increase peripheral blood neutrophil counts in MDS patients,[17] but neither has proven beneficial for long-term use. The lack of clinical benefit for G-CSF was demonstrated in a randomized clinical trial, which showed that prophylactic G-CSF did not decrease the incidence of infections or improve survival compared to standard supportive care.[18] A randomized trial of GM-CSF likewise showed no significant benefit.[19] Nonetheless, MDS patients may benefit from the short-term use of G-CSF, particularly during an infection-prone period (e.g., perioperatively), during the transient neutropenia which follows induction chemotherapy, or in the setting of antibiotic-resistant infection. As G-CSF and GM-CSF can rarely exacerbate thrombocytopenia,[18,20] these agents should be used with caution in severely thrombocytopenic patients.

In vivo and in vitro synergy on erythropoiesis has been demonstrated for rHuEPO and G-CSF. Erythroid response rates of 38–50% have been reported when these agents are combined[21,22] and responses have been lost and restored with the withdrawal and re-initiation of G-CSF, supporting their synergism.[23] Having RARS (where the response rate is 50%)[21,23,24] or

low pretreatment erythropoietin levels (≤500 U/L) and PRBC transfusion dependence of less than 2 units/month is predictive of an erythroid response to combined rHuEPO/G-CSF.[25] A randomized trial comparing G-CSF plus rHuEPO to supportive care showed that despite improvements in hematocrit and transfusion requirements, QOL parameters did not significantly improve, although the study showing this was likely underpowered to detect QOL differences.[26] No change in survival has been reported with this treatment; thus, its use should still be largely investigational. Because of its toxicity and low response rate, the combination of GM-CSF and rHuEPO is not recommended for MDS patients.[27]

### IMMUNOMODULATORY DRUGS

Both immunomodulatory therapy and IST have been tried in patients with MDS. Thalidomide is an immunomodulatory agent with numerous cytokine-altering and antiangiogenic effects.[28,29] On the basis of its significant clinical activity in multiple myeloma,[30] thalidomide has been given to MDS patients in attempts to favorably modify the bone marrow cytokine milieu and possibly impair angiogenesis. Thalidomide appears to have mostly erythropoietic activity in MDS, but it is not well tolerated. In one phase II thalidomide study, 51 of 83 patients were able to complete 12 weeks of thalidomide therapy, and 15 had an erythroid response[31] using the International Working Group response criteria. While 11 patients (13%) had a major erythroid response (a hemoglobin rise of >2 gm/dL or loss of transfusion dependence), 32 patients (38%) were removed from the study or they withdrew their consent because of excessive toxicity, progression of disease, or other medical problems. Similar results have been obtained in other trials of thalidomide in MDS, as summarized in Table 40.2. Although anemia may be significantly improved, myelosuppression is often seen, and it is difficult to predict who will respond to thalidomide. While a North American phase III trial comparing thalidomide to supportive care has been completed, its outcome has not yet been reported.

Another "immunomodulatory" agent, CC-5013 (lenalidomide), appears to have greater erythropoietic activity than does thalidomide in PRBC transfusion-dependent MDS patients. A phase I/II clinical trial of lenalidomide in MDS patients was presented at the 2003 American Society of Hematology Annual Meeting. The 33 enrolled patients had primarily low-risk MDS by IPSS score (88% were in the Low/Int-1 group) and all had significant anemia (Hgb level <9g/dL or transfusion dependent). The overall erythroid response rate was 64%, with a 58% major erythroid response rate.[32] Many patients had received, but had not responded to, thalidomide or rHuEPO therapy. The median increase in hemoglobin level was 4.4 g/dL in responding patients, and the time to treatment failure was 19–71+

| Table 40.2 | Phase II trials of thalidomide for the treatment of anemia in MDS | | | | |
|---|---|---|---|---|---|
| Reference | Number of patients | MDS subtype treated | Daily dose (mg) | ITT erythroid response rate | Drop out rate (for toxicity, POD, other) |
| (Raza, Meyer et al. 2001) | 83 | FAB-RA-36<br>RARS-13<br>RAEB-24<br>RAEBt-6<br>CMMoL-4<br>IPSS-Low-21<br>Int-1-37<br>Int-2-12<br>High-13 | 100–400 | 19%<br>(*n* = 15) | 42%<br>(*n* = 35) |
| (Musto, Falcone et al. 2002) | 25 | WHO-Ra-12<br>RAEB-I-4<br>RAEB-II-4<br>RARS-5 | 100–300 | 20%<br>(*n* = 5) | 40%<br>(*n* = 10) |
| (Strupp, Germing et al. 2002) | 34 | FAB-R-16<br>RARS-6<br>RAEB-4<br>RAEBt-5<br>CMMoL-3<br>IPSS-low-4<br>Inl-1-4<br>Int-2-9<br>High-7 | 100–500 | 56%<br>(*n* = 19) | 32%<br>(*n* = 11) |

IWG, international working group; IPSS, International Prognostic Scoring System; WHO, World Health Organization; CR, complete remission; PR, partial remission; ITT, intent to treat; POD, progression of disease; RA, refractory anemia; RARS, refractory anemia with ringed sideroblasts; RAEB, refractory anemia with excess blasts.

weeks (median not reached). In addition, lenalidomide induced major cytogenetic responses, including reversion to a normal karyotype in 10 patients. Response rates were highest in the RA subtype (82%), the IPSS Low/Int-1 risk groups (71%), in patients who never received rHuEPO (100%), and in patients with the 5q− cytogenetic abnormality (91% or 10/11 patients). Lenalidomide was well tolerated, with dose-dependent myelosuppression (neutropenia, thrombocytopenia) being the most common adverse event. Results from two recently completed, mutlicenter phase II trials, evaluating lenalidomide for 5q−-patients and for non-5q− MDS patients, will likely be reported in 2005. The apparent sensitivity of patients with the 5q− cytogenetic anomaly to lenalidomide is unexplained, as is the mechanism of action of lenalidomide or thalidomide.

### ATG AND CYCLOSPORINE
While ISTs, such as antithymocyte globulin (ATG) and cyclosporine, have remarkably altered the clinical course of patients with AA, these drugs have been of limited benefit in MDS patients. While patients with AA can be cured with IST, the response to IST in MDS patients is neither curative nor sustained beyond a year in most cases.[33] In one study, 16 of 42 patients with RA, RARS, or RAEB who were treated with 4 days of ATG became transfusion independent. The highest response rate was seen in RA patients (61%), whereas none of the patients with RARS responded.[34] Most responding patients had hypocellular marrows, and responses to ATG in both MDS and AA patients seems to be associated with expression of the HLA DR15,[35] even though patients with other HLA types also respond. Predictive models can help determine which factors in MDS patients are more likely to predict for response to ATG therapy, such as having RA, normal cytogenetics, pancytopenia, or a hypocellular bone marrow. Cyclosporine alone has also produced responses in MDS patients.[36,37]

### OTHER THERAPIES: AMIFOSTINE OR ARSENIC TRIOXIDE
Amifostine, an organic thiophosphate with antioxidant activity, was evaluated in the mid to late 1990s in MDS patients. Hematologic improvements were seen in 84% (5/18 patients) in the first amifostine trial,[38] but this response rate could not be confirmed in subsequent small phase II studies.[39–41] In general, responses were brief, and some responses were lost by the time the subsequent cycle of amifostine was due to be administered. Combinations of amifostine with other agents have also shown only modest activity.[42]

Arsenic trioxide, an FDA-approved treatment for acute promyelocytic leukemia, has also shown modest activity in MDS patients. Hematologic improvements were seen in two small early clinical trials,[43,44] and several patients had major erythroid responses with loss of transfusion dependence. Myelosuppression and other toxicities were generally mild to moderate and manageable, included grade 3 and 4 myelosuppression. In a study of arsenic trioxide and thalidomide, trilineage hematologic responses were seen in 2/28 patients, both of whom carried the inv(3)(q21q26.2) cytogenetic abnormality.[45] As our knowledge grows, the use of therapies without widespread efficacy in specific subsets of MDS patients (such as those with inv(3)(q21), if these results are confirmed by others) may be useful.

## DIFFERENTIATING AGENTS

The maturation block evident in patients with MDS has provided a rationale for more than a decade of treatments with "differentiation-inducing" agents. However, none of the clinical trials with such agents have provided clear evidence of a differentiating effect, despite the demonstration of in vitro differentiation effects on leukemia cell lines. The agents studied include retinoids, vitamin $D_3$ analogs, cytarabine (at one time thought to induce differentiation at low doses), phenylbutyrate, and hexamethylene bisacetamide. Overall, the results have been generally disappointing.[46] Low-dose cytarabine continues to be used for some MDS patients, perhaps based on a randomized study comparing low-dose cytarabine to supportive care, in which a 35% hematologic response was seen. However, in that study cytarabine did not improve survival or delay progression to acute myelocytic leukemia (AML).[47] cis-Retinoic acid was also shown to be no better than supportive care in another randomized trial.[48] A more recent trial reported hematologic improvement in 11/19 patients with the newer vitamin $D_3$ analog, calcitriol.[49]

## DEMETHYLATING AGENTS

DNA methylation is a normal mechanism of gene expression regulation, and abnormal DNA methylation patterns that can interfere with the expression of genes used for growth, differentiation, and survival are seen in MDS. It has been known for some time that hypomethylating drugs can promote in vitro cellular differentiation,[50] and that this occurs at doses much lower than those needed for maximal cytotoxic effect. The clinical trials using the DNA demethylating agents 5-azacytidine (azacitidine, Vidaza) and 5-aza-2'-deoxycytidine began decades ago, prior to a full understanding of their demethylating effects. As a result, they were initially studied as cytidine analogs, using a classic phase I design to determine their maximally tolerated dose in leukemia patients. Subsequent trials in MDS patients used lower, more tolerable doses, with the goal of inducing differentiation and minimizing toxicity, which manifested itself primarily as myelosuppression in the earlier, high-dose trials.

Low-dose 5-azacytidine was first used to treat MDS by the Cancer and Leukemia Group B (CALGB) in the 1980s. Small studies evaluated 5-azacytidine at a dose of 75 mg/m$^2$/day by either continuous intravenous infusion or subcutaneous injection for 7 days each month and found a 49% or 50% response rate, respectively; both showed a complete remission (CR) rate of 12%.[51,52] In a subsequent, multicenter, randomized, phase III trial, 191 patients with MDS of all subtypes were randomized to receive either 5-azacytidine given subcutaneously at a dose of 75 mg/m$^2$/day for 7 days per month with supportive care, or supportive care alone.[53] Patients on the supportive care arm were permitted to crossover to the 5-azacytidine arm after 4 months for worsening disease or persistent severe cytopenias. The overall response rate (CR + PR) on the 5-azacytidine arm was 23% (7% CR), with a median response duration of 15 months and a median time on treatment of 9.1 months. Hematologic improvement was seen in 37% of the patients. Responses were seen in all MDS subtypes, with a median time to best response of 93 days. Moreover, the median time to AML transformation or death was longer for patients randomized to receive 5-azacytidine (21 months) than those in the supportive care arm (12 months). A nonsignificant difference in median survival was detected (20 months vs. 14 months, $p = 0.10$), but a 6-month landmark analysis (to eliminate the confounding effect of the 49 crossover patients) detected an improvement in survival (18 months vs. 11 months, $p = 0.03$). Treatment with 5-azacytidine was also associated with significant improvements in QOL parameters, including fatigue, dyspnea, and psychological well-being.[54] 5-Azacytidine was approved by the FDA in May 2004 for all MDS subtypes based on this data, but treatment for the RA or RARS patients was approved only for those with moderate to severe neutropenia (ANC <1000/μL), thrombocytopenia (< 50,000/μL), or transfusion-dependent anemia.

The FDA approval of 5-azacytidine represents the first agent approved for treating patients with MDSs. The CALGB study of 5-azacytidine took many years to complete and report, and a confirmatory phase III study is underway comparing 5-azacytidine to several conventional therapies (supportive care, low-dose cytarabine, or intensive, AML-like therapies). The recent approval of 5-azacytidine in the United States suggests that this trial will primarily enroll patients in Europe. As the IPSS was not devised when the first phase III 5-azacytidine trial was started, this trial may better define which MDS patients have the highest likelihood of responding to 5-azacytidine.

Three large phase II studies of low-dose 5-aza-2'-deoxycitidine (decitabine) have been conducted in Europe, and the results recently summarized. Of 169

MDS patients treated with intravenous doses of 45–50 mg/m²/day for 3 days every 6 weeks (either 50 mg/m²/day by continuous i.v. infusion over 3 days, or 15 mg/m² every 8 h for 3 days for a total of 9 doses), 20% had a CR, 10% had a partial remission (PR), and the overall response rate was 49% (including hematologic improvement).[55] An early (after one cycle) and often dramatic rise in the platelet count was frequently seen, and was predictive of a subsequent trilineage response.[56] On the basis of these positive results, a multicenter, phase III study was opened in the United States and Canada, which completed accrual in 2003. A total of 160 patients were randomized to receive decitabine 15 mg/m² every 8 h over 3 days (total 45 mg/m²/day) plus supportive care, or supportive care alone, with no crossover allowed. Data from this trial was reported at the 2004 annual American Society of Hematology meeting with benefit seen in the IPSS high-risk and Int-2 risk patients, but not the Int-1 risk patients.[57] Among the key questions are whether decitabine and 5-azacytidine work equally well in the same types of patients, or whether some MDS patients would benefit more from one versus the other drug. In the absence of FDA approval of decitabine, however, such questions are not yet clinically relevant. An oral formulation of decitabine is in preclinical trials, and new hypomethylating agents (e.g., zebularine)[58] may also make their way into clinical trials.

These agents appear to induce hypomethylation by irreversibly binding and "trapping" DNA methyltransferases so that the next round of DNA replication produces a demethylated base at a site that was previously methylated. Although it is clear that these agents have clinical activity in MDS, demethylation of specific genes (e.g., the CDK inhibitors p15, p16, p21) has not been definitively correlated with clinical responses. Therefore, the specific mechanism by which hypomethylation induces responses in MDS remains unclear. Identifying biological correlates of clinical responses will help define the mechanism of action of these agents, and will identify predictors of hematologic responses in this heterogeneous disease. A common side effect of low-dose decitabine and 5-azacytidine is some degree of myelosuppression, which suggests that even at lower does, cytotoxicity may be important for the clinical responses seen in MDS.

Future studies with the demethylating agents 5-azacytidine and decitabine will hopefully improve our understanding of how these drugs improve the cytopenias and bone marrow function in MDS. These agents will also be combined with other therapies in an attempt to improve the CR rate and duration, which may include maintenance therapy. Attractive combinations include the use of hypomethylating agents with other drugs that also have an impact on gene regulation, such as all-*trans* retinoic acid (ATRA), vitamin D analogs, or histone deacetylase inhibitors such as SAHA, depsipeptide, phenylbutyrate, or valproic acid. Mouse models are finally being developed for MDS (e.g., see Ref. 4) and they may prove useful for such preclinical studies.

### NOVEL AGENTS AND COMBINATIONS

Improvements in our understanding of the pathobiology of MDS will help to generate new therapeutic approaches. As new agents are developed, some will be appropriate for low-risk patients, and given the

| Table 40.3 | Clinical trials of hypomethylating agents in MDS | | | | |
|---|---|---|---|---|---|
| Reference | Phase of trial | Number of patients | Dose | Response rate | Comments |
| 51 | II | 43 | 5-aza 75 mg/m² CI × 7 days | CR 12% PR/ HI 37% | |
| 52 | II | 67 | 5-aza 75 mg/m² subcutaneous × 7 days | CR 12% PR/ HI ~ 35% | |
| 53 | III | 191 | 5-aza | CR 7% PR 16% HI 37% | Median time to AML or death: 21 months for 5-aza vs. 14 months for SC (with crossover) |
| Wijermans et al Leukemia 1997 | I/II | 29 | DAC 120–150 mg/m² C.I. | CR 28% PR/HI 26% | Median survival = 46 weeks (actuar) |
| Wijermans et al JCO 2000 | II | 66 | DAC | CR 20% PR 4% HI 24% | |

GR, complete remission, PR, partial remission.

paucity of available treatments for MDS, patients should be referred for appropriate clinical trials whenever possible.Low-intensity therapies, such as histone deacetylase inhibitors, farnesyl transferase inhibitors, and tyrosine kinase inhibitors, are being tested in advanced MDS and AML, but may be evaluated in lower risk MDS as well. In Chapter X, such novel approaches to treating MDS will be discussed in detail.

## HIGH-INTENSITY THERAPY: CHEMOTHERAPY OR STEM CELL TRANSPLANTATION

Intensive chemotherapy treatment for MDS has generally produced complete remission rates of 40–50%, which is lower than the response rates seen in the younger patients with de novo AML. Furthermore, remission durations are generally brief (5–15 months), and given the treatment-related mortality of ~25–50% and the time required to recover to baseline function for survivors of such therapy, the use of AML-like therapies has been limited. Although some patients have achieved complete hematologic and cytogenetic remissions, no survival benefit has yet been shown for intensive chemotherapy. Several new combinations have been studied for advanced MDS, which include the topoisomerase I inhibitor topotecan.[59,60] These combinations are unlikely to produce a significant improvement in survival unless followed by allogeneic stem cell transplants. In general, these treatments should be reserved for higher risk patients enrolled in clinical trials, given the uncertain risk–benefit ratio.

Allogeneic stem cell transplant is the only potentially curable treatment for MDS. Although it appears that the associated short-term and long-term risks of transplant are generally acceptable for high-risk MDS patients, the optimal timing for transplanting patients

with low-risk disease is not established. Furthermore, it is not clear how pretransplant therapies or the degree of pretransplant cytoreduction impacts on the disease-free survival of MDS patients.

## TREATMENT OPTIONS—OVERVIEW

The choice of therapy, and the decision to undergo treatment, must be tailored to the individual patient. In general, the factors that govern these decisions include patient age, performance status, and medical comorbidities, as well as the patient's risk-aversion profile and the severity of the disease at presentation. MDSs are not curable without stem cell transplantation. However, the combination of advanced age and limited donor availability renders the vast majority of patients with MDS ineligible for such therapy. Intensive antileukemic chemotherapy may alter the natural history of MDS in some patients, but candidates for this therapy must be selected carefully to avoid excessive risk in this aging, medically vulnerable population.

Although supportive care remains a mainstay of treatment for many patients with low-risk, largely asymptomatic disease, the ability to impact the natural history of this disease in symptomatic (and possibly asymptomatic) patients now and in the future is exciting. Given the current state of the field, and paucity of curable options, patients with MDS should be treated on clinical protocols, if at all possible.

## COMPREHENSIVE TREATMENT STRATEGY FOR MDS

The clinical problems that MDS patients experience can be broken down into three basic categories. While anemia is the major problem for some patients, others have potentially life-threatening neutropenia or thrombocytopenia. Patients in both categories may be at high risk for developing AML. These scenarios are discussed below.

| Table 40.4   Treatment strategy for patients with MDS |
|---|
| Three clinical issues to consider if predominant problem is |
| (1) anemia: Consider rHuEPO +/− G-CSF, 5-azacytidine, ATG, (ce-5013 if FDA-approved), or Thalidomide (in a clinical trial); |
| (2) severe neutropenia or thrombocytopenia: Consider stem cell transplantation early. Alternatively (or pretransplant), consider 5-azacytidine (or decitabine, if available), ATG, or AML-like regimens; |
| (3) points 1 or 2 and/or increased blasts (at risk for leukemic progression): Consider Stem cell transplant, 5-azacytidine (or possibly decitabine). |
| Considerations for stem cell transplant candidates: patients with fewest precent blasts do best; not known if pre-stem cell transplant treatment is of benefit. |

1. *Anemia only*: These patients often have relatively good-risk disease, and are most suitable for low-intensity approaches or supportive care alone. rHuEPO should be tried for patients with symptomatic anemia; it works best in those with little or no transfusion requirements and relatively low serum erythropoietin levels. The doses required are higher than those used to treat chemotherapy-associated anemia. Patients with RARS, in particular, may benefit from combining G-CSF with rHuEPO, as there appears to be synergistic effects on erythropoiesis. Lenalidomide has shown significant activity in transfusion-dependent patients with a del(5q) cytogenetic abnormality, and also in those with a normal karyotype. Thalidomide has modest stimula-

tory activity on red blood cell production, but its activity seems inferior to lenalidomide. 5-Azacytidine has received FDA approval for RBC-transfusion-dependent patients. Although it has greater side effects than rHuEPO, its use may forestall the development of iron overload and thus may benefit certain high-risk patient subsets. Heavily transfused patients are appropriate candidates for investigational therapies and in rare instances, even stem cell transplantation. The timing for such treatment should be determined in consultation with a transplant physician.

2. *Neutropenia/thrombocytopenia*: Patients with mild to moderate, uncomplicated neutropenia and/or thrombocytopenia can often be observed; however, such patients should be evaluated on an individual basis. Patients with life-threatening neutropenia or thrombocytopenia warrant active treatment and not simply supportive care (such as platelet transfusions and antibiotics), even though some such patients may be assigned to a "low-risk" IPSS subcategory. 5-Azacytidine can induce trilineage responses and along with decitabine (an investigational agent in phase III testing) can induce rapid and impressive improvements in peripheral blood counts. Patients with severe cytopenias (even without an increase in bone marrow (BM) blasts) should be considered for allogeneic stem cell transplantation before they have life-threatening infectious or bleeding complications. Whether patients with cytopenias and no increase in BM blasts will have superior outcomes with reduced intensity stem cell transplantation is not known, but hopefully will be addressed in future clinical trials. Patients with severe cytopenias who are not eligible for a stem cell transplant should receive a series of low- or high-intensity therapies (e.g., AML-like treatment regimens) in clinical trials whenever possible.

3. *Patients at great risk for progressing to AML*: Patients with increased BM blasts and/or poor risk cytogenetics have a high likelihood of transforming to AML, and AML arising in a patient with MDS has an extremely poor prognosis. Thus, allogeneic stem cell transplant should be considered for such poor prognosis MDS patients as soon as possible. Many MDS patients will not be suitable transplant candidates based on their performance status, other complicating medical problems, age, or lack of a suitable donor. Improvements in unrelated donor transplantation may provide more hope for these patients in the future. A major risk for these patients post-stem cell transplant is disease relapse. Whether using 5-azacytidine, or standard AML induction therapy, to reduce the BM blast count prior to transplantation will improve transplant outcomes, is not known. It is a vitally important question to address. Patients who are not eligible for a stem cell transplant should be treated with 5-azacytidine, or with investigational therapy in the setting of a clinical trial.

## ACKNOWLEDGMENTS

The authors are supported by grants from the Leukemia Lymphoma Society (VK, SN), the NIH P01 CA05826 (CCPP) (SN), and the Rosemary Breslin Research fund. The authors thank Heather Hewitt and Ellie Park, for assisting in the preparation of this work, our colleagues at Memorial Sloan-Kettering Cancer Center, and the Myelodysplastic Syndrome Foundation.

## REFERENCES

1. Bennett JM, et al.: Proposals for the classification of the acute leukaemias. French–American–British (FAB) co-operative group. *Br J Haemato l* 33(4):451–458, 1976.
2. Bennett JM: World Health Organization classification of the acute leukemias and myelodysplastic syndrome. *Int J Hemato l* 72(2):131–133, 2000.
3. Greenberg P, et al.: International scoring system for evaluating prognosis in myelodysplastic syndromes. *Blood* 89(6):2079–2088, 1997.
4. Cleeland CS, et al.: Identifying hemoglobin level for optimal quality of life: results of an incremental analysis [abstract]. *Proc Am Soc Clin Oncol* 18:574a, 1999. Abstract 2215.
5. Saif MW, Hopkins JL, Gore SD: Autoimmune phenomena in patients with myelodysplastic syndromes and chronic myelomonocytic leukemia. *Leuk Lymphoma* 43(11):2083–2092, 2002.
6. Anderson LJ, et al.: Cardiovascular T2-star (T2*) magnetic resonance for the early diagnosis of myocardial iron overload. *Eur Heart J* 22(23):2171–2179, 2000.
7. Telfer PT, et al.: Hepatic iron concentration combined with long-term monitoring of serum ferritin to predict complications of iron overload in thalassaemia major. *Br J Haematol* 110(4):971–977, 2000.
8. Olivieri NF, et al.: Survival in medically treated patients with homozygous beta-thalassemia. *N Engl J Med* 331(9):574–578, 1994.
9. Dodd RY, Notari EPt, Stramer SL: Current prevalence and incidence of infectious disease markers and estimated window-period risk in the American Red Cross blood donor population. *Transfusion* 42(8):975–979, 2002.
10. *West Nile Virus Viremic Blood Donor Activity in the United States* (reported to CDC as of September 21, 2004). Available at: http://www.cdc.gov/ncidod/dvbid/west-nile/surv&control104Maps_Viremic.htm
11. Hellstrom-Lindberg E: Efficacy of erythropoietin in the myelodysplastic syndromes: a meta-analysis of 205 patients from 17 studies. *Br J Haematol* 89(1):67–71, 1995.
12. Aoki I, et al.: Responsiveness of bone marrow erythropoietic stem cells (CFU-E and BFU-E) to recombinant

human erythropoietin (rh-Ep) in vitro in aplastic anemia and myelodysplastic syndrome. *Am J Hematol* 35(1):6–12, 1990.

13. Jacobs A, et al.: Circulating erythropoietin in patients with myelodysplastic syndromes. *Br J Haematol* 73(1):36–39, 1989.

14. Casadevall N: Update on the role of epoetin alfa in hematologic malignancies and myelodysplastic syndromes. *Semin Oncol* 25(3 suppl 7):12–18, 1998.

15. Anonymous: A randomized double-blind placebo-controlled study with subcutaneous recombinant human erythropoietin in patients with low-risk myelodysplastic syndromes. Italian Cooperative Study Group for rHuEpo in Myelodysplastic Syndromes. *Br J Haematol* 103(4):1070–1074, 1998.

16. Bennett CL, et al.: Pure red-cell aplasia and epoetin therapy. *N Engl J Med* 351(14):1403–1408, 2004.

17. Harmenberg J, Hoglund M, Hellstrom-Lindberg E: G- and GM-CSF in oncology and oncological haematology. *Eur J Haematol Suppl* 55:1–28, 1994.

18. Greenberg P, et al.: Phase III randomized multicenter trial of G-CSF vs. observation for myelodysplastic syndromes (MDS). *Blood* 82(suppl 1):196a, 1993.

19. Willemze R, et al.: A randomized phase-I/II multicenter study of recombinant human granulocyte-macrophage colony-stimulating factor (GM-CSF) therapy for patients with myelodysplastic syndromes and a relatively low risk of acute leukemia. EORTC Leukemia Cooperative Group. *Ann Hematol* 64(4):173–180, 1992.

20. Schuster MW, et al.: Granulocyte-macrophage colony-stimulating factor (GM-CSF) for myelodysplastic syndrome (MDS): results of a multi-center randomized trial. *Blood* 76:318a, 1990.

21. Hellstrom-Lindberg E, et al.: Treatment of anemia in myelodysplastic syndromes with granulocyte colony-stimulating factor plus erythropoietin: results from a randomized phase II study and long-term follow-up of 71 patients. *Blood* 92(1):68–75, 1998.

22. Negrin RS, et al.: Treatment of the anemia of myelodysplastic syndromes using recombinant human granulocyte colony-stimulating factor in combination with erythropoietin. *Blood* 82(3):737–743, 1993.

23. Negrin RS, et al.: Maintenance treatment of the anemia of myelodysplastic syndromes with recombinant human granulocyte colony-stimulating factor and erythropoietin: evidence for in vivo synergy. *Blood* 87(10):4076–4081, 1996.

24. Remacha AF, et al.: Erythropoietin plus granulocyte colony-stimulating factor in the treatment of myelodysplastic syndromes. Identification of a subgroup of responders. The Spanish Erythropathology Group. *Haematologica* 84(12):1058–1064, 1999.

25. Hellstrom-Lindberg E, et al.: Erythroid response to treatment with G-CSF plus erythropoietin for the anaemia of patients with myelodysplastic syndromes: proposal for a predictive model. *Br J Haematol* 99(2):344–351, 1997.

26. Casadevall N, et al.: Health, economic, and quality-of-life effects of erythropoietin and granulocyte colony-stimulating factor for the treatment of myelodysplastic syndromes: a randomized, controlled trial. *Blood* 104(2):321–327, 2004.

27. Thompson JA, et al.: Effect of recombinant human erythropoietin combined with granulocyte/macrophage colony-stimulating factor in the treatment of patients with myelodysplastic syndrome. GM/EPO MDS Study Group. *Blood* 95(4):1175–1179, 2000.

28. D'Amato RJ, et al.: Thalidomide is an inhibitor of angiogenesis. *Proc Natl Acad Sci* USA 91(9):4082–4085, 1994.

29. Moreira AL, et al.: Thalidomide exerts its inhibitory action on tumor necrosis factor alpha by enhancing mRNA degradation. *J Exp Med* 177(6):1675-1680, 1993.

30. Singhal S, et al.: Antitumor activity of thalidomide in refractory multiple myeloma. *N Engl J Med* 341(21):1565–1571, 1999.

31. Raza A, et al.: Thalidomide produces transfusion independence in long-standing refractory anemias of patients with myelodysplastic syndromes. *Blood* 98(4):958–965, 2001.

32. List AF, et al.: Efficacy and safety of CC5013 for treatment of anemia in patients with myelodysplastic syndromes (MDS) [abstract]. *Blood* 102(11):184a, 2003. Abstract 641.

33. Biesma DH, van den Tweel JG, Verdonck LF: Immunosuppressive therapy for hypoplastic myelodysplastic syndrome. *Cancer* 79(8):1548–1551, 1997.

34. Molldrem JJ, et al.: Antithymocyte globulin for patients with myelodysplastic syndrome. *Br J Haematol* 99(3):699–705, 1997.

35. Saunthararajah Y, et al.: HLA-DR15 (DR2) is overrepresented in myelodysplastic syndrome and aplastic anemia and predicts a response to immunosuppression in myelodysplastic syndrome. *Blood* 100(5):1570–1574, 2002.

36. Catalano L, et al.: Prolonged response to cyclosporin-A in hypoplastic refractory anemia and correlation with in vitro studies. *Haematologica* 85(2):133–138, 2000.

37. Jonasova A, et al.: Cyclosporin A therapy in hypoplastic MDS patients and certain refractory anaemias without hypoplastic bone marrow. *Br J Haematol* 100(2):304–309, 1998.

38. List AF, et al.: Stimulation of hematopoiesis by amifostine in patients with myelodysplastic syndrome. *Blood* 90(9):3364–3369, 1997.

39. Bowen DT, et al.: Poor response rate to a continuous schedule of Amifostine therapy for 'low/intermediate risk' myelodysplastic patients. *Br J Haematol* 103(3):785–787, 1998.

40. Invernizzi R, et al.: Clinical and biological effects of treatment with amifostine in myelodysplastic syndromes. *Br J Haematol* 118(1):246–250, 2002.

41. Grossi A, et al.: Amifostine in the treatment of low-risk myelodysplastic syndromes. *Haematologica* 85(4):367–371, 2000.

42. Raza A, et al.: Patients with myelodysplastic syndromes benefit from palliative therapy with amifostine, pentoxifylline, and ciprofloxacin with or without dexamethasone. *Blood* 95(5):1580–1587, 2000.

43. List AF, et al.: Arsenic trioxide in patients with myelodysplastic syndromes (MDS): preliminary results of a phase II clinical study [abstract]. *J Clin Oncol* 22(14S), 2004. Abstract 6512.

44. Vey N, et al.: Trisenox™ (arsenic trioxide) in patients with myelodysplastic syndromes (MDS): preliminary results of a phase I/II study [abstract]. In: *Abstracts and Program of the 9th Congress of the European Hematology Association*, 2004 June 10–13(. Abstract #467.

45. Raza A, et al.: Arsenic trioxide and thalidomide combination produces multi-lineage hematological responses

in myelodysplastic syndromes patients, particularly in those with high pre-therapy EVI1 expression. *Leuk Res* 28(8):791–803, 2004.

46. Morosetti R, Koeffler HP: Differentiation therapy in myelodysplastic syndromes. *Semin Hematol* 33(3): 236–245, 1996.

47. Miller KB, et al.: The evaluation of low-dose cytarabine in the treatment of myelodysplastic syndromes: a phase-III intergroup study. *Ann Hematol* 65(4):162–168, 1992.

48. Koeffler HP, et al.: Randomized study of 13-cis retinoic acid v placebo in the myelodysplastic disorders. *Blood* 71(3):703–708, 1988.

49. Mellibovsky L, et al.: Vitamin D treatment in myelodysplastic syndromes. *Br J Haematol* 100(3):516–520, 1998.

50. Jones PA, Taylor SM: Cellular differentiation, cytidine analogs and DNA methylation. *Cell* 20(1):85–93, 1980.

51. Silverman LR, et al.: Effects of treatment with 5-azacytidine on the in vivo and in vitro hematopoiesis in patients with myelodysplastic syndromes. *Leukemia* 7 (suppl 1): 21–29, 1993.

52. Silverman LR, Holland JC, et al.: Azacytidine (azaC) in myelodysplastic syndromes (MDS), CALGB studies 8421 and 8921 (abstract). *Ann Hematol* 68(suppl 1):12a, 1994.

53. Silverman LR, et al.: Randomized controlled trial of azacitidine in patients with the myelodysplastic syndrome: a study of the cancer and leukemia group B. *J Clin Oncol* 20(10):2429–2440, 2002.

54. Kornblith AB, et al.: Impact of azacytidine on the quality of life of patients with myelodysplastic syndrome treated in a randomized phase III trial: a Cancer and Leukemia Group B study. *J Clin Oncol* 20(10):2441–2452, 2002.

55. Wijermans PW, Luebbert M, Verhoef G: Low dose Decitabine for elderly high risk MDS patients: who will respond? [abstract] *Blood* 100(11):96a, 2002. Abstract 355.

56. van denBosch J, et al.: The effects of 5-aza-2'-deoxycytidine (Decitabine) on the platelet count in patients with intermediate and high-risk myelodysplastic syndromes. *Leuk Res* 28(8):785–790, 2004.

57. Saba H, et al.: First report of the phase III North American trial of Dectabine in advanced myelodysplastic syndrome (MDS) [abstract]. *Blood* 104(11):23a, 2004. Abstract 67.

58. Cheng JC, et al.: Inhibition of DNA methylation and reactivation of silenced genes by zebularine. *J Natl Cancer Inst* 95(5):399–409, 2003.

59. Beran M, et al.: Results of topotecan single-agent therapy in patients with myelodysplastic syndromes and chronic myelomonocytic leukemia. *Leuk Lymphoma* 31(5–6):521–531, 1998.

60. Beran M, et al.: Topotecan and cytarabine is an active combination regimen in myelodysplastic syndromes and chronic myelomonocytic leukemia. *J Clin Oncol* 17(9):2819–2830, 1999.

# Chapter **41**

# APLASTIC ANEMIA AND STEM CELL FAILURE

*Jaroslaw P. Maciejewski*

## INTRODUCTION

### HISTORY

Dramatic disappearance of the marrow and profound cytopenia seemingly occurring without prodromal signs have stimulated the research of generations of physicians and scientists since the initial descriptions of aplastic anemia (AA) in the last decades of the nineteenth century. The almost inevitable fatal outcome of severe AA made it a subject of research by renowned hematologists. Later, its illustrative features allowed insights into stem cell function, regulation of blood cell production, and the role of immune system in the regulation of hematopoiesis. Research into the causes of AA has led to the description of cellular elements of blood, and later to the introduction of stem cell transplantation as a means of replacing a defective stem cell compartment. Today, the longer survival of patients with AA uncovers new instructive aspects of the disease and provides new therapeutic challenges. These aspects include the evolution of clonal diseases, such a myelodysplastic syndromes (MDS) and paroxysmal nocturnal hemoglobinuria (PNH).

### EPIDEMIOLOGY AND DEMOGRAPHICS

AA can occur at any age, but the peak incidence is in early adulthood. It is not clear whether the often described second peak in the sixth to seventh decades of life may be a result of the diagnostic overlap of AA and MDS that affects older individuals and can mimic AA, especially if the marrow is hypocellular.[1-3] The incidence of AA in the United States and Europe is comparable at around $4/10^6$ individuals.[4-6] In East Asia, the incidence of AA appears to be significantly higher, an early observation made by Dr Dameshek. This endemic occurrence of AA in the Far East led to many theories as to how this disease relates to PNH, also more prevalent in this part of the world, and to the search for geographically related epidemiologic factors, such as endemic pathogens. The extensive epidemiologic studies performed in Thailand did not yield specific clues, but disproved speculations as to

the role of hepatitis viruses in the etiology of classic idiopathic AA.[7] AA has been described in Africa and India, where it may be also more prevalent than in the West, but exact epidemiologic studies are not available. In the United States, AA does not appear to show an ethnic predilection.

## PATHOPHYSIOLOGY

### STEM CELL FAILURE IN AA
#### Direct and indirect stem cell injury

Iatrogenic bone marrow failure induced by chemotherapeutic drugs or radiation is perhaps the best example of a direct injury to hematopoietic stem cells. While stem cells, due to their dormant nature, may be more resistant to certain cytotoxic drugs, clearly a dose–response relationship with the degree of stem cell damage can be established. Noniatrogenic direct stem cell injury is less well characterized. If a putative inciting agent directly destroys stem cells, causing a permanent depletion, the clinical presentation of cytopenia may be delayed, precluding recognition of the causative agent. Regardless of the mechanism, direct stem cell damage is most likely random and can become obvious when certain critically low stem cell numbers are reached. None of these viral agents has been directly implicated in the pathogenesis of idiopathic AA. In the case of drugs and chemical agents most notoriously implicated in the pathogenesis of AA, the direct toxicity as a mechanism of injury is also in question. However, the most compelling evidence exists that the mechanisms of stem cell damage in AA are indirectly mediated by the cells of the immune system (see below).[8-10]

#### Quantitative defect

Theoretically, failed blood cell production in AA could be attributed to a defect restricted to the progenitor cell compartment and/or involve a stem cell. Low numbers of hematopoietic progenitors, as measured by colony assays or by flow cytometry, have been a consistent finding in AA.[11–16] Both the more committed as well as the immature (CD34+c-kit− or CD34+CD38−) progenitor cells are depleted.[15] Hematopoietic progenitor cells from AA show decreased sensitivity to trophic signals,[13] and colony formation by AA bone marrow cells remains unresponsive in vitro and in vivo, even to high levels of circulating hematopoietic growth factors present in most patients.[17–19] Unlike in murine models, measurement of more immature progenitor and stem cells is not easily accomplished in humans.

The hematopoietic recovery following successful immunosuppression demonstrates that some stem cells must be spared from the pathologic process. Serial studies were conducted to determine the numbers of stem cells during the course of disease; a profound defect in the numbers may persist for a long time upon hematopoietic recovery, e.g., following successful immunosuppression.[20,21] In most patients, a residual numeric defect may be permanent despite a full recovery of the blood counts. Complete reconstitution of the numbers may be found only in a minority of patients who sustained a complete remission.[20] Nevertheless, serial studies suggested that at least partial recovery of stem cells is possible, and a highly depleted stem cell pool can sustain seemingly normal blood cell counts (Figure 41.1).

## Qualitative defect

In multiple studies stromal function has been found to be unaffected in AA.[22–24] The defect of the stem cells, rather than that of supporting stroma, has been elegantly demonstrated in experiments in which CD34+ cells from AA patients showed poor growth on allogeneic normal stromal layers, while normal CD34+ cells planted on the stroma derived from AA patients showed normal growth properties.[19,22] Clinically, stem cell transplantation is a highly successful therapy in AA, but stromal elements remain of host origin following transplantation.[25] Damage to the stem cell compartment in acquired AA is likely the main cause for the quantitative defect by all measures used to quantitate early hematopoietic cells. The number of colony-forming cells or long-term culture-initiating cells (LTC-IC) assayed from purified CD34+ population derived from AA patients is lower than that observed with normal CD34+ cells.[12,21,26] A decreased proportion of cycling cells has also been described in AA,[11] suggesting that a blockade in cell cycling may precede apoptosis.[27,28] Alternatively, quiescent cells are resistant to apoptotic stimuli, and cycling cells may be selectively inhibited or killed, effectively turning off all active stem cells.

## Apoptosis, telomere shortening, and genetic damage

In AA, an abundance of trophic signals and a relative lack of efficacy of hematopoietic growth factors argue against their deficiency as a mechanism of apoptosis.[17] However, an increased apoptotic fraction within CD34+

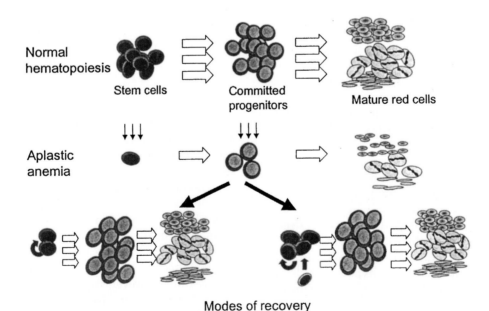

**Figure 41.1** *Fate of hematopoietic stem cell compartment in aplastic anemia. Under normal circumstances, within the stem cell compartment, a certain number of cycling stem cells maintain supplies of committed progenitor cells that produce mature blood cells. In immune-mediated aplastic anemia, all stages of hematopoietic development are affected but the decrease of the stem cell numbers is the essential lesion, explaining involvement of all blood cell lineages. After successful treatment (e.g., with immunosuppression), removal of inhibitory stimuli may allow the remaining stem cells to compensate their numeric deficiency with increased production of committed progenitor cells, and, as a result, normal or seminormal blood cell counts can be maintained (right portion). However, a limited regeneration of stem cells may be possible (either within the compartment itself or through recruitment from the more pluripotent pool) and the normal blood cell production is restored (left)*

cell populations derived from AA has been demonstrated.[29–31] In addition to proapoptotic cytokines and growth factors withdrawal, apoptosis in AA may be mediated by nitric oxide or oxygen radicals secreted by CD34[+] cells in paracrine fashion.[32,33]

Frequent evolution of clonal disease[34,35] suggests that the process leading to the depletion of stem cells may promote acquisition of stem cell damage, and the expansion of the dysplastic clone may be the result of a clonal escape, possibly due to a different susceptibility to depletion mechanisms between normal and mutated stem cells. It is also possible that the depletion of normal stem cells may more likely facilitate the recruitment of a preexisting defective (under normal circumstances quiescent) stem cell (known as the oligoclonality theory). Alternatively, some of the proposed proapoptotic signals may serve as potential DNA-damaging agents. The putative mechanisms may involve generation of reactive oxygen and nitrogen species capable of damaging the DNA.

In true stem cells, self-renewal does not result in telomere shortening, but upon recruitment and commitment the telomere length progressively declines with each division.[36–38] In general, shorter telomeres, measured by various methods, were reported in AA.[38–40] While patients with chronic moderate AA showed short telomeres, in acute severe cytopenia, shortening of the telomeres may not be evident due to the blocking of stem cell cycling. Upon recovery, due to the recruitment of new stem cells, telomeres of the progeny may provide longer measurements again, or, if the stem cell number operating at a given time is small (and normal cell counts maintained), telomere shortening may be more pronounced. In general, once a critical telomere length is reached, chromosomes may become unstable. Such a mechanism could explain the evolution of clonal karyotypic defects in AA, but shortened chromosomes were not consistently found in AA patients who evolved into myelodysplasia.

### CLASSIFICATION OF AA BASED ON ETIOLOGY AND PATHOPHYSIOLOGIC MECHANISMS

AA may have diverse causes that allow for clinically useful classification (Table 41.1). While iatrogenic AA is uncommon, it can be easily recognized. The most common is the idiopathic form of AA, and most parts of this chapter deal with this classical AA entity. Congenital bone marrow failure syndromes can evolve to AA; they will not be discussed in detail here.

#### Drug- and chemical-induced AA

Drugs and chemicals have been implicated as etiologic agents in AA for many decades. Benzene has served as a model chemical implicated in AA.[41–43] Intermittent exposure may be at least or even more toxic than chronic exposure. The mechanism of benzene toxicity is not entirely clear, and several metabolites may be

| Table 41.1 | Classification of aplastic anemia by etiology |
|---|---|
| **Aplastic anemia** | |
| Acquired aplastic anemia | Inherited aplastic anemia |
| *Idiopathic aplastic anemia* | Fanconi anemia |
| Pregnancy | Dyskeratosis congenita |
| Paroxysmal nocturnal hemoglobinuria | Reticular dysgenesis |
| | Schwachman anemia |
| *Secondary* | Genetic primary non-hematologic syndromes |
| Drugs | |
|   Iatrogenic/cytotoxic | |
|   Idiosyncratic | |
| Radiation | |
|   Iatrogenic | |
|   Accidental | |
| Viruses | |
| Pancytopenia of autoimmune diseases | |

involved. Consequently, genetic polymorphisms of the catabolic pathways may constitute predisposition factors for the development of benzene toxicity. In addition to direct toxicity comparable to that of some cytotoxic agents, other mechanisms, including stromal damage or even immune mediated effects, can be involved. Other aromatic hydrocarbons are also cited as causes of AA. Similarly, pesticides and insecticides have often been reported as causes of AA, but the rigorous systematic epidemiologic studies are scarce or showed mixed results. Overall, the proportion or cases attributable to specific pesticides or aromatic hydrocarbons is relatively small, especially given the ubiquitous nature of these chemicals in the modern world.

Medical drugs have been frequently implicated as causes of AA.[6] Cytotoxic agents may serve as a prototype, and a patient's medical history should make a diagnosis obvious. Of importance are drugs used for treatment of unrelated disorders. Chloramphenicol and AA as well as aminopyridine and agranulocytosis are the best examples of agents recognized to be associated with an increased risk of disease.[44–46] In general, drug reactions can be classified into dose-related effects and idiosyncratic reactions, in which occurrence is rare and not dose dependent. The list of drugs that have been implicated in causing AA is long, but all of them can account only for a fraction of cases (around 15%). The most comprehensive epidemiologic study performed in Europe identified agents that were associated with the occurrence of AA, but for most of the cases the stratified risk estimate was relatively low. The highest risk was found for some nonsteroidal anti-inflammatory drugs (NSAIDs) (piroxicam), gold, antithyroid agents, and allopurinol. Even for chloramphenicol, notoriously implicated in AA (at the peak of its usage 30% of all cases), the increase in the risk is modest (13-fold, or about 1/20,000). In general, agranulocytosis and mild pancytopenia are more common drug reactions than severe AA. The list of commonly implicated agents is provided in Table 41.2.

**Table 41.2** Drugs most commonly implicated in aplastic anemia

Dose-dependent marrow cytopenia
  Chemotherapy
Drug that may cause idiosyncratic association but low
  probability
  Chloramphenicol
  NSAID
  Anticonvulsants (e.g., carbamazepine)
  Antithyroid
  Gold, D-penicilinamine
  Sufonamides
  Carbonic anhydrase inhibitors
Very rare associations
  Antibiotics
  Allopurinol
  Psychotropic (e.g., phenothiazines)
  Cardiovascular drugs
  Lithium
  Sedatives (e.g., chlorpromazine)

## Radiation

Bone marrow aplasia is a well-known toxicity of ionizing radiation. Myeloablation using γ-radiation is used therapeutically as a conditioning regimen for stem cell transplantation. The bone marrow is affected directly by γ-rays, and secondarily by α- and β-particles. Certain cell types, such as lymphocytes, are very sensitive and are killed directly, while hematopoietic progenitors require cell division for severe damage; thus, mitotically active cells are most sensitive. The onset and severity of pancytopenia is dose dependent. However, the regeneration capacity of the irradiated marrow is remarkable, likely due to the presence of quiescent, more resistant stem cells. While the exact LD50 dose is not precisely known in humans, 1.5–2 Gy of whole body radiation can induce marrow aplasia. The dose of 4.5 Gy (Shields–Warren number) has been estimated to constitute the LD50.[11,47] The estimation of marrow toxicity is hampered by the toxicity to other organ systems that may limit survival. At doses at LD50, bone marrow toxicity limits survival.

## Viruses

In many respects, clinical and pathophysiologic features of AA suggest a possible infectious etiology. Most commonly, viruses have been implicated. Over the years, many of the suggested agents have been excluded as etiologic factors. The search for AA agents has been extensive. Hepatitis B and A were proven not to be the causative agent for typical AA. Similarly, cytomegalovirus (CMV), although certainly capable of producing bone marrow suppression under certain clinical circumstances, such as following stem cell transplantation, is not responsible for idiopathic AA. Certain serologic CMV types have been implicated in transplantation-refractory AA, but these studies have not found application to explain typical AA.[48–50] A series of cases clearly

attributable to Epstein–Barr virus (EBV) has been described, but again, EBV is a rare cause of AA.[51] The best evidence for a viral etiology exists in a specific hepatitis/AA syndrome, in which severe AA follows with a 3–6 months latency. So far, a specific agent of this non-A, non-B, non-C hepatitis has not been found.[52]

## Immune-mediated bone marrow failure in AA

That AA is an immune-mediated disease has been concluded from the successes of immunosuppressive (IS) therapy. Despite progress in laboratory investigations, most experimental evidence supporting an autoimmune attack in AA remains indirect, and this clinical observation provides the strongest evidence for an autoimmune pathophysiology of this disease. The inciting events for the immune reaction in AA include viral infections that, through molecular mimicry, lead to the breach of tolerance toward antigens residing on hematopoietic stem cells. In addition, cross-reactive antigens could also be generated by chemical modification or conjugation with drugs. Finally, neoantigens created by transcription of mutated fused genes may induce an immune reaction with effector cells that are unable to selectively kill abnormal cells, and mediate depletion of normal elements as well (Figure 41.2).

Experimental evidence supports an immunologic mechanism in AA (for review see[8–10]) (Figure 41.3). A role for T cells in AA was first suggested by coculture and depletion experiments, in which inhibition of hematopoietic colony formation was associated with this lymphocyte population.[53,54] Later, an inverted CD4/CD8 ratio,[27] activated cytotoxic lymphocytes (CTL) as detected by the expression of HLA-DR[55] and CD25,[56] and skewing of the variable β-chain (Vβ)repertoire of the T-cell receptor (TCR) were found, consistent with expansion of autoimmune T-cell clones.[57–65]

The damage to the stem cells can be mediated by a variety of mechanisms, including direct cell-mediated killing by CTL as well as cytokine-transduced inhibition (Figure 41.2). In addition to interferon γ (IFNγ) and tumor necrosis factor α (TNFα), Fas ligand or TNF-ralated inhibitory ligand (TRAIL) appears to play an important role as effector cytokines in the hematopoietic inhibition in AA.[29,66–68] Such mechanisms may be restricted not only to the original targets, but also may include bystander cells. Ultimately, these factors may result in apoptosis of stem cells.

## Genetic predisposition and congenital AA

Several rare congenital syndromes can present as AA or evolve to a clinical picture consistent with AA. Defect in the DNA repair machinery may lead to stem cell damage, but the pathophysiologic mechanism leading to pancytopenia is not clear. In some studies, immune mechanisms such as excessive production of TNFα have been implicated.[41,42] Fanconi anemia is the most common differential diagnostic consideration that should be excluded in all children and younger

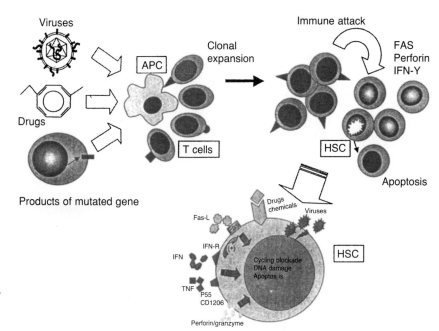

**Figure 41.2** *Immune mechanisms in AA. APC: antigen presenting cell; HSC: hematopoietic stem cells*

patients. Due to the variable presentation of Fanconi anemia, patients may show initially normal counts, and AA evolves progressively. Dysmorphic features and short stature may not be obvious. Dyskeratosis congenita is another congenital syndrome that may present with pancytopenia. Classically, leukoplakia and nail abnormalities are present.

## CLINICAL FEATURES OF AA

### PRESENTATION

Most patients with AA present with symptoms of anemia or bleeding due to deficient red blood cell and platelet production. Infection associated with low neutrophil numbers is not a common initial presentation. Often, AA is uncovered incidentally; patients may remain asymptomatic for a long time due to the latent onset of anemia. Consequently, the latency period and the onset of the disease are difficult to determine. In some cases, when AA is discovered early, a follow-up blood examination will reveal progressive worsening of cytopenia.

### DEFINITION, DIAGNOSIS, AND DIFFERENTIAL DIAGNOSIS
#### Definitions and classification

According to the useful definition of the AA Working Party, AA is defined by bone marrow cellularity (usually <10%) and a decrease in two out of three blood lineages. Cytopenia secondary to other hematologic diseases and systemic conditions has to be excluded. The issue of the requirement of normal cytogenetics is a subject of some controversy, especially that in a proportion of patients, cytogenetic analysis may not be informative. Most experts believe that the presence of karyotypic abnormalities at presentation is consistent

with the diagnosis of MDS, excluding idiopathic AA. According to the severity classification proposed by Camitta[69] (Table 41.3), patients with moderately depressed counts have an excellent prognosis even if untreated, while those with severely affected blood counts have poor survival in the absence of therapy.

### Differential diagnosis

A large number of conditions may mimic AA in all or some of its aspects and features, and depending on the clinical circumstances, some alternate diagnoses have to be excluded (Figure 41.4). Several systemic diseases can present with an aplastic bone marrow; bone marrow biopsies can be hypocellular in up to 10% of patients with MDS.[1–3] In addition, marrow aplasia can be encountered in hairy cell leukemia, or be iatrogenic. Discrimination of AA and MDS may be particularly challenging if hypocellularity precludes proper morphologic evaluation and cytogenetic examination is not informative. Clues may be provided by presence of micromegakaryocytes, myeloid dysplasia, and residual blasts.

| Table 41.3 | Classification of aplastic anemia by severity |
|---|---|
| **Aplastic anemia** | |
| Severe aplastic anemia | Moderate aplastic anemia |
| Bone marrow cellularity, 10% Depression of at least two out of three hematopoietic linegages: ANC,500/uL Transfusion dependence with absolute reticulocyte count (ARC), 60,000/uL Platelets count | Decreased bone marrow cellularity Depression of at least two out of three hematopoietic lineages not fulfilling the severity criteria as specified in the right column |

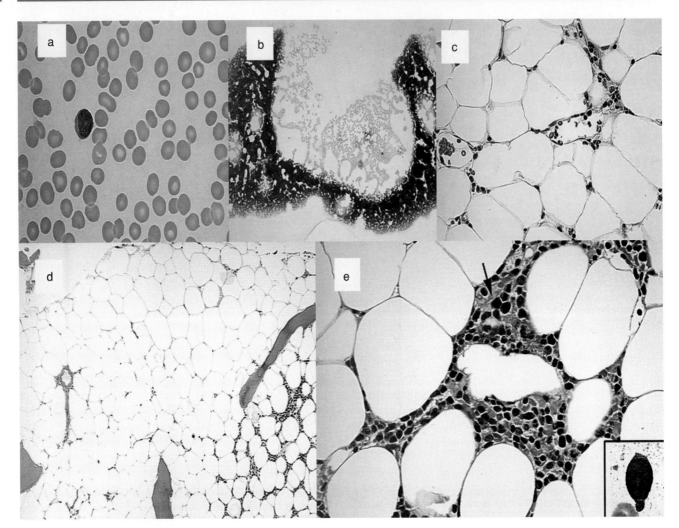

**Figure 41.3**   *Bone marrow finding in AA. (a) Peripheral blood smear from a patient with aplastic anemia demonstrates severe pancytopenia with normocytic to slightly macrocytic anemia, neutropenia, and thrombocytopenia (peripheral blood, Wright–Giemsa stain, original magnification ×100). (b) Bone marrow touch imprints may be helpful in excluding mimics of aplastic anemia, such as hairy cell leukemia, which can result in a dry tap. This low-power image of a touch imprint reflects the overall hypocellularity encountered in aplastic anemia (bone marrow biopsy touch imprint, Wright–Giemsa stain, original magnification ×10). (c) Bone marrow biopsy in aplastic anemia illustrates severe panhypoplasia with only rare scattered lymphocytes and plasma cells (bone marrow core biopsy, hematoxylin–eosin stain, original magnification ×40). (d) Because marrow cellularity may vary geographically within the biopsy, with the area immediately subjacent to the cortex often being hypocellular, it is essential to obtain an adequately sized core biopsy when evaluating for possible aplastic anemia (bone marrow core biopsy, hematoxylin–eosin stain, original magnification ×10). (e) Hypocellular MDS can mimic aplastic anemia. In this biopsy, mature myeloid elements are reduced, and the presence of occasional mononuclear cells consistent with blasts (arrow) can be a subtle feature. Marrow aspirate smear (inset) showed 9% myeloid blasts with dysplastic changes in erythroid precursors (bone marrow core biopsy, hematoxylin–eosin stain, original magnification ×40; inset: bone marrow aspirate, Wright–Giemsa stain, original magnification ×100) (courtesy of Dr. Karl Theil, Cleveland Clinic)*

## Diagnostic procedures

Diagnostic procedures include blood counts and a differential, and a bone marrow aspiration and biopsy (Figure 41.5). A reticulocyte count should always be obtained to assess severity and establish that anemia is related to the deficient marrow red blood cell production. The marrow exam should include cytogenetic evaluation. The presence of even small numbers of blasts strongly questions the correctness of the AA diagnosis. The residual erythropoiesis may be mega-loblastic; overt dysplasia of the myeloid series should not be seen in typical AA. Megakaryocytes are most typically absent or severely decreased in number. Routine flow cytometry of blood is not indicated, but may be helpful in excluding T-cell lymphoprolifera-tive syndromes and B-cell malignancies, especially hairy cell leukemia. Due to a common association and possible prognostic considerations, the presence of PNH should be investigated by flow cytometry on both red blood cells and granulocytes, which provide

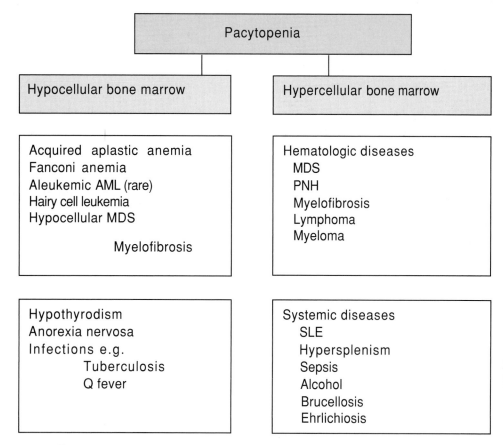

**Figure 41.4** *Differential diagnosis of idiopathic aplastic anemia and pancytopenia*

a much more sensitive and, unlike erythrocytes, transfusion-independent assessment of the size of the PNH clone. In younger patients, Fanconi anemia should be excluded by diaminobenzidine (DAB) testing. Splenomegaly and lymphadenopathy are atypi-

cal and always herald the presence of an alternative diagnosis or additional disorder.

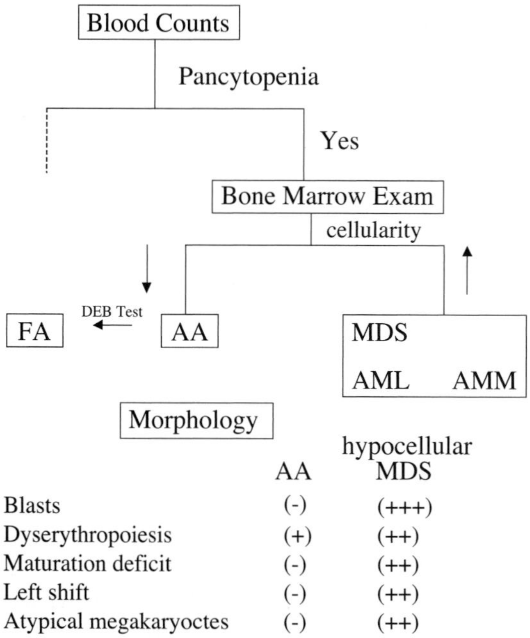

### DISTINCT CLINICAL ENTITIES

#### AA/paroxysmal nocturnal hemoglobinuria syndrome

Recent studies using a sensitive flow cytometric method have demonstrated that a glycosyl phosphatidyl inositol (GPI) deficient clone can be present in up to 1/3 of all patients with AA at presentation.[70,71] While in most of these patients PNH clones are tiny in size, in a significant minority of patients significantly expanded GPI-deficient PNH clones are present. These patients, unlike those with a primary hemolytic form of PNH, may have hypocellular bone marrow and low reticulocyte count. It has been hypothesized that the autoimmune attack responsible for the stem cell depletion in AA generates permissive conditions under which an otherwise dormant PNH clone can evolve.[72,73] The finding of a large proportion of PNH cells may be a significant feature, as administration of antithymocyte globulin (ATG) may be associated with a precipitation of a major hemolytic episode.

#### AA/hepatitis syndrome

AA/hepatitis syndrome has been described as a rare but instructive variant of this disease clearly pointing to a viral etiology of some cases of AA.[52,74] Despite extensive laboratory investigation, such a virus has not been

| | AA | hypocellular MDS |
|---|---|---|
| Blasts | (-) | (+++) |
| Dyserythropoiesis | (+) | (++) |
| Maturation deficit | (-) | (++) |
| Left shift | (-) | (++) |
| Atypical megakaryoctes | (-) | (++) |

**Figure 41.5** *Diagnostic algorithm in aplastic anemia*

found. It appears that the often fulminant hepatitis initiating the disease is caused by a non-A, non-B, non-C hepatitis virus. The hepatitis is associated with jaundice and an often pronounced rise in transaminases. It can result in fulminant liver failure. In patients who survive the hepatitic phase, transaminases, decrease and a latency period characterized by a period of a relative well-being follows. After a variable time period (often several months), pancytopenia develops with a clinical picture typical of severe AA. ATG therapy is effective and can often result in a complete remission. The time course of the syndrome is highly suggestive of virally induced hepatitis, which upon clearance of virus results in induction of cross-reactive T-cell response directed against hematopoietic stem cells.

### Chronic moderate AA

In contrast to severe AA, AA with moderately depressed counts has a favorable prognosis and often does not require therapy. The definition of moderate AA is difficult, as it may represent a transition stage of severe AA. A sufficient observation period (>3 months) with chronically and not progressively depressed counts makes the diagnosis of moderate AA. Over time the blood counts may decline, with evolution to a severe AA. It remains unclear whether moderate AA represents a separate entity, a number of nosologic entities such as unrecognized congenital bone marrow failure syndromes or a stage/variant of typical AA.

### AA in pregnancy

Pregnancy seems to predispose to AA, but this issue remains controversial. In fact, one of the first cases of AA documented in the early writings on this disease was a young pregnant woman.[75] The mechanism that triggers AA in pregnancy remains unclear, but AA often resolves with the termination of pregnancy and can recur during subsequent pregnancies. Even if the initial presentation of AA was not associated with pregnancy, women with a recent history of successfully treated AA should be counseled to not get pregnant. Successful pregnancies have been described, and in the majority of case series most of the women had good outcomes.[76] The therapy of pregnancy-associated AA depends on the gestational age of the fetus. The pregnancy of a women with severe AA may be terminated if it is close to term. Earlier in pregnancy, supportive measures are most commonly used. ATG has also been administered to women with severely depressed counts, especially low absolute neutrophil count (ANC). Overall, the prognosis for the mother and baby is good.

## THERAPY

### *IMMUNOSUPPRESSIVE THERAPY*

IS therapy remains the most important primary treatment modality for the major portion of patients affected by this disease. The most common IS regimens combine equine ATG (at 40 mg/kg/day for 4 days) with cyclosporine A (CsA) (12–15 mg/kg in a divided dose b.i.d.) given for at least 3 months, but usually for 6 months (Figure 41.6). Steroids are usually added to counteract the serum sickness intrinsic to ATG therapy. Rabbit ATG (3.5 mg/kg/d × 5d) is likely as effective as horse ATG, but its efficacy has not been compared in a randomized trial.[77] The response rate to horse ATG ranges from 70 to 80%, with a 5-year survival of 80–90%.[12,78–81] ATG appears to be superior to CsA,[82,83] and the combination of ATG and CsA provides better results than ATG alone or CsA alone.[84,85] Intense immunosuppression with ATG/CsA has also been administered with good success in elderly patients.[86] The addition of granulocyte colony-stimulating factor (G-CSF) may improve neutropenia, but does not increase survival.[87] Patients who respond have excellent survival, while those who are refractory have less favorable survival, with counts at 3 months post-ATG therapy having a good correlation with long-term prognosis. Most patients who are destined to respond do so by that time, and subsequent improvement may occur in additional one fourth of patients. Newer IS regimens may employ other agents, such as mycofenolate mofetil and, in the context of CsA toxicity, Dacluzimab Zenapax [anti-IL-2 receptor (CD25) monoclonal antibody], but the efficacy of these agents is not known. Refractory patients may be re-treated with multiple courses of ATG. Repeated ATG may result in salvage of a significant proportion of patients. In one study of patients refractory to horse ATG, rabbit ATG resulted in a 50% response rate and excellent long-term survival.[77] No good prognostic factors are available with regard to the response to ATG, with the exception of the presence of HLA-DR15 alleles and the PNH clone, both of which correlate with good responsiveness to immunosuppression.[88]

High-dose cyclophosphamide has been advocated as an effective first-line therapy alternative to ATG.[89] High response rates were reported to be associated with prevention of relapse, and also with clonal disease. However, prolonged cytopenia has resulted in an excessive toxicity related to neutropenic complications in a randomized trial between ATG/CsA and cyclophosphamide/CsA, resulting in a termination of the study.[90,91] Long-term follow-up of patients treated with cyclophosphamide showed that relapse and clonal disease can occur after this type of therapy.[91,92] It seems that high-dose cyclophosphamide does not constitute advancement over ATG/CsA, and should be used only in selected cases or in the context of clinical trials.

### *OTHER THERAPIES*
### Hematopoietic growth factors

Hematopoietic growth factors should not be used in the primary setting. Some patients will show an improvement of neutropenia with G-CSF, but severe

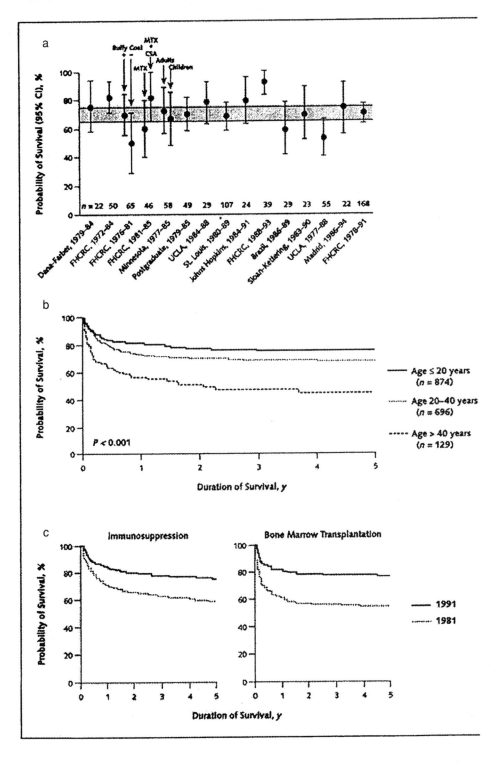

**Figure 41.6** *Results of immunosuppression and stem cell transplantation in aplastic anemia. (a) Allogeneic stem cell transplantation. Data are presented from individual hospital series in peer-reviewed publications from 1991 to 1997. The shaded area represents the 5-year probability of survival (with the same confidence intervals) of patients reported to the International Bone Marrow Transplant Registry (IBMTR) during this period. (b) The continuing influence of age on survival, as reflected in IBMTR data. (c) Comparative probability of survival after immunosuppression and stem cell transplantation. The data are for patients reported to the Working Party on Severe Aplastic Anemia of The European Group for Blood and Marrow Transplantation in the 1980s and 1990s. CSA = cyclosporine; FHCRC = Fred Hutchinson Cancer Research Center; MTX = methotrexate; UCLA = University of California, Los Angeles (Adapted with permission from Ref. 9)*

neutropenia due to a typical AA is mostly refractory. In combination with an ATG/CsA regimen, G-CSF can improve neutropenia (neutrophil response), and response to this therapy constitutes an early positive prognostic factor with respect to future response.[87] However, no survival advantage has been reported.[87] Dose escalation does not appear to be beneficial.[93]

### Anabolic steroids

Anabolic steroids have been widely used as therapy of AA, prior to the advent of IS therapy.[94,95] Currently,

androgens are mostly used as a salvage therapy for refractory patients. Historically, response rates to androgens were clearly observed, and were reported to be 30–60%. The androgens in current use include oxymethylone and danazol. Danazol has a relatively low virilizing potential.

### STEM CELL TRANSPLANTATION

AA was the first disease treated successfully with stem cell transplantation. The most common conditioning regimen was established early and includes cyclophosphamide and ATG. For graft-versus-host disease (GvHD) prophylaxis, methotrexate, together with CsA, appears to produce better results than CsA alone.[96] Improvement in the general care and treatment of GvHD rendered stem cell transplantation a much safer procedure and made transplantation a curative treatment option for more patients.

### MATCHED SIBLING DONOR TRANSPLANTATION

Allogeneic transplantation is available to only a minority of patients (around 30%). With the general improvement in the outcomes of stem cell transplantation, the overall survival (OS) for matched sibling donor transplantation has been as good as 85–90% (Figure 41.6).[96,97] Even better results were reported in children, in whom stem cell transplantation appears to be more effective in improving survival than does immunosuppression,[98] making this procedure a treatment of choice for children with severe AA and a matched sibling donor. However, the typical decrease in the OS is observed with increasing age of the recipient, making the therapeutic decision for older patients a challenge. Children and young adults with a matched sibling donor should be offered stem cell transplantation as a first therapeutic option.

### UNRELATED ALLOGENIC STEM CELL TRANSPLANTATION

The survival rates in patients who undergo a matched unrelated stem cell transplantation of approximately 35% are by far less impressive than those performed from matched sibling donors.[97] In one report from 1996, the OS was around 54%.[99] Various methods, including modified conditioning regimens and T-cell depletion, have been used to improve results,[100,101] but relatively little progress has been made in comparison to matched sibling donor transplantation.[97] Most deaths occur due to GvHD, graft failure, and opportunistic infections. More recent results, and those obtained in children, are more favorable.[102,103]

## COMPLICATIONS AND LONG-TERM PROGNOSIS

In general, patients successfully treated with immunosuppression have an excellent prognosis, while nonresponders who cannot undergo stem cell transplantation have a poor survival. In recent years, the survival of chronically pancytopenic patients improved, likely due to advances in supportive care. Conversion of severe AA into moderate disease appears to be sufficient to significantly improve the long-term prognosis. The most common complications of AA include relapse and evolution of clonal disease. These complications occur in patients treated with immunosuppression. Recipients of allogeneic grafts show a different set of long-term com-

plications, including cataracts, thyroid disorders, and secondary cancers.[100]

### RELAPSE

The relapse rate following IS therapy may be substantial. For ATG/CsA, it may be as high as 35% in 7 years.[12,81] In general, relapse has a good prognosis and survival of relapsed patients is not significantly shortened.[81] Patients with falling blood counts can receive a trial of CsA. If unsuccessful in rescuing the counts, a repeated course of ATG should be given. The response rates are likely comparable to those seen in the initial course of ATG. In some instances, rabbit ATG can be used instead of horse ATG, but it is unclear whether this measure helps to avoid more dramatic allergic reactions. High-dose cyclophosphamide (see above) has been suggested to prevent subsequent relapses.

### EVOLUTION OF CLONAL DISEASE

With the introduction of IS therapy, the survival of AA patients who are not treated with stem cell transplantation has improved significantly.[9] With long-term systematic observation, evolution of AA to other hematologic diseases has been frequently recognized as a serious late complication. Historically, the development of PNH was considered the most common clonal complication of AA. Although the appearance of PNH clones is often already observed at first presentation of bone marrow failure,[70,71] manifest PNH develops in a much smaller but significant proportion of patients. MDS is another common clonal disease occurring in the context of AA.

### EVOLUTION OF MDS

#### Theories of MDS evolution in the context of the pathophysiology of AA

A fundamental question in the evolution of clonal disease in AA is whether its pathophysiology is intrinsic to the natural history of AA, and now only observed, as patients survive longer, due to effective therapies. Alternatively, clonal evolution may be secondary to the treatment of AA, as a complication of IS therapy, or more recently, due to chronic growth factor administration. Theoretically, inhibition of immune surveillance could lead to the uncontrolled outgrowth of abnormal clones. However, MDS has occurred in AA treated with androgens only,[104,105] arguing against the theory that the clonal evolution to MDS is a consequence of immunosuppression. In addition, patients with primary MDS have been treated with IS agents and no acceleration of the disease has been observed.[36,106,107] While prolonged G-CSF treatment was linked by Japanese investigators to the evolution of monosomy 7,[105,108–110] there was no increased risk observed in a randomized study of ATG and CsA with and without G-CSF[111] or in the analysis of the European Group for Blood and Marrow Transplantation (EBMT) data.[112] In a National Institutes of Health (NIH) study,[34] many of the AA patients who developed cytogenetic abnormalities received hematopoietic growth factors, mainly as support or as salvage therapy after unsuccessful immunosuppression, and refractory disease itself may be the underlying risk factor for clonal evolution.

### Diagnosis of evolution, its frequency, and timing

The relationship between AA, a disease dominated by an immune pathophysiology similar to other organ-specific autoimmune diseases, and MDS, usually viewed as a premalignant process, remains unclear in many clinical and pathophysiologic aspects. Aberrant differentiation of hematopoietic precursor cells, increased numbers of myeloblasts, and marrow hypercellularity are all characteristic of MDS, but persistent bone marrow hypocellularity in AA may preclude reliable morphologic analysis. Clinical similarities between MDS and AA are most obvious in the hypocellular form of dysplasia, and clinical distinction is often not possible.

The development of MDS in the setting of diagnosed AA has been described in several studies, but these vary significantly in their design, and especially in case definition,[12,109,113-118] exemplifying diverse views with respect to the criteria required for the diagnosis of both MDS and AA. In historical studies of AA, patients with abnormal cytogenetics and hypoplastic marrows at presentation were often included,[119-122] and in some institutions, abnormal cytogenetic studies are compatible with a primary diagnosis of AA.[104,122-124]

Most commonly, abnormal cytogenetics was felt to exclude a diagnosis of AA, regardless of marrow morphology; in a series from the NIH involving 122 patients treated with intensive immunosuppression consisting of ATG and CsA, all patients showed a normal karyotype at presentation, and 14 subsequently developed karyotypic abnormalities, with a risk of about 21% at 10 years. Only two patients were diagnosed as having a late MDS by marrow morphology alone, with normal chromosomes.[119] In an early study from Seattle, an abnormal karyotype was reported in 7 of 183 AA patients, but only 3 of these developed after immunosuppression.[104] The differences in the diagnostic criteria are also obvious, such as in a recent analysis by the EBMT AA Working Party, in which karyotypic abnormalities occurred in 23 of 170 patients, but in 4 cases chromosomal changes were present at first diagnosis[119] and would be classified as MDS at other institutions. Similarly, in a recent British series of 13 patients with AA and abnormal cytogenetics, only 2 presented with normal karyotype and later developed an abnormality.[123] In a study of 159 children with AA from Japan, the authors identified 6 patients with the diagnosis of "AA with cytogenetic abnormalities."[122] In another cohort compiled of 100 patients from the GITMO (Gruppo Italiano Trapianto di Midollo Osseo) and EBMT study involving anti lym-

phocyte globulin (ALG), CsA, prednisone, and G-CSF, during a median follow-up of 1424 days, 11 patients developed cytogenetic abnormalities.[125] In the interval of 11 years, 8% of patients enrolled in the randomized ATG +/− CsA study developed MDS or AML.[126]

The evolution of an abnormal karyotype has also been reported in children. In a series of 114 pediatric patients from Europe, 7 developed chromosomal abnormalities but the aberrant clone was retrospectively found in 2 at presentation,[127] decreasing the true evolution rate in this study to 5/114. Among 40 Japanese pediatric patients treated with G-CSF and CsA, 11 showed clonal evolution, mainly to monosomy 7.[109] Recently, the same group reported on the development of MDS or AML in 5 of 41 children treated with immunosuppression for their hepatitis-associated AA.[128]

After clonal evolution, marrow morphology was characterized by a predominance of hypercellularity (41%) and patchy biopsy cellularity (27%), while continued hypocellularity was found in 1/3 of the patients. Frank dysplasia, including changes in megakaryocyte morphology, was found in 15 of 29 patients, and a left shift in myeloid differentiation was observed in 12. However, in 9 of 29 patients, there were no morphologic changes suggestive of MDS.[34] While the entity of AA with cytogenetic abnormalities may exist, the new appearance of a karyotypically abnormal clone in the course of AA warrants the change of current diagnosis of AA to MDS. In a recent NIH analysis, patients with AA were followed with periodic cytogenetic analyses of marrows, and evolution of abnormal karyotypes was identified in 29 patients (a total of 189 patients were analyzed), allowing for the estimation of the evolution rate of 14% in 5 years and 20% in 10 years, respectively.[34] While the detection of a new cytogenetic abnormality is a stringent diagnostic sign, it may not reflect the total rate of MDS evolution in AA. In primary MDS, the proportion of patients with a normal karyotype is 40–60%, and by analogy, it is possible that also in post-AA, MDS can evolve without overt chromosomal damage.

### Risk factors

As various types of MDS and clonal abnormalities may have different underlying pathophysiologies, it may be difficult to identify specific risk factors for progression to clonal disease. For example, monosomy 7 appears to evolve in primary refractory patients or those with incomplete responses to immunosuppression, while trisomy 8 was observed in patients whose counts improved adequately.[34] A similar clinical observation was made for the 13q− abnormality.[129] In another study, a similar distribution of clonal evolution between responders and nonresponders and monosomy 7 was observed in both groups of patients.[127]

## Chromosomal abnormalities

The most commonly found cytogenetic abnormalities following AA were aberrations of chromosome 7 and trisomy 8. For example, in a study from Seattle, monosomy 7 was found in three and trisomy 8 in two of seven patients with karyotypic abnormalities[104] and, in a Dutch series, in three of five AA patients who evolved to MDS.[114] In a recent report from Japan, a series of 9 patients with 13q− following otherwise typical AA was reported[129]; in the NIH experience, 13q− was also reported in several of the 29 patients who developed an abnormal karyotype after AA.[34] In agreement with the Japanese report, both patients showed stable counts and a good response to immunosuppression. In a study of children in Japan, monosomy 7 occurred at the highest frequency,[130] and in children reported from Germany and Austria, monosomy 7 was present in two of seven patients, while trisomy 8 was encountered once.[127] In a long-term update of the NIH ATG/CsA trial, aberrations of chromosome 7 were present in 10 and trisomy 8 in 2 out of 13 patients.[81] All other abnormalities appear to occur more randomly, and given the overall low number of patients reported, it is difficult to establish individual frequencies.

There are no predictive factors to identify patients at risk for the clonal evolution of myelodysplasia. In retrospect, blood counts of patients at the time of the cytogenetic evolution to trisomy 8 were significantly higher than those of patients with monosomy 7. Additionally, even after evolution to trisomy 8, sustained improved blood counts were often dependent upon continued CsA administration. Patients with monosomy 7 and those with complex karyotypes usually (but not always) had a poor response to immunosuppression and persistent pancytopenia.[34]

Although the appearance of a cytogenetic abnormality in a patient with AA is strong evidence of clonal evolution to MDS, in some studies a high proportion of apparently transient chromosomal changes would diminish the diagnostic and prognostic implications of new cytogenetic findings. Conversion to a normal karyotype is not a frequent event, and may also be a function of the frequency of marrow examinations. In our previously published study,[34] such an event was observed in only 2 of 29 patients, but since publication of this report another patient reverted (unpublished observation). It is likely that abnormal clones may be recruited and contribute to blood production for limited periods of time.

## Prognosis

MDS, evolving from AA, and primary MDS differ in the distribution of specific cytogenetic abnormalities. In primary MDS, aberration of chromosome 5 is generally cited as the most frequent abnormality, present in 10–37% of all patients,[131–136] but this chromosome is only rarely affected in AA patients. 20q− and −Y also are more often abnormal in primary MDS in comparison to AA.[131,133] Conversely, monosomy 7, most prominent in the late evolution of MDS from AA, occurs in a minority of primary MDS (6.5–11%).[12,131,134–138] Trisomy 8 appears to have a comparable incidence among cytogenetic abnormalities evolving from AA and in primary MDS (6–20%[131–138]).

Clearly, the diagnosis of MDS in the course of AA has prognostic significance. Most obvious modifiers include the presence of blasts, a hypercellular bone marrow, certain types of defects, and recurrence or persistence of profound cytopenia, all constituting unfavorable prognostic markers. For example, in one report, AA patients who developed secondary chromosomal abnormalities had a mortality rate of about 27% with a mean follow-up after evolution of 29 months (from the initial diagnosis, the total observation interval was 70 months). All but two deaths were related to AML.[34] Response to immunosuppression in patients with aplasia and abnormal karyotypes may be as high as 50%,[122] and certain karyotypic abnormalities (trisomy 8, 13q−) may favorably respond to immunosuppression. While the low numbers of patients reported preclude generalization, no individual abnormality predicted unresponsiveness. However, certain types of chromosomal defects are less likely to benefit from immunosuppression, including monosomy 7, complex karyotypes or 5q− syndrome. A stem cell transplantation may be the only therapeutic option for patients affected.

## EVOLUTION OF PAROXYSMAL NOCTURNAL HEMOGLOBINURIA

### Theories of PNH evolution in the context of AA

The mechanisms of the selective advantage of the PNH clone has been the subject of intense research, but no conclusive results have been obtained. The simplest model to explain how the PIG-A mutation accounts for the ability of the PNH clone to expand predicts that PIG-A mutant cells enjoy an intrinsic growth advantage. Surprisingly, clinical observation and much experimental data do not support this hypothesis.[73] Most obviously, PNH does not behave like leukemia. PNH stem cells are capable of producing mature cells of all lineages and respond to many physiologic stimuli. PNH progenitor and stem cells do not accumulate. In same patients, the proportion of PNH cells remains stable for years,[70] suggesting that GPI-deficient and normal hematopoiesis may coexist and that PNH cells do not simply displace normal cells. The presence of PNH cells in normal adults is also difficult to reconcile with this model, given the rarity of this disease. The differential susceptibility to apoptosis of PNH cells has been reported by several groups,[56,139,140] but their results have not been confirmed by others.[141,142] Appropriate controls with primary cells are difficult in such experiments, while cell lines may not reflect the situation in vitro.

## Clinical features

A PNH clone can be present in a significant proportion of patients with AA at presentation, but most patients harbor small clones without clinical significance. The presence of PNH clones constitutes a positive prognostic factor for the response to immunosuppression. The behavior of the PNH clone in the course of the disease and following therapy is erratic. In some patients, the clonal size does not change, while a clinical PNH can evolve in up to 10% of AA patients over the period of 10 years. Currently, there are no good predictive factors, and most of the current data are derived from an older cohort of patients. It remains unclear whether AA patients who developed PNH did have minor PNH clones detectable at presentation, or whether their PNH developed truly de novo. PNH can be a disabling chronic complication of AA and is associated with hemolysis, transfusion dependence, and thrombotic complications.

## REFERENCES

1. Elghetany MT, Hudnall SD, Gardner FH: Peripheral blood picture in primary hypocellular refractory anemia and idiopathic acquired aplastic anemia: an additional tool for differential diagnosis. *Haematologica* 82:21–24, 1997.

2. Barrett J, Saunthararajah Y, Molldrem J: Myelodysplastic syndrome and aplastic anemia: distinct entities or diseases linked by a common pathophysiology? *Semin Hematol* 37:15–29, 2000.

3. Tuzuner N, Cox C, Rowe JM, Watrous D, Bennett JM: Hypocellular myelodysplastic syndromes (MDS): new proposals. *Br J Haematol* 91:612–617, 1995.

4. Szklo M, Sensenbrenner L, Markowitz J, et al.: Incidence of aplastic anemia in metropolitan Baltimore: a population-based study. *Blood* 66:115–119, 1985.

5. Mary JY, Baumelou E, Guiguet M: Epidemiology of aplastic anemia in France: a prospective multicentric study. The French Cooperative Group for epidemiological study of aplastic anemia. *Blood* 75:1646–1653, 1990.

6. Kaufman D, Kelly JP, Levy M, Shapiro S: The drug etiology of agranulocytosis and aplastic anemia. New York: Oxford University Press; 1991.

7. Issaragrisil S, Kaufman D, Thongput A, et al.: Association of seropositivity for hepatitis viruses and aplastic anemia in Thailand. *Hepatology* 25:1255–1257, 1997.

8. Young N, Maciejewski JP: Aplastic anemia. In: Hoffman R, Benz EJJ, Shattil SJ, et al. (eds.) *Hematology: Basic Principles and Practice.* Philadelphia: Churchill Livingstone; 2000:297–330.

9. Young NS: Acquired aplastic anemia. *Ann Intern Med* 136:534–546, 2002.

10. Arseniev L, Tischler HJ, Battmer K, et al.: Treatment of poor marrow graft function with allogeneic CD34+ cells immunoselected from G-CSF-mobilized peripheral blood progenitor cells of the marrow donor. *Bone Marrow Transplant* 14:791–797, 2002.

11. Baverstock KF, Ash PJ: A review of radiation accidents involving whole body exposure and the relevance to the LD50/60 for man. *Br J Radiol* 56:837–844, 1983.

12. Castro-Malaspina H, Harris RE, Gajewski J, et al.: Unrelated donor marrow transplantation for myelodysplastic syndromes: outcome analysis in 510 transplants facilitated by the National Marrow Donor Program. *Blood* 99:1943–1951, 2002.

13. Novitzky N, Jacobs P: In aplastic anemia progenitor cells have a reduced sensitivity to the effects of growth factors. *Eur J Haematol* 63:141–148, 1999.

14. Bacigalupo A, Piaggio G, Podesta M, et al.: Collection of peripheral blood hematopoietic progenitors (PBHP) from patients with severe aplastic anemia (SAA) after prolonged administration of granulocyte colony-stimulating factor. *Blood* 82:1410–1414, 1993.

15. Manz CY, Nissen C, Wodnar-Filipowicz A: Deficiency of CD34+ c-kit+ and CD34+38- hematopoietic precursors in aplastic anemia after immunosuppressive treatment. *Am J Hematol* 52:264–274, 1996.

16. Scopes J, Bagnara M, Gordon-Smith EC, Ball SE, Gibson FM: Haemopoietic progenitor cells are reduced in aplastic anaemia. *Br J Haematol* 86:427–430, 1994.

17. Marsh JC: Hematopoietic growth factors in the pathogenesis and for the treatment of aplastic anemia. *Semin Hematol* 37:81–90, 2000.

18. Wodnar-Filipowicz A, Yancik S, Moser Y, et al.: Levels of soluble stem cell factor in serum of patients with aplastic anemia. *Blood* 81:3259–3264, 1993.

19. Marsh JC, Gibson FM, Prue RL, et al.: Serum thrombopoietin levels in patients with aplastic anaemia. *Br J Haematol* 95:605–610, 1996.

20. Chang KL, O'Donnell MR, Slovak ML, et al.: Primary myelodysplasia occurring in adults under 50 years old: a clinicopathologic study of 52 patients. *Leukemia* 16:623–631, 2002.

21. Podesta M, Piaggio G, Frassoni F, et al.: The assessment of the hematopoietic reservoir after immunosuppressive therapy or bone marrow transplantation in severe aplastic anemia. *Blood* 91:1959–1965, 1998.

22. Marsh JC, Chang J, Testa NG, Hows JM, Dexter TM: In vitro assessment of marrow "stem cell" and stromal cell function in aplastic anaemia. *Br J Haematol* 78:258–267, 1991.

23. Novitzky N, Jacobs P: Immunosuppressive therapy in bone marrow aplasia: the stroma functions normally to support hematopoiesis. *Exp Hematol* 23:1472–1477, 1995.

24. Novitzky N, Jacobs P: Marrow stem cell and stroma cell function in aplastic anaemia. *Br J Haematol* 79:531–533, 1991.

25. Laver J, Jhanwar SC, O'Reilly RJ, Castro-Malaspina H: Host origin of the human hematopoietic microenvironment following allogeneic bone marrow transplantation. *Blood* 70:1966–1968, 1987.

26. Rizzo S, Scopes J, Elebute MO, et al.: Stem cell defect in aplastic anemia: reduced long term culture-initiating cells (LTC-IC) in CD34+ cells isolated from aplastic anemia patient bone marrow. *Hematol J* 3:230–236, 2002.

27. Selleri C, Sato T, Anderson S, Young NS, Maciejewski JP: Interferon-gamma and tumor necrosis factor-alpha suppress both early and late stages of hematopoiesis and induce programmed cell death. *J Cell Physiol* 165:538–546, 1995.

28. Selleri C, Maciejewski JP, Sato T, Young NS: Interferon-gamma constitutively expressed in the stromal microenvironment of human marrow cultures mediates potent hematopoietic inhibition . *Blood* 87:4149–4157, 1996.

29. Kojima S, Matsuyama T, Kato S, et al.: Outcome of 154 patients with severe aplastic anemia who received transplants from unrelated donors: the Japan Marrow Donor Program. *Blood* 100:799–803, 2002.

30. Killick SB, Cox CV, Marsh JC, Gordon-Smith EC, Gibson FM: Mechanisms of bone marrow progenitor cell apoptosis in aplastic anaemia and the effect of anti-thymocyte globulin: examination of the role of the Fas-Fas-L interaction. *Br J Haematol* 111:1164–1169, 2000.

31. Ismail M, Gibson FM, Gordon-Smith EC, Rutherford TR: Bcl-2 and Bcl-x expression in the CD34$^+$ cells of aplastic anaemia patients: relationship with increased apoptosis and upregulation of Fas antigen. *Br J Haematol* 113:706–712, 2001.

32. Maciejewski JP, Selleri C, Sato T, et al.: Nitric oxide suppression of human hematopoiesis in vitro. Contribution to inhibitory action of interferon-gamma and tumor necrosis factor-alpha. *J Clin Invest* 96:1085–1092, 1995.

33. Chung IJ, Lee JJ, Nam CE, et al.: Increased inducible nitric oxide synthase expression and nitric oxide concentration in patients with aplastic anemia. *Ann Hematol* 82:104–108, 2003.

34. Maciejewski JP, Risitano A, Sloand EM, Nunez O, Young NS: Distinct clinical outcomes for cytogenetic abnormalities evolving from aplastic anemia. *Blood* 99:3129–3135, 2002.

35. Maciejewski JP, Selleri C: Evolution of clonal cytogenetic abnormalities in aplastic anemia. *Leuk Lymphoma* 45:433–440, 2004.

36. Brummendorf TH, Dragowska W, Lansdorp PM: Asymmetric cell divisions in hematopoietic stem cells. *Ann N Y Acad Sci* 872:265–272, 1999.

37. Brummendorf TH, Rufer N, Holyoake TL, et al.: Telomere length dynamics in normal individuals and in patients with hematopoietic stem cell-associated disorders. *Ann N Y Acad Sci* 938:293–303, 2001.

38. Brummendorf TH, Maciejewski JP, Mak J, Young NS, Lansdorp PM: Telomere length in leukocyte subpopulations of patients with aplastic anemia. *Blood* 97:895–900, 2001.

39. Ball SE, Gibson FM, Rizzo S, et al.: Progressive telomere shortening in aplastic anemia. *Blood* 91:3582–3592, 1998.

40. Lee JJ, Kook H, Chung IJ, et al.: Telomere length changes in patients with aplastic anaemia. *Br J Haematol* 112:1025–1030, 2001.

41. Young N: Drugs and chemicals. Young NS, Alter BP (eds.) *Aplastic Anemia, Acquired and Inherited.* Philadelphia: WB Sunders; 1994:100.

42. Smith MT: Overview of benzene-induced aplastic anaemia. *Eur J Haematol Suppl* 60:107–110, 1996.

43. Ross D: Metabolic basis of benzene toxicity. *Eur J Haematol Suppl* 60:111–118, 1996.

44. Aksoy M, Dincol K, Akgun T, Erdem S, Dincol G: Haematological effects of chronic benzene poisoning in 217 workers. *Br J Ind Med* 28:296–302, 1971.

45. Smick KM, Condit PK, Proctor RL, Sutcher V: Fatal aplastic anemia. An epidemiological study of its relationship to the drug chloramphenicol. *J Chronic Dis* 17:899–914, 1964.

46. Keiser G, Bolli P, Buchegger U: Hematologic side effects of chloramphenicol and thiamphenicol. *Schweiz Med Wochenschr* 102:1595–1598, 1972.

47. Mole RH: The LD50 for uniform low LET irradiation of man. *Br J Radiol* 57:355–369, 1984.

48. Torok-Storb B, Bolles L, Iwata M, et al.: Increased prevalence of CMV gB3 in marrow of patients with aplastic anemia. *Blood* 98:891–892, 2001.

49. Fries BC, Khaira D, Pepe MS, Torok-Storb B: Declining lymphocyte counts following cytomegalovirus (CMV) infection are associated with fatal CMV disease in bone marrow transplant patients. *Exp Hematol* 21:1387–1392, 1993.

50. Fries BC, Chou S, Boeckh M, Torok-Storb B: Frequency distribution of cytomegalovirus envelope glycoprotein genotypes in bone marrow transplant recipients. *J Infect Dis* 169:769–774, 1994.

51. Baranski B, Armstrong G, Truman JT, et al.: Epstein–Barr virus in the bone marrow of patients with aplastic anemia. *Ann Intern Med* 109:695–704, 1988.

52. Brown KE, Tisdale J, Barrett AJ, Dunbar CE, Young NS: Hepatitis-associated aplastic anemia. *N Engl J Med* 336:1059–1064, 1997.

53. Hoffman R, Zanjani ED, Lutton JD, Zalusky R, Wasserman LR: Suppression of erythroid-colony formation by lymphocytes from patients with aplastic anemia. *N Engl J Med* 296:10–13, 1977.

54. Takaku F, Suda T, Mizoguchi H, et al.: Effect of peripheral blood mononuclear cells from aplastic anemia patients on the granulocyte-macrophage and erythroid colony formation in samples from normal human bone marrow in vitro—a cooperative work. *Blood* 55:937–943, 1980.

55. Barcena A, Muench MO, Song KS, Ohkubo T, Harrison MR: Role of CD95/Fas and its ligand in the regulation of the growth of human CD34(++)CD38(−) fetal liver cells. *Exp Hematol* 27:1428–1439, 1999.

56. Horikawa K, Nakakuma H, Kawaguchi T, et al.: Apoptosis resistance of blood cells from patients with paroxysmal nocturnal hemoglobinuria, aplastic anemia, and myelodysplastic syndrome. *Blood* 90:2716–2722, 1997.

57. Abe M, Shintani Y, Eto Y, et al.: Potent induction of activin A secretion from monocytes and bone marrow stromal fibroblasts by cognate interaction with activated T cells. *J Leukoc Biol* 72:347–352, 2002.

58. Zeng W, Nakao S, Takamatsu H, et al.: Characterization of T-cell repertoire of the bone marrow in immune-mediated aplastic anemia: evidence for the involvement of antigen-driven T-cell response in cyclosporine-dependent aplastic anemia. *Blood* 93:3008–3016, 1999.

59. Karadimitris A, Manavalan JS, Thaler HT, et al.: Abnormal T-cell repertoire is consistent with immune process underlying the pathogenesis of paroxysmal nocturnal hemoglobinuria. *Blood* 96:2613–2620, 2000.

60. Zeng W, Maciejewski JP, Chen G, Young NS: Limited heterogeneity of T cell receptor BV usage in aplastic anemia. *J Clin Invest* 108:765–773, 2001.

61. Kook H, Risitano AM, Zeng W, et al.: Changes in T-cell receptor VB repertoire in aplastic anemia: effects of different immunosuppressive regimens. *Blood* 99:3668–3675, 2002.

62. Mauritzson N, Albin M, Rylander L, et al.: Pooled analysis of clinical and cytogenetic features in treatment-related and de novo adult acute myeloid leukemia and myelodysplastic syndromes based on a consecutive series of 761 patients analyzed 1976–1993 and on 5098 unselected cases reported in the literature 1974–2001. *Leukemia* 16:2366–2378, 2002.

63. Plasilova M: Paroxysmal nocturnal hemoglobinuria—in the search for disease-specific T-cell clones. *Blood* 100: 167A, 2002.

64. Risitano A, Maciejewski JP: TCR sequencing. The molecular signature of autoimmunity in aplastic anemia. *Blood* 100:155A, 2002.

65. Plasilova M, Risitano A, Maciejewski JP: Application of the molecular analysis of the T cell receptor repertoire in the study of immune-mediated hematologic disease. *Hematol J* 8:173–181, 2003.

66. Campisi J: Cellular senescence as a tumor-suppressor mechanism. *Trends Cell Biol* 11:S27–S31, 2001.

67. Sloand E, Maciejewski JP, Tisdale J, Follman D, Young NS: Intracellular interferon-y (IFN-y) in circulating and marrow T Cells detected by flow cytometry and the response to immunosuppressive therapy in patients with aplastic anemia. *Blood* 100:3129–3135, 2002.

68. Dufour C, Corcione A, Svahn J, et al.: Interferon gamma and tumour necrosis factor alpha are overexpressed in bone marrow T lymphocytes from paediatric patients with aplastic anaemia. *Br J Haematol* 115: 1023–1031, 2001.

69. Camitta BM, Rappeport JM, Parkman R, Nathan DG: Selection of patients for bone marrow transplantation in severe aplastic anemia. *Blood* 45:355–363, 1975.

70. Maciejewski JP, Rivera C, Kook H, Dunn D, Young NS: Relationship between bone marrow failure syndromes and the presence of glycophosphatidyl inositol-anchored protein-deficient clones. *Br J Haematol* 115:1015–1022, 2001.

71. Dunn DE, Tanawattanacharoen P, Boccuni P, et al.: Paroxysmal nocturnal hemoglobinuria cells in patients with bone marrow failure syndromes. *Ann Intern Med* 131:401–408, 1999.

72. Young NS: The problem of clonality in aplastic anemia: Dr Dameshek's riddle, restated. *Blood* 79:1385–1392, 1992.

73. Alvarez S, MacGrogan D, Calasanz MJ, Nimer SD, Jhanwar SC: Frequent gain of chromosome 19 in megakaryoblastic leukemias detected by comparative genomic hybridization. *Genes Chromosomes Cancer* 32:285–293, 2001.

74. Hibbs JR, Frickhofen N, Rosenfeld SJ, et al.: Aplastic anemia and viral hepatitis. Non-A, Non-B, Non-C? *JAMA* 267:2051–2054, 1992.

75. Tichelli A, Socie G, Marsh J, et al.: Outcome of pregnancy and disease course among women with aplastic anemia treated with immunosuppression. *Ann Intern Med* 137:164–172, 2002.

76. Choudhry VP, Gupta S, Gupta M, Kashyap R, Saxena R: Pregnancy associated aplastic anemia—a series of 10 cases with review of literature. *Hematology* 7:233–238, 2002.

77. Di Bona E, Rodeghiero F, Bruno B, et al.: Rabbit antithymocyte globulin (r-ATG) plus cyclosporine and granulocyte colony stimulating factor is an effective treatment for aplastic anaemia patients unresponsive to a first course of intensive immunosuppressive therapy.

Gruppo Italiano Trapianto di Midollo Osseo (GITMO). *Br J Haematol* 107:330–334, 1999.

78. Frickhofen N, Heimpel H, Kaltwasser JP, Schrezenmeier H: Antithymocyte globulin with or without cyclosporin A: 11-year follow-up of a randomized trial comparing treatments of aplastic anemia. *Blood* 101:1236–1242, 2003.

79. Nakao S, Takami A, Takamatsu H, et al.: Isolation of a T-cell clone showing HLA-DRB1*0405-restricted cytotoxicity for hematopoietic cells in a patient with aplastic anemia. *Blood* 89:3691–3699, 1997.

80. Murphy KM, Levis M, Hafez MJ, et al.: Detection of FLT3 internal tandem duplication and D835 mutations by a multiplex polymerase chain reaction and capillary electrophoresis assay. *J Mol Diagn* 5:96–102, 2003.

81. Rosenfeld S, Follmann D, Nunez O, Young NS: Antithymocyte globulin and cyclosporine for severe aplastic anemia: association between hematologic response and long-term outcome. *JAMA* 289:1130–1135, 2003.

82. Marsh J, Schrezenmeier H, Marin P, et al.: Prospective randomized multicenter study comparing cyclosporin alone versus the combination of antithymocyte globulin and cyclosporin for treatment of patients with nonsevere aplastic anemia: a report from the European Blood and Marrow Transplant (EBMT) Severe Aplastic Anaemia Working Party. *Blood* 93:2191–2195, 1999.

83. Gluckman E, Esperou-Bourdeau H, Baruchel A, et al.: Multicenter randomized study comparing cyclosporine-A alone and antithymocyte globulin with prednisone for treatment of severe aplastic anemia. *Blood* 79:2540–2546, 1992.

84. Coakley G, Brooks D, Iqbal M, et al.: Major histocompatility complex haplotypic associations in Felty's syndrome and large granular lymphocyte syndrome are secondary to allelic association with HLA-DRB1 *0401. *Rheumatology (Oxford)* 39:393–398, 2000.

85. Frickhofen N, Kaltwasser JP: Immunosuppressive treatment of aplastic anemia: a prospective, randomized multicenter trial evaluating antilymphocyte globulin (ALG) versus ALG and cyclosporin A. *Blut* 56:191–192, 1988.

86. Tichelli A, Socie G, Henry-Amar M, et al.: Effectiveness of immunosuppressive therapy in older patients with aplastic anemia. European Group for Blood and Marrow Transplantation Severe Aplastic Anaemia Working Party. *Ann Intern Med* 130:193–201, 1999.

87. Gluckman E, Rokicka-Milewska R, Hann I, et al.: Results and follow-up of a phase III randomized study of recombinant human-granulocyte stimulating factor as support for immunosuppressive therapy in patients with severe aplastic anaemia. *Br J Haematol* 119: 1075–1082, 2002.

88. Maciejewski JP, Follmann D, Nakamura R, et al.: Increased frequency of HLA-DR2 in patients with paroxysmal nocturnal hemoglobinuria and the PNH/aplastic anemia syndrome. *Blood* 98:3513–3519, 2001.

89. Brodsky RA, Sensenbrenner LL, Smith BD, et al.: Durable treatment-free remission after high-dose cyclophosphamide therapy for previously untreated severe aplastic anemia. *Ann Intern Med* 135:477–483, 2001.

90. Tisdale JF, Dunn DE, Geller N, et al.: High-dose cyclophosphamide in severe aplastic anaemia: a randomised trial. *Lancet* 356:1554–1559, 2000.

91. Tisdale JF, Maciejewski JP, Nunez O, Rosenfeld SJ, Young NS: Late complications following treatment for severe aplastic anemia (SAA) with high-dose cyclophosphamide (Cy): follow-up of a randomized trial. *Blood* 100:4668–4670, 2002.

92. Tisdale JF, Dunn DE, Maciejewski J: Cyclophosphamide and other new agents for the treatment of severe aplastic anemia. *Semin Hematol* 37:102–109, 2000.

93. Locasciulli A, Bruno B, Rambaldi A, et al.: Treatment of severe aplastic anemia with antilymphocyte globulin, cyclosporine and two different granulocyte colony-stimulating factor regimens: a GITMO prospective randomized study. *Haematologica* 89:1054–1061, 2004.

94. Hirota Y: Effects of androstanes on aplastic anemia—a prospective study. *Nippon Ketsueki Gakkai Zasshi* 44:1341–1359, 1981.

95. Najean Y, Haguenauer O: Long-term (5 to 20 years) Evolution of nongrafted aplastic anemias. The Cooperative Group for the Study of Aplastic and Refractory Anemias. *Blood* 76:2222–2228, 1990.

96. Locatelli F, Bruno B, Zecca M, et al.: Cyclosporin A and short-term methotrexate versus cyclosporin A as graft versus host disease prophylaxis in patients with severe aplastic anemia given allogeneic bone marrow transplantation from an HLA-identical sibling: results of a GITMO/EBMT randomized trial. *Blood* 96:1690–1697, 2000.

97. Bacigalupo A, Oneto R, Bruno B, et al.: Current results of bone marrow transplantation in patients with acquired severe aplastic anemia. Report of the European Group for Blood and Marrow transplantation. On behalf of the Working Party on Severe Aplastic Anemia of the European Group for Blood and Marrow Transplantation. *Acta Haematol* 103:19–25, 2000.

98. Kojima S, Horibe K, Inaba J, et al.: Long-term outcome of acquired aplastic anaemia in children: comparison between immunosuppressive therapy and bone marrow transplantation. *Br J Haematol* 111:321–328, 2000.

99. Margolis D, Camitta B, Pietryga D, et al.: Unrelated donor bone marrow transplantation to treat severe aplastic anaemia in children and young adults. *Br J Haematol* 94:65–72, 1996.

100. Horowitz MM: Current status of allogeneic bone marrow transplantation in acquired aplastic anemia. *Semin Hematol* 37:30–42, 2000.

101. Margolis DA, Casper JT: Alternative-donor hematopoietic stem-cell transplantation for severe aplastic anemia. *Semin Hematol* 37:43–55, 2000.

102. Georges GE, Storb R: Stem cell transplantation for aplastic anemia. *Int J Hematol* 75:141–146, 2002.

103. Kojima S, Inaba J, Yoshimi A, et al.: Unrelated donor marrow transplantation in children with severe aplastic anaemia using cyclophosphamide, anti-thymocyte globulin and total body irradiation. *Br J Haematol* 114:706–711, 2001.

104. Appelbaum FR, Barrall J, Storb R, et al.: Clonal cytogenetic abnormalities in patients with otherwise typical aplastic anemia. *Exp Hematol* 15:1134–1139, 1987.

105. Varma N, Varma S, Movafagh A, Garewal G: Unusual clonal cytogenetic abnormalities in aplastic anemia. *Am J Hematol* 49:256–257, 1995.

106. Molldrem JJ, Leifer E, Bahceci E, et al.: Antithymocyte globulin for treatment of the bone marrow failure associated with myelodysplastic syndromes. *Ann Intern Med* 137:156–163, 2002.

107. Selleri C, Maciejewski JP, Catalano L, et al.: Effects of cyclosporine on hematopoietic and immune functions in patients with hypoplastic myelodysplasia: in vitro and in vivo studies. *Cancer* 95:1911–1922, 2002.

108. Kaito K, Kobayashi M, Katayama T, et al.: Long-term administration of G-CSF for aplastic anaemia is closely related to the early evolution of monosomy 7 MDS in adults. *Br J Haematol* 103:297–303, 1998.

109. Yamazaki E, Kanamori H, Taguchi J, et al.: The evidence of clonal evolution with monosomy 7 in aplastic anemia following granulocyte colony-stimulating factor using the polymerase chain reaction. *Blood Cells Mol Dis* 23:213–218, 1997.

110. Bessho M, Hotta T, Ohyashiki K, et al.: Multicenter prospective study of clonal complications in adult aplastic anemia patients following recombinant human granulocyte colony-stimulating factor (lenograstim) administration. *Int J Hematol* 77:152–158, 2003.

111. Kojima S, Hibi S, Kosaka Y, et al.: Immunosuppressive therapy using antithymocyte globulin, cyclosporine, and danazol with or without human granulocyte colony-stimulating factor in children with acquired aplastic anemia. *Blood* 96:2049–2054, 2000.

112. Bacigalupo A, Brand R, Oneto R, et al.: Treatment of acquired severe aplastic anemia: bone marrow transplantation compared with immunosuppressive therapy—the European Group for Blood and Marrow Transplantation experience. *Semin Hematol* 37:69–80, 2000.

113. Paquette RL, Tebyani N, Frane M, et al.: Long-term outcome of aplastic anemia in adults treated with antithymocyte globulin: comparison with bone marrow transplantation. *Blood* 85:283–290, 1995.

114. de Planque MM, Kluin-Nelemans HC, van Krieken HJ, et al.: Evolution of acquired severe aplastic anaemia to myelodysplasia and subsequent leukaemia in adults. *Br J Haematol* 70:55–62, 1988.

115. Jameel T, Anwar M, Abdi SI, et al.: Aplastic anemia or aplastic preleukemic syndrome? *Ann Hematol* 75:189–193, 1997.

116. Young NS, Maciejewski JP: Aplastic anemia. In: Hoffman R (ed.) *Hematology: Basic Priciples and Practice*. Philadelphia: Churchill Livingstone; 1995:297–331.

117. Doney K, Leisenring W, Storb R, Appelbaum FR: Primary treatment of acquired aplastic anemia: outcomes with bone marrow transplantation and immunosuppressive therapy. Seattle Bone Marrow Transplant Team. *Ann Intern Med* 126:107–115, 1997.

118. Socie G, Henry-Amar M, Bacigalupo A, et al.: Malignant tumors occurring after treatment of aplastic anemia. European Bone Marrow Transplantation—Severe Aplastic Anaemia Working Party. *N Engl J Med* 329:1152–1157, 1993.

119. Socie G, Rosenfeld S, Frickhofen N, Gluckman E, Tichelli A: Late clonal diseases of treated aplastic anemia. *Semin Hematol* 37:91–101, 2000.

120. Anthony DD, Heeger PS, Haqqi TM: Immunization with TCR Vbeta10 peptide reduces the frequency of type-II collagen-specific Th1 type T cells in BUB/BnJ (H-2q) mice. *Clin Exp Rheumatol* 19:385–394, 2001.

121. Gaschet J, Lim A, Liem L, et al.: Acute graft versus host disease due to T lymphocytes recognizing a single

HLA-DPB1*0501 mismatch. *J Clin Invest* 98:100–107, 1996.

122. Ohga S, Ohara A, Hibi S, et al.: Treatment responses of childhood aplastic anaemia with chromosomal aberrations at diagnosis. *Br J Haematol* 118:313–319, 2002.

123. Geary CG, Harrison CJ, Philpott NJ, et al.: Abnormal cytogenetic clones in patients with aplastic anaemia: response to immunosuppressive therapy. *Br J Haematol* 104:271–274, 1999.

124. Mikhailova N, Sessarego M, Fugazza G, et al.: Cytogenetic abnormalities in patients with severe aplastic anemia. *Haematologica* 81:418–422, 1996.

125. Bacigalupo A, Bruno B, Saracco P, et al.: Antilymphocyte globulin, cyclosporine, prednisolone, and granulocyte colony-stimulating factor for severe aplastic anemia: an update of the GITMO/EBMT study on 100 patients. European Group for Blood and Marrow Transplantation (EBMT) Working Party on Severe Aplastic Anemia and the Gruppo Italiano Trapianti di Midolio Osseo (GITMO). *Blood* 95:1931–1934, 2000.

126. Frickhofen N, Heimpel H, Kaltwasser JP, Schrezenmeier H: Antithymocyte globulin with or without cyclosporin A: 11-year follow-up of a randomized trial comparing treatments of aplastic anemia. *Blood* 101:1236–1242, 2003.

127. Fuhrer M, Burdach S, Ebell W, et al.: Relapse and clonal disease in children with aplastic anemia (AA) after immunosuppressive therapy (IST): the SAA 94 experience. German/Austrian Pediatric Aplastic Anemia Working Group. *Klin Padiatr* 210:173–179, 1998.

128. Ohara A, Kojima S, Okamura J, et al.: Evolution of myelodysplastic syndrome and acute myelogenous leukaemia in children with hepatitis-associated aplastic anaemia. *Br J Haematol* 116:151–154, 2002.

129. Ishiyama K, Karasawa M, Miyawaki S, et al.: Aplastic anaemia with 13q-: a benign subset of bone marrow failure responsive to immunosuppressive therapy. *Br J Haematol* 117:747–750, 2002.

130. Kojima S, Ohara A, Tsuchida M, et al.: Risk factors for evolution of acquired aplastic anemia into myelodysplastic syndrome and acute myeloid leukemia after immunosuppressive therapy in children. *Blood* 100:786–790, 2002.

131. Michalova K, Musilova J, Zemanova Z: Cytogenetic abnormalities in 532 patients with myeloid leukemias and myelodysplastic syndrome. The Czechoslovak MDS Cooperative Group. *Czech Med* 13:133–144, 1990.

132. Sole F, Espinet B, Sanz GF, et al.: Incidence, characterization and prognostic significance of chromosomal abnormalities in 640 patients with primary myelodysplastic syndromes. Grupo Cooperativo Espanol de Citogenetica Hematologica. *Br J Haematol* 108:346–356, 2000.

133. Vila L, Charrin C, Archimbaud E, et al.: Correlations between cytogenetics and morphology in myelodysplastic syndromes. *Blut* 60:223–227, 1990.

134. Bernasconi P, Alessandrino EP, Boni M, et al.: Karyotype in myelodysplastic syndromes: relations to morphology, clinical evolution, and survival. *Am J Hematol* 46:270–277, 1994.

135. Knapp RH, Dewald GW, Pierre RV: Cytogenetic studies in 174 consecutive patients with preleukemic or myelodysplastic syndromes. *Mayo Clin Proc* 60:507–516, 1985.

136. Suciu S, Kuse R, Weh HJ, Hossfeld DK: Results of chromosome studies and their relation to morphology, course, and prognosis in 120 patients with de novo myelodysplastic syndrome. *Cancer Genet Cytogenet* 44:15–26, 1990.

137. Pedersen B: MDS and AML with trisomy 8 as the sole chromosome aberration show different sex ratios and prognostic profiles: a study of 115 published cases. *Am J Hematol* 56:224–229, 1997.

138. Kennedy B, Rawstron A, Carter C, et al.: Campath-1H and fludarabine in combination are highly active in refractory chronic lymphocytic leukemia. *Blood* 99:2245–2247, 2002.

139. Chen R, Nagarajan S, Prince GM, et al.: Impaired growth and elevated fas receptor expression in PIGA(+) stem cells in primary paroxysmal nocturnal hemoglobinuria. *J Clin Invest* 106:689–696, 2000.

140. Brodsky RA, Vala MS, Barber JP, Medof ME, Jones RJ: Resistance to apoptosis caused by PIG-A gene mutations in paroxysmal nocturnal hemoglobinuria. *Proc Natl Acad Sci USA* 94:8756–8760, 1997.

141. Yamamoto T, Shichishima T, Shikama Y, et al.: Granulocytes from patients with paroxysmal nocturnal hemoglobinuria and normal individuals have the same sensitivity to spontaneous apoptosis. *Exp Hematol* 30:187–194, 2002.

142. Ware RE, Nishimura J, Moody MA, et al.: The PIG-A mutation and absence of glycosylphosphatidylinositol-linked proteins do not confer resistance to apoptosis in paroxysmal nocturnal hemoglobinuria. *Blood* 92:2541–2550, 1998.

Chapter **42**

# ALLOGENEIC STEM CELL TRANSPLANTATION FOR MYELODYSPLASTIC SYNDROME AND APLASTIC ANEMIA

*Vikram Mathews and John F. DiPersio*

## ALLOGENEIC STEM CELL TRANSPLANTATION FOR MYELODYSPLASTIC SYNDROMES

### INTRODUCTION

Myelodysplastic syndrome (MDS) is a heterogeneous group of clonal hematopoietic disorders characterized by ineffective hematopoiesis, marrow dysplasia, and variable rates of transformation to acute myeloid leukemia predominantly affecting older patients (mean age 69 years).[1] With the aging of the population and increased awareness, the incidence and prevalence of MDS has been steadily increasing over the last 20 years.[2] In the United States, the estimated incidence of MDS is between 3.5 and 12.6 per 100,000 new.[3] MDS is associated with several subtypes diagnosed each year. The older FAB classification[4] of MDS has been replaced by the WHO classification.[5] The diagnostic subtypes have a significant bearing both for treatment and on prognosis. The blast percentage, the cytogenetic findings, and number of cytopenias at diagnosis are important in prognostication. Together these parameters have been used to generate a scoring system termed the International Prognostic Scoring System (IPSS).[6] The IPSS has a bearing not only in the overall prognosis of a patient with a diagnosis of MDS, but is also a useful predictor of transplantation outcomes.[7,8] In spite of there being significant progress in the understanding of the pathophysiology of MDS, which has translated into novel therapeutic interventions, allogeneic stem cell transplantation (SCT) still remains the only therapy that has curative potential in this condition. This was first demonstrated as early as 1984.[9] The epidemiology, molecular biology, pathology, and clinical features have been addressed in detail in Chapters 41–43.

### ALLOGENEIC SCT IN MDS

Various therapeutic options exist for the management of a newly diagnosed patient with MDS. In addition to the subtype and IPSS score at diagnosis, the age and performance status of the patient are important determinants of feasible therapeutic options. In spite of significant improvements in supportive care and the increasing therapeutic options that are available (Chapter 44 and 48), an allogeneic SCT remains the only option that has curative potential, leading to the recommendation that all patients who are eligible for a transplant procedure and have an available donor should be considered for this procedure.[10] However, in reality this therapeutic option is limited to a small fraction of patients with this diagnosis, as the majority of patients are over 65 years, with additional comorbidities and poor performance status. Even when other adverse factors are not present, this group of older patients is perceived as being unable to tolerate a standard myeloablative conditioning regimen.

Since MDS has significant variability in the natural history and response to therapy, no single therapeutic algorithm can be applied to this group of patients; rather, therapy has to be tailored to the individual patient. For patients eligible to undergo an allogeneic SCT, the factors that have a bearing on transplant outcome have to be weighed against the risks involved. In this chapter we look at some of these factors and provide a broad overview of the role of an allogeneic SCT in the management of MDS.

### EFFECT OF AGE ON OUTCOME

Intuitively, older patients should do poorly following an allogeneic SCT. Most studies have shown that recipient age is an important prognostic factor for nonrelapse mortality (NRM).[11] In a majority of the large trials using a myeloablative regimen with related[7,12–14] and unrelated donors,[12,15–17] this holds true. However, in one large study by Deeg et al.[8] that used targeted busulfan levels in a myeloablative conditioning regimen, in a multivariate analysis, there was no significant effect of age (up to 66 years) on relapse-free survival (RFS). The data on the use of nonmyeloabative transplants for older patients is still evolving and could potentially improve the outcome of older patients undergoing an allogeneic SCT.

### EFFECT OF IPSS SCORE ON OUTCOME

IPSS scores have been shown to have a bearing on the outcome following an allogeneic SCT.[7,8] In the more recent publication by Deeg et al.,[8] the 3-year RFS was 80% for patients with low-risk MDS (IPSS score 0), which progressively decreased with increasing scores to 29% among patients with an IPSS score higher than 2 (Figure 42.1). Earlier studies had shown a similar correlation with cytogenetic risk groups and posttransplant outcomes in patients with MDS. Nevill et al.[18] showed a 7-year event-free survival of 51%, 40%, and 6% in the good-, intermediate-, and poor-risk cytogenetic risk groups, respectively. Since the IPSS score includes additional parameters of percentage of blasts in the bone marrow and number of cytopenias at diagnosis,

which are important independent adverse factors,[14] it is likely to be a more robust system to predict outcome following an allogeneic SCT.

IPSS score also has an important bearing on decision making with regards to proceeding with an allogeneic stem cell transplant. In the low-risk group with a median survival of 11.8 years in patients younger than 60 years,[6] one would opt for supportive care or a nonintensive low-risk therapy rather than subject such an individual to the risk of treatment-related mortality (TRM) following an allogeneic SCT. On the other hand, a patient with an IPSS score >2, who has a median survival of a few months[6], is a candidate for an allogeneic SCT provided a donor is available and his or her performance status permits the procedure to be done.

### EFFECT OF TIME TO TRANSPLANT FROM DIAGNOSIS

While an allogeneic SCT is the only curative therapeutic option in the management of MDS, it is also associated with the highest TRM. NRM caused by infections, graft-versus-host disease (GVHD), and organ toxicity in large series of patients undergoing an allogeneic SCT varies from 30–54%.[16,18,19] It would not be appropriate to expose low-risk MDS patients to these risks. However, MDS is for the most part a continuously evolving disease process with an inexorable progression to acute leukemia, and an allogeneic SCT done in a more advanced stage of the disease process is associated with significantly worse outcomes.[7,8] The optimal time has been a matter of controversy, especially for the low- and intermediate-risk MDS. A recent publication by Cutler et al.[20] attempted to address this issue by applying a statistical technique called a Markov model to predict long-term outcomes under conditions of uncertainty. In patients with low- or intermediate-risk MDS, delayed transplantation by a fixed time interval (2–2.5 years) and prior to leukemia transformation maximized overall survival. This survival advantage was even more prominent in patients younger than 40 years in this risk group. For intermediate 2 and the high-risk group, immediate transplantation improved overall survival.

### ROLE OF INDUCTION CHEMOTHERAPY PRIOR TO AN ALLOGENEIC SCT

The majority of published studies have shown that patients in remission or with a lower percentage of bone marrow blasts have a lower relapse rate and an improved outcome. In the European Group for Blood and Marrow Transplantaton (EBMT) series, outcomes were significantly better for patients in first remission compared to the patients with active disease at the time of transplant.[12] Other groups have failed to demonstrate this benefit of remission induction prior to an allogeneic SCT,[8,14,21,22] suggesting that it would be preferable to take patients with high-risk MDS directly to an allogeneic SCT if they were eligible for this procedure. These studies are limited by being

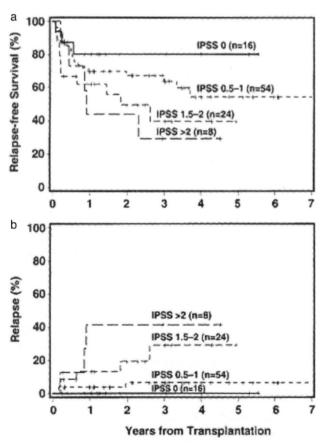

**Figure 42.1** *Impact of IPSS score on outcome. The + indicates censored patient; in 7 patients, an IPSS score could not be assigned. (a) Relapse-free survival. (b) CI of relapse. (Reprinted from Ref. 8, used with permission.)*

**Table 42.1**  Studies comparing the effect of chemotherapy prior to transplant

| Study | No. of patients | High-risk MDS (%) | Prior chemotherapy | TRM (%) | DFS (%) | OS (%) | |
|---|---|---|---|---|---|---|---|
| de Witte et al.[12] | 885 | 51 | + (111) | 37 | 44 | 49 | |
| | | | − (440) | 45 | 32 | 39 | $p < 0.001$ |
| Deeg et al.[8] | 109 | 37 | NS | 12 | 56 (HLA - identical sibling) | NS | no benefit of prior chemotherapy |
| | | | | | 59 (MUD) | NS | |
| Sutton et al.[14] | 71 | 77 | + (13) | 50 | 15 | 15 | no significant |
| | | | − (15) | 30 | 20 | 20 | difference |
| Anderson et al.[21] | 66 | 100 | + (20) | NS | 15 | NS | no significant |
| | | | − (46) | NS | 24 | NS | difference |

DFS – disease free survival; TRM – treatment related mortality; NS – not stated; OS – overall survival; MUD – matched unrelated donor transplant.

single center small retrospective analyses of heterogeneous groups of patients. The data from some studies addressing this issue are summarized in Table 42.1. The study by Copelan et al. suggests that the outcome in patients receiving induction therapy is in fact worse than those taken to transplant directly as a result of increased regimen related toxicity (RRT) compared to the group taken directly to a transplant.[22] This issue needs to be further evaluated, especially in the setting of newer, less toxic remission induction agents, preferably as a prospective study. On the basis of the available data, it would be reasonable to take patients with a low percentage of bone marrow blasts directly to transplant, while patients with a bone marrow blast percentage closer to that of a diagnosis of acute myelocytic leukemia would probably benefit from induction therapy prior to a transplant. These recommendations must also be based on the age, motivations, and comorbidities of the patient.

### CONDITIONING REGIMENS FOR ALLOGENEIC SCT IN MDS

Standard myeloablative conditioning regimens (both total body irradiation (TBI) based and non-TBI based) are associated with significant RRT, and contribute to NRM. As the majority of patients with a diagnosis of MDS are above the age of 60 years, they are less likely to tolerate these regimens. New nonmyeloablative regimens are being explored with the hope of being able to offer an allogeneic SCT, its graft-versus-leukemia effect, and the potential for cure to this older population.

#### Myeloablative conditioning regimens

In the 1980s, using a cyclophosphamide/TBI (Cy/TBI) ablative regimen resulted in a disease-free survival of 30–40% in patients with high-risk MDS.[23] In an effort to study if further intensification of the conditioning regimen would improve the outcome, busulfan was added to this regimen and compared with historical controls using Cy/TBI alone. The results showed that there was a decrease in relapse risk, but no significant

difference in survival with significantly more NRM (68% vs 36%).[24] From these early studies it appears that further intensification of the conditioning regimen is not a solution to improve the outcome in this disease. In the setting of unrelated matched donor transplants it has been shown that use of non-TBI-based conditioning regimens (Bu/Cy) is associated with improved outcomes both in the low- and high-risk MDS groups.[16] Overall, there has been a move toward the use of non-TBI-based conditioning regimens for allogeneic SCT in MDS. Oral busulfan with pharmacologic targeting and intravenous busulfan reduce the incidence of RRT and NRM and improve transplant outcomes.[16,25,26] Recent data published by Deeg et al. using targeted busulfan levels with cyclophosphamide have shown promising results even in an older patient population with low- and high-risk MDS.[8] The data from some of the largest series using myeloablative regimens are summarized in Table 42.2.

#### Nonmyeloablative conditioning regimens

In view of the older age group of patients with a diagnosis of MDS and the inability of a significant proportion of these patients to receive a standard myeloablative conditioning regimen, in the 1990s reduced intensity conditioning (RIC) or non-myeloablative conditioning regimens for an allogeneic SCT were actively pursued. It was hoped that this approach would reduce the RRT and NRM in this population. The most commonly used RIC regimen is a combination of fludarabine with either melphalan or low-dose TBI. Results from some of the largest series published[27–32] are summarized in Table 42.3. In a majority of these studies, the NRM was lower with myeloablative regimens but was associated with higher relapse rates, which was especially noted in the EBMT study.[30] More recently a publication from the MD Anderson Cancer Center showed a similar correlation with an increased risk of relapse in the group receiving a less intensive conditioning regimen when comparing two

**Table 42.2** Summary of data from some large series of patients with MDS who underwent a related matched, sibling allogeneic SCT using a myeloablative conditioning regimen

| Study | No. of patients | Age (median) | High-Risk MDS (%) | Preparative regimen | NRM (%) | DFS (%) at 3 years | OS (%) |
|---|---|---|---|---|---|---|---|
| Sutton et al.[14] | 71 | 37 | 100 | TBI based | 39 | 32 | 32 |
| Appelbaum et al.[7] | 251 | 38 (1-66) | 57 | TBI based, 69% | 42 | 41 | NS |
| de Witte et al.[12] | 885 | NS | 52 | NS | 43 | 31 | 46 |
| Sierra et al.[13] | 452 | 38 (2-64) | 60 | TBI based, 40% | 37 | 40 | 42 |

DFS – diseasefree survival; NRM – nonrelapse mortality; NS – not stated; OS – overall survival; TBI – total body irradiation.

reduced intensity regimens,[31] suggesting that more intensive conditioning may be required. There are a number of ongoing clinical trials addressing this issue, and the optimal regimen remains to be defined.

### PERIPHERAL BLOOD VERSUS BONE MARROW AS A SOURCE OF STEM CELLS

The use of G-CSF mobilized peripheral blood stem cells (PBSCs) has been associated with improved outcome compared to marrow. A retrospective analysis of the EBMT data of 234 patients with a diagnosis of MDS undergoing an HLA identical sibling transplant showed an improved 2-year survival of 50% with PBSC versus 39% with bone marrow and also reduced TRM and relapses.[33] Similar reduced relapse risk and improved overall outcome was also noted in the studies published by Deeg et al.[8] and Canizo et al.[34]

### ROLE OF ALTERNATE DONOR SOURCES

A related HLA-identical sibling is the ideal donor for an allogeneic stem cell transplant. Unfortunately only 25–30% of patients are likely to have an HLA-identical sibling. In this older population, an HLA-matched sibling may not be eligible as a donor because of age and comorbidities. Alternative donor sources include a matched unrelated donor (MUD), matched or mismatched cord blood, or a haploidentical donor. Analysis of MUD transplants under the auspices of the National Marrow Donor Program (NMDP) shows comparable results to that of an HLA identical related transplant.[16] The data with cord blood transplants is preliminary, but it has the potential to be a significant alternative source, especially with mismatched cord blood.[35,36] There is insufficient data with haploidentical transplants in this condition to recommend it outside of a clinical trial.

### CONCLUSION

An allogeneic stem cell transplant remains the only therapy with a curative potential in the management of a patient with a diagnosis of MDS. However, the risks associated with an allogeneic transplant in this older population have to be weighed against the benefits. Statistical models predict that delaying an allogeneic stem cell transplant for patients in the low-risk MDS group is associated with maximal life expectancy. Myeloablative regimens are associated with a lower risk of relapse in patients with high-risk MDS. Recent data using myeloablative regimens with targeted buslfan levels hold promise in both reducing the RRT

**Table 42.3** Summary of data of patients with MDS who underwent an HLA-identical (related and unrelated) allogeneic SCT using a nonmyeloablative conditioning regimen

| Study | No. of patients | Age (median) | High-risk MDS (%) | MUD (%) | Preparative regimen | NRM (%) | DFS (%) at 2 years | OS (%) |
|---|---|---|---|---|---|---|---|---|
| Giralt[11] | 26 | 57 | 100 | 33 | FM or FAI | 43 | 27 | 31 |
| Paker et al.[29] | 23 | 48 | 78 | 70 | FB-Campath | 26 | 39 | 48 |
| Stuart et al.[32] | 77 | 59 | 44 | 50 | F-TBI | NS | NS | 24(high risk) 40(low risk) |
| Martino et al.[30] | 194 | 54 | NS | 0 | various | 30 | 46 at 1 year | 55 at 1 year |
| De Lima et al.[31] | 26 | NS | NS | NS | FM or FAI | 30 | Relapse risk 61% with FAI vs 30% with FM* | |

DFS – disease-free survival; NRM – nonrelapse mortality; NS – not stated; OS – overall survival; TBI – total body irradiation; FAI – fludarabine, cytarabine, and idarubincin; FM – fludarabine and melphalan; FB – fludarabine and busulfan.
* Combined data of patients with diagnosis of MDS and acute myeloid leukemia.

and the risk of relapse. Preliminary data with non-myeloablative regimens show a definite reduction in NRM, though the high risk of relapse is of some concern, especially in patients in the high-risk group of MDS. Ongoing clinical trials may help identify an optimal nonmyeloablative regimen. Cytokine mobilized PBSC transplants appear to be superior to marrow transplants in this setting. Published data suggest that outcomes with MUD stem cell transplant are comparable to that with an HLA-identical related donor. Preliminary data with mismatched cord blood transplants are exciting, but remain to be validated.

## ALLOGENEIC SCT FOR APLASTIC ANEMIA

### INTRODUCTION

Acquired aplastic anemia (AA) is a rare but potentially fatal bone marrow failure syndrome characterized by pancytopenia. It can be acquired secondary to exposure to radiation, drugs, chemicals, and infections, or as part of an autoimmune disorder. However, most commonly it is idiopathic in origin. Inherited disorders such as Fanconi anemia, dyskeratosis congenital, and Shwachman's syndrome as well as acquired disorders such as paroxysmal nocturnal hemoglobinuria can lead to AA, and are not discussed in this chapter.

AA can present with varying severity. The International AA Study Group has established criteria for the diagnosis of severe aplastic anemia (SAA).[37] For the diagnosis of SAA, the bone marrow cellularity should be less than 25% of expected and two out of the following three criteria should be present (1) ANC $<0.5 \times 10^9$/lt; (2) platelets $<20 \times 10^9$/lt; and (3) reticulocytes $<1\%$. Very severe aplastic anemia (VSAA) is defined as for SAA but with an ANC $<0.2 \times 10^9$/lt. Patients not fulfilling criteria for SAA or VSAA have nonsevere AA.

Allogeneic stem cell transplant is a curative option in patients with this diagnosis. It is reserved for the treatment of patients with SAA or VSAA. It can also be considered for patients with nonsevere AA who have failed immunosuppressive therapy. An approach to the treatment of patients with a diagnosis of AA is outlined in Chapter 45.

### EFFECT OF AGE ON OUTCOME

Long-term survival for patients with AA undergoing an HLA-identical sibling transplant varies from 75% to 90%.[38–41] In most studies, patient age has a significant bearing on the outcome following an allogeneic stem cell transplant. There is some controversy as to the upper age limit at which an HLA-identical related allogeneic SCT would be offered as an initial therapy, with most recommendations putting the upper age limit as 40 years[42]; the study by Bacigalupo et al. showed that the outcomes were significantly worse for those older than 30 years.[41] Following failure of standard immunosuppressive therapy this option could be offered to all patients who have a donor and have no other contraindication to undergo an allogeneic SCT.

### CONDITIONING REGIMEN

Currently, the combination of cyclophosphamide and antithymocyte globulin (ATG) is considered the best conditioning regimen for patients with a diagnosis of AA undergoing an HLA-identical related transplant.[38,40,43,44] In a majority of studies, use of irradiation was associated with lower rejection rates but significantly higher TRM. A recent retrospective analysis by Ades et al. illustrates this[40] (Figure 42.2). In the setting of alternate donors, such as MUD SCT, the optimal regimen remains to be defined. A publication by Deeg et al. suggests that cyclophoshamide with ATG may not be sufficient in this setting.[45] The same group used escalating doses of TBI with cyclophosphamide

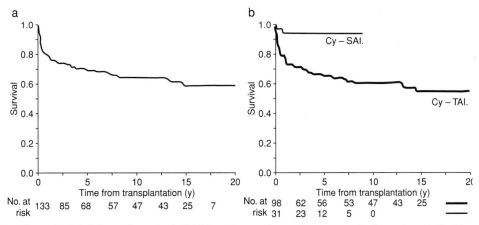

**Figure 42.2** *Overall survival. (a) Overall survival of 133 patients who underwent transplantation at the Hospital St. Louis (median follow-up of 13.6 years). (b) Overall survival according to the conditioning regimen with cyclophosphamide plus either antithymocyte globulin (Cy-ATG) or thoracoabdominal irradiation (Cy-TAI). (Reprinted from Ref. 40, used with permission.)*

and ATG and concluded that the addition of 2-Gy TBI to cyclophosphamide and ATG was associated with the best result of 67% survival at 2 years.[46] Use of Fludarabine-based and other RIC, both in the setting of related and alternate donors, remains to be evaluated in large studies.

### CYTOKINE MOBILIZED PBSC VERSUS BONE MARROW

In the setting of AA, there are no randomized control trials that have studied the benefit or disadvantages of one over the other source of stem cells. As with other allogeneic SCT, cytokine mobilized PBSC transplants are associated with faster engraftment, yet it is unclear if this translates to a superior outcome. Marsh et al. report that in personal communications the retrospective analysis of both European Blood and Marrow Transplant Group and the International Blood and Marrow Transplant Registry have shown significantly worse survival with PBSC versus bone marrow transplants (60% vs. 75%).[47] In the setting of transplanting

patients with SAA who have received multiple transfusions prior to their transplant, it has been reported that the use of PBSC improves the outcome.[48]

### ALTERNATIVE DONOR SCT

#### MUD transplants

Using the NMDP, around 70% of Caucasian patients are likely to find an HLA-matched donor; for other ethnic groups the chances are much lower. Retrospective analysis of the NMDP data reported a 2-year survival of 29% for 31 patients with SAA.[49] Better results were published from the Milwaukee group and the Fred Hutchinson Cancer Center Group, with 2-year survivals of 58% and 67%, respectively, using a more intensive conditioning regimen.[46,50] MUD transplants as first-line therapy remain experimental, and are associated with high morbidity and mortality. Guidelines from a group of experts suggest that it be reserved for patients who have failed two courses of immunosuppressive therapy.[51]

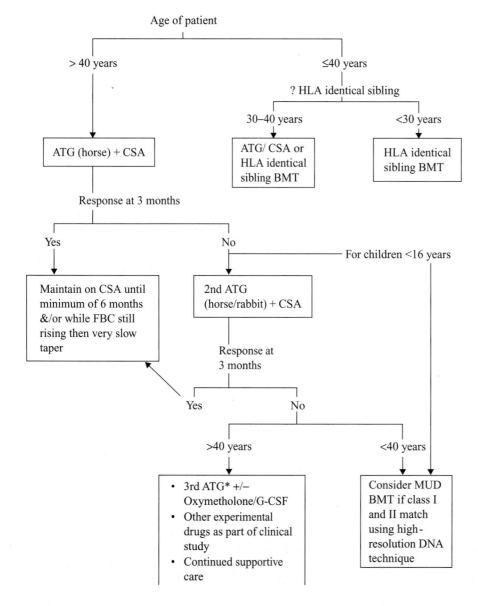

**Figure 42.3** *Algorithm for appropriate management of a patient with severe aplastic anemia (SAA) or very severe aplastic anemia (VSAA). BMT, bone marrow transplantation; G-CSF, granulocyte colony-stimulating factor; MUD, matched unrelated donor transplantation. (Reprinted from Ref. 42, used with permission.)*

## Partially matched family donor

The chance of having a one antigen mismatched family donor is 5–7% in North America and Europe.[47] Usually these transplants are done as a last resort in patients who have been clinically deteriorating with a poor performance status. The results in his setting have been dismal, with a high mortality from graft failure, GVHD, and infection.[52,53]

## Other donors

There is insufficient data with cord blood and haploidentical donors to recommend this as a standard approach for patients with SAA. Umbilical cord blood has been used in a small number of patients.[54,55] Its use is limited to small recipients because of the low number of stem cell progenitors. Recent recommendations suggest that it be considered for patients who have failed immunosuppressive therapy and are eligible for an allogeneic SCT.[51]

## CONCLUSION

An allogeneic SCT is a curative therapeutic option for patients with a diagnosis of SAA or VSAA. All patients below the age of 40 years who have an HLA-identical related donor should be considered for this procedure as first-line therapy. In this group of patients the outcome of an allogeneic SCT is superior to that of immunosuppressive therapy, with a 75–90% chance of long-term survival. In addition, unlike with immunosuppressive therapy, there is a much lower risk of late relapses and development of clonal disorders. Conditioning regimens for patients undergoing an HLA-identical related donor should preferably be free of irradiation, and it appears that cyclophoshamide combined with ATG is optimal in this setting. Preliminary retrospective analyses suggest that for HLA-identical related transplants for AA, the use of PBSC is associated with a worse outcome compared to bone marrow. Alternate donors should not be considered for front-line therapy and should be limited to patients who have failed immunosuppressive therapy. For alternate donor transplants, the use of cyclophosphamide with ATG as a conditioning regimen is probably inadequate and further intensification is justified to reduce the risk of graft rejection and improve outcomes. Figure 42.3 outlines an algorithm that could be used to decide on the appropriate management of a patient with SAA or VSAA.

## REFERENCES

1. Bowen D, et al.: Guidelines for the diagnosis and therapy of adult myelodysplastic syndromes. *Br J Haematol* 120(2):187–200, 2003.
2. Aul C, et al.: Increasing incidence of myelodysplastic syndromes: real or fictitious? *Leuk Res* 22(1):93–100, 1998.
3. Anderson J: Allogeneic hematopoietic cell transplantation for myelodysplastic and myeloproliferative disorders. In: Thomas E, Blume KG, Formans SJ (eds.) *Hematopoietic Cell Transplantation.* Malden, MA: Blackwell Science;1999:872–886.
4. Bennett JM, et al.: Proposals for the classification of the myelodysplastic syndromes. *Br J Haematol* 51(2): 189–199, 1982.
5. Harris NL, et al.: The World Health Organization classification of neoplastic diseases of the hematopoietic and lymphoid tissues. Report of the Clinical Advisory Committee meeting, Airlie House, Virginia, November, 1997. *Ann Oncol* 10(12):1419–1432, 1999.
6. Greenberg P, et al.: International scoring system for evaluating prognosis in myelodysplastic syndromes. *Blood* 89(6):2079–2088, 1997.
7. Appelbaum FR, Anderson J: Allogeneic bone marrow transplantation for myelodysplastic syndrome: outcomes analysis according to IPSS score. *Leukemia* 12 (suppl 1):S25–S29, 1998.
8. Deeg HJ, Storer B, Slattery JT, et al.: Conditioning with targeted busulfan and cyclophosphamide for hemopoietic stem cell transplantation from related and unrelated donors in patients with myelodysplastic syndrome. *Blood* 100(4):1201–1207, 2000.
9. Appelbaum FR, et al.: Allogeneic marrow transplantation in the treatment of preleukemia. *Ann Intern Med* 100(5):689–693, 1984.
10. Greenberg P, Bishop M, Deeg J: Practice guidelines for myelodysplastic syndromes. *Oncology* 12:53–80, 1998.
11. Giralt S: Bone marrow transplant in myelodysplastic syndromes: new technologies, same questions. *Curr Hematol Rep* 3(3):165–172, 2004.
12. de Witte T, et al.: Haematopoietic stem cell transplantation for patients with myelo-dysplastic syndromes and secondary acute myeloid leukaemias: a report on behalf of the Chronic Leukaemia Working Party of the European Group for Blood and Marrow Transplantation (EBMT). *Br J Haematol* 110(3):620–630, 2000.
13. Sierra J, et al.: Bone marrow transplantation from HLA-identical siblings as treatment for myelodysplasia. *Blood* 100(6):1997–2004, 2002.
14. Sutton L, et al.: Factors influencing outcome in de novo myelodysplastic syndromes treated by allogeneic bone marrow transplantation: a long-term study of 71 patients Societe Francaise de Greffe de Moelle. *Blood* 88(1):358–365, 1996.
15. Anderson JE, et al.: Unrelated donor marrow transplantation for myelodysplasia (MDS) and MDS-related acute myeloid leukaemia. *Br J Haematol* 93(1):59–67, 1996.
16. Castro-Malaspina H, et al.: Unrelated donor marrow transplantation for myelodysplastic syndromes: outcome analysis in 510 transplants facilitated by the National Marrow Donor Program. *Blood* 99(6): 1943–1951, 2002.
17. de Witte T, et al.: Genotypically nonidentical related donors for transplantation of patients with myelodysplastic syndromes: comparison with unrelated donor transplantation and autologous stem cell transplantation. *Leukemia* 15(12):1878–1884, 2001.
18. Nevill TJ, et al.: Cytogenetic abnormalities in primary myelodysplastic syndrome are highly predictive of

outcome after allogeneic bone marrow transplantation. *Blood* 92(6):1910–1917, 1998.

19. Runde V, et al.: Bone marrow transplantation from HLA-identical siblings as first-line treatment in patients with myelodysplastic syndromes: early transplantation is associated with improved outcome. Chronic Leukemia Working Party of the European Group for Blood and Marrow Transplantation. *Bone Marrow Transplant* 21(3):255–261, 1998.

20. Cutler CS, et al.: A decision analysis of allogeneic bone marrow transplantation for the myelodysplastic syndromes: delayed transplantation for low risk myelodysplasia is associated with improved outcome. *Blood*, 2004.

21. Anderson JE, et al.: Stem cell transplantation for secondary acute myeloid leukemia: evaluation of transplantation as initial therapy or following induction chemotherapy. *Blood* 89(7):2578–2585, 1997.

22. Copelan EA, et al.: Analysis of prognostic factors for allogeneic marrow transplantation following busulfan and cyclophosphamide in myelodysplastic syndrome and after leukemic transformation. *Bone Marrow Transplant* 25(12):1219–1222, 2000.

23. Appelbaum FR, et al.: Bone marrow transplantation for patients with myelodysplasia. Pretreatment variables and outcome. *Ann Intern Med* 112(8):590–597, 1990.

24. Anderson JE, et al.: Allogeneic marrow transplantation for myelodysplastic syndrome with advanced disease morphology: a phase II study of busulfan, cyclophosphamide, and total-body irradiation and analysis of prognostic factors. *J Clin Oncol* 14(1):220–226, 1996.

25. Slattery JT, Risler LJ: Therapeutic monitoring of busulfan in hematopoietic stem cell transplantation. *Ther Drug Monit* 20(5):543–549, 1998.

26. Andersson BS, et al.: Allogeneic stem cell transplantation (BMT) for AML and MDS following i.v. busulfan and cyclophosphamide (i.v. BuCy). *Bone Marrow Transplant* 25 (suppl 2):S35–S38, 2000.

27. Giralt S, et al.: Melphalan and purine analog-containing preparative regimens: reduced-intensity conditioning for patients with hematologic malignancies undergoing allogeneic progenitor cell transplantation. *Blood* 97(3):631–637, 2000.

28. Shimoni A, et al.: Allogeneic hematopoietic transplantation for acute and chronic myeloid leukemia: non-myeloablative preparative regimens and induction of the graft-versus-leukemia effect. *Curr Oncol Rep* 2(2):132–139, 2000.

29. Parker JE, et al.: Allogeneic stem cell transplantation in the myelodysplastic syndromes: interim results of outcome following reduced-intensity conditioning compared with standard preparative regimens. *Br J Haematol* 119(1):144–154, 2002.

30. Martino R, vBA, Jacobelli S, et al.: Reduced intensity conditioning regimens for allogeneic stem cell transplants from HLA identical siblings in adults with MDS: a comparison with standard myeloablative regimens. A study of the EBMT Chronic Leukemia Working Party (EBMT-CLWP) [abstract]. *Blood* 102:642, 2003. Abstract.

31. De Lima M, et al.: Non-ablative versus reduced intensity conditioning regimens in the treatment of acute myeloid leukemia and high-risk myelodysplastic syndrome. Dose is relevant for long-term disease control after allogeneic hematopoietic stem cell transplantation. *Blood*, 2004.

32. Stuart JS, Cao TM, Sandmaier BM et al.: Efficacy of non-myeloablative allogeneic transplant for patients with MDS and myeloproliferative disorders [abstract]. *Blood* 102:644, 2003. Abstract.

33. Guardiola P, et al.: Retrospective comparison of bone marrow and granulocyte colony-stimulating factor-mobilized peripheral blood progenitor cells for allogeneic stem cell transplantation using HLA identical sibling donors in myelodysplastic syndromes. *Blood* 99(12):4370–4378, 2002.

34. del Canizo, MC, et al.: Peripheral blood is safer than bone marrow as a source of hematopoietic progenitors in patients with myelodysplastic syndromes who receive an allogeneic transplantation. Results from the Spanish registry. *Bone Marrow Transplant* 32(10):987–992, 2003.

35. Ooi, J, et al.: Unrelated cord blood transplantation for adult patients with advanced myelodysplastic syndrome. *Blood* 101(12):4711–4713, 2003.

36. Ooi, J, et al.: Unrelated cord blood transplantation for adult patients with myelodysplastic syndrome-related secondary acute myeloid leukaemia. *Br J Haematol* 114(4):834–836, 2001.

37. Camitta, BM, et al.: Severe aplastic anemia: a prospective study of the effect of early marrow transplantation on acute mortality. *Blood* 48(1):63–70, 1976.

38. Storb R, et al.: Long-term follow-up of allogeneic marrow transplants in patients with aplastic anemia conditioned by cyclophosphamide combined with antithymocyte globulin. *Blood* 89(10):3890–3891, 1997.

39. Passweg JR, et al.: Bone marrow transplantation for severe aplastic anemia: has outcome improved? *Blood* 90(2):858–864, 1997.

40. Ades L, Mary J-Y, Robin M, et al.: Long-term outcome after bone marrow transplantation for severe aplastic anemia. *Blood* 103(7):2490–2497, 2004.

41. Bacigalupo A, et al.: Treatment of acquired severe aplastic anemia: bone marrow transplantation compared with immunosuppressive therapy—The European Group for Blood and Marrow Transplantation experience. *Semin Hematol* 37(1):69–80, 2000.

42. Marsh JC, Ball SE, Darbyshire P, et al.: Guidelines for the diagnosis and management of acquired aplastic anaemia. *Br J Haematol* 123(5):782–801, 2003.

43. Storb R, et al.: Cyclophosphamide combined with antithymocyte globulin in preparation for allogeneic marrow transplants in patients with aplastic anemia. *Blood* 84(3):941–949, 1994.

44. Storb R, et al.: Cyclophosphamide and antithymocyte globulin to condition patients with aplastic anemia for allogeneic marrow transplantations: the experience in four centers. *Biol Blood Marrow Transplant* 7(1):39–44, 2001.

45. Deeg HJ, et al.: Cyclophosphamide plus ATG conditioning is insufficient for sustained hematopoietic reconstitution in patients with severe aplastic anemia transplanted with marrow from HLA-A, B, DRB matched unrelated donors. *Blood* 83(11):3417–3418, 1994.

46. Deeg HJ, et al.: Marrow transplantation from unrelated donors for patients with severe aplastic anemia who have failed immunosuppressive therapy. *Biol Blood Marrow Transplant* 5(4):243–252, 1999.

47. Killick SB, Marsh JC: Aplastic anaemia: management. *Blood Rev* 14(3):157–171, 2000.

48. Herrera-Garza J, et al.: High-dose peripheral blood stem cell transplant for multitransfused severe aplastic anaemia patients without antithymocyte globulin in the conditioning regimen. *Bone Marrow Transplant* 24(8): 845–848, 1999.

49. Kernan NA, et al.: Analysis of 462 transplantations from unrelated donors facilitated by the National Marrow Donor Program. *N Engl J Med* 328(9):593–602, 1993.

50. Margolis D, et al.: Unrelated donor bone marrow transplantation to treat severe aplastic anaemia in children and young adults. *Br J Haematol* 94(1):65–72, 1996.

51. Schrezenmeier H, Bacigalupo A, Aglietta M, et al. Consensus document for treating aplastic anaemia. Consensus document of a group of international experts. In: Schrezenmeier H, Bacigalupo, A (eds.) *Aplastic Anaemia, Pathophysiology and Treatment.* Cambridge: Cambridge Univ. Press;2000:308–315.

52. Bacigalupo A, et al., Bone marrow transplantation for severe aplastic anemia from donors other than HLA identical siblings: a report of the BMT Working Party. *Bone Marrow Transplant* 3(6):531–535, 1988.

53. Hows JM, et al.: Histocompatible unrelated volunteer donors compared with HLA nonidentical family donors in marrow transplantation for aplastic anemia and leukemia. *Blood* 68(6):1322–1328, 1986.

54. Gluckman E, et al.: Outcome of cord-blood transplantation from related and unrelated donors. Eurocord Transplant Group and the European Blood and Marrow Transplantation Group. *N Engl J Med* 337(6):373–381, 1997.

55. Barker JN, et al.: Survival after transplantation of unrelated donor umbilical cord blood is comparable to that of human leukocyte antigen-matched unrelated donor bone marrow: results of a matched-pair analysis. *Blood* 97(10):2957–2961, 2001.

# Chapter 43

# DEFINITION OF RESPONSE, PROGNOSIS, AND FOLLOW-UP OF MYELODYSPLASTIC SYNDROMES

## Miguel A. Sanz and Guillermo F. Sanz

## INTRODUCTION

The myelodysplastic syndromes (MDS) have heterogeneous clinical characteristics, morphologic features, cytogenetics, and clinical outcomes that can make management of patients with these disorders difficult. This clinical and prognostic heterogeneity can complicate the planning of therapy. The different therapeutic goals for patients with MDS vary according to age, performance status, the severity of cytopenia and its associated complications, risk of progression to acute myeloid leukemia (AML), and other factors, such as socioeconomic status.

The clinical objectives may differ according to the patient's age or other factors. For example, older patients or those with poor physical health might be unable to withstand aggressive treatment compared to younger patients in better health who can more easily overcome the complications associated with high-intensity therapies. Similarly, the therapeutic goals also differ depending on the patient's risk of progressing to AML. In general, the main objectives for low-risk patients are to improve cytopenias and their associated complications, and quality of life (QOL); in contrast, the main goal for high-risk patients, especially younger patients, is to achieve complete remission (CR) and then to eradicate the malignant clone through chemotherapy and possibly stem cell transplantation.

Because a variety of strategies can be used to treat patients with MDS according to prognosis and chance of a cure, and because the goals of treatment may vary, physicians should evaluate the responses in the context of these goals. Therefore, a consensus should be reached on the use of reliable MDS prognostic classification schemes and on standardized response criteria when designing clinical trials and evaluating different treatment options.

This chapter reviews the state of the art on the assessment of responses to treatment, prognosis, and follow-up of patients with MDS.

## RESPONSE CRITERIA

In the past, the treatment for the vast majority of patients with MDS consisted of supportive care to mitigate cytopenia-related complications, which involved mainly red blood cell (RBC) transfusions and growth factor use to avoid symptomatic anemia. Only patients who progressed to AML were treated more aggressively, usually with chemotherapy similar to that used to treat AML; these patients were then assessed using the same criteria as those to assess the response to therapy for patients with AML.

The algorithm used to treat patients with MDS has become much more complex recently for several reasons. First, reliable prognostic classification systems have been developed to best determine the natural history of MDS (discussed further below) and to identify different prognostic subgroups. Second, several therapies have been developed that influence outcome and QOL in each identifiable prognostic subgroup. Third, the responses are now evaluated according to the goals of each therapeutic approach. Thus, clinicians and investigators encounter greater variability in the definitions of the responses to MDS than in the past, making it difficult to interpret and compare results between clinical trials.

To resolve this variability in the response criteria, an international working group of investigators with expertise in MDS has achieved a consensus to establish standardized response criteria for clinical trials involving patients with MDS[1-3] (Table 43.1). This working group looked for clinically relevant, practical, and

**Table 43.1    Measurement of response/treatment effect in MDS**

ALTERING DISEASE NATURAL HISTORY

1. Complete remission (CR)

    *Bone marrow evaluation:* Repeat bone marrow showing less than 5% myeloblasts with normal maturation of all cell lines, with no evidence for dysplasia.[a] When erythroid precursors constitute less than 50% of bone marrow nucleated cells, the percenage of blasts is based on all nucleated cells; when there are 50% or more erythroid cells, the percentage blasts should be based on the nonerythroid cells.

    *Peripheral blood evaluation* (absolute values must last at least 2 months)[b]:

       Hemoglobin greater than 11 g/dL (untransfused, patient not on erythropoietin)

       Neutrophils 1500/mm$^3$ or more (not on a myeloid growth factor)

       Platelets 100 000/mm$^3$ or more (not on a thrombopoetic agent)

       Blasts, 0%

       No dysplasia[a]

2. Partial remission (PR) (absolute values must last at least 2 months):

    All the CR criteria (if abnormal before treatment), except:

    *Bone marrow evaluation:* Blasts decreased by 50% or more over pretreatment, or a less advanced MDS FAB classification than pretreatment. Cellularity and morphology are not relevant.

3. Stable disease

    Failure to achieve at least a PR, but with no evidence of progression for at least 2 months.

4. Failure

    Death during treatment or disease progression characterized by worsening of cytopenias, increase in the percentage bone marrow blasts, or progression to an MDS FAB subtype more advanced than pretreatment.

5. Relapse after CR or RR—one or more of the following:

    a) Return to pretreatment bone marrow blast percentage

    b) Decrement of 50% or greater from maximum remission/response levels in granulocytes or platelets

    c) Reduction in hemoglobin concentration by at least 2g/dL or transfusion dependence[c]

6. Disease progression

    a) For patients with less than 5% blasts: a 50% or more increase in blasts to more than 5% blasts

    b) For patients with 5–10% blasts: a 50% or more increase to more than 10% blasts

    c) for patients with 10–20% blasts: a 50% or more increase to more than 20% blasts

    d) For patients with 20–30% blasts: a 50% or more increase to more than 30% blasts

    e) One or more of the following: 50% or greater decrement from maximum remission/response levels in granulocytes or platelets, reduction in hemoglobin concentration by at least 2 g/dL, or transfusion dependence[c]

7. Disease transformation

    Transformation to AML (30% or more blasts)

8. Survival and progression-free survival (see Table 43.2)

CYTOGENETIC RESPONSE

    (Requires 20 analyzable metaphases using conventional cytogenetic techniques.)

    *Major:* No detectable cytogenetic abnormality, if preexisting abnormality was present.

    *Minor:* 50% or more reduction in abnormal metaphases.

    Fluorescent in situ hybridization may be used as a supplement to follow a specifically defined cytogenetic abnormality.

QUALITY OF LIFE

    Measured by an instrument such as the FACT Questionnaire.

    Clinically useful improvement in specific domains:

       Physical

       Functional

       Emotional

       Social

       Spiritual

HEMATOLOGIC IMPROVEMENT (HI)

(Improvements must last at least 2 months in the absence of ongoing cytotoxic therapy.)[b]

Hematologic improvement should be described by the number of individual, positively affected cell lines (e.g. HI-E; HI-E + HI-N; HI-E + HI-P + HI-N).

1. Erythroid response (HI-E)

    *Major response:* For patients with pretreatment hemoglobin less than 11 g/dL, greater than 2 g/dL increase in hemoglobin; for RBC transfusion-dependent patients, transfusion independence.

    *Minor response:* For patients with a pretreatment hemoglobin less than 11 g/dL, 1–2 g/dL increase in hemoglobin; for RBC transfusion-dependent patients, 50% decrease in transfusion requirements.

2. Platelet response (HI-P)

    *Major response:* For patients with a pretreatment platelet count less than 100 000/mm$^3$, an absolute increase of 30 000/mm$^3$ or more; for platelet transfusion-dependent patiens, stabilization of platelet count and platelet transfusion independence.

*Minor response*: For patients with a pretreatment platelet count less than 100 000/mm³, a 50% or more increase in platelet count with a net increase greater than 10 000/mm³ but less than 30 000/mm³.

3. Neutrophil response (HI-N)

*Major response*: For absolute neutrophil count (ANC) less than 1500/mm³ before therapy, at least a 100% increase, or an absolute increase of more than 500/mm³, whichever is greater.

*Minor response*: for ANC less than 1500/mm³ before therapy, ANC increase of at least 100%, but absolute increase less than 500/mm³.

4. Progression/relapse after HI: One or more of the following: a 50% or greater decrement from maximum response levels in granulocytes or platelets, a reduction in hemoglobin concentration by at least 2 g/dL, or transfusion dependence.[c]

For a designated response (CR, PR, HI), all relevant response criteria must be noted on at least two successive determinations at least 1 week apart after an appropriate period following therapy (e.g., 1 month or longer).

[a]The presence of mild megaloblastoid changes may be permitted if they are thought to be consistent with treatment effect. However, persistence of pretreatment abnormalities (e.g., pseudo-Pelger-Hüet cells, ringed sideroblasts, dysplastic megakaryocytes) is not consistent with CR.

[b]In some circumstances, protocol therapy may require the initiation of further treatment (e.g., consolidation, maintenance) before the 2-month period. Such patients can be included in the response category into which they fit at the time the therapy is started.

[c]In the absence of another explanation such as acute infection, gastrointestinal bleeding, hemolysis and so on.

Adapted from Cheson BD, Bennett JM, Kantarjian H, et al.: Report of an international working group to standardize response criteria for myelodysplastic syndroms. *Blood* 96:3671–3674, 2000; used with permission.

reproducible definitions of responses that could be used easily by investigators and clinicians from different institutions. The working group defined the response categories to best evaluate the major therapeutic goals of therapy in MDS: (1) controlling symptoms resulting from cytopenia; (2) improving QOL, including minimizing the toxicity of therapy; and (3) altering the natural history of the disease by improving overall survival or decreasing progression to AML.

## PROGNOSIS OF MDS

As stated previously, the clinical and prognostic heterogeneity of MDS confers an additional difficulty when planning therapy. Some patients experience prolonged survival and remain symptom-free for many years, whereas others die within a few weeks or months after diagnosis. Overall, the median survival is nearly 19 months and the risk of AML evolution is 35% at 5 years.[3a] Most patients die as a consequence of cytopenia-associated complications, in the presence or absence of AML transformation. However a significant number of patients die of causes unrelated to the disorder. Although the French–American–British (FAB) classification[4] has been relatively effective in categorizing MDS patients, it has some limitations in the clinical setting. These limitations include the wide range of marrow blast percentages in patients classified as having refractory anemia (RA) with excess blasts (RAEB) or chronic myelomonocytic leukemia, the failure to consider some important biologic determinants such as marrow cytogenetics, and the degree and number of cytopenias. These well-accepted problems in categorizing patients with MDS have led to the development of many additional risk-based stratification systems, which are reviewed critically in this chapter.

## PROGNOSTIC FACTORS

Studies on prognostic factors in MDS have identified several patient and disease characteristics that are highly associated with survival or leukemic transformation, or both (Table 43.2). Although a number of characteristics may influence the prognosis of MDS, the percentage of bone marrow (BM) blasts, cytogenetic pattern, and number and extent of cytopenias are currently considered the most powerful prognostic factors in these disorders.[3a,5,6]

### BM blasts

Increased BM blast percentage has generally been associated with poorer prognosis for survival and with leukemic transformation in MDS patients. A Spanish group showed,[7] and others have confirmed,[8,9] that adding an extra cutoff point of 10% to the generally accepted 5 and 20% FAB criteria clearly improved the prognostic value of this variable.

### Cytogenetics

Several series have reported the prognostic impact on survival and leukemic risk of several types of marrow chromosomal abnormalities, although only recently has this variable been shown to have independent prognostic value.[8–11] Sequential cytogenetic studies are valuable tools during follow-up.[12,13] The appearance of chromosomal abnormalities in a patient with a previously normal karyotype or the emergence of additional aberrations is associated with disease progression and shorter survival. This finding may be of particular value in patients with RA and RA with ringed sideroblasts (RARS). However, it should be stressed that chromosomal stability does not preclude the development of AML. In fact, the majority of MDS patients do not show chromosomal changes at the time of acute leukemic transformation.[3a,13]

**Table 43.2**   Prognostic factors identified in patients with MDS

| Characteristic | Unfavorable value |
| --- | --- |
| **Clinical** | |
| Age | Advanced (60 years) |
| Sex | Male |
| Systemic symptoms | Presence |
| Etiology | Therapy related |
| **Hematologic** | |
| In peripheral blood | |
| Platelets | Lower counts |
| Hemoglobin | Lower level |
| Neutrophils | Neutropenia |
| Leukocytes | Leukopenia or leukocytosis |
| Blasts | Presence |
| In bone marrow | |
| Blasts | Higher percentage |
| Micromegakaryocytes | Presence |
| Basophilia/eosinophilia | Higher percentage |
| Dysplasia | Multilineal (2/3 lines)[a] |
| **Marrow biopsy findings** | |
| Cellularity | Increased |
| ALIP[b] | Presence |
| Dysmegakaryopoiesis | Severe |
| Fibrosis | Presence |
| **FAB classification** | RAEB, RAEBT[c] |
| **Biochemical parameters** | |
| LDH | Increased |
| β-2-microglobulin | Increased |
| **Cytogenetics[d]** | Complex (>2 abnormalities) |
| | Monosomy 7/del(7q) |
| **Molecular genetics** | |
| N-RAS mutation | Presence |
| p53 deletion | Presence |
| FMS mutation | Presence |
| p15 methylation | Presence |
| WT1 expression | Higher |
| VEGFR-1 expression | Higher |
| **Marrow culture studies** | |
| Number of colonies | Lower |
| Number of clusters | Higher |
| Colony-to-cluster ratio | Low |
| Leukemic pattern | Presence |
| **Immunophenotype** | |
| CD34-positive cells | Higher proportion |
| Immature-to-mature cell ratio | Increased |
| CD7-positive blasts in marrow | Higher percentage |
| **Marrow apoptosis** | Increased |

[a] As defined by the WHO classification.
[b] ALIP denotes abnormal localization of immature precursors.
[c] RAEBT denotes refractory anemia with excess blasts in transformation.
[d] Favorable categories are normal karyotype, and del(5q), del(20q), and −Y as single abnormalities.

### Cytopenias

Of various peripheral blood cell counts, platelet counts and hemoglobin level have a greater prognostic weight than neutrophil counts.[7] Several studies have demonstrated that the greater the severity and the higher the number of cytopenias, the worse the survival and the higher the risk of leukemic evolution.[7,9]

### Other characteristics

Other variables with prognostic value, but of lesser importance, include age (which reflects a poorer tolerance to cytopenia-associated complications and the impact of other comorbid conditions associated with older age rather than a more aggressive clinical course)[7,9]; FAB classification[7]; gender (worse prognosis for male patients, which may be explained to some extent by the greater life expectancy of women in industrialized countries)[7]; percentage of blasts in peripheral blood[7]; presence of immature myeloid precursors and nucleated RBCs in peripheral blood[7]; degree of multilineage dysplasia in RA and RARS (as in the recent World Health Organization [WHO] proposals of classification of MDS[14])[15–21]; marrow basophilia or eosinophilia,[22] serum lactate dehydrogenase (LDH) level (which may provide an indirect measure of ineffective hematopoiesis and leukemic burden)[23]; and some BM biopsy findings, such as abnormal location of immature myeloid precursors (ALIP), hypercellularity, and fibrosis.[5,6,24] Other characteristics, such as serum β-2-microglobulin level,[25] in vitro growth pattern of granulocyte-macrophage progenitors,[26] plasma soluble interleukin 2 receptor level,[27] plasma levels of soluble vascular endothelial growth factor receptor 1,[28] and magnetic resonance imaging pattern[29] have been also implicated in MDS prognosis. Several flow cytometry parameters have been shown to influence the outcome of disease,[30] including the expression of CD7, CD10, and CD15 by BM blasts,[31] and the number of CD34-positive cells in the peripheral blood.[32] A prognostic scoring system based exclusively on flow cytometry data has been reported to predict the outcome after allogeneic stem cell transplantation.[33]

The recent progress in understanding the biology of MDS has led to studies of new prognostic parameters to predict outcome. A greater degree of apoptosis in the BM, as measured by different techniques, has been associated with longer survival and time to develop AML.[34–45] Mutations of *ras*, *fms*, and *p53* genes, which reflect genomic instability, occur more frequently in patients with poor prognosis and are associated with shorter survival and a higher risk of leukemia.[46,47] The level of expression of WT1, measured by real-time quantitative polymerase chain reaction (PCR), has a strong direct relationship with the percentage of blasts in the BM and the presence of chromosomal abnormalities.[48] Telomere stability, another marker of genomic instability, is frequently impaired in high-risk MDS. Patients with shortened terminal restriction fragments, measured by the PCR-based twin reversed arterial perfusion assay, have a significantly lower hemoglobin level, higher percentage of BM blasts, higher incidence of cytogenetic abnormalities, and a higher risk of leukemic transformation.[37] The incidence of inactivation by methylation of the p15 gene is higher in patients with ≥10% BM blasts and increases with progression to AML.[49,50] Preliminary evidence suggests that gene profiling could also have prognostic value in MDS patients.[51,52] Information on the prognostic relevance of these new biological factors, however, is still scarce. Further studies that include a larger number of cases and multivariate analyses are needed before this evidence can be accepted and used in the clinical management of patients.

### PROGNOSTIC SCORING SYSTEMS

Research on prognostic factors has led to the development of several scoring systems, some of which incorporate cytogenetic factors.[3a,5,6]

### Scoring systems without karyotype analyses

Table 43.3 shows the main prognostic scoring systems proposed for MDS that do not include cytogenetic factors. The Bournemouth score was the first proposed scoring system. Patients were assigned to one of three risk groups based on the number of cytopenias present and the proportion of blasts in the BM.[53] The main criticism of this system is the emphasis on blood cytopenias in relation to the proportion of blasts in the BM.[7] The scoring system proposed by the Spanish group uses the proportion of BM blasts, platelet count, and age.[7] This system is easy to use and has been demonstrated to predict survival in

other series, including untreated patients and patients treated with granulocyte colony-stimulating factor or AML-type chemotherapy.[6,55,56] The Goasguen score uses only two cytopenias (hemoglobin and platelets) and blasts in the BM,[54] and the Düsseldorf score includes these same variables and the serum LDH concentration.[23]

### Scoring systems with karyotype analyses

Table 43.4 shows the main prognostic scoring systems proposed for MDS that include cytogenetic factors. The Lille group was the first to incorporate cytogenetics in a prognostic score of MDS,[8] though only cases with complex abnormalities were considered as a high-risk group. An International MDS Risk Analysis Workshop was convened to improve the clinical and prognostic utility of scoring systems, to better define the cytogenetic risk categories, and to develop a consensus prognostic risk-based analysis system. This workshop published the International Prognostic Scoring System (IPSS) in 1997.[9] The IPSS includes the proportion of blasts in the BM, cytogenetics, and number of cytopenias. Combining the risk scores for these three major variables allows patients to be stratified into four distinctive risk groups according to both survival and AML evolution; the risk scores are low (0 points), intermediate-1 (0.5–1.0 points), intermediate-2 (1.5–2.0 points), and high (≥2.5 points). The overall median survival was 5.7, 3.5, 1.2, and 0.4 years for low-, intermediate-1-, intermediate-2-, and high-risk patients, respectively (Figure 43.1). The time taken for 25% of the patients in each of the four risk groups to evolve toward acute leukemia was 9.4, 3.3, 1.1, and 0.2 years, respectively. Survival of low-risk patients was strongly related to age, with median survival times of 11.8 years in patients ≤60 years of age, 4.8 years in

**Table 43.3** Prognostic scoring systems without karyotype analyses for patients with MDS

| Scoring system | 0 | 1 | 2 | Risk group | Score |
|---|---|---|---|---|---|
| Bournemouth[53] | | | | | |
|   Hemoglobin (g/dL) | >10 | ≤10 | | | |
|   Neutrophils (×10⁹/L) | >2.5 and ≤16 | ≤2.5 and >16 | | Low | 0 or 1 |
|   Platelets (×10⁹/L) | ≥100 | <100 | | Intermediate | 2 or 3 |
|   Marrow blasts (%) | <5 | ≥5 | | High | 4 |
| Spanish[7] | | | | | |
|   Marrow blasts (%) | <5 | 5–10 | 11–30 | Low | 0 or 1 |
|   Platelets (×10⁹/L) | ≥100 | 51–100 | ≤50 | Intermediate | 2 or 3 |
|   Age (years) | ≤60 | >60 | | High | 4 or 5 |
| Goasguen[54] | | | | | |
|   Hemoglobin (g/dL) | >10 | ≤10 | | Low | 0 |
|   Platelets (×10⁹/L) | >100 | ≤100 | | Intermediate | 1 or 2 |
|   Marrow blasts (%) | <5 | ≥5 | | High | 3 |
| Düsseldorf[23] | | | | | |
|   Marrow blasts (%) | <5 | ≥5 | | low (A) | 0 |
|   Platelets (×10⁹/L) | >100 | ≤100 | | Intermediate (B) | 1 or 2 |
|   Hemoglobin (g/dL) | >9 | ≤9 | | High (C) | 3 or 4 |
|   LDH (U/L) | ≤200 | >200 | | | |

**Table 43.4**  Main prognostic scoring systems with karyotype analyses for patients with MDS

| Scoring system | Points | | | | | Risk group | Score |
|---|---|---|---|---|---|---|---|
| | 0 | 0.5 | 1 | 1.5 | 2 | | |
| **Lille[8a]** | | | | | | | |
| Marrow blasts (%) | <5 | | 5–10 | | 11–30 | Low | 0 |
| Karyotype[b] | Good | | poor | | | Intermediate | 1 or 2 |
| Platelets (×10⁹/L) | >75 | | <75 | | | High | 3 or 4 |
| **IPPS[9]** | | | | | | Low | 0 |
| Marrow blasts (%) | <5 | 5–10 | | 11–20 | 21–30 | Intermediate-1 | 0.5–1 |
| Karyotype[c] | Good | Intermediate | Poor | | | Intermediate-2 | 1.5–2 |
| Cytopenias[d] | 0 or 1 | 2 or 3 | | | | High | 2.5–3.5 |

[a] For leukemic risk, only blasts in BM and karyotype are considered.
[b] Good, normal, single abnormalities; poor, complex (≥2) abnormalities.
[c] Good, normal, del(5q) only, del(20q) only, −Y only; intermediate, +8, single miscellaneous, double abnormalities; poor, very complex (>2) abnormalities, chromosome 7 abnormalities.
[d] Cytopenias, hemoglobin <10 g/dL, platelets <100 × 10⁹/L, neutrophils <1.8 × 10⁹/L

patients of 61–70 years, and 3.9 years in patients >70 years of age.[9]

Scoring systems, particularly the IPSS, are useful for defining the outcome and for designing and accurately analyzing therapeutic trials in patients with MDS. The IPSS has proven its value in several series of untreated patients,[10,57–60] and in series of patients treated with intensive chemotherapy[61] or stem cell transplantation.[62] Because of its clinical value and simplicity, the IPSS has gained universal acceptance and is now used to decide the most appropriate therapy in an individual patient and to design clinical trials in patients with MDS.

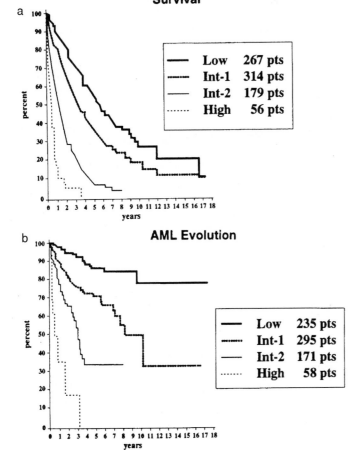

# International MDS Risk Classification

**Figure 43.1**  Surival (a) and freedom from AML evolution (b) of MDS patients related to their classification by the IPSS for MDS: low, intermediate-1, (Int-1), Int-2, and high (Kaplan-Meier curves). (Adapted from Greenberg P, Cox C, LeBeau MM, et al.: International scoring system for evaluating prognosis in myelodysplastic syndromes. Blood 89:2079–2088, 1997; used with permission)

## FOLLOW-UP

The clinical and analytical follow-up of patients with MDS depends primarily on their individual prognosis, based on the IPSS scoring system, and the approach chosen for their treatment. Physicians should also consider that the therapy of patients with MDS is always investigational, as no therapy outside of stem cell transplantation is curative. Whenever possible, patients should be included in well-designed clinical trials aimed at evaluating new therapeutic interventions and conducted according to the standards of good clinical practice. In all cases, follow-up evaluations must include serial physical examination; blood analyses, including whole blood counts, and blood biochemistry; and BM aspirates and biopsies. A careful morphologic review of peripheral blood and BM slides is mandatory to evaluate the cellularity, the percentage of blast cells, and the presence and degree of dysplasia of the different hematopoietic cell lines, which may signal the progression to a more advanced morphologic MDS subtype or the occurrence of AML transformation.

Periodic cytogenetic studies are also required to assess the appearance of new chromosomal abnormalities and the evolution of the malignant clone. In addition to conventional cytogenetics, the use of fluorescence in situ hybridization techniques is strongly recommended, because these highly sensitive tests can detect hidden chromosomal aberrations that influence the outcome.[63] For this purpose, the use of probes for ruling out numerical and/or structural abnormalities of chromosomes 5, 7, 8, 11 and 20 should be considered. As stated previously, the frequency of invasive techniques should depend on the prognosis, type of therapy, and good clinical judgment. Performing a BM aspirate and biopsy annually seems appropriate for low-risk patients with stable blood cell counts who are not enrolled in a clinical trial. In all instances, a sudden deterioration of cytopenias or the appearance or increase of blasts in the blood should prompt a complete BM evaluation. For patients included in clinical trials, the timing of BM examinations will be determined by the trial specifications. Obviously, in patients undergoing intensive chemotherapy, BM aspirates with or without a core biopsy should be performed after each cycle of treatment. The international consensus criteria for evaluating responses must be strictly adhered to in all cases.

## REFERENCES

1. Cheson BD, Bennett JM, Kantarjian H, et al.: Report of an international working group to standardize response criteria for myelodysplastic syndromes. *Blood* 96:3671–3674, 2000.
2. Cheson BD, Bennett JM, Kantarjian H, et al.: Myelodysplastic syndromes standardized response criteria: further definition. *Blood* 98:1985, 2001.
3. Cheson BD, Greenberg PL, Bennett JM, et al.: Clinical application and proposal for modification of the international working group (IWG) response criteria in myelodysplasia. *Blood* 108:419–425, 2006.
3a. Sanz GF, Sanz MA, Vallespi T: Etiopathogeny, prognosis and therapy of myelodysplastic syndromes. *Hematol Cell Ther* 39:277–294, 1997.
4. Bennett JM, Catovsky D, Daniel MT, et al. (FAB Co-operative Group): Proposals for the classification of the myelodysplastic syndromes. *Br J Haematol* 51:189–199, 1982.
5. Sanz GF, Sanz MA, Greenberg PL: Prognostic factors and scoring systems in myelodysplastic syndromes. *Haematologica* 83:358–368, 1998.
6. Greenberg PL, Sanz GF, Sanz MA: Prognostic scoring systems for risk assessment in myelodysplastic syndromes. *Forum (Genova)* 9:17–31, 1999.
7. Sanz GF, Sanz MA, Vallespí T, et al.: Two regression models and a scoring system for predicting survival and planning treatment in myelodysplastic syndromes: a multivariate analysis of prognostic factors in 370 patients. *Blood* 74:395–408, 1989.
8. P, Hebbar M, Lai JL, et al.: Cytogenetic analysis has strong independent prognostic value in de novo myelodysplastic syndromes and can be incorporated in a new scoring system: a report on 408 cases. *Leukemia* 7: 1315–1323, 1993.
9. Greenberg P, Cox C, LeBeau MM, et al.: International scoring system for evaluating prognosis in myelodysplastic syndromes. *Blood* 89:2079–2088, 1997.
10. Sole F, Espinet B, Sanz GF, et al.: Incidence, characterization and prognostic significance of chromosomal abnormalities in 640 patients with primary myelodysplastic syndromes. Grupo Cooperativo Espanol de Citogenetica Hematologica. *Br J Haematol* 108:346–356, 2000.
11. Vallespi T, Imbert M, Mecucci C, et al.: Diagnosis, classification, and cytogenetics of myelodysplastic syndromes. *Haematologica* 83:258–275, 1998.
12. Ghaddar HM, Stass SA, Pierce S, Estey E: Cytogenetic evolution following the transformation of myelodysplastic syndrome to acute myelogenous leukemia: implications on the overlap between the two diseases. *Leukemia* 10:1649–1653, 1994.
13. White AD, Culligan DJ, Hoy TG, et al.: Extended cytogenetic follow-up of patients with myelodysplastic syndrome. *Br J Haematol* 81:499–502, 1992.
14. Brunning RD, Head D, Bennett JM, et al.: Myelodysplastic syndromes: introduction. In: Jaffe ES, Harris NL, Stein H, Vardiman JW (eds.) *Tumours of Haematopoietic and Lymphoid Tissues.* Lyon, France: IARC Press; 2001:63–67.
15. Gattermann N, Aul C, Schneider W: Two types of acquired idiopathic sideroblastic anaemia (AISA). *Br J Haematol* 74:45–52, 1990.
16. Rosati S, Mick R, Xu F, et al.: Refractory cytopenia with multilineage dysplasia: further characterization of an

"unclassifiable" myelodysplastic syndrome. *Leukemia* 10:20–26, 1996.

17. Matsuda A, Jinnai I, Yagasaki F, et al.: Refractory cytopenia with severe dysplasia: clinical significance of morphological features in refractory anemia. *Leukemia* 12:482–485, 1998.

18. Germing U, Gattermann N, Strupp C, et al.: Validation of the WHO proposals for a new classification of primary myelodysplastic syndromes: a retrospective analysis of 1600 patients. *Leuk Res* 24:983–992, 2000.

19. Lee JH, Lee JH, Shin YR, et al.: Application of different prognostic scorings systems and comparison of the FAB and WHO classifications in Korean patients with myelodysplastic syndromes. *Leukemia* 17:305–313, 2003.

20. Cermak J, Michalova K, Brezinova J, et al.: A prognostic impact of separation of refractory cytopenia with multilineage dysplasia and 5q- syndrome from refractory anemia in primary myeleodysplastic syndrome. *Leuk Res* 27:221–229, 2003.

21. Howe RB, Porwit-MacDonald A, Wanat R, et al.: The WHO classification of MDS does make a difference. *Blood* 103:3265–3270, 2004.

22. Matsushima T, Handa H, Yokohama A, et al.: Prevalence and clinical characteristics of myelodysplastic syndrome with bone marrow eosinophilia or basophilia. *Blood* 101:3386–3390, 2003.

23. Aul C, Gattermann N, Heyll A, et al.: Primary myelodysplastic syndromes: analysis of prognostic factors in 235 patients and proposals for an improved scoring system. *Leukemia* 6:52–59, 1992.

24. Verburgh E, Achten R, Maes B, et al.: Additional prognostic value of bone marrow histology in patients subclassified according to the International Prognostic Scoring System for myelodysplastic syndromes. *J Clin Oncol* 21:273–282, 2003.

25. Gatto S, Ball G, Onida F, et al.: Contribution of B-2 microglobulin levels to the prognostic stratification of survival in patients with myelodysplastic syndromes. *Blood* 102:1622–1625, 2003.

26. Raymakers R, De Witte T, Loziasse J, et al.: In vitro growth pattern and differentiation predict for progression of myelodysplastic syndromes to acute nonlymphocytic leukemia. *Br J Haematol* 78:35–41, 1991.

27. Yosoke N, Ogata K: Plasma soluble interleukin-2 receptors in patients with myelodysplastic syndromes. *Leuk Lymphoma* 28:171–176, 1997.

28. Hu Q, Dey AL, Yang Y, et al.: Soluble vascular endothelial growth factor receptor 1, and not receptor 2, is an independent prognostic factor in acute myeloid leukemia and myelodysplastic syndromes. *Cancer* 100:1884–1891, 2004.

29. Tagaki S, Tanaka O, Origasa H, et al.: Prognostic significance of magnetic resonance imaging of femoral marrow in patients with myelodysplastic syndromes. *J Clin Oncol* 17:277–283, 1999.

30. Benesch M, Deeg HJ, Wells D, et al.: Flow cytometry for diagnosis and assessment of prognosis in patients with myelodysplastic syndromes. *Hematology* 9:171–177, 2004.

31. Ogata K, Nakamura K, Yokose N, et al.: Clinical significance of phenotypic features of blasts in patients with myelodysplastic syndrome. *Blood* 100:3887–3896, 2002.

32. Fuchigami K, Mori H, Matsuo T, et al.: Absolute numbers of circulating CD34+ cells is abnormally low in refractory anemias and extremely high in RAEB and RAB-t; novel pathologic features of myelodysplastic syndromes identified by highly sensitive flow cytometry. *Leuk Res* 24:163–174, 2000.

33. Wells DA, Benesch M, Loken MR, et al.: Myeloid and monocytic dyspoiesis as determined by flow cytometric scoring in myelodysplastic syndromes correlates with the IPSS and with outcome after hemopoietic stem cell transplantation. *Blood* 102:394–403, 2003.

34. Raza A, Gezer S, Mundle S, et al.: Apoptosis in bone marrow biopsy samples involving stromal and hematopoietic cells in 50 patients with myelodysplastic syndromes. *Blood* 86:268–276, 1995.

35. Tsoplou P, Kouraklis-Symeonidis A, Thanopoulou A, et al.: Apoptosis in patients with myelodysplastic syndromes: differential involvement of marrow cells in "good" versus "poor" prognosis patients and correlation with apoptosis-related genes. *Leukemia* 13:1554–1563, 1999.

36. Gupta P, Niehans GA, LeRoy SC, et al.: Fas ligand expression in the bone marrow in myelodysplastic syndromes correlates with FAB subtype and anemia, and predicts survival. *Leukemia* 13:44–53, 1999.

37. Ohyashiki JH, Iwama H, Yahata N, et al.: Telomere stability is frequently impaired in high-risk groups of patients with myelodysplastic syndromes. *Clin Cancer Res* 5: 1155–1160, 1999.

38. Shimazaki K, Ohshima K, Suzumiya J, et al.: Evaluation of apoptosis as a prognostic factor in myelodysplastic syndromes. *Br J Haematol* 110:584–590, 2000.

39. Parker JE, Mufti GJ, Rasool F, et al.: The role of apoptosis, proliferation, and the Bcl-2-related proteins in the myelodysplastic syndromes and acute myeloid leukemia secondary to MDS. *Blood* 96:3932–3938, 2000.

40. Zang DY, Goodwin RG, Loken MR, et al.: Expression of tumor necrosis factor-related apoptosis-inducing ligand, Apo2L, and its receptors in myelodysplastic syndromes: effect on in vitro hemopoiesis. *Blood* 98:3058–3065, 2001.

41. Ramos F, Fuertes-Nuñez M, Suarez-Vilela D, et al.: What does apoptosis have to do with clinical features in myelodysplastic syndrome? *Haematologica* 87:381–391, 2002.

42. Allampallam K, Shetty V, Mundle S, et al.: Biological significance of proliferation, apoptosis, cytokines, and monocyte/macrophage cells in bone marrow biopsies of 145 patients with myelodysplastic syndromes. *Int J Hematol* 75:289–297, 2002.

43. Boudard D, Vasselon C, Bertheas MF, et al.: Expression and prognostic significance of Bcl-2 family proteins in myelodysplastic syndromes. *Am J Hematol* 70:115–125, 2002.

44. Albitar M, Manshouri T, Shen Y, et al.: Myelodysplastic syndrome is not merely "preleukemia." *Blood* 100:791–798, 2002.

45. Ohyashiki K, Iwama H, Yahata N, et al.: Telomere dynamics in myelodysplastic syndromes and acute leukemic transformation. *Leuk Lymphoma* 42:291–299, 2001.

46. Padua RA, Guinn BA, Al-Shabah AI, et al.: RAS, FMS and p53 mutations and poor clinical outcome in myelodysplastic syndromes. *Leukemia* 12:887–892, 1998.

47. Kita-Sasai Y, Horiike S, Misawa S, et al.: International prognostic scoring system and TP53 mutations are independent prognostic indicators for patients with myelodysplastic syndromes. *Br J Haematol* 115:309–312, 2001.

48. Cilloni D, Gottardi E, Messa F, et al.: Significant correlation between the degree of WT1 expression and the International Prognostic Scoring System score in patients with myelodysplastic syndromes. *J Clin Oncol* 21:1988–1995, 2003.

49. Quesnel B, Guillerm G, Vereecque R, et al.: Methylation of the p15 (INK4b) gene in myelodysplastic syndromes is frequent and acquired during disease progression. *Blood* 91:2985–2990, 1998.

50. Tien H-F, Tang J-L, Tsay W, et al.: Methylation of the p15[INK4B] gene in myelodysplastic syndrome: it can be detected early at diagnosis or during disease progression and is highly associated with leukaemic transformation. *Br J Haematol* 112:148–154, 2001.

51. Hofmann W-K, de Vos S, Komor M, et al.: Characterization of gene expression of CD34+ cells from normal and myelodysplastic bone marrow. *Blood* 100:3553–3560, 2002.

52. Ueda M, Ota J, Yamashita Y, et al.: DNA microarray analysis of stage progression mechanism in myelodysplastic syndrome. *Br J Haematol* 123:288–296, 2003.

53. Mufti GJ, Stevens JR, Oscier DG, et al.: Myelodysplastic syndromes: a scoring system with prognostic significance. *Br J Haematol* 59:425–433, 1985.

54. Goasguen JE, Garand R, Bizet M, et al.: Prognostic factors of myelodysplastic syndromes—a simplified 3-D scoring system. *Leuk Res* 14:255–260, 1990.

55. Wattel E, Hecquet B, Grahek D, et al.: Long term survivors in myelodysplastic syndromes: a report on 63 cases and comparison with short and intermediate survivors. *Leuk Res* 17:733–739, 1993.

56. Bernstein SH, Brunetto VL, Davey FR, et al.: Acute myeloid leukemia-type chemotherapy for newly diagnosed patients without antecedent cytopenias having myelodysplastic syndrome as defined by French–American–British criteria: a Caner and Leukemia Group B study. *J Clin Oncol* 14:2486–2494, 1996.

57. Lee JJ, Kim HJ, Chung IJ, et al.: Comparisons of prognostic scoring systems for myelodysplastic syndromes: a Korean multicenter study. *Leuk Res* 23:425–432, 1999.

58. Pfeilstocker M, Reisner R, Nosslinger T, et al.: Cross-validation of prognostic scores in myelodysplastic syndromes on 386 patients from a single institution confirms the importance of cytogenetics. *Br J Haematol* 106:455–463, 1999.

59. Belli C, Acevedo S, Bengio R, et al.: Detection of risk groups in myelodysplastic syndromes. A multicenter study. *Haematologica* 87:9–16, 2002.

60. Zhao WL, Xu L, Wu W, et al.: The myelodysplastic syndromes: analysis of prognostic factors and comparison of prognostic systems in 128 Chinese patients from a single institution. *Hematol J* 3:137–144, 2002.

61. De Witte T, Suciu S, Verhoef G, et al.: Intensive chemotherapy followed by allogeneic or autologous stem cell transplantation for patients with myelodysplastic syndromes (MDSs) and acute myeloid leukemia following MDS. *Blood* 98:2326–2331, 2001.

62. Appelbaum FR, Anderson J: Allogeneic bone marrow transplantation for myelodysplastic syndrome: outcomes analysis according to IPSS score. *Leukemia* 12(suppl 1): S25–S29, 1998.

63. Bernasconi P, Cavigliano PM, Boni M, et al.: Is FISH a relevant prognostic tool in myelodysplastic syndromes with a normal chromosome pattern on conventional cytogenetics? A study on 57 patients. *Leukemia* 17:2107–2112, 2003.

# Chapter 44

# TREATMENT OF RELAPSED OR REFRACTORY MYELODYSPLASTIC SYNDROMES AND NEW FRONTIERS IN MYELODYSPLASTIC SYNDROME THERAPY

*Huma Qawi, Naomi Galili, and Azra Raza*

## INTRODUCTION

Myelodysplastic syndrome (MDS) is not a single disease, but rather a group of disorders affecting the bone marrow. Therefore, no single approach is likely to be of universal benefit to all patients. In fact, one way to consider the complexity of MDS is to think of it as being to the bone marrow what pneumonia is to the lungs—the response of an organ to a variety of assaults, such as aging, toxic exposure, infections, and autoimmunity. Among infections of the lungs alone, pneumonia could be the result of a variety of possible pathogens, including bacteria, viruses, tuberculous, or fungal agents. Similarly, MDS is the response of the bone marrow to a variety of unknown insults and cannot be treated as a single disease. Until recently, there was no approved treatment for MDS, but as of May 2004, 5-azacytidine (a methyltransferase inhibitor) has been approved by the Food and Drug Administration (FDA) in the United States for use in all subtypes of MDS. Most patients who will then fall in the category of relapsed or refractory disease will include those who have received some sort of supportive care (SC) in the form of transfusions or growth factors, and most likely, a trial of 5-azacytidine. Subsequent treatment options would depend upon the type of MDS and general condition of this predominantly elderly group of patients. For those with high-risk disease, the danger comes from a rapid transformation toward acute leukemia, while for those with low-risk disease, it is the deepening profundity of cytopenias, which pose a potentially lethal threat of bleeding or infection. This chapter will outline the new types of treatments that have emerged to treat these patients and summarize some of the clinical responses already seen in preliminary clinical trials.

## HIGH-RISK MDS

High-risk MDS, for this discussion, refers to patients belonging to the intermediate-2 (int-2) or high-risk International Prognostic Scoring System (IPSS) categories. As blast cells in these patients are continuously increasing and the probability of transforming into acute myeloid leukemia (AML) is high, therapeutic intervention is essential. Chemotherapeutic agents have traditionally been used, especially busulfan, VP-16, topotecan, and low-dose cytosine arabinoside alone or in combination.[1] More recently, a better understanding of the molecular mechanisms underlying the evolution of malignancy has produced new classes of drugs that have proved to be quite successful. These drugs, in addition to DNA methyltransferase inhibitors, include histone deacetylase (HDAC) inhibitors, farnesyl transferase inhibitors (FTIs), tyrosine kinase inhibitors (TKIs), and arsenic trioxide (ATO). The cellular targets of these drugs are varied and include, either singly or in combination, the chromatin structure of the MDS cell, cytoplasmic regulatory proteins that are essential for cell proliferation, survival, and cell death, and cellular receptors that respond to cytokines of the bone marrow microenvironment.

### DNA METHYLTRANSFERASE INHIBITORS

Gene silencing due to hypermethylation is the most common epigenetic modification in human malignancies.[2] Unlike genetic changes involving mutations or deletions, this modification is potentially reversible, making it attractive as a therapeutic target. Hypermethylation of the chromatin is caused by an increase in DNA methyltransferase I activity; this enzyme covalently links a methyl group to the 5-position of cytosine of CpG residues typically found in gene promoter regions (CpG islands). Normally, unmethylated CpG islands are protected from hypermethylation. This protection is lost in neoplastic cells due to the increase in DNA methyltransferase activity. The methylated promoters bind specific proteins, which then recruit transcriptional corepressors. These complexes lead to transcriptional silencing through chromatin remodeling. DNA hypermethylation of promoter regions of tumor suppressor genes leads, ultimately, to uncontrolled cell proliferation. Several of the DNA methyltransferase inhibitors are S-phase specific, making inhibitors of these agents the logical agents for cancer therapy. In the late 1960s, 5-azacytidine (Aza-C) was developed as an antitumor agent for the treatment of AML.[3] Aza-C, an analog of cytosine, is incorporated into the DNA but, unlike cytosine, cannot be methylated at position 5. In addition, Aza-C binds directly to and inhibits methyltransferase. The drug also exerts cytotoxic and cell-differentiating properties by unknown mechanisms. Most recently, as described below, Aza-C has received attention as a therapeutic agent for MDS, leading to the recent full FDA approval for Aza-C on May 19, 2004, for MDS patients of all subtypes. This is the very first agent to be fully approved by the FDA for the treatment of MDS.

The pivotal phase III study for Aza-C was a randomized controlled Cancer and Leukemia Group B (CALGB) trial carried out in 191 patients with MDS of all subtypes.[4] Half of the patients received Aza-C 75 mg/m$^2$ subcutaneously for 7 days every 4 weeks for a minimum of 16 weeks, and half received only SC. A 60% overall response was found in patients on the treatment arm (7% complete response (CR), 16% partial response (PR), and 37% with hematologic improvement (HI)), with trilineage responses in 23% of patients. Only 5% of those on the observation arm showed hematologic improvement (P < 0.001). Furthermore, when a subset of 49 patients from the observation arm crossed over to the treatment arm, a 47% response was achieved, once again with 10% achieving a CR, 4% a PR, and 33% with clinical improvement. The median duration of response was 15 months, but the most striking observation in this study was the significantly longer median time to transformation to acute leukemia and longer median survival in patients receiving treatment: 21 months, versus 12 months for the observation-only patients. Patients initially treated with Aza-C showed a median survival of 18 months in comparison to 14 months for the early crossover arm, and 11 months for those crossed over after 6 months or not crossed over at all.

Aza-C is a pro-drug for 5-aza-2′-deoxycitadine (decitabine, DAC), a pyrimidine nucleoside analog that has completed a phase III clinical trial. Aza-C is first converted to DAC before incorporation into DNA. It then binds and irreversibly inhibits DNA methyltransferase. DAC is a strong inhibitor of DNA methylation, and like Aza-C has been used for the treatment of high-risk MDS. In a phase II trial by Wijermans et al., 66 MDS patients received DAC 45 mg/m$^2$/day every 8 h for 3 days every 6 weeks, for a maximum of 6 cycles.[5]

The overall response rate was 49%, with a 64% response rate in those with an IPSS high-risk score. There were 34 CRs, with a median response duration of 31 weeks. However, there was an 8% toxic death rate, with a delayed onset of cytopenias. In a subsequent study using the same drug regime, 16 out of 50 patients with clonal cytogenetic abnormalities developed normal karyotypes after treatment with DAC,[6] responses lasting for a median of 7.5 months. This study also noted correlation of cytogenetic responses to survival.

Saba et al. have recently shown responses and better tolerance in a phase III multicenter trial of 170 MDS patients treated with DAC.[7] DAC was administered at 15 mg every 8 h for 3 days every 6 weeks. The response rate by International Working Group (IWG) criteria was 35% (10% CR, 15% PR, and 10% HI) for DAC versus 0% for SC (P < 0.001). Time to response was 100 days, and the median duration was estimated at >9 months. There were no significant differences in mortality rates on treatment, and no treatment-related deaths. As expected, grade III-IV toxicity (mainly hematologic) occurred more in DAC patients than in SC patients. Most patients tolerated the treatment well; discontinuation due to toxicity as primary reason was reported in 9% of DAC patients.

The correlation between methylation status and clinical response, however, is not yet clear. The suppressor genes p15 and p16 inhibit cyclin-dependent kinases and are frequently hypermethylated in hematologic neoplasias, including AML and MDS. Bone marrow mononuclear cells from patients with high-risk MDS were examined for p15/INK-4B and p16 methylation status during treatment with DAC.[8] Hypermethylation of the 5′ p15 region was detected in 15 of 23 (65%) patient samples examined. After treatment, 9 of 12 patient samples showed a decrease in methylation, which was associated with clinical responses in these patients. However, response to the drug was also seen in patients without hypermethylation. Thus, DAC may work by multiple mechanisms, and direct clinical correlation to methylation status cannot be assumed at this time.

More recently, a phase I trial of prolonged exposure to lower doses of DAC was conducted in 50 patients, mostly with AML/MDS.[9] Patients were given four different doses of DAC: 5 mg, 10 mg, 15 mg, and 20 mg/m$^2$/day i.v. over 1 h for 10 days. All doses were well tolerated and responses were noted even in the lowest doses. There was a 65% response rate at the 15 mg/m$^2$ dose with no increase in response after dose escalation or prolongation to 15 and 20 days. In this study, there was no correlation noted between p15 methylation at baseline or after therapy and response to DAC. Hence, DAC appears to be an effective therapy for MDS with manageable toxicity, and its role in light of the recent FDA approval for Aza-C remains to be determined.

### HISTONE DEACETYLASE INHIBITORS

Chromatin remodeling is part of the epigenetic changes seen during neoplastic transformation. While promoter hypermethylation is associated with silencing of tumor suppressor genes, it is not the only modification that controls chromatin condensation and promoter activity. Posttranslational modifications, such as acetylation, methylation, and phosphorylation of histone proteins comprising the chromatin nucleosomes, are responsible for formation of complexes that control gene expression. Typically, acetylation of the lysine residues in the histone "tail" by acetyltransferases (HAT) leads to "open" transcriptionally active chromatin, whereas deacetylation, dependent on histone deacetylases (HDAC), leads to "closed" inactive chromatin. HDAC activity is associated with promoter methylation, and it is the combination of both that contributes to promoter inactivation.[10] As therapeutic reactivation of tumor suppressor genes has gained the attention of drug companies, multiple HDAC inhibitors have been investigated. Since HDAC inhibitors are often cell-cycle and tissue specific, these agents have been found to exert pleiotropic effects.

Butyrate is an acetylating agent that has been used to induce expression of fetal hemoglobin in sickle cell anemia and thalassemia, but proved unsuccessful for the treatment of AML in phase II trials.[11] Sodium phenylbutyrate (PB), a derivative thought to be deliverable in oral form, has been shown to induce histone acetylation, p21 expression, G1 cell-cycle arrest, and apoptosis in vitro.[12] In a trial conducted by Gore et al.,[13] PB was given for 7/28 or 21/28 days to MDS and AML patients, with improvement in thrombocytopenia and neutropenia seen in a small number of patients. A dose-limiting toxicity of reversible encephalopathy was due to accumulation of phenylacetate. Currently, oral forms of PB are being investigated. Valproic acid, an oral antiepileptic agent, SAHA (suberoylanilide hydroxamic acid), and FK 228 (with FDA approval for cutaneous T-cell lymphoma) are newer HDAC inhibitors currently undergoing clinical trials.

As chromatin remodeling involves a balance between CpG methylation and histone modification, a phase I trial of sequential administration of Aza-C and PB was initiated in MDS. The dose de-escalation trial of varying doses of Aza-C followed by a 7-day continuous infusion of PB was well tolerated, with significant clinical responses.[14] Additional studies combining DAC with valproic acid are underway, with monitoring of methylation, acetylation, and gene re-expression.

### FARNESYL TRANSFERASE INHIBITORS (FTIS)

The family of Ras proteins are components of multiple cellular pathways essential for cell proliferation, growth, and survival. Addition of the carbon farnesyl group to these cytoplasmic proteins allows them to be transported to the cell membrane, where they are integral to signal transduction pathways. The enzyme farnesyl transferase mediates the farnesylation process. Ras mutations are found in <20% of MDS patients, but are more common in chronic myelomonocytic leukemia (CMMoL). Ras, however, may be activated by other proteins that similarly require farnesylation, and therefore its expression

may be controlled by multiple mechanisms. Small molecules that can selectively and competitively inhibit farnesyl transferase (FTIs) have been developed for clinical use, and two, tipifarnib (R115777) and lonafarnib (SCH66336), have been studied in high-risk MDS.

A phase I trial of R115777 in 21 MDS patients of all subtypes, reported by Kurzrock et al.,[15] established the maximum tolerated dose of 600 mg b.i.d. Of note, only two of the six responders had Ras mutations, and no correlation between Ras mutation status and response was detected in this initial study. In a phase II trial by the same group,[16] 28 MDS patients were given R115777 600 mg twice a day, 4 weeks on, 2 weeks off, to increase exposure to the drug. There were two complete responses, both of which did not possess a Ras mutation. Eleven of 27 patients discontinued treatment due to toxicity, with more than 60% of patients experiencing myelosuppression, fatigue, and nausea. The phase II study therefore concluded that lower doses should be used in future trials. A separate phase II study done in patients with poorrisk AML or MDS using 600 mg b.i.d. every 4–6 weeks yielded responses in 12 of 30 patients (2 CRs and 8 PRs), with stabilization of disease in 12 patients.[17]

List et al. conducted a phase I study of continuous dosing of lonafarnib (SCH66336) in advanced CML, MDS, CMMoL, or AML.[18] Twenty-nine percent of patients showed clinical improvement, and doselimiting toxicity was diarrhea and hypokalemia at 300 mg b.i.d. In a phase II trial by Feldman et al.,[19] 67 MDS patients with RAEB/RAEB-T or CMMoL were given lonafarnib 200 mg b.i.d. and a 29% response was seen. There were two complete responses, and 10 patients showed hematologic improvement. In this study, 26% of patients discontinued therapy due to grade III and IV toxicities. Current phase III trials are being conducted with lower doses of single-agent FTIs for longer periods of time, which may be useful for previously untreated patients and those with minimal residual disease. There is limited data to suggest a synergistic effect with chemotherapy,[20] but identifying specific molecular targets within the cell cycle may lead to useful combinations of FTIs and chemotherapeutic agents, each affecting a different stage of the cycle.

### TYROSINE KINASE RECEPTOR INHIBITORS (RTKI)

These agents inhibit signaling pathways activated by ligand binding to vascular endothelial growth factor (VEGF) receptors (VEGFRs) and other type III receptors, including c-kit, Flt-3, platelet-derived growth factor receptor β (PDGFRβ), and basic fibroblast growth factor (bFGF). By selectively mimicking ATP, these molecules impair autophosphorylation of the tyrosine kinase domain of the receptor (RTK). SU5416 is a small, lipophilic, highly protein-bound, synthetic RTK inhibitor of VEGFR-2. SU5416 binds to the ATP domain on the kinase, affecting VEGF-dependent cell proliferation. In a human colon cancer xenograft model, this molecule inhibits tumor metastases, microvessel formation, and proliferation. Like other

RTKIs, SU5416 also targets c-kit (expressed in AML blasts in 60–80% patients) and Flt-3 (mutated in about 30% of AML patients), prompting clinical studies for the treatment of AML and MDS.

A multicenter phase II study was conducted in patients with refractory AML ($n = 33$) or MDS ($n = 22$), all of whom received 145 mg/m$^2$ of SU5416 twice weekly i.v. for a median of 9 weeks.[21] Eleven patients could not complete 4 weeks of therapy (mainly due to disease progression). Three patients had a partial response and one had a hematologic response. Phase I and II studies are ongoing with SU11248 and two other RTKIs, PTK/ZK and AG13736, alone or in combination with chemotherapy.[22–24]

### Imatinib mesylate (Gleevec)

The first FDA-approved and best known TKI, imatinib mesylate, has been shown to be potent for the inhibition of the BCR/ABL tyrosine kinase in chronic myeloid leukemia (CML). Like other RTKIs, imatinib also inhibits two other tyrosine kinases, PDGFR and c-kit, at similar concentrations. A small percentage of CMMOL patients express PDGFR fusion genes involving four partner genes. This is now a distinct phenotype classified by the World Health Organization (WHO) as CMMoL-Eos, with reciprocal translocations on chromosome 5q33. Imatinib interacts with the ATP-binding pocket of PDGFRβ kinase associated with the translocation [e.g., t(5;12)(q33;p13)], much like its interaction with BCR/ABL in CML.

Four patients with CMMoL harboring a t(5;12), three of whom had the associated fusion gene *ETV6/PDGFRβ*, were treated with imatinib.[25] Hematologic responses were achieved within 4 weeks of starting treatment, and normal counts were maintained for up to 1 year. Even more impressive was the disappearance of the translocation t(5;12) by 12 weeks in three patients and by 36 weeks in the fourth patient.

Raza et al. treated 16 CMMoL patients lacking translocations of the *PDGFRβ* gene with imatinib. No responses were seen,[26] further confirming the specificity of the drug for this target. Another phase II study of 18 MDS, CMMoL, and AML patients, all lacking the fusion gene, showed no responses.[27] Although c-kit is expressed in over 80% of AML and MDS patients and imatinib is thought to inhibit c-kit, in this study no responses were achieved. These results were also seen in some solid tumors, where imatinib has failed to show any significant responses as monotherapy, despite the expression of c-kit.

### PROTEOSOME INHIBITORS (PS-341, BORTEZOMIB)

Proteosomes are enzymes that mediate many critical cellular regulatory signals by degradation of the regulatory proteins or their inhibitors and, therefore, are potential therapeutic targets for cancer. Activity of several proteins shown to be overexpressed in MDS, such as nuclear factor κB (NF-κB), AP1, and E2F1, is partly dependent upon the 26S proteosome that can be selectively inhibited by bortezomib (formerly PS-341). This agent has been approved in 2003 for use in patients with relapsed multiple myeloma, and is currently being investigated in MDS trials.

Thirty-two patients with MDS were treated with bortezomib at Rush University Medical Center.[28] All patients were treated at 1.5 mg/m$^2$ once weekly for 4 weeks followed by a 2-week recovery. Twenty patients received at least two cycles; five patients (25%) had stable disease and seven (35%) showed a partial response. Further studies in MDS with bortezomib are awaited.

### DNA TOPOISOMERASE I INHIBITOR: TOPOTECAN (HYCAMTIN)

Topotecan binds to DNA topoisomerase I and stabilizes the complex formed between topoisomerase I and DNA, which leads to DNA strand breakage and cell death. This agent has been successfully used as a single-agent treatment and in combination for patients with AML and MDS. The noncumulative and reversible nature of its hematologic cytotoxicity is attractive for induction therapy.

The activity of single-agent topotecan was evaluated by Beran et al. in 60 patients with MDS or CMMoL.[29] The dose used was 2 mg/m$^2$ by continuous infusion for 5 days every 4–6 weeks for 2 courses, and then at 1-2 mg/m$^2$ for 5 days every 4–8 weeks for a maximum of 12 courses. Thirty-one percent of patients achieved a CR, including 8/11 with cytogenetic remissions. Those with no previous treatments had higher CRs (43%), but overall there were significant toxicities. These included severe mucositis and diarrhea, febrile neutropenia in 85%, and 47% patients had documented infections, with a mortality rate of 20% in the first 4 weeks. The median survival was 10.5 months, with a median remission duration of 7.5 months.

The same group used a combined regimen of topotecan at a lower dose (1.25 mg/m2) with cytarabine (1.0 mg/m$^2$) in patients with MDS and CMMoL.[30] Fifty-six percent of patients had complete responses overall, with up to 72% CR in those with poor-prognosis karyotypes and secondary MDS. This regimen was much better tolerated, with fewer hematologic and nonhematologic toxicities. Lower response rates (33% CR and 38% PR) with topotecan and cytarabine have been reported in more recent trials.[31] Forty-five MDS patients were treated at Rush University in Chicago, in a phase II trial using a combination of topotecan and thalidomide.[32] Topotecan 2.0 mg/m$^2$ was given for 5 days every 21 days for three to five cycles, with thalidomide starting at 100 mg/day (maximum dose 300 mg) for a year. This lower dose of topotecan was well tolerated; only four patients discontinued therapy due to toxicity, and three patients died of infection/progressive disease. Of 38 evaluable patients, 20% had HI and 29% had stable disease. Responses were seen in all subtypes, and one third of patients showed a >50% reduction in bone marrow blasts.

### ARSENIC TRIOXIDE

Arsenic trioxide (ATO), the active ingredient in Fowler's solution, has been used to lower white blood cell counts since 1878. It remained in use until the advent of radiation therapy and the use of modern chemotherapeutic drugs. The drug re-emerged as an antileukemia agent in the 1990s, with the report from Chinese investigators that remissions of up to 90% were seen in patients with acute promyelocytic leukemia (APL).[33] The FDA approved ATO for use in relapsed/refractory APL in September 2001.

ATO has a wide spectrum of biologic activity, which makes it an ideal drug to use in the treatment of MDS. ATO binds to proteins with available sulfhydryl groups, causing disruption of the membrane potential of the mitochondria, releasing cytochrome c with subsequent activation of caspase effectors, and initiation of apoptosis. ATO has antiangiogenic properties, resulting in suppression of VEGF synthesis from myeloid cells, as well as significant antiproliferative activity, in part related to modulating cytokine release and interfering with cell-cycle progression. In addition, ATO can promote histone acetylation through activation of the mitogen-activated protein kinase (MAPK) signaling pathway, and can promote differentiation by modulating gene expression. It is also known to inhibit DNA methyltransferase, an important epigenetic target, as discussed above.

List et al. conducted a phase II study in which 53 MDS patients (median age 69) with both low/int-1 and int-2/high-risk groups received ATO 0.25 mg/kg, Monday to Friday for two consecutive weeks every 28 days. Response was evaluated every 8 weeks.[34] Hematologic responses were observed in 7 of 28 evaluable patients (25%). Responses were maintained for 2 months and often noted after 8–22 weeks after starting treatment. Immunosuppression was the primary adverse effect, although a small number of patients suffered from cardiac and pulmonary toxicities.

Similar results were reported by another group, who treated MDS patients on a slightly different regimen.[35] Here, ATO was given as a 1-h i.v. infusion, with a loading dose of 0.30 mg/kg/day for 5 days, and maintenance with 0.25 mg/kg/day twice weekly for 15 weeks or more. Patients were evaluated at 8 weeks. Eighty-one patients were enrolled with a median age of 67 years, of all IPSS groups. Hematologic responses, mostly erythroid, were achieved in 13 of 50 evaluable patients. There was a 5/19 (26%) response in low-risk and 8/31 (26%) response in high-risk patients. Once again, responses were seen after 6–22 weeks. Forty-four patients had stable disease for up to 6 months while on study.

### Combinations of ATO with other agents

Combining ATO with the antiangiogenic agent thalidomide, Raza et al. has recently shown that several MDS patients harboring an inv(3)(q21q26.2) abnormality achieved trilineage responses.[36] This suggested that perhaps a gene(s) on chromosome 3 may be interacting with ATO to inhibit clonal proliferation. The human *EVI-1* gene, located at chromosome 3q25-q28, has been shown to inhibit transcription of *GATA-1*

target genes and impair responsiveness of erythroid precursors to erythropoietin.[36] This suggested that perhaps EVI-1 deregulation has a role in the pathogenesis of MDS and/or response to this therapeutic regime. EVI-1 was found to be abnormally expressed in five patients, with three out of five patients responding especially well to therapy.[37] Accordingly, EVI-1 expression may be a useful preselection criterion for therapy with ATO +/− thalidomide.)

## LOW-RISK MDS

Patients with low-risk MDS should be considered for therapy only if they are receiving frequent transfusions or their disease is showing progression with increasing severity of cytopenias, appearance of new cytogenetic abnormalities, rise in blasts, or multiple incidents of bleeding and infection. At this point, it is appropriate to consider placing such a patient on an experimental protocol. The hallmark of MDS is proliferation in the presence of excessive intramedullary programmed cell death. The presence of an excess of proinflammatory cytokines, especially tumor necrosis factor α (TNFα), an increase in microvessel density (MVD) with clear evidence of neoangiogenesis, and a poorly defined immunologic component have all been demonstrated in a subset of MDS patients. These biologic insights suggested experimental therapeutic approaches, including antiangiogenic therapies, anticytokines (especially anti-TNF), cytoprotection, and immune modulation.

### ANGIOGENESIS

There is considerable increase in MVD in the bone marrow of patients with MDS.[38] The most extensively studied cytokine thought to be responsible for the development of neovascularization is VEGF.[39] Others, such as TNFα and bFGF are also involved, but VEGF appears to be the major player. VEGF and its type III receptor are overexpressed by myeloblasts and monocytes derived from the malignant clone. The increase in MVD in the bone marrow is associated with a higher percentage of blasts, which in turn correlates with increased levels of VEGF, TNFα, and bFGF. This has been shown in MVD studies where ALIPs (abnormal localized immature precursors) within the bone marrows of MDS patients express higher levels of VEGF and VEGFR, specifically VEGFR-1. VEGF has multiple activities: stimulating release of proteases from endothelial cells resulting in degradation of the extracellular matrix; recruiting mediators of apoptosis, such as TNFα and soluble Fas (CD95) ligand; and activating cell adhesion molecules. VEGF also stimulates engraftment of myeloid leukemic and hematopoietic stem cells and regulates maturation of receptor-positive cells, thus stimulating endothelial cell maturation while inhibiting hematopoietic precursor, osteoblast, and dendritic cell maturation. VEGF deregulation can thus have severe repercussions on effective hematopoiesis.

## *ANTIANGIOGENESIS AGENTS*

Many of the agents described in the above sections, such as the FTIs, TKIs, and ATO, exhibit multiple modes of action, including regulation of VEGF activity.

Thalidomide is an antiangiogenesis agent that inhibits cellular response to VEGF and proliferation of cells that express the VEGF receptor, and also has significant anti-TNF properties. Thalidomide and its analogs are described below. Other agents that have shown activity in a subset of low-risk patients include matrix metalloprotease inhibitors, which block the end results of VEGF's paracrine effects, i.e., extracellular matrix degradation, and the monoclonal antibody to VEGF, bevacizumab.

### Thalidomide

Thalidomide was used in the sixties as a sedative and antiemetic agent. Severe teratogenic effects, however, led to its removal from the market. It has been reintroduced over the last decade for the treatment of ENL (erythema nodosum leprosum) and received FDA approval for this indication in 1998. It is currently used in combination with dexamethasone, in place of conventional chemotherapy, for the initial management of multiple myeloma. The drug has been found to have multiple mechanisms of action that would make it an ideal therapeutic agent in various cancers, especially melanoma, multiple myeloma, and MDS. These include accelerating degradation of TNFα RNA message; potent inhibition of angiogenesis via its action on VEGF and bFGF, and inhibition of the transcriptional regulator NF-κB.[40–42] In addition, thalidomide alters cellular adhesion and stimulates the Th1 immune response, possibly enhancing an antitumor response.[43] Thus, thalidomide shows anti-TNFα, antiangiogenic, and immune-modulatory properties.

A phase II trial was conducted at Rush University Medical Center in which 83 MDS patients of all subtypes were given thalidomide 100 mg once a day escalating to a target dose of 400 mg a day.[44] The overall response rate was 19%. Fifty-one patients were evaluable at 12 weeks, of whom 16 (almost 30%) had an erythroid response using the IWG criteria, 2/3 of which were major responses, most of those becoming transfusion independent or achieving a >50% reduction in transfusion requirements. Improvement in thrombocytopenia or neutropenia was less significant. The most common reason patients were unable to complete the trial was due to toxicities, namely neuropathy, constipation, fatigue, and fluid retention at a dose beyond 200 mg a day. For 10 of the 16 responders, the median time to response was 16–20 weeks, and the majority of responders had lower risk disease: refractory anemia (RA) or refractory anemia with ringed sideroblasts (RARS), or a low or int-1 IPSS.

The North Central Cancer Treatment Group study, N998B, was a phase II multicenter trial with more aggressive dose escalation to 1000 mg/day of thalidomide, and was closed early due to excessive grade III toxicities in more than 85% of patients at a median interval of less than 2.5 months.[45] In those patients who tolerated treatment, median time to response was once again not reached until 16 weeks. A national, randomized phase III, placebo-controlled trial to assess overall clinical benefit of low-dose thalidomide in MDS patients with low-risk disease is nearing completion.

### Thalidomide analogs

***Lenalidomide (Revlimid)*** A more potent analog of thalidomide, CC-5013 or lenalidomide, is currently under investigation. CC-5013 is an oral immunomodulatory derivative (ImiD) of thalidomide that lacks the neurotoxicity of its parent compound, but shows 100-fold higher anti-TNF activity and 50–2000-fold higher potency for stimulating T-cell proliferation. In addition, CC5013 has antiangiogenic and antiapoptotic properties. It inhibits VEGF signaling in endothelial cells and myeloblasts, increasing adhesion of hematopoietic progenitors to bone marrow stroma, which results in sustained growth arrest and preferential extinction of myelodysplastic clones.[46] It also downregulates adhesion molecules and apoptosis inhibitory proteins, thereby increasing receptor-induced apoptosis.

The safety and efficacy of lenalidomide was studied in 45 patients with MDS with RBC transfusion-dependent disease or symptomatic anemia.[47] Patients received treatment with one of three CC5013 doses: 10 or 25 mg daily or 10 mg/day for 21 days every 4 weeks. Patients were assessed at 8 and 16 weeks according to IWG criteria. Thirty-three patients were evaluable for response after completing 8 weeks or more of therapy. Most patients (88%) were in the low/int-1 risk group. Twenty-one (64%) patients achieved an erythroid response, 19 of which were major responses; major cytogenetic responses (>50%) were achieved in 11 of 17 informative patients, with restoration of normal cytogenetics in 10. Erythroid responses were higher in those with RA or low/int-1 IPSS score or del(5q31-33). In this subset of patients with del(5q), there was also resolution of megakaryocytic dysplasia, but not a significant reduction in bone marrow blast percentage. MVD as well as bone marrow and plasma VEGF levels were decreased in responders. Multicenter phase II trials have completed in patients with 5q− syndrome and non 5q− low/int-1 MDS.

### Soluble TNFα receptor (etanercept)

Etanercept is a dimer formed of the two monomers of the extracellular p75 TNF receptor fused to the Fc portion of human type 1 immunoglobulin. It neutralizes the TNFα levels by competitive binding.[48]

Raza et al. administered etanercept at a dose of 25 mg twice weekly for 12 weeks to 20 patients.[49] Eighteen patients were evaluated, and while the drug was well tolerated there were no complete responders. Improvements in absolute neutrophil count (ANC) and platelets were seen in some patients, especially those with normal cytogenetics and a hypercellular bone marrow, but no improvement in the erythroid series could be documented with this approach. However, etanercept combined with thalidomide was effective in improving the cytopenia of some patients with MDS. Once again, the responses were restricted to 30–40% of MDS patients.

## Infliximab

Infliximab is a chimeric human–murine monoclonal antibody capable of neutralizing both free and membrane-bound TNFα. It has been used as a TNF suppressor in MDS patients.[50] Infliximab was given to 37 low-risk MDS patients in two cohorts: 5 and 10 mg/kg intravenously every 4 weeks for four cycles. Twenty-eight patients completed the four cycles. Infliximab successfully produced a variety of responses in about 20% of low- to intermediate-risk MDS patients, including multilineage responses.

## Matrix metalloprotease inhibitors (MMPis)

These compounds result in antiangiogenesis by inhibiting the matrix metalloproteases (zinc-dependent endopeptidases) of the extracellular matrix, thereby altering integrin-mediated cell adhesion. MMPis also promote local release of the proteoglycan-(membrane)-bound forms of VEGF, TNFα, and soluble Fas ligand. AG3340 is a potent, oral selective MMPi.

AG3340 (Prinomastat) was administered to 34 MDS patients of all subtypes in a phase II multicenter randomized trial.[51] Patients were given either 5 mg or 15 mg daily and those who responded after 16 weeks were continued on therapy. Of 28 evaluable patients, 4 had major erythroid responses, with a median time to response of 12 weeks and median duration of response of 29+ weeks, being sustained for over a year after the end of treatment. The higher dose caused increased arthralgias and myalgias and the benefit appeared to be more significant in those patients with a lower risk disease.

## Bevacizumab

Bevacizumab is a recombinant, anti-VEGF, humanized monoclonal antibody recently approved for the treatment of metastatic colon cancer. Neutralization of VEGF has also been shown to inhibit TNFα production by the bone marrow. There is only limited experience in MDS, with a phase II study[52] in which bevacizumab was given at a dose of 10 mg/kg every 2 weeks for 4 months, with major hematologic responses occurring in 2 of 10 evaluable patients, after 4 months of treatment.

## CYTOPROTECTIVE AGENTS
### Aminothiols

Organic thiols neutralize free radicals generated in tissues exposed to cytotoxic drugs. Amifostine is a phosphorylated aminothiol initially developed as a radioprotective agent at the Walter Reed Army Institute in the 1970s. Following administration, amifostine is phosphorylated by tissue alkaline phosphatase, an enzyme with greater activity in normal tissue than in tumor tissue. Active free thiol thus accumulates in the normal tissue, neutralizing the destructive free radicals. Thus, amifostine has been used as a radio- and cytoprotective agent for the treatment of solid tumors. In addition, amifostine protects primitive hematopoietic progenitors from chemotherapy-induced toxicity and stimulates hematopoiesis in preclinical models and in vitro studies.[53]

List et al. conducted a phase I/II study of 18 MDS patients with dose escalation of amifostine up to 400 mg/m² three times a week or 740 mg/m² weekly for 3 weeks.[54] Single or multilineage responses were seen in 83% of patients receiving three times weekly doses, which were optimized at 200 mg/m²: 14 patients had a neutrophil response, 6 had improvement in thrombocytopenia, and 5 patients had a 50% reduction in red cell transfusion requirements. Raza et al. reported the use of amifostine in combination with pentoxifylline (P), ciprofloxacin (C), and dexamethasone (D) in 35 MDS patients.[55] Pentoxifylline is a xanthine derivative that interferes with the activity of proapoptotic cytokines, such as TNFα, IL-1β, and tumor growth factor β (TGFβ). Ciprofloxacin was added as a pharmacologic inhibitor of the hepatic metabolism of pentoxifylline and dexamethasone to downregulate mRNA translation of TNFα. Twenty-nine patients completed at least 12 weeks of treatment; most patients had low- to intermediate-risk MDS. Pentoxifylline was given at 800 mg three times a day, ciprofloxacin 500 mg twice a day, and dexamethasone 4 mg a day for 4 weeks was added to partial and nonresponders at 12 weeks. Amifostine was given at 200, 300, and 400 mg/m² (i.v. or s.q.) doses three times a week along with daily PCD therapy. An improvement in cytopenias was observed in 76% of patients, and 50% of patients had a >50% decrease in transfusion requirements. However, there was no correlation seen between response rate and the dose of amifostine given.

### VITAMIN D

Vitamin D is a potent inhibitor of proliferation and induces cellular differentiation and maturation in vitro. Low levels of vitamin D have been found in some cases of AML and MDS. Bone marrow biopsies of several MDS patients with low normal levels of vitamin D showed depressed bone turnover without osteoporosis or osteomalacia. These findings are suggestive of osteoclast dysfunction, with a decrease in osteoblast recruitment and function.

There have been reported cases of improvement in blood counts after treatment with vitamin D, with some benefit reported in AML patients, accompanied, however, with toxic levels of vitamin D and hypercalemia.[56] Vitamin D may also induce cell differentiation through oncogene regulation, as leukemia cell lines showed a decrease in c-myc RNA levels after exposure to the drug calcitriol (a vitamin D derivative) in vitro. Blockage of cell differentiation is not characteristic of low-risk MDS, and vitamin D response in these patients is thought to be mediated by antiapoptotic effects, as observed in neoplastic cell lines.[57]

Nineteen patients with low- to intermediate-risk MDS were treated with vitamin D analogs: 5 patients received 266 µg of calcifediol three times a week, and the other 14 received calcitriol (1,25(OH)2D3), the most active analog of this hormone, with escalating doses from 0.25 to 0.75 µg/day.[58] With a mean follow-up of 26 months, there was 1 response in the calcifediol group and 10 responses (2 major responses) on calcitriol. Hypercalcemia was not observed, but no correlation was found between baseline levels of vitamin D levels and the presence of response.

### IMMUNOMODULATION
### Antithymocyte globulin/cyclosporine

Antithymocyte globulin (ATG) is derived from the serum of either rabbits or horses immunized with human thoracic duct lymphocytes. ATG suppresses cytotoxic and potentially inhibitory T lymphocytes, and also has an indirect effect on hematopoiesis through augmentation of hematopoietic growth factor release from T cells and stromal cells. ATG stimulates cellular differentiation, and has been successfully used to treat patients with aplastic anemia (AA).

Hypoplastic MDS, although a distinct entity from AA, has some pathophysiologic similarities, specifically T-cell-mediated immune suppression of hematopoiesis. There is evidence of an increase in cytotoxic T-cell activity, a higher percentage of CD8+ cells, as well as skewing of T-cell receptor Vβ complimentarity-determining region 3 (CDR3). This immune dysfunction in MDS is also found in low-risk MDS patients, with fewer than 10% blasts. It is reasonable, therefore, to treat hypocellular MDS patients with the same immunomodulation therapy that has been used for patients with AA, i.e., ATG and cyclosporine. These patients showed favorable responses, especially patients with HLA-DR2, HLA-DR15, or those with a paroxysmal nocturnal hemoglobinuria (PNH) phenotype (i.e., CD55 and CD59 negative). Other factors that are predictive for response to ATG are thought to be bone marrow cellularity <30%, shorter duration of red cell transfusions, and age <60 years. This therapy has recently been extended to RA and RAEB-1 patients in several small trials.

In a trial by Molldrem et al., unselected MDS patients with RA and refractory anemia with excess blasts (RAEB) were given rabbit ATG 40 mg/kg/day for 4 days, with an overall response rate of 44%.[59] Higher responses of 64% were seen in patients with RA, 81% of whom maintained transfusion independence for a median of 36 months. This included 48% of those with severe thrombocytopenia and 55% of those with severe neutropenia. A follow-up with a total of 61 patients was reported in 2002, with an overall response of 34%.[60]

Subsequently, in a study of a select group of 30 patients with low-risk MDS and <10% blasts, horse ATG 1.5 vials/10kg/day was given for 5 days.[61] Ten of 20 evaluable patients responded and became transfusion independent, with a median duration of response of 15.5 months, and 62% of the RA patients responded. Only one patient had normal counts at the 6-month follow-up, and there was no relationship between age, gender, cytogenetic clone, bone marrow cellularity, and response.

In a trial of 32 unselected MDS patients (RA, RAEB/RAEB-T, or CMMoL) treated with ATG, cyclosporine, and prednisone, only one CR and four PRs were achieved (OR 16%).[62] Another small phase II trial of eight MDS patients treated with ATG and prednisone showed no responses; although three patients had the HLA-DR15 allele, this did not improve responses, and toxicities were significant.[63] The role of ATG therefore remains limited to patients with hypocellular MDS, especially those with specific phenotypic features, as described above.

## FUTURE OF EXPERIMENTAL THERAPY IN MDS

A number of single agents belonging to different classes of drugs have now been found to be of benefit for subsets of MDS patients. Targeted therapies, such as imatinib for patients with fusion proteins resulting from abnormalities of 4(q12) or t(5;12), and lenalidomide in patients with 5q–, are likely to remain restricted to small subsets of MDS patients. For the vast majority of both low- and high-risk patients, the challenge is to match the right drug with the individual needs of the patient. While ever-evolving biologic insights are providing a better and more healthy rationale for specific therapies, the ability to administer a single drug as a result of such insights is still a faraway dream. In AML, both ara-C and anthracyclines as single agents produced complete responses in approximately 30% of patients. It was only when the two drugs were combined in the so-called 7 + 3 regimen that we began to see the synergy and additive effects, with remission rates in the 60–70% range. Applying the same lessons to MDS, it is clear that while we are finally starting to witness responses to single-agent therapy in subsets of patients, the future lies in developing combination trials. As a general rule, it would be worthwhile to consider combining agents that target the clone of MDS cells with those that target the bone marrow microenvironment, so that both the seed and the soil are simultaneously affected. Examples of future combination trials would be the use of agents like DNA methyltransferase inhibitors, FTIs, TKIs, and arsenic with antiangiogenic, anti-TNF, and immunemodulatory drugs. In the final analysis, it is an exciting time to be involved in translational research in MDS as the last two decades have taken us from having nothing to offer our patients save supportive care, to having almost an embarrassment of riches. One drug has already been approved for use in this disease, and several others are approaching approval.

## REFERENCES

1. Kantarjian H, Beran M, Cortes J, et al.: Long-term follow-up results of the combination of topotecan and cytarabine and other intensive chemotherapy regimens in myelodysplastic syndrome. *Cancer* 106(5):1099–1109, 2006.

2. Herman JG, Baylin SB: Gene silencing in cancer in association with promoter hypermethylation. *N Engl J Med* 349(21):2042–2054, 2003.

3. Saiki JH, McCredie KB, Vietti TJ, et al.: 5-azacytidine in acute leukemia. *Cancer* 42(5):2111–2114, 1978.

4. Silverman LR, Demakos EP, Peterson BL, et al.: Randomized controlled trial of azacitidine in patients with the myelodysplastic syndrome: a CALGB study. *J Clin Oncol* 20:2429–2440, 2002.

5. Wijermans P, Lubbert M, Verhoef G, et al.: Low-dose 5-aza-2'-deoxycitidine, a DNA hypomethylating agent, for the treatment of high-risk myelodysplastic syndrome: a multicenter phase II study in elderly patients. *J Clin Oncol* 18:956–962, 2000.

6. Lubbert M, Wijermans P, Kunzmann R, et al.: Cytogenetic responses in high-risk myelodysplastic syndrome following low-dose treatment with the DNA methylation inhibitor 5-aza-2'-deoxycytidine. *Br J Haematol* 114: 349–357, 2001.

7. Kantarjian H, Issa JP, Rosenfeld CS, et al.: Decitabine improves patient outcomes in myelodysplastic syndromes: results of a phase III randomized study. *Cancer* 106(8):1794–1803, 2006.

8. Daskalakis M, Nguyen TT, Nguyen C, et al.: Demethylation of a hypermethylated P15/INK4B gene in patients with myelodysplastic syndrome by 5-aza-2'-deoxycytidine (decitabine) treatment. *Blood* 100:2957–2964, 2002.

9. Issa JP, Garcia-Manero G, Giles FJ, et al.: A phase I study of low-dose prolonged exposure schedules of the hypomethylating agent 5-aza-2'-deoxycytidine (decitabine) in hematopoietic malignancies. *Blood* 103:1635–1640, 2004.

10. Cameron EE, Bachman KE, Myohanen S, Herman JG, Baylin SB: Synergy of demethylation and histone deacetylase inhibition in the re-expression of genes silenced in cancer. *Nat Genet* 21(1):103–107, 1999.

11. Miller AA, Kurschel E, Osieka R, Schmidt CG: Clinical pharmacology of sodium butyrate in patients with acute leukemia. *Eur J Cancer Clin Oncol* 23:1283–1287, 1987.

12. DiGiuseppe JA, Weng L-J, Yu KH, et al.: Phenylbutyrate-induced G1 arrest and apoptosis in myeloid leukemia cells: structure–function analysis. *Leukemia* 13;1243–1253, 1999.

13. Gore SD, Weng LJ, Figg WD, et al.: Impact of the prolonged infusions of the putative differentiating agent sodium phenylbutyrate on myelodysplastic syndromes and acute myeloid leukemia. *Clin Cancer Res* 8:963–970, 2002.

14. Miller CB, Herman JG, Baylin SB, et al.: A phase I dose-deescalation trial of combined DNA methyltransferase/histone deacetylase inhibition in myeloid malignancies. *Blood* 99(suppl 1), 2001.

15. Kurzrock R, Kantarjian HM, Cortes JE, et al.: Farnesyltransferase inhibitor R115777 in myelodysplastic syndrome: clinical and biologic activities in the phase I setting. *Blood* 102:4527–4534, 2003.

16. Kurzrock R, Albitar M, Cortes J, et al.: Phase II study of R115777, a farnesyltransferase inhibitor, in myelodysplastic syndrome. *J Clin Oncol* 22:1287–1292, 2004.

17. Lancet JE, Karp JE, Gotlib G, et al.: Zarnestra (R115777) in previously untreated poor-risk AML and MDS: preliminary results of a phase II trial. *Blood* 11(100):560a, 2002. Abstract 2200.

18. List AF, DeAngelo D, O'Brien S, et al.: Phase I study of continuous oral administration of lonafarnib (Sarasar) in patients with advanced hematologic malignancies. *Blood* 100(11):789a, 2002. Abstract 3120.

19. Feldman EJ, Cortes J, Holyoake TL, et al.: Continuous oral lonafarnib (Sarasar) for the treatment of patients with myelodysplastic syndrome. *Blood* 102:421a, 2003.

20. Lancet JE, Karp JE: Farnesyltransferase inhibitors in hematologic malignancies: new horizons in therapy. *Blood* 102:3880–3889, 2003.

21. Giles FJ, Stopeck AT, Silverman LR, et al.: SU5416, a small molecule tyrosine kinase receptor inhibitor, has its biologic activity in patients with refractory acute myeloid leukemia or myelodysplastic syndromes. *Blood* 102:795–901, 2003.

22. Foran J, Paquette R, Copper M, et al.: A phase I study of repeated oral dosing with SU11248 for the treatment of patients with acute myeloid leukemia who have failed or are not eligible for conventional therapy. *Blood* 100:558a, 2002. Abstract 2195.

23. Mufti G, List AF, Gore SD, Ho AYL: Myelodysplastic syndrome: ASH education book. *Hematology* 176–199, 2003.

24. Roboz GJ, Giles FJ, List AF, et al.: Phase I trial PTK/787/ZK222584 (PTK/ZK), an inhibitor of vascular endothelial growth factor receptor tyrosine kinases in AML and MDS. *Proc Am Soc Clin Oncol* 22:568, 2003. Abstract 2284.

25. Apperley JF, Gardembas M, Melo JV, et al.: Response to Imatinib mesylate in chronic myeloproliferative diseases with rearrangements of platelet-derived growth factor receptor beta. *N Engl J Med* 347:481–487, 2002.

26. Raza A, Lisak L, Dutt D, et al.: Gleevec (imatinib mesylate) in 16 patients with chronic myelomonocytic leukemia (CMMoL). *Blood* 98(11):273b, 2001. Abstract 4829.

27. Cortes JE, Giles F, O'Brien S, et al.: Treatment with imatinib mesylate in patients with refractory or relapsed acute myeloid leukemia (AML), high-risk myelodysplastic syndrome (MDS), or myeloproliferative disorders. *Blood* 100(11):800a, 2002. Abstract 3160.

28. Raza A, Lisak L, Tahir S, et al.: Myelodysplastic syndrome patients show a variety of hematologic responses to proteosome inhibitor Bortezomib (PS 341). *Blood* 100 (11):338b, 2002. Abstract 4906.

29. Beran M, Estey, E, O'Brien S, et al.: Results of topotecan single-agent therapy in patients with myelodysplastic syndromes and chronic myelomonocytic leukemia. *Leuk Lymphoma* 31:521–531, 1998.

30. Beran M, Estey E, O'Brien S, et al.: To evaluate the efficacy and safety of the combination of topotecan and cytarabine in patients with MDS and CMML. *J Clin Oncol* 17:2819–2830, 1999.

31. Weihrach MR, Staib P, Seiberlich, et al.: Phase I/II clinical study of topotecan and cytarabine in patients with myelodysplastic syndrome, chronic myelomonocytic leukemia and myeloid leukemia. *Leuk Lymphoma* 45(4):699–704, 2004.

32. Lisak L, Tahir S, Billmeier J, et al.: Topotecan and thalidomide is an effective treatment in a subset of patients with high risk myelodysplastic syndromes. *Proc Am Soc Clin Oncol* 22:578, 2003. Abstract 2324.

33. List A, Beran M, DiPersio J, et al.: Opportunities for Trisenox (arsenic trioxide) in the treatment of myelodysplastic syndromes. *Leukemia* 17, 1499–1507, 2003.

34. List AF, Schiller GJ, Mason J, et al.: Trisenox (arsenic trioxide) in patients with myelodysplastic syndromes (MDS): preliminary findings in a phase 2 clinical study. *Blood* 102(11):423a, 2003. Abstract 1539.

35. Nobert V, Dreyfus F, Guerci A, et al.: Trisenox (arsenic trioxide) in patients with myelodysplastic syndromes (MDS): preliminary results of a phase I/II study. *Blood* 102(11):422a, 2003. Abstract 1536.

36. Raza A, Buonamici S, Lisak L, et al.: Arsenic trioxide and thalidomide combination produces multi-lineage hematological responses in myelodysplastic syndrome patients, particularly those with high pre-therapy EVI-1 expression. *Leuk Res* 28(8):791–803, 2004.

37. Candoni A, Silvestri F, Buonamici S, et al.: Targeted therapies in myelodysplastic syndromes: ASH 2003. *Semin Hematol* 41(2 suppl 4):13–20, 2004.

38. Korkolopoulou P, Apostolidou E, Pavlopoulos PM, et al.: Prognostic evaluation of the microvascular network in myelodysplastic syndromes. *Leukemia* 15(9):1369–1376, 2001.

39. Bellamy WT, Richter L, Sirjani D, et al.: Vascular endothelial cell growth factor is an autocrine promoter of abnormal localized immature myeloid precursors and leukemia progenitor formation in myelodysplastic syndromes. *Blood* 97:1427–1434, 2001.

40. Sampaio EP, Sarno EN, Galilly R, Cohn ZA, Kaplan G: Thalidomide selectively inhibits tumor necrosis factor alpha production by stimulated human monocytes. *J Exp Med* 173(3):699–703, 1991.

41. Moreira AL, Sampaio EP, Zmuidzinas A, Frindt P, Smith KA, Kaplan G: Thalidomide exerts its inhibitory action on tumor necrosis factor alpha by enhancing mRNA degradation. *J Exp Med* 177(6):1675–1680, 1993.

42. Majumdar S, Lamothe B, Aggarwal BB: Thalidomide suppresses NF-kappa B activation induced by TNF and H202, but not that activated by ceramide, lipopolysaccharides, or phorbol ester. *J Immunol* 168(6):2644–2651, 2002.

43. Haslett PA, Corral LG, Albert M, Kaplan G: Thalidomide costimulates primary human T lymphocytes, preferentially inducing proliferation, cytokine production, and cytotoxic responses in the CD8+ subset. *J Exp Med* 187(11):1885–1892, 1998.

44. Raza A, Meyer P, Dutt D, et al.: Thalidomide produces transfusion independence in long-standing refractory anemias of patients with myelodysplastic syndromes. *Blood* 98:958–965, 2001.

45. Morena-Aspitia A, Geyer S, Li C-Y, et al.: N998B: Multicenter phase II trial of thalidomide (Thal) in adult patients with myelodysplastic syndrome (MDS). *Blood* 100(11):96a, 2002. Abstract 354.

46. Dredge K, Horsfall R, Robinson SP, et al.: Orally administered lenalidomide (CC-5013) is anti-angiogenic in vivo and inhibits endothelial cell migration and Akt phosphorylation in vitro. *Microvasc Res* 69(1–2):56–63, 2005.

47. List AF, Kurtin S, Glinsmann-Gibson B, et al.: Efficacy and safety of CC5013 for treatment of anemia in patients with myelodysplastic syndromes (MDS). *Blood* 102(11):184a, 2003. Abstract 641.

48. Raza A: Anti-TNF therapies in rheumatoid arthritis, Crohn's disease and myelodysplastic syndromes. *Micosc Res Tech* 50(3);229–235, 2000.

49. Raza A, Lisak L, Tahir S, et al.: Combination of thalidomide and etanercept (tumor necrosis factor receptor or TNFR) effective in improving the cytopenias of some patients with myelodysplastic syndromes (MDS). *Blood* 100(11):340b, 2002. Abstract 4914.

50. Raza A, Candoni A, Khan U, et al.: Remicade as TNF suppressor in patients with myelodysplastic syndromes. *Leuk Lymphoma* 45(10):2099–2104, 2004.

51. List AF, Kurtin SE, Callander N, et al.: Randomized, double-blind phase II study of the matrix metalloprotease (MMP) inhibitor, AG3340 (Prinomastat) in patients with myelodysplastic syndrome (MDS). *Blood* 100(11):789a, 2002. Abstract 3119.

52. Gotlib J, Jamieson CHM, List A, et al.: Phase II study of bevacizumab (anti-VEGF humanized monoclonal antibody) in patients with myelodysplastic syndrome (MDS). *Blood* 102:425a, 2003.

53. Raza A.: *Experimental Approaches and Novel Therapies*. New York: Springer Verlag; 1998:42–45.

54. List AF, Brasfield F, Heaton K, et al.: Stimulation of hematopoiesis by amifostine in patients with myelodysplastic syndrome. *Blood* 90:3364–3369, 1997.

55. Raza A, Qawi H, Lisak L, et al.: Patients with myelodysplastic syndromes benefit from palliative therapy with amifostine, pentoxifylline, and ciprofloxacin with or without dexamethasone. *Blood* 95:1580–1587, 2000.

56. Koeffler HP, Hirji K, Itri L, et al.: 1,25-dihydroxyvitamin D3: in vitro and in vivo effects on human preleukemic and leukemic cells. *Cancer Treat Rep* 69:1399–1405, 1985.

57. Xu HM, Jones CG, Fernandez CE, et al.: 1,25-dihydroxyvitamin D3 protects HL60 cells against apoptosis but down-regulates the expression of bcl-2 gene. *Exp. Cell Res* 209:367–374, 1993.

58. Mellibovsky L, Diez A, Perez-Vila E, et al.: Vitamin D treatment in myelodysplastic syndromes. *Br J Haematol* 100:516–520, 1998.

59. Molldrem JJ, Caples M, Mavroudis D, et al.: Antithymocyte globulin for patients with myelodysplastic syndrome. *Br J Haematol* 99;699–705, 1997.

60. Molldrem JJ, Leiffer E, Bahceci E, et al.: Anti-thymocyte globulin for the treatment of the bone marrow failure associated with myelodysplastic syndromes. *Ann Intern Med* 137;156–163, 2002.

61. Killick B, Mufti G, Cavenagh JD, et al.: A pilot study of antithymocyte globulin (ATG) in the treatment of patients with 'low-risk' myelodysplasia. *Br J Haematol* 120:679–684, 2003.

62. Yazji S, Giles FJ, Tsimberidou A-M, et al.: Antithymocyte globulin (ATG)-based therapy in patients with myelodysplastic syndromes. *Leukemia* 17:2101–2106, 2003.

63. Steensma DP, Dispenzieri A, Moore SB, et al.: Antithymocyte globulin has limited efficacy and substantial toxicity in unselected anemic patients with myelodysplastic syndrome. *Blood* 101:2156–2158, 2003.

# Section 2
# CHRONIC MYELOPROLIFERATIVE DISEASES

## Chapter 45
# EPIDEMIOLOGY, RISK FACTORS, AND CLASSIFICATION

*Hanspreet Kaur, Deepjot Singh, and Alan Lichtin*

## INTRODUCTION

Chronic myeloproliferative disorders (CPMDs) are characterized by the chronic proliferation of one or more of the three hematopoietic cell lines or by marrow stromal cells, in various proportions. Polycythemia vera (PV), idiopathic myelofibrosis (IMF), chronic myelogenous leukemia (CML), and essential thrombocytosis (ET) have been traditionally classified as "chronic myeloproliferative disorders."[1] These disorders are believed to originate from a clonal transformation of a multipotent hematopoietic progenitor cell, resulting in an overproduction of one or more of the myeloid (i.e., granulocytic, erythroid, and megakaryocytic) lineages in the absence of a defined stimulus.[2] In contrast to the ineffective erythropoiesis observed in the myelodysplastic syndromes, the proliferating cells show relatively normal maturation, with a resultant increase in granulocytes, red blood cells, and/or platelets in the peripheral blood. Other features shared by these disorders include splenomegaly and hepatomegaly from extramedullary hematopoiesis; marrow hypercellularity, megakaryocytic hyperplasia, and dysplasia; chromosomal abnormalities of chromosomes 1, 8, 9, 13, and 20; leukemic skin infiltrates, and spontaneous transformation into acute blast phase or bone marrow failure due to myelofibrosis or ineffective erythropoiesis.[3–6] The diagnosis of

individual entities is therefore complicated by their overlapping features. The presence of the *BCR/ABL* fusion gene in association with characteristic morphologic and clinical findings permits an unequivocal diagnosis of CML. However, no specific chromosomal or molecular markers exist uniformly for the other conditions. Diagnosis of the other conditions is made on the basis of clinical, laboratory, and morphologic findings, which can be misleading. For example, approximately 10% of patients in one study of IMF actually had PV, while many patients initially diagnosed as ET had PV, instead.[7–8]

As CML is discussed in detail in Chapters 16–22, we will concentrate on the Philadephia (Ph)-chromosome-negative CMPDs.

## CLASSIFICATION

The classification of CMPDs is based on the lineage of the predominant proliferating cells and the prominence of marrow fibrosis, taken together with a constellation of clinical and laboratory features.

The World Health Organization (WHO) classification system[6] identifies seven conditions under the category of CMPDs, as shown in Table 45.1.

Tefferi[9] classified ET, PV, and IMF as CPMDs. The CMPDs, in turn, are members of a broader class of

**Table 45.1** WHO classification of chronic myeloproliferative diseases

Chronic myelogenous leukemia [Ph chromosome, t (9;22) (q34;q11), *BCR/ABL* positive]
Chronic neutrophilic leukemia
Chronic eosinophilic leukemia (and the hypereosinophilic syndrome)
Polycythemia vera
Chronic idiopathic myelofibrosis (with extramedullary hematopoiesis)
Essential thrombocythemia
Chronic myeloproliferative disease, unclassifiable

Adapted from Jaffe et al.[6]

"clonal" stem cell processes operationally designated as the chronic myeloid disease groups (CMDs).

The classification of chronic myeloid disorders is shown in Table 45.2. The classification system is somewhat arbitrary, as features may overlap between myelodysplastic syndrome (MDS) and CMPD. The identification of specific disease-causing mutations similar to the Ph chromosome in CML is hoped to pave the path toward a molecular classification system of CMDs.

## EPIDEMIOLOGY

The CMPDs are primarily seen in the adult population, with a peak in the fifth to seventh decades of life. The combined annual incidence of the CMPDs is approxi-

**Table 45.2** Operational classification of chronic myeloid disorders

Chronic myeloid leukemia
Myelodysplastic syndrome
   IPSS—low risk
   IPSS—intermediate risk 1
   IPSS—intermediate risk 2
   IPSS—high risk
Chronic myeloproliferative disease
   Essential thrombocythemia
   Polycythemia vera
   Myelofibrosis with myeloid metaplasia
Atypical chronic myeloid disorder
   Chronic neutrophilic leukemia
   Chronic eosinophilic leukemia
   Hypereosinophilic syndrome
   Chronic basophilic leukemia
   Juvenile myelomonocytic leukemia
   Chronic myelomonocytic leukemia
   Transient myeloproliferative/leukemia syndrome of Down syndrome
   Systemic mast cell disease
   Otherwise undefined myeloproliferative disorder

IPSS, International Prognostic Scoring System.

mately 6–9/100,000 people.[6] The first epidemiologic data were based on a large population study published by Prochazka and Markowe.[10] The incidence of PV in Europe and North America is similar, with eight to ten cases per million individuals per year.[11] PV varies from 2 cases per million individuals per year in Japan to 13 per million per year in Australia.[6]

In a population-based study in Olmsted County, Minnesota, from 1935 to 1989, the age- and sex-adjusted incidence rate of PV was 1.9/100,000 person-years.[12] In the same county, in another population-based study from 1976 to 1995, the authors reported an approximate annual incidence of 2.5, 2.3, and 1.3 per 100,000 for ET, PV, and de novo agnogenic myeloid metaplasia (AMM), respectively. In a report from the United Kingdom, from 1984 to 1993, 2376 cases of CMPDs, including ET, PV, and AMM, were reported.[13] The standardized incidence rate was 2.27/100,000 person-years for all three conditions. The incidence rate per 100,000 for PV, ET, and AMM was 0.92, 0.79, and 0.57, respectively. Although in adults the true incidence of chronic idiopathic fibrosis is not known, it is estimated to be between 0.5 and 1.5 per 100,000 individuals per year.[9,14] The true incidence for chronic neutrophilic leukemia (CNL) is unknown, as fewer than 100 cases have been reported.[6] In a study of 660 cases of chronic leukemias of myeloid origin, not one single case of CNL was observed.[15] Chronic eosinophilic leukemia (CEL) and hypereosinophilic syndrome (HES) are rare diseases. As it is often difficult to distinguish between the two, the true incidence of these conditions is unknown. It appears that approximately 10–20% of all cases of CPMDs may be unclassifiable.[6]

PV appears to be more common in men than in women, with reported male-to-female ratios ranging from 1.2 to 2.2 in various studies.[11–13,16] In the 1000 cases of ET in a study by McNally et al., there was no difference between the sexes. An age-specific (30–50 years) female preponderance in ET was seen, however. More males were affected by AMM. Males are more commonly affected by CEL and HES than females, with a male-to-female ratio of around 9:1 in HES.[6]

CMPDs are diseases of older individuals, with low rates until age 50, and a peak in incidence from 60 to 80 years of age.[11,13,16] The maximum incidence of PV exceeded 20/100,000 person-years in the Olmsted County data. The median age of presentation is similar in ET, PV, and AMM, being 55–65 years. The mean age at diagnosis of PV has been increasing steadily since the 1920s.[13,16,17] A few cases of PV diagnosed under the age of 40 have been reported.[18] The age-specific mortality calculated by Prochazka and Markowe[10] showed a sharp increase beginning in the early 40s, with the age-specific mortality reaching a maximum in the 75- and 84-year age group. CNL has been reported in both adolescents and older adults.[19,20] HES may present at any age, though its peak incidence is in the fourth decade of life.[21]

Racial and ethnic factors influence the incidence of PV. PV is significantly less common in blacks than in whites. It is also more common in individuals of Jewish origin (Ashkenazi) than of non-Jewish origin.[11,22,23]

Familial occurrence of PV has been reported, with a 6% incidence of patients enrolled in the protocols of the Polycythemia Vera Study Group, and in some sporadic cases.[24,25]

## RISK FACTORS

There is no strong evidence that supports the association of the CMPDs with environmental exposures. A number of toxic agents, including lead, saponin, and benzene, and the Rauscher and feline leukemia virus, antigen–antibody complexes, and ionizing radiation have been shown to cause AMM in experimental animals.[26] The extramedullary hematopoiesis is believed to be a result of a normal response of mesenchymal cells to tissue injury. Some reported associations with AMM include exposure to toluene and benzene.[27,28] An increased incidence of AMM was seen in patients receiving thorotrast.[29] The victims of the atomic bombing in Hiroshima had an 18 times more risk of AMM than that of the remainder of the Japanese population, with symptoms appearing at an average age of 6 years after the exposure, lending credence to the thought that radiation or nuclear exposure is a risk factor for developing AMM.[30]

## REFERENCES

1. Dameshek W: Some speculations on the myeloproliferative syndromes. *Blood* 6:372, 1951.
2. Adamson JW, Fialkow PJ, Murphy S, et al.: Polycythemia vera: stem-cell and probable clonal origin of the disease. *N Engl J Med* 295:913, 1976.
3. Swolin B, Weinfeld A, Westin J: A prospective long-term cytogenetic study in polycythemia vera in relation to treatment and clinical course. *Blood* 72:386, 1988.
4. Diez-Martin JL, Graham DL, Petitt RM, et al.: Chromosome studies in 104 patients with polycythemia vera. *Mayo Clinic Proc* 66:287, 1991.
5. Berk PD, Goldberg JD, Silverstein MN, et al.: Increased incidence of acute leukemia in polycythemia vera associated with chlorambucil therapy. *N Engl J Med* 304:441, 1981.
6. Jaffe ES, Harris NL, Stein H, et al. (eds.): *World Health Organization Classification of Tumors: Pathology and Genetics of Tumours of Haematopoietic and Lymphoid Tissues.* Lyon, France: IARC Press; 2001:15.
7. Linman J, Bethell F: Agnogenic myeloid metaplasia. *Am J Med* 22:107, 1957.
8. Gunz F: Hemorrhagic thrombocythemia: a critical review. *Blood* 15:706, 1960.
9. Tefferi A: Chronic myeloid disorders: classification and treatment overview. *Semin Hematol* 38(1 suppl 2):1, 2001.
10. Prochazka AV, Markowe HLJ: The epidemiology of polycythemia vera in England and Wales 1968–1982. *Br J Cancer* 53:59, 1986.
11. Modan B: An epidemiological study of polycythemia vera. *Blood* 26:257, 1965.
12. Ania BJ, Suman VJ, Sobell JL, et al.: Trends in the incidence of polycythemia vera among Olmstead County, Minnesota, residents, 1935–1989. *Am J Hematol* 47:89, 1994.
13. McNally RJQ, Roman RE, Cartwright RA: Age and sex distribution of haematological malignancies in the UK. *Hematol Oncol* 15:173, 1997.
14. Mesa RA, Silverstein MN, Jacobsen SJ, et al.: Population-based incidence and survival figures in essential thrombocythemia and agnogenic myeloid metaplasia: an Olmsted County study, 1976–1995. *Am J Hematol* 61:10, 1999.
15. Shepherd PC, Ganesan TS, Galton DA: Haematological classification of the chronic myeloid leukaemias. *Baillieres Clin Haematol* 1:887, 1987.
16. Berlin NI: Diagnosis and classification of the polycythemias. *Semin Hematol* 12:339, 1975.
17. Osgood EE: Polycythemia vera: age relationships and survival. *Blood* 26:243, 1965.
18. Najean Y, Mugnier P, Dresch C, et al.: Polycythemia vera in young people: an analysis of 58 cases diagnosed before 40 years. *Br J Haematol* 67:285, 1987.
19. You W, Weisbrot IM: Chronic neutrophilic leukemia. Report of two cases and review of the literature. *Am J Clin Path* 72:233, 1979.
20. Zittoun R, Rea D, Ngoic LH, Ramond S: Chronic neutrophilic leukemia. A study of four cases. *Ann Hematol* 68:55, 1994.
21. Weller PF, Bubley GJ: The idiopathic hypereosinophilic syndrome. *Blood* 83:2759, 1994.
22. Damon A, Holub DA: Host factors in polycythemia *vera*. *Ann Intern Med* 49:43, 1958.
23. Chaiter Y, Brenner B, Aghai E, et al.: High incidence of myeloproliferative disorders in Ashkenazi Jews in northern Israel. *Leuk Lymphoma* 7:251, 1992.
24. Brubaker LH, Wsasserman LR, Goldberg JD, et al.: Increased prevalence of polycythemia vera in parents of patients on polycythemia study group protocols. *Am J Hematol* 16:367, 1984.
25. Inaba T, Shimazaki C, Hirai H, et al.: Familial polycythemia vera in father and daughter. *Am J Hematol* 51:172, 1996.
26. Wasserman LR, Berk PD, Berlin N (eds.): *Polycythemia Vera and the Myeloproliferative Disorders.* Philadelphia: WB Saunders; 1995.
27. Honda Y, Delzell E, Cole P: An updated study of mortality among workers at a petroleum manufacturing plant. *J Occup Environ Med* 37:194, 1995.
28. Hu H: Benzene-associated myelofibrosis. *Ann Intern Med* 106:171, 1987.
29. Visfeldt J, Andersson M: Pathoanatomical aspects of haematological disorders among Danish patients exposed to thorium dioxide. *APMIS* 103:29, 1995.
30. Anderson RE, Hioshino T, Yammamoto T: Myelofibrosis with myeloid metaplasia in survivors of the atomic bomb in Hiroshima. *Ann Inter Med* 60:1, 1964.

# Chapter 46

# MOLECULAR BIOLOGY, PATHOLOGY, AND CYTOGENETICS

*Claire N Harrison*

## INTRODUCTION

The term myeloproliferative disease (MPD) was first used in 1951 by Dameshek[1] to unify the conditions chronic myeloid leukemia (CML), polcythemia vera (PV), and idiopathic myelofibrosis (MF). This group of entities later included essential thrombocythemia (ET). The revised WHO classification[2] also includes some newer entities and recognizes an overlap between myeloproliferative and myelodysplastic disorders (MPD/MDS) (Table 46.1). The WHO classification of these disorders interestingly does not include systemic mastocytosis, which now resides in a new group "mast cell diseases." All these disorders have a predisposition to developing acute leukemia (usually myeloid) and/or MF to a variable extent.

This chapter focuses upon the chronic MPDs, with the exception of CML, and the overlap between MPD/MDS disorders and mastocytosis. For each disorder in turn pathology, cytogenetics, and molecular biology will be discussed. The molecular basis of many of these conditions is becoming increasingly apparent and this has the potential to revise diagnostic pathways and to force the review of classification. For example, the V617F JAK2 mutation discovered in 2005 is present in up to 95% of PV and 50% of ET and MF, respectively.[3–7]

The WHO classification places more emphasis, than do previous diagnostic criteria, upon pathology, in particular on features of the bone marrow trephine most especially megakaryocyte morphology (Figure 46.1). This remains to be fully validated, and although it is currently undergoing revision, a more substantial revision may be required in the light of rapid advances in molecular knowledge (this is reviewed in detail in the Idiopathic Myelofibrosis Molecular Biology section and Figure 46.2). When all MPDs (excluding CML) are considered, cytogenetic abnormalities in order of frequency are $-Y$, $+8$, $+9$, $-7$, del(20)(q11q13), del (13)(q12q14), del(5)(q13q33), and del(12)(p12). Conventional cytogenetics remain the evaluation of choice, but for rarer specific abnormalities (e.g., FIP1L1 PDGFRα) either RTPCR or FISH would be required. Deletion of chromosome 20q is probably one of the best characterized abnormalities in MPD and although a minimal common deleted region has been identified, no genes have yet been classified. For the common Philadelphia negative MPDs as discussed in this chapter, the most consistent and highly prevalent molecular abnormality akin to *BCR/ABL* for CML is V617F JAK2.[3–7] The discovery of thrombopoietin triggered further interest in this and other cytokines in MPDs, and much molecular research has relatively fruitfully focussed in this field. Indeed a recent mutation in the cognate receptor cMPL has been identified in a small proportion of patients with ET and MF but thus far not PV.[8,9] A pathogenic theme for the common MPDs in particular is that somatic mutations at a stem cell level result in at least two key events—hypersensitivity

| Table 46.1 | WHO classification of chronic myeloproliferative diseases |
|---|---|

Chronic myeloproliferative disease
- Chronic myeloid leukemia
- Chronic neutrophilic leukemia
- Chronic eosinophilic leukemia (and hypereosinophilic syndrome)
- Polycythemia vera
- Chronic idiopathic myelofibrosis (with myeloid metaplasia)
- Essential thrombocythemia
- Mastocytosis
- Chronic myeloproliferative disease unclassifiable

Mixed myelodysplastic/myeloproliferative disorders
- Chronic myelomonocytic leukemia
- Atypical chronic myeloid leukemia
- Juvenile myelomonocytic leukemia

Myelodysplastic/myeloproliferative disease, unclassifiable

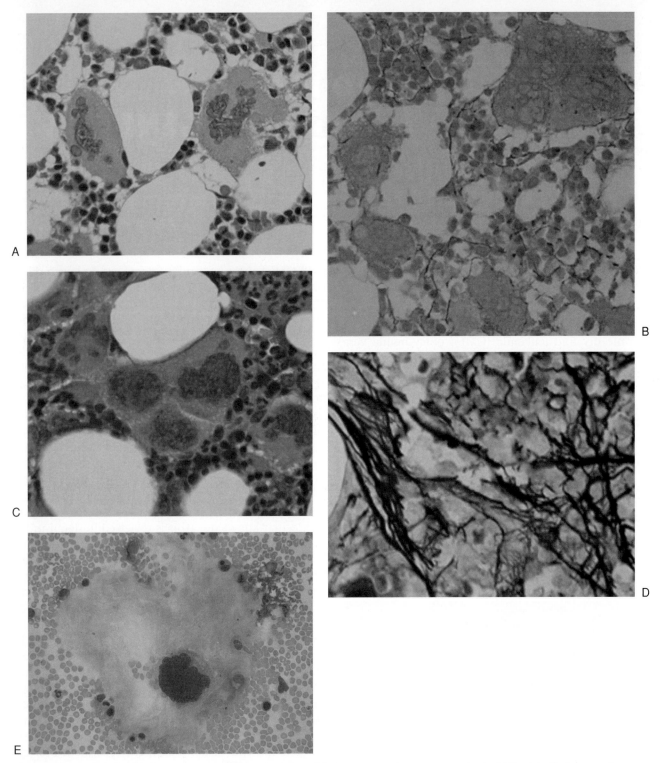

**Figure 46.1**  *Examples of marrow  pathology features. (A) Large megakaryocyte typical of ET with distinct nuclear morphology; (B) Scanty reticulin in such cases; (C) Megakaryocyte morphology said to be more in keeping with MF indistinct nuclear morphology and clustering; (D) Dense reticulin formation; (E) Large megakaryocytes demonstrating emperipolesis.*

to proliferative signals and resistance to inhibitory ones.

## POLYCYTHEMIA VERA

The dominant feature of polycythemia vera (PV), also termed polcythemia rubra vera or primary proliferative polycythemia, is the excessive production of erythrocytes frequently accompanied by increases in other hematopoietic lineages. To achieve a diagnosis of PV it is important to exclude potential causes of a secondary erythrocytosis. Clinical evaluation, pathology, cytogenetics, and the determination of erythropoietin levels or demonstration of spontaneous erythroid colonies are all potentially useful. Probably the most important diagnostic feature is now the presence of detectable V617F as it is only detected in myeloid disorders (principally MPDs and occasionally leukemias[10]) and an elevated hematocrit.

### PATHOLOGY OF PV

The blood film may show evidence of iron deficiency, neutrophilia, and basophilia and occasionally immature myeloid precursors are seen. The aspirate is usually hypercellular with increases of erythroid, granulocytic, and megakaryocytic lineages. The megakaryocytes are bigger and nuclear lobation is increased. The trephine biopsy (Figure 46.1) demonstrates a similar extent of hypercellularity. Often reticulin is increased and may be significantly increased in 10%[11] Erythropoiesis is morphologically normal but abnormalities of megakaryocyte morphology are common. Megakaryocytes are not only increased but they also have abnormal morphology. Both large and small forms are seen and emperipolesis is prominent.[12] Iron stores are commonly reduced or absent. Up to one-third of patients with PV progress to florid MF in the later stages of their disease, and the pathological features are then indistinguishable from primary MF.

### CYTOGENETICS

The most common cytogenetic result in PV at diagnosis is a normal study; less frequently, the following abnormalities may occur: +8, +9 (may occur concurrently); del(20)(q11q13) is also relatively common. A number of other abnormalities occur more rarely—del(1)(p11), del(3)(p11p14), t(1;6)(q11,p21), and t(1;9)(q10p10).[13] Recent studies suggest that abnormalities of chromosome 9p may be the most common abnormality in PV.[14] This may arise due to uniparental disomy resulting in loss of heterozygosity and occurs in up to 30% of PV.[15] This is the location of the *JAK2* gene and mitotic recombination is the mechanism for progressing from heterozygous to homozygous V617F JAK2.[3,5]

### MOLECULAR BIOLOGY

The marked prevalence of the mutation V617F in JAK2 kinase in PV (85–95%)[3–7] implies that it is most likely to be involved in the pathogenesis of this condition.

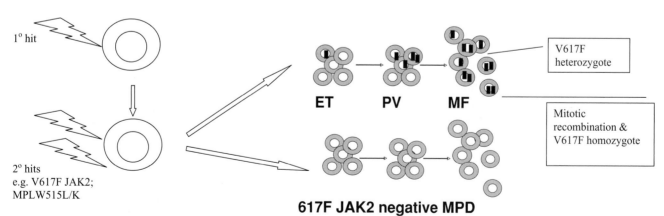

**V617F JAK2 positive MPD**

1° hit

2° hits
e.g. V617F JAK2;
MPLW515L/K

ET     PV     MF

V617F
heterozygote

Mitotic
recombination &
V617F homozygote

**617F JAK2 negative MPD**

**Figure 46.2**  *Proposed scheme for molecular pathogenesis and classification of chronic MPDs. A primary hit or hits affect a hematopoietic stem cell and may cause a "pre-MPD stem cell." Second hits are likely to include V617FJAK2 and MPLW515L/K and other as yet unidentified mutations. A continuum through ET to advanced disease is proposed where a potential drive to progression is load of V617F JAK2 due to mitotic recombination and clonal dominance but is likely to also include other genetic events.*

This is also supported by transplantation studies in mice who rapidly develop the phenotype of PV and later also develop fibrosis.[4] Here a single point mutation converts a highly conserved valine to a bulky phenylalanine which is thought to stoichiometrically affect the interaction between the kinase and pseudokinase domains of JAK2 (reviewed in Refs. 16 and 17). Studies[4-6] have shown that the JAK2 mutation causes cytokine independent activation of JAK-STAT, P13K-AKT and ERK pathways, these are involved in erythropoeitin receptor signaling. The current status of knowledge in relation to the role of Janus kinases in hemopoiesis and hematological malignancy has recently been reviewed.[16] This mutation potentially explains many of the features previously reported in PV including hypersensitivity to a number of other cytokines, granulocyte-macrophage colony-stimulating factor, stem cell factor, interleukin-3 and insulin-like growth factor 1, and reduced expression of cMPL.[18] In addition to the constitutive activity of STAT3 reported in a proportion of PV patients,[19] the mRNA for polycythemia rubra vera 1 (PRV-1) is elevated in granulocytes of PV patients[20]; overexpression of PRV-1 correlates strongly with endogenous colony formation in PV, ET, and MF[21,22] and also with V617F.[23]

## ESSENTIAL THROMBOCYTHEMIA

The predominant feature of ET is a marked, otherwise unexplained, thrombocytosis accompanied in a proportion of patients by thrombotic and/or hemorrhagic features. In the long term, a proportion of patients develop MF (less commonly than PV) and acute myeloid leukemia. The evaluation of patient involves excluding other conditions such as the other MPDs, MDS, or a reactive thrombocytosis especially for those 50% of the patients in whom the V617F JAK2 mutation is not detectable.

### PATHOLOGY

It is important to scrutinize the blood film when establishing a diagnosis of ET. Here platelets are increased and often larger, hypogranular forms are seen as are megakaryocyte nuclei; a neutrophilia may also be present. Features of MDS, MF, iron deficiency, or hyposplenism (may be present in ET due to splenic infarction) should be excluded. The aspirate shows increased numbers of large, hyperlobated megakaryocytes and platelet drifts may be prominent. Trephine biopsy appearances are variable in ET; the marrow is not always hypercellular but megakaryocytes are always increased (Figure 46.1). The extent to which megakaryocyte morphology can be used to ascertain a definitive diagnosis of ET, where the megakaryocytes are enlarged and mature, or furthermore to discriminate between true ET and a prefibrotic phase of MF[24] (a subgroup with a worse prognosis)[25] is unclear. The atypical features include immature megakaryocytes with clustering, cloud-like nuclei, erythroid hypoplasia, and increased and dysplastic granulopoiesis (Figure 46.1). It would be very attractive to be able to further subdivide patients prognostically; however, megakaryocyte morphology is notoriously difficult to reproducibly assess, and thus far there has been no evaluation of interobserver variation. The prognostic and diagnostic significance of varied reticulin density or scoring in ET remains similarly unclear.

### CYTOGENETICS

Almost 95% of ET patients will have normal cytogenetics.[26] Abnormalities when present are highly variable; MF or progression to leukemia is reported in association with del(13)(q12q14)[27] but it is not clear that this abnormality is predictive of progression. It is important to use FISH or RTPCR at diagnosis in ET to exclude the presence of BCR/ABL, where the correct diagnosis would be CML.

### MOLECULAR BIOLOGY

ET is a clinically heterogeneous disorder which is reflected in molecular analyses in these patients. Indeed a significant proportion of ET patients do not have clonal hemopoiesis as assessed using X-chromosome inactivation patterns and this subgroup may be at a lower risk of thrombotic complications.[28,29] These findings may also reflect technical limitations or a low disease burden undetectable against a polyclonal background.

The V617F JAK2 mutation is detected in 50% of patients with ET[3,30,31] and painstaking analysis of progenitors suggests that in ET it is highly unusual to detected homozygosity for V617F JAK2.[32] The majority of ET patients negative for V617F JAK2 mutation have features characteristic of an MPD.[33] The V617F positive ET patients share features in common with PV patients including higher hemoglobins and white cell counts[30,34] but have features that constrain erythropoiesis such as low erythropoietin levels and iron stores.[34] A small proportion of ET patients appear to have one of two mutations in cMPL in the juxtamembrane domain of the intracytoplasmic tail[9,35] in mouse models this recapitulates the clinical features of ET and MF.[9]

Most patients with V617F JAK2 negative ET or MF will continue to be V617F JAK2 negative as suggested by most published data thus far[36,37]; potential candidates for molecular aetiology in V617F JAK2 negative ET are manifold.

There is an emerging evidence for a V617F JAK2 negative subclinical pre-MPD phase most powerful of which is that in patients previously noted to be V617F JAK2 positive when a leukemic clone emerges it is frequently V617F negative.[36] An alternative explanation for V617F JAK2 negative leukemia occurring in these patients is that V617F JAK2 must be lost to induce a block upon differentiation; however, experiments to investigate loss of heterozygosity in the appropriate chromosomal region suggest this is not the case. Most of these patients had received hydroxyurea alone not multiple therapies so transformation of a normal stem cell seemed improbable. Further data suggesting a disparity between size populations of clonal myeloid cells (as judged by X-chromosome inactivation patterns) and V617JAK2 positive cells also suggests a pre-V617F clone[38,39]; where clonality is judged by loss of heterozygosity at 20q this data is most convincing[38] as there are significant problems in interpreting clonality using XCIPs in V617F JAK2 positive disease.[36]

## CHRONIC IDIOPATHIC MF

Chronic idiopathic MF or MF with myeloid metaplasia is a rare condition in which myeloproliferation is associated with increased fibroblast proliferation neoangiogenesis and extramedullary hemopoiesis. MF may occur in later phases of the other MPDs namely ET, PV, and CML and this reflects the continuum and substantial overlap of clinical features in the MPDs, and given the prevalence of V617F JAK2 mutation adds weight to the need to reconsideration of disease classification as discussed later.

### PATHOLOGY

Bone marrow features of this condition are variable. Cellularity ranges from being increased to markedly reduced or near absent normal hematopoiesis. Fibrosis ranges from a focal increase of reticulin to coarse parallel reticulin, the presence of collagen, and osteogenesis or new bone formation (Figure 46.2). Dense fibrosis is also associated with dilated marrow sinusoids and intrasinusoidal hematopoiesis. Variable systems of reticulin grading are in routine use and a unified system is required to inform future studies. Megakaryocyte morphology is a key to identify the newly proposed diagnostic entity prefibrotic MF. In prefibrotic MF there is at most a borderline increase in reticulin, reduced erythropoisis, and increased granulocytic and megakaryocyte proliferation, and reactive lymphoid follicles may also be apparent. Significant megakaryocyte abnormalities (as discussed in ET)[40] are a key to differentiating this entity from ET. Yet to be delineated is whether or not this is a distinct disease entity and whether hematopathologists can reliably establish this diagnosis. The spleen is a common site of extramedullary hematopoiesis in MF and variable patterns of infiltration by myeloid precursors are identified, from diffuse to nodular or a predominance of myeloid precursors.[41]

Blood film appearances are important in making the diagnosis of MF. The most characteristic include leucoerythroblastic features with teardrop poikilocytes; dysplastic features may be present in granulocytes and platelets. In the early stages of MF, these features may be either absent or not prominent.[42] Increased CD34+ cells and an elevated LDH may also be demonstrated.

### CYTOGENETICS

Conventional cytogenetic evaluation of patients with MF often fails presumably because of marrow fibrosis precluding obtaining sufficient cells on aspiration. Fibrosis was shown to be a secondary process as fibroblasts in culture were either cytogenetically normal or had clones that differed from the marrow.[43] A normal karyotype is at least as frequent as an abnormal one; furthermore some studies suggest an associated prognostic significance.[44] In a larger study reported by Tefferi[45] 90% of abnormalities were either +8, +9, del(20)(q11q13), del (13)(q12q14), and del(12)(p12) or involved chromosomes 1 or 7. Here only +8 or del(12)(p12) appeared to be independent prognostic indicators.

Of interest is the fact that chromosome 13 abnormalities (del(13)(q12q14) or translocations involving this region) appear to be consistently present both in primary MF and, most likely, as a second event in MF which evolves in the other MPDs.[46,47] The del(13)(q12q14) potentially results in the loss of RB, a well-characterized tumor suppressor gene, and this has indeed been demonstrated but only in a proportion of patients with MF.[48]

### MOLECULAR BIOLOGY

The cause of markedly enhanced fibroblast proliferation and collagen synthesis in MF could relate to an array of humoral factors that may be released from hemopoietic cells, including both the megakaryocytes and monocytes. The fibroblasts themselves rarely display intrinsic alteration and are hence regarded as "effector cells." Megakaryocytes and platelets may influence fibroblast proliferation by virtue of their increased content, release, and abnormal packaging of alpha granule contents PDGF, PF-4, TGFβ, b-FGF, and calmodulin.[49] The subcellular location of P-selectin in megakaryocytes and platelets is abnormal and may correlate with emperipoiesis, which causes disruption of the megakaryocyte organelles and causes the leakage of α–granule contents.[50] Monocytes have also been implicated in the stimulation of fibrosis. They are activated following contact with protein components of the extracellular matrix via adhesion molecules, particularly CD44, subsequently resulting in enhanced monocyte CD25 expression and increased production of TGFβ and interleukin-1. The potential role for monocytes or macrophages or indeed other genetic factors in the pathogenesis of MF is supported by animal models. At a cellular level attention has focused upon growth factor pathway anomalies and the recent identification of V617F JAK2 and MPLW515L/K[8,9] is in keeping with this. The aetiology of MF without JAK2 or cMPL mutations is unclear but the patients have all the features associated with MPD and while one publication[51] suggests they may have superior prognosis this has not been identified in all studies.[52]

Probably the next major issue in MPDs is whether it is still relevant to subdivide V617F JAK2 positive or indeed negative disease into the three different entities (PV, ET, or MF) or is it preferable to regard the MPDs as a continuum of conditions akin to the different phases of CML. Here advanced MF or AML would represent advanced phase and ET with PV chronic phase. Unlike CML the rate of progression, if at all, of patients along this continuum is slow and patients may of course present at any point of the spectrum.

This proposal is contentious but is recently strengthened by several pieces of evidence from translational research. For example, Scott et al.[32] found that none of the patients studied with ET had V617F JAK2 homozygous colonies, while such colonies were detected in all the PV patients ($p <$ 0.0001) and two ET patients after polycthemic transformation. This suggests that a fundamental difference between ET and PV might be the mitotic recombination events that generate daughter cells homozygous for V617F JAK2. Evidence that total "load" of V617F JAK2 increases between the entities ET, PV, and MF (and post-polycythemic MF) has also been reported by other groups. For example Moliterno[53] reports the median neutrophil JAK2 V617F allele percentage was greater in PV than in ET ($p = <0.001$), and that allele percentages greater than 63% were restricted to PV and MF. Similarly, Passamonti[54] recently reported in 66/90 MPD patients that significant differences in quantity of V617F JAK2 occur between PV and ET ($p = 0.01$), or PV and prefibrotic MF ($p = .005$); fibrotic MF and prefibrotic MF ($p = 0.001$) and postpolycythemic MF having higher levels than PV ($p < 0.001$). This data accords with data from the group at the Mayo Clinic groups.[55]

These findings could be extrapolated to a model of the relationship between the V617F JAK2 positive MPDs and disease progression as shown in Figure 46.1. The challenges for this model are why the majority of ET patients do not transform to PV, which may relate to a genetic predisposition to undergo mitotic recombination, as well as to elucidate the additional genetic hits causing disease progression and why some patients progress more rapidly than others who do not progress at all.

## CHRONIC EOSINOPHILIC LEUKEMIA/ HYPEREOSINOPHILIC SYNDROME

Myeloproliferative hypereosinophilic diseases are defined by a persistent (>6 months) unexplained eosinophilia greater than $1.5 \times 10^9$/L, a hypercellular bone marrow with eosinophilia, and tissue damage. They are discriminated from idiopathic hypereosinophilic syndrome by the presence of tissue damage, although this may indeed be artificial as tissue damage may be subclinical or occur in the future. While investigating these patients, a reactive cause of eosinophilia such as allergies, parasitic infections, and other malignancies (e.g., on detection of phenotypically abnormal T lymphocytes[56]) should be assiduously excluded. Eosinophil morphology varies from normal to include abnormalities such as degranulation, cytoplasmic vacuolation, hypolobulation, or hyperlobulation. The presence of Chronic eosinophilic leukemia (CEL) is suggested by increased proportion of blasts, hepatosplenomegaly, raised serum tryptase, vitamin B12, and a cytogenetic abnormality. In some patients the diagnosis will only be apparent after transformation to acute myeloid leukemia.

The detection of cytogenetic abnormalities is useful in discriminating CEL from a reactive eosinophilia. Abnormalities involving 5q33 or 8p11 are most frequent and clonality has been demonstrated even in patients with normal cytogenetics by X-chromosome inactivation patterns.[57] Abnormalities of 5q33, especially t(5;12)(q33;p13), produce the fusion oncogene TEL-PDGFRβ with constitutive activation of the kinase domain of PDGFRβ originally cloned by Golub.[58] Variable morphological features have been described from chronic myelomonocytic leukemia (CMML)-like to atypical CML, as reviewed by Bain.[59] Two other translocations involving the PDGFRβ gene are t(5;7)(q33;q11.2) and t(5;10)(q33;21.2). Rarer translocations associated with 8p11 involve the fibroblast growth factor receptor-1 (FGFR1) most commonly fusing with the ZNF198 gene of 13q12 generating t(8;13)(q11;q12); they are frequently associated with non-Hodgkin's lymphomas and have a particular tendency to leukemic transformation.[60–63]

Recently, a novel tyrosine kinase, FIP1L1-PDGFRα, has been described in 9/16 patients with hypereosinophilic syndrome[64] and 3/5 with systemic mastocytosis.[65] This is generated by microdeletion of CHIC2 and is only detectable by RTPCR or FISH; conventional cytogenetics is unhelpful. Patients with FIP1L1-PDGFRα and eosinophilia have been reported to show a dramatic response to imatinib mesylate[64,66] as have several with activated PDGFRB fusion tyrosine kinases.[67,68]

## CHRONIC NEUTROPHILIC LEUKEMIA

Chronic neutrophilic leukemia is a very rare disorder; just over 140 cases are reported but many of these may not fulfil the diagnostic criteria.[69] It is characterized by a leucocytosis in excess of $25 \times 10^9/L$ (lack of eosinophilia, basophilia, and few myeloid precursors), absent *bcr/abl*, and bone marrow myeloid hyperplasia without prominent blasts. A rarer form of CML bears some morphological similarities for CNL but has a variant *bcr/abl* (BCRe19/ABLa2). Hepatosplenomegaly may be present and in 20% of the cases an associated neoplasm has been reported. Cytogenetics are normal in the majority (90%). There have been no comprehensive studies of molecular biology. One of the difficulties in making a diagnosis of CNL is in differentiating it from a leukemoid reaction, here clonality may be helpful in females who have normal cytogenetics. As a leukemoid reaction is reported in association with myeloma or monoclonal gammopathy of uncertain significance, it would be wise to exclude these entities.

## MASTOCYTOSIS

There is a spectrum of MPDs described by the term mastocytosis in which the characteristic feature is the presence of mast cells with abnormal growth kinetics and their accumulation in organs (Table 46.2). A detailed discourse of all these mast cell disorders is beyond the scope of this chapter; the reader is directed to a recent chapter/review for further information.[70]

### PATHOLOGY

The major feature of systemic mastocytosis is the finding of compact dense multifocal mast cell infiltrates in a bone marrow trephine biopsy. These are most usefully identified by means of staining for mast cell tryptase. Such infiltrates may also be identified in other organs and lymph nodes. The individual morphology of the mast cells is also important. Typically they are spindle shaped, but may demonstrate atypia, including nuclear lobulation, smaller or absent granules, and a primitive nuclear chromatin pattern; they also aberrantly express CD2 and CD25.[32–35,37] Reticulin is usually increased, and collagen and new bone formation may be seen. "Pseudo-granulomas" may also be apparent and commonly are associated with eosinophils, lymphocytes (sometimes lymphoid nodules), and plasma cells in addition to the mast cell infiltrate.

The determination of serum tryptase level may be a useful index of burden of mast cells and is usually elevated in systemic mastocytosis. For patients with mast cell leukemia, the infiltrate comprises immature mast cell precursors which may also be identified in the blood film. It is perhaps somewhat of an anomaly that this entity appears with the MPD in the WHO classification rather than with the acute myeloid leukemias.

### CYTOGENETICS AND MOLECULAR BIOLOGY

The most important cytokine in mast cell development from CD34+ progenitors is stem cell factor, or KIT ligand. In a high proportion of cases of systemic mastocytosis, a mutation Asp-816-Val is often detectable in *c-kit*, which is the receptor for stem cell factor and is a valuable diagnostic marker.[71–73] This mutation is not always confined to mast cells but is sometimes demonstrable in other hematopoietic cells, including CD34+ cells. Cytogenetic abnormalities are variable and include +8, +9, del (5)(q), del (7)(q), monosomy 7, and del(20)(q).[74]

## CHRONIC MPD, UNCLASSIFIABLE

These patients have an MPD but cannot readily be classified with an individual disease entity sometimes as they display distinctive features of two MPD. This is a very heterogeneous group.

## MYELOPROLIFERATIVE/MYELODYSPLASTIC DISORDERS

### CHRONIC MYELOMONOCYTIC LEUKEMIA

CMML has features both of myelodysplasia and myeloproliferation. In the WHO classification it has migrated from the MDS catergory into the MPD/MDS disorders. To differentiate CMML from atypical CML, evaluation of the proportion of granulocytic precursors and the blood film to identify anormal monocytes are useful. The bone marrow is hypercellular and displays varying degrees of dysplasia and a monocytic infiltrate. Cytogenetic abnormalities are common (20–50%) but again none are specifically associated with CMML. Those patients with abnormal karyotypes are more likely to have advanced disease and to transform to acute leukemia.[75]

| Table 46.2 | WHO classification of mast cell disorders |
|---|---|

■ Cutaneous mastocytosis
■ Indolent systemic mastocytosis
■ Systemic mastocytosis with associated clonal haematologic non-mast cell lineage disease (including AML, MDS, MPD, CMML, NHL)
■ Aggressive systemic mastocytosis
■ Mast cell leukemia
■ Mast cell sarcoma
■ Extracutaneous mastocytoma.

Monosomy 7 is common, as are +8, der(12p) presenting as a terminal deletion or translocation, −Y.[75] Abnormalities of chromosome 5 (−5, 5q−, t(5;12)(q31p13)) are less common in CMML than in myelodysplasia.

### JUVENILE MYELOMONOCYTIC LEUKEMIA

This condition usually occurs in children less than 5 years old and encompasses conditions previously termed "juvenile chronic myeloid leukemia," infantile monosomy 7 syndrome, and other myelodysplastic/myeloproliferative diseases of childhood.

Juvenile myelomonocytic leukemia is particularly associated with monosomy 7.[76] In approximately 25–33%, other cytogenetic abnormalities (+8 and abnormalities of chromosome 7) also occur. Furthermore, there is an increased incidence in Down's syndrome and neurofibromatosis. Some 15% of children with JMML have features of neurofibromatosis, these and others without these features have abnormalities of the *NF 1* gene. Mutations of the *RAS* oncogene are present in 15–30%, but these patients do not, to date, have *NF 1* abnormalities.[77] A further factor of genetic interest includes an occasional tendency for familial cases and increased expression of hemoglobin F.

### ATYPICAL CML

Atypical CML is a rare condition that occurs in older patients and has a worse prognosis than CML. The blood film demonstrates a neutrophilia and an increase in myeloid precursors sometimes with dysplastic features; monocytosis is more pronounced than either eosinophilia or basophilia. The bone marrow features resemble CML, but an increase in monocytes is the feature which suggests atypical rather than typical CML. In common with CMML, karyotypic abnormalities are frequent in atypical CML, occurring in 30–80%,[78] +8 being the most frequent. Interestingly, a fusion gene between PDGFRβ and H4 has been reported in at least one patient.[79]

## MYELOPROLIFERATIVE/MYELODYSPLASTIC UNCLASSIFIED

Patients who display features of both myeloproliferative and myelodysplastic conditions are assigned to this diagnostic entity. A proportion will evolve and change diagnostic catergory with time. No specific cytogenetic abnormalities are reported in this diagnostic entity other than those already discussed for the other MPDs.

## SUMMARY

The MPDs and MDS/MPDs are an expanding population of largely clinically defined disorders for which thus far we lack a clear understanding of their pathogenesis and molecular biology. It seems hopeful that we may be able to expand our knowledge greatly in the future by harnessing emerging sophisticated technologies such as proteomics and microarray methods. A global culture of cooperation, identifying and sharing data from rare kindreds with apparently clonal inherited MPDs, is also likely to significantly advance knowledge in this field.

### REFERENCES

1. Dameshek W: Some speculations on the myeloproliferative syndromes. *Blood* 6:372–375, 1951.
2. Vardiman JW, Harris NL, Brunning RD: The World Health Organization (WHO) classification of the myeloid neoplasms. *Blood* 100(7):2292–2302, 2002.
3. Baxter EJ, Scott LM, Campbell PJ, et al.: Acquired mutation of the tyrosine kinase JAK2 in human myeloproliferative disorders. *Lancet* 365(9464):1054–1061, 2005.
4. James C, Ugo V, Le Couedic JP, et al.: A unique clonal JAK2 mutation leading to constitutive signalling causes polycythaemia vera. *Nature* 434(7038):1144–1148, 2005.
5. Kralovics R, Passamonti F, Buser AS, et al.: A gain-of-function mutation of JAK2 in myeloproliferative disorders. *N Engl J Med* 352(17):1779–1790, 2005.
6. Levine RL, Wadleigh M, Cools J, et al.: Activating mutation in the tyrosine kinase JAK2 in polycythemia vera, essential thrombocythemia, and myeloid metaplasia with myelofibrosis. *Cancer Cell* 7(4):387–397, 2005.
7. Zhao R, Xing S, Li Z, et al.: Identification of an acquired JAK2 mutation in Polycythemia vera. *J Biol Chem* 286(24):22788–22792, 2005.
8. Pardanani AD, Levine RL, Lasho T, et al.: MPL515 mutations in myeloproliferative and other myeloid disorders: a study of 1182 patients. *Blood*. In press.
9. Pikman Y, Lee BH, Mercher T, et al.: MPLW515L is a novel somatic activating mutation in myelofibrosis with myeloid metaplasia. *PLoS Med* 3(7):e270, 2006.
10. Scott LM, Campbell PJ, Baxter EJ, et al.: The V617F JAK2 mutation is uncommon in cancers and in myeloid malignancies other than the classic myeloproliferative disorders. *Blood* 106(8):2920–2921, 2005.
11. Ellis JT, Peterson P, Geller SA, Rappaport H: Studies of the bone marrow in polycythemia vera and the evolution of myelofibrosis and second hematologic malignancies. *Semin Hematol* 23(2):144–155, 1986.
12. Thiele J, Galle R, Sander C, Fischer R: Interactions between megakaryocytes and sinus wall. An ultrastructural study on bone marrow tissue in primary (essential) thrombocythemia. *J Submicrosc Cytol Pathol* 23(4):595–603, 1991.
13. Dewald GW, Wright PI: Chromosome abnormalities in the myeloproliferative disorders. *Semin Oncol* 22(4):341–354, 1995.

14. Najfeld V, Montella L, Scalise A, Fruchtman S: Exploring polycythaemia vera with fluorescence in situ hybridization: additional cryptic 9p is the most frequent abnormality detected. *Br J Haematol* 119(2):558–566, 2002.

15. Kralovics R, Guan Y, Prchal JT: Acquired uniparental disomy of chromosome 9p is a frequent stem cell defect in polycythemia vera. *Exp Hematol* 30(3): 229–236, 2002.

16. Khwaja A: The role of Janus kinases in haemopoiesis and haematological malignancy. *Br J Haematol* 134(4):366–384, 2006.

17. Kaushansky K: On the molecular origins of the chronic myeloproliferative disorders: it all makes sense. *Blood* 105(11):4187–4190, 2005.

18. Moliterno AR, Hankins WD, Spivak JL: Impaired expression of the thrombopoietin receptor by platelets from patients with polycythemia vera. *N Engl J Med* 338(9): 572–580, 1998.

19. Roder S, Steimle C, Meinhardt G, Pahl HL: STAT3 is constitutively active in some patients with Polycythemia rubra vera. *Exp Hematol* 29(6):694–702, 2001.

20. Temerinac S, Klippel S, Strunck E, et al.: Cloning of PRV-1, a novel member of the uPAR receptor superfamily, which is overexpressed in polycythemia rubra vera. *Blood* 95(8):2569–2576, 2000.

21. Kralovics R, Buser AS, Teo SS, et al.: Comparison of molecular markers in a cohort of patients with chronic myeloproliferative disorders. *Blood* 102(5):1869–1871, 2003.

22. Liu E, Jelinek J, Pastore YD, Guan Y, Prchal JF, Prchal JT: Discrimination of polycythemias and thrombocytoses by novel, simple, accurate clonality assays and comparison with PRV-1 expression and BFU-E response to erythropoietin. *Blood* 101(8):3294–3301, 2003.

23. Goerttler PS, Steimle C, Marz E, et al.: The Jak2V617F mutation, PRV-1 overexpression, and EEC formation define a similar cohort of MPD patients. *Blood* 106(8): 2862–2864, 2005.

24. Thiele J, Kvasnicka HM, Zankovich R, Diehl V: Relevance of bone marrow features in the differential diagnosis between essential thrombocythemia and early stage idiopathic myelofibrosis. *Haematologica* 85(11):1126–1134, 2000.

25. Annaloro C, Lambertenghi DG, Oriani A, et al.: Prognostic significance of bone marrow biopsy in essential thrombocythemia. *Haematologica* 84(1):17–21, 1999.

26. Chromosomal abnormalities in acute lymphoblastic leukemia: structural and numerical changes in 234 cases. *Cancer Genet Cytogenet* 4(2):101–110, 1981.

27. Sessarego M, Defferrari R, Dejana AM, et al.: Cytogenetic analysis in essential thrombocythemia at diagnosis and at transformation. A 12-year study *Cancer Genet Cytogenet* 43(1):57–65, 1989.

28. Harrison CN, Gale RE, Machin SJ, Linch DC: A large proportion of patients with a diagnosis of essential thrombocythemia do not have a clonal disorder and may be at lower risk of thrombotic complications. *Blood* 93(2): 417–424, 1999.

29. Shih LY, Lin TL, Lai CL, et al.: Predictive values of X-chromosome inactivation patterns and clinicohematologic parameters for vascular complications in female patients with essential thrombocythemia. *Blood* 100(5): 1596–1601, 2002.

30. Cheung B, Radia D, Pantelidis P, Yadegarfar G, Harrison C: The presence of the JAK2 V617F mutation is associated with a higher haemoglobin and increased risk of thrombosis in essential thrombocythaemia. *Br J Haematol* 132(2):244–245, 2006.

31. Wolanskyj AP, Lasho TL, Schwager SM, et al.: JAK2 mutation in essential thrombocythaemia: clinical associations and long-term prognostic relevance. *Br J Haematol* 131(2):208–213, 2005.

32. Scott LM, Scott MA, Campbell PJ, Green AR: Progenitors homozygous for the V617F JAK2 mutation occur in most patients with polycythemia vera, but not essential thrombocythemia. *Blood* 108(7):2435–2437, 2006.

33. Campbell PJ, Green AR: Management of polycythemia vera and essential thrombocythemia. *Hematology (Am Soc Hematol Educ Program )* 201–208, 2005.

34. Campbell PJ, Scott LM, Buck G, et al.: Definition of subtypes of essential thrombocythaemia and relation to polycythaemia vera based on JAK2 V617F mutation status: a prospective study. *Lancet* 366(9501):1945–1953, 2005.

35. Pardanani AD, Levine RL, Lasho T, et al.: MPL515 mutations in myeloproliferative and other myeloid disorders: a study of 1182 patients. *Blood*. In press.

36. Campbell PJ, Baxter EJ, Beer PA, et al.: Mutation of JAK2 in the myeloproliferative disorders: timing, clonality studies, cytogenetic associations and role in leukemic transformation. *Blood*. In press.

37. Wolanskyj AP, Lasho TL, Schwager SM, et al.: JAK2 mutation in essential thrombocythaemia: clinical associations and long-term prognostic relevance. *Br J Haematol* 131(2):208–213, 2005.

38. Kralovics R, Teo SS, Li S, et al.: Acquisition of the V617F mutation of JAK2 is a late genetic event in a subset of patients with myeloproliferative disorders. *Blood* 108(4): 1377–1380, 2006.

39. Rumi E, Passamonti F, Pietra D, et al.: JAK2 (V617F) as an acquired somatic mutation and a secondary genetic event associated with disease progression in familial myeloproliferative disorders. *Cancer* 107(9):2206–2211, 2006.

40. Thiele J, Kvasnicka HM, Fischer R, Diehl V: Clinicopathological impact of the interaction between megakaryocytes and myeloid stroma in chronic myeloproliferative disorders: a concise update. *Leuk Lymphoma* 24(5–6):463–481, 1997.

41. Mesa RA, Li CY, Schroeder G, Tefferi A: Clinical correlates of splenic histopathology and splenic karyotype in myelofibrosis with myeloid metaplasia. *Blood* 97(11): 3665–3667, 2001.

42. Thiele J, Kvasnicka HM, Werden C, Zankovich R, Diehl V, Fischer R: Idiopathic primary osteo-myelofibrosis: a clinico-pathological study on 208 patients with special emphasis on evolution of disease features, differentiation from essential thrombocythemia and variables of prognostic impact. *Leuk Lymphoma* 22(3–4):303–317, 1996.

43. Wang JC, Lang HD, Lichter S, Weinstein M, Benn P: Cytogenetic studies of bone marrow fibroblasts cultured from patients with myelofibrosis and myeloid metaplasia. *Br J Haematol* 80(2):184–188, 1992.

44. Demory JL, Dupriez B, Fenaux P, et al.: Cytogenetic studies and their prognostic significance in agnogenic myeloid metaplasia: a report on 47 cases. *Blood* 72(3): 855–859, 1988.

45. Tefferi A, Mesa RA, Schroeder G, Hanson CA, Li CY, Dewald GW: Cytogenetic findings and their clinical relevance in myelofibrosis with myeloid metaplasia. *Br J Haematol* 113(3):763–771, 2001.

46. ez-Martin JL, Graham DL, Petitt RM, Dewald GW: Chromosome studies in 104 patients with polycythemia vera. *Mayo Clin Proc* 66(3):287–299, 1991.

47. Emilia G, Sacchi S, Temperani P, Longo R, Vecchi A: Progression of essential thrombocythemia to blastic crisis via idiopathic myelofibrosis. *Leuk Lymphoma* 9(4–5): 423–426, 1993.

48. Juneau AL, Kaehler M, Christensen ER, et al.: Detection of RB1 deletions by fluorescence in situ hybridization in malignant hematologic disorders. *Cancer Genet Cytogenet* 103(2):117–123, 1998.

49. Le Bousse-Kerdiles MC, Martyre MC: Involvement of the fibrogenic cytokines, TGF-beta and bFGF, in the pathogenesis of idiopathic myelofibrosis. *Pathol Biol (Paris)* 49(2):153–157, 2001.

50. Schmitt A, Drouin A, Masse JM, Guichard J, Shagraoui H, Cramer EM: Polymorphonuclear neutrophil and megakaryocyte mutual involvement in myelofibrosis pathogenesis. *Leuk Lymphoma* 43(4):719–724, 2002.

51. Campbell PJ, Griesshammer M, Dohner K, et al.: The V617F mutation in JAK2 is associated with poorer survival in idiopathic myelofibrosis. *Blood* 107(5):2098–2100, 2005.

52. Tefferi A, Lasho TL, Schwager SM, et al.: The JAK2(V617F) tyrosine kinase mutation in myelofibrosis with myeloid metaplasia: lineage specificity and clinical correlates. *Br J Haematol* 131(3):320–328, 2005.

53. Moliterno AR, Williams DM, Rogers O, Spivak JL: Molecular mimicry in the chronic myeloproliferative disorders: reciprocity between quantitative JAK2 V617F and Mpl expression. *Blood*. In press.

54. Passamonti F, Rumi E, Pietra D, et al.: Relation between JAK2 (V617F) mutation status, granulocyte activation, and constitutive mobilization of CD34+ cells into peripheral blood in myeloproliferative disorders. *Blood* 107(9):3676–3682, 2006.

55. Tefferi A, Lasho TL, Schwager SM, et al.: The clinical phenotype of wild-type, heterozygous, and homozygous JAK2V617F in polycythemia vera. *Cancer* 106(3): 631–635, 2006.

56. Simon HU, Plotz SG, Dummer R, Blaser K: Abnormal clones of T cells producing interleukin-5 in idiopathic eosinophilia. *N Engl J Med* 341(15):1112–1120, 1999.

57. Chang HW, Leong KH, Koh DR, Lee SH: Clonality of isolated eosinophils in the hypereosinophilic syndrome. *Blood* 93(5):1651–1657, 1999.

58. Golub TR, Barker GF, Lovett M, Gilliland DG: Fusion of PDGF receptor beta to a novel ets-like gene, tel, in chronic myelomonocytic leukemia with t(5;12) chromosomal translocation. *Cell* 77(2):307–316, 1994.

59. Bain BJ: Eosinophilic leukaemias and the idiopathic hypereosinophilic syndrome. *Br J Haematol* 95(1):2–9, 1996.

60. Macdonald D, Aguiar RC, Mason PJ, Goldman JM, Cross NC: A new myeloproliferative disorder associated with chromosomal translocations involving 8p11: a review. *Leukemia* 9(10):1628–1630, 1995.

61. Reiter A, Sohal J, Kulkarni S, et al.: Consistent fusion of ZNF198 to the fibroblast growth factor receptor-1 in the t(8;13)(p11;q12) myeloproliferative syndrome. *Blood* 92(5):1735–1742, 1998.

62. Abruzzo LV, Jaffe ES, Cotelingam JD, Whang-Peng J, Del DV Jr., Medeiros LJ: T-cell lymphoblastic lymphoma with eosinophilia associated with subsequent myeloid malignancy. *Am J Surg Pathol* 16(3):236–245, 1992.

63. Xiao S, Nalabolu SR, Aster JC, et al.: FGFR1 is fused with a novel zinc-finger gene, ZNF198, in the t(8;13) leukaemia/lymphoma syndrome. *Nat Genet* 18(1):84–87, 1998.

64. Cools J, DeAngelo DJ, Gotlib J, et al.: A tyrosine kinase created by fusion of the PDGFRA and FIP1L1 genes as a therapeutic target of imatinib in idiopathic hypereosinophilic syndrome. *N Engl J Med* 348(13):1201–1214, 2003.

65. Pardanani A, Ketterling RP, Brockman SR, et al.: CHIC2 deletion, a surrogate for FIP1L1-PDGFRA fusion, occurs in systemic mastocytosis associated with eosinophilia and predicts response to imatinib mesylate therapy. *Blood* 102(9):3093–3096, 2003.

66. Pardanani A, Elliott M, Reeder T, et al.: Imatinib for systemic mast-cell disease. *Lancet* 362(9383):535–536, 2003.

67. Wilkinson K, Velloso ER, Lopes LF, et al.: Cloning of the t(1;5)(q23;q33) in a myeloproliferative disorder associated with eosinophilia: involvement of PDGFRB and response to imatinib. *Blood* 102(12):4187–4190, 2003.

68. Apperley JF, Gardembas M, Melo JV, et al.: Response to imatinib mesylate in patients with chronic myeloproliferative diseases with rearrangements of the platelet-derived growth factor receptor beta 1. *N Engl J Med* 347(7):481–487, 2002.

69. Reilly JT: Chronic neutrophilic leukaemia: a distinct clinical entity? *Br J Haematol* 116(1):10–18, 2002.

70. Valent P, Akin C, Sperr WR, Horny HP, Metcalfe DD: Mast cell proliferative disorders: current view on variants recognized by the World Health Organization. *Hematol Oncol Clin North Am* 17(5):1227–1241, 2003.

71. Longley BJ, Tyrrell L, Lu SZ, et al.: Somatic c-KIT activating mutation in urticaria pigmentosa and aggressive mastocytosis: establishment of clonality in a human mast cell neoplasm. *Nat Genet* 12(3):312–314, 1996.

72. Longley BJ Jr., Metcalfe DD, Tharp M, et al.: Activating and dominant inactivating c-KIT catalytic domain mutations in distinct clinical forms of human mastocytosis. *Proc Natl Acad Sci U S A* 96(4):1609–1614, 1999.

73. Akin C, Kirshenbaum AS, Semere T, Worobec AS, Scott LM, Metcalfe DD: Analysis of the surface expression of c-kit and occurrence of the c-kit Asp816Val activating mutation in T cells, B cells, and myelomonocytic cells in patients with mastocytosis. *Exp Hematol* 28(2):140–147, 2000.

74. Bain BJ: Systemic mastocytosis and other mast cell neoplasms. *Br J Haematol* 106(1):9–17, 1999.

75. Chronic myelomonocytic leukemia: single entity or heterogeneous disorder? A prospective multicenter study of 100 patients. Groupe Francais de Cytogenetique Hematologique. *Cancer Genet Cytogenet* 55(1):57–65, 1991.

76. Sieff CA, Chessells JM, Harvey BA, Pickthall VJ, Lawler SD: Monosomy 7 in childhood: a myeloproliferative disorder. *Br J Haematol* 49(2):235–249, 1981.

77. Emanuel PD: Myelodysplasia and myeloproliferative disorders in childhood: an update. *Br J Haematol* 105(4):852–863, 1999.

78. Martiat P, Michaux JL, Rodhain J: Philadelphia-negative (Ph-) chronic myeloid leukemia (CML): comparison with Ph+ CML and chronic myelomonocytic leukemia.

The Groupe Francais de Cytogenetique Hematologique. *Blood* 78(1):205–211, 1991.

79. Kulkarni S, Heath C, Parker S, et al.: Fusion of H4/D10S170 to the platelet-derived growth factor receptor beta in BCR-ABL-negative myeloproliferative disorders with a t(5;10)(q33;q21). *Cancer Res* 60(13):3592–3598, 2000.

# Chapter 47
# CLINICAL FEATURES AND MAKING THE DIAGNOSIS

*Richard T. Silver*

## INTRODUCTION

Under normal circumstances, the marrow progenitor cells respond selectively to differing but specific stimuli. Examples include the rise in white blood cell (WBC) count that occurs during a bacterial infection or the elevation of the platelet count after hemorrhage. Reactions such as these are self-limited, for the marrow reverts to its normal status once the stimulus subsides. Myeloproliferative disorders (MPDs), on the other hand, comprise a group of diseases in which pluripotent stem cells proliferate more or less *en masse*, at least at the onset of the illness. In the hematology literature, opinions differ as to which diseases should be included in the MPD group, but based upon improvements in clinical diagnosis and refinements in cytogenetics, and molecular biology, the diseases of major clinical importance include chronic myeloid leukemia (CML), polycythemia vera (PV), essential thrombocythemia (ET) and agnogenic myeloid metaplasia (AMM). In general, the diagnostic difficulties associated with the MPDs relate to their clinical symmetry ("clinical mimicry") and, except for CML, the lack of clinically applicable clonal markers. Thus, they share similar clinical and hematologic features. Their origin from a multipotent hematopoietic stem cell leads to clonal dominance over normal hematopoietic progenitor cells, giving rise to increased production of one or more of the formed elements of the blood. As examples, in PV, although an increased red blood cell (RBC) mass is the *sine qua non* at diagnosis, such patients often have an increase in the WBC count and/or platelet count. Physical examination of a patient with an MPD often reveals an enlarged spleen and biochemical abnormalities such as elevation in the serum values of uric acid, vitamin $B_{12}$, and $B_{12}$-binding protein. A biochemical marker that can be of value in distinguishing one MPD from another is the concentration of leukocyte alkaline phosphatase found in the cytoplasm of neutrophils. It is typically absent in patients with CML, increased in PV and ET, and variably increased, normal, or decreased in AMM. Although cytogenetic abnormalities are seen in all patients with the MPDs, the only consistent cytogenetic abnormality, the Philadelphia (Ph) chromosome, occurs in CML, sharply distinguishing it from the others. To a varying degree, increased reticulin fibers are present in the bone marrow in all the MPDs, and as the disease progresses, fibroblastic proliferation becomes evident (probably a reactive phenomenon).

Only recently has it been appreciated that the megakaryocytes are morphologically abnormal in the myeloproliferative diseases, and biologically, are central to the genesis of the fibrosis that occurs in the marrows of patients with MPDs. An experienced hematopathologist may suspect the appropriate clinical diagnosis by studying the structural characteristics of the megakaryocytes in a bone marrow biopsy from a patient with an MPD, as their appearance differs among the four diseases.

Acute leukemia develops as an end result of all the MPDs. In decreasing order of frequency, it occurs in CML, AMM, PV, and rarely in ET.[1,2] Acute leukemia may be a natural evolution of the disease, as is seen most often in CML, or it may also be related to the drugs used in treating the primary illness.[1,2]

## CHRONIC MYELOID LEUKEMIA

CML develops with an insidious onset of symptoms and signs, which may include fatigue, anemia, splenomegaly, and leukocytosis marked by an increase in neutrophils, eosinophils, and basophils. The median age of onset is 50 years[1,2] the peak incidence occurs between 50 and 60 years.[1,2] The frequency increases with age. CML occurs equally in males and females.[1]

There are three phases of the disease: the first, a chronic phase, lasts 30–40 months; the second is a transitional phase called the accelerated phase; and the terminal blast or acute ("blast crisis") phase, in which the disease resembles acute leukemia. In some patients, there is no transitional phase, and the disease transforms abruptly into an acute phase.

## CHRONIC PHASE OF CML

In the chronic phase, the WBC count approximates 200,000/dL. The myelocyte is the predominating cell in both peripheral blood and marrow. Myeloblasts are rare. Basophilia and eosinophilia are common. There may be slight anemia, which is normocytic and normochromic. The platelet count may be normal, decreased, or increased, but more than half of the patients have platelet counts greater than 1 million/μL;[2] however, thrombotic phenomena are rare.[3] The bone marrow is hypercellular, with a striking increase in granulocytic cells. Cells resembling Gaucher cells (sea-blue histiocytes) are observed in about 10% of cases.[4] Megakaryocytes are smaller than normal. Reticulin, in biopsy sections, is increased. Collagen stains may show fibrosis. Of unique importance is the presence of the Ph chromosome, demonstrated in approximately 95% of all CML patients. Those patient with phenotypic characteristics of CML but locking the ph chromosome must have marrow or blood specimens examined for the molecular abnormality, the BCR-ABL oncogene, which is present in all cases. By definition, those patients in whom the BCR-ABL oncogene cannot be found are considered to have an "atypical myeloproliferative disease" or "atypical CML."

The blast crises are divided into two general types, myeloid and lymphoid. Biphenotypic or mixed lymphoblastic–myeloblastic crises also have been observed.[5] Lymphoid blast crisis occurs in 20–30% of patients. The cells often resemble those seen in acute lymphocytic leukemia and contain terminal deoxynucleotidyl transferase.[6] (Terminal deoxynucleotidyl transferase is found mainly in poorly differentiated normal and malignant lymphoid cells of T-cell and B-cell origin and is lost as these lymphocytes differentiate and mature). Myeloid blast crisis may mimic acute myeloid leukemia. Megakaryoblastic[7] and erythroblastic[8] transformations and blast crises marked by basophilia also have been reported.

### MAKING THE DIAGNOSIS

Although the complete blood count and bone marrow findings in CML cases may be classic, less marked phenotypic presentations may mimic other myeloproliferative diseases, especially AMM. The diagnosis rests on the demonstration of the Ph chromosome in the bone marrow, the (9;22) translocation in the marrow or peripheral blood by FISH (fluorescent in situ hybridization) studies, or by reverse transcriptase analysis by polymerase chain reaction (RT-PCR) of the marrow or blood for the molecular abnormality, the BCR-ABL oncogene.

## POLYCYTHEMIA VERA (PV)

Polycythemia is defined as an increase in the volume of circulating RBCs per kilogram of body weight or, equivalently, an increase in the RBC mass. Clinically, this is expressed as an absolute increase in the number of RBCs, usually but not always accompanied by corresponding increases in the hemoglobin and hematocrit (though the hematocrit may be affected by plasma volume). Polycythemia may occur as a primary disease of unknown cause (polycythemia vera) or as a secondary manifestation of other illnesses. The diagnosis of PV is made only after other causes of secondary polycythemia have been excluded (Table 47.1).

The terms erythremia and erythrocytosis are often used to refer to primary and secondary polycythemia, respectively. Others use erythremia as a classification for patients whose only abnormality is an increased RBC volume. Both terms are superfluous and confusing, and therefore are not recommended. The term "relative" polycythemia is also a misnomer and its use should be discontinued. Similarly, "false" polycythemia is a confusing term; it is not polycythemia because the RBC volume per kilogram of body weight is normal. In this instance, the increased hematocrit is related to a decrease in plasma volume (whereas in true polycythemia, the plasma volume is usually increased, but it may also be decreased). Other terms referring to false or relative polycythemia include

| Table 47.1    Clinical classification of the polycythemias |
|---|
| *Secondary polycythemia* |
| (1) Related to inadequate oxygen delivery to tissues with respect to need |
|    (1.1) Due to decreased arterial oxygen tension |
|       (1.1.1) With physiologic or anatomic cardiopulmonary abnormalities: |
|          ■ abnormalities of lungs, chest bellows, or ventilatory |
|          ■ control mechanisms |
|          ■ right-to-left vascular shunts |
|       (1.1.2) Without physiologic or anatomic cardiopulmonary abnormalities: |
|          ■ low oxygen tension, i.e., high altitudes |
|          ■ impaired oxygen-carrying capacity of hemoglobin |
|    (1.2) Due to decreased blood flow—congestive heart failure |
| (2) Unrelated to inadequate oxygen delivery and need, and associated with benign or malignant lesions of the following: |
|    ■ kidney—cysts, hydronephrosis, adenoma, hyper-nephroma |
|    ■ cerebellum—hemangioblastoma |
|    ■ uterus—myoma |
|    ■ liver—hepatoma, hamartoma |
|    ■ other—adrenal (pheochromocytoma), lung |
| *Familial polycythemias (normal hemoglobin function)* |
| *Primary polycythemia (polycythemia vera)* |

| Table 47.2 | Relation of absolute erthrocytosis (AE) to hematocrit (Hct)[10] |
| --- | --- |
| Hct (%) | % of patients with AE |
| 50–52 | 18 |
| 56–58 | 65 |
| >60 | 100 |

stress polycythemia, stress erythrocytosis, pseudopolycythemia, and benign polycythemia. Likewise, these terms should be discarded. As it is not possible to predict an increased RBC mass by a single hematocrit determination, particularly in the lower range of increased hematocrit values, a chromium-51 RBC mass (volume) determination is mandatory. For hematocrit values more than 60%, it is not necessary to determine a Cr[51] RBC mass[2,9] (Table 47.2).

*Polycythemia vera* is a disease characterized not only by proliferation of erythroid progenitors (which results in the increased RBC mass), but also by early myeloid cells and megakaryocytes. An increasing number of cases are now being detected prior to the development of symptoms through the use of routine screening blood counts. The median age in one series of more than 100 patients is about 50 years, and nearly 40% of the patients are seen while in their 30s and 40s.[10] Other series report an older age group.[12,13] Symptoms related to hypervolemia and hyperviscosity are usually accentuated by an increase in platelet count. Headaches, lightheadedness, vertigo, and blurred vision may occur. A most troublesome symptom is pruritus, worse after a hot bath or shower, and called "aquagenic pruritus." Spontaneous bruising, peptic ulcers, and gastrointestinal hemorrhage are seen as the disease progresses. Secondary gout and uric acid kidney stones are relatively frequent, occurring in about 10% of the patients.[11]

Untreated patients are also at risk for both thrombotic and hemorrhagic events,[14] but in our series, thrombosis predominates (cerebrovascular, cardiovascular, and lower extremity, especially). Erythromelalgia (painful fingertips and toes) is frequent. A serious thrombotic event occurring in about 10% of patients with PV is the Budd–Chiarri syndrome, due to hepatic vein thrombosis.[14] This is marked by hepatosplenomegaly, ascites, edema of the lower extremities, and other consequences of portal vein obstruction.

On physical examination, about 60% of the patients in our series have had an enlarged spleen, usually 1–2 cm below the left costal margin. The complexion is usually normal, but in more advanced cases it may be dusky.

Laboratory studies reveal, in addition to the increased RBC mass (for men, RBC ≥36cm³/kg; in women ≥32cm³/kg), an elevated WBC (above 10,000/μL) in approximately 60% of patients and an increased platelet count above 400,000/μL in 75% of patients.[9] Examination of the peripheral blood smear shows a higher percentage of neutrophils, and an increased number of basophils and eosinophils. Evidence of iron deficiency exists, particularly in the bone marrow. Because of occult gastrointestinal or other internal bleeding, anemia may initially mask the diagnosis of polycythemia. Iron deficiency is manifested by a low serum iron and increased ferritin values.

As the disease progresses, extramedullary hematopoiesis (i.e., hematopoiesis in sites other than the bone marrow) occurs, often accompanied by myelofibrosis in the bone marrow. The end stage of PV is morphologically indistinguishable from that of AMM [primary myelofibrosis with myeloid metaplasia (MMM)].

Unlike CML, in PV there is no unique or specific cytogenetic marker of the disease. However, the recently, repeated molecular, abnormality, the V617F (JAK2), is of great importance SNCE 95% or more patients abnormality.[14] However, newer and more easily performed laboratory tests have demonstrated monoclonality in a number of patients with PV. Certain karyotypic changes are seen in approximately 20% of patients with PV. The most common abnormalities involve chromosomes 20 (20q(), or 9, trisomy of chromosome 8, and deletions of chromosomes 5 or 7[15] (see Chapter 46).

Recently, it has been shown that there is impaired expression of the thrombopoietin receptor, Mpl, in the platelets of patients with PV and ET.[16,17] Another genetic marker, the *PRV-1* gene, has been reported to be overexpressed in the RNA of peripheral blood granulocytes of both patients with PV and patients with ET.[18] Testing of these markers may also be valuable for diagnosis in the future, though it is too early to use these genetic markers in practice. A schema suggested for the evaluation of patients suspected of PV is shown in Table 47.3.

| Table 47.3 | Suggested evaluation of a patient with polycythemia |
| --- | --- |
| History (family history important to exclude hemoglobinopathies and familial polycythemias) |
| Physical examination, including neurologic and pelvic examinations |
| Complete blood count, reticulocyte count, platelet count, serum uric acid |
| Urinalysis |
| Red blood cell volume with Cr[51] |
| JAK2 determination |
| Serum erythropoietin |
| Arterial oxygen saturation |
| Bone marrow aspiration and biopsy with stains for iron, reticulin, and collagen |
| Chest X-ray, electrocardiogram |
| Optional: |
|   – Leukocyte alkaline phosphatase determination |
|   – Hemoglobin electrophoresis |
|   – Vitamin $B_{12}$ and vitamin $B_{12}$-binding capacity |

**Table 47.4** Criteria for the diagnosis of polycythemia vera (Polycythemia Vera Study Group Criteria)

| | |
|---|---|
| $A_1$ Increased RBC mass<br>Men $\geq$36 cm$^3$ / kg<br>Women $\geq$32 cm$^3$/kg | $B_1$ Thrombocytosis, platelets<br>>600,000/cells/mm$^3$ |
| $A_2$ Arterial oxygen $\geq$92% | $B_2$ WBC count<br>$\geq$12,000/mm$^3$ in absence<br>of fever or infarction |
| $A_3$ Splenomegaly | $B_3$ Leukocyte alkaline<br>phosphatase score >100<br>$B_4$ Elevated serum vitamin $B_{12}$<br>(>900 pg/mL) or elevated<br>unsaturated vitamin $B_{12}$-<br>binding capacity >2200<br>pg/mL |

The diagnosis is acceptable if $A_1$, $A_2$, and $A_3$ are present:
  (1)    $A_1$    +    $A_2$    +    $A_3$
  or, in the absence of splenomegaly,

  (2)    A1    1    +    A2 and any two of column B

**Table 47.5** Suggested diagnostic criteria, polycythemia vera

Must have*
  (a) Increased RBC mass or Hct $\geq$60% in men,
      58% in women
  (b) Absence of any cause of secondary erythrocytosis
      or familial polycythemia (assumes serum eythro
      poietin level not increased)
And any three of the following:
  (c) Palpable splenomegaly
  (d) serum erythropoietin <5U/mL
  (e) Platelets $\geq$400,000/$\mu$L
  (f) WBC $\geq$12,000/$\mu$L
  (g) Bone marrow biopsy

      (i) Cellularity, reticulin, fibrosis
      (ii) Megakaryocyte abnormalities

* Please see text regarding JAK2 expression

Until recently, the diagnosis of PV was made after all causes of secondary polycythemia had been excluded (Table 47.1). The most commonly used criteria for the diagnosis of PV had been those of the Polycythemia Vera Study Group (PVSG).[11] These criteria were established for diagnosing patients with active polycythemia entering a therapeutic trial comparing the value of phlebotomy only, chlorambucil, or P-32.[11] For historical purposes, the PVSG diagnostic criteria are shown in Table 47.4. Note that the RBC mass determination was used *both* for establishing the existence of polycythemia per se and as a criterion for diagnosing PV. Categories $B_2$, $B_3$, and $B_4$ all reflect an increase in WBCs and their progenitors. (Yet in our series, only 60% of patients had a leukocytosis).

There are many other limitations of these criteria, which were, in fact, appreciated by the PVSG. Nevertheless, in the ensuing 40 years they have been used, and/or cited in the literature, for diagnosing patients with PV at least 270 times.[11,18] Other limitations of the criteria include the following: (1) the increase in RBC mass should be used to establish whether or not a patient is polycythemic, and not as a diagnostic criterion; (2) the abnormalities seen on bone marrow biopsy characteristic of PV are not mentioned: these are panhyperplasia, absent iron stores, increased reticulin fibers, and morphologic abnormalities of the megakaryocytes[19]; (3) determination of the serum erythropoietin level is not required.

### MAKING THE DIAGNOSIS

A more contemporary approach to the diagnosis of PV is outlined in Table 47.5. It includes the demonstration of an increased RBC mass, particularly for patients with only a modest increase in hematocrit. It is not possible to predict an increased RBC mass from a single hematocrit value, except for a hematocrit more than 60% in men and 58% in women. A careful history, physical examination, and screening laboratory studies, including oxygen saturation values, should exclude polycythemia due to inadequate oxygen delivery to tissues with respect to need; a serum erythropoietin value should be elevated in those cases where the polycythemia is associated with a benign or malignant tumor. As always, an accurate history is important. It should exclude familial polycythemias.

A proactive approach to the diagnosis of PV is shown in Table 47.5. Splenomegaly occurs in about 60% of patients, an elevated WBC in 60%, increased platelets in 75%. In PV, the serum erythropoietin most often, but not always, is less than 5U/mL. A bone marrow biopsy is helpful, both for establishing the diagnosis and for baseline purposes in order to follow the progress of the disease. Due attention should be paid to cellularity (panhyperplasia), iron stores (which should be diminished or absent), reticulin content and fibrosis, and abnormal megakaryocyte morphology.

## ESSENTIAL THROMBOCYTHEMIA (ET)

By far the most common cause of thrombocytosis in general medical practice is a reactive or secondary process. This is related to acute or occult bleeding, infection, or malignant diseases. Thus, a careful history, physical examination, and appropriate laboratory studies should establish the cause of secondary thrombocytosis in the majority of cases.

Thrombocytosis may be associated with the myelodysplastic 5q− syndrome, which is characterized by deletion of the long arm of chromosome 5 (see Chapter X). In addition to thrombocytosis, these patients will often have anemia and immature granulocytes including myeloblasts in the peripheral blood and/or bone marrow. Thus, cytogenetic studies are crucial in excluding this diagnosis.

In the absence of causes of secondary thrombocytosis, a diagnosis of ET may be considered when a patient is found with an increased platelet count (≥400,000/μL), symptoms of thrombosis (usually), or hemorrhage. ET is a disease characterized by an increased platelet count owing to proliferation of an abnormal clone of megakaryocytes unresponsive to normal control mechanisms governing platelet production.

ET affects young and middle-aged women and men. Recurrent thromboses and, paradoxically, bleeding are the cardinal features. Although some patients, particularly younger ones, remain asymptomatic for long periods, approximately 50% of patients with ET are first seen as emergencies because of an episode of vascular occlusion that may be either arterial, venous, or both.

In our center, most younger patients present with thromboses rather than hemorrhage. Variable symptoms and signs include transient ischemic attacks, stroke, thrombosis of the splenic and/or hepatic veins, and evidence of peripheral circulatory impairment characterized by digital cyanosis, erythromelalgia, and pain and burning owing to microvascular clogging of small vessels by platelets. Clinical bleeding is manifested by easy bruising, bleeding of mucosal surfaces, epistaxis, unexplained hemorrhage, and postoperative hemorrhage.

Aside from the physical findings related to the aforementioned, physical examination of the asymptomatic patient is usually unremarkable. About one third of asymptomatic patients have splenomegaly, which is only modest in degree (1–3 cm below the left costal margin).

The peripheral smear shows clusters and clumps of megakaryocytes and giant platelets. Granulocyte and RBC morphology is essentially normal. The WBC is slightly increased in a minority of patients. Cytogenetic abnormalities (not related to the Ph chromosome diagnostic of CML) are present in only a few patients with ET. The overall significance of cytogenetic abnormalities in terms of clinical course and prognosis is unclear.

Sometimes, an often unrecognized and curious laboratory abnormality may lead to the diagnosis of ET in asymptomatic patients. When a routine electrolyte panel is submitted for analysis, an artificially abnormal high potassium value may be found. This is due to loss of potassium released from large numbers of platelets, which occurs during clotting in vitro. This abnormality is not associated with any deleterious clinical effect. This spuriously high potassium value is known as pseudohyperkalemia. If a potassium determination is required from a patient with ET, a plasma sample, wherein unclotted blood is submitted for laboratory analysis, will avoid this problem.

As in PV, abnormalities of the MpL receptor abnormality[16,17] and the *PRV-1* gene occur in ET.[18] As yet, the practical clinical use of these two tests remains to be established. Abnormal JAK2 expression has been observed in approximately 50% of patients with ET. It has been suggested that the course of JAK2 (+) patient may be more aggresive than JAK2 (−) patients but it is too soon to rely in this statement as fact.[19] Thus, ET is largely based on exclusion of secondary reactive causes of thrombocytosis.

Recently, in ET, the morphologic changes in marrow megakaryocytes have been appreciated.[20] Thus, all patients with a presumptive diagnosis of ET should have a marrow biopsy performed. In reactive thrombocytosis, the number of megakaryocytes is slightly-to-moderately increased, but size and nuclear lobulation remain normal; there is no tendency for megakaryocytes to cluster together. Megakaryocytes in ET, increased in number, are scattered or loosely grouped within the bone marrow. ET megakaryocytes are characterized by large, giant-sized megakaryocytes and exhibit deeply lobulated staghorn-like nuclei. Sheets and clumps of platelets may be associated with masses of platelet debris.

The platelet abnormality occurring in ET cannot be quantified by any measure of platelet dysfunction; despite a great deal of research, the pathophysiologic basis for excessive bleeding and thrombosis is not clearly understood. The results of in vitro platelet function tests are variable and show impaired or absent epinephrine-induced platelet aggregation. There is no exact correlation between the platelet count and thrombosis or hemorrhage, although in general, the higher the platelet count, the greater is the likelihood of these events occurring.

The diagnostic criteria for ET are shown in Table 47.6. These criteria are based on modified criteria proposed originally by the Polycythemia Vera Study Group (PVSG) and the World Health Organization.[21] All criteria must be fulfilled to make a diagnosis of ET. Note that collagen fibrosis of the marrow in 1/3 of the marrow was allowed by the PVSG. Permitting this degree of fibrosis may confuse ET with early cases of AMM (MMM).

### MAKING THE DIAGNOSIS

The platelet count of reactive thrombocytosis accompanying inflammation, bleeding, cancer, or infection is rarely elevated to the degree seen in ET. A Serum, ferretin level is helpful in excluding iron deficiency (bleeding as a cause of thrombocytosis). Thrombosis never occurs in secondary thrombocytosis. All patients considered to have ET should have cytogenetic or molecular studies performed to exclude CML, a disease that can present in a patient with an increased platelet count and only a modest elevation of the WBC. For patients with borderline or moderately elevated RBC values, a $Cr^{51}$ RBC mass study is mandatory to exclude PV. JAK2

**Table 47.6** Suggested diagnostic criteria, essential thrombocythemia

1. Sustained platelet count greater than $400 \times 10^3/L$

2. No cause for a reactive thrombocytosis due to inflammation, infection, bleeding, neoplasia, prior splenectomy

3. Hematocrit less than 40% or normal red blood cell (RBC) mass

4. Stainable iron in the marrow or normal RBC mean corpuscular volume

5. No Ph chromosome or *bcr/abl* gene rearrangement

6. Bone marrow biopsy specimen showing proliferation mainly of the megakaryocytic lineage with increased numbers of enlarged, mature megakaryocytes with nuclei resembling staghorns

7. Collagen fibrosis of the bone marrow absent. Reticulin fibrosis minimal or absent

8. No significant splenomegaly or leukoerythroblastic blood film

9. No evidence of a myelodysplastic syndrome

positivity is helpful in diagnosis in about half the patient seen.

## AGNOGENIC MYELOID METAPLASIA (AMM)—MYELOFIBROSIS WITH MYELOID METAPLASIA (MMM)

AMM (also known as idiopathic MMM), is characterized initially by a hypercellular bone marrow, extramedullary hematopoiesis, splenomegaly, and a leukoerythroblastic peripheral blood picture. The disease can be defined as the causally unknown (agnogenic) proliferation of hematopoietic cells (myeloid cells) in organs or tissues that are not usually involved in blood cell formation (metaplasia). *Extramedullary hematopoiesis* is a term meaning that this blood cell formation occurs outside the medullary or bone marrow cavity. Leukoerythroblastic anemia means that WBCs and RBCs of varying degrees of immaturity are seen in the peripheral blood.

AMM occurs primarily in older patients. Nearly two thirds of the cases occur between the ages of 50 and 70, about equally in men and in women. Symptoms and signs depend upon the stage of disease when the patient is first encountered. Most often, symptoms are related to anemia and/or an enlarged spleen. Otosclerosis, which can be a presenting symptom in advanced cases, causes deafness in about 10% of patients.

Symptoms and signs depend upon the stage of disease when the patient is first seen. Classically, the spleen is enlarged, the degree depending upon the severity and/or duration of the disease. About a fourth of the patients are asymptomatic and seek medical attention solely because an enlarged spleen is found on routine physical examination, or because of an abnormal peripheral blood smear. Those patients who become symptomatic suffer from fatigue, symptoms related to an enlarged spleen, gout due to elevated uric acid levels, and constitutional symptoms such as weight loss, night sweats, fatigue, and peripheral edema. The latter represent advanced symptoms. Pressure of a large spleen on the stomach may lead to delayed gastric emptying and early satiety.[21] Myeloid metaplasia may occur in unusual sites, such as the pulmonary, gastrointestinal, and central nervous systems. Although extramedullary hematopoiesis occurs frequently in the lymph nodes, it rarely accounts for significant nodal enlargement.

Splenomegaly may be found only on radiographic or sonographic examination when it cannot be appreciated clinically.

The hemoglobin ranges between 9 and 13 g/dL. The WBC count is elevated in about half of the patients, normal in one third, and low in the remainder. Examination of the peripheral blood smear discloses a shift toward granulocytic immaturity, including a few myeloblasts and promyelocytes. Significant changes in the RBCs include variation in size and shape and teardrop-shaped forms (though teardrop forms are not specific for AMM). Large fragments and clumps of megakaryocytes and large platelets may be seen. Nucleated RBCs are noted in advanced cases. The platelet count may be increased, normal, or low, depending upon the stage of disease.

The bone marrow aspirate in almost every patient yields a "dry tap," even when the marrow biopsy is highly cellular. Recently, a prefibrotic stage of AMM without splenomegaly has been defined, with the diagnosis based on bone marrow findings (see below). Thus, unless a marrow examination is performed when the patient is initially seen, the clinical diagnosis may be confused with ET. A bone marrow biopsy shows panhypercellularity in the early stages of the disease and, most strikingly, increased numbers of morphologically atypical megakaryocytes appearing in clusters.[18,22] These changes occur when there is little fibrosis, and have been labeled "the prefibrotic state."[22] Previously, such patients had been incorrectly thought to have ET.[22] Often the nuclear segmentation with hypolobulation of the megakaryocytes gives rise to a bulbous or open nuclear appearance. Megakaryocytes in AMM are more atypical than those in other subtypes of MPDs, and consequently present the major discriminating diagnostic hallmark. As the disease progresses, there is a striking increase in reticulin and collagen fibrosis. In advanced stages, overt collagen and fibrous osteosclerosis is noted. Special silver stains demonstrate an increase in the amount of reticulin fibers even before the classic increase in collagen tissue occurs.

Obviously, the true morphologic diagnosis of myeloid metaplasia (or equivalently, extramedullary hematopoiesis) rests upon the demonstration of this process in the spleen and/or the liver; however, rarely are the risks justified to make the diagnosis by biopsy of either of these organs.

As the disease progresses, the spleen gradually enlarges, as may the liver. Anemia becomes more severe and is complicated both by iron deficiency owing to bleeding from esophageal varices and by relative folic acid deficiency. The high portal blood flow due to the enlarged spleen may cause "forward liver failure," portal hypertension, and ascites. Thrombosis of the hepatic vein and development of the Budd–Chiari syndrome have been recognized. Eventually, the spleen may occupy the entire abdomen. Ascites may develop.

## MAKING THE DIAGNOSIS

The clinical diagnosis of AMM is highly unlikely in the absence of a palpable spleen. Examination of the peripheral blood smear is very important, as typical teardrop RBCs, immature granulocytes, nucleated erythroid cells and abnormalities of platelet and megakaryocytic morphology are seen in the blood film. The diagnosis of early myelofibrosis requires an experienced hematopathologist, but as the disease advances, the degree of fibrosis and osteosclerosis makes the disease readily apparent. As in ET, about 50% of patients express abnormality of JAK2 in the periferal blood or marrow.[23]

In about 20% of patients with CML, significant fibrosis is noted when the patient is first encountered.[2] Therefore, appropriate cytogenetic and molecular tests to exclude CML should be performed in patients with AGM.

## REFERENCES

1. Silver RT: Chronic myeloid leukemia. *Hematol Oncol Clin North Am* 17(5):1159, 2003.
2. Silver RT: Chronic myeloid leukemia in Cancer Medicine. In: *Holland-Frei*, Vol. 2. Hamilton, London: BV Decker Inc; 2003:2117–2124.
3. Silver RT: Anagrelide is effective in treating patients with hydroxyurea-resistant thrombocytosis in patients with chronic myeloid leukemia. *Leukemia* 19(1):39, 2005.
4. Dosik H, Rosner F, Sawitsky A: Acquired lipidosis: Gaucher-like cells and "blue" cells in chronic granulocytic leukemia. *Semin Hematol* 9(3):309, 1972.
5. Silver RT: Importance of correlating TdT positivity in blast phase CML with cytogenetics. *Proc Am Soc Oncol* 592, 1981.
6. McCaffery R, Smoler DE, Baltimore D: Terminal deoxynucleotidyl transferase in a case of childhood acute lymphoblastic leukemia. *Proc Natl Acad Sci U S A* 70:521, 1973.
7. Bain B, Catovsky D, O'Brien M: Megakaryoblastic transformation of chronic granulocytic leukemia. *J Clin Pathol* 30:235, 1977.
8. Rosenthal S, Canellos GP, Gralnick HR: Erythroblastic transformation of chronic granulocytic leukemia. *Am J Med* 63:116, 1977.
9. Michallet M, Maloisel F. Delain M. et al.: Pegylated recombinent interferon alpha-2b vs recombinant interferon alpha-2b for the initial treatment of chronic-phase chronic myelogenous leukemia: a phase III study. *Leukemia* 18(2):309–15, Feb 2004.
10. Pearson TC: Apparent polycythemia. *Blood Rev* 5:205, 1991.
11. Berlin NI: Polycythemia vera. *Hematol Oncol Clin North Am* 17(5):1191, 2003.
12. Tefferi A: Polycythemia vera: a comprehensive review and clinical recommendations. *Mayo Clin Proc* 78:174, 2003.
13. Gruppo Igaliano Studio Polycythemia. Polycythemia vera: the natural history of 1213 patients followed for 20 years. *Ann Intern Med* 123:656, 1995.
14. Kralovics R, Passamonti F, Buser AS, Teoss, Tiedt R Passweg JR, Tichelli A, Cazzola M, Skoda R. *New Eng J Med* 352:1779–1790, 2005.
15. Najfeld V, Montella L, Scalise A, et al.: Exploring polycythemia vera with FISH: additional cryptic 9p is the most frequent abnormality detected. *Br J Haematol* 119(2):558, 2002.
16. Moliterno AR, Hankins WD, Spivak JL: Impaired expression of the thrombopoietin receptor by platelets from patients with polycythemia vera. *N Engl J Med* 338(9):572, 1998.
17. Horikawa Y, Matsumura I, Hashimoto K, et al.: Markedly reduced expression of platelet c-mpl receptor in essential thrombocythemia. *Blood* 90(10):4031.
18. Temerinac S, Klippel S, Strunck E, et al.: Cloning of PRV-1, a novel member of the uPAR receptor superfamily, which is overexpressed in polycythemia rubra vera. *Blood* 95(8):2569, 2000.
19. Jones AV, Kreil S, Zoi K, et al.: Widespread occurence of the JAK2 V617F mutation in chronic myeloproliferative disorders. *Blood.* 106(6):2162–8, Sep 15 2005.
20. Michiels JJ: Bone marrow histopathology and biological markers as specific clues to the differential diagnosis of essential thrombocythemia, polycythemia vera and pre-fibrotic agnogenic myeloid metaplasia. *Hematol J* 5(2): 93, 2004.
21. Thiele J, Kvasnicka HM: Chronic myeloproliferative disorders with thrombocythemia: a comparative study of two classifications systems (VSG, WHO) on 839 patients. *Ann Hematol* 82: 148, 2003.
22. Silverstein MN, Wollaeger EE, Baggenstoss AH: Gastrointestinal and abdominal manifestations of agnogenic myeloid metaplasia. *Arch Intern Med* 131:532, 1973.

# Chapter 48

# TREATMENT APPROACH TO POLYCYTHEMIA VERA AND ESSENTIAL THROMBOCYTHEMIA

## Steven M. Fruchtman and Celia L. Grosskreutz

## POLYCYTHEMIA VERA

### INCIDENCE AND CLINICAL PRESENTATION

The incidence of polycythemia vera (PV) is slightly higher in men than in women (2.8 vs 1.3 cases per 100,000 per year).[1] The mean age at diagnosis is 62 years (range, 20–85).[2]

The clinical presentation of patients with PV can be nonspecific, and may include headaches (48%), weakness (47%), dizziness (43%,) pruritus (43%), and excessive sweating (33%). Most patients are asymptomatic and come to a hematologist's attention based on a "routine" complete blood count (CBC).

Erythromelalgia (burning pain in the feet and hands accompanied by erythema, pallor, or cyanosis) is common in PV and is considered to be secondary to microvascular thrombotic complications (also seen in essential thrombocythemia, ET). It is more common when platelet counts are above 400,000/μL.[3]

Venous and arterial thrombosis are also common in PV patients and are related to increased blood viscosity and other unknown factors. Major thrombotic events can happen in 15% of the patients and include cerebrovascular accidents, myocardial infarction, superficial thrombophlebitis, deep venous thrombosis, pulmonary emboli, Budd–Chiari syndrome, and mesenteric thrombosis.[4]

Gastrointestinal symptoms of peptic ulcer disease are common and can be attributed to histamine release from tissue basophils and from Helicobacter pylori.[5]

On physical exam, patients often will have splenomegaly (70%), facial plethora (67%), and hepatomegaly (40%).

Laboratory abnormalities may include elevated hematocrit and red blood cell mass in almost all patients, platelet count >400,000/μL (in 60%), and a white blood cell (WBC) count >12,000/μL (in 40%). Bone marrow cellularity is increased in 90% of cases, and iron storage is absent in 95%.

### SURVIVAL

Survival in symptomatic patients without treatment is estimated to be between 6 and 18 months, and with appropriate therapy >10 years. However, the mean survival is influenced by the age at diagnosis. Thus, younger patients diagnosed and managed appropriately can have longer survivals. The main causes of death are thrombosis (29%), hematologic malignancies in those treated in previous eras with alkylating agents (23%), nonhematologic malignancies (16%), hemorrhage (7%), and myelofibrosis with myeloid metaplasia (3%).[6]

### DIAGNOSIS

The diagnosis of PV can be made with great confidence if the proposed modified criteria are used, as shown in Table 48.1.[7] Despite its inclusion in Table 48.1, the need for routine red cell mass determination

| Table 48.1 Proposed modified criteria for the diagnosis of polycythemia vera |
| --- |
| A1 Raised red cell mass (>25% above mean normal predicted value, or PCV ≥0.60 in males or 0.56 in females) |
| A2 Absence of cause of secondary erythrocytosis |
| A3 Palpable splenomegaly |
| A4 Clonality marker, i.e., acquired abnormal marrow karyotype |
| B1 Thrombocytosis (platelet count >400 × 10⁹/L) |
| B2 Neutrophil leucocytosis (neutrophil count >10 × 10⁹/L; >12.5 × 10⁹/L in smokers) |
| B3 Splenomegaly demonstrated on isotope or ultrasound scanning |
| B4 Characteristic BFU-E growth or reduced serum erythropoietin |

A1 + A2 + A3 or A4 establishes PV; A1 + A2 + two of B establishes PV .

**Table 48.2    Common causes of secondary erythrocytosis**

**Congenital**
　Mutant high-oxygen-affinity hemoglobin
　Congenital low 2,3-diphosphoglycerate
　Autonomous high erythropoietin production

**Acquired**
　Arterial hypoxemia (high altitude, cyanotic congenital
　　heart disease, chronic lung disease)
　Other causes of impaired tissue oxygen delivery (smoking)
　Renal lesions (renal tumors, cysts diffuse parenchymal
　　disease, hydronephrosis, renal artery stenosis, renal
　　transplantation)
　Endocrine lesions (adrenal tumors)
　Miscellaneous tumors (cerebellar hemangioblastoma,
　　uterine fibroids, bronchial carcinoma)
　Drugs (androgens)
　Hepatic lesions (hepatoma, cirrhosis, hepatitis)

is controversial. Its major utility is in the evaluation of border line elevations of hematocrit. It is important to exclude secondary causes of erythrocytosis (Table 48.2) related to increased erythropoietin, which may be physiologically appropriate (e.g., high altitude, smoking) or physiologically inappropriate (e.g., erythropoietin-secreting tumors). Thus, the measurement of serum erythropoietin is helpful in the differential diagnosis. PV patients have low or normal erythropoietin production secondary to a negative feedback mechanism. In contrast, patients with secondary erythrocytosis typically have elevated erythropoietin levels.

### TREATMENT

The aim of treatment is to prevent thromboses by reducing the elevated red cell mass, often with phlebotomy. Some patients require cytoreductive drugs to control the number of circulating blood elements, while others benefit from low-dose aspirin. The only potentially curative therapy is allogeneic stem cell transplantation. This is a consideration only in patients who develop high-risk postpolycythemic myeloid metaplasia with myelofibrosis, or transformation to acute leukemia.

### Phlebotomies

Phlebotomies of 250–500 mL as frequently as every other day should be performed until a hematocrit of between 40 and 45% is obtained. In older adults and in those with compromised hemodynamic status, only 250–300 mL should be removed each session, with a frequency of not more than twice a week. Once a normal hematocrit is achieved, a blood count should be checked every 4–8 weeks, and phlebotomy should be performed whenever the hematocrit is greater than 45% in men and 42% in women.[8]

### Myelosuppression

Phlebotomy will not be able to control leukocytosis, hyperuricemia, hypermetabolism, pruritus, and the complication of splenomegaly that are seen in PV patients. Patients treated with phlebotomy alone have a higher incidence of serious thrombotic complications during the first 3 years of therapy when compared to patients treated with myelosuppression.[6] Thus, older patients who are more prone to thrombotic disease should be treated with myelosuppression in addition to phlebotomy. Recent data from the European Collaboration Low Dose Aspirin Trial in PV (ECLAP) suggest that low-dose aspirin may also prevent certain thrombotic complications.[9]

*Hydroxyurea* HU is an antimetabolite that prevents DNA synthesis by inhibiting ribonucleoside reductase. The initial dose is 15 mg/kg daily orally, and subsequent adjustment of the dose is based on initial weekly blood counts for a month, to control the hematocrit without causing leukopenia or thrombocytopenia. If the WBC count falls below 3500 cells/mm$^3$ or the platelet count falls to less than 100,000/ mm$^3$, HU is withheld until these elements normalize, and then is reinstituted at 50% of the prior dose. When the peripheral blood count is maintained within an acceptable range on a stable dose of HU, the interval between blood counts is lengthened to every 2 weeks, and then to every 4 weeks.

For patients who require frequent phlebotomies or who have platelet counts greater than 600,000/mm$^3$, the dose of HU can be increased by 5 mg/kg daily at monthly intervals, with frequent monitoring until control is achieved. The majority of patients will be controlled with doses between 500 and 1000 mg daily. Supplemental phlebotomy is preferable to increased myelosuppression to control the hematocrit.

In emergency situations, particularly in those presenting with signs of decreased cerebral perfusion in the setting of an elevated hematocrit or marked thrombocytosis, more rapid control of disease may be crucial.

In these emergency situations, daily phlebotomy to a hematocrit of 45% should be accompanied by a loading dose of HU of 30 mg/kg/day for 7 days, followed by a maintenance dose of 15 mg/kg daily. Besides the requirement for close observation to prevent excessive marrow suppression, acute toxicity of HU is rare; occasionally, rash, fever, nausea, and oral or lower extremity ulcerations may be seen. The leukemogenic potential of HU is an issue that remains unsettled, though most evidence indicate it has little or no potential to induce leukemia.[10,11] This has prompted trials with other agents considered safe for long-term use, such as interferon-α (IFN-α) and anagrelide.

*Interferon-a* IFN-α is a biologic response modifier that suppresses the proliferation of hematopoietic progenitors. In PV patients, IFN-α reduces the hematocrit to below 45% in 60% of the patients. It is also highly effective in controlling the platelet counts. The initial dose of IFN-α is 3 million units three times per week subcutaneously. Full response usually requires 6 months to a year of treatment. The major side effects are flu-like symptoms, fever, and joint pain that can be controlled with acetaminophen. Liver function abnormalities and depression are also seen. IFN-α does not cross the placenta, and thus may be used in pregnant women who have a need for myelosuppression, although the majority of pregnant women do not have an indication for marrow suppression and the CBC may normalize during pregnancy. It can aid in the treatment of pruritus.[12]

*Anagrelide* It is an oral quinazoline derivative that has a profound effect on the maturation of megakaryocytes, resulting in a reduction of platelet production. It controls thrombocytosis in 66% of patients with PV or ET. Time to response is between 17 and 25 days. It is also reported to cause a minimal decrease in hematocrit. The initial dose should be 0.5 mg orally twice daily. Typically, steady state doses are 2.2–2.5 mg daily. The most significant side effects include palpitations, fluid retention, dizziness, and headaches; these are related to the drug's vasodilatory and inotropic properties. They can be minimized by initially starting with a low dose, such as 0.5 mg twice daily, and gradually increasing the dose until control of the platelet count is achieved. Patients with lactose intolerance may have diarrhea due to packaging of anagrelide with lactose. Patients with PV treated with anagrelide in one study developed acute leukemia at a rate of 2.6% (13 of 455). However, all the patients were previously exposed to other cytoreductive agents. There were no patients who transformed to acute leukemia who were exposed only to anagrelide.[13]

### Antithrombotic therapy

Low-dose *aspirin*, 80–100 mg daily, seems reasonable to recommend, in addition to cytoreduction, for patients who have a prior history of thrombosis or cardiovascular disease.[9] In addition, aspirin is effective for the treatment of erythromelalgia and other microvascular, neurologic, and ocular disturbances.

In patients with PV who continue to have thrombotic or vascular symptoms, despite aspirin and good control of the hematocrit and platelet count with phlebotomy and myelosuppression, *clopidogrel* 75 mg daily or *ticlopidine* 250 mg orally twice daily should be considered.[14]

## ESSENTIAL THROMBOCYTHEMIA

### INCIDENCE AND CLINICAL PRESENTATION

The incidence of essential thrombocythemia (ET) has been reported to be 2.38 patients/100,000 population/year. ET and PV appear to have approximately a 1:4 relative incidence,[15] but ET may have been underdiagnosed until the recent introduction of routine platelet counts included in the CBC. ET affects primarily middle-aged people, with an average age at diagnosis of 50–60 years. In several reports, a higher prevalence in females bas been noted.

The presenting symptoms of patients with ET are variable. Many patients (12–67%) reach medical attention fortuitously, as a result of an extreme degree of thrombocytosis detected when obtaining a routine blood cell count. Most patients present with symptoms related to small- or large-vessel thrombosis or minor bleeding. Neurologic complications are common, with headaches being the most common and paresthesias of the extremities second.[16,17] Transient neurologic symptoms seen in ET include unsteadiness, dysarthria, dysphoria, motor hemiparesis, scintillating scotomas, amaurosis fugaz, vertigo, dizziness, migraine-like symptoms, syncope, and seizures.

Erythromelalgia refers to a syndrome of redness and burning pain in the extremities, and is usually preceded by paresthesias. It is caused by microvascular circulatory insufficiency. Cold is reported to provide relief to these symptoms, while heat intensifies them.

Symptoms related to coronary artery disease or transient ischemic attacks may precede or accompany the onset of erythromelalgia.[16] Thrombosis of large veins and arteries in patients with ET still occurs commonly,[18] particularly in the arteries of the legs (30%), the coronary arteries (18%), the renal arteries (10%), and splenic and hepatic veins (Budd–Chiari syndrome) (7%).

Spontaneous abortion during the first trimester of pregnancy was found in 43% of ET patients, compared with 15% expected in the general population, and is due to placental thrombosis leading to placental infarction.[19]

Hemorrhagic problems plague some patients with ET; the primary site of bleeding is the gastrointestinal tract. Other sites of bleeding may be the skin, eyes, urinary tract, gums, tooth sockets (following extraction), or brain. The syndrome of hemorrhagic thrombocythemia is closely correlated with a significant increase of platelet counts in excess of $1000 \times 10^6$/L, and is associated with pseudohyperkalemia.[3,16] It is also associated with the development of acquired von Willebrand deficiency due to the absorption of von Willebrand multimers by the platelets and megakaryocytes.

Constitutional symptoms, such as weight loss, sweating, low-grade fever, and pruritus, can occur in 20–30% of the patients, and can be improved with the initiation of myelosuppressive therapy. Splenomegaly is detectable in 40–50% of patients, and 20% have hepatomegaly.

### CRITERIA FOR DIAGNOSIS OF ET

1. Platelet count >600,000/mm³ on two different occasions, separated by a 1-month interval.[20]
2. Hemoglobin level ≥13 g/dL or normal red cell mass (males <36 mL/kg and females <32 mL/kg).
3. Stainable iron in marrow or normal iron studies.
4. Collagen fibrosis of marrow:
   (a) absent or

(b) <1/3 biopsy area without both splenomegaly and leukoerythroblastic reaction.

5. Absence of the Philadelphia chromosome or the fusion *bcr/abl* gene by polymerase chain reaction; absence of clonal cytogenetics abnormalities associated with myelodysplastic disorders.

6. Absence of identifiable cause of reactive thrombocytosis.

## LABORATORY FINDINGS

Laboratory findings include platelet count in the range of 450,000–1,000,000/mm³, leukocytosis, basophilia, and the presence of megathrombocytes in the peripheral smear. Marrow cellularity is increased in 90% of the patients, with bizarre megakaryocytes with nuclear pleomorphisms and clustering of megakaryocytes. Enlargement of megakaryocytes with multilobulated nuclei, and their tendency to cluster in small groups along sinuses, is the hallmark of ET.[21] The bone marrow may also appear normal.

Bleeding times are prolonged in 10–20% of the patients. Platelet aggregation studies are frequently abnormal, most often demonstrating impaired aggregation in response to epinephrine, ADP, and collagen, but not to arachidonic acid and ristocetin.[22] Laboratory features of acquired von Willebrand syndrome (simulating type II vW factor deficiency) are associated with a platelet count >1000 × 10⁹/L. An enhanced thrombotic risk in ET patients has been associated with a reduction in the concentration of protein S, antithrombin III, protein C, and resistance to activated protein C resulting from an associated genetic defect in factor V,[23] along with patients who have both ET and acquired anticardiolipin antibodies.

## TREATMENT

The optimal therapy for patients with ET remains uncertain. Certain concepts, however, apply to all patients. One is that the precise and correct diagnosis is of utmost importance, and that all patients with ET should stop smoking to minimize the risk factors associated with atherosclerotic disease and thrombosis. Indiscriminant use of high doses of nonsteroidal anti-inflammatory drugs, especially in those patients with extreme elevations in platelet numbers ≥1,500,000, should be avoided because this practice can lead to an increased risk of hemorrhage. Use of such agents is particularly common in the older age group in which ET is common. Finally, cytoreductive agents such as those that have been used in the past and have more recently been shown to increase the rate of leukemic transformation must be avoided.[24]

In a randomized trial of high-risk patients, cytoreductive therapy has been shown to lessen the chance of developing additional thrombotic events.[25] High-risk patients include patients older than 60 years and patients with a history of a previous thrombotic episode,

including erythromelalgia, transient ischemic attacks, or large vessel thrombosis. Until a pharmacologic agent is available that is well tolerated and is proven safe for long-term use, no myelosuppressive therapy is an acceptable alternative in asymptomatic patients younger than 60 years. If a patient has a platelet count ≥1,500 × 10⁹/L and the acquired von Willebrand syndrome, platelet reduction therapy is also indicated to avoid the high risk of hemorrhage. Patients with this syndrome should avoid the use of aspirin.

In those patients requiring platelet reduction therapy, the choice between the use of anagrelide, IFN-α, and HU therapy is based upon patient age, ease of administration, comorbidities, and drug-related toxicity. In patients older than 60 years, HU therapy is the treatment of choice, while in younger patients, who may require myelosuppression, we prefer to initiate therapy with anagrelide. If a patient cannot tolerate anagrelide, we then start therapy with HU. Although we remain concerned about the leukemogenic potential of HU, whether or not there is an increased risk is controversial; clearly, the risk is less than that with alkylating agents or ³²P. Those patients who initially receive HU and no longer respond to this agent or suffer toxicity and require another agent should not receive long-term ³²P or melphalan therapy. This sequence of administration is associated with an extremely high risk of leukemic transformation. Those patients who have had a trial of HU and require further treatment should receive either anagrelide or IFN-α. Doses of each of these agents required for disease control will, of course, be dependent on the target platelet level.

Strict control to a platelet count ≤450 × 10⁹/L may lead to greater protection from thrombosis than merely reduction to a level ≤600 × 10⁹/L. There are no randomized trials to support this approach, but the available anecdotal information is compelling, and this objective may be easier to achieve with anagrelide or IFN-α than agents from previous eras, as neutropenia can be avoided.[26] Our success in achieving this goal is dependent on the ability of the patient to tolerate the agents used. In the younger patient, if such strict control is not achievable due to poor compliance or toxicity associated with the agents used, we are satisfied with continuing therapy and accepting a higher platelet number in the 600 × 10⁹/L range. In these patients, the addition of low-dose aspirin (81 or 100 mg/day) should be considered; it is less clear to us if those patients who achieve better platelet control with cytoreductive therapy should also be so treated. However, if one examines recent studies from Europe in PV trying to address this question, the approach of combining aspirin with cytoreduction in patients requiring cytoreduction appears to minimize thrombotic complications.[9] In patients who suffer from thrombotic episodes, particularly episodes involving the microcirculation or large vessels, we administer low-dose aspirin (81 mg/day). This dose of aspirin may increase the number of bleeding episodes to a modest degree, but is effective in treatment of thrombotic events, which are the major cause of mortality.

HU can be started at a dose of 1 g/day and then adjusted to achieve a target platelet count ($<350 \times 10^9$/L), with care to avoid the development of significant leukopenia. Anagrelide is initiated at 0.5 mg b.i.d. and increased by 0.5 mg/day every 5–7 days, if platelet counts do not begin to drop. The usual dose to achieve platelet number control is 2.0–2.5 mg/day. There are patients who do not tolerate either HU or anagrelide. In this patient group, IFN-α therapy is initiated at 3 million units three times per week subcutaneously. Another choice for therapy is busulfan at 4 mg/day for 2-week courses every time the platelet count rises above the normal range. Busulfan therapy is reserved for patients older than 60 years, and those refractory or intolerant to other approaches. Busulfan can precipitously drop platelet numbers, and thus patients receiving this therapy should be monitored closely.

We do not routinely treat patients younger than 40 years with cytoreduction, unless they already have had thrombohemorrhagic symptoms, have significant risk factors for atherosclerotic disease, or have other comorbidities. Serious complications even in young, otherwise healthy, patients with prolonged platelet counts of $>2.0 \times 10^6$/mm$^3$ are unusual. However, these marked elevations of platelet numbers can be anxiety-provoking situations for both patient and clinician; thus they may receive cytoreduction with anagrelide.

In certain situations, even in young, low-risk patients, treatment should be instituted. Surgery can increase the risk of thrombosis and use of anti-inflammatory agents can increase the risk of bleeding postoperatively. Under these circumstances, the platelet count should be lowered to the normal range. In pregnant patients with ET, low-dose aspirin therapy is the first treatment option, except in the third trimester of pregnancy, when prostaglandin inhibitors should be avoided. If the patient develops symptoms as a result of thrombosis within the vasculature, platelet reduction therapy is necessary and IFN-α therapy is the treatment of choice. As IFN does not cross the placenta, it likely will not be teratogenic. HU, anagrelide, and busulfan have been successfully used to treat myeloproliferative disorders during pregnancy, but they are probably teratogenic if used during the first trimester. If such agents are needed, they should be instituted after the first trimester, but ideally should be avoided.

In a patient with ET and a serious acute hemorrhagic event, the site of bleeding should be immediately determined and antiplatelet aggregating agents stopped. Although the platelet count may be high, these platelets should be considered to be qualitatively abnormal, leading to defective hemostasis. The patient may be suffering from acquired von Willebrand syndrome. In patients with acquired von Willebrand syndrome, DDAVP or Factor VIII concentrates containing von Willebrand factor can be used in the setting of a bleeding episode. If acquired von Willebrand syndrome is not present, the transfusion of normal platelets is suggested. In those patients with persistent hemorrhage, immediate reduction of the platelet count can be achieved by plateletpheresis. HU at 2–4 g/day for 3–5 days should be administered immediately, then reduced to 1 g/day. Any patient receiving HU should be monitored for the onset of granulocytopenia and/or thrombocytopenia. Reduction of platelet counts is usually observed within 3–5 days of HU treatment. Anagrelide can also be employed in this scenario, at a dose of at least 2 mg/day, and increased as required to control platelet numbers.

In contrast, patients with acute arterial thrombosis require immediate institution of platelet antiaggregating agents. Aspirin at a dose of 81 mg/day is suggested. Patients with erythromelalgia or transient ischemic attacks will have a rapid cessation of symptoms following the use of low-dose aspirin. In a patient with a life-threatening arterial thrombosis, the platelet count should be lowered with either a combination of apheresis and HU or with HU alone, depending on the severity of the event. Surgical intervention may also be required. If the arterial thrombosis involves the microcirculation and is not life threatening (transient ischemic attacks or erythromelalgia), immediate low-dose aspirin therapy is indicated and platelet reduction therapy (HU, anagrelide, or IFN-α) can be initiated using standard dose and schedule.[13,27-35]

## REFERENCES

1. Ania BJ, Suman VJ, Sobell JL, et al.: Trends in the incidence of polycythemia vera among Olmsted County, Minnesota residents, 1935–1989. *Am J Hematol* 47:89–93, 1994.
2. Berlin NI: Diagnosis and classification of the polycythemias. *Semin Hematol* 12:339–351, 1975.
3. Michiels JJ: Erythromelalgia and vascular complications in polycythemia vera. *Semin Thromb Hemost* 23:441–454, 1997.
4. De Stefano V, Teofili L, Leone G, et al.: Spontaneous erythroid colony formation as the clue to an underlying myeloproliferative disorder in patients with Budd–Chiari syndrome or portal vein thrombosis. *Semin Thromb Hemost* 23:411–418, 1997.
5. Torgano G, Mandelli C, Massaro P, et al.: Gastroduodenal lesions in polycythaemia vera: frequency and role of Helicobacter pylori. *Br J Haematol* 117:198–202, 2002.
6. Berk PD, Wasserman LR, Fruchtman SM, et al.: Treatment of polycythemia vera: a summary of clinical trials conducted by the polycythemia vera study group. In: Wasserman LR, Berk PD, Berlin NI (eds.) *Polycythemia*

*Vera and the Myeloproliferative Disorders.* Philadelphia, PA: Saunders; 1995:166.

7. Pearson TC: Diagnosis and classification of erythrocytoses and thrombocytoses. *Baillieres Clin Haematol* 11:695–720, 1998.

8. Streiff MB, Smith B, Spivak JL: The diagnosis and management of polycythemia vera in the era since the Polycythemia Vera Study Group: a survey of American Society of Hematology members' practice patterns. *Blood* 99:1144–1149, 2002.

9. Landolfi R, Marchioli R, Kutti J, et al.: Efficacy and safety of low-dose aspirin in polycythemia vera. *N Engl J Med* 350:114–124, 2004.

10. Fruchtman SM, Mack K, Kaplan ME, et al.: From efficacy to safety: a Polycythemia Vera Study group report on hydroxyurea in patients with polycythemia vera. *Semin Hematol* 34:17–23, 1997.

11. How safe is hydroxyurea in the treatment of polycythemia vera? *Haematologica* 84:673–674, 1999.

12. Berlin N, Berlin NI: Polycythemia vera. *Hematol Oncol Clin North Am* 17:1191–1210, 2003.

13. Fruchtman SM, Petitt RM, Gilbert HS, et al.: Anagrelide: analysis of long term safety and leukemogenic potential in myeloproliferative diseases (MPDs). Presented at: Annual Meeting of the American Society of Hematology; 2002; Philadelphia, PA.

14. Cuisset T, Frere C, Quilici J, et al.: Behefit of a 600 mg loading dose of clopidogrel on platelet reactivity and clinical outcomes in patients with non-ST-segment elevation acute coronary syndrome undergoing coronary stenting. *J Am Coll Cardiol* 48:1339–1345, 2006.

15. Mesa RA, Silverstein MN, Jacobsen SJ, et al.: Population-based incidence and survival figures in essential thrombocythemia and agnogenic myeloid metaplasia: an Olmsted County Study, 1976–1995. *Am J Hematol* 61:10–15, 1999.

16. Michiels JJ, van Genderen PJ, Lindemans J, et al.: Erythromelalgic, thrombotic and hemorrhagic manifestations in 50 cases of thrombocythemia. *Leuk Lymphoma* 22(suppl 1):47–56, 1996.

17. Michiels JJ, van Genderen PJ, Jansen PH, et al.: Atypical transient ischemic attacks in thrombocythemia of various myeloproliferative disorders. *Leuk Lymphoma* 22(suppl 1):65–70, 1996.

18. Johnson M, Gernsheimer T, Johansen K: Essential thrombocytosis: underemphasized cause of large-vessel thrombosis. *J Vasc Surg* 22:443–447, 1995; discussion 448–449.

19. Griesshammer M, Heimpel H, Pearson TC: Essential thrombocythemia and pregnancy. *Leuk Lymphoma* 22(suppl 1):57–63, 1996.

20. Murphy S, Peterson P, Iland H, et al.: Experience of the Polycythemia Vera Study Group with essential thrombocythemia: a final report on diagnostic criteria, survival, and leukemic transition by treatment. *Semin Hematol* 34:29–39, 1997.

21. Georgii A, Buhr T, Buesche G, et al.: Classification and staging of Ph-negative myeloproliferative disorders by histopathology from bone marrow biopsies. *Leuk Lymphoma* 22(suppl 1):15–29, 1996.

22. Finazzi G, Budde U, Michiels JJ: Bleeding time and platelet function in essential thrombocythemia and other myeloproliferative syndromes. *Leuk Lymphoma* 22(suppl 1):71–78, 1996.

23. Ruggeri M, Gisslinger H, Tosetto A, et al.: Factor V Leiden mutation carriership and venous thromboembolism in polycythemia vera and essential thrombocythemia. *Am J Hematol* 71:1–6, 2002.

24. Cortelazzo S, Finazzi G, Ruggeri M, et al.: Hydroxyurea for patients with essential of thrombocythemia and a high risk of thrombosis. *NEJM* 332:1132–1136, 1995.

25. Ruggeri M, Finazzi G, Tosetto A, et al.: No treatment for low-risk thrombocythemia results from a prospective study. *Br J Haem* 103:772–777, 1998.

26. Fruchtman SM, Pettit R, Gilbert H, et al.: Anagrelide therapy significantly reduces desease related symptoms in patients with myeloproliferative disorders. *Blood* 102(a), 2003.

27. Wright CA, Tefferi A: A single institutional experience with 43 pregnancies in essential thrombocythemia. *Eur J Haematol* 66:152–159, 2001.

28. van Genderen PJ, Mulder PG, Waleboer M, et al.: Prevention and treatment of thrombotic complications in essential thrombocythaemia: efficacy and safety of aspirin. *Br J Haematol* 97:179–184, 1997.

29. Finazzi G, Ruggeri M, Rodeghiero F, et al.: Second malignancies in patients with essential thrombocythaemia treated with busulphan and hydroxyurea: long-term follow-up of a randomized clinical trial. *Br J Haematol* 110:577–583, 2000.

30. Finazzi G, Barbui T: Efficacy and safety of hydroxyurea in patients with essential thrombocythemia. *Pathol Biol (Paris)* 49:167–169, 2001.

31. Finazzi G, Ruggeri M, Rodeghiero F, et al.: Efficacy and safety of long-term use of hydroxyurea in young patients with essential thrombocythemia and a high risk of thrombosis. *Blood* 101:3749, 2003.

32. Hanft VN, Fruchtman SR, Pickens CV, et al.: Acquired DNA mutations associated with in vivo hydroxyurea exposure. *Blood* 95:3589–3593, 2000.

33. Storen EC, Tefferi A: Long-term use of anagrelide in young patients with essential thrombocythemia. *Blood* 97:863–866, 2001.

34. Elliott MA, Tefferi A: Interferon-alpha therapy in polycythemia vera and essential thrombocythemia. *Semin Thromb Hemost* 23:463–472, 1997.

35. Tomer A: Effects of anagrelide on in vivo megakaryocyte proliferation and maturation in essential thrombocythemia. *Blood* 99:1602–1609, 2002.

# Chapter 49

# APPROACH TO CHRONIC IDIOPATHIC MYELOFIBROSIS (WITH EXTRAMEDULLARY HEMATOPOIESIS)

*Ruben A. Mesa and Ayalew Tefferi*

Chronic idiopathic myelofibrosis (CIMF) is a chronic myeloproliferative disorder first described in 1879 by Gustav Heuck[1] with a report of two patients with massive splenomegaly, constitutional symptoms, and intramedullary fibrosis. This disorder was further defined as a distinct entity in the twentieth century as agnogenic myeloid metaplasia[2] (AMM). AMM was subsequently categorized as a subset of myelofibrosis with myeloid metaplasia (MMM).[3] The diagnosis of MMM includes patients with a de novo presentation (i.e., AMM) as well as those who progressed from a previous chronic myeloproliferative disorder (specifically essential thrombocythemia or polycythemia vera[4]) to the disorders of postthrombocythemic (PTMM) and postpolycythemic myeloid metaplasia (PPMM), respectively.[3] As the clinical presentation, prognosis, and management are indistinguishable for both de novo CIMF and the secondary states of PTMM and PPMM, we will refer to MMM as one disease.

MMM is a clonal[5] hematopoietic stem disorder, resulting in two major processes. The first process is a myeloproliferation that is manifest by an intramedullary expansion of one or more myeloid lineages, resulting frequently in either leukocytosis and/or thrombocytosis. Additionally, an increase in circulating immature myeloid cells is observed which can accumulate in the spleen, liver, or other organs and lead to extramedullary hematopoiesis. The second is a prominent, polyclonal reactive process within the marrow, which leads to fibroblast proliferation, deposition of collagen (types I and III) and other connective tissues (i.e., fibronectin and proteoglycans), neoangiogenesis,[6] osteosclerosis, reticulin fibrosis, and ineffective hematopoiesis.

## INITIAL ASSESSMENT

### CLINICAL PRESENTATION

Patients with MMM have a tremendous degree of variability in symptoms, exam findings, and laboratory abnormalities. Typically, patients present in the seventh decade of life (median age 67[7]), although MMM can be diagnosed at any age. Symptoms related to MMM can be broken down into one of three main categories.

### MYELOPROLIFERATIVE SYMPTOMS

Increases in circulating mature (i.e., neutrophils) and immature (i.e., myelocytes, metamyelocytes, myeloblasts, etc.) myeloid cells occur in varying degrees in MMM. These cells have a propensity for accumulation in the reticuloendothelial system, particularly in the spleen and liver.[8] These organs expand to accommodate the burden of myeloid cells, and the resulting hepatosplenomegaly may lead to pain, early satiety, sequestration of erythrocytes and platelets, and portal hypertension.[9] Extramedullary hematopoiesis also can occur in the lungs (leading to pulmonary hypertension[10]), abdomen, spine,[11] and pericardium.[12]

### CYTOPENIAS

Cytopenias of varying severity are characteristic of MMM and are multifactorial. Anemia is the most common cytopenia and can be caused by (1) ineffective hematopoiesis, (2) decreased marrow production capability because of the severity of the reactive fibrosis, (3) splenic sequestration, (4) myelosuppression from MMM therapy (i.e., from hydroxyurea), (5) hemolysis, or (6) bleeding from the gastrointestinal tract (e.g., from varices resulting from portal hypertension). Thrombocytopenia also occurs in MMM, although it is less common than anemia at presentation, and may result from the same factors that cause anemia, as well as from consumption through disseminated intravascular coagulation.

### CONSTITUTIONAL SYMPTOMS

These include hypermetabolic symptoms of fever, night sweats, and unintentional weight loss. In addition, mild-to-overwhelming fatigue may occur frequently in excess of what would be anticipated with respect to the degree of the patient's anemia. Lastly, bone pain (thought to result from intramedullary expansion from myeloproliferation) may occur and may be severe.

## EVALUATION OF PROGNOSIS

MMM is a disease with a wide degree of prognostic variability, with most patients eventually expiring from their disease in the absence of leukemic transformation (LT). Several prognostic factors have been examined, with the most useful being the Lille criteria for MMM,[13] which include the presence or absence of anemia (hemoglobin <10 g/dL) or extremes of leukocyte count (<4 or >30 × 10^9/L). The Lille criteria modeled median survival in MMM patient groups of 93, 26, and 13 months, respectively, based on the presence of 0, 1, or 2 abnormalities. Additional negative prognostic factors include increasing age,[14] increased circulating myeloblasts at diagnosis,[15] increased peripheral blood CD34+ cell count,[16] and abnormal karyotypic analysis[14] (especially trisomy 8 and deletions of the "p" arm of chromosome 12).

## HEMATOPOIETIC STEM CELL TRANSPLANTATION

### MYELOABLATIVE ALLOGENEIC STEM CELL TRANSPLANT

Allogeneic hematopoietic stem cell transplantation is the only therapy that has the potential to be curative in MMM (see Table 49.1). Guardiola and colleagues[26] performed myeloablative allogeneic transplants in 55 MMM patients (median age 42). The 5-year survival was approximately 50%, with a 27% 1-year transplant-related mortality and 33% experiencing grade III–IV acute graft-versus-host disease (GvHD). Subsequent trials have confirmed the potential for long-term complete response with allogeneic stem cell transplant, but at the cost of significant short- and long-term risk, particularly in older patients (see Table 49.1).

Deeg and colleagues[23] reported data on 56 patients with MMM receiving allogeneic stem cell transplantation (with a range of mainly busulfan-based conditioning regimens) and showed a 3-year survival of 58% (highest with "targeted" busulfan conditioning). Several patients demonstrated sustained absence of obvious features of diseases (splenomegaly or intramedullary fibrosis). Nonrelapse mortality was 18/56 (32%), with 68 and 59% incidences of acute (grades II–IV) and chronic GvHD (extensive in 90% of those afflicted), respectively. Posttransplant mortality was highest in those with poor Lille prognosis,[13] karyotypic abnormalities, and severe marrow fibrosis.

### NONMYELOABLATIVE STEM CELL TRANSPLANT IN MMM

Allogeneic transplant with reduced intensity conditioning regimens have recently shown promise in the therapy of MMM.[21] A series by Rondelli and colleagues[24] of 20 "high-risk" MMM patients (by Lille criteria[27]) with a median age of 54 years underwent reduced intensity conditioning allogeneic transplant. Survival was 90% at 18 months, with a 10% transplant-related mortality (both from complications of GvHD). Chronic GvHD (>grade II) was present in 50% of evaluable patients. Significant clinical improvement was noted in many, but extent and duration of remission have not yet been published.

### AUTOLOGOUS STEM CELL TRANSPLANT IN MMM

Autologous stem cell transplantation has the advantage of use in (1) older patients, (2) those without an HLA match, and (3) those who would not tolerate an allogeneic transplant. A multicenter, pilot, study of 21 MMM patients who received an autologous stem cell (mobilized with granulocyte colony-stimulating factor) transplant[25] was recently published with several interesting findings. The procedure was overall surprisingly well tolerated (transplant-related mortality 3/21; 1< day 100), with improvements seen in both cytopenias and myeloproliferative symptoms.

## MEDICAL SURGICAL AND RADIOTHERAPEUTIC OPTIONS IN CIMF

No therapy, other than perhaps stem cell transplant, has been shown to impact the survival of MMM patients. Thus, nontransplant management strategies are palliative in orientation and goal. When palliative therapy is appropriate, it is necessary to identify which disease manifestations truly affect quality of life (see Figure 49.1). Currently, there has been only modest success with palliating myeloproliferative and cytopenia-associated symptoms, with no real success in either improving MMM-associated constitutional symptoms or preventing blastic transformation.

**Table 49.1    Published results for hematopoietic stem cell transplantation in MMM**

| Reference | Disease | Graft | N | Age median (range) | Conditioning | Mortality <Day 100 | NRM | GvHD | Results |
|---|---|---|---|---|---|---|---|---|---|
| 17 | AMM | Allo (6 ALT) | 55 | 42 (4–53) | Varied | NR | 27% | 60% acute, 27/45 chronic | 22/55 had CR Adverse prognostic anemia, osteosclerosis, abnormal karyotype, increasing age |
| 18 | MMM | Allo | 66 | NR | Varied | NR | NR | NR | 5-year survival 14% (age >45 years); 62% (age <45) Delayed engraftment if pre-HSCT anemia Osteosclerosis associated with GvHD |
| 19 | MMM | Allo | 50 | 43 (10–66) | NR | NR | NR | NR | 50% 5-year disease-free survival "Better" outcomes for patients >45 than seen by Guardiola et al. |
| 20 | PPMM PTMM | Allo (8 ALT) | 19 | 43 (18–59) | Varied | 27% | 37% | 47% | 47% with sustained CR (median 41 months after HSCT) |
| 21 | MMM | Allo (RIC) | 4 | 48–58 | Fludarabine/ mel phalan | 0 | 0 | 25%, 75% | 1/4 with acute GvHD 3/4 with chronic GvHD |
| 22 | MMM | Allo | 25 | 48 (46–50) | Cy-TBI (n = 23) Bu-Cy (n = 2) | 20% | 48% | 52% acute, 58% chronic | 36% VOD 20% long-term CR (median 35 months follow-up) |
| 23 | MMM | Allo | 56 | 43 (10–66) | BuCy (n = 44) Bu-TBI (n = 7) Cy-TBI (n = 5) | 14.3% | NR | 68% acute, 59% chronic | "Targeted Bu-Cy" 76% survival 53% alive without fibrosis (>1 year posttransplant) |
| 24 | MMM | Allo (RIC) | 20 | 54 (27–68) | Varied | 0% | 10% | 25% acute, 50% chronic | 10% TRM 90% survival at 18 months Long-term remission rate not clear |

*table continues*

**Table 49.1    continued**

| Reference | Disease | Graft | N | Age median (range) | Conditioning | Mortality <Day 100 | NRM | GvHD | Results |
|---|---|---|---|---|---|---|---|---|---|
| 25 | MMM | Auto | 21 | 59 (45–75) | Oral busulfan | 5% | 14% | NA | Anemia response 10/17 Platelet response 4/8 Spleen response 7/10 |

HSCT, hematopoietic stem cell transplantation; NRM, nonrelapse mortality; GvHD, graft-versus-host disease; AMM, agnogenic myeloid metaplasia; MMM, myelofibrosis with myeloid metaplasia; PPMM, postpolycythemic myeloid metaplasia; PTMM, postthrombocythemic myeloid metaplasia; VOD, veno-occulsive disease; Allo, allogeneic stem cell transplant; ALT, alternative donor (i.e., matched unrelated, haploidentical); Bu, busulfan; Cy, cyclophosphamide; TBI, total body irradiation.

## THERAPY OF CYTOPENIAS

### TRANSFUSIONS

Direct replacement of red blood cells through transfusion is the cornerstone of palliating anemia-related symptoms in MMM. Currently, there are no data to support the routine use of iron chelation therapy for prevention of secondary iron overload in these transfusion-dependent individuals. Indeed, there are no data demonstrating definitive end-organ toxicity from iron overload in MMM patients. Unfortunately, the poor prognosis associated with transfusion dependence in MMM results in a short survival duration, making concerns over long-term effects of iron overload moot.

Platelet transfusions in MMM are less frequently required, but lead to alloimmunization more rapidly than erythrocyte transfusions. Therefore, platelet transfusions in MMM should be limited to hemorrhagic episodes or thrombocytopenia severe enough that risks of spontaneous bleeding are unacceptable (platelet counts $<10 \times 10^9$/L or higher in clinical scenarios, such as fever).

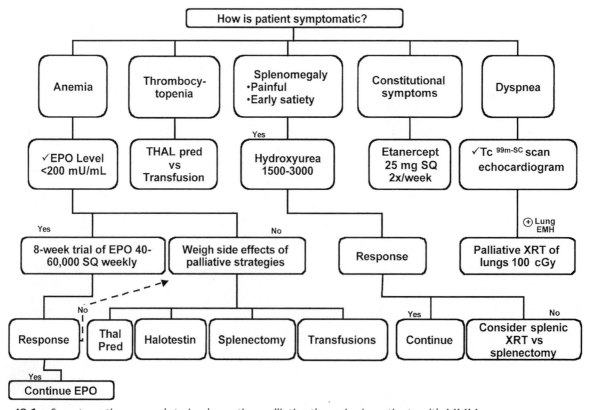

**Figure 49.1** *Symptomatic approach to implementing palliative therapies in patients with MMM*

## ERYTHROPOIETIN

The administration of exogenous erythropoietin has been occasionally helpful for MMM-associated anemia. Rodriguez et al.[28] described their experience and conducted a meta-analysis of patients with MMM treated with erythropoietin. A response rate of 33% was seen, with doses of up to 600 units/kg/week being required. Patients with serum erythropoietin levels of <125 mU/mL had the highest likelihood of response. Responses to exogenous erythropoietin most frequently occurred within 2–3 months, with responses ranging from mild decreases in transfusion dependence to complete transfusion independence.

## ANDROGENS

Androgens have been beneficial for the treatment of MMM-associated anemia. Various androgen formulations have been used in MMM patients, including nandrolone,[29] oxymetholone, and danazol.[30,31] Doses of danazol in the range of 600–800 mg/day led to responses in four out of seven patients (treated from 3 to 6 months) with MMM anemia in a report by Cervantes et al.[30] In this study, responders had either previously been splenectomized, or had only modest splenomegaly. In addition, it has been suggested that MMM patients with karyotypic abnormalities are less likely to respond to palliative androgen therapy.[29]

## THALIDOMIDE

Initial pilot studies with thalidomide in MMM were dose escalating, starting with 100 mg of thalidomide per day[32–40] (see Table 49.2). The published trials of thalidomide as single-agent therapy in MMM had several interesting findings. First, the activity observed in these trials was mainly manifest in the improvement of cytopenias (anemia and thrombocytopenia), with less frequent improvement in splenomegaly. In addition, patients with MMM did poorly with dose escalation, and in fact did not tolerate the agent well even at doses of 200 mg/day of thalidomide. Finally, a subset of MMM patients can experience unwanted myeloproliferation with thalidomide therapy.[43] Interestingly, myeloproliferation has even been observed in patients without prior identified myeloproliferative disorders.[44]

In excess of 100 patients with MMM have been reported in the literature to have received thalidomide as single-agent therapy for their disease. These trials (outlined in Table 49.2) demonstrate that thalidomide does appear to be reproducibly active in improving anemia and thrombocytopenia in approximately 30–40% of patients, with more modest relief from symptomatic hepatosplenomegaly. Subsequent trials using low-dose thalidomide (50 mg/day) appear to retain the activity but with less toxicity (see Table 49.2). Additionally, the combination of 50 mg/day of thalidomide with a corticosteroid taper[41] has resulted in improvements in the toxicity profile, decreases in toxicity dropout, and equivalent if not superior efficacy. Responses, when obtained, to thalidomide can be durable even after discontinuation of the drug. In a recent report[45] of long-term outcomes with thalidomide among initial responders, 35% (7 of 20 patients)

**Table 49.2** Published clinical trials of thalidomide in CIMF

| Author | Reference | N | Min | Max | Anemia response (%) | Platelet response (%) | Spleen response (%) |
|---|---|---|---|---|---|---|---|
| **Single-agent thalidomide trials** | | | | | | | |
| Elliott et al. | 34 | 15 | *50 | 400 | 20 | 80 | 7 |
| Barosi et al. | 32 | 21 | 100 | 400 | 43 | 66.7 | 20 |
| Canepa et al. | 33 | 10 | 200 | 800 | 30 | 30 | 30 |
| Pozzato et al. | 39 | 6 | 100 | NR | 50 | NR | 0 |
| Piccaluga et al. | 38 | 12 | 100 | 600 | 25 | 25 | 16.7 |
| Grossi et al. | 35 | 7 | 50 | 150 | 43 | 57 | 72 |
| Merup et al. | 37 | 15 | 200 | 800 | 0 | 0 | 0 |
| Strupp et al. | 40 | 16 | 100 | 400 | 60 | 71 | 23 |
| Marchetti et al. | 36 | 63 | 50 | 400 | 22 | 22 | 19 |
| **Combination thalidomide trials** | | | | | | | |
| Mesa et al. (THAL+ PRED) | 41 | 21 | 50 | 50 | 62 | 75 | 19 |
| Visani et al. (THAL + EPO) | 42 | 1 | 100 | 400 | 100 | NA | 100 |

Min, minimum thalidomide dose; Max, maximum thalidomide dose.
*Note*: Several trials include patients with PPMM and PTMM, respectively.

maintained a hematologic response for 16–31 months after discontinuation of thalidomide and keeping off all other therapies for MMM. Recent trails with linalidomide show similar results with less toxicity.

## THERAPY OF MYELOPROLIFERATIVE SYMPTOMS

The palliation of symptomatic extra-medullary hematopoiesis (EMH) in MMM is accomplished through either nonspecific myelosuppressive drug therapy (in an attempt to decrease the contributory circulating myeloid progenitor pool) or targeted cytoreduction, using either radiotherapy or surgery.

### SPLENOMEGALY

The surgical removal of the spleen is one of the oldest acknowledged therapies for MMM[46] (see Table 49.3), yet has only been palliative in benefit with significant risks (bleeding and infection) of perioperative and long-term complications (i.e., thrombocytosis). If splenectomy is only palliative and risky in MMM, should any MMM patient be splenectomized? In a recent retrospective review from our institutional experience with 223 splenectomized MMM patients, we found that patients with certain surgical indications were more likely to experience clinical benefit.[9] Specifically, patients whose primary indication for splenectomy was painful splenomegaly experienced durable symptomatic relief and occasional improvement in refractory anemia. However, we found only marginal benefit in patients splenectomized to ameliorate portal hypertension, and adverse outcomes in patients splenectomized for thrombocytopenia. The latter group also experienced increased morbidity and mortality with the procedure. Additionally, postoperative risks of significant thrombocytosis were associated with increased preoperative platelet counts. Therefore, our current recommendations are to offer palliative splenectomy to individuals with refractory, severely symptomatic, splenomegaly (unresponsive to hydroxyurea) with aggressive postoperative control of thrombocytosis (with platelet-lowering agents +/− platelet apheresis).

### Hydroxyurea

Hydroxyurea is a useful, oral, well-tolerated, nonspecific myelosuppressive agent that can reduce the leukocytosis and occasional thrombocytosis associated with MMM.[77] The reduction of leukocytosis in MMM is clinically useful only if it is extreme and symptomatic, or if the reduction in leukocytosis leads to a significant reduction in splenomegaly (seen in approximately 25% of patients). Occasionally, substantial doses of hydroxyurea (2–3 g/day) are needed to achieve a meaningful reduction in splenomegaly. Hydroxyurea may potentially exacerbate anemia or thrombocytopenia (if present), but supplemental exogenous erythropoietin may

| Table 49.3 | Reports of therapeutic splenectomy in CIMF/MMM | | | |
|---|---|---|---|---|
| Study | Reference | Year | Number of patients | Mortality (%) |
| Hickling | 47 | 1937 | 27 | 56 |
| Bukh and With | 48 | 1945 | 1 | 0 |
| Green et al. | 49 | 1953 | 5 | 0 |
| Videbaek | 50 | 1956 | 3 | 0 |
| Jensen | 46 | 1964 | 6 | 16 |
| Gomes et al. | 51 | 1967 | 15 | 27 |
| Schwartz et al. | 52 | 1970 | 12 | 8 |
| Morgenstern | 53 | 1971 | 20 | 15 |
| Milner et al. | 54 | 1973 | 13 | 0 |
| Silverstein and Remine | 55 | 1974 | 29 | 24 |
| Gale et al. | 56 | 1974 | 7 | 0 |
| Mulder et al. | 57 | 1977 | 19 | 5 |
| Cabot et al. | 58 | 1978 | 19 | 5 |
| Little | 59 | 1978 | 8 | 0 |
| Silverstein and Remine | 60 | 1979 | 50 | 10 |
| Benbassat and Ligumski | 61 | 1979 | 321 | 7.5 |
| Jarvinen et al. | 62 | 1982 | 30 | 6.7 |
| Coon and Liepman | 63 | 1982 | 34 | 12 |
| Musser et al. | 64 | 1984 | 17 | 18 |
| Sharp et al. | 65 | 1985 | 12 | 8 |
| Dotevall et al. | 66 | 1987 | 1 | 0 |
| Benbassat et al. | 67 | 1990 | 307 | 13 |
| Brenner et al. | 68 | 1988 | 34 | 15 |
| Schmitz et al. | 69 | 1992 | 1 | 0 |
| Barosi et al. | 70 | 1993 | 71 | 8 |
| Lafaye et al. | 71 | 1994 | 39 | 13 |
| Jameson et al. | 72 | 1996 | 3 | 0 |
| Mittelman et al. | 73 | 1997 | 8 | 0 |
| Bohner et al. | 74 | 1997 | 7 | NR |
| Barosi et al. | 75 | 1998 | 87 | NR |
| Tefferi et al. | 9 | 2000 | 223 | 9 |
| Akpek et al. | 76 | 2001 | 26 | 11 |

be used to ameliorate the associated anemia. Complications of hydroxyurea may include lower extremity ulceration[78] and undesired myelosuppression exacerbating underlying cytopenias.

## Alkylating agents

Melphalan is an orally bioavailable alkylating agent with myelosuppressive properties. The action of alkylating agents in MMM includes a direct, nonspecific myelosuppression, and therefore they may potentially palliate symptoms associated with myeloproliferation.[79] A clinical trial was recently reported in MMM using low doses of melphalan.[80] Over a 7-year period, 104 patients with MMM were treated with 2.5 mg of oral melphalan three times a week. The agent was active, with 66% of patients achieving a response after a median of 7 months of therapy. The greatest impact was on myeloproliferative manifestations. However, the major reason for study discontinuation was blastic transformation in 26% of the study cohort, as high as 48% in pretreated patients. Thus, the long-term use of melphalan in MMM may increase the risk of LT and should be used only in appropriate circumstances (e.g., the older patient who needs myelosuppression and is not a candidate for/or has not responded to hydroxyurea).

## 2-Chlorodeoxyadenosine

Therapeutic splenectomy in MMM may result in extreme thrombocytosis, leukocytosis, and accelerated hepatomegaly.[81] Palliative benefit from the purine nucleoside analog 2-chlorodeoxyadenosine (2-CdA) has been reported to provide beneficial cytoreduction in such instances.[81] The agent has been used successfull in MMM in either of two common schedules (0.10 mg/kg intravenously by continuous infusion for 7 days or 5 mg/m² intravenously over 2 h for five consecutive days per cycle). 2-CdA (after a median of one to two cycles) responses were observed in 55, 50, 55, and 40% of patients for hepatomegaly, thrombocytosis, leukocytosis, and anemia, respectively. Cytopenias were frequent, but usually transient and without clinical consequence. Responses were sustained for a median of 6 months after discontinuation of the treatment.

## Other agents

Recent clinical trials with novel therapies, such as lenalidomide (Revlimid®), the farnesyltransferase inhibitor tipifarnib[82] and the oral vascular endothelial growth factor inhibitor PTK787[83] have demonstrated preliminary benefits in reducing MMM-associated organomegaly. Durability and overall efficacy of these agents for the disorder have not yet been reported.

## Splenic Radiation

Several reports (see Table 49.4) have described the palliative benefit to external beam radiation in improving symptomatic splenomegaly in MMM.[88,89] The Mayo Clinic experience[88] described a group of 23 MMM patients who received a median radiation course of 277 cGy in a median of eight fractions. An objective decrease in spleen size was noted in 94% of patients; however, 44% of patients experienced posttreatment cytopenias (26% were severe and 13% fatal). In addition, splenic radiation seemed to increase morbidity and mortality of subsequent splenectomy when undertaken. Splenic radiation is effective for palliating MMM-associated splenomegaly but should be limited to patients with adequate platelet counts, and to those who are not likely to be splenectomized.

## NONSPLENIC EXTRAMEDULLARY HEMATOPOIESIS

Myeloid progenitors are sensitive to the cytotoxic effects of external beam radiotherapy (XRT); therefore, it is reasonable to hypothesize that judicious use of radiotherapy may reduce symptomatic aggregations of extramedullary hematopoiesis. Indeed, palliative radiotherapy has been used successfully in a variety of settings in MMM (see Table 49.4).

### LUNGS

The sequestration of myeloid precursors into the pulmonary parenchyma can lead to symptomatic pulmonary hypertension in MMM.[10] We have recently reported our experience with single-fraction, low-dose (100 cGy) external beam radiation to the lungs for palliating MMM-associated pulmonary hypertension.[94] A total of seven patients at our institution have experienced a palliative benefit from pulmonary XRT demonstrated by improved performance status, decreased pulmonary artery pressures on echocardiography, and less EMH on lung ⁹⁹ᵐTc sulfur colloid scans.

### LIVER

The experience with palliative radiotherapy for MMM-associated hepatomegaly has been less positive than for the spleen.[91] Though responses can be achieved with irradiating the liver, they are not durable. In addition, the exacerbation of underlying cytopenias (which are invariably present) are problematic. Indeed, routine irradiation of the liver is not recommended, and if cytoreduction is required then medical therapy (i.e, hydroxyurea) should be considered.

## THERAPY OF CONSTITUTIONAL SYMPTOMS

MMM is variably associated with a wide range of constitutional symptoms. The most common of these is fatigue, which can range from mild to debilitating. Patients may also suffer from hypercatabolic symptoms, manifested as night sweats, fevers, and significant loss of lean body mass. Lastly, patients occasionally suffer from bone pain that can be severe. There have not been many therapeutic agents, either tested or reported, to significantly palliate these problems. Indeed, these symptoms frequently can be the most debilitating and frustrating to arise in MMM patients.

**Table 49.4**   XRT for palliating extramedullary hematopoiesis in patients with MMM

| Reference | Patients (n) | Dose (cGy) | Fractions | Response/Comments |
|---|---|---|---|---|
| *Radiation to the spleen* | | | | |
| 84 | 39 | | | ■ 63% response rate |
| 85 | 14 | 600 | 9 | ■ 95% response rate |
| | | | | ■ Significant cytopenias in 57% |
| 86 | 25 | | | ■ 88% with symptomatic decrease in splenomegaly |
| 87 | 10 | 150–300 | 6–10 | ■ Responses in 90% |
| | | | | ■ Cytopenias common |
| 88 | 23 | 277 | 7.5 | ■ 93.9% decrease in spleen size |
| | | | | ■ Median duration of response 6 months |
| | | | | ■ Toxicities: cytopenias, complicated subsequent splenectomy |
| 89 | 15 | 980 | 22 | ■ 59% response rate |
| | | | | ■ Toxicities: cytopenias |
| 90 | 4 | 450 | 9 | ■ All patients with a palliative response |
| | | | | ■ Toxicities: cytopenias |
| *Radiation to the liver* | | | | |
| 91 | 14 | 150 | 6 | ■ 35% with transient reduction in hepatomegaly |
| | | | | ■ 62% with significant cytopenias |
| *Radiation to the abdomen for ascites* | | | | |
| 92 | 1 | 1000 | 10 | ■ Case report of response for ascites |
| | | | | ■ Cytopenias worsened with therapy |
| 93 | 4 | 200 | 7 | ■ Good responses for ascites |
| | | | | ■ Resolution of ureteral obstruction |
| *Radiation to the lungs* | | | | |
| 94 | 4 | 100 | 1 | ■ 75% experienced improvement in pulmonary hypertension |
| | | | | ■ Durable responses achieved with little toxicity |
| 95 | 1 | 200 | 4 | ■ Case report with good durable response |
| 93 | 2 | 125 | 5 | ■ Resolution of dyspnea and pleural effusions |
| *Radiation for paraspinal/intraspinal EMH* | | | | |
| 93 | 5 | 100–1000 | 1–5 | ■ Excellent and prompt responses to therapy in 4/5 |

Tumor necrosis factor α (TNF-α) is a cytokine implicated both in the pathogenesis of MMM, as well as in being profibrogenic[96] and potentially a direct inhibitor of hematopoiesis,[97] and a cause of MMM-associated constitutional symptoms (fatigue and cachexia).[98] Etanercept (Enbrel, Immunex, Seattle, WA) is an inhibitor of TNF-α Based on its activity and safety, it was piloted in MMM.[99] Twenty-two patients with MMM were prospectively treated with twice-weekly subcutaneous injections of etanercept (25 mg per injection) for up to 24 weeks. The drug was well tolerated and was successful in improving MMM-associated constitutional symptoms in 60% of those enrolled. However, only modest benefit was observed in either improving peripheral cytopenias or reducing splenomegaly (20%).

## LEUKEMIC TRANSFORMATION OF MMM

Leukemic transformation of MMM occurs in approximately 10–15% of patients,[100] and is usually fatal. A recent series of 91 consecutive MMM patients[101] who underwent LT reported that transformation was usually clinically heralded by organomegaly, worsening constitutional symptoms, anemia, thrombocytopenia, and leukocytosis. At the diagnosis of MMM, these patients had frequently presented with typical disease-related features, but about half had an increase in circulating myeloblasts. All episodes of LT were acute myeloid leukemia, with all French–American–British subtypes represented except M3. Additionally, 91% of patients displayed an abnormal karyotype. LT from MMM was usually fatal, with 89 patients (98%) having expired of disease or therapy a median of 2.6 months (range 0–24.2) after LT. Supportive care alone or noninduction chemotherapy had similar outcomes in 48 patients and 19 patients, respectively (median survival <3 months in both groups). Induction chemotherapy in 24 patients (26%) had a 33% mortality with no complete remissions achieved [median survival 3.4 months (range 0.9–24.3)]. However, a subset of patients (n = 10; 41%) reverted their marrow to a chronic phase of MMM after induction. Salvage regimens for nonresponders were overall unsuccessful. The outcome of LT in MMM with current therapies is dismal. Either supportive care alone or appropriate clinical trials should be considered.

## ESTABLISHING A THERAPEUTIC PLAN FOR MMM

The wide range of prognosis and symptomatology in MMM is a significant issue as we decide on the aggressiveness of therapy. Management of this complex disorder should diminish short-term morbidity from the disease with an eye on long-term goals.

### SHORT-TERM MANAGEMENT GOALS

In the short term, our goal with MMM is to diminish the immediate possible morbidities at presentation, with the least amount of expense and toxicity from therapy. Therefore, the patient who presents with asymptomatic or minimally symptomatic disease may most appropriately be observed (see Figure 49.1). To date, no survival benefit has been demonstrated for reduction of asymptomatic splenomegaly, reduction of asymptomatic leukocytosis, or improvements in mild anemia (i.e., hemoglobin >11 g/dL).

### LONG-TERM MANAGEMENT GOALS

Establishment of a long-term plan is again crucial in this disease. Specifically, upon presentation, it is reasonable to assess whether a stem cell transplant will ever be appropriate for a particular patient. If the patient is a transplant candidate, but currently is stable and at low risk, observation or minimally toxic therapies may be used as short-term interventions, with consideration of the transplant at time of progression.

## SUMMARY

The current management of MMM is problematic, as there are limited options that have been shown to impact survival and disease course. Allogeneic stem cell transplantation, although potentially curative in some patients, is not an option for many patients because of older age, lack of donors, and comorbidities. Useful palliative options exist for treating symptoms from the disease, but have overall not improved survival for the disease. Active investigations into novel agents for the therapy of MMM with thalidomide analogs such as lenalidomide and others ongoing. Improved understanding of pathogenetic mechanism of disease or disease progression may hopefully yield therapeutic targets of greater specificity and efficacy.

## REFERENCES

1. Heuck G: Zwei falle von Leukamie mit eigenthumlichem blut-resp knochenmarksbefund. *Arch Pathol Physiol Klinische Med* 78:475–496, 1879.

2. Jackson H, Lemon H: Agnogenic myeloid metaplasia of the spleen: a syndrome simulating other more definite hematologic disorders. *N Engl J Med* 222:985–994, 1940.

3. Tefferi A: Myelofibrosis with myeloid metaplasia. *N Engl J Med* 342:1255–1265, 2000.

4. Hirsch E: Generalized osteosclerosis with chronic polycythemia vera. *Arch Pathol* 19:91–97, 1935.

5. Jacobsen R, Salo A, Fialkow P: Agnogeneic myeloid metaplasia: a clonal proliferation of hematopoietic stem cells with secondary myelofibrosis. *Blood* 51:189, 1978.

6. Mesa RA, Hanson CA, Rajkumar SV, Schroeder G, Tefferi A: Evaluation and clinical correlations of bone marrow angiogenesis in myelofibrosis with myeloid metaplasia. *Blood* 96:3374–3380, 2000.

7. Mesa RA, Silverstein MN, Jacobsen SJ, Wollan PC, Tefferi A: Population-based incidence and survival figures in essential thrombocythemia and agnogenic myeloid metaplasia: an Olmsted County study, 1976—1995. *Am J Hematol* 61:10–15, 1999.

8. Mesa RA, Li CY, Schroeder G, Tefferi A: Clinical correlates of splenic histopathology and splenic karyotype in myelofibrosis with myeloid metaplasia. *Blood* 97:3665–3667, 2001.

9. Tefferi A, Mesa RA, Nagorney DM, Schroeder G, Silverstein MN: Splenectomy in myelofibrosis with myeloid metaplasia: a single-institution experience with 223 patients. *Blood* 95:2226–2233, 2000.

10. Dingli D, Utz JP, Krowka MJ, Oberg AL, Tefferi A: Unexplained pulmonary hypertension in chronic myeloproliferative disorders. *Chest* 120:801–808, 2001.

11. Koch CA, Li CY, Mesa RA, Tefferi A: Nonhepatosplenic extramedullary hematopoiesis: associated diseases, pathology, clinical course, and treatment. *Mayo Clin Proc* 78:1223–1233, 2003.

12. Tefferi A, Elliot MA: Serious myeloproliferative reactions associated with the use of thalidomide in myelofibrosis with myeloid metaplasia. *Blood* 96:4007, 2000.

13. Dupriez B, Morel P, Demory JL, et al.: Prognostic factors in agnogenic myeloid metaplasia: a report on 195 cases with a new scoring system [see comments]. *Blood* 88:1013–1018, 1996.

14. Tefferi A, Mesa RA, Schroeder G, Hanson CA, Li CY, Dewald GW: Cytogenetic findings and their clinical relevance in myelofibrosis with myeloid metaplasia. *Br J Haematol* 113:763–771, 2001.

15. Cervantes F, Pereira A, Esteve J, et al.: Identification of "short-lived" and "long-lived" patients at presentation of idiopathic myelofibrosis. *Br J Haematol* 97:635–640, 1997.

16. Barosi G, Viarengo G, Pecci A, et al.: Diagnostic and clinical relevance of the number of circulating CD34(+) cells in myelofibrosis with myeloid metaplasia. *Blood* 98:3249–3255, 2001.

17. Guardiola P, Anderson JE, Bandini G, et al.: Allogeneic stem cell transplantation for agnogenic myeloid metaplasia: a European Group for Blood and Marrow Transplantation, Societe Francaise de Greffe de Moelle, Gruppo Italiano per il Trapianto del Midollo Osseo,

and Fred Hutchinson Cancer Research Center Collaborative study. *Blood* 93:2831–2838, 1999.

18. Guardiola P, Anderson JE, Gluckman E: Myelofibrosis with myeloid metaplasia. *N Engl J Med* 343:659, 2000; discussion: 659–660.

19. Deeg HJ, Appelbaum FR: Stem-cell transplantation for myelofibrosis. *N Engl J Med* 344:775–776, 2001.

20. Jurado M, Deeg H, Gooley T, et al.: Haemopoietic stem cell transplantation for advanced polycythaemia vera or essential thrombocythaemia. *Br J Haematol* 112:392–396, 2001.

21. Devine SM, Hoffman R, Verma A, et al.: Allogeneic blood cell transplantation following reduced-intensity conditioning is effective therapy for older patients with myelofibrosis with myeloid metaplasia. *Blood* 99:2255–2258, 2002.

22. Daly A, Song K, Nevill T, et al.: Stem cell transplantation for myelofibrosis: a report from two Canadian centers. *Bone Marrow Transplantation* 32:35–40, 2003.

23. Deeg HJ, Gooley TA, Flowers ME, et al.: Allogeneic hematopoietic stem cell transplantation for myelofibrosis. *Blood* 102:3912–3918, 2003.

24. Rondelli D, Barosi G, Bacigalupo A, et al.: Non-myeloablative allogeneic HSCT in high risk patients with myelofibrosis. *Blood* 102:695a, 2003.

25. Anderson JE, Tefferi A, Craig F, et al.: Myeloablation and autologous peripheral blood stem cell rescue results in hematologic and clinical responses in patients with myeloid metaplasia with myelofibrosis. *Blood* 98:586–593, 2001.

26. Guardiola P, Esperou H, Cazalshatem D, et al.: Allogeneic bone marrow transplantation for agnogenic myeloid metaplasia. *Br J Haematol* 98:1004–1009, 1997.

27. Dupriez B, Morel P, Demory J, et al.: Prognostic factors in agnogenic myeloid metaplasia: a report on 195 cases with a new scoring system [see comments]. *Blood* 88:1013–1018, 1996.

28. Rodriguez JN, Martino ML, Dieguez JC, Prados D: rHuEpo for the treatment of anemia in myelofibrosis with myeloid metaplasia. Experience in 6 patients and meta-analytical approach. *Haematologica* 83:616–621, 1998.

29. Besa E, Nowell P, Geller N, Gardner F: Analysis of the androgen response of 23 patients with agnogenic myeloid metaplasia: the value of chromosomal studies in predicting response and survival. *Cancer* 49:308, 1982.

30. Cervantes F, Hernandez-Boluda JC, Alvarez A, Nadal E, Montserrat E: Danazol treatment of idiopathic myelofibrosis with severe anemia. *Haematologica* 85:595–599, 2000.

31. Levy V, Bourgarit A, Delmer A, et al.: Treatment of agnogenic myeloid metaplasia with danazol—a report of four cases. *Am J Hematol* 53:239–241, 1996.

32. Barosi G, Grossi A, Comotti B, Musto P, Gamba G, Marchetti M: Safety and efficacy of thalidomide in patients with myelofibrosis with myeloid metaplasia. *Br J Haematol* 114:78–83, 2001.

33. Canepa L, Ballerini F, Varaldo R, et al.: Thalidomide in agnogenic and secondary myelofibrosis. *Br J Haematol* 115:313–315, 2001.

34. Elliott MA, Mesa RA, Li CY, et al.: Thalidomide treatment in myelofibrosis with myeloid metaplasia. *Br J Haematol* 117:288–296, 2002.

35. Grossi A, Gavazzi S, Biscardi M, et al.: Thalidomide therapy effects on angiogenic growth factors (VEGF, TGF-Beta) and KDR expression in myeloid metaplasia with myelofibrosis. *Blood* 100:a4939, 2002.

36. Marchetti M, Barosi G, Balestri F, et al.: Low-dose thalidomide ameliorates cytopenias and splenomegaly in myelofibrosis with myeloid metaplasia: a phase II trial. *J Clin Oncol* 22:424–431, 2004.

37. Merup M, Kutti J, Birgergard G, et al.: Negligible clinical effects of thalidomide in patients with myelofibrosis with myeloid metaplasia. *Med Oncol* 19:79–86, 2002.

38. Piccaluga PP, Visani G, Pileri SA, et al.: Clinical efficacy and antiangiogenic activity of thalidomide in myelofibrosis with myeloid metaplasia. A pilot study. *Leukemia* 16:1609–1614, 2002.

39. Pozzato G, Zorat F, Nascimben F, Comar C, Kikic F, Festini G: Thalidomide therapy in compensated and decompensated myelofibrosis with myeloid metaplasia. *Haematologica* 86:772–773, 2001.

40. Strupp C, Germing U, Scherer A, et al.: Thalidomide for the treatment of idiopathic myelofibrosis. *Eur J Haematol* 72:52–57, 2004.

41. Mesa RA, Steensma DP, Pardanani A, et al.: A phase 2 trial of combination low-dose thalidomide and prednisone for the treatment of myelofibrosis with myeloid metaplasia. *Blood* 101:2534–2541, 2003.

42. Visani G, Mele A, Malagola M, Isidori A, Finelli C, Piccaluga P: Sequential combination of thalidomide and erythropoietin determines transfusion independence and disease control in idiopathic myelofibrosis previously insensitive to both drugs as single agents. *Leukemia* 17:1669, 2003.

43. Tefferi A, Elliott MA: Serious myeloproliferative reactions associated with the use of thalidomide in myelofibrosis with myeloid metaplasia. *Blood* 96:4007, 2002.

44. Kyrtsonis MC, Kokoris SI, Kontopidou FN, Siakantaris MP, Kittas C, Pangalis GA: Development of a myeloproliferative disorder in a patient with monoclonal gammopathy of undetermined significance secreting immunoglobulin of the M class and treated with thalidomide and anti-CD20 monoclonal antibody. *Blood* 97:2527–2528, 2001.

45. Mesa RA, Elliott MA, Faoro L, Tefferi A: Durable and unmaintained remissions with thalidomide-based drug therapy in myelofibrosis with myeloid metaplasia: long term outcome analysis of 2 prospective trials. *Blood* 102:a104, 2003.

46. Jensen M: Splenectomy in myelofibrosis. *Acta Med Scand* 175:533–544, 1964.

47. Hickling RA: Splenectomy in myeloid metaplasia. *Q J Med* 30:253, 1937.

48. Bukh H, With TK: Splenectomy in chronic non-leukemic myeloid splenomegaly with a report of osteosclerosis. *Acta Chir Scand* 92:507–532, 1945.

49. Green TW, Conley C, Ashburn LI, Peters HR: Splenectomy for myeloid metaplasia of the spleen. *N Engl J Med* 248:211–219, 1953.

50. Videbaek A: Fibrosis and sclerosis of the bone marrow. *Acta Haematol* 15:235–245, 1956.

51. Gomes MR, Silverstein MN, Remine WH: Splenectomy for agnogenic myeloid metaplasia. *Surg Gynecol Obstet* 125:106–108, 1967.

52. Schwartz SI, Bernard RP, Adams JT, Bauman AW: Splenectomy for hematologic disorders. *Arch Surg* 101:338–347, 1970.

53. Morgenstern L: Splenectomy for massive splenomegaly due to myeloid metaplasia. *Am J Surg* 122:288–293, 1971.

54. Milner GR, Geary CG, Wadsworth LD, Doss A: Erythrokinetic studies as a guide to the value of splenectomy in primary myeloid metaplasia. *Br J Haematol* 25:467–484, 1973.

55. Silverstein MN, Remine WH: Sex, splenectomy, and myeloid metaplasia. *JAMA* 227:424–426, 1974.

56. Gale D, Sacks P, Lynch S, Bothwell TH, Bezwoda W, Stevens K: The place of splenectomy in haematological disorders. *S Afr Med J* 48:1240–1245, 1974.

57. Mulder H, Steenbergen J, Haanen C: Clinical course and survival after elective splenectomy in 19 patients with primary myelofibrosis. *Br J Haematol* 35:419–427, 1977.

58. Cabot EB, Brennan MF, Rosenthal DS, Wilson RE: Splenectomy in myeloid metaplasia. *Ann Surg* 187:24–30, 1978.

59. Little JM: A prospective study of 100 splenectomies. *Aust N Z J Surg* 48:390–397, 1978.

60. Silverstein MN, Remine WH: Splenectomy in myeloid metaplasia. *Blood* 53:515–518, 1979.

61. Benbassat J PS, Ligumski M: Splenectomy in patients with agnogenic myeloid metaplasia: an analysis of 321 published cases. *Br J Haematol* 42:207–214, 1979.

62. Jarvinen H, Kivilaakso E, Ikkala E, Vuopio P, Hastbacka J: Splenectomy for myelofibrosis. *Ann Clin Res* 14:66–71, 1982.

63. Coon WW, Liepman MK: Splenectomy for agnogenic myeloid metaplasia. *Surg Gynecol Obstet* 154:561–563, 1982.

64. Musser G, Lazar G, Hocking W, Busuttl W: Splenectomy for hematologic disease. *Ann Surg* 200:40–45, 1984.

65. Sharp P, Grace CS, Rozenberg MC, Ham JM: Splenectomy for massive splenomegaly. *Aust N Z J Surg* 55:489–492, 1985.

66. Dotevall A, Kutti J, Wadenvik H, Westin J: A retrospective analysis of a consecutive series of patients splenectomized for various hematologic disorders. *Acta Haematol* 77:38–44, 1987.

67. Benbassat J, Gilon D, Penchas S: The choice between splenectomy and medical treatment in patients with advanced agnogenic myeloid metaplasia. *Am J Hematol* 33:128–135, 1990.

68. Brenner B, Nagler A, Tatarsky I, Hashmonai M: Splenectomy in agnogenic myeloid metaplasia and postpolycythemic myeloid metaplasia. A study of 34 cases. *Arch Intern Med* 148:2501–2505, 1988.

69. Schmitz N, Suttorp M, Schlegelberger B, Weber-Matthiesen K, Tiemann M, Sonnen R: The role of the spleen after bone marrow transplantation for primary myelofibrosis. *Br J Haematol* 81:616–618, 1992.

70. Barosi G, Ambrosetti A, Buratti A, et al.: Splenectomy for patients with myelofibrosis with myeloid metaplasia: pretreatment variables and outcome prediction. *Leukemia* 7:200–206, 1993.

71. Lafaye F, Rain JD, Clot P, Najean Y: Risks and benefits of splenectomy in myelofibrosis: an analysis of 39 cases. *Nouv Rev Fr Hematol* 36:359–362, 1994.

72. Jameson JS, Thomas WM, Dawson S: Splenectomy for haematologic disease. *J R Coll Surg Edinb* 41:307–311, 1996.

73. Mittelman MKS, Zeidman A: Splenectomy for hematologic disease—a single institution experience. *Haematologica* 28:185–198, 1997.

74. Bohner H, Tirier C, Rotzcher VM: Indications for and results of splenectomy in different hematologic disorders. *Langenbecks Arch Chir* 382:79–82, 1997.

75. Barosi G, Ambrosetti A, Centra A, et al.: Splenectomy and risk of blast transformation in myelofibrosis with myeloid metaplasia. Italian Cooperative Study Group on Myeloid with Myeloid Metaplasia. *Blood* 91:3630–3636, 1998.

76. Akpek G, McAneny D, Weintraub L: Risks and benefits of splenectomy in myelofibrosis with myeloid metaplasia: a retrospective analysis of 26 cases. *J Surg Oncol* 77:42–48, 2001.

77. Lofvenberg E, Wahlin A: Management of polycythaemia vera, essential thrombocythaemia and myelofibrosis with hydroxyurea. *Eur J Haematol* 41:375–381, 1988.

78. Best PJ, Daoud MS, Pittelkow MR, Petitt RM: Hydroxyurea-induced leg ulceration in 14 patients [see comments]. *Ann Intern Med* 128:29–32, 1998.

79. Manoharan A, Pitney WR: Chemotherapy resolves symptoms and reverses marrow fibrosis in myelofibrosis. *Scand J Haematol* 33:453–459, 1984.

80. Petti MC, Latagliata R, Spadea T, et al.: Melphalan treatment in patients with myelofibrosis with myeloid metaplasia. *Br J Haematol* 116:576–581, 2002.

81. Tefferi A, Silverstein MN, Li CY: 2-Chlorodeoxyadenosine treatment after splenectomy in patients who have myelofibrosis with myeloid metaplasia. *Br J Haematol* 99:352–357, 1997.

82. Mesa RA, Camoriano JK, Geyer SM, et al.: A phase 2 consortium (P2C) trial of R115777 (Zarnestra) in myelofibrosis with myeloid metaplasia: interim analysis of 18 patients. *Blood* 102:a3428, 2003.

83. Giles FJ, List AF, Roboz GJ, et al.: Phase I/II study of PTK787/ZK 222584 (PTK/ZK), a novel, oral VEGF-receptor inhibitor, in patients with myelofibrosis with myeloid metaplasia. *Blood* 102:a3431, 2003.

84. Silverstein MN: Control of hypersplenism and painful splenomegaly in myeloid metaplasia by irradiation. *Int J Radiat Oncol Biol Phys* 2:1221–1222, 1977.

85. Greenberger JS, Chaffey JT, Rosenthal DS, Moloney WC: Irradiation for control of hypersplenism and painful splenomegaly in myeloid metaplasia. *Int J Radiat Oncol Biol Phys* 2:1083–1090, 1977.

86. Slanina J, Vondraczek A, Wannenmacher M: Symptomatic irradiation therapy of the spleen in advanced osteomyelosclerosis. *Dtsch Med Wochenschr* 111:1144–1150, 1986.

87. Wagner H Jr, McKeough PG, Desforges J, Madoc-Jones H: Splenic irradiation in the treatment of patients with chronic myelogenous leukemia or myelofibrosis with myeloid metaplasia. Results of daily and intermittent fractionation with and without concomitant hydroxyurea. *Cancer* 58:1204–1207, 1986.

88. Elliott MA, Chen MG, Silverstein MN, Tefferi A: Splenic irradiation for symptomatic splenomegaly associated with myelofibrosis with myeloid metaplasia. *Br J Haematol* 103:505–511, 1998.

89. Bouabdallah R, Coso D, Gonzague-Casabianca L, Alzieu C, Resbeut M, Gastaut JA: Safety and efficacy of splenic irradiation in the treatment of patients with idiopathic myelofibrosis: a report on 15 patients. *Leuk Res* 24:491–495, 2000.

90. McFarland JT, Kuzma C, Millard FE, Johnstone PA: Palliative irradiation of the spleen. *Am J Clin Oncol* 26:178–183, 2003.

91. Tefferi A, Jimenez T, Gray LA, Mesa RA, Chen MG: Radiation therapy for symptomatic hepatomegaly in myelofibrosis with myeloid metaplasia. *Eur J Haematol* 66:37–42, 2001.

92. Leinweber C, Order SE, Calkins AR: Whole-abdominal irradiation for the management of gastrointestinal and abdominal manifestations of agnogenic myeloid metaplasia. *Cancer* 68:1251–1254, 1991.

93. Koch C, Li C, Mesa R, Tefferi A: Nonhepatosplenic extrameduallry hematopoiesis: associated diseases, pathology, clinical course, and treatment. *Mayo Clin Proc* 78:1223–1233, 2003.

94. Steensma DP, Hook CC, Stafford SL, Tefferi A: Low-dose, single-fraction, whole-lung radiotherapy for pulmonary hypertension associated with myelofibrosis with myeloid metaplasia. *Br J Haematol* 118:813–816, 2002.

95. Weinschenker P, Kutner JM, Salvajoli JV, et al.: Whole-pulmonary low-dose radiation therapy in agnogenic myeloid metaplasia with diffuse lung involvement. *Am J Hematol* 69:277–280, 2002.

96. Battegay EJ, Raines EW, Colbert T, Ross R: TNF-alpha stimulation of fibroblast proliferation. Dependence on platelet-derived growth factor (PDGF) secretion and alteration of PDGF receptor expression. *J Immunol* 154:6040–6047, 1995.

97. Rusten LS, Jacobsen SE: Tumor necrosis factor (TNF)-alpha directly inhibits human erythropoiesis in vitro: role of p55 and p75 TNF receptors. *Blood* 85:989–996, 1995.

98. Dinarello CA, Cannon JG, Wolff SM, et al.: Tumor necrosis factor (cachectin) is an endogenous pyrogen and induces production of interleukin 1. *J Exp Med* 163:1433–1450, 1986.

99. Steensma DP, Mesa RA, Li CY, Gray L, Tefferi A: Etanercept, a soluble tumor necrosis factor receptor, palliates constitutional symptoms in patients with myelofibrosis with myeloid metaplasia: results of a pilot study. *Blood* 99:2252–2254, 2002.

100. Cervantes F, Tassies D, Salgado C, Rovira M, Pereira A, Rozman C: Acute transformation in nonleukemic chronic myeloproliferative disorders: actuarial probability and main characteristics in a series of 218 patients. *Acta Haematol* 85:124–127, 1991.

101. Mesa RA, Tefferi A: Survival and outcomes to therapy in leukemic transformation of myelofibrosis with myeloid metaplasia: a single institution experience with 91 patients. *Blood* 102:a3414, 2003.

# Chapter 50

# MANAGEMENT OF CHRONIC MYELOMONOCYTIC LEUKEMIA AND OTHER RARE MYELOPROLIFERATIVE DISORDERS

*Miloslav Beran*

## CHRONIC MYELOMONOCYTIC LEUKEMIA

### INTRODUCTION

Chronic myelomonocytic leukemia (CMML) is a clonal bone marrow disorder of stem cells. The distinguishing feature is a persistent absolute monocytosis (blood monocytes greater than $1 \times 10^9$/L). Studies of the disease's natural history reveal heterogeneity in pathology, clinical features, and the outcome of untreated patients, as measured by duration of survival. The recent World Health Organization (WHO) reclassification of CMML and its inclusion as a separate entity in the groups of myeloproliferative/myelodysplastic disorders reflects two major pathologic features that appear with varying prominence in individual patients: cellular proliferation, which involves predominantly white blood cell (WBC) lineage and is often associated with organ infiltration and organomegaly, and maturation defects characterized by marrow dysplasia, which may involve all cell lineages, and result in anemia, thrombocytopenia, and rarely neutropenia.[1] Either proliferative or dysplastic features may predominate in the clinicopathologic profile of individual patients, and the predominance may change during the course of the disease, usually from dysplastic to proliferative. Whether CMML should be categorized into dysplastic and proliferative entities based on the arbitrarily chosen "cutoff" for WBC at $13 \times 10^9$/L, or whether these features could be viewed as various stages of the same disease, is still being discussed[2,3] and was recently reviewed.[3] It is tempting to speculate that different cellular regulatory pathways may be activated as a consequence of the presence of different primary or secondary molecular lesions. However, as will be discussed later in this chapter, these basic features do have some relevance in the current treatment of individual patients. These features are only marginally associated with prognosis and survival.[3,4]

### ASSESSMENT OF PROGNOSIS

Because optimal CMML management is still being developed and a multitude of investigational options are available, the ability to assess the risk-to-benefit ratio of any particular treatment for individual patients is important. This assessment has been facilitated by the identification of both disease- and patient-related variables associated with outcome, as measured by survival. In turn, these variables have led to the development of prognostic scoring systems for CMML that allow identification of patients with various life expectancies and risks of succumbing to the disease if untreated.[4]

The most significant variables negatively associated with survival, as determined by a multivariate analysis of a large number of patients with well-defined CMML, are the degree of anemia; the presence of circulating immature WBC; the absolute blood lymphocyte count; an increased percentage of bone marrow blasts; and an abnormal karyotype.[4] Although age was not a significant prognostic variable in that multivariate analysis, the goals of optimal management are modified by age-related considerations (e.g., quality of life vs potentially limited prolongation of survival), and age should always be considered, along with auxiliary medical problems and patients' wishes, in choosing the approach for optimal management.

### PRETREATMENT EVALUATION

Continuous development of investigational treatments, identification of prognostic variables, and the recent success of targeted therapy with imatinib mesylate in selected CMML patients with specific chromosomal alterations associated with activation of receptor tyrosine kinases (RTKs, see below), all support the need for an extended initial evaluation. In addition to clinical assessment and the standard laboratory tests used to establish a diagnosis, the pretreatment workup should include bone marrow aspiration, biopsy, and cytogenetic analysis. Information on $\beta_2$-microglobulin and plasma lactate dehydrogenase (LDH) concentrations are useful because high plasma levels are associated with a worse prognosis.[4] In patients up to 65–70 years old, HLA tissue typing of patients and their siblings should be considered, given the possibility of a reduced-intensity conditioning regimen and allogeneic stem cell transplantation (SCT). Both karyotyping and molecular screening for the BCR/ABL translocation are therapeutically relevant, as they have prognostic implications and are necessary to exclude BCR/ABL-positive disease with monocytosis and to identify rare cases with specific translocations involving genes coding for RTK.[5–8] (This is discussed in detail elsewhere.) Cells from patients with translocations involving platelet-derived growth factor receptor (PDGFR)β may be further evaluated by molecular assays to verify such molecular abnormalities, and result in abnormally functioning RTK sensitive to TK inhibitors, such as imatinib mesylate.[5–8] In myeloproliferative disorders (MPD), including CMML, translocations involving PDGFRβ [such as t(5;12)] frequently appear to be associated with marrow dysplasia and blood eosinophilia.[8] In the absence of an abnormal karyotype, the possibility of a cryptic translocation involving the 5q33 region may mandate further molecular screening using, for example, polymerase chain reaction (PCR) and specific primers.

Ideally, the final therapeutic decision is made on the basis of both the patient's clinical status and the prognostically significant features of the disease.[4] With the exception of SCT in certain patients, however, the available treatment modalities rarely, if ever, result in the eradication of CMML. The relative rarity of the disease, lack of agreement on a "standard of care," and lack of uniform criteria for patient response hamper initiation of well-designed randomized clinical trials needed to answer such questions. This said, numerous treatment modalities, which are all by definition investigational, provide various levels of disease control and improvements in quality of life.

### TREATMENT OPTIONS

Traditionally, the management of CMML has focused on disease-associated clinical symptoms, symptoms associated with marrow failure (i.e., anemia and thrombocytopenia), and symptoms of increased myeloproliferation (i.e., increased WBC count, organomegaly, and hypermetabolic state). For this purpose, an intuitive stratification into "dysplastic" CMML, resembling myelodysplastic syndrome (MDS), and "proliferative" CMML, resembling MPD, seems practical.[2–4] MDS CMML is primarily managed with supportive care, and cytotoxic therapy is added when signs of proliferative disease, characterized by an increased WBC count and/or organ involvement or constitutional symptoms, appear. MPD CMML is managed with cytotoxic therapy plus supportive care.

### Supportive care

In elderly patients who have low-risk or intermediate-1-risk CMML at the time of diagnosis, as assessed with the MD Anderson Prognostic Score (MDAPS),[4] the median survival times from presentation are 24 and 18 months, respectively.[4] For such patients, supportive care similar to that given for patients with low-risk MDS and participation in clinical trials using low-toxicity agents are recommended. Severe anemia (hemoglobin concentration <10 g/dL) or transfusion-dependent anemia may be treated with weekly doses of erythropoietin of 40,000–60,000 units for a trial period of 6–8 weeks, with pretreatment assessment of endogenous erythropoietin levels and monitoring of treatment by weekly evaluation of reticulocyte count and hemoglobin concentration. Unlike in MDS,[9] the benefit of such treatment in CMML is not well documented. Growth factors such as granulocyte-colony-stimulating factor and granulocyte-macrophage colony-stimulating factor should be used cautiously because of their propensity to induce an unwanted monocytic response. Their use should be limited to febrile patients, particularly those with documented infection and severe neutropenia, not responding to antibiotics. To avoid allosensitization, platelet transfusions should be administered on the basis of symptoms of clinically significant hemorrhage rather than on platelet counts; an exception to this rule is the use of prophylactic transfusions in patients enrolled in clinical trials. Routine use of prophylactic platelet transfusions is not recommended. Whether associated with leukocytosis or not, severe thrombocytopenia usually signals advanced disease and indicates a need for reassessment of the patient's risk status and change in therapeutic strategy.

### Established single-agent oral chemotherapy

In patients who have CMML with a significant myeloproliferative component, high WBC count, or organomegaly, treatment with single-agent chemotherapy has been the standard of care. Oral agents such as busulfan, 6-mercaptopurine, hydroxyurea, and oral etoposide have been used empirically with some success, but a prospective randomized study conclusively determined the superiority of hydroxyurea over etoposide in terms of overall survival in patients with mostly advanced proliferative disease (i.e., splenomegaly, mild thrombocytopenia, and increased bone marrow blasts): 24 months for hydroxyurea versus 9 months for etoposide.[10] This is the only prospective randomized study to date that has compared two treatment regimens in patients with CMML. Although neither regimen induced complete remission (CR) or affected the natural history of the disease, the results supported the idea of using hydroxyurea plus supportive care as the "standard-of-care" arm in any future randomized trials. No randomized study comparing "treatment" with supportive care has ever been reported in CMML.

Agents currently approved by the Food and Drug Administration for the management of CMML (defined as a subcategory of MDS by FAB classification) are 5-azacytidine (Vidaza®) and 2'-deoxy-5'-azacytidine (Dacogen®). One major reason for the lack of clinical trials specifically designed for CMML is the French–American British classification which recognized CMML as a subcategory of MDS, and guided the enrollment of patients with CMML into MDS trials. The identification of CMML as a separate disease entity,[1] together with the availability of a prognostic risk assessment developed specifically for CMML,[4] should facilitate future design of CMML-specific trials.

### Other chemotherapeutic agents

Not much is known about the effectiveness of other cytoreductive agents in managing CMML as assessed in phase I/II trials. For example, three separate studies with the anthracycline idarubicin suggested that it has limited activity, with no significant responses observed in CMML patients who were treated daily with intermediate dosages.[11,12]

In the first trial of *oral etoposide (VP-16)*, 10 consecutive patients with CMML were treated with 100 mg of etoposide orally, daily for 3 days (50 mg in "nonproliferative" disease), followed by a "maintenance" dose of 50 mg twice weekly. Clinical benefit, observed in seven patients, included improvement of anemia, thrombocytopenia, and extramedullary disease. Diminished benefit was noted in patients with increased blasts in the blood and bone marrow.[13] A second etoposide trial used 50 mg orally, daily for 21 days every 4 weeks.[14] Twelve of 17 patients with CMML experienced hematologic responses, three after failing treatment with hydroxyurea. The median duration of hematologic responses was 9+ months (range 4–49+ months). Responses consisted of control of leukocytosis in 12 patients, normalization of platelet counts in 2 thrombocytopenic patients, and resolution of anemia in 1 case. Two of six patients with splenomegaly had >50% reduction in spleen size.[15]

The use of *cladribine* (2-chlorodeoxyadenosine-2 CdA, or *2-CdA*) to manage CMML was prompted by the drug's proven efficacy in indolent lymphoproliferative disorders and by the observation of decrease in monocyte counts in patients with lymphoproliferative disorders treated with cladribine. An initial trial of cladribine at 0.1 mg/kg/day for 5–7 days in four patients[15] resulted in a rapid decrease in monocyte counts. These results were subsequently confirmed in seven patients given cladribine in a dosing schedule of 0.2 mg/m² daily for 5 days every 3 weeks for a total of three cycles.[16] With this regimen, one patient attained a CR lasting 4 months and three patients exhibited partial responses (PRs) lasting 3–6 month. Although the overall response of 55% was encouraging, no further trials were conducted.

*Cytarabine* (*cytosine arabinoside*, or *ara-C*), administered subcutaneously at low dosages of 10–20 mg daily for 10–21 days, was studied extensively in the management of MDS and to a lesser degree of CMML during the 1980s and early 1990s. The initial enthusiasm was sparked by speculation on the ability of cytarabine to induce terminal differentiation of malignant hematopoietic cells. Although the contribution of differentiation to the treatment outcome was never proven and the effect was attributed to the cytotoxic action of the drug, the effectiveness of the regimen was well documented. In small studies using cytarabine to manage CMML, the CR rates varied from 0 to 25%, and a review of data from 80 patients noted 9 CRs and a calculated CR rate of 14%.[17] Thus, the efficacy of cytarabine was modest and, ultimately, the treatment outcomes were viewed skeptically. Because of the small numbers of patients in the reported trials, the associated myelosuppression, and the lack of information on response durations, the value of cytarabine in the management of CMML is poorly documented. However, the activity of low-dose cytarabine is probably comparable to that of other single agents, such as 5-azacytidine, decitabine, and topotecan, in terms of effect on the bone marrow and CR rates. Its future use may more likely lie in combination with other agents, as documented for high-dose cytarabine plus topotecan.[18]

### Topoisomerase I inhibitors

Among studies using recently developed agents, encouraging results have been obtained with the topoisomerase I inhibitor topotecan in a phase II study of 30 patients with diagnosis of CMML, both previously treated and untreated. Topotecan was given as a continuous intravenous infusion at the maximal tolerated dosage (MTD) of 10 mg/m² over 5 days every 4–8 weeks.[19,20] Topotecan induced a CR in almost one-third of the patients, and for the first time, CRs due to a single agent were characterized by karyotypic conversion of bone marrow from abnormal to diploid.[19,20] This result suggested that topotecan has a differential effect on normal and CMML cells. The median CR duration was 7.5 months (range 1–31 months), and median survival was 10.5 months.[20] In this single-arm study, the impact on survival could not be documented.[19,20]

An oral preparation of topotecan with satisfactory bioavailability was investigated in two studies using three regimens.[21–23] Given over 17 days at dosages varying from 0.8 to 1.9 mg/m²/day, 5 days on, 2 days off for three cycles, oral topotecan induced CRs in two of seven patients with CMML.[21] The dose-limiting toxicity was nausea and vomiting, and the MTD was 1.4 mg/m²/day. In a phase II study, 1.2 mg/m² of topotecan was given orally either twice daily for 5 days or once daily for 10 days, and both schedules delivered the same total dose.[22,23] Ten patients with CMML were included. Although no patients achieved a CR, seven exhibited a response.[23] The duration of responses was not reported, and the impact of the treatment with oral topotecan on the natural history of the disease is unknown.

Another orally bioavailable topoisomerase I inhibitor, 9-nitro-20-(S)-camptothecin, was studied in a phase II study as a continuous daily administration at doses adjusted according to each patient's tolerance. The study group included 23 patients with CMML; responses were observed in 10 (1 CR, 4 PRs, and 5 hematologic improvements [HI]).[60]

The optimal administration schedule for increasing the rate and duration of responses remains to be defined for both topotecan and 9-nitro-20-(S) -camptothecin. At present, topotecan administered intravenously at the MTD appears to be the more effective agent against CMML, with the highest documented frequency of complete hematologic and cytogenetic remissions.[19,20] The potential value of these topoisomerase I inhibitors would be best appreciated in a randomized trial comparing them with hydroxyurea, analogous to the trial that compared hydroxyurea and etoposide.[10] The use of topoisomerase I inhibitors to manage CMML might be more effective in combination therapy than as single agents.[18]

### 2-Deoxycytidine analogs (hypomethylating agents)

The role of 5-azacytidine and 5-aza-2'-deoxycytidine (decitabine) in the treatment of MDS and, to a lesser degree, in MPD has been investigated for well over a decade. Besides their cytotoxic activity, these agents induce hypomethylation of genes involved in regulating proliferation and differentiation, particularly tumor suppressor genes that are frequently hypermethylated in malignant disorders and presumably also in CMML.[24] This hypomethylating effect is believed to be particularly active at relatively low doses. The effectiveness of both 5-azacytidine[25] and decitabine[26,27] in managing MDS is well documented, but their efficacy and usefulness in managing CMML are less clear.

In the randomized trial comparing subcutaneous 5-azacytidine (75 mg/m²/day for 7 days every 4 weeks) with supportive care, seven patients with CMML were included in each group.[25] The responses were not analyzed in detail by disease category, but the responses of CMML patients were reported to be "similar" to those with high-risk MDS [refractory anemia with excess blasts (RAEB) and refractory anemia with excess blasts in transformation (RAEBt)]: 8% CR, 15% PR, and 38% HI. Three monthly courses were needed to obtain the best response. Compared with supportive care, the 5-azacytidine regimen provided a significant delay in the disease progression and some survival advantage in patients with MDS; whether these benefits also applied to the small cohort with CMML is unknown.[25]

The effectiveness of decitabine in managing CMML can be assessed from European clinical trials of this agent. In one study of 66 patients with high-risk MDS,[26] subjects were treated with decitabine (15 mg/m² given as an intravenous infusion over 4 h every 8 h for 3 days,

for a cumulative dose of 135 mg/m² over 3 days) every 6 weeks for a maximum of six courses. The study included nine patients with CMML; the cases were classified by the International Prognostic Scoring System, suggesting that all nine belonged to the category of MDS CMML.[2,4] Four (44%) of the nine patients responded: 1 CR, 1 PR, and 2 HI.[26] The actuarial median response duration for the entire study cohort of 66 patients was 31 weeks, and it increased from 26 weeks in patients with HI to 39 weeks for patients with a PR to 36 weeks for those with a CR; no information was provided specifically for the nine patients with CMML.[26] In a subsequent review, the results of three separate studies of 124 patients, including 16 with CMML, revealed cytogenetic CR in two patients with CMML.[27] The response rates and durations were not specifically reported for the CMML patients, however.[27] Together, these results suggest a role for both 5-azacytidine and decitabine in managing CMML, but because reports on their effectiveness in treating CMML are sporadic, no conclusion can be reached. Further study and new assessments based on larger and more formal investigations are required before an accurate evaluation can be made.

### Agents targeting fusion RTKs

Discovery of unique chromosomal abnormalities and underlying molecular changes of RTKs causatively associated with CMML or atypical chronic myelogenous leukemia (aCML)[5–8] suggested potential therapeutic agents targeting the molecular basis of these disorders. The proof of principle was provided by documentation of activity of imatinib mesylate in the management of MPD, including CMML, characterized by activation of the *PDGFRβ* gene by its fusion to *tel* oncogene, a process rendering the PDGFRβ TK permanently activated and responsible for the dysregulated cell growth.[7] After the publication of encouraging results on the in vitro inhibitory activity of imatinib mesylate on PDGFRβ TK,[28] four patients with t(5;12)(q33;q13) and PDGFRβ fused with either TEL(ETV6) (three patients) or an unknown partner (one patient), all with elevated WBC counts and eosinophilia, were treated with 400 mg of imatinib orally, daily. All four patients achieved a CR and the levels of fusion transcripts decreased significantly, even becoming negative in one patient.[5] Responses occurred as early as 1 month, but could be delayed up to 9 months, suggesting disease heterogeneity and the need for prolonged treatment in some cases. Similar responses to imatinib were reported for a CMML patient with the *RAB5EP/PDGFRβ* fusion gene underlying a t(5;17)(q33;p13.3) who achieved a molecular CR 6 weeks after the start of imatinib therapy.[6] Further CRs were reported for a CMML patient with t(5;12)(q33;p13)[29] and for a patient with aCML and a t(5;10)(q33;q22).[30] This concept supported a trial in which imatinib was given to patients with CMML in the expectation of potential activity through as-yet-undetected imatinib-sensitive pathways. So far, the results have been uniformly negative in 19 patients with CMML,[31,32] seven with aCML,[31] and eight with MDS.[32] Thus, imatinib continues to be indicated for trial use in patients with documented rare karyotypic abnormalities that lead to production of imatinib-sensitive fusion TKs. Most patients achieved response within 6 weeks of the initiation of treatment with 400 mg imatinib mesylate daily and continued the treatment in remission. With only preliminary experience, duration of the responses and the optimal treatment schedule are unknown. Although data on the association between the progression of CMML and aCML into more aggressive disease and decreased effectiveness or loss of response to imatinib have been restricted to those from single-case observations (M. Beran, personal observation), this association is analogous to the limited activity of imatinib in advanced BCR-ABL-positive CML.[33]

### Farnesyltransferase inhibitors

The *ras* oncogene is positioned at the crossroads of cellular signaling pathways, and its role in the neoplastic process is well appreciated.[34,35] Mutations in codons 12, 13, or 62 of *ras* significantly affect its physiological role and result in a permanently activated state, causing dysregulated proliferation. CMML is the hematologic malignancy with the highest frequency of ras mutations; in the largest reported cohort of patients, the prevalence of the *N-ras* and *K-ras* mutations was 38%,[4] and the presence of the mutation appeared to negatively influence patients' prognosis and response to therapy.[36] These findings made CMML an attractive target for treatment that blocks ras activity by inhibiting the enzyme farnesyltransferase, which is essential for posttranslational ras modification and attainment of its functional state.[34,35]

Of several farnesyltransferase inhibitors being investigated, tipifarnib (R115777, Zarnestra) and lonafarnib (SH66366, Sarasar) were explored in studies that included a limited number of patients with CMML. In a phase I study, an oral preparation of tipifarnib was administered to 10 patients; two showed a PR and one exhibited an HI, although those responses were transient.[37,38] In a phase I/II study, tipifarnib was given to patients with MPD, including seven patients with aCML and two with CMML.[39] At an initial oral dosage of 300 mg twice daily for 21 days every 4 weeks, clinical responses were noted in three of the seven patients with aCML and none of the patients with CMML.[39] Finally, in the phase II study, lonafarnib, administered orally at 200–300 mg daily until disease progressed or unacceptable toxicity occurred, was investigated in 35 patients with CMML.[40] Among the 25 patients evaluable for response, one achieved a CR and seven exhibited HI, mostly in a single lineage; one patient became independent of red blood cell transfusions.[40]

Orally administered farnesyltransferase inhibitors represent a new category of "targeting" agents; they are only in the early stages of clinical investigations in CMML. However, because the responses to treatment in the malignancies investigated so far, including CMML, do not appear to be influenced by the *ras* mutational status, and because the responses have correlated poorly with the degree of inhibition of farnesyltransferase,[37,38] processes other than farnesylation may be targeted by these agents. Their role as single agents in the treatment of CMML remains uncertain.

### Miscellaneous agents

The presence of increased angiogenesis in CMML[41] stimulated interest in the potential use of angiogenesis inhibitors for managing this disease. A limited number of patients with CMML have been treated with thalidomide. Of seven patients with CMML treated with 100–400 mg thalidomide orally, daily in two studies,[42,43] only one experienced a minor and transient improvement in platelet counts. Because of its poorly predictable adverse effects and the seeming lack of activity, future use of thalidomide in treating patients with CMML is unlikely. Other antiangiogenic and immunomodulating agents, including derivatives of thalidomide that have both antiangiogenic and immunomodulatory properties, are in early stages of clinical development. Phase I/II studies are including patients with CMML.

### Intensive chemotherapy using combination regimens

The first patients with CMML who were treated with combination chemotherapy used to manage acute myelogenous leukemia (AML) were probably those whose initial diagnosis was AML that was later reclassified as MDS or CMML. In later trials in patients with AML, patients with CMML were occasionally included, along with RAEB and RAEBt, as all three categories were considered high-risk MDS. More often than not, little information was given on the clinical and hematologic status of CMML patients, and in such prospective studies, selection bias toward treating younger patients with advanced disease was likely. With few exceptions, treatment regimens consisted of cytarabine (given at standard dosages for 5–7 days) plus anthracycline or anthracenedione antibiotics (daunorubicin, mitoxantrone, or idarubicin). A review of six such studies conducted between 1980 and 1995 identified only 35 patients with CMML, 11 (31%; 95% confidence interval 15.9–47.0%) of whom achieved a CR.[18] Duration of remission and overall survival, when reported, tended to be short and there was no convincing evidence that addition of anthracyclines to cytarabine improved the outcome.

Unfortunately, in most clinical trials, the responses of the CMML cohort were not evaluated separately, further clouding their interpretation. From the results of studies with at least some data available, it may be concluded that such treatments are feasible and that in a portion of patients with CMML, a CR can be obtained, although at the expense of substantial morbidity and even mortality.

Further information on the role of intensive combination chemotherapy was obtained from a series of clinical trials that used chemotherapy of increasing intensity to manage CMML. One such trial used a combination of two single agents with documented effectiveness in CMML and low cardiotoxicity: topotecan, administered as a continuous intravenous infusion at 1.25 mg/m$^2$ over 24 h, daily for 5 days, and cytarabine, as a 2-h infusion at a dosage of intermediate intensity, 1 g/m$^2$/day, for 5 days.[18] Patients who did not experience a CR after the first course of therapy received a second course and a dose adjustment when indicated. Patients who experienced a CR were eligible for postremission chemotherapy. In this prospective phase II study, patients with CMML, RAEB, and RAEBt were registered separately, and treatment outcome was evaluated separately for each disease. Among the 27 patients with CMML who enrolled in the study, 12 (44%; 95% confidence interval 25–65) achieved a CR.[11] Analysis by disease stage showed a CR rate of 62% in CMML patients with <5% bone marrow blasts (corresponding to CMML I by WHO criteria) and 29% in those with >5% bone marrow blasts (CMML II by WHO criteria). As was the case for the RAEB and RAEBt patients, the response rates were not affected by the presence of diploid or abnormal karyotypes, or by primary or secondary CMML. In most CMML patients with an abnormal karyotype, conversion to diploid status was observed. Responses did not differ in patients treated immediately on diagnosis and in those with up to 6 months' history of antecedent hematologic disorder. At a median follow-up of 7 months, the median duration of CR was 33 weeks and the median survival time was 42 weeks.[18] Although the presence of an abnormal karyotype had no significant effect on the response rate, its presence appeared to be associated with a shorter response duration. As with any myelosuppressive treatment, neutropenia-associated fever and infections were the most frequently reported complications during treatment and were observed in 50% of the patients. With supportive care and close surveillance, the mortality rate in the CMML cohort was 10%; all deaths were related to infectious causes.[18]

Most, if not all, combination chemotherapy regimens used to manage CMML included cytarabine as the most active agent. In an attempt to develop an alternative treatment and explore the reported effectiveness of etoposide in CMML,[13,14] a group of 17 patients with CMML was treated with a combination of etoposide (100–200 mg/m$^2$ daily for 5 days) and carboplatinum (continuous intravenous infusion, 200 mg daily for 3–5 days). Of the 17 patients enrolled, 14 were classified by WHO criteria as having CMML I and 3 as having CMML II; 14 had platelet counts of <100 × 10$^9$/L, all 17 were anemic (10 with hemoglobin concentrations less than 10 g/dL), 13 had "proliferative" CMML, and 10 had an abnormal karyotype. Despite the severe myelosuppression and marrow aplasia characteristically caused by

this regimen, five (29%) CMML patients achieved a CR with a median duration of 16 weeks (range 3–22 weeks),[44] indicating that although intensive combination chemotherapy without cytarabine resulted in a CR in one-third of patients, the benefit, as measured by CR duration, was not durable. Achieved at the price of high toxicity and risk of death, the results were not better than those obtained in another study by the same institution with the single-agent topotecan.[19,20] This conclusion led to questioning of the benefit of intensification of chemotherapy in managing CMML.

One comparison of chemotherapy regimens of various intensities used to manage CMML over a 15-year time period[44] included 23 CMML patients treated with a combination of various high-intensity regimens containing high-dose cytarabine plus fludarabine, anthracycline antibiotics (idarubicin and liposomal daunorubicin), or both. Compared with a less intensive topotecan plus cytarabine regimen, no further improvement in the CR rate was achieved, likely because the more intensive regimens induced higher mortality. CR duration remained short, as did overall survival.[44] Because of the limited size of the CMML cohorts treated with various regimens, identification of covariates associated with response and response duration was inconclusive so far. A trend for lower CR rates was noted for patients with more than 5% marrow blasts (CMML-II and for patients with abnormal karyotype.[18] A recent update of the results from the topotecan plus cytarabine regimen, then including 39 patients with CMML, confirmed the earlier results, as did a review of high-dose cytarabine-based regimens updated to 30 patients.[44]

Taken together, these results indicate that although complete hematologic and cytogenetic responses can be obtained in up to 40% of CMML patients, response durations are limited. Only occasional patients remain disease free at 3 years. Further intensification of induction chemotherapy appears to increase mortality and morbidity without leading to an improved response rate and response duration. Topotecan plus cytarabine yields the best results in terms of morbidity, mortality, response rates, and response durations. Whether similar results could be obtained with less intensive regimens (e.g., standard- or low-dose cytarabine plus topotecan, or anthracycline antibiotics at presumably lower toxicity) remains to be investigated in controlled clinical trials. The benefit of postremission chemotherapy, in terms of both intensity and duration, remains unanswered. Responding patients enjoy a better quality of life and prolonged survival, but the effect of the treatment on survival may be related to the natural history of the disease. To date, no treatment regimen positively impacts the natural history of the disease or extends expected survival. As is the case with every management approach in CMML, the value of combination chemotherapy on patient survival will be determined only in a randomized trial against best standard of care; e.g., supportive care (plus hydroxyurea in patients with proliferative disease).

Should chemotherapy be considered at all in the management of CMML, and if so, which regimen should be chosen? No consensus is currently available, but several observations may guide such decision making. At present, the regimen of topotecan plus cytarabine appears to be the best studied, most effective, and least toxic. More than 80% of patients who achieve a CR do so after a single course of this treatment. Although additional complete responses may be achieved with further courses, these responses are obtained with an increased risk for complications, at a higher cost, and tend to be shorter. Thus, one course of this regimen (and possibly other combination regimens) may segregate patients who will likely benefit from additional chemotherapy from those who will not. Supportive care or investigational treatment in the setting of clinical trials may be an alternative option, particularly for high-risk CMML patients. Thus, CMML patients with clinical symptoms or a high-risk prognostic score (e.g., MDAPS)[4] may be candidates for such trials. Another candidate group for chemotherapy may be patients with HLA-matched donors who are considered for allogeneic SCT. Because CMML is resistant to chemotherapy, the frequency of relapses in patients with active disease who receive SCT is high.[46–48] Cytoreduction, and particularly induction of CR, before the SCT may improve the outcome.

### Allogeneic stem cell transplantation

Only two studies report results obtained with allogeneic SCT in adult patients with CMML.[46,47] The outcome of such patients was traditionally included in studies of allogeneic SCT in patients with MDS, of which CMML has been considered a subcategory. Recent WHO classification established CMML as a separate category[1]; the effect of the reclassification on the prognostic impact of SCT is not yet appreciated.

In a European study,[46] 50 patients with CMML underwent SCT at 43 centers; 44 of the donors were HLA matched (38 siblings, six unrelated donors, and one nonsibling relative), and six were partially mismatched. At a median age of 44 years (range 19–63 years), this patient group was clearly selected with respect to age; 40% had karyotypic abnormalities and 36% had between 5 and 29% marrow blasts at the time of transplantation. The median time from diagnosis to SCT was 9 months. Two patients (4%) failed to engraft, and the treatment-associated mortality was high (47%). Median follow-up was 29 months (range 1–59 months); the 5-year estimated overall survival rate was 21%, the disease-free survival rate 16%, and the 5-year estimated probability of relapse 61%.[46] No significant associations with outcome were identified, although transplantation early in the disease might have had a positive influence.[46] The probability of relapse was higher in patients without graft-versus-host disease

(51%) than in those with this disease (29%), and the probability of relapse was higher in patients who received T-cell-depleted grafts (61%) than in those who did not (45 %), suggesting a favorable graft-versus-leukemia effect.

Another study[47] reported results for 21 patients with de novo CMML (12 with "proliferative" disease and nine with nonproliferative disease) who underwent SCT. The cohort consisted of both adults and children (median age 47 years). Twelve of the donors were HLA-identical siblings, four were matched unrelated donors, and five were mismatched donors. Before SCT, only two patients had received intensive combination chemotherapy after progression to AML. After SCT, five patients died of organ failure, two died of chronic graft-versus-host disease, and five relapsed and died. The cumulative relapse rate at 3 years was 25%, and 0.7–8.1 years after transplantation (median 6.9 years), nine (43%) of the patients were still alive.[47] The small size of the patient cohort limited the significance of covariates associated with outcome. SCT later in the course of disease and signs of disease acceleration (e.g., more than 5% marrow blasts), but not abnormal karyotype or proliferative disease, appeared to influence the outcome negatively: four of the five patients who relapsed had an increased percentage of marrow blasts at the time of transplantation.

Finally, a European study of SCT in 43 patients with childhood CMML[48] revealed a 5-year event-free survival rate of 31% (38% in patients who received cells from HLA-matched siblings). However, the relapse rate of 58% suggested resistant disease. The major obstacles of the few studies that have examined the effect of SCT on patients with CMML were the toxicity of the procedure and resistant disease. Additional results, including those for a few CMML patients in reports on MDS, are scattered in the literature, and no critical review is currently available. References to some recent studies are found in a review on the role of SCT in MDS[49] and MPD.[50–52] The conclusion that can be drawn is that SCT is feasible and occasionally "curative" only in younger patients, even though the procedure is associated with considerable morbidity and mortality, and young people make up a small proportion of patients with CMML. This interpretation is compromised by the small number of study patients to date and the heterogeneity of CMML.

Newer transplantation approaches attempt to avoid the excessive toxicity of current conditioning regimens by using lower doses of immunosuppressive drugs (e.g., fludarabine or antithymocyte globulin) and myelosuppressive drugs.[53,54] In patients with MDS, the reduced-intensity regimen results in full engraftment and recovery with less immediate toxicity,[53] thereby extending eligibility for SCT to older persons. The approach relies on the graft-versus-leukemia effect more than ablation of malignant cells by the conditioning regimen, though its success in patients with relatively resistant high-risk CMML is unclear. Because of the high frequency of relapses[46] in patients receiving standard cytoreductive regimens,[46] it seems reasonable, at least for patients with high-risk CMML, to attempt induction of CR immediately before transplantation. The claimed advantage of SCT in low-risk patients and those transplanted early after diagnosis is based on results of retrospective studies or phase II clinical trials with small numbers of CMML patients who are highly selected,[46,47] which complicates interpretation of the results. The absence of randomized studies leaves open the question of whether a delay of transplantation until disease progression would compromise the outcome. For MDS, modeling of the expected outcome of early transplantation suggested an advantage for patients with high-risk disease, whereas patients with low-risk disease benefited from delayed transplantation.[55] In both situations, delay until progression to leukemia resulted in the worst outcome.[55] Thus, patients with low-risk and intermediate-risk disease (by, e.g., MDAPS) may be best treated by supportive care and can be encouraged to participate in investigational clinical trials. Patients with intermediate-risk and high-risk CMML should be considered for SCT if a suitable donor is available. Although many treatment centers prefer a direct transplant procedure, an induction attempt followed by SCT may be a better choice in light of the high relapse rate in such patients and the availability of effective and safe induction therapy.

## ATYPICAL CHRONIC MYELOGENOUS LEUKEMIA

### INTRODUCTION

This category was recently introduced by the WHO classification into the subgroup of myelodysplastic/myeloproliferative disorders.[1] To some extent, it is still a diagnosis of exclusion and includes patients with predominantly overproduction of neutrophils and various degrees of dysplasia in one or more hematopoietic lineages. The most important feature, differentiating aCML from CML is the absence of the BCR/ABL translocation or any variant translocations present in CML. This makes the diagnostic category of aCML similar, if not identical, to that of BCR/ABL-negative CML.[56] Minor distinguishing features include absence of basophilia, older age, more frequent presentation with lower WBC counts, thrombocytopenia, and anemia.[56–60] Separation from CMML is less stringent: Both disorders share the proliferative and dysplastic marrow feature, high median age, and a lack of distinguishing cytogenetic or molecular features. The presence of absolute monocytosis ($>1\times 10^9$/L monocytes) in CMML in association with relative monocytosis ($>8$–10% monocytes on blood smear[2,56,58,60]) separates CMML from aCML. aCML is a rare disease, and in the past cases were included in the category of Ph- negative CML. As about one-half of Ph-negative CML cases are BCR/ABL positive,[60,61] it was difficult to assess characteristic features, prognosis, and response to therapies. Assuming that BCR/ABL-negative cases of CML and aCML are, if not identical, then clinicopathologically very similar entities, information on characteristics, prognostic variables, and outcome of this rare disorder(s) can be based on an analysis of 76 patients.[56] The median survival of patients was 24 months and progression into acute leukemia occurred in 30%. Chromosomal abnormalities were found in 30% of patients, with trisomy 8 being the most frequent, while monosomy 7 was not observed. Complex chromosomal abnormalities were rare. Multivariate analysis identified age >65 years, hemoglobin <10 g/dL, and WBC $>50 \times 10^9$/L as variables associated with poor survival. Younger patients with better blood counts had a median survival of 38 months, compared to 9 months for older patients with compromised counts.[56] The overall prognosis is worse and survival shorter in patients with a CML (Bcr/Abl-negative CML) compared to Ph'-positive CML.[58,59,61] In at least one study, the survival seems not significantly affected by treatment.[56]

The outcome is, however, similar to that in CMML.[3,4,56,59,61] No study has demonstrated the importance of the single objective distinguishing feature of monocytosis as being associated with a different outcome. A detailed analysis of factors associated with outcome in 485 patients (CMML, 304; BCR/ABL-negative CML, 74; Ph-negative, BCR/ABL unknown, 107) found that a diagnosis of CMML indeed confers a significantly shorter median survival (12.6 months) than BCR/ABL-negative CML [21.4 months and Ph-negative, BCR/ABL unknown CML (18.3 months)]. This finding provided, for the first time, the empirical support for separating aCML from CMML.[45]

### TREATMENT

Similar to patients with CMML, the most therapeutically relevant diagnostic tests are karyotype analyses, which should be completed with additional testing for the presence of *BCR/ABL* fusion gene or gene transcripts by fluorescence in situ hybridization (FISH) and, preferably, by molecular testing using PCR. The BCR/ABL-negative CML/aCMLs are rare and only recently defined diseases. No clinical trial has ever been conducted to assess the effectiveness of any specific treatment. Traditionally, the primary goal of therapeutic interventions has been to control myeloproliferation manifested by leukocytosis, or thrombocytosis, and amelioration of anemia, thrombocytopenia, and systemic clinical symptoms associated with the disease (i.e., fatigue, weigh loss, night sweats, cough, bone pain, and organomegaly). In asymptomatic patients with moderate leukocytosis without anemia or thrombocytopenia, it may be prudent to observe the patient with appropriate hematologic follow-up to assess the rate of disease progression.

Younger patients who may be potential candidates for allogeneic SCT should initiate tissue typing of family members and search for a potential stem cell donor. Exceptions to this "observe-and-wait" approach are the rare patients with documented balanced translocations involving RTKs, who are amenable to treatment with TK inhibitors, such as imatinib mesylate, as discussed in the Section "Chronic Myelomonocytic Leukemia".

### Cytoreductive agents

Hydroxyurea and busulfan are the agents most frequently reported as treatment choices in patients with diseases resembling aCML.[62] Both can be used either on a daily schedule with the dose adjusted to the desired leukocyte blood count, or alternatively, on a cyclical schedule aiming initially for resolution of systemic symptoms and reduction of the leukocyte count. Due to its more rapid onset of action and lack of delayed effect on the bone marrow, hydroxyurea is more suitable for continuous, daily maintenance treatment. Busulphan's effects on the bone marrow are less predictable and may be delayed and cumulative, resulting in a prolonged bone marrow suppression. Therefore, its cyclical use is preferable. Although not formally documented in clinical studies, anemia and thrombocytopenia often persist in aCML patients with well-controlled leukocytosis, either as a consequence of the disease itself, treatment-associated myelosuppression, or both. Careful dose titration is therefore recommended for hydroxyurea and particularly for busulphan. An unfavorable response of these patients to busulfan has been considered by some a characteristic feature of aCML,[62] and even treatment with hydroxyurea often yields only partial and transient disease control.[62,63] The effectiveness of both agents is particularly limited in the management of organomegaly.

Analysis of the impact of the effects of various treatments after referral to a tertiary cancer center failed to document significant differences in the survival of treated and untreated patients.[56]

In patients with splenomegaly, splenectomy may result in a temporary alleviation of anemia and thrombocytopenia, provided that the bone marrow remains functional and the cytopenias are not a consequence of disease evolution. Therefore, a bone marrow aspiration, biopsy, and karyotyping should be part of the preoperative evaluation. A recent report on the value of splenectomy in 12 patients with CMML showed improvement of thrombocytopenia in 4 of 11, and a modest improvement of anemia in 2 of 9 patients. None of the anemic patients achieved transfusion independence.[64] There are no reports in aCML, but it is reasonable to expect similar results. Thus, splenectomy should be viewed as a palliative measure, particularly in patients with clinical symptoms, including pain due to splenomegaly. Of the remaining options to reduce splenomegaly, splenic irradiation is ineffective in myeloid malignancies and intensive intravenous chemotherapy using, e.g., cytarabine, although effective as a palliative treatment, it is invariably associated with bone marrow suppression. (M. Beran, unpublished observation, 2003).

The effectiveness of both oral drugs is particularly limited in control of hepatosplenomegaly. Analysis of the impact of treatment after referral to one tertiary cancer center failed to document significant differences in the survival between treated and untreated patients.

### Interferon α

There are no prospective data on the efficacy of interferon α (IFN-α) in treating aCML. IFN-α has been used, however, in Ph-negative CML, and a retrospective analysis of some of these patients revealed the absence of the BCR-ABL abnormality, rendering the diagnosis similar to aCML. In one report, two of six patients with BCR-ABL-negative CML achieved a CR, while four patients failed to respond.[63] In another study involving Ph-negative CML, 21 patients were treated with a daily subcutaneous dose of up to 5 million units/m² of IFN-α.[61] Seven of seven (100%) patients with BCR/ABL-positive disease responded, while five of six (83%) patients with BCR/ABL-negative CML and six of eight (75%) patients with CMML failed to respond. The outcome of the two latter groups was worse as well.[61] This experience suggests a limited role for IFN-α in aCML. In patients presenting with low platelet counts, the known platelet-lowering effect of INF-α treatment may further aggravate thrombocytopenia.

Recent availability of pegylated IFN, a pharmacologic formulation providing a slow release of the agent with weekly administration, has renewed interest in reexamining the efficacy of IFN-α in MPD, including aCML. In the absence of better choices, this treatment may be offered as an investigational alternative to hydroxyurea or for patients failing hydroxyurea therapy.

### Combination chemotherapy

In individual cases, complete responses to combination chemotherapy that included cytarabine have been reported. Although limited information is available, it appears that responses are lower than in CMML and that this approach should be saved for cases evolving into AML. Complete responses may be obtained in a minority of patients with such "secondary" AML or blast phase of aCML and, as in similar cases of AML secondary to MDS and CMML, the responses are short, and long-term disease-free survival is rarely obtained. Intensive chemotherapy may be considered as a cytoreductive approach before allogeneic SCT.

### Allogeneic stem cell transplantation

There are no reports summarizing the experience with SCT in aCML, and the lack of experience is reflected in a recent review of the results of SCT in MPD.[65] With no curative option and generally poor control of aCML with currently available modalities, SCT should be considered in younger patients with available HLA-matched donors and particularly in those presenting with unfavorable risk factors.[56] As with other rare disorders, the preferable use of investigational treatment modalities should be in the context of clinical trials.

## HYPEREOSINOPHILIC SYNDROME AND CHRONIC EOSINOPHILIC LEUKEMIA

### INTRODUCTION

Recognition of heterogeneity in hypereosinophilic syndrome (HES) is important as identification of the exact pathologic mechanisms becomes relevant to the design of treatment strategies and the overall management of individual patients. This importance is best illustrated by seminal discoveries of the unique therapeutic efficacy of imatinib mesylate in a subset of patients with HES[66–72] and by the identification of the FIP1L1-PDGFRα TK as the molecular basis in a subpopulation of patients and as a therapeutic target of imatinib[69,73] and potentially other small-molecule TK inhibitors.[74]

Although hypereosinophilia may have any number of causes, the clinical symptoms and organ damage appear to be related to the pathologic consequences of the chronically elevated eosinophils.[75,76] Because the benign and malignant disorders are not yet always distinguishable, treatment of patients with hypereosinophilia is aimed primarily at suppressing eosinophil counts (particularly in symptomatic patients); the ultimate goal is to prevent or limit organ damage.

A therapeutically relevant classification of HES plus chronic eosinophilic leukemia (CEL) is emerging, still largely under development and dictated by the exclusion criteria spelled out in the most recent WHO classification[76] and by other criteria. Eradication of symptoms and prevention of eosinophil-triggered organ damage remain the primary overall concerns, but in a subcategory of patients, the choice of treatment is now based on the likely underlying molecular mechanism(s). Recognition of therapeutically important features of HES suggests a need for closely integrated diagnostic workup with therapeutic decision making.

### DIAGNOSTIC AND TREATMENT PARADIGMS

The diagnosis of HES or CEL requires exclusion of reactive causes of eosinophilia. According to WHO criteria,[76] reactive causes include infections, hypersensitivity and allergic diseases, immune system disorders, metabolic abnormalities, and diseases of the connective tissue, heart, lungs, skin, and gastrointestinal systems. CEL remains, to a degree, a poorly defined entity.[77] The most characteristic feature distinguishing CEL from HES is the presence of karyotypic abnormalities in the myeloid cells or presence of increased blast cells in the bone mar-

row (5–19%) or blood (more than 2%).[76] Differential diagnoses further include malignant disorders in which eosinophilia is either reactive (e.g., secondary to tumor-producing hematopoietic growth factors) or where eosinophils are part of the hematopoietic malignant clone [e.g., CML, AML with inv(16) or t(8;21), MDS with t(1;7), hematologic malignancies involving rearrangement of transcription factor ETV6, MPD with t(5;12)(q33;p13), hematologic malignances associated with rearrangement of 5q chromosome in the area coding for genes regulating eosinophilic growth factors, and other rare hematologic malignancies].

For the remaining cases which fulfill the original criteria for HES,[78] the WHO criteria,[76] and other criteria,[77,79] further screening should include complete bone marrow examination, including histologic examination, karyotype analysis, FIP1L1-PDGFRα by PCR or FISH, and documentation of disease and eosinophil clonality by FISH or molecular methods. Abnormal T-lymphocyte subsets may be identified immunophenotypically as immature T cells (CD3[+], CD4[−], and CD8[−]) or aberrant T cells (CD3[−] and CD4[+]),[80,81] with or without rearrangement of T-cell receptor genes.[80–83] The usefulness of determining interleukin 5 (IL-5) and other cytokines plasma concentrations is unknown. Association of eosinophilia with systemic mastocytosis[84,85] supports the determination of plasma tryptase concentrations. Assessment of splenomegaly, hepatomegaly, abnormal marrow function (e.g., anemia, thrombocytopenia, marrow fibrosis, and dysplasia), and elevated plasma concentrations of tryptase helps define "myeloproliferative variant" and thus influences therapeutic decisions.[86] The final pretreatment assessment should focus on identifying and grading the involvement of cardiovascular, pulmonary, neurologic, dermatologic, and other systems known to be involved in patients with hypereosinophilia, and should help guide the risk-to-benefit ratio of a particular therapeutic approach. This consideration is particularly important with the use of novel, investigational treatments that were pioneered using imatinib mesylate.

### MANAGEMENT

Because the eosinophils produce end-organ damage through their activation, regardless of the cause of eosinophilia,[75] the primary aim of hypereosinophilia management is to reduce the number of eosinophils. The secondary, though no less important, goal is to reduce or correct the already incurred damage. The treatment selected is dictated by the status of the disease at diagnosis and identification of the cause of hypereosinophilia, and consists of nonspecific measures as well as treatment tailored to patients with a particular subcategory of HES.

End-organ damage does not always correlate with the degree of eosinophilia[75,87]; therefore, assessment of successful therapy should not be limited to monitoring eosinophil counts, but should also involve regular evaluation of organ status and function (e.g., echocardiograms every 6 months to assess the presence and extent of cardiac disease). The same approach applies to reassessment of the original diagnosis because the evolution of the disease (e.g., clonal evolution in HES) may require timely changes in the management strategy.

## Corticosteroids

For patients with symptomatic HES and evidence of end-organ damage or clinical symptoms, such as cough, dyspnea, myalgia, or neurologic deficits, the first treatment of choice is the daily administration of systemic corticosteroids (1 mg/kg). In most cases, this treatment results in a rapid reduction of eosinophilia, organ infiltration with eosinophils, suppression of the inflammatory process, and prevention of further organ damage. Whether such treatment ameliorates existing organ damage is uncertain.[88–91] In patients positive for FLIP1-PDGFRα, imatinib mesylate would be an alternative and probably preferable treatment. Documentation of clonal HES (FLIP1-PDGFRα, abnormal karyotype), CEL, or clonal hematologic disorder with eosinophilia on the diagnostic sample or on a subsequent follow-up examination would require reconsideration of this approach plus additional agents or change of therapy.

## Hydroxyurea and other single-agent chemotherapy

For steroid-resistant HES patients and particularly in patients with "myeloproliferative" HES or CEL, hydroxyurea is a first-line agent that effectively reduces eosinophil counts, organ infiltration, and hepatosplenomegaly, and thus likely delays end-organ damage.[89–91] The initial dose of 1–2 g of hydroxyurea per day is often sufficient to bring the eosinophil count to within the normal range. Subsequent maintenance dosing requires monitoring to avoid myelosuppression and cytopenias.

Other cytotoxic agents have occasionally been used empirically, mostly for patients with proliferative HES and evidence of end-organ damage. Case reports of successful treatment include use of cyclophosphamide in HES with recurrent eosinophilic colitis,[92] vincristine,[78,93,94] and, in hydroxyurea-resistant HES, cytosine arabinoside (100 mg/m² given subcutaneously or intravenously) daily for 5 days plus prednisone 100 mg orally, daily, for 5 days, every month (M. Beran, unpublished observations, 2003). Ameliorated clinical symptoms and suppressed eosinophilia were reported with each of the above treatments. The effect of chemotherapy on the natural course of the disease remains unknown.

## Immunosuppresive agents

The use of hydroxyurea may be less effective in managing T-cell-mediated HES than other types of HES. T-cell-mediated HES is characterized by the expansion of immunophenotypically abnormal T cells (CD3⁺, CD4⁻,

CD8⁻, or CD3⁻, CD4⁺) and, in some cases, by a clonal rearrangement of the T-cell receptor genes.[81,82] Development of T-cell lymphoma and Sezary syndrome in this group of HES patients indicated the neoplastic potential of such T cells.[82] These T-cells have a helper type 1 or 2 cytokine profile, and secretion of eosinophil production-stimulating factors may be a pathogenetic mechanism underlying the "lymphocytic" variant of HES.[83] Some patients respond well to treatment with T-cell suppressive agents, such as cyclosporin A[95,96] or cladribine in combination with steroids.[97]

## Interferon α

The success of using IFN-α in managing Ph-positive CML[98] and clinicopathological similarities between CML and HES (particularly its proliferative variant) have prompted trials of IFN-α in the management of HES. The first report of a successful response in a patient with HES was followed by a series of mostly case reports, some associated with literature reviews.[99–107] The initial dose of IFN-α varied between 1 and 5 million units/m² subcutaneously, daily, 5 days/week, and was adjusted according to the patient's tolerance. As with most of the trials in this patient population, the estimations of response rates, duration of responses, and the effect on existing end-organ damage or prevention of its development were plagued by the limited size of the treated population, the disease's heterogeneity, the limited follow-up, and the lack of a control population treated with the "standard of care" (i.e., steroids plus hydroxyurea).

## Imatinib mesylate

The pathologic features of some cases of HES are reminiscent of those of other MPD, such as BCR/ABL-positive CML. The groundbreaking success of targeted treatment of CML with imatinib mesylate[28] prompted its empirical use in patients with HES who failed other therapies. The first reported patient treated with imatinib mesylate achieved a complete response after only 2 weeks of treatment at 100 mg a day,[66] a fraction of the standard dose used for treatment of CML.[28] This observation, followed by reports of similar responses in additional patients with HES,[67–72] ushered in what appears to be a new era of HES management and reclassification.

This clinical success prompted a search for an imatinib mesylate target in patients with HES, leading to the seminal discovery of a new fusion gene, the product of which is the molecular basis of HES in some patients. Deletion of an 800-kilobase part of the PDGFRα gene leads to fusion of its 5′ end to the 3′ end of a new gene FIP1L1 on chromosome 4.[69–73,77,79,86,108] The FIP1L1/PDGFRα gene product, an intracellular protein with TK function, is unique because it is autophosphorylated due to deletion of the portion of PDGFRα gene coding for the juxtamembrane portion of the PDGFRα receptor known to inhibit phosphorylation of the ATP-binding site, and thus promotes uncontrolled growth. The most convincing documentation that the FIP1L1-PDGFRα TK is a target of imatinib was imatinib's loss of inhibitory action in cells with acquired mutation (T671I) in the TK domain of the *FIP1L1/PDGFRα* fusion gene, which implies that the mutation confers resistance to imatinib mesylate.[69,74]

The clinical experience with imatinib mesylate in managing HES and CEL can be summarized as follows: In most responding patients, daily oral doses of 100 mg effectively induced complete responses. The median time to response was 4 weeks, but responses were seen within the first 2 weeks of treatment. In only a few cases, increasing the imatinib dose to 400 mg was required for response.[71] The adverse effects were minimal and similar to those experienced by patients with Ph-positive CML.[28,33] The exceptions were two cases of congestive heart failure, both in responding patients, ensuing shortly after initiation of imatinib treatment.[72,108] Administration of steroids resulted in the resolution of symptoms in both cases, raising the question of whether steroids should be used during initial therapy with imatinib (with or without monitoring of troponin levels), particularly in patients with existing cardiac involvement. All HES and CEL patients with the FLIP1L1/PDGFRα abnormality responded regardless of the disease stage, and no cases of primary resistance have been reported.[69,109] In one study, however, four of nine patients who achieved a complete response with imatinib had no detectable FIP1L1-PDGFRα.[69] This observation not only indicated the presence of other imatinib targets but also argued in favor of an empirical trial of imatinib in patients with HES or CEL. Such a trial would ensure that no patient missed a potential therapeutic benefit, contribute further to a therapeutically meaningful classification of HES and CEL, and provide clinical feedback and guidance for ongoing translational research.

The complete responses were associated with normalization of eosinophil counts and normalization of hematologic parameters with resolution of clinical symptoms.[69,109] Among 41 patients with HES or CEL included in seven reports, 29 (71%) achieved CRs and one achieved a PR.[109] Of six patients monitored for FLIP1L1-PDGFRα transcripts, molecular remissions were documented in five after 1–12 months of treatment with 400 mg imatinib daily.[71] The treatment effect on end-organ damage is unknown because the experience is limited. No amelioration of cardiac disease was noted in three patients at the time they achieved CR,[71] but the clearing of interstitial pulmonary infiltrates,[71,110] normalization of pulmonary function tests,[71] and a major improvement in the bone marrow fibrosis of responding HES patients was encouraging.[71,109]

What is the optimal treatment strategy for patients with HES and CEL and FIP1L1/PDGFRα? Although the clinical experience with imatinib mesylate is limited, these disease categories are clearly highly sensitive to the agent. Thus, the starting daily dose of 100 mg is recommended after the expression level of the fusion transcripts has been determined, if possible with PCR. In HES patients with cardiac disease, use of prophylactic oral steroids during the first week of treatment should be considered. Because the median time to optimal response was 4 weeks, failure to respond should prompt consideration of dose escalation. The benefit of dose escalation is supported by experience in a limited number of HES cases and is corroborated by extensive experience on dose response to imatinib in patients with Ph-positive CML.[111,112] For patients who achieve CRs, the treatment strategy developed for CML should be adapted; they could continue on the same daily dose and be monitored for minimal residual disease by PCR every 3–6 months and for degree of end-organ damage (e.g., heart damage every 6 months with cardiac sonography). In patients with CRs but positive for minimal residual disease, after 6–12 months, dose escalation according to clinical tolerance is an option worth to investigate.

A similar treatment approach should be used for imatinib-mesylate-responsive patients lacking FIP1L1/PDGFRα. Hematologic status, and end-organ damage and function must be monitored.

Recently, a lemtuzumab (Campath-1H™) has shown remarkable activity in patients with FIP1LI/PDGFRα-negative HES. Normalization of absolute eosinophil counts was observed in 8 of 9 patients within 4 weeks of treatment with weekly cycles of alemtuzumab.[113] The mechanism of action is likely by direct interaction with CD52 target antigen on eosinophils. Although dosing and maintenance must be optimized and safety of the treatment documented, the preliminary results justify further clinical investigation.

### Allogeneic stem cell transplantation

The use of allogeneic SCT in patients with HES or CEL remains at the exploratory stage and is limited to selected cases with aggressive disease. Successful engraftment using standard myeloablative regimens and disease-free survival between 8 months and 5 years have been reported.[114–117] Recently, the concept of nonmyeloablative SCT has been applied to a few HES patients, who achieved engraftment after reduced-intensity conditioning.[118,119] Follow-up of those patients has not exceeded 12 months, so the potential advantage of this less toxic approach is not yet evident. Nonmyeloablative SCT is worth attempting in selected symptomatic patients who fail standard treatments, including imatinib mesylate. Because of transplantation-related complications (e.g., serious infections and acute or chronic graft-versus-host disease), and the likely bias inherent in patient selection, the major challenge will be to determine the benefit of SCT in a limited number of candidates for this treatment.

## REFERENCES

1. Vardiman JW, Harris NL, Banning R: The World Health Organization (WHO) classification of the myeloid neoplasms. *Blood* 100:2292, 2002.

2. Bennett JM, Catovsk D, Daniel TM, et al.: The chronic myeloid leukaemias: guidelines for distinguishing chronic granulocytic, atypical chronic myeloid, and chronic myelomonocytic leukaemia. Proposals by the French–American–British Cooperative Leukaemia Group. *Br J Haematol* 87:746, 1994.

3. Onida F, Beran M: Chronic myelomonocytic leukemia: myeloproliferative variant. *Curr Hematol Rep* 3:218, 2004.

4. Onida F, Kantarjian HM, Smith TL, et al.: Prognostic factors and scoring systems in chronic myelomonocytic leukemia: a retrospective analysis of 213 patients. *Blood* 99:840, 2002.

5. Apperley JF, Gardembas M, Melo JV, et al.: Response to imatinib mesylate in patients with chronic myeloproliferative diseases with rearrangements of the platelet-derived growth factor receptor beta. *N Engl J Med* 347:481, 2002.

6. Magnusson MK, Meade KE, Nakamura R, et al.: Activity of STI571 in chronic myelomonocytic leukemia with a platelet-derived growth factor beta receptor fusion oncogene. *Blood* 100:1088, 2002.

7. Anastasiadou E, Schwaller J: Role of constitutively activated protein tyrosine kinases in malignant myeloproliferative disorders: an update. *Curr Opin Hematol* 10:40, 2003.

8. Steer EJ, Cross NCP: Myeloproliferative disorders with translocation of chromosome 5q31-35: role of the platelet-derived growth factor receptor beta. *Acta Haematol* 107:113, 2002.

9. Hellstrom-Lindberg E: Efficacy of erythropoetin in the myelodysplastic syndromes: a meta analysis of 205 patients from 17 studies. *Br J Haematol* 89:67, 1995.

10. Wattel E, Guerci A, Hecquet B, et al.: A randomized trial of hydroxyurea versus VP-16 in advanced chronic myelomonocytic leukemia. *Blood* 88:2480, 1996.

11. Greenberg BR, Reynolds RD, Charron CB, et al.: Treatment of myelodysplastic syndromes with daily oral idarubicin: a phase I–II study. *Cancer* 71:1989, 1993.

12. Lowenthal RM, Lambertenghi-Deliliers G: Oral idarubicin as treatment for advanced myelodysplastic syndrome. *Haematologica* 76:398, 1991.

13. Oscier DG, Worsley A, Hamblin T, et al.: Treatment of chronic myelomonocytic leukemia with low dose etoposide. *Br J Haematol* 72:468, 1989.

14. Doll DC, Kasper LM, Taetle R, et al.: Treatment with low-dose oral etoposide in patients with myelodysplastic syndromes. *Leuk Res* 22:9, 1998.

15. Tilman M, Saben A, Hakimian D, et al.: 2-chlorodeoxyadenosine (2-CDA) in the treatment of myelomonocytic leukemias. *Proc Am Soc Clin Oncol* 14:340a, 1995. Abstract 1022.

16. Krieger O, Uaspara H, Girschkofsky D, et al.: 2-Chlorodeoxadenosine (2-CDA) in the therapy of high risk CMML. *Br J Haematol* 96(suppl 2):231, 1996. Abstract 867.

17. Seymour J, Cortes J.: Chronic myelomonocytic leukemia. In: Talpaz M, Kantarjian H (eds.) *Medical Management of Chronic Myelogenous Leukemia.* New York: Marcel Dekker, Inc; 1999:43.

18. Beran M, Estey E, O'Brien S, et al.: Topotecan and cytarabine is an active combination regimen in myelodysplastic syndromes and chronic myelomonocytic leukemia. *J Clin Oncol* 17:2819, 1999.

19. Beran M, Kantarjian H, O'Brien S, et al.: Topotecan, a topoisomerase I inhibitor, is active in the treatment of myelodysplastic syndrome and chronic myelomonocytic leukemia. *Blood* 88:2473, 1996.

20. Beran M, Estey E, O'Brien S, et al.: Results of topotecan single agent therapy in patients with myelodysplastic syndromes and chronic myelomonocytic leukemia. *Leuk Lymphoma* 31:521, 1998.

21. Beran M, O'Brien S, Thomas DA, et al.: Phase I study of oral topotecan in hematologic malignancies. *Clin Cancer Res* 15:4084, 2003.

22. Grinblatt DL, Daohai Y, Klein C, et al.: Two schedules of oral topotecan for myelodysplastic syndromes (MDS)—CALGB Study 19803. *Proc Am Soc Clin Oncol* 20:303a, 2001. Abstract 1209.

23. Grinblatt DL, Yu D, Hars V, et al.: Relationship of response to oral topotecan (topo) for myelodysplastic syndromes (MDS) with IPSS group and cytogenetics—CALGB Study 19803. *Blood* 100: Abstract 3137, 2002.

24. Santini V, Kantarjian HM, Issa JP: Changes in DNA methylation in neopasia: pathophysiology and therapeutic implications. *Ann Intern Med* 134:573, 2001.

25. Silverman LR, Demakos EP, Peterson BL, et al.: Randomized controlled trial of azacitidine in patients with the myelodysplastic syndrome: a study of the cancer and leukemia group B. *J Clin Oncol* 15:2429, 2002.

26. Wijermans P, Lubbert M, Verhoef G, et al.: Low-dose 5-aza-2'deoxycytidine, a DNA hypomethylating agent, for the treatment of high-risk myelodysplastic syndrome: a multicenter phase II study in elderly patients. *J Clin Oncol* 18:956, 2000.

27. Lubbert M, Wijermans P, Kunzmann R, et al.: Cytogenetic responses in high risk myelodysplastic syndromes following low-dose treatment with the DNA methylation inhibitor 5-aza-2'-deoxycytidine. *Br J Haematol* 114:349, 2001.

28. Drucker BJ, Tamura B, Buchdunker E, et al.: Effects of a selective inhibitor of the abl tyrosine kinase on the growth of Bcr-Abl positive cells. *Nat Med* 2:561, 1996.

29. Issa JP, Garcia-Manero G, Giles FJ, et al.: Phase I study of low-dose prolonged exposure schedules of the hypomethylating agent 5-aza-2'-deoxycitidine (decitabine) in hematopoeitic malignancies. *Blood* 103:1635, 2004.

30. Garcia JL, Font de Mora J, Hermandez JM, et al.: Imatinib mesylate elicits positive clinical response in atypical chronic myeloid leukemia involving the platelet-derived growth factor receptor beta. *Blood* 102:2699, 2003.

31. Cortes J, Giles F, O'Brien S, et al.: Results of imatinib mesylate therapy in patients with refractory or recurrent acute myeloid leukemia, high risk myelodysplastic syndrome, and myeloproliferative disorders. *Cancer* 97:2760, 2003.

32. Raza A, Lisak L, Dutt D, et al.: Gleevac (imatinib mesylate) in 16 patients with chronic myelomonocytic leukemia (CMMoL). *Blood* 96(suppl 1): Abstract 4829, 2000.

33. Talpaz M, Silver RT, Drucker R, et al.: Imatinib induces durable hematologic and cytogenetic responses in patients with accelerated phase chronic myeloid leukemia: results of a phase 2 study. *Blood* 99:1928, 2002.

34. Rebollo A, Martinez AC: Ras proteins: research advances and new functions. *Blood* 94:2971, 1999.

35. Le DT, Shannon KM: Ras processing as a therapeutic target in hematological malignancies. *Curr Opin Hematol* 9:308, 2002.

36. Onida F, Gatto S, Scappini B, et al.: Significance of ras point mutations for prognosis and response to treatment in chronic myelomonocytic leukemia: analysis of 112 patients. *Proc Am Soc Clin Oncol* 20: Abstract 1048, 2002.

37. Kurzrock R, Sebti SM, Kantarjian HM, et al.: Phase I study of a farnesyl transferase inhibitor, R115777, in patients with myelodysplastic syndrome [abstract]. *Blood* 98:623a, 2001.

38. Kurzrock R, Kantarjian H, Cortes JE, et al.: Farnesyl transferase inhibitor R115777 in myelodysplastic syndrome: clinical and biological activities in the phase I setting. *Blood* 102:4527, 2003.

39. Gotlib J, Loh M, Vattikuti S, et al.: Phase I/II Zarnestra™ (farnesyl transferase inhibitor (FTI) R11577, Tipifarnib) in patients with myeloproliferative disorders (MPDs): preliminary results. *Blood* 100: Abstract 3153, 2002.

40. Feldman E, Cortes J, Holyoake T, et al.: Continuous oral lonafarnib (Sarasar™) for the treatment of patients with myelodysplastic syndrome. *Blood* 102: Abstract 1531, 2003.

41. Verstovsek S, Estey E, Manshouri T, et al.: Clinical relevance of vascular endothelial growth factor receptors 1 and 2 in acute myeloid leukemia and myelodysplastic syndrome. *Br J Haematol* 188:151, 2002.

42. Raza A, Meyer P, Dutt D, et al.: Thalidomide produces transfusion independence in long-standing refractory anemias of patients with myelodysplastic syndromes. *Blood* 98:958, 2001.

43. Strupp C, Germing U, Aivado M, et al.: Thalidomide treatment of patients with myelodysplastic syndromes. *Leukemia* 16:1, 2002.

44. Beran M, Onida F, Cortes J, et al.: Chemotherapy of increasing intensity in the treatment of chronic myelomonocytic leukemia (CMML). *Blood* 98: Abstract 2614, 2001.

45. Beran M, Shen Y, Onida F, et al.: Prognostic significance of monocytosis in patients with myeloproliferative disorders. *Leuk Lymph* 47:417, 2006

46. Kroger N, Zabelina T, Guardiola P, et al.: Allogeneic stem cell transplantation of adult chronic myelomonocytic leukemia: a report on behalf of the Chronic Leukemia Working Party of the European Group for Blood and Bone Marrow Transplantation (EBMT). *Br J Haematol* 118:67–73, 2002.

47. Zang DY, Deeg HJ, Gooley T, et al.: Treatment of chronic myelomonocytic leukemia by allogeneic bone marrow transplantation. *Br J Haematol* 110:217, 2000.

48. Locatelli F, Niemeyer CH, Angelucai E, et al.: Allogeneic bone marrow transplantation for chronic myelomonocytic leukemia in childhood. A report from the European Working Group on Myelodysplastic Syndromes in Childhood. *J Clin Oncol* 15:566, 1997.

49. Cuger S, Sacks N: Bone marrow transplantation for myelodysplastic syndrome—who? when? and which? *Bone Marrow Transplant* 30:199, 2002.

50. Benesch M, Deeg HJ: Hematopoeitc stem cell transplantation for acute patients with myelodysplastic syndromes and myeloproliferative disorders. *Mayo Clin Proc* 78:891, 2003.

51. Maziarz RT, Mesa RA: Allogeneic stem cell transplantation for chronic myeloproliferative disorders and myelodysplastic syndrome: the question is "when?" *Mayo Clin Proc* 78:941, 2003.

52. Przepiorka S, Giralt S, Khouri I, et al.: Allogeneic marrow transplantation for myeloproliferative disorders other than chronic myelogenous leukemia: review of forty cases. *Am J Hematol* 57:24, 1998.

53. Alzea EP, Kim HT, Cutter C, et al.: AML and MDS treated with nonmyeloablative stem cell transplantation: overall and progression-free survival comparable to myeloablative transplantation. *Blood* 102: Abstract 266, 2003.

54. Giralt S, Anagnastopoulos A, Shahjahauau M, et al.: Nonablative stem cell transplantation for older patients with acute leukemias and myelodysplastic syndromes. *Semin Hematol* 39:57, 2002.

55. Cutler C, Lee S, Greenberg P, et al.: A decision analysis of allogeneic stem cell transplantation for MDS: delayed transition for low risk MDS is associated with improved outcome. *Blood* 104:579, 2002.

56. Onida F, Ball G, Kantarjian HM, et al.: Characteristics and outcome of patients with Philadelphia chromosome negative, bcr/abl negative chronic myelogenous leukemia. *Cancer* 95:1673, 2002.

57. Pugh WC, Pearson M, Vardiman JW, et al.: Philadelphia chromosome-negative chronic myelogenous leukaemia: a morphological reassessment. *Br J Haematol* 60:457, 1985.

58. Kantarjian HM, Keating MJ, Walkers RS, et al.: Clinical and prognostic features of Philadelphia chromosome-negative chronic myelogenous leukemia. *Cancer* 58:2023, 1986.61. Costello R, Sainty D, Lafage-Pochitaloff M, et al.: Clinical and biological aspects of Philadelphia-negative/BCR-negative chronic myeloid leukemia. *Leuk Lymphoma* 25:225, 1997.

59. Martiat P, Michaux JL, Rodhain J: Philadelphia-negative (Ph−) chronic myeloid leukemia (CML): comparison with Ph+ CML and chronic myelomonocytic leukemia. The Groupe Francais de Cytogenetique Hematologique. *Blood* 78:205, 1991.

60. Cortes J, O'Brien S, Beran M, et al.: Efficacy of a topoisomerase I inhibitor, 9-nitro-20-(S)-camptothecin (9-NC, RFS2000) in chronic myelomonocytic leukemia (CMML) and high-risk myelodysplastic syndromes (MDS). *Blood* 98: Abstract 2602, 2001.

61. Kantarjian HM, Shtalrid M, Kurzrock R, et al.: Significance and correlations of molecular analysis result in patients with Philadelphia-chromosome-negative chronic myelogenous leukemia and chronic myelomonocytic leukemia. *Am J Med* 85:639, 1988.

62. Spiers ASD: Management of the chronic leukemias: special considerations in the elderly patient. Part III: Rarer chronic myeloid leukemias. *Hematology* 7:1, 2002.

63. Kurzrock R, Kantarjian H, Shtalrid M, et al.: Philadelphia chromosome-negative chronic myelogenous leukemia without breakpoint cluster region

rearrangement: a chronic myeloid leukemia with a distinct clinical course. *Blood* 75:445, 1990.

64. Steensma DP, Tefferi A, Li CY: Clinical outcomes and pathological patterns after splenectomy for chronic myelomonocytic leukemia (CMML). *Blood* 102: Abstract 4907, 2003.

65. Benesch M, Deeg HJ: Hematopoeitic cell transplantation for adult patients with myelodysplastic syndromes and myeloproliferative disorders. *Mayo Clin Proc* 78:981, 2003.

66. Schaller JL, Burkland GA: Case report: rapid and complete control of idiopathic hypereosinophilia with imatinib mesylate. *Med Gen Med* 3:9, 2001.

67. Ault P, Cortes J, Koller C, et al.: Response of idiopathic hypereosinophilic syndrome to treatment with imatinib mesylate. *Leuk Res* 26:881, 2002.

68. Cortes J, Ault P, Koller C, et al.: Efficacy of imatinib mesylate in the treatment of idiopathic hypereosinophilic syndrome. *Blood* 101:4714, 2003.

69. Cools J, De Angelo DJ, Gotlib J, et al.: A tyrosine kinase created by fusion of the *PDGFRA* and *FIP1L1* genes as a therapeutic target of imatinib in idiopathic hypereosinophilic syndrome. *N Engl J Med* 348:1201, 2003.

70. Salem Z, Zalloua PA, Chehal A, et al.: Effective treatment of hypereosinophilic syndrome with imatinib mesylate. *Hematol J* 4:410, 2003.

71. Klion AD, Robyn J, Akin C, et al.: Molecular remission and reversal of myelofibrosis in response to imatinib mesylate treatment in patients with the myeloproliferative variant of hypereosinophilic syndrome. *Blood* 103:473, 2004.

72. Pitini V, Arrigo C, Azzarello D, et al.: Serum concentration of cardiac troponin T in patients with hypereosinophilic syndrome treated with imatinib is predictive of adverse outcomes. *Blood* 102:3456, 2003.

73. Griffin JH, Leung J, Bruner RJ, et al.: Discovery of a fusion kinase in EOL-1 cells and idiopathic hypereosinophilic syndrome. *Proc Natl Acad Sci U S A* 100:7830, 2003.

74. Cools J, Stover EH, Boulton CL, et al.: PKC412 overcomes resistance to imatinib in a murine model of FIP1L1-PDGFRalpha-induced myeloproliferative disease. *Cancer Cell* 3:4509, 2003.

75. Brito-Babapulle, F: The eosinophilias, including the idiopathic hypereosinophilic syndrome. *Br J Haematol* 121:203-233, 2003.

76. Bain B, Pierre R, Imbert M, et al.: Chronic eosinophilic leukemia and the hypereosinophilic syndrome. In: Jaffe ES, Harris NL, Stein H, Vardiman JW (eds.) *Tumours of Haematopoetic and Lymphoid Tissues.* Lyon, France: World Health Organization of Tumours, IARC Press; 2001:29.

77. Oliver JW, Deol I, Morgan DL, et al.: Chronic eosinophilic leukemia and hypereosinophilic syndromes. Proposal for classification, literature review and report of a case with unique chromosomal abnormality. *Cancer Genet Cytogenet* 107:111–117, 1998.

78. Chusid MJ, Dale DC, West BC, et al.: The hypereosinophilic syndrome: analysis of fourteen cases and review of the literature. *Medicine* 54:1, 1975.

79. Brito-Babapulle E: Clonal eosinophilic disorders and the hypereosinophilic syndrome. *Blood Rev* 11:129-145, 1997.

80. Roufosse F, Cogan E, Goldman M: The hypereosinophilic syndrome revisited. *Ann Rev Med* 54:169, 2003.

81. Cogan E, Schandene L, Crusiaux A, et al.: Brief report: clonal proliferation of type 2 helper T cells in a man with the hypereosinophilic syndrome. *N Eng J Med* 330:535, 1994.

82. Simon HU, Yousefi S, Dommann-Scherrer CC, et al.: Expansion of cytokine-producing CD4-DC8-T cells associated with abnormal Fas expression and hypereosinophilia. *J Exp Med* 183:1071, 1996.

83. Simon HU, Plotz SG, Dummer R, et al.: Abnormal clones of T-cells producing interleukin 5 in idiopathic hypereosinophilia. *N Engl J Med* 341:1112, 1999.

84. Pardanani A, Elliott M, Reeder T, et al.: Imatinib for systemic mast-cell disease. *Lancet* 362:535, 2003.

85. Pottier P, Planchon B, Grossi O: Complete remission with imatinib mesylate (Glivec) of an idiopathic hypereosinophilic syndrome associated with a cutaneous mastocytosis after failure of interferon-alpha. *Rev Med Interne* 24:542, 2003.

86. Klion AD, Noel P, Akin C et al.: Elevated serum tryptase levels identify a subset of patients with a myeloproliferative variant of idiopathic hypereosinophilic syndrome associated with tissue fibrosis, poor prognosis and imatinib responsiveness. *Blood* 101:4660–4666, 2003.

87. Ommen SR, Seward JB, Tajik AJ: Clinical and echocardiographic features of the hypereosinophilic syndrome. *Am J Cardiol* 86:110, 2000.

88. Hayashi S, Isobe M, Okubo Y, et al.: Improvement of eosinophilic heart disease after steroid therapy: successful demonstration by endomyocardial biopsied specimens. *Heart Vessels* 14:104, 1999.

89. Fauci AS, Harley JB, Roberts WC, et al.: NIH Conference: the idiopathic hypereosinophilic syndromes. Clinical, pathophysiological and therapeutic considerations. *Ann Intern Med* 97:78, 1982.

90. Weller PF, Bubley GJ: The idiopathic hypereosinophilic syndrome. *Blood* 83:2759, 1994.

91. Parillo JE, Fauci AS, Wolff SM: Therapy of the hypereosinophilic syndrome. *Ann Intern Med* 89:167, 1978.

92. Lee JH, Lee JW, Jang CS, et al.: Successful cyclophosphamide therapy in recurrent eosinophilic colitis associated with hypereosinophilic syndrome. *Yonsei Med J* 43:267, 2002.

93. Cofrancesco E, Cortellaro M, Pogliani E, et al.: Response to vincristine treatment in a case of idiopathic hypereosinophilic syndrome with multiple clinical manifestations. *Acta Haematol* 72:21, 1984.

94. Sakamoto K, Erdreich-Epstein A, deClerck Y, et al.: Prolonged clinical response to vincristine treatment in two patients with hypereosinophilic syndrome. *Am J Pediatr Hematol Oncol* 14:348, 1992.

95. Nadarajah S, Krafchick B, Roifman C, et al.: Treatment of hypereosinophilic syndrome in a child using cyclosporine: implication for a primary T cell abnormality. *Paediatrics* 99:630, 1997.

96. Zabel P, Schlaak M: Cyclosporin for hypereosinophilic syndrome. *Ann Hematol* 62:230, 1991.

97. Ueno NT, Zhao S, Robertson LE, et al.: 2 Chlorodeoxyadenosive therapy for idopathic hypereosinophilic syndrome. *Leukaemia* 11:1386, 1997.

98. Kantarjian HM, Smith TL, O'Brien S, et al.: Prolonged survival in chronic myelogenous leukemia after cytogenetic response to interferon-alpha therapy. *Ann Intern Med* 122:254, 1995.
99. Butterfield JH, Gelich GJ: Response of six patients with idiopathic hypereosinophilic syndrome to interferon alpha. *J Allergy Clin Immunol* 94:1318, 1994.
100. Baratta L, Afeltra A, Delfino M, et al.: Favorable response to high-dose interferon-alpha in idiopathic hypereosinophilic syndrome with restrictive cardiomyopathy—case report and literature review. *Angiology* 53:465, 2002.
101. Luciano L, Catalano L, Sarrantonio C, et al.: AlphaINF-induced hematologic and cytogenetic remission in chronic eosinophilic leukemia with t(1;5). *Haematologica* 84:651, 1999.
102. Ceretelli S, Capochiani E, Petrini M: Interferon-alpha in the idiopathic hypereosinophilic syndrome: consideration of five cases. *Ann Hematol* 77:161, 1998.
103. Canonica GW, Passalacqua G, Pronzato C, et al.: Effective long term alpha interferon treatment for hypereosinophilic syndrome. *J Allergy Clin Immunol* 96:131, 1995.
104. Schoffski P, Ganser A, Pascheberg U, et al.: Complete haematological and cytogenetic response to interferon alpha-2a of a myeloproliferative disorder with eosinophilia associated with a unique t(4;7) aberration. *Ann Hematol* 79:95, 2000.
105. Yamada O, Kitahara K, Imamura K, et al.: Clinical and cytogenetic remission induced by interferon-alpha in a patient with chronic eosinophilic leukaemia associated with a unique t(3:9:5) translocation. *Am J Haematol* 58:137, 1998.
106. Malbrain ML, Van den Bergh H, Zachee P: Further evidence for the clonal nature of the idiopathic hypereosinophilic syndrome: complete haematological and cytogenetic remission induced by interferon-alpha in a case with a unique chromosomal abnormality. *Br J Haematol* 92:176, 1996.
107. Zielinski RM, Lawrence WD: Interferon a for the hypereosinophilic syndrome. *Ann Intern Med* 113:716, 1990.
108. Pardanani A, Reeder T, Porrata LF, et al.: Imatinib therapy for hypereosinophilic syndrome and other eosinophilic disorders. *Blood* 101:3391, 2003.
109. Gotlib J, Cools J, Malone JM III, et al.: The FIP1L1-PAGFRalpha fusion tyrosine kinase in hypereosinophilic syndromes and chronic eosinophilic leukemia: implications for diagnosis, classification and management. *Blood* 103:2879, 2004.
110. Pardanani A, Ketterlin RP, Brockman SR, et al.: CHIC2 deletion, a surrogate for FIP1L1-PDGFRA fusion, occurs in systemic mastocytosis associated with eosinophilia and predicts response to imatinib mesylate therapy. *Blood* 102:3093, 2003.
111. Kantarjian HM, Sawyers CL, Hochhaus A, et al.: Hematologic and cytogenetic responses to imatinib mesylate in chronic myelogenous leukemia. *N Engl J Med* 346:645, 2002.
112. Cortes J, Giles F, O'Brien S, et al.: Result of high-dose imatinib mesylate in patients with Philadelphia-positive chronic myelogenous leukemia after failure to interferon-a. *Blood* 102:83, 2003.
113. Quintas-Cardama A, Tefferi A, Corter J, et al.: Alemtuzumab (Campath-1H™) is effective therapy for hypereosinophilic syndrome (HES). Submitted to ASH, abstract, 2006.
114. Vazquez L, Caballero D, Canizo DC, et al.: Allogeneic peripheral blood cell transplantation for hypereosinophilic syndrome with myelofibrosis. *Bone Marrow Transplant* 25:217, 2000.
115. Chockalingam A, Jalil A, Shadduck RK, et al.: Allogeneic peripheral blood stem cell transplantation for hypereosinophilic syndrome with severe cardiac dysfunction. *Bone Marrow Transplant* 23:1093, 1999.
116. Fukushima T, Kuriyama K, Ito H, et al.: Successful bone marrow transplantation for idiopathic hypereosinophilic syndrome. *Br J Haematol* 90:213, 1995.
117. Sadoun A, Lacotte L, Delwail V, et al.: Allogeneic bone marrow transplantation for hypereosinophilic syndrome with advanced myelofibrosis. *Bone Marrow Transplant* 19:741, 1997.
118. Juvonen E, Volin L, Kopenen A, et al.: Allogeneic blood stem cell transplantation following non-myeloablative conditioning for hypereosinophilic syndrome. *Bone Marrow Transplant* 29:457, 2002.
119. Ueno NT, Anagnostopoulos A, Rondon G, et al.: Successful non-myeloablative allogeneic transplantation for treatment of idiopathic hypereosinophilic syndrome. *Br J Haematol* 119:131, 2002.

# Section 1
# NON-HODGKIN'S LYMPHOMA

## Chapter 51
## THE CLASSIFICATION OF NON-HODGKIN'S LYMPHOMA

*P.G. Isaacson*

## INTRODUCTION

The aim of a lymphoma classification is to provide a means of communication between those with a special interest in this group of diseases. The classification must be reproducible and clinically relevant, so that the results of treatment can be compared worldwide, and sufficiently flexible to allow the incorporation of new data. Finally, the classification should be histopathologically based since it is the histopathologist who, almost always, makes the initial diagnosis. Traditionally, Hodgkin's disease (Hodgkin's lymphoma) and non-Hodgkin's lymphomas have been classified separately. This is a reflection of the specific identifying cell and limited morphological range of Hodgkin's disease as well as its distinctive clinical features. In comparison, the clinicopathological features of the non-Hodgkin's lymphomas are much more wide ranging and less distinct for any given entity. Not surprisingly, therefore, there have been only two classifications of Hodgkin's disease proposed since 1925 compared to more than 25 classifications of non-Hodgkin's lymphoma that have appeared in the same period.

To the early pathologists, the histological appearances of all non-Hodgkin's lymphomas were alike, consisting of replacement of the normal lymph node architecture by sheets of small or sometimes larger cells with dark-staining nuclei. It was clear, however, that not all cases behaved alike; the survival of patients

with non-Hodgkin's lymphoma varied from a few months to many years. Pathologists were, therefore, under an increasing pressure from their clinical colleagues to predict the natural course of an individual case. Initial therapeutic success with Hodgkin's disease was followed by the emergence of more effective means of therapy for the non-Hodgkin's lymphomas. These therapies were not homogeneously effective in all the non-Hodgkin's lymphomas and the results clearly varied according to their histology. Consequently, clinicians began to demand much more precise and clinically relevant histological diagnoses. In 1966, in response to this, Rappaport formulated the first clinically relevant histological classification of non-Hodgkin's lymphomas. Broadly speaking, the Rappaport classification divided lymphomas into those composed of small cells and those composed of large cells. Each of these groups could be further subdivided into those with a follicular (or nodular) growth pattern and those that were diffuse. The follicular and small-celled tumors were clinically less aggressive; a better survival could, therefore, be predicted and, importantly, less potent and less toxic therapy was suitable for these cases. The converse applied to cases with a diffuse growth pattern, especially if composed of large cells. As histological techniques improved, allowing finer morphological discrimination between cells, more detailed classifications emerged. In parallel with these improvements it was becoming possible to establish the immunophenotype of lymphoma cells using immunohistochemical techniques. It soon became evident that the lymphoma cells were closely related to normal lymph node cells and that the cells of many non-Hodgkin's lymphomas recapitulated the cytology of normal lymphocytes, particularly the B cells of the follicle center. It was also clear, however, that there were an alarmingly wide variety of lymphoid neoplasms and a whole host of classifications based on these new concepts soon emerged. This caused so much confusion that a series of special international meetings were convened to decide on a single clinically relevant classification that could be used throughout the world. In the absence of any consensus, The United States National Cancer Institute convened a study to evaluate the competing classifications and the result was the compromise "Working Formulation for Clinical Use."[1] It was stressed at the time that this "formulation," although based on histopathology, was a system for translation between the competing classifications and not a classification in its own right. However, it was rapidly accepted as such by pathologists, particularly in the United States where it became the classification of choice. The working formulation divided lymphomas into three grades based on their clinical behavior, according to their response to therapy prevalent in the late nineteen sixties and early seventies. Imprecise collective morphological terms such as "large cell" and "mixed small and large cell" were used to characterize individual entities. The result was that different clinicopathological entities were lumped together and as new entities were described, they merely became absorbed into this rather rigid system. The Working Formulation was incapable of incorporating the rapidly expanding amount of immunophenotypic data on which pathologists were, nevertheless, increasingly relying for lymphoma diagnosis. The Working Formulation thus soon lost its main reason for existence, namely its clinical relevance.

The majority of European pathologists never accepted the Working Formulation and preferred to use the Kiel classification. This classification and its updated editions[2] were based on immunophenotypic data dividing lymphomas into B- and T-cell types and, thereafter, into individual entities based principally on the similarity of their cells to normal lymphocyte variants. The lymphomas were designated low or high grade according to their cytological characteristics, rather than their predetermined clinical behavior and in keeping with established schemes for other tumors. Unlike the Working Formulation, the Kiel Classification had a sound biological basis and could easily be updated and maintain its clinical relevance. Criticisms that could be leveled at the Kiel Classification included overreliance on establishing the normal cell counterpart for each type of lymphoma, illogical oversplitting of some entities, and failure specifically to include extranodal lymphomas.

The use of different lymphoma classifications on either side of the Atlantic and the inherent defects in each contradicted the basic requirement of a classification, namely that it should provide a language for international communication, and threatened a return to the chaos of the 1970s. Moreover, new techniques and new concepts were emerging that urgently required incorporation into the principles underlying lymphoma classification. Developments in immunohistochemistry meant that a cell lineage could confidently be assigned to most lymphomas and that many distinctive functional properties of the neoplastic cells could be determined. Distinctive molecular genetic properties of the different disorders also began to emerge and some of these could be identified using simple immunohistochemical techniques. Another important development was the recognition that many lymphomas arose in extranodal sites and that the site of origin was often a significant clinical determinant.

## THE REVISED EUROPEAN AMERICAN LYMPHOMA CLASSIFICATION

In 1991 a group of pathologists from both sides of the Atlantic and the Far East formed an International Lymphoma Study Group that met annually to discuss research. Not surprisingly, this group soon began to address issues of lymphoma classification as outlined above and the need for a new approach to classification soon became evident. Of three alternative approaches that emerged, to update either the Working Formulation or the Kiel classification or to produce an entirely new classification, a decision was made to adopt the latter course. The basis for what was to become the Revised European American Lymphoma (REAL) Classification[3] was the construction of a list of neoplastic lymphoproliferative disorders each defined as far as possible according to a set of five properties, namely morphology (histology), immunophenotype, genotype, normal cell counterpart, and clinical features. The degree to which these properties contribute to the classification of each entity varies. In some cases, such as mantle cell lymphoma, each property is highly distinctive, perhaps reflecting its basic distinctive genotype,[4] while for others such as nasal-type natural killer (NK)-cell lymphoma[5] clinical features together with immunophenotype are the most important.

## THE WORLD HEALTH ORGANIZATION CLASSIFICATION

In 1995, the World Health Organization (WHO), the Society for Hematopathology and the European Association for Haematopathology undertook a joint project to produce a comprehensive classification of all hematologic neoplasms including those of myeloid lymphoid and histiocytic lineage. Since the REAL classification had only recently been proposed and was in the process of clinical evaluation, the task proposed for lymphoid neoplasms was to update and revise the REAL classification with input from additional experts in order to broaden the consensus. The formation of the steering committee and 10 subcommittees, each charged with the review of a specific group of neoplasms, involved 52 expert histopathologists and hematologists. In recognition of the importance of clinical relevance, a clinical advisory committee of 35 experts in the fields of leukemia and lymphoma from around the world was convened. The subcommittees and the clinical advisory committee met separately, the former on many occasions, and recommendations were fed to the steering committee prior to a joint meeting of all committee members that was held in November 1997 at Airlie House in Virginia. The aim of this final meeting was to reach agreement on particular controversies most of which had arisen consequent to actual use or, in effect, field testing of the REAL classification, to ensure that there was common ground between pathologists and clinicians and to agree on the final format. The agenda of the Airlie House meeting comprised a series of topics and questions that had been proposed by members of the subcommittee and the clinical advisory committee. In the case of the lymphomas, discussion of these topics served to refine and update the REAL classification, which could then be subsumed into the WHO scheme.

## THE BASIS OF THE REAL AND WHO CLASSIFICATIONS

### MORPHOLOGY

Morphology remains the mainstay of lymphoma diagnosis since it is, in effect, the collective expression of the immunophenotype, genotype, and normal cell counterpart. Once an entity has been defined on the basis of its collective properties, morphology on its own is often sufficient for a definitive diagnosis. However, lymphomas of identical morphology, but arising in different sites, may constitute different disease entities and some single disease entities may be morphologically heterogeneous. For example, anaplastic large cell lymphoma (ALCL) arising in lymph nodes behaves much more aggressively than the morphologically identical tumor arising in the skin,[6] while the cytological features of enteropathy-type T-cell lymphoma are highly variable and do not influence its clinical behavior.[7] Histological grade alone, which should not be confused with clinical aggressiveness, is no longer considered a basis for the separation of lymphomas into broad groups. Many entities may transform from low- to high-grade morphology as part of

their natural history and can present de novo as either low- or high-grade lesions.

### IMMUNOPHENOTYPE

The immunophenotype of lymphomas was first used in the Kiel classification for broad grouping of lymphomas into B-cell and T-cell types. With the inclusion of the NK-cell lymphomas into the T-cell group, this distinction remains a fundamental consideration in the REAL classification and serves as a primary step in the separation of the lymphomas into two broad groups. Within these broad groupings the detailed immunophenotype is useful in helping to define individual entities but in only a few instances does a combination of immunophenotypic properties alone serve to define an entity that cannot be distinguished by other means. This is true of mantle cell lymphoma where the defining genotype, t(11;14), results in expression of cyclin D1, the defining immunophenotype.

### GENOTYPE

With increasing recognition that cancer is a genetic disease, the genotype of lymphomas is assuming greater significance in their classification. For some entities such as follicular lymphoma, [t(14;18)], and mantle cell lymphoma, [t(11;14)], the genotype is indeed the defining property. However, genotyping is beyond the capability of most laboratories and, fortunately, the genotype finds expression as reproducible morphological and/or immunophenotypic features that allow confident and reproducible diagnoses.

### NORMAL CELL COUNTERPART

The normal cell counterpart, although not always known, is a useful aid to classification as it helps to characterize the morphology and phenotype of the lymphoma and, importantly, to understand its clinical behavior which may relate to the physiologic pathways of the normal cell. This property is more significant for B-cell lymphomas than for T-cell lymphomas largely because more is known about the B-cell subtypes and their functional characteristics.

### CLINICAL FEATURES

The inclusion of clinical features, including the site of origin, aggressiveness, and prognosis as an integral and practical part of the definition of lymphomas as distinct diseases is one of the more novel aspects of the REAL and WHO classifications.

### SITE OF ORIGIN

Neither the Working Formulation nor the Kiel classification acknowledged that a significant percentage of lymphomas do not arise in lymph nodes. Extranodal lymphoma accounts for some 25% of all cases in the United States,[8] while in the Far East the percentage is much higher amounting to 45% in Japan and 60% in Korea.[9] The site of origin of lymphomas is of considerable importance and the distribution of lymphoma types shows a markedly different bias in different sites. Thus, extranodal Hodgkin's disease is altogether rare and follicular lymphoma, one of the commonest nodal tumors, occurs only infrequently as a primary tumor in the gastrointestinal tract despite its high content of native lymphoid tissue.[10] In some organs and/or tissues, such as the skin, gastrointestinal tract and, to a lesser extent the spleen, lymphomas specifically characteristic of that site alone occur. Examples include cutaneous follicle center cell lymphoma,[11] enteropathy-type T-cell lymphoma,[12] and splenic marginal zone lymphoma (SMZL).[13] For clinical purposes it is sometimes useful to group together the lymphomas that arise in specific sites and to approach the diagnosis of lymphoma arising in those sites in this way rather than in the purest sense of an overall lymphoma classification. This is best exemplified by lymphomas arising in the gastrointestinal tract[10] and the skin.[11] However, the use of entirely separate classifications for lymphomas arising at different extranodal sites is to be discouraged.[14]

### CLINICAL AGGRESSIVENESS

The REAL and WHO classifications clearly distinguish between histological grade and clinical aggressiveness. Histological grade is based on cell and especially nuclear size, density of nuclear chromatin, and the proliferation fraction determined by immunostaining with Ki-67. Low-grade lymphomas are composed of small cells with dense nuclear chromatin and a low proliferation fraction; the converse is true for high-grade tumors. The REAL and WHO classifications, unlike the Kiel classification, do not separate lymphomas according to grade in recognition of the fact that low-grade lymphomas may transform to high-grade tumors without changing the disease "entity." Histological grade mostly correlates with clinical aggressiveness, but this is not always the case. Mantle cell lymphoma is histologically low grade but clinically aggressive[15] as are some T-cell lymphomas such as angioimmunoblastic T-cell lymphoma.[16] The Working Formulation and the Kiel classification both stressed the fundamental importance of "grade" in determining treatment, although using the term to mean different things. The REAL and WHO classifications instead stress the disease entity. Thus, not all "low-grade" B-cell lymphomas are necessarily treated alike as exemplified by hairy cell leukemia, for which highly specific therapy has evolved.[17] It is likely that as the different entities become more sharply defined and are recognized clinically, more disease-specific therapies will emerge.

### PROGNOSIS

Clinical aggressiveness is often confused with prognosis but does not have the same meaning. For example, ALCL, a high-grade neoplasm, is clinically aggressive but has a good prognosis since it responds excellently to therapy.[18] A variety of prognostic factors within each disease influence the clinical outcome. One of these is histological grade, but clinical features are also important. The more important of these have been collected together to form the International Prognostic Index (IPI),[19] the measurement of which is a powerful predictor of clinical outcome in any given patient.

## THE STRUCTURE OF THE WHO CLASSIFICATION

As in the Kiel classification, the lymphomas, defined according to the principles described above, are firstly divided broadly into B- and T-cell groups (Table 51.1). A modification is the inclusion of lymphomas with a NK-cell phenotype in the T-cell group. In each of these two groups the precursor cell, or lymphoblastic, lymphomas are separated from the larger group of peripheral cell tumors. The order in which the different entities are cited is not fixed and can be changed according to the convenience of the user. For example, the B-cell lymphomas can be grouped into those with peripheral blood involvement, plasma cell neoplasms, extranodal lymphomas, nodal lymphomas, and lymphoproliferative disorders of uncertain malignant potential. The T/NK-cell lymphomas are often similarly grouped into those that tend to involve the peripheral blood, cutaneous lymphomas, other extranodal lymphomas, nodal lymphomas, and a single entity of uncertain lineage.

### HODGKIN'S LYMPHOMA

Given the increasing evidence that Hodgkin's disease is a B-cell neoplasm,[20,21] the authors of the REAL classification took the decision to include Hodgkin's disease in the lymphoma classification albeit as a separate table. This concept was continued in the WHO classification with the modification that Hodgkin's disease is now designated as Hodgkin's lymphoma (HL). There is, however, still a preference for maintaining the "Hodgkin" eponym since in this way, the unique features of HL, including, importantly, its specific therapy and good prognosis will continue to be recognized. Not surprisingly, the classification of this disorder is little changed from those of Jackson and Parker, and Lukes and Collins. The only changes in its classification are the implicit recognition that lymphocyte-predominant HL is a different disorder from classical HL and the addition of the entity "lymphocyte-rich HL." The intention is that the inclusion of this new category will serve to prevent misdiagnosis of these cases as lymphocyte-predominant HL especially when they present with nodular or follicular histology.[22] It could be argued that Hodgkin's lymphoma eventually will be listed in the table of B-cell lymphomas.

**Table 51.1** The World Health Organization classification of lymphoid malignancies

| *B-cell neoplasms* | *T and putative NK-cell neoplasms* |
|---|---|
| Precursor B-cell neoplasm | Precursor T-cell neoplasm |
| B-cell lymphoblastic lymphoma/leukemia | T-lymphoblastic lymphoma/leukemia |
| Mature B-cell neoplasms | Mature T-cell and NK-cell neoplasms |
| Chronic lymphocytic leukemia/small lymphocytic lymphoma | T-cell prolymphocytic leukemia |
| Prolymphocytic leukaemia | T-cell large granular lymphocytic leukemia |
| Lymphoplasmacytic lymphoma | Aggressive NK-cell leukemia |
| Splenic marginal zone lymphoma | Adult T-cell lymphoma/leukemia (HTLV-1+) |
| Hairy cell leukaemia | Mycosis fungoides and Sezary syndrome |
| Plasma cell myeloma | Extranodal T/NK-cell lymphoma, nasal type |
| Monoclonal gammopathy of undetermined significance | Enteropathy-type T-cell lymphoma |
| Solitary plasmacytoma of bone | Angioimmunoblastic T-cell lymphoma |
| Extraosseous plasmacytoma | Peripheral T-cell lymphoma unspecified |
| Primary amyloidosis | Hepatosplenic T-cell lymphoma |
| Heavy chain diseases | Subcutaneous panniculitis-like T-cell lymphoma |
| Extranodal marginal zone lymphoma of mucosa-associated lymphoid tissue (MALT-lymphoma) | Blastic NK-cell lymphoma |
| Nodal marginal zone lymphoma | Angioimmunoblastic T-cell lymphoma |
| Follicular lymphoma | Peripheral T-cell lymphoma, unspecified |
| Mantle cell lymphoma | Systemic anaplastic large cell lymphoma |
| Diffuse large B-cell lymphoma | T-cell proliferations of uncertain malignant potential |
| Mediastinal (thymic) large B-cell lymhoma | Primary cutaneous CD30 positive lymphoproliferative disorders |
| Intravascular large B-cell lymphoma | |
| Primary effusion lymphoma | *Hodgkin's lymphoma* |
| Burkitt lymphoma | Nodular lymphocyte predominance |
| B-cell proliferations of uncertain malignant potential | Classical |
| Lymphomatoid granulomatosis | Nodular sclerosis |
| Posttransplant lymphoproliferative disorder, polymorphic | Lymphocyte rich (nodular) |
| | Mixed cellularity |
| | Lymphocyte depletion |

## REPRODUCIBILITY AND CLINICAL RELEVANCE

The value of any lymphoma classification is only as good as its histopathological reproducibility and its clinical relevance. In this respect, the validity of the REAL and WHO classifications had already been tested to a certain extent prior to their publication since many of the entities had been subject to detailed clinicopathological analysis in the medical literature. Shortly after its publication, moreover, the reproducibility and clinical relevance of the REAL classification were formally evaluated.

### THE LYMPHOMA CLASSIFICATION PROJECT

Shortly after its publication, an international study was convened to determine whether the REAL classification could be readily applied by a group of six expert hematopathologists who, with one exception, were not associated with the original proposal.[22] The aims of the project were to judge whether the classification could be used in practice, to test its interobserver reproducibility, to assess the need for immunophenotyping in making a diagnosis (one of the criticisms following its publication having been that the REAL classification was not cost effective in this respect!), to determine whether the constituent diseases were clinically distinctive either at presentation or in terms of clinical

outcome, and to determine the relevant frequency of these diseases in the study populations. The participating pathologists, assisted by clinicians and statisticians, studied 1400 cases of lymphoma comprising 80–210 cases in each of eight centers in North America, Europe, Asia, and Africa.

The participants found that the REAL classification was highly practical, allowing the ready classification of 95% of cases. Interobserver reproducibility was greater than 85% for most entities, which was a substantial improvement over previous studies using other classifications where reproducibility was frequently in the region of only 60% or less. Immunophenotyping was not necessary for the classification of certain diseases including follicular lymphoma and small lymphocytic lymphoma/chronic lymphocytic leukemia but essential for the classification of T-cell lymphomas and particularly helpful for some B-cell disorders including mantle cell lymphoma and diffuse large B-cell lymphoma (DLBCL).

In undertaking clinicopathological correlation, the Lymphoma Classification Project showed that the different diseases recognized by the REAL classification did indeed differ in terms of clinical presentation and survival, supporting the contention that they were distinct biological entities. However, an important finding of the study was that classification is not the only predictor of clinical outcome of any individual case. In this respect, the power of the IPI was confirmed. For example, patients with follicular lymphoma and an IPI score of 1–3 have a median survival of 7–10 years, while the median survival for the minority with an IPI of 4 or 5 is significantly reduced to 1.5 years.[23]

## THE RELATIVE FREQUENCY OF THE DIFFERENT LYMPHOMAS

Inevitably, in any discussion of lymphoma classification there tends to be greater emphasis on the rare and difficult conditions than is necessarily warranted by their frequency. Because of epidemiologic differences and regional bias, it is difficult to generalize about the distribution of different lymphomas. Extrapolating from previous studies that preceded the REAL classification, and the results of the Lymphoma Classification Project (Table 51.2), it is possible to obtain some sort of perspective. Thus, in North America and Europe, B-cell lymphomas account for approximately 85% of all lymphomas. The Lymphoma Classification Project found that, together, large B-cell lymphoma (30.6%), follicular lymphoma (22.1%), mucosa-associated lymphoid tissue (MALT) lymphoma (7.6%), lymphocytic lymphoma/chronic lymphocytic leukemia (6.7%), and mantle cell lymphoma (6.0%) comprised 73% of all lymphomas. Given that Asian and African patients were represented by only two of the eight centers, these relative incidence figures are less valid for Asia or Africa where overall there is a much lower frequency of follicular lymphoma and, in parts of Asia, a higher frequency of T-cell lymphoma.

## UPDATING THE WHO CLASSIFICATION

Previous experience, especially with the Working Formulation, has shown that lymphoma classification is necessarily a constantly moving target. New concepts and consequently newly recognized diseases are constantly arising and demand to be included in current classifications. The REAL classification recognized this both tacitly and overtly by the inclusion of provisional entities. The question of how to address the problem of updating the classification was left hanging, however. In this respect it was a fortunate coincidence that, shortly after the publication of the REAL classification, the WHO commenced the ambitious project with the aim of formulating a new comprehensive classification of both lymphoma and leukemia. In terms of the lymphomas, the WHO classification project has essentially addressed the immediate problem of updating and refining the REAL classification. However, the problem of continuous updating of the WHO classification still remains to be addressed.

### GENE EXPRESSION PROFILING

The profound effect of the advent of immunohistochemistry on lymphoma classification, outlined above, is likely to be repeated once the new gene array techniques[24] move out of the academic research area into diagnostic pathology laboratories. This technique permits automated, semiquantitative comparative analysis of the expression of thousands of genes (the entire human genome) from RNA extracted from a small sample of fresh tissue. By simultaneous analysis of a large number of cases of lymphoma, those with identical and distinctive patterns of either overexpression or underexpression of certain genes can be identified and recognized (i.e., classified) as distinctive diseases. The power of this technique, with regard to lymphoma classification, was first demonstrated in a series of DLBCLs[25] (see below) and it is likely that as more studies are completed considerable changes in lymphoma classification will follow. Unlike previous changes in lymphoma classification, however, the broad principles of the WHO classification are unlikely to change.

## ISSUES RELATING TO INDIVIDUAL ENTITIES IN THE WHO CLASSIFICATION

As with any new classification, when the WHO lymphoma classification was presented to the hematologists and oncologists[26] who would be using it in the clinic, several contentious issues arose that deserve special consideration and clarification.

### PRECURSOR CELL NEOPLASMS

With respect to the relationship of the solid precursor cell tumors with the leukemias, the FAB terms L1, L2, and L3 are no longer relevant, since L1 and L2 do not predict immunophenotype or clinical behavior and L3 is equivalent to Burkitt lymphoma (BL) in a leukemic phase. Lymphoblastic lymphomas and leukemias are the same disease in different stages.

| Table 51.2    Relative incidence of non-Hodgkin's lymphomas (Non-Hodgkin's Lymphoma Classification Project) | |
|---|---|
| Diffuse large B cell | 30.6% |
| Follicular | 22.1% |
| Marginal zone B-cell of MALT type | 7.6% |
| Peripheral T cell | 7.0% |
| Small B lymphocytic | 6.7% |
| Mantle cell | 6.0% |
| Primary mediastinal large B cell | 2.4% |
| Others | 17.6% |

## THE MATURE B-CELL LEUKEMIAS

The term "mature" is preferable to "peripheral" to describe the majority of the lymphomas. Chronic lymphocytic leukemia and lymphocytic lymphoma are clearly the same disease although they tend to be seen by different clinicians. However, prolymphocytic leukemia is distinctly different.

## FOLLICULAR LYMPHOMA

Grading of follicular lymphoma is a contentious issue but it is now agreed that grading should be carried out according to the method proposed by Berard,[27] which described 3 grades based on the number of large cells (centroblasts) per high-power field. Grade 3 follicular lymphoma is divided into 3a and 3b, the latter used for tumors comprising sheets of centroblasts. In practice, only grade 3 (greater than 15 centroblasts per high-power field) is clinically significant being indicative of more aggressive disease that may require doxorubicin-containing therapy.[28] The presence and percentage of diffuse areas should also be commented on although the clinical significance of this point is not yet clear.

## CUTANEOUS FOLLICLE CENTER LYMPHOMA

This controversial and poorly defined skin tumor[25] tends to occur in the upper half of the body and appears to be unrelated to follicular lymphoma but is, rather, a variant of DLBCL. Its importance lies in its remarkably indolent clinical behavior.

## MARGINAL ZONE LYMPHOMAS

Three separate entities comprise this group of lymphomas. The first two, marginal zone lymphoma of MALT and nodal marginal zone lymphoma +/− monocytoid B cells, are closely related but the third, "SMZL," is a quite different disease.

## MARGINAL ZONE LYMPHOMA OF MUCOSA-ASSOCIATED LYMPHOID TISSUE

This type of lymphoma arises in extranodal sites and recapitulates the histology of the Peyer's patch.[29] The stomach is the commonest site. MALT lymphomas are, by definition, low grade. Transformation to a diffuse large B-cell (high-grade) lymphoma can occur and this phenomenon is clinically significant and should be documented in the histology report. However, the term "high-grade MALT lymphoma" should not be used for these cases. In particular, DLBCLs arising de novo at extranodal sites where MALT lymphomas occur, such as the stomach, should not be called high-grade MALT lymphomas since this terminology may bias the clinician toward inappropriate therapy.

## NODAL MARGINAL ZONE LYMPHOMA +/− MONOCYTOID B CELLS

The lymph node histology of this entity is identical to that of the lymph nodes involved by MALT lymphoma[30] so that the possibility of a cryptic MALT lymphoma should always be born in mind when a diagnosis of nodal marginal zone lymphoma is entertained.

## SPLENIC MARGINAL ZONE LYMPHOMA

The constituent cells of SMZL bear only passing resemblance to splenic marginal zone cells and do not share their immunophenotype.[31] Patients typically present with splenomegaly often accompanied by anemia and thrombocytopenia. Peripheral blood involvement is often, but not always, present and in some of these cases the circulating neoplastic lymphocytes have a villous appearance. These cases were previously termed "splenic lymphoma with villous lymphocytes."[32] The use of this somewhat imprecise term will not only fail to include those cases without circulating villous lymphocytes but, more importantly, tends to include other cases of B-cell lymphoma with peripheral blood spillover since the cells of various lymphomas may sometimes adopt a villous appearance, either real or artifactual, in the peripheral blood. This is an important consideration since SMZL tends to respond favorably to splenectomy alone in contrast to its poor response to chemotherapy.[33]

## DLBCL AND BURKITT-LIKE LYMPHOMA

The classification of large B-cell lymphomas as a single group has been controversial. Various morphologic subtypes have been recognized including centroblastic, immunoblastic, anaplastic, and T-cell rich but the clinical significance of subclassifying DLBCL in this way is of doubtful significance and they do not appear to constitute separate diseases. There are, however, three rare large B-cell lymphomas that do appear to merit the designation as distinct diseases namely primary mediastinal (thymic) large B-cell lymphoma,[33] intravascular lymphoma,[34] and primary effusion lymphoma.[35] There is little doubt that within the category of DLBCL there are at least several more distinct entities that might benefit from different therapies. Their recognition is one of the challenges faced by hematopathologists, and gene profiling techniques have already shown great promise in this area. The original study using this technique[25] showed that it was possible to recognize two major clinically significant groups of DLBCL, those derived, respectively, from germinal center cells and so-called activated B cells. Subsequently, a third group has been recognized[36] and a further study has vindicated the separate classification of mediastinal large B-cell lymphoma.[37]

The borderline between DLBCL and BL is not always clear-cut. The WHO clinical advisory meeting took the decision that those DLBCL with Burkitt-like morphology that did not strictly conform to that of BL, but with c-myc rearrangement and a proliferation fraction of 100%, are best termed "atypical BL" and should receive therapy tailored for BL. Thus, they represent a subtype of BL, the others being endemic BL, nonendemic BL, and immunodeficiency-associated BL.

## MATURE T- AND NK-CELL LYMPHOMAS

Clinical syndromes rather than cytomorphological features form the principal basis for the identification of real diseases within this difficult group. Several provisional disorders listed in the REAL classification are now recognized as defined entities but, despite many attempts to recognize distinct diseases, most T-cell lymphomas end up being classified as "T-cell lymphoma unspecified." This is clearly unsatisfactory and is partly due to the rarity of T-cell lymphomas as a whole. It is to be hoped that the adoption of the new principles of classification will, as new data accumulate perhaps with the aid of gene profiling, lead to the rationalization of this group.

## ANAPLASTIC LARGE-CELL LYMPHOMA

Previously defined on the basis of its cytology and expression of CD30, it has become clear that more than one "real" disease can exhibit these features. The discovery of the t(2;5) translocation, which results in the expression of anaplastic lymphoma kinase (ALK) protein, has helped to define a form of T/null-cell ALCL that tends to occur in children and young adults and which, although aggressive, carries a good prognosis with appropriate therapy.[38] It seems likely that the somewhat similar, but t(2;5) (ALK) negative, cases are a different disorder, but this awaits confirmation. Again, gene profiling is likely to give us the answer. It is clear, however, that primary cutaneous ALCL,[39] which is always ALK negative and, moreover, lacks a cytotoxic phenotype, is an entirely different entity.

Cutaneous ALCL is closely related to the benign disorder lymphomatoid papulosis and the term "cutaneous lymphoproliferative disorder"[40] has been suggested for those cases with overlapping features. Whether such a term is appropriate in a lymphoma classification is a moot point and in recognition of this, this entity is included under the subheading "T-cell neoplasm of uncertain malignant potential."

## CONCLUSIONS

The WHO classification of lymphoid neoplasms represents a major step forward in our understanding of these tumors. Moreover, in building on the REAL classification, it has pointed the way to practical methods of further updating, which will be essential if the classification is to endure and to continue to serve the needs of clinicians. Implicit in the classification are signposts for further research, particularly with respect to DLBCL and T-cell lymphoma, unspecified. The formulation of the WHO classifications must be counted as a considerable achievement. By contrast with previous attempts to classify this difficult group of tumors, a large number of pathologists, 19 for the REAL classification and over 50 for the WHO scheme, have been involved, and to have achieved consensus within this group is remarkable! Perhaps even more remarkable is to have maintained this consensus in presenting such radically new concepts to the clinicians who treat patients with lymphoma.

## REFERENCES

1. Non-Hodgkin's lymphoma pathologic classification project: National Cancer Institute sponsored classifications of non-Hodgkin's lymphomas: summary and description of a Working Formulation for clinical usage. *Cancer* 49:2112–2135, 1982.
2. Stansfeld A, Diebold J, Kapanci Y, et al.: Updated Kiel classification for lymphomas. *Lancet* 1:292, 1988.
3. Harris NL, Jaffe ES, Stein H, et al.: A revised European-American classification of lymphoid neoplasms: a proposal from the International Lymphoma Study Group. *Blood* 84:1361–1392, 1994.
4. Banks P, Chan J, Cleary M, et al: Mantle cell lymphoma: a proposal for unification of morphologic, immunologic, and molecular data. *Am J Surg Pathol* 16:637–640, 1992.
5. Jaffe ES, Chan JKC, Su IJ, et al.: Report of the workshop on nasal and related extranodal angiocentric T/NK cell lymphomas: definitions, differential diagnosis, and epidemiology. *Am J Surg Pathol* 20:103–111, 1996.
6. de Bruin PC, Beljaards RC, van Heerde P, et al.: Differences in clinical behaviour and immunophenotype between primary cutaneous and primary nodal anaplastic large cell lymphoma of T-cell or null cell phenotype. *Histopathology* 23:127–135, 1993.
7. Isaacson PG: Gastrointestinal lymphomas of T- and B-cell types. *Mod Pathol* 12:151–158, 1999.
8. Greiner TC, Medeiros LJ, Jaffe ES: Non-Hodgkin's lymphoma. *Cancer* 75:370–380, 1995.
9. Ko YH, Kim CW, Park CS, et al.: REAL classification of malignant lymphomas in the Republic of Korea: incidence of recently recognized entities and changes in clinicopathologic features. Hematolymphoreticular Study Group of the Korean Society of Pathologists. Revised European-American lymphoma. *Cancer* 83:806–812, 1998.
10. Isaacson PG, Norton AJ: Extranodal lymphomas: malignant lymphoma of the gastrointestinal tract. In: *Extranodal Lymphomas.* Edinburgh: Churchill Livingstone; 1994:15–65.
11. Willemze R, Kerl H, Sterry W, et al.: EORTC classification for primary cutaneous lymphomas: a proposal from the Cutaneous Lymphoma Study Group of the European Organization for Research and Treatment of Cancer. *Blood* 90:354–371, 1997.
12. Wright DH: Enteropathy associated T-cell lymphoma. *Cancer Surv* 30:249–261, 1997.
13. Isaacson PG: Primary splenic lymphoma. *Cancer Surv* 30:193–212, 1997.
14. Jaffe ES, Sander CA, Flaig MJ: Cutaneous lymphomas: a proposal for a unified approach to classification using the REAL/WHO Classification. *Ann Oncol* 11 (suppl 1): 17–21, 2000.

15. Campo E, Raffeld M, Jaffe ES: Mantle-cell lymphoma. *Semin Hematol* 36:115–127, 1999.

16. Jaffe ES: Angioimmunoblastic T-cell lymphoma: new insights, but the clinical challenge remains (editorial). *Ann Oncol* 6:631–632, 1995.

17. Kraut EH, Grever MR, Bouroncle BA: Long-term follow-up of patients with hairy cell leukaemia after treatment with 2'-deoxycoformycin. *Blood* 79:111–1120, 1994.

18. Brugieres L, Delay MC, Pacquement H, et al.: CD30(+) anaplastic large-cell lymphoma in children: analysis of 82 patients enrolled in two consecutive studies of the French Society of Pediatric Oncology. *Blood* 92:3591–3598, 1998.

19. Shipp MA: Prognostic factors in aggressive non-Hodgkin's lymphoma: who has "high-risk" disease? *Blood* 83:1165–1173, 1994.

20. Kuppers R, Rajewsky K, Zhao M, et al.: Hodgkin's disease: clonal Ig gene rearrangements in Hodgkin and Reed-Sternberg cells picked from histological sections. *Ann N Y Acad Sci* 764:523–524, 1995.

21. Marafioti T, Hummel M, Anagnostopoulos I, et al.: Origin of nodular lymphocyte-predominance Hodgkin's disease from a clonal expansion of highly mutated germinal-center B cells. *N Engl J Med* 337:453–458, 1997.

22. Lymphoma Classification Project. A clinical evaluation of the International Lymphoma Study Group classification of non-Hodgkin's lymphoma. *Blood* 89:3909–3918, 1997.

23. Ashton-Key M, Thorpe PA, Allen JP, et al.: Follicular Hodgkin's disease. *Am J Surg Pathol* 19:1294–1299, 1995.

24. Staudt LM: Gene expression profiling of lymphoid malignancies. *Annu Rev Med* 53:303–318, 2002.

25. Willemze R, Meijer CJLM, Sentis HJ, et al.: Primary cutaneous large cell lymphomas of follicular center cell origin. *J Am Acad Dermatol* 16:518–526, 1987.

26. Coiffier B, Anderson J, Armitage J, et al.: Clinical prognostic factors are stronger predictors of outcome in non-Hodgkin's lymphoma (NHL) than pathologic subtype. *Blood* 88:293a, 1996.

27. Harris NL, Jaffe ES, Diebold J, et al.: Lymphoma Classification-from controversy to consensus: the REAL and WHO Classification of lymphoid neoplasms. *Ann Oncol* 11(suppl 1):3–10, 2000.

28. Mann R, Berard C: Criteria for the cytologic subclassification of follicular lymphomas: a proposed alternative method. *Hematol Oncol* 1:187–192, 1982.

29. Martin AR, Weisenberger DD, Chan WC, et al.: Prognostic value of cellular proliferation and histologic grade in follicular lymphoma. *Blood* 85:3671–3678, 1995.

30. Isaacson PG: Extranodal lymphomas: the MALT concept. *Verh Dtsch Ges Pathol* 76:14–23, 1992.

31. Nizze H, Cogliatti SB, von Schilling C, et al.: Monocytoid B-cell lymphoma: morphological variants and relationship to low grade B-cell lymphoma of the mucosa-associated lymphoid tissue. *Histopahtology* 18:403–414, 1991.

32. Mollejo M, Menarguez J, Lloret E, et al.: Splenic marginal zone lymphoma: a distinctive type of low-grade B-cell lymphoma. A clinicopathological study of 13 cases. *Am J Surg Pathol* 19:1146–1157, 1995.

33. Catovsky D, Matutes E: Splenic lymphoma with circulating villous lymphocytes/splenic marginal zone lymphoma. *Semin Hematol* 36:148–154, 1999.

34. Catovsky D: Current approach to the biology and treatment of chronic lymphoid malignancies other than CLL. *Hematol Cell Ther* 38:S63–S66, 1996.

35. Aisenberg AC: Primary large cell lymphoma of the mediastinum. *Semin Oncol* 26:251–258, 1999.

36. Alizadeh AA, Eisen MB, Davis RE, et al.: Distinct types of diffuse large B-cell lymphoma identified by gene expression profiling. *Nature* 403:503–511, 2000.

37. Rosenwald A, Wright G, Chan WC, et al.: The use of molecular profiling to predict survival after chemotherapy for diffuse large-B-cell lymphoma. *N Engl J Med* 346:1937–1947, 2002.

38. Falini B, Bigerna B, Fizzotti M, et al.: ALK expression defines a distinct group of T/null lymphomas ("ALK lymphomas") with a wide morphological spectrum. *Am J Pathol* 53:875–886, 1998.

39. Paulli M, Berti E, Rosso R, et al.: CD30/Ki-1 positive lymphoproliferative disorders of the skin. Clinicopathologic correlation and statistical analysis of 86 cases: a multicentric study from the EORTC cutaneous lymphoma project group. *J Clin Oncol* 13:1343–1354, 1996.

40. Willemze R, Beljaards RC: Spectrum of primary cutaneous CD30 (Ki-1)-positive lymphoproliferative disorders. A proposal for classification and guidelines for management and treatment. *J Am Acad Dermatol* 28:973–980, 1993.

# Chapter 52

# PATHOLOGY AND MOLECULAR GENETICS OF NON-HODGKIN'S LYMPHOMA

*James R. Cook and Eric D. Hsi*

## B-CELL LYMPHOMAS

### INTRODUCTION

The B-cell lymphomas can be thought to arise from normal B-cell counterparts and therefore can be placed in the context of normal B-cell development. This model serves as a framework for understanding the origin of these lymphomas (Figure 52.1). In this section, we will present the typical histopathologic, immunophenotypic, and molecular genetic features of the B-cell lymphomas.

### SMALL LYMPHOCYTIC LYMPHOMA

*General:* Small lymphocytic lymphoma (SLL) represents approximately 7% of non-Hodgkin's lymphomas (NHLs)[1] and presents in adulthood with a median age

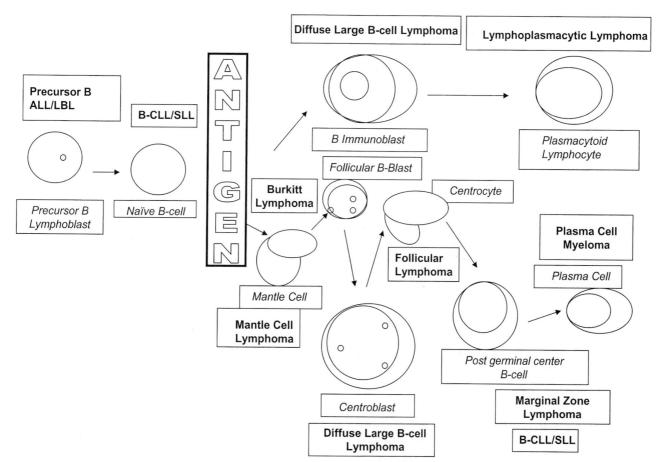

**Figure 52.1** *Schema of B-cell development and lymphoma. (Modified from Ref. 109, with permission of the International Agency for Research on Cancer.)*

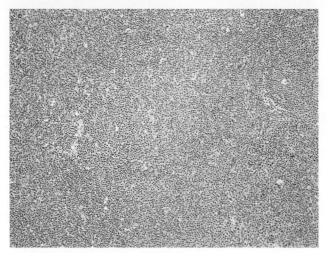

**Figure 52.2** *SLL, low magnification shows a diffuse infiltrate of small lymphocytes with a central pale area representing a proliferation center*

| Table 52.1 | Frequency of chromosomal abnormalities[a] |
|---|---|
| Aberration | Percentage of cases |
| 13q deletion | 55 |
| 11q deletion | 18 |
| Trisomy 12 | 16 |
| 17p deletion | 7 |
| 6q deletion | 6 |
| Trisomy 8q | 5 |
| t(14q32) | 4 |
| Trisomy 3q | 3 |
| Normal | 18 |

[a]Defined by FISH, some cases may have more than one abnormality.

of 65 years and a 2:1 male predominance. It is the tissue equivalent of chronic lymphocytic leukemia (CLL).

*Pathology:* SLL is a diffuse process that effaces lymph node architecture with a small lymphoid infiltrate. The cells have condensed chromatin, round nuclear contours, and scant cytoplasm. As in CLL, intermediate-sized lymphocytes with slightly open chromatin and a small central nucleolus (paraimmunoblasts) are always present and oftentimes aggregate to form proliferation centers (Figures 52.2 and 52.3). Increased numbers of paraimmunoblasts can be seen in biopsies and this does not constitute a transformation of SLL. Only when sheets of large cells are present does one consider a large cell transformation of SLL to diffuse large B-cell lymphoma (a form of Richter syndrome)

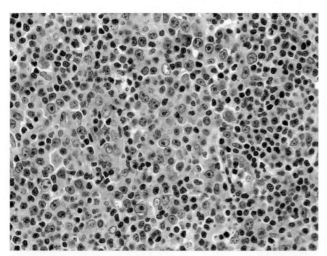

**Figure 52.3** *SLL, high magnification shows the detail of a proliferation center. Nucleolated cells (paraimmunoblasts) are present in increased numbers*

*Immunophenotype:* The immunophenotype of SLL is identical to CLL and the cells express CD5, CD19, CD20, CD23, and restricted surface immunoglobulin.

*Molecular genetics:* SLL has monoclonally rearranged immunoglobulin heavy (*IGH*) chain genes, which can be detected by PCR or Southern blot methods. Much has been learned regarding the cytogenetic abnormalities that have prognostic significance.[2] Table 52.1 shows the most common abnormalities and their frequency. Cases with del 13q and trisomy 12 have relatively good prognosis compared to those cases with del 11q or del 17p.[2] *IGH* mutational status has also been shown to be an important predictor of outcome. Cases of CLL with unmutated *IGH* have a relatively poor prognosis compared to those with mutated *IGH* (>2% deviation from germline sequences).[3,4] Recent expression arrays studies have shown excellent (but not 100%) correlation between *ZAP-70* expression (present in unmutated SLL/CLL) and *IGH* mutational status.

### MANTLE CELL LYMPHOMA

*General:* Mantle cell lymphoma (MCL) represents approximately 6% of lymphomas.[1] It generally presents in middle-aged to older adults with a median age of approximately 60 and a male predominance. Stage 3 or 4 involvement is common at presentation and bone marrow involvement is seen in more than half the patients at presentation. Although nodal disease is most common, primarily extranodal disease involving Waldeyer's ring or the gastrointestinal tract does occur.[5]

*Pathology:* Nodular, mantle zone, and diffuse architectural patterns of infiltration can occur. In the mantle zone pattern, the lymphomatous infiltrate surrounds reactive germinal centers. In the nodular pattern, the infiltrate replaces normal follicles. The diffuse pattern is most common. The infiltrate is very monotonous and is composed of small lymphocytes with slightly irregular nuclei, condensed chromatin, and inconspicuous cytoplasm (Figure 52.4). Mitotic

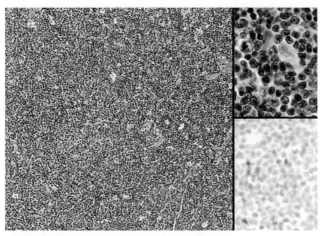

**Figure 52.4** *MCL, low magnification shows a diffuse infiltrate of small lymphocytes. Inset (upper right) shows the high magnification appearance with an epithelioid histiocyte in the center. The lower inset show cyclin D1 expression*

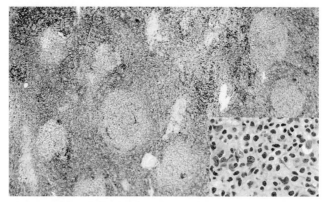

**Figure 52.5** *Follicular lymphoma demonstrating a nodular architecture. The inset shows the cytologic features with predominantly small cleaved cells in this case*

figures, unusual in other low-grade B-cell lymphomas, are commonly seen in MCL. Epithelioid histiocytes are frequently admixed in the infiltrate, imparting a "mottled" look at low to intermediate magnification.

The blastoid variant is an aggressive variant of MCL and is characterized histologically by intermediate-sized cells. A fine blast-like chromatin can be seen in some cases resembling lymphoblastic lymphoma. Other cases have a more pleomorphic appearance and more closely resemble large cell lymphoma.[6] Mitotic figures (>20/10 hpf) are seen and associated with a poor prognosis.[5]

*Immunophenotype:* The characteristic immunophenotype of MCL is CD5+, CD10−, CD19+, CD20+(bright), CD23−, FMC7+, surface Ig light chain restricted, and cyclin D1+.[7]

*Molecular genetics:* Expression of cyclin D1 is seen in the vast majority of cases and is a consequence of the t(11;14)(q13;q32) that helps define this lymphoma. Only rare cases of MCL may lack this translocation.[8] This translocation can be detected by standard cytogenetics or FISH. PCR assays exist but because of the variability in breakpoints these are not as widely used in clinical laboratories as FISH. Blastoid mantle cell lymphomas have characteristic (although not specific) additional genetic abnormalities such as *TP53* mutation, deletion of *P16*, deletion of *P21*, and tetraploidy.[9–11]

### FOLLICULAR LYMPHOMA

*General:* Follicular lymphoma is the second most common NHL after diffuse large B-cell lymphoma and comprises approximately 22% of lymphomas.[1] It occurs in older adults with a median age of 59 years and female predominance.[1] Most patients have disseminated disease at presentation, with only 33% of patients having stage 1 or 2 disease. Bone marrow is involved in 40% of patients. This lymphoma generally has a long relapsing and remitting disease course with

a 5 year overall survival of 72% but a failure-free survival of only 40%.[1]

*Pathology:* The hallmark of follicular lymphoma is the follicular architecture. The follicles are occupied by neoplastic cells recapitulating the normal lymphoid follicle. The lymphoma cells are neoplastic centrocytes (cleaved cells) and centroblasts (large noncleaved cells) in varying proportions, which determines the cytologic grade (Figure 52.5). Lymphoma cells are also seen between the neoplastic follicles when these areas are closely inspected and can also be a useful diagnostic feature. Cytologic grades are determined according to Mann and Berard (Table 52.2).[12]

The WHO classification suggests that overall and failure-free survival does correlate with cytologic grade, although conflicting data exists.[13,14] Evolution of treatment regimens will likely impact the importance of grading.

Diffuse areas can be seen in follicular lymphoma in varying proportions. The WHO recommends reporting the proportion of diffuse areas (see Table 52.1). The amount of diffuse component may indicate a worse prognosis, particularly with grade 3 lymphoma,[15] and any diffuse component of sheets of large cells is best considered diffuse large B-cell lymphoma. A diffuse

| Table 52.2 | Cytologic grading of follicular lymphoma |
|---|---|
| Grade | Centroblasts/hpf (average of 10 fields, 0.159 mm²/hpf = 40 × objective, 18 mm ocular field of view) |
| 1 | 0–5 |
| 2 | 6–15 |
| 3 | >15 |
| 3a | Centrocytes admixed with centroblasts |
| 3b | Sheets of centroblasts |

Diffuse areas are reported as follows: Follicular = greater than 75% follicular pattern; follicular and diffuse = 25–75% follicular; focally follicular = less than 25% follicular.

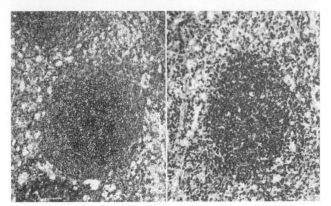

**Figure 52.6**   *Immunostains in the case shown in Figure 52.5 demonstrate expression of CD20 (left) and bcl-2 (right). The case also expressed CD10 and bcl-6 (not shown)*

variant of low-grade follicular lymphoma is recognized by the WHO classification.

*Immunophenotype:* Follicular lymphomas are CD5−, CD10+, CD19+, and CD20+ B-cells. Light chain restriction can usually be demonstrated; however, a minority of cases may lack detectable surface immunoglobulin.[16] Bcl-6 is also expressed in a great majority of follicular lymphomas and is a useful marker when the differential includes other B-cell lymphomas with a nodular pattern such as that may occur in nodular mantle cell lymphoma.[17] Bcl-2 is overexpressed in 85% of follicular lymphomas and expression can be useful in distinguishing follicular hyperplasia (negative) from follicular lymphoma (positive) (Figure 52.6). Expression levels depend on cytologic grade, with nearly 100% of grade 1 lymphomas expressing bcl-2, while only 75% of grade 3 lymphomas express this oncoprotein.[18]

*Molecular genetics:* Follicular lymphoma is typically characterized by t(14;18)(q32;q21). It can be found in approximately 80–90% of follicular lymphomas.[19] This brings the *BCL2* gene under the influence of *IGH* and results in overexpression of this antiapoptotic protein. The breakpoints in the *BCL2* gene are clustered in the major and minor breakpoint regions of *BCL2*.[20] Thus, PCR assays can be designed to detect this translocation. These can detect t(14;18)(q32;q21) in approximately 60–70% of cases of follicular lymphoma.[19] Additional probe sets can be used to detect other less common breakpoints and improve detection of this translocation.[21] FISH probes flanking breakpoints have a higher detection rate and are a preferred method for detection of this translocation.[22]

**Variant follicular lymphomas**

Primary cutaneous follicular lymphomas have been somewhat controversial, probably due to lack of consistent definition. Many studies, when adhering to WHO classification criteria, report a low percentage

(<30%) of cases harboring a t(14;18)(q32;q21) and also low rate of expression of bcl-2 protein, compared to nodal follicular lymphoma. These lymphomas are very indolent and have an excellent prognosis.[23] Pediatric follicular lymphomas are also a peculiar subset of follicular lymphomas. Although histopathologic features are essentially identical to adult cases, those occurring in children are usually bcl-2 protein negative and lack a *BCL2/IGH* translocation.[24]

### EXTRANODAL MARGINAL ZONE B-CELL LYMPHOMA OF MUCOSA-ASSOCIATED LYMPHOID TISSUE

*General:* Mucosa-associated lymphoid tissue (MALT) lymphomas are extranodal lymphomas that commonly involve mucosal sites in adults with a median age of 61 years.[1] These are often associated with autoimmune disorders such as Sjögren syndrome and Hashimoto thyroiditis. These lymphomas comprise approximately 7.6% of NHLs. The most common site is the gastrointestinal tract (51%) with the stomach accounting for the great majority of those cases. Other common sites include lung (10%), orbit (12%), skin (9%), salivary gland (6%), and thyroid (5%).[25]

Gastric MALT lymphomas can serve as a prototype of antigen driven lymphomas with *Helicobacter pylori* present in up to 90% of cases.[26] Subsequent studies have shown the organism is responsible for antigen stimulation of the lymphoma, which is dependent on T-cell help while B-cells react to autoantigens.[27–29] Treatment for *Helicobacter* is now part of the therapy in gastric MALT lymphomas and can, in some cases, cause regression and cure of disease.[30]

Most (66%) patients present with low stage (1 or 2) disease but up to 30% may have disseminated disease at diagnosis.[1,31] This is an indolent lymphoma with a 5 year survival of 85%.[31]

*Pathology:* MALT lymphomas recapitulate normal MALT in that they can have an organized architecture in mucosal sites with hyperplastic germinal centers, expansion of marginal zone cells, and superficial plasma cell differentiation. Occasionally, the plasma cell differentiation can be extreme, mimicking a plasmacytoma. Using a gastric MALT lymphoma as the example, the mucosa is infiltrated by a dense lymphoid infiltrate consisting of small lymphocytes with round to slightly irregular contours and moderate amounts of pale cytoplasm (marginal zone cells or "centrocyte-like" cells). Nucleoli are inconspicuous. There are admixed larger centroblastic cells present and plasma cells vary in number

The marginal zone cells can infiltrate epithelium and destroy the glandular structures. These are termed lymphoepithelial lesions (LELs) and are a hallmark of this disease (Figure 52.7). Marginal zone cells can invade the reactive germinal centers in a process termed follicular colonization.

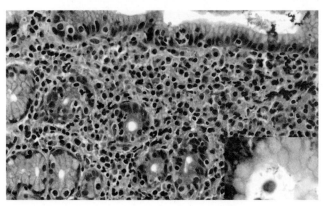

**Figure 52.7**  *Gastric MALT lymphoma with LELs (left center). The inset shows H. pylori organisms in Giemsa staining*

*Immunophenotype:* MALT lymphoma cells express CD19, CD20, and surface immunoglobulin. They lack CD5 and CD10. CD43, an antigen not normally expressed on B-cells can be seen in up to approximately 60% of cases.[32] Cytoplasmic immunoglobulin can be detected in minority (20%) of cases. Cases with t(11;18)(q21;q21) and t(1;14)(p22;q32) express nuclear bcl-10.[33]

*Molecular genetics:* Much has been learned about the molecular genetics of MALT lymphomas. A t(11;18)(q21;q21) is the most common recurrent cytogenetic abnormality in MALT lymphomas, occurring in approximately 20% of MALT lymphomas. The frequency varies by site, being most common in lung (38%) and stomach (25%) and uncommon in the salivary gland and thyroid (Table 52.3).[34,35]

This translocation results in a fusion of the *API2* and *MLT1* genes that appears to activate NFκB.[36] Detection of this translocation has clinical significance since those cases of gastric MALT lymphoma with the t(11;18)(q21;q21) do not respond to anti-*Helicobacter* therapy and are associated with infection by CAG-A+ strains of the organism. A t(14;18)(q32;q21) resulting in an *IGH/MLT1* translocation has also been recently described in MALT lymphomas, particularly in those MALT lymphomas with low incidence of *API2/MLT1*.[37]

Another recurrent translocation is seen in MALT lymphomas. The t(1;14)(p22;q32) is an uncommon translocation in MALT lymphoma. It juxtaposes *IGH*

| Table 52.3  Frequency of API2/MLT1 translocation in MALT lymphoma | |
| --- | --- |
| Site | Frequency |
| Lung | 38% |
| Stomach | 24% |
| Conjunctiva | 19% |
| Orbit | 14% |
| Skin, salivary, thyroid | Rare |

and *BCL10* genes, resulting in nuclear expression of bcl-10. Recently, bcl-10 has been shown to interact with MLT1 protein. These two proteins are also capable of activating NFκB via IKB kinase (IKK) activation. Thus, it appears that both these translocations have a common mechanism of action, namely to activate NFκB, which may play a major role in lymphomagenesis.[38]

### SPLENIC MARGINAL ZONE LYMPHOMA

*General:* Splenic marginal zone lymphoma (SMZL) is an uncommon lymphoma and probably accounts for less than 3% of lymphomas. The median age at diagnosis is 68 years with a slight male predominance.[39] It presents with splenomegaly and peripheral blood involvement is common. The appearance in the peripheral blood accounts for the term splenic lymphoma with villous lymphocytes. Adenopathy is uncommon and a small monoclonal gammopathy is present in up to two-thirds of patients.[40]

*Pathology:* Peripheral blood morphology is variable. The cells are small with moderate amounts of pale cytoplasm and short cytoplasmic projections that may aggregate at opposite ends of the cells. Nucleoli are inconspicuous. At times the cells lack noticeable projections and have a more monocytoid or plasmacytic appearance.

In the spleen, there is expansion of the white pulp. Marginal zones may be expanded and a nodular appearance can be seen from replacement of the pre-existing follicles. The cells have a variable appearance with small lymphocytes having scant cytoplasm often seen at the centers of the nodules and monocytoid B-cells with more abundant cytoplasm present at the edges of the nodules (Figures 52.8 and 52.9). Transformed centroblastic cells are present and there may be plasmacytic differentiation. There is always extension into red pulp that can be highlighted by immunohistochemistry. Hilar lymph nodes are usually

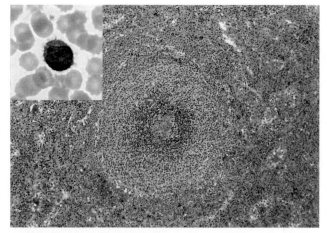

**Figure 52.8**  *Splenic marginal zone lymphoma. Low magnification shows expansion of the white pulp with prominent marginal zones. The inset (upper left) shows a circulating lymphoma cells with villous cytoplasmic projections*

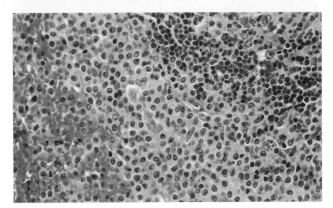

**Figure 52.9** *Splenic marginal zone lymphoma. High magnification shows the characteristic cytologic features of small cells with abundant pale cytoplasm. The upper right corner shows part of a germinal center surrounded by a thin rim of mantle cells*

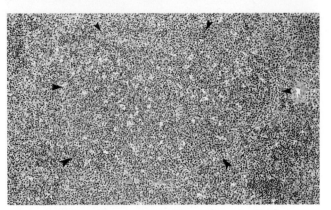

**Figure 52.10** *Nodal marginal zone B-cell lymphoma showing a germinal center (arrows) that is ill-defined and being infiltrated by lymphoma cells*

involved with replacement of the germinal centers but patent sinuses.[41,42] Bone marrow involvement is often in a sinusoidal distribution but the pattern is not entirely specific.[43,44]

*Immunophenotype:* The immunophenotype is CD5−, CD10−, CD19+, CD20+, CD22+, CD25−/+, CD103−, bcl-2+, bcl-6−, surface Ig+.[17,45,46]

*Molecular genetics:* Recent studies have show frequent deletion of 7q31-32 in SMZL.[47] Other common abnormalities include gain of 3q and abnormalities of chromosomes 1, 8, and 14.[48] Note that translocations of *MLT1* seen in extranodal marginal zone lymphomas of MALT type are not seen in SMZL, thus further supporting the contention that these are unrelated disorders.[49] Cases with chromosomal losses, including del 7q, may identify cases with a poor survival.[50] *IGH* mutational analysis shows, as in CLL, heterogeneity within SMZL and cases. Unmutated SMZL appeared to have a shorter overall survival and del 7q31 was overrepresented in this group.[50]

### NODAL MARGINAL ZONE LYMPHOMA

*General:* Nodal marginal zone lymphoma is an uncommon lymphoma, comprising approximately 2% of NHL. There is a slight female predominance (M:F = 0.7) and the median age at diagnosis is 58 years. Forty percent of patients have marrow involvement at presentation and the overall survival is approximately 55% at 5 years.[1] In order to make this diagnosis, patients should not have previous or concurrent extranodal marginal zone lymphoma of MALT type.

*Pathology:* The lymph node is altered by an infiltrate of marginal zone cells. These cells are small with condensed chromatin, slightly irregular nuclei, and variable amounts of pale cytoplasm. The cells, therefore, can vary between centrocyte-like cells and monocytoid B-cells. Plasmacytic differentiation can be seen in some cases. The infiltrate expands the interfollicular areas with preservation of reactive germinal centers

(Figures 52.10 and 52.11). Colonization of the follicles can occur and impart a nodular appearance to the lymphoma. Two subtypes have been suggested, a MALT type and splenic type, based on resemblance to these two lymphomas.[51]

*Immunophenotype:* This lymphoma expresses CD19, CD20, and surface immunoglobulin. CD5 or CD10 are not expressed. Some cases express IgD and this has been suggested as a differentiating characteristic between the splenic type (positive) and the MALT type (negative).[51]

*Molecular genetics:* Little is known regarding the molecular genetics of this lymphoma. It has been shown that these lymphomas do not contain *MLT1* translocations, supporting the concept that these lymphomas are distinct from MALT lymphomas.[34]

### LYMPHOPLASMACYTIC LYMPHOMA

*General:* Lymphoplasmacytic lymphoma (LPL) is an uncommon lymphoma (1% of lymphomas) that presents equally in men and women. The median age at diagnosis is 63 years.[1] A subset of patients, approximately 25%, present clinically with Waldenstrom macroglobulinemia. The overall survival at 5 years is 59%.[1]

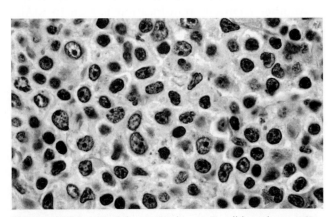

**Figure 52.11** *Nodal marginal zone B-cell lymphoma. At high magnification, the cytologic features of the lymphoma cells surrounding the follicle in Figure 10*

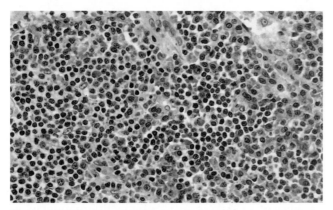

**Figure 52.12** *Lymphoplasmacytic lymphoma consisting of a diffuse infiltrate of small lymphocytes and plasma cells*

*Pathology:* The morphologic features of LPL are variable. Cytologically, the lymphoma is composed of small lymphocytes with plasmacytoid features and plasma cells that are part of the neoplasm. Dutcher bodies (intranuclear cytoplasmic intrusions) can be seen. Recently, three morphologic patterns have been described. In one, there are open sinuses with small follicles. In the second, there are hyperplastic germinal centers, and in the third there is diffuse effacement of the lymph node (Figure 52.12). Epithelioid histiocytes are commonly seen.

*Immunophenotype:* The lymphoma cells express CD19 and CD20 with surface immunoglobulin. Cytoplasmic immunoglobulin is expressed in the plasmacytic cells and heavy chain is usually IgM, although other can be seen uncommonly. Presence of CD5 should prompt consideration of CLL/SLL.

*Molecular genetics:* Relatively little is known regarding the molecular genetics of LPL. Immunoglobulin genes are clonally rearranged. Initials studies have suggested a t(9;14)(p13;q32) translocation; however, recent studies suggest this is not a common occurrence.[52]

### DIFFUSE LARGE B-CELL LYMPHOMA

*General:* Diffuse large B-cell lymphoma (DLBCL) is the most common NHL. It occurs most commonly in adults with a median age of 64 years and a slight male predominance. Unlike indolent lymphomas, only 17% of patients have bone marrow involvement.[1] This lymphoma is potentially curable with a cure rate of approximately 35% with anthracycline-based therapies.[53]

*Pathology:* DLBCL is characterized by a diffuse infiltrate of large cells. Size can be gauged by histiocyte or endothelial cells within the tissue. DLBCL cells are typically larger than these cells. The cytologic features can be variable. Many cases have a predominance of centroblasts with vesicular chromatin and multiple small nucleoli. The nucleus can be round or lobulated. Some cells resemble immunoblasts with prominent central nucleoli. Cytoplasm is generally moderate in amount.

Occasional cases are composed of large centrocytes with open chromatin. Mitotic figures are variably prominent. In some case, partial involvement of the lymph node can be seen. Rare cases will involve interfollicular areas.

Extranodal DLBLCs appear similar to nodal cases. Some may represent transformation of MALT lymphomas. A variant of DLBLC, primary mediastinal DLBCL, typically has lobulated cells and sclerosis. Another variant, intravascular DLBCL involves vessels only.

*Immunophenotype:* The vast majority of DLBCLs express pan-B-cell antigens such as CD19 and CD20. Surface immunoglobulin is expressed in most cases but may be lacking in some.[54] Expression of bcl-2 and high Ki-67 index have been associated with poor prognosis in DLBCL.[55,56] Bcl-6 expression has been suggested to be indicative of a more favorable outcome.[57] Recent expression array studies have shown that phenotyping with CD10, Bcl-6, and MUM-1 can help identify the germinal center type of DLBLC (Figure 52.13).[58]

*Molecular genetics:* Rearranged B-cell receptor genes are present. Recurrent genetic abnormalities can be found. For example, the t(14;18)(q21;q32), characteristic of FL, can be seen in approximately 20% of DLBLC.[59] BCL6 rearrangements are also common and can be found in approximately 30% of cases.[60] Much progress has been made in understanding gene expression patterns in DLBCL by using microarrays.[61–63] These studies have allowed distinction of prognostic subgroups within DLBCL, which are independent of the International Prognostic Index. Germinal center-like DLBCL (having expression patterns similar to germinal center B-cells) appear to have a favorable prognosis compared to the activated B-cell like DLBCL (having expression patterns similar to activated B-cells). Distillation of this complex data to practical clinical laboratory assays is beginning. Genetic expression models

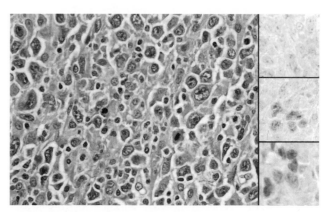

**Figure 52.13** *Diffuse large B-cell lymphoma. Sheets of centroblastic cells are present. Immunostains show the cells lack CD10 (top inset), but express bcl-6 (middle inset) and MUM1(bottom inset). This phenotype is consistent with a nongerminal center-type DLBCL, associated with a worse outcome compared the germinal center-type DLBCL*

using expression data from just a few genes[62–64] or immunohistochemical staining for three genes[58] have been shown to be prognostically significant. Using a model of weighted gene expression, investigators showed that just six genes yielded prognostic information independent of the IPI in two independent data sets. Three genes (*BCL2*, *SCYA3*, and *CCND2*) were associated with worse prognosis and three genes (*LMO2*, *BCL6*, and *FN1*) were associated with good prognosis.[64]

### BURKITT LYMPHOMA

*General:* Burkitt lymphoma (BL) is a highly aggressive B-cell lymphoma that can present as a lymphoma or acute leukemia. It often occurs in extranodal sites. Three clinical variants are recognized. The endemic form occurs in Africa, where it is the most common childhood malignancy. Epstein–Barr virus (EBV) is present in virtually 100% of cases. The sporadic form occurs in the developed world and children and younger adults. It is uncommon and represents about 1% of lymphomas with a median age of 31 years and male predominance.[1] EBV is present in approximately 30% of cases. Immunodeficiency-associated BL is seen typically in HIV infected patients, where it often occurs early in the course of infection (sometimes as the AIDS defining illness). Its incidence appears to be decreasing in the era of more effective retroviral therapy.[65] EBV is seen in approximately 40% of cases.[66]

*Pathology:* Burkitt lymphoma shows a starry sky pattern at low magnification because of the numerous tingible body macrophages that are present in the infiltrate containing apoptotic debris. The lymphoma cells are intermediate in size and uniform in appearance with vesicular chromatin and multiple inconspicuous nucleoli. There is a thin rim basophilic cytoplasm. The individual cells may show a retraction artifact around the cells. Mitoses are frequent and apoptosis of individual cells is present (Figure 52.14). Imprint morphol-

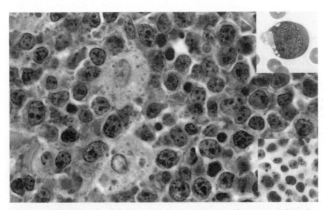

**Figure 52.14** *Burkitt lymphoma. Sheets of intermediately sized cells (compared to tingible body macrophage nuclei in left center) are seen with multiple inconspicuous nucleoli. The upper right inset shows lymphoma cells with basophilic cytoplasm and distinct vacuoles. The bottom inset is a Ki-67 antigen immunostain showing an extremely high proliferative fraction*

ogy shows uniform cells with deeply basophilic cytoplasm and cytoplasmic vacuolization, which stains positively with oil-red O. In HIV-associated cases, plasmacytoid differentiation may be seen.

*Immunophenotype:* The immunophenotype is that of a mature B-cell expressing CD19, CD20, CD10, and surface immunoglobulin. The cells are negative for precursor-B-cell blast markers such as CD34 or TdT. Bcl-2 is also absent in most cases. Ki-67 is expressed in more than 90% of cells as a result of the underlying molecular genetic abnormality (described below).

*Molecular genetics:* Burkitt lymphoma is defined by the presence of a *C-MYC* translocation with immunoglobulin genes. Cytogenetically, this can be t(8;14)(q24;q32) or the variant translocations t(2;8)(p11;q24) or t(8;22)(q24;q11). These can be detected by FISH techniques and place *C-MYC* under the control of the immunoglobulin gene promoters, which leads to overexpression of *C-MYC*. This, in turn, causes expression of genes important in cell cycle such that virtually 100% of cells are cycling. Breakpoints in the immunoglobulin genes appear to vary depending on the type of BL. In endemic cases, the breakpoint is in the joining region suggesting transformation at the early B-cell stage, while in sporadic cases it involves the heavy chain switch region, suggesting a later B-cell stage of development at transformation.[67] EBV viral genome can be detected in EBV positive cases and is clonally integrated, consistent with infection prior to malignant transformation.[68]

While *C-MYC* translocations are present in BL, it should be noted that it is not specific for this lymphoma since *C-MYC* translocation can occur as a secondary event in other types of lymphomas.

### LYMPHOMATOID GRANULOMATOSIS

*General:* Lymphomatoid granulomatosis (LYG) is a rare lymphoproliferative disorder typically involving lung and other extranodal sites such as skin, kidney, and central nervous system. It is an angiodestructive and angioproliferative lesion that only recently has been understood to be an EBV driven B-cell lymphoproliferative disorder. A previous term in the literature that likely represent LYG is angioimmunoproliferative lesion. Patients present with respiratory symptoms such as cough, chest pain, and dyspnea. Constitutional "B" symptoms are also common. This presents in adults with a median age of 40 years and a male predominance.[69] Patients with immunodeficiency states are at increased risk for LYG.[70–72] The clinical course is variable and spontaneous regression of some low-grade lesions may occur. Treatment with multiagent chemotherapy and interferon has been used with some success.[73]

*Pathology:* LYG appears as a polymorphous lymphoid infiltrate with necrosis. The cells are, for the most part, small to intermediate in size with angulated nuclei. The infiltrate is angiocentric and infiltration of the vasculature occurs. Destruction of the vessels may contribute to the necrosis. Rare larger atypical transformed cells are present with the appearance of immunoblasts or sometimes demonstrating more atypia. Mitotic figures are present to varying degrees. A three-tier histologic grading scheme has been proposed[74] based upon the number of proliferating large B-cells.[75] Grade 3 lesions correspond to an overt large cell lymphoma.

*Immunophenotype:* Immunophenotyping shows the majority of small lymphocytes are T-cells with a CD4 predominance compared to CD8. The large cell are now shown to be CD20+ B-cells.

*Molecular genetics:* In situ hybridization (ISH) shows that the large B-cells are EBV-positive in the higher grade lesions.[69,76] Gene rearrangement studies are often negative due to the low level of neoplastic B-cells in the infiltrate. Higher grade lesions more frequently have monoclonal *IGH* rearrangements. Grading is aided by EBER ISH. Grade 1 lesions have less than 5 cells/hpf. Grade 2 has 5–20 cells and grade 3 tumors have numerous EBV-positive cells that can form sheets.

### PRIMARY EFFUSION LYMPHOMA

*General:* Primary effusion lymphoma is a rare type of large B-cell lymphoma that occurs most frequently in HIV-infected patients. It usually presents in patients as an effusion in the absence of lymphadenopathy or mass. Pericardial, pleural, or peritoneal cavities may be involved. The lymphoma is highly associated with HHV-8 and most, but not all, cases are EBV-positive. It is an aggressive lymphoma with short survival.[77,78]

*Pathology:* On Wright stain the cells are pleomorphic. Some cells may have features of immunoblasts with large nuclei and prominent nucleoli. Others are more anaplastic with multilobated nuclei and/or multinucleation. The cytoplasm is deeply basophilic. Vacuoles may be present. Histologic sections, when a mass is present, show similar cells.[77,78]

*Immunophenotype:* The cells are usually negative for pan B-cell antigens such as CD19 and CD20 but show expression of plasmacytic differentiation such as CD38 and CD138. CD30 is often expressed as is epithelial membrane antigen. Surface and cytoplasmic immunoglobulin are not detectable.[77,78]

*Molecular genetics:* IGH is rearranged, as expected. The HHV-8 viral genome encodes for several genes that may be involved in lymphomagenesis such as cyclin genes, cytokines, and molecules important in regulating apoptosis and nuclear transcription factors.[79–82]

## T-CELL AND NK-CELL MALIGNANCIES

### INTRODUCTION

Like their B-cell counterparts, several types of T-cell and NK-cell lymphomas are currently recognized as distinct clinicopathologic entities. Importantly,

approximately half of T-cell lymphomas do not appear to represent any of the currently defined clinicopathologic categories, and are instead classified as members of a heterogeneous group of lymphomas designated "peripheral T-cell lymphoma, unspecified" (see below). Establishing a diagnosis of a specific type of T-cell or NK-cell lymphoma is heavily dependent upon integration of the associated clinical data. Knowledge of the clinical findings is especially important for the cutaneous T-cell lymphomas. Close cooperation between the clinician and pathologist is therefore essential for the most precise diagnosis.

### PERIPHERAL T-CELL LYMPHOMA, UNSPECIFIED

*General:* The designation "peripheral T-cell lymphoma, unspecified" (PTCLU) encompasses a heterogeneous group of mature T-cell neoplasms that do not meet criteria for one of the more distinct clinicopathologic entities described below. Overall, PTCLU accounts for approximately half of all mature T-cell lymphomas.[83] In most cases, patients present primarily with nodal disease, although extranodal presentations also occur, including those with primary cutaneous disease.

*Pathology:* The histologic findings in PTCLU are very diverse. There is usually extensive effacement of the normal lymph node architecture by a diffuse proliferation of the malignant cells (Figure 52.15). Some cases consist of small- to intermediate-sized cells with only minimal cytologic atypia, such that distinction from T-zone hyperplasia can be difficult by morphology alone. In most cases, however, the malignant cells are intermediate to large in size, with irregular nuclear contours and vesicular chromatin.[83] Frequently, the malignant cells exhibit prominent pale to clear cytoplasm. A subset of cases will include large, Reed–Sternberg-like cells, creating a differential diagnosis that includes Hodgkin's lymphoma.

*Immunophenotype:* In general, cases of PTCLU will express one or more T-cell antigens. Frequently,

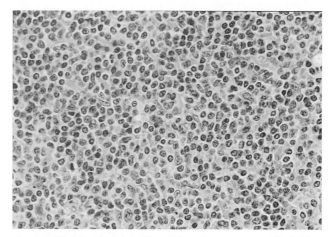

**Figure 52.15** *Peripheral T-cell lymphoma, unspecified. This case displays a diffuse infiltrate of small- to intermediate-sized cells with pale cytoplasm admixed with occasional large transformed cells*

however, the phenotype is aberrant, with loss of at least one T-cell antigen. Such cases often require extensive immunophenotypic studies with numerous antibodies to confirm a T-cell lineage. CD30 may be expressed on a subset of the malignant cells in some cases.[83]

*Molecular genetics:* Clonal T-cell receptor rearrangements are usually detectable by PCR and/or Southern blot studies. Most cases of PTCLU will display a complex karyotype by classical cytogenetic studies, but specific, recurrent karyotypic abnormalities have not been identified. Genomic profiling studies have identified a complex pattern of recurrent chromosomal gains and losses,[84] but the diagnostic significance of such changes remains to be determined.

### ANAPLASTIC LARGE CELL LYMPHOMA

*General:* Anaplastic large cell lymphoma (ALCL) represents approximately 3% of all NHL in adults, but 10–30% of NHL in childhood.[85] Typically, the disease presents in systemic fashion with involvement of lymph nodes and possibly extranodal sites, including skin, bone, soft tissue, and other sites. This systemic form of disease must be distinguished from cases that present with disease limited to the skin (see section on CD30+ lymphoproliferative disorders of the skin below). Most patients will present at advanced stage (stage 3 or 4). Detection of ALK rearrangements (see below) are of importance due to the superior outcome of ALK+ ALCL compared to ALK − ALCL.[86]

*Pathology:* Although the morphologic features of ALCL are variable, essentially all cases will contain varying numbers of large cells with eccentrically placed, band- or horseshoe-shaped nuclei, often with a punctate area of eosinophilic cytoplasm located adjacent to the nucleus.[85] These large cells are known as "hallmark cells," because their morphology is characteristic of ALCL (Figure 52.16). Variants of ALCL, termed "lymphohistiocytic variant ALCL" and "small cell variant ALCL," have also been described.

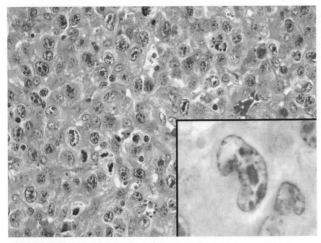

**Figure 52.16** *Anaplastic large cell lymphoma. Sheets of large, pleomorphic cells are present. The inset shows a characteristic "hallmark cell" with a band-shaped nucleus and central, punctate eosinophilic cytoplasm*

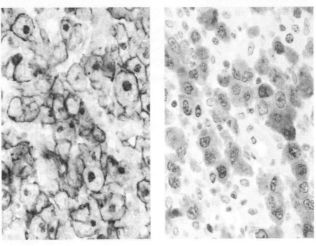

**Figure 52.17** *Anaplastic large cell lymphoma. Immunostains of the case shown in Figure 52.16 demonstrate the large cells to be positive for CD30 (left panel) and ALK (right panel)*

The marked nuclear pleomorphism seen in routine histologic sections of ALCL leads to a wide differential diagnosis. In some cases, the malignant cells resemble the Reed–Sternberg cells of Hodgkin's lymphoma. In other cases, the cells resemble metastatic carcinoma, especially in cases with only partial effacement, where the malignant cells may be confined to the lymph node sinuses.

*Immunophenotype:* The large cells will be strongly positive for CD30 and recent studies have indicated the vast majority of cases will express clusterin.[87,88] Most cases will also express cytotoxic proteins such as granzyme B or TIA1. The expression of other T-cell antigens is quite variable, although most cases will express at least one T-cell antigen. In some cases, no detectable T-cell antigens will be identified, leading to the designation "null cell." The T-cell origin of these latter cases is only revealed by the presence of monoclonal T-cell receptor rearrangements. In the majority of cases, ALK protein can be detected by immunohistochemistry as a result of a balanced translocation involving the *ALK* gene at 2p23 (Figure 52.17) The ALK-positive cases are also typically positive for EMA.

*Molecular genetics:* In approximately 60–80% of cases overall, and in an even greater percentage of cases arising in childhood, a balanced translocation is present involving the *ALK* gene at 2p23.[85,89] In roughly 75% of such cases, the translocation is t(2;5)(p23;q35) involving *ALK* and *NPM*. In the remaining 25% of translocations, one of a large number of other translocation partner genes is involved instead of *NPM*, such as *TPM3* (1q25), *TFG* (3q35), *ATIC* (2q25), or *CLTC* (17q23). Other translocation partner genes have also been described.

Translocations involving the *ALK* gene generally lead to aberrant expression of the ALK protein, which can be detected by immunohistochemistry. ALK translocations are best detected at the molecular level

FISH probes, which are capable of detecting rearrangement of the ALK gene, regardless of the partner gene present.[90]

### ANGIOIMMUNOBLASTIC T-CELL LYMPHOMA

*General:* Angioimmunoblastic T-cell lymphoma (AITL) accounts for 1–2% of NHL.[91] Initially thought to represent an abnormal immune reaction, molecular studies have demonstrated this process to represent a clonal malignancy.[92] Patients typically present at high stage with adenopathy, hepatosplenomegaly, and, often, bone marrow involvement. Systemic symptoms such as fever and pruritis are common. Laboratory abnormalities such as circulating immune complexes and hemolytic anemia are also seen.

*Pathology:* Lymph nodes involved by AITL show architectural effacement by a proliferation of small- to intermediate-sized lymphocytes with pale to clear cytoplasm and variable numbers of large transformed cells.[92] Regressively transformed germinal centers are often present and there is a characteristic proliferation of arborizing vessels (Figure 52.18). Increased numbers of follicular dendritic cells are characteristic of AITL, often associated with the vascular proliferation.

*Immunophenotype:* The malignant cells are typically CD4+, and recent studies have shown most cases of AITL to coexpress CD10.[93,94] Expression of other T-cell antigens is variable. Most cases also display scattered large, EBV-positive B-cells that may give rise to secondary B-cell lymphomas in a subset of patients.

*Molecular genetics:* Clonal T-cell rearrangements are detectable by PCR or Southern blot studies in at least 75% of cases. Clonal B-cell populations may also be detected in some cases, likely corresponding to accompanying EBV-positive B-cells.[91] Recurring cytogenetic abnormalities include trisomy 3, trisomy 5, and gains of the X chromosome, although none of these represent specific findings.[95]

### ENTEROPATHY-TYPE T-CELL LYMPHOMA

*General:* Enteropathy-type T-cell lymphoma (ETL) is a neoplasm of intraepithelial lymphocytes that is often associated with celiac disease. While in some cases there is a history of celiac disease since childhood, in most cases of ETL, celiac disease is diagnosed either concurrently with or shortly before diagnosis of the lymphoma.[96] Prior to diagnosis of an overt lymphoma, some patients will experience a period of refractory celiac disease and/or intestinal ulcers (ulcerative jejunitis). Establishing a diagnosis from small endoscopic mucosal biopsies can be very difficult, and excision of a full-thickness intestinal biopsy specimen may be required for a definitive diagnosis.

*Pathology:* One or more ulcerating mass lesions are present in the jejunum or ileum. Occasionally, other parts of the GI tract may also be involved. Histologically, the tumor cells display a variable appearance. In most cases, the infiltrate is composed of medium-sized lymphocytes with round to irregular nuclei, vesicular chromatin, and variable amounts of cytoplasm.[97] Small cell variants and cases with markedly anaplastic features have also been described. Areas of uninvolved intestinal mucosa often show features of celiac disease (villous blunting, crypt hypertrophy, and increased numbers of intraepithelial lymphocytes).

*Immunophenotype:* The neoplastic cells in ETL typically demonstrate expression of CD3, CD7, CD103, and cytotoxic proteins such as TIA1 or granzyme B.[96,98] The tumor cells are usually negative for CD5, CD4, and CD8, although in some cases a CD8 positive, CD56 positive phenotype is present.[99]

*Molecular genetics:* A monoclonal T-cell population is present, and may be detected by PCR or Southern blot studies. Biopsies of refractory sprue or ulcerative jejunitis may contain monoclonal T-cell populations with clonal rearrangements identical to the overt lymphoma, suggesting these may represent precursor lesions.[100] PCR studies alone therefore are not sufficient to distinguish between refractory sprue and ETL. Interestingly, most patients display the HLA DQA1*0501, DQB1*0201 genotype that is associated with celiac disease.[101]

### EXTRANODAL NK/T-CELL LYMPHOMA OF NASAL TYPE

*General:* Extranodal NK/T-cell lymphoma of nasal type (or "NK/T-cell lymphoma") is most prevalent in Asia, Mexico, and South America, but occurs in other ethnic groups as well.[102,103] The term "NK/T-cell" reflects the finding that while the majority of cases appear to represent neoplasms of NK cells, a subset are thought to be of T-cell type. In some cases, it may not be possible to distinguish with certainty whether the neoplastic cells represent T-cells or NK-cells. Most commonly, this

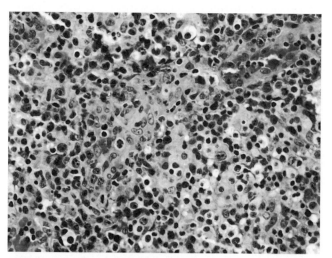

**Figure 52.18** *Angioimmunoblastic T-cell Lymphoma. The lymph node is effaced by a diffuse proliferation of intermediate to large lymphocytes with pale cytoplasm. There is an accompanying vascular proliferation*

lymphoma arises within the nasal cavity, but essentially identical cases may occur at other extranodal sites including skin, testis, soft tissue, and GI tract.

*Pathology:* The morphologic findings in NK/T-cell lymphoma are somewhat variable. In most cases, a diffuse proliferation of small- to intermediate-sized lymphoid cells are present, but some cases display numerous large, even anaplastic, lymphoid cells.[102-104] A characteristic feature of this neoplasm is that the proliferation often centers around and infiltrates vessel walls. There is often associated vascular destruction and extensive necrosis, which in some cases can obscure the malignant infiltrate.

*Immunophenotype:* The malignant cells in NK/T-cell lymphoma typically display a CD2+, CD56+, surface CD3−, and cytoplasmic CD3ε+ phenotype. There is consistent expression of cytotoxic proteins such as granzyme B and TIA1.[102,105] Nearly all cases are EBV-positive, especially those arising in the nasal cavity, and in Asian patients. The association with EBV may be somewhat less strong in Western populations and in cases arising at nonnasal sites.[105-107]

*Molecular genetics:* Most cases represent malignancies of true NK cells and so lack clonal rearrangements of the T-cell receptor genes. In a subset of cases, however, clonal rearrangements may be detected, consistent with a true T-cell origin. In EBV positive cases, clonality of the episomal EBV DNA can also usually be demonstrated. The most frequent cytogenetic abnormality is del(6q), although this abnormality is also found in many other forms of lymphoma. There is currently little information available regarding other possible recurrent cytogenetic abnormalities.[108]

### HEPATOSPLENIC T-CELL LYMPHOMA

*General:* Hepatosplenic T-cell lymphoma (HSTL) is a rare systemic lymphoma that generally presents with involvement of the liver, spleen, and bone marrow.[109] Initially described as a lymphoma of γδ-type T-cells, it is now known that some otherwise identical cases consist of αβ T-cells. Importantly, it should be realized that other types of T-cell lymphoma may consist of γδ-type T-cells and such cases should not be categorized as HSTL solely because of the type of T-cell receptor expressed.

*Pathology:* There is typically splenomegaly, and histologic sections of the spleen display prominent red pulp infiltration by a proliferation of intermediate-sized lymphoid cells. The white pulp is characteristically uninvolved.[109,110] Similarly, the liver displays a striking infiltrate of the hepatic sinusoids by similar appearing cells, with sparing of the portal tracts. The bone marrow is also usually involved, and displays clusters of intermediate-sized lymphoid cells within the sinusoids.[110,111]

*Immunophenotype:* Typical cases display an immature cytotoxic T-cell phenotype with expression of TIA1, but not perforin or granzyme B. Most cases are positive for CD2 and CD3, but are negative for CD4, CD5, and CD8.[109,110] Expression of other T-cell associated antigens is variable. Most cases express the γδ T-cell receptor, although occasional αβ T-cell receptor positive cases are well described.[109,112] Many cases show co-expression of CD56. There is no association with EBV.

*Molecular genetics:* Many cases appear to be associated with a recurrent cytogenetic abnormality, isochromosome 7q.[109,110] The exact incidence of i(7q) in HSTL has not yet been clarified, although it is clear that not all cases contain this abnormality. Monoclonal T-cell receptor rearrangements may be detected by PCR or Southern blot studies.

### MYCOSIS FUNGOIDES/SÉZARY SYNDROME

*General:* Mycosis fungoides (MF) is defined as a primary cutaneous T-cell lymphoma that clinically presents with patches and plaques and histologically displays an epidermotropic infiltrate of small- to intermediate-sized cells with atypical, cerebriform nuclei.[113] Although some have used the term "cutaneous T-cell lymphoma (CTCL)" synonymously with MF, this practice is to be strongly discouraged because many other types of T-cell lymphoma may also present with primary cutaneous disease. Within the spectrum of MF is a clinical variant condition designated "granulomatous slack skin" characterized by folds of atrophic skin, usually within the axilla or groin. Sezary syndrome is also regarded as a variant of MF and is characterized by peripheral blood involvement by malignant T-cells with cerebriform nuclei, usually associated with adenopathy and erythroderma.

*Pathology:* The skin lesions of MF are histologically characterized by an epidermal infiltrate of small- to intermediate-sized cells with irregular, cerebriform nuclei. The presence of such cells in small clusters, known as "Pautrier's microabscesses," is very characteristic of the disease, but in most cases the epidermal infiltrate is present predominantly as scattered, single atypical cells.[114] The dermal component may be variable, ranging from a sparse, often band-like, infiltrate in earlier lesions to an extensive collection of malignant cells filling the dermis in advanced stages (Figures 52.19 and 52.20). In a variant form of MF, known as "pagetoid reticulosis," the dermal component is characteristically absent. Some cases of MF are associated with follicular mucinosis, a condition of mucinous changes within a hair follicle accompanied by an infiltrate of malignant cells within the follicular epithelium. The variant known as granulomatous slack skin typically shows a granulomatous infiltrate within the infiltrate, where the admixed lymphocytes include a population of cerebriform cells, similar to those seen in typical MF. In Sezary syndrome, cerebriform malignant cells are present within the peripheral blood.

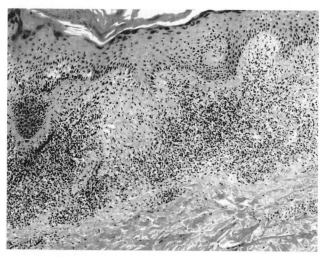

**Figure 52.19** *Mycosis fungoides. At low power, a band-like lymphocytic infiltrate is seen in the upper dermis*

In more advanced disease, there is frequently involvement of lymph nodes, and several schemes have been proposed to grade the extent of nodal involvement. The WHO classification recommends a modification of earlier criteria [113,115,116] to divide cases into three grades of lymph node involvement. In grade I cases, there is no definitive morphologic evidence of nodal involvement. Such cases may show dermatopathic lymphadenopathy and scattered cerebriform cells, but clusters of atypical cells are not present. In grade II cases, clusters of atypical, cerebriform cells focally efface the lymph node architecture. Lastly, grade III cases demonstrate complete effacement of the nodal architecture by a diffuse infiltrate of malignant cells. Importantly, this scheme is intended to quantitate lymph node involvement with a previous diagnosis of MF, and should not be definitively applied to patients without prior, biopsy-proven MF.

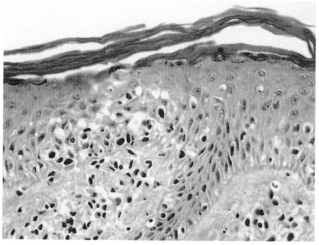

**Figure 52.20** *Mycosis fungoides. At high power, collections of atypical lymphocytes are identified in the epidermis*

*Immunophenotype:* Typically, the malignant cells of MF are positive for T-cell antigens including CD3, CD2, CD5, and, usually, CD4. Occasional cases may lack CD4 and express CD8, especially in the variant form known as pagetoid reticulosis. Most cases display aberrant loss of the CD7 antigen. The finding of CD7 loss must be interpreted with caution, however, as some inflammatory dermatoses also contain significant populations of CD7– T-cells.

*Molecular genetics:* T-cell receptor gene rearrangements are generally detectable by PCR and/or Southern blot studies. Information regarding the cytogenetic findings in MF is limited by the difficulties of successful karyotypic analysis of small skin biopsies. Analysis of peripheral blood lymphocytes in patients with Sezary syndrome generally display complex karyotypes,[117] but specific recurrent abnormalities have not been identified. Recent comparative genomic hybridization studies have suggested losses of chromosomes 1p and 17p may be common.[118]

### PRIMARY CUTANEOUS CD30-POSITIVE LYMPHOPROLIFERATIVE DISORDERS

*General:* The category of primary cutaneous CD30+ lymphoproliferative disorders includes a spectrum of cases that range from primary cutaneous anaplastic large cell lymphomas (C-ALCL) at one end to cases of lymphomatoid papulosis (LYP) at the other.[119,120] Cases designated as C-ALCL are clinically characterized by single or localized skin lesions and are histologically composed of sheets of large, atypical CD30 positive lymphocytes. There may be partial or complete spontaneous regression, but frequent cutaneous relapses generally occur. In contrast, cases designated as LYP present clinically as multiple papules that display spontaneous regression and histologically contain an inflammatory infiltrate with varying numbers of atypical CD30 positive lymphocytes. The clinical course is benign, but chronic, often lasting over many years. Lastly, some cases are designated as "borderline lesions" because there is a discrepancy between the clinical and histologic findings (e.g., a clinical appearance most consistent with LYP, but histology displaying sheets of CD30+ cells, suggestive of C-ALCL). In the absence of complete clinical information, many pathologists prefer to designate these disorders simply as "CD30+ lymphoproliferative disorder."

*Pathology:* In C-ALCL, there is a diffuse dermal infiltrate of intermediate to large lymphoid cells that resemble those found in cases of systemic ALCL.[119,121] In some cases, multinucleate or binucleate cells are present, creating a differential diagnosis that includes Hodgkin's lymphoma. Any accompanying inflammatory infiltrate is usually quite mild.

The histologic findings in LYP are quite variable.[119,120] The most frequent pattern, which has been designated type A LYP, consists of a wedge-shaped dermal infiltrate composed of varying numbers of large, atypical lymphoid cells admixed with neutrophils, eosinophils, histiocytes, and small lymphocytes. Much less commonly (<10% of LYP), the histologic findings may resemble those of mycosis fungoides (so-called type B LYP). In these latter cases, an infiltrate of cerebriform small lymphocytes is present. Some individuals may display a mixture of both Type A and Type B lesions.

*Immunophenotype:* In both C-ALCL and LYP, the neoplastic cells are CD30+ and display variable loss of associated T-cell antigens. Most cases are CD4+, although occasional CD8+ cases may also occur. The majority of cases will also express cytotoxic proteins, such as TIA1 and granzyme B. Expression of ALK protein, if it occurs at all in these disorders, is rare. The finding of ALK expression therefore strongly suggests secondary cutaneous involvement by a systemic ALCL rather than primary cutaneous disease.

*Molecular genetics:* Clonally rearranged T-cell receptors may be identified in the majority of cases of both C-ALCL and LYP. Genotypic studies therefore do not assist in differentiating between C-ALCL and LYP. In some patients, different T-cell receptor clones may be identified in different lesions of LYP.[122] In other LYP patients, however, the same T-cell receptor clone can be identified in multiple lesions over time. For example, in one report, single-cell analysis identified the same T-cell receptor clone in different biopsies taken over 4 years apart.[123] There is currently little data available regarding cytogenetic abnormalities within C-ALCL and LYP.

### SUBCUTANEOUS PANNICULITIS-LIKE T-CELL LYMPHOMA

*General:* Subcutaneous panniculitis-like T-cell lymphoma (SPTCL) is an uncommon form of lymphoma (<1% of all NHLs) composed of cytotoxic T-lymphocytes.[124–126] Patients typically present with multiple subcutaneous nodules, most commonly on the extremities and trunk. Frequently, SPTCL may be accompanied by a hemophagocytic syndrome with associated fevers, cytopenias and hepatosplenomegaly.[125] This area is undergoing change in definitions depending on whether the tumor cells express γδ-type or αβ-type T-cell receptor.

*Morphology:* There is typically a diffuse infiltrate of small- to intermediate-sized lymphocytes throughout the subcutaneous tissues, often without sparing of the lobular septae.[125,126] The infiltrate may extend into the dermis as well, although the dermal component is usually relatively minor (particularly in the αβ-type). Areas of vascular invasion may be present, and there is frequent necrosis (particularly in the γδ-type). Characteristically, the malignant cells tightly ring individual adipocytes. There may be accompanying histiocytes, especially in areas of fat necrosis.

*Immunophenotype:* The malignant cells express cytotoxic molecules including TIA1, granzyme B and perforin. Most cases are CD8+ and express the αβ T-cell receptor.[124,125] Approximately 25% of cases, however, express the γδ T-cell receptor. Many of these latter cases lack expression of both CD4 and CD8 and are positive for CD56. There is no association with EBV. It is these γδ-type lymphomas that appear to have an aggressive clinical course. The αβ-type appears to have an indolent course and is currently the only type accepted as SPTCL in the recently published WHO-EORTC classification of cutaneous lymphomas.[127] The γδ-type is now classified as a provisional entity (primary cutaneous γδ-T-cell lymphoma).

*Molecular genetics:* Rearrangements of the T-cell receptor are usually detectable by PCR and/or Southern blot studies. EBV is absent. Currently, no characteristic cytogenetic abnormalities have been identified.

### BLASTIC NK-CELL LYMPHOMA

*General:* Blastic NK-cell lymphoma is a rare neoplasm characterized by a blastoid morphology and tendency to involve the skin and peripheral blood. There may also be systemic nodal involvement.[126,128] The cell of origin and most appropriate nomenclature for this neoplasm have been subjects of controversy, and this malignancy is incompletely characterized at present. This neoplasm is classified as a natural killer lymphoma in the WHO system, due largely to the characteristic expression of CD56. More recently, however, studies have suggested this neoplasm is derived from DC2 cells, a type of dendritic cells.[129–131]

*Pathology:* In cutaneous blastic NK-cell lymphoma, there is typically a diffuse infiltrate of intermediate-sized cells with dispersed chromatin. In many cases, the tumor cells infiltrate the dermis in a single-file pattern.[126,128]

*Immunophenotype:* The neoplastic cells are characteristically positive for CD56, CD4, and CD123. Some cases may be at least partially positive for CD34, TdT, and/or CD68.[126,128] Other T-cell associated antigens are typically negative. There is no association with EBV.

*Molecular genetics:* The T-cell receptor genes are in the germline configuration. Characteristic, recurrent cytogenetic abnormalities have not been identified to date.

### REFERENCES

1. The Non-Hodgkin's Lymphoma Classification Project. A clinical evaluation of the International Lymphoma Study Group classification of non-Hodgkin's lymphoma. *Blood* 89:3909–3918, 1997.

2. Dohner H, Stilgenbauer S, Benner A, et al.: Genomic alterations and survival in chronic lymphocytic leukemia. *N Engl J Med* 343:1910–1916, 2000.

3. Hamblin TJ, Davis Z, Gardiner A, et al.: Unmutated Ig V(H) genes are associated with a more aggressive form of chronic lymphocytic leukemia. *Blood* 94:1848–1854, 1999.

4. Damle RN, Wasil T, Fais F, et al.: Ig V gene mutation status and CD38 expression as novel prognostic indicators in chronic lymphocytic leukemia. *Blood* 94:1840–1847, 1999.

5. Argatoff LH, Connors JM, Klasa RJ, et al.: Mantle cell lymphoma: a clinicopathologic study of 80 cases. *Blood* 89:2067–2078, 1997.

6. Ott G, Kalla J, Hanke A, et al.: The cytomorphological spectrum of mantle cell lymphoma is reflected by distinct biological features. *Leuk Lymphoma* 32:55–63, 1998.

7. Diaz de Leon E, Alkan S, Huang JC, et al.: Utility of an immunohistochemical panel (CD5, CD10, CD20, CD23, CD43, and Cyclin D1) in parafffin-embedded tissues for the differentiation fo b-cell non-Hodgkin's lymphomas of small lymphocytes. *Mod Pathol* 11:1046–1051, 1998.

8. Fu K, Weisenburger DD, Greiner TC, et al.: Cyclin D1-negative mantle cell lymphoma: a study of 9 cases. *Mod Pathol* 17:248A, 2004.

9. Greiner TC, Moynihan MJ, Chan WC, et al.: p53 mutations in mantle cell lymphoma are associated with variant cytology and predict a poor prognosis. *Blood* 87:4302–4310, 1996.

10. Ott G, Kalla J, Ott MM, et al.: Blastoid variants of mantle cell lymphoma—frequent bcl-1 rearrangements at the major translocation cluster regions and tetraploid chromosome clones. *Blood* 89:1421–1429, 1997.

11. Pinyol M, Hernandez L, Cazorla M, et al.: Deletions and loss of expression of p16(ink4a) and p21(waf1) genes are associated with aggressive variants of mantle cell lymphomas. *Blood* 89:272–280, 1997.

12. Mann RB, Berard CW: Criteria for the cytologic subclassification of follicular lymphomas: a proposed alternative method. *Hematol Oncol* 1:187–192, 1983.

13. Chau I, Jones R, Cunningham D, et al.: Outcome of follicular lymphoma grade 3: is anthracycline necessary as front-line therapy? *Br J Cancer* 89:36–42, 2003.

14. Jaffe ES, Harris NL, Stein H, et al.: *Tumours of Haematopoeitic and Lymphoid Tissues.* Lyon, France: IARC Press; 2001.

15. Hans CP, Weisenburger DD, Vose JM, et al.: A significant diffuse component predicts for inferior survival in grade 3 follicular lymphoma, but cytologic subtypes do not predict survival. *Blood* 101:2363–2367, 2003.

16. Ngan B, Warnke A, Cleary ML: Variability of immunoglobulin expression in follicular lymphoma. An immunohistologic and molecular genetic study. *Am J Pathol* 135:1139–1144, 1989.

17. Raible MD, Hsi ED, Diaz de Leon E, et al.: bcl-6 protein expression in follicle center cell lymphomas: a marker for distinguishing these lymphomas from other low grade-lymphoproliferative disorders. *Am J Clin Pathol* 112:101–107, 1999.

18. Gaulard P, d'Agay MF, Peuchmaur M, et al.: Expression of the bcl-2 gene product in follicular lymphoma. *Am J Pathol* 140:1089–1095, 1992.

19. Horsman DE, Gascoyne RD, Coupland RW, et al.: Comparison of cytogenetic analysis, southern analysis, and polymerase chain reaction for the detection of t(14; 18) in follicular lymphoma. *Am J Clin Pathol* 103:472–478, 1995.

20. Seto M, Jaeger U, Hockett RD, et al.: Alternative promoters and exons, somatic mutation and deregulation of the Bcl-2-Ig fusion gene in lymphoma. *EMBO J* 7:123–131, 1988.

21. Albinger-Hegyi A, Hochreutener B, Abdou MT, et al.: High frequency of t(14;18)-translocation breakpoints outside of major breakpoint and minor cluster regions in follicular lymphomas: improved polymerase chain reaction protocols for their detection. *Am J Pathol* 160:823–832, 2002.

22. Vaandrager JW, Schuuring E, Raap T, et al.: Interphase FISH detection of BCL2 rearrangement in follicular lymphoma using breakpoint-flanking probes. *Genes Chromosomes Cancer* 27:85–94, 2000.

23. Mirza I, Macpherson N, Paproski S, et al.: Primary cutaneous follicular lymphoma: an assessment of clinical, histopathologic, immunophenotypic, and molecular features. *J Clin Oncol* 20:647–655, 2002.

24. Lorsbach RB, Shay-Seymore D, Moore J, et al.: Clinicopathologic analysis of follicular lymphoma occurring in children. *Blood* 99:1959–1964, 2002.

25. Thieblemont C, Bastion Y, Berger F, et al.: Mucosa-associated lymphoid tissue gastrointestinal and non-gastrointestinal lymphoma behavior: analysis of 108 patients. *J Clin Onco* 15:1624–1630, 1997.

26. Wotherspoon AC, Ortiz-Hidalgo C, Falzon MR, et al.: *Helicobacter pylori*-associated gastritis and primary B-cell gastric lymphoma. *Lancet* 338:1175–1176, 1991.

27. Hussell T, Isaacson PG, Crabtree JE, et al.: *Helicobacter pylori*-specific tumour-infiltrating T cells provide contact dependent help for the growth of malignant B cells in low- grade gastric lymphoma of mucosa-associated lymphoid tissue. *J Pathol* 178:122–127, 1996.

28. Hussell T, Isaacson PG, Crabtree JE, Spencer J: The response of cells from low-grade B-cell gastric lymphomas of mucosa-associated lymphoid tissue to *Helicobacter pylori.* *Lancet* 342:571–574, 1993.

29. Greiner A, Marx A, Heesemann J, et al.: Idiotype identity in a MALT-type lymphoma and B cells in *Helicobacter pylori* associated chronic gastritis. *Lab Invest* 70:572–578, 1994.

30. Fischbach W, Goebeler-Kolve ME, Dragosics B, et al.: Long term outcome of patients with gastric marginal zone B cell lymphoma of mucosa associated lymphoid tissue (MALT) following exclusive *Helicobacter pylori* eradication therapy: experience from a large prospective series. *Gut* 53:34–37, 2004.

31. Thieblemont C, Berger F, Dumontet C, et al.: Mucosa-associated lymphoid tissue lymphoma is a disseminated disease in one third of 158 patients analyzed *Blood* 95:802–806, 2000. [Erratum, *Blood* 95(8):2481, 2000].

32. Hsi ED, Zukerberg LR, Schnitzer B, et al.: Development of extrasalivary gland lymphoma in myoepithelial sialadenitis. *Mod Pathol* 8:817–824, 1995.

33. Liu H, Ye H, Dogan A, et al.: T(11;18)(q21;q21) is associated with advanced mucosa-associated lymphoid tissue lymphoma that expresses nuclear BCL10. *Blood* 98:1182–1187, 2001.

34. Remstein ED, James CD, Kurtin PJ: Incidence and subtype specificity of API2-MALT1 fusion translocations in extranodal, nodal, and splenic marginal zone lymphomas. *Am J Pathol* 156:1183–1188, 2000.

35. Ye H, Liu H, Attygalle A, et al.: Variable frequencies of t(11;18)(q21;q21) in MALT lymphomas of different sites: significant association with CagA strains of H. pylori in gastric MALT lymphoma. *Blood* 102:1012–1018, 2003.

36. Zhou H, Du MQ, Dixit VM: Constitutive NF-kappaB activation by the t(11;18)(q21;q21) product in MALT lymphoma is linked to deregulated ubiquitin ligase activity. *Cancer Cell* 7:425–431, 2005.

37. Streubel B, Lamprecht A, Dierlamm J, et al.: T(14;18)(q32;q21) involving IGH and MALT1 is a frequent chromosomal aberration in MALT lymphoma. *Blood* 101:2335–2339, 2003.

38. Cavalli F, Isaacson PG, Gascoyne RD, et al.: MALT Lymphomas. *Hematology* 241–258, 2001.

39. Mulligan SP, Matutes E, Dearden C, et al.: Splenic lymphoma with villous lymphocytes: natural history and response to therapy in 50 cases. *Br J Haematol* 78: 206–209, 1991.

40. Melo JV, Hegde U, Parreira A, et al.: Splenic B cell lymphoma with circulating villous lymphocytes: differential diagnosis of B cell leukaemias with large spleens. *J Clin Pathol* 40:642–651, 1987.

41. Hammer RD, Glick AD, Greer JP, et al.: Splenic marginal zone lymphoma. A distinct B-cell neoplasm. *Am J Surg Pathol* 20:613–626, 1996.

42. Isaacson PG, Matutes E, Burke M, et al.: The histopathology of splenic lymphoma with villous lymphocytes. *Blood* 84:3828–3834, 1994.

43. Costes V, Duchayne E, Taib J, et al.: Intrasinusoidal bone marrow infiltration: a common growth pattern for different lymphoma subtypes. *Br J Haematol* 119: 916–922, 2002.

44. Labouyrie E, Marit G, Vial JP, et al.: Intrasinusoidal bone marrow involvement by splenic lymphoma with villous lymphocytes: a helpful immunohistologic feature. *Mod Pathol* 10:1015–1020, 1997.

45. Matutes E, Morilla R, Owusu-Ankomah K, et al.: The immunophenotype of splenic lymphoma with villous lymphocytes and its relevance to the differential diagnosis with other B-cell disorders. *Blood* 83:1558–1562, 1994.

46. Lima M, dos Anjos Teixeira M, Queiros ML, et al.: BCL-2 oncoprotein (p26) in splenic lymphoma with villous lymphocytes: a comparative study with other chronic B-cell disorders. *Am J Hematol* 56:122–125, 1997.

47. Gruszka-Westwood AM, Hamoudi R, Osborne L, et al.: Deletion mapping on the long arm of chromosome 7 in splenic lymphoma with villous lymphocytes. *Genes Chromosomes Cancer* 36:57–69, 2003.

48. Sole F, Salido M, Espinet B, et al.: Splenic marginal zone B-cell lymphomas: two cytogenetic subtypes, one with gain of 3q and the other with loss of 7q. *Haematologica* 86:71–77, 2001.

49. Remstein ED, James CD, Kurtin PJ: Incidence and subtype specificity of API2-MALT1 fusion translocations in extranodal, nodal, and splenic marginal zone lymphomas. *Am J Pathol* 156:1183–1188, 2000.

50. Algara P, Mateo MS, Sanchez-Beato M, et al.: Analysis of the IgV(H) somatic mutations in splenic marginal zone lymphoma defines a group of unmutated cases with frequent 7q deletion and adverse clinical course. *Blood* 99:1299–1304, 2002.

51. Campo E, Miquel R, Krenacs L, et al.: Primary nodal marginal zone lymphomas or splenic and MALT type. *Am J Surg Pathol* 23(1):59–68, 1999.

52. Cook JR, Aguilera NI, Reshmi-Skarja S, et al.: Lack of PAX5 rearrangements in lymphoplasmacytic lymphomas: reassessing the reported association with t(9;14). *Hum Pathol* 35:447–454, 2004.

53. Fisher RI, Gaynor ER, Dahlberg S, et al.: Comparison of a standard regimen (CHOP) with three intensive chemotherapy regimens for advanced non-Hodgkin's lymphoma. *N Engl J Med* 328:1002–1006, 1993.

54. Li S, Eshleman JR, Borowitz MJ: Lack of surface immunoglobulin light chain expression by flow cytometric immunophenotyping can help diagnose peripheral B-cell lymphoma. *Am J Clin Pathol* 118:229–234, 2002.

55. Gascoyne RD, Adomat SA, Krajewski S, et al.: Prognostic significance of Bcl-2 protein expression and Bcl-2 gene rearrangement in diffuse aggressive non-Hodgkin's lymphoma. *Blood* 90:244–251, 1997.

56. Miller TP, Grogan TM, Dahlberg S, et al.: Prognostic significance of the Ki-67-associated proliferative antigen in aggressive non-Hodgkin's lymphomas: a prospective Southwest Oncology Group trial. *Blood* 83:1460–1466, 1994.

57. Lossos IS, Jones CD, Warnke R, et al.: Expression of a single gene, BCL-6, strongly predicts survival in patients with diffuse large B-cell lymphoma. *Blood* 98:945–951, 2001.

58. Hans CP, Weisenburger DD, Greiner TC, et al.: Confirmation of the molecular classification of diffuse large B-cell lymphoma by immunohistochemistry using a tissue microarray. *Blood* 103:275–282, 2004.

59. Huang JZ, Sanger WG, Greiner TC, et al.: The t(14;18) defines a unique subset of diffuse large B-cell lymphoma with a germinal center B-cell gene expression profile. *Blood* 99:2285–2290, 2002.

60. Lo Coco F, Ye BH, Lista F, et al.: Rearrangements of the BCL6 gene in diffuse large cell non- Hodgkin's lymphoma. *Blood* 83:1757–1759, 1994.

61. Alizadeh AA, Eisen MB, Davis RE, et al.: Distinct types of diffuse large B-cell lymphoma identified by gene expression profiling. *Nature* 403:503–511, 2000.

62. Rosenwald A, Wright G, Chan WC, et al.: The use of molecular profiling to predict survival after chemotherapy for diffuse large-B-cell lymphoma. *N Engl J Med* 346:1937–1947, 2002.

63. Shipp MA, Ross KN, Tamayo P, et al.: Diffuse large B-cell lymphoma outcome prediction by gene-expression profiling and supervised machine learning. *Nat Med* 8:68–74, 2002.

64. Lossos IS, Czerwinski DK, Alizadeh AA, et al.: Prediction of survival in diffuse large-B-cell lymphoma based on the expression of six genes. *N Engl J Med* 350:1828–1837, 2004.

65. Levine AM, Seneviratne L, Espina BM, et al.: Evolving characteristics of AIDS-related lymphoma. *Blood* 96:4084–4090, 2000.

66. Diebold J, Raphael M, Prevot S, et al.: Lymphomas associated with HIV infection. *Cancer Surv* 30:263–293, 1997.

67. Neri A, Barriga F, Knowles DM, et al.: Different regions of the immunoglobulin heavy-chain locus are involved in chromosomal translocations in distinct patho-genetic forms of Burkitt lymphoma. *Proc Natl Acad Sci USA* 85:2748–2752, 1988.

68. Neri A, Barriga F, Inghirami G, et al.: Epstein-Barr virus infection precedes clonal expansion in Burkitt's and acquired immunodeficiency syndrome-associated lymphoma. *Blood* 77:1092–1095, 1991.

69. Nicholson AG, Wotherspoon AC, Diss TC, et al.: Lymphomatoid granulomatosis - evidence that some cases represent epstein-barr virus-associated b-cell lymphoma. *Histopathology* 29:317–324, 1996.

70. Haque AK, Myers JL, Hudnall SD, et al.: Pulmonary lymphomatoid granulomatosis in acquired immunode-ficiency syndrome: lesions with Epstein-Barr virus infection. *Mod Pathol* 11:347–356, 1998.

71. Ilowite NT, Fligner CL, Ochs HD, et al.: Pulmonary angiitis with atypical lymphoreticular infiltrates in Wiskott-Aldrich syndrome: possible relationship of lymphomatoid granulomatosis and EBV infection. *Clin Immunol Immunopathol* 41:479–484, 1986.

72. Cohen ML, Dawkins RL, Henderson DW, et al.: Pulmonary lymphomatoid granulomatosis with immunodeficiency terminating as malignant lymphoma. *Pathology* 11:537–550, 1979.

73. Jaffe ES, Wilson WH: Lymphomatoid granulomatosis: pathogenesis, pathology and clinical implications. *Cancer Surv* 30:233–248, 1997.

74. Lipford EH, Jr, Margolick JB, Longo DL, et al.: Angiocentric immunoproliferative lesions: a clinico-pathologic spectrum of post-thymic T-cell prolifera-tions. *Blood* 72:1674–1681, 1988.

75. Guinee DG Jr, Perkins SL, Travis WD, et al.: Proliferation and cellular phenotype in lymphomatoid granulomatosis: implications of a higher proliferation index in B cells. *Am J Surg Pathol* 22:1093–1100, 1998.

76. Guinee D, Jr, Jaffe E, Kingma D, et al.: Pulmonary lym-phomatoid granulomatosis. Evidence for a proliferation of Epstein-Barr virus infected B-lymphocytes with a prominent T-cell component and vasculitis. *Am J Surg Pathol* 18:753–764, 1994.

77. Ansari MQ, Dawson DB, Nador R, et al.: Primary body cavity-based AIDS-related lymphomas. *Am J Clin Pathol* 105:221–229, 1996.

78. Nador RG, Cesarman E, Chadburn A, et al.: Primary effusion lymphoma: a distinct clinicopathologic entity associated with the Kaposi's sarcoma-associated herpes virus. *Blood* 88:645–656, 1996.

79. Cannon ML, Cesarman E: The KSHV G protein-coupled receptor signals via multiple pathways to induce tran-scription factor activation in primary effusion lym-phoma cells. *Oncogene* 23:514–523, 2004.

80. An J, Sun Y, Rettig MB: Transcriptional coactivation of c-Jun by the KSHV-encoded LANA. *Blood* 103:222–228, 2004.

81. An J, Sun Y, Sun R, et al.: Kaposi's sarcoma-associated herpesvirus encoded vFLIP induces cellular IL-6 expres-sion: the role of the NF-kappaB and JNK/AP1 pathways. *Oncogene* 22:3371–3385, 2003.

82. Cesarman E, Nador RG, Bai F, et al.: Kaposi's sarcoma-associated herpesvirus contains G protein-coupled receptor and cyclin D homologs which are expressed in Kaposi's sarcoma and malignant lymphoma. *J Virol* 70:8218–8223, 1996.

83. Ralfkiaer E, Muller-Hermelink HK, Jaffe ES: Peripheral T-cell lymphoma, unspecified. In: Jaffe ES, Harris NL, Stein H, et al. (eds.) *Tumours of the Haematopoietic and Lymphoid Tissues.* Lyons, France: IARC Press; 2001.

84. Zettl A, Rudiger T, Konrad MA, et al.: Genomic profil-ing of peripheral T-cell lymphoma, unspecified, and anaplastic large T-cell lymphoma delineates novel recurrent chromosomal alterations. *Am J Pathol* 164:1837–1848, 2004.

85. Delsol G, Ralfkiaer E, Stein H, et al.: Anaplastic large cell lymphoma. In: Jaffe ES, Harris NL, Stein H, et al. (eds.) *Tumours of the Haematopoietic and Lymphoid System.* Lyon, France: IARC Press; 2001.

86. Falini B, Pileri S, Zinzani PL, et al.: ALK+ lymphoma: clinico-pathological findings and outcome. *Blood* 93:2697–2706, 1999.

87. Lae ME, Ahmed I, Macon WR: Clusterin is widely expressed in systemic anaplastic large cell lymphoma but fails to differentiate primary from secondary cuta-neous anaplastic large cell lymphoma. *Am J Clin Pathol* 118:773–779, 2002.

88. Wellmann A, Thieblemont C, Pittaluga S, et al.: Detection of differentially expressed genes in lym-phomas using cDNA arrays: identification of clusterin as a new diagnostic marker for anaplastic large-cell lymphomas. *Blood* 96:398–404, 2000.

89. Drexler HG, Gignac SM, von Wasielewski R, et al.: Pathobiology of NPM-ALK and variant fusion genes in anaplastic large cell lymphoma and other lymphomas. *Leukemia* 14:1533–1559, 2000.

90. Cataldo KA, Jalal SM, Law ME, et al.: Detection of t(2;5) in anaplastic large cell lymphoma: comparison of immunohistochemical studies, FISH, and RT-PCR in paraffin-embedded tissue. *Am J Surg Pathol* 23:1386–1392, 1999.

91. Jaffe E, Ralfkiaer E: Angioimmunoblastic T-cell lym-phoma. In: Jaffe E, Harris N, Stein H, et al. (eds.) *Tumours of Haematopoietic and Lymphoid Tissues.* Lyon, France: IARC Press; 2001.

92. Ferry JA: Angioimmunoblastic T-cell lymphoma. *Adv Anat Pathol* 9:273–279, 2002.

93. Attygalle A, Al Jehani R, Diss TC, et al.: Neoplastic T cells in angioimmunoblastic T-cell lymphoma express CD10. *Blood* 99:627–633, 2002.

94. Attygalle A, Diss TC, Isaacson PG, et al.: CD10 expres-sion in extranodal dissemination of angioimmunoblas-tic T-cell lymphoma. *Am J Surg Pathol* 15:964, 2002.

95. Lepretre S, Buchonnet G, Stamatoullas A, et al.: Chromosome abnormalities in peripheral T-cell lym-phoma. *Cancer Genet Cytogenet* 117:71–79, 2000.

96. Isaacson PG, Wright D, Ralfkiaer E, et al.: Enteropathy-type T-cell lymphoma. In: Jaffe ES, Harris NL, Stein H, et al. (eds.) *Tumours of Haematopoietic and Lymphoid Tissues.* Lyons, France: IARC Press; 2001.

97. Chott A, Dragosics B, Radaszkiewicz T: Peripheral T-cell lymphomas of the intestine. *Am J Pathol* 141:1361–1371, 1992.

98. Spencer J, Cerf-Bensussan N, Jarry A, et al.: Enteropathy-associated T cell lymphoma (malignant histiocytosis of the intestine) is recognized by a mono-clonal antibody (HML-1) that defines a membrane

molecule on human mucosal lymphocytes. *Am J Pathol* 132:1–5, 1988.

99. Chott A, Haedicke W, Mosberger I, et al: Most CD56+ intestinal lymphomas are CD8+CD5-T-cell lymphomas of monomorphic small to medium size histology. *Am J Pathol* 153:1483–1490, 1998.

100. Bagdi E, Diss TC, Munson P, et al.: Mucosal intra-epithelial lymphocytes in enteropathy-associated T-cell lymphoma, ulcerative jejunitis, and refractory celiac disease constitute a neoplastic population. *Blood* 94:260–264, 1999.

101. Howell WM, Leung ST, Jones DB, et al.: HLA-DRB, -DQA, and -DQB polymorphism in celiac disease and enteropathy-associated T-cell lymphoma. Common features and additional risk factors for malignancy. *Hum Immunol* 43:29–37,1995.

102. Chan JKC, Jaffe ES, Ralfkiaer E: Extranodal NK/T-cell lymphoma, nasal type. In: Jaffe ES, Harris NL, Stein H, et al. (eds.) *Tumours of the Haematopoietc and Lymphoid System.* Lyons, France: IARC Press, 2001.

103. Cheung MM, Chan JK, Wong KF: Natural killer cell neoplasms: a distinctive group of highly aggressive lymphomas/leukemias. *Semin Hematol* 40:221–232, 2003.

104. Kinney MC: The role of morphologic features, phenotype, genotype, and anatomic site in defining extranodal T-cell or NK-cell neoplasms. *Am J Clin Pathol* 111:S104–S118, 1999.

105. Chan JK, Sin VC, Wong KF, et al.: Nonnasal lymphoma expressing the natural killer cell marker CD56: a clinicopathologic study of 49 cases of an uncommon aggressive neoplasm. *Blood* 89:4501–4513, 1997.

106. Martin AR, Chan WC, Perry DA, et al.: Aggressive natural killer cell lymphoma of the small intestine. *Mod Pathol* 8:467–472, 1995.

107. Petrella T, Delfau-Larue MH, Caillot D, et al.: Nasopharyngeal lymphomas: further evidence for a natural killer cell origin. *Hum Pathol* 27:827–833, 1996.

108. Wong KF, Zhang YM, Chan JK: Cytogenetic abnormalities in natural killer cell lymphoma/leukaemia–is there a consistent pattern? *Leuk Lymphoma* 34:241–250, 1999.

109. Jaffe E, Harris N, Stein H, et al.: *Tumours of Haematopoietic and Lymphoid Tissues.* Lyon, France: IARC Press; 2001.

110. Belhadj K, Reyes F, Farcet JP, et al.: Hepatosplenic gammadelta T-cell lymphoma is a rare clinicopathologic entity with poor outcome: report on a series of 21 patients. *Blood* 102:4261–4269, 2003.

111. Vega F, Medeiros LJ, Bueso-Ramos C, et al.: Hepatosplenic gamma/delta T-cell lymphoma in bone marrow. A sinusoidal neoplasm with blastic cytologic features. *Am J Clin Pathol* 116:410–419, 2001.

112. Macon WR, Levy NB, Kurtin PJ, et al.: Hepatosplenic alphabeta T-cell lymphomas: a report of 14 cases and comparison with hepatosplenic gammadelta T-cell lymphomas. *Am J Surg Pathol* 25:285–296, 2001.

113. Ralfkiaer E, Jaffe ES: Mycosis fungoides and Sezary syndrome. In: Jaffe ES, Harris NL, Stein H, et al. (eds.) *Tumours of the Haematopoietic and Lymphoid Tissues.* Lyons, France: IARC Press; 2001.

114. Willemze R, Kerl H, Sterry W, et al.: EORTC classification for primary cutaneous lymphomas: a proposal from the Cutaneous Lymphoma Study Group of the European Organization for Research and Treatment of Cancer. *Blood* 90:354–371, 1997.

115. Colby TV, Burke JS, Hoppe RT: Lymph node biopsy in mycosis fungoides. *Cancer* 47:351–359, 1981.

116. Scheffer E, Meijer CJ, van Vloten WA: Dermatopathic lymphadenopathy and lymph node involvement in mycosis fungoides. *Cancer* 45:137–148, 1980.

117. Thangavelu M, Finn WG, Yelavarthi KK, et al.: Recurring structural chromosome abnormalities in peripheral blood lymphocytes of patients with mycosis fungoides/Sezary syndrome. *Blood* 89:3371–3377, 1997.

118. Mao X, Lillington D, Scarisbrick JJ, et al.: Molecular cytogenetic analysis of cutaneous T-cell lymphomas: identification of common genetic alterations in Sezary syndrome and mycosis fungoides. *Br J Dermatol* 147:464–475, 2002.

119. Ralfkiaer E, Delsol G, Willemze R, et al.: Primary cutaneous CD30-positive T-cell lymphoproliferative disorders. In: Jaffe ES, Harris NL, Stein H, et al. (eds.) *Tumours of the Haematopoietic and Lymphoid Tissues.* Lyons, France: IARC Press; 2001.

120. Willemze R, Meijer CJ: Primary cutaneous CD30-positive lymphoproliferative disorders. *Hematol Oncol Clin North Am* 17:1319–1332, 2003.

121. Kadin ME, Carpenter C: Systemic and primary cutaneous anaplastic large cell lymphomas. *Semin Hematol* 40:244–256, 2003.

122. Weiss LM, Wood GS, Trela M, et al.: Clonal T-cell populations in lymphomatoid papulosis. Evidence of a lymphoproliferative origin for a clinically benign disease. *N Engl J Med* 315:475–479, 1986.

123. Steinhoff M, Hummel M, Anagnostopoulos I, et al.: Single-cell analysis of CD30+ cells in lymphomatoid papulosis demonstrates a common clonal T-cell origin. *Blood* 100:578–584, 2002.

124. Jaffe ES, Ralfkiaer E: Subcutaneous panniculitis-like T-cell lymphoma. In: Jaffe ES, Harris NL, Stein H, et al. (eds.) *Tumours of Haematopoietic and Lymphoid Tissues.* Lyons, France: IARC Press; 2001.

125. Jaffe ES, Krenacs L, Raffeld M: Classification of cytotoxic T-cell and natural killer cell lymphomas. *Semin Hematol* 40:175–184, 2003.

126. Santucci M, Pimpinelli N, Massi D, et al.: Cytotoxic/natural killer cell cutaneous lymphomas. Report of eortc cutaneous lymphoma task force workshop. *Cancer* 97:610–627, 2003.

127. Willemze R, Jaffe ES, Burg G, et al.: WHO-EORTC classification for cutaneous lymphomas. *Blood* 105:3768–3785, 2005.

128. Chan JKC, Jaffe ES, Ralfkiaer E: Blastic NK-cell lymphoma. In: Jaffe ES, Harris NL, Stein H, et al. (eds.) *Tumours of the Haematopoietic and Lymphoid Tissues.* Lyons, France: IARC Press; 2001.

129. Bene MC, Feuillard J, Jacob MC: Plasmacytoid dendritic cells: from the plasmacytoid T-cell to type 2 dendritic cells CD4+CD56+ malignancies. *Semin Hematol* 40:257–266, 2003.

130. Feuillard J, Jacob MC, Valensi F, et al.: Clinical and biologic features of CD4(+)CD56(+) malignancies. *Blood* 99:1556–1563, 2002.

131. Jacob MC, Chaperot L, Mossuz P, et al.: CD4+ CD56+ lineage negative malignancies: a new entity developed from malignant early plasmacytoid dendritic cells. *Haematologica* 88:941–955, 2003.

# Chapter 53

# TREATMENT APPROACH TO FOLLICULAR LYMPHOMAS

*Bruce D. Cheson*

## CLASSIFICATION AND PROGNOSIS

The follicular lymphomas are the second most common subtype of indolent non-Hodgkin's lymphoma (NHL), representing about 25–30% of NHL. In the working formulation, these tumors were subclassified into follicular small cleaved cell, follicular mixed small and large cell, and follicular large cell, based on the number of larger cells per high-powered field.[1] In the more recent Revised European American Lymphoma[2] and the subsequent, universally adopted World Health Organization (WHO) classifications,[3,4] the nomenclature became grade I, grade II, and grade III, respectively. Grade III has been further subdivided into grade III A or grade III B, reflecting the presence of centroblasts (III A) or sheets of centroblasts (III B). A clinically meaningful difference in outcome between grade I and II has not been uniformly demonstrable.[5–8]

The conduct of clinical trials has been facilitated by the availability of prognostic scoring systems[9,10] and standardized response criteria.[11] The International Prognostic Index, originally developed for diffuse large B-cell lymphoma,[9] can distinguish risk groups in patients with follicular lymphoma as well.[12,13] However, better separation among the prognostic subsets may be afforded by the new Follicular Lymphoma International Prognostic Index[10] that uses stage, age, number of involved nodal sites, lactate dehydrogenase (LDH), and hemoglobin to identify low- (0–1 adverse factor), intermediate- (2 factors), or high-risk (≥3 factors) patients.

## THERAPY

### LIMITED-STAGE DISEASE

Only about 10–15% of patients present with limited-stage (stage I and nonbulky stage II) disease. For these patients, radiation therapy may result in prolonged disease-free survival. Whether or not they are cured is controversial, since relapses occur even after 10–20 years.[14] Prolonged progression-free survival without therapy in some series suggests that watchful waiting may be an appropriate option.[15]

### ADVANCED-STAGE DISEASE

Patients with advanced follicular NHL are characterized by an indolent clinical course with a median survival of 6–10 years.[16,17] Nevertheless, early intervention with treatment in patients with asymptomatic, nonbulky disease has not been associated with a prolongation of survival.[18,19] As a result, a watch-and-wait approach has been routinely recommended until treatment is clinically indicated on the basis of disease-related symptoms, massive or progressive lymphadenopathy or hepatosplenomegaly, potential organ compromise, or bone marrow involvement resulting in peripheral blood cytopenias.

### Standard chemotherapy

When treatment is indicated, no particular chemotherapy regimen has clearly prolonged the survival of patients with advanced-stage follicular NHL compared with another. Extensive experience with single alkylating agents alone or combined with vincristine and prednisone [e.g., cyclophosphamide, vincristine, and prednisone (CVP)], or CVP with adriamycin [cyclophosphamide, hydroxydaunomycin (doxorubicin), Oncovin (vincristine), and prednisone (CHOP)] failed to demonstrate a major difference in outcome.[17,20] Thus, until recently, a single alkylating agent or CVP was the standard. The use of CHOP is often reserved for patients for whom there is a concern of histologic conversion, or at the time of such conversion. Single-agent fludarabine is an active agent in previously treated and untreated patients,[21–26] and fludarabine-based combinations with cyclophosphamide or mitoxantrone demonstrated high response rates in phase II trials.[27,28] The regimen of fludarabine plus mitoxantrone has been reported to induce a higher complete response rate than that of CHOP, and with more molecular remissions, but with a similar overall response rate and time to progression.[29]

## Interferon therapy

Interferon (IFN) has modest single-agent activity in the treatment of patients with low-grade NHL,[30-32] leading to a series of phase III trials. IFN was approved by the Food and Drug Administration (FDA) for "low-grade" NHL in combination with aggressive chemotherapy largely based on a study from the Groupe d'Etude Lymphomes Folliculaire,[33] including 242 evaluable patients with follicular NHL and a high tumor burden. They were treated with doxorubicin, cyclophosphamide, teniposide, and prednisone for a year either alone or with concurrent IFN, which was continued out to 18 months. There was an advantage in response rate for the combined modality arm (85% vs 69%). At a median of 6-year follow-up, the progression-free survival was 2.9 years and 1.5 years, and the overall survival was not reached versus 5.6 years for the IFN-containing arm and the chemotherapy-alone arm, respectively.[34]

However, at least 10 randomized trials have evaluated the role of IFN either during induction,[35] as a maintenance,[36-39] or in both settings[33,40-43] with remarkably inconsistent results.

Rohatiner and colleagues[44] conducted a meta-analysis of these trials. In the five studies in which chemotherapy was considered to be "less intensive," defined as not including an anthracycline or anthracene agent,[38,40-43] there was no evidence of any benefit from IFN. In the five trials of "more intensive" treatment,[34-37,39] there was no improvement in the response rate when IFN was added to chemotherapy, but there was an overall prolongation of time to disease progression and survival, limited to patients with either a complete or partial response to their induction regimen. The conclusion was that IFN played a role in responsive patients who were receiving more intensive chemotherapy.

Nevertheless, given the disparate results of the various trials, the toxicity of this agent, and the availability of effective monoclonal antibodies, there is no clear role for IFN in the current management of follicular lymphoma.

## Monoclonal antibody therapy

An increasing number of monoclonal antibodies are either commercially available or available in clinical trials for follicular NHL (Table 53.1).

*Single-agent rituximab therapy* The treatment paradigm for the approach to indolent B-cell malignancies has been revolutionized by the availability of active monoclonal antibodies and related agents. Rituximab has become an integral component of the therapy of most patients with follicular NHL. The original studies of this chimeric anti-CD20 monoclonal antibody were conducted in patients with relapsed and refractory follicular and low-grade NHL. In the pivotal trial including 166 patients treated with a dose of 375 mg/m$^2$

**Table 53.1** Unconjugated monoclonal antibodies for follicular NHL

| Antibody | Target | Status |
|---|---|---|
| Rituximab | CD20 | Commercial |
| Alemtuzumab | HLA-DR | Commercial |
| Galiximab (IDEC-114) | CD80 | Phase II |
| Humanized anti-CD20 | CD20 | Phase I/II |
| Bevacizumab (Avastin) | VEG-F | Commercial* |
| Anti-CD40 | CD40 | Phase I |
| Anti-TRAIL | Trail 1,2 | Phase I |
| Epratuzumab | CD52 | ? |
| Apolizumab (Hu1D10) | CD22 | ? |

"*", for colorectal cancer; "?", future uncertain.

weekly for 4 weeks,[45] responses were induced in 48% of patients, including 6% complete remissions, with an about 13-month duration of response. This antibody has been widely adopted because of its activity and favorable toxicity profile. Most adverse reactions occur during the infusion and consist primarily of fevers, chills, with occasional hypotension. Premedication includes acetaminophen and diphenhydramine. Demerol may be indicated for rigors. Hydrocortisone may also help ameliorate these toxicities. Delayed myelosuppression, especially neutropenia, has been observed, although the etiology of this phenomenon is unclear.

Attempts to improve on the activity of rituximab have included increasing the dose, dose density, or number of infusions, using it earlier in the course of the disease, combining it with chemotherapy or other biologics, maintenance therapy, and identifying patients more likely to experience a response. Administration of eight weekly infusions instead of the standard four neither increased the response rate nor clearly prolonged the time to progression.[46] In chronic lymphocytic leukemia, administration of higher doses or schedules involving three doses per week was not clearly associated with meaningful clinical benefit.[47,48] Pursuing such an approach is, therefore, not warranted in follicular NHL.

The activity of rituximab correlates with the extent of prior treatment. When rituximab is used as initial therapy, response rates have been greater than 70% compared with the 50–58% in relapsed/refractory patients[49,50]; however, the duration of response has been disappointing.

*Rituximab and chemotherapy combinations* The large number of studies that have been conducted with rituximab in combination with chemotherapy suggest that results with the combination are superior to what would be expected with either chemotherapy or rituximab alone. These observations support the in vitro studies suggesting that monoclonal antibodies such as rituximab can sensitize lymphoma

**Table 53.2** Rituximab + chemotherapy regimens, for follicular NHL

| Author | Patients | Other drug(s) | RR (CR)% |
|---|---|---|---|
| Czuczman[53] | 38 | CHOP | 100(63) |
| Hiddemann[55] | 205 | CHOP | 97(20) |
| Marcus[56] | 162 | CVP | 81(40) |
| Czuczman[57] | 40 | Flu | 91(83) |
| Martinelli[58] | 29 | CLB | 90(50) |
| Sacchi[59] | 39 | Flu/Cy | 97(74) |
| Gregory[60] | 41 | FM | 97(45) |
| Vitolo[61] | 59 | FND | 95(90) |
| Zinzani[62] | 47 | FN | 87(59) |
| Rummel[63] | 35 | Bendamustine | 97(71) |

cells to the effects of subsequent chemotherapy.[51,52] Czuczman et al.[53] were the first to report a combined modality experience with 38 patients, 31 of whom were previously untreated, who received CHOP plus rituximab. The overall response rate was 100% with 58% complete remissions and a median time to progression of 8.3 years.[54] However, comparable response rates can be achieved with a variety of other chemotherapy-rituximab regimens (Table 53.2).[55–63] Any differences in complete or overall response rates among the various regimens may be explained by a number of factors including patient selection or the point in time when response is assessed, as maximal responses may occur several months following therapy. Nevertheless, the relative duration of responses among these various regimens has not been compared.

Recent randomized trials have shown superiority for rituximab-containing regimens over chemotherapy alone. However, the optimal approach to such combinations is unknown. In some of these studies, the antibody has been combined with the chemotherapy. The German Low Grade Lymphoma Study Group conducted a randomized study of 394 patients who were allocated to either CHOP or rituximab plus CHOP (R-CHOP), with a secondary randomization to a variety of postremission therapies including INF or stem cell transplantation (SCT).[55] There was no advantage from rituximab in overall response rate (97% vs 93%), but the combination was associated with a longer event-free survival and a trend toward a longer overall survival. The variety of postremission therapies makes these data difficult to interpret. Marcus and coworkers[56] randomized 322 patients with either intermediate- or poor-risk follicular NHL to either CVP alone or with rituximab (CVP-R). The dose of drugs was lower than usually used at only 750 mg/m$^2$ with prednisolone 40 mg/m$^2$. The overall response rates and complete response rates were significantly higher with CVP-R at 81 and 40% versus 57 and 10% for CVP alone. The median time to treatment failure with CVP-R was 27 months compared with 7 months for CVP at a median follow-up of 18 months. In addition, the median time to progression was not reached for CVP-R compared with 113 months for CVP alone.

***Maintenance therapy with rituximab*** Maintenance rituximab therapy has also been evaluated in an attempt at prolonging the time to disease progression and, possibly, survival.[50,64,65] In several trials, rituximab has been used as a single-agent for induction followed by the same agent as maintenance. Hainsworth et al.[50] treated 62 patients with follicular and low-grade NHL, using four weekly doses of rituximab followed by four additional doses every 6 months for 2 years. The time to progression of 32 months was longer than expected. In a randomized trial, Ghielmini et al.[64] reported previously treated (n = 128) and previously untreated patients (n = 57) who received four weekly doses of rituximab followed by a randomization to no further therapy or to maintenance consisting of a single infusion of rituximab every 2 months for a total of 8 months. At a median follow-up of 35 months, the median event-free survival was 23 months for the prolonged treatment group compared with 12 months in those allocated to no further treatment. This advantage was greatest in the chemotherapy-naïve patients.

About 40% of patients who have experienced an initial response to rituximab lasting at least six months respond a second time with a duration at least as long as the initial response.[66] Thus, whether maintenance is associated with an outcome that is superior to retreatment is an important question. Hainsworth et al.[67] conducted a study in which patients who were treated with an initial 4 weeks of rituximab were then randomized to maintenance therapy as previously published[50] or retreatment upon recurrence; although response rates and time to progression favored the maintenance arm, the time to which another treatment other than rituximab was required was similar (31 months vs 27 months). The ongoing Eastern Cooperative Oncology Group (ECOG) "RESORT" trial is comparing treatment until relapse with retreatment at the time of recurrence. Therefore, at the present time, the preferable approach is not clear.

Investigators from ECOG recently presented the early results from a trial exploring the role of rituximab maintenance following induction chemotherapy.[65] The initial study design had included a randomization during induction between CVP (cyclophosphamide 1000 mg/m$^2$ with prednisone 100 mg/m$^2$ every 3 weeks for six to eight cycles, determined by the rapidity of the response) and fludarabine plus cyclophosphamide; however, the latter arm was discontinued because of excessive toxicity. Rituximab maintenance was started 4 weeks after the completion of the chemotherapy, and four weekly infusions were delivered every 6 months for 2 years. After CVP, approximately 15% of patients attained a

CR with an overall response rate of 79%. Rituximab improved the response rate in 22% of patients, while an improvement in response was noted in 8% of patients receiving no further therapy. Progression-free survival was 4.5 for the maintenance arm versus 1.5 years for observation at a median follow-up of only 1.2 years, with a trend in favor of the maintenance arm in overall survival ($p = .06$). Van Oers et al. randomized 461 patients with relapsed or refractory follicular lymphoma to CHOP or R-CHOP with a secondary randomization to rituximab maintenance or observation. Maintenance was associated with a longer time to progression with a suggestion of a survival advantage.[67a]

### Patient selection for antibody therapy

In the future, the optimal treatment may be determined by clinical and biological characteristics of individual patients. Patient characteristics that appear to predict those patients more likely to respond to rituximab therapy include polymorphisms for FcRgammaIII, which represents the binding site on natural killer cells for the rituximab antibody,[68] and DNA microarray signatures.[69] Moreover, in large B-cell NHL the benefit of rituximab appears to be limited to patients whose tumors overexpress the *bcl-2* gene.[70] Whether these observations will determine which patients will receive rituximab remains to be seen.

### Other monoclonal antibodies

A number of other unconjugated antibodies are being evaluated in clinical trials for follicular NHL (Table 53.1).

***Alemtuzumab*** Alemtuzumab (Campath-1H) is a humanized anti-CD52 monoclonal antibody with activity in chronic lymphocytic leukemia as well as T-cell lymphomas; however, its single-agent activity in indolent B-cell NHL has been disappointing.[71,72]

***Epratuzumab*** Epratuzumab is a humanized IgG1 monoclonal antibody directed against the CD22 antigen, expressed on a variety of lymphomas. In a dose-escalation study of epratuzumab in 55 patients with indolent NHL, no dose-limiting toxicities were identified.[73] The overall response rate was 24% in those with follicular histologies. In a subsequent trial, both epratuzumab and rituximab were administered using an empiric schedule with each weekly for 4 weeks. The response rate and duration were disappointing, suggesting that a inferior dose and schedule of this combination was used.[74]

***Anti-CD80 (Galiximab)*** CD80 is an immune costimulatory molecule present on the surface of NHL cells. Galiximab (IDEC-114) is a macaque-human chimeric anti-CD80 antibody with in vivo antilymphoma properties. In phase I trials, the antibody was well tolerated except for mild fatigue, nausea, and headaches. Moreover, single-agent activity was approximately 15%.[75] Based on preclinical data suggesting synergy, a phase I/II study of the combination of galiximab and rituximab was conducted, and a response rate of 58.3% was reported.[76] This combination has been evaluated as the initial therapy for patients with follicular lymphoma in a Cancer and Leukemia Group B phase II trial and results are pending.

***Apolizumab*** Apolizumab (Hu1D10, Remitogen) is a humanized monoclonal antibody directed against a polymorphic determinant of HLA-DR, found on both normal B-cells and in about half of patients with lymphoid malignancies. Limited activity and excessive toxicities have halted its development (U. Hegde, T. White, M. Stetler-Stevenson et al., unpublished data, 2002).[77,78]

***Humanized anti-CD20*** Several humanized anti-CD20 monoclonal antibodies are in clinical trials.[79] Potential advantages are activation of different pathways enhancing cell kill, and a shorter infusion time. Whether there will be any clinical benefit remains to be determined.

### Radioimmunotherapy (RIT)

Two radioimmunoconjugates are currently commercially available; Y-90 ibritumomab tiuxetan (Zevalin) and I-131 tositumomab (Bexxar). The clinical trials thus far conducted with radioimmunoconjugates have demonstrated greater activity than their cold antibody, and are useful in patients who have relapsed after or who are refractory to rituximab.

***Y-90 ibritumomab tiuxetan*** Y-90 ibritumomab tiuxetan has a murine rituximab conjugated to the isotope.[80] The Y-90 ibritumomab tiuxetan regimen takes about 8 days to administer. On the first day, a dose of cold rituximab at 250 mg/m² is administered to bind nontumor CD20 sites and to facilitate better biodistribution. Because Y-90 is a beta emitter, it cannot be used for imaging; thus, indium-111-labeled ibritumomab is substituted for biodistribution studies performed at days 2–3, and if needed, 6–7 to ensure appropriate localization of the isotope. On days 7–8, another low dose of cold antibody is delivered followed by 0.4 mCi/kg of Y-90 ibritumomab tiuxetan (not to exceed 32 mCi) for patients with platelet counts of at least 150,000/mm³. The dose is reduced to 0.3 mCi in patients with a platelet count of 100–149,000/mm³.[81]

In the initial phase I/II trial,[82] the overall response rate in 32 patients with follicular/low-grade NHL was 82%, including 26% complete remissions. Response could be predicted by tumor grade, tumor burden, whether or not the bone marrow was involved with lymphoma, and the extent of that bone marrow involvement. The median time to progression was 12.9+ months with a median response duration of 11.7+ months. The major toxicity was myelosuppression, with median granulocyte and platelet nadirs of 1100/mm$^3$ and 49,500/mm$^3$, respectively.

The additive benefit of the radioisotope is supported by the activity of radioimmunotherapy in rituximab failures. Y-90 ibritumomab tiuxetan induces responses in 74% of these patients with 15% complete remissions.[83] How radioimmunotherapy compares with unconjugated antibody therapy has been addressed in a randomized trial in which 143 patients, with relapsed CD20-positive NHL without previous rituximab exposure, received either rituximab or Y-90 ibritumomab tiuxetan.[84] Whereas the response rates were higher with Y-90 ibritumomab tiuxetan (80%) than with rituximab (56%), there was no difference between the arms in time to disease progression. Responses to this agent may be quite durable with 24% of responders having a time to progression longer than 3 years and some responses in excess of 5 years.[85]

*I-131 tositumomab* I-131 tositumomab is a conjugate of the murine anti-CD20 antibody tositumomab and I-131. It is approved for use in patients with relapsed/refractory follicular or transformed NHL. As with Y-90 ibritumomab tiuxetan, treatment occurs over about a week. Thyroid protection is required with I-131 tositumomab because of the radioactive iodine. I-131 is a gamma emitter, and dosimetry is required to provide patient-specific dosing. In a multicenter pivotal trial,[86] 65% of the 60 heavily pretreated patients with NHL responded including 20% CR. The response rate in the subset with follicular histologies was 81%. Response rates and response duration were significantly higher than from the last chemotherapy. The response rate has been 63% with 29% complete responses in rituximab-refractory patients.

### Newer approaches to radioimmunotherapy

A number of approaches are under investigation to increase the activity of radioimmunotherapy. Multiple dosing and retreatment are being studied in clinical trials. Radioimmunotherapy is also being used earlier in the course of the disease. I-131 tositumomab has been administered to 76 previously untreated patients, of which 97% responded, including 63% complete remissions, and with almost 59% free of progression at 5 years for all patients, and this endpoint was not yet reached for those who achieved a CR.[87] A similar study is under way with Y-90 ibritumomab tiuxetan. I-131 tositumomab can be safely administered after CHOP chemotherapy, and it converts some partial responses to complete responses.[88] A randomized phase III of R-CHOP followed by I-131 tositumomab compared to R-CHOP is ongoing within the Southwest Oncology Group and the Cancer and Leukemia Group B. A variety of sequences of chemotherapy and radioimmunotherapy are under investigation.

RIT has also been used in the stem cell transplant setting. Gopal and coworkers compared their results with follicular lymphoma patients who received high-dose I-131 tositumomab with those treated using various high-dose chemotherapy regimens and found better overall survival and progression-free survival, with lower toxicity in the RIT-treated population.[89]

### Toxicities of radioimmunotherapy

The major complications of radioimmunotherapy are infusional reactions during the administration of the cold antibody, especially the rituximab, and myelosuppression that occurs around 7–9 weeks after therapy. Febrile neutropenia or infections that require hospitalization are uncommon events. There is little in the way of alopecia, nausea, vomiting, or mucositis. Because of the radioactive iodine, I-131 tositumomab therapy is associated with hypothyroidism in fewer than 10% of patients.

As a result of the treatment associated with myelosuppression, exclusionary criteria for the use of radioimmunotherapy include >25% bone marrow involvement, a hypocellular bone marrow (<15% cellular), platelets <100,00/mm$^3$, neutrophils <1500/mm$^3$, extensive prior radiation therapy, and prior stem cell transplant, the latter because the safety in this setting is unknown, and pregnancy or lactation. Thus, review of a bone marrow biopsy is essential prior to radioimmunotherapy.

One of the major concerns with RIT is the potential for the development of secondary acute myelogenous leukemia or myelodysplastic syndrome. The reported risk is about 1.5% with Y-90 ibritumomab tiuxetan, and 6.3% with I-131 tositumomab. However, the development of this secondary malignancy likely relates to the type and extent of prior treatment, as many patients have cytogenetic abnormalities suggestive of myelodysplasia prior to receiving radioimmunotherapy. In addition, there have been no cases of myelodysplastic syndrome in patients receiving radioimmunotherapy as their initial treatment.[87] Moreover, based on reviews of the literature, the risk may not be greater than expected from chemotherapy alone.[86,90,91]

Whether these myelotoxic agents will compromise the ability to safely deliver subsequent therapies has been another area of concern. Preliminary reports with both Y-90 ibritumomab tiuxetan and I-131 tositumomab suggest that patients can tolerate additional therapies; however, response and toxicity data are not yet available.[92,93]

Y-90 ibritumomab tiuxetan and I-131 tositumomab appear to have comparable activity, and their relative toxicity is being tested in a large phase III trial. Current research is directed at trying to combine or sequence radioimmunotherapy with chemotherapy and other biologicals.

## NEW AGENTS

### ANTISENSE OLIGONUCLEOTIDES

Antisense oligonucleotides are chemically modified single-strand DNA molecules with a nucleotide sequence that is complementary to the target mRNA and, therefore, are capable of inhibiting expression of the target gene. Bcl-2 upregulation is thought to be responsible for maintaining the viability of tumor cells, as well as inducing a form of multidrug resistance. The *bcl-2* gene is a rational target in follicular NHL because it is overexpressed in most tumors.

Oblimersen sodium (Genasense, Genta Incorporated, Berkeley Heights, NJ) is a phosphorothioate oligonucleotide consisting of 18 modified DNA bases (i.e., 18-mer) that targets the first six codons of Bcl-2 mRNA to form a DNA/RNA duplex. This agent is the first antisense molecule to be widely tested in the clinic for the treatment of human tumors.

In the single phase I study of oblimersen in 21 patients with NHL,[94] one patient attained a complete response, which lasted unmaintained for longer than 3 years. Combinations of oblimersen with fludarabine, bortezomib, rituximab, and other agents are in development.

### VACCINES

Several vaccines are currently in clinical trials for follicular NHL. Most of these are directed against the idiotype of the hypervariable region of the immunoglobulin light chain. Interest in this approach has been stimulated by a number of nonrandomized studies, such as one from Stanford in which 49% of patients with follicular NHL reacted to their own idiotype conjugated to keyhole limpet hemocyanin (KLH) by exhibiting a cellular and humoral immune response. Those patients capable of mounting such a response had a time to tumor progression of 7.9 years compared to 1.3 years for those who could not.[95] The results of the three randomized trials will determine if there is clinical benefit from this approach.

### NEW CHEMOTHERAPY DRUGS
#### Bendamustine

Bendamustine is a bifunctional compound with both an alkylating nitrogen mustard group and a purine-like benzimidazole ring. It was first synthesized in 1963 in the German Democratic Republic and has been used extensively in Germany since then. Bendamustine has demonstrated activity in indolent and aggressive NHL, Hodgkin's lymphoma, chronic lymphocytic leukemia, and multiple myeloma.[96–99] In vitro and clinical data also support a beneficial interaction with rituximab. In a study of 63 patients with relapsed/refractory indolent NHL or mantle cell lymphoma, the response rate to this combination was 94% with 71% complete remissions.[63] This combination was extremely well tolerated. To better characterize the activity of this agent and to provide broader experience with the agent, it is now being studied alone and in combination with rituximab in phase II trials in the United States.

#### Bortezomib

Bortezomib (PS-341; Velcade) is a potent, reversible inhibitor of the 26S proteasome, an enzyme important in the intracellular degradation of proteins including those involved in cell cycle regulation, transcription factor activation, apoptosis, and cell trafficking. A primary target for this agent is nuclear factor kappa B (NF-κB). Bortezomib is the first proteasome inhibitor to be studied in the clinic, and has recently been approved by the FDA for the treatment of relapsed/refractory multiple myeloma.[100] The rationale for a study in NHL is that NF-κB is overexpressed in a number of histologies. In reports from Goy et al.[101] and O'Connor et al.,[102] responses were noted in patients with follicular NHL and, notably, mantle cell lymphoma.

### STEM CELL TRANSPLANTATION

The experience with SCT for low-grade NHL is limited because of the older age of the population, the relatively long natural history of the disease, the tendency for peripheral blood and bone marrow involvement, and the fact that most patients have already received extensive prior therapy at the time a transplant is considered. Autologous SCT for low-grade NHL has generally been disappointing with no evidence of cure.[103–106] However, in a recently published study,[107] patients who responded to three cycles of salvage chemotherapy were randomized to either three more cycles or high-dose therapy with autologous stem cell support. Only 89 patients were randomized; nevertheless, a benefit for transplantation was observed in both progression-free and overall survival, but with no plateau on the survival curve.

Serious complications of autologous SCT for NHL include up to a 20% actuarial risk of myelodysplastic syndrome and acute myelogenous leukemia,[108–111] and the outcome of those patients is extremely poor.

Allogeneic SCT has been used infrequently in follicular NHL because of an excessive treatment-related mortality.[112,113] In an analysis of the 81 patients from the International Bone Marrow Transplant Registry,[112] transplanted at a median age of 41 years, 56% had never achieved a complete remission and the projected survival at 3 years was 46%, with 43% disease-free survival. The median follow-up was only 23 months. However, the transplant-related mortality was 44%. Chemosensitivity prior to transplant was the strongest predictor of outcome.

As a result, the long-term outcome of autologous and allogeneic transplants have been comparable because of the early mortality with allogeneic transplants and the late relapses with autologous SCT.[114,115] More recently, benefit has been suggested for submyeloablative SCT; however, longer follow-up is required to better assess the impact of this therapy.[116–118]

## HISTOLOGIC TRANSFORMATION OF FOLLICULAR LYMPHOMA

Patients with a follicular lymphoma have a relatively constant risk over time of transforming into a more aggressive histology, most often a diffuse large B-cell lymphoma.[16,119,120] The frequency of this occurrence varies among series from fewer than 20%[16] to at least 30%.[119] The difference among studies reflects a number of factors, including the duration of follow-up, the definition of what is called "transformed lymphoma," and the method of surveillance. In studies in which patients had lymph nodes routinely rebiopsied, the likelihood of identifying transformation is greater. Patients with histologic transformation are a clinically diverse group; some exhibit no clinical effects at the time this diagnosis is identified by a lymph node biopsy, whereas others present with the recent onset of fever, sweat, weight loss, rapidly progressive lymphadenopathy and splenomegaly, and a markedly elevated serum LDH. The outcome of patients with histologic transformation is better in patients identified prior to the development of these signs and symptoms.[120] In general, aggressive chemotherapy is recommended and, if a complete remission is achieved, autologous SCT is a potentially effective treatment option.[121] Activity has also been reported with radioimmunotherapy.[84,86]

## SUMMARY

After decades of clinical research using various combinations of nonspecific cytotoxic drugs, there is now a wealth of new approaches for patients with follicular NHL. The availability of an expanding menu of novel targeted agents provides great promise for therapeutic advances. These include monoclonal antibodies such as rituximab, radioimmunotherapeutics, anti-idiotype vaccines, antisense oligonucleotides, and proteasome inhibitors. Clearly, higher complete and overall response rates are achieved with antibody–chemotherapy combinations than with chemotherapy alone; however, whether an eventual prolongation in survival will be achieved remains to be demonstrated by longer follow-up. As there is still no consensus as to the optimal initial therapy, a clinical trial remains the preferred option (Figure 53.1). The potential for cure will result from the rational development of multiple targeted agents with individualized treatment selection based on specific molecular and biologic findings.

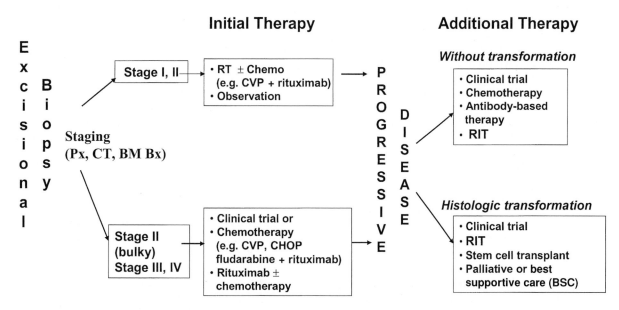

**Figure 53.1** *Suggested paradigm for the management of patients with follicular NHL*

## REFERENCES

1. The Non-Hodgkin's Lymphoma Pathologic Classification Project: National Cancer Institute sponsored study of classifications of non-Hodgkin's lymphomas. *Cancer* 449:2112–2135, 1982.

2. Harris NL, Jaffe ES, Stein H, et al.: A revised European–American classification of lymphoid neoplasms: a proposal from the International Lymphoma Study Group. *Blood* 84:1361–1392, 1994.

3. Harris NL, Jaffe ES, Diebold J, et al.: World Health Organization classification of neoplastic diseases of the hematopoietic and lymphoid tissues: report of the clinical advisory committee meeting—Airlie House, Virginia. *J Clin Oncol* 17:3835–3849, 1999.

4. Jaffe ES, Harris NL, Stein H, et al.: Tumours of haematopoietic and lymphoid tissues. In: *World Health Organization Classification of Tumours: Pathology & Genetics.* Lyon, France: IARC Press, 2001.

5. Ott G, Katzenberger T, Lohr A, et al.: Cytomorphologic, immunohistochemical, and cytogenetic profiles of follicular lymphoma: 2 types of follicular lymphoma grade 3. *Blood* 99:3806–3812, 2002.

6. Chau I, Jones R, Cunningham D, et al.: Outcome of follicular lymphoma grade 3: is anthracycline necessary as front-line therapy? *Br J Cancer* 89:36–42, 2003.

7. Hans CP, Weisenburger DD, Vose JM, et al.: A significant diffuse component predicts for inferior survival in grade 3 follicular lymphoma, but cytologic subtypes do not predict survival. *Blood* 101:2363–2367, 2003.

8. Hsi ED, Mirza I, Lozanski G, et al.: A clinicopathologic evaluation of follicular lymphoma grade 3A versus grade 3B reveals no survival differences. *Arch Pathol Lab Med* 128:863–868, 2004.

9. Shipp MA, Harrington DP, Anderson JR, et al.: Development of a predictive model for aggressive lymphoma: the International Non-Hodgkin's Lymphoma Prognostic Factors Project. *N Engl J Med* 329:987–994, 1993.

10. Solal-Céligny P, Roy P, Colombat P, et al.: Follicular lymphoma international prognostic index. *Blood* 104:1258–1265, 2004.

11. Cheson BD, Horning SJ, Coiffier B, et al.: Report of an International Workshop to standardize response criteria for non-Hodgkin's lymphomas. *J Clin Oncol* 17:1244–1253, 1999.

12. Löpez-Guillermo A, Montserrat E, Bosch F, et al.: Applicability of the International Prognostic Index for aggressive lymphomas in patients with low-grade lymphoma. *J Clin Oncol* 12:1343–1348, 1994.

13. Hermans J, Krol ADG, van Groningen K, et al.: International prognostic index for aggressive non-Hodgkin's lymphoma is valid for all malignancy grades. *Blood* 86:1460–1463, 1995.

14. Mac Manus M, Hoppe RT: Is radiotherapy curative for stage I and II low-grade follicular lymphoma? Results of a long-term follow-up study of patients treated at Stanford University. *J Clin Oncol* 14:1282–1290, 1996.

15. Advani R, Rosenberg SA, Horning SJ: Stage I and II follicular non-Hodgkin's lymphoma: long-term follow-up of no initial therapy. *J Clin Oncol* 22:1454–1459, 2004.

16. Horning SJ, Rosenberg SA: The natural history of initially untreated low-grade non-Hodgkin's lymphoma. *N Engl J Med* 311:1471–1475, 1984.

17. Dana BW, Dahlberg S, Nathwani BN, et al.: Long-term follow-up of patients with low-grade malignant lymphomas treated with doxorubicin-based chemotherapy or chemoimmunotherapy. *J Clin Oncol* 11:644–651, 1993.

18. Young RC, Longo DL, Glatstein E, et al.: The treatment of indolent lymphomas: watchful waiting v aggressive combined modality treatment. *Semin Hematol* 25:11–16, 1988.

19. Brice P, Bastion Y, Lepage E, et al.: Comparison of low-tumor-burden follicular lymphomas between an initial no-treatment policy, prednimustine, or interferon alfa: a randomized study from the Group D'Etude des Lymphomes Folliculares. *J Clin Oncol* 15:1110–1117, 1997.

20. Kimby E, Björkholm M, Gahrton G, et al.: Chlorambucil/prednisone vs. CHOP in symptomatic low-grade non-Hodgkin's lymphomas: a randomized trial from the Lymphoma Group of Central Sweden. *Ann Oncol* 5:567–571, 1994.

21. Hochster HS, Kim K, Green MD, et al.: Activity of fludarabine in previously treated non-Hodgkin's low-grade lymphoma: results of an Eastern Cooperative Oncology Group study. *J Clin Oncol* 10:28–32, 1992.

22. Redman JR, Cabanillas F, Velasquez WS, et al.: Phase II trial of fludarabine phosphate in lymphoma: an effective new agent in low-grade lymphoma. *J Clin Oncol* 10:790–794, 1992.

23. Zinzani PL, Lauria F, Rondelli D, et al.: Fludarabine: an active agent in the treatment of previously-treated and untreated low-grade non-Hodgkin's lymphoma. *Ann Oncol* 4:575–578, 1993.

24. Pigaditou A, Rohatiner AZS, Whelan JS, et al.: Fludarabine in low-grade lymphoma. *Semin Oncol* 20:24–27, 1993.

25. Hiddemann W, Unterhalt M, Pott C, et al.: Fludarabine single-agent therapy for relapsed low-grade non-Hodgkin's lymphomas: a phase II study of the German Low-grade Non-Hodgkin's Lymphoma Study Group. *Semin Oncol* 20:28–31, 1993.

26. Solal-Céligny P, Brice P, Brousse N, et al.: Phase II trial of fludarabine monophosphate as first-line treatment in patients with advanced follicular lymphoma: a multicenter study by the Groupe d'Etude des Lymphomes de l'Adulte. *J Clin Oncol* 14:514–519, 1996.

27. Flinn IW, Byrd JC, Morrison C, et al.: Fludarabine and cyclophosphamide with filgrastim support in patients with previously untreated indolent lymphoid malignancies. *Blood* 96:71–75, 2000.

28. Velasquez WS, Lew D, Grogan TM, et al.: Combination of fludarabine and mitoxantrone in untreated stages III and IV low-grade lymphoma: S9501. *J Clin Oncol* 21:1996–2003, 2003.

29. Zinzani PL, Pulsoni A, Perrotti A, et al.: Fludarabine plus mitoxantrone with and without rituximab versus CHOP with and without rituximab as front-line treatment for patients with follicular lymphoma. *J Clin Oncol* 22:2654–2661, 2004.

30. Merigan TC, Sikora K, Breeden JH, et al.: Preliminary observations on the effect of human leukocyte interferon in non-Hodgkin's lymphoma. *N Engl J Med* 299:1449–1553, 1978.

31. Foon KA, Sherwin SA, Abrams PG, et al.: Treatment of advanced non-Hodgkin's lymphoma with recombinant leukocyte A interferon. *N Engl J Med* 311:1148–1152, 1984.

32. O'Connell MJ, Colgan JP, Oken MM, et al.: Clinical trial of recombinant leukocyte A interferon as initial therapy for favorable histology non-Hodgkin's lymphomas and chronic lymphocytic leukemia. An Eastern Cooperative Oncology Group pilot study. *J Clin Oncol* 4:128–136, 1986.

33. Solal-Céligny P, Lepage E, Brousse N, et al.: Recombinant interferon alfa-2b combined with a regimen containing doxorubicin in patients with advanced follicular lymphoma. *N Engl J Med* 329:1608–1614, 1993.

34. Solal-Céligny P, Lepage E, Brousse N, et al.: A doxorubicin-containing regimen with or without interferon alpha-2b for advanced follicular lymphomas: final analysis of survival and toxicity in the GELF 86 trial. *J Clin Oncol* 16:2332–2338, 1998.

35. Smalley RV, Andersen JW, Hawkins MJ, et al.: Interferon alfa combined with cytotoxic chemotherapy for patients with non-Hodgkin's lymphoma. *N Engl J Med* 327:1336–1341, 1992.

36. Avilés A, Duque G, Talavera A, et al.: Interferon alpha 2b as maintenance therapy in low grade malignant lymphoma improves duration of remission and survival. *Leuk Lymphoma* 20:495–499, 1996.

37. Unterhalt M, Hermann R, Koch P, et al.: Long term interferon alpha maintenance prolongs remission duration in advanced low grade lymphomas and is related to the efficacy of initial cytoreductive therapy. *Blood* 88:453a, 1996. Abstract 1801.

38. Hagenbeek A, Carde P, Meerwaldt JH, et al.: Maintenance of remission with human recombinant interferon alfa-2a in patients with stages III and IV low-grade malignant non-Hodgkin's lymphoma. *J Clin Oncol* 16:41–47, 1998.

39. Fisher RI, Dana BW, LeBlanc M, et al.: Alpha-interferon consolidation following intensive chemotherapy does not prolong the failure-free survival of patients with low grade non-Hodgkin's lymphoma: results of SWOG-8809, a randomized phase III study. *J Clin Oncol* 18:2010–2016, 2000.

40. Chisesi T, Congiu M, Contu A, et al.: Randomized study of chlorambucil (CB) compared to interferon (alfa-2b) in low-grade non-Hodgkin's lymphoma: an interim report of a randomized study. *Eur J Cancer* 27:S31–S33, 1991.

41. Price CGA, Rohatiner AZS, Steward W, et al.: Interferon alfa-2b in addition to chlorambucil in the treatment of follicular lymphoma: preliminary results of a randomized trial in progress. *Eur J Cancer* 27:S34–S36, 1991.

42. Peterson BA, Petroni G, Oken MM, et al.: Cyclophosphamide versus cyclophosphamide plus interferon alfa-2b in follicular low grade lymphomas: a preliminary report of an intergroup trial (CALGB 8691 and EST 7486). *Proc Am Soc Clin Oncol* 12:366, 1993. Abstract 1240.

43. Arranz R, García-Alfonso P, Sobrino P, et al.: Role of interferon alfa-2b in the induction and maintenance treatment of low-grade non-Hodgkin's lymphoma: results from a prospective, multicenter trial with double randomization. *J Clin Oncol* 16:1538–1546, 1998.

44. Rohatiner AZS, Gregory W, Peterson B, et al.: A meta-analysis (MA) of randomised trials evaluating the role of interferon (IFN) as treatment for follicular lymphoma (FL). *Proc Am Soc Clin Oncol* 17:4a, 1998. Abstract 11.

45. McLaughlin P, Grillo-López AJ, Link BK, et al.: Rituximab chimeric anti-CD20 monoclonal antibody therapy of relapsed indolent lymphoma: half of patients respond to a four-dose treatment program. *J Clin Oncol* 16:2825–2833, 1998.

46. Piro LD, White CA, Grillo-López AJ, et al.: Extended rituximab (anti-CD20 monoclonal antibody) therapy for relapsed or refractory low-grade or follicular non-Hodgkin's lymphoma. *Ann Oncol* 10:655–661, 1999.

47. O'Brien SM, Kantarjian H, Thomas DA, et al.: Rituximab dose-escalation trial in chronic lymphocytic leukemia. *J Clin Oncol* 19:2165–2170, 2001.

48. Byrd JC, Murphy T, Howard RS, et al.: Rituximab using a thrice weekly dosing schedule in B-cell chronic lymphocytic leukemia and small lymphocytic lymphoma demonstrates clinical activity and acceptable toxicity. *J Clin Oncol* 19:2153–2164, 2001.

49. Colombat P, Salles G, Brousse N, et al.: Rituximab (anti-CD20 monoclonal antibody) as single first-line therapy for patents with follicular lymphoma with a low tumor burden: clinical and molecular evaluation. *Blood* 97:101–106, 2001.

50. Hainsworth JD, Lichty S, Burris HA III, et al.: Rituximab as first-line and maintenance therapy for patients with indolent non-Hodgkin's lymphoma. *J Clin Oncol* 20:4261–4267, 2002.

51. Demidem A, Lam T, ALas S, et al.: Chimeric anti-CD20 (IDEC-C2B8) monoclonal antibody sensitizes a B cell lymphoma cell line to cell killing by cytotoxic drugs. *Cancer Biother Radiopharm* 12:177–186, 1997.

52. Johnson TA, Press OW: Synergistic cytotoxicity of iodine-131-anti-CD20 antibodies and chemotherapy for treatment of B-cell lymphomas. *Int J Cancer* 85:104–112, 2000.

53. Czuczman MS, Grillo-López AJ, White CA, et al.: Treatment of patients with low-grade B-cell lymphoma with the combination of chimeric anti-CD20 monoclonal antibody and CHOP chemotherapy. *J Clin Oncol* 17:268–276, 1999.

54. Czuczman M, Grillo-López AJ, LoBuglio AF, et al.: Patients with low-grade NHL treated with rituximab + CHOP experience prolonged clinical and molecular remission. *Blood* 102: Abstract 1493, 2003.

55. Hiddemann W, Dreyling M, Forstpointner R, et al.: Combined immuno-chemotherapy (R-CHOP) significantly improves time to treatment failure in first line therapy of follicular lymphoma—results of a prospective randomized trial of the German Low Grade Lymphoma Study Group (GLSG). *Blood* 102: Abstract 352, 2003.

56. Marcus R, Imrie K, Belch A, et al.: An international multi-centre, randomized, open-label phase III trial comparing rituximab added to CVP chemotherapy to CVP chemotherapy alone in untreated stage III/IV follicular non-Hodgkin's lymphoma. *Blood* 102: Abstract 87, 2003.

57. Czuczman MS, Fallon A, Mohr A, et al.: Phase II study of rituximab plus fludarabine in patients (pts) with

low-grade follicular lymphoma (LGL): final report. *Blood* 98:601a, 2001. Abstract 2518.

58. Martinelli G, Laszlo D, Mancuso P, et al.: Rituximab plus chlorambucil in low-grade non Hodgkin's lymphomas (NHL): clinical results of a phase II study. *Blood* 100:777a, 2002. Abstract 3073.

59. Sacchi S, Tucci A, Merli F, et al.: Phase II study with fludarabine and cyclophosphamide plus rituximab (FC+R) in relapsed follicular lymphoma patients. *Blood* 100: 572a, 2002. Abstract 2246.

60. Gregory SA, Venugopal P, Adler S, et al.: Combined fludarabine, mitoxantrone and rituximab achieves a high response rate as initial treatment for advanced low grade non-Hodgkin's lymphoma (LGNHL). *Blood* 100:362a, 2002. Abstract 1401.

61. Vitolo U, Boccomini C, Ladetto M, et al.: High clinical and molecular response rate in elderly patients with advanced stage follicular lymphoma treated at diagnosis with a brief chemo-immunotheraepy FND + rituximab. *Blood* 100:359a, 2002. Abstract 1392.

62. Zinzani PL: A multicenter randomized trial of fludarabine and mitoxantrone (FM) plus rituximab versus CHOP plus rituximab as first-line treatment in patients with follicular lymphoma. *Blood* 100:93a, 2002. Abstract 344.

63. Rummel MJ, Kim SZ, Chow KU, et al.: Bendamustine and rituximab act synergistically in vitro and are effective in the treatment of relapsed or refractory indolent and mantle cell lymphomas. *Blood* 102:104a, 2003. Abstract 353.

64. Ghielmini M, Schmitz SF, Cogliatti SB, et al.: Prolonged treatment with rituximab in patients with follicular lymphoma significantly increases event-free survival and response duration compared with weekly × 4 schedule. *Blood* 103:4416–4423, 2004.

65. Hochster HS, Weller E, Ryan T, et al.: Results of E1496: A phase III trial of CVP with or without maintenance rituximab in advanced indolent lymphoma (NHL). *Proc Am Soc Clin Oncol* 22:558s, 2004. Abstract 6502.

66. Davis TA, Grillo-López AJ, White CA, et al.: Rituximab anti-CD20 monoclonal antibody therapy in non-Hodgkin's lymphoma: safety and efficacy of retreatment. *J Clin Oncol* 18:3135–3143, 2000.

67. Hainsworth JD, Litchy S, Greco FA: Scheduled rituximab maintenance therapy versus rituximab retreatment at progression in patients with indolent non-Hodgkin's lymphoma (NHL) responding to single-agent rituximab: a randomized trial of the Minnie Pearl Cancer Research Network. *Blood* 102: Abstract 231, 2003.

67a. Van Oers MHJ, Van Glabbeke M, Teodorovic I, et al.: Chimeric anti-CD20 monoclonal antibody (Rituximab; Mabthera) in remission induction and maintenance treatment of relapsed/resistant follicular non-Hodgkin's lymphoma. Final analysis of a phase III randomized intergroup clinical trial. *Blood* 106(Part 1): 107a (abstract 353), 2005.

68. Weng WK, Levy R: Two immunoglobulin G fragment C receptor polymorphisms independently predict response to rituximab in patients with follicular lymphoma. *J Clin Oncol* 21:3940–3947, 2003.

69. Bohen SP, Troyanskaya OG, Alter O, et al.: Variation in gene expression patterns in follicular lymphoma and

response to rituximab. *Proc Natl Acad Sci USA* 100: 1926–1930, 2003.

70. Mounier N, Briere J, Gisselbrecht C, et al.: Rituximab plus CHOP (R-CHOP) overcomes bcl-2-associated resistance to chemotherapy in elderly patients with diffuse large B-cell lymphoma (DLBCL). *Blood* 101:4279–4284, 2003.

71. Keating MJ, Flinn I, Jain V, et al.: Therapeutic role of alemtuzumab (CAMPATH-1H) in patients who have failed fludarabine: results of a large international study. *Blood* 99:3554–3561, 2002.

72. Lundin J, Österborg A, Brittinger G, et al.: CAMPATH-1H monoclonal antibody therapy for previously treated low-grade non-Hodgkin's lymphomas: a phase II multicenter study. *J Clin Oncol* 16:3257–3263, 1998.

73. Leonard JP, Coleman M, Ketas JC, et al.: Phase I/II trial of epratuzumab (humanized anti-CD22 antibody) in indolent non-Hodgkin's lymphoma. *J Clin Oncol* 21: 3051–3059, 2003.

74. Emmanouilides C, Leonard J, Schuster SJ, et al.: Multicenter, phase 2 study of combination antibody therapy with epratuzumab plus rituximab in recurring low-grade NHL. *Blood* 102: Abstract 233, 2003.

75. Czuczman M, Witzig TE, Vose JM, et al.: Results of a phase I/II multicenter trial of galiximab (IDEC-114, anti-CD80 antibody) therapy for relapsed or refractory follicular lymphoma. *Blood* 102:647–648a, 2003. Abstract 2393.

76. Gordon LI, Moore JO, Cheson BD, et al.: Phase I results from a multicenter trial of galiximab (anti-CD80 antibody, IDEC-114) in combination with rituximab for the treatment of follicular lymphoma. *Blood* 102:307b, 2003. Abstract 4951.

77. Link BK, Wang H, Byrd JC, et al.: Phase I trial of humanized 1D10 (Hu1D10) monoclonal antibody targeting class II molecules in patients with relapsed lymphoma. *Proc Am Soc Clin Oncol* 19:24a, 2000. Abstract 86.

78. Link BK, Kahl B, Czuczman M, et al.: A phase II study of Remitogen™ (Hu1D10), a humanized monoclonal antibody in patients with relapsed or refractory follicular, small lymphocytic, or marginal zone/MALT B-cell lymphomas. *Blood* 98:606a, 2001. Abstract 2540.

79. Stein R, Qu Z, Chen S, et al.: Characterization of a new humanized anti-CD20 monoclonal antibody, IMMU-106, and its use in combination with the humanized anti-CD22 antibody, epratuzumab, for the therapy of non-Hodgkin's lymphoma. *Clin Cancer Res* 10: 2868–2878, 2004.

80. Cheson BD: Radioimmunotherapy of non-Hodgkin's lymphomas. *Blood* 101:391–398, 2003.

81. Wiseman GA, Gordon LI, Multani PS, et al.: Ibritumomab tiuxetan radioimmunotherapy for patients with relapsed or refractory non-Hodgkin's lymphoma and mild thrombocytopenia: a phase II multicenter trial. *Blood* 99:4336–4342, 2002.

82. Witzig TE, White CA, Wiseman GA, et al.: Phase I/II trial of IDEC-Y2B8 radioimmunotherapy for treatment of relapsed or refractory CD20(+) B-cell non-Hodgkin's lymphoma. *J Clin Oncol* 17:3793–3803, 1999.

83. Witzig TE, Flinn IW, Gordon LI, et al.: Treatment with ibritumomab tiuxetan radioimmunotherapy in patients with rituximab-refractory follicular non-Hodgkin's lymphoma. *J Clin Oncol* 20:3262–3269, 2002.

84. Witzig TE, Gordon LI, Cabanillas F, et al.: Randomized controlled trial of yttrium-90-labeled ibritumomab tiuxetan radioimmunotherapy versus rituximab immunotherapy for patients with relapsed or refractory low-grade, follicular, or transformed B-cell non-Hodgkin's lymphoma. *J Clin Oncol* 20:2453–2463, 2002.

85. Gordon LI, Molina A, Witzig T, et al.: Durable responses after ibritumomab tiuxetan radioimmunotherapy for CD20+ B-cell lymphoma: long-term follow-up of a phase 1/2 study. *Blood* 103:4429–4431, 2004.

86. Kaminski MS, Zelenetz AD, Press OW, et al.: Pivotal study of Bexxar (Iodine I-131 tositumomab) for chemotherapy-refractory low-grade or transformed low-grade B-cell non-Hodgkin's lymphomas. *J Clin Oncol* 19:3918–3928, 2001.

87. Kaminski MS, Tuck M, Regan D, et al.: High response rate and durable remissions in patients with previously untreated, advanced-stage, follicular lymphoma treated with tositumomab and iodine I-131 tositumomab (Bexxar©). *Blood* 100:356a, 2002. Abstract 1381.

88. Press OW, Unger JM, Braziel RM, et al.: A phase 2 trial of CHOP chemotherapy followed by tositumomab/iodine I 131 tositumomab for previously untreated follicular non-Hodgkin's lymphoma: Southwest Oncology Group protocol S9911. *Blood* 102:1606–1612, 2003.

89. Gopal AK, Gooley TA, Maloney DG, et al.: High-dose radioimmunotherapy versus conventional high-dose therapy and autologous stem cell transplantation for relapsed follicular non-Hodgkin lymphoma: a multivariable cohort analysis. *Blood* 102:2351–2357, 2003.

90. Bennett JM, Kaminski MS, Knox SJ, et al.: Assessment of treatment-related myelodysplastic syndromes (tMDS) and acute myeloid leukemia (tAML) in patients with low-grade non-Hodgkin's lymphoma (LG-NHL) treated with tositumomab and iodine-131 tositumomab (the Bexxar therapeutic regimen). *Blood* 102: Abstract 91, 2003.

91. Witzig TE, White CA, Gordon LI, et al.: Safety of yttrium-90 ibritumomab tiuxetan radioimmunotherapy for relapsed low-grade, follicular, or transformed non-Hodgkin's lymphoma. *J Clin Oncol* 21:1263–1270, 2003.

92. Kaminski M, Bahm V, Estes J, et al.: Tolerance of treatment subsequent to frontline Bexxar™ (tositumomab and iodine I131 tositumomab) in patients (Pts) with follicular lymphoma. *Blood* 98:603a, 2001. Abstract 2526.

93. Ansell SM, Ristow KM, Habermann TM, et al.: Subsequent chemotherapy regimens are well tolerated after radioimmunotherapy with [90]Yttrium ibritumomab tiuxetan for non-Hodgkin's lymphoma. *J Clin Oncol* 20:3885–3890, 2002.

94. Waters JS, Webb A, Cunningham D, et al.: Phase I and pharmacokinetic study of bcl-2 antisense oligonucleotide therapy in patients with non-Hodgkin's lymphoma. *J Clin Oncol* 18:1809–1811, 2000.

95. Hsu FJ, Caspar C, Czerwinski D, et al.: Tumor-specific idiotype vaccines in the treatment of patients with B-cell lymphoma—long term results of a clinical trial. *Blood* 89:3129–3135, 1997.

96. Kath R, Blumenstengel K, Fricke HJ, et al.: Bendamustine monotherapy in advanced and refractory chronic lymphocytic leukemia. *J Cancer Res Clin Oncol* 127:48–54, 2001.

97. Schwänen C, Karakas T, Begmann L: Bendamustine in the treatment of low-grade non-Hodgkin's lymphomas. *Onkologie* 23:318–324, 2000.

98. Weidmann E, Kim SZ, Rost A, et al.: Bendamustine is effective in relapsed or refractory aggressive non-Hodgkin's lymphoma. *Ann Oncol* 13:1285–1289, 2002.

99. Bremer K: High rates of long-lasting remissions after 5-day bendamustine chemotherapy cycles in pre-treated low-grade non-Hodgkin's lymphomas. *J Cancer Res Clin Oncol* 128:603–609, 2002.

100. Richardson PG, Barlogie B, Berenson JR, et al.: A phase 2 study of bortezomib in relapsed, refractory myeloma. *N Engl J Med* 348:2609–2617, 2003.

101. Goy A, Younes A, McLaughlin P, et al.: A phase II study of proteasome inhibitor bortezomib in relapsed or refractory B-cell non-Hodgkin's lymphoma. *J Clin Oncol* 23:667–675, 2005.

102. O'Connor OA, Wright J, Moskowitz C, et al.: Phase II clinical experience with the novel proteasome inhibitor bortezomib in patients with indolent non-Hodgkin's lymphoma and mantle cell lymphoma. *J Clin Oncol* 23:676–684, 2005.

103. Freedman AS, Nadler LM: Which patients with relapsed non-Hodgkin's lymphoma benefit from high-dose therapy and hematopoietic stem-cell transplantation? *J Clin Oncol* 11:1841–1843, 1993.

104. Freedman AS, Gribben JG, Neuberg D, et al.: High-dose therapy and autologous bone marrow transplantation in patients with follicular lymphoma. *Blood* 88: 2780–2786, 1996.

105. Rohatiner AZS, Johnson PWM, Price CGA, et al.: Myeloablative therapy with autologous bone marrow transplantation as consolidation therapy for recurrent follicular lymphoma. *J Clin Oncol* 12:1177–1184, 1994.

106. Freedman AS, Neuberg D, Mauch P, et al.: Long-term follow-up of autologous bone marrow transplantation in patients with relapsed follicular lymphoma. *Blood* 94:3325–3333, 1999.

107. Schouten HC, Qian W, Kvaloy S, et al.: High-dose therapy improves progression-free survival and survival in relapsed follicular non-Hodgkin's lymphoma: results from the randomized European CUP trial. *J Clin Oncol* 21:3918–3927, 2003

108. Darrington DL, Vose JM, Anderson JR, et al.: Incidence and characterization of secondary myelodysplastic syndrome and acute myelogenous leukemia following high-dose chemoradiotherapy and autologous stem-cell transplantation for lymphoid malignancies. *J Clin Oncol* 12:2527–2534, 1994.

109. Miller JS, Arthur DC, Litz CE, et al.: Myelodysplastic syndrome after autologous bone marrow transplantation: an additional late complication of curative cancer therapy. *Blood* 83:3780–3788, 1994.

110. Stone RM, Neuberg D, Soiffer R, et al.: Myelodysplastic syndrome as a late complication following autologous bone marrow transplantation for non-Hodgkin's lymphoma. *J Clin Oncol* 12:2535–2542, 1994.

111. Friedberg JW, Neuberg D, Stone RM, et al.: Outcome in patients with myelodysplastic syndrome after autologous bone marrow transplantation for non-Hodgkin's lymphoma. *J Clin Oncol* 17:3128–2135, 1999.

112. van Besien KW, Khouri IF, Giralt S, et al.: Allogeneic bone marrow transplantation for refractory and recurrent low-grade lymphoma: the case for aggressive management. *J Clin Oncol* 13:1096–1102, 1995.

113. van Besien K, Sobocinski KA, Rowlings PA, et al.: Allogeneic bone marrow transplantation for low-grade lymphoma. *Blood* 92:1832–1836, 1998.

114. Ratanatharathorn V, Uberti J, Karanes C, et al.: Prospective comparative trial of autologous versus allogeneic bone marrow transplantation in patients with non-Hodgkin's lymphoma. *Blood* 84:1050–1055, 1994.

115. Haioun C, Lepage E, Gisselbrecht C, et al.: Comparison of autologous bone marrow transplantation with sequential chemotherapy for intermediate-grade and high-grade non-Hodgkin's lymphoma in first complete remission: a study of 464 patients. *J Clin Oncol* 12:2543–2551, 1994.

116. Khouri IF, Keating M, Körbling M, et al.: Transplant-lite: induction of graft-versus malignancy using fludarabine-based nonablative chemotherapy and allogeneic blood progenitor-cell transplantation as treatment for lymphoid malignancies. *J Clin Oncol* 16:2817–2824, 1998.

117. Khouri IF, Saliba RM, Giralt SA, et al.: Nonablative allogeneic hematopoietic transplantation as adoptive immunotherapy for indolent lymphoma: low incidence of toxicity, acute graft-versus-host disease, and treatment-related mortality. *Blood* 98:3595–3599, 2001.

118. Faulkner RD, Craddock C, Byrne JL, et al.: BEAM-alemtuzumab reduced-intensity allogeneic stem cell transplantation for lymphoproliferative diseases: GVHD, toxicity and survival in 65 patients. *Blood* 103:428–434, 2004.

119. Hubbard SM, Chabner B, DeVita VT Jr, et al.: Histologic progression in non-Hodgkin's lymphoma. *Blood* 59:258–264, 1982.

120. Yuen AR, Kamel OW, Halpern J, et al.: Long-term survival after histologic transformation of low-grade follicular lymphoma. *J Clin Oncol* 13:1726–1733, 1995.

121. Schouten HC, Bierman PJ, Vaughn WP, et al.: Autologous bone marrow transplantation in follicular non-Hodgkin's lymphoma before and after histologic transformation. *Blood* 74:2579–2584, 1989.

# Chapter 54

# TREATMENT APPROACH TO DIFFUSE LARGE B-CELL LYMPHOMAS

*Sonali M. Smith and Koen van Besien*

## INTRODUCTION

Non-Hodgkin's lymphoma (NHL) is the fifth most common malignancy in the United States, with 53,400 new cases and 23,400 deaths in 2003.[1] The overall incidence of NHL rose by 80% over the past 3 decades, for reasons that are not entirely clear.[2,3] Diffuse large B-cell lymphoma (DLBCL) is the most common histologic subtype of NHL. It accounts for almost one-third of cases and is considered the prototype for aggressive lymphomas.

DLBCL is a chemosensitive disease. Approximately half of the patients are cured with front-line anthracycline-based chemotherapy. However, many others will relapse after initial response and become candidates for potentially curative transplantation strategies. Patients with refractory disease, those who relapse following transplant and those who are not candidates for transplantation, have no true curative options and most will ultimately die of lymphoma. The factors determining clinical outcome are increasingly complex, and are discussed in detail below.

## INITIAL PRESENTATION

DLBCL may occur in all age groups, but the incidence increases with age. The median age at presentation is 63 years, with a slight male preponderance.[4] Children with DLBCL comprise only 700–800 cases per year in the United States, and tend to present with widespread disease, high-grade disease, and frequent extranodal involvement.[5] Most adult patients with DLBCL also present with symptoms. Symptoms may include a rapidly enlarging lymph node, B symptoms (fevers, night sweats, >10% loss of body weight) or other constitutional symptoms, or paraneoplastic syndromes. Approximately 30–40% of the patients have an extranodal site of involvement,[3,4] and DLBCL can occur in nearly every body site. Several sites merit their own

diagnostic categories in the WHO classification due to unique clinical and/or pathologic features. These include primary effusion lymphoma (PEL), intravascular DLBCL, and primary mediastinal lymphoma (PMBL); PMBL is discussed later. PEL and intravascular large B-cell lymphoma are extremely rare subtypes with a uniformly poor prognosis.[6] PEL typically occurs in the setting of immunodeficiency and has been clearly linked to human herpesvirus 8 (HHV-8) infection. No mass can be identified, and the malignant cells instead accumulate in body cavities such as the pleural, peritoneal, or pericardial spaces. Intravascular diffuse large B-cell lymphoma is characterized by widely disseminated circulating malignant cells that frequently occlude small vessels. Diagnosis is often delayed due to heterogeneous presentations, and the pathologic features are often not appreciated until the time of autopsy.

## DIAGNOSIS AND INITIAL EVALUATION

The diagnosis of DLBCL requires adequate tissue for histologic, flow cytometric, and immunohistochemical studies. Histopathologic examination reveals a diffuse growth pattern of medium- to large-sized cells that replace the normal nodal architecture. Several morphologic variants exist (centroblastic, immunoblastic, T-cell/histiocyte rich, anaplastic)[6] but do not currently influence initial treatment strategies. The classic immunophenotype of DLBCL is $CD20^+$, $CD22^+$, $CD19^+$, $CD79a^+$, and with surface and cytoplasmic immunoglobulin expression in the majority of cases. Less commonly, CD5 or CD10 may be expressed,[6] necessitating differentiation from other NHL subtypes. Molecular studies such as immunoglobulin gene rearrangement studies may be needed to confirm the diagnosis in cases with weak or absent surface markers or in cases with pleomorphic morphology. Other immunohistochemical stains for markers such as Pax5 and MUM1 can identify a B-cell process and a post-germinal center process, respectively.[7] Cytogenetics may also be performed on lymph node or bone marrow biopsy samples. Three recurring chromosomal abnormalities have been described: t(14;18) in 30% of cases, 3q27 in 30–40% of cases, and t(8;14) in occasional cases. However, cytogenetic analysis is currently used merely to support a diagnosis of DLBCL and is not used to subclassify the disease or guide treatment.

Once the diagnosis is established, the initial evaluation consists of staging and clinical assessment. The initial staging procedures should include imaging (most commonly CT scan or MRI) of the chest, abdomen, and pelvis, and a bone marrow aspirate and core biopsy. In many centers, bilateral bone marrow biopsies are preferred, but a single biopsy of good quality may be acceptable. An international collaboration suggests that an aggregate bone marrow biopsy of at least 2 cm is sufficient if only one side is sampled.[8] A test of cardiac function in anticipation of anthracycline-based therapy is usually recommended as well.

Gallium scintigraphy (Ga-67) or positron emission tomography (PET) with [18]fluorine fluorodeoxyglucose provide complementary information. Although neither of these tests is part of the standard response criteria,[8] they are commonly used to provide a baseline and to aid in the evaluation of residual masses following the end of treatment. Both are extremely sensitive imaging tools that can be used as part of routine staging to evaluate response to treatment, to evaluate residual masses following treatment, and to predict risk of relapse after completion of treatment. Gallium imaging has been used for many years, but, more recently, PET scanning has received increasing interest because of its convenience of use and its greater sensitivity. Several groups have used PET to assess residual masses in Hodgkin's lymphoma and NHL following treatment. It is now fairly well established that residual PET positivity after completion of treatment correlates with an increased risk for recurrence in aggressive lymphoma, and should at the very least lead to increased surveillance for relapse.[9,10] The optimal management of patients who have residual PET positivity after completion of treatment is not determined. Other studies suggest that PET positivity midway through treatment is a strong predictor for treatment failure.[11,12] Again, the optimal management of such patients remains undetermined.

In staging patients with newly diagnosed DLBCL, an important question is when to obtain a lumbar puncture and when to consider central nervous system (CNS) prophylaxis. In contrast to high-grade lymphomas such as Burkitt's or Burkitt-like subtypes, the risk of CNS involvement for intermediate grade lymphomas appears to be low at approximately 1–2%.[13,14] However, CNS relapse carries a grim prognosis and is uniformly fatal with less than 25% of the patients sur-viving the first year following diagnosis.[14] The median time to death following diagnosis is only 5 months.[13] There are many reports linking clinical risk factors at diagnosis to an increased risk of CNS relapse, including blood and bone marrow involvement, testicular involvement, bulky retroperitoneal disease, sinus involvement, epidural involvement, and elevated lactate dehydrogenase (LDH). Therefore, we have recommended a lumbar puncture as part of the initial evaluation in patients with any of these characteristics.

## PATHOLOGIC AND PROGNOSTIC FEATURES

Over the past several decades, DLBCL is increasingly understood to be a heterogenous disease with widely variable clinical outcomes. The Ann Arbor staging system (Table 54.1) provides a measure of tumor burden, and is an essential, though no longer sufficient, determinant of prognosis and treatment. Approximately 40% of patients present with localized disease (stage I and II) and the rest have disseminated disease at initial presentation.[15] In general, the prognosis of early-stage patients is better than that of patients with advanced disease. Still, the prognosis of individual patients is not accurately predicted by the Ann Arbor stage alone. In 1993, an international task force developed a model, called the International Prognostic Index (IPI), that can be easily implemented for individual patients, using readily available clinical, laboratory, and radiographic features.[15] This study analyzed over 2000 patients receiving anthracycline-based treatment for clinical features potentially predictive of outcome and identified five that retained independent prognostic

**Table 54.1**  Ann Arbor (Cotswold revision) staging system for malignant lymphomas

| Ann Arbor staging for malignant lymphomas | |
| --- | --- |
| Stage I | Involvement of a single lymph node region or a lymph node structure of a single extralymphatic site |
| Stage II | Involvement of two or more lymph node regions on the same side of the diaphragm or localized contiguous involvement of an extralymphatic site and lymph node organ |
| Stage III | Involvement of lymph node regions on both sides of the diaphragm |
| Stage IV | Diffuse or disseminated involvement of one or more extranodal organs or tissues, with or without associated lymph node involvement |

A: absence of B symptoms
B: presence of B symptoms (fevers, night sweats, weight loss > 10% of body weight)
E: extranodal disease or extension from known nodal site of disease
X: bulky disease (> 1/3 widening of the mediastinum at T5-T6 or maximum size of nodal mass > 10 cm)

**Table 54.2** The International Prognostic Index

| Adverse factor | | Risk group | Number of factors present | 5-year DFS (%) | 5-year OS (%) |
|---|---|---|---|---|---|
| Age | > 60 years | Low | 0–1 | 70 | 73 |
| PS | ≥ 2 | Low/Intermediate | 2 | 50 | 51 |
| LDH | > Normal | High/Intermediate | 3 | 49 | 43 |
| Extranodal sites | ≥2 | High | 4–5 | 40 | 26 |
| Stage | III–IV | | | | |

significance. These include age ≥60 years, tumor stage, B symptoms, serum LDH level, and the presence of more than one extranodal site of involvement. The IPI is essentially a scoring system in which these five clinical features are tallied to categorize patients into one of four prognostic groups that correlate with both relapse-free survival (RFS) and overall survival (OS) (Table 54.2). Moreover, patients with low-risk disease consistently attain complete response more frequently than the patients with higher risk disease. In addition to providing prognostic guidance at an individual patient level, the IPI provides a common language for clinical trials to allow homogeneity when comparing patient groups. For now, the IPI remains the most clinically useful tool to predict prognosis.

Recent research highlights the clinical and molecular heterogeneity of this most common form of NHL even further, via gene expression profiles and microarray technology. Microarray analysis of gene expression involves the simultaneous evaluation of thousands of genes by hybridizing complementary DNA to the mRNA in a cell of interest. In an elegant pilot study by Alizadeh and colleagues,[16] normal and malignant lymphoid cells were analyzed on a "lymphochip" microarray that included nearly 18,000 genes of interest. These genes were all of putative importance in normal B-cell development and/or in the progression to neoplasia. The authors identified two molecular signatures, germinal center B cell like (GC) and activated B cell like (ABC). They then applied the lymphochip to 40 patients with previously untreated DLBCL and compared the genetic signature with the clinical outcome. The OS for all patients at 5 years was 52%; however, the OS for patients with the GC pattern of gene expression was 76% as compared to only 16% for patients with the ABC pattern ($p < 0.01$). Even more powerful is their finding that patients within the low-risk IPI group could be further separated, in terms of prognosis, by the gene expression pattern. In summary, their data suggest that DLBCL comprises at least two distinct diseases differentiated by the expression pattern of hundreds of genes. A larger multicenter study confirms these findings, validates the significance of these two molecular signatures, and identifies a probable third signature (labeled "Type 3") of genetic importance.[17]

Most recently, Lossos and colleagues evaluated 36 genes identified by microarray analysis that predicted survival.[18] Using quantitative real-time polymerase chain reaction (RT-PCR) in 66 frozen patient samples, they ranked the genes by their ability to predict survival and identified the six most powerful genes: *LMO2*, *BCL6*, *FN1*, *CCND2*, *SCYA3*, and *BCL2*. They then developed a prognostic model based on the weighted expression of these six genes, which is potentially a simpler approach to determine prognosis than is the use of microarrays. It is likely that similar reports will eventually allow further ability to predict survival at an individual patient level using readily available techniques such as immunohistochemistry or flow cytometry. In addition to its potential clinical utility, microarray technology also aids in the understanding of lymphoma biology by identifying genes and genetic pathways that determine growth rate, responsiveness to therapy, or other important clinical parameters.

## INITIAL THERAPY OF LOCALIZED DLBCL

Approximately 30–40% of DLBCL patients present with stage I or II disease,[15] often referred to as localized or limited-stage disease. Many localized cases involve extranodal sites with or without regional lymph node involvement. Historically, early-stage DLBCL was treated with irradiation alone. However, this led to unsatisfactory 5-year progression-free survival (PFS) rates of approximately 50% for patients with stage I disease and 20% for patients with stage II disease.[19–21] A retrospective review with greater than 10 years of follow-up by the British National Lymphoma Investigation with subgroup analysis shows that the elderly fared especially poorly with radiation alone, underscoring the negative prognostic connotation of advanced age and supporting the need for systemic therapy even in clinically localized disease.[22]

The most common current strategy is to use combined modality treatment with anthracycline-based chemotherapy followed by radiotherapy. However, the optimal number of chemotherapy cycles is unknown, and several investigators have questioned whether or not radiation therapy (RT) can be eliminated entirely. There are now several phase III studies addressing this issue. A Southwest Oncology Group (SWOG) trial[23] randomized 401 patients with nonbulky stage I and II diseases to cyclophosphamide, doxorubicin, vincristine, prednisone (CHOP) × 8 versus CHOP × 3 plus RT; 75%

of the patients in this series had DLBCL, and 37% had primary extranodal disease. Initial results with a median follow-up of 4.4 years showed that combined modality therapy (CMT) was superior in terms of PFS (77% vs 64%, $p = 0.03$) and OS (82% vs 72%, $p = 0.02$). A recent update, however, shows that the PFS and OS curves of the chemotherapy only arm and the combined modality arm converge at 7–9 years.[24]

The authors also introduced the application of a stage-modified IPI for early-stage DLBCL. This stage-modified IPI included four components: age >60 years, stage II (as opposed to stage I), increased LDH, and poor performance status. As in the IPI, a point was assigned for the presence of each of these parameters. They found that even apparently localized NHL has widely variable outcomes, and that a stage modified IPI provided important prognostic information. For example, patients with 0–1 risk factor had a 5-year PFS and OS of 77% and 82%, respectively, as compared to only 34% and 45% for patients with more than two risk factors. Using the stage modified IPI, the authors conclude that limited CHOP (three cycles) plus involved field radiation therapy is appropriate for patients with stage I or nonbulky stage II disease, but that patients with adverse risk factors may not benefit from shortened chemotherapy plus radiation.

Another phase III randomized study by the Eastern Cooperative Oncology Group (ECOG) compared CHOP times eight cycles with or without consolidative low-dose radiation (30 Gy) for patients achieving complete remission.[25] All partial responders received 40 Gy to residual masses. Nearly two-thirds of patients in this series had stage II or IIE disease. Sixty-one percent of eligible patients achieved a complete remission with CHOP and were subsequently randomized. With a median follow-up of 6 years, patients randomized to radiation enjoyed an improved disease-free survival (73% vs 56%, $p = 0.05$), failure-free survival (75% vs 56%, $p = 0.06$), and time to progression (80% vs 67%, $p = 0.06$). However, there was no difference in OS.

The Groupe d'Etude des Lymphomes de l'Adulte (GELA) also addressed the ability to eliminate RT entirely in a group of elderly patients with minimal risk factors.[26] In this study, presented in abstract form, 455 eligible patients older than 60 years were randomized to CHOP times four cycles with or without 40-Gy RT. All patients had good prognosis disease. In the preliminary presentation of this trial, there is no difference in event-free survival (EFS) or OS with 49 months median follow-up. Furthermore, in patients older than 69 years, radiotherapy actually increased toxicity. The authors suggest that CHOP times four cycles may be sufficient for this favorable subgroup.

In summary, combined modality therapy with limited cycles of anthracycline-based chemotherapy has been the accepted standard treatment for patients with limited-stage DLBCL. Newer information, such as the lack of a survival benefit with continued follow-up and the potential to cure patients with prolonged chemotherapy, is challenging the role of radiation. Mature follow-up and final publication of the randomized controlled trials mentioned above are certain to guide future treatment selection. Our standard approach is to deliver three or four cycles of CHOP-rituximab (CHOP-R) chemotherapy followed by involved field radiation for patients with minimal risk factors (i.e., stage I or nonbulky stage II), and to deliver six cycles of CHOP-R for others with early-stage DLBCL. The results of the GELA study suggest that involved field radiation may not be necessary or beneficial for all patients. This study has only been reported in abstract form, and until its definitive publication, our treatment recommendations are not guided by its results. More recent data regarding the use of rituximab in patients with DLBCL will be discussed below.

## INITIAL THERAPY OF ADVANCED DLBCL

Nearly 3 decades ago, CHOP chemotherapy was introduced: cyclophosphamide 750 mg/m$^2$ on day 1, adriamycin 50 mg/m$^2$ on day 1, vincristine 1.4 mg/m$^2$ on day 1 (maximum 2 mg), and prednisone 100 mg daily on days 1–5.[27] This early report, in the era prior to routine radiographic follow-up, demonstrated a previously undescribed overall clinical response rate of over 90% in a heterogeneous group of lymphoma patients. It quickly became the standard against which other regimens were measured. During the subsequent 2 decades, alternative combinations were proposed that appeared more intense and more effective than CHOP in phase II and/or single institution studies. These include combinations such as m-BACOD (low-dose methotrexate, bleomycin, doxorubicin, cyclophosphamide, vincristine, dexamethasone), ProMACE-CytaBOM (prednisone, doxorubicin, cyclophosphamide, etoposide alternating with cytarabine, bleomycin, vincristine, and methotrexate), and MACOP-B (methotrexate, doxorubicin, cyclophosphamide, vincristine, prednisone, and bleomycin) among others. However, a definitive phase III, randomized, controlled trial conducted by the SWOG and the ECOG demonstrated that CHOP was equally efficacious and less toxic than these second-generation regimens.[28] Specifically, 899 eligible patients with bulky stage II, stage III, or stage IV aggressive lymphomas were randomized to either CHOP, m-BACOD, ProMACE-CytaBOM, or MACOP-B. There was no significant difference in either EFS (44% at 3 years) or OS (52–54% at 3 years). Furthermore, CHOP had the lowest number of deaths due to toxicity. With 6 years of follow-up, the PFS and OS curves continue to overlap for all treatment groups.[29] CHOP remained the gold standard during most of the nineties. A recent meta-analysis of nearly 2000 patients enrolled on randomized controlled trials of CHOP versus second-generation regimens confirms these findings as well.[30] The authors report that newer regimens did not confer a statistically significant survival advantage at 5 years as compared to CHOP.

But several recently published randomized studies show that some dose-intensive regimens are indeed superior to CHOP and constitute one of the several exciting developments in the treatment of lymphoma. Promising strategies include the addition of targeted therapies to CHOP, the addition of other chemotherapeutic agents to CHOP, shortening the cycle length to increase dose intensity, and the use of infusional chemotherapy that allow dose escalation. The use of hematopoietic growth factors such as filgrastim and peg-filgrastim has substantially facilitated dose intensification in the modern era. Also, the IPI or similar prognostic models are routinely used in patient selection for recent trials. It is typically patients with high IPIs that are assigned to more dose-intense strategies, and such patients may be destined to benefit more.

### RITUXIMAB IN DLBCL

Perhaps the most radical change in the treatment of aggressive lymphomas has been the addition of the monoclonal antibody, rituximab. Rituximab is a murine/human chimeric monoclonal antibody against the CD20 antigen present on both normal mature and malignant B cells. The function of CD20 is unknown, but the binding of rituximab to its target leads to cell death via antibody dependent cell-mediated cytotoxicity, complement dependent cytotoxicity, and apoptosis. Rituximab has an excellent safety profile, with the most common adverse events (flushing, rash, pruritus, hypotension) being limited to the duration of infusion. Rarely, anaphylaxis has been described. Several phase II studies showed that rituxan had modest single agent activity in large cell lymphoma.[31,32] On the basis of in vitro data suggesting that rituximab sensitizes cells to chemotherapy, several groups have pursued front-line therapy in combination with CHOP and reported promising response and survival rates.[33,34] A pivotal phase III study performed by a French–Belgian cooperative group, the GELA, confirmed these promising findings.[35] This multicenter, randomized controlled trial compared CHOP versus CHOP-R in 399 patients older than 60 years with DLBCL. The median age was 69 years and nearly 90% of patients had diffuse large B cell as the presenting histology. The original report, with 2-year follow-up, showed CHOP-R to be superior in terms of complete remission rate (76% vs 63%, $p = 0.005$), 2-year EFS (57% vs 38%, $p < 0.001$), and 2-year OS (70% vs 57, $p = 0.007$). Longer follow-up of 3 years continues to demonstrate an advantage for patients receiving rituximab: EFS 53% versus 35%, $p = 0.00008$ and OS 62% versus 51%, $p = 0.008$.[36] The GELA study was the first randomized study of large cell lymphoma in more than 10 years to show an advantage for the investigational arm. This, as well as the extremely favorable safety profile for rituximab, resulted in a great degree of enthusiasm and widespread adoption of the CHOP-R regimen as the new standard.

More recent studies have confirmed these promising results in other subgroups of patients, such as those with early-stage disease and those younger than 60 years. In addition, considerable attention was devoted to an analysis of rituximab's contribution to clinical outcome by the British Colombia Cancer Agency.[37] Due to governmental regulation, rituximab was not approved for use in front-line aggressive lymphomas in British Columbia, until March 2001. Sehn and colleagues thus compared the 18-month survival of 142 patients treated prior to this date to 152 patients treated after this date. Only 9% of the patients treated for DLBCL prior to March 2001 had received rituximab with CHOP, and only 15% of the patients treated for DLBCL after March 2001 had not received rituximab. The results show an impressive improvement in PFS in the rituximab era in both elderly and young patients.

More recently, the enthusiasm over CHOP-R has been tempered somewhat by the results of a multicenter phase III randomized controlled trial in the United States. In this intergroup study, over 600 older patients with DLBCL were randomized to CHOP with or without rituximab.[38] The rituximab was scheduled to be given on five occasions during six cycles of CHOP therapy; in addition, a second randomization with maintenance rituximab ($375 \text{ mg/m}^2$ weekly times four doses, repeated every 6 months times four) was incorporated. With a median follow-up of almost 3 years, there was no significant difference in overall response rate or OS. However, patients receiving rituximab, either as part of CHOP or as part of maintenance, enjoyed a prolonged time to treatment failure. Rituximab maintenance did not further improve time to treatment failure (TTF) in patients who had already received rituximab with their CHOP chemotherapy. There is considerable debate over how to interpret these results. Some claim that the study was flawed because of an insufficient intensity of rituximab administration. Others argue that the benefits of rituximab may not be as great as originally thought.

Finally, there may be subsets of patients who benefit to a greater magnitude with rituximab. In a follow-up analysis of the GELA data, Mounier and colleagues report that CHOP-R confers an improved OS in patients with bcl-2 overexpression (67% vs 48%, $p = 0.004$) but not in patients lacking bcl-2 overexpression (72% vs 67%, $p = $ NS).[39] They also show that the benefit of rituximab is greater in patients with a low IPI score than in patients with higher-risk disease. Finally, some data suggest that genetic polymorphisms in the Fcγ IIIA receptor of lymphocytes predicts for inherent sensitivity versus resistance to rituximab.[40,41]

Thus, the optimal incorporation of rituximab into existing therapies continues to be refined. All in all, it appears that the addition of rituximab improves the outcome of patients with large cell lymphoma with minimal toxicity. Despite remaining questions about the magnitude of its effect in specific subgroups of patients, it is likely to be widely used.

## DOSE INTENSIFICATION

The GELA recently published results of a multicenter prospective phase III study comparing CHOP to a second-generation regimen that was initiated in 1993.[42] Over 600 older patients were randomized to either ACVBP (intensified doxorubicin, intensified cyclophosphamide, vindesine, bleomycin, prednisone, intrathecal methotrexate) or standard CHOP treatment. All patients received growth factor prophylaxis. The complete remission rates did not differ between the two groups, and ACVBP was associated with a significant increase in hematologic and nonhematologic toxicity and treatment-related deaths. But with a median follow-up of 68 months, the ACVBP patients had a longer EFS (39% vs 29%, $p = 0.005$), longer disease-free survival (62% vs 44%, $p = 0.0002$), and an improvement in OS (46% vs 38%, $p = 0.036$) at 5 years. This study was conducted at the same time as the influential, but negative, SWOG randomized study comparing CHOP to second-generation regimens. Explanations for these discrepant results include the possibility that the ACVBP regimen is superior to the investigational regimens tested in the SWOG study, or that patient selection was more geared to patients with advanced disease in the GELA study.

## VARIATIONS IN CYCLE LENGTH WITH DOSE INTENSIFICATION OF CHOP

The original cycle length of 21 days for CHOP was based on the average time needed for hematopoietic recovery. However, the introduction of effective hematopoietic stem cell growth factors such as filgrastim, sargramostin, and peg-filgrastim allow a shortening of cycle length with the goal of increased drug intensity. A phase II SWOG study demonstrated that the drugs in CHOP could be both intensified (CHOP-DI) and the cycle duration could be shortened safely in a group of over 100 patients with aggressive and high-grade lymphomas.[43] CHOP-DI led to an improved OS at 5 years as compared to a historical control group; however, the main endpoint of the study was PFS, and no difference between the CHOP-DI patients and historical control patients could be demonstrated.

Two large German multicenter phase III randomized studies (NHL-B1 and NHL-B2) also address the issue of cycle shortening with or without the addition of etoposide to CHOP. The design for each study was a four-armed randomized (2 × 2 factorial) controlled trial in both younger (18–60 years) and older (61–75 years) patients.[44,45] The following regimens were delivered for a total of six cycles: CHOP-21 (the standard arm), CHOP-14, CHOEP-21 (CHOP with addition of etoposide 100 mg/m[2] on days 1 through 3), and CHOEP-14. All patients on the shortened cycle arms received growth factor support whereas for the 3-weekly regimens the growth factor support was at the physician's discretion. The NHL-B2 trial for older patients included both favorable prognosis patients (defined by normal LDH at diagnosis) and unfavorable prognosis patients (defined by an increased LDH at diagnosis). By contrast, the NHL-B1 study for younger patients included only favorable prognosis patients. Young patients with elevated LDH were enrolled on a competing trial. The NHL-B2 trial for older patients randomized 689 patients and, with a median follow-up of 58 months, shows that CHOP-14 significantly improved the EFS and OS compared with CHOP-21. The addition of etoposide did not improve these endpoints, and, when given in an every 14-day schedule, substantially increased the hematologic and nonhematologic toxicity. In the NHL-B1 study for young patients, shortening the cycle leneth did improve the OS at 5 years. The addition of etoposide substantially improved the complete response rate and the EFS; in contrast to the trial in older patients, CHOEP-21 and CHOEP-14 were successfully delivered without excessive toxicity. The authors suggest that CHOEP should be the preferred regimen for this population. However, these trials were designed before the routine addition of rituximab, and it remains to be seen if rituximab is able to overcome the need to intensify CHOP, either with or without etoposide.[46]

## INFUSIONAL REGIMENS

Another means of intensifying CHOP is the use of infusional administration. Infusional regimens are based on the premise that prolonged exposure of antineoplastic agents breeds less drug resistance as compared to brief, but higher, doses of chemotherapy. The infusional regimen EPOCH (etoposide, prednisone, vincristine, cyclophosphamide, adriamycin) is highly active in aggressive lymphomas. It was first tested in a group of relapsed and refractory patients, all of whom had failed front-line CHOP-like regimens.[47] Despite the fact that all patients had previously received these same agents, the overall response rate exceeded 70% in patients with aggressive lymphomas. Furthermore, the authors discovered significant variability in serum drug concentrations between patients. This formed the basis for their subsequent investigation of dose-adjusted EPOCH (DA-EPOCH) in which chemotherapy drug doses are escalated or de-escalated each cycle based on the neutropenic nadir and neutropenic duration during the previous cycle; this type of patient-specific therapy could theoretically allow maximal use of each agent. In a group of 49 evaluable patients with previously untreated DLBCL, 92% achieved a complete response, and there was a PFS of 70% and OS of 73% at 5 years.[48] Most recently, the addition of rituximab to DA-EPOCH was tested in a cooperative group setting. DA-EPOCH-R will be the investigational arm in a large, randomized, prospective Cancer and Leukemia Group B study for advanced lymphoma.

### AUTOLOGOUS TRANSPLANTATION AS CONSOLIDATION TREATMENT IN NEWLY DIAGNOSED PATIENTS IN FIRST REMISSION

Transplantation in DLBCL is usually reserved for relapsed patients, but many have investigated its role in consolidation of response to first-line regimens. The results appear to be highly dependent on patient selection and timing of transplantation. Two prospective randomized trials evaluated autologous transplantation in patients with a slow response (i.e., less than a complete remission) to standard front-line regimens.[49,50] A randomized Dutch study assessed 106 patients with previously untreated intermediate grade lymphoma receiving CHOP chemotherapy.[49] After three cycles, 69 patients had achieved a PR and were randomized to receive either three more cycles of CHOP or to proceed to an autologous stem cell transplantation. The authors found no advantage of high-dose chemotherapy with autologous transplantation over CHOP in terms of overall response rate, EFS, disease-free survival, or OS. The Italian study compared either DHAP (dexamethasone, cytarabine, cisplatin) versus high-dose chemotherapy with BEAC (carmustine, etoposide, cytarabine, cyclophosphamide) and autologous stem cell transplant in partial remitters following two-thirds of an anthracycline-containing regimen.[50] However, only 49 patients were randomized, which was insufficient to detect a statistically meaningful difference between the two arms. A third prospective randomized study, performed by the German High-Grade non-Hodgkin's Lymphoma Study Group, evaluated the role of high-dose chemotherapy in patients achieving at least a minor response following two cycles of CHOEP (CHOP plus etoposide) as compared to three more cycles of CHOEP followed by involved field radiation.[51] It also failed to identify an advantage of transplantation following abbreviated induction. Furthermore, even patients with high-intermediate and high-risk lymphoma did not appear to benefit from early transplant in this trial.

In contrast, the French–Belgian LNH87-2 trial retrospectively applied the IPI and identified 236 high-intermediate and high-risk patients who were randomized to either more chemotherapy or autologous transplantation after achieving complete remission.[52] Both DFS and OS favored the autologous arm (55% vs 39%, $p = 0.02$; and 64% vs 49%, $p = 0.04$, respectively) in these higher risk subgroups. A study from Milan also evaluated the benefit of autologous transplantation as part of initial treatment for patients with adverse prognostic features (stage III/IV disease and large tumor bulk) in a prospective randomized trial.[53] This study was restricted to patients with classic DLBCL (no discordant lymphomas) and those without bone marrow involvement. With a median follow-up of 55 months, they found significantly improved CR rates, FFP, RFS and EFS, and borderline improved OS for those undergoing autologous transplantation compared to the control group who received MACOP-B. The most recent study in favor of consolidative autologous transplant in first remission was published by the GOELAMS in 2004.[54] Nearly 200 consecutive eligible patients were randomized to receive either standard CHOP for 8 cycles, or CEEP (cyclophosphamide, epirubicin, vindesine, prednisone) for 2 cycles followed by high dose methotrexate/cytarabine, and BEAM (BCNU, etoposide, cytarabine, melphalan) with autologous stem cell transplant. Patients randomized to the transplant arm enjoyed a prolonged PFS, but there was no statistical advantage in terms of complete remission rate or OS except for the high intermediate IPI risk group in which the transplant arm enjoyed a superior OS (74% vs 44%, $p = 0.001$). The authors conclude that high intermediate IPI risk group patients should receive an autologous transplant as part of front-line therapy.

In summary, the role of autologous transplantation as part of initial management in aggressive lymphomas remains unclear. A meta-analysis of 11 randomized trials concludes that there may be a benefit to transplant for patients with high-risk disease, who are younger and who are transplanted in complete remission.[55] It should be emphasized that none of the above studies included rituximab and that this may influence the outcome. Certain subgroups, such as those with intermediate and high-intermediate IPI scores, may derive benefit when transplanted in first complete remission, whereas a recent randomized multi-institutional investigation by the EORTC has convincingly shown that high-dose chemotherapy and autologous transplantation in first remission does not confer benefit for patients with low or low-intermediate IPI scores.[56] Autologous transplantation after shortened induction regimens and for patients in partial remission seems not to be of benefit. Dose intensification continues to be investigated in an ongoing intergroup randomized study in the United States.[57]

### CNS PROPHYLAXIS

It is not clear which, if any, subgroup of patients should receive CNS prophylaxis and exactly what that prophylaxis should consist of. Although the IPI correlates with a higher incidence of CNS recurrence, even patients with low-intermediate risk disease may have CNS relapse.[58] A French group has shown that CNS prophylaxis with systemic and intrathecal methotrexate may decrease the incidence of CNS relapse compared with reported incidence in the literature,[13] but most investigators agree that prospectively designed studies delineating the optimal prophylactic and treatment strategy are still needed.

## OUR CURRENT APPROACH TO TREATMENT OF DLBCL

Patients with early stage (I–II) disease are treated with CHOP-R for three to six cycles, depending on the stage-adjusted IPI. Those with 0–1 risk factors are given three cycles of CHOP-R followed by radiation. This is generally a very well-tolerated approach. For those with a stage-adjusted IPI >1, we prefer to administer six cycles of chemotherapy with CHOP-R. Radiation therapy is not routinely administered for such patients, but is considered for those with residual masses, especially if those masses are PET positive.

Patients with advanced disease are staged with CT scans and a bilateral bone marrow biopsy. We include a PET scan in our initial staging work-up and will routinely restage patients after four cycles of treatment. Modifications in treatment strategy will be considered for those with residual PET positivity after four cycles. A lumbar puncture is a part of the staging work-up for those with IPI greater than 2, those with testicular lymphoma, those with lymphoma in the head and neck area, and those with large cell lymphoma in the bone marrow. We currently do not have guidelines for prophylactic intrathecal treatment. Our patients with advanced stage lymphoma are treated with CHOP-R for six cycles at 21-day intervals. We will consider CHOP-R-14 with G-CSF support for patients with an increased LDH. We do not usually recommend autologous transplant in first remission, unless there is major concern for residual disease after completion of treatment, usually based on the presence of residual PET positivity. Our recommendations are admittedly somewhat guided by empiricism. Continued accrual to prospective studies is indicated, especially for patients with unfavorable prognostic features.

## PRIMARY MEDIASTINAL B-CELL LYMPHOMA

Primary mediastinal B-cell lymphoma (PMBL) is a distinct subtype of diffuse large cell lymphoma originating from thymic B cells. It was first described nearly 25 years ago[59,60] and is now recognized as a unique entity based on clinical, immunophenotypic, and genotypic features. PMBL accounts for approximately 5% of all aggressive lymphomas and affects mainly young adults. The median age at presentation is in the third decade, with a slight female predilection. Most patients present with significant symptoms, including shortness of breath, superior vena cava syndrome, phrenic nerve palsy, cough, or chest pain, all due to local aggressiveness and invasion of other mediastinal and thoracic structures. Up to 80% of patients have disease limited to the thorax at presentation[61]; the bone marrow is only rarely involved. Despite their young age and apparently localized initial presentation, only a third of patients are alive at 5 years, and recurrences typically involve distant extranodal sites such as the kidney or CNS.

Histologic examination reveals a massive diffuse proliferation along with significant fibrosis. Similar to other DLBCLs, PMBL expresses CD19, CD20, and CD45 with variable expression of surface immunoglobulin and HLA molecules. Cytogenetic analysis shows several recurring abnormalities: gains of chromosome 9p in 50% of cases,[62] trisomy 12q31 in 31% of cases, and trisomy 2p in occasional cases.[63] Molecular features include amplification of the *rel* gene and overexpression of the *mal* gene, with absence of bcl-2, bcl-6, and myc expression. Recently, the gene expression pattern via microarray analysis of PMBL was shown to more closely resemble Hodgkin's lymphomas rather than NHLs.[64] The clinical implications of this finding are yet to be defined, and PMBL continues to be treated similar to other DLBCLs.

In addition to unique epidemiologic and pathologic features, PMBL presents its own treatment challenges. Despite the initial supradiaphragmatic localization, there is difficulty in assigning patients a stage. Some consider PMBL to be stage II, whereas others feel that IVE is more appropriate due to invasion of mediastinal or intrathoracic structures.[61] This could lead to heterogeneity when comparing patient populations between trials and published reports. Regardless of the staging, a full course of anthracycline-based treatment is initially offered, similar to advanced stage, aggressive lymphomas. However, up to a third of patients have primary refractory disease, and consolidative measures should therefore be considered. Mediastinal irradiation to the primary mass is commonly used. A report from the MD Anderson Cancer Center suggests that RT prevents local relapse,[65] a finding supported by several European studies.[66,67] In a multicenter Italian study, patients remaining gallium avid after MACOP-B converted to gallium negative after consolidative RT and few patients relapsed. However, other authors have shown that RT adds little to disease control. Lazzarino and colleagues retrospectively reported on 99 evaluable patients and found that the relapse rate did not significantly differ between patients receiving RT and those who did not.[61] Furthermore, 11 of 12 relapses in the RT group were intrathoracic. A French group reported that patients achieving only a PR to front-line chemotherapy did not further respond to RT.[68] High-dose chemotherapy followed by autologous stem cell rescue in first remission has also been proposed, with very promising phase II data.[63]

At relapse, patients with PMBL are considered for autologous stem cell transplantation. In general, this population may do better as compared to the general group of aggressive lymphoma patients, partly due to their younger age and partly due to less common bone marrow involvement. Popat and colleagues[69] report a series of patients with recurrent or refractory DLBCL treated with high-dose chemotherapy and found that having PMBL was a favorable prognostic feature. Sehn and colleagues[70] also performed a retrospective analysis of 35 patients with PMBL treated with high-dose cyclophosphamide, carmustine, and etoposide (CBV) plus autologous bone marrow transplant (ABMT). Patients with primary refractory disease had 58% long-term disease-free survival and patients with relapsed disease had 27% long-term disease-free survival. The strongest predictor of PFS was chemotherapy responsiveness immediately before transplant. But even in chemo-therapy-refractory patients, 33% long-term survival was observed.

## TREATMENT OF RELAPSED AND REFRACTORY DLBCL

More than half of all DLBCL patients initially entering remission with combination chemotherapy will relapse. The standard treatment approach for such patients is to deliver salvage chemotherapy followed by consolidative autologous stem cell transplantation in patients demonstrating chemosensitivity.[71a] Patients with chemorefractory disease and patients relapsing following an autologous stem cell transplant have an overall poor prognosis and should be considered for allogeneic stem cell transplantation or for clinical trials with investigational agents. The role of autologous and allogeneic transplant in the management of relapsed and refractory aggressive lymphomas is discussed elsewhere in chapters 64 and 65.

The optimal salvage regimen is not known, and there are no phase III, prospective, randomized trials comparing various combinations. Most of the data is from phase II trials, and the choice of treatment is often influenced by both patient features and physician preferences. Some commonly used regimens include DHAP,[71a] ESHAP[71b] (etoposide, methylprednisolone, cytarabine, cisplatin), ICE[72] (ifosfamide, carboplatin, etoposide), IE[73] (ifosfamide, etoposide), MINE[73,74] (mesna, ifosfamide, mitoxantrone, etoposide) and EPOCH[48,75] (etoposide, prednisone, vincristine, cyclophosphamide, doxorubicin), among others. The DHAP regimen is one of the first salvage regimens to be designed. In the Parma trial, patients with relapsed lymphomas receiving DHAP had an overall response rate of 58%, but the 5-year EFS and OS of patients not subsequently transplanted were only 12% and 32%, respectively.[71a]

Ifosfamide-based regimens are gaining in popularity, partly due to the ability to dose-escalate the ifos-famide, and also because they are excellent stem cell mobilizing regimens.[72,73] Overall response rates are over 60%, although the complete response rate is only 24%.[73] The major advantage to improving salvage regimens is to demonstrate chemosensitivity, since this is arguably the most crucial characteristic-determining outcome following autologous stem cell transplantation in aggressive lymphomas. Of the ifosfamide-based salvage regimens for aggressive lymphomas, extensive data have been published on the ICE (ifosfamide, carboplatin, etoposide) regimen developed at the Memorial Sloan Kettering Cancer Center (MSKCC).[73–78] In an initial publication, investigators at MSKCC treated 163 consecutive transplant-eligible patients with relapsed or refractory aggressive NHL with 3 cycles of the ICE regimen. The overall response rate was 66%, allowing 89% of patients to proceed to a planned autologous stem cell transplant. There was minimal nonhematologic toxicity, although a third of patients had greater than grade 3 thrombocytopenia. All patients received growth factor support during each cycle of treatment. There are several other high-dose ifosfamide-based regimens that are in widespread use,[72,73] and all appear to be effective at stem cell mobilization. However, despite high activity, none of these regimens are curative unless followed by a consolidative transplant procedure.

The addition of rituximab to salvage regimens appears to substantially improve the response rate. For example, Kewalramani and colleagues show that the overall response rate and complete response rate increases to 81% and 55%, respectively, when adding rituximab to the ICE regimen.[79] Although not specifically demonstrated for large cell lymphoma, rituximab also serves as an "in vivo purge" during stem cell collection[80,81] and is likely to be an important component of most pretransplant salvage regimens for CD20-positive malignancies.

There are a multitude of promising investigational agents being pursued for the treatment of lymphomas. These include proteosome inhibitors (bortezomib or Velcade), anti-Bcl-2 agents (oblimersen sodium or Genasense), antiangiogenic agents, liposomal formulations of standard chemotherapeutic agents (liposomal vincristine, liposomal doxorubicin), newer monoclonal antibodies (epratuzamab), and radiolabeled monoclonal antibodies (ibritumomab tiuxetan or Zevalin, tositumomab or Bexxar). Phase II and III studies are ongoing, and several of the most active agents in preliminary studies are being incorporated into front-line regimens.

## SUMMARY

Significant advances in our understanding of DLBCL have been made in the past decade. Assessment of prognosis by use of the IPI is now in widespread use and facilitates treatment decisions. More recently, microarray technology has refined our ability to formulate prognosis, has generated interesting hypotheses regarding the biology of the disease, and will hopefully allow the design of better treatment strategies for the various subgroups in the near future. DLBCL is a largely chemosensitive disease, and CHOP chemotherapy has long represented an acceptable standard. But relapses are still common and salvage regimens and transplantation are important components of treatment for relapsed disease. The impact of the monoclonal antibody, rituximab, in both front-line and relapsed regimens is encouraging, and may change the long-term outcome of this disease. Recent data also has revived interest in dose intensity as a further way of improving treatment for large cell lymphoma. Ongoing research and development of new agents is critical, and the next decade promises to provide even more effective options for our patients.

## REFERENCES

1. Jemal A, Murray T, Samuels A, et al.: Cancer statistics, 2003. *CA Cancer J Clin* 53:5–26, 2003.
2. Chiu BC, Weisenburger DD: An update of the epidemiology of non-Hodgkin's lymphoma. *Clin Lymphoma* 4: 161–168, 2003.
3. Groves FD, Linet MS, Travis LB, et al.: Cancer surveillance series: non-Hodgkin's lymphoma incidence by histologic subtype in the United States from 1978 through 1995. *J Natl Cancer Inst* 92:1240–1251, 2000.
4. Diebold J, Anderson JR, Armitage JO, et al.: Diffuse large B-cell lymphoma: a clinicopathologic analysis of 444 cases classified according to the updated Kiel classification. *Leuk Lymphoma* 43:97–104, 2002.
5. Raetz E, Perkins S, Davenport V, et al.: B large-cell lymphoma in children and adolescents. *Cancer Treat Rev* 29:91–98, 2003.
6. Jaffe ES, Harris NL, Stein H, et al.: World Health Organization Classification of Tumours. In: *Tumours of Haematopoietic and Lymphoid Tissues.* Lyon, France: IARC Press; 2001.
7. de Leval L, Harris NL: Variability in immunophenotype in diffuse large B-cell lymphoma and its clinical relevance. *Histopathology* 43:509–528, 2003.
8. Cheson BD, Horning SJ, Coiffier B, et al.: Report of an international workshop to standardize response criteria for non-Hodgkin's lymphomas. NCI Sponsored International Working Group. *J Clin Oncol* 17:1244, 1999.
9. de Wit M, Bohuslavizki KH, Buchert R, et al.: 18FDG-PET following treatment as valid predictor for disease-free survival in Hodgkin's lymphoma. *Ann Oncol* 12:29–37, 2001.
10. Mikhaeel NG, Timothy AR, Hain SF, et al.: 18-FDG-PET for the assessment of residual masses on CT following treatment of lymphomas. *Ann Oncol* 11(suppl 1): 147–150, 2000.
11. Jerusalem G, Beguin Y, Fassotte MF, et al.: Whole-body positron emission tomography using 18F-fluorodeoxyglucose for posttreatment evaluation in Hodgkin's disease and non-Hodgkin's lymphoma has higher diagnostic and prognostic value than classical computed tomography scan imaging. *Blood* 94:429–433, 1999.
12. Jerusalem G, Beguin Y, Fassotte MF, et al.: Persistent tumor 18F-FDG uptake after a few cycles of poly-chemotherapy is predictive of treatment failure in non-Hodgkin's lymphoma. *Haematologica* 85:613–618, 2000.
13. Haioun C, Besson C, Lepage E, et al.: Incidence and risk factors of central nervous system relapse in histologically aggressive non-Hodgkin's lymphoma uniformly treated and receiving intrathecal central nervous system prophylaxis: a GELA study on 974 patients. Groupe d'Etudes des Lymphomes de l'Adulte. *Ann Oncol* 11: 685–690, 2000.
14. van Besien K, Ha CS, Murphy S, et al.: Risk factors, treatment, and outcome of central nervous system recurrence in adults with intermediate-grade and immunoblastic lymphoma. *Blood* 91:1178–1184, 1998.
15. A predictive model for aggressive non-Hodgkin's lymphoma: The International Non-Hodgkin's Lymphoma Prognostic Factors Project. *N Engl J Med* 329:987–994, 1993.
16. Alizadeh AA, Eisen MB, Davis RE, et al.: Distinct types of diffuse large B-cell lymphoma identified by gene expression profiling. *Nature* 403:503–511, 2000.
17. Rosenwald A, Wright G, Chan WC, et al.: The use of molecular profiling to predict survival after chemotherapy for diffuse large-B-cell lymphoma. *N Engl J Med* 346:1937–1947, 2002.
18. Lossos IS, Czerwinski DK, Alizadeh AA, et al.: Prediction of survival in diffuse large-B-cell lymphoma based on the expression of six genes. *N Engl J Med* 350:1828–1837, 2004.
19. Chen MG, Prosnitz LR, Gonzalez-Serva A, et al.: Results of radiotherapy in control of stage I and II non-Hodgkin's lymphoma. *Cancer* 43:1245–1254, 1979.
20. Kaminski MS, Coleman CN, Colby TV, et al.: Factors predicting survival in adults with stage I and II large-cell lymphoma treated with primary radiation therapy. *Ann Intern Med* 104:747–756, 1986.
21. Sweet DL, Kinzie J, Gaeke ME, et al.: Survival of patients with localized diffuse histiocytic lymphoma. *Blood* 58:1218–1223, 1981.
22. Spicer J, Smith P, Maclennan K, et al.: Long-term follow-up of patients treated with radiotherapy alone for early-stage histologically aggressive non-Hodgkin's lymphoma. *Br J Cancer* 90:1151–1155, 2004.
23. Miller TP, Dahlberg S, Cassady JR, et al.: Chemotherapy alone compared with chemotherapy plus radiotherapy for localized intermediate- and high-grade non-Hodgkin's lymphoma. *N Engl J Med* 339:21–26, 1998.
24. Miller TP, LeBlanc M, Spier CM, et al.: CHOP alone compared to CHOP plus radiotherapy for early stage aggressive non-Hodgkin's lymphomas: update of the Southwest Oncology Group (SWOG) randomized trial. *Blood* 98:724a, 2001.
25. Horning SJ, Weller E, Kim K, et al.: Chemotherapy with or without radiotherapy in limited-stage diffuse aggressive non-Hodgkin's lymphoma: Eastern Cooperative Oncology Group study 1484. *J Clin Oncol* 22: 3032–3038, 2004.

26. Fillet G, Mounier N, Thieblemont C, et al.: Radiotherapy is unnecessary in elderly patients with localized aggressive non-Hodgkin's lymphoma: results of the GELA LNH 93-4 study. *Blood* :337a, 2002.

27. McKelvey EM, Gottlieb JA, Wilson HE, et al.: Hydroxyldaunomycin (Adriamycin) combination chemotherapy in malignant lymphoma. *Cancer* 38:1484–1493, 1976.

28. Fisher RI, Gaynor ER, Dahlberg S, et al.: Comparison of a standard regimen (CHOP) with three intensive chemotherapy regimens for advanced non-Hodgkin's lymphoma. *N Engl J Med* 328:1002–1006, 1993.

29. Fisher RI, Shah P: Current trends in large cell lymphoma. *Leukemia* 17:1948–1960, 2003.

30. Messori A, Vaiani M, Trippoli S, et al.: Survival in patients with intermediate or high grade non-Hodgkin's lymphoma: meta-analysis of randomized studies comparing third generation regimens with CHOP. *Br J Cancer* 84:303–307, 2001.

31. Coiffier B, Haioun C, Ketterer N, et al.: Rituximab (anti-CD20 monoclonal antibody) for the treatment of patients with relapsing or refractory aggressive lymphoma: a multicenter phase II study. *Blood* 92: 1927–1932, 1998.

32. Tobinai K, Igarashi T, Itoh K, et al.: Japanese multicenter phase II and pharmacokinetic study of rituximab in relapsed or refractory patients with aggressive B-cell lymphoma. *Ann Oncol* 15:821–830, 2004.

33. Vose JM, Link BK, Grossbard ML, et al.: Phase II study of rituximab in combination with chop chemotherapy in patients with previously untreated, aggressive non-Hodgkin's lymphoma. *J Clin Oncol* 19:389–397, 2001.

34. Vose JM, Link BK, Grossbard ML, Czuczman M, Grillo-Lopez A, Fisher RI: Long-term update of a phase II study of rituximab in combination with CHOP chemotherapy in patients with previously untreated, aggressive non-Hodgkin's lymphoma. *Leuk Lymphoma* 46:1569–1573, 2005.

35. Coiffier B, Lepage E, Briere J, et al.: CHOP chemotherapy plus rituximab compared with CHOP alone in elderly patients with diffuse large-B-cell lymphoma. *N Engl J Med* 346:235–242, 2002.

36. Coiffier B: Effective immunochemotherapy for aggressive non-Hodgkin's lymphoma. *Semin Oncol* 31:7–11, 2004.

37. Sehn LH, Donaldson J, Chhanabhai M, et al.: Introduction of combined CHOP-rituximab therapy dramatically improved outcome of diffuse large B-cell lymphoma (DLBC) in British Columbia (BC). *Blood* 102:88a, 2003.

38. Habermann TM, Weller EA, Morrison VA, et al.: Rituximab-CHOP versus CHOP alone or with maintenance rituximab in older patients with diffuse large B-cell lymphoma. *J Clin Oncol* 24:3121–3127, 2006.

39. Mounier N, Briere J, Gisselbrecht C, et al.: Rituximab plus CHOP (R-CHOP) overcomes bcl-2–associated resistance to chemotherapy in elderly patients with diffuse large B-cell lymphoma (DLBCL). *Blood* 101:4279–4284, 2003.

40. Dall'Ozzo S, Tartas S, Paintaud G, et al.: Rituximab-dependent cytotoxicity by natural killer cells: influence of FCGR3A polymorphism on the concentration-effect relationship. *Cancer Res* 64:4664–4669, 2004.

41. Cartron G, Dacheux L, Salles G, et al.: Therapeutic activity of humanized anti-CD20 monoclonal antibody and polymorphism in IgG Fc receptor FcgammaRIIIa gene. *Blood* 99:754–758, 2002.

42. Tilly H, Lepage E, Coiffier B, et al.: Intensive conventional chemotherapy (ACVBP regimen) compared with standard CHOP for poor-prognosis aggressive non-Hodgkin lymphoma. *Blood* 102:4284–4289, 2003.

43. Blayney DW, LeBlanc ML, Grogan T, et al.: Dose-intense chemotherapy every 2 weeks with dose-intense cyclophosphamide, doxorubicin, vincristine, and prednisone may improve survival in intermediate- and high-grade lymphoma: a phase II study of the Southwest Oncology Group (SWOG 9349). *J Clin Oncol* 21: 2466–2473, 2003.

44. Pfreundschuh M, Trumper L, Kloess M, et al.: Two-weekly or 3-weekly CHOP chemotherapy with or without etoposide for the treatment of elderly patients with aggressive lymphomas: results of the NHL-B2 trial of the DSHNHL. *Blood* 104:634–641, 2004.

45. Pfreundschuh M, Trumper L, Kloess M, et al.: Two-weekly or 3-weekly CHOP chemotherapy with or without etoposide for the treatment of young patients with good-prognosis (normal LDH) aggressive lymphomas: results of the NHL-B1 trial of the DSHNHL. *Blood* 104: 626–633, 2004.

46. Coiffier B, Salles G: Immunochemotherapy is the standard of care in elderly patients with diffuse large B-cell lymphoma. *Blood* 104:1584-1585. [Author reply 1585–1586.]

47. Gutierrez M, Chabner BA, Pearson D, et al.: Role of a doxorubicin-containing regimen in relapsed and resistant lymphomas: an 8-year follow-up study of EPOCH. *J Clin Oncol* 18:3633–3642, 2000.

48. Wilson WH, Grossbard ML, Pittaluga S, et al.: Dose-adjusted EPOCH chemotherapy for untreated large B-cell lymphomas: a pharmacodynamic approach with high efficacy. *Blood* 99:2685–2693, 2002.

49. Verdonck LF, van Putten WL, Hagenbeek A, et al.: Comparison of CHOP chemotherapy with autologous bone marrow transplantation for slowly responding patients with aggressive non-Hodgkin's lymphoma. *N Engl J Med* 332:1045–1051, 1995.

50. Martelli M, Vignetti M, Zinzani PL, et al.: High-dose chemotherapy followed by autologous bone marrow transplantation versus dexamethasone, cisplatin, and cytarabine in aggressive non-Hodgkin's lymphoma with partial response to front-line chemotherapy: a prospective randomized italian multicenter study. *J Clin Oncol* 14:534–542, 1996.

51. Kaiser U, Uebelacker I, Abel U, et al.: Randomized study to evaluate the use of high-dose therapy as part of primary treatment for "aggressive" lymphoma. *J Clin Oncol* 20:4413–4419, 2002.

52. Haioun C, Lepage E, Gisselbrecht C, et al.: Survival benefit of high-dose therapy in poor-risk aggressive non-Hodgkin's lymphoma: final analysis of the prospective LNH87-2 protocol—a groupe d'Etude des lymphomes de l'Adulte study. *J Clin Oncol* 18:3025–3030, 2000.

53. Gianni AM, Bregni M, Siena S, et al.: High-dose chemotherapy and autologous bone marrow transplantation compared with MACOP-B in aggressive B-cell lymphoma. *N Engl J Med* 336:1290–1297, 1997.

54. Milpied N, Deconinck E, Gaillard F, et al.: Initial treatment of aggressive lymphoma with high-dose

chemotherapy and autologous stem-cell support. *N Engl J Med* 350:1287–1295, 2004.

55. Strehl J, Mey U, Glasmacher A, et al.: High-dose chemotherapy followed by autologous stem cell transplantation as first-line therapy in aggressive non-Hodgkin's lymphoma: a meta-analysis. *Haematologica* 88:1304–1315, 2003.

56. Kluin-Nelemans HC, Zagonel V, Anastasopoulou A, et al.: Standard chemotherapy with or without high-dose chemotherapy for aggressive non-Hodgkin's lymphoma: randomized phase III EORTC study. *J Natl Cancer Inst* 93:22–30, 2001.

57. Fisher RI: Autologous bone marrow transplantation for aggressive non-Hodgkin's lymphoma: lessons learned and challenges remaining. *J Natl Cancer Inst* 93:4–5, 2001.

58. Bos GM, van Putten WL, van der Holt B, et al.: For which patients with aggressive non-Hodgkin's lymphoma is prophylaxis for central nervous system disease mandatory? Dutch HOVON Group. *Ann Oncol* 9:191–194, 1998.

59. Miller JB, Variakojis D, Bitran JD, et al.: Diffuse histiocytic lymphoma with sclerosis: a clinicopathologic entity frequently causing superior venacaval obstruction. *Cancer* 47:748–756, 1981.

60. Lichtenstein AK, Levine A, Taylor CR, et al.: Primary mediastinal lymphoma in adults. *Am J Med* 68:509–514, 1980.

61. Lazzarino M, Orlandi E, Paulli M, et al.: Treatment outcome and prognostic factors for primary mediastinal (thymic) B-cell lymphoma: a multicenter study of 106 patients. *J Clin Oncol* 15:1646–1653, 1997.

62. Joos S, Otano-Joos MI, Ziegler S, et al.: Primary mediastinal (thymic) B-cell lymphoma is characterized by gains of chromosomal material including 9p and amplification of the REL gene. *Blood* 87:1571–1578, 1996.

63. van Besien K, Kelta M, Bahaguna P: Primary mediastinal B-cell lymphoma: a review of pathology and management. *J Clin Oncol* 19:1855–1864, 2001.

64. Savage KJ, Monti S, Kutok JL, et al.: The molecular signature of mediastinal large B-cell lymphoma differs from that of other diffuse large B-cell lymphomas and shares features with classical Hodgkin lymphoma. *Blood* 102:3871–3879, 2003.

65. Nguyen LN, Ha CS, Hess M, et al.: The outcome of combined-modality treatments for stage I and II primary large B-cell lymphoma of the mediastinum. *Int J Radiat Oncol Biol Phys* 47:1281–1285, 2000.

66. Bieri S, Roggero E, Zucca E, et al.: Primary mediastinal large B-cell lymphoma (PMLCL): the need for prospective controlled clinical trials. *Leuk Lymphoma* 35:139–146, 1999.

67. Zinzani PL, Martelli M, Magagnoli M, et al.: Treatment and clinical management of primary mediastinal large B-cell lymphoma with sclerosis: MACOP-B regimen and mediastinal radiotherapy monitored by (67)Gallium scan in 50 patients. *Blood* 94:3289–3293, 1999.

68. Haioun C, Gaulard P, Roudot-Thoraval F, et al.: Mediastinal diffuse large-cell lymphoma with sclerosis: a condition with a poor prognosis. *Am J Clin Oncol* 12:425–429, 1989.

69. Popat U, Przepiork D, Champlin R, et al.: High-dose chemotherapy for relapsed and refractory diffuse large B-cell lymphoma: mediastinal localization predicts for a favorable outcome. *J Clin Oncol* 16:63–69, 1998.

70. Sehn LH, Antin JH, Shulman LN, et al.: Primary diffuse large B-cell lymphoma of the mediastinum: outcome following high-dose chemotherapy and autologous hematopoietic cell transplantation. *Blood* 91:717–723, 1998.

71a. Philip T, Guglielmi C, Hagenbeek A, et al.: Autologous bone marrow transplantation as compared with salvage chemotherapy in relapses of chemotherapy-sensitive non-Hodgkin's lymphoma. *N Engl J Med* 333:1540–1545, 1995.

71b. Velasquez WS, McLaughlin P, Tucker S, et al.: ESHAP–an effective chemotherapy regimen in refractory and relapsing lymphoma: a 4-year follow-up study. *J Clin Oncol* 12:1169–1176, 1994.

72. Moskowitz CH, Bertino JR, Glassman JR, et al.: Ifosfamide, carboplatin, and etoposide: a highly effective cytoreduction and peripheral-blood progenitor-cell mobilization regimen for transplant-eligible patients with non-Hodgkin's lymphoma. *J Clin Oncol* 17:3776–3785, 1999.

73. van Besien K, Rodriguez A, Tomany S, et al.: Phase II study of a high-dose ifosfamide-based chemotherapy regimen with growth factor rescue in recurrent aggressive NHL. High response rates and limited toxicity, but limited impact on long-term survival. *Bone Marrow Transplant* 27:397–404, 2001.

74. Celik I, Kars A, Guler N, et al.: Phase II trial of MINE as a front-line therapeutic modality in intermediate- and high-grade non-Hodgkin's lymphomas. *Eur J Cancer* 34:759–760, 1998.

75. Jermann M, Jost LM, Taverna C, et al.: Rituximab-EPOCH, an effective salvage therapy for relapsed, refractory or transformed B-cell lymphomas: results of a phase II study. *Ann Oncol* 15:511–516, 2004.

76. Zelenetz AD, Hamlin P, Kewalramani T, et al.: Ifosfamide, carboplatin, etoposide (ICE)-based second-line chemotherapy for the management of relapsed and refractory aggressive non-Hodgkin's lymphoma. *Ann Oncol* 14 (suppl 1):i5–i10, 2003.

77. Moskowitz C: Risk-adapted therapy for relapsed and refractory lymphoma using ICE chemotherapy. *Cancer Chemother Pharmacol* 49 (suppl 1):S9–S12, 2002.

78. Hamlin PA, Zelenetz AD, Kewalramani T, et al.: Age-adjusted International Prognostic Index predicts autologous stem cell transplantation outcome for patients with relapsed or primary refractory diffuse large B-cell lymphoma. *Blood 102*:1989–1996, 2003.

79. Kewalramani T, Zelenetz AD, Nimer SD, et al.: Rituximab and ICE as second-line therapy before autologous stem cell transplantation for relapsed or primary refractory diffuse large B-cell lymphoma. *Blood* 103:3684–3688, 2004.

80. Magni M, Di Nicola M, Devizzi L, et al.: Successful in vivo purging of CD34-containing peripheral blood harvests in mantle cell and indolent lymphoma: evidence for a role of both chemotherapy and rituximab infusion. *Blood* 96:864–869, 2000.

81. Flinn IW, O'Donnell PV, Goodrich A, et al.: Immunotherapy with rituximab during peripheral blood stem cell transplantation for non-Hodgkin's lymphoma. *Biol Blood Marrow Transplant* 6:628–632, 2000.

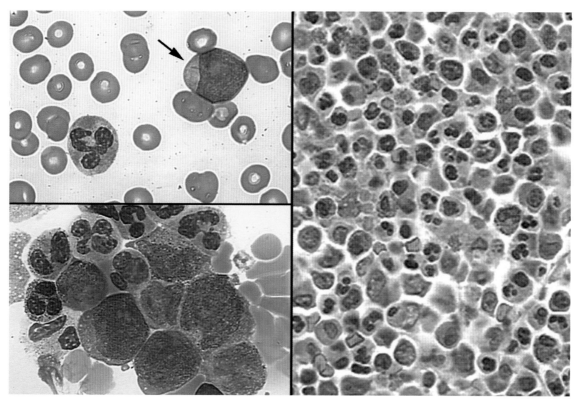

**PLATE 1** *Acute myeloid leukemia with t(8;21)(q22;q22): Peripheral blood smear shows a blast with an Auer rod (arrow) and a neutrophil with characteristic salmon-colored cytoplasmic granules (upper left); bone marrow aspirate shows blasts admixed with maturing myeloid cells (bottom left); and bone marrow biopsy is hypercellular with blasts admixed with maturing myeloid cells and eosinophils. (Wright–Giemsa stain, left panels; hematoxylin–eosin stain, right panel)*

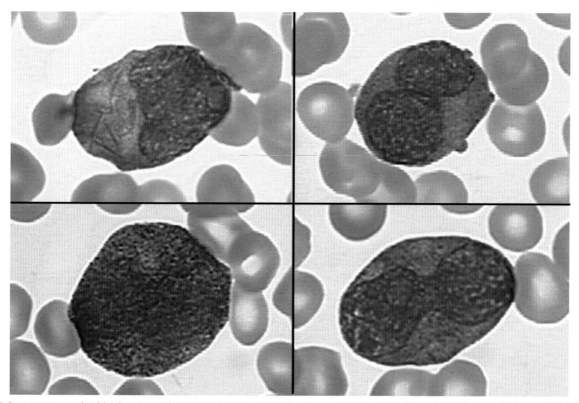

**PLATE 2** *Acute myeloid leukemia with t(15;17)(q22;q21): Features of blasts include multiple Auer rods (upper left), hyper-granular cytoplasm (lower left), and bilobed nuclei (upper and lower right panels). This leukemia is often associated with a low white blood cell count, and characteristic blasts containing multiple Auer rods may require a careful search to identify. (Wright–Giemsa stain)*

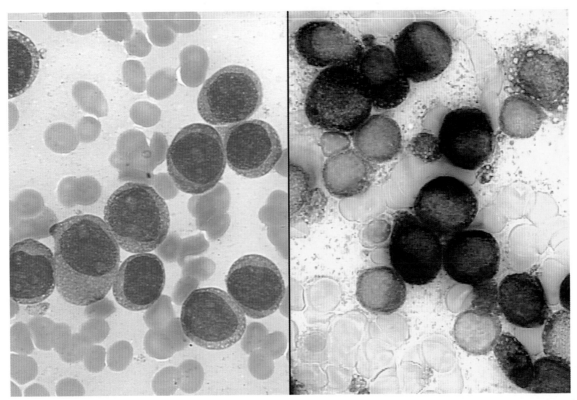

**PLATE 3** *Acute monoblastic leukemia: Blasts have moderate amounts of cytoplasm and nuclei with one to two nucleoli (left panel). Monocytic differentiation is demonstrated in the blasts by positive cytochemical stain for nonspecific esterase as shown by red-brown cytoplasmic staining (right panel). (Wright–Giemsa stain, left panel; nonspecific esterase stain [α-naphthyl butyrate], right panel)*

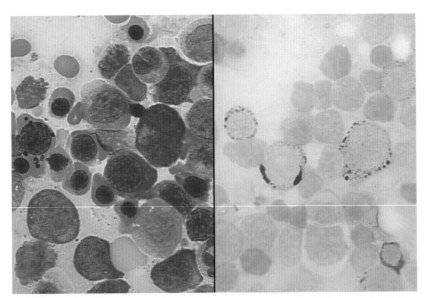

**PLATE 4** *Acute erythroleukemia: An increase in erythroid elements with dysplastic features including megaloblastoid chromatin and nuclear fragmentation is evident in this bone marrow aspirate smear (left panel). PAS stain is useful to identify abnormal "blocklike" cytoplasmic staining in immature erythroid precursors (right panel). (Wright–Giemsa stain, left panel; PAS stain, right panel)*

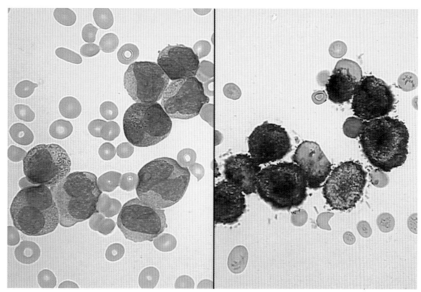

**PLATE 5** *Acute myeloid leukemia with t(15;17)(q22;q21): The hypogranular variant is often associated with an elevated white blood count with most blasts having lightly granular to almost agranular cytoplasm, but still retaining the typical bilobed nucleus (left panel). A cytochemical stain for myeloperoxidase (right panel) demonstrates intense cytoplasmic positivity as shown by blue-black granules. (Wright–Giemsa stain, left panel; myeloperoxidase stain, right panel)*

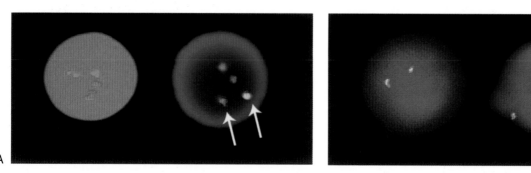

A                          B

**PLATE 6** *FISH techniques: (a) It shows a BCR/ABL dual fusion probe set applied to interphase nuclei. Nucleus at left shows two normal signals for the BCR locus at 22q11.2 (green) and two normal signals for the ABL locus at 9q34 (red). Nucleus at right shows one normal BCR locus (green), one normal ABL locus (red), and two fusion signals (arrows) with juxtaposition of red and green signals, reflecting the rearranged chromosomes 9 and 22. (b) It shows an MLL break apart probe set applied to interphase nuclei. In this probe set, the 5' region flanking MLL is labeled in green and the 3' region flanking MLL is labeled in red. Nucleus at left shows two fusion signals, reflecting the normal (unrearranged) MLL loci at 11q23. Nucleus at right shows one normal (unrearranged) MLL locus. The separation of the green (5' MLL) and red (3' MLL) signals (arrows) shows that rearrangement of this locus has occurred.*

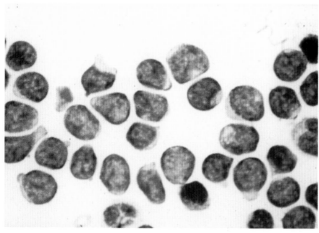

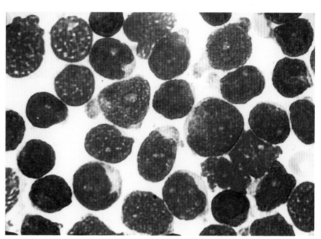

**PLATE 7** *L1—uniform small peripheral lymphoid blasts with minimal to moderate cytoplasm, effaced chromatin, and occasional to more numerous nucleoli.*

**PLATE 8** *L2—variable-sized peripheral blood lymphoblasts with variable chromatin pattern and more frequent nucleoli.*

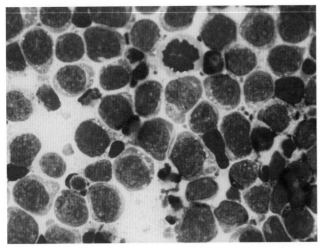

**PLATE 9** *L3—Burkitt leukemia in bone marrow with uniform blast forms, cytoplasmic vacuoles, and increased mitoses.*

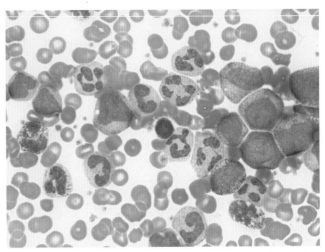

**PLATE 10** *A peripheral blood film of a patient with classical CML.*

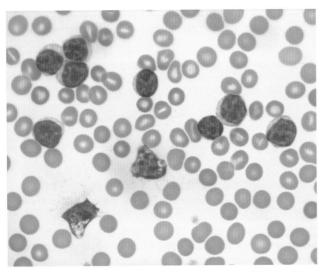

**PLATE 11** *Typical peripheral blood smear in CLL showing small cells with clumped nuclear chromatin and occasional smudge cells.*

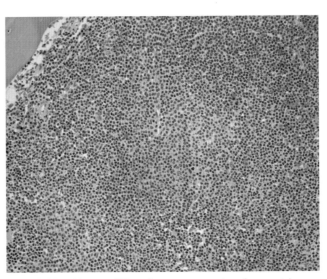

**PLATE 13** *Heavy, diffuse bone marrow involvement in CLL. A growth center can be identified in the biopsy.*

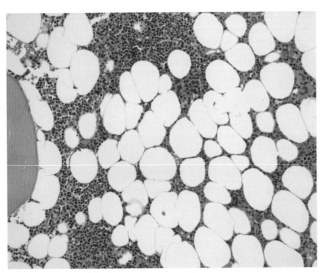

**PLATE 12** *Bone marrow showing minimal nodular pattern of involvement.*

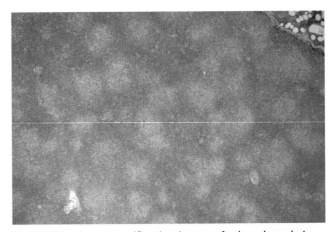

**PLATE 14** *Low magnification image of a lymph node in CLL with "pseudo-follicular" pattern.*

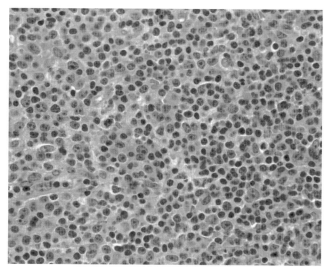

**PLATE 15** *Higher magnification of the same lymph node showing growth centers with increased prolymphocytes and paraimmunoblasts.*

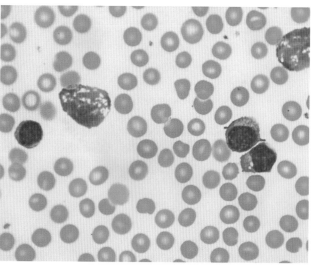

**PLATE 16** *Peripheral blood smear with "atypical" CLL. Cells have slightly less clumped chromatin and more flowing cytoplasm.*

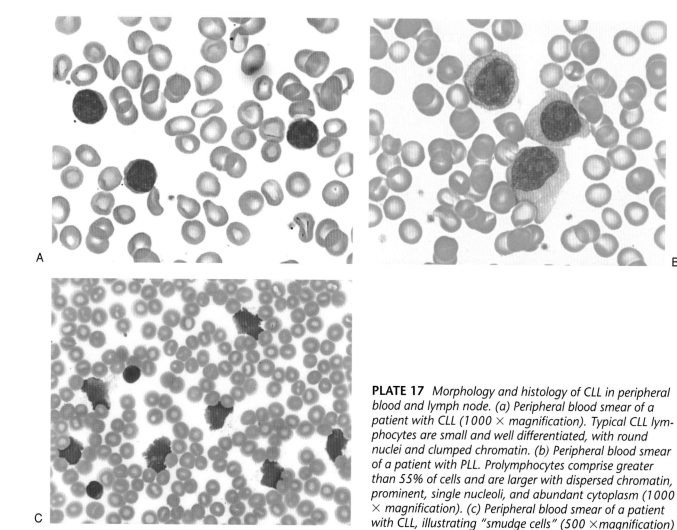

A

B

C

**PLATE 17** *Morphology and histology of CLL in peripheral blood and lymph node. (a) Peripheral blood smear of a patient with CLL (1000 × magnification). Typical CLL lymphocytes are small and well differentiated, with round nuclei and clumped chromatin. (b) Peripheral blood smear of a patient with PLL. Prolymphocytes comprise greater than 55% of cells and are larger with dispersed chromatin, prominent, single nucleoli, and abundant cytoplasm (1000 × magnification). (c) Peripheral blood smear of a patient with CLL, illustrating "smudge cells" (500 ×magnification)*

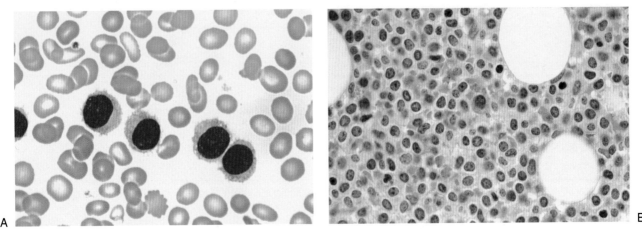

**PLATE 18** *(a) Peripheral smear of a patient with hairy-cell leukemia, demonstrating classic feature of the hairy cells, including bean-shaped nucleus, homogenous, ground-glass chromatin, and abundant pale blue cytoplasm with "hairy" projections. Presence of leukocytosis is atypical for HCL. (b) Bone marrow trephine biopsy of a patient with hairy-cell leukemia, showing diffuse infiltration of hairy cells with abundant pale cytoplasm.*

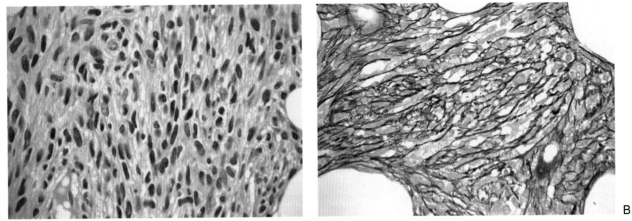

**PLATE 19** *(a) Bone marrow trephine biopsy showing hairy cells with spindle shape nuclei. (b) Bone marrow trephine biopsy stained for reticulin, demonstrating extensive fibrosis surrounding the individual hairy cells, typical for HCL.*

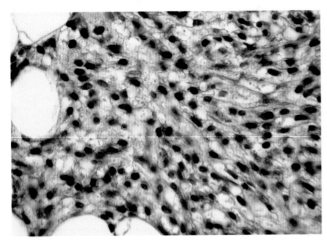

**PLATE 20** *Immunohistochemistry stain (MB2) of bone marrow trephine biopsy indicating that hairy cells are of B-cell origin.*

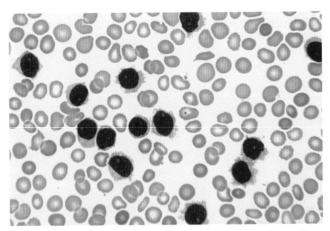

**PLATE 21** *Peripheral smear of a patient with hairy-cell variant, demonstrating abundant cytoplasm with irregular borders and visible nucleoli (in contrast to HCL).*

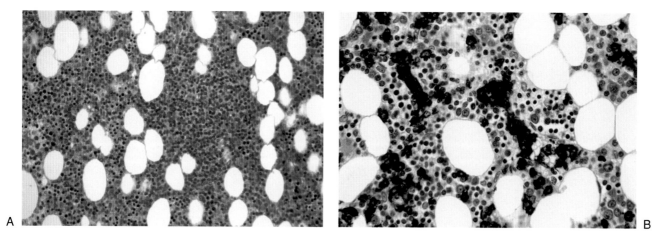

**PLATE 22** *Bone marrow trephine biopsy of a patient with splenic marginal zone lymphoma showing (a) focal lymphoid aggregates and (b) immunostaining for CD20 delineates intrasinusoidal and interstitial infiltration by lymphocytes.*

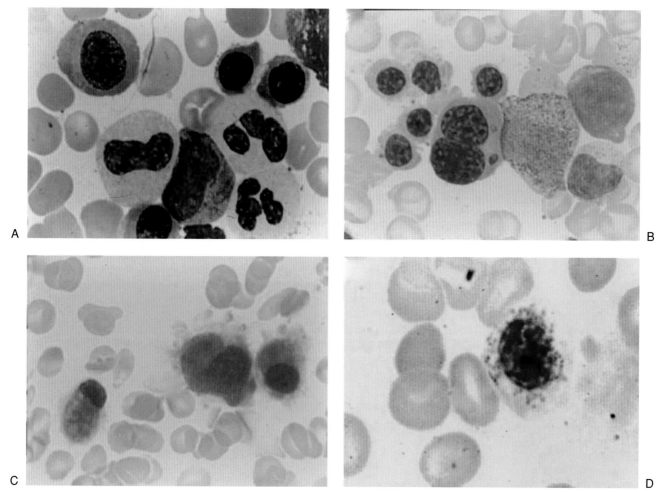

**PLATE 23** *Bone marrow: (A) megaloblastoid erythroid precursor, pseudo-Pelger-Huët neutrophils (bilobed and hypogranular), and a myeloblast with Auer rods; (B) dysplastic erythroid precursors, bi-nucleated erythroid precursor, and a myeloblast; (C) mononuclear and micromegakaryocytes; (D) Prussian blue stain of the bone marrow showing a ring sideroblast.*

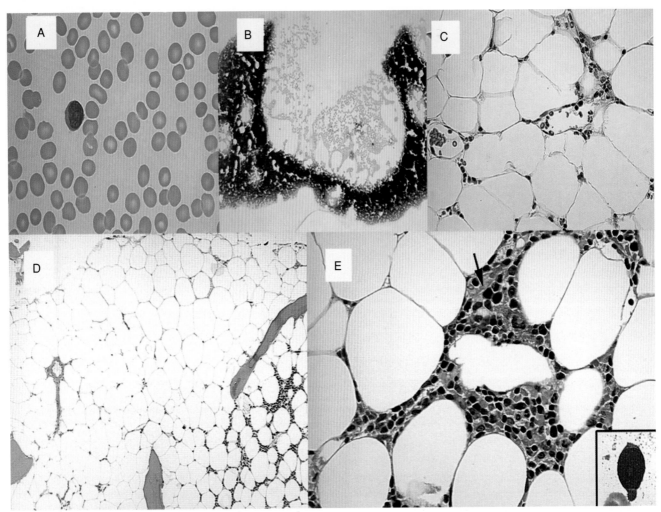

**PLATE 24** *Bone marrow finding in AA. (a) Peripheral blood smear from a patient with aplastic anemia demonstrates severe pancytopenia with normocytic to slightly macrocytic anemia, neutropenia, and thrombocytopenia (peripheral blood, Wright–Giemsa stain, original magnification ×100). (b) Bone marrow touch imprints may be helpful in excluding mimics of aplastic anemia, such as hairy cell leukemia, which can result in a dry tap. This low-power image of a touch imprint reflects the overall hypocellularity encountered in aplastic anemia (bone marrow biopsy touch imprint, Wright–Giemsa stain, original magnification ×10). (c) Bone marrow biopsy in aplastic anemia illustrates severe panhypoplasia with only rare scattered lymphocytes and plasma cells (bone marrow core biopsy, hematoxylin–eosin stain, original magnification ×40). (d) Because marrow cellularity may vary geographically within the biopsy, with the area immediately subjacent to the cortex often being hypocellular, it is essential to obtain an adequately sized core biopsy when evaluating for possible aplastic anemia (bone marrow core biopsy, hematoxylin–eosin stain, original magnification ×10). (e) Hypocellular MDS can mimic aplastic anemia. In this biopsy, mature myeloid elements are reduced, and the presence of occasional mononuclear cells consistent with blasts (arrow) can be a subtle feature. Marrow aspirate smear (inset) showed 9% myeloid blasts with dysplastic changes in erythroid precursors (bone marrow core biopsy, hematoxylin–eosin stain, original magnification ×40; inset: bone marrow aspirate, Wright–Giemsa stain, original magnification ×100)*

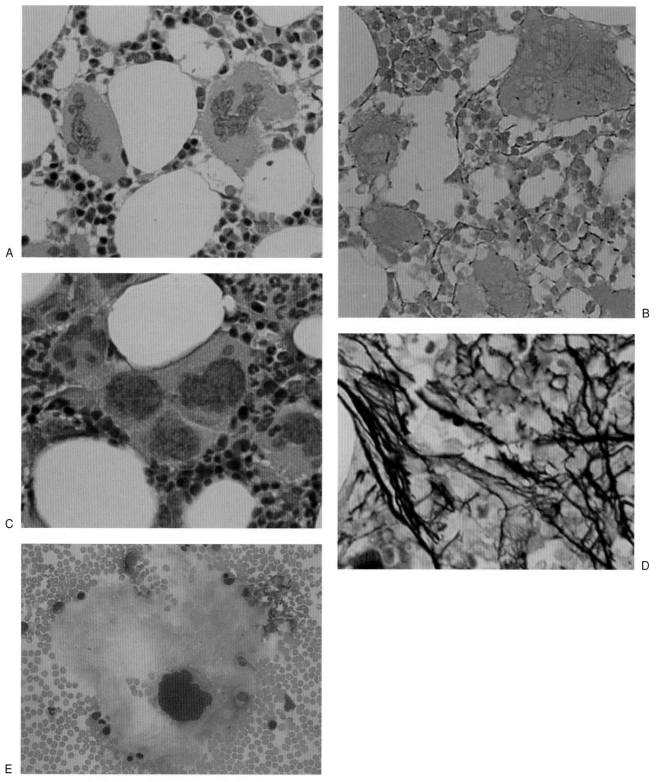

**PLATE 25** *Illustration of the histological features of ET and MF. (a) Trephine biopsy from ET patient with normal cellularity and increased numbers of large megakaryocytes, with abundant cytoplasm, and deeply lobated and hyperlobated nuclei. (b) Reticulin preparation from a case showing scanty normal distribution of reticulin fibers. (c) A patient with MF: the cellularity is increased and megakaryocytes are smaller and clustered together. Their nuclei are hyperchromatic with "cloud-like" lobulation.(d) Reticulin preparation from case c, showing dense parallel thick fibers. (e) Giant megakaryocyte in a bone marrow aspirate from an ET patient showing emperipolesis.*

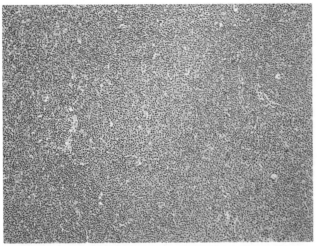

PLATE 26   SLL, low magnification shows a diffuse infiltrate of small lymphocytes with a central pale area representing a proliferation center.

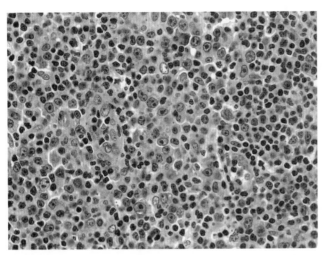

PLATE 27   SLL, high magnification shows the detail of a proliferation center. Nucleolated cells (paraimmunoblasts) are present in increased numbers.

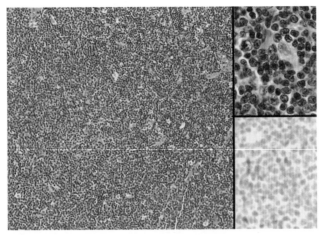

PLATE 28   MCL, low magnification shows a diffuse infiltrate of small lymphocytes. Inset (upper right) shows the high magnification appearance with an epithelioid histiocyte in the center. The lower inset show cyclin D1 expression.

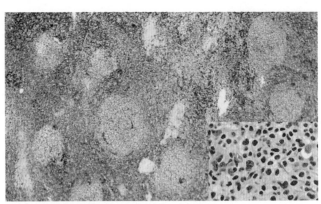

PLATE 29   Follicular lymphoma demonstrating a nodular architecture. The inset shows the cytologic features with predominantly small cleaved cells in this case.

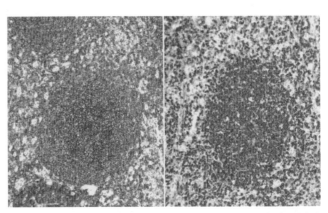

PLATE 30   Immunostains in the case shown in Figure 52.5 demonstrate expression of CD20 (left) and bcl-2 (right). The case also expressed CD10 and bcl-6 (not shown).

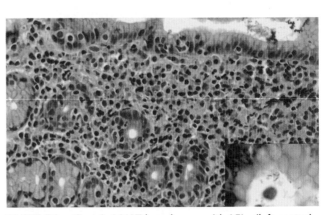

PLATE 31   Gastric MALT lymphoma with LELs (left center). The inset shows H. pylori organisms in Giemsa staining.

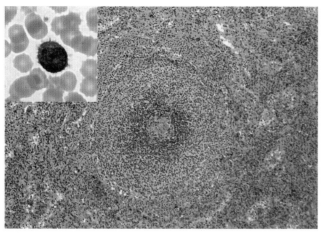

PLATE 32 *Splenic marginal zone lymphoma. Low magnification shows expansion of the white pulp with prominent marginal zones. The inset (upper left) shows a circulating lymphoma cells with villous cytoplasmic projections.*

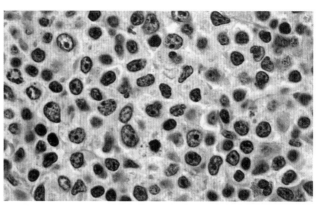

PLATE 35 *Nodal marginal zone B-cell lymphoma. At high magnification, the cytologic features of the lymphoma cells surrounding the follicle in figure 10.*

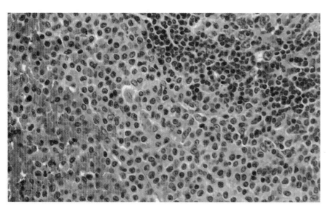

PLATE 33 *Splenic marginal zone lymphoma. High magnification shows the characteristic cytologic features of small cells with abundant pale cytoplasm. The upper right corner shows part of a germinal center surrounded by a thin rim of mantle cells.*

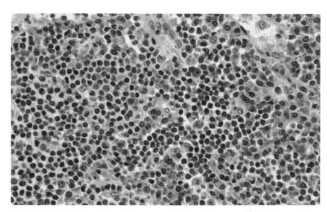

PLATE 36 *Lymphoplasmacytic lymphoma consisting of a diffuse infiltrate of small lymphocytes and plasma cells.*

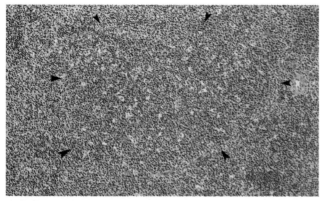

PLATE 34 *Nodal marginal zone B-cell lymphoma showing a germinal center (arrows) that is ill-defined and being infiltrated by lymphoma cells.*

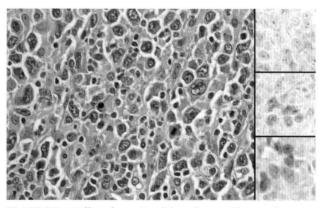

PLATE 37 *Diffuse large B-cell lymphoma. Sheets of centroblastic cells are present. Immunostains show the cells lack CD10 (top inset), but express bcl-6 (middle inset) and MUM1(bottom inset). This phenotype is consistent with a nongerminal center-type DLBCL, associated with a worse outcome compared the germinal center-type DLBCL.*

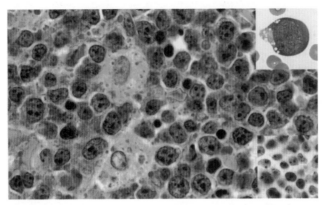

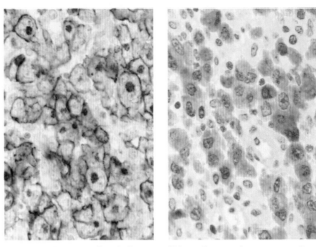

**PLATE 38** *Burkitt lymphoma. Sheets of intermediately sized cells (compared to tingible body macrophage nuclei in left center) are seen with multiple inconspicuous nucleoli. The upper right inset shows lymphoma cells with basophilic cytoplasm and distinct vacuoles. The bottom inset is a Ki-67 antigen immunostain showing an extremely high proliferative fraction.*

**PLATE 41** *Anaplastic large cell lymphoma. Immunostains of the case shown in Figure 52.16 demonstrate the large cells to be positive for CD30 (left panel) and ALK (right panel).*

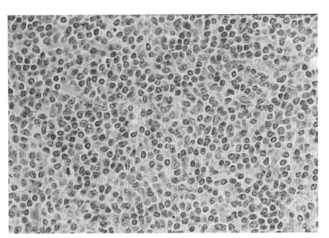

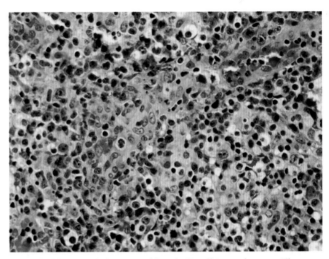

**PLATE 39** *Peripheral T-cell lymphoma, unspecified. This case displays a diffuse infiltrate of small- to intermediate-sized cells with pale cytoplasm admixed with occasional large transformed cells.*

**PLATE 42** *Angioimmunoblastic T-cell Lymphoma. The lymph node is effaced by a diffuse proliferation of intermediate to large lymphocytes with pale cytoplasm. There is an accompanying vascular proliferation.*

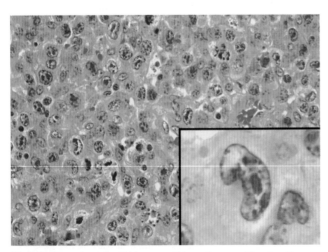

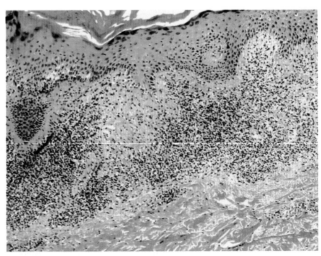

**PLATE 40** *Anaplastic large cell lymphoma. Sheets of large, pleomorphic cells are present. The inset shows a characteristic "hallmark cell" with a band-shaped nucleus and central, punctate eosinophilic cytoplasm.*

**PLATE 43** *Mycosis fungoides. At low power, a band-like lymphocytic infiltrate is seen in the upper dermis.*

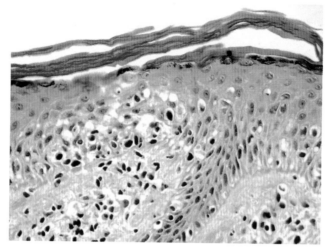

**PLATE 44** *Mycosis fungoides. At high power, collections of atypical lymphocytes are identified in the epidermis.*

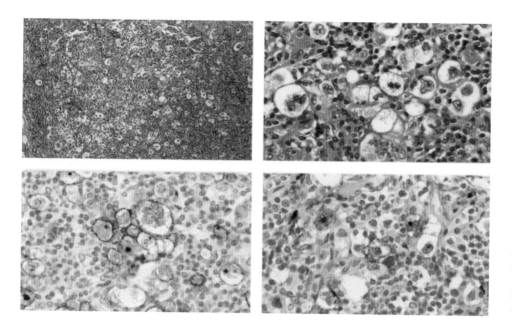

**PLATE 45** *Nodular sclerosis Hodgkin's lymphoma. The lymph node is effaced by a lymphoid proliferation that is separated into nodules by dense collagenous bands of fibrosis (upper left). The nodules contain numerous Reed-Sternberg cells and mononuclear variants (upper right). The neoplastic cells are positive for CD30 (lower left) and CD15 (lower right)*

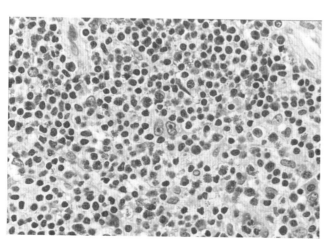

**PLATE 46** *Mixed cellularity Hodgkin's lymphoma. A binucleate Reed-Sternberg cell is seen surrounded by small lymphocytes, eosinophils, and plasma cells*

**PLATE 47** *Lymphocyte-rich classical Hodgkin's lymphoma. At low power, there is a lymphoid-rich infiltrate with a predominantly diffuse growth pattern. A residual germinal center is seen (center right)*

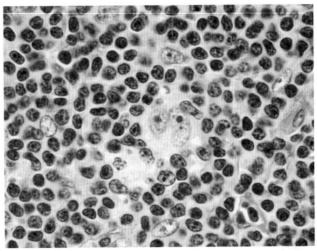

**PLATE 48** *Lymphocyte-rich classical Hodgkin's lymphoma. At high power, a binucleate Reed-Sternberg cell is present surrounded by numerous small lymphocytes*

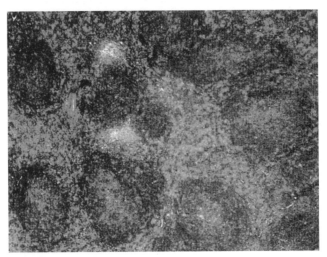

**PLATE 49** *Nodular lymphocyte predominant Hodgkin's lymphoma. A nodular proliferation of lymphocytes and histiocytes is present*

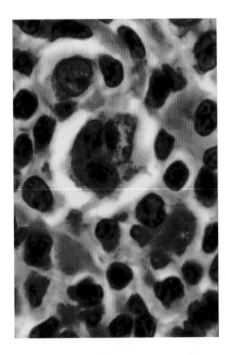
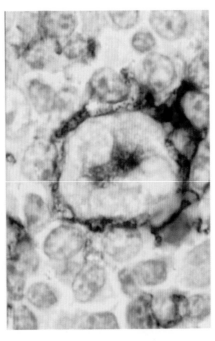

**PLATE 50** *Nodular lymphocyte predominant Hodgkin's lymphoma. The neoplastic cells in nLPHL show multiple nuclear lobes with vesicular chromatin and prominent nucleoli (left). There is strong expression of CD20 (right)*

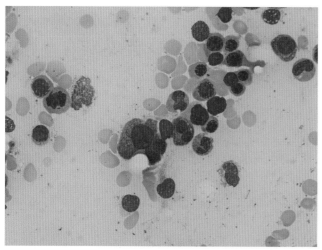

**PLATE 51** *Bone marrow aspirate of a patient with myeloma. Needle-shaped, azurophilic crystalline inclusions in cytoplasm of plasma cells representing Ig inclusion material*

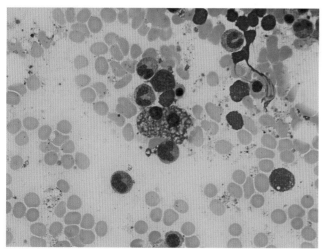

**PLATE 52** *Bone marrow aspirate of a patient with myeloma. Mott cells are plasma cells with multiple bluish cytoplasmic inclusion bodies*

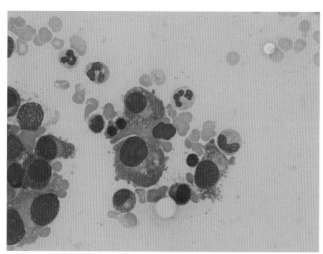

**PLATE 53** *Bone marrow aspirate of a patient with IgA myeloma. "Flame" cells are typically associated with IgA myeloma. They are plasma cells which stain eosinophilic pink in the periphery of the cytoplasm due to the accumulation of Ig*

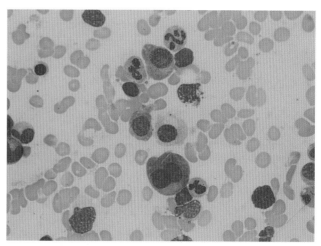

**PLATE 54** *Binucleated plasma cell in a patient with myeloma*

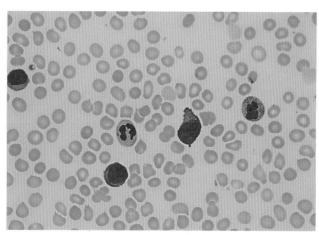

**PLATE 55** *Plasmablasts with prominent nucleoli in a patient with plasma cell leukemia*

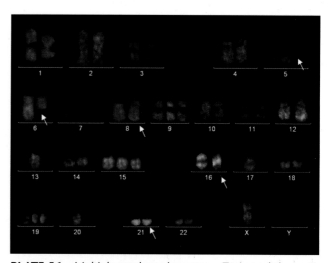

**PLATE 56** *Multiple myeloma karyotype: Top panel shows G-banded karyotype with extra copies of chromosomes 5, 7, 9, 15, and 19, loss of the Y chromosome, monosomy 13, and complex unbalanced rearrangements involving chromosomes 16, 17, and 20. The complex der(16) and cryptic t(8;21) were identified only on M-FISH (shown in the bottom panel). The t(8;21) breakpoint on 8q is at the site of the MYC gene*

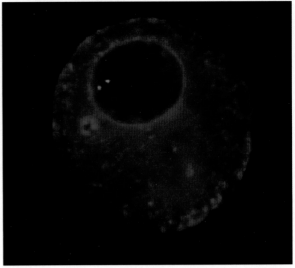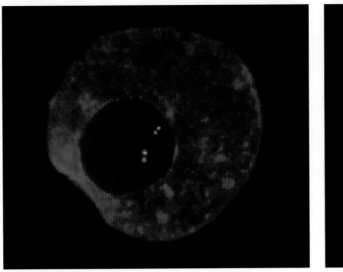

A

B

**PLATE 57** *FISH showing (a) normal plasma cell with two copies of chromosome 13 (two probes for each copy), and (b) plasma cell in myeloma with deletion of one copy of chromosome 13*

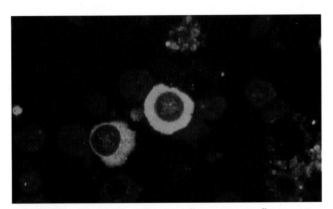

**PLATE 58** *Circulating plasma cells as seen on florescent microscopy after staining for cytoplasmic immunoglobulin light chains*

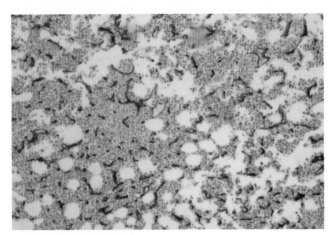

**PLATE 59** *Increased bone marrow microvessels in myeloma bone marrow as visualized by immunohistochemical staining for CD34*

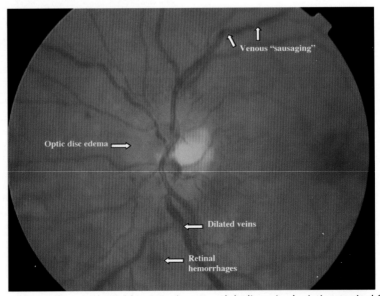

**PLATE 60** *Ocular exam of a patient with Waldenström's macroglobulinemia depicting typical findings of hyperviscosity*

# Chapter 55

# TREATMENT APPROACH TO MANTLE CELL LYMPHOMA

*Ellie Guardino, Kristen N. Ganjoo, and Ranjana Advani*

## INTRODUCTION

Mantle cell lymphoma (MCL) is a distinct entity of lymphoma in the WHO classification[1] and represents approximately 5–6% of all non-Hodgkin's lymphomas.[2] The incidence of MCL is 2–3 per 100,000/year and occurs with at a median age of 65 years. Classical nodal and extra-nodal MCL is associated with overexpression of Cyclin D1 from the presence of the t(11;14) (q13; q32) translocation juxtaposing the *BCL1* gene and the immunoglobulin heavy chain locus.[3–5] MCL exhibits a strong tendency toward extranodal involvement, especially the gastrointestinal tract,[6] bone marrow, and spleen. The approach to staging is similar to aggressive lymphomas, and also includes colonoscopy due to a high incidence of lower GI tract involvement.[7] MCL has moderate chemosensitivity, with complete responses to conventional chemotherapy ranging from 20% to 60%.[8–10] Despite this, the disease has a dismal outcome and tends to recur following conventional therapy, with a median survival of 3 years.[11–13]

## HISTOLOGY

MCL comprises a group of lymphoma subtypes previously classified as centrocytic lymphoma, lymphocytic lymphoma, or diffuse small-cleaved cell lymphoma.[14–16] Two morphologic subtypes of MCL are now classified: classic or typical MCL, which comprises 90%, and the blastoid variant, which is found in 10% of cases.[15] The malignant cell type of the classic or typical MCL is composed of morphologically small- to medium-sized lymphocytes with irregular nuclei and condensed chromatin, while the blastoid variant resembles lymphoblasts with medium size rounded nuclei, dispersed chromatin, and scant cytoplasm.[16] The blastoid variant has a high mitotic index compared to the classic MCL and has a worse prognosis than the classic form, with a median survival of <2 years.[17] Architecturally, three different patterns are recognized: mantle-zone pattern with the malignant cells surrounding normal germinal centers, nodular pattern, and diffuse pattern with loss of germinal centers.

## IMMUNOPHENOTYPE

MCL is thought to arise from naïve pregerminal center B cells in the primary follicles or mantle zone of secondary follicles. It has an immunophenotype of a mature B cell,[15,16,18–21] expressing CD19, CD20, CD22, CD79A, IgM, and/or IgD. MCL express lambda light chain more often than kappa light chain. Additionally, these malignant cells are CD5+, CD43+, but CD23−, and CD10−, which differentiates them from chronic lymphocytic leukemia. Most cases display an unmutated immunoglobulin chain locus.[22,23] Recent studies have now shown that 25–30% of MCL carry mutations in the IgV$_H$, a feature of postgerminal center cells.[22,24,25]

Some patients may present with peripheral lymphocytosis with a t(11;14) translocation, extra-nodal disease, and may have a different clinical course than that for classical MCL. In a study that looked at the clinical course in 80 MCL patients with circulating t(11;14) lymphocytes, IgV$_H$ genes were unmutated in 90% of nodal MCL patients, while only 44% of the extra-nodal patients had unmutated IgV$_H$ genes.[26] Interestingly, long-term survivors in this study were all found in the extra-nodal group with IgV$_H$ gene mutation. The authors suggested that mutated IgV$_H$ genes found in the extra-nodal asymptomatic MCL group may be of use to identify patients who have more indolent disease and for whom early intensive treatment is not indicated. Further studies are warranted before adopting this management approach for extra-nodal MCL.

### GENETICS/CYTOGENETICS

MCL is associated with the t(11;14)(q13;q32) the ataxia telangiectasia mutation and the 11q deletion. The t(11;14) juxtaposes the Cyclin D1 gene to the B-cell immunoglobulin transcription enhancer, which results in the overexpression of Cyclin D1.[16] This results in deregulation of the G1 phase of the cell cycle. While Cyclin D1 overexpression is a hallmark of MCL, it is also observed in a variety of other hematologic and nonhematologic malignancies, and the precise role that Cyclin D1 overexpression plays in the development of MCL is not understood. This translocation is found in more than 95% of MCL cases. Up to 50% of the breakpoints on 11q13 occur within a restricted area called the major translocation cluster, and this region is used to amplify genomic DNA by PCR as a diagnostic method. Using the PCR assay as a molecular diagnostic tool for MCL detects the rearrangement in only 35%of patients.[16] New PCR methods are being investigated that examine the Cyclin D1/Cyclin D3 ratio by real-time PCR, and these have shown improved specificity for the diagnosis of MCL.[27] PCR has also been used for molecular follow-up studies of MCL[16,28]

Fluorescence in situ hybridization (FISH) can show the t(11;14) translocation with a greater sensitivity of >95%. Another benefit of FISH is that it can be performed on archival cytologic material.[29]

Additional diagnostic approaches for MCL are under investigation. Microarray data suggests that there may be a disease-specific signature, including signatures for apoptosis, cell cycle, and cell signaling [30]. Transgenic animal studies have shown that CCND1 gene overexpression alone cannot induce lymphoma and that other oncogenic factors, such as c-myc, are needed.[31] Cyclin D1 overexpression is the only one mechanism responsible for deregulating the G1 phase of the cell cycle in MCL. Other mechanisms include hypermethylation and inactivation of p16[INK4a], TP53 mutations, and loss of p27[Kip1].[32–35] Microarray analysis has shown that MCL exhibits alterations in the expression of apoptosis-related molecules, with an overall pattern of antiapoptosis[36] and a low MCL apoptotic rate.[37] In addition, MCL cells have been shown to express low or absent levels of Fas and thus may have prolonged survival.[38] Additionally, the myeloid cell leukemia 1 (Mcl-1) gene, a member of the BCL-2 gene family, and its protein product promotes cell survival and Mcl-1-positive MCL tumors have been shown to have a higher frequency of blastoid/large-cell morphology, and higher Ki67 immunolabelling.[39] Using RNA expression profiling, Rosenwald et al. have identified a set of 48 genes that stratify MCL patients into subsets that differ by more than 5 years in median survival.[5] These recent elucidations in the biology of this disease, we hope, will in turn result in better diagnostics, prognostics, and treatments for MCL.

## PROGNOSTIC FACTORS

Tumor-associated prognostic features are related to the morphologic pattern—the mantle zone variant tends to behave more indolently while the blastoid variant is aggressive.[40] Clinical prognostic factors for MCL include poor performance status, anemia, splenomegaly, and advanced age.[23] Mutations in p53, abnormalities in the CDK inhibitors p16–p21, a high Ki67 staining index, unmutated IgV$_H$ gene, elevated β2M, and overexpression of topo II$\alpha$ are all usually associated with aggressive behavior.

## TREATMENT APPROACHES

Prognosis remains poor in MCL, and patients who respond to treatment usually relapse. There is currently no standard treatment for the disease. Conventional treatment of MCL results in response rates of 20–60%. The disease invariably recurs and the median survival in this disease is approximately 3 years. Therapeutic options are continually being refined as the clinical methods of classifying MCL evolve and as the biology elucidates the histologic and cytogenetic characteristics of MCL subtypes.

### CHEMOTHERAPY

Currently, the initial treatment for MCL is similar to that for other aggressive lymphomas. An anthracycline-based approach is the standard even though randomized clinical studies have not proven a survival advantage with anthracycline-containing regimens over nonanthracycline-containing regimens.[41–43] Meusers and colleagues reported the results of a randomized study comparing CVP (cyclophosphamide, vincristine, and prednisone) to CHOP (cyclophosphamide, adriamycin, vincristine, and prednisone) chemotherapy in 63 MCL patients.[42] No significant difference was found in response rate and overall survival (OS). A second randomized study compared two anthracycline-containing regimens with CVP.[41] The response rate was better with the anthracycline regimens, but the median survival was equal in both groups. A third randomized study compared PmM (prednimustine, mitoxanthrone) with CVP.[43] The response rate and the event-free survival (EFS) were better with PmM, but the median overall response rate (ORR) was the same in both groups.

The most commonly used regimen is CHOP. With this the complete response (CR) rate is 20–80%, median failure-free survival (FFS) is 10–16 months, and median OS is 3 years. Several approaches have been used to intensify CHOP. In one phase II prospective study of 28 patients with aggressive MCL, complete responses following four cycles of CHOP chemotherapy were seen in only 7%. In the same study, the addition of Dexamethasone, Cytarabine, Cisplatin (DHAP) to CHOP in a sequential fashion demonstrated a complete response in 84% of the remaining patients compared to CHOP alone.[44]

The MD Anderson group has used an intensive leukemic regimen, hyper-CVAD (high-dose methotrexate and cytosine arabinoside in combination with a dose intense CHOP-like combination: hyper-fraction-ated cyclophosphamide, vincristine, doxorubicin, and dexamethasone), for up to 8 cycles. Several reports by the MD Anderson investigators have been published with this regimen. The number of cycles of therapy have varied between four and eight depending on whether or not autologous stem cell transplant (ASCT) was done as part of primary treatment, and several reports have also included patients for whom this reg-imen was used as salvage therapy. In one report of patients >65 years treated with hyper-CVAD as pri-mary treatment,[45] the ORR was 92% (95% C.I. 73–99) with a CR rate of 68% (95% C.I. 46–85). At a median follow-up of 17 months, the median FFS for the entire group was 15 months. Hematologic toxicity was sig-nificant, but only 5% of the cycles were associated with grade 3 infection. In another study of 45 patients with advanced stage MCL (50% previously treated), subjects received four cycles of hyper-CVAD and those who achieved a CR went on to ASCT. The ORR was 93.5% (CR, 38%, and partial remission (PR), 55.5%).[46] The previously untreated patients had a 3 year OS and EFS of 92% and 72%, respectively. This was higher than CHOP or CHOP-like treated historical controls at this institution, who had a 3-year OS and EFS of 25% and 17%, respectively. A similar observation has been reported in a study comparing hyper-CVAD induction chemotherapy with CHOP or CHOP-like induction followed by ASCT, with superiority being shown in the hyper-CVAD induction group.[47] Both of these reports should be viewed with caution as they are ret-rospective in nature, treatment groups were not well matched, and all of the patients received ASCT after hyper-CVAD treatment. Despite the lack of random-ized studies evaluating the different treatment regi-mens for MCL, it appears that the newer approaches (i.e., hyper-CVAD or DHAP) may result in superior ORR compared to CHOP or CHOP-like therapy. Whether the improved remission rates translate into improved survival is unclear as the median follow-up of all these studies is short (<3 years). Patients should be enrolled on clinical trials in order to evaluate these new approaches.

### ROLE OF ANTIBODY THERAPY AND OTHER IMMUNOTHERAPIES

MCL is a B-cell malignancy that expresses CD20. The anti-CD20 antibody, rituximab, has been stud-ied as a single agent in MCL with response rates of 20–40%.[28,48–50]

In vitro and clinical observations in patients with follicular NHL suggest that the effect of rituximab might be enhanced by the synergistic effect of chemotherapy. Based on these observations, rituximab and CHOP (R-CHOP) induction therapy in patients with newly diagnosed MCL has been evaluated[51] In a phase II trial, 40 previously untreated patients with stage II through IV MCL were treated with six cycles of R-CHOP. Forty-eight percent of patients achieved a complete response (CR)/CR unconfirmed (CRu), and 48% of patients obtained a partial response (PR), with an ORR of 96%. However, 28 of the 40 patients have already relapsed or developed progressive disease with a median PFS of 16.6 months. Twenty-five patients had PCR-detectable BCL-1/IgH or clonal IgH products in peripheral blood or bone marrow at diagnosis and nine of these had no evidence of PCR-detectable disease in peripheral blood or bone marrow after R-CHOP ther-apy. Despite molecular remissions, patients had similar clinical outcomes and PFS. R-CHOP has also been eval-uated in a prospective randomized study by the German lymphoma study group (GLSG). Previously untreated patients with advanced disease were ran-domly assigned to receive conventional CHOP or R-CHOP. In early responders who achieved a CR after four cycles, no further induction was given. All other responding patients received six cycles of CHOP or R-CHOP followed by alpha-interferon maintenance ther-apy or a myeloablative consolidation followed by ASCT depending on the patient's age. One hundred and twenty two patients were evaluated prior to transplant, and R-CHOP was reported to result in a significantly superior CR rate compared to CHOP alone (34% vs. 7% $p = 0.00024$). Also, the addition of rituximab improved the ORR by approximately 20% in comparison to chemotherapy alone (94 % vs. 75%, $p = 0.005$). The time to treatment failure was significantly longer in the R-CHOP group, but time to progression was not signif-icantly different.[52]

Rituximab has also been evaluated in combination with other agents. The GLSG has also reported prelimi-nary results of a prospective randomized trial of ritux-imab in combination with FCM (fludarabine, cyclophos-phamide, mitoxantrone) compared to FCM alone in patients with relapsed or refractory MCL 54. A total of four courses were given. An ORR of 62% versus 43% was observed in favor of the RFCM group, with a signifi-cantly longer OS ($p < 0.005$) [53–56]

These two randomized trials of the GLSG suggest that both in previously treated and relapsed MCL, CR rates were increased by approximately 30% and ORR by 20% with combined immunochemotherapy.

The MD Anderson group has evaluated rituximab with hyper-CVAD. Compared to prior studies with Hyper-CVAD alone, rituximab 375 mg/m² was added on day 1 of the first 6 courses and ASCT was not given to patients who achieved a CR within six courses of treatment. Seventy-seven previously untreated patients, median age 62, all with stage IV disease were treated with R-hyper-CVAD.[57] Fifty six patients received at least six cycles and were used as the denominator for response assessment. The CR rate was 90%. At a median follow-up of 14 months, the 2-year FFS and OS were 72% and 90%, respectively. In a subset analysis evaluat-ing outcome according to age, patients <65 years treated with R-hyper-CVAD without ASCT did not have a significantly different outcome compared to historical controls who received the same hyper-CVAD regiment with ASCT. In patients >65 years, there was a trend favoring the R-hyper-CVAD. These reports suggest that the addition of rituximab to standard induction regimens appears to result in improved response rates. Again, longer follow-up is required to assess if any impact has been made on survival.

### TRANSPLANTATION

Stem cell transplantation can improve survival in other NHLs. This treatment has also been applied to MCL with mixed results.[58-60] Most studies have used this approach in patients with relapsed or refractory disease.

There is emerging data suggesting that ASCT used earlier in the course of disease has a greater benefit.[58] Dreger et al. examined the impact of ASCT on the prognosis of MCL in two prospective studies with 46 patients. ASCT in these studies was not curative but, if given as intensive first line treatment, prolonged the time to progression.[61] More recently, a study evaluating 28 patients who underwent B cell purged ASCT following CHOP induction showed DFS and OS of 31 months and 50 months, respectively. At 5 years, 20 of 28 patients died and only 4 had no evidence of disease.[62] Another prospective study evaluated 21/28 patients with newly diagnosed stage III or IV MCL who achieved a CR with induction therapy and then received ASCT. The 3 year EFS and OS were 83% and 90%, respectively.[44] Another trial used dose-escalating CHOP chemotherapy for induction followed by ASCT. These patients were not required to have a CR to go on to ASCT, and only 11 of 41 patients had a CR. Twenty-four of the transplant patients achieved or maintained a CR, and the 4-year OS and FFS rates were 51% and 15%, respectively with a median FFS of 2.5 years, similar to conventional chemotherapy.[63,64] Interestingly, 80% of the patients who achieved an initial CR prior to transplant were alive without disease at 4 years.

Retrospective studies have reached similar conclusions. A retrospective study done in Finland showed similar DFS data with ASCT to prospective trials.[65] Retrospective data supported the use of ASCT early in disease.[66] Specifically, an analysis of the European Blood and Bone Marrow Transplant registries of 195 MCL patients treated with ASCT reported on OS/PFS at 2-year and 5-year were 76%/55% and 50%/33%, respectively. Patients who were transplanted in first CR were 33% less likely to die from MCL than patients with chemosensitive disease who were transplanted later. Another study evaluating the effect of early transplant in MCL was a retrospective analysis of 69 patients at Stanford and City of Hope who underwent ASCT with or without ex vivo graft purging.[67] Patients who were in first CR at the time of transplant (39%) had an estimated 3- and 5- year OS/DFS rates of 93%/74% and 77%/50%, respectively. In comparison, the OS/DFS rates at 3- and 5- years for patients who were not in 1st

remission at the time of transplant were 64%/51% and 39%/21%. The median time to relapse in the group transplanted in first CR was 32 months compared to 10.5 months. Additionally, the relapse rate was lower: 19% versus 50%. Together, these studies clearly demonstrate the need for good induction regimens for MCL. Alternatively, the subset of MCL that is chemoresponsive may represent the only subset that benefits significantly from ASCT.

Hyper-CVAD induction treatment for MCL in combination with transplant has also been evaluated.[46] After four courses of hyper-CVAD, 45 patients were consolidated with high-dose cyclophosphamide, total-body irradiation, and autologous or allogeneic blood or marrow stem-cell transplantation (43/45 patients had Ann Arbor stage IV disease). For the 25 previously untreated patients, the OS and (EFS) rates at 3 years were 92% (95% CI, 80 to 100) and 72% (95% CI, 45 to 98) compared with 25% (95% CI, 12 to 62; $P = .005$) and 17% (95% CI, 10 to 43; $P = .007$), respectively, for the previously treated patients. When compared with a historic control group who received a CHOP-like regimen, untreated patients in the study had a 3-year EFS rate of 72% versus 28% ($P = .0001$) and a better OS rate (92% v 56%; $P = .05$).

Another recent study using hyper-CVAD induction followed by ASCT in patients with MCL[68] resulted in 5-year DFS and OS of 43% and 77%, respectively. The patients in the study had untreated MCL, with <10% MCL in the marrow at the time of ASCT and other favorable characteristics and only patients who had achieved a CR went on to transplant.

Thus, it appears that at least for patients with chemosensitive disease, ASCT as consolidation following chemotherapy induction may be associated with an improved outcome. The optimal induction regimen has not been addressed in a randomized study. A retrospective analysis by Conde et al. evaluated the induction regimens used for MCL.[47,63] An international database of 119 patients with MCL who had received ASCT between 1988 and 2002 was evaluated. The induction regimens were primarily hyper-CVAD and CHOP-like therapy, and 50/119 patients had CR at transplant. The conditioning regimens varied and the CR rate after transplant was 87%. The estimated OS and DFS were impressive at 50% and 32%, respectively. There was a median DFS of 38 months and 50% survival rate at 10 years in this study. Comparing the induction regimens, it was found that hyper-CVAD was superior in this analysis to CHOP or CHOP-like regimens; however, the patients who received hyper-CVAD had fewer adverse prognostic features (bulky disease, advanced stage, high LDH). Despite these differences, the authors report that in the hyper-CVAD group the DFS at 4-years was 68% compared to 33% in patients treated with CHOP or CHOP-like therapy. It should be noted that none of these regimens employed rituximab along with the induction chemotherapy. Retrospective data from MD

Anderson suggests that R-hyper-CVAD was equivalent in outcome when compared to hyper-CVAD followed by ASCT. This suggests that more effective induction regimens that use immunotherapy upfront may be good alternative strategies. It is imperative to enroll patients in well designed prospective clinical trials to evaluate the role of these newer therapies.

Methods to assess molecular remission posttransplant have been evaluated and appear to be predictive of a prolonged disease-free survival.[69] Sixteen patients with MCL treated with ASCT were examined using PCR based strategies to evaluate residual tumor cells posttransplant. Molecular remission in this group was found in only 12.5%. There is a suggestion that cyclin D1/IgH-probe fusion fluorescence in situ hybridization analysis may provide additional information for evaluating the character of circulating MCL cells in peripheral blood and MRD.[70] Although this type of methodology needs to evolve fully, these types of methods may aid in the evaluation of response to different induction and high-dose therapy.

### ROLE OF PURGING

MCL is particularly resistant to purging.[71] The efficacy of immunological purging was assessed by using polymerase chain reaction (PCR) for minimal residual disease (MRD) on 26 MCL patients undergoing transplant. All patients had MRD detected by PCR after transplant irrespective of prior history of bone marrow involvement. This study demonstrated that reinfusion of stem cells with MRD was associated with a poor outcome. In addition, one study demonstrated that despite using anti-B-cell monoclonal antibody for ex vivo purging of the autograft, 88% of the autografts still had evidence of lymphomatous contamination.[62] The use of in vivo purging using rituximab is promising, with evidence of clinical and molecular remissions.[72,73] Gianni et al treated 28 patients with MCL younger than 60 years who completed at least 6 cycles of CHOP-like chemotherapy. Patients were treated with three cycles of cisplatin or doxorubicin-based debulking chemotherapy followed by high-dose sequential therapy with rituximab and ASCT. The 54-month OS and EFS rates were 89% and 79%, respectively as compared to rates for historical controls of 42% and 18%. Interestingly, clinical and molecular remission was found in 20/20 patients tested following in vivo purging, but not following debulking chemotherapy or following mobilization. Another study showed PCR negativity following transplant and in vivo purging with rituximab.[74] In this study, patients were treated with chemotherapy and subsequently received high-dose cytosine arabinoside and rituximab as in-vivo purging. Twelve patients were evaluable for molecular remission. Ten of the 12 patients achieved PCR negativity posttransplant.

Two studies have suggested that posttransplant rituximab increases the clinical and molecular response rate of MCL patients receiving ASCT.[75,76] In one study of advanced stage MCL, all patients who received posttransplant rituximab were alive without clinical or molecular relapse at 239 days posttransplant.[75] The treatment was well tolerated and encouraging, albeit longer follow-up is needed.

Cumulatively, these approaches employing rituximab either in vivo for purging or posttransplant suggest that molecular and clinical remission may play a role in the long term outcome. Again, none of these studies have a long enough follow-up to assess the impact on OS.

### ALLOGENEIC TRANSPLANTATION

Allogeneic transplantation has only been evaluated in patients with refractory MCL, and it has been shown to induce durable remissions in some cases.[77] Twenty MCL patients underwent allogeneic transplant using a myeloablative regimen at the University of Nebraska.[78] Nine of 20 patients are alive and disease-free 1–9 years posttransplant. A trial investigating nonmyeloablative transplant in 18 patients with MCL who had failed multiple prior chemotherapies, including 28% who had failed prior ASCT, has been published. CR was achieved in 17 of 18 patients, and with a median follow-up of 26 months the estimated 3-year survival rate and current PFS was 85.5% and 82%, respectively.[77]

### RADIOIMMUNOTHERAPY

Radioimmunotherapy (RIT) is an attractive therapeutic option for patients with NHL, as these are radiosensitive tumors. The two clinically available radioimmunoconjugates are iodine [131]I tositumomab (Bexxar) and ibritumomab tiuxetan (Zevalin) using yttrium-90. These have been used extensively in patients with indolent lymphoma, but little experience is available in MCL.

In a study from Seattle, Gopal and colleagues examined the role of [131]I-radiolabeled (Tositumomab) in relapsed MCL.[79] The antibody dose was 1.7 mg/kg body weight, and the normal amount of [131]I was calculated to deliver 20–25 Gy to vital normal organs. The treatment was followed 10 days later by administration of high-dose etoposide (30–60 mg/kg), cyclophosphamide (60–100 mg/kg), and infusion of cryopreserved autologous stem cells. A total of 16 patients were treated with a median number of 3 prior therapies and 7 with chemotherapy resistant disease. In 11 patients with measurable disease the CR and OS were 91% and 100%, respectively. Fifteen patients were alive at the time of evaluation and 12 had no progression of lymphoma at 6–57 months from transplant and 16–97 months from diagnosis. The ORR at 3 years from transplant was estimated at 93% and PFS at 61%. These results are encouraging and warrant further investigation.

The role of RIT in the upfront management of MCL is also being assessed. In an ongoing trial, the Eastern Cooperative Oncology Group is evaluating radioimmunotherapy after R-CHOP induction chemotherapy. While R-CHOP may be an effective induction regimen for MCL, it is not sufficient for durable remission. In this trial, patients who respond to R-CHOP are treated with $^{90}$Yttrium-ibritumomab (Zevalin).

### OTHER IMMUNOTHERAPIES

Interferon may offer another immunotherapeutic option in MCL. Phase II studies have demonstrated a potential for longer progression-free survival with the addition of maintenance Interferon-α.[80,81] This warrants further investigation in randomized trials. In addition, idiotype vaccines as adjuvant to immunotherapy are under investigation.[82,83]

### NEWER AGENTS

Bortezomib is a potent and specific proteosome inhibitor that down regulates the NF-kB pathway. Recently, two studies have reported encouraging activity with this agent in patients with relapsed/refractory MCL.[84,85] Fifty-three percent of patients (8/15) had a response, with a median duration of 3 months. One relapsed MCL patient was retreated and achieved a second PR lasting 4+ months.[85] The mechanism of antitumor activity in MCL is not known, though the biology of MCL provides some clues. Reduced expression of P27 and loss of normal P53 function are both associated with a poor prognosis in MCL. The intracellular levels of P27 and P53 are both modulated by proteosomal degradation[86,87] It is possible that inhibition of the proteosome by bortezomib may contribute to its activity in MCL.

Thalidomide in combination with rituximab was evaluated in relapsed/refractory MCL patients, and impressive antitumor activity has been reported.[88,89] In one study, 16 patients with relapsed/refractory MCL were treated with rituximab at 375 mg/m$^2$ for four weekly doses concomitantly with thalidomide. Eighty-one percent (13/16) experienced an objective response with 5 achieving a CR (31%). The median PFS was 20.4 months (95% CI, 17.3–23.6), and estimated 3-year survival was 75%.[88] There were three severe adverse events: two thromboembolic and one grade IV neutropenia. The encouraging antitumor effect warrants further investigation in MCL.

## SUMMARY AND FUTURE DIRECTIONS

MCL is an aggressive lymphoma that generally presents in advanced stages and has a median survival of about 3 years. Despite response to chemotherapy, the disease typically recurs within 1 year of therapy. Improved induction therapy using intensive regimens appear to increase the time to progression. Rituximab and radiolabeled anti-CD20 monoclonal antibodies have shown encouraging results when added to chemotherapy and stem cell transplantation. Rituximab also appears to improve clinical and molecular responses in patients when used for posttransplant consolidation and in vivo purging. Nonmyeloablative transplant is being evaluated as another promising treatment option which will be useful in the older patient population. As the field evolves, defining a MCL molecular signature, which identifies alterations in gene sets which are associated with molecular, phenotypic and clinical distinctions in this disease, will impact treatment decisions.[30,90] By using molecular profiling, we may be able to identify subsets of patients with indolent or aggressive MCL or subsets of genes that predict treatment responses.[30,91–93]

As the optimal approach to the management of patients with MCL is still evolving, it is critical that these patients are enrolled in clinical trials to identify better treatment options.

### REFERENCES

1. Jaffe ES: *World Health Organization Classification of Tumours: Tumours of the Haemopoitic and Lymphoid Tissues.* Lyon, France: IARC Press; 2001.
2. Velders GA: Mantle-cell lymphoma: a population-based clinical study. *J Clin Oncol* 14:1269–1274, 1996.
3. Li JY: Detection of translocation t (11;14)(q13;q32) in mantle cell lymphoma by fluorescence in situ hybridization. *Am J Pathol* 154:1449–1452, 1999.
4. Sola B: Expression of cyclins D-type in B-chronic lymphoproliferative disorders. *Leukemia* 14:1318–1319, 2000.
5. Rosenwald A: The proliferation gene expression signature is a quantitiative integrator of oncogenic events that predicts survival in mantle cell lymphoma. *Cancer Cell* 3:185–197, 2003.
6. Romaguera JE: Frequency of gastrointestinal involvement and its clinical significance in mantle cell lymphoma. *Cancer* 97:586–589, 2003.
7. NCCN Guidelines version 1.2004. National Comprehensive Cancer Network Inc., 2004.
8. Bosch F: Mantle cell lymphoma: presenting features, response to therapy and prognostic factors. *Cancer* 82:567–575, 1998.
9. Gressin R: Treatment of mantle-cell lymphomas with the VAD +/-chlorambucil regimen with or without subsequent high-dose therapy and peripheral blood stem-cell transplantation. *Ann Oncol* 8(suppl 1): S103–S106, 1997.
10. Zucca E: Patterns of survival in mantle cell lymphoma. *Ann Oncol* 6:257–262, 1995.

11. Kauh J: Mantle cell lymphoma: clinicopathologic features and treatments. *Oncology* 17:879–881, 2003.

12. Shivdassani R: Intermediate lymphocytic lymphoma: clinical and pathologic features of a recently characterized subtype of non-Hodkin's lymphoma. *J Clin Oncol* 11:802–811, 1993.

13. Jacobsen E: An update on the role of high-dose therapy with autologous or allogeneic stem cell transplantation in mantle lymphoma. *Curr Opin Oncol* 16:106–113, 2004.

14. Zucca E: European Lymphoma Task Force (ELTF): report of the workshop of mantle cell lymphoma (MCL). *Ann Oncol* 5:507–511, 1994.

15. Swerdlow SH: Mantle cell Lymphoma. In: *World Health Organization Classification of Tumours: Pathology and Genetics of Tumours of Haematopoietic and Lymphoid Tissues*. Lyon, France: IARC Press; 2001: 168–170.

16. Bertoni F: Molecular basis of mantle cell lymphoma. *Br J Haematol* 124:130–140, 2004.

17. Zucca E: Management of rare forms of lymphoma. *Curr Opin Oncol* 10:377–384, 1998.

18. Campo E: Mantle cell lymphoma. *Semin Hematol* 36:115–127, 1999.

19. Lai R: Pathologic diagnosis of mantle cell lymphoma. *Clin Lymphoma* 1:197–206, 2000.

20. Pileri S: The pathologist's view point. Part II-aggressive lymphomas. *Haematologica* 85:1308–1321, 2000.

21. Dreyling M: Mantle cell lymphoma. In: *Annual of Lymphoid Malignancies* 1:61–68, 2001.

22. Walsh SH: Mutated VH genes and preferential VH3-21 use define new subsets of mantle cell lymphoma. *Blood* 101:4047–4054, 2003.

23. Lenz G: Mantle cell lymphoma: established therapeutic options and future directions. *Ann Hematol* 2003.

24. Thorselius M: Somatic hypermutation and V(H) gene useage in mantle cell lymphoma. *Eur J Haematol* 68:217–224, 2002.

25. Camacho FI: Molecular heterogeneity in MCL, defined by the use of specific VH genes and the frequency of somatic mutations. *Blood* 101: 4042–4046, 2003.

26. Orchard J: A sub-set of t(11;14) lymphoma with mantle cell features displays mutated IgVH genes and includes patients with good prognosis, non-nodal disease. *Blood* 101(12):4975–4981, 2003.

27. Jones CD: Cyclin D1/Cyclin D3 ratio by real-time PCR improves specificity for the diagnosis of mantle cell lymphoma. *J Mol Diagn* 6(2):84–89, 2004.

28. Ghielmini M: The effect of rituximab on patients with follicular and mantle-cell lymphoma. Swiss Group for Clinical Cancer Research (SAKK). *Ann Oncol* 11:123–126, 2000.

29. Bentz JS: Rapid detection of the t(11;14) translocation in mantle cell lymphoma by interphase fluorescence in situ hybridization on archival cytopathologic material. *Cancer* 102:124–131, 2004.

30. Martinez N: The molecular signature of mantle cell lymphoma reveals multiple signals favoring cell survival. *Cancer Res* 63:8226–8232, 2003.

31. Bodrug SE: Cyclin D1 transgene impedes lymphocyte maturation and collaborates in lymphomagenesis with the myc gene. *EMBO J* 13:2124–2130, 1994.

32. Pinyol M: Deletions and loss of expression of p16 INK4 and p21 Waf1 genes are associated with aggressive variants of mantle cell lymphomas. *Blood* 86:272–280, 1997.

33. Quintanilla-Martinez L: Mantle cell lymphomas lack expression of p27kip1, a cyclin-dependent kinase inhibitor. *Am J Pathol* 153:175–182, 1998.

34. Chiarle R: Increased proteasome degradation of cyclin-dependent kinase inhibitor p27 is associated with a decreased overall survival in mantle cell lymphoma. *Blood* 95:619–626, 2000.

35. Greiner TC: P53 mutations in mantle cell lymphoma are associated with variant cytology and predict a poor prognosis. *Blood* 87:4302–4310, 1996.

36. Hoffman WK: Altered apoptosis pathways in mantle cell lymphoma detected by oligonucleotide microarray. *Blood* 98:787–794, 2001.

37. Hermann M: Differential expression of apoptosis, Bcl-x and c-Myc in normal and malignant lymphoid tissues. *Eur J Haematol* 59: 20–30, 1997.

38. Clodi K: Unbalanced expression of Fas and CD40 in mantle cell lymphoma. *Br J Haematol* 103:217–219, 1998.

39. Khoury JD: Expression of Mcl-1 in mantle cell lymphoma is associated with high-grade morphology, a high proliferative state, and p53 overexpression. *J Pathol* 199:90–97, 2003.

40. Majlis A: Mantle cell lymphoma: correlation of clinical outcome and biologic features with three histologic variants. *J Clin Oncol* 15, 1664–1671, 1997.

41. Teodorovic I: Efficacy of four different regimens in 64 mantle-cell lymphoma cases: Clinicopathologic comparison with 498 other non- Hodgkin's lymphoma subtypes. European Organization for the Research and Treatment of Cancer Lymphoma Cooperative Group. *J Clin Oncol* 13:2819–2826, 1995.

42. Meusers P: Multicentre randomized therapeutic trial for advanced centrocytic lymphoma: anthracycline does not improve the prognosis. *Hematol Oncol* 7:365–380, 1989.

43. Unterhalt M: Prednimustine, mitoxanthrone (PmM) vs cyclophosphamide, vincristine, prednisone (COP) for the treatment of advanced low-grade non-Hodgkin's lymphoma. German Low-Grade Lymphoma Study Group. *Leukemia* 10:836–843, 1996.

44. Lefrere F: Sequential chemotherapy by CHOP and DHAP regimens followed by high-dose therapy with stem cell transplantation induces a high rate of complete response and improves event-free survival in mantle cell lymphoma: a prospective study. *Leukemia* 16:587–593, 2002.

45. Romaguera JE: Untreated aggressive mantle cell lymphoma: results with intensive chemotherapy without stem cell transplant in elderly patients. *Leuk Lymphoma* 39:77–85, 2000.

46. Khouri IF: Hyper-CVAD and high-dose methotrexate/ cytarabine followed by stem-cell transplantation: an active regimen for aggressive mantle-cell lymphoma. *J Clin Oncol* 16:3803–3809, 1998.

47. Conde E: Autologous stem cell transplantation (ASCT) for mantle cell lymphoma (MCL). *Blood* 100:2529a, 2002. [Abstract]

48. Foran JM: European phase II study of rituximab (chimeric anti-CD20 monoclonal antibody) for patients

with newly diagnosed mantle-cell lymphoma and previously treated mantle-cell lymphoma, immunocytoma, and small B-cell lymphocytic lymphoma. *J Clin Oncol* 18:317–324, 2002.

49. Tobinai K: Monoclonal antibody therapy for B-cell lymphoma: clinical trials of an anti-CD20 monoclonal antibody for B-cell lymphoma in Japan. *Int J Hematol* 76:411–419, 2002.

50. Nguyen DT: IDEC-C2B8 anti-CD20 (rituximab) immunotherapy in patients with low-grade non-Hodgkin's lymphoma and lymphoproliferative disorders: evaluation of response on 48 patients. *Eur J Haematol* 62:76–82, 1999.

51. Howard OM: Rituximab and CHOP induction therapy for newly diagnosed mantle-cell lymphoma: molecular complete responses are not predictive of progression-free survival. *J Clin Oncol* 20:1288–1294, 2002.

52. Hiddemann W: Effect of addition of rituximab to front line therapy with cyclophosphamide, doxorubicin, vincristine, and prednisone (CHOP) on the remission rate and time to treatment failure (TTF) compared to CHOP alone in mantle cell lymphoma (MCL). *Proc of ASCO* 556, 2004. Abstract 6501.

53. Dreyling MH: Combined immuno-chemotherapy (R-FCM) results in superior remission and survival rates in recurrent follicular and mantle cell lymphoma. Final Results of a Prospective Randomized Trial of the German Low Grade Lymphoma Study Group (GLSG). In *ASH Annual Meeting*, Orlando, FL, Dec 2003. Abstrract 351.

54. Forstpointner R: Increased response rate with rituximab in relapsed and refractory follicular and mantle cell lymphomas—results of a prospective randomized study of the German Low-Grade Lymphoma Study Group. *Dtsch Med Wochensch* 127(43):2253–2258, 2002.

55. Hiddemann W: The addition of Rituximab to combination chemotherapy (CT) significantly improves the treatment of mantle cell lymphoma (MCL): results of two prospective randomized studies by the german low grade study group (GLSG). *Blood* 100(suppl):229, 2002.

56. Hiddemann W: Rituximab plus chemotherapy in follicular and mantle cell lymphomas. *Semin Oncol* 30(1, suppl 2):16–20, 2003.

57. Romaguera J: R-HyperCVAD without transplant in Mantle Cell Lymphoma. In *American Society of Hematology Annual Meeting*, 2001.Abstr 3030.

58. Ketterer N: Intensive therapy with peripheral stem cell transplantation in 16 patients with mantle cell lymphoma. *Ann Oncol* 8:701–704, 1997.

59. Haas R: Myeloablative therapy with blood stem cell transplantation is effective in mantle cell lymphoma. *Leukemia* 10:1975–1979, 1996.

60. Decaudin D: Efficacy of autologous stem cell transplantation in mantle cell lymphoma: a 3 year follow-up study. *Bone Marrow Transplant* 25:251–256, 2000.

61. Dreger P: The impact of autologous stem cell transplantation on the prognosis of mantle cell lymphoma: a joint analysis of two prospective studies with 46 patients. *Hematol J* 1: 87–94, 2000.

62. Freedman AS: High-dose chemoradiotherapy and anti-B-cell monoclonal antibody-purged autologous bone marrow transplantation in mantle-cell lymphoma: no evidence for long-term remission. *J Clin Oncol* 16:13–18, 1998.

63. Jacobsen E: An update on the role of high-dose therapy with autologous or allogeneic stem cell transplantation in mantle cell lymphoma. *Curr Opin Oncol* 16(2): 106–113, 2004.

64. Andersen NS: Primary treatment with autologous stem cell transplantation in mantle cell lymphoma: outcome related to remission pretransplant. *Eur J Hematol* 71:73–80, 2003.

65. Oinonen R: Autologous stem cell transplantation in patients with mantle cell lymphoma. *Leuk Lymphoma* 43:1229–1237, 2002.

66. Vandenberghe E: Outcome of autologous transplantation for mantle cell lymphoma: a study by the European blood and bone marrow transplant and autologous blood and marrow transplant registries. *Br J Haematol* 120:793–800, 2003.

67. Molina A: Autologous stem cell transplantation (ASCT) for mantle cell lymphoma (MCL): a report of 69 patients from City of Hope (COH) and Stanford. *Blood* 100:680a, 2002. [Abstract]

68. Khouri I: Nonablative allogeneic stem-cell transplantation for advanced/recurrent mantle-cell lymphoma. *J Clin Oncol* 21:4407–4412, 2003.

69. Corradini P: Long-term follow-up of indolent lymphoma patients treated with high-dose sequential chemotherapy and autografting: evidence that durable molecular and clinical remission frequently can be attained only in follicular subtypes. *J Clin Oncol* 22:1460–1468, 2004.

70. Gu J: Evaluation of peripheral blood involvement of mantle cell lymphoma by fluorescence in situ hybridization in comparison with immunophenotypic and morphologic findings. *Mod Pathol* 17:553–560, 2004.

71. Andersen NS: Failure of immunologic purging in mantle cell lymphoma assessed by polymerase chain reaction detection of minimal residual disease. *Blood* 90:4212–4221, 1997.

72. Magni M: Successful in vivo purging of CD34- containing peripheral blood harvests in mantle cell and indolent lymphoma: evidence for a role of both chemotherapy and rituximab infusion. *Blood* 96: 864–869, 2000.

73. Gianni AM: Long-term remission in mantle cell lymphoma following high-dose sequential chemotherapy and in vivo rituximab-purged stem cell autografting. *Blood* 102:749–755, 2003.

74. Geisler CH: Mantle cell lymphoma (MCL): increased clinical and molecular response rates adding Ara-C and rituximab to CHOP + BEAM and autologous stem cell transplantation. Results of the 1$^{st}$ and 2$^{nd}$ Nordic MCL protocols. *Blood* 100:253a, 2002. [Abstract]

75. Mangel J: Immunotherapy with rituximab following high-dose therapy and autologous stem-cell transplantation for mantle cell lymphoma. *Semin Oncol* 29:56–59, 2002.

76. Brugger W: Treatment of follicular and mantle cell lymphoma with rituximab after high-dose chemotherapy and autologous blood stem cell transplantation: a multicenter phase II study. *Blood* 100:253a, 2002. [Abstract]

77. Khouri IF: Long-term follow-up of autologous stem cell transplantation in patients with diffuse mantle cell lymphoma in first disease remission: the prognostic value of beta2-microglobulin and the tumor score. *Cancer* 98:2630–2635, 2003.

78. Deshpande A: The Baidasle/cheson/Kauh et al. article reviewed. *Oncology* 17(6):896–898, 2003.

79. Gopal AK: High-dose chemo-radiotherapy with autologous stem cell support for relapsed mantle cell lymphoma. *Blood* 99:3158–3162, 2002.

80. Teodorovic I: Efficacy of four different regimens in 64 mantle-cell lymphoma cases: clinicopathologic comparison with 498 other non-Hodgkin's lymphoma subtypes. European Organization for the Research and Treatment of Cancer Lymphoma Cooperative Group. *J Clin Oncol* 13:2819-2826, 1995.

81. Hiddemann W: Mantle-cell lymphomas have more widespread disease and a slower response to chemotherapy compared with follicle-center lymphomas: results of a prospective comparative analysis of the German Low-Grade Lymphoma Study Group. *J Clin Oncol* 16: 1922–1930, 1998.

82. Wilson WH: Idiotype vaccine following EPOCH-rituxan treatment in untreated MCL. *Blood* 100:60:608a, 2002. [Abstract]

83. Leonard J: Personalized recombinant idiotype vaccination after chemotherapy as initial treatment for MCL. *Blood* 100:4792a, 2002. [Abstract]

84. O'Connor OA: Marked clinical activity of the novel proteosome inhibitor bortezomib in patients with relapsed follicular (RL) and mantle cell lymphoma (MCL). In: *ASCO Annual Meeting*, 2004. Abstract 6582.

85. Goy A: Update on a phase (ph) 2 study of bortezomib in patients (pts) with relapsed or refractory indolent or aggressive non-hodgkin's lymphoma (NHL). 2004 ASCO Annual Meeting, and its deregulation in cancer. *J Cell Physiol* 183:10–17, 2000. [Abstract 6581]

86. Slingerland J: Regulation of the cdk inhibitor p27 and its deregulation in cancer. *J Cell Physiol* 183(1):10–17, 2000.

87. Kubbutat MH: Regulation of p53 stability by Mdm2. *Nature* 15(387):299–303, 1997.

88. Kaufmann H: Anti-tumor activity of rituximab plus thalidomide in patients with relapsed/refractory mantle cell lymphoma. *Blood*, First Edition Paper: DOI 10:1182, 2004.

89. Drach J: Durable remissions after rituximab plus thalidomide for relapsed/refractory mantle cell lymphoma. In: *ASCO Annual Meeting*, 2004, Abstract 6583.

90. Thieblemont C: Small lymphocytic lymphoma, marginal zone B-cell lymphoma, and mantle cell lymphoma exhibit distinct gene-expression profiles allowing molecular diagnosis. *Blood* 103:2727–2737, 2004.

91. Hoffman WK: Altered apoptosis pathways in mantle cell lymphoma detected by oligonucleotide microarray. *Blood* 98:787–794, 2001.

92. Bennaceur-Griscelli A: High level of glutathione-S-transferase expression in mantle cell lymphomas. *Clin Cancer Res* 10:3029–3034, 2004.

93. Schrader C: Topoisomerase IIa expression in mantle cell lymphoma: a marker of cell proliferation and a prognostic factor for clinical outcome. *Leukemia* 1–7, 2004.

94. Behr TM: High-dose myeloablative radioimmunotherapy of mantle cell non-Hodgkin lymphoma with the iodine 131-labeled chimeric anti-CD20 antibody C2B8 and autologous stem cell support. *Cancer* 94:1363–1372, 2002.

# Chapter 56

# TREATMENT APPROACH TO HIGH-GRADE NON-HODGKIN'S LYMPHOMAS

*John W. Sweetenham*

The development of the Revised European American Lymphoma Classification and the subsequent World Health Organization (WHO) Classification of tumors of the hematopoietic and lymphoid tissues has resulted in a departure from the traditional "grading" of non-Hodgkin's lymphomas (NHLs) intrinsic to older lymphoma classifications, particularly the Working Formulation.[1] Despite this, the designation of high-grade NHL is generally considered to encompass Burkitt's lymphoma and precursor B-cell and T-cell lymphoblastic lymphoma/leukemia. Additionally, the entity of "atypical" Burkitt/Burkitt-like lymphoma, used to identify a group of aggressive B-cell NHLs with features in common with Burkitt's lymphoma (BL) and diffuse large B-cell NHL (DLBCL), is also included in this group of diseases.

## PRECURSOR B- AND T-CELL LYMPHOBLASTIC LYMPHOMA

### INTRODUCTION

Precursor T-cell and B-cell lymphoblastic leukemia and lymphoma are malignant diseases of lymphoblasts. Historically, the term lymphoblastic lymphoma (LBL) has been used to describe these diseases when they present with prominent nodal involvement and less clinically apparent involvement of the bone marrow or peripheral blood. LBL has been recognized as a distinct entity in most lymphoma classifications including the Working Formulation and Kiel classifications. However, since it is now clear that precursor LBL and leukemia are identical morphologically, and at the immunophenotypic and genotypic levels, they are recognized as a single entity in the WHO classification of lymphoid malignancies. Despite this, the clinical management of patients with predominantly nodal involvement has developed separately from that for lymphoblastic leukemias, and as a result, the treatment approach for LBL is different from that previously adopted for acute lymphoblastic leukemia (ALL). This is further confounded by the fact that the clinical distinction between LBL and ALL has varied between centers and between publications, making the literature on this subject difficult to interpret.

### FREQUENCY

LBL is a rare disease, comprising 2% of all NHLs.[2] Eighty-five to ninety percent of adult cases are of T-cell origin and occur most frequently in adolescent and young adult males.[3-6] The median age for patients with LBL is around 20 years, with most series reporting male predominance. There has been no apparent change in the incidence of LBL in recent years.

### CLINICAL FEATURES

LBL has a peak incidence in the second and third decades. Characteristic presenting features include male predominance, mediastinal involvement, occurring in 60–70% of patients, reflecting the thymic origin of the malignant cells in LBL, and pleural and pericardial effusions, sometimes with resulting cardiac tamponade. Symptoms and signs of superior vena caval obstruction may be present. Mediastinal masses are uncommon in patients with B-cell LBL. Peripheral lymph node involvement is present in 60–80% of the patients at diagnosis, most commonly in cervical, supraclavicular, and axillary regions.

LBL commonly involves the bone marrow and central nervous system (CNS). The frequency of bone marrow involvement at presentation is difficult to determine from published series in view of the variable distinction between LBL and ALL. In a recent prospective study from Europe, 21% of the adult patients with LBL had bone marrow involvement at presentation.[7] Leukemic overspill is also common, but the frequency is obscured by inconsistent distinction between LBL and ALL.

CNS involvement is uncommon at presentation, occurring in approximately 5–10% of the patients. Typical manifestations of CNS involvement include meningeal involvement with a pleocytosis in the cerebrospinal fluid, or cranial nerve involvement, characteristically involving ophthalmic or facial nerves. Several reports suggest that CNS involvement at presentation is more common in patients with bone marrow involvement. Although CNS involvement at presentation is uncommon, it is a frequent site of relapse in the absence of adequate prophylaxis, when the incidence of relapse has been reported to be as high as 31%.[8] Other less common sites of involvement include the liver, spleen, and subdiaphragmatic lymph nodes, as well as bone, skin, and testes.

### PATHOLOGY AND PATHOGENESIS

Precursor T- and B-cell LBLs are neoplasms of lymphoblasts of T- and B-cell lineage, respectively. Morphologically, they are very similar, comprising small- to medium-sized blast cells with little cytoplasm, inconspicuous nucleoli, and moderately condensed to dispersed chromatin.[4] Convoluted nuclei are sometimes seen, but this has no clinical significance. Extensive mitotic figures are usually seen and widespread apoptosis is a common feature. The presence of apoptotic bodies being phagocytosed by macrophages produces the "starry sky" pattern typical of high-grade NHLs. Although this appearance is more characteristic of BL, it occurs relatively frequently in lymphoblastic disease, and in most cases, there are clear morphologic distinctions between the two entities. Additionally, immunohistochemical and cytogenetic features of the two diseases are distinct, so that diagnostic confusion is rare. However, the distinction of lymphoblastic disease from other NHLs subtypes can be obscured in poorly processed or fixed tissue specimens. Additionally, lymphocyte-rich thymomas have similar morphologic features, but can usually be distinguished on the basis of the epithelial distribution characteristic of thymoma.

The typical immunophenotype for T- and B-cell LBL is summarized in Table 56.1.[9–13] Most cases of T-cell disease have clonal rearrangement of T-cell receptor genes, most commonly δ, although this finding is not specific to T-cell lineage, and may also be seen in B-cell disease. Chromosomal translocations involving T-cell receptor genes have little value diagnostically, although they provide important information regarding the pathogenesis of lymphoblastic disease (see below).

One-third of patients have chromosomal translocations involving the α and δ T-cell receptors (14q11.2), the β receptor (7q35), or the γ receptor (7p14-15).[14] These translocations typically result in high levels of coexpression of T-cell receptor genes with transcription factor genes (*TAL1/SCL, TAL2* and *LYL1*, and *HOX11/TLX1*).[15–17] These patterns of gene expression

| Table 56.1 | Immunophenotype of precursor lymphoblastic leukemia/lymphoma. Summarized from references 9–13 | |
| --- | --- | --- |
| **T cell (85–90%)** | | **B cell (10–15%)** |
| | TdT | |
| | CD99 | |
| | CD34 | |
| | sIg | |
| CD7 | | CD79a |
| CD5 | | CD19 |
| CD2 | | CD20+/− |
| sCD3⁻ | | |
| cCD3⁺ | | |
| CD4 +/− | | |
| CD8 +/− | | |

also characterize different stages in thymocyte maturation which, according to recent microarray studies, may identify specific molecular subtypes of lymphoblastic disease.[18] As an example, samples with gene expression profiles associated with TAL1 or LYL1 expression are similar to late cortical thymocytes, have relatively high expression of *bcl-2*, and demonstrate higher levels of drug resistance and a poorer prognosis.

### PROGNOSTIC FACTORS

Determining prognostic factors in lymphoblastic disease has been difficult, partly because of the rarity of this disease, and the limited sample size in most published reports, and partly because of the variable criteria for distinguishing between LBL and lymphoblastic leukemia.

Retrospective studies of patients with LBL have identified adverse clinical prognostic factors for overall and disease-free survival.[19–21] Few of these have been consistent across different series.

Coleman et al.[8] identified favorable and unfavorable risk groups in a series of 44 patients treated at Stanford University on the basis of Ann Arbor stage IV, bone marrow or CNS involvement, and serum lactate dehydrogenase (LDH) level <300 IU/L (normal = 200 IU/L). Patients with these factors were considered poor risk, with a 5-year freedom from relapse of only 19%. Good-risk patients, who lacked these factors, had a 5-year freedom from relapse rate of 94%.

The applicability of the International Prognostic Index (IPI) for aggressive NHLs has also been investigated. A retrospective series of 62 patients from France concluded that the IPI did not have prognostic significance in adults with LBL.[22] Similarly, a retrospective analysis of 26 patients with LBL was reported by the

Non-Hodgkin's Lymphoma Classification Project.[23] The number of IPI risk factors was not predictive of overall or failure-free survival.

The utility of the IPI was also investigated in a European randomized trial in adult patients,[7] representing the only prospectively collected data set in an unselected population. This study showed a statistically significant trend for lower overall survival with an increasing number of adverse factors according to the age-adjusted IPI ($p = 0.016$). However, although there was a clearly inferior survival in patients with three adverse factors, there was little distinction between those with zero, one, or two factors, and the value of the IPI as a prognostic model remains unclear.

Data regarding immunophenotypic and genetic risk factors in precursor lymphoblastic disease have been exclusively derived from patients with lymphoblastic leukemias. In adult patients with T-cell ALL, expression of T-cell antigens including CD1, CD2, CD4, and CD5 has been associated with a favorable prognosis. In the Cancer and Leukemia Group B 8364 study, overall and disease-free survival correlated with the number of T-cell antigens expressed. [24]

Gene expression profiles have identified subtypes of precursor T-cell lymphoblastic disease characterizing different stages in thymocyte maturation, which may identify prognostic subgroups.[18] Patients with *HOX11* expression show a pattern of gene expression corresponding to the early cortical thymocyte. This group has a favorable clinical outcome. These cells are apparently developmentally arrested at a stage at which they are particularly sensitive to drug-induced apoptosis.

In contrast, those samples with gene expression profiles associated with *TAL1* or *LYL1* expression resemble late cortical and early pro-T thymocytes, respectively, and show more drug resistance and correspondingly higher levels of *bcl-2*.

For patients with B-cell disease, most studies have been reported from childhood B-cell ALL series. Translocations involving the *MLL* gene at 11q23 predict for unfavorable outcome, as does the t(9;22)(q34;q11.2). Hyperdiploid karyotype, trisomy 4, 10, and 17 are favorable risk factors.

### TREATMENT

Studies conducted in the 1960s in LBL used chemotherapy regimens developed for the treatment of less clinically aggressive types of NHL.[4,5,22,25,26] These studies reported poor outcomes. For example, Nathwani et al. reported results in 95 patients (children and adults) treated on various protocols that did not include CNS prophylaxis.[4] Patients with leukemic involvement were included in these series. The complete response rate was 24%, and the median survival was 17 months, with less than 10% of patients alive and disease free at 5 years. Similar results were reported for other similar chemotherapy regimens.

The use of intensive chemotherapy and radiation protocols in childhood LBL resulted in substantial improvements in outcome. Long-term disease-free survival rates between 60 and 80% were reported for children treated with regimens such as LSA$_2$L$_2$. A randomized trial in childhood LBL, comparing LSA$_2$L$_2$ with COMP (cyclophosphamide, vincristine, methotrexate, prednisone) demonstrated a 2-year actuarial failure-free survival of 76% for the LSA$_2$L$_2$ arm compared with only 26% for those receiving COMP ($p = 0.0002$).[27]

Subsequently, chemotherapy/radiotherapy regimens similar in design to LSA$_2$L$_2$, adapted from those in adult ALL, have been applied to adult patients with LBL.[8,19,20,28–30] Most of these regimens are characterized by intensive remission induction chemotherapy, CNS prophylaxis, a phase of consolidation chemotherapy, and a prolonged maintenance phase, often lasting for 12–18 months.

Results from some of these regimens are summarized in Table 56.2. A recent study from MD Anderson Cancer Center has explored the use of hyperCVAD (fractionated cyclophosphamide, vincristine, doxorubicin, and dexamethasone, alternating with high-dose methotrexate and cytosine arabinoside) in 33 adult patients with LBL. Intrathecal CNS prophylaxis was given and mediastinal radiation was recommended (although not always given) to all patients with mediastinal presentations. They reported a 91% complete remission rate, and 3-year actuarial progression-free and overall survival rates of 66 and 70%, respectively.[31]

Since all of these series are small, differences in reported outcomes are unlikely to be significant. Results from the unselected patient series reported by the Non-Hodgkin's Lymphoma Classification Project are inferior to this, with a reported 5-year actuarial overall survival of only approximately 20%.[32] This may reflect selection bias in the clinical series.

### RADIATION THERAPY

In addition to the use of prophylactic cranial radiation for prevention of CNS disease, some protocols have included mediastinal radiation for patients who present with isolated or bulky mediastinal disease. The benefit of this approach is unknown. A report from MD Anderson Cancer Center described 47 patients over an 18-year period who received mediastinal radiation as a component of their initial induction therapy.[33] The use of mediastinal irradiation was associated with a lower incidence of mediastinal relapse, but had no effect on failure-free or overall survival. The 5-year overall and progression-free survival rates of 66 and 64% reported in this series are comparable to many other regimens that do not include mediastinal radiation.

### STEM CELL TRANSPLANTATION AS CONSOLIDATION THERAPY IN FIRST REMISSION

Several groups have investigated of the role of high-dose therapy with autologous or allogeneic stem cell

**Table 56.2    Results of intensive combination chemotherapy regimens in adults with lymphoblastic lymphoma**

| Reference | Regimen | Number of patients | Response rate | Failure-free survival/relapse-free survival | Overall survival |
|---|---|---|---|---|---|
| Coleman[8] | ALL-type protocols, intensified CNS prophylaxis in the second | 44 | 100% (95% CR, 5% PR) | 3-year FFS = 56% | 3 years = 56% |
| Slater[19] | Various ALL protocols | 51 | 80% CR for non leukemic; 77% CR for leukemic | N/A | 5-year actuarial OS = 45% |
| Bernasconi[20] | Various ALL protocols | 31 | 77% | 3-year RFS = 45% | 3-year = 59% |
| Morel[21] | CHOP plus various ALL protocols | 80 | 82% CR | 46% at 30 months | 51% at 30 months |
| Levine[28] | Modified LSA$_2$L$_2$ | 15 | 73% CR 27% PR | 5-year actuarial FFS = 35% | 5-year actuarial OS = 40% |
| Weinstein[29] | APO | 21 | 95% CR | 3-year actuarial FFS = 58% | 5-year actuarial OS = 69% |
| Hoelzer[30] | Two ALL-type protocols, including CNS and mediastinal irradiation | 45 | 93% CR | 7-year actuarial DFS = 62% | 7-year actuarial OS = 51% |

ALL, acute lymphoblastic leukemia; FFS, failure-free survival; RFS, relapse-free survival; OS, overall survival; CR, complete remission; PR, partial remission.

transplantation in first remission, in an attempt to reduce the relatively high rate of relapse after induction therapy.[23,34–36]

Reported results of this approach, summarized in Table 56.3, have appeared superior to those achieved with conventional dose consolidation and maintenance chemotherapy. Long-term disease-free survival in most of these series has been between 60 and 80%, but most of these studies have conducted survival analyses from the date of stem cell transplantation, and have therefore selected for patients who respond to initial induction therapy, and who are likely to represent a more favorable group. Very few of these studies have included a true intent to treat analysis. One such study

has been reported by Jost et al. in which all patients were followed from the date of diagnosis. The 3-year actuarial overall and event-free survival rates were 48 and 31%, respectively.[35] These results are comparable to those reported for conventional dose first-line therapy.

A small randomized trial has compared the use of high-dose therapy and autologous stem cell transplantation with conventional dose consolidation and maintenance therapy as postremission therapy in adult patients with LBL.[7] This study included 119 adult patients who were treated with intensive induction therapy, 111 of whom were assessable for response. The overall response rate was comparable to other series, at 82%. However, of 98 patients eligible

**Table 56.3    Results of first remission stem cell transplantation in adults with lymphoblastic lymphoma**

| Reference | Induction therapy/High-dose regimen/stem cell source | Number of patients | Failure-free survival/relapse-free survival | Overall survival |
|---|---|---|---|---|
| Bouabdallah[23] | Various ALL-type induction regimens/High-dose cyclophosphamide and TBI/allogeneic and autologous BMT | 62 (30 received bone marrow transplant in first CR) | 5 year EFS = 58% | 5 year OS = 60% |
| Verdonck[34] | CHOP or ALL-like induction/high-dose cyclophosphamide and TBI/autologous BMT | 9 | 6/9 in long-term remission | 6/9 long-term survivors |
| Jost[35] | MACOP-B or VACOP-B induction/high-dose cyclophosphamide and TBI or CBV/autologous BMT | 20 | 3-year EFS = 31% | 3-year OS = 48% |
| Sweetenham[36] | Multiple induction and high-dose regimens/ autologous BMT | 105 | 6-year PFS = 63% | 6-year OS = 64% |

ALL, acute lymphoblastic leukemia; EFS, even-free survival; OS, overall survival; PFS, pregression-free survival.

for randomization, only 65 were actually randomized. The 3-year actuarial relapse-free survival rate was 24% for patients receiving conventional consolidation and maintenance therapy, compared with 55% for those receiving high-dose therapy and autologous stem cell transplantation ($p = 0.065$). The corresponding values for overall survival were 45 and 56% ($p = 0.71$). The fact that there was a nonsignificant trend for improved relapse-free survival in the transplant arm, but no difference in overall survival, may be due to the fact that some patients who relapsed after conventional dose consolidation therapy were "rescued" by high-dose therapy in second remission.

The role of allogeneic transplantation in first relapse is also unclear. Limited prospectively collected data are available. These were reported in the context of the European randomized trial mentioned above. In this study 12 patients with HLA-identical sibling donors were treated with allogeneic transplantation in first remission. The 3-year actuarial overall survival of 58% for this group is comparable to results in patients receiving autologous transplants. A recent study from the International Bone Marrow Transplant Registry compared outcomes for autologous and allogeneic stem cell transplantation in adult patients with LBL.[37] This study included a subset of patients undergoing transplantation in first remission, although this subset was not analyzed separately. Patients undergoing allogeneic transplantation in this series had a lower relapse rate following transplant, but this was offset by a much higher rate of nonrelapse mortality, resulting in equivalent overall survival in both groups. At present there are, therefore, no data to suggest that allogeneic transplantation is the optimal approach.

### STEM CELL TRANSPLANTATION FOR RELAPSED OR REFRACTORY DISEASE

The use of conventional dose chemotherapy regimens as salvage therapy produces response rates of less than 10% and median overall of only around 9 months.[8,19–21] Some studies have investigated the role of autologous stem cell transplantation in this situation.

In a retrospective study from Europe, 41 patients underwent high-dose therapy and autologous stem cell transplantation in second complete remission.[36] The 3-year actuarial progression-free survival and overall survival for this group were 30 and 31%, respectively. The sensitivity of the disease to conventional dose therapy given prior to the transplant was predictive of outcome. The 5-year actuarial overall survival for those with chemosensitive relapse was 31% compared with 18% for those with chemorefractory disease.

Since patients in chemosensitive relapse have a superior outcome compared to those with chemorefractory relapse, all relapsing patients should receive conventional dose salvage therapy in an attempt to induce a second remission prior to high-dose therapy. However, even in those patients with refractory disease, the reported long-term disease-free survival of 18% is superior to that achieved with conventional dose salvage, and these patients should also be offered high-dose therapy.

In view of the relatively young age of adult patients with LBL, it is anticipated that their regimen-related mortality after allogeneic transplantation is likely to be relatively low. If a graft-versus-lymphoma effect exists in this disease, then the low relapse rate observed in patients who survive allogeneic transplantation might result in improved overall survival compared with autologous transplantation. A retrospective, case-controlled analysis from the European Group for Blood and Marrow Transplantation (EBMT) comparing autologous with allogeneic stem cell transplantation reported a lower relapse rate for patients receiving allogeneic compared with autologous stem cell transplantation (2% vs 48%, respectively, $p = 0.035$).[38] However, progression-free survival for both groups was equivalent because of the higher procedure-related mortality in the allogeneic group. Although one other series has reported a superior outcome for patients receiving HLA-matched allogeneic transplants, this was also a small retrospective series.[23] Patients proceeding to allogeneic transplant are likely to be favorable in terms of age, performance status, and time in remission prior to transplant–all factors that might bias for improved survival.

The study mentioned above, from the International Bone Marrow Transplant Registry, compared outcomes for autologous and allogeneic stem cell transplantation in adult patients with LBL. No difference in survival was observed.[37]

## BURKITT'S LYMPHOMA

BL is a rare tumor of mature B cells, thought to be of germinal center origin. Clinically, it is a highly aggressive disease, with frequent extranodal presentation, which may present as an acute leukemia. It is composed of monomorphic medium-sized B cells with numerous mitotic figures and basophilic cytoplasm. Single translocations involving the c-myc oncogene are always present in this disease, and may help to distinguish it from other aggressive B-cell lymphomas. Variant cases of BL, designated as atypical BL, Burkitt-like lymphoma, and BL with plasmacytoid differentiation are also recognized.

### FREQUENCY

Three distinct clinical variants of BL are recognized, each of which has a distinct morphology and biologic behavior.

### Endemic Burkitt's lymphoma

The original description of BL was based on this subtype of the disease, which occurs in equatorial Africa, where it is the most common childhood tumor.[39] It shows male predominance and a peak incidence at 4–7 years. The areas of peak incidence appear to coincide with the distribution of endemic malaria.[40]

### Sporadic Burkitt's lymphoma

This variant is seen throughout the world, and has a peak incidence in children and young adults, with a median age of about 30 years. It comprises between 1 and 2% of all NHLs in the United States of America and Western Europe.[41]

### Burkitt's lymphoma in association with immunodeficiency

This variant is primarily seen in patients with acquired immunodeficiency syndrome (AIDS), and may also occur in other immune compromised patients, including those who receive immunosuppressive therapy following solid organ or stem cell transplantation.[42]

### CLINICAL FEATURES

The clinical characteristics of BL differ between endemic and sporadic cases, although there is some overlap between these two entities. Frequent extranodal sites of involvement are seen in all cases. The classical presentation of endemic BL, with a jaw tumor, is seen in 50% to 70% of endemic cases, but less than 10% of sporadic BL.[39,43,44]

The majority of cases (around 90%) of sporadic BL present with abdominal masses, frequently involving the ileocecal region.[45] Common presenting symptoms therefore include abdominal pain and distension, change in bowel habit, nausea and vomiting, and occasionally, gastrointestinal bleeding or perforation. Abdominal obstruction secondary to intussusception may also occur. Retroperitoneal disease is common, and may result in extradural extension and spinal cord compression. Other frequent sites of involvement in sporadic BL include bone marrow (20%), pleural effusions (20%), and CNS disease (15%). Breast involvement, although uncommon, is associated with onset of the disease at puberty, or during pregnancy and lactation, and is typically bilateral, and often very bulky.[46,47]

CNS disease most commonly presents either with cranial nerve palsies or with cerebrospinal fluid pleocytosis.[48] Numbness of the lip and chin, associated with compression of the inferior alveolar nerve is relatively frequent in patients with bone marrow disease, presumably because this nerve passes through the mandible. Although this is not, in itself, indicative of CNS disease, it is a well-documented risk factor for involvement of the CNS.[49]

### PATHOLOGY AND PATHOGENESIS

#### Classical Burkitt's lymphoma

This pattern is seen in almost all cases of endemic BL, most cases of sporadic BL, and many cases of immunodeficiency-associated disease. Affected tissues are diffusely infiltrated by monomorphic, medium-sized cells. A distinct "starry sky" pattern can be seen as a result of the presence of benign macrophages ingesting nuclear debris resulting from the apoptotic death of the lymphoma cells. A very high proliferation rate is characteristic of BL. "Squaring off" of the cytoplasm is a common feature, especially using mercury-based fixatives such as B5.[1]

### Variant BL with plasmacytoid differentiation

This variant is most commonly seen in BL associated with HIV infection. Pleomorphism in nuclear shape and size is more common than in classical BL. Nuclei are often slightly eccentric, and nucleoli are frequently single and central, giving the appearance of plasmacytoid immunoblasts.[1,50] This results in a morphology that has some features of diffuse large B-cell lymphoma.

### Atypical Burkitt's and Burkitt-like lymphoma

*Atypical* BL is characterized by a very high proliferation fraction (close to 100% Ki-67 or MIB-1 positive) in association with evidence of the presence of *c-myc* translocation.[1,51] It differs from classical BL morphologically in that there is greater nuclear pleomorphism and nucleoli are more prominent, but present in lower numbers. The atypical morphologic features are probably related more to tissue processing artifact than to true biologic differences, and all other features of this entity are identical to classical BL, with the typical immunophenotype, including presence of CD10, absence of *bcl-2*, and cytogenetic or molecular evidence of a *myc* translocation as a single genetic abnormality.

Cases designated as *Burkitt-like* lymphoma are biologically distinct from classical BL, and have some features more consistent with diffuse large B-cell lymphoma.[1,52] As such they represent "gray zone" cases. Although these cases usually show a diffuse pattern of lymph node infiltration, cases with a follicular pattern are sometimes seen. High mitotic rates and a starry sky pattern are common, but large centroblasts are nearly always present. These cases usually have a lower proliferation rate by MIB-1 or Ki-67, and may either lack *c-myc* translocations or show *c-myc* and *bcl-2* rearrangements in the same cells.

The typical immunophenotype for BL is summarized in Table 56.4. Tumor cells in classical and atypical BL are mature B cells that express CD19, CD20, CD22, and Cd79a, along with surface IgM, commonly with light chain restriction. Their germinal center origin is confirmed by frequent expression of CD10 and *bcl-6*.

All cases of BL have a translocation of *myc* at band q24 from chromosome 8 either to the Ig heavy chain region on chromosome 14 [t(8;14)] or to the light chain loci on chromosome 22q11 [t(8;22)] or chromosome 2q11 [t(2;8)].[1] For those cases with t(8;14) translocations,

| Table 56.4 | Immunophenotype and genetic/molecular features of Burkitt's lymphoma and variants | | |
|---|---|---|---|
| | Classical Burkitt's lymphoma | Atypical Burkitt's lymphoma | Burkitt-like lymphoma |
| CD10 | ++ | ++ | +/− |
| Bcl-2 | − | − | ++/− |
| Bcl-6 | ++ | ++ | +/− |
| Cytogenetics | t(8;14) or t(2;8) or t(8;22) | t(8;14) or t(2:8) or t(8;22) | Variable. Myc translocation may be present and may coexist with Bcl-2 translocation |
| Molecular features | Myc rearrangement | Myc rearrangement | Bcl-2 +/−, myc =/− |

the breakpoint varies between sporadic and endemic cases. In endemic cases, the breakpoint is at the heavy chain joining region, characteristic of a relatively early B cell. In sporadic cases, the translocation affects the Ig switch region, which characterizes a later stage of B-cell development.[53] The *myc* gene becomes constitutively expressed with the result that the cells progress through the cell cycle. This is thought to be the critical event in lymphomagenesis in this disease, although *myc* activation also activates various target genes that are involved in the regulation of apoptosis.

### The role of Epstein–Barr virus

The Epstein–Barr virus (EBV) is known to be an important factor in the development of endemic BL, where it is present in the majority of tumor cells. It is thought that the development of the lymphoma in this case is preceded by a long period of polyclonal B-cell activation secondary to multiple infective events, including the presence of EBV as well as malaria. Subsequent abnormal T-cell regulation of EBV infected cells may then lead to the development of lymphoma.[44,54]

In contrast to endemic disease, the incidence of EBV in sporadic BL is less, at about 30% in immunocompetent patients, and about 25–40% in those who are immunosuppressed.[42,55] Although EBV is implicated in the etiology of BL, its exact role remains unclear.

### TREATMENT

The treatment of BL is largely based upon the use of dose-intensive, multiagent chemotherapy regimens, which incorporate high-dose systemic methotrexate and cytosine arabinoside for control of potential CNS as well as systemic disease. Most of the regimens developed in the last 5–10 years have initially been used in pediatric populations, and subsequently adapted for treatment of adults. Overall, modern regimens have been highly effective, with long-term remissions reported in over 90% of the patients, even with advanced and apparently poor risk disease. Risk stratification has gained increasing importance in terms of determining therapy of appropriate intensity.

Several models for risk stratification have been developed in recent years. These are summarized in Table 56.5. For adults with BL, the risk factors described for patients entered into the NCI-89-C-41 protocol have been most widely applied.[58] In the original description of this regimen in adults, patients with high-risk disease received alternating cycles of cyclophosphamide, vincristine, doxorubicin, methotrexate (CODOX-M) and ifosfamide, etoposide, cytosine, arabinoside (IVAC) therapy (see below) whereas those with low-risk disease received a less intensive treatment protocol including CODOX-M chemotherapy only. In a subsequent European trial of a modified version of this protocol, similar risk stratification was used, in which low-risk patients were defined as having a normal LDH level, WHO performance status of 0 or 1, Ann Arbor stage I or II, and no residual tumor masses >10 cm in diameter.[59] All other patients were regarded as high risk. The most widely used regimens for BL have initially been introduced in pediatric populations, and subsequently adapted for adults, usually with comparable results. Details of reports of some of these regimens are summarized in Table 56.6. Most of these regimens are highly myelosuppressive, with high rates of neutropenia and infectious complications, and require support with hematopoietic growth factors. Common aspects of these regimens include intensive induction therapy with multiple chemotherapy agents, relatively short treatment duration, absence of any proven benefit from prolonged or maintenance therapy, and the use of CNS prophylaxis and therapy. In view of the high proliferation rate of these tumors, the importance of rapid initiation of cycles of chemotherapy as early as possible after hematopoietic recovery has been realized, and the use of nonmyelosuppressive drugs at the time of neutrophil nadir to maintain dose intensity is also a principle of several regimens.

The use of radiation therapy, even as a method of CNS treatment or prophylaxis, has been largely abandoned in the absence of data from randomized trials demonstrating its benefit compared with high-dose systemic methotrexate of cytarabine, coupled with

**Table 56.5    Pregnostic risk factors for adult Burkitt's lymphoma**

| Berlin–Frankfurt–Munich (BFM) group[56] | | LMB group[57] | | National Cancer Institute[58] | |
|---|---|---|---|---|---|
| Risk group | Features | Risk group | Features | Risk group | Features |
| 1 | Complete surgical resection | A | Complete surgical resection stage I or abdominal stage II | Low risk | Stage I or II and LDH <150% of normal |
| 2 | Incomplete surgical resection: Stage I and II Stage III with LDH <500 IU/L | B | All patients not in groups A or C | High risk | All other patients |
| 3 | Incomplete surgical resection: Stage III with LDH 500–999 IU/L Stage V or B-cell leukemia with LDH<1000 IU/L; CNS negative | C | Central nervous system involvement or bone marrow involvement with ≥25% blasts | | |
| 4 | Incomplete surgical resection: Stage III and LDH >999 IU/L Stage IV or B-cell leukemia and LDH > 999 IU/L ±CNS | | | | |

LDH, lactate dehydrogenase; CNS, central nervous system.

intrathecal therapy or prophylaxis. Despite this, some groups continue to use radiation therapy, although at reduced doses, as a component of CNS prophylaxis or treatment.[63] No agreed standard of care exists for the initial treatment of BL. Most regimens in common use have features as described above.

Results of these regimens have improved progressively over the last 20 years. Pediatric patients with limited-stage disease, generally defined as stage I or II, completely resected abdominal disease, have long-term disease-free survival rates of 90–100% when treated with combination chemotherapy regimens described above.

In adult patients, some single center studies have reported similar results. In the study from the National Cancer Institute, using the NCI 89-C-41 protocol in an adult population, all patients with limited-stage disease, treated with three cycles of the CODOX-M regimen, achieved long-term disease-free survival, although patient numbers in this series were small.[58] In a subsequent multicenter study of a modified NCI 89-C-41 protocol in Europe, including an older, less selected patient population, the 2-year actuarial event-free survival was 83%.[59]

Results from most other groups using comparable chemotherapy have been similar. No single combination has emerged as being superior and any intensive multiagent regimen with the characteristics described above, such as those included in Table 56.6, can be considered acceptable.

**Table 56.6    Results of intensive combination chemotherapy regimens in adults with Burkitt's lymphoma**

| First author & reference | Regimen | Number of patients | Response rate | Failure-free survival/ relapse-free survival | Overall survival |
|---|---|---|---|---|---|
| Soussain et al[60] | Various LMB protocols | 65 | 89% CR | N/A | 74% at 3 years |
| McMaster et al[61] | Novel intensive chemotherapy-only regimen | 20 | 85% CR | 60% at 5 years | 60% at 5 years |
| Magrath et al[58] | NCI 89-C-41 | 39 | 95% CR | 92% at 2 years | 92 % at 2 years |
| Mead et al[59] | Modified NCI 89-C-41 | 52 | 87% OR (77% CR) | 65% at 2 years | 73% at 2 years |
| Thomas et al [62] | Hyper-CVAD | 26 | 81% | N/A | 49% at 3 years |

CR, complete remission.

## STEM CELL TRANSPLANTATION AS CONSOLIDATION THERAPY IN FIRST REMISSION

There have been only a limited number of studies addressing the role of high-dose therapy and autologous or allogeneic stem cell transplantation in first remission in this disease. This is mainly a result of the effectiveness of intensive induction chemotherapy regimens with high survival rates as documented above. In view of these excellent results, there is little rationale for the use of early stem cell transplantation.

The largest reported series of patients with Burkitt's or Burkitt-like NHL undergoing autologous stem cell transplantation was reported by the EBMT.[64] This retrospective, registry-based study included 70 patients receiving high-dose therapy in first complete remission after induction chemotherapy. Various induction chemotherapy regimens had been used. The actuarial 3-year progression-free and overall survival rates were 72 and 73%, respectively.

In an intention to treat analysis by Jost et al., patients with LBL and BL received a brief duration induction chemotherapy regimen followed by high-dose therapy and autologous stem cell transplantation for responding patients.[35] The estimated 3-year event-free and overall survival were 31 and 48%, respectively, indicating the inadequacy of the initial induction therapy in this group. There is no evidence at present to suggest an improvement in survival with first remission transplantation for patients in remission after intensive induction chemotherapy regimens.

## STEM CELL TRANSPLANTATION FOR RELAPSED OR REFRACTORY DISEASE

The outcome for patients with relapsed or primary refractory Burkitt's and Burkitt-like lymphoma is poor, with reported median survival duration of only 6 months after conventional dose second-line chemotherapy regimens. Very few series have specifically addressed the role of high-dose therapy in this context. The study from the EBMT included 32 patients with relapsed and refractory disease. For those with chemosensitive relapses, long-term progression-free survival of 37% was reported, suggesting that transplant strategies may benefit this group. By contrast, patients with resistant relapses or primary refractory disease progressed rapidly, with most having relapse within 6 months of autologous transplantation.[64]

Very few reports have specifically addressed the role of allogeneic transplantation for Burkitt's and Burkitt-like lymphoma. There are anecdotal reports suggesting a possible graft-versus-lymphoma effect on this disease, but few comparative data with autologous stem cell transplantation. A matched analysis from the EBMT included 71 patients with BL receiving allogeneic transplants from a variety of donors, who were matched with 416 patients receiving autologous transplants.[38] No differences in either relapse rates or overall survival were reported according to stem cell source. At present, there is no evidence to suggest that allogeneic transplantation is associated with superior outcome, and its use should probably be reserved for patients with bone marrow or peripheral blood involvement or those treated on trial protocols.

## REFERENCES

1. Jaffe ES, Harris NL, Stein H, et al.: *Tumors of the haematopoietic and lymphoid tissues. World Health Organization.* Lyon, France: IARC Press; 2001.
2. The non-Hodgkin's Lymphoma Classification Project: A clinical evaluation of the International Lymphoma Study Group classification of non-Hodgkin's lymphomas. *Blood* 89:3909–3918, 1997.
3. Rosen PJ, Feinstein DI, Pattengale PK, et al.: Convoluted lymphocytic lymphoma in adults: a clinicopathological entity. *Ann Intern Med* 89:319–324, 1978.
4. Nathwani BN, Diamond LW, Winberg CD, et al.: Lymphoblastic lymphoma: A clinicopathologic study of 95 patients. *Cancer* 48:2347–2357, 1978.
5. Murphy SB: Management of childhood non-Hodgkin's lymphoma. *Cancer Treat Rep* 61:1161–1173, 1977.
6. Warnke RA, Weiss LM, Chan JKC, et al.: Tumors of the lymph nodes and spleen. In: *Atlas of Tumor Pathology.* Washington, DC: Armed Forces Institute of Pathology; 1995.
7. Sweetenham JW, Santini G, Qian W, et al.: High-dose therapy and autologous stem-cell transplantation versus conventional dose consolidation/maintenance therapy as post-remission therapy for adult patients with lymphoblastic lymphoma: results of a randomized trial of the European Group for Blood and Marrow Transplantation and the United Kingdom Lymphoma Group. *J Clin Oncol* 19:2927–2936, 2001.
8. Coleman NC, Picozzi VJ, Cox RS, et al.: Treatment of lymphoblastic lymphoma in adults. *J Clin Oncol* 4:1626–1637, 1986.
9. Griffith RC, Kelly DR, Nathwani BN, et al.: A morphologic study of childhood lymphoma of the lymphoblastic type: the Pediatric Oncology Group experience. *Cancer* 1987; Cossman J, Chused TM, Fisher RI, et al.: Diversity of immunologic phenotypes of lymphoblastic lymphoma. *Cancer Res* 43:4486–4490, 1983.
10. Sheibani K, Nathwani BN, Winberg CD, et al.: Antigenically defined subgroups of lymphoblastic lymphoma: relationship to clinical presentation and biological behavior. *Cancer* 60:183–190, 1987.
11. Link MP, Stewart SJ, Warnke RA, et al.: Discordance between surface and cytoplasmic expression of the Leu-4(T3) antigen I thymocytes and in blast cells from childhood T lymphoblastic malignancies. *J Clin Invest* 76:248–253, 1985.
12. Chilosi M, Pizzolog G: Review of terminal deoxynucleotidyl transferase: biological aspects, methods of detection, and selected diagnostic applications. *Appl Immunohistochem* 3:209–221, 1995.
13. Borowitz M Ferrando AA, Neuberg D, Staunton J, et al.: Gene expression signatures define novel oncogenic pathways in T cell acute lymphoblastic leukemia. *Cancer Cell* 1:75–87, 2002.

14. Bonowitz MJ: Immunologic markers in childhood acute lymphoblastic leukemia. *Hematol Oncol Clin North Am* 4:743–765, 1990.

15. Okuda T, Fisher R, Downing JR: Molecular diagnostics in pediatric acute lymphoblastic leukemia. *Mol Diagn* 1:139–151, 1996.

16. Finger LR, Kagan J, Christopher G, et al. Involvement of the TCL5 gene on human chromosome 1 in T-cell leukemia and melanoma. *Proc Natl Acad Sci USA* 86:5039–5043, 1989.

17. Mellentin JD, Smith SD, Cleary ML: Lyl-1, A novel gene altered by chromosomal translocation in T-cell leukemia, codes for a protein with helix-loop-helix DNA binding motif. *Cell* 58:77–83, 1989.

18. Xia Y, Brown L, Yang CY, et al.: TAL2, a helix-loop-helix gene activated by the t(7;9)(q34;q32) translocation in human T-cell leukemia. *Proc Natl Acad Sci USA* 88:11416–11420, 1989.

19. Slater DE, Mertelsmann R, Koriner B, et al.: Lymphoblastic lymphoma in adults. *J Clin Oncol* 4:57-67, 1986.

20. Bernasconi C, Brusamolino E, Lazzarino M, et al.: Lymphoblastic lymphoma in adult patients; clinico-pathological features and response to intensive multi-agent chemotherapy analogous to that used in acute lymphoblastic leukemia. *Ann Oncol* 1:141–160, 1990.

21. Morel P, Lepage E, Brice P, et al.: Prognosis and treatment of lymphoblastic lymphoma in adults: A report on 80 patients. *J Clin Oncol* 10:1078–1085, 1992.

22. Voakes JB, Jones SE, McKelvey EM: The chemotherapy of lymphoblastic lymphoma. *Blood* 57:186–188, 1981.

23. Bouabdallah R, Xerri L, Bardou V-J, et al.: Role of induction chemotherapy and bone marrow transplantation in adult lymphoblastic lymphoma: a report on 62 patients from a single center. *Ann Oncol* 9:619–625, 1998.

24. Czuczman MS, Dodge RK, Stewart CC, et al.: Value of imunophenotype in intensively treated adult acute lymphoblastic leukemia: Cancer and Leukemia Group B study 8364. *Blood* 93:3931–3939, 1999.

25. Colgan JP, Anderson J, Habermann TM, et al.: Long-term follow-up of a CHOP-based regimen with maintenance chemotherapy and central nervous system prophylaxis in lymphoblastic non-Hodgkin's lymphoma. *Leuk Lymphoma* 15:291–296, 1994.

26. Kaiser U, Uebelacker I, Havemann K: Non-Hodgkin's lymphoma protocols in the treatment of patients with Burkitt's lymphoma and lymphoblastic lymphoma: a report on 58 patients. *Leuk Lymphoma* 36:101–108, 1999.

27. Anderson JR, Wilson JF, Jenkin RDT, et al.: Childhood non-Hodgkin's lymphoma. The results of a randomized therapeutic trial comparing a 4-drug regimen (COMP) with a 10-drug regimen (LSA₂L₂). *New Engl J Med* 308:559–565, 1983.

28. Levine AM, Forman SJ, Meyer PR, et al.: Successful therapy of convoluted T-lymphoblastic lymphoma in the adult. *Blood* 61:92–99, 1983.

29. Weinstein HJ, Cassady JR, Levey R: Long-term results of the APO protocol (vincristine, doxorubicin [adriamycin] and prednisone) for the treatment of mediastinal lymphoblastic lymphoma. *J Clin Oncol* 1:537–541, 1983.

30. Hoelzer D, Gokbuget N, Digel W, et al.: Outcome of adult patients with T-lymphoblastic lymphoma treated according to protocols for acute lymphoblastic leukemia. *Blood* 99:4379–4385, 2002.

31. Thomas DA, O'Brien S, Cortes J, et al.: Outcome with the hyper-CVAD regimens in lymphoblastic lymphoma. *Blood* 104:1624–1630, 2004.

32. Armitage JO, Weisenberger DD: New approach to classifying non-Hodgkin's lymphomas: Clinical features of the major histologic subtypes. *J Clin Oncol* 16:2780–2795, 1998.

33. Dabaja BS, Ha CS, Thomas DA, et al.: The role of local radiation therapy for mediastinal disease in adults with T-cell lymphoblastic lymphoma. *Cancer* 94:2738–2744, 2002.

34. Verdonck LF, Dekker AW, deGast GC, et al.: Autologous bone marrow transplantation for adult poor risk lymphoblastic lymphoma in first remission. *J Clin Oncol* 4:644–646, 1992.

35. Jost LM, Jacky E, Dommann-Scherrer C, et al.: Short-term weekly chemotherapy followed by high dose therapy with autologous bone marrow transplantation for lymphoblastic and Burkitt's lymphomas in adult patients. *Ann Oncol* 6:445–451, 1995.

36. Sweetenham JW, Santini G, Pearce R, et al.: High-dose therapy and autologous bone marrow transplantation for adult patients with lymphoblastic lymphoma: Results from the European Group for Bone Marrow Transplantation. *J Clin Oncol* 12:1358–1365, 1994.

37. Levine JE, Harris RE, Loberiza FR, et al.: A comparison of allogeneic and autologous bone marrow transplantation for lymphoblastic lymphoma. *Blood* 101:2476–2482, 2003.

38. Chopra R, Goldstone AH, Pearce R, et al.: Autologous versus allogeneic bone marrow transplantation for non-Hodgkin's lymphoma: a case controlled analysis of the European Bone Marrow Transplant Group registry data. *J Clin Oncol* 10:1690–1695, 1992.

39. Burkitt D: A sarcoma involving the jaws in African children. *Br J Surg* 46:218–223, 1958.

40. Dalldorf G, Linsell CA, Marnhart FE, et al.: An epidemiological approach to the lymphomas of African children and Burkitt's sarcoma of the jaws. *Perspect Biol Med* 7:435–449, 1964.

41. Wright D, McKeever P, Carter R: Childhood non-Hodgkin's lymphomas in the United Kingdom: findings from the UK Children's Cancer Study Group. *J Clin Pathol* 50:128–134, 1997.

42. Raphael M, Gentilhomme O, Tulliez M, et al.: Histopathologic features of high grade non-Hodgkin's lymphomas in acquired immunodeficiency syndrome. *Arch Pathol Lab Med* 115:15–20, 1991.

43. Burkitt DP: General features and facial tumours. In: Burkitt DP, Wright DH (eds.) *Burkitt's lymphoma*. Edinburgh and London: Livingstone; 1970.

44. Wright DH: Burkitt's lymphoma: a review of the pathology, immunology and possible aetiological factors. In: Sommers SC (ed.), *Pathology Annual*. New York: Appleton-Century-Crofts;1971:249–261.

45. Levine PH, Kamaraju LS, Connelly RR, et al.: The American Burkitt's Lymphoma Registry: eight years' experience. *Cancer* 49:1016–1022, 1982.

46. Shepherd JJ, Wright DH: Burkitt's tumour presenting as bilateral swelling of the breast in women of childbearing age. *Br J Surg* 54:776–780, 1967.

47. Hugh JC, Jackson FI, Hanson J, et al.: Primary breast lymphoma. An immunohistologic study of 20 new cases. *Cancer* 66:2602–2611, 1990.

48. Ziegler JL, Magrath IT. Burkitt's lymphoma. In: Ioachim HL, (ed.) *Pathobiology Annual*. New York: Appleton Century Croft, 1974:129–142.

49. Landesberg R, Yee H, Datikashvili M, et al.: Unilateral mandibular lip anesthesia the sole presenting symptom of Burkitt's lymphoma: case report and review of the literature. *J Oral Maxillofac Surg* 59:322–326, 2001.

50. Hui PK, Feller AC, Lennert K: High-grade non-Hodgkin's lymphoma of B-cell type. I: Histopathology. *Histopathology*12:127–143, 1988.

51. Spina D, Leoncini L, Megha T, et al.: Cellular kinetic and phenotypic heterogeneity in and among Burkitt's and Burkitt-like lymphomas. *J Pathol* 182:145–150, 1997.

52. Braziel RM, Arber DA, Slovak ML, et al.: The Burkitt-like lymphomas: a Southwest Oncology Group study delineating phenotypic, genotypic, and clinical features. *Blood* 97:3713–3720, 2001.

53. Yano T, Sander CA, Clark HM, et al.: Clustered mutations in the second exon of the MYC gene in sporadic Burkitt's lymphoma. *Oncogene* 8:2741-2748, 1993.

54. Facer CA, Playfair JH: Malaria, Epstein-Barr Virus and the genesis of lymphomas. *Adv Cancer Res* 53:33–72, 1989.

55. Gutierrez MI, Bhatia K, Barriga F, et al.: Molecular epidemiology of Burkitt's lymphoma from South America: differences in breakpoint location and Epstein Barr Virus association from tumors in other World regions. *Blood* 79:3261–3266,1992.

56. Reiter A, Schrappe M, Tiemann M, et al.: Improved treatment results in childhood B-cell neoplasms with tailored intensification of therapy: a report of the Berlin-Frankfurt-Munich NHL-BFM 90. *Blood* 94:3294–3306, 1999.

57. Patte C, Michon J, Frappaz D, et al.: Therapy of Burkitt and other B-cell acute lymphoblastic leukemia and lymphoma: experience with the LMB protocols of the SFOP (French Paediatric Oncology Society) in children and adults. *Balliere's Clin Hamatol* 2: 339–348, 1994.

58. Magrath I, Adde M, Shad A, et al.: Children and adults with small non-cleaved cell lymphoma have a similar excellent outcome when treated with the same chemotherapy regimen. *J Clin Oncol* 14:925–934, 1996.

59. Mead GM, Sydes MR, Walewski J, et al.: An international evaluation of CODOX-M and CODOX-M alternating with IVAC in adult Burkitt's lymphoma: results of United Kingdom Lymphoma Group LY06 study. *Ann Oncol* 13:1264–1274, 2002.

60. Soussain C, Patte C, Ostronoff M, et al.: Small non-cleaved cell lymphoma and leukemia in adults. A retrospective study of 65 adults treated with the LMB pediatric protocols. *Blood* 85:664–674, 1995.

61. McMaster M, Greer JP, Greco A, et al.: Effective treatment of small-noncleaved cell lymphoma with high-intensity, brief duration chemotherapy. *J Clin Oncol* 9:941–946, 1991.

62. Thomas DA, Cortes J, O'Brien S, et al.: Hyper-CVAD program in Burkitt's type adult acute lymphoblastic leukemia. *J Clin Oncol* 17:2461–2470, 1999.

63. Rizzieri DA, Johnson JL, Niedzwiecki D, et al.: Intensive chemotherapy with and without cranial radiation for Burkitt leukemia and lymphoma. *Cancer* 100:1438–1448, 2004.

64. Sweetenham JW, Pearce R, Taghipour G, et al.: Adult Burkitt's and Burkitt-like non-Hodgkin's lymphoma–outcome for patients treated with high-dose therapy and autologous stem cell transplantation in first remission or at relapse: results from the European Group for Blood and Marrow Transplantation. *J Clin Oncol* 14:2465–2472, 1996.

# Chapter 57

# TREATMENT APPROACH TO MARGINAL ZONE AND MALT LYMPHOMAS

*Emanuele Zucca*

The term *marginal zone lymphoma* (MZL) is believed to be derived from B cells normally present in the marginal zone and was proposed in the Revised European–American Lymphoma (REAL) classification[1] to take account of three apparently related lymphoma subtypes, namely the extranodal "low-grade B-cell lymphoma of mucosa-associated lymphoid tissue (MALT)" usually named MALT lymphoma, the nodal "monocytoid B-cell lymphoma," and the "primary splenic MZL with or without villous lymphocytes". At that time, the available cytogenetic data seemed to suggest that all three of these lymphomas share similar cytogenetic alterations, but several important cytogenetic and molecular genetic observations have later revealed the distinctiveness of these lymphoid neoplasms, and each is now considered a separate subtype in the World Health Organization (WHO) classification.[2–4]

While splenic and nodal MZL are very rare disorders, each comprising less than 1% of lymphomas,[5] the extranodal MZL of MALT type is not uncommon. In a survey of more than 1400 non-Hodgkin's lymphomas from nine institutions in the United States of America, Canada, the United Kingdom, Switzerland, France, Germany, South Africa, and Hong Kong, this entity represented approximately 8% of the total number of cases, including both the most common gastrointestinal (GI) and the less usual non-GI localizations.[5]

## EXTRANODAL MARGINAL ZONE LYMPHOMA OF MALT

### DISEASE FEATURES
#### Pathology
Primary gastric MALT lymphoma is the most common and best studied MALT lymphoma but the histologic features of extranodal B-cell MZL (MALT lymphomas) are similar regardless of the site of origin.[2,6,7] The most striking feature of MALT lymphoma is the presence of a variable number of lymphoepithelial lesions defined by evident invasion and partial destruction of mucosal glands by the tumor cells. The morphology of MALT lymphoma cells is heterogeneous. Marginal zone cells are the predominant component and are small-to-medium-size cells with irregularly shaped nuclei (centrocytelike cells). Other cell types comprise monocytoid cells and small B lymphocytes. A degree of plasma cell differentiation is often present. Any of these cytologic aspects can predominate, or they can coexist within the same case. The B cells of MALT lymphoma show the immunophenotype of the normal marginal zone B cells present in spleen, Peyer's patches, and in lymph nodes. Therefore, the tumor B cells express surface immunoglobulins and pan-B antigens (CD19, CD20, and CD79a), and the marginal-zone-associated antigens CD35 and CD21 but lack of CD5, CD10, CD23, and cyclin D1 expression. A number of nonneoplastic, reactive T cells are often present. Scattered transformed large blast cells are also usually found. Their prognostic significance is not fully understood, but only when solid or sheetlike proliferations of large cells are present should the lymphoma be considered to have transformed. The resulting tumor cannot reliably be distinguished from other diffuse large B-cell lymphomas. Therefore, the current recommendation is that such cases be defined as diffuse large B-cell lymphoma, avoiding the term "high-grade" MALT lymphomas.[2]

Certain histologic features appear to indicate that the MALT lymphoma B cells might be or have been involved in an immune response: the presence of tumor lymphocytes in the germinal centers of nonneoplastic follicles (follicular colonization), the presence of scattered transformed blasts, the often prominent plasma cell differentiation, and the often rich T-cell nonneoplastic component. MALT lymphoma usually arises in mucosal sites where lymphocytes are not normally present and where a MALT is acquired in response to either chronic infectious conditions or autoimmune processes: *Helicobacter pylori* gastritis, Hashimoto's thyroiditis, and Sjögren syndrome.[8] Sequence analysis of the immunoglobulin genes expressed by the MALT lymphoma B cells shows a pattern of somatic hypermutation and intraclonal variation, suggesting that the tumor cell has undergone antigen selection in germinal centers and that they continue to be at least partially driven by direct antigen stimulation.[9–12]

### Epidemiology and etiology

A significant association has been reported in epidemiologic studies between *H. pylori* infection and gastric lymphomas with either low-grade or high-grade histology.[13] In vitro experiments have demonstrated that the neoplastic cells of gastric MALT lymphoma proliferate in a strain-specific response to *H. pylori* and that this response is dependent on T-cell activation by the microorganism.[14] The presence of the B-cell clone that will become predominant in the transformation to MALT lymphoma has been demonstrated in the chronic *H. pylori* gastritis that preceded the lymphoma.[15] More than 20 studies have reported regressions of gastric MALT lymphoma in more than half of the treated patients after antibiotic eradication of *H. pylori*.[16] The association of *H. pylori* with gastric MALT lymphoma has led to the hypothesis that the microorganism may provide the antigenic stimulus for sustaining the growth of the lymphoma in the stomach. However, the tumor-derived immunoglobulin usually does not recognize *H. pylori* but does recognize various autoantigens.[17]

Besides *H. pylori*, other infectious agents have been associated to particular extranodal marginal zone B cell lymphomas. *Borrelia burgdorferi* may be implicated in the pathogenesis of at least a subset of cutaneous marginal zone B cell lymphomas. The microorganism can be found in skin lymphomas, and a complete remission can be achieved with adequate antibiotic therapy alone.[18–20]

Ferreri et al.[21] demonstrated the presence of *Chlamydia psittaci* in about 80% of ocular adnexa MZL and showed that antibiotics therapy aimed to the *C. psittaci* can be followed by histologic regression of these MZL.

*Campylobacter jejuni* has been associated with the immunoproliferative small intestine disease (IPSID, also known as alpha-chain disease) that is now considered an extranodal MZL, more frequent in Middle East, especially in the Mediterranean area.[22]

Since the 1970s, it was already known that early stage IPSID may regress after antibiotic therapies eliminating unknown organism(s),[23] but only in 2004 has this lymphoma been linked to a specific pathogen.[22]

All these data, together with the pattern of somatic hypermutation and ongoing mutations of the immunoglobulin genes, strongly associate the origin of extranodal MZLs, with a background of chronic antigenic stimulation associated with infectious conditions and/or autoimmune conditions. It can be postulated that interaction of host T cell and antigen-presenting cells with bacterial antigens or with cross-reactive autoantigens leads to a cascade of complex events, which finally results in autonomous clonal B-cell expansion and proliferation.

However, extranodal MZLs are relatively rare, while *H. pylori* infection is extremely common, being present in the stomach of one half of the world population.[24] Therefore, both bacterial and host factors have to interact to cause lymphoma. Polymorphisms affecting genes involved in inflammatory responses and antioxidative capacity may be part of the genetic background for the MALT lymphomagenesis in individual *H. pylori* infected persons.[25] The persistent antigenic stimulation may render the clone more susceptible to genetic alterations that can result in neoplastic transformation and tumor progression. Free radicals are likely to play a role in the development of B-cell genomic damage in the chronic gastritis, and their presence is increased in the presence of the CagA-positive strains of *H. pylori*.[26]

### Genetic abnormalities

The most common aberration is the t(11;18)(q21;q21), which results in a fusion of the apoptosis inhibitor gene *API2* with the *MALT1* gene.[27–29] The t(11;18) is present in 30–50% of extranodal MZL of MALT type, but not in nodal MZL lymphoma and splenic MZL.[30] It is usually the sole cytogenetic alteration. The frequency of the t(11;18) in MALT lymphoma is site related: more frequent in the GI tract and in the lung, less common in conjunctiva and orbit, and absent or almost absent in salivary glands, thyroid, liver, and skin.[26,31]

The t(1;14)(p22;q32) is much more rare, and it deregulates the expression of the survival-related gene *BCL10*, highly expressed in the nucleus of the neoplastic B cells of MALT lymphomas carrying this translocation.[32,33] Interestingly, nuclear expression of *BCL10* is also present in the t(11;18)-positive MALT lymphomas, indicating that nuclear localization of *BCL10* can occur as the consequence of two apparently independent cytogenetic events.[26,30,34] In MALT lymphomas without these translocations, as well as in nonneoplastic germinal center and marginal zone B cells, *BCL10* is expressed only in the cytoplasm.[35]

The t(14;18)(q32;q21) translocation, cytogenetically identical to the one involving *BCL12* in follicular lymphoma but involves MALT1 (which is localized about 5 Mb centromeric of *BCL12* on 18q21), has been described in approximately 20% of MALT lymphomas.[31,36,37] This translocation appears to be more common in lymphomas of ocular adnexa, liver, and skin than in GI tract and lung. In contrast to t(11;18), it is often associated with additional genetic abnormalities, such as trisomies of chromosome 3 and 12.

The three seemingly disparate translocations that target *BCL10* and MALT1 appear to affect the same signaling pathway, resulting in the constitutive activation of nuclear factor kappa B (NF-κB), a transcription factor with a central role in immunity, inflammation, and apoptosis.[38,39] This activation of the NF-κB pathway seems critical to lymphoma antigen-independent growth and progression.[40] Other cytogenetic abnormalities have also been reported but their pathogenetic role is unclear.[6]

## Clinical features

The presenting symptoms of MALT lymphomas are nonspecific and mainly related to their anatomic location. Few patients present with elevated lactate dehydrogenase (LDH) or β2-microglobulin levels.[41,42] Constitutional B symptoms are exceedingly uncommon.[41]

MALT lymphoma usually remains localized for a prolonged period within the tissue of origin, but involvement of multiple mucosal sites is not uncommon, being reported in up to one-third of cases. It has been postulated that this dissemination may be due to specific expression of special homing receptors or adhesion molecules on the surface of most MALT lymphoma cells and normal B cells of MALT.[43-45] Bone marrow involvement is reported in up to 20% of cases.[6] Within the stomach, low-grade MALT lymphoma is often multifocal and this may explain the report of relapses in the gastric stump after surgical excision. When regional lymph nodes are involved, MALT lymphoma cells tend to localize in the marginal zone without disturbing the lymph node architecture. Gastric MALT lymphoma can often disseminate to the splenic marginal zone where it is usually undetectable by conventional histopathology. The incidental discovery of secondary small intestinal MALT lymphoma during gastrectomy for MALT lymphoma has been reported too, and concomitant GI and non-GI involvement is found in approximately 10% of cases.

## DIAGNOSIS AND STAGING OF GASTRIC MALT LYMPHOMA

The stomach is the most common and best studied organ involved with MALT lymphoma and it will be helpful to discuss the clinical aspects of diagnosis, staging, and treatment of gastric MALT lymphoma separately from all other sites.

The most common presenting symptoms of gastric MALT lymphoma are dyspepsia, epigastric pain, nausea, and chronic manifestations of GI bleeding, such as anemia. The upper GI complaints often lead to an endoscopy that usually reveals nonspecific gastritis or peptic ulcer with mass lesions being unusual.[41]

The best staging system is still controversial.[46] We use the modification of the Blackledge staging system recommended at an international workshop.[47,48]

The initial staging procedures should include a gastroduodenal endoscopy with multiple biopsies from each region of the stomach, duodenum, gastroesophageal (GE)

junction, and from any abnormal-appearing site. The presence of active *H. pylori* infection must be determined by histochemistry and breath test. Endoscopic ultrasound is recommended to evaluate the presence of perigastric lymph nodes and the depth of infiltration of the gastric wall. A deep infiltration is associated with a higher risk of lymph node involvement, and a lower response rate with antibiotic therapy alone.[49-52] Presentation with multiple MALT localizations is more frequent in patients with non-GI lymphoma, in which about one-fourth of cases have been reported to present with involvement of multiple mucosal sites or nonmucosal sites such as bone marrow.[53,54]

Regardless of the presentation site, initial workup should include complete blood counts, basic biochemical studies (including LDH and β2-microglobulin), computed tomography of the chest, abdomen, and pelvis, and a bone marrow biopsy. Indeed, although the disease remains usually localized in the stomach, systemic dissemination and bone marrow involvement should be assessed at presentation, since prognosis is worse with advanced-stage disease or with unfavourable International Prognostic Index (IPI) score.[41]

## TREATMENT OF MALT LYMPHOMA

### *H. pylori* eradication in gastric MALT lymphoma

The regression of gastric MALT lymphoma after antibiotic eradication of *H. pylori* was first reported in 1993 by Wotherspoon and colleagues, who described the efficacy of antibiotic therapy in six patients with superficially invasive gastric MALT lymphoma.[55] Several groups thereafter confirmed the efficacy of antibiotics in inducing apparently durable lymphoma remissions in 60–100% of patients with localized *H. Pylori*-positive gastric MALT lymphoma.[42,49,50,52,56-58] The histologic remission can usually be documented within 6 months from the *H. pylori* eradication but sometimes the period required is more prolonged and the therapeutic response may be delayed up to more than 1 year.[41]

It is now generally accepted that eradication of *H. pylori* with antibiotics should be employed as the sole initial treatment of localized (i.e., confined to the gastric wall) MALT lymphoma. Actually, this is at present the best studied therapeutic approach with more than 20 reported studies.[59,60] Any of the highly effective antibiotic regimens proposed[61,62] can be used. Several effective anti-*H. pylori* programs are available and any of them can be used.[61-63] It is expected that following 10–14 days of antibiotic treatment, *H. pylori* will be eradicated in 85–90% of the patients.[63] Our regimen of choice is a 10-day triple therapy with a proton-pump inhibitor (e.g., omeprazole 20 mg b.i.d., pantoprazole 40 mg once daily, esomeprazole 40 mg once daily, or others), amoxicillin (1 g b.i.d.), and clarithromycin (500 mg b.i.d.). Metronidazole (500 mg b.i.d.) can replace amoxicillin in penicillin-allergic individuals, but metronidazole resistance is common and can reduce the treatment efficacy. After treatment, strict endoscopic follow-up is recommended, with multiple biopsies taken at 2–3 months to document *H. pylori* eradication and, subsequently, at least twice per year for 2 years to monitor the histologic regression of the lymphoma. In cases of unsuccessful *H. pylori* eradication, a second-line anti-Helicobacter therapy should be attempted with alternative triple- or quadruple-therapy regimens of proton-pump inhibitors plus antibiotics. However, it is still unknown whether *H. pylori* eradication will definitely cure the lymphoma; therefore, long-term follow-up of antibiotic-treated patients is mandatory. Some cases of documented tumor recurrence following *H. pylori* reinfection have been reported, suggesting that residual dormant tumor cells can be present despite clinical and histologic remission. Relapses have also been documented without *H. pylori* reinfection, indicating the emergence of B-cell lymphoma clones that are no longer antigen dependent.[56,58]

Several studies of postantibiotic molecular follow-up demonstrated a long-term persistence of monoclonal B cells after histologic regression of the lymphoma in about half of the cases, suggesting that *H. pylori* eradication does not eradicate the lymphoma clone.[58,64] Therefore, histologic evaluation of posttreatment gastric biopsies remains to be a fundamental follow-up procedure. Unfortunately, the interpretation of residual lymphoid infiltrate can be very difficult, and there are no uniform criteria for the definition of histologic remission. Wotherspoon in 1993 proposed a simple score to express the degree of confidence in the diagnosis of MALT lymphoma on small gastric biopsies.[55] This scoring system has been used to evaluate the response to therapy in some trials, but many investigators found it difficult to apply in this setting and other criteria have been proposed.[56] The lack of standardized and reproducible criteria can affect the comparison of the results from different clinical trials. A novel histologic grading system has been proposed by Copie-Bergman and colleagues.[65] This system classifies the histologic features in posttreatment gastric biopsies as "complete histologic remission," "probable minimal residual disease," "responding residual disease," and "no change." It may become a useful tool but its reproducibility still needs to be confirmed on larger series.

The efficacy of antibiotic therapy is reduced in locally advanced disease, and as mentioned before, endoscopic ultrasound can be useful to predict the lymphoma response to *H. pylori* eradication. The response rate is 70–90% for the mucosa-confined lymphomas, but then decreases markedly and progressively for the tumors infiltrating the submucosa, the muscularis propria, and the serosa. In cases with documented nodal involvement, a response is unlikely.[50,52] The t(11;18) translocation is absent in gastric MALT lymphomas showing complete regression,[66] but present in 77% of nonresponsive tumors, including 68% of those with the disease confined to the gastric wall.[67] Therefore, this translocation can be a valuable molecular marker to predict the therapeutic response of gastric MALT lymphoma to *H. pylori* eradication[30,67,68] and in addition to routine histology and immunohistochemistry, fluorescence in situ hybridization analysis for detection of t(11;18) may be useful for identifying disease that is unlikely to respond to antibiotic therapy.

### Management of *H. Pylori*-negative or antibiotic-resistant patients

No definite guidelines exist for the management of the subset of *H. pylori*-negative cases or for the patients who fail antibiotic therapy. A choice can be made among conventional oncologic modalities but there are no published randomized studies to help with the decision. In two retrospective series of patients with gastric low-grade MALT lymphoma, no statistically significant difference was apparent in survival between patients who received different initial treatments, including antibiotics against *H. pylori*, chemotherapy, surgery with or without additional chemotherapy, or radiation therapy.[42,69]

Excellent disease control using radiation therapy alone has been reported by several institutions supporting the approach that modest-dose involved-field radiotherapy (30 Gy given in 4 weeks radiation to the stomach and perigastric nodes) is the treatment of choice for patients with stage I–II MALT lymphoma of the stomach without evidence of *H. pylori* infection or with persistent lymphoma after antibiotics.[70,71] Surgery has been widely and successfully used in the past, but the precise role for surgical resection should now be redefined in view of the promising results of a more conservative approach.[41]

Patients with systemic disease should be considered for systemic chemotherapy and/or immunotherapy with anti-CD-20 monoclonal antibodies. Only a few compounds and regimens have been tested specifically in MALT lymphomas. Oral alkylating agents (either cyclophosphamide or chlorambucil, with median treatment duration of 1 year) can result in a high rate of disease control.[72,73] More recent phase II studies demonstrated some antitumor activity of the purine analogs fludarabine[74] and cladribine (2-CdA),[75] possibly associated with an increased risk of secondary myelodysplastic syndrome,[76] and of a combination regimen of chlorambucil/mitoxantrone/prednisone.[77] The activity of the anti-CD20 monoclonal antibody rituximab has also been shown in a phase II study to have a response rate of about 70%,[78] and it may represent an additional option for the treatment of systemic disease. Rituximab is active in gastric MALT lymphomas resistant or refractory to antibiotics, or not associated with *H. pylori* infection. Different from the setting of antibiotic therapy, the t(11;18)(q21;q21) translocation seems not to be a predictive marker of response to rituximab.[79]

## Management of non-gastric localizations

The stomach is the most common and best studied site of involvement, but MALT lymphomas have also been described in various non-GI sites, such as salivary gland, thyroid, skin, conjunctiva, orbit, larynx, lung, breast, kidney, liver, prostate, and even in the intracranial dura.[53,54,80] One-fourth of non-GI MALT lymphomas have been reported to present with involvement of multiple mucosal sites or nonmucosal sites such as bone marrow.[53,54] Nevertheless, despite presenting so often with stage IV disease, they usually have a quite indolent course regardless of treatment type (5-year survival of 90%). The rate of histologic transformation seems much lower than that in follicular lymphomas. Patients at high risk according to the IPI, and those with lymph node involvement at presentation, but not those with involvement of multiple MALT sites, have a worse outcome. Localization may have prognostic relevance. In a radiotherapy study from Toronto,[70] gastric and thyroid MALT lymphomas had better outcome, whereas distant failures were common for other sites, however, despite relapse, the disease most often maintained an indolent course.

In a multicentric retrospective survey of 180 non-gastric cases observed over a long period of time, patients were treated according to the current policy of each institution at the time of diagnosis, and the presence of organ-specific problems presumably had a role in the choice of treatment. This study showed no evidence of a clear advantage for any type of therapy.[53]

In general, the considerations regarding the treatment of H. pylori-negative cases can be applied. Radiation therapy is the best studied approach[81] and is the treatment of choice for localized lesions. The optimal management of disseminated MALT lymphomas is less clearly defined. The treatment choice should be "patient tailored," taking into account the site, the stage, and the clinical characteristics of the individual patient. The anti-CD20 antibody rituximab has shown clinical activity,[78] and the efficacy of its combination with chemotherapy is being explored in a randomized study of the International Extranodal Study Group. The finding that C. psittaci is associated with MALT lymphoma of the ocular adnexa may provide the rationale for the antibiotic treatment of localized lesions and preliminary encouraging results have been reported, but this approach remains investigational and will need to be confirmed by larger clinical studies.

## SPLENIC MARGINAL ZONE LYMPHOMA

### DISEASE FEATURES
#### Pathology

The disease is characterized by a lymphoid infiltrate in the splenic white pulp that grows in a nodular patter replacing preexisting follicles.[4,82] A variable degree of red pulp infiltration is also often present. Small lymphocytes are predominant in central areas, while medium-size cells resembling splenic marginal zone lymphocytes are present in the periphery. Plasmacytic differentiation as well as, rarely, clusters of plasma cells can be present.

The neoplastic cells show typical positivity for surface (and sometimes cytoplasmic) immunoglobulins and pan-B antigens (CD19, CD20, and CD22); they usually coexpress CD11c, and lack CD5, CD10, and CD23 expression.

Up to two-thirds of the patients with splenic MZL present the characteristic circulating villous lymphocytes, with short cytoplasmic projections. When these are more than 20% of the lymphocyte count, the term "splenic lymphoma with villous lymphocytes" is commonly used.[83]

Bone marrow is usually involved, even in cases with no circulating neoplastic cells. The pattern of infiltration is typically nonparatrabecular, intrasinusoidal only. However, this pattern of bone marrow involvement can be found also in other small-cell lymphomas.[84–86]

When biopsied, the liver is usually involved with a nodular infiltration of portal tracts, and hilar splenic lymph node involvement is common. According to the WHO classification, the peripheral lymph node involvement is typically absent.[87] Transformation to a diffuse large B-cell lymphoma occurs in about 15% of the cases.[88]

### Genetic abnormalities

Sequence analysis of the immunoglobulin genes expressed by the splenic marginal zone B cells shows that approximately half of the cases bear unmutated and half have mutated immunoglobulin heavy-chain genes,[89,90] suggesting the possibility that this lymphoma subtype derives from different B-cell subsets than those normally present in the marginal zone. Cases with unmutated IgH genes may have a poorer prognosis and are more commonly associated with the presence of chromosome 7q loss,[89] but it has to be underscored that the 7q deletions are relatively common in hematologic malignancies and not specific for splenic MZL. Gain of chromosome 3 appears to be another common abnormality.[91,92] The t(9;14)(p13;q32) translocation which juxtaposes the IgH locus to the PAX5 gene[93,94] has also been reported; however, its frequency is controversial.[95] Using cDNA microarray, Thieblemont et al. have compared the gene expression profile of splenic MZL, mantle cell lymphoma, and small lymphocytic lymphoma.[96] The gene coding for the serine threonine kinase AKT1 was the most representative among the gene clusters specific for splenic MZL; its possible role in the pathogenesis of splenic MZL needs to be further clarified.

### Association with infectious agents
Despite relevant geographic variations, hepatitis C virus (HCV) seems to be involved in splenic MZL and nodal MZL

lymphomagenesis.[97–101] Of great interest, some patients with splenic lymphoma with villous lymphocyes and HCV infection achieved a lymphoma remission after treatment with interferon alfa with or without concomitant ribavirin.[101,102] This suggests a strict relationship between HCV and splenic MZL, indicating the necessity to search for HCV infection in patients affected by this lymphoma subtype. Analogous to the *H. Pylori* infection in the gastric MZL, it appears that HCV may be responsible for an antigen-driven stimulation of the lymphoma clone. Prospective studies are warranted to confirm this interesting finding.

An association with malaria and with Epstein–Barr virus infection, both acting as strong polyclonal B-cell activators, has been shown in tropical Africa.[103–105] Tropical splenic lymphoma appears as a form of splenic MZL, characterized by a high percentage of circulating villous lymphocytes, unmutated immunoglobulin genes, and a predilection for middle-age women.

### Clinical features

Most patients are over 50 with a similar incidence in males and females.[87] The disease usually presents with massive splenogamy, which produces abdominal discomfort and pain. Diagnosis is often made at splenectomy performed to establish the cause of unexplained spleen enlargement. B symptoms are present in 25–60% of cases; anemia, thrombocytopenia, or leukocytosis are reported in approximately 25% of cases. Autoimmune hemolytic anemia is not uncommon, being found in up to 15% of patients. Splenic hilar lymph nodes appear to be involved in about 25% of cases, but peripheral lymph node involvement is typically absent. Approximately 30% of cases have liver involvement.[106–110] Nearly all patients have bone marrow involvement, often accompanied by involvement of peripheral blood (defined as the presence of absolute lymphocytosis of more than 5%).[109] Because of the high frequency of bone marrow or liver involvement, about 95% of cases are classified as Ann Arbor stage IV. Serum paraproteinemia is observed in about 10–25% of cases,[107–109] most frequently of IgM type posing the problem of the differential diagnosis with lymphoplasmacytic lymphoma/Waldenstrom macroglobulinemia.[82,111]

In advanced stages of either splenic, nodal, or extranodal MZL, a precise diagnosis can be very difficult in cases presenting with concomitant splenic, extranodal, and nodal involvement.[108,112]

### TREATMENT OF SPLENIC MARGINAL ZONE LYMPHOMA

The clinical course is usually indolent with 5-year overall survival ranging from 65 to 80%, and most cases can be safely managed with an initial wait-and-see policy.[107,109,110] When treatment is needed, this is usually because of large symptomatic splenomegaly or cytopenias. Splenectomy appears to be the treatment of choice; it allows a reduction/disappearance of circulating tumor lymphocytes, and recovery of the lymphoma-associated cytopenia.[106,107,110,112,113] The benefit of splenectomy often persists for several years, and time to next treatment can be longer than 5 years in cases where lymphocytosis persists and or progresses after splenectomy.[112] Adjuvant chemotherapy after splenectomy may result in higher rate of complete responses; however, there is no evidence of a survival benefit.[112]

Chemotherapy alone may be considered for patients who require treatment but have a contraindication to splenectomy, and also for the patient with clinical progression after spleen removal. Alkylating agents and fludarabine have been reported to be active and can be used as single agents or in combination. The anti-B-cell monoclonal antibody, rituximab, alone or in combination with chemotherapy, is capable—according to a few case reports—to induce good responses in cases refractory to standard chemotherapy.[112,114,115] Treatment of HCV infection with interferon alpha alone or in combination with ribavirin may be helpful for the patients with splenic lymphoma with villous lymphocyte and HCV infection.[102,116]

## NODAL MARGINAL ZONE LYMPHOMA

### DISEASE FEATURES
#### Pathology

In contrast with mucosa-based extranodal MALT lymphoma, nodal MZL is typically lymph node based. The tumor cell morphology is heterogeneous and resembles the lymph node involvement of extranodal and splenic MZL. The marginal zone and interfollicular areas are infiltrated by marginal zone B cells, monocytoid B cells, or small B lymphocytes. Plasma cell differentiation can be present, as well as some large cells.[3,117–120]

#### Genetic abnormalities

No specific genomic alteration is known to occur in nodal MZL. The most common alterations, such as gain of 3q, are also present in extranodal and splenic MZL.

Analysis of the IgH genes suggest a prevalence of cases with mutated IgH genes, but, similarly to splenic MZL, unmutated cases do exist.[121–123] These data are in accordance with the different normal B-cell populations resident within the marginal zone, which comprise both naïve and postgerminal center B cells.[124]

As noted, both nodal and splenic MZL have been associated with HCV infection.[97,98,100,101,125–127]

#### Clinical features

The clinical data are sparse and have been largely drawn from pathologic series rather than clinical centers.[128,129] Nodal MZL is a disease of older people, with median age at presentation in the sixth decade, and affects both sexes, with an unusual (albeit slight) female predominance. The most common presenting feature is a localized adenopathy, most often in the neck.

## TREATMENT OF NODAL MARGINAL ZONE LYMPHOMA

There is at present no consensus about the best treatment, individual cases being managed differently according to site and stage. Indeed, there are very few studies comparing nodal MZL with the other low-grade B-cell lymphomas. Treatment options may include single-agent chlorambucil or fludarabine, or combination chemotherapy regimens (such as the cyclophos- phamide, vincristine, and prednisone or cyclophos- phamide, hydroxydaunomycin (doxorubicin), Oncovin (vincristine), and prednisone). Rituximab may also have some efficacy,[130] and anti-HCV treatment may induce lymphoma regression in some HCV-infected patients.[116] Autologous transplantation has been used in younger patients with adverse prognostic factors and high number of large cells subtypes.[108] However, no prospective studies have been conducted so far, and treatment decision should be based on the histologic and clinical features of the individual patient.[117,127]

## REFERENCES

1. Harris NL, Jaffe ES, Stein H, et al.: A revised European–American classification of lymphoid neoplasms: a proposal from the International Lymphoma Study Group. *Blood* 84:1361–1392, 1994.
2. Isaacson PG, Muller-Hermelink HK, Piris MA, et al.: Extranodal marginal zone B-cell lymphoma of mucosa-associated lymphoid tissue (MALT lymphoma). In: Jaffe ES, Harris NL, Stein H, et al. (eds.) *World Health Organization Classification of Tumours: Pathology and Genetics of Tumours of Haematopoietic and Lymphoid Tissues*. Lyon, France: IARC Press; 2001:157–160.
3. Isaacson PG, Nathwani BN, Piris MA, et al.: Nodal marginal zone B-cell lymphoma. In: Jaffe ES, Harris NL, Stein H, et al. (eds.) *World Health Organization Classification of Tumours: Pathology and Genetics of Tumours of Haematopoietic and Lymphoid Tissues*. Lyon, France: IARC Press; 2001:161.
4. Isaacson PI, Piris MA, Catovsky D, et al.: Splenic marginal zone lymphoma. In: Jaffe ES, Harris NL, Stein H, et al. (eds.) *World Health Organization Classification of Tumours: Pathology and Genetics of Tumours of Haematopoietic and Lymphoid Tissues*. Lyon, France: IARC Press, 2001:135–137.
5. The Non-Hodgkin's Lymphoma Classification Project: A clinical evaluation of the International Lymphoma Study Group classification of non-Hodgkin's lymphoma. *Blood* 89:3909–3918, 1997.
6. Cavalli F, Isaacson PG, Gascoyne RD, et al.: MALT lymphomas. *Hematology Am Soc Hematol Educ Program* 241–258, 2001.
7. Pozzi B, Cerati M, Capella C: MALT lymphoma: pathology. In: Bertoni F, Zucca E (eds.) *MALT Lymphomas*. Georgetown, TX: Landes Bioscience/Kluwer Academic, 2004:17–45.
8. Isaacson P, Wright DH: Extranodal malignant lymphoma arising from mucosa-associated lymphoid tissue. *Cancer* 53:2515–2524, 1984.
9. Qin Y, Greiner A, Trunk MJ, et al.: Somatic hypermutation in low-grade mucosa-associated lymphoid tissue-type B-cell lymphoma. *Blood* 86:3528–3534, 1995.
10. Du M, Diss TC, Xu C, et al.: Ongoing mutation in MALT lymphoma immunoglobulin gene suggests that antigen stimulation plays a role in the clonal expansion. *Leukemia* 10:1190–1197, 1996.
11. Bertoni F, Cazzaniga G, Bosshard G, et al.: Immunoglobulin heavy chain diversity genes rearrangement pattern indicates that MALT-type gastric lymphoma B cells have undergone an antigen selection process. *Br J Haematol* 97:830–836, 1997.
12. Zucca E, Bertoni F, Roggero E, et al.: Autoreactive B cell clones in marginal-zone B cell lymphoma (MALT lymphoma) of the stomach. *Leukemia* 12:247–249, 1998.
13. Parsonnet J, Hansen S, Rodriguez L, et al.: Helicobacter pylori infection and gastric lymphoma. *N Engl J Med* 330:1267–1271, 1994.
14. Hussell T, Isaacson PG, Crabtree JE, et al.: Helicobacter pylori-specific tumour-infiltrating T cells provide contact dependent help for the growth of malignant B cells in low-grade gastric lymphoma of mucosa-associated lymphoid tissue. *J Pathol* 178:122–127, 1996.
15. Zucca E, Bertoni F, Roggero E, et al.: Molecular analysis of the progression from Helicobacter pylori-associated chronic gastritis to mucosa-associated lymphoid-tissue lymphoma of the stomach. *N Engl J Med* 338:804–810, 1998.
16. Zucca E, Cavalli F: Are antibiotics the treatment of choice for gastric lymphoma? *Curr Hematol Rep* 3:11–16, 2004.
17. Hussell T, Isaacson PG, Crabtree JE, et al.: Immunoglobulin specificity of low grade B cell gastrointestinal lymphoma of mucosa-associated lymphoid tissue (MALT) type. *Am J Pathol* 142:285–292, 1993.
18. Garbe C, Stein H, Dienemann D, et al.: Borrelia burgdorferi-associated cutaneous B cell lymphoma: clinical and immunohistologic characterization of four cases. *J Am Acad Dermatol* 24:584–590, 1991.
19. Kutting B, Bonsmann G, Metze D, et al.: Borrelia burgdorferi-associated primary cutaneous B cell lymphoma: complete clearing of skin lesions after antibiotic pulse therapy or intralesional injection of interferon alfa-2a. *J Am Acad Dermatol* 36:311–314, 1997.
20. Roggero E, Zucca E, Mainetti C, et al.: Eradication of Borrelia burgdorferi infection in primary marginal zone B-cell lymphoma of the skin. *Hum Pathol* 31:263–268, 2000.
21. Ferreri AJ, Guidoboni M, Ponzoni M, et al.: Evidence for an association between Chlamydia psittaci and ocular adnexa lymphomas. *J Natl Cancer Inst* 96:586–594, 2004.
22. Lecuit M, Abachin E, Martin A, et al.: Immunoproliferative small intestinal disease associated with Campylobacter jejuni. *N Engl J Med* 350:239–48, 2004.
23. Zucca E, Roggero E, Bertoni F, et al.: Primary extranodal non-Hodgkin's lymphomas. Part 1: Gastrointestinal, cutaneous and genitourinary lymphomas. *Ann Oncol* 8:727–737, 1997.

24. Parsonnet J: *Helicobacter pylori*: the size of the problem. *Gut* 43(suppl 1):S6–S9, 1998.

25. Rollinson S, Levene AP, Mensah FK, et al.: Gastric marginal zone lymphoma is associated with polymorphisms in genes involved in inflammatory response and antioxidative capacity. *Blood* 102:1007–1011, 2003.

26. Ye H, Liu H, Attygalle A, et al.: Variable frequencies of t(11;18)(q21;q21) in MALT lymphomas of different sites: significant association with CagA strains of *H. pylori* in gastric MALT lymphoma. *Blood* 102:1012–1018, 2003.

27. Auer IA, Gascoyne RD, Connors JM, et al.: t(11;18)(q21;q21) is the most common translocation in MALT lymphomas. *Ann Oncol* 8:979–985, 1997.

28. Ott G, Katzenberger T, Greiner A, et al.: The t(11;18)(q21;q21) chromosome translocation is a frequent and specific aberration in low-grade but not high-grade malignant non-Hodgkin's lymphomas of the mucosa-associated lymphoid tissue (MALT-) type. *Cancer Res* 57:3944–3948, 1997.

29. Dierlamm J, Baens M, Wlodarska I, et al.: The apoptosis inhibitor gene *API2* and a novel *18q* gene, MLT, are recurrently rearranged in the t(11;18)(q21;q21) associated with mucosa-associated lymphoid tissue lymphomas. *Blood* 93:3601–3609, 1999.

30. Liu H, Ye H, Dogan A, et al.: T(11;18)(q21;q21) is associated with advanced mucosa-associated lymphoid tissue lymphoma that expresses nuclear BCL10. *Blood* 98:1182–1187, 2001.

31. Murga Penas EM, Hinz K, Roser K, et al.: Translocations t(11;18)(q21;q21) and t(14;18)(q32;q21) are the main chromosomal abnormalities involving MLT/MALT1 in MALT lymphomas. *Leukemia* 17:2225–2229, 2003.

32. Zhang Q, Siebert R, Yan M, et al.: Inactivating mutations and overexpression of BCL10, a caspase recruitment domain-containing gene, in MALT lymphoma with t(1; 14)(p22;q32). *Nat Genet* 22:63–68, 1999.

33. Willis TG, Jadayel DM, Du MQ, et al.: Bcl10 is involved in t(1;14)(p22;q32) of MALT B cell lymphoma and mutated in multiple tumor types. *Cell* 96:35–45, 1999.

34. Kuo SH, Chen LT, Yeh KH, et al.: Nuclear expression of BCL10 or nuclear factor kappa B predicts *Helicobacter pylori*-independent status of early-stage, high-grade gastric mucosa-associated lymphoid tissue lymphomas. *J Clin Oncol* 22:3491–3497, 2004.

35. Ye H, Dogan A, Karran L, et al.: BCL10 expression in normal and neoplastic lymphoid tissue: nuclear localization in MALT lymphoma. *Am J Pathol* 157: 1147– 1154, 2000.

36. Sanchez-Izquierdo D, Buchonet G, Siebert R, et al.: MALT1 is deregulated by both chromosomal translocation and amplification in B-cell non-Hodgkin lymphoma. *Blood* 101:4539–4546, 2003.

37. Streubel B, Lamprecht A, Dierlamm J, et al.: T(14;18)(q32;q21) involving IGH and MALT1 is a frequent chromosomal aberration in MALT lymphoma. *Blood* 101:2335–2339, 2003.

38. Lucas PC, Yonezumi M, Inohara N, et al.: Bcl10 and MALT1, independent targets of chromosomal translocation in malt lymphoma, cooperate in a novel NF-kappa B signaling pathway. *J Biol Chem* 276: 19012–19019, 2001.

39. Ho L, Davis RE, Conne B, et al.: MALT1 and the API2-MALT1 fusion act between CD40 and IKK and confer NF-κB dependent proliferative advantage and resistance against FAS-induced cell death in B cells. *Blood* 2004.

40. Isaacson PG, Du MQ: MALT lymphoma: from morphology to molecules. *Nat Rev Cancer* 4:644–653, 2004.

41. Zucca E, Bertoni F, Roggero E, et al.: The gastric marginal zone B-cell lymphoma of MALT type. *Blood* 96: 410–419, 2000.

42. Pinotti G, Zucca E, Roggero E, et al.: Clinical features, treatment and outcome in a series of 93 patients with low-grade gastric MALT lymphoma. *Leuk Lymphoma* 26:527–537, 1997.

43. Dogan A, Du M, Koulis A, et al.: Expression of lymphocyte homing receptors and vascular addressing in low-grade gastric B-cell lymphomas of mucosa-associated lymphoid tissue. *Am J Pathol* 151:1361–1369, 1997.

44. Drillenburg P, van der Voort R, Koopman G, et al.: Preferential expression of the mucosal homing receptor integrin alpha 4 beta 7 in gastrointestinal non-Hodgkin's lymphomas. *Am J Pathol* 150:919–927, 1997.

45. Drillenburg P, Pals ST: Cell adhesion receptors in lymphoma dissemination. *Blood* 95:1900–1910, 2000.

46. de Jong D, Aleman BM, Taal BG, et al.: Controversies and consensus in the diagnosis, work-up and treatment of gastric lymphoma: an international survey. *Ann Oncol* 10:275–280, 1999.

47. Blackledge G, Bush H, Dodge OG, Crowther D: A study of gastro-intestinal lymphoma. *Clin Oncol* 5:209–219, 1979.

48. Rohatiner A, d'Amore F, Coiffier B, et al.: Report on a workshop convened to discuss the pathological and staging classifications of gastrointestinal tract lymphoma. *Ann Oncol* 5:397–400, 1994.

49. Sackmann M, Morgner A, Rudolph B, et al.: Regression of gastric MALT lymphoma after eradication of *Helicobacter pylori* is predicted by endosonographic staging. MALT Lymphoma Study Group. *Gastroenterology* 113:1087–1090, 1997.

50. Ruskone-Fourmestraux A, Lavergne A, Aegerter PH, et al.: Predictive factors for regression of gastric MALT lymphoma after anti-*Helicobacter pylori* treatment. *Gut* 48:297–303, 2001.

51. Eidt S, Stolte M, Fischer R: Factors influencing lymph node infiltration in primary gastric malignant lymphoma of the mucosa-associated lymphoid tissue. *Pathol Res Pract* 190:1077–1081, 1994.

52. Steinbach G, Ford R, Glober G, et al.: Antibiotic treatment of gastric lymphoma of mucosa-associated lymphoid tissue. An uncontrolled trial. *Ann Intern Med* 131:88–95, 1999.

53. Zucca E, Conconi A, Pedrinis E, et al.: Nongastric marginal zone B-cell lymphoma of mucosa-associated lymphoid tissue. *Blood* 101:2489–495, 2003.

54. Thieblemont C, Dumontet C, Salles G, et al.: Mucosa-associated lymphoid tissue (MALT)-lymphoma are disseminated disease in 1/3 of the patients. *Ann Oncol* 10(suppl 3):25, 1999.

55. Wotherspoon AC, Doglioni C, Diss TC, et al.: Regression of primary low-grade B-cell gastric lymphoma of mucosa-associated lymphoid tissue type after eradication of *Helicobacter pylori*. *Lancet* 342:575–577, 1993.

56. Neubauer A, Thiede C, Morgner A, et al.: Cure of *Helicobacter pylori* infection and duration of remission of low-grade gastric mucosa-associated lymphoid tissue lymphoma. *J Natl Cancer Inst* 89:1350–1355, 1997.

57. Nakamura S, Matsumoto T, Suekane H, et al.: Predictive value of endoscopic ultrasonography for regression of gastric low grade and high grade MALT lymphomas after eradication of *Helicobacter pylori*. *Gut* 48:454–460, 2001.

58. Bertoni F, Conconi A, Capella C, et al.: Molecular follow-up in gastric mucosa-associated lymphoid tissue lymphomas: early analysis of the LY03 cooperative trial. *Blood* 99:2541–2544, 2002.

59. Stolte M, Bayerdorffer E, Morgner A, et al.: Helicobacter and gastric MALT lymphoma. *Gut* 50(suppl 3): III19–III24, 2002.

60. Ahmad A, Govil Y, Frank BB: Gastric mucosa-associated lymphoid tissue lymphoma. *Am J Gastroenterol* 98: 975–986, 2003.

61. Malfertheiner P, Megraud F, O'Morain C, et al.: Current European concepts in the management of *Helicobacter pylori* infection—the Maastricht Consensus Report. The European Helicobacter Pylori Study Group (EHPSG). *Eur J Gastroenterol Hepatol* 9:1–2, 1997.

62. Howden CW, Hunt RH: Guidelines for the management of *Helicobacter pylori* infection. Ad Hoc Committee on Practice Parameters of the American College of Gastroenterology. *Am J Gastroenterol* 93:2330–2338, 1998.

63. Graham DY, Rakel RE, Fendrick AM, et al.: Practical advice on eradicating *Helicobacter pylori* infection. *Postgrad Med* 105:137–148, 1999.

64. Thiede C, Wundisch T, Alpen B, et al.: Persistence of monoclonal B cells after cure of *Helicobacter pylori* infection and complete histologic remission in gastric mucosa-associated lymphoid tissue B-cell lymphoma. *J Clin Oncol* 19:1600–1609, 2001.

65. Copie-Bergman C, Gaulard P, Lavergne-Slove A, et al.: Proposal for a new histological grading system for post-treatment evaluation of gastric MALT lymphoma. *Gut* 52:1656, 2003.

66. Alpen B, Neubauer A, Dierlamm J, et al.: Translocation t(11;18) absent in early gastric marginal zone B-cell lymphoma of MALT type responding to eradication of *Helicobacter pylori* infection. *Blood* 95:4014–4015, 2000.

67. Liu H, Ruskon-Fourmestraux A, Lavergne-Slove A, et al.: Resistance of t(11;18) positive gastric mucosa-associated lymphoid tissue lymphoma to *Helicobacter pylori* eradication therapy. *Lancet* 357:39–40, 2001.

68. Liu H, Ye H, Ruskone-Fourmestraux A, et al.: T(11;18) is a marker for all stage gastric MALT lymphomas that will not respond to *H. pylori* eradication. *Gastroe nterology* 122:1286–1294, 2002.

69. Thieblemont C, Dumontet C, Bouafia F, et al.: Outcome in relation to treatment modalities in 48 patients with localized gastric MALT lymphoma: a retrospective study of patients treated during 1976–2001. *Leuk Lymphoma* 44:257–262, 2003.

70. Tsang RW, Gospodarowicz MK, Pintilie M, et al.: Localized mucosa-associated lymphoid tissue lymphoma treated with radiation therapy has excellent clinical outcome. *J Clin Oncol* 21:4157–4164, 2003.

71. Schechter NR, Portlock CS, Yahalom J: Treatment of mucosa-associated lymphoid tissue lymphoma of the stomach with radiation alone. *J Clin Oncol* 16: 1916–1921, 1998.

72. Hammel P, Haioun C, Chaumette MT, et al.: Efficacy of single-agent chemotherapy in low-grade B-cell mucosa-associated lymphoid tissue lymphoma with prominent gastric expression. *J Clin Oncol* 13:2524–2529, 1995.

73. Levy M, Copie-Bergman C, Traulle C, et al.: Conservative treatment of primary gastric low-grade B-cell lymphoma of mucosa-associated lymphoid tissue: predictive factors of response and outcome. *Am J Gastroenterol* 97:292–297, 2002.

74. Zinzani PL, Stefoni V, Musuraca G, et al.: Fludarabine containing chemotherapy as frontline treatment of nongastrointestinal mucosa-associated lymphoid tissue lymphoma. *Cancer* 100:2190–2194, 2004.

75. Jager G, Neumeister P, Brezinschek R, et al.: Treatment of extranodal marginal zone B-cell lymphoma of mucosa-associated lymphoid tissue type with cladribine: a phase II study. *J Clin Oncol* 20:3872–3877, 2002.

76. Jager G, Hofler G, Linkesch W, et al.: Occurrence of a myelodysplastic syndrome (MDS) during first-line 2-chloro-deoxyadenosine (2-CDA) treatment of a low-grade gastrointestinal MALT lymphoma. Case report and review of the literature. *Haematologica* 89:ECR01, 2004.

77. Wohrer S, Drach J, Hejna M, et al.: Treatment of extranodal marginal zone B-cell lymphoma of mucosa-associated lymphoid tissue (MALT lymphoma) with mitoxantrone, chlorambucil and prednisone (MCP). *Ann Oncol* 14:1758–1761, 2003.

78. Conconi A, Martinelli G, Thieblemont C, et al.: Clinical activity of rituximab in extranodal marginal zone B-cell lymphoma of MALT type. *Blood* 102:2741–2745, 2003.

79. Martinelli G, Laszlo D, Ferreri AJ, et al.: Clinical activity of rituximab in gastric marginal zone non-Hodgkin's lymphoma resistant to or not eligible for anti-*Helicobacter pylori* therapy. *J Clin Oncol* 23:1979–1983, 2005.

80. Thieblemont C, Bastion Y, Berger F, et al.: Mucosa-associated lymphoid tissue gastrointestinal and nongastrointestinal lymphoma behavior: analysis of 108 patients. *J Clin Oncol* 15:1624–1630, 1997.

81. Schechter NR, Yahalom J: Low-grade MALT lymphoma of the stomach: a review of treatment options. *Int J Radiat Oncol Biol Phys* 46:1093–1103, 2000.

82. Piris MA, Mollejo M, Chacon I, et al.: Splenic marginal zone B-cell lymphoma. In: Mauch PM, Armitage J, Coiffier B, et al. (eds.) *Non-Hodgkin's Lymphomas*. Philadelphia, PA: Lippincott Williams & Wilkins; 2004:275–282.

83. Isaacson PG, Matutes E, Burke M, et al.: The histopathology of splenic lymphoma with villous lymphocytes. *Blood* 84:3828–3834, 1994.

84. Schenka AA, Gascoyne RD, Duchayne E, et al.: Prominent intrasinusoidal infiltration of the bone marrow by mantle cell lymphoma. *Hum Pathol* 34:789–791, 2003.

85. Kent SA, Variakojis D, Peterson LC: Comparative study of marginal zone lymphoma involving bone marrow. *Am J Clin Pathol* 117:698–708, 2002.

86. Audouin J, Le Tourneau A, Molina T, et al.: Patterns of bone marrow involvement in 58 patients presenting primary splenic marginal zone lymphoma with or without circulating villous lymphocytes. *Br J Haematol* 122:404–412, 2003.

87. Isaacson PG: Splenic marginal zone B cell lymphoma. In: Mason DY, Harris NL (eds.) *Human Lymphoma: Clinical Implications of the REAL Classification.* London: Springer-Verlag; 1999:7.1–7.6.

88. Camacho FI, Mollejo M, Mateo MS, et al.: Progression to large B-cell lymphoma in splenic marginal zone lymphoma: a description of a series of 12 cases. *Am J Surg Pathol* 25:1268–1276, 2001.

89. Algara P, Mateo MS, Sanchez-Beato M, et al.: Analysis of the IgV(H) somatic mutations in splenic marginal zone lymphoma defines a group of unmutated cases with frequent 7q deletion and adverse clinical course. *Blood* 99:1299–1304, 2002.

90. Tierens A, Delabie J, Malecka A, et al.: Splenic marginal zone lymphoma with villous lymphocytes shows ongoing immunoglobulin gene mutations. *Am J Pathol* 162:681–689, 2003.

91. Dierlamm J: Genetic abnormalities in marginal zone B-cell lymphoma. *Haematologica* 88:8–12, 2003.

92. Gazzo S, Baseggio L, Coignet L, et al.: Cytogenetic and molecular delineation of a region of chromosome 3q commonly gained in marginal zone B-cell lymphoma. *Haematologica* 88:31–38, 2003.

93. Iida S, Rao PH, Nallasivam P, et al.: The t(9;14)(p13;q32) chromosomal translocation associated with lymphoplasmacytoid lymphoma involves the *PAX-5* gene. *Blood* 88:4110–4117, 1996.

94. Ohno H, Ueda C, Akasaka T: The t(9;14)(p13;q32) translocation in B-cell non-Hodgkin's lymphoma. *Leuk Lymphoma* 36:435–445, 2000.

95. Cook JR, Aguilera NI, Reshmi-Skarja S, et al.: Lack of PAX5 rearrangements in lymphoplasmacytic lymphomas: reassessing the reported association with t(9;14). *Hum Pathol* 35:447–454, 2004.

96. Thieblemont C, Nasser V, Felman P, et al.: Small lymphocytic lymphoma, marginal zone B-cell lymphoma, and mantle cell lymphoma exhibit distinct gene-expression profiles allowing molecular diagnosis. *Blood* 103:2727–2737, 2004.

97. Gisbert JP, Garcia-Buey L, Pajares JM, et al.: Prevalence of hepatitis C virus infection in B-cell non-Hodgkin's lymphoma: systematic review and meta-analysis. *Gastroenterology* 125:1723–1732, 2003.

98. Chan CH, Hadlock KG, Foung SK, et al.: V(H)1-69 gene is preferentially used by hepatitis C virus-associated B cell lymphomas and by normal B cells responding to the E2 viral antigen. *Blood* 97:1023–1026, 2001.

99. Zucca E, Roggero E, Maggi-Solca N, et al.: Prevalence of *Helicobacter pylori* and hepatitis C virus infections among non-Hodgkin's lymphoma patients in Southern Switzerland. *Haematologica* 85:147–153, 2000.

100. Luppi M, Negrini R: MALT lymphoma: epidemiology ad infectious agents. In: Bertoni F, Zucca E (eds.) *MALT lymphomas.* Georgetown, TX: Landes Bioscience/Kluwer Academic, 2004:1–16.

101. Arcaini L, Paulli M, Boveri E, et al.: Splenic and nodal marginal zone lymphomas are indolent disorders at high hepatitis C virus sero prevalence with distinct presenting features but similar morphologic and phenotypic profiles. *Cancer* 100:107–115, 2004.

102. Hermine O, Lefrere F, Bronowicki JP, et al.: Regression of splenic lymphoma with villous lymphocytes after treatment of hepatitis C virus infection. *N Engl J Med* 347:89–94, 2002.

103. Bates I, Bedu-Addo G, Rutherford T, et al.: Splenic lymphoma with villous lymphocytes in tropical West Africa. *Lancet* 340:575–577, 1992.

104. Bates I, Bedu-Addo G, Jarrett RF, et al.: B-lymphotropic viruses in a novel tropical splenic lymphoma. *Br J Haematol* 112:161–166, 2001.

105. Bedu-Addo G, Bates I: Causes of massive tropical splenomegaly in Ghana. *Lancet* 360:449–454, 2002.

106. Catovsky D, Matutes E: Splenic lymphoma with circulating villous lymphocytes/splenic marginal-zone lymphoma. *Semin Haematol* 36:148–154, 1999.

107. Troussard X, Valensi F, Duchayne E, et al.: Splenic lymphoma with villous lymphocytes: clinical presentation, biology and prognostic factors in a series of 100 patients. Groupe Francais d'Hematologie Cellulaire (GFHC). *Br J Haematol* 93:731–736, 1996.

108. Berger F, Felman P, Thieblemont C, et al.: Non-MALT marginal zone B-cell lymphomas: a description of clinical presentation and outcome in 124 patients. *Blood* 95:1950–1956, 2000.

109. Chacon JI, Mollejo M, Munoz E, et al.: Splenic marginal zone lymphoma: clinical characteristics and prognostic factors in a series of 60 patients. *Blood* 100:1648–1654, 2002.

110. Thieblemont C, Felman P, Berger F, et al.: Treatment of splenic marginal zone B-cell lymphoma: an analysis of 81 patients. *Clin Lymphoma* 3:41–47, 2002.

111. Berger F, Isaacson PG, Piris MA, et al.: Lymphoplasmacytic Lymphoma/Waldenstroem macroglobulinemia. In: Jaffe ES, Harris NL, Stein H, et al. (eds.) *World Health Organization Classification of Tumours: Pathology and Genetics of Tumours of Haematopoietic and Lymphoid Tissues.* Lyon, France: IARC Press; 2001:135–137.

112. Thieblemont C, Felman P, Callet-Bauchu E, et al.: Splenic marginal-zone lymphoma: a distinct clinical and pathological entity. *Lancet Oncol* 4:95–103, 2003.

113. Mulligan SP, Matutes E, Dearden C, et al.: Splenic lymphoma with villous lymphocytes: natural history and response to therapy in 50 cases. *Br J Haematol* 78:206–209, 1991.

114. Arcaini L, Orlandi E, Scotti M, et al.: Combination of rituximab, cyclophosphamide, and vincristine induces complete hematologic remission of splenic marginal zone lymphoma. *Clin Lymphoma* 4:250–252, 2004.

115. Paydas S, Yavuz S, Disel U, et al.: Successful rituximab therapy for hemolytic anemia associated with relapsed splenic marginal zone lymphoma with leukemic phase. *Leuk Lymphoma* 44:2165–2166, 2003.

116. Vallisa D, Bernuzzi P, Arcaini L, et al.: role of anti-hepatitis C virus (HCV) treatment in HCV-related, low-grade, B-cell, non-Hodgkin's lymphoma: a Multicenter Italian experience. *J Clin Oncol* 23:468–473, 2005.

117. Berger F, Traverse-Glehen A, Salles G: Nodal marginal zone B-cell lymphoma. In: Mauch PM, Armitage J, Coiffier B, et al. (eds.) *Non-Hodgkin's Lymphomas.* Philadelphia, PA: Lippincott Williams & Wilkins; 2004:361–365.

118. Feller AC, Diebold J: *Histopathology of Nodal and Extranodal Non-Hodgkin's Lymphomas.* 3rd ed. Berlin: Springer-Verlag; 2004.

119. Armitage JO, Cavalli F, Longo DL: *Text Atlas of lymphomas.* London: Martin Dunitz; 1999.

120. Grogan TM: Does nodal marginal zone lymphoma exist? In: Mason DY, Harris NL (eds.) *Human Lymphoma: Clinical Implications of the REAL Classification.* London: Springer-Verlag; 1999:18.1–18.5.

121. Marasca R, Vaccari P, Luppi M, et al.: Immunoglobulin gene mutations and frequent use of VH1-69 and VH4-34 segments in hepatitis C virus-positive and hepatitis C virus-negative nodal marginal zone B-Cell lymphoma. *Am J Pathol* 159:253–261, 2001.

122. Conconi A, Bertoni F, Pedrinis E, et al.: Nodal marginal zone B-cell lymphomas may arise from different subsets of marginal zone B lymphocytes. *Blood* 98: 781–786, 2001.

123. Camacho FI, Algara P, Mollejo M, et al.: Nodal marginal zone lymphoma: a heterogeneous tumor: a comprehensive analysis of a series of 27 cases. *Am J Surg Pathol* 27:762–771, 2003.

124. Martin F, Kearney JF: Marginal-zone B cells. *Nat Rev Immunol* 2:323–335, 2002.

125. Karavattathayyil SJ, Kalkeri G, Liu HJ, et al.: Detection of hepatitis C virus RNA sequences in B-cell non-Hodgkin lymphoma. *Am J Clin Pathol* 113:391–398, 2000.

126. Thalen DJ, Raemaekers J, Galama J, et al.: Absence of hepatitis C virus infection in non-Hodgkin's lymphoma. *Br J Haematol* 96:880–881, 1997.

127. Arcaini L, Paulli M, Boveri E, et al.: Marginal zone-related neoplasms of splenic and nodal origin. *Haematologica* 88:80–93, 2003.

128. Nathwani BN, Anderson JR, Armitage JO, et al.: Marginal zone B-cell lymphoma: a clinical comparison of nodal and mucosa-associated lymphoid tissue types. Non-Hodgkin's Lymphoma Classification Project. *J Clin Oncol* 17:2486–2492, 1999.

129. Sheibani K, Burke JS, Swartz WG, et al.: Monocytoid B-cell lymphoma. Clinicopathologic study of 21 cases of a unique type of low-grade lymphoma. *Cancer* 62: 1531–1538, 1988.

130. Koh LP, Lim LC, Thng CH: Retreatment with chimeric CD 20 monoclonal antibody in a patient with nodal marginal zone B-cell lymphoma. *Med Oncol* 17: 225–228, 2000.

Chapter

# Chapter 58

# TREATMENT APPROACH TO PRIMARY CENTRAL NERVOUS SYSTEM LYMPHOMAS

*Tamara N. Shenkier and Joseph M. Connors*

## DEFINITION

Primary central nervous system lymphoma (PCNSL) is a non-Hodgkin's lymphoma (NHL) confined to the craniospinal axis without evidence of systemic spread. It should be distinguished from nodal or extranodal NHL that has disseminated to the CNS, which is a different clinical entity. In this chapter, we will discuss the epidemiology, pathology, clinical presentation, diagnosis, and treatment of PCNSL in immunocompetent patients. PCNSL that develops in the context of acquired immunosuppression will be discussed in Chapters 66 and 67.

## EPIDEMIOLOGY

In the past, PCNSL has been reported to represent about 1–2% of all NHL and 5% of all brain tumors.[1] However, these numbers do not reflect the rising incidence of this condition in the past three decades. Much of this rise has been due to the AIDS epidemic, but a two- to threefold rise has also been seen in the immunocompetent population.[2] Some population-based studies suggest this increase is a result of improved detection due to the widespread availability of computed tomographic (CT) scans and magnetic resonance imaging (MRI) and due to better diagnostic techniques, such as stereotactic biopsy. However, a recent Surveillance, Epidemiology and End Results (SEER) analysis refuted this hypothesis.[3] It is reported that the age-adjusted incidence increased from 0.15 to 0.48 per 100,000 person-years from 1973 to 1997. This increase was seen in all age groups and both genders and outpaced the increased incidence of systemic NHL for this period sixfold. Furthermore, if this increase were due to ascertainment bias, there would have been an increased rate of glioma over time, which was not seen. Although the rate of increase of PCNSL has lev-

eled off in the last decade, it appears that the true incidence is increasing.

## PATHOLOGY

The vast majority of PCNSL in immunocompetent patients are Epstein Barr virus (EBV) negative diffuse large B-cell lymphomas (DLBCL). Other histologies, such as T-cell and small lymphocytic lymphoma, are rare.[2,4,5] Unlike other NHLs, it appears that the histological classification of PCNSL does not have prognostic or clinical importance.[6] PCNSL usually grows in an angiocentric pattern with sheets of cells that infiltrate adjacent brain parenchyma. Perivascular reactive T-cells are seen in 30% of cases. The CNS is normally devoid of lymphoid tissue; therefore, the site of the cell of origin from which PCNSL develops is likely extraneural. This cell possesses a specific tropism for the nervous system. Both molecular genetic and immunophenotypic studies have suggested that the cell of origin is from the germinal center as BCL6 proto-oncogene mutations or BCL6 protein expression have been reported in the majority of cases.[7,8] Further evidence for this theory is the high proportion of somatic mutations in the clonally rearranged immunoglobulin heavy chains (VH genes) from PCNSL specimens.[9] More recent studies have demonstrated a unique immunophenotype and gene expression signature which is distinct from nodal diffuse large B cell lymphoma and which may have both prognostic and potential therapeutic implications.[10,11]

## CLINICAL CHARACTERISTICS

### PRESENTATION

Most patients present with an acute or subacute manner with one of several clinical scenarios: symptoms of raised intracranial pressure (such as headache, nausea, vomiting, drowsiness, or visual abnormalities);

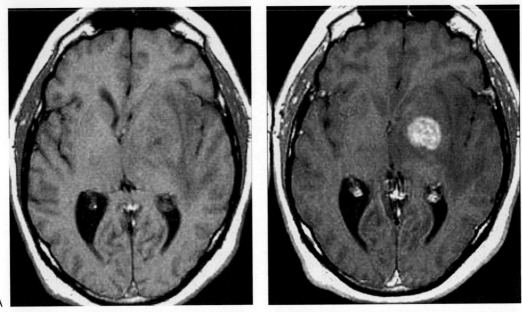

**Figure 58.1**    *An example of the MRI features of PCNSL. Pre- and postgadolinium T1 MRI images showing an isodense lesion in the region of the left basal ganglia and thalamus. There is a mass effect with compression of the left lateral ventricle and moderate surrounding edema. The lesion enhances homogenously postcontrast*

progressive focal neurological deficits or, if the frontal lobes are involved or there is diffuse parenchymal infiltration, cognitive and behavioral abnormalities.[12] Unlike other primary brain tumors, seizures are uncommon, because PCNSL usually affects subcortical structures.

Central structures apart from the brain parenchyma are often affected. The eye itself is a direct extension of the brain, and 10–20% of patients with PCNSL have ocular involvement at diagnosis.[13,14] Ocular lymphomas can involve the vitreous, retina, choroid, or optic nerve itself, and cause blurred vision, floaters, or maybe clinically silent. The process may begin unilaterally, but eventually bilateral involvement develops. The majority of patients, who present with ocular lymphoma alone, will eventually develop cerebral involvement. Concomitant involvement of the leptomeninges can be seen in 15% of patients, but is rarely the sole site of disease.

Several large retrospective studies have described the clinical characteristics of patients with PCNSL.[5,15,16] The median age at diagnosis is about 60 years, with a wide range of 12–85 years. There is a slight male predominance, and two-third of patients present with a poor performance status. One-third of patients have elevated serum lactate dehydrogenase (LDH). One-third of patients have involvement of deep structures, including the cerebellum, basal ganglia, corpus callosum, and brain stem. Brain lesions are multifocal in 30–40% of patients, and even when the tumor is seemingly localized by MRI, microscopic disease involves radiologically normal brain tissue at autopsy.[17] Therefore, PCNSL should be considered disseminated within the CNS at diagnosis.

## DIAGNOSIS

There is no single radiologic pattern of PCNSL that is pathognomonic, but several distinctive neuroimaging features can strongly suggest the diagnosis. CT scans show iso or hyperdense lesions that homogeneously enhance in 90% of cases.[18] The neuroimaging technique of choice is MRI, which demonstrates an intense signal on nonenhanced T1 imaging and dense, diffuse enhancement in 90% of cases after administration of gadolinium contrast (Figure 58.1). The lesions usually have indistinct borders and less associated cerebral edema than primary gliomas or metastatic tumors.[1] They may be multiple in 30–35% of cases, are frequently periventricular in location and usually involve corpus callosum, thalamus, or basal ganglia. Experience with positron emission tomography (PET) in immunocompetent patients with PCNSL is progressively growing, but does not appear to distinguish PCNSL from other malignant brain tumors.[19] The use of PET in predicting response to therapy has not yet been addressed in PCNSL.

The best method to diagnose PCNSL is stereotactic biopsy of an enhancing mass lesion. Subtotal resection is not necessary therapeutically and is usual only performed when the diagnosis of lymphoma is in doubt. In some cases, the diagnosis is established by examination of a vitrectomy specimen from the eye or cytopathology or flow cytometry of cerebrospinal fluid (CSF), obviating the need for a brain biopsy. One distinctive feature of PCNSL is that corticosteroids given to relieve high intracranial pressure can have a potent acute antitumor effect that removes all CT or MRI signs of the lesions, sometimes prior to histologic diagnosis.[18] However, without further treatment patients whose tumors have regressed will inevitably relapse. Therefore, whenever possible, steroids should be withheld until a diagnostic biopsy has been obtained.

### STAGING AND PROGNOSIS

Once the diagnosis is established, usually by stereotactic biopsy of a cerebral lesion, further staging is required. All patients should have a contrast-enhanced brain MRI scan, chest radiography, testing for human immunodeficiency virus (HIV 1 and 2), routine hematology, and routine chemistry including serum LDH, protein electrophoresis, creatinine, and liver enzymes. As intraocular involvement and leptomeningeal infiltration are detected in a significant minority of cases, tests to ascertain the presence or absence of disease in these sites are warranted. Indirect ophthalmoscopy and slit-lamp examination should be employed for the evaluation of intraocular disease, and lumbar puncture is recommended in patients in whom the test can be done safely (i.e. those with no evidence of severe raised intracranial pressure). The CSF should be evaluated for protein, cytopathology and sent for flow cytometry. Any patient who presents with seemingly isolated intraocular or leptomeningeal disease should have a contrast-enhanced brain MRI to rule out concomitant intracerebral lesions.

There is controversy regarding how extensively patients with PCNSL should be evaluated for evidence of systemic lymphoma. Some advocate that staging of patients with PCNSL should be similar to that of systemic NHL. However, tests outside the CNS usually yield negative results; the disease is confined to the CNS in more then 95% of patients.[20] Although the inclusion of patients who have not had complete staging workup in prospective clinical trials has been reported to have led to unreliable conclusions, the omission of bone marrow examination and CT scanning of the chest, abdomen, and pelvis has not led to any change in overall outcome or pattern of relapse in a 13-year retrospective population-based study in British Columbia.[21–23] Recently standardized guidelines for the baseline evaluation and response assessment of PCNSL have been published. In the context of clinical trials, adherence to these standards is critical to ensure comparability between studies.[24]

Prospective studies have consistently shown that age less than 60 years and superior performance status are related to better OS.[25,26] In a recent study, three additional factors also carried adverse prognostic significance: elevated serum LDH, elevated CSF protein concentration, and involvement of deep structures of the brain (such as brainstem, basal ganglia, cerebellum, and corpus callosum).[27] The overall 2-year survival for patients with 0–1, 2–3, and 4–5 factors were approximately 80, 50, and 20%, respectively. This five factor model has not yet been validated in a separate independent cohort of patients and is not yet in wide clinical use.

## PRIMARY TREATMENT

The diffuse nature of PCNSL and the existence of the blood–brain barrier (BBB) have accounted for the lack of success of treatment approaches, including those used for primary brain tumors (e.g. surgical resection and irradiation) and systemic lymphoma (e.g. CHOP (cyclophosphamide, doxorubicin, vincristine, and prednisone) based chemotherapy). The best treatment modality for PCNSL has not yet been identified.

### CORTICOSTEROIDS

Corticosteroids, which are part of the treatment of systemic NHL, have a role in the treatment of PCNSL, by reducing tumor-associated edema and causing lysis of malignant lymphocytes. Although initial responses may be as high as 40%, complete and durable responses are rare.[28] Neither the specific type nor the optimal dose of corticosteroids has been established. Occasionally, the clinical and radiographic features are highly suggestive of PCNSL, and the tumor has regressed following corticosteroids, making tissue confirmation impossible. The initial response to corticosteroids appears to predict for outcome.[29] Those patients with an excellent clinical and radiographic response following corticosteroids alone have a better long-term outcome than nonresponders.

### SURGERY

Surgery is required to confirm the histologic diagnosis, but has no therapeutic role. The median survival of patients treated with supportive care alone is 1–3 months, compared to 4–5 months for those who undergo surgical resection.[30] Furthermore, because PCNSL is often multifocal and deep within the brain, resection is technically difficult. Extensive surgery should be reserved for the occasional patient who requires urgent intervention because of acute neurologic deterioration due to cerebral herniation.

### WHOLE BRAIN IRRADIATION

Whole-brain irradiation (WBXRT) at doses of 40–50 Gy delivered with conventional fractions was the standard of care for years. Despite initial high response rates (60–70%), local relapse is common, and the median survival of treated patients is only 12–18 months.[31,32] The reason for local relapse after excellent response remains unclear, especially since irradiation produces local control in 80–90% of cases of localized DLCL.[33] To assess the impact of increasing the dose of irradiation, the Radiation Therapy Oncology Group (RTOG) conducted a phase II prospective study of

PCNSL patients treated with 40 Gy WBXRT plus a 20 Gy boost to the involved area.[34] Despite this approach, most relapses still occurred in the brain, and the local control rate was only 39%. Seventy-nine percent of these recurrences were in the region that received 60 Gy. The median survival was 12 months.

Not only is WBXRT of 40–50 Gy only modestly effective, but it leads to unacceptable neurotoxicity in a significant proportion of patients, especially when combined with chemotherapy. Because of this problem, investigators have studied modifications of the dose or volume of irradiation. The RTOG recently reported a study using a methotrexate-based regimen in combination with 45 Gy WBXRT. The protocol was modified during the trial to deliver 36 Gy in a hyperfractionated scheduled to those patients who achieved a complete response to chemotherapy.[35] There was no difference in local relapse or survival between those who received the lower and higher doses of irradiation, and the rate of neurotoxicity was the same. In contrast, when the dose of WBXRT was reduced from 45to 30.6 Gy in two consecutive series of patients who achieved a complete response to chemotherapy, the 3-year OS was compromised for patients younger than 60 years (92% vs. 60% $p = 0.04$).[36] Another study assessed the outcome for patients treated with focal irradiation instead of WBXRT.[37] Patients treated with margins less than 4 cm had higher out-field recurrences compared to those treated with >4 cm margins (83% vs. 22% $p = 0.008$).

In summary, these data demonstrate that a boost to the tumor bed does not improve local control, but partial irradiation compromises it. In order to achieve the optimal benefit from irradiation, WBXRT should be administered. However, the optimal dose and fractionation of irradiation when combined with effective chemotherapy is not yet defined. The threshold at which local control is maintained and neurotoxicity is minimized remains to be determined.

### CHEMOTHERAPY IN COMBINATION WITH WBXRT

Chemotherapy in combination with WBXRT, or combined modality therapy, has been used to treat PCNSL for over two decades. Initially, chemotherapy regimens used to treat systemic NHL were employed. Systemic administration of CHOP or CHOD (with dexamethasone), either before or after WBXRT, has been studied in two phase II and one randomized phase III trial.[26,38,39] In the phase II, trials the reported median survivals of 10 and 13 months were no better than historical controls using WBXRT alone, and were associated with high toxicity and a 15% mortality. The randomized trial of WBXRT followed by CHOP or no further treatment showed no difference in failure-free or OS between the two arms, although the study was terminated early due to poor accrual. These data demonstrate that there is no role for CHOP-type therapy in the treatment of PCNSL.

The BBB is a unique obstacle to the successful treatment of brain tumors because high-molecular-weight or polar compounds cannot cross an intact BBB. Although there is partial disruption of the BBB in PCNSL, early successful treatment with corticosteroids effectively reconstitutes the barrier.[40] Successful inroads to treating PCNSL include selection of drugs with physicochemical properties, such as lipid solubility and low molecular weight, which can permeate an intact BBB. One such drug is methotrexate (MTX), an antimetabolite that can penetrate the intact BBB when given intravenously at doses over 1 g/m².[41] High-dose MTX refers to systemically administered MTX, infused over 4–6 h, at doses higher than 1 g/m² and usually over 3.5 g/m², followed by folinic acid rescue. It plays a modest role in the treatment of systemic lymphoma, but has become the most important single agent in the treatment of PCNSL. The optimal schedule, dose, and regimen have not been established, but many mature phase II trials of combined modality therapy with MTX-based regimens have been published. These data are summarized in Table 58.1 and report higher median survivals than those seen with WBXRT alone. As is the case with phase II trials in general, single institutions report better outcomes than multi institutional trials. The reasons for these differences may be treatment-related, such as less familiarity with the chemotherapy protocol, but may also include referral bias, in that only a select number of patients are fit enough to travel to a specific center for experimental treatment.

Most of these trials used intrathecal and systemic chemotherapy to prevent leptomeningeal relapse or treat occult disease. Since intravenously infused, rapidly administered MTX in doses above 3 g/m² can achieve cytotoxic CSF levels, it is unclear whether the addition of intrathecal chemotherapy is necessary. Furthermore complications arise from the placement of an Ommaya reservoir. A recent case-controlled retrospective study concluded that patients who received 3.5 g/m² of MTX did not have improved disease control or survival with the additional administration of intrathecal chemotherapy.[42] However, this conclusion did not apply to patients with overt positive CSF cytology.

Several large retrospective series have examined outcomes according to treatment.[5,15] They provide long-term follow-up on a heterogeneously treated group of patients. One study of 466 patients in which only 6%, who had been treated with MTX-containing combined modality regimens. Those patients who received at least two cycles of chemotherapy had a median survival of 22 months, compared to 17 months for those treated with WBXRT alone. This difference was not significant. In the series from the International Extranodal Lymphoma Study Group (IELSG), about half of the patients were treated with high-dose MTX-containing regimens prior to WBXRT.

**Table 58.1** Results of combined modality treatment for PCNSL using MTX-based regimens

| Chemotherapy (Systemic) | | IT chemo | Institution | Median Age (yr) | N | WBXRT dose Gy (boost) | Median PFS (months) | Median OS (months) | 5y% | Comments | Reference |
| Pre XRT | Post XRT | | | | | | | | | | |
|---|---|---|---|---|---|---|---|---|---|---|---|
| MTX 1g/m² × 2 | 3 g/m² ara-C ×2 | Yes | Single | 58 | 31 | 40 (14) | 40 | 42 | 22 | 5 yr CSS 60% (if < 50y) | 70, 82 |
| MTX 3.5g/m² ×5 + vincristine procarbazine | 3 g/m² ara-C ×2 | Yes | Single | 65 | 52 | 45 | Not reached | 60 | 50 | Median OS 33mo (if ≥ 60y) Not reached (if ≤ 60y) | 46 |
| MTX 3.5g/m² | | No | Single | | 25 | 30 (variable) | 32 | 33 | | | 83 |
| C5R including MTX 3g/m² ×2 ara-C 500 mg/m² + CHOP type | | Yes | Single | 51 | 25 | 20 (30) | | | 56 | Median FU 24 months | 43 |
| MTX 2.5g/m² × 5 + vincristine procarbazine | | Yes | Multi | 57 | 102 | a) 45 b) 36 | 24 | 36 | 32 | Median OS 22 mo (if > 60y) 50 mo (if < 60 yr) | 35 |
| MTX 1 g/m² × 2 | | Only in 3 pts with + CSF | Multi | 58 | 46 | 45 (5.4) | 40 | 33 | | | 49 |
| MTX 3 g/m² × 2 + Teniposide carmustine | | yes | Multi | 51 | 52 | 40 | | 46 | 58 (3 yr%) | 10% toxic deaths | 44 |

XRT = irradiation; MTX = methotrexate; FU = follow-up; WBXRT = whole brain irradiation; PFS = progression-free survival; OS = overall survival; ara-C = cytarabine; IT = intrathecal; CSS = cause specific survival.

The overall 2-year survival was 37%, but rose to 60% for those patients who received MTX as part of their primary therapy. In addition, a multivariate analysis suggested that for those patients treated with MTX, the addition of high-dose cytarabine also contributed to a survival benefit. However, due to the heterogeneous treatment approach and multicenter nature of the study, one cannot determine the optimal chemotherapy approach for this disease based on these data. The observation of a better prognosis with cytarabine should be interpreted with caution as it may not be attributable to treatment itself but to other known or unknown prognostic factors affecting the selection of the treatment. We studied the outcomes for 122 patients with PCNSL treated with three consecutive therapeutic approaches over 13 years in British Columbia. The median OS was 17 months. When analyzed by intention-to-treat, outcomes had not changed over time. However, those patients who received MTX, regardless of age and performance status, had a median OS of 31 months.[23]

The results of phase II studies and the retrospective series will not be corroborated by a phase III randomized trial, because expert opinion has determined that, based on the available data, MTX-based chemotherapy should be administered along with WBXRT. The median survival of patients treated with this approach ranges from 33 to 60 months, compared to 12–18 months for those given WBXRT alone. Although a selection bias cannot be excluded, it likely does not account for all of the benefit attributed to MTX. However, there are many outstanding issues regarding the use of MTX in combined modality treatment including the optimal dose of MTX, duration of treatment, and best chemotherapy regimen. Studies have used doses ranging from 1 to 8 $g/m^2$. Our data and the IELSG series showed no difference in outcome according to dose. Most studies and ongoing protocols use 3–4 $g/m^2$. Although one retrospective study suggested that cytarabine contributed independently to outcome,[5] there has been no randomized comparison of different chemotherapy regimens. In general, the more intensive multiagent protocols, such as C5R[43] and MBVP,[44] have reported higher acute treatment-related morbidity and mortality compared to simpler protocols.

### NEUROTOXICITY

Although the acute toxicity from simple MTX-based combined modality treatment is acceptable, delayed neurotoxicity resulting from the combined effects of MTX and WBXRT is a serious problem that limits the overall efficacy of these regimens. The condition is termed "leukoencephalopathy," and is characterized by diffuse white matter abnormalities, cortical atrophy, and ventricular dilatation.[45] Clinically, patients present with a progressive and irreversible neurological syndrome of cognitive impairment, ataxia, and

incontinence, which develops a median of 9–16 months following treatment. The incidence of neurotoxicity seems to be related to several variables one of which is the use of WBXRT. One study reported that surviving patients older than 60 years who received WBXRT following MTX-based chemotherapy had a 83% risk of leukoencephalopathy, compared to 17% in those who were not irradiated.[46] Only 6% of patients under age 60 years who were irradiated developed this complication. However a trial from Germany in which complete responders to induction chemotherapy were randomized to WBXRT or not reported equivalent rates of neurotoxicity in older and younger participants (19% and 21%, respectively). Moreover, the rates did not differ between those who received WBXRT and those who did not.[47] Other studies have reported a 22–26% incidence of this problem.[48,49] Subtler forms of this condition are not as well documented, but one study reported that only 20% of patients aged 40–60 years at diagnosis, who were alive and disease free at 4 years, were capable of working.[48] Finally, it is unclear whether there is an independent contribution of intrathecally administered chemotherapy to the development of leukoencephalopathy. In one trial of combined modality treatment, there was no significant difference in the rate of neurotoxicity between those who received intrathecal chemotherapy and those who did not.[42]

In an effort to reduce leukoencephalopathy, current treatment strategies are focusing on using chemotherapy alone and deferring WBXRT for responders, especially in older patients. Since cognitive impairment often is present at diagnosis in PCNSL, this approach will not entirely prevent chronic neurological symptoms. However this complication has been reported less commonly in those patients treated with chemotherapy alone.[47,50–52]

### CHEMOTHERAPY ALONE

Chemotherapy approaches have included using MTX as a single agent, combining MTX with other drugs that penetrate the BBB, and administering high-dose chemotherapy and stem cell rescue in patients who respond to induction MTX-based regimens. These studies are outlined in Table 58.2 and demonstrate a wide range of OS. The striking difference compared to combined modality treatment appears to be the minimal neurotoxicity.

While the majority of studies have focused on using combinations of chemotherapy agents that penetrate the BBB, other investigators developed administration strategies that improve drug delivery to the brain. With the patient under general anesthesia, the femoral artery is catheterized and an osmotic agent, mannitol, can be used to temporarily disrupt the BBB. This is followed by the intravenous and intraarterial infusion of chemotherapy, and is repeated monthly for up to 12 cycles in responding patients.[59] One

Table 58.2  Results of selected trials of MTX based chemotherapy alone in the treatment of PCNSL

| Chemotherapy (Systemic) | | IT chemo | Institution | Median Age (yr) | N | Median PFS (mo) | Median OS (mo) | Comments | Neurotoxicity | Reference |
| --- | --- | --- | --- | --- | --- | --- | --- | --- | --- | --- |
| MTX dose | Other drugs | | | | | | | | | |
| 8 g/m² × 4<br>3.5 g/m² × 13 | None | No | Multi | 59 | 59 | 12.8 | 55.4 | | No | 53 |
| 8 g/m² × 8<br>3.5 g/m² × indefinite | None | No | Single | 63 | 31 | 16.7 | 30.4 | | No | 54 |
| 8 g/m² × 6 | None | No | Multi | 60 | 37 | 13.7 for responders | | CR 30%<br>PD 38% | | 55 |
| 1 g/m² × 3 | Lomustine procarbazine steroids | Yes | Multi | 72 | 50 | 8 | 14 | | 8% | 56 |
| 5 g/m² × 2 | cytarabine ifosphosphamide vincristine cyclophosphamide vindesine | Yes | Multi | 62 | 65 | 21 | 50 | <60 yr estimated 2y OS = 80% >60 yr median OS = 34 months | 3% | 57 |
| 3.5 g/m² × 5<br>+<br>3 g/m²/d × 2 cytarabine | Responders<br>BEAM + ASCT | No | Multi | 53 | 28 (14 completed BEAM + ASCT | 5.6 (all)<br>9.3 (BEAM) | not reached | one acute toxic death | minimal | 58 |

CR = complete response; OS = overall survival; IT = intrathecal; PD = progressive disease; PFS = progression-free survival; MTX = methotrexate; BEAM + ASCT = carmustine, etoposide, cytarabine, melphalan + autologous stem cell transplant.

center treated 74 patients this way over 15 years and reported a median OS of 40 months and a 5-year OS of 42%. Ten patients experienced significant acute morbidity and mortality, but no cases of neurocognitive impairment were seen in surviving patients. There have been no randomized trials comparing conventionally administered chemotherapy to that delivered with BBB disruption. In view of this as well as the procedural complexities and acute toxicity associated with this approach, this technique has not been widely adopted.

Ongoing clinical trials are focused on adding additional agents to MTX such as thiotepa, ifosfamide, or rituximab.[57,60,61] Rituximab is a chimeric anti CD20 monoclonal antibody that improves the survival of patients with systemic diffuse large B cell lymphoma when administered with CHOP.[62] Because of its physicochemical characteristics, it does not penetrate an intact BBB. Despite this, several studies are currently exploring it's use in the treatment of PCNSL.[61] In addition to trying to enhance efficacy, current trials are also attempting to reduce the toxicity of combined modality treatment by either reducing the dose of WBXRT or deferring it entirely for patients who achieve a complete response to systemic therapy.[63,64]

## SPECIAL THERAPEUTIC CIRCUMSTANCES

### INTRAOCULAR LYMPHOMA

When intraocular lymphoma (IOL) is present at diagnosis, there is usually concomitant cerebral involvement. If WBXRT is being used in the primary treatment, the eyes should also be included in the irradiation field. The long term side-effects of orbital irradiation include the development of cataracts, retinal detachment, and optic nerve atrophy. High-dose intravenous MTX alone can achieve therapeutic concentrations in the vitreous humour.[65] One study reported a complete response in four of five patients with IOL treated with this approach.[66] This suggests that orbital XRT can be deferred in patients with stable visual findings who receive MTX. One approach is to assess for persistent disease after four cycles of chemotherapy. If IOL is still detected, then orbital irradiation can be administered.

It is rare for patients to present with IOL alone. Ninety percent of these patients will eventually relapse in the brain, and any treatment approach should keep this in mind. Chemotherapy alone, with orbital and/or WBXRT reserved for persistent or progressive disease, is an attractive option that minimizes toxicity.

### LEPTOMENINGEAL LYMPHOMA

Leptomeningeal involvement is seen in about 15% of patients diagnosed with PCNSL. The presentation is commonly clinically silent and only detectable by cytological examination of the CSF. Less frequently, there can be overt cranial nerve or nerve root symptoms that are easily visible as gadolinium enhancement of the leptomeninges on MRI examination. Leptomeningeal disease is usually present with intracerebral involvement, but in 1–2% of cases it is the sole site of PCNSL.

The treatment depends on the extent of the disease. If bulky disease is present and symptomatic, localized irradiation to the spinal cord or skull base should be employed but chemotherapy, delivered either intrathecally or intravenously, is required to take care of disease disseminated throughout the CSF. Systemic chemotherapy with 8 g/m² of MTX does penetrate the CSF and achieves prolonged cytotoxic CSF concentrations at least comparable to those from intrathecal administration.[67] Intrathecal administration of MTX or cytarabine usually requires insertion of a ventricular reservoir because the drugs are given twice a week, due to the short half life in the CSF. A sustained release form of liposomal cytarabine, administered every 2 weeks, has been compared to conventional cytarabine for the treatment of lymphomatous meningitis.[68] Those patients who received the sustained release formulation had a higher response rate (71 vs 15%) and greater improvement in performance status than those who were treated with conventional cytarabine.

If leptomeningeal involvement is clinically silent and detected only by cytological examination of the CSF, it is unclear whether or not intrathecal chemotherapy needs to be given when chemotherapy regimens that include high-dose intravenous MTX are employed as primary treatment.[42,66] One approach is to follow such patients carefully and withhold intrathecal treatment if the patient is improving and the CSF cytology clears after four cycles of MTX.

### SPINAL LYMPHOMA

True intramedullary spinal cord lymphoma, in contrast to epidural disease, is very rare. Intracerebral, intraocular, and leptomeningeal disease should be ruled out with the staging investigations described in the section above. If the lymphoma is confined to the spine, combined modality treatment with MTX-containing chemotherapy and localized irradiation is recommended.

## TREATMENT FOR RELAPSED OR REFRACTORY DISEASE

The majority of patients with PCNSL relapse following primary treatment, and a significant minority have progressive disease during primary treatment. One retrospective study of 173 patients concluded that patients whose overall condition is suitable to receive salvage therapy have significantly prolonged survival compared to those who are given no further treatment (14 vs 2 months).[69] Although this improved survival may be largely due to patient, rather than treatment-related factors, fit patients should be offered salvage treatment. However, there are no standard recommendations for second-line therapy as most studies are small case series of heterogeneously treated patients. The choice of treatment depends on the patient's prior treatment, the site of relapse (brain, ocular, leptomeningeal, spinal, systemic, or a combination), and the disease-free interval.

Patients who relapse in the brain following WBXRT (either alone or as part of combined modality treatment) should be offered chemotherapy. MTX can be administered to those who did not receive it during first line therapy, although neurotoxicity remains a concern with this sequence of therapy. Several chemotherapy options have been reported to be useful for those who progress or relapse soon after MTX-based combined modality treatment. These include high-dose cytarabine (3g/m²),[70] PCV (procarbazine, lomustine, and vincristine),[71] thiotepa, temozolamide,[72] and topotecan.[73,74] High-dose chemotherapy with thiotepa, busulfan, and cyclophosphamide followed by autologous peripheral blood stem cell (PBSC) infusion can result in 64% survival at 3 years, but was too toxic for patients over 60 years of age. Of the 22 patients who were treated with this approach, 14 had received CYVE (cytarabine and etoposide) to ascertain chemosensitivity prior to high-dose treatment.[75] There are ongoing studies using rituximab intravenously for relapsed disease.[76,77]

WBXRT can be used at progression or relapse if it was not part of the initial therapy. One study reported an overall response of 76 % and a median survival of 6.8 months with this strategy while another reported a median survival of 11 months.[78,79] However WBXRT mat not be essential as some patients with a long disease-free interval after receiving MTX alone as their primary treatment can be effectively retreated with the same chemotherapy regimen. In one study, 9 of 11 patients achieved a second complete response after reinduction.[80]

Patients who have an isolated intraocular relapse following treatment with chemotherapy alone should be treated with ocular XRT. Since these patients are also at high risk of relapse in the brain, WBXRT can be considered, but it may be deferred until intracerebral progression is demonstrated. The report of high-dose chemotherapy and PBSC rescue described above included eleven patients with intraocular involvement, four of whom had isolated ocular disease and demonstrated its feasibility in this group. For patients whose eyes have been previously irradiated, intravitreal MTX is also an option.[81]

Patients who relapse in the leptomeninges can be managed with spinal cord irradiation, intrathecal or systemic chemotherapy as described in the Leptomeningeal Lymphoma section above.

## SUMMARY

There are still several unresolved issues regarding the optimal management of PCNSL. The need for WBXRT, especially in patients over 60 years old, remains controversial and the best compromise between disease control and delayed neurotoxicity has not been identified. PCNSL is a chemosensitive disease but the optimal systemic regimen has yet to been defined. Other controversial issues include the role of intrathecal chemotherapy for primary treatment and the optimal salvage treatment for refractory and relapsed disease.

## REFERENCES

1. Fine HA, Loeffler JS: Primary central nervous system lymphoma. In: Canellos G, Lister TA, Sklar JL (ed.) *The Lymphomas*. Philadelphia, W.B. Saunders, 1998, 481–494.

2. Cote TR, Manns A, Hardy CR, et al.: Epidemiology of brain lymphoma among people with or without acquired immunodeficiency syndrome. AIDS/Cancer Study Group. *J Natl Cancer Inst* 88:675–679, 1996.

3. Olson JE, Janney CA, Rao RD, et al.: The continuing increase in the incidence of primary central nervous system non-Hodgkin lymphoma: a surveillance, epidemiology, and end results analysis. *Cancer* 95:1504–1510, 2002.

4. Camilleri-Broet S, Martin A, Moreau A, et al.: Primary central nervous system lymphomas in 72 immunocompetent patients: pathologic findings and clinical correlations. Groupe Ouest Est d'etude des Leucenies et Autres Maladies du Sang (GOELAMS). *Am J Clin Pathol* 110: 607–612, 1998.

5. Ferreri AJ, Reni M, Pasini F, et al.: A multicenter study of treatment of primary CNS lymphoma. *Neurology*. 58: 1513–1520, 2002.

6. Shenkier TN, Blay JY, O'Neill BP, et al.: Primary CNS lymphoma of T-cell origin: a descriptive analysis from the international primary CNS lymphoma collaborative group. *J Clin Oncol* 23:2233–2239, 2005.

7. Braaten KM, Betensky RA, de Leval L, et al.: BCL-6 expression predicts improved survival in patients with primary central nervous system lymphoma. *Clin Cancer Res* 9:1063–1069, 2003.

8. Larocca LM, Capello D, Rinelli A, et al.: The molecular and phenotypic profile of primary central nervous system lymphoma identifies distinct categories of the disease and is consistent with histogenetic derivation from germinal center-related B cells. *Blood* 92:1011–1019, 1998.

9. Thompsett AR, Ellison DW, Stevenson FK, et al.: V(H) gene sequences from primary central nervous system

lymphomas indicate derivation from highly mutated germinal center B cells with ongoing mutational activity. *Blood* 94:1738–1746, 1999.

10. Camilleri-Broet S, Criniere E, Broet P, et al.: A uniform activated B-cell-like immunophenotype might explain the poor prognosis of primary central nervous system lymphomas: analysis of 83 cases. *Blood* 107(1):190–196, 2006.

11. Rubenstein JL, Fridlyand J, Shen A, et al.: Gene expression and angiotropism in primary CNS lymphoma. *Blood* 107(9):3716–3723, 2006.

12. Behin A, Hoang-Xuan K, Carpentier AF, et al.: Primary brain tumours in adults. *Lancet* 361:323–331, 2003.

13. Ferreri AJ, Blay JY, Reni M, et al.: Relevance of intraocular involvement in the management of primary central nervous system lymphomas. *Ann Oncol* 13:531–538, 2002.

14. Hormigo A, DeAngelis LM: Primary ocular lymphoma: clinical features, diagnosis, and treatment. *Clin Lymphoma* 4:22–29, 2003.

15. Hayabuchi N, Shibamoto Y, Onizuka Y: Primary central nervous system lymphoma in Japan: a nationwide survey. *Intern J Radiat Oncol BiolPhys* 44:265–272, 1999.

16. Bataille B, Delwail V, Menet E, et al.: Primary intracerebral malignant lymphoma: report of 248 cases. *J Neurosurg* 92:261–266, 2000.

17. Lai R, Rosenblum MK, DeAngelis LM: Primary CNS lymphoma: A whole-brain disease? *Neurology* 59:1557–1562, 2002.

18. Fine HA, Mayer RJ: Primary central nervous system lymphoma. *Ann Intern Med* 119:1093–1104, 1993.

19. Roelcke U, Leenders KL: Positron emission tomography in patients with primary CNS lymphomas. *J NeuroOncol* 43:231–236, 1999.

20. Herrlinger U: Primary CNS lymphoma: findings outside the brain. *J NeuroOncol* 43:227–230, 1999.

21. Ferreri AJ, Reni M, Villa E: Therapeutic management of primary central nervous system lymphoma: lessons from prospective trials. *Ann Oncol* 11:927–937, 2000.

22. O'Neill BP, Dinapoli RP, Kurtin PJ, et al.: Occult systemic non-Hodgkin's lymphoma (NHL) in patients initially diagnosed as primary central nervous system lymphoma (PCNSL): how much staging is enough? *J Neurooncol* 25:67–71, 1995.

23. Shenkier TN, Voss N, Chhanabhai M, et al.: The treatment of primary central nervous system lymphoma in 122 immunocompetent patients. *Cancer* 103(5): 1008–1017, 2005.

24. Abrey LE, Batchelor TT, Ferreri AJ, et al.: Report of an international workshop to standardize baseline evaluation and response criteria for primary CNS lymphoma. *J Clin Oncol* 23:5034–5043, 2005.

25. Corry J, Smith JG, Wirth A, et al.: Primary central nervous system lymphoma: age and performance status are more important than treatment modality. *Int J Radiat Oncol BiolPhys* 41:615–620, 1998.

26. Mead GM, Bleehen NM, Gregor A, et al.: A medical research council randomized trial in patients with primary cerebral non-Hodgkin lymphoma: cerebral radiotherapy with and without cyclophosphamide, doxorubicin, vincristine, and prednisone chemotherapy. *Cancer* 89:1359–1370, 2000.

27. Ferreri AJ, Blay JY, Reni M, et al.: Prognostic scoring system for primary CNS lymphomas: the International Extranodal Lymphoma Study Group experience. *J Clin Oncol* 21:266–272, 2003.

28. Pirotte B, Levivier M, Goldman S, et al.: Glucocorticoid-induced long-term remission in primary cerebral lymphoma: case report and review of the literature. *J Neurooncol* 32:63–69, 1997.

29. Mathew BS, Carson KA, Grossman SA. Initial response to glucocorticoids: an important prognostic factor in patients with primary CNS lymphoma (PCNSL) *Proc Am Soc Clin Oncol* 21:76a; 2002.

30. Henry JM, Heffner RR Jr, Dillard SH, et al.: Primary malignant lymphomas of the central nervous system. *Cancer* 34:1293–1302, 1974.

31. Nelson DF: Radiotherapy in the treatment of primary central nervous system lymphoma (PCNSL). *J Neurooncol* 43:241–247, 1999.

32. Laperriere NJ, Cerezo L, Milosevic MF, et al.: Primary lymphoma of brain: results of management of a modern cohort with radiation therapy. *Radiother Oncol* 43: 247–252, 1997.

33. Shenkier TN, Voss N, Fairey R, et al.: Brief chemotherapy and involved-region irradiation for limited-stage diffuse large-cell lymphoma: an 18-year experience from the British Columbia Cancer Agency. *J Clin Oncol* 20: 197–204, 2002.

34. Nelson DF, Martz KL, Bonner H, et al.: Non-Hodgkin's lymphoma of the brain: can high dose, large volume radiation therapy improve survival? Report on a prospective trial by the Radiation Therapy Oncology Group (RTOG): RTOG 8315. *Int J Radiat Oncol Biol Phys* 23:9–17, 1992.

35. DeAngelis LM, Seiferheld W, Schold SC, et al.: Combination chemotherapy and radiotherapy for primary central nervous system lymphoma: Radiation Therapy Oncology Group Study 93-10. *J Clin Oncol* 20:4643–4648, 2002.

36. Bessell EM, Lopez-Guillermo A, Villa S, et al.: Importance of radiotherapy in the outcome of patients with primary CNS lymphoma: an analysis of the CHOD/BVAM regimen followed by two different radiotherapy treatments. *J Clin Oncol* 20:231–236, 2002.

37. Shibamoto Y, Hayabuchi N, Hiratsuka J, et al.: Is whole-brain irradiation necessary for primary central nervous system lymphoma? Patterns of recurrence after partial-brain irradiation. *Cancer* 97:128–133, 2003.

38. Schultz C, Scott C, Sherman W, et al.: Preirradiation chemotherapy with cyclophosphamide, doxorubicin, vincristine, and dexamethasone for primary CNS lymphomas: initial report of radiation therapy oncology group protocol 88-06. *J Clin Oncol* 14:556–564, 1996.

39. O'Neill BP, O'Fallon JR, Earle JD, et al.: Primary central nervous system non-Hodgkin's lymphoma: survival advantages with combined initial therapy? *Int J Radiat Oncol Biol Phys* 33:663–673, 1995.

40. Ott RJ, Brada M, Flower MA, et al.: Measurements of blood-brain barrier permeability in patients undergoing radiotherapy and chemotherapy for primary cerebral lymphoma. *Eur J Cancer* 27:1356–1361, 1991.

41. Balis FM, Poplack DG: Central nervous system pharmacology of antileukemic drugs. *Am J Pediatr Hematol Oncol* 11:74–86, 1989.

42. Khan RB, Shi W, Thaler HT, et al.: Is intrathecal methotrexate necessary in the treatment of primary CNS lymphoma? *J Neurooncol* 58:175–178, 2002.

43. Blay JY, Bouhour D, Carrie C, et al.: The C5R protocol: A regimen of high-dose chemotherapy and radiotherapy in primary cerebral non-Hodgkin's lymphoma of patients with no known cause of immunosuppression. *Blood* 86(8):2922–2929, 1995.

44. Poortmans PMP, Kluin-Nelemans HC, Haaxma-Reiche H, et al.: High-dose methotrexate-based chemotherapy followed by consolidating radiotherapy in Non-AIDS-related primary central nervous system lymphoma: European Organization for Research and Treatment of Cancer Lymphoma Group Phase II Trial 20962. *J Clin Oncol* 21:4483–4488, 2003.

45. Filley CM, Kleinschmidt-DeMasters BK: Toxic leukoencephalopathy. *N Engl J Med* 345:425–432, 2001.

46. Abrey LE, Yahalom J, DeAngelis LM: Treatment for primary CNS lymphoma: the next step. *J Clin Oncol* 18:3144–150, 2000.

47. Korfel A, Martus P, Nowrousian MR, et al.: Response to chemotherapy and treating institution predict survival in primary central nervous system lymphoma. *British J Haematol* 128(2):177–183, 2005.

48. Blay JY, Conroy T, Chevreau C, et al.: High-dose methotrexate for the treatment of primary cerebral lymphomas: analysis of survival and late neurologic toxicity in a retrospective series. *J Clin Oncol* 16:864–871, 1998.

49. O'Brien P, Roos D, Pratt G, et al.: Phase II multicenter study of brief single-agent methotrexate followed by irradiation in primary CNS lymphoma. *J Clin Oncol* 18:519, 2000.

50. Sandor V, Stark-Vancs V, et al.: Phase II trial of chemotherapy alone for primary CNS and intraocular lymphoma. *J Clin Oncol* 16(9):3000–3006, 1998.

51. Fliessbach K, Helmstaedter C, et al.: Neuropsychological outcome after chemotherapy for primary CNS lymphoma: a prospective study. *Neurology* 64(7):1184–1188, 2005.

52. Batchelor T, Carson K, et al.: Treatment of primary CNS lymphoma with methotrexate and deferred radiotherapy: a report of NABTT 96-07. *J Clin Oncol* 21(6):1044–1049, 2003.

53. Batchelor T, Carson K, et al.: Treatment of primary CNS lymphoma with methotrexate and deferred radiotherapy: a report of NABTT 96-07. *J Clin Oncol* 21(6):1044–1049, 2003.

54. Guha-Thakurta N, Damek D, et al.: Intravenous methotrexate as initial treatment for primary central nervous system lymphoma: response to therapy and quality of life of patients. *J Neurooncol* 43(3):259–268, 1999.

55. Herrlinger U, Schabet M, et al.: German Cancer Society Neuro-Oncology Working Group NOA-03 multicenter trial of single-agent high-dose methotrexate for primary central nervous system lymphoma. *Ann Neurol* 51(2):247–252, 2002.

56. Hoang-Xuan K, Taillandier L, et al.: Chemotherapy alone as initial treatment for primary CNS lymphoma in patients older than 60 years: a multicenter phase II study (26952) of the European Organization for Research and Treatment of Cancer Brain Tumor Group. *J Clin Oncol* 21(14):2726–2731, 2003.

57. Pels H, Schmidt-Wolf IGH, et al.: Primary central nervous system lymphoma: results of a pilot and phase II study of systemic and intraventricular chemotherapy with deferred radiotherapy. *J Clin Oncol* 21(24):4489–4495, 2003.

58. Abrey LE, Moskowitz CH, et al.: Intensive methotrexate and cytarabine followed by high-dose chemotherapy with autologous stem-cell rescue in patients with newly diagnosed primary CNS lymphoma: an intent-to-treat analysis. *J Clin Oncol* 21(22):4151–4156, 2003.

59. McAllister LD, Doolittle ND, Guastadisegni PE, et al.: Cognitive outcomes and long-term follow-up results after enhanced chemotherapy delivery for primary central nervous system lymphoma. *Neurosurgery* 46:51–60; 2000. [Discussion 60–61]

60. Ferreri AJ, Dell'Oro S, et al.: MATILDE regimen followed by radiotherapy is an active strategy against primary CNS lymphomas. *Neurology* 66(9):1435–1438, 2006.

61. El Kamar FG, Deangelis LM, Yahalom J, et al.: Combined immunochemotherapy with reduced dose whole brain radiotherapy (WBRT) for newly diagnosed patients with primary CNS lymphoma (PCNSL). *American Society of Clinical Oncology*, New Orleans, 2004, abstr 1518.

62. Coiffier B, Lepage E, Briere J, et al.: CHOP Chemotherapy plus Rituximab compared with chop alone in elderly patients with diffuse large-b-cell lymphoma. *N Engl J Med* 346:235–242, 2002.

63. Batchelor T, Loeffler JS: Primary CNS lymphoma. *J Clin Oncol* 24(8):1281–1288, 2006.

64. Pels H, Schlegel U: Primary central nervous system lymphoma. *Curr Treat Opt Neurol* 8(4):346–357, 2006.

65. Henson JW, Yang J, Batchelor T: Intraocular methotrexate level after high-dose intravenous infusion. *J Clin Oncol* 17:1329, 1999.

66. Batchelor T, Carson K, O'Neill A, et al.: Treatment of primary CNS lymphoma with methotrexate and deferred radiotherapy: A Report of NABTT 96-07. *J Clin Oncol* 21:1044–1049, 2003.

67. Glantz MJ, Cole BF, Recht L, et al.: High-dose intravenous methotrexate for patients with nonleukemic leptomeningeal cancer: is intrathecal chemotherapy necessary? *J Clin Oncol* 16:1561–1567, 1998.

68. Glantz MJ, LaFollette S, Jaeckle KA, et al.: Randomized trial of a slow-release versus a standard formulation of cytarabine for the intrathecal treatment of lymphomatous meningitis. *J Clin Oncol* 17:3110–3116, 1999.

69. Reni M, Ferreri AJ, Villa E: Second-line treatment for primary central nervous system lymphoma. *Br J Cancer* 79:530–534, 1999.

70. Abrey LE, DeAngelis LM, Yahalom J: Long-term survival in primary CNS lymphoma. *J Clin Oncol* 16:859–863, 1998.

71. Herrlinger U, Brugger W, Bamberg M, et al.: PCV salvage chemotherapy for recurrent primary CNS lymphoma. *Neurology* 54:1707–1708, 2000.

72. Reni M, Ferreri AJ, Landoni C, et al.: Salvage therapy with temozolomide in an immunocompetent patient with primary brain lymphoma. *J Natl Cancer Inst* 92: 575–576, 2000.

73. Reni M, Mason W, et al.: Salvage chemotherapy with temozolomide in primary CNS lymphomas: preliminary results of a phase II trial. *Eur J Cancer* 40(11):1682–1688, 2004.

74. Fischer L, Thiel E, et al.: Prospective trial on topotecan salvage therapy in primary CNS lymphoma. *Ann Oncol* 17(7):1141–1145, 2006.

75. Soussain C, Suzan F, Hoang-Xuan K, et al.: Results of intensive chemotherapy followed by hematopoietic

stem-cell rescue in 22 patients with refractory or recurrent primary CNS lymphoma or intraocular lymphoma. *J Clin Oncol* 19:742–749, 2001.

76. Pels H, Schulz H, et al.: Treatment of CNS lymphoma with the anti-CD20 antibody rituximab: experience with two cases and review of the literature. *Onkologie* 26(4):351–354, 2003.

77. Enting RH, Demopoulos A, et al.: Salvage therapy for primary CNS lymphoma with a combination of rituximab and temozolomide. *Neurology* 63(5):901–903, 2004.

78. Sharis C, Hochberg FH, Thornton AF, et al.: Is there a role for cranial radiotherapy after primary high dose intravenous methotrexate in primary central nervous system lymphoma? {abstr 2098}. *Int J Radiat Oncol Biol Phys* 45(3):327, 2004.

79. Nguyen PL, Chakravarti A, et al.: Results of whole-brain radiation as salvage of methotrexate failure for immunocompetent patients with primary CNS lymphoma. *J Clin Oncol* 23(7):1507–1513, 2005.

80. Chon B, Hochberg F, Loeffler J, et al.: Methotrexate reinduction in patients with relapsed primary central nervous system lymphoma. *Neuro-Oncology* 3:356, 2001, abstr 357.

81. Fishburne BC, Wilson DJ, Rosenbaum JT, et al.: Intravitreal methotrexate as an adjunctive treatment of intraocular lymphoma. *Arch Ophthalmol* 115:1152–1156, 1997.

82. DeAngelis L, Yahalom J, Thaler H, et al.: Combined modality therapy for primary CNS lymphoma. *J Clin Oncol* 10:635–643, 1992.

83. Glass J, Gruber ML, Cher L, et al.: Preirradiation methotrexate chemotherapy of primary central nervous system lymphoma: long-term outcome. *J Neurosurg* 81:188–195, 1994.

# Chapter 59

# TREATMENT APPROACH TO CUTANEOUS LYMPHOMAS

## Christiane Querfeld, Timothy M. Kuzel, Joan Guitart, and Steven T. Rosen

Cutaneous lymphomas comprise both T- and B-cell subtypes and represent a heterogeneous group of non-Hodgkin's lymphomas. There are no standard guidelines for the treatment of these entities. However, precise diagnosis and identification of prognostic features is critical in determing therapy.[1] Select subtypes can be cured, while prolongation of life and effective palliation can be achieved in the majority of patients.

## TREATMENT OF PRIMARY CUTANEOUS B-CELL LYMPHOMA

The classification of primary cutaneous B-cell lymphoma (PCBCL) remains controversial with separate and distinct terminology promoted by the Working Formulation, the Revised European–American Lymphoma (REAL) classification, the World Health Organization (WHO) and the European Organization for Research and Treatment of Cancer (EORTC).[2–4] Most long-term follow-up data are based on studies according to the EORTC (Table 59.1). The varied classification schemes make it difficult to interpret the literature concerning treatment.

PCBCLs are characterized by a favorable prognosis with a tendency to remain localized to a limited area of the skin and a low risk of extracutaneous spread. Compared to cutaneous T-cell lymphoma (CTCL), experience with treatment of PCBCL is more limited and focuses on follicle center cell lymphoma (FCCL). The optimum treatment for marginal zone lymphoma (MZL)/immunocytoma (IC), large B-cell lymphoma of the leg (LBCL of the leg), and the provisional entities remains controversial. Traditional treatment approaches, including surgical excision, local radiation, and/or chemotherapy, are most commonly used, but relapses occur frequently. Antibiotics may be used as a first-line treatment of *Borrelia burgdorferi*-associated primary cutaneous B-cell lymphoma.[5,6] Biologic therapies, such as interferon alpha and rituximab, a chimeric monoclonal antibody directed against

CD20 cell surface marker, have been incorporated into treatment strategies.[7,8] In select patients with relapsing and refractory disease, autologous or allogeneic transplantation is appropriate.

### RADIATION THERAPY

PCBCL are highly radiosensitive, and radiation therapy is often the preferred therapy for solitary or localized grouped lesions. There are few retrospective studies available on radiotherapy of PCBCL, and they include small numbers of patients. Prospective trials have not been reported. Reported complete remission rates range from 92 to 100%, with 5-year survival rates ranging from 67 to 100%.[9–12] However, cutaneous recurrences are common, and were observed in 16–67% of patients.

In a recent retrospective study, 34 patients with PCBCL treated with radiotherapy were identified and classified according to EORTC and WHO criteria.[9] Twenty-six patients were treated with electron beam radiation, six patients with orthovoltage radiation, and one patient each with photon beam radiation and combination of photon and electron beam radiation. The authors note that a 2- to 3-cm margin added to the radiation site is generally used at their institution, although exact data were not available. All patients achieved a complete response (CR) to initial treatment. Five-year relapse-free survival ranged from 62 to 73% for follicle center cell (FCC) by EORTC/diffuse large B-cell lymphoma (DLBCL) by WHO, FCC by EORTC/follicular lymphoma (Fol) by WHO, and MZL by EORTC and WHO, with a 5-year overall survival of 100%. Patients with LBCL of the leg by EORTC/leg DLBCL by WHO showed worse results, with a 5-year relapse-free survival of 33% and a 5-year overall survival of 67%. However, only three patients were classified as leg DLBCL. The less favorable prognosis of the anatomic site leg seems to be consistent with previously published data and EORTC classification.[2,13] Eight of 13 relapses were confined to the skin and 5 developed extracutaneous spread. The

**Table 59.1** The WHO-EORTC classification for primary cutaneous lymphomas and associated frequency and 5-year survival[a]

| WHO-EORTC | Frequency (%) | 5-year survival (%) |
|---|---|---|
| **Cutaneous T-cell and NK-cell lymphoma** | | |
| *Indolent* | | |
| Mycosis fungoides | 44 | 88 |
| ■ Follicular MF | 4 | 80 |
| ■ Pagetoid reticulosis | <1 | 100 |
| ■ Granulomatous Slack Skin | <1 | 100 |
| CD30[+] lymphoproliferative diseases | | |
| ■ Anaplastic large cell lymphoma | 8 | 95 |
| ■ Lymphomatoid Papulosis | 12 | 100 |
| Subcutaneous panniculitis-like T-cell lymphoma | 1 | 82 |
| CD4[+] small/medium pleomorphic T-cell lymphoma | 2 | 72 |
| *Aggressive* | | |
| Sézary syndrome | 3 | 24 |
| Cutaneous peripheral T-cell lymphoma, unspecified | 2 | 16 |
| ■ Cutaneous aggressive CD8[+] T-cell lymphoma | <1 | 18 |
| ■ Cutaneous γ/δ T-cell lymphoma | <1 | – |
| Cutaneous NK/T-cell lymphoma, nasal-type | <1 | – |
| **Cutaneous B-cell lymphoma** | | |
| *Indolent* | | |
| Follicle center cell lymphoma | 11 | 95 |
| Marginal zone lymphoma | 7 | 99 |
| *Intermediate clinical behavior* | | |
| Large B-cell lymphoma of the leg | 4 | 55 |
| Cutaneous diffuse large B-cell lymphoma, other | <1 | 50 |
| Intravascular large B-cell lymphoma | <1 | 65 |

[a]Data from Willemze R, Jaffe ES, Burg G, et al.: WHO-EORTC classification for cutaneous lymphomas. *Blood* 105:3768–3785, 2005.

median radiation dose was 40 Gy, and ranged from 20 to 48 Gy. Patients receiving doses less than 36 Gy showed an increased risk of recurrence.

Eich et al. retrospectively examined 35 patients with PCBCL, mostly with FCCL.[10] Four patients were identified with LBCL of the leg. They treated 32 patients with electron beam radiation (5–12 MeV), 2 with photon beam radiation (5 MV), and 1 with a combination thereof (5 MeV, 6 MV). Thirty-four patients achieved a CR after initial treatment. However, cutaneous relapses occurred in 31% of patients, mostly at nonirradiated sites. Five-year relapse-free survival of all patients was 50%, with a 5-year overall survival of 75%. Median dose to target was 45 Gy, and ranged from 27 to 54 Gy with a median fractionated dose of 1.8 Gy. Reported radiation margins ranged from 2 on the head to 5 cm on the trunk and extremities. Treatment was generally well tolerated with documented grade I reactions in 30 patients (86%) according to EORTC criteria[14] and teleangiectasia in 3 patients after a median of 3 years.

Kirova et al. reported 25 patients treated with initial radiation, with similar results.[11] All patients were treated with electron beam therapy delivered with electrons of 8-MeV energy and total doses ranging from 30 to 40 Gy. Depending on the extent of skin disease, either extended field or localized field irradiation was used. A healthy skin margin of at least 2.5 cm was included in the radiation field. The CR rate was 92%, with a 5-year overall survival of 75%. The 5-year disease-free survival was 75%. Relapses occurred between 2 months and 13 years in 16% of the patients, primarily in unirradiated sites. Side effects were usually grade I reactions at presentation, with occurrence of skin cancer in one patient after 10 years.

Rijlaarsdam et al. reported 55 patients with FCCL. Forty patients received radiation therapy.[12] Thirty-one were treated with electron beam, eight with photon beam equipment, and one with orthovolt radiation. Doses ranged from 30 to 40 Gy with 2-cm safety margins. All patients achieved CR. The reported relapse rate was 20% (8 patients). Four patients had leg involvement. A better estimated 5-year survival rate of 89% for all patients was reported, which might be related to the indolent nature of FCCL. Three patients with tumors on the legs died of disease.

### SURGERY

Except for anecdotal case reports of successful treatment of PCBCL with surgical excision, no studies have proven its efficacy. Local recurrences are frequently observed in more than 50% of patients; therefore, combinations of surgery, radiotherapy, or chemotherapy are frequently used.[15,16] Surgical excision can be considered for small, localized lesions; however, the advantage over radiotherapy is unknown.

### CHEMOTHERAPY

Systemic chemotherapy has been used in the treatment of PCBCL, especially for patients with multifocal or extensive lesions or with LBCL of the leg, as they are to be considered at higher risk of developing systemic involvement.[2] Several studies have shown the high efficacy of multiagent chemotherapy, with CR rates in up to 89% of the cases.[17] The cyclophosphamide, doxorubicin, vincristine, and prednisone

(CHOP) regimen has been found to be superior to cyclophosphamide, vincristine, and prednisone (COP) by some investigators.[14,17]

Rijaarsdam et al. reported a small, nonrandomized trial that included only 15 patients with FCCL treated with initial polychemotherapy.[14] Eleven patients received six cycles of CHOP and four patients received COP. CR occurred in 14 of 15 patients, with an estimated 5-year survival rate of 93%. All 4 patients treated with COP relapsed, whereas only 2 of 11 patients treated with CHOP relapsed. A study by Santucci et al. of 65 patients with PCBCL included 6 patients treated with COP or COP with bleomycin (COP-B). CR occurred in all six patients; however, four of them relapsed within 2–14 months.[18]

A follow-up study of 81 patients, in which 46 with PCBCL were treated with CHOP or COP, showed a CR rate of 89% and a 5-year survival of 97%, with a relapse-free survival of 70%. However, the relapse rate was 33%, and 55% in patients with LCBCL of the leg.[17]

Recently, Sarris et al. evaluated the outcome after doxorubicin-based polychemotherapy versus radiotherapy for patients with cutaneous DLBCL diagnosed according to the Working Formulation.[19] Ten patients received radiation and 33 received doxorubicin-based chemotherapy followed by radiation in 25 cases. The latter included eight patients with FCCL. The CR rate was 90% for radiation, 88% for doxorubicin-based chemotherapy, and 100% for combined modality. The 12-year progression-free survival of 71% was significantly higher in patients treated with chemotherapy/combined modality therapy compared with radiotherapy alone, in which it was 0%. Twelve-year overall survival was 77% in patients treated with chemotherapy/combined modality therapy versus 25% in patients treated with radiotherapy. In this series, the majority of patients had lesions on the head, neck, and trunk.

In contrast, Bekkenk et al. (as previously noted) found in a limited number of patients with multifocal FCCL or MZ/IC no difference in outcome and prognosis after treatment with either radiation or chemotherapy.[20] Polychemotherapy consisted of six cycles of either CHOP or COP therapy in nine patients with FCCL. Five patients received electron beam radiation, with a target dose of 40 Gy. All patients achieved a CR, with a median relapse-free survival of 36 months. Eight patients were diagnosed with MZ/IC. Two of them received CHOP or COP, respectively; one patient was treated with Chlorambucil, three with radiation or surgical excision, and two patients with topical steroids. Only the patient treated with CHOP achieved a CR. Cutaneous relapses occurred in two patients with FCCL treated with chemotherapy and in all patients with MZ/IC. One patient with FCCL developed extracutaneous disease.

### PERIPHERAL STEM CELL TRANSPLANTATION

The prognostic value of stem-cell transplantation in larger series of patients with primary CBCL has not been evaluated. Responses to high-dose therapy (HDT) followed by autologous stem cell transplantation (ASCT) have been reported to be effective in CBCL.[21] A series of 14 patients with cutaneous lymphomas treated with HDT/ASCT included three patients with disseminated and relapsed FCCL/DLBL. Eight patients, seven with CTCL, relapsed. Six of these patients relapsed within 4 months. No relapse occurred in patients with FCCL/DLBL, with a disease-free follow-up time of 15 months, 36 months, and 5 years, respectively.

### RECOMMENDED TREATMENT APPROACH FOR PRIMARY CUTANEOUS B-CELL LYMPHOMA

The clinical course and prognosis of CBCL is excellent and significantly differs from systemic lymphomas. Our approach to treatment strategies depends on the number and localization of lesions and the patient's age and health condition. The toxicity of treatment should not outweigh the cosmetic and functional disability of the disease. We prefer initial observation for patients with unifocal or multifocal lesions. If cosmetic consequences are a concern, we use local therapies such as radiation, intralesional steroid injection, and surgery or rituximab. We reserve systemic doxorubicin-based chemotherapy with or without rituximab for recurrent multilesional or disseminated cutaneous or extracutaneous tumors or LBCL of the leg.

## TREATMENT OF PRIMARY CUTANEOUS T-CELL LYMPHOMA

No treatment cures patients with the indolent forms of CTCLs, such as mycosis fungoides (MF)/ Sézary syndrome (SS) and lymphomatoid papulosis (LyP). Prognosis and survival of patients with CTCL remains dependent upon overall clinical staging and response to therapy. Over the last decade, various effective treatment modalities and novel treatment approaches have been developed for patients with MF/SS, which are based on an increased understanding of the pathobiology of the disease. However, experience with patients with other rare CTCL is limited, and the selection of treatment strategies remains more difficult.

### TREATMENT OF EARLY STAGE MYCOSIS FUNGOIDES

Treatment of MF/SS includes topical and systemic therapies that can be administered alone or in combination. In early stage IA to IIA MF, the disease is mostly limited to the upper dermis, with prominent epidermotropism that can be treated successfully with topical modalities. Multiagent chemotherapy regimens, used early in the course, demonstrated no survival benefit.[22] Various topical treatment options exist for early stages.

### TOPICAL STEROIDS

Although widely used, limited data are available regarding the use of topical steroids in early stage MF. In an investigational trial, 79 patients were treated daily with topical class I-III steroids.[23] Thirty-two (63%) stage T1 patients and seven (25%) stage T2 patients achieved complete clearing. Thirteen patients (40%) with stage T1 and two patients (29%) with stage T2 relapsed; however, the median observation time was only 9 months. Reported side effects were minor skin irritation in 2 patients, reversible skin atrophy in 1 patient, and reversible depression of serum cortisol levels in 10 patients.

### TOPICAL CHEMOTHERAPY

Topical nitrogen mustard has been used for management of MF since 1959.[24] Many investigators have demonstrated the efficacy of topical nitrogen mustard in patch and/or plaque disease of MF.[25] A recent update of 203 patients with MF (clinical stage I–III) treated with topical nitrogen mustard demonstrated CR rates of 76–80% for patients with stage IA and 35–68% for those with stage IB disease.[26] Fewer than 10% of patients developed progression of disease. Most common side effects were irritant contact dermatitis. No secondary malignancies related to therapy were reported. Topical Carmustine (BCNU) showed similar results, with an 86% CR rate; however, patients may develop progressing teleangiectasias from treatment.[27] Mild leukopenia occurred in 3.7% of the patients.

### TOPICAL RETINOIDS

Topical retinoid application may be an effective approach in early stage MF. They exert their effects through two basic types of nuclear receptors: the retinoic acid (RAR) and rexinoid (RXR) receptor family. No comparison of different retinoids has been evaluated. In a dose-escalating phase I/II trial of the RXR-specific retinoid bexarotene, 0.1–1.0%, the CR rate was 21%, with an overall response rate of 63%.[28] Side effects were restricted to the application site and consisted of mild to moderate irritation, with erythema in 73% of the cases. Bexarotene 1% gel was approved by the Food and Drug Administration (FDA) as a therapy for stages IA through IIA MF.

### PHOTOTHERAPY/PHOTOCHEMOTHERAPY

Ultraviolet (UV) light of different wavelengths has been used for many years. UVA (320–400 nm) and UVB (290–320 nm) are most common. Treatment combination with UVA and photosensitizing compounds (psoralens) is termed PUVA. PUVA has been used since 1976 in the treatment of various dermatological diseases including CTCL, and is one of our preferred treatment options in early stage MF.[29] It is extremely effective at clearing patch and plaque disease; however, the impact of maintenance therapy remains uncertain. Several studies confirm high remission rates in early stages of MF, with reported complete remissions in up to 71.4% of patients.[29–32] Long-term remissions have been reported for PUVA. We evaluated follow-up data of 66 patients with early stage disease who achieved CR after PUVA monotherapy, and showed that 50% of the patients maintained CR with a median of 84 months, and 50% of the patients relapsed with a median disease-free interval of 39 months. Median follow-up time was 94 months.[32] Reported short-term side effects were most commonly nausea and erythema. About 30% of patients developed skin malignancies, such as squamous or basal cell carcinoma.

The efficacy of UVB is more limited to patch stage, while PUVA is also effective in clearing plaques. The effects of UVB phototherapy were retrospectively evaluated in 37 patients with MF limited to patch/plaque disease.[33] Seventy-one percent achieved a CR, with a median duration of 22 months. Eighty-three percent of patients with disease limited to patches achieved remission, whereas none of the patients with plaque disease achieved remission. Narrowband (NB)-UVB is considered to be less carcinogenic and may be an alternative treatment option in early stage MF. In three small retrospective analyses, patients with clinical stage IA/IB and parapsoriasis and treated with NB-UVB showed CR rates between 54.2 and 83%.[34–36] However, remission times were short and a maintenance schedule has been difficult to establish. Long-wave ultraviolet A (UVA1) has likewise shown efficacy in single case reports.[37]

### TOTAL SKIN ELECTRON BEAM THERAPY

Recently published data of the therapeutic efficacy of total skin electron beam therapy (TSEB) from centers with extensive experience showed 40–98% complete remission rates among patients with stage IA and MF IB, with approximately 50% of patients with clinical stage IA and 25% of patients with clinical stage IB remaining in long-term remission.[38] TSEB treatment in early stages remains controversial because of its potential toxicity. Side effects can be significant, and consist of erythema, edema, scaling, ulceration, and irreversible loss of skin adnexa. TSEB may be repeated for palliative effects, although at reduced doses. Adjuvant therapy including PUVA, photopheresis, and INF-α may improve the duration of response.

### RECOMMENDED TREATMENT APPROACH FOR EARLY STAGE MYCOSIS FUNGOIDES

Nonrandomized clinical trials have not suggested that any one skin-directed therapy is preferable. Treatment choice should be made with the patient's preference and practitioner's skill in mind. Our philosophy regarding the management of patients is to maximize benefits while minimizing side effects. Therefore, we advocate the use of topical monotherapy. If patients fail to respond, we switch to a different topical therapy. Our first-line treatment for early stage patients is PUVA or NB-UVB therapy. However, in cases of refractory early stages we consider combination therapy such as PUVA or NB-UVB with low-dose systemic bexarotene or INF-α.

### TREATMENT OF ADVANCED STAGE MYCOSIS FUNGOIDES/SÉZARY SYNDROME

Patients may ultimately progress into more aggressive and advanced disease with either cutaneous or extracutaneous tumor manifestations. Treatment goals in advanced stages should be to reduce tumor burden, to relieve symptoms, to decrease the risk of transformation into aggressive lymphoma, and to preserve quality of life. Standard methods include mono- or polychemotherapy, extracorporeal photopheresis, interferons, retinoids, monoclonal antibodies, recombinant toxins, combination therapy, and high-dose chemotherapy with allogeneic stem cell transplant.

### SYSTEMIC CHEMOTHERAPY

Systemic chemotherapy should be restricted to patients with advanced stage disease or with multiple relapsed and refractory plaques and tumors. Established treatment options include single-agent or multiagent chemotherapy such as steroids, methotrexate, chlorambucil, vincristine, doxorubicin, cyclophosphamide, etoposide, and alkylators. Combination chemotherapy with CHOP or CHOP-like therapies has been shown to achieve higher response rates of approximately 70–80%.[39] Eighty-one patients (46 primary CBCL and 35 CTCL) were treated with COP or CHOP regimens. The overall response rate was 40% in CTCL patients, with a CR in 23% of patients. The median response duration was 5.7 months and median survival was 19 months. A phase II trial with the etoposide, vincristine, doxorubicin, cyclophosphamide, and oral prednisone (EPOCH) regimen in 15 patients with refractory CTCL resulted in an overall response rate of 80%.[40] Twenty-seven percent of patients achieved a CR, and 53% of patients achieved a partial response (PR) with a median duration of 8 months and an overall survival of 13.5 months. Grade 3 or 4 hematologic toxicity occurred in eight patients (61%).

Among single-agent chemotherapies, liposomal doxorubicin, pentostatin, and gemcitabine have been effective. An investigational trial with a limited number of patients demonstrated efficacy of pegylated liposomal doxorubicin monotherapy, with an overall response rate of 80% and a CR in 6 of 10 patients (60%).[41] Recent published multicenter data of pegylated doxorubicin in 34 patients with recurrent or recalcitrant CTCL revealed a response rate of 88.2%.[42] Twenty-seven patients (79.4%) achieved a CR with a median duration of 12 months, ranging from 9.5 to 44 months. Adverse effects were seen in 14 patients and were generally mild compared with other chemotherapy regimen. Only six patients experienced grade 3 or 4 toxicity.

Studies of purine analogs, such as pentostatin (2-deoxycoformycin), fludarabine, and 2-chlorodeoxyadenosine (2-CdA), have demonstrated significant initial response rates of up to 100%. However, most responses were short lived and were accompanied by harmful side effects related to prolonged immunosuppression.[43–45] Pentostatin has been evaluated in 28 heavily pretreated patients with MF/SS who were treated on a dose-escalating phase II trial, with doses ranging from 3.75 to 5.0 mg/m²; a CR was achieved in 25% of patients.[46] Most patients developed granulocytopenia with significant lowering of CD4 counts, nausea, and neutropenic fever. Kuzel et al. investigated 2-CdA in 21 patients with relapsed/refractory MF/SS.[47] Three patients (14%) attained a CR, with a median duration of 4.5 months and a range of 2.5–16 months. Gemcitabine, a novel pyrimidine antimetabolite, was investigated at two centers in a phase II trial at a dosage of 1.2 g/m² in 44 patients with clinical stage IIB–IV MF/SS.[48] Twelve percent of patients achieved a CR, and 26% of patients achieved a PR, with a median duration of 15 months and 10 months, respectively.

Temozolomide, a new oral alkylating agent, is being evaluated in a phase II trial of patients with relapsed MF and SS. Patients with MF/SS have been shown to have low levels of DNA repair enzyme $O^6$ alkylguanine DNA alkyltransferase (AGT) and may be particularly sensitive to this alkylator.[49] Preliminary data have been reported with a more than 50% decrease in tumor burden in 5 of 22 patients with MS/SS (26%), lasting for a median duration of 4 months.[50] Twelve of 16 patients tested did not express AGT. Patients with AGT expression did not respond to treatment.

### BIOLOGIC RESPONSE MODIFIERS

The ratio of T-helper cell type 1 ($T_h1$) and type 2 ($T_h2$) has been hypothesized to be critical for disease progression. In advanced stages there is a dominant $T_h2$ cytokine profile leading to an impaired host antitumor response.[51] Treatments such as biologic response modifiers target the reconstitution of immune function for disease control. Currently, immune-modifying treatment options such as bexarotene, immunomodulatory cytokines such as interferon-alpha (INF-α), and interleukin 2 and 12 (IL-2, IL-12), and extracorporeal photopheresis (ECP) are used to treat MF/SS.

### INTERFERON-ALPHA

INF-α was first reported in 1984 by Bunn et al. for the treatment of advanced and heavily pretreated MF/SS, with an overall response rate of 45%.[52] Papa et al. showed response rates between 70% for advanced stage III–IV and 80% for early stage patch/plaque disease.[53] Olsen et al. showed, in an investigational trial of 3 versus 36 MU daily of INF α-2a in 22 patients with clinical stage I–IV MF/SS, an overall response rate of 38% in low-dose-treated patients compared to 79% in high-dose-treated patients.[54] Side effects were dose related and were most commonly flu-like symptoms. The development of neutralizing antibodies has been associated with INF-α therapy, with variable impact on response rates.[55] They appear to be higher in patients treated with INF α-2a compared to INF α-2b. The combination therapy IFN-α and PUVA resulted in high response rates in more than 90% of patients and showed superiority to other combinations.[56,57]

## RETINOIDS

The therapeutic efficacy of some retinoids, such as isotretinoin, etretinate, and acitretin in CTCL, has been confirmed in several small, monotherapy studies.[58–61] Response rates range from 44 to 67%, with CR rates from 21 to 35%. They seem to be equally effective, with median response duration around 8 months. Common effects consisted of skin and mucous membrane dryness. Oral bexarotene is a USFDA approved synthetic retinoid for refractory CTCL that selectively binds to RXR. In two multicenter phase II–III clinical trials it has been tested in early and advanced stages of CTCL patients.[62,63] Reported response rates in early stages were between 45 and 54%. An overall response rate was observed in 94 patients with advanced disease, with only 4% complete responders, and with a median duration of 10 months. At the recommended dose of 300 mg/m² daily, it is associated with significant side effects, such as hyperlipidemia, hypothyroidism, and cytopenias. Retrospective comparison data suggest that there may be little difference in efficacy between bexarotene (RXR-specific retinoid) and agents such as all-*trans* retinoic acid (RAR-specific retinoid), but clear differences in toxicity exist.[64]

## EXTRACORPOREAL PHOTOCHEMOTHERAPY

ECP is a leukapheresis-based method in which 8-MOP treated blood mononuclear cells are exposed to UVA and returned to the patient. It is performed on two consecutive days every month. Although the mechanism of action is not completely understood, induction of apoptosis with subsequent release of tumor antigens leading to a systemic antitumor response against the malignant T-cell clone is suspected.[65,66] In 1987 Edelson et al. published the first report on the efficacy of ECP in a cohort of 41 refractory CTCL patients. Thirty-seven patients (73%) achieved a response, with a CR in 24% of patients.[67] In the same year the FDA approved ECP for advanced and refractory CTCL. There have been several confirmatory studies reported on ECP monotherapy, with overall response rates between 50 and 73% for patients with MF/SS.[67–70] Ideal candidates for ECP are patients with

SS with a short duration of disease without previous intense therapies, low tumor burden, modest numbers of circulating atypical cells, near normal counts of circulating CD8+ T lymphocytes, and exaggerated CD4 to CD8 ratio.[68–70] The results in patients with marked immunosuppression or tumor lesions were disappointing, but provided the rationale for combining treatments. Synergistic effects have been reported with INF-α, retinoids, and TSEB.[70–73] A retrospective study of 47 patients with advanced stage III–IV disease treated with ECP or with ECP combination therapy with INF-α, retinoids, or sargramostim reported an overall response rate of 79%.[71] The overall response rate in patients who received combination therapy was 84%, with a CR in 26% of patients. The median survival for the patients undergoing combination therapy was 74 months. The effect of ECP as adjuvant therapy was evaluated in patients with advanced stage T3 and T4 disease who achieved a CR after TSEB treatment. Significantly better overall survival at 3 years was reported with adjuvant doxorubicin/cyclophosphamide (75%) or with adjuvant ECP (100%) compared to those with TSEB therapy (50%) alone.[73]

## TARGETED MODALITIES

### Denileukin diftitox (Ontak)

Denileukin diftitox (IL-2 receptor specific fusion protein combined with diphtheria toxin) targets selectively the IL-2 receptor on malignant and activated T cells. In phase I/II and III trials it showed favorable 30[74] to 37%[75] response rates in CTCL patients. These trials were limited to patients with CD25 expression (alpha chain of IL-2R) in more than 20% of malignant T cells. The quality of life in responding patients was significantly improved.[76] However, adverse effects including acute transfusion-related events such as fever, rash, chills, myalgias, and vascular leak syndrome (VLS) have been reported. VLS occurred in 27% of the patients, which may be diminished by premedication with steroids.[77]

### Alemtuzumab (Campath-1H)

Alemtuzumab is a humanized monoclonal antibody directed against the lymphocyte surface antigen CD52, which is abundantly expressed on normal and most malignant T lymphocytes.[78] Alemtuzumab is currently the focus of many clinical trials in hematologic malignancies and has been used in the treatment of lymphomas and lymphoid leukemias. A published phase II trial of alemtuzumab in 22 patients with advanced MF/SS demonstrated a clinical response in 55% of the cases, with 32% complete remissions, including some SS patients clearing effectively circulating Sézary cells.[79] Median response duration was 12 months, and ranged from 5 to 32 months. The compound is associated with significant hematologic toxicity and infectious complications consisting of reactivation of cytomegalovirus, herpes zoster, miliary tuberculosis, and pulmonary aspergillosis.

## PERIPHERAL STEM CELL TRANSPLANT

Autologous and allogeneic stem cell transplantation (SCT) is a well-established treatment option for various hematologic diseases, though there is limited experience in CTCL. A few retrospective studies have reported on autologous SCT leading to complete remissions in the majority of patients treated; however, most patients relapse rapidly.[80,81] The duration of remission does not seem to be related to stage of the disease or absence of a detectable T-cell clone in the harvest.[82] However, it is now suggested that a greater T-cell depletion of the harvest may be associated with a greater risk of rapid relapse, perhaps by compromising the immune antitumor response.[82,83]

Allogeneic transplants are known to achieve more durable complete remissions, most likely due to an immunologic graft-versus-lymphoma effect. Response durations as long as 6 years posttransplant have been reported, suggesting that it may be a curative option.[84] It does, however, carry a higher risk of treatment-related mortality, including life-threatening infections and graft-versus-host disease (GVHD). Molina et al. followed six patients with advanced and refractory MF/SS who received donor-related allogeneic SCT (four patients) and donor-unrelated SCT (two patients).[85] All patients achieved a CR, with mild GVHD. Five patients remained disease free from 3 to 65 months posttransplant, and one patient died of GVHD 16 months posttransplant. Guitart et al. reported on allogeneic SCT therapy in patients with advanced stages of MF/SS who had not responded to standard treatment options.[86] A sustained CR was achieved in two patients with disease-free duration time of 15 months and $4\frac{1}{2}$ years, respectively, posttransplant. There was no evidence of GVHD. One patient with advanced and refractory stage IVA and large cell transformation on histology relapsed after 9 months with limited cutaneous recurrence and remained alive more than 6 years posttransplant.

## TREATMENT OF CD30⁺ LYMPHOPROLIFERATIVE DISORDERS

CD30⁺ cutaneous lymphoproliferative disorders include LyP presenting with chronic, recurrent, and self-healing skin eruptions and CD30⁺ LTCL.[87] Their common phenotypic hallmark is the CD30⁺ T lymphocyte that morphologically resembles Reed–Sternberg cells. Reported treatment modalities are doxycycline, PUVA, NB-UVB, methotrexate, INF-α, topical steroid and bexarotene formulations, and radiation.[88–91] However, none of these treatments alter the natural course of disease; therefore, the short-term benefits should be weighed against the potential harmful side effects. Observation in patients with few lesions is recommended, whereas in patients with more disseminated disease low-dose methotrexate or UV light treatment might be effective in clearing disease.[92]

Primary cutaneous CD30⁺ LTCL presenting with solitary or localized cutaneous nodules appear to have a favorable prognosis, as confirmed in several studies.[93] Spot radiation for solitary or localized lesions is the preferred treatment, with systemic chemotherapy reserved for cases with large tumor burden and/or extracutaneous involvement.[94,95] Therapy regimens include doxorubicin-based (doxorubicin with CHOP or CHOP-like) chemotherapy, INF-α, or oral bexarotene.

## TREATMENT OF SMALL- AND MEDIUM-SIZED PLEOMORPHIC T-CELL LYMPHOMA AND CD30⁻ LARGE T-CELL LYMPHOMA

Patients with CD30⁻ LTCL or small/medium-sized PTCL usually present with solitary, localized, or generalized plaques, nodules, or tumors without spontaneous regression.[96] Both entities do not express CD30 with absence of a $T_h2$ cytokine profile in CD30⁻ LTCL.[97] In CD30⁻ LTCL, large cells comprise over 30% of the dermal infiltrate and might resemble classical MF undergoing large cell transformation. Multiagent systemic chemotherapy is recommended in most cases, with radiotherapy limited to localized disease, although abbreviated responses are often seen with a high relapse rate. This was supported by Bekkenk et al., who reported on 82 patients with CD30⁻ peripheral T-cell lymphoma.[96] Forty-six patients were diagnosed with a primary cutaneous CD30⁻ LTCL. Most patients with solitary or localized skin lesions were treated with radiation, whereas patients presenting with multifocal skin lesions or with extracutaneous involvement were treated with doxorubicin-based chemotherapy. A complete remission was achieved in 12 (63%) of 19 patients treated with radiotherapy and in 5 (27%) of 18 patients treated with doxorubicin-based chemotherapy. Complete remissions were generally short lived, with a median duration of 6 months for radiotherapy-treated patients and 10 months for patients treated with doxorubicin-based chemotherapy. Twelve of 19 patients (63%) with small/medium-sized PTCL reached a complete remission, including 10 (83%) of 12 treated with radiotherapy and 2 (40%) of 5 patients treated with doxorubicin-based chemotherapy. The median response duration for the complete responders was 58 months. Patients with small- or medium-sized PTCL had a significantly better prognosis, with a 5-year overall survival rate of 45% compared to 12% in patients with primary cutaneous CD30⁻ LTCL.

## CONCLUSION

Primary cutaneous lymphomas encompass a spectrum of clinical and histologic variants, characterized by skin-homing lymphocytes. Awareness of their unique clinical behavior provides a stage-dependent treatment approach and minimizes unnecessary interventions. Systemic progression in CBCL is uncommon and 5-year survival rates are excellent, although relapses occur frequently. Treatment considerations for CBCL mostly rely on retrospective studies and are based on clinical presentation and morphologic evaluation. Histologic characterization of B-cell lymphomas in extranodular locations, such as the skin, can be problematic (i.e., small vs large cleaved cells), and does not appear to have the same predictive power compared to their nodal counterparts. Current clinical trials focus mainly on patients with MF/SS, as these patients represent the majority of cutaneous lymphomas. Skin-directed therapies are reserved for early stages.[98] Immune-modifying therapies have emerged for the treatment of advanced and/or refractory stages. They have the potential to reconstitute immune function while augmenting host antitumor response.

Combined immunomodulatory regimens may result in sustained remission of disease. Our gold standard for advanced stages is the combined use of PUVA and INF-α at a dose of up to 9 MU thrice weekly or as tolerated. Systemic single-agent or multiagent chemotherapies should be reserved for more advanced and refractory disease. Clinical trials are ongoing to refine protocols for combination therapy to improve efficacy and minimize toxicity. Advances in molecular biology technology may allow selective targeting of both B- and T-cell-mediated effects. Investigational agents, such as histone-deacetylase inhibitors, and the novel T-cell costimulatory agents, such as deoxynucleotide CpG7909 (cytosine-phosphorothiolated guanine-containing oligonucleotides) and lenalidomide, are being evaluated in phase I/II trials.

## REFERENCES

1. Querfeld C, Guitart J, Kuzel TM, Rosen ST: Primary cutaneous lymphomas: a review with current treatment options. *Blood Rev* 17:131, 2003.
2. Willemze R, Jaffe ES, Burg G, et al.: WHO-EORTC classification for primary cutaneous lymphomas. *Blood* 105:3768, 2005.
3. Sander CA, Flaig MJ, Jaffe ES: Cutaneous manifestations of lymphoma: a clinical guide based on the WHO classification. *Clin Lymphoma* 2:86, 2001.
4. Chan JKC, Banks PM, Cleary ML, et al.: A revised European–American classification of lymphoid neoplasms proposed by the International Lymphoma Study Group. A summary version. *Am J Clin Pathol* 103:543, 1995.
5. Hofbauer GF, Kessler B, Kempf W, et al.: Multilesional primary cutaneous diffuse large B-cell lymphoma responsive to antibiotic treatment. *Dermatology* 203:168, 2001.
6. Kutting B, Bonsmann G, Metze D, et al.: Borrelia burgdorferi-associated primary cutaneous B cell lymphoma: complete clearing of skin lesions after antibiotic pulse therapy or intralesional injection of interferon alfa-2a. *J Am Acad Dermatol* 36:311, 1997.
7. Bonnekoh B, Schulz M, Franke I, Gollnick H: Complete remission of a primary cutaneous B-cell lymphoma of the lower leg by first-line monotherapy with the CD20-antibody rituximab. *J Cancer Res Clin Oncol* 128:161, 2002.
8. Mounier N, Briere J, Gisselbrecht C, et al.: Rituximab plus CHOP (R-CHOP) overcomes bcl-2–associated resistance to chemotherapy in elderly patients with diffuse large B-cell lymphoma (DLBCL). *Blood* 101:4279, 2003.
9. Smith BD, Glusac EJ, McNiff JM, et al.: Primary cutaneous B-cell lymphoma treated with radiotherapy: a comparison of the European Organization for Research and Treatment of Cancer and the WHO classification systems. *J Clin Oncol* 15:634, 2004.
10. Eich HT, Eich D, Micke O, et al.: Long-term efficacy, curative potential, and prognostic factors of radiotherapy in primary cutaneous B-cell lymphoma. *Int J Radiat Oncol Biol Phys* 55:899, 2003.
11. Kirova YM, Piedbois Y, Le Bourgeois JP: Radiotherapy in the management of cutaneous B-cell lymphoma. Our experience in 25 cases. *Radiother Oncol* 52:15, 1999.
12. Rijlaarsdam JU, Toonstra J, Meijer OW, et al.: Treatment of primary cutaneous B-cell lymphomas of follicle center cell origin: a clinical follow-up study of 55 patients treated with radiotherapy or polychemotherapy. *J Clin Oncol* 14:549–555, 1996.
13. Vermeer MH, Geelen FA, van Haselen CW, et al.: Primary cutaneous large B-cell lymphomas of the legs. A distinct type of cutaneous B-cell lymphoma with an intermediate prognosis. Dutch Cutaneous Lymphoma Working Group. *Arch Dermatol* 132:1304, 1996.
14. Cox JD, Stetz J, Pajak TF: Toxicity criteria of the Radiation Therapy Oncology Group (RTOG) and the European Organization for Research and Treatment of Cancer (EORTC). *Int J Radiat Oncol Biol Phys* 31:1341, 1994.
15. Cerroni L, Arzberger E, Pütz B, et al.: Primary cutaneous follicle center cell lymphoma with follicular growth pattern. *Blood* 95:3922, 2000.
16. Sah A, Barrans SL, Parapaia LA, et al.: Cutaneous B-cell lymphoma: pathological spectrum and clinical outcome in 51 consecutive patients. *Am J Hematol* 75:195, 2004.
17. Fierro MT, Quaglino P, Savoia P, et al.: Systemic polychemotherapy in the treatment of primary cutaneous lymphomas: a clinical follow-up study of 81 patients treated with COP or CHOP. *Leuk Lymphoma* 31:583, 1998.
18. Santucci M, Pimpinelli N, Arganini L: Primary cutaneous B-cell lymphoma: a unique type of low-grade lymphoma. *Cancer* 67:2311, 1991.
19. Sarris A, Braunschweig I, Medeiros LJ, et al.: Primary cutaneous non-Hodgkin's lymphoma of Ann Arbor stage I: preferential cutaneous relapses but high cure rate with doxorubicin-based therapy. *J Clin Oncol* 19:398, 2001.
20. Bekkenk MW, Vermeer MH, Geerts ML, et al.: Treatment of multifocal primary cutaneous B-cell lymphoma: a clinical follow-up study of 29 patients. *J Clin Oncol* 17:2471, 1999.
21. Ingen-Housz-Oro S, Bachelez H, Verola O, et al.: High-dose therapy and autologous stem cell transplantation

in relapsing cutaneous lymphoma. *Bone Marrow Transplant* 33:629, 2004.

22. Rosen ST, Foss FM: Chemotherapy for mycosis fungoides and the Sézary syndrome. *Hematol Oncol Clin North Am* 9:1109, 1995.

23. Zackheim HS, Kashani-Sabet M, Amin S: Topical corticosteroids for mycosis fungoides. *Arch Dermatol* 134:949, 1998.

24. Haserick J, Richardson J, Grant DJ: Remission of lesions in mycosis fungoides following topical application of nitrogen mustard. *Cleve Clin Q* 26:144, 1959.

25. Vonderheid EC, Tan ET, Kantor AF, et al.: Long-term efficacy, curative potential, and carcinogenicity of topical mechlorethamine chemotherapy in cutaneous T cell lymphoma. *J Am Acad Dermatol* 20:416, 1989.

26. Kim YH, Martinez G, Varghese A, Hoppe RT: Topical nitrogen mustard in the management of mycosis fungoides: update of the Stanford experience. *Arch Dermatol* 139:165, 2003.

27. Zackheim HS: Topical carmustine (BCNU) for patch/plaque mycosis fungoides. *Semin Dermatol* 13:202, 1994.

28. Breneman D, Duvic M, Kuzel T, Yocum R, Truglia J, Stevens VJ: Phase 1 and 2 trial of bexarotene gel for skin-directed treatment of patients with cutaneous T-cell lymphoma. *Arch Dermatol* 138:325, 2002.

29. Gilchrest BA, Parish JA, Tanenbaum L, Haynes HA, Fitzpatrick TB: Oral methoxypsoralen photochemotherapy of mycosis fungoides. *Cancer* 38:683, 1976.

30. Rosenbaum MM, Roenigk HH Jr, Caro WA, Esker A: Photochemotherapy in cutaneous T cell lymphoma and parapsoriasis en plaques. Long-term follow-up in forty-three patients. *J Am Acad Dermatol* 13:613, 1985.

31. Herrmann JJ, Roenigk HH, Hurria A, et al.: Treatment of mycosis fungoides with photochemotherapy (PUVA): long-term follow-up. *J Am Acad Dermatol* 33:234, 1995.

32. Querfeld C, Rosen ST, Kuzel TM, et al.: Long-term follow-up of patients with early stage cutaneous T-cell lymphoma who achieved complete remission on psoralen plus UV-A monotherapy. *Arch Dermatol* 141:305, 2005.

33. Ramsay DL, Lish KM, Yalowitz CB, Soter NA: Ultraviolet-B phototherapy for early-stage cutaneous T-cell lymphoma. *Arch Dermatol* 128:931, 1992.

34. Diederen PV, van Weelden H, Sanders CJ, et al.: Narrowband UVB and psoralen-UVA in the treatment of early-stage mycosis fungoides: a retrospective study. *J Am Acad Dermatol* 48:215, 2003.

35. Gathers RC, Scherschun L, Malick F, et al.: Narrowband UVB phototherapy for early-stage mycosis fungoides. *J Am Acad Dermatol* 47:191, 2002.

36. Hofer A, Cerroni L, Kerl H, Wolf P: Narrowband (311-nm) UV-B therapy for small plaque parapsoriasis and early-stage mycosis fungoides. *Arch Dermatol* 135:1377, 1999.

37. Plettenberg H, Stege H, Megahed M, et al.: Ultraviolet A1 (340–400 nm) phototherapy for cutaneous T-cell lymphoma. *J Am Acad Dermatol* 41:47, 1999.

38. Jones G, Wilson LD, Fox-Goguen L: Total skin electron beam radiotherapy for patients who have mycosis fungoides. *Hematol Oncol Clin North Am* 17:1421, 2003.

39. Fierro MT, Quaglino P, Savoia P, Verrone A, Bernengo MG: Systemic polychemotherapy in the treatment of primary cutaneous lymphomas: a clinical follow-up study of 81 patients treated with COP or CHOP. *Leuk Lymphoma* 31:583, 1998.

40. Akpek G, Koh HK, Bogen S, et al.: Chemotherapy with etoposide, vincristine, doxorubicin, bolus cyclophosphamide, and oral prednisone in patients with refractory cutaneous T-cell lymphoma. *Cancer* 86:1368, 1999.

41. Wollina U, Graefe T, Karte K: Treatment of relapsing or recalcitrant cutaneous T-cell lymphoma with pegylated liposomal doxorubicin. *J Am Acad Dermatol* 42:40, 2000.

42. Wollina U, Dummer R, Brockmeyer NH, et al.: Multicenter study of pegylated liposomal doxorubicin in patients with cutaneous T-cell lymphoma. *Cancer* 98:993, 2003.

43. Betticher DC, Frey MF, von Rohr A, et al.: High incidence of infections after 2-chlorodeoxyadenosine (2-CDA) therapy in patients with malignant lymphomas and chronic and acute leukaemias. *Ann Oncol* 5:57, 1994.

44. Cummings FJ, Kim K, Neiman RS, et al.: Phase II trial of pentostatin in refractory lymphomas and cutaneous T-cell disease. *J Clin Oncol* 9:565, 1991.

45. Grever MR, Bisacia E, Scarborough DA, et al.: An investigation of 2'-deoxycoformycin in the treatment of cutaneous T-cell lymphoma. *Blood* 61:279, 1983.

46. Kurzrock R, Pilat S, Duvic M: Pentostatin therapy of T-cell lymphomas with cutaneous manifestation. *J Clin Oncol* 17:3117, 1999.

47. Kuzel TM, Hurria A, Samuelson E, et al.: Phase II trial of 2-chlorodeoxyadenosine for the treatment of cutaneous T-cell lymphoma. *Blood* 87:906, 1996.

48. Zinzani PL, Baliva G, Magagnoli M, et al.: Gemcitabine treatment in pretreated cutaneous T-cell lymphoma: experience in 44 patients. *J Clin Oncol* 18:2603, 2000.

49. Dolan ME, McRae BL, Ferries-Rowe E, et al.: $O^6$-Alkylguanine-DNA alkyltransferase in cutaneous T-cell lymphoma: implications for treatment with alkylating agents. *Clin Cancer Res* 5:2059, 1999.

50. Rosen ST, Guitart J, Martone B, et al.: Phase II trial of temozolomide for treatment of mycosis fungoides/Sézary syndrome. *Proc ASCO* Abstract 406, 2002.

51. Rook AH, Lessin SR, Jaworsky C, et al.: Immunopathogenesis of cutaneous T-cell lymphoma. Abnormal cytokine production by Sézary cells. *Arch Dermatol* 129:486–489, 1993.

52. Bunn PA, Foon KA, Ihde DC, et al.: Recombinant leukocyte A interferon: an active agent in advanced cutaneous T-cell lymphomas. *Ann Intern Med* 101:484, 1984.

53. Papa G, Tura S, Mandelli F, et al.: Is interferon alpha in cutaneous T-cell lymphoma a treatment of choice? *Br J Haematol* 79:S48, 1991.

54. Olsen EA, Rosen ST, Vollmer RT, et al.: Interferon alfa-2a in the treatment of cutaneous T cell lymphoma. *J Am Acad Dermatol* 20:395, 1989.

55. Itri LM, Sherman MI, Palleroni AV, et al.: Incidence and clinical significance of neutralizing antibodies in patients receiving recombinant interferon-alpha 2a. *J Interferon Res* 9:S9, 1989.

56. Kuzel TM, Roenigk HH, Samuelson E, et al.: Effectiveness of interferon alfa-2a combined with photochemotherapy for mycosis fungoides and Sézary syndrome. *J Clin Oncol* 13:257, 1995.

57. Rupoli S, Barulli S, Guiducci B, et al.: Low dose inter-feron-α2b combined with PUVA is an effective treatment of early stage mycosis fungoides: results of a multicenter study. *Hematologica* 84:809, 1999.

58. Kessler JF, Jones SE, Levine N, et al.: Isotretinoin and cutaneous helper T-cell lymphoma (mycosis fungoides). *Arch Dermatol* 123:201, 1987.

59. Thomsen K, Molin L, Volden G, et al.: 13-cis-retinoic acid effective in mycosis fungoides. A report from the Scandinavian Mycosis Fungoides Group. *Acta Derm Venereol* 64:563, 1984.

60. Molin L, Thomsen K, Volden G, et al.: Oral retinoids in mycosis fungoides and Sezary syndrome: a comparison of isotretinoin and etretinate. A study from the Scandinavian Mycosis Fungoides Group. *Acta Derm Venereol* 67:232, 1987.

61. Thomsen K, Hammar H, Molin L, Volden G: Retinoids plus PUVA (RePUVA) and PUVA in mycosis fungoides, plaque stage. A report from the Scandinavian Mycosis Fungoides Group. *Acta Derm Venereol* 69:536, 1989.

62. Duvic M, Martin AG, Kim Y, et al.: Phase 2 and 3 clinical trial of oral bexarotene (Targretin capsules) for the treatment of refractory or persistent early-stage cutaneous T-cell lymphoma. *Arch Dermatol* 137:581, 2001.

63. Duvic M, Hymes K, Heald P, et al.: Bexarotene is effective and safe for treatment of refractory advanced-stage cutaneous T-cell lymphoma: Multinational phase II-III trial results. *J Clin Oncol* 19:2456, 2001.

64. Querfeld C, Rosen ST, Guitart J, et al.: Comparison of selective RAR and RXR retinoid mediated efficacy, tolerance, and survival in refractory cutaneous T-cell lymphoma. *J Am Acad Dermatol* 51:25, 2004.

65. Yoo EK, Rook AH, Elenitsas R, et al.: Apoptosis induction by ultraviolet light A and photochemotherapy in cutaneous T-cell lymphoma: relevance to mechanism of therapeutic action. *J Invest Dermatol* 107:235, 1996.

66. Rook AH, Suchin KR, Kao DMF, et al.: Photopheresis: clinical applications and mechanisms of action. *J Invest Dermatol Symp Proc* 4:85, 1999.

67. Edelson R, Berger C, Gasparro F, et al.: Treatment of cutaneous T-cell lymphoma by extracorporeal photochemotherapy. Preliminary results. *N Engl J Med* 316:297, 1987.

68. Heald PW, Perez MI, Christensen I, et al.: Photopheresis therapy of cutaneous T-cell lymphoma: the Yale-New Haven Hospital experience. *Yale J Biol Med* 62:629, 1989.

69. Koh HK, Davis BE, Meola T, Lim HW: Extracorporeal photopheresis for the treatment of 34 patients with cutaneous T-cell lymphoma (CTCL). *J Invest Dermatol* 102:567, 1994.

70. Gottleib SL, Wolfe JT, Fox FE, et al.: Treatment of cutaneous T-cell lymphoma with extracorporeal photophoresis monotherapy and in combination with recombinant interferon alpha: a 10-year experience at a single institution. *J Am Acad Dermatol* 35:946, 1996.

71. Suchin KR, Cucchiara AJ, Gottleib SL, et al.: Treatment of cutaneous T-cell lymphoma with combined immunomodulatory therapy: a 14-year experience at a single institution. *Arch Dermatol* 138:1054, 2002.

72. Wilson LD, Jones GW, Kim D, et al.: Experience with total skin electron beam therapy in combination with extracorporeal photopheresis in the management of patients with erythrodermic (T4) mycosis fungoides. *J Am Acad Dermatol* 43:54, 2000.

73. Wilson LD, Licata AL, Braverman IM, et al.: Systemic chemotherapy and extracorporeal photochemotherapy for T3 and T4 cutaneous T-cell lymphoma patients who have achieved a complete response to total skin electron beam therapy. *Int J Radiat Oncol Biol Phys* 32:987, 1995.

74. LeMaistre CF, Saleh MN, Kuzel TM, et al.: Phase I trial of a ligand fusion-protein (DAB389IL-2) in lymphomas expressing the receptor for interleukin-2. *Blood* 91:399, 1998.

75. Olsen E, Duvic M, Frankel A, et al.: Pivotal phase III trial of two dose levels of denileukin diftitox for the treatment of cutaneous T-cell lymphoma. *J Clin Oncol* 19:376, 2001.

76. Duvic M, Kuzel TM, Olsen EA, et al.: Quality-of-life improvements in cutaneous T-cell lymphoma patients treated with denileukin diftitox (ONTAK®). *Clin Lymphoma* 2:222, 2002.

77. Foss FM, Bacha P, Osann KE, et al.: Biological correlates of acute hypersensitivity events with DAB(389)IL-2 (denileukin diftitox, ONTAK) in cutaneous T-cell lymphoma: decreased frequency and severity with steroid premedication. *Clin Lymphoma* 1:298, 2001.

78. Dearden CE, Matutes E, Catovsky D: Alemtuzumab in T-cell malignancies. *Med Oncol* 19:S27, 2002.

79. Lundin J, Hagberg H, Repp R, et al.: Phase II study of alemtuzumab (anti-CD52 monoclonal antibody, Campath-1H) in patients with advanced mycosis fungoides/Sezary syndrome. *Blood* 101:4267, 2003.

80. Bigler RD, Crilley P, Micaily B, et al.: Autologous bone marrow transplantation for advanced stage mycosis fungoides. *Bone Marrow Transplant* 7:133, 1991.

81. Sterling JC, Marcus R, Burrows NP, Roberts SO: Erythrodermic mycosis fungoides treated with total body irradiation and autologous bone marrow transplantation. *Clin Exp Dermatol* 20:73, 1995.

82. Olavarria E, Child F, Woolford A, et al.: T-cell depletion and autologous stem cell transplantation in the management of tumour stage mycosis fungoides with peripheral blood involvement. *Br J Haematol* 114:624, 2001.

83. Russell-Jones R, Child F, Olavarria E, et al.: Autologous peripheral blood stem cell transplantation in tumor-stage mycosis fungoides: predictors of disease-free survival. *Ann N Y Acad Sci* 941:147, 2001.

84. Koeppel MC, Stoppa M, Resbeut D, et al.: Mycosis fungoides and allogenic bone marrow transplantation. *Acta Derm Venereol* 74:331, 1994.

85. Molina A, Arber D, Murata-Collins JL, et al.: Clinical, cytogenetic and molecular remissions after allogeneic hematopoietic stem cell transplantation for refractory Sézary syndrome and tumor-stage mycosis fungoides. *Blood* 98:409A, 2001.

86. Guitart J, Wickless S, Oyama Y, et al.: Long-term remission after allogeneic hematopoietic stem cell transplantation for refractory cutaneous T-cell lymphoma. *Arch Dermatol* 138:1359, 2002.

87. Liu HL, Hoppe RT, Kohler S, et al.: CD30+ cutaneous lymphoproliferative disorders: the Stanford experience in lymphomatoid papulosis and primary cutaneous anaplastic large cell lymphoma. *J Am Acad Dermatol* 49:1049, 2003.

88. Paul M, Krowchuk P, Hitchcock M, Jorizzo J: Lymphomatoid papulosis: successful weekly pulse superpotent topical corticosteroid therapy in three pediatric patients. *Pediatr Dermatol* 13:501, 1996.

89. Vonderheid E, Sajjadian A, Kadin M: Methotrexate is effective therapy for lymphomatoid papulosis and other primary cutaneous CD30-positive lymphoproliferative disorders. *J Am Acad Dermatol* 34:470, 1996.

90. Wyss M, Dummer R, Dommann S, et al.: Lymphomatoid papulosis-treatment with recombinant interferon alpha-2a and etretinate. *Dermatology* 190: 288, 1995.

91. Krathen RA, Ward S, Duvic M: Bexarotene is a new treatment option for lymphomatoid papulosis. *Dermatology* 206:142, 2003.

92. Bekkenk MW, Geelen FA, van Voorst Vader PC, et al.: Primary and secondary cutaneous CD30⁺ lymphoproliferative disorders: a report from the Dutch Cutaneous Lymphoma Group on the long-term follow-up data of 219 patients and guidelines for diagnosis and treatment. *Blood* 95:3653, 2000.

93. French LE, Shapiro M, Junkins-Hopkins JM, et al.: Regression of multifocal, skin-restricted, CD30-positive large T-cell lymphoma with interferon alfa and bexarotene therapy. *J Am Acad Dermatol* 45:914, 2001.

94. Beljaards RC, Meijer CJ, van der Putte SC, et al.: Primary cutaneous T-cell lymphoma: clinicopathological features and prognostic parameters of 35 cases other than mycosis fungoides and CD30-positive large cell lymphoma. *J Pathol* 172:53, 1994.

95. Vermeer MH, Tensen C, van der Stoop PM, et al.: Absence of T$_h$2 cytokine messenger expression in CD30-negative primary cutaneous large T-cell lymphomas. *Arch Dermatol* 137:901, 2001.

96. Bekkenk MW, Vermeer MH, Jansen PM, et al.: Peripheral T-cell lymphomas unspecified presenting in the skin: analysis of prognostic factors in a group of 82 patients. *Blood* 102:2213, 2003.

97. Hoque SR, Child FJ, Whittaker SJ, et al.: Subcutaneous panniculitis-like T-cell lymphoma: a clinicopathological, immunophenotypic and molecular analysis of six patients. *Br J Dermatol* 148:516, 2003.

98. Trautinger F, Knobler R, Willemze R, et al.: EORTC consensus recommendations for the treatment of mycosis fungoides/Sezary syndrome. *Eur J Cancer* 42:1014, 2006.

# Chapter 60

# MATURE T-CELL NON-HODGKIN'S LYMPHOMA: DIAGNOSIS AND THERAPY

## Nam H. Dang and Fredrick Hagemeister

T-cell lymphoid malignancies are a heterogeneous group of relatively rare diseases that are defined as distinct entities by a constellation of laboratory and clinical characteristics, including morphologic features, immunophenotypes, genetic abnormalities, clinical manifestations, and responses to treatment. The mature T- and natural killer (NK)-neoplasms as defined by the World Health Association (WHO) classification account for approximately 10% of all lymphoid malignancies.[1] However, the incidences of certain subtypes vary considerably by race and geography, with non-AIDS-related T-cell malignancies occurring much more frequently in the Far East than in North America. For example, in the Non-Hodgkin's Lymphoma Classification Project,[2] 9.4% of all cases of non-Hodgkin's lymphoma (NHL) (129 of 1378) were classified as peripheral T-cell lymphomas (PTCL), 33 (2.4%) of which were anaplastic large-cell lymphomas (ALCL). The frequencies of the remaining subtypes of PTCL (96 of 1378, 7%) ranged from 1.5% (Vancouver) to 18.3% (Hong Kong). Although the reason for this observed difference in frequencies is not clear for most subtypes, such variability is related in some situations to an association between a specific virus and the T-cell malignancy, such as the linkage between Epstein–Barr virus (EBV) and with NK/T-cell lymphoma and human T-cell lymphotropic virus 1 (HTLV-1) with adult T-cell leukemia/lymphoma (ATLL).

## CLASSIFICATION AND CLINICOPATHOLOCIAL FEATURES

In the past, classification of T-cell lymphoid malignancies has been controversial, with no internationally accepted schema. The previously accepted morphology-based Working Formulation relied on morphology alone, and did not consider T-cell malignancies as separate and distinct entities. Rather, T-cell lymphomas that occurred infrequently and generally had a poor prognosis were included in different pathologic subtypes (diffuse-mixed, large cell, and lymphoblastic) and were treated like their B-cell counterparts.[3] Subsequently, the Revised European–American classification of lymphoid neoplasms (REAL)[4] has subdivided all lymphomas into B-cell and T-cell lymphomas to avoid the confusion created by the Working Formulation. The REAL classification further subdivides T-cell lymphoid malignancies into two major groups based on the T-cell maturation stage: precursor T-cell neoplasms and peripheral T-cell neoplasms. Furthermore, the peripheral T- and NK-cell neoplasms are subdivided into additional categories, with some provisional subtypes. Thus, the REAL classification was a major advance in the characterization of lymphoid malignancies, because it recognized that the site of disease presentation is a significant aspect of disease biology, with extranodal T-cell lymphomas being inherently different from nodal subtypes. Following the publication of the REAL classification in 1994, new findings regarding some categories of lymphoma clarified the status of entities that were listed as provisional in the REAL classification, particularly among the T-cell lymphomas. The currently used WHO classification is based on the principles established by the REAL classification and incorporates minor additional modifications.[1,5] Besides the precursor T-cell neoplasms, this classification includes 14 subgroups among the mature T- and NK-cell malignancies. Since the site of disease presentation represents a key aspect of disease biology and clinical course, an attempt is made to give it a more prominent role in subgroup characterization, leading to the classification of disease subtypes as being primarily leukemic, nodal, extranodal, or cutaneous (Table 60.1).

### PREDOMINANTLY LEUKEMIC GROUP

There are four subtypes in the predominantly leukemic group. Comprising up to 20% of all prolymphocytic leukemia and 1% of chronic lymphocytic

**Table 60.1**  Mature T- and NK-cell neoplasms in the proposed WHO classification system

**Predominantly leukemic malignant neoplasms**
  T-cell prolymphocytic leukemia
  T-cell large granular lymphocytic leukemia
  NK-cell leukemia
  Sézary syndrome

**Predominantly nodal malignant neoplasms**
  Peripheral T-cell lymphoma, unspecified
  Angioimmunoblastic T-cell lymphoma
  Adult T-cell leukemia/lymphoma
  Anaplastic large-cell lymphoma

**Predominantly extranodal malignant neoplasms**
  Nasal NK/T-cell lymphoma
  Enteropathy-type intestinal T-cell lymphoma
  Subcutaneous panniculitislike T-cell lymphoma
  Hepatosplenic gamma/delta T-cell lymphoma

**Predominantly cutaneous malignant neoplasms**
  Mycosis fungoides
  CD30+ lymphoproliferative disease (primary cutaneous anaplastic large-cell lymphoma)

NK, natural killer; WHO, World Health Organization.
Adapted from Jaffe et al.[5]

leukemia (CLL) cases, T-cell prolymphocytic leukemia (T-PLL) and CLL present clinically as overt leukemia but are often associated with involvement of lymph nodes, liver, spleen, bone marrow, skin, and mucosal surfaces. It is an aggressive disease with the median survival of patients being less than 1 year, and is rarely curable with available therapy. Cytologically, the leukemic cells are small-to-medium sized with irregular nuclei, prominent nucleoli, and abundant, nongranular cytoplasm. Immunophenotypic analysis reveals that most tumor cells express CD4, along with CD2, CD3, CD5, CD7, and the alpha/beta T-cell receptor (TCR). Molecular studies have demonstrated rearrangement of the $TCR\beta$ and $TCR\gamma$ genes, with the $TCR\delta$ gene usually deleted and the $Ig$ heavy- and light-chain genes usually in the germline configuration. A characteristic chromosomal abnormality occurring in approximately two-thirds of T-PLL/CLL patients is inv 14 (q11;q32), with trisomy 8 also having been reported.[4,6–10]

Large granular lymphocytic leukemia (LGLL) is divided into two subtypes, T- and NK-cell leukemias. Patients with LGLL tend to be older than 50 years of age and often have multiple episodes of recurrent infections occurring over years, as well as fatigue or bleeding. Furthermore, autoimmune diseases such as rheumatoid arthritis are often associated with LGLL, particularly T-LGLL. Physical examination may reveal mild hepatosplenomegaly and lymphadenopathy, while laboratory studies often show lymphocytosis, neutropenia, anemia, and/or thrombocytopenia. The T-cell subtype usually has more adverse features, such as anemia and splenomegaly. While the clinical course is usually indolent, some cases are quite aggressive. In particular, cases associated with EBV infection may exhibit an aggressive behavior. The circulating lymphoid cells are small with cytoplasmic granules, and may resemble B-CLL. The malignant cells of T-LGLL are often CD2+, CD3+, alpha/beta TCR+, CD8+, CD16+, CD25−, CD56−, and CD57+. However, the NK-cell tumors are CD2+, CD3−, alpha/beta TCR−, CD8+, CD16+, CD25−, CD56+, and CD57+. T-LGLL cells have rearrangements of the $TCR\gamma$, $TCR\alpha$, and $TCR\beta$ genes, while NK-cell tumors do not have $TCR$ gene rearrangements. In both types, the $Ig$ genes are often in the germline configuration.[4,11–14] Recently, expression of the ectopeptidase CD26/dipeptidyl peptidase IV has been associated with an aggressive clinical behavior in T-LGLL.[15]

Sezary syndrome (SS) is the leukemic variant of mycosis fungoides (MF), although it can occasionally arise de novo. Patients usually present with multiple cutaneous plaques or nodules, generalized erythroderma, lymphadenopathy, and circulating tumor cells (Sezary cells) in the peripheral blood. SS has an aggressive clinical course, with an expected survival being typically less than 2 years, particularly in the presence of extracutaneous disease. The malignancy is composed of small cells with cerebriform nuclei, and they usually express CD2, CD3, alpha/beta TCR, CD4, and CD5, with variable expression of CD25 and with one-third of cases being CD7+.[4,16] Furthermore, CD26 is typically absent on the tumor cell surface, a fact that can be utilized to detect presence of tumor cells in the peripheral blood.[17]

### PREDOMINANTLY NODAL GROUP

Peripheral T-cell lymphoma, unspecified (PTCL), is the most common of all the T-cell neoplasms. However, this subtype is less well defined than the other T-cell malignancies and has protean manifestations. While comprising less than 15% of all lymphomas in most European and US studies, it is more common in Japan and other Asian countries. Most patients with PTCL are adults who have generalized lymphadenopathy and involvement of other extranodal sites, including bone marrow, skin, liver, spleen, lung, and Waldeyer's ring, with accompanying pruritis, eosinophilia, and hemophagocytic syndrome. PTCLs are generally aggressive neoplasms and require combination chemotherapy, although current treatments usually result in relatively short duration of response and poor overall survival. The neoplastic lymphoid cells vary in size, ranging from atypical small cells to medium-sized or large tumor cells with irregular nuclei and abundant clear cytoplasm. These tumor cells display a mature T-cell phenotype, expressing such pan-T-cell antigens as CD2, CD3, CD5, CD7, CD4 or CD8, and alpha/beta TCR, while B-cell surface antigens are generally lacking. Molecular studies show rearrangements of the $TCR\beta$ and $TCR\gamma$ genes in most instances, while the $Ig$ genes are usually in germline configuration.[4,18–27]

Angioimmunoblastic T-cell lymphoma is a relatively rare disorder with distinctive clinical behavior and generally poor outcome. This entity is part of a spectrum of clinical conditions ranging from angioimmunoblastic lymphadenopathy with dysproteineimia (AILD) to malignant lymphoma. Patients with AILD are at risk of developing malignant lymphomas that may be of either T-cell or B-cell lineage, while clonal populations of T cells may also be seen in AILD cases without overt histologic evidence of malignant lymphoma. Furthermore, investigators have reported cases of de novo lymphomas that have histologic features similar to those of lymphomas arising from an AILD background. Patients with angioimmunoblastic T-cell lymphoma often exhibit systemic disease with generalized lymphadenopathy, fever, weight loss, malaise, and skin rash. They tend to be older males with nodal and extranodal disease and numerous adverse risk factors. Laboratory studies reveal anemia (often positive for direct Coombs' test), eosinophilia, and polyclonal hypergammaglobulinemia. Although occasional remissions or protracted remissions have been reported (usually in the setting of AILD and not angioimmunoblastic T-cell lymphoma), the disease is considered aggressive, with infectious complications and progression to high-grade lymphomas. Morphologically, this disease is characterized by the presence of a mixture of small lymphocytes and large, atypical lymphoid cells with abundant and clear cytoplasm. Other characteristics include obliteration of the lymph node architecture, burned out germinal centers, and arborizing proliferation of small blood vessels. Tumor cells tend to be mature CD4[+] T cells expressing T-cell-associated antigens, with TCR gene rearrangement seen in most cases of angioimmunoblastic T-cell lymphoma. Nonrandom and clonal chromosomal abnormalities, particularly those involving chromosomes 3 or 5, have been detected, and EBV infection is often associated with the disease.[2,4,28–38]

ATLL is a clinicopathological entity closely associated with infection by the human T-cell leukemia/lymphoma retrovirus HTLV-1, which is transmitted either by infected cells via semen, blood products, needles, breast milk, or by transplacental migration, with an incubation period ranging from 20 to 30 years. HTLV-1 is endemic in the Caribbean basin, southeastern United States, and southwestern Japan. HTLV-1 infection is demonstrated by the presence of serum antibodies or by molecular detection of the virus through the polymerase chain reaction (PCR) technique or Southern blot hybridization. Occurring mainly in adults, ATLL presents with one of four clinical subtypes. Acute ATLL represents the most common subtype: patients generally have widespread adenopathy, hepatosplenomegaly, skin lesions, peripheral blood and cerebrospinal fluid involvement, lytic bone lesions, and hypercalcemia that may develop in the absence of bone lesions. Patients with this disorder

have a median survival duration of less than 1 year. Lymphomatous ATLL is the second most common disease subtype, with a slightly better prognosis than that reported for the acute form. Patients usually present with lymphadenopathy and involvement of visceral organs without hepatosplenomegaly or hypercalcemia. Chronic ATLL is associated with an absolute lymphocytosis and cytologically abnormal circulating cells, skin lesions, visceral involvement, and lymphadenopathy, with survival rates of more than 2 years. Finally, patients with smoldering ATLL have chronic disease for years with skin lesions, and minimal disease involvement in the peripheral blood and visceral organs. Morphologically, the circulating cells are of medium size, with basophilic cytoplasm and irregular, multilobulated nuclei. ATLL cells have a mature T-cell phenotype, expressing alpha/beta TCR, CD4, and other pan-T-cell antigens. Of note is that the tumor cells usually express high levels of CD25 on the cell surface, which may be a target for therapeutic interventions. Molecular studies show TCR gene rearrangements, and the Ig genes are often in germline configuration.[4,39–42]

Primary nodal anaplastic large T/null-cell lymphoma (ALCL) presents as a systemic disease affecting children and adults involving lymph nodes and extranodal sites, including the skin. Considered aggressive lymphomas, these tumors require treatment with combination chemotherapy, with response and survival rates that are similar to those for diffuse aggressive large B-cell lymphomas. Although patients with these lymphomas are potentially curable, late relapses have been observed. The neoplastic cells are large blastic cells with pleomorphic nuclei, prominent nucleoli, and abundant cytoplasm. The malignant cells are often cohesive and are preferentially found within lymph node sinuses. Tumor cells classically express the activation antigen CD30, while many cases also express such activation markers as CD25, CD26, CD38, as well as the proliferation antigens CD71 and Ki-67. The systemic form of ALCL also expresses epithelial membrane antigen. The T-cell variant expresses pan-T-cell antigens such as CD2, CD3, CD5, CD7, and CD4, and lacks B-cell antigens. On the other hand, null-cell ALCL lacks immunophenotypic and molecular evidence of B- or T-cell lineage. While T-cell ALCL usually exhibits TCR gene rearrangement, there is a high rate of lineage promiscuity, since immunoglobulin genes are also found to be rearranged in T-cell ALCL, while B-cell tumors often have TCR gene arrangement. A key feature on a subset of systemic ALCL is the occurrence of chromosomal translocations involving chromosome 5q35, usually as t(2;5)(p23;q35). This chromosomal translocation juxtaposes the anaplastic lymphoma kinase (ALK) gene on chromosome 2p23 with the nucleophosmin (NPM) nucleolar phosphoprotein gene on 5q35, and is often found with the systemic form of T-cell ALCL, although it is not limited to this subset. Besides the classic t(2;5), other translocations may also activate the *ALK* gene and participate in the pathogenesis of ALCL.[4,43–57]

### PREDOMINANTLY EXTRANODAL GROUP

Extranodal NK/T-cell lymphoma or angiocentric lymphoma is a unique clinicopathological entity associated with EBV infection that usually presents with destructive nasal or midline facial tumor. Affecting both children and adults, it is a rare disease in the United States and Europe, and is more common in Asia. Other organ involvement is common; sites include the nasal cavity, upper respiratory tract, lung, skin, kidney, and central nervous system, with lymph node involvement being relatively rare. The clinical course may be indolent or aggressive, and is at least partly dependent on the number of large lymphoid cells present. It is also commonly associated with a hemophagocytic syndrome thought to be induced by cytokine production by tumor cells leading to activation of benign histiocytes, resulting in fever, hepatosplenomegaly, pancytopenia, and hemolysis. Although the disease is often localized at presentation, chemotherapy is generally administered in conjunction with radiotherapy. However, the relapse rate is high, and overall prognosis is generally poor. In one report, although patients with angiocentric lymphoma tended to be younger than patients with other T-cell lymphomas and had favorable prognostic features, they failed to go into remission with anthracycline-based combination chemotherapy.[23] Others have reported that angiocentric nasal lymphoma typically occurs in young females (median age 49 years) at extranodal sites, but with few adverse risk factors and with limited-stage disease.[2] The disease is characterized morphologically by an angiocentric and angioinvasive infiltrate composing of a mixture of atypical lymphoid cells admixed with normal lymphocytes, plasma cells, and histiocytes. These tumors tend to accumulate greater numbers of large atypical lymphoid cells, and with fewer inflammatory cells over time, potentially indicating an increasingly worse clinical behavior. There is a propensity for invasion and destruction of blood vessels with prominent ischemic necrosis of tumor and normal tissues. Immunophenotypically, the tumors cells express pan-T-cell antigens CD2 and CD7, while C3 is often absent. While they may be CD4+ or CD8+, angiocentric lymphoma cells often express the NK-cell-associated antigen CD56. Immunoglobulins and B-cell antigens are negative. Molecular studies show that *TCR* and *Ig* genes are usually germ line, while EBV genomes are usually detected by Southern blot, PCR, and in situ hybridization techniques.[4,58–66]

A subset (10–25%) of primary intestinal lymphomas has a T-cell phenotype, also known as enteropathy-type intestinal T-cell lymphoma. This disease tends to occur in adults with a history of gluten-sensitive enteropathy or celiac disease, although it can occasionally be found in patients without a history of enteropathy. Patients usually present with weight loss, abdominal pain, and jejunal involvement, and are typically diagnosed at the time of emergency surgery for small bowel perforation. The clinical course is often aggressive with associated poor survival rates, and death usually occurs from intestinal perforation due to chemotherapy-refractory malignant ulcers. Postmortem examination often reveals multiple jejunal ulcers that are associated with perforation, and a distinct mass may be absent. Histologic studies show that the uninvolved intestine may have blunting of villi, as is commonly seen in celiac disease. Tumors are found diffusely and contain a mixture of small, medium, and large lymphoid cells. Immunophenotypically, tumor cells are CD3+, CD4−/CD8− or CD4−/CD8+, CD7+, CD30+, CD103+, and are negative for B-cell antigens. Molecular studies show *TCR* gene rearrangement, with *Ig* genes being germline.[4,67–70]

Subcutaneous panniculitislike T-cell lymphoma usually presents with single or multiple subcutaneous nodules, affecting most often the extremities and trunk. The clinical course may be indolent with spontaneously waxing and waning skin lesions or may be very aggressive. Most patients are adults and usually exhibit fever, pancytopenia, and hepatosplenomegaly at diagnosis. A significant number of patients present initially with a hemophagocytic syndrome causing systemic symptoms, while others may develop a hemophagocytic syndrome during the course of their illness, with usually a fatal outcome. Bone marrow studies may be instrumental in establishing the diagnosis of disease-associated hemophagocytic syndrome. Histologically, the tumors involve the subcutaneous tissue, with infiltration of the neoplastic cells in the adipose tissue leading to coagulative necrosis. Tumor cells consist of a mixture of small and large cells, and accrual of large cells can occur over time. Immunophenotypically, the tumor cells have a mature T-cell immunophenotype, expressing CD8 and other pan-T-cell antigens. *TCR* genes are rearranged, while *Ig* genes are the germline configuration.[4,71,72]

Hepatosplenic gamma/delta T-cell lymphoma is a rare disease found in young adults, often males, who present with marked hepatosplenomegaly and bone marrow involvement, with no or minimal lymphadenopathy, and infrequently, skin lesions. The disease is usually refractory to current treatment, with its clinical course being quite aggressive and with a high rate of disease relapse and death. These tumors are composed of medium-size lymphoid cells with irregular nuclear contours, condensed chromatin, and small nucleoli. There is sinusoidal infiltration in the liver, while the red pulp of the spleen is involved, and the white pulp is spared. The tumor cells usually express CD2, CD3, CD7, and the TCR gamma/delta chains, while CD5 is absent. *TCR* genes are also typically rearranged.[4,73,74]

## PROGNOSTIC FACTORS

### INTERNATIONAL PROGNOSTIC INDEX

Several investigators have described the clinical aggressiveness of various subgroups of T-cell lymphomas and have correlated disease behavior with various factors at presentation. In the Non-Hodgkin's Lymphoma Classification Project analysis, there was a wide spectrum of clinical behavior for different T-cell lymphoma subsets (Table 60.2). Patients with anaplastic large T-cell lymphomas have the best 5-year survival rate (77%), while those with other T-cell subsets such as PTCL have much worse outcomes (25% 5-year survival).[75] In a recent analysis of the 96 non-ALCL PTCL cases diagnosed within the Non Hodgkin's Lymphoma Classification Project, the frequency of PTCL varied from 1.5 to 18.3% according to country of origin. Seventy percent of the patients in this study had received combination chemotherapy which contained doxorubicin, resulting in 5-year failure-free and overall survival rates of 20 and 26%, respectively. Performance status and International Prognostic Index (IPI) scores at presentation strongly correlated with 5-year overall and failure-free survival results. However, other components of the IPI, such as age, clinical stage, serum lactate dehydrogenase (LDH), and the presence of extranodal involvement, were not statistically correlated with disease outcome. There were no statistically significant differences for the overall and failure-free survival rates among various major T-cell subtypes. Of note is the fact that within the PTCL, "not-otherwise-specified" category (PTCL, NOS), the number of transformed blast counts per 10 high-power fields was statistically significant for both overall and failure-free survival.[2] Although the IPI project did not allow analysis of the influence of immunophenotype on overall survival results, investigators have used the IPI to predict outcome for T-cell lymphomas. For example, Rüdiger et al.[2] demonstrated that IPI scores (0–2 features vs 3–5 features) separated T-cell lymphomas into groups with significantly different overall survival and failure-free survival rates. Gisselbrecht et al.[22] reported that 45% of patients with T-cell lymphomas had three or more adverse prognostic factors when stratified by their IPI score compared with only 37% of those with B-cell lymphomas. Furthermore, these investigators could still separate patients with T-cell lymphomas into groups with significantly different survival rates, using the IPI system. Results for each IPI group were also significantly worse for those with T-cell tumors compared to those for patients with B-cell lymphomas who had the same IPI scores, respectively, particularly for those with IPI scores of 2 or more. Melnyk et al.[23] found that response and survival rates for patients with T-cell lymphomas were better for those with low rather than high IPI scores. In addition, Lopez-Guillermo et al.[76] reported that patients with PTCL and low plus low/intermediate IPI scores had significantly better survival rates than those with high plus intermediate/high-risk scores. In the study of Ansell et al.,[77] the IPI strongly predicted survival results when all patients were included in the analysis, and when patients were separated into cohorts of 60 years and younger and older than 60 years, the age-adjusted IPI also significantly predicted outcome. While hepatic and bone marrow involvement were also significant prognostic factors by univariate analysis, only the IPI remained significant by multivariate analysis. IPI scores also predicted overall survival rates for patients with T-cell lymphomas in the study reported by Reiser et al.,[78] as did elevated LDH, B-symptoms, and extranodal involvement; however, the presence of bulky disease (>7.5 cm), advanced-stage III/IV disease and bone marrow involvement did not. Armitage and Weisenburger[79] separated patients with PTCL into groups according to IPI, and found differences in survival rates for those with IPI scores of 0 and 1 as compared to those with IPI scores of 2 or greater, although these differences were not statistically significant. IPI scores also did not predict outcomes for patients with anaplastic large T-cell lymphomas.[79]

### T-CELL PHENOTYPE

The T-cell phenotype is an important adverse prognostic factor all by itself. Except for CD30+ anaplastic large T-cell lymphomas, patients with T-cell lymphomas have significantly lower response rates and shorter disease-free and overall survival results than do those with B-cell lymphomas.[22,23,80] Gisselbrecht et al.[22]

**Table 60.2**  REAL classification of lymphoma entities according to clinical aggressiveness

| Subgroup | 5-Year overall survival rate (%) |
|---|---|
| Anaplastic large T/null cell | 77 |
| Marginal zone, MALT | 74 |
| Follicular | 72 |
| Lymphoplasmacytic | 59 |
| Marginal zone, nodal | 57 |
| Small lymphocytic | 51 |
| Primary mediastinal large B cell | 50 |
| Burkitt-like | 47 |
| Diffuse large B cell | 46 |
| Burkitt's | 44 |
| Mantle cell | 27 |
| Lymphoblastic, T cell | 26 |
| Peripheral T cell | 25 |

MALT, mucosa-associated lymphoid tissue; REAL, Revised European–American Classification of Lymphoid Neoplasms.
Adapted from The Non-Hodgkin's Lymphoma Classification Project.[75]

showed that patients with non-ALCL T-cell tumors have more disseminated disease, B symptoms, bone marrow involvement, hepatosplenomegaly, and skin involvement than do those with B-cell lymphomas with comparable histologic grades. Furthermore, patients with T-cell lymphomas are more likely to be anemic, and have hypereosinophilia, hypergammaglobulinemia, and increased $\beta_2$-microglobulin levels. On the other hand, T-ALCL patients are more likely to have localized disease with more favorable IPI scores, with better remission and overall survival rates, than those with non-ALCL T-cell or B-cell lymphomas. Complete remission (CR) rates were 63% for B-NHL, 54% for T-NHL (72% for ALCL and 49% for non-ALCL T-NHL). Five-year survival rates were 52% for B-NHL, and 41% for T-NHL (64% for ALCL and 35% for non-ALCL T-NHL). Five-year event-free survival rates were 42% for B-NHL and 33% for T-NHL. Five adverse factors significantly influenced survival outcome by multivariate analysis: age greater than 60 years, disseminated stage, elevated LDH, performance status, and non-ALCL T-cell lymphoma histology. Coiffier et al.[80] compared patients with PTCL and B-cell diffuse large-cell lymphoma, and found that PTCL patients were more likely to have an aggressive presentation with advanced-stage and B symptoms. While there was no difference in response rates between the two groups, patients with T-cell lymphomas had higher relapse rates (43% vs 29%), shorter freedom-from-relapse results (median: 34 months vs outcome not reached), and shorter overall survival rates (median: 42 months vs 50 months). Multivariate analysis demonstrated that the T-cell phenotype was an independent adverse prognostic factor. Comparing patients with ALCL and non-ALCL PTCL, Lopez-Guillermo et al.[76] showed that ALCL histology was an important variable predicting favorable results, with CR rates of 69% for those with ALCL and 45% for those with other PTCL; median survival results were 65 months for ALCL and 20 months for other PTCL; and 4-year survival probabilities were 62% for ALCL and 32% for other PTCL. In another series containing 560 cases of aggressive lymphomas (68 patients with T-cell and 492 with B-cell lymphomas) at MD Anderson Cancer Center, the T-cell phenotype was an independent adverse prognostic factor, with T-cell tumors having worse outcomes than B-cell lymphomas of comparable IPI or MD Anderson Prognostic Tumor Score Index. Patients with T-cell lymphomas were more likely to have advanced disease, B symptoms, and other poor prognostic features compared to those with B-cell lymphomas, including elevated LDH or $\beta_2$-microglobulin levels. However, age and extranodal disease distributions were not significantly different between these two groups. Compared to their B-cell counterparts, T-cell lymphomas had lower CR rates (65% for T-cell and 76% for B-cell lymphomas), shorter 5-year failure-free survival (38% for T-cell and 56% for B-cell lymphomas), and lower overall survival (38% for T-cell and 63% for B-cell lymphomas). Consistent with other studies, patients with ALCL had higher response and survival rates. There was a significantly greater number of deaths in patients with non-ALCL tumors more than 3 years after treatment, many of which were due to late relapses.[23]

## TREATMENT MODALITIES

### CONVENTIONAL CHEMOTHERAPY

Treatment of the non-ALCL T-cell lymphomas with conventional chemotherapy designed for B-cell lymphomas has had only limited success. Common anthracycline-containing regimens result in low response rates and short durations of remission, and the vast majority of patients develop resistant disease. For example, Armitage et al. evaluated 134 cases of PTCL diagnosed at three centers from 1973 to 1986: 80 patients had been treated with intensive regimens such as CHOP [cyclophosphamide, hydroxydaunorubicin (doxorubicin), Oncovin (vincristine), and prednisone] with or without bleomycin, CAP-BOP (cyclophosphamide, doxorubicin, procarbazine, bleomycin, vincristine, and prednisone), COMLA (cyclophosphamide, vincristine, methotrexate, and cytosine arabinoside), and MACOP-B (methotrexate, doxorubicin, cyclophosphamide, vincristine, prednisone, and bleomycin).[21] While the median survival was 17 months and the 4-year survival was 28% for all 134 patients, for the 80 patients who received intensive combination chemotherapy, 50% achieved a CR, with the 4-year durability of remission being 41% and the overall survival of this intensively treated group being 45%. However, the 4-year disease-free survival for those with stage IV disease, comprising 50% of the patients, was only 10%. Ansell et al.[77] evaluated 78 patients seen at the Mayo Clinic with T-cell lymphomas from 1985 to 1995; most received doxorubicin-containing regimens, including CHOP, ProMACE-CytaBOM (methotrexate, prednisone, doxorubicin, cyclophosphamide, etoposide, cytarabine, bleomycin, and vincristine), and m-BACOD (methotrexate, bleomycin, doxorubicin, cyclophosphamide, vincristine, and dexamethasone). The median overall survival duration for the 78 patients on study was 22 months (range 1–105 + months). The median survival for high-risk IPI patients was 6 months, compared to 15 months for high-intermediate IPI patients, and 24 months for low-intermediate IPI patients, and the median survival for the low-risk group was not reached; the differences in survival rates were statistically significant. There were no significant differences in response rates among the T-cell subtypes, and univariate analysis showed no statistically significant survival differences among various T-cell subgroups. Rüdiger et al. studied 96 cases of non-ALCL PTCL evaluated in the Non-Hodgkin's Lymphoma Classification Project, 70% of whom had received doxorubicin-containing regimens. The 5-year overall survival was 26%, and the failure-free survival was 20%.[2] Physicians from French and Belgian centers evaluated 288 PTCL patients (60 cases of T-ALCL and 228 cases of non-ALCL PTCL) treated with anthracycline-containing regimens, including m-BACOD (methotrexate, bleomycin, doxorubicin, cyclophosphamide, vincristine, and dexamethasone), ACVB (doxorubicin, cyclophosphamide, vindesine, bleomycin, and prednisone), and NCVB (mitoxantrone, cyclophosphamide, vindesine, bleomycin, and prednisone), followed by consolidation and maintenance therapies or autologous transplantation in many cases. The CR rates were 54% for all patients, 72% for those with ALCL, and 49% for those with non-ALCL T-cell lymphomas, and 5-year survival rates were 41, 64, and 35%, respectively. Five factors adversely and significantly influenced survival by multivariate analysis: age greater than 60 years, advanced stage, elevated LDH, performance status, and non-ALCL T-cell lymphoma.[22] Lopez-Guillermo et al.[76] evaluated 174 T-cell lymphomas from Spanish institutions; 30 were ALCL and the rest consisted of PTCL unspecified, angioimmunoblastic T-cell, angiocentric, intestinal T-cell, and hepatosplenic gamma/delta T-cell lymphomas. Most patients received CHOP-like therapy. CR rates were 69% for ALCL cases and 45% for other PTCL subtypes, with a median survival of 65 months for ALCL and 20 months for other PTCL, and 4-year survival probabilities of 62 and 32%, respectively. From MD Anderson Cancer Center, Melnyk et al. evaluated 68 T-cell lymphoma patients treated from 1984 to 1995 with anthracycline-containing regimens such as CHOP–bleomycin alternating with DHAP (dexamethasone, cisplatin, and cytarabine), CHOP–bleomycin alternating with CMED (cyclophosphamide, etoposide, methotrexate, and dexamethasone), CHOP–bleomycin alternating with OPEN (vincristine, etoposide, mitoxantrone, and prednisone), or alternating triple therapy consisting of ASHAP (cytarabine, doxorubicin, cisplatin, and methylprednisolone), MBACOS (doxorubicin, cyclophosphamide, vincristine, bleomycin, methylprednisolone, and methotrexate), and MINE (mesna, ifosfamide, mitoxantrone, and etoposide).[23] Similar to reports of others, the CR rate was 65%, the 5-year failure-free survival rate was 38%, and overall survival result was 38%, and those with ALCL had better results. Interestingly, a significant number of deaths in patients with non-ALCL T-cell lymphomas occurred 3 years after treatment, many of whom died due to late relapses.

Other investigators also have reported that T-ALCL has a better prognosis than non-ALCL cases. Compared to the non-T-ALCL PTCL, the 33 T/null (indeterminant)-ALCL patients in the Non-Hodgkin's Lymphoma Classification Project were significantly younger, less likely to have advanced-stage disease or bone marrow involvement, more likely to have favorable IPI score, and importantly, had greater survival results. The estimated 5-year overall survival for all T/null-ALCL patients in this series was 75% and the failure-free survival was 56%, and most (81%) of these patients had been treated for curative intent with doxorubicin-containing regimens. Patients with ALK+ and ALK− disease had no significant differences in clinical features or survival.[81] However, in a study reported by the British Columbia Cancer Agency and the University of Nebraska Medical Center, which evaluated 57 patients with systemic T/null ALCL treated with doxorubicin-containing multiagent chemotherapy protocols for curative intent, the 5-year overall survival rate was 57% (56% for 32 cases of T-ALCL and 83% for 25 cases of null-ALCL).[82] ALK protein expression was an independent predictor of survival, as there was a statistically significant survival difference between the ALK+ (31 cases) and ALK− (26 cases) groups. For the ALK+ cases, the 5-year overall survival was 93% and the 5-year failure-free survival was 88%, while the 5-year overall survival was 37% and the 5-year failure-free survival was 37% for the ALK− cases. Finally, in a retrospective study involving patients with systemic T/null ALCL from multiple European institutions, the majority of whom received doxorubicin-containing regimens, showed that the ALK+ subgroup had an overall survival of 71% compared to only 15% for the ALK- subset. Ten-year disease-free survival rates were 82% for the ALK+ group and 28% for the ALK− subset.[83]

Studies evaluating treatment for other specific T-cell lymphoma subtypes that are non-ALCL generally have reported disappointing responses, duration of response and survival rates. T-prolymphocytic leukemia (T-PLL) is relatively resistant to conventional chemotherapy, as demonstrated by a study involving 78 patients with T-PLL.[7] Thirty-two patients had received alkylating agents and nine (28%) experienced transient partial remissions (PRs). Five of 15 patients (33%) had responded to CHOP, with 1 CR lasting 3 months. However, of the 31 patients treated with pentostatin, 15 experienced responses (3 CRs, lasting 8, 10, and 12 months, and 12 PRs), of which 8 responses were in 15 patients treated with pentostatin as first-line therapy. Chott et al. reported results for 27 patients with intestinal T-cell lymphoma; only 7 of 14 treated with multiagent chemotherapy completed therapy. Twenty of these 27 patients have died, and 17 died within 6 months from diagnosis. The overall median survival was 4 months, and patients with stage I had better survival rates than other patients.[67] In another study with 45 patients with hepatosplenic gamma/delta T-cell lymphoma, most of whom were treated with alkylating agents, CHOP or CHOP-like therapies, second- or third-generation regimens for high-grade lymphomas, and autologous or allogeneic stem cell or peripheral stem cell transplantation, CRs were obtained in five and relapses were common and early in the treatment course. Thirty-six patients were dead at the time of this study, with a median survival of only 8 months (range 0–42 months).[84] However,

Matutes et al. reported results for 15 patients with ATLL who received alpha-interferon and zidovudine (AZT), 11 of whom had previously received anthracycline-containing chemotherapy regimens. Seven patients had progressive disease, and eight were in remission at the time of study completion. When starting alpha-interferon and AZT, four patients had progressive disease, eight were in partial/complete remission, and three untreated patients had active disease. PRs lasting 2+ to 44+ months (median duration 10 months) occurred in 10 (67%) patients, four (26%) had no responses, and one was not evaluable. Eight patients died 3–41 months from diagnosis. Median survival for all 15 patients was 18 months; survival for nonresponders ranged from 4 to 20 months (median 6 months), and the 6 patients with PR were alive 8–82 months from diagnosis, with 55% of all patients alive at 4 years. This study therefore suggested that this combination may improve the outcome of ATLL and help maintain responses, and should be studied in other populations.[85]

Standard treatments for nasal NK/T-cell lymphoma are unsatisfactory. In a retrospective analysis of Chinese patients with primary NHL of the nose and nasopharynx, many of whom received CHOP, CEOP (cyclophosphamide, epirubicin, vincristine, and prednisone) or ProMACE-CytaBOM, with or without radiation, patients with NK/T-cell lymphoma had very poor results.[86] Compared to patients with T-cell (24 patients, 21.3%) or B-cell (38 patients, 33.6%) phenotypes, those with NK/T-cell lymphoma (51 patients, 45.1%) had the highest male-to-female ratio, more frequent involvement of the nasal cavity alone, a higher risk of skin dissemination, more frequent development of hemophagocytic syndrome, and worse prognosis. The CR rate for NK/T-cell disease was 56%, compared to 69.6 and 76.3% for T-cell and B-cell phenotypes, respectively. The 5-year actuarial disease-free survival rates were 25.1% for NK/T-cell disease, 41.9% for T-cell phenotype, and 40.9% for B-cell phenotype. The 5-year actuarial overall survival was 31.1% for NK/T-cell phenotype, 57.7% for T-cell phenotype, and 35% for B-cell phenotype. The median overall survival was 12.5 months for NK/T-cell phenotype, 93.4 months for T-cell phenotype, and 17 months for B-cell phenotype. In another study, investigators treated patients with localized nasal NK/T-cell lymphoma with four cycles of CHOP and involved-field radiation therapy, obtaining a response of 58% and an estimated overall 3-year survival of 59%. In fact, only 35% of patients completed the planned sequential chemoradiotherapy due to disease progression during chemotherapy. These results led to the authors' conclusion that better treatments were needed for localized nasal NK/T-cell lymphoma.[87]

### HIGH-DOSE CHEMOTHERAPY/STEM CELL TRANSPLANT

Several groups have examined the impact of high-dose chemotherapy on T-cell lymphomas. Investigators at

MD Anderson Cancer Center performed a retrospective analysis of 36 patients with relapsed or refractory PTCL who received high-dose chemotherapy and autologous (29 patients) or allogeneic (7 patients) hematopoietic transplantation.[88] The 3-year overall survival rate was 36%, and progression-free survival (PFS) rate was 28%. The 3-year probabilities of survival for the autologous and allogeneic groups were 39 and 29%, respectively, while the PFS rates at 3 years were 32 and 14%, respectively. The pretransplant serum LDH level was the most important prognostic factor for both overall survival and PFS results. Furthermore, patients with an IPI score of ≤1 had better overall survival, but not PFS rates, than those with greater IPI scores. At a median follow-up of 43 months, 13 patients (36%) were still alive with no evidence of disease. These data were comparable to published studies of high-dose chemotherapy for relapsed or refractory B-cell lymphomas, and suggested that stem cell transplant should be considered for selected patients with T-cell lymphomas. In a study reported by Vose et al., 41 patients with relapsed intermediate- or high-grade lymphomas (17 cases of T-cell and 24 cases of B-cell lymphomas) underwent high-dose therapy and autologous transplantation for salvage therapy. Comparable results were obtained for B- and T-cell lymphomas.[89] The T-cell patients had a slightly higher CR rate that was not statistically significant (59% compared to 42%), with the durations of response being similar (50% at 30 months, with no late relapses). The 2-year overall survival rates for both groups were also similar, being 35% for T-cell lymphomas and 30% for B-cell lymphomas, as were the 2-year disease-free survival rates (28% for the T-cell group and 17% for the B-cell patients). Predictors of poor outcome for both groups of patients were poor performance status, bulky tumor, and high LDH levels. A study involving 40 patients with relapsed T-cell lymphomas from Norway and Sweden also examined the role of high-dose therapy with autologous stem cell transplantation.[90] All patients had chemosensitive disease and had received anthracycline-containing regimens, mainly CHOP, VACOP-B (etoposide, doxorubicin, cyclosphophamide, vincristine, prednisone, and bleomycin), or MACOP-B (methotrexate, doxorubicin, cyclophosphamide, vincristine, prednisone, and bleomycin), prior to transplantation. At the time of stem cell transplant, 17 patients were in first PR or CR, and 23 were in second or third PR or CR. Conditioning regimens included BEAM (carmustine, etoposide, cytarabine, and melphalan) in 15 patients, BEAC (carmustine, etoposide, cytarabine, and cyclophosphamide) in 14, BEAC without etoposide and total body irradiation (TBI) in 1, cyclophosphamide and TBI in 8, and melphalan and mitoxantrone in 2. There were three (7.5%) treatment-related deaths; however, 32 patients (80%) achieved or maintained a CR after stem cell transplant, with relapses occurring in 16 patients, all within 2 years following transplantation.

**Table 60.3    Results of phase II trials with pentostatin in T-cell lymphoma**

| Study | Lymphoma type | Number of patients | Partial remissions | Complete remissions | Overall response rate (%) |
|---|---|---|---|---|---|
| Smyth et al.[93] | Lymphoblastic lymphoma | 7 | 2 | 2 | 57 |
| Lofters et al.[94] | Adult T-cell leukemia | 6 | 1 | 0 | 17 |
| Yamaguchi et al.[95] | Adult T-cell leukemia | 5 | 2 | 0 | 40 |
| Greiner et al.[96] | Cutaneous T-cell lymphoma | 18 | 5 | 2 | 39 |
| Monfardini et al.[97] | Low-grade lymphoma | 18 | 3 | 0 | 17 |
|  | T-cell high- and | 12 | 1 | 1 | 8 |
|  | intermediate-grade | 7 | 1 | 0 | 14 |
|  | lymphoma |  |  |  |  |
| Mercieca et al.[98] | Sézary syndrome | 20 | 9 | 3 | 60 |
|  | T-cell non-Hodgkin's lymphoma | 27 | 5 | 0 | 19 |
|  | Adult T-cell leukemia | 25 | 1 | 2 | 12 |
|  | Cutaneous T-cell lymphoma (no Sézary syndrome) | 13 | 0 | 0 | 60 |
| Ho et al.[99] | Sézary syndrome and mycosis fungoides | 19 | 4 | 1 | 26 |
| Dearden et al.[100] | Adult T-cell leukemia | 20 | 1 | 2 | 15 |
|  | Cutaneous T-cell lymphoma | 13 | 6 | 1 | 54 |
| Cummings et al.[101] | Non-Hodgkin's lymphoma | 25 | 4 | 0 | 16 |
|  | Hodgkin's disease | 3 | 1 | 0 | 33 |
|  | Cutaneous T-cell lymphoma | 8 | 4 | 0 | 50 |
| Duggan et al.[102] | Non-Hodgkin's lymphoma | 76 | 7 | 5 | 16 |
| Ho et al.[103] | Sézary syndrome and mycosis fungoides | 46 | 17 | 1 | 39 |
| Kurzrock et al.[104] | Sézary syndrome | 14 | 6 | 4 | 71 |
|  | Mycosis fungoides | 6 | 3 | 1 | 66 |
|  | Peripheral T-cell lymphoma | 3 | 2 | 1 | 100 |
| Grever et al.[105] | Cutaneous T-cell lymphoma | 21 | 4 | 2 | 29 |

Adapted from Verstovsek et al.[106]

The 3-year overall, event-free, and relapse-free survival rates were 58, 48, and 56%, respectively. As expected, patients with ALCL had better outcomes than did other histologies (79 and 44%, respectively). Furthermore, these data appeared similar to those reported for stem cell transplant for relapsed high-grade B-cell lymphomas.[91] Others have studied allogeneic HLA-matched sibling transplantation with combined marrow and CD34+-enriched peripheral blood stem cell transplantation after cytoreductive chemotherapy and TBI for refractory cutaneous T-cell lymphoma (CTCL), suggesting that this approach may be potentially beneficial for selected patients.[92]

## PURINE ANALOGS

The purine analogs pentostatin (deoxycoformycin), fludarabine, and cladribine (2-chlorodeoxyadenosine/2-CdA) are a group of structurally similar drugs that are active agents in the therapy of T-cell lymphomas. T-cells have high levels of adenosine deaminase (ADA), a key enzyme involved in purine metabolism, and as ADA inhibitors, these drugs produce DNA damage and impairment of DNA repair. As single agents, the purine analogs are relatively well tolerated, with myelosuppression being usually mild, although it tends to be more severe with cladribine than with pentostatin. Of note is the fact that these agents produce lymphopenia and immunosuppression, occasionally resulting in the development of opportunistic infections.

Several studies have demonstrated that pentostatin has activity against T-cell lymphoma (Table 60.3). Investigators at the Royal Marsden Hospital in London demonstrated that pentostatin has activity in postthymic mature T-cell malignancies. Mercieca et al.[98] obtained an overall response rate of 32% for 145 patients treated with pentostatin for a variety of mature T-cell tumors, most of whom had disease considered relapsed or refractory to anthracycline-containing regimens or alkylating agents. The median overall duration of response was 6 months, ranging from 3 to 66 months. For the 55 patients with T-PLL, 5 achieved a CR and 20 achieved a PR, lasting from 3 to 16 months (median 6 months), for an overall response rate of 45%. For the 16 patients with SS, 3 experienced a CR and 7 had PRs, ranging from 3 to 66 months (median 9 months), for an overall response rate of 62%. However, 13 patients with other types of CTCL, including 5 with MF, did not respond to pentostatin. Nonetheless, of the four patients with circulating Sézary cells without skin involvement, two (50%) had PRs in terms of improvement in peripheral lymphocytosis and bone marrow function. Two of the five patients with LGLL leukemia also achieved a CR, one lasting 18 months and the other lasting 12 months. However, other subsets of T-cell disease in this study had lower response rates to pentostatin. Two of the 25 patients with ATLL achieved a CR, one lasting 33 months and the other died of an opportunistic infection while still in CR 5 months after stopping drug treatment; another achieved a PR lasting 5 months, with an overall response rate of 12%. Meanwhile, 27 patients with PTCL were treated, with 5 PRs and no CR, for an overall response rate of 19%. The duration of response was from 3 to 28 months, with a median response duration of 9 months. There was no statistically significant difference in the response rates of previously untreated patients compared to those for patients previously treated with one or more regimens (35% vs 29%, respectively), with histologic subtype being the single most important factor influencing results.

Other investigators have studied pentostatin for patients with relapsed CTCL or PTCL with prominent cutaneous manifestations.[104] Of the 24 patients evaluable for response, six (25%) patients had CR and 11 (46%) patients had PR. Ten of 14 (71%) patients with SS, four of six (66%) with tumor stage MF, and three of three with PTCL responded. Although the median response duration of the patients with tumor-stage MF was only 2 months (range 1–2 months) and 3.5 months for SS patients, there were two SS patients with prolonged responses lasting greater than 1 year. One of the three PTCL patients had an ongoing CR at 20 months. The most common side effect observed in these patients who had received a median of three prior therapies (range 1–12) was significant lowering of CD4 counts, and several subsequently developed herpes zoster infection.

Recently, investigators at MD Anderson Cancer Center treated 14 patients with relapsed noncutaneous T-cell lymphomas with pentostatin, and reported details regarding its lymphopenic effects.[107] One patient (7%) had a CR and six (43%) had PRs, with the median PFS result for responders being 6 months (range 2–15 months). A significant reduction in circulating CD26+ T lymphocytes was observed in treated patients, potentially associated with immunosupression. In one patient with PR, the decrease in the levels of CD26+ T lymphocytes was associated with genital herpes reactivation, while resolution of this opportunistic infection was associated with a recovery in CD26+ T-cell levels, once pentostatin was discontinued. Since CD4+CD26+ T lymphocytes are memory helper T cells, the selective loss of CD26+ T cells in lymphoma patients treated with pentostatin has important clinical implications, and may partly explain the relatively high incidence of opportunistic infections observed in patients receiving this agent.

The other purine analogs, cladribine and fludarabine, also have activity in T-cell lymphomas, although relatively limited data are available. One study involving 25 patients with relapsed or refractory cutaneous T-cell lymphoproliferative disorders (24 MF or SS and 1 Ki-1 + ALCL) showed that 2-CdA treatment resulted in a 24% response rate, with 3 patients (12%) having a CR with a median duration of 4.5 months (range 2.5–16 months) and three patients having a PR with a median duration of 2 months (range 2–4 months). The most significant toxicities were myelosuppression and infection, with opportunistic infections occurring in a significant percentage of patients.[108,109] Another study also demonstrated 2-CdA activity in T-cell lymphomas, as 22 patients with such varied diagnoses as T-LGLL, T-PLL, T-CLL, SS, MF, and PTCL who were treated with 2-CdA had a response rate of 41%. Four responders (18%) had CRs (1 T-PLL, 1 MF, and 2 T-LGLL) while five patients (23%) had PRs (2 T-CLL, 1 SS, and 2 PTCL). All patients with PR and one CR patient developed relapses at a median of 7 months (range 5–26 months), while three patients with CR remain in remission at 30+, 36+, and 54+ months. The median overall survival was 12 months, and the main toxicities were fever and infection.[110] To date, there is only limited published data to suggest that fludarabine has single-agent activity in certain subsets of T-cell lymphoma, particularly MF.[111,112]

Several investigators have studied purine-analog-containing combination therapies for T-cell tumors. In a phase II study of 41 patients with advanced MF/SS, the combination of pentostatin and intermittent high-dose recombinant interferon alfa-2a resulted in CR in two and PR in 15 patients, for an overall response rate of 41%. The PFS duration for responders was 13.1 months, and common toxicities for this combination included opportunistic infection and interferon-related constitutional symptoms.[113] The combination of fludarabine and interferon alfa-2a was also tested in another phase II trial of 35 patients with advanced MF/SS, with 4 CRs and 14 PRs for an overall response rate of 51%.[114] The median PFS duration for responders was 5.9 months, with three of the CRs still in remission after 18–35 months. Significant toxicities included constitutional symptoms, neutropenia, and infections. Another study with 12 patients with advanced refractory primary CTCL demonstrated that treatment with the combination of fludarabine and cyclophosphamide resulted in 1 CR and 4 PRs for an overall response rate of 42%. The mean duration of response was 10 months, with bone marrow toxicity being the common and significant side effect.[115] Finally, the combination of fludarabine, mitoxantrone, and dexamethasone has produced 1 CR that has lasted 15 months after treatment cessation in a patient with aggressive subcutaneous panniculitislike T-cell lymphoma.[116]

### GEMCITABINE

Gemcitabine is a novel pyrimidine antimetabolite with clinical activity and a low-toxicity profile in solid tumors and selected T-cell hematologic malignancies. A phase II study involving 44 previously treated patients with either MF ($n = 30$) or PTCL with exclusive skin involvement ($n = 14$) treated with gemcitabine reported 5 (11.5%) CRs and 26 (59%) PRs, for an overall response rate of 70.5%.[117] Responses varied by histology: three of 30 (10%) MF patients attained a CR and 18 of 30 (60%) had PRs, while two of 14 (14.5%) PTCL patients had CRs and eight of 14 (57%) achieved PRs. The median duration of CR was 15 months (range 6–22 months) and of PR was 10 months (range 2–15 months). Treatment was generally well tolerated, and hematologic toxicities were mild. Gemcitabine was also found to be effective and well-tolerated therapy for relapsed or refractory T-cell malignancies in another study involving 10 patients with various histologies.[118] There were 2 CRs and 4 PRs, for an overall response rate of 60%, with a median duration of response of 13.5 months.

A pivotal, multicenter phase III trial was then performed to evaluate the activity of denileukin diftitox in patients with CD25$^+$ CTCL.[119] Patients were randomized to receive denileukin diftitox given at a dose of either 9 µg/kg/day for 5 days every 3 weeks or 18 µg/kg/day for 5 days every 3 weeks, with no steroid premedication. Thirteen of 36 patients receiving the higher dose had an objective response, as compared to eight of 35 patients in the lower dose cohort. Overall, 20% of patients had PRs while 10% had CRs, with the mean duration of response being 6.9 months. There were CRs in both groups, with the 3 CRs in the lower dose group having early stage (IB) disease, while the 3 CRs in the higher dose group had stage IIB or higher disease, suggesting a role for the higher dose in patients with advanced-stage disease (Table 60.4). An increase in the titer of antidenileukin diftitox antibodies was seen in most patients, which did not have a significant effect on antitumor efficacy. Regarding tumor CD25 status, 58% of all skin samples of CTCL patients met the inclusion criteria of having greater than 20% CD25 positivity on tumor cell surface. However, in multiple instances, the results from multiple biopsies taken from the same patient showed a wide range of CD25 expression. Side effects included acute hypersensitivity-type events related to drug administration, associated with dypsnea, back pain, hypotension, chest tightness, pruritus, and flushing. Transient elevation of liver enzymes was also seen, as well as rashes and

**Table 60.4** Denileukin diftitox in cutaneous T-cell lymphoma—results from pivotal phase III trial[119]

| | | DAB$_{389}$ IL-2 dose | | | | |
|---|---|---|---|---|---|---|
| | | 9 µg/kg/day | | 18 µg/kg/day | | All |
| Stage | N | Response | n | Response | n | Response |
| | | Response in phase III CTCL trial | | | | |
| All | 35 | 8 (23%) | 36 | 13 (36%) | 71 | 21 (30%) |
| ≤IIA | 14 | 6 (43%) | 12 | 4 (33%) | 26 | 10 (38%) |
| ≥IIB$^a$ | 21 | 2 (10%) | 24 | 9 (38%) | 45 | 11 (24%) |
| | | Response by stage in phase III CTCL trial | | | | |
| | | n = 35 | | n = 36 | | |
| CR | | 3 | | 4 | | |
| | | IB (3) | | IB (1) | | |
| | | | | IIB (2) | | |
| | | | | IVA (1) | | |
| PR | | 5 | | 9 | | |
| | | IB (1) | | IB (2) | | |
| | | IIA (2) | | IIA (1) | | |
| | | IIB (1) | | IIB (3) | | |
| | | IVA (1) | | III (2) | | |
| | | | | IVA (1) | | |

CTCL, cutaneous T-cell lymphoma.
$^a$Logistic regression favoring high dose for stage ≥IIB ($P = 0.07$).
Adapted from Foss FM.[120]

flulike symptoms. A vascular leak syndrome, associated with hypotension, edema, and hypoalbuminemia, was also noted in approximately 25% of patients. Most side effects were transient and tended to occur early in treatment. Steroid premedication was not used in the pivotal trial to avoid ambiguity in interpreting efficacy; however, in a subsequent study with 15 CTCL patients, which allowed for the use of intravenous steroids, there was a higher response rate (60%) with denileukin diftitox with a substantial decrease in adverse effects.[121] The improvement in patient's tolerability associated with concurrent steroid administration may have led to greater patient compliance and treatment completion, potentially resulting in better response rate; in the pivotal phase III trial, many patients discontinued therapy prior to completing four cycles due to toxicity and were deemed nonresponders. Therefore, steroid premedication may ultimately lead to greater patient compliance and higher response rates with this drug. Besides its efficacy in CTCL, denileukin diftitox also has activity in other T-cell lymphomas and deserves further study in these diseases.[122,123]

### CAMPATH-1H/ANTI-CD52 ANTIBODY

CD52 is a nonmodulating glycosylphosphatidylinositol-linked protein that is expressed, in abundance, on normal and malignant B and T lymphocytes, monocytes, macrophages, and eosinophils, but not on hematopoietic progenitor cells.[124,125] Given the high expression of CD52 on the surface of malignant cells, specific antibody targeting this antigen may serve as appropriate novel therapy for these CD52-expressing tumors. Campath-1H is a genetically engineered human IgG1 anti-CD52 monoclonal antibody, consisting of the hypervariable regions of the parental rat antibody inserted into the framework domains of normal human immunoglobulin *IgG1* genes. As a humanized antibody, Campath-1H may work through a number of mechanisms, including complement-mediated lysis, antibody-dependent cell cytotoxicity, and apoptosis. Different cell types express different levels of CD52 on their surface, which may explain in part the observed variation in their sensitivity to Campath-1H-mediated lysis.[126] Campath-1H treatment is generally well tolerated, with the most significant toxicity being prolonged lymphopenia associated with opportunistic infections, especially in heavily pretreated patients.

Prior to the development of Campath-1H, a predecessor antibody, the rat antibody Campath-1G caused clearance of malignant cells from the blood and bone marrow in various lymphoid malignancies, suggesting potential clinical applications for anti-CD52 antibody therapy.[127] In a subsequent phase II study involving 39 patients with T-PLL, all but two patients of whom had received prior therapy with a variety of agents, investigators obtained an overall response rate of 76%, with 60% CR and 16% PR.[128] The median disease-free interval was 7 months (range 4–45 months). Clearance of tumor cells from the blood and bone marrow was generally rapid but did not cause tumor lysis syndrome. Disease resolution from skin, spleen, and lymph nodes also occurred in approximately half of the affected patients, although those with bulky lymph node masses, serous effusions, or hepatic or central nervous system involvement had more resistant disease. There was a statistically significant difference in survival for patients achieving a CR (median 16 months) as compared to partial responders (median 9 months) or nonresponders (median 4 months). Meanwhile, 12 patients were retreated with Campath-1H following relapse, with five (42%) achieving a second CR and one achieving PR, with responses lasting 5–6 months. Seven patients received high-dose therapy with autologous stem cell support, and stem cells harvested from these patients were free of T-PLL cells as documented by flow cytometry and PCR studies. Three of these patients remained alive in CR at 5, 7, and 15 months following autograft. Four additional patients underwent allogeneic stem cell transplants, with three being alive in CR up to 24 months following allograft. As expected, major toxicities were prolonged lymphopenia and opportunistic infections. In a retrospective analysis of compassionate use of the drug for relapsed or refractory T-PLL, 76 patients treated with Campath-1H had an overall response rate of 51% including a 39.5% CR rate, with the median duration of CR being 8.7 months (range 0.13+ to 44.4 months) and median time to progression for all patients being 4.5 months (range 0.1–45.4 months).[129] These figures are very favorable in this population whose response rate to first-line chemotherapy was only 32%, with a 6% CR rate and a median time to progression of only 2.3 months (range 0.2–28.1 months). Specific organ CRs varied: 39% in the bone marrow, 33% in the spleen, 32% in lymph nodes, 30% in the liver, and 43% in the skin. Campath-1H also had activity in patients with advanced CTCL. A phase II multicenter study was done in Europe, which enrolled previously treated patients with low-grade NHLs, including CTCL.[130] Out of the eight patients with MF, there were four responders (50%), including 2 CRs. This response rate was higher than the 14% response rate (six of 42 patients had PR) seen with the B-cell lymphoma patients under study. Among the four responding MF patients, the median time to progression was 10 months (range 2–14 months). Consistent with previous findings, the most pronounced antitumor effect was seen in blood, bone marrow, and skin, while there was low response with bulky lymph nodes and splenomegaly.

## CONCLUSION

T-cell lymphoid malignancies represent a heterogeneous group of relatively rare diseases that are defined as distinct entities by a constellation of laboratory and clinical features, including morphologic features, immunophenotype, genetic features, clinical manifestation, and clinical course. Recent classification attempts have considered mature T-cell malignancies as separate entities, with site of disease presentation being an important part of disease behavior. Excluding rare exceptions such as ALCL, our knowledge regarding disease pathophysiology, prognostic factors, and disease-specific molecular features is still incomplete, due to their relative rarity and heterogeneity. Also, except for ALCL and certain CTCL, T-cell tumors often have systemic involvement, are generally aggressive, and are relatively refractory to currently available treatments. Therefore, there is an urgent need to identify novel molecular targets on T-cell malignancies for future therapy, which may also serve as potential prognostic markers for selected disease subsets. For most T-cell lymphoid malignancies, available treatment modalities have included conventional combination chemotherapy, often with anthracycline-containing regimens, resulting in rather disappointing results in terms of response rate, response duration, and overall survival. Other agents with published activities include the purine analogs and gemcitabine, and these drugs need further study. Recent efforts have focused on the use of targeted therapy, especially the fusion protein denileukin diftitox and the monoclonal Campath-1H/anti-CD52 antibody, which have definite activity in various subsets of T-cell tumors. Other investigational agents including monoclonal antibodies targeting cell surface antigens are under development in various clinical trials at the present time. However, in view of the unsatisfactory outcomes seen in most cases of T-cell lymphoid malignancies, novel therapies should be explored in large, prospective randomized trials involving multiple institutions, and patients with these malignancies should be enrolled on these trials as the first choice of therapy. Potential combinations involving established chemotherapy regimens with emerging targeted therapies that exhibit novel mechanisms of action and nonoverlapping toxicities should also be considered for the treatment of T-cell lymphoid malignancies to improve clinical outcomes.

## REFERENCES

1. Jaffe ES, Harris NL, Diebold J, et al.: World Health Organization classification of neoplastic diseases of the hematopoietic and lymphoid tissues. A progress report. *Am J Clin Pathol* 111(suppl 1):S8–S12, 1999.
2. Rüdiger T, Weisenburger DD, Anderson JR, et al.: Peripheral T-cell lymphoma (excluding anaplastic large-cell lymphoma): results from the Non-Hodgkin's Lymphoma Classification Project. *Ann Oncol* 13: 140–149, 2002.
3. The Non-Hodgkin's Lymphoma Pathologic Classification Project: National Cancer Institute sponsored study of classifications of non-Hodgkin's lymphomas: summary and description of a working formulation for clinical usage. *Cancer* 49:2112–2135, 1982.
4. Harris NL, Jaffe ES, Stein H, et al.: A revised European–American classification of lymphoid neoplasms: a proposal from the International Lymphoma Study Group. *Blood* 84:1361–1392, 1994.
5. Jaffe ES, Krenacs L, Raffeld M: Classification of T-cell and NK-cell neoplasms based on the REAL classification. *Ann Oncol* 8(suppl 2):S17–S24, 1997.
6. Brito-Babapulle V, Pomfret M, Matutes E, et al.: Cytogenetic studies on prolymphocytic leukemia. II: T-cell prolymphocytic leukemia. *Blood* 70:926–931, 1987.
7. Matutes E, Brito-Babapulle V, Swansbury J, et al.: Clinical and laboratory features of 78 cases of T-prolymphocytic leukemia. *Blood* 78:3269–3274, 1991.
8. Matutes E, Garcia TJ, O'Brien M, et al.: The morphological spectrum of T-prolymphocytic leukaemia. *Br J Haematol* 64:111–124, 1986.
9. Hanson CA, Bockenstedt PL, Schnitzer B, et al.: S100-positive, T-cell chronic lymphoproliferative disease: an aggressive disorder of an uncommon T-cell subset. *Blood* 78:1803–1813, 1991.
10. Knowles DM: Immunophenotypic and antigen receptor gene rearrangement analysis in T cell neoplasia. *Am J Pathol* 134:761–785, 1989.
11. McKenna RW, Arthur DC, Gajl-Peczalska KJ, et al.: Granulated T-cell lymphocytosis with neutropenia: malignant or benign chronic lymphoproliferative disorder? *Blood* 66:259–266, 1985.
12. Loughran TP Jr: Clonal diseases of large granular lymphocytes. *Blood* 82:1–14, 1993.
13. Pelicci PG, Allavena P, Subar M, et al.: T-cell receptor (alpha, beta, gamma) gene rearrangements and expression in normal and leukemic large granular lymphocytes/natural killer cells. *Blood* 70:1500–1508, 1987.
14. Sheridan W, Winton EF, Chan WC, et al.: Leukemia of non-T lineage natural killer cells. *Blood* 72:1701–1707, 1988.
15. Dang NH, Aytac U, Sato K, et al.: T-large granular lymphocyte lymphoproliferative disorder: expression of CD26 as a marker of clinically aggressive disease and characterization of marrow inhibition. *Br J Haematol* 121:857–865, 2003.
16. Lutzner M, Edelson R, Schein P, et al.: Cutaneous T-cell lymphomas: the Sezary syndrome, mycosis fungoides, and related disorders. *Ann Intern Med* 83:534–552, 1975.
17. Jones D, Dang NH, Duvic M, et al.: Absence of CD26 expression is a useful marker for diagnosis of T-cell lymphoma in peripheral blood. *Am J Clin Pathol* 115:885–892, 2001.
18. Haioun C, Gaulard P, Bourquelot P, et al.: Clinical and biological analysis of peripheral T-cell lymphomas: a single institution study. *Leuk Lymphoma* 7:449–455, 1992.
19. Armitage JO, Vose JM, Linder J, et al.: Clinical significance of immunophenotype in diffuse aggressive non-Hodgkin's lymphoma. *J Clin Oncol* 7:1783–1790, 1989.

20. Cheng AL, Chen YC, Wang CH, et al.: Direct comparisons of peripheral T-cell lymphoma with diffuse B-cell lymphoma of comparible histological grades—should peripheral T-cell lymphoma be considered separately? *J Clin Oncol* 7:725–731, 1989.

21. Armitage JO, Greer JP, Levine AM, et al.: Peripheral T-cell lymphoma. *Cancer* 63:158–163, 1989.

22. Gisselbrecht C, Gaulard P, Lepage E, et al.: Prognostic significance of T-cell phenotype in aggressive non-Hodgkin's lymphomas. *Blood* 92:76–82, 1998.

23. Melnyk A, Rodriguez A, Pugh WC, et al.: Evaluation of the revised European–American lymphoma classification confirms the clinical relevance of immunophenotype in 560 cases of aggressive non-Hodgkin's lymphoma. *Blood* 89:4514–4520, 1997.

24. Picker LJ, Weiss LM, Medeiros LJ, et al.: Immunophenotypic criteria for the diagnosis of non-Hodgkin's lymphoma. *Am J Pathol* 128:181–201, 1987.

25. Suchi T, Lennert K, Tu LY, et al.: Histopathology and immunohistochemistry of peripheral T-cell lymphomas: a proposal for their classification. *J Clin Pathol* 40:995–1015, 1987.

26. Weiss LM, Crabtree GS, Rouse RV, et al.: Morphologic and immunologic characterization of 50 peripheral T-cell lymphomas. *Am J Pathol* 118:316–324, 1985.

27. Weiss LM, Trela MJ, Cleary ML et al.: Frequent immunoglobulin and T-cell receptor gene rearrangements in "histiocytic" neoplasms. *Am J Pathol* 121:369–373, 1985.

28. Frizzera G, Moran EM, Rappaport H: Angioimmunoblastic lymphadenopathy with dysproteinaemia. *Lancet* 1:1070–1073, 1974.

29. Lukes RJ, Tindle BH: Immunoblastic lymphadenopathy. A hyperimmune entity resembling Hodgkin's disease. *N Engl J Med* 292:1–8, 1975.

30. Feller AC, Griesser H, Schilling CV, et al.: Clonal gene rearrangement patterns correlate with immunophenotype and clinical parameters in patients with angioimmunoblastic lymphadenopathy. *Am J Pathol* 133:549–556, 1988.

31. Pangalis GA, Moran EM, Nathwani BN, et al.: Angioimmunoblastic lymphadenopathy. Long-term follow-up study. *Cancer* 52:318–321, 1983.

32. Weiss LM, Strickler JG, Dorfman RF, et al.: Clonal T-cell populations in angioimmunoblastic lymphadenopathy and angioimmunoblastic lymphadenopathy-like lymphoma. *Am J Pathol* 122:392–397, 1986.

33. Nathwani BN, Rappaport H, Moran EM, et al.: Malignant lymphoma arising in angioimmunoblastic lymphadenopathy. *Cancer* 41:578–606, 1978.

34. Lipford EH, Smith HR, Pittaluga S, et al.: Clonality of angioimmunoblastic lymphadenopathy and implications for its evolution to malignant lymphoma. *J Clin Invest* 79:637–642, 1987.

35. Godde-Salz E, Feller AC, Lennert K: Chromosomal abnormalities in lymphogranulomatosis X (LgrX)/angioimmunoblastic lyphadenopathy (AILD). *Leuk Res* 11:181–190, 1987.

36. Anagnostopoulos I, Hummel M, Finn T, et al.: Heterogeneous Epstein–Bar virus infection patterns in peripheral T-cell lymphoma of angioimmunoblastic lymphadenopathy type. *Blood* 80:1804–1812, 1992.

37. Weiss LM, Jaffe ES, Liu XF, et al.: Detection and localization of Epstein–Barr viral genomes in angioimmunoblastic lymphadenopathy and angioimmunoblastic lymphadenopathy-like lymphoma. *Blood* 79:1789–1795, 1992.

38. Abruzzo LV, Schmidt K, Weiss LM, et al.: B-cell lymphoma after angioimmunoblastic lymphadenopathy: a case with oligoclonal gene rearrangements associated with Epstein–Barr virus. *Blood* 82:241–246, 1993.

39. Shimamoto Y, Suga K, Shibata K, et al.: Clinical importance of extraordinary integration patterns of human T-cell lymphotropic virus type I proviral DNA in adult T-cell leukemia/lymphoma. *Blood* 84:853–858, 1994.

40. Waldmann TA, White JD, Goldman CK, et al.: The interleukin-2 receptor: a target for monoclonal antibody treatment of human T-cell lymphotrophic virus I-induced adult T-cell leukemia. *Blood* 82:1701–1712, 1993.

41. Shimoyama M: Diagnostic criteria and classification of clinical subtypes of adult T-cell leukaemia- lymphoma. A report from the Lymphoma Study Group (1984–87). *Br J Haematol* 79:428–437, 1991.

42. van Krieken JH, Elwood L, Andrade RE et al.: Rearrangement of the T-cell receptor delta chain in T-cell lymphomas with a mature phenotype. *Am J Pathol* 139:161–168, 1991.

43. Kadin ME, Sako D, Berliner N, et al.: Childhood Ki-1 lymphoma presenting with skin lesions and peripheral lymphadenopathy. *Blood* 68:1042–1049, 1986.

44. Agnarsson BA, Kadin ME: Ki-1 positive large cell lymphoma. A morphologic and immunologic study of 19 cases. *Am J Surg Pathol* 12:264–274, 1988.

45. Bitter MA, Franklin WA, Larson RA, et al.: Morphology in K-1 (CD30)—positive non-Hodgkin's lymphoma is correlated with clinical features and the presence of a unique chromosomal abnormality, t(2,5)(p23, q35). *Am J Surg Pathol* 14:305–316, 1990.

46. Greer JP, Kinney MC, Collins RD, et al.: Clinical features of 31 patients with Ki-1 anaplastic large-cell lymphoma. *J Clin Oncol* 9:539–547, 1991.

47. Penny RJ, Blaustein JC, Longtine JA, et al.: Ki-1-positive large cell lymphomas, a heterogenous group of neoplasms. Morphologic, immunophenotypic, genotypic, and clinical features of 24 cases. *Cancer* 68:362–373, 1991.

48. Stein H, Mason DY, Gerdes J, et al.: The expression of the Hodgkin's disease associated antigen Ki-1 in reactive and neoplastic lymphoid tissue: evidence that Reed–Sternberg cells and histiocytic malignancies are derived from activated lymphoid cells. *Blood* 66:848–858, 1985.

49. Herbst H, Tippelmann G, Anagnostopoulos I, et al.: Immunoglobulin and T-cell receptor gene rearrangements in Hodgkin's disease and Ki-1-positive anaplastic large cell lymphoma: dissociation between phenotype and genotype. *Leuk Res* 13:103–116, 1989.

50. Piris M, Brown DC, Gatter KC, et al.: CD30 expression in non-Hodgkin's lymphoma. *Histopathology* 17:211–218, 1990.

51. Delsol G, Al Saati T, Gatter KC, et al.: Coexpression of epithelial membrane antigen (EMA), Ki-1, and interleukin-2 receptor by anaplastic large cell lymphomas. Diagnostic value in so-called malignant histiocytosis. *Am J Pathol* 130:59–70, 1988.

52. Kaneko Y, Frizzera G, Edamura S, et al.: A novel translocation, t(2;5) (p23;q35), in childhood phagocytic large

T-cell lymphoma mimicking malignant histiocytosis. *Blood* 73:806–813, 1989.

53. Lopategui JR, Sun LH, Chan JK, et al.: Low frequency association of the t(2;5) (p23;q35) chromosomal translocation with CD30+ lymphomas from American and Asian patients. A reverse transcriptase-polymerase chain reaction study. *Am J Pathol* 146:323–328, 1995.

54. Mason DY, Bastard C, Rimokh R, et al.: CD30-positive large cell lymphomas ("Ki-1 lymphoma[") are associated with a chromosomal translocation involving 5q35. *Br J Haematol* 74:161–168, 1990.

55. Falini B, Bigerna B, Fizzotti M, et al.: ALK expression defines a distinct group of T/null lymphomas ("ALK lymphomas") with a wide morphological spectrum. *Am J Pathol* 153:875–886, 1998.

56. Benharroch D, Meguerian-Bedoyan Z, Lamant L, et al.: ALK-positive lymphoma: a single disease with a broad spectrum of morphology. *Blood* 91:2076–2084, 1998.

57. Hernandez L, Pinyol M, Hernandez S, et al.: TRK-fused gene (TFG) is a new partner of ALK in anaplastic large cell lymphoma producing two structurally different TFG-ALK translocations. *Blood* 94(9):3265–3268, 1999.

58. Katzenstein AL, Carrington CB, Liebow AA: Lymphomatoid granulomatosis: a clinicopathologic study of 152 cases. *Cancer* 43:360–373, 1979.

59. DeRemee RA, Weiland LH, McDonald TJ: Polymorphic reticulosis, lymphomatoid granulomatosis. Two diseases or one? *Mayo Clin Proc* 53:634–640, 1978.

60. Lipford EH Jr, Margolick JB, Longo DL, et al.: Angiocentric immunoproliferative lesions: a clinicopathologic spectrum of post-thymic T-cell proliferations. *Blood* 72:1674–1681, 1988.

61. Simrell CR, Margolick JB, Crabtree GR, et al.: Lymphokine-induced phagocytosis in angiocentric immunoproliferative lesions (AIL) and malignant lymphoma arising in AIL. *Blood* 65:1469–1676, 1985.

62. Medeiros LJ, Peiper SC, Elwood L, et al.: Angiocentric immunoproliferative lesions: a molecular analysis of eight cases. *Hum Pathol* 22:1150–1157, 1991.

63. Nakamura S, Suchi T, Koshikawa T, et al.: Clinicopathologic study of CD56 (NCAM)-positive angiocentric lymphoma occurring in sites other than the upper and lower respiratory tract. *Am J Surg Pathol* 19:284–296, 1995.

64. Chan JK, Ng CS, Lau WH, et al.: Most nasal/nasopharyngeal lymphomas are peripheral T-cell neoplasms. *Am J Surg Pathol* 11:418–429, 1987.

65. Harabuchi Y, Yamanaka N, Kataura A, et al.: Epstein–Barr virus in nasal T-cell lymphomas in patients with lethal midline granuloma. *Lancet* 335:128–130, 1990.

66. Kanavaros P, Lescs MC, Briere J, et al.: Nasal T-cell lymphoma: a clinicopathologic entity associated with peculiar phenotype and with Epstein–Barr virus. *Blood* 81:2688–2695, 1993.

67. Chott A, Dragosics B, Radaszkiewicz T: Peripheral T-cell lymphomas of the intestine. *Am J Pathol* 141: 1361–1371, 1992.

68. Isaacson P, Wright DH: Intestinal lymphoma associated with malabsorption. *Lancet* 1:67–70, 1978.

69. Murray A, Cuevas EC, Jones DB, et al.: Study of the immunohistochemistry and T-cell clonality of enteropathy-associated T-cell lymphoma. *Am J Pathol* 146:509–519, 1995.

70. Wright DH, Jones DB, Clark H, et al.: Is adult-onset coeliac disease due to a low-grade lymphoma of intraepithelial T lymphocytes? *Lancet* 337:1373–1374, 1991.

71. Gonzalez CL, Medeiros LJ, Braziel RM, et al.: T-cell lymphoma involving subcutaneous tissue. A clinicopathologic entity commonly associated with hemophagocytic syndrome. *Am J Surg Pathol* 15:17–27, 1991.

72. Burg G, Dummer R, Wilhelm M, et al.: A subcutaneous delta-positive T-cell lymphoma that produces interferon gamma. *N Engl J Med* 325:1078–1081, 1991.

73. Farcet JP, Gaulard P, Marolleau JP, et al.: Hepatosplenic T-cell lymphoma: sinusal/sinusoidal localization of malignant cells expressing the T-cell receptor gamma delta. *Blood* 75:2213–2219, 1990.

74. Gaulard P, Bourquelot P, Kanavaros P, et al.: Expression of the alpha/beta and gamma/delta T-cell receptors in 57 cases of peripheral T-cell lymphomas. Identification of a subset of gamma/delta T-cell lymphomas. *Am J Pathol* 137:617–628, 1990.

75. The Non-Hodgkin's Lymphoma Classification Project: A clinical evaluation of the International Lymphoma Study Group classification of non-Hodgkin's lymphoma. *Blood* 89:3909–3918, 1997.

76. Lopez-Guillermo A, Cid J, Salar A, et al.: Peripheral T-cell lymphomas: initial features, natural history, and prognostic factors in a series of 174 patients diagnosed according to the R.E.A.L. classification. *Ann Oncol* 9:849–855, 1998.

77. Ansell SM, Habermann TM, Kurtin PJ, et al.: Predictive capacity of the International Prognostic Factor index in patients with peripheral T-cell lymphoma. *J Clin Oncol* 15:2296–2301, 1997.

78. Reiser M, Josting A, Soltani M, et al.: T-cell Non-Hodgkin's lymphoma in adults: clinicopathological characteristics, response to treatment and prognostic factors. *Leuk Lymphoma* 43:805–811, 2002.

79. Armitage JO, Weisenburger DD: New approach to classifying non-Hodgkin's lymphomas: clinical features of the major histologic subtypes. *J Clin Oncol* 16: 2780–2795, 1998.

80. Coiffier B, Brousse N, Peuchmaur M, et al.: Peripheral T-cell lymphomas have a worse prognosis than B-cell lymphomas: a prospective study of 361 immunophenotyped patients treated with the LNH-84 regimen. *Ann Oncol* 1:45–50, 1990.

81. Weisenburger DD, Anderson JR, Diebold J, et al.: Systemic anaplastic large-cell lymphoma: results from the non-Hodgkin's lymphoma classification project. *Am J Hematol* 67:172–178, 2001.

82. Gascoyne RD, Aoun P, Wu D, et al.: Prognostic significance of anaplastic lymphoma kinase (ALK) protein expression in adults with anaplastic large cell lymphoma. *Blood* 93:3913–3921, 1999.

83. Falini B, Pileri S, Zinzani PL, et al.: ALK+ Lymphoma: clinico-pathological findings and outcome. *Blood* 93:2697–2706, 1999.

84. Weidmann E: Hepatosplenic T cell lymphoma. A review on 45 cases since the first report describing the disease as a distinct lymphoma entity in 1990. *Leukemia* 14:991–997, 2000.

85. Matutes E, Taylor GP, Cavenagh J, et al.: Interferon α and zidovudine therapy in adult T-cell leukaemia lymphoma:

response and outcome in 15 patients. *Br J Haematol* 113: 779–784, 2001.

86. Cheung MMC, Chan JKC, Lau WH, et al.: Primary non-Hodgkin's lymphoma of the nose and nasopharynx: clinical features, tumor immunophenotype, and treatment outcome in 113 patients. *J Clin Oncol* 16:70–77, 1998.

87. Kim WS, Song SY, Ahn YC, et al.: CHOP followed by involved field radiation: is it optimal for localized nasal natural killer/T-cell lymphoma? *Ann Oncol* 12:349–352, 2001.

88. Rodriguez J, Munsell M, Yazji S, et al.: Impact of high-dose chemotherapy on peripheral T-cell lymphomas. *J Clin Oncol* 19:3766–3770, 2001.

89. Vose JM, Peterson C, Bierman PJ, et al.: Comparison of high-dose therapy and autologous bone marrow transplantation for T-Cell and B-Cell non-Hodgkin's lymphomas. *Blood* 76:424–431, 1990.

90. Blystad AK, Enblad G, Kvaloy S, et al.: High-Dose therapy with autologous stem cell transplantation in patients with peripheral T cell lymphomas. *Bone Marrow Transplant* 27:711–716, 2001.

91. Philip T, Guglielmi C, Hagenbeek A, et al.: Autologous bone marrow transplantation as compared with salvage chemotherapy in relapses of chemotherapy-sensitive non-Hodgkin's lymphoma. *N Engl J Med* 333: 1540–1545, 1995.

92. Guitart J, Wickless SC, Oyama Yu, et al.: Long-term remission after allogeneic hematopoietic stem cell transplantation for refractory cutaneous T-cell lymphoma. *Arch Dermatol* 138:1359–1365, 2002.

93. Smyth JF, Prentice HG, Proctor S, et al.: Deoxycoformycin in the treatment of leukemias and lymphomas. *Ann N Y Acad Sci* 451:123–128, 1985.

94. Lofters W, Campbell M, Gibbs WN, et al.: 2'-Deoxycoformycin therapy in adult T-cell leukemia/lymphoma. *Cancer* 60:2605–2608, 1987.

95. Yamaguchi K, Yul LS, Oda T, et al.: Clinical consequences of 2'-deoxycoformycin treatment in patients with refractory adult t-cell leukemia. *Leuk Res* 10: 989–993, 1986.

96. Greiner D, Olsen EA, Petroni G: Pentostatin (2'-deoxycoformycin) in the treatment of cutaneous T-cell lymphoma. *J Am Acad Dermatol* 36:950–955, 1997.

97. Monfardini S, Sorio R, Cavalli F, et al.: Pentostatin (2'-deoxycoformycin, dCF) in patients with low-grade (B-T-Cell) and intermediate-and high-grade (T-cell malignant lymphomas: phase II study of the EORTC Early Clinical Trials Group. *Oncology* 53:163–168, 1996.

98. Mercieca J, Matutes E, Dearden C, et al.: The Role of pentostatin in the treatment of T-Cell malignancies: analysis of response rate in 145 patients according to disease subtype. *J Clin Oncol* 12:2588–2593, 1994.

99. Ho AD, Thaler J, Willemze R, et al.: Pentostatin (2'-deoxycoformycin) for the treatment of lymphoid neoplasms. *Cancer Treat Rev* 17:213–215, 1990.

100. Dearden C, Matutes E, Catovsky D: Deoxycoformycin in the treatment of mature T-cell leukemias. *Br J Cancer* 64:903–906, 1991.

101. Cummings FJ, Kyungmann K, Neiman RS, et al.: Phase II trial of pentostatin in refractory lymphomas and cutaneous T-cell disease. *J Clin Oncol* 9:565–571, 1991.

102. Duggan DB, Anderson JR, Dillman R, et al.: 2'Deoxycoformycin (pentostatin) for refractory non-Hodgkin's lymphoma: a CALGB phase II study. *Med Pediatr Oncol* 18:203–206, 1990.

103. Ho AD, Suciu S, Stryckmans P, et al.: Pentostatin in T-cell malignancies, an EORTC phase II trial. *Proc Am Soc Clin Oncol* 18:13a, 1999.

104. Kurzrock R, Pilat S, Duvic M: Pentostatin therapy of T-cell lymphomas with cutaneous manifestations. *J Clin Oncol* 17:3117–3121, 1999.

105. Grever MR, Chapman RA, Ratanatharathorn V, et al: An investigation of deoxycoformycin in advanced cutaneous T cell lymphoma (CTCL). *Blood* 66(suppl 1):215a, 1986.

106. Verstovek S, Cabanillas F, Dang NH: CD26 in T-cell lymphomas: a potential clinical role? *Oncology* 14(suppl 2):17–23, 2000.

107. Dang NH, Hagemeister FB, Duvic M, et al.: Pentostatin in T-non-Hodgkin's lymphomas: efficacy and effect on CD26+ T lymphocytes. *Oncol Rep* 10:1513–1518, 2003.

108. Kong LR, Samuelson E, Rosen ST, et al.: 2-Chlorodeoxyadenosine in cutaneous T-cell lympho-proliferative disorders. *Leuk Lymphoma* 26:89–97, 1997.

109. Kuzel TM, Hurria A, Samuelson E, et al.: Phase II trial of 2-chlorodeoxyadenosine for the treatment of cutaneous T-cell lymphoma. *Blood* 87:906–911, 1996.

110. O'Brien S, Kurzrock R, Duvic M, et al.: 2-chlorodeoxyadenosine therapy in patients with T-cell lymphoproliferative disorders. *Blood* 84:733–738, 1994.

111. Von Hoff DD, Dahlberg S, Hartstock RJ, et al.: Activity of fludarabine monophosphate in patients with advanced mycosis fungoides: a Southwest Oncology Group study. *J Natl Cancer Inst* 82: 1353–1355, 1990.

112. Redman JR, Cabanillas F, Velasquez WS, et al.: Phase II trial of fludarabine phosphate in lymphoma: an effective new agent in low-grade lymphoma. *J Clin Oncol* 10:790–794, 1992.

113. Foss FM, Ihde DC, Breneman DL, et al.: Phase II study of pentostatin and intermittent high-dose recombinant interferon alfa-2a in advanced mycosis fungoides/sézary syndrome. *J Clin Oncol* 10: 1907–1913, 1992.

114. Foss FM, Ihde DC, Linnoila IR, et al.: Phase II trial of fludarabine phosphate and interferon alfa-2a in advanced mycosis fungoides/sezary syndrome. *J Clin Oncol* 12:2051–2059, 1994.

115. Scarisbrick JJ, Child JF, Clift A, et al.: A trial of fludarabine and cyclophosphamide combination chemotherapy in the treatment of advanced refractory primary cutaneous T-cell lymphoma. *Br J Dermatol* 144: 1010–1015, 2001.

116. Au WY, Ng WM, Choy C, et al.: Aggressive subcutaneous panniculitis-like T-cell lymphoma: complete remission with fludarabine, mitoxantrone and dexamethasone. *Br J Dermatol* 143:408–410, 2000.

117. Zinzani PL, Baliva G, Magagnoli M, et al.: Gemcitabine treatment in pretreated cutaneous t-cell lymphoma: experience in 44 Patients. *J Clin Oncol* 18:2603–2606, 2000.

118. Sallah S, Wan JY, Nguyen NP: Treatment of refractory T-cell malignancies using gemcitabine. *Br J Haematol* 113:185–187, 2001.

119. Olsen E, Duvic M, Frankel A, et al.: Pivotal phase III trial of two dose levels of denileukin diftitox for the treatment of cutaneous T-cell lymphoma. *J Clin Oncol* 19:376–388, 2001.

120. Foss FM: DAB$_{389}$IL-2 (ONTAK): a novel fusion toxin therapy for lymphoma. *Clin Lymphoma* 1:110–116, 2000.

121. Foss FM, Bacha P, Osann KE, et al.: Biological correlates of acute hypersensitivity events with DAB(389)IL-2 (denileukin diftitox, ONTAK) in cutaneous T-cell lymphoma: decreased frequency and severity with steroid premedication. *Clin Lymphoma* 1:298–302, 2001.

122. Talpur R, Apisarnthanarax N, Ward S, et al.: Treatment of refractory peripheral t-cell lymphoma with denileukin diftitox (ONTAK®). *Leuk Lymphoma* 43:121–126, 2002.

123. McGinnis KS, Shapiro M, Junkins-Hopkins JM, et al.: Denileukin diftitox for the treatment of panniculitic lymphoma. *Arch Dermatol* 138:740–742, 2002.

124. Gilleece MH, Dexter TM: Effect of Campath-1H antibody on human hematopoietic progenitors in vitro. *Blood* 82:807–812, 1993.

125. Treumann A, Lifely MR, Schneider P, et al.: Primary structure of CD52*. *J Biol Chem* 270:6088–6099, 1995.

126. Ginaldi L, De Martinis M, Matutes E, et al.: Levels of expression of CD52 in normal and leukemic b and t Cells: correlation with in vivo therapeutic responses to Campath-1H. *Leuk Res* 22:185–191, 1998.

127. Dyer MJS, Hale G, Hayhoe FGJ, et al.: Effects of CAMPATH-1 antibodies in vivo in patients with lymphoid malignancies: influence of antibody isotype. *Blood* 73:1431–1439, 1989.

128. Dearden CE, Matutes E, Cazin B, et al.: High remission rate in T-cell prolymphocytic leukemia with CAMPATH-1H. *Blood* 98:1721–1726, 2001.

129. Keating MJ, Cazin B, Coutré S, et al.: Campath-1H treatment of T-Cell prolymphocytic leukemia in patients for whom at least one prior chemotherapy regimen has failed. *J Clin Oncol* 20:205–213, 2002.

130. Lundin J, Österborg A, Brittinger G, et al.: CAMPATH-1H monoclonal antibody in therapy for previously treated low-grade non-Hodgkin's lymphomas: a phase II multicenter study. *J Clin Oncol* 6:3257–3263, 1998.

# Chapter 61

# TREATMENT APPROACH TO HIV-RELATED LYMPHOMAS

*Mark Bower*

## INTRODUCTION

Acquired immunodeficiency syndrome (AIDS) following infection with human immunodeficiency virus (HIV) was brought to the world's attention in 1981, with the first case reports of *Pneumocystis carinii* pneumonia (PCP) in homosexual men in Los Angeles. These reports were quickly followed by descriptions of Kaposi's sarcoma (KS) in similar patient groups. There followed a cornucopia of opportunistic infections and isolated reports of high-grade B-cell non-Hodgkin's lymphomas (NHL), both primary cerebral lymphomas and systemic NHL. By 1985, high-grade B-cell NHL was included along with KS as an AIDS-defining illness by the Centers for Disease Control (CDC), following the publication of a series of 90 homosexual men with NHL.[1] A number of other cancers occur at an increased frequency in people with HIV infection, including Hodgkin's lymphoma, anal cancer, lung cancer, and testicular seminoma[2,3]; however, these malignancies have not been included in the definition of AIDS. In addition, an increased incidence of multicentric Castleman's disease (MCD) has been found in people with HIV, following the recognition of an association between MCD and AIDS-associated KS.[4,5] Studies by the World Health Organization have shown that by December 2003, over 20 million people had died of AIDS and 42 million people were living with the virus. The number of people newly infected with HIV is approximately 6 million per year.[6]

Dramatic improvements in the antiviral therapy of HIV infection occurred in the second half of the 1990s which have altered the natural history of HIV infection in those economies where these medicines are widely available. The introduction of highly active antiretroviral therapy (HAART) has led to a fall in the incidence of both opportunistic infection and AIDS-associated malignancies. The development of effective antiretroviral therapies commenced with the introduction of nucleoside reverse transcriptase inhibitors

starting with zidovudine in 1987. In the last 8 years, three new classes of antiretroviral agents have been introduced: protease inhibitors (PIs) (saquinavir, indinavir, ritonavir, nelfinavir, and lopinavir), non-nucleoside reverse transcriptase inhibitors (nevirapine, delavirdine, and efavirenz), and fusion inhibitors (enfuvirtide). The introduction of the first two classes in the late 1990s led to the use of combination HAART. HAART has had an enormous impact on the treatment of HIV in terms of overall survival, incidence of opportunistic infections, and quality of life. In randomized studies, HAART led to a dramatic decline in the mortality and morbidity of HIV.[7] However, only 1 million of the estimated 42 million people infected with HIV worldwide are receiving HAART, as the majority of affected people live in developing countries. In addition, even in the established market economies with access to medical treatment, many individuals remain undiagnosed and consequently do not receive HAART.

## AIDS-RELATED SYSTEMIC LYMPHOMA

### EPIDEMIOLOGY OF AIDS-RELATED LYMPHOMA IN ERA OF HAART

NHLs are associated with both congenital and iatrogenic immunosuppression, and so it was perhaps not surprising that an increased incidence was demonstrated early in the AIDS epidemic. Registry linkage studies in the pre-HAART era found that the incidence of NHL in HIV-positive individuals was 60–200 times higher than in the matched HIV-negative population[8,9] and the relative risk was even greater for primary cerebral lymphomas. Following the introduction of HAART, the incidence of both KS and primary cerebral lymphoma has fallen significantly in both registry linkage and cohort studies.[10–12] In contrast the effects on systemic NHL are less clear although some cohort studies suggest a modest nonsignificant decline in the incidence,[13–15] including in the hemophilia population.[16]

An international meta-analysis of 20 cohort studies compared the incidence of systemic NHL between 1992–1996 and 1997–1999. This meta-analysis confirmed an overall reduction in the incidence of both primary cerebral lymphoma (rate ratio = 0.42) and systemic immunoblastic lymphoma (rate ratio = 0.57) but not Burkitt's lymphoma (rate ratio = 1.18).[17]

### PREDICTORS OF AIDS-RELATED LYMPHOMA

Genetic, infectious, and immunologic factors influence the development of AIDS-related lymphoma. For example, germline chemokine and chemokine receptor gene variants have been found to influence the chance of developing these tumors.[18,19] Acyclovir has mild activity against Epstein–Barr in vivo, and one case–control study has shown that administration of high-dose acyclovir (≥800 mg/day) for ≥1 year was associated with a significant reduction in the incidence of NHL.[20]

An analysis of a cohort of over 8000 HIV-positive patients has identified three factors in multivariate analysis that are significantly associated with the development of NHL: age, nadir CD4 cell count, and no prior HAART.[21] As the CD4 count falls, the development of lymphoma becomes more likely, and this may explain the declining incidence of NHL since the introduction of HAART, as it is thought that the immune restoration that accompanies HAART protects against the development of AIDS-related lymphoma. Nonetheless, the risk of lymphoma persists even among patients who are on HAART and have no detectable HIV viremia.[22]

### CLINICAL PRESENTATION OF AIDS-RELATED LYMPHOMA

The majority of patients with systemic AIDS-related lymphomas present with advanced stage disease and B symptoms. Extranodal disease, bone marrow involvement, and leptomeningeal disease are all common features. Hepatic involvement occurs in up to 25% patients, while one in five patients has bone marrow involvement by NHL. In addition, HIV infection itself is associated with trilineage abnormalities of hematopoiesis[23,24] and the poor hematologic reserves add to the myelotoxicity of cytotoxic chemotherapy. Central nervous system (CNS) involvement by systemic AIDS-associated NHL is frequent; leptomeningeal disease is present at diagnosis in 3–10% and is significantly associated with both Burkitt's lymphoma and paraspinal or paranasal involvement.[25–28]

In the published series from our institution (Chelsea & Westminster Hospital, London) that compared the clinical characteristics of 99 AIDS-related lymphomas presenting prior to 1996 and 55 that presented between 1996 and 1999, there were no differences in the stage at presentation, presence of B symptoms, bone marrow infiltration, or performance status between the two groups. However, the patients who developed lymphoma in the HAART era were less likely to have had a prior AIDS diagnosis, were older, and had higher CD4 cell counts at the time of lymphoma diagnosis.[29] Thus, although there has been a change in the immunologic parameters of lymphoma patients, this would seem to reflect changes in the population at risk rather than any alteration of the biology of the lymphomas. A further analysis of patients who presented with lymphoma in the era of HAART compared those who were receiving HAART at the time of lymphoma diagnosis ($n = 17$) with those who were not ($n = 34$). Again there were no significant differences between the stages or disease sites at presentation but the CD4 cell counts at lymphoma diagnosis were higher in those on HAART.

### TREATMENT OF AIDS-RELATED LYMPHOMA IN THE ERA OF HAART

During the 1980s, conventional chemotherapy schedules were used at full dosages for patients with better prognostic factors. However, marked toxicity and an increased incidence of opportunistic infections lead to modifications of the standard lymphoma regimens, such as the modified methotrexate, bleomycin, doxorubicin, cyclophosphamide, vincristine, dexamethasone (mBACOD) schedule used by the AIDS clinical trials group (ACTG).[30] The subsequent development of hematopoetic growth factors allowed more myelotoxic schedules to be studied. Full-dose mBACOD with granulocyte-macrophage colony-stimulating factor (GM-CSF) support was compared with low-dose mBACOD in ACTG-142, a randomized trial. The median survival in the low-dose arm was 7.7 months and was 6.8 months in the standard-dose arm. There was no difference in either response or survival duration; however, an increased incidence of neutropenic sepsis was recorded in the full-dose arm (Table 61.1). Of note, more patients had active lymphoma at the time of death in the low-dose arm of the study, suggesting that the enhanced anti-tumor activity of the standard schedule was being offset by the greater toxic deaths.[27] A number of phase II trials were conducted in this era with complete remission (CR) rates of 14–68% but the median survival in unselected patients never exceeded 1 year (Table 61.2).

The only other randomized controlled trial of treatment for AIDS-related systemic NHL was also conducted predominantly in the pre-HAART era. The European Intergroup Study devised a risk stratified trial in which patients were allocated into one of three prognostic groups on the basis of CD4 count $<100 \times 10^6$/L, a prior AIDS-defining diagnosis, and an eastern co-operative oncology group (ECOG) performance status score $>1$. In the good prognosis group, 188 patients were randomized between ACVB/LNH84 (doxorubicin, cyclophosphamide, vindesine, bleomycin, and prednisolone) and CHOP (cyclophosphamide, doxorubicin, vincristine, and prednisolone) regimens. Complete

**Table 61.1**    Table of phase III chemotherapy trials

| Regimen | Patients treated | Median CD4 count (per mm³) | Complete remission (%) | Median survival (months) | HAART | References |
|---|---|---|---|---|---|---|
| ACTG-142 low-dose mBACOD arm | 94 | 100 | 41 | 9 | None | 27 |
| ACTG-142 full-dose mBACOD arm | 98 | 107 | 52 | 8 | None | 27 |
| European Intergroup Study good prognosis ACVB arm | 80 | 200 | 66 | | 51% 2-year OS | 31 |
| European Intergroup Study good prognosis CHOP arm | 79 | | 60 | | 43% 2-year OS | 31 |
| European Intergroup Study moderate prognosis CHOP arm | 59 | 60 | 63 | | 35% 2-year OS | 31 |
| European Intergroup Study moderate prognosis half-dose CHOP arm | 51 | | 39 | | 28% 2-year OS | 31 |

**Table 61.2**    Table of Phase II chemotherapy studies from the pre-HAART era

| Regimen | Patients treated | Median CD4 count (per mm³) | Complete remission (%) | Median survival (months) | HAART | References |
|---|---|---|---|---|---|---|
| HD ara-C/HD MTX | 9 | 173 | 33 | 6 | None | 32 |
| COMP and ProMACE-MOPP | 83 | | 33 | 5 | None | 33 |
| COMET-A | 38 | 164 | 58 | 5 | None | 34 |
| COMLA, mBACOD, CHOP | 27 | 169 | 46 | 11 | None | 34 |
| L-17, NHL-7, CHOP | 30 | | 56 | 6 | None | 35 |
| LNH-84 | 141 | 227 | 63 | 9 | None | 36 |
| Low-dose mBACOD | 35 | 150 | 35 | 4 | None | 30 |
| Oral chemo | 38 | 84 | 34 | 7 | None | 37 |
| CHOP | 60 | 103 | 54 | 13 | None | 38 |
| CHOP | 21 | <200 | 19 | 5 | None | 39 |
| CHOP | 38 (good risk) | | 68 | 21 | | 40 |
| CHOP | 18 (poor risk) | | 28 | 5 | | 40 |
| PVB | 12 (poor risk) | | | 2 | | 40 |
| CEOP | 18 | | 44 | 9 | None | 41 |
| MACOP-B | 8 | 79 | 50 | 4 | None | 42 |
| CHVm-P | 37 | 35 | 14 | | None | 43 |
| EACBOPM-P | 30 | | 33 | 8 | None | 44 |
| ACVB | 32 | | 56 | 9 | None | 45 |

HD are-C/HDMTX, high dose cytarabine/high dose methotrexate; COMP, cyclophosphamide, vincristine, methotrexate and prednisolone; Pro MACE-MOPP, Prednisolone, methotrexate, doxorubicin, cyclophosphamide, etoposide/mustine, vincristine, procarbazine and prednisolone; COMET-A, cyclophosphamide, Oncovin, methotrexate, leucovorin, etoposide, cytarabine; COMLA, cyclophosphamide, Oncovin, methotrexate, leucovorin, cytarabine; LNH-84, high-dose methotrexate plus leucovorin, ifosfauride, etoposide, asparaginase, and cytarabine; PVB, prednisolone, vincristine, bleomycin; CEOP, cyclophosphamide, etoposide, vincristine, prednisolone; MACOP-B, methotrexate, doxorubicin, cyclophosphamide, vincristine, prednisone, bleomycin; CHVm-p, cyclophosphamide, doxorubicin, teniposide, prednisone, vincristine, bleomycin; EACBOPM-P, etoposide, doxorubicin, cyclophosphamide, bleomycin, vincristine, methotrexate, prednisone

**Table 61.3** Table of phase II trials with historical controls

| Regimen | Patients treated | Median CD4 count (per mm³) | Complete remission (%) | Median survival (months) | HAART | References |
|---|---|---|---|---|---|---|
| CHOP | 41 | 163 | 34 | 7 | None | 46 |
| CHOP + HAART | 17 | 200 | 75 | NYR | 100% | 46 |
| CHOP | 80 | 146 | 36 | 7 | None | 47 |
| CHOP + HAART | 24 | 190 | 50 | NYA | 100% | 47 |

NYR, not yet reached

response rates were 65% and 56%, respectively, and there was no difference in overall survival, suggesting that as with other studies in high-grade lymphoma, nonmyeloablative dose intensification offers little benefits as first-line treatment. One hundred and thirty-nine patients with intermediate-risk disease (one adverse factor) were randomized to receive either full-dose CHOP or half-dose CHOP. Patients treated with full-dose CHOP had a significantly higher complete response rate (59% compared to 35%), although this did not translate into an improved overall survival. It should be remembered that the majority of patients were enrolled onto this study prior to the widespread use of HAART and that only around a quarter of the patients were receiving HAART at entry. The poor-risk group was randomized between half-dose CHOP and vincristine and prednisolone, but recruitment to this arm is incomplete.[31]

A number of groups have recently described an improvement in the overall survival for these patients compared to historical controls since the introduction of HAART. In two studies, the outcome of treatment with CHOP chemotherapy has been compared in the pre-and post-HAART eras, and improved CR rates and overall survivals have been demonstrated[46] (Table 61.3). However, in many series, there has been no change in the lymphoma response rates and the improvements in survival duration may be related to reduced deaths from opportunistic infections among patients who achieve durable tumor remissions[48–51] (Tables 61.3 and 61.4).

Infusional chemotherapy for high-grade lymphoma was pioneered at the Albert Einstein Cancer Center in New York, using the combination of cyclophosphamide, doxorubicin, and etoposide (CDE) administered as a 96-h continuous infusion for up to six courses at 4-weekly intervals, together with granulocyte colony-stimulating factor (G-CSF).[59] Early reports of a selected group of 25 patients with AIDS-related lymphomas who were treated with CDE and didanosine reported an impressive median survival of 18.4 months, and this schedule was widely heralded as a breakthrough in the management of AIDS related lymphoma (ARL).[60] The same schedule was then combined with saquinavir, with similar results, although there was more mucositis with the PI.[61] A large multicenter phase II trial of infusional CDE has been conducted by the Eastern Cooperative Oncology Group, and the results have been far less impressive as is so often the case following encouraging initial single-center studies[62] (Table 61.5).

At the National Cancer Institute, EPOCH (etoposide, prednisolone, vincristine, cyclophosphamide, and doxorubicin) has been developed which omits all

**Table 61.4** Table of phase II trials in post;–HAART era

| Regimen | Patients treated | Median CD4 count (per mm³) | Complete remission (%) | Median survival (months) | HAART (%) | References |
|---|---|---|---|---|---|---|
| BEMOP/CA | 30 | 262 | 60 | 24 | 33 | 52 |
| Hyper-CVAD (BL only) | 13 | 77 | 92 | >30 | 69 | 53 |
| LNHIV-91 | 52 | 276 | 71 | 15 | | 54 |
| Rituximab-CDE | 30 | 132 | 86 | NYR | 100 | 55 |
| Rituximab-CHOP | 61 | 171 | 80 | NYR | | 56 |
| CIOD | 14 | >100 | 93 | 35 | | 57 |
| Modified CHOP | 40 | 138 | 30 | | 100 | 58 |
| CHOP | 25 | 122 | 48 | | 100 | 58 |

BEMOP/CA, bleomycin, etoposide, methotrexate, vincristine, prednisolone, cyclophosphamide, doxorubicin; Hyper-CVAD, fractionated cyclophosphamide, vincristine, doxorubicin, dexamethasone; BL, Burkitt lymphoma; LNHIV-91, 3-4 cycles of ACVBP (doxorubicine, cyclophsphamide, Vindesine, bleomycin, prednisolone) followed by 3 cycles of CVM (Cyclophosphamide, etoposide, methotrexate); CIOD, cyclophosphamide, idarubicin, vincristine, prednisolone

| Table 61.5 | Table of phase II infusional chemotherapy studies | | | | | |
|---|---|---|---|---|---|---|
| Regimen | Patients treated | Median CD4 count (per mm$^3$) | Complete remission (%) | Median survival (months) | HAART | References |
| CDE | 62 | 70 | 53 | 18 | 12/62 (19%) | 59–61 |
| CDE (ECOG) | 48 | 78 | 46 | 8 | None | 62 |
| EPOCH | 39 | 198 | 74 | NYA | Interrupted | 63 |

HAART for the duration of the chemotherapy. Initial reports have been encouraging with a complete response rate of 79%. However, there was a dramatic fall in CD4 cell count during chemotherapy, and even on restarting the HAART at the end of chemotherapy this took 12 months to recover to baseline levels[64] (Table 61.5). This phase II study has been expanded to 39 selected patients[63] and is currently under investigation in a multicenter study under the auspices of the AIDS malignancy consortium. As there are no comparative studies, it is difficult to recommend an optimal gold standard therapy, and there are advocates of conventional CHOP as well as supporters of infusional therapies.

The use of infusional chemotherapy requires G-CSF support, and this is also frequently necessary with CHOP in this patient group in view of the high frequency of myelodysplasia. Although it was considered a possibility that GM-CSFs could stimulate HIV replication, there is no evidence that the use of these agents results in a rise in HIV viremia or progression of HIV disease.

The high rate of leptomeningeal disease at presentation, which may be asymptomatic,[30] led to the widespread use of staging lumbar punctures and the use of prophylactic intrathecal chemotherapy for patients considered to be at high risk of relapse in the cerebrospinal fluid (CSF). The prophylactic administration of intrathecal chemotherapy to patients with these risk factors but without meningeal disease at presentation prevented meningeal relapse in 81%.[25]

Chemotherapy results in a decline in CD4 cell counts in both immunocompetent and immunocompromised patients,[65,66] and prophylaxis to prevent opportunistic infections, particularly in this patient group, requires careful attention. It is well established in the management of HIV infection that prophylaxis should commence against PCP when the CD4 cell count falls below 200/mm$^3$ and against *Mycobacterium avium* complex (MAC) when it falls below 50/mm$^3$ (Ref. 67).

The prolonged T-cell depletion recorded following EPOCH[64] was previously demonstrated for patients receiving chemotherapy in the pre-HAART era.[68] The concomitant use of chemotherapy and HAART has been widely practiced, and a study in patients with ARL has demonstrated that when used together the CD4 cell count declines by 50% during chemotherapy but recovers rapidly within 1 month of completing chemotherapy. The CD8 and natural killer (CD16 and CD56) cell counts follow a similar profile, while the B-cell (CD19) count recovers more slowly but is restored to prechemotherapy levels by 3 months. There was no change in the HIV mRNA viral load during chemotherapy.[69] In view of the decline in CD4 cell count by 50%, PCP prophylaxis should commence at CD4 cell counts of 400/mm$^3$ and MAC at CD4 counts of 100/mm$^3$.

The improved survival described since the introduction of HAART and the preservation of immune function suggest that the combination of chemotherapy with HAART is an important step forward in the management of AIDS-related lymphomas.[46,47,58,69] However, there are both toxicity and pharmacokinetic drawbacks to the concomitant administration of chemotherapy and HAART. As mentioned in the first series describing the use of saquinavir with CDE, there was an increased incidence of mucositis[61] and more anemia in another series including patients receiving concomitant PIs.[47] The PI class of antiretrovirals may modify the metabolism of cytotoxic drugs via inhibition of the CYP3A4 enzyme, and indeed pharmacokinetic studies have demonstrated a modest delay in the clearance of cyclophosphamide in patients receiving indinavir, compared to historical controls, although no increase in hematologic toxicity was observed.[58] We have recently compared CDE-chemotherapy-induced toxicity among patients receiving concomitant PI or PI-sparing HAART regimens (chiefly non-nucleoside reverse transcriptase inhibitor [NNRTI] based). The concomitant administration of PIs was associated with a significantly higher rate of grade III–IV infections and grade III–IV neutropenia, although there was no difference in survival between the groups.[70]

### OUTCOMES IN THE ERA OF HAART

The CR rates for regimens using the combination of chemotherapy and HAART are 48–92% and the published 2-year overall survivals are 48–60%.[46,47,53,58,71] These response rates and survival duration statistics are starting to approach those seen in the general population with advanced-stage high-grade lymphoma. Indeed, while the prognostic factors for survival in the pre-HAART era were predominantly immunologic (prior AIDS-defining illness and CD4 cell count),[34,72] a more recent analysis of prognostic factors in AIDS-related lymphoma closely resembles that for the general population, with the International Prognostic

Index being an equally valuable guide in both circumstances.[73,74]

### FUTURE DEVELOPMENTS FOR AIDS-RELATED LYMPHOMAS

The improvements in the treatment of HIV infection have led to a more aggressive management strategy for AIDS-related lymphomas, and this has resulted in better outcomes. Further refinements mirror those seen in immunocompetent patients with high-grade lymphoma, including the addition of anti-CD20 antibodies to first-line therapy and the use of high-dose chemotherapy with autologous stem cell transplantation at first relapse.

As almost all AIDS-related NHL express CD20, several groups have explored the role of rituximab, humanized monoclonal antibody to CD20, either alone or as an adjunct to chemotherapy in the management of AIDS-related NHL.[55,75] CD20 antigen is a hydrophobic transmembrane protein that is located on pre-B and mature B lymphocytes. It is also expressed in greater than 90% B-cell NHLs including systemic AIDS-related NHLs, but it is not expressed on hematopoietic stem cells, pro-B cells, normal plasma cells, or other normal tissues. Rituximab efficiently lyses AIDS-related NHL cells in vitro via complement-dependent cytotoxicity and antibody-dependent cellular cytotoxicity.[76] Early trials are encouraging,[77] although profound and prolonged B-cell lymphopenia has been observed following rituximab.[78] Indeed, rituximab has been administered with CDE in a phase II pilot trial with concomitant HAART, and the 2-year overall survival was 80%[55] and achieved a complete response rate of 80% when used in combination with CHOP.[56] However, in a randomized phase III study of CHOP with or without rituximab that enrolled 142 patients, preliminary results have been disappointing with no difference in response rate or duration between the trial arms. Moreover, there was a higher incidence of neutropenic sepsis and death among those receiving rituximab.[79] Patients have also undergone successful autologous stem cell transplantation for AIDS-related lymphomas despite predictions that adequate harvesting would prove difficult due to myelodysplasia.[80–85]

## PRIMARY CEREBRAL LYMPHOMA

Primary CNS lymphoma (PCL) is defined as an NHL that is confined to the craniospinal axis without systemic involvement. This diagnosis is rare in immunocompetent patients but occurs more frequently in patients with both congenital and acquired immunodeficiency. AIDS-related PCL occurs equally frequently across all ages and transmission risk groups, and the tumors are high-grade B-cell diffuse large cell or immunoblastic NHLs. The presence of Epstein–Barr virus (EBV) is a universal feature of HIV-associated PCL but EBV is not found in other PCLs.[86,87] EBV may be detected by immunocytochemical staining of biopsy tissue or by polymerase chain reaction (PCR) amplification of CSF using EBV-specific oligonucleotide primers.

### EPIDEMIOLOGY OF HIV-ASSOCIATED PRIMARY CEREBRAL LYMPHOMA

Registry linkage studies confirmed a markedly increased relative risk of PCL among patients with AIDS, with an incidence as high as 2–6% in one early report.[88] This high incidence of PCL was confirmed by both cohort and linkage studies. Patients who develop PCL generally have advanced immunosuppression and for the most part have had a prior AIDS-defining illness. Shortly after the introduction of HAART, a decline in the incidence of PCL was recognized by many clinicians, and a meta-analysis of cohort studies that compare the pre- and post-HAART eras confirmed a significant decline (relative risk 0.42: 99% confidence interval 0.24–0.75).[17] Indeed this fall is more dramatic than that seen for systemic AIDS-related lymphomas and PCL is associated with more severe immunosuppression than systemic AIDS-related lymphoma.

### CLINICAL PRESENTATION AND DIFFERENTIAL DIAGNOSIS

The commonest causes of cerebral mass lesions in HIV-seropositive patients are toxoplasmosis and primary cerebral lymphoma and the differential diagnosis often proves difficult. Both diagnoses occur in patients with advanced immunodeficiency (CD4 cell counts $<50 \times 10^6$/L) and present with headaches and focal neurologic deficits. Clinical features that favor PCL include a more gradual onset over 2–8 weeks and the absence of a fever. CT and MRI scanning usually reveal solitary or multiple ring enhancing lesions with prominent mass effect and edema. Again, these features occur in both diagnoses, although PCL lesions are usually periventricular while toxoplasmosis more often affects the basal ganglia. Thus, the combination of clinical findings and standard radiologic investigations rarely provide a definitive diagnosis. Moreover, toxoplasma serology (IgG) is falsely negative in 10–15% of patients with cerebral toxoplasmosis. More than 85% patients with cerebral toxoplasmosis will respond clinically and radiologically to 2 weeks of anti-toxoplasma therapy, and this has become the cornerstone of the diagnostic algorithm for cerebral masses in severely immunodeficient patients.

In these patients, it has been a standard practice to commence empirical anti-toxoplasmosis treatment for 2 weeks duration, and resort to a brain biopsy if there is no clinical or radiologic improvement. This strategy avoids the routine use of brain biopsy in these patients who frequently have a very poor performance status and prognosis. Although this algorithm avoids early surgical intervention, it is relatively ineffective in diagnosing PCL early, and may compromise the outcome of therapy in these patients. In addition, there is a disinclination to treat patients with radiotherapy or chemotherapy empirically based exclusively on the failure of anti-toxoplasmosis treatment without a definitive histologic diagnosis.

The discovery that all HIV-associated PCLs are associated with EBV infection has led to the development of a PCR method that can detect EBV DNA in the CSF. This has become established as a diagnostic test with a high sensitivity (83–100%) and specificity (>90%).[89–91] In addition, radionuclide imaging by [201]thallium single photon emission computed tomography ([201]Th-SPECT) or [18]F-fluorodeoxyglucose positron emission tomography (FDG-PET) is able to differentiate between PCL and cerebral toxoplasmosis. PCLs are thallium avid and demonstrate increased uptake on PET scanning; however, although both techniques have high specificity for PCL, neither are highly sensitive and thus cannot be used alone but, in combination with PCR, are emerging as a diagnostic alternative to brain biopsy. The application of PCR and [201]Th-SPECT in the diagnosis of contrast-enhancing brain lesions in 27 patients was shown to result in a positive and a negative predictive value of 100% and 88%, respectively, which supports their combined value as an alternative to brain biopsy.[91] Further studies are now required to compare effectiveness of PCR with [201]Th-SPECT or FDG-PET.

### TREATMENT OF HIV-ASSOCIATED PRIMARY CEREBRAL LYMPHOMA

The standard treatment modality is whole brain irradiation, but the median survival time is just 2.5 months or less. Although patients who were treated with radiotherapy or chemotherapy lived longer than those who received best supportive care only, no randomized studies have been conducted and it remains uncertain whether therapy improves survival.[92] There is an increasing enthusiasm for the treatment of PCL in immunocompetent patients with both radiotherapy and chemotherapy, and recent results have been encouraging. The use of chemotherapy for PCL is limited by the poor penetration of cytotoxics into brain parenchyma due to the blood–brain barrier and the toxicity, especially myelosuppression, of these agents in patients with advanced immunosuppression and poor performance status. Combination chemotherapy prolongs survival in immunocompetent patients with PCL but at the cost of severe myelotoxicity. Single-agent chemotherapy with intravenous high-dose methotrexate and folinic acid rescue was studied in AIDS patients with PCL in the context of a prospective uncontrolled study that included 15 patients. The results showed a complete response in 47% of patients, a median survival of 19 months, a low relapse rate of

approximately 14%, and no evidence of neurologic impairment nor treatment-limiting myelotoxicity.[93] A controlled trial of intravenous methotrexate versus whole brain irradiation is needed to confirm these encouraging results. Now that antiretroviral therapies are improving survival, it may be necessary to reassess currently available diagnostic and treatment modalities aiming to cure HIV-associated PCL.

## HIV-ASSOCIATED HODGKIN'S LYMPHOMA

As with other AIDS-related malignancies, oncogenic viruses are thought to play a central role in the pathogenesis of HD. Single-cell PCR amplification methods can identify EBV in the Reed–Sternberg cells in approximately 10–70% HD, and in patients with HIV-associated HD, EBV is found in the Reed–Sternberg cells in nearly all cases.[94] There are also differences in the histopathology of HD between the immunocompetent population and the people with HIV. Two histopathological subtypes occur at a higher frequency in people with HIV: these are mixed cellularity (approximately 40%) and lymphocyte depleted (approximately 20%).[95,96] In the HIV-negative population, these subtypes occur at 24% and 3–6%, respectively, and are associated with a worse prognosis compared to the more common nodular sclerosing and lymphocyte-predominant subtypes. Mixed cellularity subtype is more common in developing countries and in the elderly,[96,97] and immune dysfunction and epidemiologic differences of EBV are thought to be responsible for this; however, their prognosis is still better than the HIV-seropositive population.

### EPIDEMIOLOGY OF HIV-ASSOCIATED HODGKIN'S LYMPHOMA

Although HD occurs quite frequently in patients with HIV, both illnesses affect similar age groups, and there was debate as to whether the incidence is increased in people with HIV. Cohort studies from San Francisco[98] and New York[99] early in the HIV epidemic failed to identify an increased risk, and to this day HD is not an AIDS-defining diagnosis. However, subsequent subgroup analysis of the New York data suggested that there was an increased incidence of HD among intravenous drug users (IVDU) with HIV. Moreover, the Italian Cooperative group for AIDS-related tumors described 35 patients with HIV and HD and almost all of these patients were IVDU.[100]

More recent cohort studies, including the San Francisco City Clinic cohort[101] and multicenter AIDS cohort study (MACS),[102] report a relative risk of 19 compared to the age-adjusted general population. The most comprehensive data to date come from large linkage studies across the United States and Puerto Rico, which gave a relative risk of 7.6.[103] This figure has been repeated in other large linkage studies and is significantly lower than that for NHL in patients with HIV. The difference between the early small cohorts and these later large cohorts is probably due to the small number of HD cases seen rather than due to a real change in incidence over time. Since the introduction of HAART, the incidence of some AIDS-related malignancies such as KS and primary cerebral lymphoma has fallen while of others such as systemic NHL appears to be unchanged. There are as yet no reports that describe the effect of HAART usage on the incidence of HD.

### CLINICAL PRESENTATION OF HIV-ASSOCIATED HODGKIN'S LYMPHOMA

HIV-seropositive patients with HD generally present with more advanced-stage disease than do seronegative patients. In the seven reported series, 70–85% of seropositive patients present with Ann Arbor stage III or IV, while less than half of the immunocompetent patients with HD will have stage III/IV disease at presentation.[95,96,104–108] Moreover, B symptoms occur in 70–100% of HIV-seropositive patients with HD, although it may be impossible to distinguish the relative contributions of HIV and HD to these symptoms. Extranodal HD also occurs more commonly (up to 70%) than in the HIV-negative population. The bone marrow is the most commonly involved extranodal site affecting 50% of patients; other extranodal sites include skin, liver, and occasionally the CNS. Furthermore, there is a lower incidence of mediastinal involvement in the HIV-seropositive population (13%) compared to the general population with HD (70%).[95] The mixed cellularity histologic subtype, which is more common in HIV-positive patients, does not affect the mediastinum as commonly as the other types; nevertheless, the histologic differences do not account for all the difference observed in mediastinal disease.

The median CD4 cell count at diagnosis of HD is between 128 and 306/μL in the published series all of which pre-date the HAART era. This is higher than the median CD4 cell count reported in the pre-HAART era for high-grade NHL. At presentation of HD, 50–90% of patients had been previously diagnosed with HIV, while 4–46% (median 11%) had a prior AIDS-defining diagnosis. Thus HD tends to present at an earlier stage of immunosuppression than NHL, and it is intriguing that HD is not a feature of iatrogenic immunosuppression in allograft transplant recipients, although post-transplant NHL is a well-recognized entity.

### TREATMENT OF HIV-ASSOCIATED HODGKIN'S LYMPHOMA

Since most patients will present with relatively preserved immune function and no prior AIDS-defining illness, clinicians have generally adopted a similar approach to the first-line therapy in HIV-seropositive patients as for the general population. Most patients have advanced disease at presentation and are therefore candidates for combination chemotherapy. In the general population, HD is associated with a complex immunologic deficit. At the time of HD diagnosis, the CD4 cell count and function is often normal but becomes depressed during the progression of the disease, resulting in an increased incidence of opportunistic infections compared to other malignancies. It is hardly surprising that when the immunosuppressive effect of HIV is added to this, opportunistic infections become a major source of morbidity during chemotherapy.

The published series of HD in patients with HIV include a total of 359 patients. In all the series, there is a similar predominance of advanced-stage disease and mixed cellularity histology. The chemotherapy schedules that have been used, although not consistent in any series, have been mainly MOPP (mustine, vincristine, procarbazine, and prednisolone), ABVD (doxorubicin, bleomycin, vinblastine, and dacarbazine), or an alternating hybrid of the two (MOPP/ABVD). In these unrandomized, uncontrolled series, no regimen has been shown to produce higher response rates or longer response durations or survival. The CR rates ranged between 44% and 79% with a median of 58%, while the median survival was 11 months with a range between 10 and 18 months. The largest study consisted of 114 patients,[105] the median age was 29 years, 79% were IVDU, and the median CD4 count was 275/μL. The combination of MOPP and ABVD showed some benefit over MOPP alone (CR rate 68% vs 38%); however, this has not been reported in other series. These response rates and overall survivals are considerably worse than the results published for HD in the general population, where response rates exceed 80% and the median survival exceeds 10 years.

A major portion of poor survival in HIV-seropositive patients with HD is due to infectious complications. In the published series, 45–75% of patients developed opportunistic infections during chemotherapy. In one study, 71% of patients became neutropenic during treatment.[109] Concurrent G-CSF has been used in two studies, but this has no demonstrated benefit on toxicity or mortality.[96,108] After 1 year, 55% of patients had developed an AIDS-defining diagnosis (usually an opportunistic infection), and 3 years after HD had been diagnosed 71% of patients had AIDS compared to only 24% of a matched seropositive population.[95] It has been proposed that chemotherapy may be responsible for the progression of immunosuppression; however, this may be a less important factor following the introduction of HAART. Indeed the incidence of opportunistic infection during chemotherapy for HD was only 13% among patients concomitantly receiving zidovudine monotherapy. It remains to be seen whether HAART will further reduce the infectious complications and progressive immunosuppression during and following chemotherapy for HD.

The prognostic factors for overall survival in patients with HIV and HD identified in the pre-HAART era relate chiefly to immunosuppression rather than HD. Poor prognostic factors at presentation included a low CD4 count (0% 18-month survival if less than 300/μL), prior AIDS-defining diagnosis, anemia, and a poor performance status.[95] These variables are similar to those for NHL in the same era; however, more recent data for NHL from the late 1990s have shown that the prognostic factors for HIV-associated NHL closely resemble those for NHL in the general population. It remains uncertain whether HAART will reduce the incidence or improve the outcome of HIV-associated HD. Certainly in the HAART era there is greater enthusiasm for an aggressive approach including progenitor stem cell transplantation for these patients.

## HIV-ASSOCIATED MULTICENTRIC CASTLEMAN'S DISEASE

Benjamin Castleman first described multicentric Castleman's disease (MCD) as a case record of the Massachusetts General Hospital, familiar to all the readers of the *New England Journal of Medicine*, in 1954.[110] Interest in MCD has grown in recent years with the AIDS epidemic, since there has been an increased incidence of MCD in HIV-positive patients. This followed the recognition of an association between MCD and AIDS-associated KS, again following initial publication of case reports.[4,5] Castleman's disease is divided into localized disease and MCD which is characterized by polylymphadenopathy and multiorgan involvement. The localized form is treated with surgery but the management of MCD is less clear and has a more aggressive course. Histologically, it is divided into the hyalinized vascular form and plasma variant, the former being more common in localized disease and the latter more common in MCD. MCD is associated with Kaposi's sarcoma herpesvirus (KSHV) infection, which is also known as human herpesvirus 8 (HHV-8). The virus encodes a homolog of interleukin 6 (IL-6), a proinflammatory cytokine, which is thought to mediate some of the clinical features of MCD. The diagnosis is established by biopsy and treatment is often based on case reports in the literature, as there are no randomized trials. Surgery has less of a role but splenectomy may be useful as a debulking procedure to alleviate hematologic sequelae. Systemic treatments have included chemotherapy as well as anti-herpesvirus treatment to reduce the KSHV viral load, and HAART to reduce HIV viral burden. Lately, treatment with monoclonal antibodies against both IL-6 and CD20 has been studied. The introduction of HAART has altered the natural history of HIV infection; however, its impact on MCD is difficult to ascertain.

The plasma cell variant of MCD occurs most frequently in people with HIV infection. The histologic appearances are of an intense plasmacytosis in the interfollicular areas of the nodes, with a prominent increase in capillaries and postcapillary venules, which may be hyalinized. The concentrically arranged mantle zone may produce a characteristic 'onion peel' appearance. KSHV has been demonstrated in nearly all MCD samples from HIV-positive patients and in half MCD patients without HIV infection.[111] KSHV is also present in the malignant cells of plasmablastic lymphomas that occur more frequently in patients with MCD.[112,113]

### CLINICAL FEATURES OF HIV-ASSOCIATED CASTLEMAN'S DISEASE

In general, MCD presents in the fourth or fifth decade of life but occurs earlier in people who are HIV positive. Patients often present with generalized malaise, night sweats, rigors, fever, anorexia, and weight loss. On examination, they have multiple lymphadenopathy, hepatosplenomegaly, ascites, edema, and effusions both pulmonary and pericardial. Laboratory investigations may reveal thrombocytopenia, anemia, hypoalbuminemia, and hypergammaglobulinemia. The systemic symptoms are attributed to IL-6 and can be severe enough to cause pancytopenia, organ failure, particularly respiratory and renal, as well as shock, requiring admission into intensive care units. HIV-infected patients with MCD have a greater preponderance for pulmonary complications. MCD is more likely to lead to neuropathic complications than does locally confined Castleman's disease. Patients can develop polyneuropathies, leptomeningeal and CNS infiltration, as well as myasthenia gravis.[114] The polyneuropathy is a chronic inflammatory demyelinating neuropathy and may be present as part of the rare POEMS syndrome (Crow–Fukase disease). POEMS syndrome consists of polyneuropathy, organomegaly, endocrinopathy, monoclonal gammopathy, and skin changes. Patients are diagnosed with POEMS syndrome if they have two of these clinical features as well as plasma cell dyscrasia. Not only is MCD itself potentially fatal due to organ failure, but it is also associated with a 15-fold increased incidence of NHL. The majority of these lymphomas are plasmablastic and are thought to arise from expansion of plasmablastic microlymphomas seen in MCD lesions.[112,113]

### TREATMENT OF HIV-ASSOCIATED CASTLEMAN'S DISEASE

There are no definitive gold standard treatments for MCD. No randomized trials have been conducted on account of the infrequency of the diagnosis, and often only case reports have appeared in the literature. Although surgery is the mainstay of treatment for localized Castleman's disease, with complete removal of the mediastinal lesions being curative, it has a limited role in MCD. Splenectomy, in addition to establishing the histologic diagnosis, may have a therapeutic benefit as a debulking procedure, as some of the hematologic sequelae such as thrombocytopenia and anemia may in part be due to splenomegaly. Following splenectomy, there is often resolution of the constitutive symptoms but this may be short lived, and some form of maintenance therapy is needed to prevent relapse.[115]

For immunocompetent patients, the chemotherapy regimens for MCD are based on lymphoma schedules such as CHOP. However, in the pre-HAART era, these schedules were associated with marked toxicity in HIV-positive patients, and as a consequence, other schedules were developed. In the largest published study from Paris of 20 patients, there was a partial response in 9/9 patients with single agent vinblastine; however, only 4 patients remained stable with maintenance therapy (4–6 mg/2 weeks). Four patients received upfront ABV (adriamycin, bleomycin, and vincristine), three achieving a partial remission. Intermittent treatment with cyclophosphamide achieved a partial response in a further three patients.[115] Although there is little evidence on which to base treatment strategies, in many centers combination chemotherapy is used initially to induce remission in aggressive forms of MCD. This may be followed by gentler, single-agent chemotherapy regimens, such as vinblastine or etoposide, to maintain the response.

Studies have now been undertaken to see if the addition of HAART in the treatment of MCD has any effect on morbidity and mortality. The effect of HAART has been described in seven patients with MCD and HIV infection.[116] Six patients responded to chemotherapy, and immune reconstitution was described in five patients. However, patients continued to require long-term chemotherapy to prevent further episodes of MCD. The mean survival was 48 months, which was longer than that described in the pre-HAART era patients when most patients succumbed to opportunistic infections related to HIV. In addition, there were no cases of plasmablastic lymphoma as a complication of MCD.

## REFERENCES

1. Ziegler JL, Beckstead JA, Volberding PA, et al.: Non-Hodgkin's lymphoma in 90 homosexual men. Relation to generalized lymphadenopathy and the acquired immunodeficiency syndrome. *N Engl J Med* 311(9):565–570, 1984.
2. Frisch M, Biggar RJ, Engels EA, et al.: Association of cancer with AIDS-related immunosuppression in adults. *JAMA* 285(13):1736–1745, 2001.
3. Bower M, Powles T, Nelson M, et al.: HIV-related lung cancer in the era of highly active antiretroviral therapy. *AIDS* 17(3):371–375, 2003.
4. Dickson D, Ben-Ezra JM, Reed J, et al.: Multicentric giant lymph node hyperplasia, Kaposi's sarcoma, and lymphoma. *Arch Pathol Lab Med* 109(11):1013–1018, 1985.
5. Lachant NA, Sun NCJ, Leong LA, et al.: Multicentric angiofollicular lymph node hyperplasia (Castleman's disease) followed by Kaposi's sarcoma in two homosexual males with the acquired immunodeficiency syndrome (AIDS). *Am J Clin Pathol* 83:27–33, 1985.
6. Joint United Nations Programme on HIV/AIDS. *Report on the Global HIV/AIDS Epidemic.* Geneva: UNAIDS; 2003.
7. Palella FJ Jr, Delaney KM, Moorman AC, et al.: Declining morbidity and mortality among patients with advanced human immunodeficiency virus infection. HIV Outpatient Study Investigators. *N Engl J Med* 338(13):853–860, 1998.
8. Beral V, Peterman T, Berkelman R, et al.: AIDS-associated non-Hodgkin lymphoma. *Lancet* 337(8745):805–809, 1991.
9. Biggar RJ, Rosenberg PS, Cote T: Kaposi's sarcoma and non-Hodgkin's lymphoma following the diagnosis of AIDS. Multistate AIDS/Cancer Match Study Group. *Int J Cancer* 68(6):754–758, 1996.
10. Ledergerber B, Telenti A, Egger M, et al.: Risk of HIV related Kaposi's sarcoma and non-Hodgkin's lymphoma with potent antiretroviral therapy: prospective cohort study. *Br Med J* 319:23–24, 1999.
11. Inungu J, Melendez MF, Montgomery JP: AIDS-related primary brain lymphoma in Michigan, January 1990 to December 2000. *AIDS Patient Care STDS* 16(3):107–112, 2002.
12. Kirk O, Pedersen C, Cozzi-Lepri A, et al.: Non-Hodgkin lymphoma in HIV-infected patients in the era of highly active antiretroviral therapy. *Blood* 98(12):3406–3412, 2001.
13. Buchbinder SP, Vittinghoff E, Colfax G, et al.: Declines in AIDS incidence associated with highly active anti-retroviral therapy (HAART) are not reflected in KS and lymphoma incidence. In: *Proceedings of the 2nd National AIDS Malignancy Conference*, National Cancer Institute, Bethesda, MD, 1998:S7.
14. Jacobson LP, Yamashita TE, Detels R, et al.: Impact of potent antiretroviral therapy on the incidence of Kaposi's sarcoma and non-Hodgkin's lymphomas among HIV-1-infected individuals. Multicenter AIDS Cohort Study. *J Acquir Immune Defic Syndr* 21(suppl 1):34–41, 1999.
15. Rabkin CS, Testa MA, Huang J, et al.: Kaposi's sarcoma and non-Hodgkin's lymphoma incidence trends in AIDS Clinical Trial Group study participants. *J Acquir Immune Defic Syndr* 21(suppl 1):31–33, 1999.
16. Wilde JT, Lee CA, Darby SC, et al.: The incidence of lymphoma in the UK haemophilia population between 1978 and 1999. *AIDS* 16(13):1803–1807, 2002.
17. International Collaboration on HIV and Cancer: Highly active antiretroviral therapy and incidence of cancer in

human immunodeficiency virus-infected adults. J *Natl Cancer Inst* 92:1823–1830, 2000.

18. Rabkin C, Yang Q, Goedert J, et al.: Chemokine and chemokine receptor gene variants and risk of non-Hodgkin's lymphoma in human immunodeficiency virus 1 infected individuals. *Blood* 93:1838–1842, 1999.

19. Dean M, Jacobson L, McFarlane G, et al.: Reduced risk of AIDS lymphoma in individuals heterozygous for the CCR5-delta32 mutation. *Cancer Res* 59:3561–3564, 1999.

20. Fong IW, Ho J, Toy C, et al.: Value of long-term administration of acyclovir and similar agents for protecting against AIDS-related lymphoma: case–control and historical cohort studies. *Clin Infect Dis* 30:757–761, 2000.

21. Stebbing J, Gazzard B, Mandalia S, et al.: Antiretroviral treatment regimens and immune parameters in the prevention of systemic AIDS-related non-Hodgkin's lymphoma. *J Clin Oncol* 22(11):2177–2183, 2004.

22. Gerard L, Galicier L, Maillard A, et al.: Systemic non-Hodgkin lymphoma in HIV-infected patients with effective suppression of HIV replication: persistent occurrence but improved survival. *J Acquir Immune Defic Syndr* 30(5):478–484, 2002.

23. Scadden DT, Zeira M, Woon A, et al.: Human immunodeficiency virus infection of human bone marrow stromal fibroblasts. *Blood* 76:317–322, 1992.

24. Moses AV, Williams S, Heneveld ML, et al.: Human immunodeficiency virus infection of bone marrow endothelium reduces induction of stromal hematopoietic growth factors. *Blood* 87(3):919–925, 1996.

25. Sarker D, Thirlwell C, Nelson M, et al.: Leptomeningeal disease in AIDS-related non-Hodgkin's lymphoma. *AIDS* 17(6):861–865, 2003.

26. Desai J, Mitnick R, Henry D, et al.: Patterns of central nervous system recurrence in patients with systemic human immunodeficiency virus-associated non-Hodgkin lymphoma. *Cancer* 86:1840–1847, 1999.

27. Kaplan LD, Straus DJ, Testa MA, et al.: Low dose compared with standard dose m-BACOD chemotherapy for non-Hodgkin's lymphoma associated with human immunodeficiency virus infection. *N Engl J Med* 336:1641–1648, 1997.

28. Cingolani A, Gastaldi R, Fassone L, et al.: Epstein–Barr virus infection is predictive of CNS involvement in systemic AIDS-related non-Hodgkin's lymphomas. *J Clin Oncol* 18(19):3325–3330, 2000.

29. Matthews GV, Bower M, Mandalia S, et al.: Changes in acquired immunodeficiency syndrome-related lymphoma since the introduction of highly active anti-retroviral therapy. *Blood* 96(8):2730–2734, 2000.

30. Levine AM, Wernz JC, Kaplan L, et al.: Low dose chemotherapy with central nervous system prophylaxis and zidovudine maintenance in AIDS-related lymphoma. *J Am Med Assoc* 266:84–88, 1991.

31. Tirelli U: Dose adjusted treatment in AIDS-related lymphoma. *J Acquir Immunodefic Syndr* 23:A12, 2000.

32. Gill PS, Levine AM, Krailo M, et al.: AIDS-related malignant lymphoma: results of prospective treatment trials. *J Clin Oncol* 5:1322–1328, 1987.

33. Knowles D, Chamulak G, Subar M, et al.: Lymphoid neoplasia associated with the acquired immunodeficiency syndrome (AIDS): The New York University Medical Center experience with 109 patients. *Ann Intern Med* 108:744–753, 1988.

34. Kaplan LD, Abrams DI, Feigal E, et al.: AIDS-associated non-Hodgkin's lymphoma in San Francisco. *JAMA* 261(5):719–724, 1989.

35. Lowenthal D, Strauss D, Campbell S, et al.: AIDS-related lymphoid neoplasia. The Memorial Hospital Experience. *Cancer* 61:2325–2337, 1988.

36. Gisselbrecht C, Oksenhendler E, Tirelli U, et al.: Human immunodeficiency virus-related lymphoma treatment with intensive combination chemotherapy. French-Italian Cooperative Group. *Am J Med* 95(2):188–196, 1993.

37. Remick SC, McSharry JJ, Wolf BC, et al.: Novel oral combination chemotherapy in the treatment of intermediate grade and high grade AIDS-related non-Hodgkin's lymphoma. *J Clin Oncol* 11:1691–1702, 1992.

38. Aviles A, Nambo MJ, Halabe J: Treatment of acquired immunodeficiency syndrome-related lymphoma with a standard chemotherapy regimen. *Ann Hematol* 78(1):9–12, 1999.

39. Kersten MJ, Verduyn TJ, Reiss P, et al.: Treatment of AIDS-related non-Hodgkin's lymphoma with chemotherapy (CNOP) and r-hu-G-CSF: clinical outcome and effect on HIV-1 viral load. *Ann Oncol* 9(10):1135–1138, 1998.

40. Weiss R, Huhn D, Mitrou P, et al.: HIV-related non-Hodgkin's lymphoma: CHOP induction therapy and interferon-alpha-2b/zidovudine maintenance therapy. *Leuk Lymphoma* 29(1–2):103–118, 1998.

41. Davis AJ, Goldstein D, Milliken S: Long term follow-up of CEOP in the treatment of HIV related non-Hodgkin's lymphoma (NHL). *Aust N Z J Med* 28(1):28–32, 1998.

42. Schurmann D, Grunewald T, Weiss R, et al.: Intensive treatment of AIDS-related non-Hodgkin's lymphomas with the MACOP-B protocol. *Eur J Haematol* 54(2):73–77, 1995.

43. Tirelli U, Errante D, Oksenhendler E, et al.: Prospective study with combined low-dose chemotherapy and zidovudine in 37 patients with poor-prognosis AIDS-related non-Hodgkin's lymphoma. French-Italian Cooperative Study Group. *Ann Oncol* 3(10):843–847, 1992.

44. Sawka CA, Shepherd FA, Brandwein J, et al.: Treatment of AIDS-related non-Hodgkin's lymphoma with a twelve week chemotherapy program. *Leuk Lymphoma* 8(3):213–220, 1992.

45. Gabarre J, Lepage E, Thyss A, et al.: Chemotherapy combined with zidovudine and GM-CSF in human immunodeficiency virus-related non-Hodgkin's lymphoma. *Ann Oncol* 6:1025–1032, 1995.

46. Navarro JT, Ribera JM, Oriol A, et al.: Influence of highly active anti-retroviral therapy on response to treatment and survival in patients with acquired immunodeficiency syndrome-related non-Hodgkin's lymphoma treated with cyclophosphamide, hydroxy-doxorubicin, vincristine and prednisone. *Br J Haematol* 112:909–915, 2001.

47. Vaccher E, Spina M, di Gennaro G, et al.: Concomitant cyclophosphamide, doxorubicin, vincristine, and prednisone chemotherapy plus highly active antiretroviral therapy in patients with human immunodeficiency virus-related, non-Hodgkin lymphoma. *Cancer* 91(1):155–163, 2001.

48. Antinori A, Cingolani A, Alba L, et al.: Better response to chemotherapy and prolonged survival in AIDS-related lymphomas responding to highly active anti-retroviral therapy. *AIDS* 15(12):1483–1491, 2001.

49. Besson C, Goubar A, Gabarre J, et al.: Changes in AIDS-related lymphoma since the era of highly active anti-retroviral therapy. *Blood* 98(8):2339–2344, 2001.

50. Bower M, Matthews G, Powles T, et al.: Changes in AIDS related lymphoma (ARL) in the era of highly active antiretroviral therapy (HAART). *Proc ASCO* 19:17a, 2000.

51. Chow KU, Mitrou PS, Geduldig K, et al.: Changing incidence and survival in patients with AIDS-related non-Hodgkin's lymphomas in the era of highly active anti-retroviral therapy (HAART). *Leuk Lymphoma* 41(1–2):105–116, 2001.

52. Bower M, Stern S, Fife K, et al.: Weekly alternating combination chemotherapy for good prognosis AIDS-related lymphoma. *Eur J Cancer* 36(3):363–367, 2000.

53. Cortes J, Thomas D, Rios A, et al.: Hyperfractionated cyclophosphamide, vincristine, doxorubicin, and dex-amethasone and highly active antiretroviral therapy for patients with acquired immunodeficiency syndrome-related Burkitt lymphoma/leukemia. *Cancer* 94(5):1492–1499, 2002.

54. Oksenhendler E, Gerard L, Dubreuil ML, et al.: Intensive chemotherapy (LNHIV-91 regimen) and G-CSF for HIV associated non-Hodgkin's lymphoma. *Leuk Lymphoma* 39(1–2):87–95, 2000.

55. Tirelli U, Spina M, Jaeger U, et al.: Infusional CDE with rituximab for the treatment of human immunodeficiency virus-associated non-Hodgkin's lymphoma: preliminary results of a phase I/II study. *Recent Results Cancer Res* 159:149–153, 2002.

56. Boue F, Gabarre J, Gisselbrecht C, et al.: Phase II trial of CHOP plus Rituximab in patients with HIV-associated non-Hodgkin's lymphoma. *J Clin Oncol* 24(25):4123–4128, 2006.

57. Gastaldi R, Martino P, Gentile G, et al.: High dose of idarubicin-based regimen for diffuse large cell AIDS-related non-Hodgkin's lymphoma patients: a pilot study. *Haematologica* 86(10):1051–1059, 2001.

58. Ratner L, Lee J, Tang S, et al.: Chemotherapy for human immunodeficiency virus-associated non-Hodgkin's lymphoma in combination with highly active antiretroviral therapy. *J Clin Oncol* 19(8):2171–2178, 2001.

59. Sparano JA, Wiernik PH, Strack M, et al.: Infusional cyclophosphamide, doxorubicin, and etoposide in human immunodeficiency virus- and human T-cell leukemia virus type I-related non-Hodgkin's lymphoma: a highly active regimen. *Blood* 81(10): 2810–2815, 1993.

60. Sparano JA, Wiernik PH, Hu X, et al.: Pilot trial of infusional cyclophosphamide, doxorubicin and etoposide plus didanosine and filgrastim in patients with HIV associated non-Hodgkin's lymphoma. *J Clin Oncol* 14:3026–3035, 1996.

61. Sparano JA, Wiernik PH, Hu X, et al.: Saquinavir enhances the mucosal toxicity of infusional cyclophosphamide, doxorubicin and etoposide in patients with HIV-associated non-Hodgkin's lymphoma. *Med Oncol* 15:50–57, 1998.

62. Sparano J, Lee S, Chen M, et al.: Phase II trial of infusional cyclophosphamide, doxorubicin and etoposide (CDE) in HIV-associated non-Hodgkin's lymphoma: an Eastern Cooperative Oncology Group trial (E1494). *Proc ASCO* 18:12a, 1999.

63. Little RF, Pittaluga S, Grant N, et al.: Highly effective treatment of acquired immunodeficiency syndrome-related lymphoma with dose-adjusted EPOCH: impact of antiretroviral therapy suspension and tumor biology. *Blood* 101(12):4653–4659, 2003.

64. Little R, Pearson D, Steinberg S, et al.: Dose-adjusted EPOCH chemotherapy in previously untreated HIV-associated non-Hodgkin' lymphoma. *Proc ASCO* 18:10a, 1999.

65. Hakim FT, Cepeda R, Kaimei S, et al.: Constraints on CD4 recovery postchemotherapy in adults: thymic insufficiency and apoptotic decline of expanded peripheral CD4 cells. *Blood* 90(9):3789–3798, 1997.

66. Mackall C: T-cell immunodeficiency following cyto-toxic antineoplastic therapy: a review. *Stem Cells* 18:10–18, 2000.

67. Kaplan JE, Masur H, Holmes KK: Guidelines for preventing opportunistic infections among HIV-infected persons—2002. Recommendations of the U.S. Public Health Service and the Infectious Diseases Society of America. *MMWR Recomm Rep* 51(RR-8):1–52, 2002.

68. Zanussi S, Simonelli C, D'Andrea M, et al.: The effects of antineoplastic chemotherapy on HIV disease. *AIDS Res Hum Retroviruses* 12(18):1703–1707, 1996.

69. Powles T, Imami N, Nelson M, et al.: Effects of combination chemotherapy and highly active antiretroviral therapy on immune parameters in HIV-1 associated lymphoma. *AIDS* 16:531–536, 2002.

70. Bower M, McCall-Peat N, Ryan N et al.: Protease inhibitors potentiate chemotherapy-induced neutropenia. *Blood* 104(9):2943–2946, 2004.

71. Thirlwell C, Stebbing J, Nelson M, et al.: CDE chemotherapy plus HAART for AIDS related non-Hodgkin's lymphoma. In *6th International Congress on Drug Therapy in HIV infection;* 2002; Glasgow; 2002:94.

72. Levine AM, Sullivan Halley J, Pike MC, et al.: Human immunodeficiency virus-related lymphoma. Prognostic factors predictive of *survival. Cancer* 68(11):2466–2472, 1991.

73. Rossi G, Donisi A, Casari S, et al.: The International Prognostic Index can be used as a guide to treatment decisions regarding patients with human immunodeficiency virus-related non-Hodgkin lymphoma. *Cancer* 86:2391–2397, 1999.

74. Straus DJ, Huang J, Testa MA, et al.: Prognostic factors in the treatment of human immunodeficiency virus-associated non-Hodgkin's lymphoma: analysis of AIDS Clinical Trials Group protocol 142—low-dose versus standard-dose m-BACOD plus granulocyte-macrophage colony-stimulating factor. *J Clin Oncol* 16:3601–3606, 1998.

75. Barrett J, Linn C, Saleh M: Rituximab for the treatment of AIDS-associated non-Hodgkin's lymphoma. *J Acquir Immunodefic Syndr* 21:A40, 1999.

76. Golay J, Gramigna R, Facchinetti V, et al.: Acquired immunodeficiency syndrome-associated lymphomas are efficiently lysed through complement-dependent cytotoxicity and antibody-dependent cellular cytotoxicity by rituximab. *Br J Haematol* 119(4):923–929, 2002.

77. Spina M, Sparano JA, Jaeger U, et al.: Rituximab and chemotherapy is highly effective in patients with CD20-positive non-Hodgkin's lymphoma and HIV infection. *AIDS* 17(1):137–138, 2003.

78. De Paoli P, Vaccher E, Tedeschi R, et al.: Lymphocyte subsets and viral load in patients with HIV-associated non-Hodgkin's lymphoma treated with anti-CD20 monoclonal antibody and chemotherapy. *Cancer Immunol Immunother* 50(3):157–162, 2001.

79. Kaplan LD, Scadden DT, for the AIDS malignancies consortium: No benefit from rituximab in a randomized phase III trial of CHOP with or without rituximiab for patients with HIV-associated non-Hodgkin's lymphoma: AIDS malignancies consortium study 010. *Proc ASCO* 22:564, 2003.

80. Gabarre J, Leblond V, Sutton L, et al.: Autologous bone marrow transplantation in relapsed HIV-related non-Hodgkin's lymphoma. *Bone Marrow Transplant* 18(6):1195–1197, 1996.

81. Campbell P, Iland H, Gibson J, et al.: Syngeneic stem cell transplantation for HIV-related lymphoma. *Br J Haematol* 105(3):795–798, 1999.

82. Gabarre J, Azar N, Autran B, et al.: High-dose therapy and autologous haematopoietic stem-cell transplantation for HIV-1-associated lymphoma. *Lancet* 355(9209):1071–1072, 2000.

83. Krishnan A, Molina A, Zaia J, et al.: Autologous stem cell transplantation for HIV-associated lymphoma. *Blood* 98(13):3857–3859, 2001.

84. Kentos A, Vekemans M, Van Vooren JP, et al.: High-dose chemotherapy and autologous CD34-positive blood stem cell transplantation for multiple myeloma in an HIV carrier. *Bone Marrow Transplant* 29(3):273–275, 2002.

85. Molina A, Zaia J, Krishnan A: Treatment of human immunodeficiency virus-related lymphoma with haematopoietic stem cell transplantation. *Blood Rev* 17(4):249–258, 2003.

86. MacMahon EM, Glass JD, Hayward SD, et al.: Epstein–Barr virus in AIDS-related primary central nervous system lymphoma. *Lancet* 338(8773):969–973, 1991.

87. Cinque P, Brytting M, Vago L, et al.: Epstein–Barr virus DNA in cerebrospinal fluid from patients with AIDS-related primary lymphoma of the central nervous system. *Lancet* 342:398–401, 1993.

88. Snider WD, Simpson DM, Nielsen S, et al.: Neurological complications of acquired immune deficiency syndrome: analysis of 50 patients. *Ann Neurol* 14(4):403–418, 1983.

89. Arribas J, Clifford D, Fichtenbaum C, et al.: Detection of Epstein–Barr virus DNA in cerebrospinal fluid for diagnosis of AIDS-related central nervous system lymphoma. *J Clin Microbiol* 33(6):1580–1583, 1995.

90. De Luca A, Antinori A, Cingolani A, et al.: Evaluation of cerebrospinal fluid EBV-DNA and IL-10 as markers for in vivo diagnosis of AIDS-related primary central nervous system lymphoma. *Br J Haematol* 90:844–849, 1995.

91. Castagna A, Cinque P, d'Amico A, et al.: Evaluation of contrast-enhancing brain lesions in AIDS patients by means of Epstein–Barr virus detection in cerebrospinal fluid and 201thallium single photon emission tomography. *AIDS* 11:1522–1523, 1997.

92. Bower M, Fife K, Sullivan A, et al.: Treatment outcome in presumed and confirmed AIDS-related primary cerebral lymphoma. *Eur J Cancer* 35(4):601–604, 1999.

93. Jacomet C, Girard P, Lebrette M, et al.: Intravenous methotrexate for primary central nervous system non-Hodgkin's lymphoma in AIDS. *AIDS* 11:1725–1730, 1997.

94. Uccini S, Monardo F, Stoppacciaro A, et al.: High frequency of Epstein–Barr virus genome detection in Hodgkin's lymphoma of HIV-positive patients. *Int J Cancer* 46(4):581–585, 1990.

95. Andrieu JM, Roithmann S, Tourani JM, et al.: Hodgkin's lymphoma during HIV1 infection: the French registry experience. French Registry of HIV-Associated Tumors. *Ann Oncol* 4(8):635–641, 1993.

96. Errante D, Zagonel V, Vaccher E, et al.: Hodgkin's lymphoma in patients with HIV infection and in the general population: comparison of clinicopathological features and survival. *Ann Oncol* 5(suppl 2):37–40, 1994.

97. Riyat MS: Hodgkin's lymphoma in Kenya. *Cancer* 69(4):1047–1051, 1992.

98. Biggar RJ, Horm J, Goedert JJ, et al.: Cancer in a group at risk of acquired immunodeficiency syndrome (AIDS) through 1984. *Am J Epidemiol* 126(4):578–586, 1987.

99. Biggar RJ, Burnett W, Mikl J, et al.: Cancer among New York men at risk of acquired immunodeficiency syndrome. *Int J Cancer* 43:979–985, 1989.

100. Tirelli U, Vaccher E, Rezza G, et al.: Hodgkin's lymphoma and infection with the human immunodeficiency virus in Italy. *Ann Intern Med* 108:309–310, 1988.

101. Hessol N, Katz M, Liu J, et al.: Increased incidence of Hodgkin's lymphoma in homosexual men with HIV infection. *Ann Intern Med* 117:309–311, 1992.

102. Lyter D, Bryant J, Thackeray R, et al.: Non-AIDS defining malignancies in the Multicentre AIDS Cohort Study, 1984–1996. *J Acquir Immune Defic Syndr Hum Retrovirol* 17:A13, 1998.

103. Goedert JJ, Cote TR, Virgo P, et al.: Spectrum of AIDS-associated malignant disorders. *Lancet* 351(9119):1833–1839, 1998.

104. Rubio R. Hodgkin's lymphoma associated with HIV: a clinical study of 46 cases. *Cancer* 73:2400–2407, 1994.

105. Tirelli U, Errante D, Dolcetti R, et al.: Hodgkin's lymphoma and HIV infection: clinicopathologic and virologic features of 114 patients from the Italian cooperative group on AIDS and tumors. *J Clin Oncol* 13:1758–1767, 1995.

106. Ames E, Conjalka M, Goldberg A, et al.: Hodgkin's lymphoma and AIDS: 23 new cases and a review of the literature. *Hematol Oncol Clin North Am* 5:343–356, 1991.

107. Monfardini S, Tirelli U, Vaccher E, et al.: Hodgkin's lymphoma in 63 intravenous drug users infected with human immunodeficiency virus. Gruppo Italiano Cooperativo AIDS & Tumori (GICAT). *Ann Oncol* 2(suppl 2):201–205, 1991.

108. Levine A, Cheung T, Tupule J: Preliminary results of AIDS clinical trial group phase II trial of ABVD chemotherapy with G-CSF in HIV infected patients with Hodgkin's lymphoma. *J Acquir Immun Defic Syndr Hum Retrovirol* 14:A12, 1997.

109. Strauss D: HIV associated lymphomas. *Med Clin North Am* 81:495–510, 1997.

110. Castleman B, Towne VW: Case records of the Massachusetts General Hospital: Case No. 40231. *N Engl J Med* 250(23):1001–1005, 1954.

111. Soulier J, Grollet L, Oskenhendler E, et al.: Kaposi's sarcoma-associated herpesvirus-like DNA sequences in multicentric Castleman's disease. *Blood* 86:1276–1280, 1995.

112. Du MQ, Liu H, Diss TC, et al.: Kaposi sarcoma-associated herpesvirus infects monotypic (IgM lambda) but polyclonal naive B cells in Castleman disease and associated lymphoproliferative disorders. *Blood* 97(7):2130–2136, 2001.

113. Oksenhendler E, Boulanger E, Galicier L, et al.: High incidence of Kaposi sarcoma-associated herpesvirus-related non-Hodgkin lymphoma in patients with HIV infection and multicentric Castleman disease. *Blood* 99(7):2331–2336, 2002.

114. Day JR, Bew D, Ali M, et al.: Castleman's disease associated with myasthenia gravis. *Ann Thorac Surg* 75(5):1648–1650, 2003.

115. Oksenhendler E, Duarte M, Soulier J, et al.: Multicentric Castleman's disease in HIV infection: a clinical and pathological study of 20 patients. *AIDS* 10:61–67, 1996.

116. Aaron L, Lidove O, Yousry C, et al.: Human herpesvirus 8-positive Castleman disease in human immunodeficiency virus-infected patients: the impact of highly active antiretroviral therapy. *Clin Infect Dis* 35(7): 880–882, 2002.

# Chapter **62**

# POSTTRANSPLANT LYMPHOPROLIFERATIVE DISORDERS

*Terrance Comeau and Thomas Shea*

## INTRODUCTION

The term posttransplant lymphoproliferative disorder (PTLD) is used to describe a heterogeneous group of lymphoproliferative diseases that occur in hematopoietic stem cell transplant (HSCT) and solid organ transplant (SOT) recipients. These lymphoid disorders were first documented in the 1960s and were initially called "reticulum cell sarcomas."[1] Interestingly, a subgroup of these diseases was labeled "pseudolymphomas" as these retained the ability to undergo spontaneous regression.[2] We now have a greater understanding of PTLD, a disease that most often involves B cells and usually is associated with reactivation of latent Epstein–Barr virus (EBV) infections in the setting of decreased T-cell function. The incidence of this disorder is generally reported to range from 0.8 to 20%, but is felt to be underreported due to its varied clinical presentation.[3,4] These lymphomas are seen in different settings, and, some situations are much more likely to predispose to their occurrence than others. It is imperative that transplant physicians remain cognizant of this entity, as effective therapies are now available that can lower the mortality rate from the 50–80% range seen in the early 1990s[5–8] to cure rates approaching 100% if patients are diagnosed when the tumor burden is low.[9–10]

## PATHOPHYSIOLOGY

EBV, also known as human herpesvirus 4 (HHV4), is the prototype of the gamma subfamily of potentially oncogenic herpesviruses.[11] EBV was discovered over 35 years ago by electron microscopy of cells cultured from Burkitt's lymphoma tissue by Epstein, Achong, and Barr[12]; it is ubiquitous and is known to infect over 90% of people and to persist in the body for life.[13]

Primary EBV infections occurring in early childhood are often asymptomatic. In contrast, primary infections occurring in adolescence and young adulthood often lead to the self-limiting lymphoproliferative disease called infectious mononucleosis (IM), characterized by the triad of fever, lymphadenopathy, and pharyngitis.

EBV, which usually infects humans by entering the oropharynx in saliva, replicates in epithelial cells by coupling of the viral gp 350 glycoprotein with the CD21 receptor on B cells. This leads to host cell infection and subsequent infiltration of oropharyngeal tissue. EBV-infected B cells express a pattern of EBV latent genes known as "latency III" genes. Hence, these cells express multiple viral proteins including the six nuclear proteins known as EBV nuclear antigens (EBNAs) 1, 2, 3a, 3b, 3c, and LP; integral membrane proteins known as latent membrane proteins (LMP) 1, 2a, and 2b; and two untranslated RNAs known as EBERs 1 and 2 (EBV-encoded small RNAs). EBNA1 binds to viral DNA and is responsible for the maintenance of EBV episomes in replicating B cells.[14] EBNA2 up-regulate cellular proteins that contribute to the growth and transformation of B cells. LMP1 also functions as a constitutively activated member of the tumor necrosis factor receptor superfamily that activates a number of signaling pathways in a ligand-independent manner. LMP1 can substitute for CD40 in vivo and leads to the activation of the transcription factor NF-κB (nuclear factor kappa B), which in turn results in cytokine production and B-cell proliferation. Finally, LMP2a alters B-cell receptor (BCR) signaling by mimicking the rescue signal normally delivered by this receptor, thereby enabling nontransformed B cells to survive without appropriate BCR signaling.

Normally, B cells transformed by EBV or containing replicating virus are highly immunogenic and induce an intense cytotoxic T lymphocyte (CTL) and natural killer cell response. These activated T cells, appearing in the peripheral blood as atypical lymphocytes, help control the proliferation of infected B cells. Fortunately, most EBV-infected B cells are eliminated, but some are able to persist because they down-regulate immunogenic EBV proteins, thus allowing the cells to avoid immune recognition. Eventually, the EBV genome forms an episome that remains latent in resting memory B cells. These EBV-infected cells now express only the "latency 0" gene pattern, which consists of LMP2a, the EBERs, and possibly EBNA1.[13,15] Hence, in the immunocompetent host, an equilibrium is established in which rare EBV-infected cells lacking expression of immunogenic proteins coexist with EBV-specific CTLs. EBV undergoes lytic replication in numerous B cells in the oropharynx of healthy carriers. When people become immunosuppressed after HSCT or SOT, critical T-cell control of B-cell growth is no longer present, leading to unchecked proliferation of EBV-infected cells, which may in turn result in B-cell hyperplasia or frank malignancy.[15]

The origin of EBV-infected cells in PTLD varies depending on the transplant population being studied. In SOT patients, the PTLD cells are usually of recipient origin. However, most PTLD cells in the HSCT setting are donor derived. It should be noted that primary EBV infection may also result in PTLD; this is usually seen in children.

## INCIDENCE AND RISK FACTORS

The incidence of PTLD varies depending on the type of transplant, recipient age, and type of immunosuppression used (Tables 62.1 and 62.2). The incidence of PTLD is 4 times higher in pediatric than in adult transplant recipients.[16] In SOT recipients, the incidence of PTLD varies with the type of allograft: 19% of intestinal transplants, 2–10% of heart transplants, 5–9% of heart–lung transplants, 2–8% of liver transplants, and 1–10% of renal transplants.[16] Additional risk factors for PTLD in SOT patients include high levels of immunosuppression (particularly with antithymocyte globulin), EBV seronegative recipient of a seropositive donor, development of primary EBV infection after transplant, and presence of cytomegalovirus (CMV) disease. For example, PTLDs are the most common tumors in children after organ transplant and represent over 50% of all posttransplant tumors; this is in contrast to adults where such tumors comprise only

| Table 62.2   Relative risk of PTLD in HSCT by method of T-cell depletion[19] | |
|---|---|
| Method of T-cell depletion (TCD) | Relative risk |
| No TCD | 1 |
| CAMPATH-1 monoclonal antibody | 2 |
| Elutriation/density gradient centrifugation | 2.6 |
| Lectins | 4.1 |
| Anti-T-cell monoclonal antibody | 12.3 |
| Sheep red blood cell rosetting | 15.6 |

15% of posttransplant malignancies.[17] In addition, children undergoing small intestine transplants may have an EBV-PTLD incidence as high as 32%.[18]

For patients undergoing HSCT, several risk factors have been identified to predict for the risk of PTLD in different settings. Curtis et al. evaluated over 18,000 patients who underwent allogeneic HSCT at 235 centers worldwide. The cumulative incidence of PTLD was 1% at 10 years. The incidence was found to vary markedly with time after transplant, with high rates occurring during the first 5 months, followed by a steep decline in incidence between 6 and 12 months posttransplant.[19] The high incidence of PTLD during the first 5 months after transplant is consistent with studies that show the temporal pattern of immune reconstitution in HSCT recipients. For example, Lucas et al. noted that levels of anti-EBV CTL precursors appear to return to normal by 6 months posttransplant in most patients.[20] In their multivariate analysis, Curtis et al. found that the risk of early (<1 year posttransplant) PTLD was strongly associated with unrelated or ≥2 human leukocyte antigen (HLA)-mismatched related donors, T-cell depletion methods that selectively target T cells or T + NK cells or E-rosetting, use of antithymocyte globulin for prophylaxis or treatment of acute graft-versus-host disease (GVHD), and use of the anti-CD3 monoclonal antibody 64.1 (given for therapy of acute GVHD). The cumulative incidence of PTLD for patients with 0, 1, 2, or 3–4 major risk factors were 0.5, 1.7, 8, and 22.3%, respectively. They also noted a weaker association with the occurrence of acute GVHD grades II–IV and with conditioning regimens that included total body irradiation (TBI). The risk appeared to vary by dose of fractionated TBI, with a 3.5- to

| Table 62.1   Risk factors for PTLD | |
|---|---|
| Solid organ transplant | Hematopoietic SCT |
| Allograft type (e.g., intestinal) | Type of transplant |
| High levels of immunosuppression (e.g., Antithymocyte globulin) | High levels of immunosuppression (e.g., Antithymocyte globulin) |
| EBV seronegative recipient of seropositive donor | Donor type: unrelated of ≥2 HLA-mismatched related donor |
| Presence of CMV disease | T-cell depletion |

EBV, Epstein–Barr virus; HLA, human leukocyte antigen; CMV,

4.3-fold increased risk seen for doses ≥13 Gy. The only risk factors identified for late-onset (>1-year posttransplant) PTLD were extensive chronic GVHD and TBI dose.[19] There is a suggestion that conditioning regimens containing fludarabine also may be associated with an increased risk of PTLD.[21]

Significant differences were detected among T-cell depletion techniques used. As noted above, a high risk of PTLD was observed among recipients of grafts that were T-cell depleted using monoclonal antibodies or sheep red blood cell E-rosetting techniques that selectively targeted T (or T + NK) cells. However, lower rates of PTLD were associated with methods that removed both T and B cells, such as CAMPATH-1 monoclonal antibodies, elutriation, and lectins.[19] This was also confirmed in a study by Hale and Waldmann in which 2401 recipients received grafts that were T-cell-depleted with CAMPATH-1M or 1G; the cumulative risk of PTLD was only 1.1%. They hypothesized that the depletion of B cells may reduce the viral load or virus target tissue in the interval before full recovery of T-cell function.[22] Patients receiving CD34 selected allografts do not appear to be at an increase risk of PTLD as the B-lymphocyte contamination of the isolated CD34+ cells is low.[23]

Rare cases of PTLD have been reported in recipients of autologous HSCTs.[15,24] Powell et al.[25] reported an unexpectedly high incidence of EBV-PTLD in patients undergoing CD34+ selected autologous peripheral blood stem cell transplant for neuroblastoma: 5 of 156 patients (3.5%). This is in contrast to a report by Gross et al. who reported no cases of EBV-PTLD in their review of 853 autologous stem cell transplants.[4]

Finally, EBV-negative PTLDs appear to be morphologically and clinically distinct from EBV-positive PTLDs in that they tend to have a later onset, a higher prevalence of monomorphic lymphomas, and a greater proportion derived from T cells.[19,26-28] Although EBV-negative PTLDs have distinct features and are felt to be associated with a poor prognosis, some do respond to decreased immunosuppression, similar to EBV-positive cases.[27,28]

## CLINICAL FEATURES

The presentation of PTLDs may range from an asymptomatic state to a rapidly progressive, fulminate course with a fatal outcome.[8] Hence, it is important to maintain vigilance in high-risk patients. Symptoms are varied and may be related to the EBV viral infection, B symptoms from overt lymphoma, organ dysfunction, and/or mass effect. Early symptoms may be nonspecific and may include malaise, fever, and weight loss. In children with primary EBV posttransplant, IM is the most common presentation: fever, tonsillar and adenoid hypertrophy, cervical lymphadenopathy, and hepatomegal with abnormal liver enzymes. Patients with central nervous system (CNS) involvement may present with seizures. Gastrointestinal (GI) involvement may manifest with abdominal pain, diarrhea, GI bleeding or perforation. It is important to remember that dysfunction in the organ transplanted may be an indication of involvement by PTLD. Reams et al. reported that 70% of their lung and heart–lung recipients who developed PTLD presented with thoracic organ involvement.[29] Hence, any transplant patient who experiences adenopathy, mass lesions, unexplained fever or pain, weight loss, or dysfunction of the transplanted organ should be investigated for PTLD.

## EVALUATION

Serologic testing has traditionally been used to investigate EBV-related disorders. However, such testing may be unreliable in the transplant population as a result of altered antibody production by host immunosuppression and passive transfer of antibody from blood products given in the peritransplant period. One of the most useful techniques to evaluate for EBV-PTLD is polymerase chain reaction (PCR) testing of peripheral blood, which may detect disease before the onset of clinical symptoms.[30] High EBV viral loads in high-risk patients often predict for the development of EBV-PTLD. Aalto et al. evaluated serum samples from 12 HSCT recipients who had died from PTLD using quantitative PCR (qPCR) for EBV-DNA.[31] They found that all of the PTLD patients became EBV-DNA positive with progressively rising copy numbers, and that EBV-DNA was first detectable 23 days before death, which was earlier than the onset of symptoms (which occurred 15 days before death). In their patient population, they noted that qPCR for EBV-DNA in serum was highly sensitive (100%) and specific (96%). However, Wagner et al. found that the detection of two or more levels of EBV-DNA above 4000 copies/mcg had a sensitivity of 100% for the prediction of early PTLD but a specificity of only 50%.[32] Carpentier et al. evaluated the utility of EBV early-antigen (EA) serologic testing in conjunction with peripheral blood EBV-DNA viral load testing as a marker for risk of PTLD. They found that at the EBV-DNA threshold at which PTLD occurs, the positive predictive value based on the absence of high-titer EA antibody was increased to 75%; that is, patients with high EBV-DNA load but without significant EA antibody titers had a 75% risk of developing PTLD.[33] Such testing would not be useful in patients with EBV-negative PTLD or those EBV-positive patients who do not shed large amounts of EBV into the peripheral blood.[34]

Detailed radiologic investigations including CT scans of the chest, abdomen, and pelvis are necessary to evaluate the extent of disease. Patients with GI complaints may require endoscopy with biopsy. Thoracentesis may be necessary to evaluate pleural effusions, and paracentesis to evaluate ascites. Patients with CNS signs or symptoms or abnormal head CT

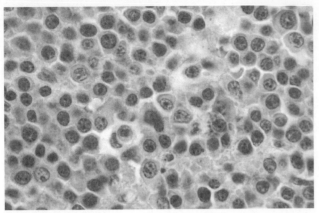

**Figure 62.1**   *PTLD: reactive plasmacytic hyperplasia-type polyclonal*

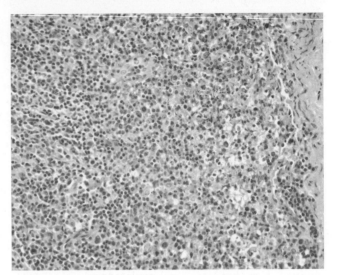

**Figure 62.3**   *PTLD: polymorphic monoclonal*

scans or MRI scans may warrant a lumbar puncture with CSF evaluation. Castellano-Sanchez et al. reported the features of 12 patients with primary CNS PTLD; by neuroimaging, most patients showed multiple (3–9) intra-axial, contrast-enhancing lesions. CNS PTLDs were noted to be uniformly high-grade lymphomas and were associated with extremely short survival periods.[35]

Tissue biopsy confirms the diagnosis of PTLD. Excisional biopsy provides adequate tissue for evaluation of cell type, clonality, virologic studies, and architectural background (Figures 62.1 to 62.8). Cytology alone has a limited role in the diagnosis of PTLD as it does not permit subclassification. Immunophenotyping by flow cytometry or immunohistochemistry should be performed to determine the cell type (B vs T) and cell marker status, which may direct therapy (e.g., CD20 expression). While the majority of these are B-cell tumors and are associated with EBV, approximately 9% of all PTLD and as many as 27% of EBV-negative tumors may be of T-cell origin.[26–28] PTLD can be confused with organ transplant rejec-

tion unless the cells are identified as B cells by B-cell markers such as CD19, CD20, CD21, or CD22. Also, PTLD may coexist with acute rejection. When the allograft itself is affected, histologic features such as plasmacytoid infiltrates, immunoblastic cells, nodular infiltrates, and serpiginous necrosis, especially in the absence of neutrophils, is suggestive of PTLD. Tumor clonality may be determined by evaluating for immunoglobulin or T-cell receptor gene rearrangements. Evaluation for viral markers should also be performed with in situ hybridization for Epstein–Barr early RNA (EBER) or immunostaining for EBV LMP.[3,16]

A formal classification system of PTLD was established by two international consensus groups (ASTS/ASTP EBV-PTLD Task Force and the Mayo Clinic organized International Consensus Development Meeting on EBV-Induced PTLD) and published in 1999.[3] They suggested that the term PTLD should be used to encompass the large spectrum of EBV lymphoproliferative processes seen after organ or stem cell transplantation.

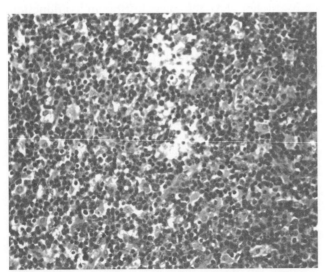

**Figure 62.2**   *PTLD: polymorphic polyclonal type*

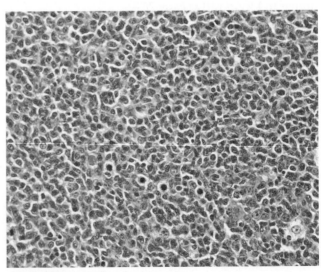

**Figure 62.4**   *PTLD: monomorphic*

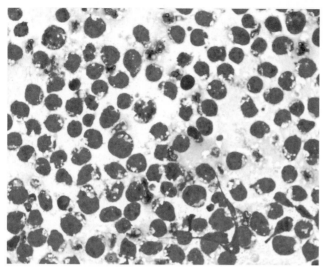

**Figure 62.5** *PTLD Burkitt's type (touch prep)*

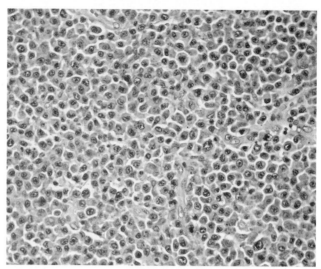

**Figure 62.7** *PTLD: plasmacytoma-like (monoclonal kappa)*

In addition, they recommended that posttransplant IM and plasma cell hyperplasia continue to be included under the heading of PTLD, but that they be clearly segregated as reactive hyperplasias. They also recommended that the term PTLD, when not further qualified, be used to refer to neoplastic forms of PTLD that are termed "polymorphic PTLD" (including polymorphic lymphoma and polymorphic B-cell hyperplasia, which can be a monoclonal lesion), or "lymphomatous" PTLD (including so-called monomorphic PTLD). Harris et al. described polymorphic PTLDs as destructive lesions that produce architectural effacement of lymph nodes but that, unlike most lymphomas, show a full range of B-cell maturation from immunoblasts to plasma cells with small- and medium-sized lymphocytes and numerous cells resembling centrocytes/cleaved follicular center cells.[36] In contrast, monomorphic PTLDs often have sufficient architectural and cytological atypia to be categorized as high-grade lymphomas. Monomorphic PTLDs are characterized by infiltrates causing nodal architectural effacement with confluent sheets of transformed cells; all or most cells are large, transformed, blastic cells with prominent nucleoli and basophilic cytoplasm.[36] Most monomorphic PTLDs fall into the category of diffuse large cell lymphomas. The consensus groups also stated that neoplastic forms of EBV-positive PTLD should ideally have (1) disruption of underlying architecture by a lymphoproliferative process, (2) presence of monoclonal or oligoclonal cell populations as revealed by cellular and/or viral markers, and (3) evidence of EBV infection in many of the cells. The demonstration of a lymphoid tumor containing unequivocal evidence of any two of these features was felt to be sufficient to establish the diagnosis of neoplastic PTLD. A working diagnosis could be made in the presence of (1) or (2) alone in the proper clinical setting. In practical terms, this eliminates all inflammatory lesions in which EBV might be demonstrated, with the exceptions of plasma cell hyperplasia and IM.

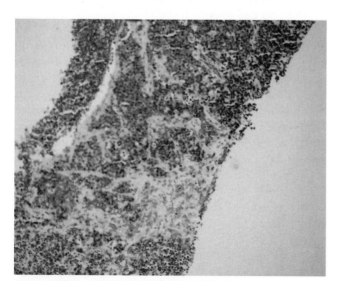

**Figure 62.6** *PTLD: Burkitt's type (EBV ISH)*

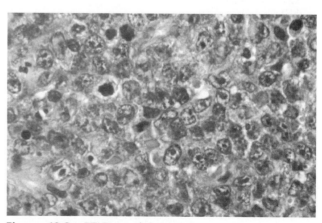

**Figure 62.8** *PTLD: myeloma type*

| Table 62.3 | Harris formulation |
|---|---|

*Early/Benign PTLD*
Plasmacytic or atypical lymphoid hyperplasia
Infectious mononucleosis-like syndrome
  – Nodal disease with preservation
  – <3 months posttransplantation
  – Polyclonal

*Polymorphic PTLD*
  – Nodal disease with effacement of lymph node architecture or extranodal disease
  – Full range of B-cell maturation
  – Monoclonal
  – Normal cytogenetics
  – No oncogene mutations

*Monomorphic PTLD (Non-Hodgkin's B- or T-Cell lymphoma)*
  – Nodal disease with effacement of lymph node architecture or invasive extranodal disease
  – Monomorphic sheets of transformed B cells
  – Monoclonal
  – Some with abnormal cytogenetics or mutations in ras or p53

*PTLD-Other*
T-cell-rich, large B-cell (Hodgkin's-like) lymphoma
  – Nodal disease
  – Background of small T-cells with superimposed Reed–Sternberg–like cells
  – Monoclonal
Plasmacytoma-like lesions
  – Nodal disease with effacement of lymph node architecture by mature plasma cells with monoclonal immunoglobulin
  – Monoclonal
Multiple myeloma

*Criteria For Evaluation of Clonality (Specify B or T Cell)*
C0 Polyclonal
C1 Monoclonal-not further categorized
  C1a Monoclonal component estimated at <50% of cells
  C1b Monoclonal component estimated at ≥50% of cells
  C1c Multiclonal or oligoclonal pattern
CX not evaluated

*Criteria For Evaluation of EBV within PTLD (detection by EBER2 or LMP1 expression)*
E0 EBV negative
E1 EBV Present-not further categorized
  E1a Nonclonal viral pattern
  E1b Clonal viral pattern
EX not evaluated

| Table 62.4 | World Health Organization categories of PTLD |
|---|---|

WHO Categories of Posttransplant lymphoproliferative disorders

Early lesions
  Reactive plasmacytic hyperplasia
  Infectious mononucleosis-like
PTLD polymorphic
  Polyclonal (rare)
  Monoclonal
PTLD monomorphic (classify according to lymphoma classification)
  B-cell lymphomas
    Diffuse large B-cell lymphoma (immunoblastic, centroblastic, anaplastic)
    Burkitt/Burkitt-like lymphoma
    Plasma cell myeloma
  T-cell lymphomas
    Peripheral T-cell lymphoma, not otherwise categorized
    Other types (Hepatosplenic, gamma-delta, T/NK)
Other types (rare)
  Hodgkin's disease–like lesions (associated with methotrexate therapy)
  Plasmacytoma-like lesions

## MANAGEMENT

The prevention and treatment of EBV-PTLD may include numerous modalities (Table 62.5), the choice of which may be dictated by certain prognostic features (Table 62.6). The survival rates of patients who develop PTLD vary widely depending on the type of transplant (SOT vs HSCT), category of PTLD (early polyclonal vs monocloncal monomorphic), and the therapy employed.[15]

### REDUCTION OF IMMUNOSUPPRESSION, SURGERY, RADIATION THERAPY

Decreasing immunosuppressive therapy is often the first step taken in the management of PTLD in the SOT setting and has proven to be efficacious in small case series reports, with response rates ranging from 23 to 89%. Tsai et al. reported one of the largest series on the outcome of 42 adult organ transplant recipients who developed PTLD and were treated with reduction in immunosuppression with or without surgical resection of all known disease: 73.8% achieved a complete remission. Of those patients who were treated with reduction in immunosuppression alone, 63% responded, with a median time to documented response of 3.6 weeks. They noted that an elevated LDH ratio, organ dysfunction, and multiorgan involvement by PTLD predicted for lack of response to reduction in immunosuppression. In patients with none of these risk factors, 89% responded to reduction in immunosuppression, while 60% with 1 risk factor responded and 0 % with 2–3 risk factors responded. However, such a maneuver is associated with the risk

Finally, they recommended that the classification system formulated by Harris et al.[36] be used (Table 62.3) with supplemental information (clonality, EBV status) appended to the histological diagnosis of PTLD. The World Health Organization (WHO) also defined several categories of PTLD (Table 62.4).

Although no specific staging system for PTLD exists, the consensus group recommended that the Ann Arbor Staging Classification with Cotswold modifications be used.

| Table 62.5 Management of PTLD |
|---|
| Monitor EBV-DNA viral load by PCR in cell-free plasma once every 1–2 weeks in high-risk transplant patients. |
| When EBV reactivation occurs, screen patients for signs and symptoms of early PTLD. |
| Obtain histologic confirmation of PTLD and perform staging studies to document extent of disease. This includes serum LDH, CT/PET scans, and bilateral bone marrow aspirate and biopsy. |
| Reduce immunosuppressive therapy as tolerated by SOT or HSCT recipient. |
| Consider surgery or radiation therapy for localized disease. |
| Patients who fail to respond to reduction in immunosuppression should be considered for therapy with rituximab if CD20 expression documented. |
| Patients who fail to respond to rituximab or who are not candidates for such therapy should be considered for cytotoxic chemotherapy. Patients with stage IV disease and those with an elevated LDH may be considered for initial combination therapy with both chemotherapy and rituximab. |
| If available, HSCT patients can be considered for adoptive immunotherapy with donor T-cells. |

SOT: Solid eagar transplant; EBV: Epstein–Barr virus; PTLD: past-transplant lymphoproliferative disorder; LDH: Grent lactate dehydrogenase; HSCT: Remotopoietic stem cell transplant.

of allograft rejection, which can be fatal in setting of heart, liver, or lung transplantation. In this study, almost all cases of acute rejection could be treated by increasing immunosuppression without compromising the initial effect of immunosuppresion on reduction of the PTLD. Tsai et al. noted that the high response rate and low rejection rate in this study suggests that one can often find a level of immunosuppression sufficient for PTLD resolution while simultaneously protecting the allograft in many patients.[37] Liver, pancreas, and kidney transplant patients are often treated with complete cessation of all immunosuppression, except for a maintenance dose of steroids to prevent an adrenal crisis, as acute rejection can be quickly identified noninvasively by following liver enzymes and serum creatinine. Severe rejection can then be aborted with reinstitution of immunosuppre-

| Table 62.6 Poor prognostic features |
|---|
| Monomorphic subtype with high state |
| High LDH |
| Multivisceral disease (4 or more sites) |
| CNS involvement |
| HSCT vs SOT |

LDH: lactate dehydrogenase; HSCT: Renatopoictic stem cell transplant; SOT: solid organ transplant.

sion and rescue of the graft. In contrast, for heart and lung transplant recipients, immunosuppression is reduced but not stopped completely. For example, drugs such as azathioprine and mycophenolate mofetil are discontinued, while drugs such as steroids, cyclosporine, or tacrolimus are maintained at a reduced dose. Patients not responding with a CR (Complete Remission) or PR (Partial Remission) by 4 weeks should be evaluated for additional therapies. Radiation therapy applied to localized PTLD may also be curative.

Unfortunately, HSCT recipients rarely benefit from a decrease in immunosuppressive therapy as endogenous immune recovery posttransplant may take several weeks to months.

### ANTI-B-CELL THERAPY

There are numerous reports that support the effectiveness of anti-B-cell therapy for the treatment of PTLD in both SOT and HSCT patients.[38,39] Benkerrou et al.[40] reported the outcome of 58 patients after SOT or HSCT with EBV-PTLD who were treated with anti-CD21 plus anti-CD24 antibodies: 61% of patients achieved a CR, with a 1-year overall survival of 46% (compared with 29% in historical controls). Several recent reports have demonstrated a benefit from the use of rituximab, a humanized monoclonal IgG1 kappa antibody against the CD20 antigen found on the surface of malignant and normal B cells, but not on other normal tissues. It has been found to mediate complement-dependent cell lysis and antibody-dependent cellular cytotoxicity.[41] Milpied et al. reported the outcome of 32 transplant recipients with PTLD who were treated with rituximab: response (CR + PR) was seen in 65% of SOT and 83% of HSCT recipients, with 73% surviving at 1 year.[42] Ganne et al. reported the outcome of eight cases of PTLD occurring after SOT. Complete remission was achieved in seven patients, and seven patients maintained functioning grafts.[43] Rituximab is often used as first-line therapy in patients with PTLD occurring after HSCT and as second-line therapy after failure of reduction in immunosuppression in SOT recipients.

Rituximab has also been used in the preemptive setting for the prevention of PTLD in high-risk patients. van Esser et al.[44] evaluated EBV reactivation by PCR viral load testing in patients undergoing allogeneic HSCT. They found that patients undergoing a T-cell depleted allogeneic HSCT were at high risk for PTLD if the plasma EBV viral load exceeded 1000 genome equivalents/milliliter (gEq/mL). Although the negative predictive value of viral load testing was 100%, the positive predictive value was only 39%, indicating that many patients were still able to mount an effective immune response and clear the viral reactivation. They suggested that monitoring the reconstitution of EBV-specific T lymphocytes may add to the predictive value of the viral load by PCR; such assays are now available and include the enumeration of EBV-specific

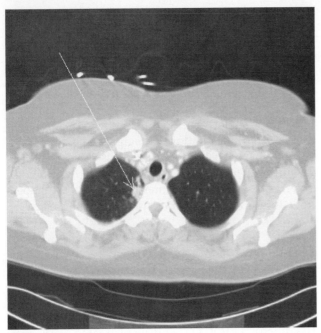

**Figure 62.9** *Pulmonary nodule*

T cells by tetramer binding or by the induction of intracellular interferon -gamma (IFN-γ) in T cells after specific stimulation.[44] In order to evaluate the prevention of EBV-PTLD by preemptive use of rituximab, van Esser et al.[9] evaluated 49 recipients of a TCD allogeneic HSCT by performing EBV viral load by PCR. Preemptive therapy with a single infusion of rituximab was given to 15 patients with an EBV viral load of 1000 gEq/mL or more. A total of 14 patients demonstrated a complete response, as defined by prevention of EBV-PTLD and complete clearance of EBV-DNA from the plasma, which was achieved after a median of 8 days.

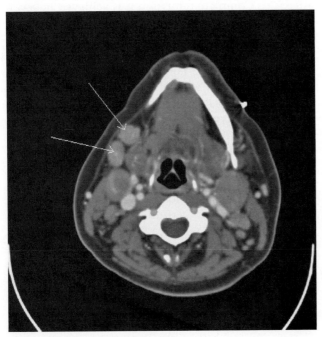

**Figure 62.10** *Neck adenopathy*

They compared this outcome with their historical cohort with the same high-risk features and showed a reduction of PTLD incidence from 49 to 18% and reduction in PTLD mortality from 26 to 0%.[9] However, not all B-cell PTLD express CD20. Kaleem et al. found that 16% of the PTLD cases they evaluated by flow cytometry showed almost complete lack of CD20 expression and several other cases showed partial and dim expression on CD20.[45]

Finally, analysis of patients with PTLD in remission after chemotherapy or withdrawal of immunosuppression has confirmed a relationship between disease activity and EBV viral load by PCR. However, Yang et al. suggest that this correlation may not exist in patients treated with rituximab. They note that EBV-infected lymphocytes in the peripheral blood differ in their sensitivity to rituximab from tumor cells of PTLD; that is, EBV-infected cells in the peripheral blood rapidly decline with therapy, whereas the response of tumor cells is variable. They caution that monitoring viral load in peripheral blood may not predict clinical response in patients with PTLD treated with rituximab.[46]

### RAPAMYCIN

Rapamycin is a macrolide antifungal antibiotic isolated from *Streptomyces hygroscopicus* that has potent immunosuppressive properties. It blocks cell cycle progression from phase G1 to S and inhibits some signal transduction pathways. Besides its inhibitory effects on normal cells of the immune system, rapamycin also inhibits proliferation of transformed cell lines, such as B cells transformed by EBV.

Garcia et al. recently reported two cases of PTLD after renal transplantation that were successfully treated with rituximab in association with rapamycin. This is a potentially useful combination as it allows for the maintenance of some degree of the immunosuppression necessary to preserve graft function while exerting anti-PTLD effects.[41]

### CHEMOTHERAPY

Chemotherapy is usually considered for use when the preceding treatment options have failed, as it may be associated with significant morbidity and mortality. Unfortunately, HSCT patients, who are more resistant to reduction in immunosuppression, are frequently in need of early chemotherapy. Patients with high LDH and multiorgan involvement are another group most likely to require such therapy. Perhaps the early identification of such risk factors may permit more rapid initiation of effective chemotherapy regimens. Anthracycline containing regimens such as CHOP and ProMACE-CytaBOM have been used in the past and may provide long-term relapse-free survival.[15] However, recent investigations in children and adults with PTLD after SOT have demonstrated a high response rate with less toxicity and mortality with low-dose combination chemotherapy. For example, Gross et al.[47] showed that low-dose cyclophosphamide/prednisone induces a high response rate (>90%) with minimal toxicity. However, the 2-year event-free survival was only 58%. To improve the long-term outcome, Orjuela et al. recently reported the results of a pilot study in which six patients with PTLD following SOT were treated with 2–6 courses of CPR (cyclophosphamide, prednisone, and rituxin) and reported an overall response rate of 100% (85% CR, 15% PR). All patients in CR survived with functioning allografts.[48] Oertel et al. reported their experience with salvage chemotherapy (carboplatin/etoposide with G-CSF support) in patients with refractory or relapsed PTLD after SOT: five of nine patients achieved a complete remission.[49]

## ADOPTIVE IMMUNOTHERAPY

Khatri et al. demonstrated the striking temporal relationship between the endogenous expansion of a TCR Vß-restricted, CD3$^+$CD8$^+$ population of MHC class I-restricted CTL and the regression of a monoclonal PTLD in a HSCT recipient. Unfortunately, the delay in recovery of such immune surveillance against transformed EBV-positive B cells results in the development of potentially fatal PTLD. T-cell immunotherapy has been reported to be efficacious in the management of PTLD in this setting.[39] O'Reilly et al. reported on 18 HSCT patients with EBV-PTLD who were treated with nonspecific donor lymphocyte infusions (DLI): 16 of 18 patients experienced eradication of PTLD. However, only 10 survived in sustained CR and 3 patients died of GVHD, a major side effect of DLI.[50] Attempts have been made to improve the efficacy and reduce the risk of GVHD by administering EBV-specific CTLs.[51] Rooney et al. detailed the outcome of 39 recipients of matched unrelated donor/partially mismatched related donor transplants who received prophylactic EBV-specific CTLs (EBVs-CTL). None of the treated HSCT recipients developed PTLD, whereas 7 of 61 controls not receiving such therapy developed PTLD.[52]

In the SOT setting, adoptive immunotherapy has also been evaluated on a limited basis. Nalesnick et al. reported the experience of seven SOT recipients with PTLD; peripheral blood mononuclear cells harvested from the patients were cultured with interleukin-2 (IL-2). The infusion of these lymphokine-activated killer cells into the four patients with EBV-positive tumors resulted in sustained involution of their tumors. Unfortunately, two patients suffered organ rejection.[53] Haque et al. reported their experience with three SOT patients whose EBV-specific cells lines were cultured from autologous T cells collected prior to transplant; the prophylactic infusion of these cells after transplant resulted in the suppression of circulating EBV-DNA levels to below pretansplant levels. Interestingly, the EBV-specific CTLs were measurable in the patients' blood for 3 months posttransplant.[54] Finally, a phase 1/2 trial with eight SOT patients who had progressive PTLD unresponsive to conventional treatment were given infusions of partly HLA-matched allogeneic EBV-specific CTLs from a frozen bank of CTLs derived from healthy blood donors. Three of the five patients who completed treatment achieved a complete remission, and the EBV load in their peripheral blood fell to undetectable levels in all patients who responded to treatment; no GVHD developed and graft function improved in three cases.[55] It was noted that tumor responses were mainly seen in those with early, localized, polyclonal disease.

EBVs-CTL therapy may not find widespread use for several reasons: it requires 2–3 weeks to generate such cells, the technology for larger scale expansion of EBV-CTLs is expensive, such technology is not available in every transplant center, and this approach is not effective in patients who develop EBV deletion mutants.[11]

## ARGININE BUTYRATE

Arginine butyrate and other histone deacetylase inhibitors induce the activity of certain genes. Exposure of EBV-positive tumor cells to butyrate results in robust induction of herpesvirus in immediate-early and early (lytic) genes, including thymidine kinase (TK), and a modest induction of lytic replication. There is now extensive experience in the administration of arginine butyrate over extended periods of time to adults and children with sickle cell anemia or β-thalassemia to therapeutically reactivate fetal globin expression. In vitro studies demonstrated that induction of EBV-TK activity was possible in EBV-immortalized B cells and that these previously ganciclovir-resistant cells were then rendered susceptible to antiviral nucleoside analogs. Faller et al. have used arginine butyrate to induce the latent viral TK gene expression and enzyme induction in tumor cells and then treated the patients with ganciclovir: 5 of 10 previously refractory patients experienced a complete clinical response and an additional 2 patients achieved a partial response.[56]

## ANTI-INTERLEUKIN 6 THERAPY

IL-6 is a cytokine that is known to promote the growth and differentiation of B cells. A phase 1–2 study was reported by Haddad et al. in which 12 SOT recipients with PTLD refractory to reduction of immunosuppression were treated with anti-IL-6: 5 of 12 patients achieved CR and 3 patients achieved a PR.[57,58]

## ANTIVIRAL THERAPY

Many studies have incorporated antiviral nucleoside analog drugs such as acyclovir and ganciclovir. The nucleosides require conversion to the monophosphate form by the viral enzyme TK. Additional phosphorylations are then performed by cellular kinases. Acyclovir or ganciclovir triphosphates are then preferentially incorporated into DNA by viral DNA polymerase, where they then act as obligate chain terminators. However, TK and viral DNA polymerase are enzymes that are only expressed during lytic infection, while EBV-PTLD is thought to result from latently infected proliferating B cells. Hence, no effect of these drugs would be expected with respect to the prevention or treatment of PTLD. Nevertheless, acyclovir is often instituted when EBV-PTLD is diagnosed, but there is scant information documenting the effectiveness of either acyclovir, ganciclovir, or newer antiviral agents such as cidofovir.[11] Despite a paucity of data supporting the merits of using antiviral therapy in this setting, the European Best Practice Expert Group on Renal Transplantation suggests that in the case of EBV-positive B-cell lymphomas, antiviral treatment with acyclovir, valacyclovir, or ganciclovir may be initiated for at least 1 month or according to the blood level of EBV replication when available.[59]

### INTERFERON ALPHA THERAPY

There are numerous case reports in the literature demonstrating the effectiveness of IFN-α in the management of EBV-PTLD after HSCT and SOT. Davis et al. reported the outcome of 14 patients with EBV-PTLD who were treated with IFN-α 3 million $U/m^2$ daily for at least 3 weeks and continued for 6–9 months in responders: 8 of 14 patients achieved a CR.[60] Patients treated with IFN-α in various studies have received additional therapies, and this makes it unclear whether IFN-α is truly an effective therapy for PTLD.[11] The toxicity and lower response rates associated with IFN-α also makes it less appealing than more recent options such as rituximab.

## SUMMARY

In conclusion, over the last decade our understanding of the pathophysiology of PTLD has enabled us to detect the disorder at a subclinical stage that permits the institution of therapies capable of improving outcome. Indeed, the high mortality reported in the 1980s and early 1990s appears to have been supplanted by much improved long-term survival rates. These improved outcomes have been based primarily on the use of antibodies such as the anti-CD20 agent rituximab for early-stage patients and combined with chemotherapy for patients with more advanced disease. Ongoing advances in our understanding of immunobiology and development of newer immunosuppressive agents may one day allow patients undergoing SOT or HSCT to avoid such a complication.

### REFERENCES

1. Starzl TE: Discussion of Murray JE, Wilson RE, Tilney NL, et al. Five years experience in renal transplantation with immunosuppressive drugs: survival, function, complications and the role of lymphocyte depletion by thoracic duct fistula. *Ann Surg* 168:416, 1968.
2. Geis WP, Iwatsuki S, Molnar Z, et al.: Pseudolymphoma in renal allograft recipients. *Arch Surg* 113:461, 1978.
3. Paya CV, Fung JJ, Nalesnik MA, et al.: Epstein–Barr virus-induced post transplant lymphoproliferative disorders. ASTS/ASTP EBV-PTLD Task Force and The Mayo Clinic Organized International Consensus Development Meeting. *Transplantation* 68:1517–1525, 1999.
4. Gross TG, Steinbuch M, DeFor T, et al.: B cell lymphoproliferative disorders following hematopoietic stem cell transplantation: risk factors, treatment and outcome. *Bone Marrow Transplant* 23:251–258, 1999.
5. Chen JM, Barr ML, Chadburn A, et al.: Management of lymphoproliferative disorders after cardiac transplantation. *Ann Thorac Surg* 56:527, 1993.
6. Raymond E, Tricottet V, Samuel D, Reynes M, Bismuth H, Misset JL: Epstein–Barr virus-related localized hepatic lymphoproliferative disorders after liver transplantation. *Cancer* 76:1344, 1995.
7. Montone KT, Litzky LA, Wurster A, et al.: Analysis of Epstein–Barr virus-associated posttransplantation lymphoproliferative disorder after lung transplantation. *Surgery* 119: 544, 1996.
8. Micallef IN, Chhanabhai M, Gascoyne RD, et al.: Lymphoproliferative disorders following allogeneic bone marrow transplantation: the Vancouver experience. *Bone Marrow Transplant* 22(10):981–987, 1998 Nov.
9. van Esser JW, Niesters HG, van der Holt B, et al.: Prevention of Epstein–Barr virus-lymphoproliferative disease by molecular monitoring and preemptive rituximab in high-risk patients after allogeneic stem cell transplantation. *Blood* 99(12):4364–4369, 2002 Jun 15.
10. Soler MJ, Puig JM, Mir M, et al.: Post transplant lymphoproliferative disease: treatment and outcome in renal transplant recipients. *Transplant Proc* 35(5):1709–1713, 2003 Aug.
11. Meijer E, Dekker AW, Weersink AJ, Rozenberg-Arska M, Verdonck LF: Prevention and treatment of Epstein–Barr virus-associated lymphoproliferative disorders in recipients of bone marrow and solid organ transplants. *Br J Haematol* 119(3):596–607, 2002 Dec.
12. Cohen JI: Epstein–Barr virus infection. *New Engl J Med* 343:481–492, 2000.
13. Wagner HJ, Rooney CM, Heslop HE: Diagnosis and treatment of posttransplantation lymphoproliferative disease after hematopoietic stem cell transplantation. *Biol Blood Marrow Transplant* 8(1):1–8, 2002.
14. Young LS, Murray PG: Epstein–Barr virus and oncogenesis: from latent genes to tumours. *Oncogene* 22(33): 5108–5121, 2003 Aug 11.
15. Loren AW, Porter DL, Stadtmauer EA, Tsai DE: Post-transplant lymphoproliferative disorder: a review. *Bone Marrow Transplant* 31(3):145–155, 2003 Feb.
16. Shroff R, Rees L: The post-transplant lymphoproliferative disorder—a literature review. *Pediatr Nephrol* 19(4):369–377, 2004 Apr.
17. Smets F, Sokal EM: Epstein–Barr virus-related lymphoproliferation in children after liver transplant: role of

immunity, diagnosis, and management. *Pediatr Transplant* 6(4):280–287, 2002 Aug.

18. Finn L, Reyes J, Bueno J, Yunis E: Epstein–Barr virus infections in children after transplantation of the small intestine. *Am J Surg Pathol* 22(3):299–309, 1998 Mar.

19. Curtis RE, Travis LB, Rowlings PA, et al.: Risk of lymphoproliferative disorders after bone marrow transplantation: a multi-institutional study. *Blood* 94(7):2208–2216, 1999 Oct 1.

20. Lucas KG, Small TN, Heller G, Dupont B, O'Reilly RJ: The development of cellular immunity to Epstein–Barr virus after allogeneic bone marrow transplantation. *Blood* 87(6):2594–2603, 1996 Mar 15.

21. Lange A, Klimczak A, Dlubek D, Dybko J: B-cell lymphoproliferative syndrome and peripheral blood CD20+ cells expansion after hematopoietic stem cell transplantation: association with fludarabine and anti-thymocyte globulin containing conditioning regimen. *Transplant Proc* 35(8):3093–3095, 2003 Dec.

22. Hale G, Waldmann H: Risks of developing Epstein–Barr virus-related lymphoproliferative disorders after T-cell-depleted marrow transplants. CAMPATH Users. *Blood* 91(8):3079–3083, 1998 Apr 15.

23. Handgretinger R, Schumm M, Lang P, et al.: Transplantation of megadoses of purified haploidentical stem cells. *Ann N Y Acad Sci* 872:351–361, 1999 Apr 30.

24. Hauke RJ, Greiner TC, Smir BN, et al.: Epstein–Barr virus-associated lymphoproliferative disorder after autologous bone marrow transplantation: report of two cases. *Bone Marrow Transplant* 21:1271–1274, 1998.

25. Powell JL, Bunin NJ, Callahan C, Aplenc R, Griffin G, Grupp SA: An unexpectedly high incidence of Epstein–Barr virus lymphoproliferative disease after CD34+ selected autologous peripheral blood stem cell transplant in neuroblastoma. *Bone Marrow Transplant* 33(6):651–657, 2004 Mar.

26. Leblond V, Davi F, Charlotte F, et al.: Posttransplant lymphoproliferative disorders not associated with Epstein–Barr virus: a distinct entity? *J Clin Oncol* 16(6):2052–2059, 1998 Jun.

27. Nelson BP, Nalesnik MA, Bahler DW, Locker J, Fung JJ, Swerdlow SH: Epstein–Barr virus-negative post-transplant lymphoproliferative disorders: a distinct entity? *Am J Surg Pathol* 24(3):375–385, 2000 Mar.

28. Leblond V, Dhedin N, Bruneel M, et al.: Identification of prognostic factors in 61 patients with posttransplantation lymphoproliferative disorders. *J Clin Oncol* (3): 772–778, 2001 Feb 19.

29. Reams BD, McAdams HP, Howell DN, Steele MP, Davis RD, Palmer SM: Posttransplant lymphoproliferative disorder: incidence, presentation, and response to treatment in lung transplant recipients. *Chest* 124(4): 1242–1249, 2003 Oct.

30. Lucas KG, Burton RL, Zimmerman SE, et al.: Semiquantitative Epstein–Barr virus (EBV) polymerase chain reaction for the determination of patients at risk for EBV-induced lymphoproliferative disease after stem cell transplantation. *Blood* 91(10):3654–3661, 1998 May 15.

31. Aalto SM, Juvonen E, Tarkkanen J, et al.: Lymphoproliferative disease after allogeneic stem cell transplantation—pre-emptive diagnosis by quantification of Epstein–Barr virus DNA in serum. *J Clin Virol* 28(3):275–283, 2003 Dec.

32. Wagner HJ, Cheng YC, Huls MH, et al.: Prompt versus pre-emptive intervention for EBV- lymphoproliferative disease. *Blood* 2004 Jan 29. Epub ahead of print.

33. Carpentier L, Tapiero B, Alvarez F, Viau C, Alfieri C: Epstein–Barr virus (EBV) early-antigen serologic testing in conjunction with peripheral blood EBV DNA load as a marker for risk of posttransplantation lymphoproliferative disease. *J Infect Dis* 188(12):1853–1864, 2003 Dec 15.

34. Tsai DE, Nearey M, Hardy CL, et al.: Use of EBV PCR for the diagnosis and monitoring of post-transplant lymphoproliferative disorder in adult solid organ transplant patients. *Am J Transplant* 2(10):946–954, 2002 Nov.

35. Castellano-Sanchez AA, Li S, Qian J, Lagoo A, Weir E, Brat DJ: Primary central nervous system posttransplant lymphoproliferative disorders. *Am J Clin Pathol* 121(2):246–253, 2004 Feb.

36. Harris NL, Ferry JA, Swerdlow SH: Posttransplant lymphoproliferative disorders (PTLD): summary of Society for Hematopathology Workshop. *Semin Diag Pathol* 14:8, 1997.

37. Tsai DE, Hardy CL, Tomaszewski JE, et al.: Reduction in immunosuppression as initial therapy for posttransplant lymphoproliferative disorder: analysis of prognostic variables and long-term follow-up of 42 adult patients. *Transplantation* 71(8):1076–1088, 2001 Apr 27.

38. Kuehnle I, Huls MH, Liu Z, et al.: CD20 monoclonal antibody (rituximab) for therapy of Epstein–Barr virus lymphoma after hemopoietic stem-cell transplantation. *Blood* 95(4):1502–1505, 2000 Feb 15.

39. Davis JE, Moss DJ: Treatment options for post-transplant lymphoproliferative disorder and other Epstein–Barr virus-associated malignancies. *Tissue Antigens* 63(4): 285–292, 2004 Apr.

40. Benkerrou M, Jais JP, Leblond V, et al.: Anti-B-cell monoclonal antibody treatment of severe posttransplant B-lymphoproliferative disorder: prognostic factors and long-term outcome. *Blood* 92:3137–3147, 1998.

41. Garcia VD, Bonamigo Filho JL, Neumann J, et al.: Rituximab in association with rapamycin for post-transplant lymphoproliferative disease treatment. *Transpl Int* 16(3):202–206, 2003 Mar. Epub 2003 Feb 13.

42. Milpied N, Vasseur B, Parquet N, et al.: Humanized anti-CD20 monoclonal antibody (Rituximab) in post transplant B-lymphoproliferative disorder: a retrospective analysis on 32 patients. *Ann Oncol* 11(suppl 1):113–116, 2000.

43. Ganne V, Siddiqi N, Kamaplath B, et al.: Humanized anti-CD20 monoclonal antibody (Rituximab) treatment for post-transplant lymphoproliferative disorder. *Clin Transplant* 17(5):417–422, 2003 Oct.

44. van Esser JW, van der Holt B, Meijer E, et al.: Epstein–Barr virus (EBV) reactivation is a frequent event after allogeneic stem cell transplantation (SCT) and quantitatively predicts EBV-lymphoproliferative disease following T-cell–depleted SCT. *Blood* 98(4):972–978, 2001 Aug 15.

45. Kaleem Z, Hassan A, Pathan MH, White G: Flow cytometric evaluation of posttransplant B-cell lymphoproliferative disorders. *Arch Pathol Lab Med* 128(2):181–186, 2004 Feb.

46. Yang J, Tao Q, Flinn IW, et al.: Characterization of Epstein–Barr virus-infected B cells in patients with

posttransplantation lymphoproliferative disease: disappearance after rituximab therapy does not predict clinical response. *Blood* 96(13):4055–4063, 2000 Dec 15.

47. Gross TG, Hinrichs SH, Winner J, et al.: Treatment of post-transplant lymphoproliferative disease (PTLD) following solid organ transplantation with low-dose chemotherapy. *Ann Oncol* 9(3):339–340, 1998 Mar.

48. Orjuela M, Gross TG, Cheung YK, Alobeid B, Morris E, Cairo MS: A pilot study of chemoimmunotherapy (cyclophosphamide, prednisone, and rituximab) in patients with post-transplant lymphoproliferative disorder following solid organ transplantation. *Clin Cancer Res* 9(10 Pt 2):3945S–3952S, 2003 Sep 1.

49. Oertel SH, Papp-Vary M, Anagnostopoulos I, Hummel MW, Jonas S, Riess HB: Salvage chemotherapy for refractory or relapsed post-transplant lymphoproliferative disorder in patients after solid organ transplantation with a combination of carboplatin and etoposide. *Br J Haematol* 123(5):830–835, 2003 Dec.

50. O'Reilly RJ, Small TN, Papadopoulos E, Lucas K, Lacerda J, Koulova L: Biology and adoptive cell therapy of Epstein–Barr virus-associated lymphoproliferative disorders in recipients of marrow allografts. *Immunol Rev* 157:195–216, 1997 Jun.

51. Gustafsson A, Levitsky V, Zou JZ, et al.: Epstein–Barr virus (EBV) load in bone marrow transplant recipients at risk to develop posttransplant lymphoproliferative disease: prophylactic infusion of EBV-specific cytotoxic T cells. *Blood* 95(3):807–814, 2000 Feb 1.

52. Rooney CM, Smith CA, Ng CY, et al.: Infusion of cytotoxic T cells for the prevention and treatment of Epstein–Barr virus-induced lymphoma in allogeneic transplant recipients. *Blood* 92:1549–1555, 1998.

53. Nalesnik MA, Rao AS, Zeevi A, et al.: Autologous lymphokine-activated killer cell therapy of lymphoproliferative disorders arising in organ transplant recipients. *Transplant Proc* 29(3):1905–1906, 1997 May.

54. Haque T, Amlot PL, Helling N, et al.: Reconstitution of EBV-specific T cell immunity in solid organ transplant recipients. *J Immunol* 160(12):6204–6209, 1998 Jun 15.

55. Haque T, Wilkie GM, Taylor C, et al.: Treatment of Epstein–Barr-virus-positive post-transplantation lymphoproliferative disease with partly HLA-matched allogeneic cytotoxic T cells. *Lancet* 360(9331):436–442, 2002 Aug 10.

56. Faller DV, Mentzer SJ, Perrine SP: Induction of the Epstein–Barr virus thymidine kinase gene with concomitant nucleoside antivirals as a therapeutic strategy for Epstein–Barr virus-associated malignancies. *Curr Opin Oncol* 13(5):360–367, 2001 Sep.

57. Durandy A: Anti-B cell and anti-cytokine therapy for the treatment of post-transplant lymphoproliferative disorder: past, present, and future. *Transpl Infect Dis* 3(2):104–107, 2001 Jun.

58. Haddad E, Paczesny S, Leblond V, et al.: Treatment of B-lymphoproliferative disorder with a monoclonal anti-interleukin-6 antibody in 12 patients: a multicenter phase 1-2 clinical trial. *Blood* 97(6):1590–1597, 2001 Mar 15.

59. BPG Expert Group on Renal Transplantation: European best practice guidelines for renal transplantation. Section IV: Long-term management of the transplant recipient. IV.6.1. Cancer risk after renal transplantation. Post-transplant lymphoproliferative disease (PTLD): prevention and treatment. *Nephrol Dial Transplant* 17(suppl 4):31–33, 35–36, 2002.

60. Davis CL, Wood BL, Sabath DE: Interferon-alpha treatment of posttransplant lymphoproliferative disorder in recipients of solid organ transplants. *Transplantation* 66:1770–1779, 1998.

# Chapter 63

# TREATMENT APPROACH TO ADULT T-CELL LYMPHOMA/ LEUKEMIA

*Karen W.L. Yee and Francis J. Giles*

## INTRODUCTION

Human T-cell leukemia virus type 1 (HTLV-1), a double-stranded RNA retrovirus, has been demonstrated to be the causative agent in the development of adult T-cell leukemia/lymphoma (ATL/L). HTLV-1 infection is endemic in the southwestern part of Japan and the Caribbean basin, with geographic clusters reported in Africa, Central and South America, the Middle East, and the southeastern United States.[1]

The majority of individuals infected with HTLV-1 are asymptomatic carriers; however, a proportion will develop either ATL/L or a chronic inflammatory syndrome [e.g., HTLV-1-associated myelopathy/tropical spastic paraparesis (HAM/TSP), polymyositis, arthropathy, infective dermatitis, and uveitis].[2–7] The lifetime risk of an HTLV-1 carrier developing either ATL or HAM/TSP is 1–5% and 1–2%, respectively.[8–11] ATL occurs only after a long latency period, ranging from 10 to 30 years, with the accumulation of additional oncogenic events.[12–14]

Four criteria need to be fulfilled in order to make the diagnosis of ATL: (1) histologically and/or cytologically proven T-cell lymphoid malignancies (i.e., usually expression of CD2, CD3, CD4, and CD5 with absent CD7 and CD8), (2) abnormal T lymphocytes consistently present in the peripheral blood, except in the lymphoma type (i.e., flower cells and/or small and mature T lymphocytes with incised or lobulated nucleus), (3) seropositivity for HTLV-1 (by indirect immunofluorescence, enzyme-linked immunosorbent assay, passive hemagglutination, or Western blot), and (4) clonal integration of proviral DNA into the cellular DNA of neoplastic T cells [by Southern blot analysis, polymerase chain reaction (PCR), or inverse PCR].[15–19]

ATL is classified into four clinical subtypes (i.e., acute, lymphoma, chronic, or smouldering) with different prognoses and outcomes (Table 63.1). Because of the heterogeneous outcomes, even within a subtype, it

may be prudent to stratify all patients into high- and low-risk groups at the time of diagnosis on the basis of the following poor prognostic features: hypercalcemia, elevated levels of serum lactate dehydrogenase, poor performance status, age over 40 years, and multiple sites of disease.[16] Patients with low-, standard high-, and extremely high risk disease had median survival times of 37, 8, and 2.4 months, respectively.[16] Other features that have been associated with a poor outcome and/or progression from smouldering or chronic ATL to acute ATL include poor performance status, increased serum creatinine, high white blood cell count, microsatellite instability, high expression of the proliferation marker Ki-67, unusual immunophenotype, integration of a defective HTLV-1 provirus, deletions of *p15* and/or *p16* genes, and high serum thymidine kinase, serum soluble interleukin 2 receptor (IL-2R), serum $\beta_2$-microglobulin, or serum parathyroid hormone-related protein levels.[16,20–30] However, none of these risk factors have been prospectively validated.

## CONVENTIONAL TREATMENT MODALITIES

### CHEMOTHERAPY

#### Chronic and smouldering ATL

Approximately 90 patients with chronic or smouldering ATL have been treated with chemotherapy.[1,24,31–34] Overall survival (OS) does not appear to be significantly improved with chemotherapy compared to historical controls (10.9–16 months vs 24.3 months, respectively),[1,32,33] with only one retrospective study showing a median survival of 37.9 months for 51 patients treated with a variety of chemotherapy regimens.[24]

#### Acute and lymphomatous ATL

Patients with acute and lymphoma subtypes of ATL have been treated with a variety of chemotherapeutic regimens, initially those used for non-Hodgkin's lymphoma, with complete response (CR) rates of 19–36%

**Table 63.1**    Clinical subtypes of adult T-cell leukemia[15]

| Features | Subtypes | | | |
| --- | --- | --- | --- | --- |
| | Smouldering ($n = 45$) | Chronic ($n = 152$) | Lymphoma ($n = 156$) | Acute[a] ($n = 465$) |
| Lymphocytes ($\times 10^9$/L) | <4 | ≥4[b] | <4 | +/− |
| Abnormal T lymphocytes in PB (%) | ≥5[c] | ≥5[c] | ≤1 | ≥5[c] |
| Flower cells | Occasional | Occasional | − | +/− |
| Hypercalcemia | − | − | +/− | +/− |
| LDH | ≤1.5 × ULN | ≤2 × ULN | +/− | +/− |
| Skin lesions | +/− | +/− | +/− | +/− |
| Lung lesions | +/− | +/− | +/− | +/− |
| Bone lesions | − | − | +/− | +/− |
| Bone marrow involvement | − | − | +/− | +/− |
| Hepatosplenomegaly | − | +/− | +/− | +/− |
| Extranodal involvement (other than specified above) | − | − | +/− | +/− |
| Lymphadenopathy | − | +/− | +[d] | +/− |
| Infections at diagnosis (%) | 35.6 | 35.5 | 11.5 | 27.5 |
| Proportion of cases (%) | 5.5 | 18.6 | 19.1 | 56.8 |
| Median survival (months) | Not reached | 24.3 | 10.5 | 6.2 |
| Projected OS$_{4y}$(%) | 62.8 | 26.9 | 5.7 | 5 |

"−," Absent; "+," present; "+/−," may be present; OS$_{4y}$, 4 year overall survival; ULN, upper limit of normal.
[a] Patients with ATL who do not fit criteria for smouldering, chronic, or lymphoma subtypes.
[b] With T lymphocytes >3.5 × $10^9$/L (including abnormal T lymphocytes).
[c] If abnormal T lymphocytes in PB <5%, patients should have biopsy-proven malignant lesion(s).
[d] Biopsy-proven; +/− no specific qualification.

Modified from Shimoyama et al. 1991.

and median survivals of 4.7–10 months.[16,35–37] Attempts to improve the response rates and OS led to the incorporation of multiple non-cross-resistant agents, extended duration of therapy, and incorporation of intrathecal chemotherapy (in an attempt to prevent meningeal recurrence), yielding CR rates of 17–44% (Table 63.2).[1,24,31–33,38–44] Responses were not durable and significantly lower for patients with ATL compared with B-cell non-Hodgkin's lymphoma or peripheral T-cell lymphoma.[38,39,42] Reported response durations were less than 8 months,[32,44] and median OS was only 5.5–13 months.

These studies[32,38,39,42,44] demonstrate the limitations of treating patients with ATL with conventional agents. The lack of good-quality responses (i.e., CRs) achieved with chemotherapy is a consequence of several factors: intrinsic resistance of ATL cells secondary to P-glycoprotein overexpression, mutations of the tumor suppressor gene *p53*, expression of the free-radical scavenger, ATL-derived factor, and abnormalities of topoisomerase II activities.[45–50]

### STEM CELL TRANSPLANTATION
#### Autologous stem cell transplantation
##### Acute and lymphomatous ATL
At least 13 patients with ATL (nine acute and four lymphoma) have received an autologous stem cell

transplantation (ASCT).[51–59] Median age was 49 years (range 33–65 years); 61.5% of patients had refractory disease, partial responses (PRs), or were in early relapse at the time of transplant. All patients achieved or maintained either a CR (92.3%) or a PR (7.7%) post-ASCT. Although disappearance of the monoclonal band by Southern blot analysis and by inverse PCR after ASCT can be demonstrated in a few cases, the durability of remission is unclear.[51,52] Clinical outcomes have been complicated by early recurrence and fatal infections, with OS of 0.47–12+ months and only 8% of patients surviving >12 months post-ASCT. CD34$^+$ selection does not improve results; Southern blot analysis of the peripheral blood stem cells (PBSCs) revealed contamination with HTLV-1-infected cells[57] and have been documented relapses despite.[52,53,57,59] ASCT does not have a role in the treatment of patients with ATL, outside of an investigational trial.

#### Allogeneic stem cell transplantation
##### Myeloablative stem cell transplantation
The disappearance of the proviral monoclonal band by Southern blot analysis and PCR after allogeneic stem cell transplant has been demonstrated; however, serial analysis was not performed to determine durability of remission.[60–64] At this time, it is unclear

**Table 63.2** Chemotherapeutic regimens for treatment of acute and lymphoma ATL

| Chemotherapy regimen | Patient characteristics | | | | | Response | | Reference |
|---|---|---|---|---|---|---|---|---|
| | N (evaluable) | Median age (range, years) | Acute subtype (%) | Prior therapy (%) | Median F/U (months) | Response rate (%) | Median OS (months) | |
| CV'P | 10 | 56.5 (44–72) | 77.8 | 0 | 6.4 | | 6.3 | 35 |
| VEPA (n = 24) vs VEPA-M (n = 30) | 54 | 27.6% ≥ 60 years[a] | | | NR | CR 17 vs 37 (Overall CR 28) | 7.5[b] | 38–40 |
| CHOP (n = 14) vs VEPA (n = 32) [LSG1/LSG2] | 46 | 56.1–57.5 (28–74) | 0 | 0 | NR | CR 35.7 vs 43.8 | 4.7 vs 7.7 | 36 |
| Single agent[c], COP, VEMP, VEPA, CHOP, MACOP-B, or other combination therapy | 717 (635) | 57.1 (24–92)[d] | NR | 0 | NR | CR 18.7 | 10[d] | 16 |
| Alternating VEPA-B, M-FEPA, and VEPP-B [LSG4] | 43 | NR | NR | NR | 56 | CR 42 | 8 | 31, 40–42 |
| VEPA, LSG4, or LSG4 + cisplatin | 110 (108)[e] | NR | 76.4 | 0 | NR | OR 67.6; CR 18.5; PR 49.1 | 5.5 vs 8.7[f] | 24, 31 |
| RCM protocol | 43 | 64 (34–78) | 65.1 | NR | NR | OR 86; CR 20.9; PR 65.1 | 6 | 43 |
| CHOP/VP-16/MCNU/mito | 83 (81) | 59 (32–74) | 54.3 | 32.1 | NR | OR 74.1; CR 35.8; PR 38.3 | 8.5 | 44 |
| Anthracycline- or mitoxantrone-based therapy[g] | 21 (16)[h] | 51 (21–74) | 61.9 | NR | NR | OR 56.3; CR 18.8; PR 37.5 | 5.5 | 1 |
| OPEC/MPEC (n = 79) or DOEP (n = 8) | 87[i] | 62 (41–87)[j] | 58.6[k] | 19.5 | 9.5 | OR 90; CR 31; PR 59 | 7.5 | 32 |
| Alternating VCAP, AMP, and VECP & IT [LSG15] | 96 (93) | 54.5 (29–69) | 60.4[l] | 0 | NR | OR 80.6; CR 35.5; PR 45.1 | 13 | 33 |
| CHOP | 22 | NR | NR | NR | NR | NR | 7.3[j] | 45 |

P = NS unless otherwise specified.

AMP, doxorubicin, ranimustine, and prednisolone; CV'P, cyclophosphamide, doxorubicin, vincristine, and prednisolone or prednisone; CHOP, cyclophosphamide, doxorubicin, vincristine, and prednisone; CHOP/VP-16/MCNU/mito, CHOP followed by etoposide, ranimustine, and mitoxantrone; COP, cyclophosphamide, vincristine, and prednisolone; DOEP, daily oral etoposide and prednisolone; F/U, follow-up; IT, intrathecal methotrexate and cytarabine; LSG4, doxorubicin, cyclophosphamide, vincristine, prednisone, vindesine, methotrexate, etoposide, procarbazine, and bleomycin; MACOP-B, methotrexate, doxorubicin, cyclophosphamide, vincristine, prednisolone, and bleomycin; M-FEPA, methotrexate, vindesine, cyclophosphamide, prednisolone, and doxorubicin; NR, not reported; OPEC/MPEC, vincristine or methotrexate, prednisolone, etoposide, and cyclophosphamide; PBSCT, peripheral blood stem cell transplant; RCM, response-oriented cyclic multidrug protocol (i.e., cyclophosphamide, prednisolone, vindesine, and ranimustine (week 1) followed by cyclophosphamide, prednisolone, methotrexate, and pirarubicin (week 2), cyclophosphamide, prednisolone, etoposide, peplomycin, and cytarabine (week 3), and cyclophosphamide, prednisolone, mitomycin C, and doxorubicin (week 4); VCAP, vincristine, cyclophosphamide, doxorubicin, and prednisolone; VEPA, vincristine, etoposide, cyclophosphamide, prednisolone, and doxorubicin; VEPA, vincristine, cyclophosphamide, prednisolone, and doxorubicin; VEPA-B, VEPA and bleomycin; VEPA-M, VEPA and methotrexate; VEPP-B, methotrexate, cyclophosphamide, procarbazine, prednisolone, and doxorubicin.

[a] Median age not reported; [b] for ATL patients treated with both VEPA and VEPA-M; [c] etoposide, interferon alpha, interferon gamma, cyclophosphamide, vincristine, prednisolone, or other single agent; [d] for all 854 patients (including 137 untreated patients); [e] includes 51 chronic and 11 smoldering subtypes; [f] for acute vs lymphoma subtype; [g] except for one acute ATL patient who received single-agent cyclophosphamide, one lymphoma subtype supportive care only, and one chronic ATL topical therapy for skin disease (two patients also received PBSCT); [h] includes one chronic subtype; [i] includes 14 chronic subtypes; [j] mean; [k] includes 10 chronic subtypes; [l] includes patients with acute (n = 14) ATL; lymphoma (n = 22), and progressive chronic (n = 14) ATL.

whether undetectable minimal residual disease is associated with improved relapse-free survival and OS.

### Chronic and smouldering ATL

The use of myeloablative matched-related donor (MRD) allogeneic stem cell transplantation has been reported in only four patients with chronic ATL (Table 63.3).[60,67,71] Median age was 40.5 years (range 33–55 years); three patients had a PR and one relapsed disease at the time of transplant. Seventy-five percent of donors were HTLV-1 seronegative. All patients achieved either a CR (75%) or a PR (25%) after transplantation.

**Table 63.3** Myeloablative allogeneic stem cell transplant for treatment of ATL

| Age (years) | Disease status at SCT | Median F/U (months) | Donor/ status HTLV-1 | Response to SCT | Disease control[a] (months) | Overall survival[a] (months) | Cause of death | Reference |
|---|---|---|---|---|---|---|---|---|
| | | | | *Acute subtype* | | | | |
| 43 | Refractory | 6.8 | MRD/NR | CR | 6.2 | 6.8 | CMV interstitial pneumonitis | 65 |
| 48 | CR | 11.8 | MRD/− | CR | 11 | 11.8 | ATL | 66 |
| 41 | CR | 23+ | MRD/− | CR | 23+ | 23+ | NA | 61 |
| 42 | CR | 13 | MRD/− | CR | 13 | 13 | ATL | 64 |
| 37 | PR | 80+ | MRD/+ | CR | 80+ | 80+ | NA | 64 |
| 38 | CR | NR | MRD/+ | CR | 3 | NR | Renal insufficiency | 67 |
| 47 | Refractory | 24+ | MRD/− | CR | 24+ | 24+ | NA | 68 |
| 46 | Relapsed | 14+ | MRD/+ | CR | 14+ | 14+ | NA | 62 |
| 38 | CR | 10.1 | MRD/+ | CR | 3.9 | 10.1 | Renal insufficiency | 60 |
| 41 | CR | 34.4+ | MRD/− | CR | 34.4+ | 34.4+ | NA | 60 |
| 37 | PR | 31.5+ | MRD/+ | CR | 31.5+ | 31.5+ | NA | 60 |
| 44 | PR | 28.7+ | MRD/− | CR | 28.7+ | 28.7+ | NA | 60 |
| 45 | CR | 15.5 | MUD/− | CR | 15.5 | 15.5 | GI bleeding | 60 |
| 42 | CR | 19.5+ | MRD/− | CR | 19.5+ | 19.5+ | NA | 60 |
| 48 | Refractory | 4.1 | MRD/− | CR | 4.1 | 4.1 | Acute GvHD | 60 |
| 47 | PR | 11.8+ | MRD/− | CR | 3.7 | 11.8+ | NA | 60 |
| 51 | Refractory | 16+ | MUD/NS | CR | 16+ | 16+ | NA | 63 |
| 36 | Relapsed | 7+ | MRD/NS | CR | 2 | 7+ | NA | 69, 70 |
| 51 | CR | 14 | MRD/+ | CR | 7 | 14 | NR | 70 |
| 47 | CR | 13 | MRD/− | CR | 13 | 13 | Chronic GvHD | 71 |
| 46 | CR | 26.8+ | MRD/+ | CR | 26.8+ | 26.8+ | NA | 71 |
| 27 | CR | 31.5+ | MRD/− | CR | 31.5+ | 31.5+ | NA | 71 |
| 46 | PD | 4.5 | MRD/+ | CR | 4.5 | 4.5 | GI bleeding due to acute GvHD | 71 |
| | | | | *Lymphomatous subtype* | | | | |
| 51 | PR | 9.3 | MRD/+ | CR | 9.3 | 9.3 | Pneumonitis | 60 |
| 15 | CR | 23.3+ | MRD/− | CR | 23.3+ | 23.3+ | NA | 71 |
| 44 | PD | 1.6 | 2-antigen mismatch related/− | CR | 1.6 | 1.6 | Acute GvHD | 71 |
| 47 | CR | 12+ | MRD/− | CR | 12+ | 12+ | NA | 71 |
| 46 | PR | 10 | MUD/− | CR | 10 | 10 | NR | 70 |
| | | | | *Chronic subtype* | | | | |
| 33 | PR | 18+ | MRD/+ | CR | 18+ | 18+ | NA | 67 |
| 33 | PR | 32.7+ | MRD/− | PR | 32.7+ | 32.7+ | NA | 60 |
| 48 | Relapsed | 15 | MRD/− | CR | NR | 15 | Chronic GvHD | 71 |
| 55 | CR | 7.7 | MRD/− | CR | NR | 7.7 | Chronic GvHD | 71 |

MRD, matched-related donor; MUD, matched unrelated donor; NA, not applicable; NR, not reported; PD, progressive disease.
[a] After stem cell transplant.

Median OS was 16.5 months (range 7.7–32.7+ months) with 50% of patients dying from graft-versus-host disease (GvHD). At the current time, the role of allogeneic transplantation in this setting remains to be defined.

### Acute and lymphomatous ATL

Results of myeloablative allogeneic transplantation have been described in 28 patients with acute ($n = 23$) and lymphomatous ($n = 5$) ATL (Table 63.3).[61–71] Median age was 44.5 years (range 15–51 years); 28.6% of patients had relapsed, refractory, or progressive disease at the time of transplant, and 21.4% had a PR. Sixty-four percent of donors were HTLV-1 seronegative. Only three patients received a matched unrelated donor (MUD) transplant, two a T-cell-depleted transplant, and one a two-antigen mismatch related transplant. All patients achieved a CR after transplantation. Median OS was 14 months (range 1.6–80+ months). Survival data, based on (i) donor HTLV-1 status, (ii) ATL subtype, and (iii) recipient status at the time of transplant, have been evaluated in patients who received an MRD, unmanipulated, allotransplant. Median OS for recipients of donor HTLV-1-seropositive stem cells was 9.7 months (range 4.5–80+ months) compared to 8.6 months (range 4.1–34.4+ months) for donor HTLV-1-seronegative stem cells; for acute subtypes, 8.4 months (range 4.1–80+ months) compared to 9.3 months (range 9.3–23.3+ months) for lymphomatous subtypes; and for patients transplanted in CR, 13 months (range 10.1–34.4+ months) compared to 9.3 months (range 9.3–80+ months) and 4.5 months (range 4.1–24+ months) for patients transplanted in PR and with progressive, relapsed, or refractory disease, respectively

### Nonmyeloablative stem cell transplantation

The importance of the host immune responses in eradicating ATL cells and controlling disease onset or recurrence is underscored by a graft-versus-leukemia effect postallogeneic transplantation,[60,61] recurrence of disease after T-cell-depleted allogeneic stem cell transplants,[64,66] and reports of ATL occurring postsolid organ transplantation.[72] Reconstituted cellular immunity, as manifested by induction of cytotoxic T lymphocytes against HTLV-1-infected cells, in ATL patients after nonmyeloablative allogeneic stem cell transplantation from HTLV-1-negative HLA-identical siblings may contribute to graft-versus-leukemia effects.[73] These data, together with the high treatment-related mortality associated with standard allogeneic transplantation, have provided the impetus for studies, using low-intensity conditioning regimens.

### Acute and lymphomatous ATL

Results of nonmyeloablative stem cell transplantation have been reported for eight patients wih ATL (five acute and three lymphoma) (Table 63.4).[70,71,74,75] Median age was 55 years (range 52–59 years); 50% of patients had either refractory or progressive disease at the time of transplantation, and 25% had a PR. A fludarabine-based regimen was used in all but two cases.[70,74] Five out of six patients achieved a CR after transplant; however, median survival was only 2.3 months (range 0.8–9+ months). The two patients who had achieved a CR at the time of transplant were still alive at 8+ and 9+

**Table 63.4**  Nonmyeloablative allogeneic stem cell transplant for treatment of ATL

| Age (years) | Disease status at SCT | Median F/U (months) | Donor/ status HTLV-1 | Response to SCT | Disease control[a] (months) | Overall survival[a] (months) | Cause of death | Reference |
|---|---|---|---|---|---|---|---|---|
| | | | | *Acute subtype* | | | | |
| 55 | CR | 9+ | MRD/− | CR | 9+ | 9+ | NA | 74 |
| 52 | PR | 0.8 | MRD/− | NR | NR | 0.8 | Interstitial pneumonitis | 71 |
| 53 | PR | 4 | Partial mismatch related/− | NR | NR | 4 | NR | 70 |
| 58 | Refractory | 1 | Partial mismatch related/+ | CR | NR | 1 | NR | 70 |
| 55 | Refractory | 2 | MRD/− | NR | NR | 2 | NR | 70 |
| | | | | *Lymphomatous subtype* | | | | |
| 59 | PD | 2.3 | NR/NR | CR | 0.4 | 2.3 | Variceal hemorrhage | 75 |
| 59 | PD | 2.3 | MUD/− | CR | 2.3 | 2.3 | GI bleeding | 71 |
| 55 | CR | 8+ | MRD/− | CR | 8+ | 8+ | NA | 70 |

MRD, matched-related donor; MUD, matched unrelated donor; NA, not applicable; NR, not reported; PD, progressive disease.
[a] After stem cell transplant.

months[70,74]; one of whom demonstrated undetectable proviral load in the peripheral blood mononuclear cells by PCR analysis.[74]

Evaluation of transplantation data is complicated by heterogeneity in patient selection, choice of conditioning regimen, source of stem cells, degree of antigen mismatch, and HTLV-1 status of donors. For both myeloablative and nonmyeloablative allogeneic stem cell transplantations, the optimal conditioning regimen, source of stem cells (bone marrow vs peripheral blood), and type of GvHD prophylaxis are unclear. The use of HTLV-1-seropositive, but disease-free, donors is also uncertain. HTLV-1-seropositive donors may improve transplantation results by providing viral-specific immunocompetent cells and preventing clonal expression of infected lymphocytes posttransplantation. However, there is a theoretical concern that recipients of stem cells from HTLV-1-seropositive donors, with oligoclonal integration in donor germline by Southern analysis,[62] will be at risk of developing or relapsing with ATL after allogeneic stem cell transplantation.

## OTHER TREATMENT MODALITIES

### RETROVIRAL AND IMMUNOMODULATORY AGENTS
**Retroviral monotherapy**
Maintenance of viral DNA load can occur through either host genome replication or viral replication through the HTLV-1 reverse transcriptase.[19] HTLV-1 replication can be inhibited by a variety of nucleoside reverse transcriptase inhibitors, including zidovudine, zalcitabine, tenofovir, and possibly, lamivudine.[76,77] Zidovudine (AZT) is a thymidine analog, which after phosphorylation is incorporated into proviral DNA causing chain termination. It is unclear whether zidovudine monotherapy has significant activity.[78]

**Interferons**
Single-agent interferon alpha has been evaluated in a small series of patients with acute, lymphomatous, and chronic ATL, with OR rates of 25–33% and CR rates of 0–25%.[79,80] There have been anecdotal reports using interferon beta and gamma to treat patients with ATL with modest activity.[81] Twelve patients have been treated with interferon alpha in combination with bestrabucil, a conjugate of chlorambucil and β-estradiol, and prednisolone.[82] Nine of the patients (75%) obtained a PR with a median response duration of 9 weeks.

**Retrovirals and interferon**
The mechanism of action of combination zidovudine and interferon alpha remains unclear. The therapeutic effects may be mediated by inhibition of HTLV-1 replication rather than a direct cytotoxic effect on leukemic cells.[83]

### Chronic or smouldering ATL
Only three patients with smouldering ($n = 1$) or chronic ($n = 2$) ATL have been treated with combination zidovudine and interferon alpha, with none achieving a CR.[84–86]

### Acute and lymphomatous ATL
AZT and interferon alpha have been used to treat over 80 patients with acute or lymphomatous ATL (Table 63.5).[84–91] The majority of patients had acute ATL and had received prior therapy. Overall response rates ranged from 14 to 89% with CR rates of 0–53%. Higher responses may be achieved in previously untreated patients.[91] Median OS remained dismal and was usually <12 months. However, it appears to be significantly increased in responders.[87,90,91]

These therapeutic outcomes have not exceeded those with recent chemotherapeutic regimens, but can be administered to patients with poor performance status[87] and may be associated with less toxicity, the major toxicities being hematologic.

### NUCLEOSIDE ANALOGS
There are currently three analogs of deoxyadenosine, i.e., fludarabine, cladribine, and pentostatin, in clinical use for the treatment of lymphoproliferative disorders. In patients with ATL, most experience has been obtained with pentostatin and the least with fludarabine.[93]

Single-agent cladribine (2-chlorodeoxyadenosine) has limited activity in patients with relapsed or refractory acute or lymphomatous ATL (OR 7%; CR 0%).[94,95] At least four studies have assessed the effectiveness of pentostatin (deoxycoformycin) monotherapy in patients with ATL.[96–99] The majority of patients had either acute or lymphomatous subtypes, and had received prior therapy. Overall response rates were 15–20% with CR rates ≤10%. The majority of studies did not report OS.[96,97,99]

Given these encouraging results, a multicenter phase II trial evaluated the efficacy of pentostatin in combination with doxorubicin, vincristine, etoposide, and prednisolone in 60 patients with previously untreated ATL (34 acute, 21 lymphoma, and 5 chronic).[100] Median age was 56 years (range 31–69 years). Fifty-nine patients were evaluable for response. Overall response was 52.5% (CR 28.8%; PR 23.7%). However, therapy was discontinued in 62.7% of patients—52.5% during induction therapy because of progressive disease and 10.2% because of toxicity. Only 17% completed the entire 10 cycles of therapy. Both median follow-up and median OS were 7.4 months. Therefore, pentostatin-containing regimens have limited activity in patients with ATL.

### ARSENIC TRIOXIDE
Treatment of HTLV-1-transformed cells and primary ATL samples with arsenic trioxide can inhibit cell

**Table 63.5   Retroviral and/or immunomodulatory agents for treatment of acute and lymphoma ATL**

| N (evaluable) | Patient characteristics | | | | Response | | | Reference |
|---|---|---|---|---|---|---|---|---|
| | Median age (range, years) | Acute subtype (%) | Prior therapy (%) | Median F/U (months) | Response rate (%) | Median disease control (months) | Median OS (months) | |
| *Interferon alpha and zidovudine* | | | | | | | | |
| 19 | 48 (16–88) | 90 | 36.8 | NR | OR 58 CR 26; PR 32 | NR | 3 | 87, 88 |
| 10 (9)[a] | 35 (23–75) | 80 | 10 | NR | OR 89 CR 22; PR 67 | EFS 12 | NR | 84, 85 |
| 7 | 28 (18–56) | 43 | 100 | NR | OR 14 CR 0; PR 14 | 9 | NR[c] | 89 |
| 15 | 54 (28–79) | 73 | 80 | NR | OR 67[d] | Response duration 10 | 18 | 90 |
| 18 (12) | 47.5 (22–68) | 61 | 83.3 | NR | OR 25 CR 8; PR 17 | Response duration 2.4 | 6 | 86 |
| 19 (17)[e] | 45 (27–75) | 79 | 31.6 | 36+ | OR 76 CR 53; PR 23 | EFS 7 | 11 | 91 |
| *Interferon alpha and arsenic trioxide* | | | | | | | | |
| 7 | 46 (28–56) | 57 | 86 | 1.5 | OR 57 CR 14; PR 43 | PFS 1.5 | 1.5 | 92 |

EFS, event-free survival; F/U, follow-up; PFS, progression-free survival; IFN, interferon; AZT, zidovudine.

[a]Includes one smouldering subtype; [b]includes two chronic subtypes; [c]all six nonresponders did not survive for >1 month; [d] at the time of study, 8 of 15 patients were in CR or PR; therefore, 10 of 15 patients achieved or maintained a response on AZT and IFN (but no further details provided); [e] 3 of these patients had been previously reported (Refs. 84 and 85).

proliferation and induce apoptosis.[101–103] A synergistic effect is achieved when arsenic is combined with interferon alpha, leading to $G_1$ cell cycle arrest, inhibition of cell proliferation, and induction of apoptosis.[101]

A phase II study assessed the efficacy of combination therapy with arsenic trioxide and interferon alpha in seven patients with relapsed or refractory ATL (four acute and three lymphoma).[92] Median age was 46 years (range 28–56 years). None of the patients completed the planned treatment because of toxicity ($n = 3$) or disease progression ($n = 4$). Median treatment duration of arsenic trioxide was 22 days (range 17–28 days) and 21 days (range 4–28 days) for interferon alpha. Overall response was 57% (CR 14%; PR 43%). Progression-free survival was 1.5 months (range <1–32+ months) with a median OS of 1.5 months (range 1–32+ months).

Experience with retinoids as a single agent or in combination with interferon alpha and zidovudine in patients with ATL has been limited. Less than 15 ATL patients have been treated,[104–109] with only 1 patient with concomitant acute promyelocytic leukemia and smouldering ATL achieving a CR.[104] It is unclear whether improved efficacy may be obtained on combining retinoids with chemotherapy or novel targeted therapies.

## TOPOSIOMERASE INHIBITORS

Conventional topoisomerase II inhibitors, such as the epipodophyllotoxins (e.g., etoposide) and the anthracyclines (e.g., doxorubicin), have been administered to patients with ATL, usually as part of a multiagent chemotherapy regimen (see above) (Table 63.2).[110]

### Irinotecan hydrochloride

Irinotecan hydrochloride (CPT-11), a camptothecin derivative, is a prodrug that is converted to the active compound SN-38, which in turn inhibits topoisomerase I. CPT-11 was evaluated in a phase II study involving 13 patients (3 acute and 10 lymphoma) with relapsed or refractory ATL.[111] Median age was 63 years (range 44–78 years). The OR rate was 38.5% (CR 7.7%; PR 30.8%) with a median response duration of 31 days. All responders had lymphoma subtype. Grade 3 or 4 toxicities included leukopenia (66.7%), thrombocytopenia (41.7%), anemia (33.3%), and diarrhea (46.2%). One treatment-related death occurred.

### Sobuzoxane

Sobuzoxane (MST-16), a topoisomerase II inhibitor, is an orally administered bis(2,6-dioxopiperazine) analog prodrug that is converted to the active metabolite ICRF-154.[112] MST-16 has been administered to 24 patients with ATL (13 acute, 8 lymphoma, and 2 chronic) in a dose-escalating phase I/II study.[113] Median age was 55 years (range 41–76 years). Twenty-five percent of patients had been previously treated. Of the 23 evaluable patients, OR rate was 43.5% (CR 8.7%; PR 34.8%); all responses occurred in previously untreated patients. Responses were observed mostly in patients who received MST-16 at doses of 1200–1600 mg/day. Median duration of responses was 282 days and 41 days for patients who achieved a CR and PR, respectively. Common grade 3 or 4 toxicities included reversible leukopenia (80%) and anemia (26.1%).

Based on the findings of the phase I/II study, MST-16 has been evaluated at a dose of 1600 mg/day.[114] Preliminary results in six patients with ATL (subtype not specified) have been presented.[114] Median age was 47 years (range 41–76 years). Only one patient had received prior therapy. Overall response rate was 66.7% (CR 33.3%; PR 33.3%) with a median response duration of 5 months. The major toxicity was myelosuppression.

## MONOCLONAL ANTIBODIES

### Anti-Tac antibodies

#### Unmodified anti-Tac monoclonal antibodies

Nineteen patients with ATL (11 acute, 4 lymphoma, and 4 chronic) were treated with an unmodified murine anti-Tac monoclonal antibody.[115] Nine patients were previously untreated. Therapy was relatively well tolerated. Three of six responding patients developed human antimurine antibodies (HAMA) against the anti-Tac antibody. An OR rate of 32% (CR 11%; PR 21%) was achieved with response durations of 9 weeks to over 3 years. Responses were seen in patients with lymphoma ($n = 2$), chronic ($n = 3$), and acute ($n = 1$) subtypes; only two were previously treated and four had soluble IL-2R levels of less than 10,000 U/mL. To overcome limitations with murine antibodies, including a short circulating half-life in humans, increased immunogenicity with repeated dosing, and relatively ineffective recruitment of host antibody-dependent cellular cytotoxicity, a humanized anti-Tac antibody (daclizumab) was developed.[116,117] Anecdotal reports of remissions in patients with chronic and smouldering forms of ATL treated with daclizumab have been observed.[118] Therefore, single-agent daclizumab is currently being evaluated in patients with ATL in a phase I/II study.

#### Radiolabeled anti-Tac monoclonal antibodies

Yttrium-90 radiolabeled murine anti-Tac antibody has been administered to 18 patients with ATL (11 acute, 2 lymphoma, and 5 chronic) in a phase I/II study.[119] Eight patients were previously untreated. Five of nine responding patients developed HAMA against the anti-Tac antibody. Grade 3 or 4 toxicities consisted of myelosuppression (67%), transient hepatotoxicity (17%), and renal toxicity (6%). An OR rate of 56% (CR 12%; PR 44%) was achieved with response durations of 1 month to over 33 months. Responses were seen in patients with chronic ($n = 3$) and acute ($n = 6$) subtypes; only three were previously treated and five had soluble IL-2R levels of less than 10,000 U/ml.

## SUPPORTIVE CARE

Patients with ATL often present with infectious complications (i.e., bacterial, fungal, protozoal, and/or viral) at diagnosis (Table 63.1).[15] Infectious complications at diagnosis were observed less frequently in the lymphoma subtype than all other subtypes ($P < 0.01$), suggesting that this subset of patients may be less immunosuppressed.[15] Several mechanisms have been reported to account for this immunodeficient state, including impaired cytotoxic function of HTLV-1-infected CD8$^+$ lymphocytes, modulation of helper T-lymphocyte responses with predominantly a T$_H$1 cytokine response, and suppressed production of T lymphocytes in the thymus in HTLV-1-infected individuals.[120–122]

Prevention of opportunistic infections is, therefore, crucial to improving survival in ATL. Prophylactic co-trimoxazole is effective in reducing the incidence of *Pneumocystis carinii* pneumonia in patients with ATL. Stool should be screened for *Strongyloides* at diagnosis, and patients with positive cultures treated. These patients may require prolonged prophylaxis against *Strongyloides*. Similarly, prophylaxis against fungal and viral infections should be considered.

## SUMMARY

There is currently no curative or proven effective therapy for ATL. Given the poor results with conventional therapies, every possible attempt should be made to enroll patients with chronic, acute, and lymphomatous ATL onto investigational clinical trials.

For patients who are not candidates or cannot be enrolled onto a clinical trial, the following approach may be considered. Because of the lack of proven effective therapy and relatively long survival, patients with smouldering ATL should be observed until signs of disease progression. In order to minimize treatment-related toxicities and mortality, patients with low-risk chronic ATL should not receive chemotherapy, but may benefit from therapy with AZT and interferon alpha or monoclonal IL-2R antibodies. For patients with high-risk chronic, acute, or lymphomatous ATL, chemotherapy with anthracycline-based regimen or combination of AZT and interferon alpha should be instituted in an attempt to achieve a CR or PR. Patients with chemosensitive disease and a suitable donor should proceed with an allogeneic transplant. For patients with no response, progressive disease, or relapsed disease, investigational agents against novel targets (previously described) should be considered. Since most patients relapse after chemotherapy or AZT and interferon alpha therapy, patients who achieve a CR and are not candidates for or do not wish to receive an allogeneic stem cell transplant, some form of maintenance therapy should be considered, such as AZT and interferon alpha (after chemotherapy), or monoclonal IL-2R antibodies. All patients should receive prophylaxis against *Pneumocystis carinii* pneumonia, and should be evaluated for prophylaxis against fungal, viral, and *Strongyloides* infections.

## REFERENCES

1. Pawson R, Richardson DS, Pagliuca A, et al.: Adult T-cell leukemia/lymphoma in London: clinical experience of 21 cases. *Leuk Lymphoma* 31:177, 1998.
2. Morgan O StC, Rodgers-Johnson P, Mora C, Char G: HTLV-I and polymyositis in Jamaica. *Lancet* 2:1184, 1989.
3. Sherman MP, Amin RM, Rodgers-Johnson PE, et al.: Identification of human T cell leukemia/lymphoma virus type I antibodies, DNA, and protein in patients with polymyositis. *Arthritis Rheum* 38:690, 1995.
4. Nishioka K, Maruyama I, Sato K, et al.: Chronic inflammatory arthropathy associated with HTLV-I. *Lancet* 1:441, 1989.
5. Sato K, Maruyama I, Maruyama Y, et al.: Arthritis in patients infected with human T lymphotropic virus type I. Clinical and immunopathologic features. *Arthritis Rheum* 34:714, 1991.
6. LaGrenade L, Hanchard B, Fletcher V, et al.: Infective dermatitis of Jamaican children: a marker for HTLV-I infection. *Lancet* 336:1345, 1990.
7. Mochizuki M, Watanabe T, Yamaguchi K, et al.: HTLV-I uveitis: a distinct clinical entity caused by HTLV-I. *Jpn J Cancer Res* 82:236, 1992.
8. Kondo T, Kono H, Miyamoto N, et al.: Age- and sex-specific cumulative rate and risk of ATLL for HTLV-1 carriers. *Int J Cancer* 43:1061, 1989.
9. Cleghorn FR, Manns A, Falk R, et al.: Effect of human T-lymphotrophic virus type I infection on non-Hodgkin's lymphoma incidence. *J Natl Cancer Inst* 87:1009, 1995.
10. Tajima K: The 4th nation-wide study of adult T-cell leukemia/lymphoma (ATL) in Japan: estimates of risk of ATL and its geographical and clinical features. The T- and B-cell Malinancy Study Group. *Int J Cancer* 45:237, 1990.
11. Maloney EM, Cleghorn FR, Morgan OS, et al.: Incidence of HTLV-I associated myelopathy/tropical spastic paraparesis (HAM/TSP) in Jamaica and Trinidad. *J Acquir Immune Defic Syndr Hum Retrovirol* 17:167, 1998.
12. Okamoto T, Ohno Y, Tsugane S, et al.: Multi-step carcinogenesis model for adult T-cell leukemia. *Jpn J Cancer Res* 80:191, 1989.
13. Osame M, Izumo S, Igata A, et al.: Blood transfusion and HTLV-I associated myelopathy. *Lancet* ii:104, 1986.
14. Chen Y-C, Wang C-H, Su I-J, et al.: Infection of HTLV type I and development of human T-cell leukemia/lymphoma in patients with hematologic neoplasms: a possible linkage to blood transfusion. *Blood* 74:388, 1989.
15. Shimoyama M, and members of The Lymphoma Study Group (1984–1987): Diagnostic criteria and classification of clinical subtypes of adult T-cell leukemia-lymphoma: a report from The Lymphoma Study Group (1984–1987). *Br J Haematol* 79:428, 1991.

16. Lymphoma Study Group (1984–1987): Major prognostic factors of patients with adult T-cell leukemia-lymphoma: a cooperative study. *Leuk Res* 15:81, 1991.

17. Uchiyama T, Yodoi J, Sagawa K, et al.: Adult T-cell leukemia: clinical and hematologic features of 16 cases. *Blood* 50:481, 1977.

18. Takemoto S, Matsuoka M, Yamaguchi K, et al.: A novel diagnostic method of adult T-cell leukemia: monoclonal integration of human T-cell lymphotropic virus type I provirus DNA detected by inverse polymerase chain reaction. *Blood* 84:3080, 1994.

19. Wattel E, Cavrois M, Gessain A, Wain-Hobson S: Clonal expansion of infected cells: a way of life for HTLV-I. *J Acquir Immune Defic Syndr Hum Retrovirol* 13(suppl 1): S92, 1996.

20. Shirono K, Hattori T, Takatsuki K: A new classification of clinical stages of adult T-cell leukemia based on prognosis of the disease. *Leukemia* 8:1834, 1994.

21. Takatsuki K: Adult T-cell leukemia. *Intern Med* 34:947, 1995.

22. Kamihira S, Sohda H, Atogami S, et al.: Phenotypic diversity and prognosis of adult T-cell leukemia. *Leuk Res* 16:435, 1992.

23. Tsukasaki K, Tsushima H, Yamamura M, et al.: Integration patterns of HTLV-I provirus in relation to the clinical course of ATL: frequent clonal change at crisis from indolenet disease. *Blood* 89:948, 1997.

24. Tsukasaki K, Ikeda S, Murata K, et al.: Characteristics of chemotherapy-induced clinical remission in long survivors with aggressive adult T-cell leukemia/lymphoma. *Leuk Res* 17:157, 1993.

25. Hayami Y, Komatsu H, Iida S, et al.: Microsatellite instability as a potential marker for poor prognosis adult T cell leukemia/lymphoma. *Leuk Lymphoma* 32:345, 1999.

26. Yamada Y, Hatta Y, Murata K, et al.: Deletions of p15 and/or p16 genes as a poor-prognosis factor in adult T-cell leukemia. *J Clin Oncol* 15:1778, 1997.

27. Sadamori N, Ikeda S, Yamaguchi K, et al.: Serum deoxythymidine kinase in adult T-cell leukemia-lymphoma and its related disorders. *Leuk Res* 15:99, 1991.

28. Kamihira S, Atogami S, Sohda H, et al.: Significance of soluble interleukin 2 receptor levels for evaluation of the progression of adult T-cell leukemia. *Cancer* 73:2753, 1994.

29. Sadamori N, Mine M, Hakariya S, et al.: Clinical significance of beta 2-microglobulin in serum of adult T cell leukemia. *Leukemia* 9:594, 1995.

30. Sadamori N, Mine M, Kasahara H: Clinical and biological significance of serum parathyroid hormone-related protein in adult T-cell leukemia. *Leuk Res* 19:229, 1995.

31. Hanada S, Utsunomiya A, Suzuki S, et al.: Treatment for adult T-cell leukemia. *Cancer Chemother Pharmacol* 40(suppl):S47, 1997.

32. Matsushita K, Matsumoto T, Ohtsubo H, et al.: Long-term maintenance combination chemotherapy with OPEC/MPEC (vincristine or methotrexate, prednisolone, etoposide and cyclophosphamide) or with daily oral etoposide and prednisolone can improve survival and quality of life in adult T-cell leukemia/lymphoma. *Leuk Lymphoma* 36:67, 1999.

33. Yamada Y, Tomonaga M, Fukuda H, et al.: A new G-CSF-supported combination chemotherapy, LSG15, for adult T-cell leukemia-lymphoma (ATL): Japan Clinical Oncology Group Study 9303. *Br J Haematol* 113:375, 2001.

34. Besson C, Panelatti G, Delaunay C, et al.: Treatment of adult T-cell leukemia-lymphoma by CHOP followed by therapy with antinucleosides, alpha interferon and oral etoposide. *Leuk Lymphoma* 43:2275, 2002.

35. Makino T, Uozumi K, Shimazaki T, et al.: Combination chemotherapy for adult T-cell leukemia (ATL) using cyclophosphamide, vindesine and prednisolone (CV'P). *J Jpn Soc Cancer Ther* 23:2657, 1988.

36. Shimamoto Y, Suga K, Shimojo M, et al.: Comparison of CHOP versus VEPA therapy in patients with lymphoma type of adult T-cell leukemia. *Leuk Lymphoma* 2:335, 1990.

37. Shapira I, Feldman J, Solomon WB: Poor survival in ATL patients treated with CHOP chemotherapy [abstract]. *Blood* 104:228b, 2004.

38. Shimoyama M, Ota K, Kikuchi M, et al.: Chemotherapeutic results and prognostic factors of patients with advanced non-Hodgkin's lymphoma treated with VEPA or VEPA-M. *J Clin Oncol* 6:128, 1988.

39. Shimoyama M, Ota K, Kikuchi M, et al.: Major prognostic factors of adult patients with advanced T-cell lymphoma/leukemia. *J Clin Oncol* 6:1088, 1988.

40. Tobinai K, Hotta T: Clinical trials for malignant lymphoma in Japan. *Jpn J Clin Oncol* 34:369, 2004.

41. Shimoyama M, Shiakawa S, members of the JCOG-LSG: Treatment outcome and prognostic factors of patients with advanced aggressive T and B lymphoma treated with 2nd generation LSG4 protocol [abstract]. *Jpn J Clin Hematol* 32:1247, 1993.

42. Tobinai K, Shimoyama M, Minato K, et al.: Japan Clinical Oncology Group phase II trial of second-generation "LSG4 protocol" in aggressive T- and B-lymphoma: a new predictive model for T- and B-lymphoma [abstract]. *Proc Am Soc Clin Oncol* 13: 378a, 1994.

43. Uozumi K, Hanada S, Ohno N, et al.: Combination chemotherapy (RCM protocol: response-oriented cyclic multidrug protocol) for the acute or lymphoma type adult T-cell leukemia. *Leuk Lymphoma* 18:317, 1995.

44. Taguchi H, Kinoshita K-I, Takatsuki K, et al.: An intensive chemotherapy of adult T-cell leukemia/lymphoma: CHOP followed by etoposide, vindesine, ranimustine and mitoxantrone with granulocyte colony-stimulating factor support. *J AIDS Hum Retrovirol* 12:182, 1996.

45. Gautenhaus RB, Wang P, Hoffman P: Induction of the WAF1/CIP1 protein and apoptosis in human T-cel leukemia virus type I-transformed lymphocytes after treatment with adriamycin by using a p53-independent pathway. *Proc Natl acad Sci U S A* 93:265, 1996.

46. Kuwazaru Y, Hamada S, Furukawa T, et al.: Expression of P-glycoprotein in adult T-cell leukemia cells. *Blood* 76:2065, 1990.

47. Sakashita A, Hattori T, Miller CW, et al.: Mutations of the p53 gene in adult T-cell leukemia. *Blood* 79:477, 1992.

48. Uittenbogaard MN, Giebler HA, Reisman D, Nyborg JK: Transcriptional repression of p53 by human T-cell leukemia virus type I Tax protein. *J Biol Chem* 270:28503, 1995.

49. Yokimozo A, Ono M, Nanri H, et al.: Cellular levels of thioredoxin associated with drug sensitivity to cisplatin, mitomycin C, doxorubicin, and etoposide. *Cancer Res* 55:4293–4297, 1995.

50. Wang J, Kobayashi M, Sakurada K, et al.: Possible roles of adult T-cell leukemia (ATL)-derived factor/thioredoxin in the drug resistance of ATL to adriamycin. *Blood* 89:2480, 1997.

51. Fujiwara H, Arima N, Akasaki Y, et al.: Interferon-α therapy following autologous peripheral blood stem cell transplantation for adult T cell leukemia/lymphoma. *Acta Haematol* 107:213, 2002.

52. Nakane M, Ohashi K, Sato Y, et al.: Molecular remission in adult T cell leukemia after autologous CD34+ peripheral blood stem cell transplantation. *Bone Marrow Transplant* 24:219, 1999.

53. Tsukasaki K, Maeda T, Arimura K, et al.: Poor outcome of autologous stem cell transplantation for adult T-cell leukemia/lymphoma: a case report and review of the literature. *Bone Marrow Transplant* 23:87, 1999.

54. Seki S, Hiraga H: Transplantation of autologous bone marrow purged by 4-hydroperoxycyclophosphamide for a patient with ATL [in Japanese; abstract]. *Jpn J Clin Hematol* 33:1482, 1992.

55. Morikawa T, Chiyoda S: Autologous bone marrow transplantation for adult T-cell leukemia/lymphoma [in Japanese; abstract]. *Jpn J Clin Hematol* 34:310, 1993.

56. Ohno E, Ohtsuka E, Ogata M, et al.: Autologous PBSCT for a patient with remission state of ATL [in Japanese; abstract]. *Jpn J Clin Hematol* 37:1091, 1996.

57. Watanabe J, Kondo H, Hatake K: Autologous stem cell transplantations for recurrent adult T cell leukemia/lymphoma using highly purified CD34+ cells derived from cryopreserved peripheral blood stem cells. *Leuk Lymphoma* 42:1115, 2001.

58. Asou N, Sakai K, Yamaguchi K, et al.: Autologous bone marrow transplantation in a patient with lymphoma type adult-T cell leukemia [in Japanese]. *Jpn J Clin Hematol* 26:229, 1985.

59. Uehira K, Suzuki R, Miura K, et al.: Transplantation of autologous CD34+ PBSC purified by the immunomagnetic bead method for a patient with ATL [in Japanese; abstract]. *Jpn J Hematol Cell Transplant* 19:80, 1996.

60. Utsunomiya A, Miyazaki Y, Takatsuka Y, et al.: Improved outcome of adult T cell leukemia/lymphoma with allogeneic hematopoietic stem cell transplantation. *Bone Marrow Transplant* 27:15, 2001.

61. Borg A, Liu Yin JA, Johnson PRE, et al.: Successful treatment of HTLV-1-associated acute adult T-cell leukaemia lymphoma by allogeneic bone marrow transplantation. *Br J Haematol* 94:713, 1996.

62. Kishi Y, Kami M, Oki Y, et al.: Successful bone marrow transplantation for adult T-cell leukemia form a donor with oligoclonal proliferation of T-cells infected with human T-cell lymphotropic virus. *Leuk Lymphoma* 42:819, 2001.

63. Ogata M, Ogata Y, Imamura T, et al.: Successful bone marrow transplantation from an unrelated donor in a patient with adult T cell leukemia. *Bone Marrow Transplant* 30:699, 2002.

64. Leclercq I, Mortreux F, Morschhauser F, et al.: Semiquantitative analysis of residual disease in patients treated for adult T-cell leukaemia/lymphoma (ATLL). *Br J Haematol* 105:743, 1999.

65. Sobue R, Yamauchim T, Miyamura K, et al.: Treatment of adult T cell leukemia with mega-dose cyclophosphamide and total body irradiation followed by allogeneic bone marrow transplantation. *Bone Marrow Transplant* 2:441, 1987.

66. Ljungman P, Lawler M, Åsjö B, et al.: Infection of donor lymphocytes with human T lymphotrophic virus type I (HTLV-I) following allogeneic bone marrow transplantation for HTLV-I positive adult T-cell leukaemia. *Br J Haematol* 88:403, 1994.

67. Obama K, Tara M, Sao H, et al.: Allogeneic bone marrow transplantation as a treatment for adult T-cell leukemia. *Int J Hematol* 69:203, 1999.

68. Tajima K, Amakawa R, Uehira K, et al.: Adult T-cell leukemia successfully treated with allogeneic bone marrow transplantation. *Int J Hematol* 71:290, 2000.

69. Ohguchi H, Sai T, Hamazaki Y, Hiwatashi K: Cyclopsorin A withdrawal causes spontaneous remission of recurrent subcutaneous tumors after allogeneic peripheral blood stem cell transplantation for adult T-cell leukemia/lymphoma [in Japanese]. *Rinsho Ketsueki* 44:102, 2003.

70. Ishikawa T: Current status of therapeutic approaches to adult T-cell leukemia. *Int J Hematol* 78:304, 2003.

71. Kami M, Hamaki T, Miyakoshi S, et al.: Allogeneic haematopoietic stem cell transplantation for the treatment of adult T-cell leukaemia/lymphoma. *Br J Haematol* 120:304, 2003.

72. Hoshida Y, Li T, Dong Z, et al.: Lymphoproliferative disorders in renal transplant patients in Japan. *Int J Cancer* 91:869, 2001.

73. Harashima N, Kurihara K, Utsunomiya A, et al.: Graft-versus-Tax response in adult T-cell leukemia patients after hematopoietic stem cell transplantation. *Cancer Res* 64:391, 2004.

74. Abe Y, Yashiki S, Choi I, et al.: Eradication of virus-infected T-cells in a case of adult T-cell leukemia/lymphoma by nonmyeloablative peripheral blood stem cell transplantation with conditioning consisting of low-dose total body irradiation and pentostatin. *Int J Hematol* 76:91, 2002.

75. Hamaki T, Kami M, Igarashi M, et al.: Non-myeloablative hematopoietic stem cell transplantation for the treatment of adult T-cell lymphoma in a patient with advanced hepatic impairment. *Leuk Lymphoma* 44:703, 2003.

76. Hill SA, Lloyd PA, McDonald S, et al.: Susceptibility of human T cell leukemia virus type I to nucleoside reverse transcriptase inhibitors. *J Infect Dis* 188:424, 2003.

77. García-Lerma JG, Nidtha S, Heneine W: Susceptibility of human T cell leukemia virus type 1 to reverse-transcriptase inhibitors: evidence for resistance to lamivudine. *J Infect Dis* 184:507, 2001.

78. Saito N, Takemori N, Hirai K, et al.: Suppression of HTLV-1-induced human leukemia cell infiltration by zidovudine. *Am J Hematol* 47:246, 1994.

79. Kamihira S, Soda H, Kinoshita K, Ichimaru M: Effect of human lymphoblast interferon in adult T-cell leukemia and non-Hodgkin's lymphoma [in Japanese]. *Gan To Kagaku Ryoho* 10:2188, 1983.

80. Ichimaru M, Kamihira S, Moriuchi Y, et al.: Clinical study on the effect of natural alpha-interferon (HLBI) in the treatment of adult T-cell leukemia [in Japanese]. *Gan To Kagaku Ryoho* 15:2975, 1988.

81. Tamura K, Makino S, Araki Y, et al.: Recombinant interferon beta and gamma in the treatment of adult T-cell leukemia. *Cancer* 59:1059, 1987.

82. Ezaki K, Hirano M, Yamada K, et al.: A combinational trial of human lymphoblastoid interferon and bestrabucil (KM 2210) for adult T cell leukemia-lymphoma. *Cancer* 68:695, 1991.

83. Bazarbachi A, Nasr R, El-Sabban ME, et al.: Evidence against a direct cytotoxic effect of alpha interferon and zidovudine in HTLV-I associated adult T cell leukemia/lymphoma. *Leukemia* 14:716, 2000.

84. Hermine O, Bouscary D, Gessain A, et al.: Brief report: treatment of adult T-cell leukemia-lymphoma with zidovudine and interferon alfa. *N Engl J Med* 332:1749, 1995.

85. Bazarbachi A, Hermine O: Treatment with a combination of zidovudine and [alpha]-interferon in naive and pretreated adult T-cell leukemia/lymphoma patients. *J Acquir Immune Defic Syndr Hum Retrovirol* 13(suppl 1): S186, 1996.

86. White JD, Wharfe G, Stewart DM, et al.: The combination of zidovudine and interferon alpha-2B in the treatment of adult T-cell leukemia/lymphoma. *Leuk Lymphoma* 40:287, 2001.

87. Gill PS, Harrington W Jr, Kaplan MH, et al.: Treatment of adult T-cell leukemia-lymphoma with a combination of interferon alfa and zidovudine. *N Engl J Med* 332:1744, 1995.

88. Gill PS, Harrington W Jr, Levine AM: Interferon alfa and zidovudine in adult T-cell leukemia-lymphoma. *N Engl J Med* 333:1286, 1995.

89. Wharfe G, Hanchard B: Zidovudine and interferon therapy for adult T-cell leukaemia/lymphoma. Results of a preliminary study at UHWI-Mona. *West Indian Med J* 45:107, 1996.

90. Matutes E, Taylor GP, Cavenagh J, et al.: Interferon α and zidovudine therapy in adult T-cell leukaemia lymphoma: response and outcome in 15 patients. *Br J Haematol* 113:779, 2001.

91. Hermine O, Allard I, Lévy V, et al.: A prospective phase II clinical trial with the use of zidovudine and interferon-alpha in the acute and lymphoma forms of adult T-cell leukemia/lymphoma. *Hematol J* 3:276, 2002.

92. Hermine O, Dombret H, Poupon J, et al.: Phase II trial of arsenic trioxide and alfa interferon in patients with relapsed/refractory adult T-cell leukemia/lymphoma. *Hematol J* 5:130, 2004.

93. Arima N, Mizoguchi H, Shirakawa S, et al.: Phase I clinical study of SH L573 (fludarabine phosphate) in patients with chronic lymphocytic leukemia and adult T-cell leukemia/lymphoma [in Japanese]. *Gan To Kagaku Ryoho* 26:619, 1999.

94. Tobinai K, Uike N, Saburi Y, et al.: Phase II study of cladribine (2-chlorodeoxyadenosine) in relapsed or refractory adult T-cell leukemia-lymphoma. *Int J Hematol* 77:512, 2003.

95. Uike N, Choi I, Tokoro A, et al.: Adult T-cell leukemia-lymphoma successfully treated with 2-chlorodeoxyadenosine. *Intern Med* 37:411, 1998.

96. Tobinai K, Shimoyama M, Inoue S, et al.: Phase I study of YK-176 (2'-deoxycoformycin) in patients with adult T-cell leukemia-lymphoma. *Jpn J Clin Oncol* 22:164, 1992.

97. Yamaguchi K, Yul LS, Oda T, et al.: Clinical consequences of 2'-deoxycoformycin treatment in patients with refractory adult T-cell leukaemia. *Leuk Res* 10:989, 1986.

98. Lofters W, Campbell M, Gibbs WN, Cheson BD: 2'-deoxycoformycin therapy in adult T-cell leukemia/lymphoma. *Cancer* 60:2605, 1987.

99. Dearden C, Matutes E, Catovsky D: Deoxycoformycin in the treatment of mature T-cell leukaemias. *Br J Cancer* 94:903, 1991.

100. Tsukasaki K, Tobinai K, Shimoyama M, et al.: Deoxycoformycin-containing combination chemotherapy for adult adult T-cell leukemia-lymphoma: Japan Clinical Oncology Group study (JCOG9109). *Int J Hematol* 77:164, 2003.

101. Bazarbachi A, El-Sabban ME, Nasr R, et al.: Arsenic trioxide and interferon-α synergize to induce cell cycle arrest and apoptosis in human T-cell lymphotropic virus type I-transformed cells. *Blood* 93:278, 1999.

102. Mahieux R, Pise-Masison C, Gessain A, et al.: Arsenic trioxide induces apoptosis in human T-cell leukemia virus type 1- and type 2-infected cells by a caspase-3-dependent mechanism involving Bcl-2 cleavage. *Blood* 98:3762, 2001.

103. Ishitsuka K, Ikeda R, Utsunomiya A, et al.: Arsenic trioxide induces apoptosis in HTLV-I infected T-cell lines and fresh adult T-cell leukemia cells through CD95 or tumor necrosis factor α receptor independent caspase activation. *Leuk Lymphoma* 43:1107, 2002.

104. Tsukasaki K, Fujimoto T, Hata T, et al.: Concomitant complete remission of APL and smouldering ATL following ATRA therapy in a patient with two diseases simultaneously. *Leukemia* 9:1797, 1995.

105. Tsukasaki K, Tomonaga M: ATRA, NF-κB and ATL. *Leuk Res* 25:407, 2001.

106. Toshima M, Nagai T, Izumi T, et al.: All-trans-retinoic acid treatment for chemotherapy-resistant acute adult T-cell leukemia. *Int J Hematol* 72:343, 2000.

107. Maeda Y, Naiki Y, Sono H, et al.: Clinical application of all-trans retinoic acid (tretinoin) for adult T-cell leukaemia. *Br J Haematol* 109:671, 2000.

108. Maeda Y, Yamaguchi T, Ueda S, et al.: All-trans retinoic acid reduced skin involvement of adult T-cell leukemia. *Leukemia* 18:1159, 2004.

109. Chan EF, Dowdy YG, Lee B, et al.: A novel chemotherapeutic regimen (interferon alfa, zidovudine, and etretinate) for adult T-cell lymphoma resulting in rapid tumor destruction. *J Am Acad Dermatol* 40:116, 1999.

110. Kojima H, Hori M, Shibuya A, et al.: Successful treatment of a patient with adult T-cell leukemia by daily oral administration of low-dose etoposide. Decrease in the amount of HTLV-I proviral DNA revealed by the polymerase chain reaction method. *Cancer* 72:3614, 1993.

111. Tsuda H, Takatsuki K, Ohno R, et al.: Treatment of adult T-cell leukaemia-lymphoma with irinotecan hydrochloride (CPT-11). *Br J Cancer* 70:771, 1994.

112. Andoh T: Bis(2,6-dioxopiperazines), catalytic inhibitors of DNA topoisomerase II, as molecular probes, cardioprotectors and antitumor drugs. *Biochimie* 80:235, 1998.

113. Ohno R, Masaoka T, Shirakawa S, et al.: Treatment of adult T-cell leukemia/lymphoma with MST-16, a new oral antitumor drug and a derivative of bis(2,6-dioxopiperazine). *Cancer* 71:2217, 1993.

114. Ichihashi T, Kiyoi H, Fukutani H, et al.: Effective treatment of adult T cell leukemia/lymphoma with a novel oral antitumor agent, MST-16. *Oncology* 49:333, 1992.

115. Waldmann TA, White JD, Goldman CK, et al.: The interleukin-2 receptor: a target for monoclonal antibody treatment of human T-cell lymphotrophic virus I-induced adult T-cell leukemia. *Blood* 82:1701, 1993.

116. Queen C, Schneider WP, Selick HE, et al.: A humanized antibody that binds to the interleukin 2 receptor. *Proc Natl Acad Sci U S A* 86:10029, 1989.

117. Junghans RP, Waldmann TA, Landolfi NF, et al.: Anti-Tac-H, a humanized antibody to the interleukin 2 receptor with new features for immunotherapy in malignant and immune disorders. *Cancer Res* 50:1495, 1990.

118. Waldmann TA: T-cell receptors for cytokines: Targets for immunotherapy of leukemia/lymphoma. *Ann Oncol* 11(suppl 1):S101, 2000.

119. Waldmann TA, White JD, Carrasquillo JA, et al.: Radioimmunotherapy of interleukin-2Rα-expressing adult T-cell leukemia with yttrium-90-labeled anti-Tac. *Blood* 86:4063, 1995.

120. Yasunaga J, Sakai T, Nosaka K, et al.: Impaired production of naïve T lymphocytes in human T-cell leukemia virus type I-infected individuals: its implications in the immunodeficient state. *Blood* 97:3177, 2001.

121. Porto AF, Neva FA, Bittencourt H, et al.: HTLV-1 decreases Th2 type of immune response in patients with strongyloides. *Parasite Immunol* 23:503, 2001.

122. Nagai M, Brennan MB, Sakai JA, et al.: CD8+ T-cells are an in vitro reservoir for human T-cell lymphotropic virus type I. *Blood* 98:1858, 2001.

# Chapter 64

# AUTOLOGOUS HEMATOPOIETIC CELL TRANSPLANTATION FOR NON-HODGKIN'S LYMPHOMA

## Ginna G. Laport and Robert S. Negrin

Non-Hodgkin's lymphoma (NHL) is the fifth most common cancer among men and women with a projected incidence of over 54,000 new cases in the United States in 2004.[1] Many patients with NHL can be cured today with frontline combination chemotherapy and/or radiotherapy. However, for patients with suboptimal responses to initial therapy or for patients with relapsed or refractory disease, salvage therapy alone is typically inadequate to achieve long-term survival.[2,3] Fortunately, high-dose chemotherapy (HDC) with autologous hematopoietic cell transplantation (AHCT) offers curative potential. Dose-intensive treatment has unequivocally been shown to be the treatment of choice for patients with relapsed, chemosensitive, intermediate-grade lymphomas, and recent data have shown that a certain subset of these patients benefit from AHCT while in first remission. Until recently, HDC had not consistently yielded durable responses for patients with relapsed indolent lymphoma but new data showing a survival advantage was recently reported.[4] However, the role of AHCT and the appropriate timing in such entities as mantle cell lymphoma (MCL), the T-cell lymphomas, and high-grade lymphomas remains controversial. This chapter will discuss the application of HDC with AHCT in NHL and review emerging advances such as the role of rituximab (RTX) for in vivo purging and posttransplant maintenance therapy and the use of radioimmunotherapy (RIT) in the preparative regimen.

## RATIONALE FOR HIGH-DOSE CHEMOTHERAPY

The rationale for high-dose cytotoxic chemotherapy stems from the steep dose-response curve of alkylating agents and radiotherapy (RT) and tumor cell response in human tumors.[5,6] Doubling the dose of alkylating agents increases tumor cell kill by a log or more and utilizing a 5- to 10-fold increase in the dose of alkylating agents overcomes the resistance of tumor cells against lower doses.[7] HDC also aims to destroy the tumor cells in an expediently timely manner to prevent the emergence of resistant clones. The observation that increasing doses of alkylating agents conferred a decreased survival of murine lymphoma cells in vivo provided initial evidence of a dose-response curve specifically in tumor cells of lymphoid origin.[8] In 1978, investigators from the National Cancer Institute were the first to report the use of HDC followed by autologous hematopoietic cell transplantation (AHCT) for patients with relapsed lymphoma.[9] These encouraging results were the initial clinical evidence that has led to the widespread application of this aggressive treatment modality.

## INTERMEDIATE/AGGRESSIVE LYMPHOMA

AHCT is curative in a subset of patients with relapsed intermediate-grade lymphoma and is considered a standard therapy for patients with chemosensitive disease at first relapse. In 1987, Philip et al. reported the prognostic significance of chemosensitivity to salvage therapy prior to autologous stem cell transplantation in patients with recurrent or refractory NHL.[10] This multi-institutional study accrued 100 patients with either primary refractory, sensitive relapse or resistant relapse. The actuarial 3-year disease-free survival (DFS) was 0% in the primary refractory group, 14% in the resistant relapse group, and 36% in the sensitive relapse group. Subsequently, the PARMA study in 1995 was the pivotal randomized phase III trial that unequivocally demonstrated the benefit of dose-intensive chemotherapy over conventional salvage treatment.[11] A total of 215 patients with intermediate-grade ($n = 163$) and high-grade ($n = 52$) NHL in first or second relapse initially received DHAP (dexamethasone, cytarabine, cisplatin) as salvage therapy.

The 109 patients who responded were randomized to autologous stem cell transplantation versus additional courses of DHAP. After 5 years of follow-up, the final analysis clearly favored the autologous stem cell transplantation arm in terms of event-free survival (46% vs 12%, $p = 0.0001$) and overall survival (53% vs 32%, $p = 0.038$). The 90 patients who did not respond to salvage therapy and who were not randomized experienced a dismal 5-year overall survival (OS) of only 11%.

Subsequent updates from the PARMA trial have retrospectively examined certain patient characteristics to identify factors of predictive value. Time to relapse (relapse within 12 months vs later than 12 months) and elevated lactate dehydrogenase (LDH) levels at relapse were features with negative prognostic value, whereas time to relapse was also a powerful prognostic factor for both OS and progression-free survival (PFS).[12] Interestingly, T-cell immunophenotype and large tumor size, frequently considered adverse prognostic factors, were not found to negatively influence outcome. The International Prognostic Index (IPI) was also used retrospectively as a prognostic model at the time of relapse and was highly predictive of both response and OS in the PARMA trial.[13] Blay et al. reported that the IPI at relapse highly correlated with OS for patients in the DHAP arm but not for patients in the transplant arm. For the DHAP-treated patients, the 5-year OS was 48% for patients with an IPI of 0 compared to 0% for patients with an IPI of 3. For patients who underwent BMT, the 5-year OS showed little variance ranging from 47 to 51% among all IPI risk groups. However, for patients with an IPI > 0, a survival advantage was seen in favor of the BMT arm when compared to the DHAP arm. Thus, patients in the low-risk group fared well regardless of the therapy administered with a median survival of 56 months after relapse in both arms.

The group from Memorial Sloan Kettering Cancer Center also evaluated the prognostic significance of the secondary age adjusted IPI in 150 patients with relapsed or primary refractory diffuse large cell lymphoma (DLCL) who received ICE (ifosfamide, carboplatin, etoposide) as second-line chemotherapy.[14] The PFS and OS were 70 and 74% for low-risk patients (0 factors) compared to 16 and 18%, $p < 0.001$, respectively, for high-risk patients at the time of relapse. Specifically, for patients with ICE-chemosensitive disease, the OS rates were 83 and 26% for the low-risk and high-risk groups, respectively ($p < 0.001$), demonstrating that high-risk patients fare poorly regardless of chemosensitivity. Thus, the secondary age-adjusted IPI appeared to hold more prognostic value compared to chemosensitivity as this clinical index may actually be more reflective of disease biology.

Gugliemi et al. examined risk factors retrospectively in 474 patients with DLCL at relapse who received various salvage regimens including chemotherapy,

surgery, and/or RT with only 20% of patients proceeding to AHCT.[15] Relapse within 12 months from diagnosis, elevated serum LDH, advanced stage, and poor performance status represented independent prognostic factors for PFS and OS for patients with chemosensitive disease and for those who proceeded to AHCT. Similar to the PARMA findings, this analysis also demonstrated that the T-cell phenotype was not a negative prognostic factor. Caballero et al. reported the results of 452 patients, who received HDC, from the GEL-TAMO Cooperative Group.[16] Approximately half of the patients had active disease with 32% being in first complete remission (CR) and 19% in second CR. The three variables that significantly influenced DFS and OS were number of prior regimens to reach first CR, disease status at transplant (first CR vs $\geq$ second CR), and total body irradiation (TBI) in the conditioning regimen. Patients who received chemotherapy only experienced significantly longer PFS and OS although a higher percentage of patients in the TBI group had progressive disease prior to AHCT. As seen in the Memorial Sloan Kettering analysis, the age-adjusted IPI at transplantation was also predictive of OS. Not surprisingly, response to transplant predicted OS with patients who achieved a CR posttransplant experiencing a 64% OS compared to 17% and 4% for partial remission (PR) and nonresponding patients, respectively.

## HIGH-DOSE CHEMOTHERAPY IN FIRST OR PARTIAL REMISSION

The application of AHCT to patients with NHL as frontline therapy has been explored by several investigators based primarily on the success of this treatment modality in the chemosensitive relapse setting (see Table 64.1). Encouraging results have been reported in some but not all studies most likely due to the fact that the published trials are heterogeneous with respect to patient selection, timing of transplantation, choice of induction and conditioning regimens, length of induction phase, remission status requirements, and nonuniform histologic subtypes.

The LNH87-2 trial by the GELA (Groupe d'Etude des Lymphomes de Adulte) group was a phase III trial that enrolled 916 patients with intermediate- and high-grade lymphoma in first CR with one or more unfavorable prognostic factors who received induction treatment using the LHN84 protocol.[24] Only those patients who achieved a CR (61%, $n = 541$) were randomized to receive sequential chemotherapy or proceed to autologous stem cell transplantation. Initial analysis revealed no difference in DFS and OS between the two consolidative treatment arms. However, a subset analysis of the higher risk population who had two or three risk factors favored the autologous stem cell

**Table 64.1** Randomized trials of autologous hematopoietic cell transplantation for newly diagnosed aggressive NHL

| Group/Year | Inclusion criteria | Age adjusted IPI | Time of randomization | No. of patients | Treatment | DFS/PFS (%) | p | OS (%) | p | Years | Comments |
|---|---|---|---|---|---|---|---|---|---|---|---|
| GOELAMS[17] 2004 | Aggressive NHL Stage 3 or 4 Stage 2 bulky | low, low int, high int | At diagnosis | 99 98 | CHOP × 8 Induction, BEAM | 37[a] 55 | 0.037 | 44[b] 74 | 0.001 | 5 | AHCT hi int risk pts |
| Italian coop group[18] 2003 | DLCL, PTCL ALCL | high int, high | At diagnosis | 75 75 | MACOPB × 12 weeks MACOPB × 8 weeks, BEAM | 65 77 | 0.21 | 65 64 | 0.95 | 5 | No difference |
| GELA[19] 2002 | DLCL, PTCL High grade NHL | hi int, high | At diagnosis | 181 189 | ACVBP × 4 + seq chemo CEOP + ECVBP + BEAM | 52 39 | 0.01 | 60 46 | 0.007 | 5 | AHCT inferior |
| German NHL group[20] 2002 | Aggressive NHL Stage II–IV High LDH | nr | Response to induction | 154 158 | CHOEP × 5 CHOEP × 3, BEAM | 49 59 | 0.22 | 63 62 | 0.68 | 3 | No difference |
| EORTC[21] 2001 | Aggressive NHL Stage II–IV | low, low int | Response to induction | 96 98 | CHVmP/BV × 5 CHVmP/BV × 3, BEAM | 56 61 | ns | 77 68 | ns | 5 | No difference |
| GELA[22] 2000 | Aggressive NHL | high int, high | CR after induction | 111 125 | LNH-84 LNH-84 + BEAM | 39 55 | 0.02 | 49 64 | 0.04 | 8 | AHCT benefits higher risk IPI |
| Milano group[23] 1997 | DLCL | high int, high | At diagnosis | 50 48 | MACOPB × 12 weeks High dose sequential | 49[b] 76 | 0.004 | 55 81 | 0.09 | 7 | Improved EFS with AHCT |

NHL: non-Hodgkin's lymphoma; GOELAMS: Groupe Ouest-Est des Leucemies et des Autres Maladies du Sang; IPI: international prognostic index; DFS: disease-free survival; OS: overall survival; int: intermediate; CHOP: cyclophospamide, doxorubicin, vincristine, prednisone; AHCT: autologous hematopoietic cell transplantation; BEAM: carmustine, etoposide, cytarabine, melphalan; coop: cooperative; DLCL: diffuse large cell lymphoma; PTCL: peripheral T-cell lymphoma; ALCL: anaplastic large cell lymphoma; MACOPB: methotrexate, doxorubicin, cyclophosphamide, vincristine, prednisone, bleomycin; GELA: Groupe d'Etude des Lymphomes de Adulte; ACVBP: doxorubicin, cyclophosphamide, vindesine, bleomycin, prednisone; CEOP: cyclophosphamide, epirubicin, vincristine, etoposide, prednisone; ECVBP: epirubicin, cyclophosphamide, vindesine, bleomycin, prednisone; LDH: lactate dehydrogenase; CHOEP: cyclophosphamide, doxorubicin, vincristine, etoposide, prednisone; EORTC: European Organization for Research and Treatment of Cancer; CHVmP/BV: cyclophosphamide, doxorubicin, Teniposide, prednisone, bleomycin, vincristine; LNH-84: doxorubicin, cyclophosphamide, vinblastine, bleomycin, bleomycin, vinblastine, bleomycin; nr: not reported; ns: not significant.

[a] event-free survival; EFS: event-free survival.

[b] overall survival for high intermediate risk patients.

transplantation arm for both DFS and OS at 8 years (55% vs 39%, $p = 0.02$ and 64% vs 49%, $p = 0.04$, respectively).[22] The LNH93-3 study, which accrued between 1993 and 1995, was a follow-up randomized trial that was eligible only to patients in the high-intermediate- or high-risk age-adjusted IPI prognostic categories.[25] With the intention of improving upon the 61% CR rate seen in the earlier trial, a novel abbreviated, intense firstline regimen that incorporated HDC at day + 60 was administered. A total of 370 patients were randomized either to receive full standard induction course or a short induction phase with a debulking course followed by two cycles of standard therapy before receiving AHCT. Patients in the transplant arm experienced both inferior OS and EFS with the early closing to accrual in 1996 due to the poor results. A final update published in 2002 reported the continued inferiority in terms of EFS and OS in the transplant arm with a 5-year median follow-up.[19] The shortened induction phase in the HDC arm was thought to contribute to the negative outcome. A recent retrospective analysis from the GELA group pooled the data of 330 patients from the LNH-87 and LNH-93 trials to estimate the prognostic effect of clinical and biologic variables. Only the patients who obtained a CR prior to transplantation were included. T-cell phenotype, more than one extranodal site, or bone marrow (BM) involvement were adverse prognostic factors for both DFS and OS. The age-adjusted IPI was of no prognostic value.[26]

Other studies utilizing abbreviated standard induction therapy also showed no benefit of HDC over standard therapy. The German High Grade Non-Hodgkin's Lymphoma Study Group randomized 312 patients all younger than 60 years and with elevated serum LDH levels who obtained at least a PR to standard therapy.[20] Both arms received consolidative involved field radiation therapy (IFRT). With a median follow-up of 46 months, there was no difference in EFS or OS between the conventional and transplant groups (EFS: 49% vs 59%, $p = 0.22$; OS: 63% vs 62%, $p = 0.68$) even among the high-intermediate- and high-risk subgroups. A phase III European Organization for Research and Treatment of Cancer trial of 194 patients with responsive disease yielded similar results.[21] With a median follow-up of 53 months, an intent to treat analysis also showed no benefit in terms of disease progression between the two treatment arms, and a subset analysis of the IPI risk groups also failed to yield an advantage for the experimental group.

As with the LNH93-3 trial, Martelli et al. also sought to assess the role of early intensification with HDC and AHCT as frontline therapy but restricted accrual to patients with intermediate-high- or high-risk patients according to the age adjusted IPI.[18] Seventy-five patients received the standard MACOP-B (methotrexate, doxorubicin, cyclophosphamide, vincristine, prednisone, bleomycin) regimen for 12 weeks or MACOP-B for 8 weeks prior to autologous HCT. An intent to treat analysis demonstrated no difference in 5-year PFS and OS. These results may be somewhat confounded by the fact that 44% of the patients in the conventional chemotherapy arm received AHCT postrelapse and 40% of the patients in the transplant arm actually did not receive a transplant for reasons including progression and patient refusal.

The recently published French GOELAMS (Groupe Ouest-Est des Leucemies et des Autres Maladies du Sang) study is the first large randomized trial that included all age-adjusted IPI risk groups except the high-risk group since it was known that the use of standard CHOP (cyclophosphamide, doxorubicin, vincristine, prednisone) in this group tended to yield poor outcomes.[17] A total of 197 patients were randomized to full course CHOP or CEEP (cyclophosphamide, epirubicin, vindesine, prednisone) for two cycles followed by an intensification regimen with high-dose methotrexate and cytarabine before proceeding to transplant. With a median follow-up of 4 years, the estimated 5-year EFS clearly favored the transplant arm over the chemotherapy arm (55% vs 37%, $p = 0.037$) but did not translate into an OS advantage except among the patients in the high-intermediate group. The patients in this particular subgroup experienced both an improved EFS (56% vs 28%, $p = 0.003$) and OS (74% vs 44%, $p = 0.001$) favoring the transplant arm (see Figures 64.1 and 64.2).

Before the IPI was widely utilized, two Italian groups conducted randomized trials enrolling patients with high risk-features such as bulky or advanced-stage disease.[23,27] There were favorable trends with regards to freedom from progression or DFS but no advantages were seen in OS. For patients who are considered slow responders to up-front chemotherapy, AHCT does not appear to benefit this group. Two randomized trials from the Netherlands and Italy failed to show a survival advantage with early AHCT.[28,29]

Based on the array of published evidence regarding AHCT for first-line therapy in aggressive NHL, it appears that patients in the high-intermediate- or high-risk age-adjusted IPI categories experience better outcomes with AHCT upfront but only when this strategy is applied after a full course of induction therapy for maximal cytoreduction. RTX was not available at the commencement of these trials so the impact of the combination of RTX with CHOP on transplant outcome has not been assessed. Thus, the potential impact of incorporating RTX in both the control and transplant arms is an area of ongoing investigation. Many of the above studies were also plagued by high dropout rates in the transplant arms and the use of transplant for salvage in the control arm, which also confounded outcome data.

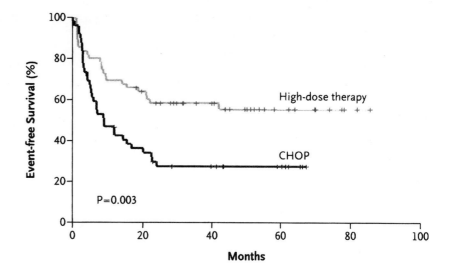

**Figure 64.1** *Event-free survival among patients with a high-intermediate risk according to the age-adjusted International Prognostic Index. (CHOP denotes cyclophosphamide, doxorubicin, vincristine, prednisone.) (Copyright 2004, Massachusetts Medical Society, from Milpied et al.[25] All rights reserved)*

## MANTLE CELL LYMPHOMA

MCL represents 5–10% of all lymphoma cases and is characterized by the t(11;14) translocation resulting in rearrangement of the *bcl-1* locus and cyclin D1 protein overexpression.[30–32] Patients with MCL typically present with advanced-stage disease and carry a median overall survival of only 3 years despite high initial response rates.[31] Thus, the absence of curative therapy has led to the increased application of HDC with AHCT as part of frontline therapy and as early salvage treatment for relapsed disease (see Table 64.2). Although numerous published studies have demonstrated high initial rates of CR, plateaus in the survival curves are yet to be convincingly demonstrated, especially for patients transplanted beyond first CR. The MD Anderson Cancer Center Group administered intensive induction therapy with the hyperCVAD (cyclophosphamide, doxorubicin, vincristine, prednisone, cytarabine, methotrexate) regimen followed by AHCT to 25 patients as frontline therapy and to 20

previously treated patients.[40] The 3-year EFS and OS rates were 72% and 92%, respectively, for the newly diagnosed patients compared to only 17 and 25% for the previously treated patients. A historical control group that received a CHOP-like regimen without AHCT had a median 3-year EFS of only 28%. The prognostic significance of remission status was also confirmed in a large retrospective analysis of 195 patients from the European Bone Marrow Transplant Group (EBMT) and Autologous Bone Marrow Transplant Registry (ABMTR).[34] The 5-year PFS and OS rates for all patients were 33 and 50%, respectively. Patients who were transplanted beyond first CR were nearly 3 times more likely to succumb to relapse than patients transplanted in first remission. The combined Stanford/City of Hope experience also demonstrated better outcomes for first CR patients as the median time to relapse was 32 months compared to 11 months for patients transplanted beyond first CR.[37] However, late relapses were seen in both groups of patients. This trial also found that the number of prior chemotherapy regimens and

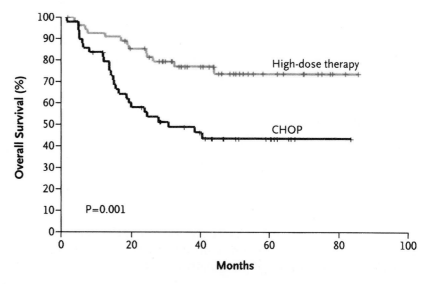

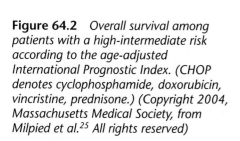

**Figure 64.2** *Overall survival among patients with a high-intermediate risk according to the age-adjusted International Prognostic Index. (CHOP denotes cyclophosphamide, doxorubicin, vincristine, prednisone.) (Copyright 2004, Massachusetts Medical Society, from Milpied et al.[25] All rights reserved)*

**Table 64.2** Autologous hematopoietic cell transplantation for mantle cell lymphoma

| Group/Year | n | Status | Regimen | PFS/EFS (%) | OS (%) | Years |
|---|---|---|---|---|---|---|
| Canadian multicenter[33] 2004 | 20 | Newly diagnosed | CHOP then CBV | 89 | 88 | 3 |
| EBMT[34] 2003 | 195 | ≥ CR1 including refractory | BEAM or BEAC or CBV or others | 33 | 50 | 5 |
| Milan group[35] 2003 | 28 | Newly diagnosed | High dose sequential | 79 | 89 | 4.5 |
| Nordic Lymphoma Group[36] 2003 | 27 | Newly diagnosed | CHOP then BEAM | 15 | 61 | 4 |
| Stanford/City of Hope[37] 2002 | 69 | CR1 > CR1 | TBI/VP/CY or CBV | 50 21 | 74 51 | 5 5 |
| French multicenter[38] 2002 | 23 | Newly diagnosed | CHOP + DHAP then TBI/ara-C/Mel | 83 | 90 | 3 |
| FHCRC[39] 2002 | 16 | Relapsed | CY/tositumomab | 61 | 93 | 3 |

PFS/EFS: progression-free survival/event-free survival; OS: overall survival; CHOP: cyclophosphamide, doxorubicin, vincristine, prednisone; CBV: cyclophosphamide, carmustine, etoposide; EBMT: European Bone Marrow Transplant Group; CR1: first complete remission; BEAM: carmustine, etoposide, cytarabine, melphalan; BEAC: carmustine, etoposide, cytarabine, cyclosphosphamide; TBI: total body irradiation, VP: etoposide; CY: cyclophosphamide; ara-C: cytarabine; Mel: melphalan; CRC: cancer research center.

the use of TBI in the preparative regimen did not improve survival which was in contrast to a French study that reported significantly improved DFS for patients who received TBI-based conditioning regimens.[41] Investigators from the University of Nebraska reported a 2-year EFS of 35% and OS of 65% in 40 MCL patients who were transplanted in either first CR, sensitive relapse or were induction failures.[42] In a multivariate analysis, patients who received three or more prior regimens had a dismal 2-year EFS of 0% compared with 45% for patients who received less than three prior therapies which was in contrast to the Stanford/City of Hope findings regarding impact of prior therapies.

The Nordic Lymphoma Group also tested an augmented CHOP induction regimen followed by AHCT as primary therapy.[36] Only patients who responded after three cycles of CHOP proceeded to transplantation. In an intent to treat analysis, the 4-year failure-free survival (FFS) and OS rates were 15% and 51%, respectively. Chemosensitivity was a favorable prognostic factor as patients transplanted in CR experienced a statistically significant improved FFS and OS compared to PR patients. Interestingly, tumor cell contamination was measured in the autografts and no correlation was seen between the number of tumor cells reinfused and outcome.

In a similar fashion, a French group also incorporated AHCT after CHOP chemotherapy but only for slow responders.[38] Patients who achieved less than a CR received DHAP for intensification before proceeding to AHCT. The 3-year EFS and OS rates were 83% and 90%, respectively, with a median follow-up of 4 years. The EFS incidence was particularly notable since patients with mantle zone histology, a known favorable prognostic factor, were excluded and a majority of patients had an increased *beta*-2 microglobulin level, a reported poor prognostic factor.[43]

Because of the continuous patterns of relapse seen in all of the above mentioned studies, alternative strategies have been explored including the use of RTX during mobilization for the purposes of in vivo purging due to the concern that autologous grafts contaminated by tumor cells can potentially contribute to relapse. The role of RTX as maintenance therapy after AHCT to eradicate minimal residual disease (MRD) is also the subject of active investigation. Magni et al. treated seven patients with four doses of RTX in combination with high-dose sequential chemotherapy with autologous stem cell support and successfully obtained polymerase chain reaction (PCR)-negative leukapheresis products.[44] The Milan Group recently published some of the most encouraging results to date in 28 previously untreated patients who received standard dose debulking chemotherapy followed by four cycles of sequential chemotherapy in which autologous stem cell support was provided after the last three cycles.[35] RTX was included in three of four cycles including the mobilization cycle. The OS and EFS rates at 54 months were 89% and 79%, respectively, with 24 of 27 evaluable patients remaining in continuous CR. These results compared much more favorably to a historical control group that had an OS of 42% and EFS of 18% and to previously published trials. This technique of combining RTX with high-dose sequential chemotherapy proved to be an effective method of in vivo purging as leukapheresis products from 20 informative patients were PCR negative.

A multicenter trial from Canada also produced similar results when RTX was incorporated during mobilization and as posttransplant maintenance therapy.[33] With an impressive 80 months of follow-up, the PFS and OS rates were 89% and 88%, respectively. The feasibility of combining radiolabeled antibody therapy with AHCT was explored by the Seattle Group.[39] Tositumomab ([131]I-labeled CD20-specific monoclonal antibody) was added to high-dose cyclophosphamide and etoposide in 16 heavily pretreated MCL patients. The CR and overall response rates were 91% and 100%, respectively, with a 3-year PFS and OS of 61% and 93%, respectively. These were unexpectedly favorable outcomes since most patients had received greater than three prior regimens or were chemorefractory at the time of transplant.

## FOLLICULAR NHL

For patients with follicular NHL, several studies have shown improved DFS but one recently published study has also shown an advantage for OS (see Table 64.3). EBMT conducted a randomized trial known as the CUP Trial in which 140 patients with relapsed follicular NHL were randomized to either chemotherapy alone, AHCT with a purged autograft using monoclonal antibodies, or AHCT with an unpurged autograft.[4] With a median follow-up of 69 months, the patients who received AHCT, purged or unpurged, showed a significantly higher 2-year PFS and OS compared to the chemotherapy patients. There was no difference between the two AHCT arms in these endpoints. OS rates at 4 years for the chemotherapy arm, unpurged AHCT arm, and purged AHCT arm were 46%, 71%, and 77%, respectively. The 2-year PFS was 26%, 58%, and 55%, respectively. There was a significant reduction in hazard rates for both PFS and OS when a comparison was performed between the chemotherapy patients and the combined groups of autologous AHCT patients (see Figures 64.3 and 64.4).

As with conventional chemotherapy, the outcome for patients who receive AHCT is related to the number of prior chemotherapy regimens received. Three retrospective studies have shown that patients with follicular lymphoma (FL) undergoing AHCT who had received more than three prior chemotherapy regimens showed inferior survival compared to patients treated with less than three prior regimens.[49,52,53]

In a large retrospective series of 904 patients from the International Bone Marrow Transplant Registry (IBMTR), 67% of patients underwent AHCT with an unpurged graft, 14% received a purged graft, and 19% received a myeloablative allogeneic HCT.[54] The 5-year OS rates of 55%, 62%, and 51%, respectively, were comparable between all three groups despite a markedly

| Table 64.3 | Autologous hematopoietic cell transplantation for follicular NHL | | | | | | | |
|---|---|---|---|---|---|---|---|---|
| Group/Year | n | Preparative regimen | Stem cell source | DFS/PFS (%) | OS (%) | Years | TRM (%) | Incidence of secondary MDS/AML (%) |
| *First Remission* | | | | | | | | |
| GITMO[45] 2002 | 80 | High dose sequential | PBPC | 67 | 84 | 4 | 2 | 4 |
| Stanford/COH[46] 2001 | 37 | TBI/VP/CY | purged BM | 70 | 86 | 10 | 5 | 5 |
| GOELAMS[47] 2000 | 27 | CY/TBI | purged BM | 55 | 64 | nr | 7 | nr |
| *Relapsed* | | | | | | | | |
| CUP (randomized)[4] 2003 | 24 | CHOP × 6 | na | 26 | 46 | 4[a] | 0 | nr |
| | 33 | CHOP × 3, CY/TBI | BM | 58 | 71 | | 9 | |
| | 32 | CHOP × 3, CY/TBI | purged BM | 55 | 77 | | 6 | |
| FHCRC[48] 2003 | 27 | tositumomab | purged BM or PBPC | 48 | 67 | 5 | 4 | 7 |
| Stanford[49] 2001 | 49 | TBI/VP/CY | purged PBPC | 44 | 60 | 4 | 10 | 7 |
| St. Bartholomew's[50] 2001 | 99 | CY/TBI | purged BM | 63 | 69 | 5 | 4 | 12 |
| Dana Farber[51] 99 | 153 | CY/TBI | purged BM | 42 | 66 | 8 | 1 | 8 |
| Nebraska[52] 1997 | 100 | CY/TBI, BEAC | BM | 44 | 65 | 4 | 8 | 2 |

DFS: disease-free survival; PFS: progression-free survival; OS: overall survival; TRM: treatment-related mortality; MDS: myelodysplastic syndrome; AML: acute myelogenous leukemia; GITMO: Gruppo Italiano Trapianto Midollo Ossseo; COH: City of Hope; PBPC: peripheral blood progenitor cell; TBI: total body irradiation; VP: etoposide; CY: cyclophosphamide; BM: bone marrow; FHCRC: Fred Hutchinson Cancer Research Center; BEAC: carmustine, etoposide, cytarabine, cyclophosphamide; nr: not reported.
[a]for overall survival only.

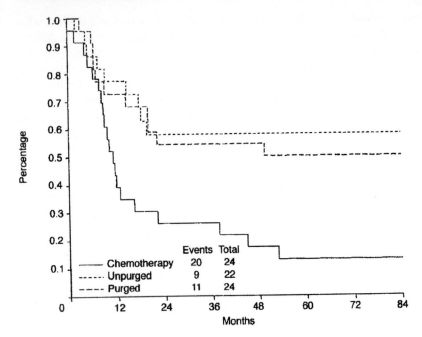

**Figure 64.3** *Progression-free survival for patients randomized to three arms in the CUP trial. (CUP denotes chemotherapy, unpurged autograft, purged autograft.) (Reprinted with permission for the American Society of Clinical Oncology from Schouten et al.[4])*

lower relapse rate among the allogeneic recipients. The lower recurrence rate in the allogeneic group was offset by a higher treatment related mortality. Negative prognostic factors included advanced age, refractory disease, high LDH, BM involvement, and a poor performance status. A direct comparison between the purged and unpurged autologous recipients revealed a significantly lower risk of recurrence among the purged recipients, which contradicted the CUP trial findings that showed no impact of purging. Patients are assigned to a treatment strategy based on the availability of an HLA-matched sibling.

In a prospective manner, several groups have evaluated the efficacy of early intensive therapy in newly diagnosed FL patients or patients in first remission. Three such trials from Stanford, Dana Farber, and the GOELAMS group utilized HDC with TBI and *ex vivo* antibody purging of the autograft.[46,47,55] With a median follow-up of 5–6 years for all three trials, the OS approached 90% in the first two trials with the latter trial reporting an OS of 64%. The latter trial accrued older patients and patients with higher tumor burdens. An Italian multicenter group transplanted 111 patients, most being in first remission and who received unmanipulated grafts.[56] Relapse-free survival and OS were superior compared to conventional chemotherapy with the patients transplanted in second CR experiencing almost a twice as

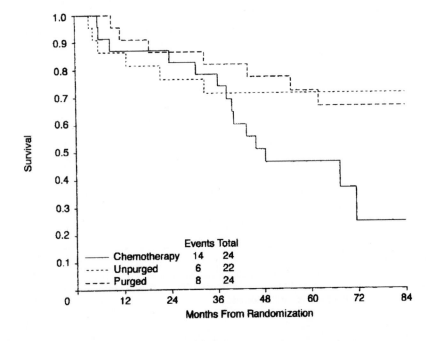

**Figure 64.4** *Overall survival for patients randomized to three arms in the CUP trial.[3] (CUP denotes chemotherapy, unpurged autograft, purged autograft.) (Reprinted with permission for the American Society of Clinical Oncology from Schouten et al.[4])*

high a relapse rate compared to first CR patients. Nearly 5% of the patients, however, developed a secondary malignancy, which is similar to the previously mentioned studies in this particular subset of patients. Another large Italian multicenter trial (Gruppo Italiano Trapianto Midollo Ossseo) with newly diagnosed FL patients reported an impressive 4-year DFS and OS of 67% and 84% with high-dose sequential chemotherapy.[45] This trial demonstrated the importance of achieving a molecular remission as the subgroup of patients who were PCR negative for either the bcl-2 translocation or the heavy chain (IgH) gene rearrangement after transplant had a projected DFS of 85%.

There has been mounting evidence confirming the prognostic relevance of molecular monitoring of MRD in indolent lymphoma patients who are known to express the bcl-2/IgH rearrangement. The attainment of PCR negativity after transplantation appears to be highly predictive of continued CR as shown in trials from Dana Farber, St Bartholomew's, University of Heidelberg, and an Italian multicenter group.[45,50,51,57] In the Heidelberg study, the relapse rate was 4.5 times higher in patients who were PCR positive in either the BM or peripheral blood at any given time posttransplantation in comparison with PCR-negative patients.[57] The Dana Farber Group demonstrated the negative impact of persistent PCR positivity in the graft after in vitro purging as the 8-year freedom from relapse was 83% in the patients who received PCR-negative grafts compared to 19% in patients who received PCR-positive grafts.[51] In contrast, the St Bartholomew's trial found no correlation between PCR status of the reinfused BM and outcome, but PCR negativity following transplantation portended a more favorable outcome.[50]

Various in vitro purging methods have been utilized to decrease or eliminate residual tumor cells from the harvest product but are typically expensive, labor intensive, and can be associated with substantial cell losses. Thus, in vivo purging is a more attractive strategy and RTX has recently emerged as a promising agent for this purpose when given concurrently with chemotherapy. Three recent studies have evaluated the effectiveness of this combination and yielded stem cell harvests with no PCR-detectable disease in the graft.[44,58,59] One such study by Magni et al. evaluated 15 patients with MCL or FL who were given two cycles of intensive chemotherapy with two doses of RTX.[44] Ninety-three percent of the patients who received RTX had PCR-negative harvests compared to only 40% of the patients who had received the identical chemotherapeutic regimen without RTX. Four other studies that incorporated RTX specifically into the mobilization regimen yielded PCR-negative harvests ranging from 60 to 100% of the products that were known to be PCR positive prior to collection.[60–63] The effect of in vivo purging on clinical outcome is still unclear but should become more evident as the data mature.

As a method to augment targeted radiation to lymphomatous sites while reducing toxicity to healthy organs, the Seattle Group explored the feasibility of administering high-dose RIT with the $^{131}$I-antiCD20 monoclonal antibody, tositumomab, with AHCT in previously treated FL patients.[48] A multivariable comparison was performed with FL patients who received conventional HDC with AHCT. The RIT regimen was well tolerated with the RIT patients experiencing significantly superior PFS and OS compared to the historical HDC patients (PFS: 48% vs 29% and OS: 67% vs 53%, respectively). The treatment-related mortality (TRM) risk of 3.7% compared favorably with the 11% TRM observed in the historical HDC group.

The occurrence of histologic transformation (HT) occurs in up to 70% of low-grade lymphoma patients and carries a median survival of 1 year or less after transformation with conventional chemotherapy.[64–66] However, this adverse prognosis may be modified by HDC with AHCT although this is controversial. Initial reports from Nebraska and the EBMT reported poor outcomes after AHCT for this subset of patients.[67,68] A more recent update from the EBMT found similar outcomes after AHCT for transformed patients compared to case-matched controls with low-grade disease or de novo high- or intermediate-grade disease.[69] Increased LDH at the time of transformation was the only adverse predictive factor for both OS and PFS. However, a TRM of 18% was seen which was similar to the 20% TRM reported from the Princess Margaret Hospital in another retrospective analysis in which TRM was closely linked to advanced age. In the Princess Margaret study, the median OS for the 35 transformed patients was a notable 58 months from the time of transformation with the best outcomes seen in patients who attained a CR prior to transplant.[70] The Stanford Group published a 4-year DFS of 49% and OS of 50% in 17 patients with HT, which was similar to the updated EBMT study.[49] Comparable outcomes after transplantation also were reported by Corradini et al. with a 10-year projected EFS of 54% for HT patients compared to 65% for patients who retained a low-grade histology.[71] Together these data suggest that patients with HT may benefit from dose-intensive chemotherapy, especially patients with chemosensitive disease, and that the occurrence of HT does not necessarily portend a poor outcome.

## PERIPHERAL T-CELL LYMPHOMA

The prognostic significance of the T-cell phenotype in NHL is controversial but it has generally been shown that patients with peripheral T-cell lymphoma (PTCL) have a worse outcome compared to patients with B-cell diffuse lymphoma[72,73] when treated with conventional chemotherapy. It has been challenging to draw definitive conclusions regarding the effect of HDC with AHCT in this patient population due to the low incidence of this subtype and the heterogeneity of the lymphomas that fall under this classification that are not always clearly delineated in published studies. Rodriguez et al. of the Spanish GEL-TAMO group (Spanish Group for Lymphoma and Autologous Transplantation) has reported the largest series to date of 115 patients with PTCL treated with AHCT.[74] The 5-year OS and DFS rates were 60% and 56%, respectively, with a median follow-up of 37 months. When the outcome of the 37 patients who were transplanted in first remission was examined separately, OS increased to 80%, which was statistically significant. The age-adjusted IPI and LDH at transplant were of relevant prognostic significance in this particular study. In contrast, the patients with refractory disease had a 0% OS which concurred with an EBMT report of 64 patients of varying remission status in which most of the 8 refractory patients experienced dismal outcomes.[75] Actuarial OS at 10 years was 70% for all patients. The Princess Margaret Group and two Scandinavian studies showed that PTCL patients of the anaplastic large cell lymphoma (ALCL) subtype tended to experience better outcomes after AHCT compared to the other histologic subtypes under PTCL.[76–78] Jantunen et al. reported a 5-year OS of 85% for ALCL patients compared to 35% for the other PTCL histologies. Song et al. from the Princess Margaret Hospital compared 36 patients with PTCL to 97 patients with B-cell DLCL and found no difference in EFS (37% vs 42%, respectively) and OS (48% vs 53%, respectively) after AHCT. Again, more favorable outcomes among the ALCL patients compared to the other PTCL patients were observed. The ALCL patients had superior survivals relative to the PTCL-not otherwise specified subgroup but similar outcomes compared to the DLCL patients. The Memorial Sloan Kettering series excluded ALCL patients and also reported no difference in EFS or OS between PTCL patients and corresponding DLCL patients.[79] The secondary age-adjusted IPI was a strong predictor for EFS as patients in the high-intermediate- or high-risk groups faired poorly regardless of chemosensitivity. An MD Anderson series of 36 PTCL patients reported the predictive relevance of the pre-transplant IPI for OS but not for PFS with pretransplant LDH affecting both PFS and OS.[80] The GEL-TAMO group also examined the impact of AHCT in 35 patients who were primary induction failures and obtained a 5-year DFS and OS of 43% and 51%, respectively, thus indicating that HDC/AHCT can rescue initial chemotherapy failures.[81] On the basis of these data, a subset of patients with PTCL may be cured with AHCT, especially those who demonstrate chemosensitive disease. The role of HDC as frontline therapy is less clear although the limited available data show encouraging results.

## HIGH-GRADE LYMPHOMA/BURKITT'S LYMPHOMA

There have been few reports and no randomized studies evaluating the role of HDC/AHCT in patients with Burkitt's lymphoma (BL). Brief duration high-intensity chemotherapy protocols currently confer survival rates approaching 70% and HDC has not improved outcome as compared to frontline therapy.[82,83] Smeland et al. reported a 65% OS for newly diagnosed BL patients treated with high-intensity chemotherapy with a comparable 71% OS seen for patients who underwent AHCT in first remission. The data from the EBMT registry concurred showing a 3-year actuarial OS of 72% for 70 adult BL patients transplanted in first CR. For patients with chemosensitive relapse and resistant disease, the OS rates were 37% and 7%, respectively.[84] The City of Hope reported similar results with a 3-year DFS and OS of 60% for 10 BL patients who received AHCT in first CR or PR.[85] Thus, patients with recurrent or refractory BL should be channeled toward an allogeneic HCT as AHCT has been generally unsuccessful in such patients.

Lymphoblastic lymphoma is a clinically aggressive disease that accounts for only 2% of the NHLs. This clinical entity is usually composed of precursor T cells, has a predilection for young males, and frequently involves the BM and/or central nervous system.[86] Because of the frequent BM involvement and its resemblance to acute lymphoblastic leukemia, allogeneic transplantation is typically recommended in most cases. However, a recent retrospective analysis from the IBMTR/ABMTR failed to find a survival advantage for 76 patients with lymphoblastic lymphoma who received an allogeneic transplant compared to 128 patients who received an autograft.[87] The 5-year OS rates were 39% vs 44%, respectively. Although the 5-year relapse rate was significantly lower in the allogeneic patients (34% vs 56%, $p = 0.004$), the 5-year TRM was higher in the allogeneic recipients (25% vs 5%). Independent of the source of stem cells, multivariate analysis revealed that BM involvement at the time of transplant and disease status beyond first remission were associated with inferior outcomes. Another retrospective analysis of 214 patients from the EBMT demonstrated superior outcomes for patients who received an autograft in first CR compared to patients transplanted in second CR or patients with resistant disease.[88] The 6-year actuarial OS rates were 63%, 31%, and 15%, respectively. The efficacy of AHCT versus conventional dose consolidation as postremission therapy was studied in a European prospective trial of 119 patients.[89] Autologous transplantation produced a trend for improved RFS but not for OS (57% and 53%, respectively) when compared to conventional dose maintenance therapy after 37 months of follow-up. Thus, both retrospective registry data and a few other series suggest that autologous transplantation can confer long-term remissions in a select group of patients.

## POSTTRANSPLANT CONSOLIDATION/ MAINTENANCE THERAPY

HDC with AHCT can cure nearly half of NHL patients with chemosensitive disease and about 30% of patients with primary refractory disease. However, relapse still accounts for the majority of deaths in this patient population with most relapses occurring in sites of previous bulk disease. IFRT as adjuvant therapy posttransplantation is a strategy that can reduce this risk. Advantages for administering IFRT posttransplantation include the ability to tailor radiation dose based on residual disease volume, which may allow use of lower radiation doses and avoid delaying HDC in patients with rapidly progressive disease. The University of Chicago group transplanted 53 patients with relapsed/refractory NHL with 6 patients receiving IFRT to sites of persistent disease after transplantation.[90] Although the sample size was small, the IFRT patients experienced significantly improved local control of persistent disease sites (100% vs 29%, $p = 0.01$) and had a lower incidence of recurrences in previously active sites. Not surprisingly, the sites at greatest risk of relapse were sites failing to achieve a CR to induction therapy regardless of subsequent response to AHCT. Vose et al. from Nebraska demonstrated that not receiving IFRT either before or after transplant was an adverse prognostic factor for OS in a series of 184 patients with NHL patients with primary refractory disease.[91] The University of Rochester group provided AHCT to 136 relapsed/refractory NHL patients.[92] Fifty-one patients received posttransplant IFRT. Of the 58 patients transplanted with bulky disease, the 30 patients who received IFRT had a 3-year EFS of 35% versus 16% ($p = 0.04$) for the 28 patients who did not receive IFRT. Bulky disease was defined as nodal or extranodal disease >2 cm in diameter or >20% of marrow involvement with lymphoma. The patients with nonbulky disease did not experience a survival advantage with IFRT as consolidation. Unfortunately, there are no comparative trials addressing the role of IFRT after transplantation but IFRT should be offered as a valuable adjunct in this setting to reduce relapse rates in sites of previous bulk disease and to confer local control in residual sites after transplantation. However, potential concerns associated with IFRT include increased incidence of pneumonitis, transient cytopenias, and an increased risk of secondary MDS/AML.[93,94]

Numerous other strategies that have been employed to reduce the relapse risk include cytokine therapy with IL-2, antibody-based therapies, and cellular therapies involving IL-2 activated products with natural killer cells or cytokine-induced killer cells.[95–99] However, the use of the anti-CD20 monoclonal antibody, RTX, as maintenance therapy after transplantation to eliminate residual tumor cells is increasingly being explored. Given its minimal toxicity profile and non-cross-resistant mechanism with chemotherapy, RTX has currently emerged as the most appealing agent for adjuvant therapy posttransplantation for patients with indolent, aggressive, and mantle cell B-cell NHL. In a German multicenter phase II study, 20 patients with newly diagnosed FL and 10 patients with MCL received four weekly doses of RTX at a median of 2 months posttransplant.[100] The addition of RTX increased both the complete clinical and molecular remission rates over time. At 6 months of follow-up, the clinical CR rate of 59% increased to 88% after 24 months of follow-up. Additionally, prior to transplantation, 22% of peripheral blood or BM samples were PCR negative. These numbers increased to 53% immediately after AHCT to 72% immediately after RTX administration and then to an impressive 100% PCR negativity at 6 months posttransplantation. These results indicated that clearance of MRD can continue for several months after RTX administration. The RTX was well tolerated with a 4% incidence of transient leukopenia and lymphocytopenia although seven patients developed pneumonia. B-cell peripheral blood counts normalized approximately 12 months after RTX consolidation therapy. Buckstein et al. administered RTX maintenance therapy to 17 patients with follicular NHL who had also received RTX prior to the mobilization regimen.[101] At a median of 1 year of follow-up, all assessable patients remained in CR and all seven patients evaluable for molecular monitoring remained bcl-2 negative at 6 months. In this study, four of 12 patients who received alpha-interferon instead of RTX for maintenance relapsed at a median follow-up of 28 months. In other published reports, Magni et al. and Ladetto et al. demonstrated the safety and feasibility of incorporating RTX for the purposes of in vivo purging and post-HSCT maintenance therapy in patients with B-cell NHL including follicular NHL.[44,58] A large ongoing trial in Europe conducted by the EBMT is evaluating the roles of both in vivo purging and maintenance therapy with RTX in a multicenter setting for FL patients in second or third remission. This trial involves a four-arm randomization to either in vivo purging and maintenance, purging without maintenance, maintenance without purging, or no RTX administration.

The Stanford Group administered four weekly infusions of RTX to 28 patients with NHL beginning 42 days after transplant with additional infusions given at 6 months.[97] All patients had rapid depletion of B cells with no increase in infection or significant adverse events except for an isolated transient neutropenia that occurred in 54% of the patients. At a median follow-up of 30 months, the EFS and OS rates were 83% and 88%, respectively. These results compare very favorably when the subgroup of 21 patients with DLCL were compared to a historical control group of DLCL patients who underwent AHCT without RTX maintenance therapy (see Figure 64.5). The 2-year EFS and OS rates were 58% and 62%, respectively, in the control group. Longer follow-up and the results of an ongoing Intergroup randomized trial will reveal the true clinical benefit of RTX maintenance therapy, but initial data speak strongly for both the safety and efficacy in the adjuvant setting.

## RISK OF SECONDARY MYELODYSPLASIA/ACUTE MYELOGENOUS LEUKEMIA AFTER AUTOGRAFTING

Secondary malignancies are a known late complication after conventional and HDC with treatment-related myelodysplastic syndrome (t-MDS) and treatment-related acute myelogenous leukemia (t-AML) being the most predominant type of secondary malignancies observed after AHCT.[102–104] This particular late effect in NHL patients following AHCT has been extensively described by numerous groups with the reported crude incidence varying from 3 to 12%

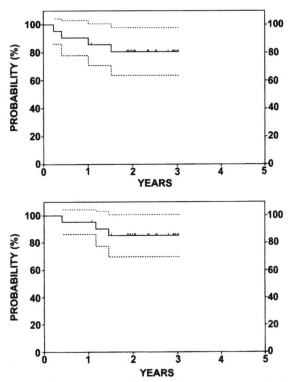

**Figure 64.5** *Event-free survival (top) and overall survival (bottom) for 21 patients with relapsed or refractory diffuse large B-cell lymphoma. Dotted lines represent 95% confidence interval. Tic marks represent censored data. (From Horwitz et al.[97] with permission. Copyright American Society of Hematology)*

and the estimated actuarial risk ranging from 3 to 19% at 5–10 years.[105–111] The median time from AHCT to diagnosis of t-MDS/t-AML is approximately 2–4 years with median survival durations following this complication being only several months. Allogeneic transplantation salvages only a minority of these patients. The most common associated cytogenetic abnormalities include aberrations of chromosome 5 and/or 7 or complex abnormalities that have a strong association with cumulative doses of alkylating agents.[112,113] Topoisomerase II inhibitors such as etoposide and doxorubicin have been associated with 11q23/21q22 abnormalities and a shorter latency period.[114,115]

It is not clear whether the antecedent chemotherapy and RT or the transplantation conditioning regimen has the greater impact in the development of t-MDS/t-AML. A case-control analysis from the ABMTR analyzed 2739 patients with NHL or Hodgkin's disease who had undergone AHCT and found that the type and intensity of prior chemotherapy contributed substantially to the development of this late complication.[111] The 7-year cumulative risk of developing t-MDS/t-AML was 3.9% with the relative risk being four to eight times higher for patients who had received large cumulative doses of mechlorethamine or chlorambucil, respectively. The dose of TBI was also important, as patients who received >13.2 Gray had a relative risk of 4.4, compared to patients who received <13.2 Gray. Prior chemotherapy was also implicated in a Danish series of NHL and HD patients, which found that HDC with AHCT did not increase the risk of leukemic complications above the level observed after conventional chemotherapy.[106] Thus, antecedent chemotherapy was the most important predictive factor. The Dana Farber Group reported a 19.8% actuarial incidence at 10 years without evidence of a plateau in 552 NHL patients who underwent AHCT with cyclophosphamide and TBI as the conditioning regimen.[109] Prior IFRT and lower number of cells infusion during transplantation were the only variables that differed between patients who did and did not develop MDS/AML.

Although there is a consensus that cumulative dose of prior chemotherapy is related to the development of t-MDS/t-AML, the contribution of TBI in the preparative regimen toward the development of this late complication remains controversial. The EBMT retrospectively studied 5000 patients with lymphoma who had undergone AHCT. Sixty-eight patients developed MDS with a median follow-up of 3 years.[110] Multivariate analysis revealed TBI in the conditioning regimen, older age at transplant and low-grade histology as independent variables predictive of MDS development. The low-grade histology patients were also more likely to have received a greater total dose of alkylating agents such as chlorambucil and cyclophosphamide prior to AHCT compared to the patients with intermediate/high-grade disease. An MD Anderson series reported that the use of TBI was independently associated with an increased risk of t-MDS/t-AML, especially when combined with high-dose cyclophosphamide and etoposide.[108] Prior fludarabine administration and BM involvement also increased this risk. The City of Hope Group did not find the use of TBI in the conditioning regimen to be of prognostic value but demonstrated that pretransplant RT did confer a higher risk, which concurred with the DFCI findings.[107] In contrast to the ABMTR analysis and the above-mentioned Danish study, pretransplant chemotherapy did not affect the risk of t-MDS/t-AML. However, for patients who received etoposide for stem cell priming, a 12.3 fold increased risk of developing t-AML with 11q23 abnormalities was seen. In summary, t-MDS and t-AML are serious consequences after AHCT. The assessment of occult cytogenetic abnormalities before hematopoietic cell mobilization or harvest should be routinely performed, especially in heavily pretreated patients who may already harbor early MDS prior to transplantation.

## CONCLUSION

Autologous transplantation has emerged as an effective therapy for patients with NHL of a variety of histologies at various points in disease treatment. Randomized clinical trials have demonstrated improved outcomes as compared to standard chemotherapy in several settings including for patients with intermediate-grade B-cell DLCL with chemosensitive relapse and for patients with high risk features in first CR. Patients who do not achieve a CR with initial induction chemotherapy also can be salvaged with AHCT. Patients with relapsed low-grade lymphoma who have not been heavily pretreated also benefit from AHCT. However, the occurrence of secondary malignancies, especially t-MDS and t-AML, is a problematic late effect that adversely impacts long-term survival rates. Newer concepts such as immunotherapy with monoclonal antibodies, cell-based therapies and nonmyeloablative allogeneic transplantation are under active investigation in an effort to further improve outcomes.

## REFERENCES

1. Jemal A, Tiwari RC, Murray T, et al.: Cancer statistics, 2004. *CA Cancer J Clin* 54:8, 2004.
2. Cabanillas F: Experience with salvage regimens at M.D. Anderson Hospital. *Ann Oncol* 2 (suppl 1):31, 1991.
3. Velasquez WS, Cabanillas F, Salvador P, et al.: Effective salvage therapy for lymphoma with cisplatin in combination with high-dose Ara-C and dexamethasone (DHAP). *Blood* 71:117, 1988.
4. Schouten HC, Qian W, Kvaloy S, et al.: High-dose therapy improves progression-free survival and survival in relapsed follicular non-Hodgkin's lymphoma: results from the randomized European CUP trial. *J Clin Oncol* 21:3918, 2003.
5. Frei E III, Cucchi CA, Rosowsky A, et al.: Alkylating agent resistance: in vitro studies with human cell lines. *Proc Natl Acad Sci USA* 82:2158, 1985.
6. Schabel FM Jr, Trader MW, Laster WR Jr, et al.: Patterns of resistance and therapeutic synergism among alkylating agents. *Antibiot Chemother* 23:200, 1978.
7. Hill RP, Stanley JA: The response of hypoxic B16 melanoma cells to in vivo treatment with chemotherapeutic agents. *Cancer Res* 35:1147, 1975.
8. Bruce WR, Meeker BE: Comparison of the sensitivity of normal hematopoietic and transplanted lymphoma colony-forming cells to tritiated thymidine. *J Natl Cancer Inst* 34:849, 1965.
9. Appelbaum FR, Deisseroth AB, Graw RG Jr, et al.: Prolonged complete remission following high dose chemotherapy of Burkitt's lymphoma in relapse. *Cancer* 41:1059, 1978.
10. Philip T, Armitage JO, Spitzer G, et al.: High-dose therapy and autologous bone marrow transplantation after failure of conventional chemotherapy in adults with intermediate-grade or high-grade non-Hodgkin's lymphoma. *N Engl J Med* 316:1493, 1987.
11. Philip T, Guglielmi C, Hagenbeek A, et al.: Autologous bone marrow transplantation as compared with salvage chemotherapy in relapses of chemotherapy-sensitive non-Hodgkin's lymphoma. *N Engl J Med* 333:1540, 1995.
12. Guglielmi C, Gomez F, Philip T, et al.: Time to relapse has prognostic value in patients with aggressive lymphoma enrolled onto the Parma trial. *J Clin Oncol* 16:3264, 1998.
13. Blay J, Gomez F, Sebban C, et al.: The International Prognostic Index correlates to survival in patients with aggressive lymphoma in relapse: analysis of the PARMA trial. Parma Group. *Blood* 92:3562, 1998.
14. Hamlin PA, Zelenetz AD, Kewalramani T, et al.: Age-adjusted International Prognostic Index predicts autologous stem cell transplantation outcome for patients with relapsed or primary refractory diffuse large B-cell lymphoma. *Blood* 102:1989, 2003.
15. Guglielmi C, Martelli M, Federico M, et al.: Risk-assessment in diffuse large cell lymphoma at first relapse. A study by the Italian Intergroup for Lymphomas. *Haematologica* 86:941, 2001.
16. Caballero MD, Perez-Simon JA, Iriondo A, et al.: High-dose therapy in diffuse large cell lymphoma: results and prognostic factors in 452 patients from the GEL-TAMO Spanish Cooperative Group. *Ann Oncol* 14:140, 2003.
17. Milpied N, Deconinck E, Gaillard F, et al.: Initial treatment of aggressive lymphoma with high-dose chemotherapy and autologous stem-cell support. *N Engl J Med* 350:1287, 2004.
18. Martelli M, Gherlinzoni F, De Renzo A, et al.: Early autologous stem-cell transplantation versus conventional chemotherapy as front-line therapy in high-risk, aggressive non-Hodgkin's lymphoma: an Italian

multicenter randomized trial. *J Clin Oncol* 21:1255, 2003.

19. Gisselbrecht C, Lepage E, Molina T, et al.: Shortened first-line high-dose chemotherapy for patients with poor-prognosis aggressive lymphoma. *J Clin Oncol* 20:2472, 2002.

20. Kaiser U, Uebelacker I, Abel U, et al.: Randomized study to evaluate the use of high-dose therapy as part of primary treatment for "aggressive" lymphoma. *J Clin Oncol* 20:4413, 2002.

21. Kluin-Nelemans HC, Zagonel V, Anastasopoulou A, et al.: Standard chemotherapy with or without high-dose chemotherapy for aggressive non-Hodgkin's lymphoma: randomized phase III EORTC study. *J Natl Cancer Inst* 93:22, 2001.

22. Haioun C, Lepage E, Gisselbrecht C, et al.: Survival benefit of high-dose therapy in poor-risk aggressive non-Hodgkin's lymphoma: final analysis of the prospective LNH87-2 protocol—a groupe d'Etude des lymphomes de l'Adulte study. *J Clin Oncol* 18:3025, 2000.

23. Gianni AM, Bregni M, Siena S, et al.: High-dose chemotherapy and autologous bone marrow transplantation compared with MACOP-B in aggressive B-cell lymphoma. *N Engl J Med* 336:1290, 1997.

24. Haioun C, Lepage E, Gisselbrecht C, et al.: Benefit of autologous bone marrow transplantation over sequential chemotherapy in poor-risk aggressive non-Hodgkin's lymphoma: updated results of the prospective study LNH87-2. Groupe d'Etude des Lymphomes de l'Adulte. *J Clin Oncol* 15:1131, 1997.

25. Gisselbrecht C, Lepage E, Morel P, et al.: Intensified phase including autologous peripheral stem cell transplantation does not improve response rate and survival in lymphoma with at least 2 adverse prognostic factors when compared to ACVB regimen. *Blood* 88:10, 1996.

26. Mounier N, Gisselbrecht C, Briere J, et al.: Prognostic factors in patients with aggressive non-Hodgkin's lymphoma treated by front-line autotransplantation after complete remission: a cohort study by the Groupe d'Etude des Lymphomes de l'Adulte. *J Clin Oncol* 22:2826, 2004.

27. Santini G, Salvagno L, Leoni P, et al.: VACOP-B versus VACOP-B plus autologous bone marrow transplantation for advanced diffuse non-Hodgkin's lymphoma: results of a prospective randomized trial by the non-Hodgkin's Lymphoma Cooperative Study Group. *J Clin Oncol* 16:2796, 1998.

28. Martelli M, Vignetti M, Zinzani PL, et al.: High-dose chemotherapy followed by autologous bone marrow transplantation versus dexamethasone, cisplatin, and cytarabine in aggressive non-Hodgkin's lymphoma with partial response to front-line chemotherapy: a prospective randomized Italian multicenter study. *J Clin Oncol* 14:534, 1996.

29. Verdonck LF, van Putten WL, Hagenbeek A, et al.: Comparison of CHOP chemotherapy with autologous bone marrow transplantation for slowly responding patients with aggressive non-Hodgkin's lymphoma. *N Engl J Med* 332:1045, 1995.

30. Raffeld M, Jaffe ES: bcl-1, t(11;14), and mantle cell-derived lymphomas. *Blood* 78:259, 1991.

31. Weisenburger DD, Armitage JO: Mantle cell lymphoma—an entity comes of age. *Blood* 87:4483, 1996.

32. Bosch F, Jares P, Campo E, et al.: PRAD-1/cyclin D1 gene overexpression in chronic lymphoproliferative disorders: a highly specific marker of mantle cell lymphoma. *Blood* 84:2726, 1994.

33. Mangel J, Leitch HA, Connors JM, et al.: Intensive chemotherapy and autologous stem-cell transplantation plus rituximab is superior to conventional chemotherapy for newly diagnosed advanced stage mantle-cell lymphoma: a matched pair analysis. *Ann Oncol* 15:283, 2004.

34. Vandenberghe E, Ruiz de Elvira C, Loberiza FR, et al.: Outcome of autologous transplantation for mantle cell lymphoma: a study by the European Blood and Bone Marrow Transplant and Autologous Blood and Marrow Transplant Registries. *Br J Haematol* 120:793, 2003.

35. Gianni AM, Magni M, Martelli M, et al.: Long-term remission in mantle cell lymphoma following high-dose sequential chemotherapy and in vivo rituximab-purged stem cell autografting (R-HDS regimen). *Blood* 102:749, 2003.

36. Andersen NS, Pedersen L, Elonen E, et al.: Primary treatment with autologous stem cell transplantation in mantle cell lymphoma: outcome related to remission pretransplant. *Eur J Haematol* 71:73, 2003.

37. Molina A, Kraft D, Carter A, et al.: Autologous stem cell transplantation for mantle cell lymphoma: a report of 69 patients from City of Hope and Stanford. *Blood* 100:182a, 2002.

38. Lefrere F, Delmer A, Suzan F, et al.: Sequential chemotherapy by CHOP and DHAP regimens followed by high-dose therapy with stem cell transplantation induces a high rate of complete response and improves event-free survival in mantle cell lymphoma: a prospective study. *Leukemia* 16:587, 2002.

39. Gopal AK, Rajendran JG, Petersdorf SH, et al.: High-dose chemo-radioimmunotherapy with autologous stem cell support for relapsed mantle cell lymphoma. *Blood* 99:3158, 2002.

40. Khouri IF, Romaguera J, Kantarjian H, et al.: Hyper-CVAD and high-dose methotrexate/cytarabine followed by stem-cell transplantation: an active regimen for aggressive mantle-cell lymphoma. *J Clin Oncol* 16:3803, 1998.

41. Milpied N, Gaillard F, Moreau P, et al.: High-dose therapy with stem cell transplantation for mantle cell lymphoma: results and prognostic factors, a single center experience. *Bone Marrow Transplant* 22:645, 1998.

42. Vose JM, Bierman PJ, Weisenburger DD, et al.: Autologous hematopoietic stem cell transplantation for mantle cell lymphoma. *Biol Blood Marrow Transplant* 6:640, 2000.

43. Khouri IF, Saliba RM, Okoroji GJ, et al.: Long-term follow-up of autologous stem cell transplantation in patients with diffuse mantle cell lymphoma in first disease remission: the prognostic value of beta2-microglobulin and the tumor score. *Cancer* 98:2630, 2003.

44. Magni M, Di Nicola M, Devizzi L, et al.: Successful in vivo purging of CD34-containing peripheral blood harvests in mantle cell and indolent lymphoma: evidence for a role of both chemotherapy and rituximab infusion. *Blood* 96:864, 2000.

45. Ladetto M, Corradini P, Vallet S, et al.: High rate of clinical and molecular remissions in follicular lymphoma

patients receiving high-dose sequential chemotherapy and autografting at diagnosis: a multicenter, prospective study by the Gruppo Italiano Trapianto Midollo Osseo (GITMO). *Blood* 100:1559, 2002.

46. Horning SJ, Negrin RS, Hoppe RT, et al.: High-dose therapy and autologous bone marrow transplantation for follicular lymphoma in first complete or partial remission: results of a phase II clinical trial. *Blood* 97:404, 2001.

47. Colombat P, Cornillet P, Deconinck E, et al.: Value of autologous stem cell transplantation with purged bone marrow as first-line therapy for follicular lymphoma with high tumor burden: a GOELAMS phase II study. *Bone Marrow Transplant* 26:971, 2000.

48. Gopal AK, Gooley TA, Maloney DG, et al.: High-dose radioimmunotherapy versus conventional high-dose therapy and autologous hematopoietic stem cell transplantation for relapsed follicular non-Hodgkin lymphoma: a multivariable cohort analysis. *Blood* 102:2351, 2003.

49. Cao TM, Horning S, Negrin RS, et al.: High-dose therapy and autologous hematopoietic-cell transplantation for follicular lymphoma beyond first remission: the Stanford University experience. *Biol Blood Marrow Transplant* 7:294, 2001.

50. Apostolidis J, Gupta RK, Grenzelias D, et al.: High-dose therapy with autologous bone marrow support as consolidation of remission in follicular lymphoma: long-term clinical and molecular follow-up. *J Clin Oncol* 18:527, 2000.

51. Freedman AS, Neuberg D, Mauch P, et al.: Long-term follow-up of autologous bone marrow transplantation in patients with relapsed follicular lymphoma. *Blood* 94:3325, 1999.

52. Bierman, PJ, Vose JM, Anderson JR, et al.: High-dose therapy with autologous hematopoietic rescue for follicular low-grade non-Hodgkin's lymphoma. *J Clin Oncol* 15:445, 1997.

53. Colombat P, Binet C, Linassier C, et al.: High dose chemotherapy with autologous marrow transplantation in follicular lymphomas. *Leuk Lymphoma* 7 (suppl):3, 1992.

54. van Besien K, Loberiza FR Jr, Bajorunaite R, et al.: Comparison of autologous and allogeneic hematopoietic stem cell transplantation for follicular lymphoma. *Blood* 102:3521, 2003.

55. Freedman AS, Gribben JG, Neuberg D, et al.: High-dose therapy and autologous bone marrow transplantation in patients with follicular lymphoma during first remission. *Blood* 88:2780, 1996.

56. Voso MT, Martin S, Hohaus S, et al.: Prognostic factors for the clinical outcome of patients with follicular lymphoma following high-dose therapy and peripheral blood stem cell transplantation (PBSCT). *Bone Marrow Transplant* 25:957, 2000.

57. Moos M, Schulz, R, Martin S, et al.: The remission status before and the PCR status after high-dose therapy with peripheral blood stem cell support are prognostic factors for relapse-free survival in patients with follicular non-Hodgkin's lymphoma. *Leukemia* 12:1971, 1998.

58. Ladetto M, Zallio F, Vallet S, et al.: Concurrent administration of high-dose chemotherapy and rituximab is a feasible and effective chemo/immunotherapy for patients with high-risk non-Hodgkin's lymphoma. *Leukemia* 15:1941, 2001.

59. Lazzarino M, Arcaini L, Bernasconi P, et al.: A sequence of immuno-chemotherapy with Rituximab, mobilization of in vivo purged stem cells, high-dose chemotherapy and autotransplant is an effective and non-toxic treatment for advanced follicular and mantle cell lymphoma. *Br J Haematol* 116:229, 2002.

60. Galimberti S, Guerrini F, Morabito F, et al.: Quantitative molecular valuation in autotransplant programs for follicular lymphoma: efficacy of in vivo purging by Rituximab. *Bone Marrow Transplant* 32:57, 2003.

61. Belhadj K, Delfau-Larue MH, Elgnaoui T, et al.: Efficiency of in vivo purging with rituximab prior to autologous peripheral blood progenitor cell transplantation in B-cell non-Hodgkin's lymphoma: a single institution study. *Ann Oncol* 15:504, 2004.

62. Goldberg S, Pecora AL, Jennis A, et al.: Rituximab permits in vivo purging and collection of tumor-free stem cells prior to autologous transplantation for B-cell non-Hodgkin's lymphoma. *Blood* 94:141a, 1999.

63. Salles G, Moullett I, Charlot C, et al.: In vivo purging with rituximab before autologous peripheral blood progenitor cells transplantation in lymphoma patients. *Blood* 94:141a, 1999.

64. Horning SJ, Rosenberg SA: The natural history of initially untreated low-grade non-Hodgkin's lymphomas. *N Engl J Med* 311:1471, 1984.

65. Gallagher CJ, Gregory WM, Jones AE, et al.: Follicular lymphoma: prognostic factors for response and survival. *J Clin Oncol* 4:1470, 1986.

66. Acker B, Hoppe RT, Colby TV, et al.: Histologic conversion in the non-Hodgkin's lymphomas. *J Clin Oncol* 1:11, 1983.

67. Schouten HC, Colombat P, Verdonck LF, et al.: Autologous bone marrow transplantation for low-grade non-Hodgkin's lymphoma: the European Bone Marrow Transplant Group experience. EBMT Working Party for Lymphoma. *Ann Oncol* 5 (suppl 2):147, 1994.

68. Schouten HC, Bierman PJ, Vaughan WP, et al.: Autologous bone marrow transplantation in follicular non-Hodgkin's lymphoma before and after histologic transformation. *Blood* 74:2579, 1989.

69. Williams CD, Harrison CN, Lister TA, et al.: High-dose therapy and autologous stem-cell support for chemosensitive transformed low-grade follicular non-Hodgkin's lymphoma: a case-matched study from the European Bone Marrow Transplant Registry. *J Clin Oncol* 19:727, 2001.

70. Chen CI, Crump M, Tsang R, et al.: Autotransplants for histologically transformed follicular non-Hodgkin's lymphoma. *Br J Haematol* 113:202, 2001.

71. Corradini P, Ladetto M, Zallio F, et al.: Long-term follow-up of indolent lymphoma patients treated with high-dose sequential chemotherapy and autografting: evidence that durable molecular and clinical remission frequently can be attained only in follicular subtypes. *J Clin Oncol* 22:1460, 2004.

72. Gisselbrecht C, Gaulard P, Lepage E, et al.: Prognostic significance of T-cell phenotype in aggressive

non-Hodgkin's lymphomas. Groupe d'Etudes des Lymphomes de l'Adulte (GELA). *Blood* 92:76, 1998.

73. Melnyk A, Rodriguez A, Pugh WC, et al.: Evaluation of the Revised European–American Lymphoma Classification confirms the clinical relevance of immunophenotype in 560 cases of aggressive non-Hodgkin's lymphoma. *Blood* 89:4514, 1997.

74. Rodriguez J, Caballero MD, Gutierrez A, et al.: High-dose chemotherapy and autologous stem cell transplantation in peripheral T-cell lymphoma: the GEL-TAMO experience. *Ann Oncol* 14:1768, 2003.

75. Fanin R, Ruiz de Elvira MC, Sperotto A, et al.: Autologous stem cell transplantation for T and null cell CD30-positive anaplastic large cell lymphoma: analysis of 64 adult and paediatric cases reported to the European Group for Blood and Marrow Transplantation (EBMT). *Bone Marrow Transplant* 23:437, 1999.

76. Blystad AK, Enblad G, Kvaloy S, et al.: High-dose therapy with autologous stem cell transplantation in patients with peripheral T cell lymphomas. *Bone Marrow Transplant* 27:711, 2001.

77. Jantunen E, Wiklund T, Juvonen E, et al.: Autologous stem cell transplantation in adult patients with peripheral T-cell lymphoma: a nation-wide survey. *Bone Marrow Transplant* 33:405, 2004.

78. Song KW, Mollee P, Keating A, et al.: Autologous stem cell transplant for relapsed and refractory peripheral T-cell lymphoma: variable outcome according to pathological subtype. *Br J Haematol* 120:978, 2003.

79. Kewalramani T, Nimer SD, Zelentz PA, et al.: Similar outcomes for chemosensitive relapsed or primary refractory peripheral T-cell lymphoma and diffuse large B-cell lymphoma treated with autologous transplantation. *Blood* 100:646a, 2002.

80. Rodriguez J, Munsell M, Yazji S, et al.: Impact of high-dose chemotherapy on peripheral T-cell lymphomas. *J Clin Oncol* 19:3766, 2001.

81. Rodriguez J, Caballero MD, Gutierrez A, et al.: High dose chemotherapy and autologous stem cell transplantation in patients with peripheral T-cell lymphoma not achieving complete response after induction chemotherapy. The GEL-TAMO experience. *Haematologica* 88:1372, 2003.

82. Smeland S, Blystad AK, Kvaloy SO, et al.: Treatment of Burkitt's/Burkitt-like lymphoma in adolescents and adults: a 20-year experience from the Norwegian Radium Hospital with the use of three successive regimens. *Ann Oncol* 15:1072, 2004.

83. McMaster ML, Greer JP, Greco FA, et al.: Effective treatment of small-noncleaved-cell lymphoma with high-intensity, brief-duration chemotherapy. *J Clin Oncol* 9:941, 1991.

84. Sweetenham JW, Pearce R, Taghipour G, et al.: Adult Burkitt's and Burkitt-like non-Hodgkin's lymphoma—outcome for patients treated with high-dose therapy and autologous stem-cell transplantation in first remission or at relapse: results from the European Group for Blood and Marrow Transplantation. *J Clin Oncol* 14:2465, 1996.

85. Nademanee A, Molina A, O'Donnell MR, et al.: Results of high-dose therapy and autologous bone marrow/stem cell transplantation during remission in

poor-risk intermediate- and high-grade lymphoma: international index high and high-intermediate risk group. *Blood* 90:3844, 1997.

86. Rosen PJ, Feinstein DI, Pattengale PK, et al.: Convoluted lymphocytic lymphoma in adults: a clinicopathologic entity. *Ann Intern Med* 89:319, 1978.

87. Levine JE, Harris RE, Loberiza FR Jr, et al.: A comparison of allogeneic and autologous bone marrow transplantation for lymphoblastic lymphoma. *Blood* 101:2476, 2003.

88. Sweetenham JW, Liberti G, Pearce R, et al.: High-dose therapy and autologous bone marrow transplantation for adult patients with lymphoblastic lymphoma: results of the European Group for Bone Marrow Transplantation. *J Clin Oncol* 12:1358, 1994.

89. Sweetenham JW, Santini G, Qian W, et al.: High-dose therapy and autologous stem-cell transplantation versus conventional-dose consolidation/maintenance therapy as postremission therapy for adult patients with lymphoblastic lymphoma: results of a randomized trial of the European Group for Blood and Marrow Transplantation and the United Kingdom Lymphoma Group. *J Clin Oncol* 19:2927, 2001.

90. Mundt AJ, Williams SF, Hallahan D: High dose chemotherapy and stem cell rescue for aggressive non-Hodgkin's lymphoma: pattern of failure and implications for involved-field radiotherapy. *Int J Radiat Oncol Biol Phys* 39:617, 1997.

91. Vose JM, Zhang MJ, Rowlings PA, et al.: Autologous transplantation for diffuse aggressive non-Hodgkin's lymphoma in patients never achieving remission: a report from the Autologous Blood and Marrow Transplant Registry. *J Clin Oncol* 19:406, 2001.

92. Rapoport AP, Lifton R, Constine LS, et al.: Autotransplantation for relapsed or refractory non-Hodgkin's lymphoma (NHL): long-term follow-up and analysis of prognostic factors. *Bone Marrow Transplant* 19:883, 1997.

93. Toren A, Nagler R, Nagler A: Involved field radiation post autologous stem cell transplantation in lymphoma patients is associated with major haematological toxicities. *Med Oncol* 15:113, 1998.

94. Emmanouilides C, Asuncion DJ, Wolf C, et al.: Localized radiation increases morbidity and mortality after TBI-containing autologous stem cell transplantation in patients with lymphoma. *Bone Marrow Transplant* 32:863, 2003.

95. Nagler A, Ackerstein A, Or R, et al.: Immunotherapy with recombinant human interleukin-2 and recombinant interferon-alpha in lymphoma patients postautologous marrow or stem cell transplantation. *Blood* 89:3951, 1997.

96. Lauria F, Raspadori D, Ventura MA, et al.: Immunologic and clinical modifications following low-dose subcutaneous administration of rIL-2 in non-Hodgkin's lymphoma patients after autologous bone marrow transplantation. *Bone Marrow Transplant* 18:79, 1996.

97. Horwitz SM, Negrin RS, Blume KG, et al.: Rituximab as adjuvant to high-dose therapy and autologous hematopoietic cell transplantation for aggressive non-Hodgkin lymphoma. *Blood* 103:777, 2004.

98. Leemhuis T, Wells S, Horn P, et al.: Autologous cytokine induced killer cells for the treatment of relapsed Hodgkin's disease and non-Hodgkin's lymphoma. *Blood* 96:839a, 2000.

99. Jensen M, Tan G, Forman S, et al.: CD20 is a molecular target for scFvFc:zeta receptor redirected T cells: implications for cellular immunotherapy of CD20+ malignancy. *Biol Blood Marrow Transplant* 4:75, 1998.

100. Brugger W: Clearing minimal residual disease with rituximab consolidation therapy. *Semin Oncol* 31:33, 2004.

101. Buckstein R, Imrie K, Spaner D, et al.: Consolidative immunotherapy with rituxan in autologous stem cell transplantation in follicular lymphoma is associated with molecular remissions. *Proc Am Soc Clin Oncol* 19:26a, 2000.

102. Pedersen-Bjergaard J, Andersen MK, Christiansen DH: Therapy-related acute myeloid leukemia and myelodysplasia after high-dose chemotherapy and autologous stem cell transplantation. *Blood* 95:3273, 2000.

103. Stone RM, Neuberg D, Soiffer R, et al.: Myelodysplastic syndrome as a late complication following autologous bone marrow transplantation for non-Hodgkin's lymphoma. *J Clin Oncol* 12:2535, 1994.

104. Darrington DL, Vose JM, Anderson JR, et al.: Incidence and characterization of secondary myelodysplastic syndrome and acute myelogenous leukemia following high-dose chemoradiotherapy and autologous stem-cell transplantation for lymphoid malignancies. *J Clin Oncol* 12:2527, 1994.

105. Micallef IN, Lillington DM, Apostolidis J, et al.: Therapy-related myelodysplasia and secondary acute myelogenous leukemia after high-dose therapy with autologous hematopoietic progenitor-cell support for lymphoid malignancies. *J Clin Oncol* 18:947, 2000.

106. Pedersen-Bjergaard J, Pedersen M, Myhre J, et al.: High risk of therapy-related leukemia after BEAM chemotherapy and autologous stem cell transplantation for previously treated lymphomas is mainly related to primary chemotherapy and not to the BEAM-transplantation procedure. *Leukemia* 11:1654, 1997.

107. Krishnan A, Bhatia S, Slovak ML, et al.: Predictors of therapy-related leukemia and myelodysplasia following autologous transplantation for lymphoma: an assessment of risk factors. *Blood* 95:1588, 2000.

108. Hosing C, Munsell M, Yazji S, et al.: Risk of therapy-related myelodysplastic syndrome/acute leukemia following high-dose therapy and autologous bone marrow transplantation for non-Hodgkin's lymphoma. *Ann Oncol* 13:450, 2002.

109. Friedberg JW, Neuberg D, Stone RM, et al.: Outcome in patients with myelodysplastic syndrome after autologous bone marrow transplantation for non-Hodgkin's lymphoma. *J Clin Oncol* 17:3128, 1999.

110. Milligan DW, Ruiz De Elvira MC, Kolb HJ, et al.: Secondary leukaemia and myelodysplasia after autografting for lymphoma: results from the EBMT. EBMT Lymphoma and Late Effects Working Parties. European Group for Blood and Marrow Transplantation. *Br J Haematol* 106:1020, 1999.

111. Metayer C, Curtis RE, Vose J, et al.: Myelodysplastic syndrome and acute myeloid leukemia after autotransplantation for lymphoma: a multicenter case-control study. *Blood* 101:2015, 2003.

112. Smith SM, Le Beau MM, Huo D, et al.: Clinical-cytogenetic associations in 306 patients with therapy-related myelodysplasia and myeloid leukemia: the University of Chicago series. *Blood* 102:43, 2003.

113. Johansson B, Mertens F, Heim S, et al.: Cytogenetics of secondary myelodysplasia (sMDS) and acute nonlymphocytic leukemia (sANLL). *Eur J Haematol* 47:17, 1991.

114. Pedersen-Bjergaard J, Andersen MK, Johansson B: Balanced chromosome aberrations in leukemias following chemotherapy with DNA-topoisomerase II inhibitors. *J Clin Oncol* 16:1897, 1998.

115. Larson RA, Le Beau MM, Ratain MJ, et al.: Balanced translocations involving chromosome bands 11q23 and 21q22 in therapy-related leukemia. *Blood* 79:1892, 1992.

# Chapter 65

# ALLOGENEIC HEMATOPOIETIC STEM CELL TRANSPLANTATION FOR NON-HODGKIN'S LYMPHOMA

*Hillard M. Lazarus*

## INTRODUCTION

### HISTORICAL PERSPECTIVE: AUTOLOGOUS STEM CELL TRANSPLANTATION

Although many non-Hodgkin's lymphoma (NHL) histologic subtypes can be cured using combination chemotherapy, many patients experience relapse or never achieve remission after initial therapy. For several decades, high-dose chemoradiation therapy and autologous stem cell transplantation (auto SCT), using either autologous bone marrow or, subsequently, autologous peripheral blood stem cells (auto PBSC), has been demonstrated to be an effective therapy for sensitive-relapse NHL patients.[1–3] This modality can also be effective in refractory relapse or even primary refractory disease states.[4,5] Some investigators have reported data supporting a recommendation for use of auto SCT in NHL patients at high risk for relapse.[6,7] Obvious benefits of auto SCT are use of self as a donor, no need for posttransplant immunosuppression and its attendant risks, and the avoidance of graft-versus-host disease (GvHD). On the other hand, this modality usually is ineffective in the setting of significant tumor bulk, cannot be offered to patients who have been subjected to extensive previous treatment limiting mobilization of blood stem cells,[8] and lacks graft-versus-lymphoma (GvL) effect. The major limitation of auto SCT is relapse after transplant, due, in part, to intrinsic lymphoma resistance to cytotoxic agents and the potential for reinfusion of occult tumor cells that may contribute to relapse.[9] In vitro purging methods indirectly have been shown to provide benefit in some patients, but the results are not conclusive.[10,11] The prognosis after relapse in auto SCT recipients is extremely poor.

## ALLOGENEIC HEMATOPOIETIC STEM CELL TRANSPLANTATION

Hematopoietic stem cell transplantation using cells collected from an allogeneic donor (allo SCT) is an option being used with increased frequency. In the past, this approach was used less often in view of limited donor availability, and high nonrelapse mortality, in part, due to GvHD. Allo SCT has the potential for improving patient outcome, as there is no infusion of lymphoma cells (normal donor) and the donor effector cells provide the potential for a GvL effect[12] (Table 65.1).

## GRAFT-VERSUS-LYMPHOMA EFFECT

Evidence for a graft-versus-malignancy or GvL effect in NHL is mixed (Table 65.2). In a review, Mollee and colleagues[13] noted the conflicting results in a number of studies, as the GvL effect was not uniform in the

**Table 65.1** Allo SCT compared to auto SCT for NHL: advantages and disadvantages

| Advantages | Disadvantages |
|---|---|
| Normality of infused stem cells | Increased non-relapse mortality |
| Grafts-versus-lymphoma effect | Increased "allogeneic-radated" morbidity |
| Avoidance of secondary AML/MDS | Age and donor restrictions |
| No graft contamination by lymphoma | Increased costs Lack of randomized trials |

AML, acute myeloid leukemia; MDS, myelodys plastic syndrome.

**Table 65.2**    Evidence of graft-versus-malignancy effect in humans

- Abrupt immunosuppression withdrawal or GvHD or flare reestablishes complete remissions
- Relapse higher in syngeneic than in allogeneic graft recipients
- GvHD protective against relapse in some patient subgroups
- T-cell depletion increases relapse rates in CML patients
- Donor lymphocyte infusions can induce complete remissions
- Allo SCT relapse rates are lower than those for auto SCT

GvHD, graft-versus-host disease; CML, chronic myeloid leukemia

intermediate- and high-grade histologic subtypes. The data for follicular NHL, a slower growing neoplasm, are more convincing. Tse and colleagues[14] recently reported the benefit of GvL across many studies in which low-grade NHL patients underwent allo SCT using either a myeloablative or reduced-conditioning regimen.

## REASONS TO CONSIDER ALLOGENEIC HEMATOPOIETIC STEM CELL TRANSPLANTATION FOR NHL

Clinicians and investigators have offered patients allo SCT rather than auto SCT for a variety of reasons, including technical considerations such as failure to collect sufficient stem cells for transplant. Alternatively, health care professionals may recommend an allo SCT for inherent biases, such as resistance to therapy and gross marrow involvement (Table 65.3). Also, some patients who relapse after an auto SCT are offered an allograft.

## MYELOABLATIVE ALLO SCT IN FAILED AUTO PBSCT

Freytes et al.[15] recently published a retrospective analysis of IBMTR data collected from 1990 to 1999 on 114 lymphoma (N = 35 Hodgkin's disease and N = 79 NHL) patients who received a myeloablative allo SCT after a failed auto SCT. Sixteen patients had low-grade

**Table 65.3**    Reasons for clinicians and investigators to consider allo SCT rather than auto SCT

- Resistance to initial therapy
- Resistance to salvage therapy
- Resistance to both initial and salvage therapy
- Bone marrow histologic (gross) involvement
- Failure to harvest auto PBSC
- Relapse after auto SCT

NHL, 52 intermediate- and high-grade, and 8 had other types such as composite, mantle-cell, and peripheral T-cell NHL. A variety of graft sources were used (61% sibling-matched; 14% haploidentical sib; 25% unrelated). Treatment-related mortality was 22% at 1 year and 25% at 5 years. Overall survival at 3 years was 33% and decreased to 24% by 5 years after allo SCT. Similarly, progression-free survival (PFS) was 25% and 5% at 3 and 5 years, respectively. Complete remission at time of transplant and use of total body irradiation (TBI) in the preparative regimen were associated with lower rates of tumor progression and higher overall survival. These results are quite disappointing, but reflect both a poor-risk patient group, as well as an emerging approach. Specifically, van Besien and colleagues[16] noted dramatic improvement in overall survival after myeloablative HLA sibling-matched allo SCT from 39% during the 1990–1993 period to 72% over 1997–1999. Readers of the literature must take into account such improvements when comparing studies, especially when not conducted during concurrent periods of time.

## MYELOABLATIVE ALLO SCT AS FIRST TRANSPLANT: AGGRESSIVE NHL

Several single-arm cohort studies have used myeloablative allo SCT for relapsed or, rarely, high-risk (for relapse) aggressive as well as low-grade NHL patients. Significantly fewer aggressive NHL patients have undergone this approach, as historically most patients have been offered auto SCT as therapy. Table 65.4 shows five series of myeloablative allo SCT for NHL.[17–21] Most patients exhibited refractory disease at time of transplant, and as a result of extensive prior therapy and anticipated complications such as GvHD, nonrelapse mortality was quite high, accounting for death in one third to one half of patients. One single-institution series reported by Stein and colleagues[20] noted only a 15% overall survival at 5 years after transplant, a reflection of advanced, heavily pretreated patients.

## MYELOABLATIVE ALLO SCT AS FIRST TRANSPLANT: LOW-GRADE (FOLLICULAR) NHL

Table 65.5 illustrates the results of seven reports in which follicular NHL patients were given myeloablative conditioning followed by infusion of allogeneic stem cells.[22–28] Aside from the IBMTR[22] and EBMTR[23] communications of registry data, all series are quite small and follow-up is somewhat limited for the slower growing (compared to aggressive) NHL subtypes. Relapse rates are low, partially explained by the more potent GvL effect in low-grade NHL (compared to aggressive histologies) observed with allo SCT; van

**Table 65.4** Single-arm cohort (enrollment >20 patients) for myeloablative allo SCT in patients with aggressive histology NHL

| References | No. of patients | Refractory at time allo SCT | Nonrelapse mortality | PFS/EFS | OS | Relapse | Comments |
|---|---|---|---|---|---|---|---|
| Dhedin et al.[17] | 73 | 37% | 32/73 (44%) | 5-year PFS 40% | 41% at 5 years | 30% at 5 years | Subgroup of 22 patients with chemosensitive relapse had 60% PFS and 13% relapse. |
| Toze et al.[18] | 92[a] | NA | 29%[a] | NA | 37%[a] | NA | Largest single-center report but includes low-grade histologies |
| Juckett et al.[19] | 21 | 29% | NA | 5-year PFS 33% | 6/21 at 39 months | 43% at 5 years | T-cell depleted marrow; 5-year PFS 40% vs 17% for chemosensitive vs refractory disease |
| Stein et al.[20] | 32 | 44% | 17/32 (53%) | 5-year EFS 11% | 16% at 5 years | NA | 10 deaths due to progressive lymphoma |
| Mitterbauer et al.[21] | 35(20)[a] | 23/35 (66%) | 48% at 5 years | NA | 35% at 5 years | 23% at 5 years | Two-institution trial |

[a]Includes low-grade histologies (a total of 35 patients reported but only 20 had aggressive NHL).
Allo SCT, allogeneic stem cell transplantation; int-grade, intermediate-grade non-Hodgkin's lymphoma; PFS, progression-free survival; EFS, event-free survival; OS, overall survival.

Besien and coworkers[29] noted that diffuse large-cell NHL was among the least sensitive to the GvL effect. In fact, in two series of allo SCT in low-grade NHL by Toze and colleagues[26] and Forrest et al.,[27] no relapses were reported; additionally, two relapses after allo SCT were reinduced into a complete remission using chemotherapy, indicating that all 16 allografts were alive in complete remission.

**Table 65.5** Selected studies using myeloablative conditioning and allo SCT for follicular NHL

| References | No. of patients | Median follow-up | PFS | OS | TRM | Relapse | Comments |
|---|---|---|---|---|---|---|---|
| Stein et al.[22] | 15 | 60 months | NS | 15% | 53% | 33% | |
| Van Besien et al.[23] | 113 | 25 months | 49 at 36 months | 49 at 36 months | 40% at 36 months | 16% | Registry data 1984–1995 |
| Peniket et al.[24] | 231 | 60 months | 43% | 51% at 48 months | 38% at 48 months | 25% | Case-matched showing high TRM but low relapses |
| Mandigers et al.[25] | 15 | 36 months | 67% | | 33% | 13% | T-cell depleted transplant |
| Toze et al.[26] | 16 | 29 months | 56% | | 25% | 0 | Four unrelated donors and 12 sibling donors |
| Forrest et al.[27] | 24 | 28 months | 78% at 28 months | 78% at 28 months | 21% | 0 | No relapses noted |
| Yakoub-Agha et al.[28] | 16 (14)[a] | 39 months | 65% at 2 years | 68% at 2 years | 5/16 | 2/14 | Two relapses after allo SCT alive at 13 and 41 months after salvage chemotherapy |

PFS, progression-free survival; OS, overall survival; VP, etoposide; BM, bone marrow; PB, peripheral blood; TRM, treatment-related mortality occuring in the first year after transplant; CR, complete remission; NS, not stated specifically; Dexa-BEAM, dexamethasone/BCNU/etoposide/cytrabine/melphalan.
[a]Two patients received nonmyeloablative allo SCT.

**Table 65.6** Comparative analyses detailing outcome of myeloablative transplantation for intermediate-and high-grade

| References | Type | No. of patients | Nonrelapse mortality | PFS/EFS | OS | Relapse or progression | Comments |
|---|---|---|---|---|---|---|---|
| Bierman et al.[10] | Allo | 626 | NA | NA | NA | NA | No direct comparison of auto vs allo SCT: allo SCT T-replete had best disease-free survial |
| | Auto | 1,758 | NA | NA | NA | NA | |
| | Twin | 58 | NA | NA | NA | NA | No direct evidence of GvL effect |
| Peniket et al.[24] | Allo | 787 | 33–42% at 4 years[a] | NA | 37–42% at 4 years[a] | NA | Retrospective analysis of huge patient numbers (registry data) TRM in allo SCT offset lower relapse rates: significantly worse outcome on auto SCT |
| | Auto | 14,687 | NA | NA | NA | NA | |
| Chopra et al.[30] | Allo | 43 | 28% | 49% | NA | 29% | Matched case–control study of registry data: inter- and high grade |
| | Auto | 43 | 14%, $p = 0.008$ | 43% ($p = $ NS) | NA | 35% | |
| Chopra et al.[30] | Allo | 49 | 24% | 57% | | 24% | Matched case–control study of registry data: lymphoblastic |
| | Auto | 49 | 10%, $p = 0.006$ | 44% | | 48% $p = 0.035$ | |
| Chopra et al.[30] | Allo | 8 | 13% | 25% | NA | 71% | Matched case–control study of registry data: Burkitt's |
| | Auto | 8 | 0 | 38% | | 63% | |
| Milpied et al.[7] | Allo | 12 | 17% | 67% | | 17% | Small series of lymphoblastic lymphomas receiving marrow grafts in first CR |
| | Auto | 13 | 0% | 70% | | 31% | |
| Levine et al.[31] | Allo | 76 | 25% | 36% | | 34% | Retrospective analysis of registry data in lymphoblastic lymphomas |
| | Auto | 128 | 5%, $p < 0.001$ | 39% | | 56%, $p = 0.004$ | |
| Bureo et al.[32] | Allo | 14 | 21% | 57% | | not reported | Small-size pediatric study |
| | Auto | 32 | 9% | 57% | | | |
| Ratanatharathorn et al.[33] | Allo | 31 | | 24% | | | Prospective, single institutional trial |
| | Auto | 35 | | 47% $p = 0.21$ | | | |
| Schimmer et al.[34] | Auto | 385 (70% aggressive) | 6% | 52% at 3 years | 62% at 3 years | 41% at 3 years, $p = 0.006$ | 1986–1997 Ontario Canada regional study; allo SCT assigned for involved marrow or inadequate marrow harvest |
| | Allo | 44 (55% aggressive) | 23% $p = 0.001$ | 71% at 3 years | 72% at 3 years | 6% at 3 years | |

GVL, graft versus lymphoma; inter-grade, intermediate-grade non-Hodgkin;s lymphoma; PFS, progression-free survival; EFS, event-free survival; OS, overall survival; CT, complete remission.
[a]Includes intermediate-, high-grade, Burkitt's and lymphoblastic NHL.

## COMPARISONS OF ALLO SCT VERSUS AUTO SCT

A number of investigations have reported trials comparing allo SCT to auto SCT for intermediate- and high-grade as well as low-grade NHL (Tables 65.6 and 65.7). Most of these studies were retrospective comparisons, often using observational databases from groups such as the IBMTR/ABMTR and the EBMTR. The reports often do not provide intricate detail regarding specific patients outcome. In several instances, the investigators reported the data using case-matched controls, and indicated hazard ratios for measures of patient outcome. In the case of intermediate- and high-grade NHL, Bierman and associates[10] recently published a combined IBMTR/EBMTR analysis involving more than 3000 NHL patients receiving stem cell transplants. A total of 2018 patients received unpurged autografts while 376 patients were given purged autografts. Further, 774 patients received T-cell replete allografts and 119 allografts that were T-cell depleted. These groups were compared to 89 syngeneic grafts. These data from this observational database analysis failed to demonstrate a GvL effect. Recipients of unpurged auto SCT, however, had a fivefold increase risk of relapse compared to the syngeneic group; further, unpurged auto SCT patients had a twofold increased relapse rate compared to purged graft recipients. In the case of low-grade NHL patients, this finding was associated with an improved overall and disease-free survival. This information provides indirect evidence that autologous tumor contamination may contribute to NHL relapse, an advantage possessed by use of an allograft.

## COMPARISONS OF ALLO SCT VERSUS AUTO SCT: INTERMEDIATE- AND HIGH-GRADE NHL

Table 65.6 shows a number of publications comparing allo SCT and auto SCT.[7,10,24,30–34] Among the earliest reports were small series by Milpied and colleagues[7] and Bureo and coworkers.[32] Chopra et al.[30] communicated one of the first matched case–control studies. The way they reported their data enabled them to evaluate various NHL subtypes. For both lymphoblastic lymphoma and intermediate- and high-grade NHL, the benefit of a reduced treatment-related mortality in auto SCT was offset by a higher relapse rate, i.e., allo SCT and auto SCT results were comparable. Subsequently, Peniket and the EBMTR[24] retrospectively analyzed data from 1982 to 1998, in which they compared 1185 allogeneic transplants (as the first transplant) for lymphoma with 14,687 autologous procedures. Patients receiving allogeneic transplants were subdivided according to histology: low-grade NHL (231 patients); intermediate-grade NHL (147 patients); high-grade NHL (255 patients); lymphoblastic NHL (314 patients); Burkitt's lymphoma (71 patients); and Hodgkin's disease (167 patients). Actuarial overall survival at 4 years from transplantation was as follows: low-grade NHL 51.1%; intermediate-grade NHL 38.3%; high-grade NHL 41.2%;

| Table 65.7 | Comparative analyses detailing outcome of myeloablative transplantation for low-grade NHL | | | | | | |
|---|---|---|---|---|---|---|---|
| References | Type | No. of patients | Nonrelapse mortality | PFS/EFS | OS | Relapse or progression | Comments |
| Verdonck et al.[35] | Allo | 15 | 27% | 70% | | 0, $p = 0.0002$ | Mixed variety of low-grade histologies 78% |
| | Auto | 18 | 0, $p$ = NR | 22%, $p = 0.015$ | | | |
| Lin et al.[36] | Allo | 25 | 28% | 41% | | NR | |
| | Auto | 62 | 3% | 35% | | NR | |
| Hosing et al.[37] | Allo | 44 | 34% | 45% at 53 months | 49% at 53 months | 19%, $p = 0.003$ | Initially more favorable outcome results in autografts but eclipsed by allografts over time |
| | Auto | 68 | 6% | 17% at 71 months | 34% at 71 months | 74% | |
| Van Besien et al.[16] | Allo | 176 | 30% at 5 years, $p < 0.001$ | 45% at 5 years, $p < 0.001$ | 51% at 5 years | 21% at 5 years, $p < 0.001$ | Retrospective registry review |
| | Auto purged | 131 | 14% at 5 years | 39% at 5 years | 62% at 5 years | 43% at 5 years | |
| | Auto unpurged | 597 | 8% at 5 years | 31% at 5 years | 55% at 5 years | 58% at 5 years | |

PFS, progression-free survival; EFS, event-free survival; OS, overall survival; NR, not reported.

lymphoblastic lymphoma 42.0%; Burkitt's lymphoma 37.1%; and Hodgkin's disease 24.7%. These outcomes are relatively poor because of the high procedure-related mortality associated with these procedures, particularly in patients with Hodgkin's disease (51.7% actuarial procedure-related mortality at 4 years). Multivariate analysis showed that for all lymphomas apart from Hodgkin's disease, status at transplantation significantly affected outcome. A matched analysis revealed that for all categories of lymphoma, overall survival was better for auto SCT than for allo SCT. Relapse rate was better in the allo SCT group for low-, intermediate- and high-grade, and lymphoblastic NHL. Allo SCT appeared superior to auto SCT in producing a lower relapse rate, but overall survival will not be superior until the toxicity of such procedures is reduced.

## COMPARISONS OF ALLO SCT VERSUS AUTO SCT: FOLLICULAR NHL

There are few trials prospectively designed to compare allo SCT versus auto SCT for follicular NHL patients. Table 65.7 illustrates the results using myeloablative preparative regimens for allo SCT as compared to auto SCT for use in follicular NHL.[16,35–37] Again, most series are small in size except for communications from registry analyses, such as the recent report by van Besien et al.[16] Treatment-related mortalities for allo SCT are approximately 30%, nearly a log-fold higher compared to auto SCT. On the other hand, relapse rates in the allo SCT group are significantly lower, approxi-

mately 20%, with no reported relapses in the small series by Verdonck.[35] Such opposing effects may not offset each other and could result in improved overall survival in those receiving allo SCT, although follow-up is short.

## CONCEPT OF REDUCED-CONDITIONING ALLO SCT

In recent years, reduced conditioning or nonmyeloablative conditioning has been used to avoid the toxic effect of the preparative regimen, yet allow donor cell engraftment to take place, and ultimately to result in a GvL effect.[38–40] These highly immunosuppressive but less toxic regimens rely upon engraftment and subsequent immunologic effect to eradicate NHL. Diaconescu and colleagues[41] at the Fred Hutchinson Cancer Research Center reported in preliminary fashion a retrospective comparison of reduced conditioning versus myeloablative conditioning for NHL patients undergoing HLA-identical allografts. They noted that despite the former group having a higher median age, higher comorbidity index, and greater likelihood of prior allograft, the treatment-related mortality at 100 days was 8.8% compared to 20.6% in the myeloablative group.

Table 65.8 shows five studies describing the data for NHL patients who underwent a reduced-conditioning allo SCT for relapse after an auto SCT.[42–46] The information presented reflects either retrospective registry analyses[42] or small single institutional studies. Mantle-cell NHL patients appeared to fare poorly in the registry

**Table 65.8** Selected studies using reduced-intensity conditioning and allo SCT for NHL relapses after auto SCT

| References | No. of patients and NHL | Nonrelapse mortality | PFS | OS | Comments |
|---|---|---|---|---|---|
| Robinson et al.[42] | N = 52 low 15 prior auto SCT (29%) | 22% at 1 years | overall PFS: 54% at 2 years | overall OS: low 65% | EBMTR retrospective study |
| | N = 62 intermediate/ high 32 prior auto SCT (52%) | 30% | 13% at 2 years | 47% at 2 years | Poor outcome in chemoresistant and non-low grade NHL |
| | N = 22 mantle cell 8 prior auto SCT (36%) | 46% | 0% at 2 years | 13% at 2 years | |
| Bertz et al.[43] | N = 20 7 prior auto SCT | 2 dead at 107 days | Alive in CR at 16, 19, 19 months | Alive at 13,16, 19,19 months | Variety of allograft donor types |
| Seropian et al.[44] | N = 21 intermediate/ high N = 7 low 11 prior auto SCT | 7% at 100 days 198% overall | 57% at 5 years | 58% at 5-years | 17 ablative and 11 nonablative; 7 in CCR from prior auto SCT |
| Branson et al.[45] | N = 38; 10 high | 20% at 14 months | 50% at 14 months | 53% at 14 months | Median follow-up 26 months |
| Escalón et al.[46] | N = 10 intermediate/ high; N = 10 low | 1 at 10 months | 95% 3-year PFS | 95% 3-year PFS | Single-center experience |

PFS, progression-free survival; OS, overall survival; CR, complete remission; CCR, coutinuous complete remission.

report due to a high treatment-related mortality (46%), but had a favorable outcome in the study from MD Anderson Cancer Center.[46] Despite the poor prognostic characteristics of an auto SCT failure, many patients remain alive in complete remission, although for the most part the follow-up period is brief. The single institution report from Escalón et al.[46] shows a strikingly excellent outcome of a 95% PFS at 3 years after allo SCT. That such patients can be treated using an initial auto SCT and subsequently salvaged using a reduced-conditioning allo SCT supports the contention of many investigators that poor-risk NHL should receive planned tandem auto SCT followed within months by a reduced-conditioning allo SCT. The rationale is that the auto SCT provides significant tumor cytoreduction allowing maximal antitumor benefit of the new donor effector cells given in the course of an allo SCT.

## REDUCED-CONDITIONING ALLO SCT AS FIRST TRANSPLANT: FOLLICULAR NHL

Data from five small studies using reduced-intensity conditioning and allo SCT as first transplant for follicular NHL are shown in Table 65.9.[47–50] In several reports, a variety of hematologic malignancy patients were treated in this fashion, and the data for follicular NHL have been culled out. The median follow-up for these series is short, but treatment-related mortality remains relatively low at approximately 20% at 1 year, except in the report by Robinson and colleagues.[50] In that study, the authors note inexplicably high treatment-related mortality and relapse rates. More patients need to be accrued to therapy and a longer duration of follow-up must be reported before stating that reduced-intensity

allo SCT changes the natural history of follicular NHL; however, the high PFS rate of approximately 70% is encouraging. The monoclonal antibody Campath-1, now being used with increased frequency, may contribute to improved patient outcome.[51] Chakraverty et al.[51] incorporated Campath-1 into the conditioning regimen for 47 matched-unrelated donor allo SCT, 29 of whom failed auto SCT. Eighty-five percent of patients attained full donor chimerism and day 100 nonrelapse mortality was 14.9%. One-year progression-free and overall survivals were 61.5 and 75.5%, respectively.

## THERAPY FOR SPECIFIC NHL SUBTYPES

NHLs are a heterogeneous group of lymphoid malignancies whose clinical behavior and response to therapy exhibit considerable variation. Mantle-cell NHL, for example, resembles a low-grade NHL morphologically, behaves aggressively, yet is incurable using conventional therapies. Use of auto SCT in mantle-cell NHL in relapse provides extremely poor prospects of attaining long-term disease-free survival.[52] Martinez et al.[53] and Grigg and colleagues[54] reported series in which allo SCT salvaged such patients, due in large part to the contribution of GvL when GvHD develops. Examples of other successful initiates already have been related earlier in this review. Further support for GvL in this context is the report from Berdeja and colleagues[55] who noted poorer survival in mantle-cell NHL patients compared to other histologic types; these patients received T-cell depleted grafts that compromise the GvL effect.

Peripheral T-cell NHL represents a less common, more resistant histologic subtype, one in which the

| Table 65.9 | Studies using reduced-intensity conditioning and allo SCT as first transplant for follicular NHL | | | | | | |
| --- | --- | --- | --- | --- | --- | --- | --- |
| References | No. of patients | Conditioning | Median follow-up | PFS | OS | Non relapse mortality at 1 year | Comments |
| Seattle[a] | 9 | Flud/TBI 200 | >12 months | 7 alive CR | 8 alive | 0 | |
| Corradini et al.[47] | 8 | TT/Flud/CY | 17 months | 5 alive CR 5, 16, 17, 25, 28 months | 5 alive CR 5, 16, 17, 25, 28 months | 1 at 8 months | Includes 4 mantle-cell NHL |
| Khouri et al.[48] | 20 | Flud/CY | 21 months | 80% | 80% | 20% | 64% cumulative incidence chronic GvHD |
| Faulkner et al.[49] | 28 | BEAM Campath | 16 months | 69% | 74% | 16% | No extensive chronic GvHD |
| Robinson et al.[50] | 28 | Flud/Alkylator (92%) BEAM Campath 8% | NS | 29% | 39% | 39% | High nonrelapse mortality and relapse |

PFS, progression-free survival; OS, overall survival; Flud, fludarabine; BEAM, BCNU/etoposide/cytarabine/melphalan;
[a] Personal communication MB Maris, Fred Hutchinson Cancer Research Center.

newer anti-B-cell monoclonal antibodies such as rituximab have no effect. Corradini et al.[56] recently reported a phase II reduced-conditioning trial in 15 relapsed and 2 primary refractory peripheral T-cell NHL patients. Patients received thiotepa, fludarabine, and cyclophosphamide followed by blood stem cells obtained from sibling-matched ($N$ = 14), sibling one-antigen mismatched ($N$ = 2), and matched-unrelated donors ($N$ = 1). Two-year nonrelapse mortality was 6% and 12 patients attained complete remission. Three-year progression-free and overall survivals were 64 and 81%, respectively.

## DONOR LYMPHOCYTE INFUSIONS

Infusions of lymphocytes obtained via apheresis collections from the patient's allogeneic stem cell donor, i.e., donor lymphocyte infusions (DLIs), have been used as effectors to provide salvage therapy for some patients who have relapsed after allo SCT. The most effective disease targets for this approach have been chronic myeloid leukemia and multiple myeloma, although other hematologic malignancies may respond.[57–61] Several small series have reported mixed results in lymphoma patients who relapsed after allo SCT.[62–64] In one of the larger series, Mandigers and associates[64] treated seven patients with low-grade NHL in relapse after an allo SCT and noted two partial and four durable complete responses lasting at least 43–89 months after infusion. DLIs appear to be more effective in lower grade rather than higher grade NHL and in the setting of low tumor volume. Infusions often are administered after cytotoxic therapy with or without monoclonal antibody therapy and after the patient has been tapered off all immunosuppressive therapy. It is unclear, however, if the GvL effect can be separated from GvHD effect using unmanipulated DLI. The most effective cell dose is not uniformly established, as the time to DLI after the transplant may play a role in efficacy and toxicity. This therapy is associated with a high incidence of GvHD and aplasia of bone marrow, resulting in a nearly 20% fatality incidence.[57,60]

## FUTURE CONSIDERATIONS

A number of potential directions to improve upon allo SCT are listed in Table 65.10. Clearly, maneuvers to reduce nonrelapse mortality are most desirable. Targeted antilymphoma regimens using radioimmunoconjugates rather than TBI have been implemented in auto SCT and are being developed for allo SCT.[65,66] Supportive care strategies, including better anti-infective agents, are being improved upon. GvHD remains a major contributor to treatment-related mortality, and the addition of sirolimus to the GvHD prophylaxis armamentarium may be extremely efficacious.[67] Other intriguing possibilities include the use of methods to enhance GvL effect, such as dendritic cell vaccines. DLI, occasionally used successfully in the setting of relapse after allo SCT in NHL, may be associated with the development of severe and fatal GvHD. Newer uses of DLI include preemptive infusion in patients at high risk for relapse (due to aggressive disease or because the allograft was T-cell depleted), or use of selective, i.e., CD8+ T-cell depleted, DLIs in an attempt to provide GvL effect without GvHD.[68–70] As discussed above, a number of investigators are using tandem auto SCT followed by allo SCT approaches. Recently, several groups have begun using novel conditioning regimens incorporating agents such as pentostatin[71] or the combination of pentostatin and extracorporeal photopheresis (ECP).[72] Chin et al.[72] reported in preliminary fashion their allo SCT reduced-intensity regimen combining lower dose TBI, pentostatin, and ECP in poor-risk patients. A total of 106 patients were enrolled using matched-related ($N$ = 76) or matched-unrelated ($N$ = 30) donor stem cell infusion. Seventy-six (72%) patients were alive without tumor 100 days after transplant. At a 15-month median follow-up, overall patient outcomes, such as chronic GvHD (47%) and relapse (23%), did not differ significantly between matched-related and matched-unrelated donors.

Some investigators have proposed improved diagnostic model approaches for low-grade and intermediate-/high-grade NHL in a manner similar to those developed for auto SCT using the International Prognostic Index.[73,74] This strategy could become a powerful tool to compare results of different treatment regimens as well as to guide clinical management.

Other areas of investigation include more selective monitoring of residual NHL to induce either GvHD and GvL, or the need to begin additional anti-NHL

---

**Table 65.10    Future directions**

- Minimizing treatment-related complications, i.e., improved supportive care, targeted preparative regimens
- Newer GvHD prevention approaches: sirolimus
- Use of new GVL maneuvers, i.e., dendritic cell vaccines
- Advanced donor lymphocyte infusion techniques, i.e., preemptive administration or selective T-cell depletion
- Strategies to improve upon engraftment in reduced-conditioning regimens
- Linkage of specific cytoreduction regimens in resistant relapses before reduced-conditioning regimens
- Develop improved prognostic scoring before transplant as done for auto SCT
- Sequential auto SCT/allo SCT
- Development of novel preparative regimens, i.e., pentostatin and extracorporeal photopheresis approaches
- Monitor tumor load after allograft for more therapy, i.e., real-time PCR assay for t [14;18]
- Expand donor pool, i.e., matched-unrelated and haploidentical donors

therapies. Chang et al.[75] evaluated tumor load using a real-time quantitative polymerase chain reaction assay for t(14;18), which they correlated with the clinical course of follicular NHL patients after stem cell transplant. None of six patients who remained in remission had samples with a tumor load >0.01% after transplant. In contrast, four of five patients (three allo SCT/two auto SCT) with relapsed/progressive disease had increasing tumor loads of >0.01% after transplant (P < 0.02). This technique likely will be validated with a greater number of cases. Finally, expansion of the donor stem cell pool will make allo SCT more available for more patients. Recent studies have demonstrated the feasibility of mismatched and haploidentical donors for allo SCT.[76–78] Sykes and colleagues[78] reported five patients with refractory NHL undergoing stem cell transplantation from haploidentical related donors sharing at least one HLA A, B, or DR allele on the mismatched haplotype. Four patients showed mixed hematopoietic chimerism with a predominance of donor lymphoid tissue and varying degrees of myeloid chimerism. Two patients exhibited antilymphoma effect and were in GvHD-free states of complete and partial clinical remission at 460 and 103 days after stem cell transplantation. Bierman and the National Marrow Donor Program[77] recently presented preliminary data in which unrelated donor stem cells were the source of cellular rescue for NHL patients undergoing allo SCT.

## SUMMARY

Allo SCT has begun to assume an increasing role in the management of NHL. This approach provides several advantages over auto SCT, including provision of a lymphoma-free graft, reduced rates of secondary myelodysplastic syndrome and leukemia, and a potentially curative GvL effect. The latter appears to be considerably more pronounced in low-grade NHL such as follicular NHL, compared to more aggressive histologies. When applied to chemosensitive patients, the lower relapse rates and reasonable long-term outcomes make allo SCT a promising therapy to pursue. Patient populations, such as those with bone marrow involvement or very high-risk disease, can be identified as having suboptimal outcomes after auto SCT and may benefit from such an approach. While the exact role of allo SCT remains to be determined, broad recommendations can be suggested for the management of patients with NHL. New approaches to allo SCT, including the use of matched-unrelated donors and reduced-intensity conditioning regimens, may expand the applicability of this potentially curative modality.

### REFERENCES

1. Phillips GL, Herzig RH, Lazarus HM, et al.: Treatment of relapsed lymphoma with cyclophosphamide, total body irradiation and autologous bone marrow transplantation. *N Engl J Med* 310:1557–1561, 1984.

2. Phillips GL, Fay JW, Herzig RH, et al.: The treatment of progressive non-Hodgkin's lymphoma with intensive chemoradiotherapy and autologous bone marrow transplantation. *Blood* 75:831–838, 1990.

3. Armitage JO: Treatment of non-Hodgkin's lymphoma. *N Engl J Med* 328:1023–1030, 1993.

4. Vose JM, Zhang MJ, Rowlings PA, et al.: Autologous transplantation for diffuse aggressive non-Hodgkin's lymphoma in patients never achieving remission: a report from the Autologous Blood and Marrow Transplant Registry. *J Clin Oncol* 19:406–413, 2001.

5. Vose JM, Rizzo JD, Tao-Wu J, et al.: Autologous transplantation for diffuse aggressive non-Hodgkin's lymphoma in first relapse or second remission. *Biol Blood Marrow Transplant* 10:116–127, 2004.

6. Haioun C, Lepage E, Gisselbrecht C, et al.: Survival benefit of high-dose therapy in poor-risk aggressive non-Hodgkin's lymphoma: final analysis of the prospective LNH87-2 protocol—a groupe d'Etude des lymphomes de l'Adulte study. *J Clin Oncol* 18:3025–3030, 2000.

7. Milpied N, Ifrah N, Kuentz M, et al.: Bone marrow transplant for adult poor prognosis lymphoblastic lymphoma in first complete remission. *Br J Haematol* 73:82–87, 1989.

8. Watts MJ, Sullivan AM, Leverett D, et al.: Back-up bone marrow is frequently ineffective in patients with poor peripheral-blood stem-cell mobilization. *J Clin Oncol* 16:1554–1560, 1998.

9. Brenner MK, Rill DR, Moen RC, et al.: Gene-marking to trace origin of relapse after autologous bone-marrow transplantation. *Lancet* 341:85–86, 1993.

10. Bierman PJ, Sweetenham JW, Loberiza FR Jr, et al.: Syngeneic hematopoietic stem-cell transplantation for non-Hodgkin's lymphoma: a comparison with allogeneic and autologous transplantation—The Lymphoma Working Committee of the International Bone Marrow Transplant Registry and the European Group for Blood and Marrow Transplantation. *J Clin Oncol* 21:3744–3753, 2003.

11. Freedman AS, Neuberg D, Mauch P, et al.: Long-term follow-up of autologous bone marrow transplantation in patients with relapsed follicular lymphoma. *Blood* 94:3325–3333, 1999.

12. Mathe G, Amiel J, Schwarzenberg L, Cattan A, Schneider M: Adoptive immunotherapy of acute leukemia: experimental and clinical results. *Cancer Res* 25:1525–1531, 1965.

13. Mollee P, Lazarus HM, Lipton J: Why aren't we performing more allografts for aggressive non-Hodgkin's lymphoma? *Bone Marrow Transplant* 31:953–960, 2003.

14. Tse WW, Lazarus HM, van Besien K: Stem cell transplantation in follicular lymphoma: progress at last? *Bone Marrow Transplant* 34:929–938, 2004.

15. Freytes CO, Loberiza FR, Rizzo JD, et al.: Myeloablative Allogeneic hematopoietic stem cell transplantation in patients who experience relapse after autologous stem cell transplantation for lymphoma: a report from the

International Bone Marrow Transplant Registry. *Blood* 104:3797–3803, 2004.

16. van Besien K, Loberiza FR Jr, Bajorunaite R, et al.: Comparison of autologous and allogeneic hematopoietic stem cell transplantation for follicular lymphoma. *Blood* 102:3521–3529, 2003.

17. Dhedin N, Giraudier S, Gaulard P, et al.: Allogeneic bone marrow transplantation in aggressive non-Hodgkin's lymphoma (excluding Burkitt and lymphoblastic lymphoma): a series of 73 patients from the SFGM database. Societ Francaise de Greffe de Moelle. *Br J Haematol* 107:154–161, 1999.

18. Toze CL, Conneally EA, Connors JM, et al.: Allogeneic hematopoietic stem cell transplantation (AlloHSCT) for non-Hodgkin's lymphoma (NHL) in Vancouver: 17-year experience of the Leukemia/BMT Program of British Columbia (BC) with related donor (RD) and unrelated (UD) donors [abstract]. *Ann Oncol* 13(suppl 2):39a, 2002.

19. Juckett M, Rowlings P, Hessner M, et al.: T cell-depleted allogeneic bone marrow transplantation for high-risk non-Hodgkin's lymphoma: clinical and molecular follow-up. *Bone Marrow Transplant* 21:893–899, 1998.

20. Stein RS, Greer JP, Goodman S, et al.: Intensified preparative regimens and allogeneic transplantation in refractory or relapsed intermediate and high grade non-Hodgkin's lymphoma. *Leuk Lymphoma* 41:343–352, 2001.

21. Mitterbauer M, Neumeister P, Kalhs P, et al.: Long-term clinical and molecular remission after allogeneic stem cell transplantation (SCT) in patients with poor prognosis non-Hodgkin's lymphoma. *Leukemia* 15:635–641, 2001.

22. Stein RS, Greer JP, Goodman S, Kallianpur A, Ahmed MS, Wolff SN: High-dose therapy with autologous or allogeneic transplantation as salvage therapy for small cleaved cell lymphoma of follicular center cell origin. *Bone Marrow Transplant* 23:227–233, 1999.

23. van Besien K, Sobocinski KA, Rowlings PA, et al.: Allogeneic bone marrow transplantation for low-grade lymphoma. *Blood* 92:1832–1836, 1998.

24. Peniket AJ, Ruiz de Elvira MC, Taghipour G, et al.: An EBMT registry matched study of allogeneic stem cell transplants for lymphoma: allogeneic transplantation is associated with a lower relapse rate but a higher procedure-related mortality rate than autologous transplantation. *Bone Marrow Transplant* 31:667–678, 2003.

25. Mandigers CM, Raemaekers JM, Schattenberg AV, et al.: Allogeneic bone marrow transplantation with T-cell-depleted marrow grafts for patients with poor-risk relapsed low-grade non-Hodgkin's lymphoma. *Br J Haematol* 100:198–206, 1998.

26. Toze CL, Shepherd JD, Connors JM, et al.: Allogeneic bone marrow transplantation for low-grade lymphoma and chronic lymphocytic leukemia. *Bone Marrow Transplant* 25:605–612, 2000.

27. Forrest DL, Thompson K, Nevill TJ, Couban S, Fernandez LA: Allogeneic hematopoietic stem cell transplantation for progressive follicular lymphoma. *Bone Marrow Transplant* 29:973–978, 2002.

28. Yakoub-Agha I, Fawaz A, Folliot O, et al.: Allogeneic bone marrow transplantation in patients with follicular lymphoma: a single center study. *Bone Marrow Transplant* 30:229–234, 2002.

29. van Besien KW, Mehra RC, Giralt SC, et al.: Allogeneic bone marrow transplantation for poor-prognosis lym-

phoma: response, toxicity and survival depend on disease histology. *Am J Med* 100:299–307, 1996.

30. Chopra R, Goldstone AH, Pearce R, et al.: Autologous versus allogeneic bone marrow transplantation for non-Hodgkin's lymphoma: a case-controlled analysis of the European Bone Marrow Transplant Group Registry data. *J Clin Oncol* 10:1690–1695, 1992.

31. Levine JE, Harris RE, Loberiza FR Jr, et al.: A comparison of allogeneic and autologous bone marrow transplant for lymphoblastic lymphoma. *Blood* 101:2476–2482, 2003.

32. Bureo E, Ortega JJ, Munoz A, et al.: Bone marrow transplantation in 46 pediatric patients with non-Hodgkin's lymphoma. Spanish Working Party for Bone Marrow Transplantation in Children. *Bone Marrow Transplant* 15:353–359, 1995.

33. Ratanatharathorn V, Uberti J, Karanes C, et al.: Prospective comparative trial of autologous versus allogeneic bone marrow transplantation in patients with non-Hodgkin's lymphoma. *Blood* 84:1050–1055, 1994.

34. Schimmer AD, Jamal S, Messner H, et al.: Allogeneic or autologous bone marrow transplantation (BMT) for non- Hodgkin's lymphoma (NHL): results of a provincial strategy. Ontario BMT Network, Canada. *Bone Marrow Transplant* 26:859–864, 2000.

35. Verdonck LF: Allogeneic versus autologous bone marrow transplantation for refractory and recurrent low-grade non-Hodgkin's lymphoma: updated results of the Utrecht experience. *Leuk Lymphoma* 34:129–136, 1999.

36. Lin TS, Elder PJ, Penza SI, et al.: Autologous stem cell transplants result in better 5-year overall, but not progression-free, survival than allogeneic transplants in patients with indolent non-Hodgkin's lymphoma. *Blood* 100 (suppl 1):644a, 2002. Abstract 2356.

37. Hosing C, Saliba RM, McLaughlin P, et al.: Long-term results favor allogeneic over autologous hematopoietic stem cell transplantation in patients with refractory or recurrent indolent non-Hodgkin's lymphoma. *Ann Oncol* 14:737–744, 2003.

38. Slavin S, Nagler A, Naparstek E, et al.: Nonmyeloablative stem cell transplantation and cell therapy as an alternative to conventional bone marrow transplantation with lethal cytoreduction for the treatment of malignant and nonmalignant hematologic diseases. *Blood* 91:756–763, 1998.

39. Khouri IF, Keating M, Korbling M, et al.: Transplant-lite: induction of graft-versus-malignancy using fludarabine-based nonablative chemotherapy and allogeneic blood progenitor-cell transplantation as treatment for lymphoid malignancies. *J Clin Oncol* 16:2817–2824, 1998.

40. McSweeney PA, Niederwieser D, Shizuru JA, et al.: Hematopoietic cell transplantation in older patients with hematologic malignancies: replacing high-dose cytotoxic therapy with graft-versus-tumor effects. *Blood* 97:3390–3400, 2001.

41. Diaconescu R, Flowers C, Storer B, et al.: Morbidity and mortality with nonmyeloablative compared to nonmyeloablative conditioning before hematopoietic cell transplantation from HLA matched related donor. *Blood* 102: 77a, 2003. Abstract 261.

42. Robinson SP, Goldstone AH, Mackinnon S, et al.: Chemoresistant or aggressive lymphoma predicts for a poor outcome following reduced-intensity allogeneic progenitor cell transplantation: an analysis from the Lymphoma Working Party of the European Group for

Blood and Bone Marrow Transplantation. *Blood* 100: 4310–4316, 2002.

43. Bertz H, Illerhaus G, Veelken H, Finke J: Allogeneic hematopoetic stem-cell transplantation for patients with relapsed or refractory lymphomas: comparison of high-dose conventional conditioning versus fludarabine-based reduced-intensity regimens. *Ann Oncol* 13: 135–139, 2002.

44. Seropian S, Bahceci E, Cooper DL: Allogeneic peripheral blood stem cell transplantation for high-risk non-Hodgkin's lymphoma. *Bone Marrow Transplant* 32: 763–769, 2003.

45. Branson K, Chopra R, Kottaridis P, et al.: Role of non-myeloablative allogeneic stem-cell transplantation after failure of autologous transplantation in patients with lymphoproliferative malignancies. *J Clin Oncol* 20: 4022–4031, 2002.

46. Escalón MP, Champlin RE, Saliba RM, et al.: Nonmyeloablative allogeneic hematopoietic transplantation: a promising salvage therapy for patients with non-Hodgkin's lymphoma whose disease has failed a prior autologous transplantation. *J Clin Oncol* 22: 2419–2423, 2004.

47. Corradini P, Tarella A, Olivieri A, et al.: Reduced-intensity conditioning followed by allografting of hematopoietic cells can produce clinical and molecular remissions in patients with poor-prognosis hematologic malignancies. *Blood* 99:75–82, 2002.

48. Khouri IF, Champlin RE: Nonmyeloablative stem cell transplantation for lymphoma. *Semin Oncol* 31:22–26, 2004.

49. Faulkner RD, Craddock C, Byrne JL, et al.: BEAM-alemtuzumab reduced-intensity allogeneic stem cell transplantation for lymphoproliferative diseases: GVHD, toxicity, and survival in 65 patients. *Blood* 103:428–434, 2004.

50. Robinson SP, Mackinnon S, Goldstone A, et al.: Higher than expected transplant-related mortality and relapse following non-myeloablative stem cell transplantation for lymphoma adversely affects progression-free survival [abstract]. *Blood* 96(suppl 1):554a, 2000.

51. Chakraverty R, Peggs K, Chopra R, et al.: Limiting transplantation-related mortality following unrelated donor stem cell transplantation by using a nonmyeloablative conditioning regimen. *Blood* 99:1071–1078, 2002.

52. Vandenberghe E, Ruiz De Elvira C, Loberiza FR, et al.: Outcome of autologous transplantation for mantle cell lymphoma: a study by the European Blood and Marrow Transplant and Autologous Blood and Marrow Transplant Registries. *Br J Haematol* 120:793–800, 2003.

53. Martinez C, Carreras E, Rovira M, et al.: Patients with mantle-cell lymphoma relapsing after autologous stem cell transplantation may be rescued by allogeneic transplantation. *Bone Marrow Transplant* 26:677–679, 2000.

54. Grigg A, Bardy P, Byron K, et al.: Fludarabine-based non-myeloablative chemotherapy followed by infusion of HLA-identical stem cells for relapsed leukemia and lymphoma. *Bone Marrow Transplant* 23:107–110, 1999.

55. Berdeja JG, Jones RJ, Zahurak MI, et al.: Allogeneic bone marrow transplantation in patients with sensitive low-grade lymphoma or mantle cell lymphoma. *Biol Blood Marrow Transplant* 7:561–567, 2001.

56. Corradini P, Dodero A, Zallio F, et al.: Graft-versus-lymphoma effect in relapsed peripheral T-cell non-Hodgkin's lymphomas after reduced intensity conditioning followed by allogeneic transplantation of hematopoietic cells. *J Clin Oncol* 22:2172–2176, 2004.

57. Kolb HJ, Schattenberg A, Goldman JM, et al.: Graft-versus-leukemia effect of donor lymphocyte transfusions in marrow grafted patients. *Blood* 86:2041–2050, 1995.

58. Porter DL, Roth MS, McGarigle C, et al.: Induction of graft-versus-host disease as immunotherapy for relapsed chronic myelogenous leukemia. *N Engl J Med* 330: 100–106, 1994.

59. van Rhee F, Lin F, Cullis JO, et al.: Relapse of chronic myeloid leukemia after allogeneic bone marrow transplant: the case for giving donor leukocyte transfusions before the onset of hematologic relapse. *Blood* 83: 3377–3383, 1994.

60. Collins R, Shpilberg O, Drobyski W, et al.: Donor leukocyte infusions in 140 patients with relapsed malignancy after allogeneic bone marrow transplantation. *J Clin Oncol* 15:433–444, 1997.

61. Lokhorst HM, Schattenberg A, Cornelissen JJ, et al.: Donor lymphocyte infusions for relapsed multiple myeloma after allogeneic stem-cell transplantation: predictive factors for response and long-term outcome. *J Clin Oncol* 18:3031–3037, 2000.

62. van Besien KW, de Lima M, Giralt SA, et al.: Management of lymphoma recurrence after allogeneic transplantation: the relevance of graft-versus-lymphoma effect. *Bone Marrow Transplant* 19:977–982, 1997.

63. Lush RJ, Haynes AP, Byrne J, et al.: Allogeneic stem-cell transplantation for lymphoproliferative disorders using BEAM-Campath (+/– fludarabine) conditioning combined with post-transplant donor-lymphocyte infusion. *Cytotherapy* 3:203–210, 2001.

64. Mandigers CM, Verdonck LF, Meijerink JP, Dekker AW, Schattenberg AV, Raemaekers JM: Graft-versus-lymphoma effect of donor lymphocyte infusion in indolent lymphomas relapsed after allogeneic stem cell transplantation. *Bone Marrow Transplant* 32:1159–1163, 2003.

65. Press OW, Eary JF, Gooley T, et al.: A phase I/II trial of iodine-131-tositumomab (anti-CD20), etoposide, cyclophosphamide, and autologous stem cell transplantation for relapsed B-cell lymphomas. *Blood* 96: 2934–2942, 2000.

66. Gopal AK, Rajendran JG, Petersdorf SH, et al.: High-dose chemo-radioimmunotherapy with autologous stem cell support for relapsed mantle cell lymphoma. *Blood* 99:3158–3162, 2002.

67. Cutler C, Antin JH: Sirolimus for GVHD prophylaxis in allogeneic stem cell transplantation. *Bone Marrow Transplant* 34:471–476, 2004.

68. Schaap N, Schattenberg A, Bar B, et al.: Induction of graft-versus-leukemia to prevent relapse after partially lymphocyte-depleted allogeneic bone marrow transplantation by pre-emptive donor leukocyte infusions. *Leukemia* 15:1339–1346, 2001.

69. Baron F, Baudoux E, Fillet G, Beguin Y: Retrospective comparison of CD34-selected allogeneic peripheral blood stem cell transplantation followed by CD8-depleted donor lymphocyte infusions with unmanipulated bone marrow transplantation. *Hematology* 7:137–143, 2002.

70. Alyea EP, Canning C, Neuberg D, et al.: CD8+ cell depletion of donor lymphocyte infusions using cd8

monoclonal antibody-coated high-density microparti—cles (CD8-HDM) after allogeneic hematopoietic stem cell transplantation: a pilot study. *Bone Marrow Transplant* 34:123–128, 2004.

71. Pavletic SZ, Bociek RG, Foran JM, et al.: Lymphodepleting effects and safety of pentostatin for nonmyeloablative allogeneic stem-cell transplantation. *Transplantation* 76:877–881, 2003.

72. Chin KM, Miller KB, Chan GW, et al.: Favorable outcomes in matched unrelated donor allogeneic stem cell transplantation using a pentostatin/extracorporeal photopheresis based reduced intensity conditioning regimen. *Blood* 102(suppl 1), 2003. Abstract 1758.

73. Hamlin PA, Zelenetz AD, Kewalramani T, et al.: Age-adjusted International Prognostic Index predicts autologous stem cell transplantation outcome for patients with relapsed or primary refractory diffuse large B-cell lymphoma. *Blood* 102:1989–1996, 2003.

74. Moskowitz CH, Nimer SD, Glassman JR, et al.: The International Prognostic Index predicts for outcome following autologous stem cell transplantation in patients with relapsed and primary refractory intermediate-grade lymphoma. *Bone Marrow Transplant* 23:561–567, 1999.

75. Chang CC, Bredeson C, Juckett M, Logan B, Keever-Taylor CA: Tumor load in patients with follicular lymphoma post stem cell transplantation may correlate with clinical course. *Bone Marrow Transplant* 32:287–291, 2003.

76. Liso A, Tiacci E, Binazzi R, et al.: Haploidentical peripheral-blood stem-cell transplantation for ALK-positive anaplastic large-cell lymphoma. *Lancet Oncol* 5: 127–128, 2004.

77. Bierman PJ, Molina A, Nelson G, et al.: Matched unrelated donor (MUD) allogeneic bone marrow transplantation for non-Hodgkin's lymphoma (NHL): results from the National Marrow Donor Program (NMDP). *Proc Am Soc Clin Oncol* 18:3a, 1999. Abstract 7.

78. Sykes M, Preffer F, McAfee S, et al.: Mixed lympho-haemopoietic chimerism and graft-versus-lymphoma effects after non-myeloablative therapy and HLA-mismatched bone-marrow transplantation. *Lancet* 353:1755–1759, 1999.

# Chapter 66

# DEFINITION OF REMISSION, PROGNOSIS, AND FOLLOW-UP IN FOLLICULAR LYMPHOMA AND DIFFUSE LARGE B-CELL LYMPHOMA

*John W. Sweetenham*

## INTRODUCTION

The emergence of new technologies impacts the care of patients with non-Hodgkin's lymphomas (NHLs). The advent of new functional imaging techniques, such as fluorodeoxyglucose positron emission tomography (FDG-PET) is being evaluated not only as a staging investigation, but also as a method for assessing response to therapy, and determining prognosis. The use of molecular techniques for the detection of residual disease after completion of therapy raises questions regarding currently used definitions of response. The prognostic significance of disease detected at the molecular level is under evaluation, as is the use of molecular studies for follow-up. The clinical prognostic factors identified by the International Prognostic Index (IPI) have provided a model for risk stratification of patients with diffuse large B-cell lymphoma (DLBCL). A similar index, the Follicular Lymphoma International prognostic Index (FLIPI), has now gained widespread use for low-grade follicular lymphoma (FL). These clinical indices have proved useful for risk stratification and for providing general prognostic information to patients with these diseases. However, there is marked variability in outcome within the risk groups identified by these prognostic models, indicating the biologic and clinical heterogeneity of these diseases. Recent gene expression profile (GEP) and tissue microarray (TMA) studies have identified patterns of gene expression and immunohistochemical features which have prognostic value independent of the IPI or FLIPI. It is likely that future prognostic models will incorporate this information.

Optimum follow up strategies for patients with NHL are unclear. The value of new (and established) imaging technologies for early detection of relapse has been systematically evaluated in only a small number of studies. The potential role of molecular techniques for early detection of subclinical relapse is also being explored.

The advent of these new techniques is therefore leading to redefinition of many of the criteria used for the assessment of prognosis, remission, and follow-up in malignant lymphomas, particularly the most common subtypes, namely DLBCL and FL.

## STANDARD RESPONSE CRITERIA IN NHL

The use of clinical response endpoints in trials in NHLs has been an intrinsic component of clinical trial design for many years. This is based largely on the observation that long-term disease-free and overall survival for patients in many clinical trials has been shown to correlate closely with the degree of clinical response. This observation holds true for first line therapy and for patients who receive second line regimens including the use of high-dose therapy and autologous stem cell transplantation (ASCT). Although a close correlation between response and event free and overall survival has been confirmed in multiple studies in aggressive NHL, results in studies in FLs and other indolent lymphomas have been less clear. Many studies have shown a correlation of clinical response with event- or failure-free survival in FLs, but in view of the indolent nature of these diseases, correlations with overall survival have been inconsistent. Additionally, in aggressive NHL, the persistence of residual masses after the completion of therapy, especially at sites of initial disease bulk, does not always indicate the presence of residual active disease. Inconsistencies in the assessment of response at sites such as the spleen and bone marrow have also added to uncertainty regarding the definition of response and comparability of results in different clinical trials.

An International Workshop to standardize response criteria for NHL was therefore developed in 1998 and published in 1999 in an attempt to provide uniform interpretation of clinical trial results across all studies.[1] This included agreed definitions of response and appropriate endpoints and follow-up schedules for use in the trial setting. The definitions provided are based primarily on clinical, radiologic, and histopathologic criteria, and they have since been modified by the inclusion of functional imaging data. A formal update of the criteria is in progress and will incorporate other data including flow cytometric analysis and molecular studies.

A summary of the response criteria is shown in Table 66.1.

The specific definitions are given next.

Complete remission (CR)

- Complete resolution of all clinically and radiologically detectable disease, all lymphoma-related symptoms, and all lymphoma-related biochemical abnormalities (such as elevated lactate dehydrogenase [LDH]).
- Lymph nodes and nodal masses must regress to normal size (defined as ≤ 1.5 cm for lymph nodes initially >1.5 cm). Lymph nodes initially measuring 1.1–1.5 cm must regress to ≤1 cm in greatest transverse diameter, or by more than 75% of the sum of the perpendicular diameters (SPD).
- If the spleen is enlarged on CT scan prior to therapy, it must regress in size and not be palpable by physical examination. Normal splenic size was not defined. Any macroscopic nodules noted in the spleen by any imaging modality must be resolved. Similar criteria apply to other organs such as the liver and kidneys.
- In view of conflicting data regarding the use of unilateral and bilateral bone marrow biopsies at staging, the workshop defined an adequate marrow evaluation as one with a minimum total biopsy length of 20 mm. If the marrow is involved at diagnosis, CR requires complete clearing of the infiltrate on repeat biopsy, which must be from the same site and the same minimum length. At the time of the initial workshop publication, since the significance of flow cytometric, molecular and cytogenetic data were not clear, these have not, to date, been incorporated into the standardized criteria (see next).

CR Unconfirmed (CR$_u$). The patients fulfill criteria for CR, with the following exceptions:

- Residual lymph node masses more than 1.5 cm in maximum transverse diameter which have regressed by more than 75% of the SPD. Individual nodes which were previously confluent must regress by more than 75% of the SPD compared with the size of the original mass.
- Indeterminate bone marrow—defined as having increased number or size of lymphoid aggregates without cytologic or architectural atypia.

Partial remission (PR)

- In SPD of the six largest nodes or nodal masses, ≥50% decrease. Where possible, these masses should be from disparate lymph node regions, be readily measurable and include mediastinal and retroperitoneal masses if these are present.
- No increase in the size of other lymph nodes, liver, or spleen.
- Splenic and liver nodules must regress by at least 50% in the SPD.
- Involvement of other organs is considered assessable but not measurable.
- Bone marrow assessment is regarded as irrelevant because it is assessable but not measurable.
- No new sites of disease.

Stable disease (SD)

- Less than PR, but more than progressive disease (PD) (see next)

Progressive disease

- More or equal to 50% increase from the nadir in SPD of any previously identified abnormal node

**Table 66.1  Response criteria for non-Hodgkin's lymphoma according to International Workshop**

| Response category | Physical examination | Lymph nodes | Lymph node masses | Bone marrow |
|---|---|---|---|---|
| CR | Normal | Normal | Normal | Normal |
| CR$_u$ | Normal | Normal | Normal | Indeterminate |
| | Normal | Normal | >75% Decrease | Normal or indeterminate |
| PR | Normal | Normal | Normal | Positive |
| | Normal | ≥50% decrease | ≥50% decrease | Irrelevant |
| | Decrease in liver/spleen | ≥50% decrease | ≥50% decrease | Irrelevant |
| Relapse/progression | Enlarging liver/spleen, new sites | New or increased | New or increased | Reappearance |

- Appearance of any new lesion during or at the end of therapy

Relapse

- Appearance of any new lesion or increase by ≥50% in the size of any previously involved site
- More or equal to 50% increase in greatest diameter of any previously identified node greater than 1 cm in short axis or in the SPD of more than one node

At the time of the initial description of these criteria, response assessment was based entirely upon physical examination, and routine radiologic and pathologic criteria.

CT scanning was considered the standard imaging modality for nodal disease. The standardized criteria require assessment by CT scan no more than 2 months after completion of therapy. Bone marrow aspirate and biopsy is considered mandatory only to confirm CR if involved initially or if new abnormalities develop in the peripheral blood count or smear.

The Workshop also defined a series of acceptable endpoints for clinical trials as documented on Table 66.2.

In most studies of aggressive NHL, remission status, defined according to these criteria, is strongly correlated with outcome. In general, a partial remission after combination chemotherapy is associated with a high risk of subsequent relapse and a low probability for long-term disease-free survival. In studies of low-grade FL, this is less clear. Although many single center studies have demonstrated that the achievement of a CR to a particular regimen is associated with superior disease-free survival and overall survival compared with patients achieving a PR, comparative trials of different regimens have typically shown that higher response rates frequently correlate with higher rates of disease-free survival or event-free survival, but this rarely correlates with improved overall survival. There are several potential explanations for this, including the effectiveness of subsequent treatments to "rescue" patients who relapse after a particular regimen. However, recent data for new first line regimens in the treatment of FL suggest that these treatments may be improving overall survival in these diseases. If these observations are confirmed, the use of refined criteria for response in FL may become central to management. If the presence of residual subclinical disease in indolent lymphomas proves predictive of subsequent relapse and survival, the potential for early treatment will require investigation.

## USE OF FUNCTIONAL IMAGING IN RESPONSE ASSESSMENT IN NHL

The use of functional imaging techniques in response assessment in NHL has now been evaluated in several studies. The potential advantage of functional imaging in this context is based on the well-documented limitation of CT-based assessments of response to therapy in NHL. This is because CT is unable to differentiate between viable tumor, fibrosis, or necrosis in a residual mass at the completion of therapy. Initial data from studies in which functional imaging has been used as an adjunct to staging have suggested that this modality may have a higher specificity and sensitivity in patients with aggressive compared with indolent lymphomas. Consequently, most data so far has been collected for patients with aggressive subtypes of NHL, particularly DLBCL. Although gallium scintigraphy has been used previously in this context, most recent data has described the use of FDG-PET. Most studies have investigated the use of this technique separately from conventional imaging techniques such as CT scanning, although some recent studies have assessed the potential addition of FDG-PET to conventional response assessment. In all cases, the studies have determined the predictive value of FDG-PET in terms of subsequent relapse and survival.

Spaepen et al. have reported results for 96 patients with various subtypes of aggressive NHL undergoing PET scans at the completion of various combination chemotherapy regimens.[2] Sixty-seven of these patients had negative PET scans at the completion of therapy, of which 80% remained in clinical CR with a median

| Table 66.2 | Definition of endpoints for clinical trials according to International Workshop | | |
|---|---|---|---|
| End point | Response category | Definition | Point of measurement |
| Overall survival | All patients | Death from any cause | Entry onto trial |
| Event-free survival | CR, CR$_u$, PR | Failure or death from any cause | Entry onto trial |
| Progression-free survival | All patients | Disease progression or death from NHL | Entry onto trial |
| Response duration | CR, CR$_u$, PR | Time to relapse or progression | First documentation of response |
| Disease-free survival | CR, CR$_u$ | Time to relapse | First documentation of response |
| Time to next treatment | All patients | Time next treatment is required | Trial entry |
| Cause-specific death | All patients | Death related to NHL | Death |

follow-up of just under 2 years. The remaining 20% of patients relapsed in a median of 316 days. All of the 29 patients with positive PET scans at the completion of therapy relapsed at a median of 105 days. A similar study by Mikhaeel reported a positive predictive value (PPV) of 100% and a negative predictive value (NPV) of 82% for PET scanning used at the completion of therapy.[3] Several other studies have now been reported, with similar results, all suggesting that FDG-PET predicts tumor viability and subsequent relapse in residual masses with 80–90% PPV, after first line and, in some cases, salvage therapy, including ASCT.[4–6]

A recent retrospective study from Juweid et al. has assessed the use of FDG-PET in combination with the International Workshop criteria (IWC) in patients with aggressive NHL in an attempt to determine whether PET scanning adds increased discrimination in outcome compared with conventional response criteria.[7] The study included 54 patients with aggressive NHL, mostly DLBCL who underwent FDG-PET and CT scanning between 1 and 16 weeks after completion of 4–8 cycles of cyclophosphamide, doxorubicin, vincristine, prednisone (CHOP)-based chemotherapy. Responses to therapy were assessed by conventional IWC and by an additional set of criteria which included PET. Based on subsequent risk of relapse, used as a surrogate for the accuracy of each methods of response assessment, IWC plus PET provided a more accurate assessment, in particular because PET was able to identify a subset of patients in PR by IWC who were PET negative, and carried a more favorable prognosis. Further studies are underway at the moment, which will probably further define the value of PET in this situation and it is likely that the IWC will be modified in the near future to integrate data from functional imaging.

Additionally, the use of functional imaging early in the course of therapy is being assessed as a method of response assessment and prediction of subsequent outcome (see the section on prognostic factors).

It is important to emphasize that most present data regarding PET scanning for response assessment relates to aggressive NHL. Few data are available for indolent subtypes of lymphoma.

## ASSESSMENT OF MOLECULAR RESPONSE AND MINIMAL RESIDUAL DISEASE

In contrast to studies of functional imaging, the use of molecular response as an endpoint has been addressed mostly in the context of FLs. Standard clinical and pathologic techniques including routine light microscopy and immunohistochemistry are capable of detecting tumor cells to the level of approximately 1 in 100 normal cells. Lower levels of disease, detected by molecular techniques, are designated as minimal residual disease (MRD). Molecular techniques can detect tumor cells to the level of 1 in 1,000,000 normal cells. Clearing of disease at the molecular level is termed molecular remission (MR). The relationship between MR and clinical outcome is unclear at present, and MR is therefore being incorporated into study endpoints in many clinical trials in FL.

Two targets for monitoring of MRD have been evaluated in FL. The t(14;18) (q32:q21) translocation is detectable in most cases of FL. It can be detected by fluorescence in situ hybridization (FISH) techniques, or by polymerase chain reaction (PCR). In the uncommon case of FL without a detectable t(14;18), the IgH gene rearrangement unique to the malignant clone, also detectable by PCR, has been used for MRD detection. Most studies exploring the role of MRD have assessed this either in peripheral blood, bone marrow, or both.

There is increasing evidence that treatment regimens which result in molecular remissions in FL are associated with prolonged clinical remissions. In a study from MD Anderson Cancer Center, 194 patients with low-grade follicular NHL and a detectable bcl-2 gene rearrangement were treated with one of three chemotherapy regimens.[8] Most patients also received interferon α as maintenance therapy. Although a correlation was observed between molecular and clinical CR rates, one-third of patients achieving clinical CRs were not in MR at the completion of therapy and one-third of patients in PR after 3–5 months eventually achieved MR. Patients achieving MR during the first year following treatment had significantly longer failure-free survival rates than those not in MR (4 year failure-free survival = 76% vs 38%; $p < 0.001$). MR was independently predictive of outcome in multivariate analysis and was also predictive within the group of patients in clinical CR. In this study, there was a concordance rate of approximately 70% between results in the peripheral blood and bone marrow, indicating that the tissue used for evaluation of MRD is an important variable. This study demonstrated that conventional dose chemotherapy regimens produce a significance MR rate in FL, a fact which has subsequently been confirmed in many other studies, especially those in which rituximab has been used as a component of first-line therapy in combination with chemotherapy.[9–11] This study also demonstrated that the achievement of both clinical CR and MR improved with time over the first 20 months of follow-up from completion of therapy, indicating that the timing of response assessment may influence the correlation between these parameters and outcome. Additionally, despite the strong correlation between achievement of MR and failure-free survival, most patients eventually progressed, indicating that MR does not equate with cure.

Several studies have now demonstrated a similar relationship between the attainment of MR and prolonged failure-free survival, and have also confirmed that the re-emergence of PCR detectable disease (or an increase in the level using quantitative PCR techniques) is correlated with subsequent clinical relapse.[12–14]

The use of MR has also been investigated in the context of patients with FL undergoing high-dose therapy and ASCT. Most of these studies have demonstrated a correlation between PCR negativity in the blood and bone marrow and subsequent disease-free survival after ASCT.[12–14] Freedman et al. reported experience in 153 patients undergoing high-dose therapy and ASCT for relapsed FL.[12] All of these patients were treated with cyclophosphamide and total body irradiation (TBI), and all had in vitro manipulation of the stem cell product with monoclonal antibodies prior to reinfusion. In this series, continued PCR negativity in the peripheral blood and marrow after ASCT correlated with continued clinical CR, an observation made in several other smaller post ASCT studies.

In summary, there are accumulating data which suggest that the achievement of MR in FL is a meaningful endpoint which correlates with clinical outcome. At present, molecular endpoints have not been incorporated into the IWC, although this is likely to change. In the meantime, the use of molecular endpoints in FL trials is essential to obtain further information on the predictive value of molecular response.

Despite encouraging data, there are several limitations to the use of molecular endpoints. The bcl-2 rearrangement can be detected in the blood of 5–10% of normal individuals (although using quantitative techniques, it is usually present at much lower levels than in the FL population).[15,16] Optimal timing for the evaluation of MR is uncertain at the moment, since PCR-detectable disease can continue to diminish and eventually disappear several months after completion of therapy.[8,17] Monoclonal antibodies such as rituximab have been shown to clear PCR-detectable disease from the blood and bone marrow more effectively than from lymph nodes, indicating that the specific therapy and the site of evaluation for MRD can both influence the molecular response.[18,19]

## PROGNOSIS AND PROGNOSTIC FACTORS

### DIFFUSE LARGE B-CELL LYMPHOMA

The clinical factors identified in the IPI for aggressive NHL have gained widespread use for risk stratification in clinical trials and are used by many clinicians to provide prognostic information for patients with these diseases.[20] The risk groups and observed relapse-free and overall survival rates are summarized in Table 66.3. The age adjusted IPI (aa-IPI) is also frequently used, especially for studies investigating dose-intensive approaches such as first remission high-dose therapy and ASCT. A stage-adjusted IPI has also been proposed for patients with limited stage disease.[21] The clinical utility of the IPI and aa-IPI has been confirmed in multiple studies of first-line therapy for aggressive NHL, and more recently, in studies for patients undergoing salvage therapy with ASCT.[22]

Although the IPI and aa-IPI have been valuable tools for risk stratification, there is marked variability in outcome within each of the IPI risk groups, reflecting the underlying biological and pathologic heterogeneity of aggressive NHL. Even in studies where entry is restricted to patients with DLBCL, this variability is still present, indicating the need for more patient-specific, biologically based risk factors.

### Molecular and immunohistochemical risk factors in DLBCL

Expression of many individual proteins detected by immunohistochemistry has been shown to have prognostic value in DLBCL. Examples of some of these are summarized in Table 66.4. The technique of GEP in which expression of thousands of genes can be investigated using cDNA or oligonucleotide probes has now been reported by several groups. The patterns of gene expression have been shown to correlate with clinical outcome and have led to the development of new prognostic models.

| Table 66.3 | Five year relapse free and overall survival rates according to the IPI and age-adjusted IPI | | |
|---|---|---|---|
| **IPI** | | | |
| Risk group | Number of adverse factors[a] | 5 year RFS (%) | 5 year OS (%) |
| Low | 0 or 1 | 70 | 73 |
| Low-intermediate | 2 | 50 | 51 |
| High-intermediate | 3 | 49 | 43 |
| High | 4 or 5 | 40 | 26 |
| **Age adjusted IPI** | | | |
| Risk group | Number of adverse factors[b] | 5 year RFS (%) | 5 year OS (%) |
| Low | 0 | 86 | 83 |
| Low-intermediate | 1 | 66 | 69 |
| High-intermediate | 2 | 53 | 46 |
| High | 3 | 58 | 32 |

RFS, relapse-free survival; OS, overall survival.
[a]Adverse risk factor for IPI are stage III or IV disease, age >60 years, elevated LDH, ECOG performance status ≥2, ≥2 extranodal sites.
[b]Adverse risk factor for age-adjusted IPI are stage III or IV disease, elevated LDH, ECOG performance status ≥2.

**Table 66.4** Examples of individual immunophenotypic features with reported prognostic significance in DLBCL

| Immunophenotype | Impact on prognosis |
| --- | --- |
| bcl-2 expression | Adverse |
| Mutated p53 | Adverse |
| High proliferative rate defined by Ki-67 | Adverse |
| Cyclin D2 positive | Adverse |
| CD 5 expression | Adverse |
| MUM-1 positive | Adverse |
| bcl-6 expression | Favorable |
| HLA class II expression | Favorable |
| Tumor infiltrating lymphocytes | Favorable |

Alizadeh et al. initially reported results using the lymphochip cDNA microarray to analyze biopsies from 44 patients with DLBCL.[23] In this study, patients with high levels of expression of genes characteristic of normal germinal center B-cells (GCB) were shown to have higher overall survival rates than those with expression profiles characteristic of activated B-cells (ABC). A study of material from 77 uniformly treated DLBCL patients reported by Shipp et al. using olignonucleotide microarrays identified a predictive model based on expression of 13 genes.[24] Rosenwald et al. subsequently described a 17-gene predictive model based on further studies using a cDNA microarray which identified four gene expression signatures characteristic of GCB, proliferating cells, reactive stromal and immune cells in the lymph node, and expression of major histocompatibility (MHC) class II antigens.[25] There was no concordance between individual genes identified in the 13- and 17-gene models previously described, possibly because the microarrays used in the studies differed and different techniques were used to develop the predictive models. The potential clinical utility of prognostic scores based on microarrays is limited by these technical differences, as well as the requirement for fresh, or optimally cryopreserved samples, and by the costs of these techniques. In an attempt to overcome some of these problems Lossos et al. have described a simplified six-gene model using quantitative RT-PCR in 66 patients with DLBCL, all treated with CHOP or related regimens.[26] Genes correlated with shorter survival were *BCL2*, *CCND2*, and *SCYA3*. Those associated with longer survival were *BCL6*, *LMO2*, and *FN1*.

Results from all of these studies have been shown to provide prognostic information which helps to refine the predictive value of the IPI. However, in view of the limitations of GEP studies outlined earlier, there has been recent interest in the use of TMAs which allow immunohistochemical analysis of protein expression from multiple tissue sections on single slides, and which can be performed on routinely fixed and paraffin-embedded clinical specimens.

A recently published study of TMAs in DLBCLs has examined expression of CD10, bcl-6, MUM1, FOXP1, cyclin D2, and bcl-2 in samples from 152 patients with DLBCL, of which 142 had previously been analyzed using GEPs.[27] Using bcl-6, CD10, and MUM1 expression, it was possible to identify samples as GCB-like or ABC-like. As shown in Table 66.5, there was a marked difference in event-free and overall survival according to phenotype, the survivals being very similar to those described for the same series classified according to GEPs. High IPI score and non-GCB phenotype were independent adverse prognostic factors in multivariate analysis. Subsequent studies have confirmed the adverse prognostic significance of non-GCB phenotype identified by TMAs.[28,29] These early results suggest that TMAs are likely to have more clinical utility than GEPs since the availability of frozen material will remain a limitation for genetic studies. A small number of immunohistochemical stains, rather than multiple stains used in TMAs may prove to have adequate predictive value in future studies. Prospective evaluation of GEPs, TMAs, and expression of individual proteins by immunohistochemistry should continue to be an integral part of new clinical trials in DLBCL in an attempt to produce more specific prognostic factors. This is particularly true since the addition of rituximab to combination chemotherapy for DLBCL. Several studies have demonstrated the superiority of rituximab/chemotherapy combinations compared with chemotherapy alone in the treatment of DLBCL. However, to date, all of the published data regarding TMAs and GEPs as prognostic tools is based on samples from patients treated with chemotherapy only. Recent reports have shown that the addition of rituximab to chemotherapy can modify the prognostic significance of certain factors. For example, the adverse prognostic effect of absent bcl-6 expression in DLBCL patients treated with CHOP does not apply to patients receiving CHOP-rituximab.[30] Two recent studies have demonstrated that the adverse prognostic significance of bcl-2 expression in DLBCL is lost in patients treated with chemotherapy/rituximab combinations.[31,32]

At present, the IPI and aa-IPI should be regarded as the standard system for identifying risk groups in DLBCL. Ongong studies of GEPs and TMAs based in samples from patients treated with rituximab-based

**Table 66.5** Tissue microarray criteria for GCB versus non-GCB derivation of DLBCL

| | CD10 | Bcl6 | MUM1 | 5 year EFS (%) | 5 year OS (%) |
| --- | --- | --- | --- | --- | --- |
| GCB | + (−) | + (−) | − | 63 | 76 |
| Non-GCB | − | − | + | 36 | 34 |

EFS, event-free survival; OS, overall survival.

combinations are in progress and are likely to refine the IPI in the future.

### "Early" functional imaging in DLBCL

The use of "early" functional imaging using FDG-PET has been shown to be predictive of prognosis in DLBCL by several groups. As previously described, FDG-PET is gaining an emerging role in the assessment of disease at the completion of therapy. However, the use of this technique at completion of therapy, although having prognostic value, is otherwise of limited clinical utility since there is no evidence to suggest that changing, or intensifying therapy for patients not in CR at the completion of primary treatment improves outcome. Functional imaging performed earlier (after one or more cycles of chemotherapy) might be a more accurate predictor of outcome than that performed at completion of chemotherapy since it may identify relatively resistant clones which are slow to respond to chemotherapy. Early detection of resistant disease might allow an early change of therapy, and even if not, might give more accurate predictive information on which to base subsequent management, including follow-up. Studies from Memorial Sloan Kettering Cancer Center have investigated the use of FDG-PET after one cycle of chemotherapy in a series of patients with NHL and Hodgkin's lymphoma and compared these results with scans performed at the completion of therapy in the same group of patients.[33] A positive FDG-PET was associated with a significantly shorter PFS at both time points. However, the PPV was higher after one cycle of therapy compared with at the completion of therapy (90% vs 83%). A similar difference was observed for the NPV (85% vs 65%) and the false negative rate (15% vs 35%) both of which also favored PET after one cycle.

A recent study from France has reported results from 90 patients with aggressive NHL treated with a variety of doxorubicin-based combination chemotherapy regimens who underwent FDG-PET after two cycles of therapy.[34] Forty-one percent of patients in this study received rituximab as a component of first-line therapy. Early FDG-PET was negative in 54 patients and positive in 36. At completion of induction therapy, 83% of patients with negative early FDG-PET had achieved clinical CR compared with 58% of those with positive FDG-PET. Significant differences were observed in 2 year event-free survival (82% vs 43%; $p < 0.0001$) and overall survival (90% vs 61%; $p < 0.006$) in favor of the FDG-PET negative group. Furthermore, the predictive value of early FDG-PET was seen in all IPI risk groups, indicating its independence from the IPI as a prognostic factor.

Early FDG-PET therefore represents another approach which may provide important prognostic information to refine the IPI. Potential limitations include the uncertainties regarding the criteria for designation of a "positive" or "negative" scan, the availability of functional imaging, and the expense of this technique. It is also possible that the predictive value of early PET may be limited to certain regimens, particularly standard regimens using fixed doses of chemotherapy. Recent studies of regimens with dynamic dose adjustments according to toxicity, such as dose-adjusted EPOCH-R (etoposide, prednisone, vincristine, cyclophosphamide, doxorubicin, rituximab)[35] have shown poor predictive value of early FDG-PET scanning, possibly because of a relatively early adjustment of dose which eradicates relatively resistant tumor clones more quickly (W.H Wilson, MD, PhD, personal communication).

## FOLLICULAR LYMPHOMA

Retrospective analyses of patients with FL have identified many clinical factors with adverse prognostic significance, including advanced age, high number of nodal sites of involvement, advanced anatomic stage, the presence of tumor bulk, and elevated LDH. The IPI described for aggressive NHL has also been applied to patients with FL, and several studies have shown it to have predictive value. The use of the IPI is limited by the fact that a relatively small number of patients have high-risk disease according to this index, limiting the patient populations for prospective studies in "poor risk" disease. Additionally, clinical factors with prognostic value in indolent lymphoma may differ substantially from those in aggressive NHL because of the biologic difference between these two entities.

The FLIPI has therefore been developed and is now regarded as the standard clinical prognostic tool for patients with low grade FL.[36] The risk groups and 5- and 10-year survival rates associated with each of these groups are summarized in Table 66.6.

A recent European study has compared the FLIPI with the IPI and also with an Italian Prognostic Index developed for FL, in a population of 465 patients with low-grade disease.[37] They demonstrated that all three indices provided useful prognostic stratification. The FLIPI identified a higher proportion of patients with high-risk disease. However, the concordance between the three indices was only 54%, indicating that as with DLBCL there is substantial biological and clinical heterogeneity within each risk group and emphasizing the need for more accurate predictors of outcome.

### MOLECULAR AN IMMUNOPHENOTYPIC PROGNOSTIC FACTORS IN FOLLICULAR LYMPHOMA

As with DLBCL, many molecular, cytogenetic, and immunohistochemical factors have been shown to have prognostic significance in small series of patients with FL.[38-40] Some of these are summarized in Table 66.7. The variability in the prognostic factors identified across many of these studies reflects selection bias into the various studies, heterogeneity of treatment

**Table 66.6**   Five year and 10 year overall survival rates for patients with FL according to FLIPI risk group

| Risk group | Number of adverse factors[a] | Distribution of patients (%) | 5 year OS (%) | 10 year OS (%) |
|---|---|---|---|---|
| Low | 0–1 | 36 | 90.6 | 70.7 |
| Intermediate | 2 | 37 | 77.6 | 50.9 |
| high | ≥3 | 27 | 52.5 | 30.5 |

OS, overall survival.
[a]Adverse risk factors for FLIPI are age ≥ 60 years, Ann Arbor stage III or IV, hemoglobin <12 g/dL, serum LDH > upper limit of normal, number of nodal sites > 4.

regimens, and the lack of consistency in the diagnosis and grading of FLs, which has been documented in many previous studies.

As with aggressive NHL, the use of GEP has recently been applied to the study of FLs in an attempt to refine prognostic groups identified by the FLIPI and IPI. The largest GEP study to date has been reported from the Leukemia and Lymphoma Molecular Profiling Project (LLMPP).[41] In this study, cDNA microarrays were performed on 191 biopsies from patients with FL for which clinical follow-up data were available. This study identified two gene expression signatures, both with high levels of genes characteristic of immune response functions. One of these signatures was associated with favorable and the other with adverse prognosis. Many of the immune response genes identified in both signatures are typically expressed in macrophages, and further studies demonstrated that the signatures with prognostic significance were expressed in cells other than the germinal center derived malignant B-cells. This study demonstrated the potential prognostic significance of the immune response in this disease, especially since the gene expression signatures had predictive value independent of the IPI.

Consistent with these observations, a recent study from British Columbia has examined the potential prognostic significance of lymphoma-associated macrophage (LAM) content in low-grade FL, using routine immuno-histochemical staining for a macrophage marker (CD68) in routinely processed and fixed clinical specimens.[42] Out of 99 evaluable patients with FL, all uniformly treated between 1987 and 1993, 87 were classified as having low LAM content and 12 as having high LAM. The median overall survival for each group was 16.3 years versus 5.0 years, respectively ($p = 0.0003$). In multivariate analysis, LAM and IPI retained independent predictive value. TMA studies are in progress for patients with FL at present and are likely to identify candidate immunohistochemical markers which will be used to construct refined prognostic models in the future.

In the meantime, clinical prognostic factors such as the FLIPI or IPI will remain the standard tool for clinical practice and clinical trials.

Few studies of functional imaging have been conducted in FL, and most suggest that the PPV and NPV of FDG-PET are relatively low, suggesting that this is unlikely to provide a useful prognostic tool in these diseases.

**Table 66.7**   Examples of morphologic, immunohistochemical, and molecular markers with prognostic significance in FL

| Marker | Impact on prognosis |
|---|---|
| Histologic grade | Higher grade carries adverse prognosis |
| Ki-67 (proliferation marker) | Higher proliferation rate carries adverse prognosis |
| Diffuse areas | Adverse |
| Loss of p53 | Adverse |
| Loss of p16 | Adverse |
| Gain of c-myc | Adverse |
| bcl-6 | Variable in different series |
| bcl-2 | Variable—site of breakpoint in rearranged bcl-2 gene has prognostic significance |

## FOLLOW-UP

Very few studies have formally addressed the optimal follow-up schedule and optimal follow-up procedures for patients with NHL. Although routine imaging techniques such as CT scanning and FDG-PET are now commonly used for the early detection of relapse, there are no published studies evaluating the utility of PET in this context, and studies of CT scanning and other imaging modalities have failed to show a high rate of early detection of relapse (although most studies were reported in the early 1990s with inferior scanning technology to that now available).[43]

Although molecular techniques such as quantitative PCR may help detect early, subclinical relapse in some subtypes of NHL, especially FL, there is no evidence at present to suggest that early treatment intervention in this context improves survival compared with the treatment of clinically detected relapse, although this may change with the increased used of monoclonal antibodies in this disease.

The International Workshop defined a recommended follow-up schedule and investigations for patients with NHL on clinical trials to establish consistency across different studies. Their recommendations were that patients should be evaluated a minimum of every 3 months after completion of treatment for 2 years, then every 6 months for 3 years, and then annually for at least a further 5 years. For patients with aggressive lymphoma, few recurrences occur beyond 10 years, although the group acknowledged that for low-grade FL, longer follow-up would be required, not only for the detection of relapse but also to monitor for late side effects of therapy such as secondary myelodysplastic syndrome or acute myeloid leukemia which have been reported with increasing frequency in the FL population.

Minimum testing recommended at each follow-up visit was for a history, full physical examination, complete blood count, and LDH. No recommendations were made regarding the appropriate intervals for imaging or other investigations.

Although this schedule has some utility for clinical trial design, follow-up schedules will to some extent be determined by the aggressiveness of the disease, the presenting prognostic factors, and the estimated risk of relapse. Investigations will be determined by the original sites and extent of disease, although at least one study in aggressive NHL has shown that over 60% of relapses occur in new sites of disease, suggesting that follow-up investigations should not be specifically directed to the original sites of disease.

As further information accumulates regarding the predictive value of PCR-based techniques, or functional imaging, these are likely to be incorporated into routine follow-up schedules. However, it is important to point out that the early detection of relapse is only helpful if effective treatment strategies are available for salvage therapy. The impact of early detection of relapse on survival is likely to be determined more by the effectiveness of salvage therapy than the ability to detect low levels of subclinical disease.

## REFERENCES

1. Cheson BD, Horning SJ, Coiffier B, et al.: Report of an International Workshop to standardize response criteria for non-Hodgkin's lymphomas. *J Clin Oncol* 17:1244–1253, 1999.
2. Spaepen K, Stroobants S, Dupont P, et al.: Prognostic value of positron emission tomography (PET with 18-fluorodeoxyglucose ([18F]FDG) after fist line chemotherapy in non-Hodgkin's lymphoma: is [18F]FDG PET a valid alternative to conventional diagnostic methods? *J Clin Oncol* 19:414–419, 2001.
3. Mikhaeel NG, Timothy AR, Hain SF, et al.: 18-FDG-PET for the assessment of residual masses on CT following treatment of lymphomas. *Ann Oncol* 11(suppl 1):147–150, 2000.
4. Vose JM, Bierman PJ, Anderson JR, et al. : Single-photon emission computed tomography gallium imaging versus computed tomography : predictive value in patients undergoing high-dose chemotherapy and autologous stem-cell transplantation for non-Hodgkin's lymphoma. *J Clin Oncol* 14:2473–2479, 1996.
5. Jerusalem G, Beguin Y, Fassotte MF, et al. : Whole body positron emission tomography using 18F-fluorodeoxyglucose for posttreatment evaluation in Hodgkin's disease and non-Hodgkin's lymphoma has higher diagnostic and prognostic value than classical computed tomography scan imaging. *Blood* 94:429–433, 1999.
6. Kostakoglu L, Goldsmith SJ: Fluorine-18 fluorodeoxyglucose positron emission tomography in the staging and follow up of lymphoma: Is it time to shift gears? *Eur J Nucl Med* 27:1564–1578, 2000.
7. Juweid ME, Wiseman GA, Vose JM, et al.: Response assessment of aggressive non-Hodgkin's lymphoma by integrated International Workshop criteria and fluorine-18-fluorodeoxyglucose positron emission tomography. *J Clin Oncol* 23:4652–4661, 2005.
8. Lopez-Guillermo A, Cabanillas F, McLaughlin P, et al.: The clinical significance of molecular response in indolent follicular lymphomas. *Blood* 91:2955–2960, 1998.
9. Zinzani PL, Pulsoni A, Perrotti A, et al.: Fludarabine plus mitoxantrone with and without rituximab versus CHOP with and without rituximab as front-line treatment for patients with follicular lymphoma. *J Clin Oncol* 22:2654–2661, 2004.
10. Vitolo U, Boccomini C, Ladetto M, et al.: High clinical and molecular response rates in elderly patients with advanced stage follicular lymphoma treated at diagnosis with a brief chemo-immunotherapy FND + rituximab. *Blood* 100:359a–360a, 2002.
11. Czuczman MS, Weaver R, Alkuzweny B, et al.: Prolonged clinical and molecular remission in patients with low-grade or follicular non-Hodgkin's lymphoma treated with rituximab plus CHOP chemotherapy: 9-year follow up. *J Clin Oncol* 22:4711–4716, 2004.
12. Freedman AS, Neuberg D, Mauch P, et al.: Long-term follow up of autologous bone marrow transplantation in patients with relapsed follicular lymphoma. *Blood* 94:3325–3333, 1999.
13. Gribben JG, Neuberg D, Freedman AS, et al.: Detection by polymerase chain reaction of residual cells with the bcl-2 translocation is associated with increased risk of relapse after autologous bone marrow transplantation for B-cell lymphoma. *Blood* 81:3449–3457, 1993.
14. Moos M, Schulz R, Martin S, et al.: The remission status before and the PCR status after high dose therapy with peripheral blood stem cell support are prognostic factors for relapse-free survival in patients with follicular non-Hodgkin's lymphoma. *Leukemia* 12:1971–1976, 1998.

15. Limpens J, Stad R, Vos C, et al.: Lymphoma-associated translocation t(14 ;18) in blood B cells of normal individuals. *Blood* 85:2528–2536, 1995.

16. Dolken G, Illerhaus G, Hirt C, et al.: BCL-2/JH rearrangements in circulating B-cells of healthy blood donors and patients with non-malignant diseases. *J Clin Oncol* 14:1333–1344, 1996.

17. Lopez-Guillermo A: molecular response assessed by PCR is the most important factor predicting failure-free survival in indolent follicular lymphoma: Update of the MDACC series. *Ann Oncol* 11(suppl 1):137–140, 2000.

18. Foran JM, Gupta RK, Cunningham D, et al.: A UK multicentre phase II study of rituximab (chimaeric anti-CD20 monoclonal antibody) in patients with follicular lymphoma, with PCR monitoring of molecular response. *Br J Haematol* 109:81–88, 2000.

19. Mandigers CM, Meijerink JP, Mensink EJ, et al.: Lack of correlation between numbers of circulating t(14;18) positive cells and response to first line treatment in follicular lymphoma. *Blood* 98:940–944, 2001.

20. The International Non-Hodgkin's Lymphoma Prognostic Factors Project. A predictive model for aggressive non-Hodgkin's lymphoma. *N Engl J Med* 329:987–994, 1993.

21. Miller TP: Limited stage lymphoma: treatment for aggressive histologies. *Hematology* 221:225–228, 2004.

22. Hamlin PA, Zelenetz AD, Kewelramani T, et al.: Age-adjusted international prognostic index predicts autologous stem cell transplantation outcome for patients with relapsed or primary refractory diffuse large B-cell lymphoma. *Blood* 102:1989–1996, 2003.

23. Alizadeh AA, Eisen MB, Davis RE, et al. : Distinct types of diffuse large B-cell lymphoma identified by gene expression profiling. *Nature* 403:503–511, 2000.

24. Shipp MA, Ross KN, Tamayo P, et al.: Diffuse large B-cell lymphoma outcome prediction by gene-expression profiling and supervised machine learning. *Nature Medicine* 8:68–74, 2002.

25. Rosenwald A, Wright G, Chan WC, et al.: The use of molecular profiling to predict survival after chemotherapy for diffuse large B-cell lymphoma. *N Engl J Med* 346:1937–1947, 2002.

26. Lossos IS, Czerwinski DK, Alizadeh AA, et al.: Prediction of survival in diffuse large B-cell lymphoma based on the expression of 6 genes. *N Engl J Med* 350:1828–1837, 2004.

27. Hans CP, Weisenberger DD, Greiner TC, et al.: Conformation of the molecular classification of diffuse large B-cell lymphoma by immunohistochemistry using a tissue microarray. *Blood* 103:275–282, 2004.

28. Saez AI, Saez AJ, Artiga MJ, et al.: Building an outcome predictor model for diffuse large B-cell lymphoma. *Am J Pathol* 164:613–622, 2004.

29. Zinzani PL, Dirnhofer S, Sabattini E, et al.: Identification of outcome predictors in diffuse large B-cell lymphoma. Immunohistochemical profiling of homogeneously treated de novo tumors with nodal presentation on tissue micro-arrays. *Haematologica* 90:341–347, 2005.

30. Winter JN, Weller E, Horning SJ, et al.: Prognostic significance of Bcl-6 protein expression in DLBCL treated with CHOP or R-CHOP: a prospective correlative study. *Blood* 107:4207–4213, 2006.

31. Mounier N, Briere J, Gisselbrecht C, et al.: Rituximab plus CHOP (R-CHOP) overcomes bcl-2 associated resistance to chemotherapy in elderly patients with diffuse large B-cell lymphoma (DLBCL). *Blood* 101:4279–4284, 2003.

32. Wilson WH, Gutierrez M, O'Connor O, et al.: The role of rituximab and chemotherapy in aggressive B-cell lymphoma: a preliminary report of dose-adjusted R-EPOCH. *Semin Oncol* 29(suppl 1):41–47, 2002.

33. Kostakoglu L, Coleman M, Leonard JP, et al.: PET predicts prognosis after one cycle of chemotherapy in aggressive lymphoma and Hodgkin's disease. *J Nuc Med* 43:1018–1027, 2002.

34. Haioun C, Itti E, Rahmouni A, et al.: [18F]fluoro-2-deoxy-D-glucose positron emission tomography (FDG-PET) in aggressive lymphoma: an early prognostic tool for predicting patient outcome. *Blood* 106:1376–1381, 2005.

35. Wilson WH, Dunleavy K, Pittaluga S, et al.: Dose-adjusted EPOCH-rituximab is highly effective in the GCB and ABC subtypes of untreated diffuse large B-cell lymphoma. *Blood* 104:49a, 2004.

36. Solal-Celigny P, Roy P, Colombat P, et al.: Follicular Lymphoma International Prognostic Index. *Blood* 104:1258–1265, 2004.

37. Perea G, Altes A, Montoto S, et al.: Prognostic indexes in follicular lymphoma : a comparison of different prognostic systems. *Ann Oncol* 16:1508–1513, 2005.

38. Hans CP, Weisenberger DD Vose JM, et al.: A significant diffuse component predicts for inferior survival in grade 3 follicular lymphoma, but cytologic subtypes do not predict survival. *Blood* 101:2363–2367, 2003.

39. Lestou VS, Gascoyne RD, Sehn L, et al. : Multicolor fluorescence in situ hybridization analysis of t(14 ;18) positive follicular lymphoma and correlation with gene expression data and clinical outcome. *Br J Haematol* 122:745–759, 2003.

40. Bilalovic N, Blystad AK, Golouh R, et al.: Expression of bcl-6 and CD10 protein is associated with longer overall survival and time to treatment failure in follicular lymphoma. *Am J Clin Pathol* 121:34–42, 2004.

41. Dave SS, Wright G, Tan B, et al.: Prediction of survival in follicular lymphoma based on molecular features of tumor-infiltrating immune cells. *New Engl J Med* 351:2159–2169, 2005.

42. Farinha P, Masoudi H, Skinnider BF, et al.: Analysis of multiple biomarkers shows that lymphoma-associated macrophage (LAM) content is an independent predictor of survival in follicular lymphoma (FL). *Blood* 106:2169–2174, 2005.

43. Radford JA, Eardley A, Woodman C, et al.: Follow-up policy after treatment for Hodgkin's disease: too many clinical visits and routine tests? A review of hospital records. *Br Med J* 314:343–346, 1997.

# Chapter 67

# TREATMENT OF TRANSFORMED NON-HODGKIN'S LYMPHOMA

*Philip J. Bierman*

## INTRODUCTION

Four patterns of histologic variation have been described for patients with non-Hodgkin's lymphoma (NHL).[1] Mixed architectural pattern refers to a single biopsy which reveals areas with both diffuse and follicular patterns. Composite lymphomas contain more than one distinct type of lymphoma (or Hodgkin's lymphoma and NHL) in the same biopsy. Discordant lymphoma refers to different types of lymphoma that occur at different locations, simultaneously. Histologic transformation (or evolution, or conversion, or progression) refers to a change in lymphoma histology that occurs during the course of a patient's disease.

Transformation is frequently unrecognized until discovered at postmortem examination. Usually, transformation refers to a change from low-grade or indolent histology to more aggressive histology, although other definitions have been used. Frequently, progression from follicular to diffuse histology is used to define transformation, and at other times transformation may be defined as an increase in the number of large cells in a biopsy.

In 1928, Maurice Richter described a patient with "chronic lymphoid leukemia" and progressive lymph node enlargement.[2] At autopsy, the lymph nodes, liver, and spleen were infiltrated by small lymphocytes and "endothelioid tumor cells" described as a "reticular cell sarcoma." Since then, the term Richter's syndrome has been used to describe the development of large-cell lymphoma in a patient with chronic lymphocytic leukemia (CLL). Retrospective series have demonstrated the occurrence of Richter's syndrome in 2–3% of CLL patients.[3,4] This syndrome has been described in CLL patients who are in remission, as well as those with active disease, and is classically associated with systemic symptoms, progressive lymphadenopathy, extranodal disease, elevated serum lactate dehydrogenase (LDH), and poor prognosis.

## EPIDEMIOLOGY

### INCIDENCE

The true incidence of histologic transformation is difficult to determine for a wide variety of reasons.[1] As noted above, there are a number of differences in the way in which transformation is defined. It may also be difficult to distinguish patients with histologic transformation from those with unrecognized discordant pathology at diagnosis. Most authors suggest that patients with evidence of transformation within 6 months of diagnosis have discordant pathology, rather than transformation.[5-7] There is also a lack of uniformity regarding patient follow-up in many series. Long-term follow-up of large cohorts is necessary to determine the true frequency of transformation, since transformation may be a late event. Many studies cite crude incidence rates instead of actuarial risk. In addition, the risk of transformation includes all patients in some series, while other reports restrict calculations to patients who have progressed and received biopsies. Accurate statistics on the risk of transformation are also impaired by a lack of standardized criteria for biopsy of suspected sites of relapse.[1] For example, peripheral nodes are more likely to be biopsied than less accessible nodes. Infrequent biopsies of suspected sites of relapse will underestimate the risk of transformation. A single biopsy of only one site of relapse may fail to identify transformation that has occurred in another location. In addition, autopsy findings may not be included in some series. Finally, results from older series may not be applicable to patients managed more recently because of refinements in lymphoma classification, ease of detecting relapse and performing biopsies, and possible influences of newer treatments.

A wide variety of situations have been described, in which changes in the histology of lymphoma occur over time.[8] Examples include progression of CLL/small lymphocytic lymphoma to diffuse large B-cell lymphoma and Hodgkin's lymphoma, progression of follicular lymphoma to diffuse large B-cell lymphoma, progression of marginal zone lymphoma to diffuse large B-cell lymphoma, and progression of mycosis fungoides to peripheral T-cell lymphoma. This chapter will focus mainly on transformation of follicular lymphomas and, to a lesser extent, on Richter's syndrome.

The frequency of NHL transformation has been examined in several series (Table 67.1). It is impossible to compare the different results due to variations in the way calculations are performed. The true rate of transformation may be overestimated, since many series perform calculations on the basis of only those patients who progress and undergo a repeat biopsy. Conversely, true rates of transformation may be underestimated, since many patients do not have repeat biopsies and few patients are examined at autopsy.

Some studies have shown a risk of transformation that plateaus after 6 or 7 years.[16,21] Other reports have shown a continuous risk of transformation without evidence of a plateau.[6,7,17] The median time to documentation of histologic transformation was 57 months for a group of low-grade lymphoma patients (follicular small cleaved cell, follicular mixed small cleaved cell and large cell, and small lymphocytic) managed with initial observation.[17] Other investigators have reported a median time from diagnosis to transformation ranging from 26 to 66 months.[6,15,16,19,22]

### RISK FACTORS

A number of prognostic factors have been analyzed for their association with transformation. In a series examining histologic progression of follicular lymphomas, it was noted that patients who transformed were more likely to have had early stage disease at initial diagnosis and were more likely to have received local radiation as primary treatment when these patients were compared to others with unchanged histology.[5] In another series, histologic transformation was found to be associated with involvement of extranodal sites of disease, stage IV disease, presence of systemic symptoms, and bulky abdominal disease at diagnosis, as well as failure to achieve a complete remission with initial therapy.[6] Lack of response to initial therapy has been associated with a higher risk of transformation in other series,[21] and it has been suggested that eradication of primary disease with initial therapy may reduce the incidence of transformation. Elevated serum $\beta_2$-microglobulin level was associated with a higher risk of transformation in one series.[21]

Other series have failed to identify risk factors associated with transformation.[7,16] It does not appear that an initial "watch-and-wait" strategy alters the risk of transformation.[17] Similarly, the risk of transformation appears to be similar when patients with follicular large-cell lymphoma are compared to patients with follicular small cleaved-cell and follicular mixed-cell lymphomas.[21] Treatment with fludarabine or other nucleoside analogs was not shown to influence the progression of CLL to large-cell lymphoma in one series,[3] although other groups have shown unexpectedly high rates of histologic transformation in patients with CLL and follicular lymphoma who were treated with fludarabine.[23] The Stanford group found that the risk of histologic conversion was not influenced whether patients were initially treated with involved-field radiation, total lymphoid or whole body irradiation, single-agent chemotherapy, or combination chemotherapy.[16]

### CLINICAL FINDINGS AND OUTCOME

In most reports, transformed lymphomas have been associated with aggressive disease and poor outcomes. Systemic symptoms and relapse at new or extranodal sites are frequently noted.[3,5–7,16,17,24,25] Other findings such as central nervous system relapse[21] and hypercalcemia[26] have also been associated with histologic transformation.

The median survival was only 4 months in a French series of patients with Richter's syndrome,[25] and only 5 months in a series of patients with Richter's syndrome from MD Anderson Cancer Center.[3] Patients who achieved remission with subsequent therapy had longer survival than those who had poorer responses ($P < 0.001$). Similar findings were noted from Stanford.[16] The median survival following documentation of histologic conversion of low-grade lymphomas was 8.5 months, as compared to 6 years for patients who continued to have indolent histology when rebiopsied ($P < 0.0001$). In this series, achievement of a complete remission after histologic conversion was also associated with a better prognosis. In another French series, the median survival following transformation of follicular lymphoma was 7 months.[21] The median survival for patients with transformation at the time of first progression was 5 months, as compared with 47 months for patients who still had follicular lymphoma at first progression ($P < 0.01$). Factors associated with improved survival following transformation were treatment with a CHOP-like (cyclophosphamide, doxorubicin, vincristine, and prednisone) regimen and normal LDH level. Another series examining outcomes in patients with nodular lymphomas noted that median survival following first repeat biopsy was 77 months for patients who retained nodular architecture, as compared to 11 months for patients with histologic progression.[5] An autopsy series from Massachusetts General Hospital showed that median survival from diagnosis was 55 months among patients who maintained a diagnosis of nodular lymphoma, as compared with 32 months for patients who progressed to a diffuse architectural pattern.[12] A series from the National Cancer Institute showed that median survival was 32

**Table 67.1**    Incidence of histologic transformation of non-Hodgkin's lymphoma

| References | Study population | Incidence | Remarks |
|---|---|---|---|
| 9 | 56 of 618 lymphomas (includes Hodgkin's lymphoma) with sequential biopsies | 13/56 = 28% | Incidence refers to cases undergoing "dedifferentiation" |
| 10 | 94 of 210 follicular lymphomas with sequential biopsies or autopsy | 28/94 = 30% | Incidence refers to cases showing transformation to diffuse architecture |
| 11 | 22 of 136 "macrofollicular" lymphomas with sequential biopsies or autopsy | 22/30 = 73% | Incidence refers to cases showing transformation to diffuse architecture |
| 12 | 18 of 65 nodular lymphomas with autopsy | 8/18 = 44% | Incidence refers to cases showing transformation to diffuse architecture |
| 13 | 30 relapsed lymphomas of 64 lymphomas with "favorable" histology | 9/30 = 30% | Incidence refers to cases showing transformation to a "higher grade" |
| 14 | Autopsy findings of 35 lymphomas with initial nodular architecture | 22/35 = 63% | Incidence refers to cases showing transformation to diffuse architecture |
| 15 | 28 of 56 nodular lymphomas with sequential biopsies | 11/28 = 39% | Incidence refers to cases showing transformation to diffuse architecture |
| 5 | 63 of 203 nodular lymphomas with sequential biopsies | 19/63 = 30% | Incidence refers to cases showing transformation to diffuse or large-cell architecture |
| 16 | 78 relapsed or refractory lymphomas of 150 with favorable histology lymphomas | 23/78 = 29% Actuarial risk = 20% at 5 years and 50% at 8 years for patients with active disease | Incidence refers to case showing transformation to "unfavorable" histology |
| 17 | 23 of 83 low-grade lymphomas initially managed with observation with sequential biopsie | 10/23 = 43% Actuarial risk = 19% at 8 years for all 83 patients | Incidence refers to case showing transformation to intermediate-grade or high-grade histology |
| 18 | Autopsy findings of 56 lymphomas with nodular architecture | 36/56 = 64% | Incidence refers to cases showing transformation to diffuse "aggressive" histology |
| 7 | 34 of 75 nodular small cleaved-cell lymphomas with sequential biopsies | 13/34 = 38% | Incidence refers to cases showing transformation to "transformed" (non-cleaved-cell) histology |
| 6 | 51 of 127 follicular low-grade lymphomas with sequential biopsies | 30/51 = 59% Actuarial risk = 30% at 5 years and 56% at 10 years for relapsed patients | Incidence refers to cases showing transformation to intermediate-grade or high-grade histology |
| 19 | 496 low-grade lymphomas | 34/496 = 7% | Incidence refers to cases showing transformation to a more aggressive histology |
| 20 | 72 of 148 follicular lymphomas with sequential biopsies or autopsy | 23/72 = 32% | Incidence refers to cases showing transformation to diffuse or large-cell architecture |
| 21 | 220 follicular lymphomas | 52/220 = 24% Actuarial risk = 22% at 5 years and 31% at 10 years for all patients, and 33% at 5 years and 51% at 10 years for patients who progressed | Incidence refers to cases showing formation to a more aggressive diffuse lymphoma |

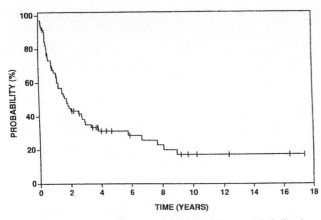

**Figure 67.1** *Overall survival of 74 patients with follicular low-grade NHL following histologic transformation. (Reprinted from Ref. 22)*

months for patients who relapsed with a nodular pattern, as compared with 17 months for those who relapsed with a diffuse pattern ($P = 0.068$).[15] The median survival among patients from Vanderbilt University with indolent lymphoma was 2.5 months for those who exhibited histologic transformation, as compared with 37.5 months for those who retained their initial histologic pattern ($P < 0.001$).[7] Median survival following histologic progression was 4 months in a series of follicular low-grade lymphomas from Denmark,[6] and 12 months in a series from Iowa.[26] The median survival following histologic transformation was approximately 1 year in a series from London.[20] In another series of 74 patients from Stanford, the median survival was 22 months following transformation (Figure 67.1).[22] Limited stage at the time of transformation ($P = 0.01$), absence of prior therapy ($P = 0.01$), and response to therapy ($P = 0.005$) were associated with longer survival after transformation. These results have been used to support the use of a "watch-and-wait" approach for the initial management of patients with low-grade follicular lymphomas. Finally, a French series examined outcomes of patients with follicular lymphomas who were treated on phase III trials.[27] The 5-year survival was estimated to be 15% for patients with subsequent transformation, as compared to 45% for those who retained follicular architecture ($P = .00001$).

These results demonstrate that histologic transformation is frequently associated with aggressive clinical behavior and poor survival. In some series, overall survival from the time of diagnosis was shorter in patients who subsequently demonstrated histologic progression.[5,7] Nevertheless, transformation may be a late event in the course of disease, and survival from the time of diagnosis may not be different when patients with unchanged histology are compared to patients who have undergone transformation.[15,16]

## ETIOLOGY OF TRANFORMATION

### DEMONSTRATION OF CLONALITY

Some "transformed" lymphomas and their preceding follicular lymphomas may be clonally unrelated.[28,29] However, evidence suggests that most transformed follicular lymphomas are derived from the same clone as the antecedent follicular lymphoma. This was shown in studies that demonstrated identical serum monoclonal proteins from a patient before and after transformation, and by studies showing cytoplasmic immunoperoxidase staining for the same protein in biopsies performed before and after transformation.[30] Investigators from Stanford examined paired lymphoma biopsies obtained before and after transformation from follicular to diffuse histology.[31] They were able to demonstrate a common clonal origin on the basis of anti-idiotype monoclonal antibody cross-reactivity, concordant immunoglobulin and *bcl-2* gene rearrangements, and sequencing of light-chain variable genes. The same group also identified identical mutations of the *bcl-6* gene in paired lymphomas that were biopsied before and after transformation.[32] Analyses of immunoglobulin $V_HDJ_H$ gene sequences[33] and bcl-2 rearrangements at other institutions[28,34,35] have also demonstrated that diffuse large B-cell lymphomas may be clonally related to antecedent follicular lymphomas.[33]

CLL and the subsequent diffuse large B-cell lymphoma are clonally related in many situations,[36–39] although the two clones may be genetically unrelated in as many as 50% of cases.[36,40,41]

### GENETIC ABNORMALITIES

Numerous molecular events have been associated with the process of transformation. Several groups have found mutations in the p53 tumor suppressor gene in transformed lymphomas.[42,43] Occasionally, p53 mutations can be identified in patients with follicular lymphoma prior to transformation, and this finding in nontranformed follicular lymphoma may be associated with a poor prognosis.[42] Mutations in the *bcl-6* gene have also been associated with progression from follicular lymphoma to diffuse large B-cell lymphoma. The Stanford group identified *bcl-6* translocations in 39% of follicular lymphomas that were known to have subsequently transformed, as compared with 14.1% in biopsies from patients that were not known to have transformed ($P = 0.0048$).[44] Rearrangements of *myc* have also been identified in transformed lymphomas and the presence of these rearrangements in follicular lymphomas may be associated with a poor prognosis and greater risk of transformation.[34] cDNA microarray analysis of transformed lymphomas has demonstrated patterns of increased expression of c-*myc* and associated targets in some specimens and decreased expression of these genes in others.[45] In addition, expression

**Table 67.2** Genetic abnormalities associated with transformation of follicular lymphoma

| Genetic abnormality | References |
|---|---|
| p53 mutation | 42, 43 |
| *myc* rearrangement/altered expression | 34, 35, 45, 49 |
| *bcl-2* mutation/dysregulation | 28, 50 |
| *bcl-6* mutation | 32, 44 |
| p15 and p16 loss/gene alteration | 46, 47, 51 |
| Cytogenetic abnormalities | |
|   del(6q) | 43, 48, 52–56 |
|   +7 | 52, 56–58 |
|   +12 | 52–54, 56, 59 |
|   Breaks in 7p | 48 |
|   del(9p21) | 46 |
|   der(18) | 52 |
|   Amplification of 13q | 60 |

Adapted from Ref. 61.

patterns of transformed lymphomas were similar to follicular lymphomas and markedly different than de novo diffuse large B-cell lymphomas. Loss or inactivation of the p15 and p16 tumor suppressor genes has also been associated with aggressive tumors and the progression of follicular lymphomas.[46,47]

Various cytogenetic abnormalities have been identified in transformed lymphomas, although the t(14;18) translocation is generally retained. Breaks involving bands 6q23-26 and 17p were associated with a significantly shorter time to transformation for follicular lymphomas ($P < 0.001$).[48]

Various genetic abnormalities associated with histologic transformation of follicular lymphomas are displayed in Table 67.2. These results suggest that histologic transformation of follicular lymphomas frequently involves acquired genetic lesions, although no common pathways have been identified.[62]

## TREATMENT OF TRANSFORMED FOLLICULAR LYMPHOMAS

### CONVENTIONAL THERAPY

Prospective treatment trials have not been performed for patients with transformed lymphomas. Most series are small and contain heterogeneous patient populations. Details of treatment are limited in many reports, and other series include patients treated in a variety of ways and patients treated in a manner that might be considered suboptimal today.

In a series from the National Cancer Institute, 50% of patients with progression from nodular to diffuse histology attained complete remissions with combination chemotherapy regimens.[5] The median duration of remission was 11 months, although one patient remained alive and in remission at 83 months follow-

ing treatment. In a series from Denmark, histologic progression from follicular low-grade histology to an intermediate- or high-grade histology was associated with a response rate below 20%.[6] In a French series, transformation was defined as progression from follicular histology to a more aggressive diffuse lymphoma.[21] The response rate was 63% in the 30 patients who were treated with CHOP-like regimens. Some of these patients were subsequently treated with high-dose therapy followed by autologous hematopoietic stem cell transplantation. Another group of 22 patients was elderly or had a poor performance status and was mostly treated with regimens that did not contain anthracyclines. The actuarial 3-year survival was 32% for patients who received anthracycline-based therapy as compared with 5% for the others ($P = 0.003$). The 13 patients with transformed lymphomas in the Vanderbilt series were treated with radiation or a variety of chemotherapy regimens that did not always include anthracyclines.[7] The median survival following histologic transformation was 2.5 months, and the outcome did not appear to be influenced by the choice of therapy. In another series from Iowa, there were no complete remissions among eight patients with transformed lymphomas who received anthracycline-based therapy, and only short remissions in a patient who received radiation therapy and one who received COPP (cyclophosphamide, vincristine, procarbazine, and prednisone).[26] In the London series of 18 patients who transformed from follicular to large-cell histology, 6 (33%) attained remissions using combination chemotherapy regimens appropriate for high-grade lymphoma.[20] Only two patients remained free of disease at 15 months and 5 years, respectively.

The Stanford group has reported the largest series of treatment results for transformed lymphomas.[22] Transformation was defined as progression from follicular low-grade histology to diffuse intermediate- or high-grade histology. Patients were mostly treated with doxorubicin-containing combination chemotherapy ($n = 43$), radiation ($n = 12$), or other chemotherapy combinations ($n = 16$). The complete remission rates were 40, 70, and 20%, respectively, although the majority of the patients receiving radiation therapy had limited-stage disease. Attainment of complete remission was significantly more likely in patients with limited disease at transformation ($p < 0.01$). The median disease-free survival was 45 months for complete responders, with a median survival of 81 months after transformation.

The MD Anderson Cancer Center has included patients with transformed lymphoma in trials of salvage therapy for NHL. The complete response rate was 50% and the partial response rate was 17% following treatment with ESHAP (etoposide, methylprednisolone, cytarabine, and cisplatin).[63] Thirty percent of these patients were projected to be alive at 3 years. A 36% complete response rate was noted when patients with transformed lymphoma were treated with ESHAP alternating with MINE (mesna, ifosfamide, mitoxantrone, and etoposide).[64]

These results confirm the poor prognosis of patients with follicular lymphoma following histologic transformation. Nevertheless, some patients are able to attain a complete response following treatment with conventional combination chemotherapy, and occasional long-term remissions have been reported. Conventional chemotherapy may also be used to achieve remission prior to the use of high-dose therapy (see below). Radiation should be considered alone or in combination with conventional therapy, especially for patients with localized disease.

### MONOCLONAL ANTIBODIES

The introduction of monoclonal antibodies has revolutionized the treatment of NHL. Rituximab, a chimeric anti-CD20 antibody, was the first monoclonal antibody approved for cancer treatment. Approximately 50% of patients with relapsed low-grade and follicular lymphomas will respond to treatment with this agent.[65] Rituximab also has substantial activity against aggressive lymphomas,[66] although it has not been extensively evaluated for transformed lymphomas. In a phase III trial comparing rituximab with $^{90}$Y ibritumomab tiuxetan (see below), three of four patients with transformed lymphomas responded to rituximab, alone.[67]

Rituximab has been combined with EPOCH (etoposide, prednisone, vincristine, cyclophosphamide, and doxorubicin) to treat 18 patients with transformed B-cell lymphomas in a trial from Switzerland.[68] The median event-free survival was 12.4 months.

More recently two anti-CD20 radiolabeled antibodies, $^{90}$Y ibritumomab tiuxetan and $^{131}$I tositumomab, have been specifically approved for the treatment of transformed B-cell NHL. The overall response rate was 56% in nine patients with transformed B-cell lymphomas who were treated with $^{90}$Y ibritumomab tiuxetan.[67] At the University of Michigan, the complete response rate was 50% and the overall response rate was 79% for patients with transformed lymphomas following treatment with $^{131}$I tositumomab.[69] The median progression-free survival was 13.9 months for responders. The outcome was similar for patients with low-grade lymphoma and significantly better than the outcome in patients with de novo aggressive lymphomas who received this treatment (Figure 67.2). The response rate was 39% for 23 patients with transformed lymphomas included in the pivotal trial of $^{131}$I tositumomab.[70] Patients had received a median of four prior chemotherapy regimens and 48% had bulky disease. The response rate was higher in patients who had transformed to follicular large-cell histology as compared to patients with diffuse histology after transformation. The multicenter trial of $^{131}$I tositumomab included 10 patients with transformed B-cell

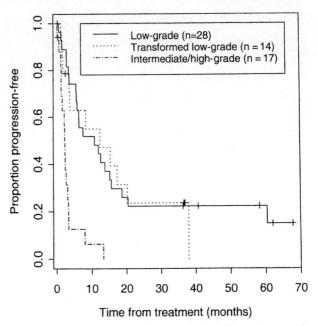

**Figure 67.2** *Progression-free survival of 59 patients with relapsed or refractory NHL following treatment with 131I tositumomab. (Reprinted from Ref. 69)*

lymphoma.[71] The complete response rate was 50%, and the overall response rate was 60%. The median response duration was 12.1 months, and these results were similar to other patients with low-grade lymphomas.

The Seattle group used a higher dose of $^{131}$I tositumomab followed by autologous stem cell transplantation to treat patients with transformed lymphomas, although individual patient results were not reported.[72]

### TRANSPLANTATION

Several reports of autologous hematopoietic stem cell transplantation for NHL have included patients with transformed lymphomas and have shown that prolonged remissions can be attained,[27,73–75] although these reports have not always provided specific details on patients with transformed histology.

A retrospective study from the University of Nebraska compared outcomes following autologous stem cell transplantation of 10 patients with transformed lymphomas and 8 patients with follicular lymphomas.[76] All patients with nontransformed lymphomas were alive between 246 and 1804 days following transplantation, while most of the patients with transformed lymphomas had early transplant-related deaths and only one was alive 99 days after transplant ($P = 0.002$). A retrospective analysis from France also examined outcomes of patients with follicular lymphoma following autologous stem cell transplantation.[77] Overall survival of the 16 patients transplanted after histologic transformation was similar to that of 44 patients with follicular lymphoma; however, failure-free survival was significantly worse for patients

| Table 67.3 | Autologous hematopoietic stem cell transplantation for transformed non-Hodgkin's lymphoma | | | |
|---|---|---|---|---|
| Reference | No. of patients | Early mortality | Results | Comments |
| 84 | 19 | 1 (5%) | Median OS 4.4 years<br>10 (53%) CCR | |
| 85 | 27 | 0 (0%) | 5-year OS 58%<br>5-year DFS 46% | 6 patients had CLL/SL |
| 86 | 35 | 7 (20%) | Median OS 33 months<br>5-year OS 37% | Includes patients with intermediate-grade lymphoma who relapsed with follicular lymphoma and patients with composite lymphoma |
| 83 | 18 | 0 (0%) | 4-year OS 61%<br>4-year EFS 38% | Includes 1 patient with CLL/SL |
| 87 | 50 | 4 (8%) | 5-year OS 51%<br>5-year PFS 30% | |

OS, overall survival; CCR, continuous complete remission; DFS, disease-free survival; CLL/SL, chronic lymphocytic leukemia/small lymphocytic lymphoma; EFS, event-free survival; PFS, progression-free survival.

with transformed lymphomas ($P = 0.04$). A small series from the European Bone Marrow Transplant Group also noted that results of autologous stem cell transplantation were poor for patients with transformed lymphomas.[78] A retrospective analysis from Dana-Farber Cancer Institute compared outcomes of autologous stem cell transplantation in 51 patients with low-grade lymphomas and 18 patients following transformation to lymphomas with diffuse architecture.[79] The 4-year disease-free survival was 23% for patients with transformed lymphomas, as compared with 47% for patients with low-grade histology, although this difference was not statistically significant ($P = 0.2$).

Other analyses have demonstrated somewhat better results of transplantation for patients with transformed lymphomas. A series from Boston found no differences in time to treatment failure when autologous transplants in 10 patients with transformed lymphomas were compared to 68 patients with intermediate- and high-grade histology who were treated with autologous transplantation.[80] A series from Sweden compared results of autologous bone marrow and stem cell transplantation of 11 patients with follicular lymphoma and 11 with transformed lymphomas.[81] No significant differences in disease-free survival were noted. The Stanford group reported that the actuarial 4-year disease-free survival and 4-year overall survival were 49 and 50%, respectively, in 17 patients with transformed lymphomas who had undergone autologous bone marrow or stem cell transplantation.[82] These results were similar to patients with follicular low-grade lymphomas and follicular large-cell lymphomas who had been transplanted. The group from Cleveland Clinic also examined results of autologous peripheral blood stem cell transplantation for patients with lymphomas that had transformed to diffuse large-cell histology.[83] The actuarial 4-year overall survival and event-free survival rates were 61 and 38%,

respectively (Table 67.3). These values were 53 and 37%, respectively, in a group of transplanted patients with de novo diffuse large-cell histology ($P = $ ns). An analysis from the European Bone Marrow Transplant Registry showed that actuarial 5-year overall survival and progression-free survival rates were 51 and 30%, respectively, in 50 patients who received autologous hematopoietic stem cell transplants for follicular lymphomas (Table 67.3; Figure 67.3).[87] No significant differences in overall survival or progression-free survival were identified when these values were compared to transplanted patients with low-grade ($P = 0.939$ and 0.673, respectively) or intermediate/high-grade histology ($P = 0.438$ and .533, respectively).

Investigators from Seattle have piloted a novel regimen combining [131]I tositumomab (see above) with high-dose etoposide and cyclophosphamide, followed

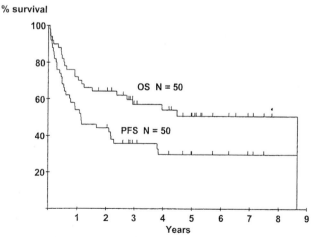

**Figure 67.3** *Overall survival (OS) and progression-free survival (PFS) of 50 patients with transformed follicular low-grade NHL following high-dose therapy and autologous hematopoietic stem cell transplantation. (Reprinted from Ref. 87)*

by autologous stem cell transplantation.[88] Patients with transformed lymphomas have been included in this trial.

Results of autologous hematopoietic stem cell transplantation in series examining transformed lymphomas are displayed in Table 67.3. These results show that transplantation can be accomplished with low transplant-related mortality and that prolonged disease-free survival can be observed. Nevertheless, it is not clear in some series that there is a plateau in progression-free survival following transplantation, and it is unknown whether patients are cured.[77,79,83–87] In addition, myelodysplastic syndromes, acute myelogenous leukemia, and second malignancies have been reported following autologous transplantation for transformed lymphomas.[85–87] Of interest is the fact that some patients have relapsed with follicular histology following autologous stem cell transplantation.[77,84,87]

Prognostic factors following autologous transplantation for transformed lymphomas have not been well characterized. The group from Dana-Farber Cancer Institute noted that 5-year overall survival following transplant was estimated at 80% for patients who underwent histologic transformation within 18 months of diagnosis, as compared with 31% for those with late transformation ($P = 0.04$).[85] The European analysis showed inferior progression-free survival following transplant for transformed lymphoma in patients with an elevated LDH level ($P = 0.0031$) and those with chemotherapy-resistant disease ($P = 0.0478$).[87] Age above 60 years has also been associated with inferior transplant outcome for transformed lymphoma.[86]

### Allogeneic transplantation

There is very little published experience with allogeneic stem cell transplantation for transformed lymphomas, although it is possible that patients might benefit from this approach, because of a graft-versus-lymphoma effect or because this approach eliminates the possibility of infusing malignant cells with the autograft. Rare patients with transformed lymphomas have been included in larger series of allogeneic transplantation for lymphoma, although it is impossible to identify results in these specific patients.[89,90] A French cooperative group analysis of allogeneic transplants for aggressive NHL included 14 patients who had transformed low-grade lymphomas or CLL out of a total of 73 cases.[91] The only patient who relapsed more than 15 months after transplant had a transformed low-grade lymphoma and relapsed with low-grade histology 7 years after transplant. A report from the University of Chicago described one patient with transformed lymphoma who was alive and well 70 months following allogeneic transplantation.[92] A report of reduced-intensity allogeneic transplantation from MD Anderson Cancer Center described two patients with transformed low-grade lymphomas who died of transplant-related complications.[93]

## TREATMENT OF RICHTER'S SYNDROME

Treatment results of Richter's syndrome are largely anecdotal or based on small series, and are subject to the same limitations discussed earlier. In a series from the University of Iowa, patients were primarily treated with chemotherapy regimens that did not contain anthracyclines, such as CVP (cyclophosphamide, vincristine, and prednisone).[4] Only one patient, who was treated with radiation, attained a complete remission and survived more than 3 months. Patients with Richter's syndrome (two with Hodgkin's lymphoma) in a French series were treated with a variety of chemotherapy regimens.[25] The median survival was 4 months, and there was no evidence of improved outcomes with anthracycline-containing regimens. Six patients, including four with localized disease treated with additional radiation, had sustained remissions between 5 and 77 months.

Thirty-three patients with Richter's syndrome at MD Anderson Cancer Center were able to receive treatment.[3] All except one were treated with systemic chemotherapy, nine received additional radiation, and one received radiation, alone. The overall response rate was 41%, and the majority of patients in this group received doxorubicin-based or fludarabine-based therapy. The overall survival was significantly better for patients who responded to therapy ($P < .001$). Four patients remained alive and in remission between 5 and 16 months. One patient relapsed with CLL more than 10 years after treatment.

The MD Anderson group has also reported results of the hyper-CVXD (cyclophosphamide, vincristine, liposomal daunorubicin, and dexamethasone) regimen in a series of 29 patients with Richter's syndrome.[94] Complete responses were obtained in 11 (38%) patients, and six had ongoing remissions between 6 and 19 months from starting therapy. The median survival was 10 months for all patients. The median survival was 19 months for those who attained a complete remission and 3 months for others ($P = 0.0008$). A regimen of fludarabine, cytarabine, cyclophosphamide, cisplatin, and granulocyte-monocyte colony-stimulating factor had little activity and significant toxicity in a cohort of patients with Richter's syndrome.[95]

Diffuse large B-cell lymphomas have also arisen in patients with lymphoplasmacytic lymphoma/Waldenström macroglobulinemia. In one series of 12 such patients, 73% died within 10 months of transformation.[96] The majority were treated with aggressive anthracycline-containing regimens. Only one patient, treated with autologous stem cell transplantation, was alive and in remission.

There were five transplant-related deaths in a series of eight patients who received allogeneic bone marrow transplants for Richter's syndrome.[97] Three patients were alive and in continuous remission between 14 and 67 months after transplant. The same institution described one patient with Richter's syndrome who was alive and in remission at least 5 months following a reduced-intensity allogeneic transplant.[93]

## SUMMARY

Histologic transformation is frequently observed when patients with follicular lymphomas have disease progression. The original and transformed lymphomas are often clonally related, although they sometimes arise from different clones. Although the literature suggests that the prognosis is poor for patients with transformed lymphomas, some patients experience long-term disease-free survival. Patients with transformed lymphomas should probably be treated with aggressive chemotherapy regimens that are used for patients with diffuse large B-cell lymphoma. Involved-field radiation therapy should also be considered for patients with localized disease. Long-term disease-free survival has also been observed following high-dose therapy and autologous hematopoietic stem cell transplantation. This approach should be considered for patients with chemotherapy-sensitive disease. There are now two radiolabeled antibodies that are specifically approved for the treatment of transformed B-cell lymphomas, and they provide another treatment option for selected patients.

## REFERENCES

1. Hoppe RT: Histologic variation in non-q's lymphomas: commentary. *Cancer Treat Rep* 65:935, 1981.
2. Richter MN: Generalized reticular cell sarcoma of lymph nodes associated with lymphatic leukemia. *Am J Pathol* 4:285, 1928.
3. Robertson LE, Pugh W, O'Brien S, et al.: Richter's syndrome: a report on 39 patients. *J Clin Oncol* 11:1985, 1993.
4. Armitage JO, Dick FR, Corder MP: Diffuse histiocytic lymphoma complicating chronic lymphocytic leukemia. *Cancer* 41:422, 1978.
5. Hubbard SM, Chabner BA, DeVita VT, et al.: Histologic progression in non-Hodgkin's lymphoma. *Blood* 59:258, 1982.
6. Ersbøll J, Schultz HB, Pedersen-Bjergaard J, et al.: Follicular low-grade non-Hodgkin's lymphoma: long-term outcome with or without tumor progression. *Eur J Haematol* 42:155, 1989.
7. Oviatt DL, Cousar JB, Collins RD, et al.: Malignant lymphomas of follicular center cell origin in humans. *Cancer* 53:1109, 1984.
8. Müller-Hermelink HK, Zettl A, Pfeifer W, et al.: Pathology of lymphoma progression. *Histopathology* 38:285, 2001.
9. Gall EA, Mallory TB: Malignant lymphoma. A clinicopathologic survey of 618 cases. *Am J Pathol* 18:381, 1942.
10. Rappaport H, Winter WJ, Hicks EB: Follicular lymphoma. A re-evaluation of its position in the scheme of malignant lymphoma, based on a survey of 253 cases. *Cancer* 9:792, 1956.
11. Wright CJE: Macrofollicular lymphoma. *Am J Pathol* 32:201, 1956.
12. Qazi R, Aisenberg AC, Long JC: The natural history of nodular lymphoma. *Cancer* 37:1923, 1976.
13. Cullen MH, Lister TA, Brearley RL, et al.: Histological transformation of non-Hodgkin's lymphoma. A prospective study. *Cancer* 44:645, 1979.
14. Risdall R, Hoppe RT, Warnke R: Non-Hodgkin's lymphoma. A study of the evolution of the disease based upon 92 autopsied cases. *Cancer* 44:529, 1979.
15. Ostrow SS, Diggs CH, Sutherland JC, et al.: Nodular poorly differentiated lymphocytic lymphoma: changes in histology and survival. *Cancer Treat Rep* 65:929, 1981.
16. Acker B, Hoppe RT, Colby TV, et al.: Histologic conversion in the non-Hodgkin's lymphomas. *J Clin Oncol* 1:11, 1983.
17. Horning SJ, Rosenberg SA: The natural history of initially untreated low-grade non-Hodgkin's lymphomas. *N Engl J Med* 311:1471, 1984.
18. Garvin AJ, Simon RM, Osborne CK, et al.: An autopsy study of histologic progression in non-Hodgkin's lymphomas. 192 cases from the National Cancer Institute. *Cancer* 52:393, 1983.
19. D'Amore F, Christensen BE, Thorling K, et al.: Incidence, presenting features and prognosis of low-grade B-cell non-Hodgkin's lymphomas. Population-based data from a Danish Lymphoma Registry. *Leuk Lymphoma* 12:69, 1993.
20. Gallagher CJ, Gregory WM, Jones AE, et al.: Follicular lymphoma: prognostic factors for response and survival. *J Clin Oncol* 4:1470, 1986.
21. Bastion Y, Sebban C, Berger F, et al.: Incidence, predictive factors, and outcome of lymphoma transformation in follicular lymphoma patients. *J Clin Oncol* 15:1587, 1997.
22. Yuen AR, Kamel OW, Halpern J, et al.: Long-term survival after histologic transformation of low-grade follicular lymphoma. *J Clin Oncol* 13:1726, 1995.
23. Cohen Y, Da'as N, Libster D, et al.: Large-cell transformation of chronic lymphocytic leukemia and follicular lymphoma during or soon after treatment with fludarabine-rituximab-containing regimens: natural history- or therapy-related complication? *Eur J Haematol* 68:80, 2002.
24. Yeshurun M, Isnard F, Garderet L, et al.: Acute liver failure as initial manifestation of low-grade non-Hodgkin's lymphoma transformation into large-cell lymphoma. *Leuk Lymphoma* 42:555, 2001.
25. Harousseau JL, Flandrin G, Tricot G, et al.: Malignant lymphoma supervening in chronic lymphocytic leukemia and related disorders. *Cancer* 48:1302, 1981.

26. Armitage JO, Dick FR, Corder MP: Diffuse histiocytic lymphoma after histologic conversion: a poor prognostic variant. *Cancer Treat Rep* 65:413, 1981.

27. Brice P, Simon D, Bouabdallah R, et al.: High-dose therapy with autologous stem-cell transplantation (ASCT) after first progression prolonged survival of follicular lymphoma patients included in the prospective GELF 86 protocol. *Ann Oncol* 11:1585, 2000.

28. Matolcsy A, Casali P, Warnke RA, et al.: Morphologic transformation of follicular lymphoma is associated with somatic mutation of the translocated *Bcl-2* gene. *Blood* 88:3937, 1996.

29. Price CGA, Tuszynski A, Watt SM, et al.: Detection of additional $J_H$/BCL2 translocations in follicular lymphoma. *Leukemia* 5:548, 1991.

30. Woda BA, Knowles DM: Nodular lymphocytic lymphoma eventuating into diffuse histiocytic lymphoma. *Cancer* 43:303, 1979.

31. Zelenetz AD, Chen TT, Levy R: Histologic transformation of follicular lymphoma to diffuse lymphoma represents tumor progression by a single malignant B cell. *J Exp Med* 173:197, 1991.

32. Lossos IS, Levy R: Higher-grade transformation of follicle center lymphoma is associated with somatic mutation of the 5' noncoding regulatory region of the *BCL-6* gene. *Blood* 96:635, 2000.

33. Matolcsy A, Schattner EJ, Knowles DM, et al.: Clonal evolution of B cells in transformation from low- to high-grade lymphoma. *Eur J Immunol* 29:1253, 1999.

34. Yano T, Jaffe ES, Longo DL, et al.: *MYC* rearrangements in histologically progressed follicular lymphomas. *Blood* 80:758, 1992.

35. Lee JT, Innes DJ, Williams ME: Sequential bcl-2 and *c-myc* oncogene rearrangements associated with the clinical transformation of non-Hodgkin's lymphoma. *J Clin Invest* 84:1454, 1989.

36. Matolcsy A, Inghirami G, Knowles DM: Molecular genetic demonstration of the diverse evolution of Richter's syndrome (chronic lymphocytic leukemia and subsequent large cell lymphoma). *Blood* 83:1363, 1994.

37. Miyamura K, Osada H, Yamauchi T, et al.: Single clonal origin of neoplastic B-cells with different immunoglobulin light chains in a patient with Richter's syndrome. *Cancer* 66:140, 1990.

38. Traweek ST, Liu J, Johnson RM, et al.: High-grade transformation of chronic lymphocytic leukemia and low-grade non-Hodgkin's lymphoma. *Am J Clin Pathol* 100:519, 1993.

39. Cherepakhin V, Baird SM, Meisenholder GW, et al.: Common clonal origin of chronic lymphocytic leukemia and high-grade lymphoma of Richter's syndrome. *Blood* 82:3141, 1993.

40. McDonnell JM, Beschorner WE, Staal SP, et al.: Richter's syndrome with two different B-cell clones. *Cancer* 58:2031, 1986.

41. Foon KA, Thiruvengadam R, Saven A, et al.: Genetic relatedness of lymphoid malignancies. Transformation of chronic lymphocytic leukemia as a model. *Ann Intern Med* 119:63, 1993.

42. Sander CA, Yano T, Clark HM, et al.: p53 mutation is associated with progression in follicular lymphomas. *Blood* 82:1994, 1993.

43. Lo Coco F, Gaidano G, Louie DC, et al.: p53 mutations are associated with histologic transformation of follicular lymphoma. *Blood* 82:2289, 1993.

44. Akasaka T, Lossos IS, Levy R: *BCL6* gene translocation in follicular lymphoma: a harbinger of eventual transformation to diffuse aggressive lymphoma. *Blood* 102:1443, 2003.

45. Lossos IS, Alizadeh AA, Diehn M, et al.: Transformation of follicular lymphoma to diffuse large-cell lymphoma: alternative patterns with increased or decreased expression of *c-myc* and its regulated genes. *Proc Natl Acad Sci U S A* 99:8886, 2002.

46. Elenitoba-Johnson KSJ, Gascoyne RD, Lim MS, et al.: Homozygous deletions at chromosome 9p21 and p15 are associated with histologic progression in follicle center lymphoma. *Blood* 91:4677, 1998.

47. Pinyol M, Cobo F, Bea S, et al.: p16$^{INK4a}$ gene inactivation by deletions, mutations, and hypermethylation is associated with transformed and aggressive variants of non-Hodgkin's lymphomas. *Blood* 91:2977, 1998.

48. Tilly H, Rossi A, Stamatoulas A, et al.: Prognostic value of chromosomal abnormalities in follicular lymphoma. *Blood* 84:1043, 1994.

49. Raghoebier S, Broos L, Kramer MHH, et al.: Histological conversion of follicular lymphoma with structural alterations of t(14;18) and immunoglobulin genes. *Leukemia* 9:1748, 1995.

50. Arcinas M, Heckman CA, Mehew JW, et al.: Molecular mechanisms of transcriptional control of bcl-2 and c-myc in follicular and transformed lymphoma. *Cancer Res* 61:5202, 2001.

51. Villuendas R, Sánchez-Beato M, Martínez JC, et al.: Loss of p16/INK4A protein expression in non-Hodgkin's lymphomas is a frequent finding associated with tumor progression. *Am J Pathol* 153:887, 1998.

52. Whang-Peng J, Knutsen T, Jaffe ES, et al.: Sequential analysis of 43 patients with non-Hodgkin's lymphoma: clinical correlations with cytogenetic, histologic, immunophenotyping, and molecular studies. *Blood* 85:203, 1995.

53. Richardson ME, Quanguang C, Filippa DA, et al.: Intermediate- to high-grade histology of lymphomas carrying t(14;18) is associated with additional nonrandom chromosome changes. *Blood* 70:444, 1987.

54. Yunis JJ, Frizzera G, Oken MM, et al.: Multiple recurrent genomic defects in follicular lymphoma. A possible model for cancer. *N Engl J Med* 316:79, 1987.

55. Offit K, Parsa NZ, Gaidano G, et al.: 6q deletions define distinct clinico-pathologic subsets of non-Hodgkin's lymphoma. *Blood* 82:2157, 1993.

56. Horsman DE, Connors JM, Pantzar T, et al.: Analysis of secondary chromosomal alterations in 165 cases of follicular lymphoma with t(14;18). *Genes Chromosomes Cancer* 30:375, 2001.

57. Armitage JO, Sanger WG, Weisenburger DD, et al.: Correlation of secondary cytogenetic abnormalities with histologic appearance in non-Hodgkin's lymphomas bearing t(14;18)(q32;q21). *J Natl Cancer Inst* 80:576, 1988.

58. Bernell P, Jacobsson B, Liliemark J, et al.: Gain of chromosome 7 marks the progression from indolent to aggressive follicle centre lymphoma and is a common

finding in patients with diffuse large B-cell lymphoma: a study by FISH. *Br J Haematol* 101:487, 1998.

59. Hough RE, Goepel JR, Alcock HE, et al.: Copy number gain at 12q12-14 may be important in the transformation from follicular lymphoma to diffuse large B cell lymphoma. *Br J Cancer* 84:499, 2001.

60. Neat MJ, Foot N, Jenner M, et al.: Localisation of a novel region of recurrent amplification in follicular lymphoma to an ~6.8 Mb region of 13q32–33. *Genes Chromosomes Cancer* 32:236, 2001.

61. Matolcsy A: High-grade transformation of low-grade non-Hodgkin's lymphomas: mechanisms of tumor progression. *Leuk Lymphoma* 34:251, 1999.

62. Nagy M, Balázs M, Ádám Z, et al.: Genetic instability is associated with histological transformation of follicle center lymphoma. *Leukemia* 14:2142, 2000.

63. Velasquez WS, McLaughlin P, Tucker S, et al.: ESHAP—an effective chemotherapy regimen in refractory and relapsing lymphoma: a 4-year follow-up study. *J Clin Oncol* 12:1169, 1994.

64. Rodriguez MA, Cabanillas FC, Velasquez W, et al.: Results of a salvage treatment program for relapsing lymphoma: MINE consolidated with ESHAP. *J Clin Oncol* 13:1734, 1995.

65. McLaughlin P, Grillo-López AJ, Link BK, et al.: Rituximab chimeric anti-CD20 monoclonal antibody therapy for relapsed indolent lymphoma: half of patients respond to a four-dose treatment program. *J Clin Oncol* 16:2825, 1998.

66. Coiffier B, Haioun C, Ketterer N, et al.: Rituximab (anti-CD20 monoclonal antibody) for the treatment of patients with relapsing or refractory aggressive lymphoma: a multicenter phase II study. *Blood* 92:1927, 1998.

67. Witzig TE, Gordon LI, Cabanillas F, et al.: Randomized controlled trial of Yttrium-90-labeled ibritumomab tiuxetan radioimmunotherapy versus rituximab immunotherapy for patients with relapsed or refractory low-grade, follicular, or transformed B-cell non-Hodgkin's lymphoma. *J Clin Oncol* 20:2453, 2002.

68. Jermann M, Jost LM, Taverna Ch., et al.: Rituximab-EPOCH, an effective salvage therapy for relapsed, refractory or transformed B-cell lymphoma: results of a phase II study. *Ann Oncol* 15:511, 2004.

69. Kaminski MS, Estes J, Zasadny KR, et al.: Radioimmunotherapy with iodine [131]I tositumomab for relapsed or refractory B-cell non-Hodgkin lymphoma: updated results and long-term follow-up of the University of Michigan experience. *Blood* 96:1259, 2000.

70. Kaminski MS, Zelenetz AD, Press OW, et al.: Pivotal study of iodine I 131 Tositumomab for chemotherapy-refractory low-grade or transformed low-grade B-cell non-Hodgkin's lymphoma. *J Clin Oncol* 19:3918, 2001.

71. Vose JM, Wahl RL, Saleh M, et al.: Multicenter phase II study of iodine-131 tositumomab for chemotherapy-relapsed/refractory low-grade and transformed low-grade B-cell non-Hodgkin's lymphoma. *J Clin Oncol* 18:1316, 2000.

72. Gopal AK, Gooley TA, Maloney DG, et al.: High-dose radioimmunotherapy versus conventional high-dose therapy and autologous hematopoietic stem cell transplantation for relapsed follicular non-Hodgkin's lymphoma: a multivariable cohort and analysis. *Blood* 102:2351, 2003.

73. López R, Martino R, Sureda A, et al.: Autologous stem cell transplantation in advanced follicular lymphoma. A single center experience. *Haematologica* 84:350, 1999.

74. van Besien K, Rodriguez A, Tomany S, et al.: Non-Hodgkin's lymphoma. Phase II study of a high-dose ifos-famide-based chemotherapy regimen with growth factor rescue in recurrent aggressive NHL. High response rates and limited toxicity, but limited impact on long-term survival. *Bone Marrow Transplant* 27:397, 2001.

75. Moskowitz CH, Nimer SD, Glassman JR, et al.: The International Prognostic Index predicts for outcome following autologous stem cell transplantation in patients with relapsed and primary refractory intermediate-grade lymphoma. *Bone Marrow Transplant* 23:561, 1999.

76. Schouten HC, Bierman PJ, Vaughan WP, et al.: Autologous bone marrow transplantation in follicular non-Hodgkin's lymphoma before and after histologic transformation. *Blood* 74:2579, 1989.

77. Bastion Y, Brice P, Haioun C, et al.: Intensive therapy with peripheral blood progenitor cell transplantation in 60 patients with poor-prognosis follicular lymphoma. *Blood* 86:3257, 1995.

78. Schouten HC, Colombat Ph., Verdonck LF, et al.: Autologous bone marrow transplantation for low-grade non-Hodgkin's lymphoma: the European Bone Marrow Transplant Group experience. *Ann Oncol* 5(suppl 1): S147, 1994.

79. Freedman AS, Ritz J, Neuberg D, et al.: Autologous bone marrow transplantation in 69 patients with a history of low-grade B-cell non-Hodgkin's lymphoma. *Blood* 77: 2524, 1991.

80. Wheeler C, Strawderman M, Ayash L, et al.: Prognostic factors for treatment outcome in autotransplantation of intermediate-grade and high-grade non-Hodgkin's lymphoma with cyclophosphamide , carmustine, and etoposide. *J Clin Oncol* 11:1085, 1993.

81. Berglund Å, Enblad G, Carlson K, et al.: Long-term follow-up of autologous stem-cell transplantation for follicular and transformed follicular lymphoma. *Eur J Haematol* 65:17, 2000.

82. Cao TM, Horning SJ, Negrin RS, et al.: High-dose therapy and autologous hematopoietic-cell transplantation for follicular lymphoma beyond first remission: the Stanford University experience. *Biol Blood Marrow Transplant* 7:294, 2001.

83. Bolwell B, Kalaycio M, Andresen S, et al.: Autologous peripheral blood progenitor cell transplantation for transformed diffuse large-cell lymphoma. *Clin Lymphoma* 3:226, 2000.

84. Foran JM, Apostolidis J, Papamichael D, et al.: High-dose therapy with autologous haematopoietic support in patients with transformed follicular lymphoma: a study of 27 patients from a single centre. *Ann Oncol* 9:865, 1998.

85. Friedberg JW, Neuberg D, Gribben JG, et al.: Autologous bone marrow transplantation after histologic transformation of indolent B cell malignancies. *Biol Blood Marrow Transplant* 5:262, 1999.

86. Chen CI, Crump M, Tsang R, et al.: Autotransplants for histologically transformed follicular non-Hodgkin's lymphoma. *Br J Haematol* 113:202, 2001.

87. Williams CD, Harrison CN, Lister TA, et al.: High-dose therapy and autologous stem-cell support for chemosensitive transformed low-grade follicular non-Hodgkin's

lymphoma: a case-matched study from the European Bone Marrow Transplant Registry. *J Clin Oncol* 19:727, 2001.

88. Press OW, Eary JF, Gooley T, et al.: A phase I/II trial of iodine-131-tositumomab (anti-CD20), etoposide, cyclophosphamide, and autologous stem cell transplantation for relapsed B-cell lymphomas. *Blood* 96:2934, 2000.

89. Robinson SP, Goldstone AH, Mackinnon S, et al.: Chemoresistant or aggressive lymphoma predicts for a poor outcome following reduced-intensity allogeneic progenitor cell transplantation: an analysis from the Lymphoma Working Party of the European Group for Blood and Bone Marrow Transplantation. *Blood* 100:4310, 2002.

90. Schimmer AD, Jamal S, Messner H, et al.: Allogeneic or autologous bone marrow transplantation (BMT) for non-Hodgkin's lymphoma (NHL): results of a provincial strategy. *Bone Marrow Transplant* 26:859, 2000.

91. Dhedin N, Giraudier S, Gaulard P, et al.: Allogeneic bone marrow transplantation in aggressive non-Hodgkin's lymphoma (excluding Burkitt and lymphoblastic lymphoma): a series of 73 patients from the SFGM database. *Br J Haematol* 107:154, 1999.

92. Dann EJ, Daugherty CD, Larson RA: Allogeneic bone marrow transplantation for relapsed and refractory Hodgkin's disease and non-Hodgkin's lymphoma. *Bone Marrow Transplant* 20:369, 1997.

93. Khouri IF, Keating M, Körbling M, et al.: Transplant-lite: induction of graft-versus-malignancy using fludarabine-based nonablative chemotherapy and allogeneic blood progenitor-cell transplantation as treatment for lymphoid malignancies. *J Clin Oncol* 16:2817, 1998.

94. Dabaja BS, O'Brien SM, Kantarjian HM, et al.: Fractionated cyclophosphamide, vincristine, liposomal daunorubicin (daunoxome), and dexamethasone (hyperCVXD) regimen in Richter's syndrome. *Leuk Lymphoma* 42:329, 2001.

95. Tsimberidou AM, O'Brien SM, Cortes JE, et al.: Phase II study of fludarabine, cytarabine (Ara-C), cyclophosphamide, cisplatin and GM-CSF (FACPGM) in patients with Richter's syndrome or refractory lymphoproliferative disorders. *Leuk Lymphoma* 43:767, 2002.

96. Lin P, Mansoor A, Bueso-Ramos C, et al.: Diffuse large B-cell lymphoma occurring in patients with lymphoplasmacytic lymphoma/Waldenström macroglobulinemia. *Am J Clin Pathol* 120:246, 2003.

97. Rodriguez J, Keating MJ, O'Brien SM, et al.: Allogeneic haematopoietic transplantation for Richter's syndrome. *Br J Haematol* 110:897, 2000.

# Chapter **68**

# NEW FRONTIERS IN NON-HODGKIN'S LYMPHOMA THERAPY

*Eric Winer, Sridar Pal, and Francine Foss*

## INTRODUCTION

A number of novel strategies have evolved for the treatment of refractory non-Hodgkin's lymphoma (NHL). Novel targeting agents that have demonstrated success in clinical trials include radiolabeled antibodies, fusion toxins, which direct cytotoxic moieties into the cell via membrane receptors, and antisense oligonucleotides, which bind to mRNA and inhibit translation of proteins in the cell. A number of agents that target specific intracellular pathways have also been developed, including bortezomib, which inhibits proteosome function, the histone deacetylase (HDAC) inhibitors, which modulate gene transcription, and gallium nitrate, which inhibits transferrin-dependent enzymatic pathways. Finally, the newer technologies have been developed to implement immunotherapeutic approaches.

## MONOCLONAL ANTIBODIES

Rituximab was the first humanized monoclonal antibody to be widely used in the treatment of patients with low- and intermediate-grade B-cell NHL. Subsequently, antibodies directed against a variety of epitopes have been developed and have demonstrated clinical efficacy. Unmodified anti-CD22 antibody as well as immunotoxin and radioimmunoconjugates of this antibody have demonstrated activity in vitro and in a limited number of patients with refractory B-cell lymphoma.[1–3] CD30, which is expressed on a subset of T-cell lymphomas, including anaplastic large cell lymphomas and Hodgkin's disease, has been an attractive target for antibody-based therapies because its expression is limited on normal cells to activated lymphocytes and natural killer cells. SGN-30, a humanized anti-CD30 antibody, has been shown to induce growth arrest and apoptosis in Hodgkin's cell lines in vitro, and a phase II clinical trial is underway to further define its clinical efficacy.[4] Alemtuzumab (Campath-1H) is a humanized mAb targeting CD52 and has recently been approved in the United States for the treatment of fludarabine-refractory B-cell chronic lymphocytic leukemia. Impressive activity has also been demonstrated in T-cell prolymphocytic leukemia and mycosis fungoides.[5] In a study of 16 patients with low- or intermediate-grade B-cell NHL who relapsed or were refractory to conventional therapy and were treated with alemtuzumab, eight (44%) achieved a clinical response, two (11%) had stable disease, and five (28%) had progressive disease. All responders had low-grade histologies.[6] Humanized anti-CD4 antibody (HuMax) is used in clinical trials in patients with relapsed and refractory cutaneous T-cell lymphoma (CTCL) and CD4-expressing peripheral T-cell lymphomas.

## FUSION TOXINS

A number of strategies have been developed to target cytotoxic proteins to tumor cells, including conjugated immunotoxins, single-chain antibody–immunotoxin conjugates, and fusion toxins. Table 68.1 summarizes in vitro and in vivo data using immunotoxins in lymphoid malignancies. The major limitation of immunotoxins, in which the toxin moiety is conjugated to a monoclonal antibody, is their ability to be internalized by the cell and translocate efficiently into the cytoplasm where they can inhibit protein synthesis. Because of their large size, conjugated immunotoxins may not be efficiently translocated into the cell and may, by nature of their epitopes, be immunogenic. Both ricin A-chain and pseudomonas exotoxin-based immunoconjugates have been developed and have demonstrated limited efficacy and significant toxicity in patients with Hodgkin's disease and NHL.[7–11]

Denileukin diftitox is a genetically engineered fusion protein combining the enzymatically active domains of diphtheria toxin and the full-length sequence of interleukin-2 (IL-2), and targets tumor cells expressing the intermediate- and high-affinity IL-2 receptors (IL-2R).[12] Denileukin diftitox has been approved for the therapy of refractory CTCL based on

**Table 68.1** Immunotoxins in lymphoma

| Immunotoxin | Activity in vitro or in clinical trials | Reference |
|---|---|---|
| Rituximab/saporin-S6 | Induced apoptosis in B-cell NHL cells in vitro, synergistic with fludarabine in vitro | Polito et al. |
| anti-CD19 (HD37-dgRTA) + anti-CD22 (RFB4-dgRTA) | In vitro study of combination immunotoxins demonstrated 100% survival in acute lymphocytic leukemia xenograft | Herrera et al. |
| anti-CD22 (RFB4-dgRTA) | Phase I study in B-cell NHL; 15 patients with refractory disease, 38% PR | Vitetta, 1991. |
| Ki-4.dgA anti-CD30 immunotoxin | Phase I study of 17 pts with refractory CD30+ lymphoma: 1 CR, 1 PR | Schnell et al. |
| anti-B4-bR | Phase II study in 16 CD19+ refractory B-cell NHL patients, no durable responses | Multani et al. |
| G28-5 sFv-PE40 | In vitro activity in B-cell NHL, targets CD40 | Francisco et al. |
| BL22 (RFB4(dsFv)-PE38) | In vitro efficacy, targets CD22 | Barth et al. |
| anti-Tac(Fv)-PE38 (LMB-2) | Phase I trial in 35 patients with CD25+ lymphoma: 7 PR (1 HD, 1 CLL, 3 hairy cell, 1 CTCL, 1 ATL) | Kreitman et al. |

CLL, chronic lymphocytic leukemia, CTCL, cutaneous T-cell lymphoma; NHL, non-Hedgkin's lymphoma.

an overall response rate of 30% in heavily pretreated patients.[13,14] Toxicities include hypersensitivity related to the infusion of protein and a low-grade vascular leak syndrome seen in 23% of patients manifested by low albumin, peripheral edema, and/or hypotension. Recent studies using steroid premedication and hydration have significantly reduced the incidence and severity of these events in patients with CTCL.[15]

Previous studies have demonstrated IL-2R expression on a variety of B-cell non-Hodgkin's lymphomas, including both low- and intermediate-grade lymphomas.[16,17] In a phase I study of escalating doses of denileukin diftitox ranging from 3 to 31 µg/kg/day × 5 days for a 21-day cycle, the expression of IL-2R was determined by immunohistochemistry as an entry criteria. Of 66 B-cell NHL patients screened, 29 expressed a component of the IL-2R (p55 or CD25, or p75 or CD122).[16] The overall response rate in 23 heavily pretreated NHL patients was 17%, including 2 of 9 patients with intermediate-grade NHL who had partial responses. On the basis of these data, a phase II study was initiated at MD Anderson Cancer Center to evaluate the efficacy of denileukin diftitox in relapsed/refractory B NHL.[18,19] All low- and intermediate-grade B-cell NHL patients were eligible, and IL-2R expression was determined based on expression of CD25 on tumor cells. Denileukin diftitox was administered at 18 µg/kg/day for 5 days every 3 weeks, for up to eight cycles. Corticosteroid premedication prior to each drug infusion was given in an attempt to reduce the incidence and severity of acute hypersensitivity. Most patients had undergone multiple prior treatments, including autologous stem cell transplants, and many had compromised bone marrow reserve. Of 29 patients treated, there were three (CR) complete response (one follicular mixed B-cell lymphoma, one B-cell DLCL, one mantle cell lymphoma), and four (PR) partial response (one SLL, three B-cell DLCL) for an overall response rate of 24%. Another study exploring the activity of denileukin diftitox in B-cellNHL was conducted by the Eastern Cooperative Oncology Group to explore the activity in IL-2R expressing and nonexpressing low-grade B-cell NHL. Studies are underway to further explore the activity of denileukin diftitox in combination with rituximab in low- and intermediate-grade refractory B-cell NHL and B-CLL.

## RADIOLABELED ANTIBODIES

Another targeting strategy for NHL has been the use of radioimmunoconjugates. Radiolabeled antibodies are capable of delivering a radiation dose to neighboring cells while minimizing doses to nonmalignant tissues. Low-dose-rate radiation continues to expose cells to radiation even after initial exposure, resulting in accumulation of cell damage leading to apoptosis in cells that may have been effectively repaired after more conventional high-dose-rate radiation.

Two radioimmunoconjugates targeting the CD20 epitope on B cells have been FDA approved for patients with B-cell NHL (Table 68.2). [131]I tositumomab (Bexxar) and [90]Y-ibritumomab tiuxetan differ in the characteristics of their radioisotope. [90]Y-ibritumomab tiuxetan consists of the high-energy β emitter [90]Yttrium

| Table 68.2 Radioimmunotherapy in non-Hodgkin's lymphoma | | |
|---|---|---|
| [131]I tositumomab | Clinical trial and response rates | Response duration |
| Kaminski et al. | 60 patients with LGL: 81% ORR, 20% CR | 6.5 months |
| Zelenitz et al. | 250 patients with LGL: 56% ORR, 30% CR | 13.5 months |
| Kaminski et al. | 76 patients with untreated LGL: 95% ORR, 74% CR | 62% 5 year PFS6 |
| Coleman et al. | 55 patients with rituximab relapsed/refractory disease who had CR | Median not reached at 3.9 years |
| Y-90 Ibritumomab tiuxetan | | |
| Witzig et al. | 34 patients Phase I/II study: 82% ORR, 26% CR | 12.9 months |
| Witzig et al. | 143 patients randomized to Y-90 Ibritumomab tiuxetan vs rituximab ORR 80% for Y-90 Ibritumomab, 30% CR | 11.2 months |
| Witzig et al. | 57 patients rituximab refractory: 74% ORR, 15% CR | 6.8 months |

LGL: low-grade lymphoma; CR: complete response; ORR: overall response rate; PFS: progression-free survival.

and has a half-life of 28 h. Beta particles deliver high energy (2.2 MeV) within a radius of approximately 5 mm, which corresponds to 100–200 cell diameters. [131]I tositumomab emits both gamma and beta particles and has a decay half-life of 8 days.[20–22]

The pivotal trial for [131]I tositumomab by Kaminski and colleagues in 2001 was a phase III nonrandomized, multicenter, single dosimetric, and therapeutic dose study in refractory/relapsed low-grade or transformed low-grade B-cell NHL.[23] The purpose of this study was to compare the efficacy of [131]I tositumomab to the last qualifying chemotherapy regimen. Sixty patients, virtually all with stage III or IV disease, were enrolled. Eighty-eight percent of patients had at least two risk factors by the International Prognostic Index.[24] The median number of prior treatments was four, and 27% of patients had prior radiation therapy. The response rate was 65% with a median duration of 6.5 months. The highest responses were seen in patients with small tumor burden (81%), patients who had not received radiotherapy (77%), and those with nontransformed low-grade NHL (81%). The only variables significantly associated with higher rate of response in a multivariate analysis were tumor burden less than 500 g and nontransformed histology.

Adverse events included fatigue (43%), fever (30%), nausea (25%), infection (25%), chills (15%), vomiting (13%), pruritis (13%), anorexia (10%), and hypotension (10%). The hematologic nadir occurred on days 43, 46, and 34 for red cells, white cells, and platelets, and median recovery occurred at 74, 78, and 73 days, respectively. In this study, five patients developed myelodysplastic syndrome 1.2–7.5 years after treatment, but all had previously received alkylating agents.[25] Two patients later developed bladder cancer, but both had previously received cyclophosphamide. An elevation of Thyroid stimulating humane (TSH) was noted in five patients, but was asymptomatic in all five.

Further analysis of a combined database from five trials using [131]I tositumomab reported a median response duration of 20.2 months in patients with transformed low-grade lymphoma.[26] The overall response rate was 56% with a median duration of response of 14.7 months. In previously untreated, advanced-stage follicular lymphoma ($n = 76$), [131]I tositumomab induced a response in 95% of patients, with 74% achieving CR.[27] Further analysis of several studies of [131]I tositumomab demonstrated "remission inversion," a longer response to radiolabeled antibody than to the last cytotoxic therapy.[28] In studies of rituximab-refractory patients, the overall response rate was 68% with 30% CR.[29,30] Retreatment with [131]I tositumomab has been reported with a 56% response rate to the second dose and a median response duration of 10.7 months. In this population, the annual incidence of myelodysplastic syndrome was 4.1%.[31] Combination studies of [131]I tositumomab with other agents such as fludarabine[32] are underway.

[90]Y-ibritumomab tiuxetan was FDA approved in the United States at a dose of 0.4 mCi/kg, with a dose reduction to 0.3 mCi/kg in patients with low platelets (100,000–150,000/mL).[22] Unlike [131]I tositumomab, [90]Y-ibritumomab tiuxetan does not require individualized dosimetry. Witzig et al. reported the superiority of [90]Y-ibritumomab tiuxetan versus rituximab in 143 patients with CD20-positive relapsed or refractory low-grade, follicular, or transformed NHL who had received a median of two previous chemotherapies and half of whom were refractory to their last therapy.[33] The response rates of [90]Y-ibritumomab tiuxetan versus rituximab were 80% versus 56%, respectively ($p = 0.002$), and complete responses were seen in 30% versus 14% ($p = 0.04$), respectively. Overall response favored the follicular lymphoma subgroup with a response rate of 86%. The time to progression estimates were similar at 11.2 months in the [90]Y-ibritumomab

tiuxetan group and 10.1 months in the rituximab group.

Combined safety data from 349 patients treated on this and four other trials showed the incidence of thrombocytopenia and neutropenia to be 61% and 57%, respectively.[33] In this group of patients, 13% received granulocyte colony-stimulating factor, 8% erythropoietin, and 22% and 20%, respectively, platelet and red blood cell transfusions. [90]Y-ibritumomab tiuxetan was approved in 2002 for use in relapsed or refractory low-grade, follicular, or transformed B-cell NHL. A long-term follow-up study has reported a time to progression of 12.6 months and response duration of 11.7 months.[34]

Other trials have further defined the use of [90]Y-ibritumomab tiuxetan in subgroups of patients. A single arm phase II study in rituximab refractory patients reported an overall response rate of 74% and complete response rate of 15%.[35] Patients with detectable levels of rituximab in their serum at the time of radiolabeled antibody administration had a lower response rate than those with nondetectable levels. Currently, multiple trials are evaluating the combination of [90]Y-ibritumomab tiuxetan as an in vivo purge prior to autologous stem cell transplantation. Thirty-one patients treated with [90]Y-ibritumomab tiuxetan have subsequently been successfully mobilized for stem cell transplantation with no increased toxicity.[36] A phase I study is evaluating sequential treatments of [90]Y-ibritumomab tiuxetan 3–6 months following initial treatment. With the use of prophylactic growth factors, retreatment with lower doses of [90]Y-ibritumomab tiuxetan in 15 patients has been safe and well tolerated.[20] Finally, investigators are still trying to determine the best time to give radioimmunotherapy. In a retrospective analysis, Emmanouilides et al. reported in a study of patients who received [90]Y-ibritumomab tiuxetan as second-line therapy that the response rate and duration were greater than those reported in more heavily pretreated patient populations.[37]

## ANTISENSE OLIGONUCLEOTIDE THERAPY

Antisense oligonucleotides (AS-ON) are short, single-stranded DNA molecules no longer than 25 bases which are complementary to a region of mRNA. When they attach by complementary base pairing, the messenger RNA is degraded, thus preventing downstream protein expression. In 1977, Paterson and colleagues demonstrated that gene expression could be modified by exogenous nucleic acids by use of single-stranded DNA in a cell-free system.[38] The following year, Zamecnik and Stephenson were able to reproduce the same results using the first synthetic oligonucleotide.[39] For several years, the field remained static due to concerns about reproducibility in more complex eukaryotic cells and the lack of acceptable targets. In 1983,

these concerns were eliminated when Simons et al. showed that antisense RNA was a naturally occurring process in eukaryotic cells and is used for regulating gene expression.[40] In the following decade, the human genome initiative has accelerated our understanding of the human genome and discovered multiple possible targets.

AS-ON exert their effect when these short sequences of single-stranded deoxyribonucleotides hybridize to selected mRNA sequences forming a heteroduplex of the mRNA and DNA. This complex engages the endogenous RNaseH cleaving the mRNA moiety, destroying the message, and releasing an intact AS-ON.[41] The molecule is then free to hybridize to another mRNA sequence. The resulting decrease in the target mRNA pool leads to a reduction in the specific encoded protein. In addition, the heteroduplex cannot appropriately dock with the normal ribosomal machinery, thereby inhibiting translation into a functional protein.[42]

To date, the most widely studied AS-ONs are targeted against Bcl-2. Bcl-2 is an antiapoptotic protein that inhibits the intrinsic apoptosis pathway. The intrinsic pathway leads to cell death by releasing caspase activating factors, such as cytochrome c, into the cytosol from the mitochondria.[43] Cytochrome c complexes with and activates apoptotic protease activating factor (APAF-1) beginning the cascade of proapoptosis proteins. The Bcl-2 protein works in a manner as yet incompletely understood to stabilize the mitochondrial membrane such that cytochrome c is not released even when stimuli are present. Elevated levels are not only associated with tumor cell resistance to normal apoptotic stimuli, but also to chemotherapeutic-induced apoptosis, suggesting a role in drug resistance.[43,44] Overexpression of Bcl-2 has been associated with a poor prognosis in patients with low-grade NHL.[44,45] The t(14;18) chromosomal translocation places the *Bcl-2* proto-oncogene under the regulation of the immunoglobulin heavy chain (IgH) Eμ enhancer, resulting in dysregulated expression of the Bcl-2 protein.[46]

Oblimersen sodium, or G3139 (Genta Inc.), is the first AS-ON molecule to be widely tested in patients. It is a fully phosphorothioated 18-mer AS-ON complementary to the first six codons of the open reading frame (ORF) of the Bcl-2 mRNA sequence. Oblimersen was identified as the most biologically active Bcl-2 antisense sequence from among a series of 40 AS-ONs designed.[47] This compound targeting positions 1–18 of the ORF reduced Bcl-2 mRNA expression to near the lower limit of detection within cancer cells.[48] Preclinical studies concerning the role of Bcl-2 in tumor cell lines and animal xenograft models have demonstrated. Oblimerson is biologically active, both as a single agent and in combination with standard chemotherapeutic agents.[48] Studies have demonstrated that AS-ON specifically downregulates Bcl-2 protein and induces apoptosis in lymphoma cell lines. Separate work by Klasa and Waters has shown that human lymphoma xenografts treated with oblimersen resulted in prolonged median survival and cured some animals.[49,50] When oblimersen was combined with other agents, such as cyclophosphamide or rituximab, the mice survived longer. These promising results lead to several clinical trials.

Two phase I trials were conducted to evaluate the safety and activity of oblimersen as a single agent in patients with NHL.[51,52] The larger included 21 patients with Bcl-2-positive relapsed NHL who received a 14-day subcutaneous infusion.[52] The median age was 54 years, nine had follicular NHL, eight had small lymphocytic NHL, three had large cell lymphoma, and one had mantle cell lymphoma. All patients had received multiple chemotherapy regimens and four patients had received high-dose chemotherapy and autologous stem cell transplantation. Oblimersen was delivered by a continuous subcutaneous infusion for 14 days at doses of 4.6–195.8 mg/m²/day. All patients experienced local skin inflammation at the sites of subcutaneous infusion. Dose limiting toxicities were observed at doses greater than 147.2 mg/m²/day and consisted of thrombocytopenia, fevers, and hypotension. Non-dose-limiting toxicities included hyperglycemia during the infusion, fatigue, and transient increases in liver enzymes, which subsequently normalized.[53] Three patients responded (one CR, two minor responses). The median overall survival for all patients was 13.4 months. The one patient in CR remained disease free at 36 months after treatment. Among the responding patients or those with stable disease, the median progression-free survival was 3.6 months. Ten of 18 patients had a significant reduction in Bcl-2 protein levels measured in peripheral blood mononuclear cells, bone marrow, in lymph node tissue. Based on this study, a dose of 110.4 mg/m²/day was recommended for further evaluation. Currently, a phase II study is underway at Royal Marsden Hospital using this dose in patients with relapsed NHL.

More recent studies have explored the use of oblimersen sodium in combination with other chemotherapeutic regimens in hopes of enhancing treatment-induced apoptosis when Bcl-2 is suppressed. In an interim analysis, a small cohort of ten chemotherapy naive patients have been treated with oblimersen and R-CHOP after failing to initially respond to six cycles of oblimersen.[54] Of these patients, two had a CR and four had a PR. The combination of these drugs did not appear to increase the toxicity of R-CHOP. Another study has combined oblimersen with rituximab in relapsed NHL. To date, 4 of 11 evaluable patients (36%) responded to the combination therapy.[18] Single-agent use of oblimersen patients with chronic lymphocytic leukemia has demonstrated activity, but a unique toxicity emerged.[55] Patients developed severe hypotension at doses well tolerated in other disease indications, and it is believed that the release of IL-8 at the time of the infusion may be responsible.[56] Additional studies are underway to further explore the activity of oblimersen in NHL and CLL.

## GALLIUM NITRATE

Gallium Nitrate is one of the Group IIIa "near-metal" salts originally evaluated for antineoplastic activity by researchers at the National Cancer Institute during a full screening of all elements of the periodic table. When initially examined by Hart and colleagues, gallium was found to be the most active of the Group IIIa elements, inhibiting greater than 90% tumor growth in six of eight subcutaneous solid tumors tested in rodents, but less effect on leukemia.[57,58] Later, phase I and phase II studies demonstrated the adverse effect of hypocalcemia, which led to FDA approval in the United States for the use of gallium nitrate for cancer-related hypercalcemia. Gallium has further been tested with encouraging results in patients with lymphoma, multiple myeloma,[59] uroepithelial cancer,[60] and ovarian cancer.[61] The kinetics of gallium were initially established by Hall and colleagues in 1971.[62] The initial half-life was 1 h, volume of distribution approximated total body water, and approximately 94% was excreted in the urine in the first 24 h.

A number of mechanisms have been proposed for the antineoplastic activity of gallium, including cellular deprivation of ferric iron by transferrin-dependent inhibition, inhibition of ribonucleotide reductase, induction of apoptosis, and interference with protein tyrosine phosphatases. Gallium binds to transferrin, although at lower affinity than iron, forming a Ga–Tf complex. It is well established that lymphoma cells express an increased number of transferrin receptors.[63] By absorbing $Ga^{3+}$ instead of $Fe^{3+}$, the cell up-regulates transferrin receptors, and therefore permits more incorporation of gallium into the cell. This inevitably starves the cell of iron, which may lead to cell death. There is also evidence that the Ga–Tf complex inhibits the intracellular release of iron, further leading to the iron deprivation.[64] This intracellular inhibition was found in vitro to be reversible by transferrin–iron complex, iron salts, or hemin.

A second mechanism of gallium is its interaction with ribonucleotide reductase. Chitambar et al.[65] demonstrated in L1201 leukemia cells that although inhibition of iron uptake indirectly inhibits the ribonucleotide reductase M2 subunit, gallium had a direct effect on the enzyme as well by inhibition of cytosine diphosphate (CDP) or (ADP). Further studies showed this interaction between gallium and ribonucleotide reductase was synergistic with hydroxyurea, a drug that also interacts with the M2 subunit of ribonucleotide reductase.[66]

Initial studies with gallium nitrate in lymphoma involved bolus administration at a dose of 700 mg/m$^2$ every 2 weeks.[67,68] The response rate was low (18%) and the toxicities included gastrointestinal toxicity, reversible renal insufficiency, and anemia. To decrease renal toxicity, Warrell et al. administered gallium nitrate by continuous 24-h i.v. infusion for 7 days every 3–5 weeks at doses of 200–400 mg/m$^2$ (Ref. 69). The maximum tolerated dose, defined by renal insufficiency, was 400 mg/m$^2$/day. In the phase II study,[69] 47 patients who had previously failed conventional chemotherapy and who had bidimensionally measurable disease were evaluated. The patient population had a median of three prior therapies and many had extranodal involvement. The overall response rate was 34% (10% for Hodgkin's lymphoma and 43% for NHL patients), with two complete responses. The median duration of response was 2.5 months.

A further trial evaluated mitoguazone 600 mg/m$^2$ i.v. on days 1 and 10, etoposide 100–125 mg/m$^2$ i.v. on days 2–4, and continuous i.v. gallium nitrate on days 1–7, given every 3–4 weeks.[70] The patient population ranged from 19–77 years, with a median of two prior therapies and all had stage III or IV disease. The overall response rate was 52% but was higher (69%) for patients with diffuse large cell lymphoma. The toxicity of this regimen, however, was significant. Eighteen patients (42%) developed neutropenic fevers and three died. Other toxicities included mucositis (47%), keratitis and conjunctivitis (26%), diarrhea (21%), renal toxicity (16%), and optic neuritis (12%), which caused transient blindness in three of the five patients affected.

A third combination regimen with gallium was based on the in vitro studies demonstrating synergy between gallium and hydroxyurea.[71] Chitambar and colleagues evaluated 14 patients with stage III or IV low- or intermediate-grade, refractory lymphoma. The age range was 53–80 years, with a median of three treatments and a median of six previous agents. Patients received doses of 200, 250, 300, or 350 mg/m$^2$ i.v. continuous infusion gallium for 7 days with either 500 mg or 1000 mg hydroxyurea concomitantly. Six of the 14 patients (43%) had a response, and the median response duration was 7 weeks. Further studies are underway to define the activity of gallium nitrate in patients with lymphoma.

## PROTEOSOME INHIBITORS

Bortezomib is a dipeptidyl boronic acid proteosome inhibitor that effectively and specifically inhibits proteosome activity. The proteosome controls the stability of numerous proteins that regulate progression through the cell cycle and apoptosis, such as cyclins, cyclin-dependent kinases, tumor suppressors, and the nuclear factor-$\kappa$B.[72] By altering the stability or activity of these proteins, proteosome inhibitors sensitize malignant cells to apoptosis. In preclinical studies, bortezomib and other proteosome inhibitors have shown activity against a variety of B-cell malignancies, including multiple myeloma, diffuse large B-cell lymphoma, mantle cell lymphoma, and Hodgkin's lymphoma.[73,74] Based on these findings, phase I clinical trials were conducted with bortezomib in various solid and hematologic malignancies. Phase II trials have been initiated for refractory chronic lymphocytic leukemia and non-Hodgkin's lymphoma.[75]

## HISTONE DEACETYLASE INHIBITORS

Histone deacetylase inhibitors are a new class of chemotherapeutic agents that induce growth arrest and apoptosis of neoplastic cells by binding to HDACs and modulating gene expression.

Depsipeptide, FR901228, is an HDAC inhibitor that has demonstrated potent in vitro and in vivo cytotoxic activity against murine and human tumor cell lines. In a phase I trial of depsipeptide conducted at the National Cancer Institute, three patients with CTCL had a partial response, and one patient with peripheral T-cell lymphoma, unspecified, had a complete response.[76] Another HDAC inhibitor, suberoylanilide hydroxamic acid (SAHA), has also demonstrated activity in patients with T-cell lymphoma. When administered intravenously in patients with advanced cancer, the maximal-tolerated dose of SAHA was 300 mg/m$^2$/day $\times$ 5 days for 3 weeks. An accumulation of acetylated histones in peripheral blood mononuclear cells and biopsied tumor tissue was demonstrated up to 4 h postinfusion. SAHA demonstrated clinical activity in patients with CTCL, and phase II clinical trials are being pursued. The activity of the HDAC inhibitors in B-cell NHL is currently under investigation.

## TUMOR VACCINES

Tumor vaccines are an active immunotherapy in which the host is induced to generate an immune response against autologous tumor cells. The different types of vaccines are quite variable and include those directed at known tumor-specific antigens, such as the idiotype vaccines and modified tumor cellular vaccines that attempt to enhance immunogenicity by introducing granuloctye macrophage colony-stimulating factor or other ligands, which improve or induce tumor antigen presentation into tumor cells. In addition, the use of primed antigen presenting cells, such as dendritic cells, to improve the immune response to the desired tumor antigens is also being explored.

B-cell lymphomas are clonal disorders with all tumor cells expressing the same tumor-specific immunoglobulin, the unique variable regions of which are termed an idiotype (Id) that can serve as a target for immunotherapy. The first clinical trial of idiotype vaccines in patients with follicular lymphoma was conducted by Dr. Levy's group at Stanford.[77,78] Thirty-two patients with follicular lymphoma in first remission were treated with autologous purified Id protein chemically linked to kehale impel (KLH) as an immunologic adjuvant. An anti-Id humoral immune response to the vaccine developed in 14 patients. Another approach has been to use antigen-loaded dendritic cells that have been harvested from the patient and primed with the purified Id protein. Timmerman et al. treated 35 follicular lymphoma patients, 25 of whom were in first remission following cytoreductive chemotherapy.[79,80] Out of the 25 patients treated in first remission, 23 demonstrated a T-cell or humoral anti-Id response to the dendritic cell vaccine. At a median follow-up of 43 months, 70% remain progression free. Response did not correlate with T-cell

response but favored those who mounted a humoral response; the difference however was not statistically significant. These data have formed the basis for two ongoing large randomized trials in patients with follicular lymphoma in first remission treated with a similar Id-KLH-pulsed dendritic cell vaccine.

Additional studies are underway to explore the use of anti-Id vaccines in patients who have been cytoreduced with chemotherapy. These studies require tumor biopsies for generation of the anti-Id vaccine, thus limiting accrual to patients with readily accessible tumor tissue. New advances in amplification and cloning of Id proteins using mammalian cells grown in tissue culture, recombinant bacteria, tobacco mosaic virus as a vector for engineering protein production in tobacco plants, naked DNA, and recombinant viruses are underway and may facilitate the availability of these therapies for an increased number of patients.

## REFERENCES

1. Amlot PL, et al.: A phase I study of an anti-CD22-deglycosylated ricin A chain immunotoxin in the treatment of B-cell lymphomas resistant to conventional therapy. *Blood* 82(9):2624–2633, 1993.

2. Cesano A, Gayko U: CD22 as a target of passive immunotherapy. *Semin Oncol* 30(2):253–257, 2003.

3. Postema EJ, et al., Final results of a phase I radioimmunotherapy trial using (186)Re-epratuzumab for the treatment of patients with non-Hodgkin's lymphoma. *Clin Cancer Res* 9(10 Pt 2):3995S–4002S, 2003.

4. Wahl AF, et al.: The anti-CD30 monoclonal antibody SGN-30 promotes growth arrest and DNA fragmentation in vitro and affects antitumor activity in models of Hodgkin's disease. *Cancer Res* 62(13):3736–3742, 2002.

5. Lundin J, et al.: CAMPATH-1H monoclonal antibody in therapy for previously treated low-grade non-Hodgkin's lymphomas: a phase II multicenter study. European Study Group of CAMPATH-1H Treatment in Low-Grade Non-Hodgkin's Lymphoma. *J Clin Oncol* 16(10):3257–3263, 1998.

6. Uppenkamp M, et al.: Monoclonal antibody therapy with CAMPATH-1H in patients with relapsed high- and low-grade non-Hodgkin's lymphomas: a multicenter phase I/II study. *Ann Hematol* 81(1):26–32, 2002.

7. Schnell R, et al.: A Phase I study with an anti-CD30 ricin A-chain immunotoxin (Ki-4.dgA) in patients with refractory CD30+ Hodgkin's and non-Hodgkin's lymphoma. *Clin Cancer Res* 8(6):1779–1786, 2002.

8. Francisco JA, et al.: In vivo efficacy and toxicity of a single-chain immunotoxin targeted to CD40. *Blood* 89(12):4493–4500, 1997.

9. Conry RM, et al.: Phase I trial of an anti-CD19 deglycosylated ricin A chain immunotoxin in non-Hodgkin's lymphoma: effect of an intensive schedule of administration. *J Immunother Emphasis Tumor Immunol* 18(4):231–241, 1995.

10. Grossbard ML, et al.: Anti-B4-blocked ricin: a phase I trial of 7-day continuous infusion in patients with B-cell neoplasms. *J Clin Oncol* 11(4):726–737, 1993.

11. Vitetta ES, et al.: Phase I immunotoxin trial in patients with B-cell lymphoma. *Cancer Res* 51(15):4052–4058, 1991.

12. Foss FM: DAB(389)IL-2 (denileukin diftitox, ONTAK): a new fusion protein technology. *Clin Lymphoma* 1 (suppl 1):S27–S31, 2000.

13. Olsen E, et al.: Pivotal phase III trial of two dose levels of denileukin diftitox for the treatment of cutaneous T-cell lymphoma. *J Clin Oncol* 19(2):376–388, 2001.

14. Foss FM, et al.: Diphtheria toxin fusion proteins. *Curr Top Microbiol Immunol* 234:63–81, 1998.

15. Foss FM:, Interleukin-2 fusion toxin: targeted therapy for cutaneous T cell lymphoma. *Ann N Y Acad Sci* 941:166–176, 2001.

16. LeMaistre CF, et al.: Phase I trial of a ligand fusion-protein (DAB389IL-2) in lymphomas expressing the receptor for interleukin-2. *Blood* 91(2):399–405, 1998.

17. LeMaistre CF: DAB(389)IL-2 (denileukin diftitox, ONTAK): other potential applications. *Clin Lymphoma* 1 (suppl 1):S37–S40, 2000.

18. Pro B, et al.: Genasense (Bcl-2 Antisense) plus rituxamb is active in patients with relapsed or refractory B-cell non-Hodgkin's lymphoma. *Blood* 102(11), 2003.

19. Walker PL, Dang NH: Denileukin diftitox as novel targeted therapy in non-Hodgkin's lymphoma. *Clin J Oncol Nurs* 8(2):169–174, 2004.

20. Wiseman G, et al.: Interim safety results of a phase I trial of sequential doses of Yttrium-90 ibritumomab tiuxetan for previously treated patients with low-grade non-Hodgkin's lymphoma. *Proc Am Soc Clin Oncol* 22:575, 2003.

21. Wiseman GA, et al.: Phase I/II 90Y-Zevalin (yttrium-90 ibritumomab tiuxetan, IDEC-Y2B8) radioimmunotherapy dosimetry results in relapsed or refractory non-Hodgkin's lymphoma. *Eur J Nucl Med* 27(7):766–777, 2000.

22. Witzig TE, et al.: Phase I/II trial of IDEC-Y2B8 radioimmunotherapy for treatment of relapsed or refractory CD20(+) B-cell non-Hodgkin's lymphoma. J Clin Oncol. 17(12):3793–3803, 1999.

23. Kaminski MS, et al.: Pivotal study of iodine I[131] tositumomab for chemotherapy-refractory low-grade or transformed low-grade B-cell non-Hodgkin's lymphomas. *J Clin Oncol* 19(19):3918–3928, 2001.

24. Shipp MA, et al.: A predictive model for aggressive non-Hodgkin's lymphoma. The International Non-Hodgkin's Lymphoma Prognostic Factors Project. *N Engl J Med* 329(14):987–994, 1993.

25. Bennett JM, et al.: Assessment of treatment-related myelodysplastic syndromes (tMDS) and acute myeloid leukemia (tAML) in patients with low-grade non-Hodgkin's lymphoma (LG-NHL) treated with tositumomab and Iodine-131 tositumomab (The BEXXAR Therapeutic Regimen) [abstract]. *Blood* 102(11):Abstract 91, 2004.

26. Zelenetz AD, Saleh M, Vose J, Younes A, Kaminski MS: Patients with transformed low grade lymphoma attain durable responses following outpatient radioimmunotherapy with tositumomab and iodine I[131] tositumomab (Bexxar) [abstract]. *Blood* 100(11):Abstract 1384, 2002.

27. Kaminski MS, et al.: High response rates and durable remissions in patients with previously untreated, advanced-stage, follicular lymphoma treated with tositumomab and iodine I-131 tositumomab (Bexxar) [abstract]. *Blood* 100(11):Abstract 1381, 2002.

28. Leonard JP, Vose JM, Younas A: Remission inversion in patients with low grade and transformed low grade NHL: duration of response following treatment with tositumomab and iodine I[131] tositumomab [Bexxar] reproducibly exceeds that produced by the preceding therapy [abstract]. *Blood* 102(11):Abstract 4802, 2002.

29. Horning SJ, Younes A, Lucas J, Podoloff D, Jain V: Rituximab treatment failures: tositumomab and iodine I[131] tositumomab (Bexxar) can produce meaningful durable responses [abstract]. *Blood* 100(11):Abstract 1385, 2002.

30. Coleman M, Kaminski MS, Knox SJ, Zelenetz AD, Vose JM, The Bexxar therapeutic regimen (Tositumomab and Iodine I[131] Tositumomab) produces durable complete remissions in heavily pretreated patients with non-Hodgkin's lymphoma (NHL), rituximab-relapsed/refractory disease, and rituximab-naive disease [abstract]. *Blood* 102(11):Abstract 89, 2003.

31. Kaminski MS, et al.: Re-treatment with tositumomab and iodine I[131] tositumomab (the Bexxar Therapeutic Regimen) in patients with non-Hodgkin's lymphoma (NHL) with previous response to the Bexxar therapeutic regimen [abstract]. *Blood* 102(11):Abstract 1478, 2003.

32. Leonard JP, et al.: Durable remissions from fludarabine followed by the iodine I-131 tositumomab Bexxar therapeutic regimen for patients with previously untreated follicular non-Hodgkin's lymphoma (NHL) [abstract]. *J Clin Oncol* 22(14S):Abstract 6518, 2004.

33. Witzig TE, et al.: Randomized controlled trial of yttrium-90-labeled ibritumomab tiuxetan radioimmunotherapy versus rituximab immunotherapy for patients with relapsed or refractory low-grade, follicular, or transformed B-cell non-Hodgkin's lymphoma. *J Clin Oncol* 20(10):2453–2463, 2002.

34. Gordon LI, et al.: Long-term follow up of a phase I/II trial of radioimmunotherapy with yttrium 90 ibritumomab tiuxetan for CD20+ B-cell non-Hodgkin's lymphoma (NHL). *Proc Am Soc Clin Oncol*, 2004.

35. Witzig TE, et al.: Treatment with ibritumomab tiuxetan radioimmunotherapy in patients with rituximab-refractory follicular non-Hodgkin's lymphoma. *J Clin Oncol* 20(15):3262–3269, 2002.

36. Nademanee A, et al.: High dose radioimmunotherapy with yttrium 90 ibritumomab tiuxetan with high dose etoposide (VP-16) and cyclophosphamide (CY) followed by autologous hematopioetic cell transplant for poor risk or relapsed B cell non-Hodgkin's lymphoma: update of a phase I/II trial. *Proc Am Soc Clin Oncol*, 2004.

37. Emmanouilides C, et al.: Improved safety and efficacy of yttrium-90 ibritumomab tiuxetan radioimmunotherapy when administered as 2nd or 3rd line therapy for relapsed low-grade, follicular, and transformed B-cell non-Hodgkin's lymphoma (NHL). *Proc Am Soc Clin Oncol* 22:595, 2003.

38. Paterson BM, Roberts BE, Kuff EL: Structural gene identification and mapping by DNA-mRNA hybrid-arrested cell-free translation. *Proc Natl Acad Sci USA*. 74(10):4370–4374, 1977.

39. Zamecnik PC, Stephenson ML: Inhibition of Rous sarcoma virus replication and cell transformation by a specific oligodeoxynucleotide. *Proc Natl Acad Sci USA* 75(1):280–284, 1978.

40. Simons RW, Kleckner N: Translational control of IS10 transposition. *Cell* 34(2):683–691, 1983.

41. Crooke ST: Molecular mechanisms of action of antisense drugs. *Biochim Biophys Acta* 1489(1):31–44, 1999.

42. Baker BF, Monica BP: Novel mechanisms for antisense-mediated regulation of gene expression. *Biochim Biophys Acta* 1489(1):3–18, 1999.

43. Reed JC: Dysregulation of apoptosis in cancer. *J Clin Oncol* 17(9):2941–2953, 1999.

44. Schmitt CA, Rosenthal CT, Lowe SW: Genetic anaylsis of chemoresistance in primary murine lymphomas. *Nat Med* 6(9):1029–1035, 2000.

45. Gascoyne RD, et al.: Prognostic significance of Bcl-2 protein expression and Bcl-2 gene rearrangement in diffuse aggressive non-Hodgkin's lymphoma. *Blood* 90(1):244–251, 1997.

46. Rabitts TH, Rabitts PH: Molecular pathology of chromosomal abnormalities and cancer genes in human tumors. In: Glover DM, Hames BD (eds.) *Oncogenes*. UK: Oxford; 1990:83–86.

47. Cotter FE, Waters J, Cunningham D: Human Bcl-2 antisense therapy for lymphomas. *Biochim Biophys Acta* 1489(1):97–106, 1999.

48. Kitada S, et al.: Investigations of antisense oligonucleotides targeted against bcl-2 RNAs. *Antisense Res Dev* 3(2):157–169, 1993.

49. Klasa RJ, et al.: Eradication of human non-Hodgkin's lymphoma in SCID mice by BCL-2 antisense oligonucleotides combined with low-dose cyclophosphamide. *Clin Cancer Res* 6(6):2492–2500, 2000.

50. Waters JS, et al.: Bcl-2 antisense oligodeoxynucleotide (ODN) (G3139) therapy exerts its antitumor action through a sequence-specific antisense effect, and not a cell-mediated immune response. *Proc Am Soc Clin Oncol* 19(14a), 2000.

51. Webb A, et al.: BCL-2 antisense therapy in patients with non-Hodgkin lymphoma. *Lancet* 349(9059):1137–1141, 1997.

52. Waters JS, et al.: Phase I clinical and pharmacokinetic study of bcl-2 antisense oligonucleotide therapy in patients with non-Hodgkin's lymphoma. *J Clin Oncol* 18(9):1812–1823, 2000.

53. Kuss B, Cotter F: Antisense—time to shoot the messenger. *Ann Oncol* 10(5):495–503, 1999.

54. Leonard J, et al.: Genasense (oblimersen sodium, G3139) is active and well-tolerated both alone and with R-CHOP in mantle cell lymphoma (MCL). *Blood* 102(11), 2003.

55. Rai KR, et al.: Genasense (Bcl-2 antisense) monotherapy in patients with relapsed or refractory chronic lymphocytic leukemia: phase 1 and 2 results. *Am S of Hematology Annual Meeting* 2002.

56. Baird ME, et al.: G3139 promotes release of IL-8 by chronic lymphocytic leukemia cells cultured in vitro: potential implications for therapeutic use. *Am S of Hematology Annual Meeting* 2001.

57. Hart MM, et al.: Toxicity and antitumor activity of gallium nitrate and periodically related metal salts. *J Natl Cancer Inst* 47(5):1121–1127, 1971.

58. Hart MM, Adamson RH: Antitumor activity and toxicity of salts of inorganic group 3a metals: aluminum, gallium, indium, and thallium. *Proc Natl Acad Sci USA* 68(7):1623–1626, 1971.

59. Niesvizkya R, et al.: Extended survival in advanced-stage multiple myeloma patients treated with gallium nitrate. *Leuk Lymphoma* 43(3):603–605, 2002.

60. Einhorn LH, et al.: Phase II trial of vinblastine, ifosfamide, and gallium combination chemotherapy in metastatic urothelial carcinoma. *J Clin Oncol* 12(11):2271–2276, 1994.

61. Dreicer R, et al.: Vinblastine, ifosfamide, gallium nitrate, and filgrastim in platinum- and paclitaxel-resistant ovarian cancer: a phase II study. *Am J Clin Oncol* 21(3):287–290, 1998.

62. Hall SW, et al.: Kinetics of gallium nitrate, a new anticancer agent. *Clin Pharmacol Ther* 25(1):82–87, 1979.

63. Esserman L, et al.: An epitope of the transferrin receptor is exposed on the cell surface of high-grade but not low-grade human lymphomas. *Blood* 74(8):2718–2729, 1989.

64. Chitambar CR, Seligman PA: Effects of different transferrin forms on transferrin receptor expression, iron uptake, and cellular proliferation of human leukemic HL60 cells. Mechanisms responsible for the specific cytotoxicity of transferrin-gallium. *J Clin Invest* 78(6):1538–1546, 1986.

65. Chitambar CR, et al.: Inhibition of ribonucleotide reductase by gallium in murine leukemic L1210 cells. *Cancer Res* 51(22):6199–6201, 1991.

66. Chitambar CR, et al.: Inhibition of leukemic HL60 cell growth by transferrin-gallium: effects on ribonucleotide reductase and demonstration of drug synergy with hydroxyurea. *Blood* 72(6):1930–1936, 1988.

67. Weick JK, et al.: Gallium nitrate in malignant lymphoma: a Southwest Oncology Group study. *Cancer Treat Rep* 67(9):823–825, 1983.

68. Keller J, et al.: Phase II evaluation of bolus gallium nitrate in lymphoproliferative disorders: a Southeastern Cancer Study Group trial. *Cancer Treat Rep* 70(10):1221–1223, 1986.

69. Warrell RP Jr, et al.: Treatment of patients with advanced malignant lymphoma using gallium nitrate administered as a seven-day continuous infusion. *Cancer* 51(11):1982–1987, 1983.

70. Warrell RP Jr, et al.: Salvage chemotherapy of advanced lymphoma with investigational drugs: mitoguazone, gallium nitrate, and etoposide. *Cancer Treat Rep* 71(1):47–51, 1987.

71. Chitambar CR, et al.: Evaluation of continuous-infusion gallium nitrate and hydroxyurea in combination for the treatment of refractory non-Hodgkin's lymphoma. *Am J Clin Oncol* 20(2):173–178, 1997.

72. Goy, A, Gilles F: Update on the proteasome inhibitor bortezomib in hematologic malignancies. *Clin Lymphoma* 4(4):230–237, 2004.

73. Orlowski RZ, et al.: Phase I trial of the proteasome inhibitor PS-341 in patients with refractory hematologic malignancies. *J Clin Oncol* 20(22):4420–4427, 2002.

74. Orlowski RZ: Bortezomib and its role in the management of patients with multiple myeloma. *Expert Rev Anticancer Ther* 4(2):171–179, 2004.

75. Pahler JC, et al.: Effects of the proteasome inhibitor, bortezomib, on apoptosis in isolated lymphocytes obtained from patients with chronic lymphocytic leukemia. *Clin Cancer Res* 9(12):4570–4577, 2003.

76. Piekarz RL, et al.: T-cell lymphoma as a model for the use of histone deacetylase inhibitors in cancer therapy: impact of depsipeptide on molecular markers, therapeutic targets, and mechanisms of resistance. *Blood* 103(12):4636–4643, 2004.

77. Kwak LW, et al.: Induction of immune responses in patients with B-cell lymphoma against the surface-immunoglobulin idiotype expressed by their tumors. *N Engl J Med* 327(17):1209–1215, 1992.

78. Hsu FJ, et al.: Tumor-specific idiotype vaccines in the treatment of patients with B-cell lymphoma—long-term results of a clinical trial. *Blood* 89(9):3129–3135, 1997.

79. Timmerman JM, Levy R: Dendritic cell vaccines for cancer immunotherapy. *Annu Rev Med* 50:507–529, 1999.

80. Timmerman JM, et al.: Idiotype-pulsed dendritic cell vaccination for B-cell lymphoma: clinical and immune responses in 35 patients. *Blood* 99(5):1517–1526, 2002.

# Section 2
# HODGKIN'S DISEASE

## Chapter 69

# HODGKIN'S LYMPHOMA: EPIDEMIOLOGY AND RISK FACTORS

*Brian J. Bolwell*

## HISTORY

The first description of Hodgkin's lymphoma (HL) occurred when Thomas Hodgkin described the clinical history and postmortem findings of seven patients who developed a massive enlargement of lymph nodes and spleen.[1] Hodgkin was not formally credited with this discovery, however, until 1865 when Sir Samuel Wilkes published a paper entitled "Cases of enlargement of lymph glands and spleen (or Hodgkin's lymphoma), with remarks."[2] Drs Carl Sternberg and Dorothy Reed are credited with the first definitive microscopic descriptions of HL.[3,4]

## DESCRIPTIVE EPIDEMIOLOGY

HL is an uncommon cancer, with approximately 8000 new cases diagnosed in the United States annually.[5] Several large epidemiologic reports have noted that males have a slightly higher incidence of HL than do females; that whites are at higher risk than are blacks; and that HL seems to be more common in patients of higher socioeconomic class than in those of lower socioeconomic class.[6–11]

HL is associated with a bimodal age-specific incidence distribution. The first peak occurs in early adulthood, beginning at ages 10–14, peaking at ages 20–24, and decreasing at age 40–44. The second peak begins at age 50 and increases over time. Forty-one percent of cases are diagnosed in patients aged 20–34.[6]

Nodular sclerosing (NS) HL accounts for the majority of histologic subtypes of HL associated with the early-age incidence peak. NS HL has an essentially unimodal age-specific incidence, with a peak in young adults aged 20–24. The age-specific incidence rate for NS HL falls off by age 40–44, then remains relatively constant between the ages 45 and 64. Mixed cellularity HL has a unimodal age distribution, its incidence increasing slowly with age. By the age of 50, mixed cellularity has been reported to be the most common histologic subtype of HL.[6] Lymphocyte-depleted HL is rare in younger patients, and progressively increases with age.

HL is more common in first-degree relatives.[12–16] Some data suggest that siblings have a two- to fivefold increased risk of developing HL; same sex siblings may have up to a ninefold risk.[16] When HL occurs in families, it is more likely to involve males. Some early reports suggested that HL may be contagious, particularly by airborne transmission, although subsequent studies conclusively refuted this possibility.[17–19] Certain HLA antigens, particularly HLA-DP, have been associated with an increased incidence of HL and with clinical outcome.[20–22]

## HODGKIN'S LYMPHOMA AND VIRUSES

### THE POSSIBLE RELATIONSHIP OF EPSTEIN–BARR VIRUS TO HODGKIN'S LYMPHOMA

A Danish population-based study published in 1974 described over 17,000 people with a history of a positive Epstein–Barr (EBV) test, to determine if these patients were at risk for the development of subsequent malignancies. A significantly higher-than-expected incidence of HL in this patient population was discovered.[23]

Since this observation, many investigators have employed increasingly sophisticated techniques attempting to determine not just a link but also a causal association between EBV and the development of HL. Between 19 and 40% of diagnosed cases of HL are generally reported to have detectable EBV viral genomes in Reed–Sternberg cells.[24] Other investigators have noted the following: pediatric cases of HL seem to have a higher proportion of EBV-associated HL than do those of adults; there is a higher incidence of mixed cellularity histologic subtype associated with EBV than of other HL histologic subtypes; and the association of EBV in HL may be stronger in less developed countries and in populations with lower socioeconomic status.[25–30]

A recent update of a vast population-based registry study from Denmark and Sweden involving over 38,000 infectious mononucleosis patients confirmed that only HL and skin cancers occurred in statistically significant increased numbers; no other cancer was associated with infectious mononucleosis/EBV.[31] The conclusion was that the increased risk of HL appears to be a specific phenomenon.

However, many questions remain. The most obvious question is why are some cases of HL EBV positive and other cases EBV negative? Additionally, whether or not the presence of EBV viral genome Reed-Sternberg cells is a proof of causality is a very open question; most of the US population has been exposed to EBV, and one recent study found that the vast majority of small EBV-positive CD30⁻ cells carried somatically mutated V-region genes, indicating that in lymph nodes of patients with HL, as in the peripheral blood of healthy individuals, EBV persists in memory B cells.[32] One might argue that EBV-negative HL is associated with other viruses; however, there is no significant evidence that this is the case.[33] Another theory suggests that EBV may be involved in all HL cases but may be undetectable only in some; EBV might infect the cell, transform it, and then it is eliminated (the hit-and-run theory), though this theory has been difficult to substantiate.

A large Danish and Swedish registry study comparing EBV-positive and EBV-negative HL has recently been published.[34] Over 17,000 patients with serologic evidence of EBV infection were compared to a cohort of over 24,000 individuals without known EBV infection. Tumor specimens from patients developing HL were tested for the presence of EBV. Fifty-five percent of tumor specimens obtained from patients with infectious mononucleosis had evidence of EBV. There was no evidence of an increased risk of EBV-negative Hodgkin's lymphoma after infectious mononucleosis. In contrast, the risk of EBV-positive Hodgkin's lymphoma was significantly increased. The estimated median incubation time from mononucleosis to EBV-positive Hodgkin's lymphoma was 4.1 years. The risk of Hodgkin's lymphoma in the seropositive cohorts remains increased for two decades. The authors concluded that a causal association between infectious-mononucleosis-related EBV infection and the development of EBV-positive Hodgkin's lymphoma was likely. The authors also emphasized that in absolute terms, the risk of Hodgkin's lymphoma after infectious mononucleosis is only approximately 1/1000 persons; thus, other cofactors to explain the ultimately etiology of EBV-positive and EBV negative HL remain to be elucidated.

### HODGKIN'S LYMPHOMA AND HIV

Although HL is not an AIDS-defining malignancy, there is a well-known increased risk for the development of HL in human immunodeficiency virus (HIV) infected individuals.[35–41] Some differences do exist between HIV associated HL and non HIV associated HL. HIV-associated HL is diagnosed at a more advanced stage than non-HIV-associated HL; has a higher incidence of extranodal involvement; and is more likely to have an underlying histology of mixed cellularity.[36–38]

One large series from France described 45 cases of HL in HIV-infected individuals. Forty-nine percent of patients presented with mixed cellularity histology, 75% with advanced stage, and 80% with B symptoms. Not only mediastinal involvement is a site of presentation in over 50% of patients with primary HL that this series described only 13% of HIV positive HL patients with mediastinal involvement. This study found that HIV-associated HL was preceded by an AIDS manifestation in only 11% of cases. Median CD4 cell count was 306/μL at diagnosis. With standard therapy, 79% of patients achieved a complete remission, but hematologic and infectious complications were frequent. Prognosis correlated with initial CD4 cell count.[35]

Another large study from Italy described 114 cases of HIV-associated HL.[41] As with other studies, the authors noted an increase in mixed cellularity histology, a high prevalence of advanced-stage disease, and extranodal involvement. The most powerful prognostic factor was the CD4 count at diagnosis; patients with a CD4 count of greater than 250/μL had a better prognosis. Eighteen patients could be studied for the presence of EBV viral genomes. Seventy-eight percent of patients were found to have EBV associated with their HL. This relationship of EBV-positive HL and HIV-associated HL was confirmed in a subsequent study, in which Reed-Sternberg cells of virtually all studied HIV-associated HL patients expressed the EBV-encoded latent membrane protein 1.[40] Therefore, the association of HIV infection with HL may be part of the complex relationship between EBV infection and the development of HL.

Historically, clinical outcomes of patients with HIV-associated HL have been poor, with patients experiencing frequent infectious complications, and a more aggressive disease process. However, a recent report from Italy described 59 patients receiving combination chemotherapy with highly active retroviral therapy (HAART) and granulocyte colony-stimulating factor (G-CSF). Patients were treated with the Stanford V combination chemotherapy, which was well tolerated in 69% of patients completing treatment without dose reduction or delay in chemotherapy administration. Complete response was achieved by 81% of patients, and 56% were alive in remission with a median follow-up of 17 months. The authors concluded that in the era of HAART and G-CSF support, the delivery of combina tion chemotherapy to HIV-infected individuals is more feasible and more effective than seen previously.[42]

## POSSIBLE ASSOCIATION OF HODGKIN'S DISEASE WITH RHEUMATOLOGIC CONDITIONS TREATED WITH METHOTREXATE

Conflicting data exist describing a possible association of the development of lymphoproliferative disorders, including HL, with rheumatoid arthritis and other connective tissue disease.[43–46] Case reports have described an association of HL with patients receiving mild doses of methotrexate to treat their underlying condition. This has lead to the question of whether such patients receiving methotrexate, particularly those with rheumatoid arthritis, are at higher risk of developing lymphomas, including HL.

Over 25 years ago, Banks et al. published a retrospective review of all patients seen at the Mayo Clinic from 1965 to 1975 with a diagnosis of both a connective tissue disorder and a lymphoid malignancy.[47] Twenty-nine patients were identified, two with HL. There was no particular pattern of the type of lymphoproliferative disorder seen. There was also no mention of treatment for the underlying rheumatologic condition. However, the authors concluded that there was little evidence of an association between the two. The Mayo Clinic subsequently updated their data, describing 16,000 patients with rheumatoid arthritis seen from 1976 to 1992 that were cross-indexed with 21,000 patients who had hematologic malignancy and received a disease-modifying antirheumatic drug.[48] Thirty-nine patients fit this definition, four of which had HL. Twelve of the thirty-nine cases received methotrexate (two with HL). The lymphoid malignancies occurred at a median of 15 years after the diagnosis of rheumatoid arthritis. There was no pattern to the lymphoproliferative disorder seen. The authors concluded that the data did not support a relationship between methotrexate and any particular type of hematologic malignancy.

A study from France analyzed 426 rheumatoid arthritis patients treated with methotrexate to determine whether or not there was an increased incidence of cancer, compared with both rheumatoid arthritis patients never treated with methotrexate (rheumatoid control) and the regional population.[49] The regional population consisted of over 800,000 individuals. After an extensive analysis, the authors concluded that methotrexate was not found to be responsible for the development of any particular type of cancer, including hematologic cancers.

The most recently published study investigating a possible association between rheumatoid arthritis patients treated with methotrexate and the development of lymphoma is a national study from France, consisting of 61 rheumatology departments treating and following 78,000 rheumatoid arthritis patients.[50] All new cases of lymphoma occurring in rheumatoid arthritis patients over a 3-year period from 1996 to 1998 were described. The incidence of the development of non-Hodgkin's lymphoma (NHL) and HL in the study group was compared to that of the general French adult population in 1998 (46 million individuals). Twenty-five new cases of lymphoid malignancy were discovered. The median age was 63 years. The median time from the diagnosis of rheumatoid arthritis to the development of a lymphoma was 16 years. The median duration of methotrexate therapy was 5 years. Of particular interest was the fact that in contrast to many case reports describing regression, and even resolution, of lymphoma when methotrexate therapy is discontinued, this report found that of 24 patients in whom methotrexate was stopped, only 3 patients developed a spontaneous remission and 2 later relapsed. The observed annual incidence of NHL in the study group did not significantly exceed the annual incidence of NHL in the general French population after adjustment for age and sex. Only seven patients developed HL, and these small numbers make any definitive conclusion problematic.

Several studies have pointed out another confounding variable concerning the possible association of lymphoproliferative disorders with methotrexate therapy for patients with rheumatologic arthritis. Any immunosuppressive therapy may increase the risk of viral infection, including EBV. Many reports have shown that patients developing HL while receiving methotrexate therapy have detectable EBV virus, and that the EBV viral genome can be detected within the malignant lymphoid cells.[51–54] It is far more likely that any association between connective tissue disorder patients receiving immunosuppressive therapy and the development of lymphoproliferative disorders, especially HL, is related to the influence of EBV rather than an inherent susceptibility of patients with rheumatoid arthritis to the development of such cancers. The overall risk of the development of HL in patients with rheumatoid arthritis, even with immunosuppressive therapy, is still extremely low.

## SUMMARY

Epidemiology data have shown that HL has a bimodal age-specific incidence peaking at ages 20–24 and decreasing after age 44. NS HL accounts for the majority of histologic subtypes associated with early-age incidence peak. HL is more common in first-degree relatives, although there is no evidence that HL is capable of airborne transmission. There is a clear association of EBV with HL in 20–40% cases. HIV has been associated with HL, but it is unclear whether the HIV virus itself plays an etiologic role in the pathogenesis of HL in these patients. There is little, if any, data to suggest that HL is associated with rheumatologic conditions treated with immunosuppressive therapy such as methotrexate.

### REFERENCES

1. Hodgkin T: On some morbid appearances of the absorbent gland and spleen. *Med Chir Trans* 17:68–97, 1832.
2. Wilkess: Cases of lardaceaous disease and some allied affection, with remarks. *Guy's Hosp Rep* 17:103, 1856.
3. Sternberg C: Uber Eine Eigenartige Unter Ben Biobe Der Pscudoleukamie Verlaufende Tuberculose Des Lymphatischen Apparates. *Z Heilk* 19:21, 1898.
4. Reed D: On the pathological changes of Hodgkin's disease, with a special reference to its relation to tuberculosis. *Johns Hopkins Hosp Rep* 10:133, 1902.
5. Jemal A, Tiwari RC, Murray T, et al.: Cancer statistics, 2004. *CA Cancer J Clin* 54:8–29, 2004.
6. Medeiros LJ, Greiner TC: Hodgkin's disease. *Cancer Suppl* 75:357–369, 1995.
7. MacMahon B: Epidemiology of Hodgkin's disease. *Cancer Res* 26:1189–1200, 1966.
8. Grufferman S, Delzell E: Epidemiology of Hodgkin's disease. *Epidemiol Rev* 6:76–106, 1984.
9. Gutensohn N, Cole P: Epidemiology of Hodgkin's disease in the young. *Int J Cancer* 19:595–604, 1977.
10. Gutensohn N, Cole P: Childhood social environment and Hodgkin's disease. *N Engl J Med* 304:135–140, 1981.
11. Abramson JH, Pridan H, Sacks MI, Avitzour M, Peritz E: A case–control study of Hodgkin's disease in Israel. *J Natl Cancer Inst* 61:307–314, 1978.
12. Lynch HT, Saldivar VA, Guirgis HA, et al.: Familial Hodgkin's disease and associated cancer. *Cancer* 38: 2041–2041, 1976.
13. Creagan ET, Fraumeni JF: Familial Hodgkin's disease. *Lancet* 547, 1972.
14. Vianna NJ, Polan AK, Davies JNP, Wolfgang P: Familial Hodgkin's disease: an environmental and genetic disorder. *Lancet* 854–857, 1974.
15. Bernard SM, Cartwright RA, Darwin CM, et al.: Hodgkin's disease: case control epidemiological study in Yorkshire. *Br J Cancer* 55:85–90, 1987.
16. Razis DV, Diamond HD, Craver LF: Familial Hodgkin's disease: its significance and implications. *Ann Intern Med* 51:933–971, 1953.
17. Vianna NJ, Polan AD: Epidemiologic evidence for transmission of Hodgkin's disease. *N Engl J Med* 289:499–502, 1973.
18. Vianna NJ, Greenwald P, Davies JNP: Extended epidemic of Hodgkin's disease in high-school students. *Lancet* 1209–1211, 1971.
19. Grufferman S, Cole P, Levitan TR: Evidence against transmission of Hodgkin's disease in high school. *N Engl J Med* 300:1006–1011, 1979.
20. Tonks S, Oza AM, Lister TA, Bodmer JG: Association of HLA-DPB with Hodgkin's disease. *Lancet* 340:968–969, 1992.
21. Bodmer JG, Tonks S, Oza AM, Lister Ta, Bodmer WF: HLA-DP based resistance to Hodgkin's disease. *Lancet* 1455–1456, 1989.
22. Oza AM, Tonks S, Lim J, Fleetwood MA, Lister A, Bodmer JG: Clinical and epidemiological study of human leukocyte antigen-DPB alleles in Hodgkin's disease. *Cancer Res* 54:5101–5105, 1994.
23. Rosdahl N, Olesen Larsen S, Clemmesen J: Hodgkin's disease in patients with previous infectious mononucleosis: 30 years' experience. *Br Med J* 2:253–256, 1974.
24. Weiss LM, Movahed LA, Warnke RA, Sklar J: Detection of Epstein–Barr viral genomes in Reed–Sternberg cells of Hodgkin's disease. *N Engl J Med* 320:502–506, 1989.
25. Ambinder RF, Browning PJ, Lorenzana I, et al.: Epstein–Barr virus and childhood Hodgkin's disease in Honduras and the United States. *Blood* 81:462–467, 1993.
26. Zhou X, Sandvej K, Li P, et al.: Epstein–Barr virus (EBV) in Chinese pediatric Hodgkin disease. *Cancer* 92: 1621–1631, 2001.
27. Boiocchi M, De Re V, Dolcetti R, Carbone A, Scarpa A, Menestrina F: Association of Epstein–Barr virus genome with mixed cellularity and cellular phase nodular sclerosis Hodgkin's disease subtypes. *Ann Oncol* 307–310, 1992.
28. Enblad G, Sandvej K, Sundström C, Pallesen G, Glimelius B: Epstein–Barr virus distribution in Hodgkin's disease in an unselected Swedish population. *Acta Oncol* 38:425–429, 1999.
29. Glaser SL, Lin RJ, Stewart SL, et al.: Epstein–Barr virus-associated Hodgkin's disease: epidemiologic characteristics in international data. *Int J Cancer* 70:375–382, 1997.
30. Weinreb M, Day P, Murray P, et al.: Epstein–Barr virus (EBV) and Hodgkin's disease in children: incidence of EBV latent membrane protein in malignant cells. *J Pathol* 168:365–369, 1992.
31. Hjalgrim HJ, Askling J, Sorensen P, et al.: Risk of Hodgkin's disease and other cancers after infectious mononucleosis. *J Nat Cancer Inst* 92:1522–1528, 2000.
32. Spieker T, Kurth J, Küppers R, Rajewsky K, Bräuninger A, Hansmann M: Molecular single-cell analysis of the

clonal relationship of small Epstein–Barr virus-infected cells and Epstein–Barr virus-harboring Hodgkin and Reed/Sternberg cells in Hodgkin disease. *Blood* 96: 3133–3138, 2000.

33. Armstron AA, Shield L, Gallagher A, Jarrett RF: Lack of involvement of known oncogenic DNA viruses in Epstein–Barr virus-negative Hodgkin's disease. *J Cancer* 77:1045–1047, 1998.

34. Hjalgrim H, Askling J, Rostgaard K, et al.: Characteristics of Hodgkin's lymphoma after infectious mononucleosis. *N Engl J Med* 349:1324–1332, 2003.

35. Andrieu JM, Roithmann S, Tourani JM, et al.: Hodgkin's disease during HIV1 infection: French Registry of HIV associated Tumors. *Ann Oncol* 4:635–641, 1993.

36. Pelstring RJ, Zellmer RB, Sulak LE, Banks PM, Clare N: Hodgkin's disease in association with human immunod-eficiency virus infection. *Cancer* 67:1865–1873, 1991.

37. Franceschi S, Dal Maso L, Arniani S: Risk of cancer other than Kaposi's sarcoma and non-Hodgkin's lymphoma in persons with AIDS in Italy. *Br J Cancer* 78:966–970, 1998.

38. Lowenthal DA, Straus DJ, Campbell Wise S, Gold JWM, Clarkson BD, Koziner B: AIDS-related lymphoid neopla-sia. *Cancer* 61:2325–2337, 1988.

39. Serraino D, Pezzotti P, Dorrucci M, Alliegro MB, Sinicco A, Rezza G: Cancer incidence in a cohort of human immunodeficiency virus seroconverters. *Cancer* 79: 1004–1008, 1997.

40. Carbone A, Gloghini A, Larocca LM, et al.: Human immunodeficiency virus-associated Hodgkin's disease derives from post-germinal center B cells. *Blood* 93: 2319–2326, 1999.

41. Tirelli U, Errante D, Dolcetti R, et al.: Hodgkin's disease and human immunodeficiency virus infection: clinico-pathologic and virologic features of 114 patients from the Italian Cooperative Group on AIDS and Tumors. *J Clin Oncol* 13:1758–1767, 1995.

42. Spina M, Gabarre J, Rossi G, et al.: Stanford V regimen and concomitant HAART in 59 patients with Hodgkin's disease and HIV infection. *Blood* 100:1984–1988, 2002.

43. Kingsmore SF, Hall BD, Allen NB, Rice JR, Caldwell DS: Association of methotrexate, rheumatoid arthritis and lymphoma: report of 2 cases and literature review. *J Rheumatol* 19:1462–1465, 1992.

44. Ellman MH, Hurwitz H, Thomas C, Kozloff M: Lymphoma developing in a patient with rheumatoid arthritis taking low dose weekly methotrexate. *J Rheumatol* 18:1741–1743, 1991.

45. Shiroky JB, Frost A, Skelton JD, Haegert DG, Newkirk MM, Neville C: Complications of immunosuppression associated with weekly low dose methotrexate. *J Rheumatol* 18:1172–1175, 1991.

46. Kamel OW, Weiss LM, van de Rijn M, Colby TV, Kingma DW, Jaffe ES: Hodgkin's disease and lymphoprolifera-tions resembling Hodgkin's disease in patients receiving long-term low-dose methotrexate therapy. *Am J Surg Pathol* 20:1279–1287, 1996.

47. Banks PM, Witrak GA, Conn DL: Lymphoid neoplasia following connective tissue disease. *Mayo Clin Proc* 54:104–108, 1979.

48. Moder KG, Tefferi A, Cohen MD, Menke DM, Luthra HS: Hematologic malignancies and the use of methotrexate in rheumatoid arthritis: a retrospective study. *Am J Med* 99:276–281, 1995.

49. Bologna C, Picot M, Jorgensen C, Viu P, Verdier R, Sany J: Study of eight cases of cancer in 426 rheumatoid arthritis patients treated with methotrexate. *Ann Rheum Dis* 56:97–102, 1997.

50. Mariette X, Cazals-Hatem D, Warszawki J, Liote F, Balandraud N, Sibilia J: Lymphomas in rheumatoid arthritis patients treated with methotrexate: a 3-year prospective study in France. *Blood* 99:3909–3915, 2002.

51. Georgescu L, Quinn GC, Schwartzman S, Paget SA: Lymphoma in patients with rheumatoid arthritis: associ-ation with the disease state or methotrexate treatment. *Semin Arthritis Rheum* 26:794–804, 1997.

52. Kamel OW, van de Rijn M, Weiss LM, et al.: Brief report: reversible lymphomas associated with Epstein–Barr virus occurring during methotrexate therapy for rheumatoid arthritis and dermatomyositis. *N Engl J Med* 328: 1317–1321, 1993.

53. Liote F, Pertuiset E, Cochand-Priollet B, et al.: Methotrexate related B lymphoproliferative disease in a patient with rheumatoid arthritis. Role of Epstein–Barr virus infection. *J Rheumatol* 22:1174–1178, 1995.

54. Bachman TR, Sawitzke A, Perkins SL, Ward JH, Cannon GW: Methotrexate-associated lymphoma in patients with rheumatoid arthritis. *Arthritis Rheum* 39:325–329, 1996.

# Chapter 70

# PROGNOSTIC FACTORS IN HODGKIN'S LYMPHOMA

## *Michel Henry-Amar*

Since the beginning of the twentieth century, the concept has emerged that Hodgkin's lymphoma evolves through successive clinical stages associated with increasing disease spread and worsening clinical outcome. The validity of this concept has progressively been confirmed leading to the conception of staging classifications based on anatomic extent of the disease. In 1971, a consensus was reached at the Ann Arbor Workshop on the Staging of Hodgkin's lymphoma.[1] Thereafter, the so-called Ann Arbor classification was universally adopted and its prognostic significance confirmed through numerous publications, in particular one in which more than 14,000 cases from 20 cooperative groups or institutions were combined.[2] It is still used for the evaluation of patients presenting with the disease.

As time and data accumulated, it became obvious that the Ann Arbor staging could not be the sole prognostic tool in daily practice. In 1988, a modification of the Ann Arbor classification was advised by specialists attending the Cotswolds meeting in England.[3] The major modification concerned the designation of the disease extent and bulk. However, this classification is not generally used.

A variety of other clinical and biological characteristics have been used and claimed to be of prognostic significance. Some of these characteristics, combined with others, have been applied to retrospective series and demonstrated their prognostic value. They are presently used by several cooperative groups or institutions in the design of clinical trials. An extensive review of the literature has been published by Specht and Hasenclever in 1999.[4] Therefore, we will focus on the definition of prognostic factors and end points. We will also give examples specific for early and advanced stages. We will then discuss some issues that develop when using prognostic factors in the management of Hodgkin's lymphoma.

## METHODOLOGICAL ISSUES

### DEFINITION AND USE OF PROGNOSTIC FACTORS

Prognostic factors are variables measured in individuals that offer a partial explanation of the heterogeneity observed in the outcome of a given disease.[5] Prognostic factors may be used to predict the outcome of Hodgkin's lymphoma on a population (or a group of patients) basis, but not for individual patients.[6] Prognostic factors can be used to define risk groups, thus playing a role in treatment selection. In the setting of a clinical trial, they can be used in the definition of eligibility criteria and for stratification before randomization. In the analysis of a trial's results, prognostic factors may allow adjustments to improve the value of statistical comparisons made. However, the use of prognostic factors will never justify the comparison of treatments described by nonrandomized studies.[7,8]

### TYPES

Prognostic factors can be tumor related or patient related. Tumor-related factors reflect the type of the tumor, the extent of the disease, and the characteristics related to the tumor growth. These characteristics can be measured on the tumor itself or may be surrogate measures such as serum markers. Patient-related factors more often correspond to demographic characteristics or patient physiologic reserve, such as performance status. Generally speaking, tumor as well as patient-related factors are important for outcome although one may keep them separate, especially when they are used in the selection of treatment.

Usually, prognostic factors are grouped according to the point in time at which they are recorded.[6] Their values should be known at the point from which prognosis (i.e., time to response or more generally time to event) is measured. Such prognostic factors for which a single value is available (measured at diagnosis, before the start of treatment) are called fixed covariates. Other prognostic factors may be available only during treatment (e.g., received dose intensity, acute toxicity), or after the treatment is completed, or the study is closed (e.g., response to treatment, time to response). These prognostic factors are called time-dependent covariates.[5] Their use is generally a source of difficulties because time-dependent covariates may be affected by the treatment and such variables should never be used in statistical adjusted comparisons between treatments.

## END POINTS

Prognostic factors that correlate with an outcome variable must have clearly defined end points.[9] These may relate to treatment efficacy, such as response to therapy, acute toxicity, or treatment failure within a given time; they may also relate to long-term results, such as relapse-free survival for patients who reach a complete remission, disease-free survival, treatment failure-free survival, overall or cause-specific survival, or cumulative probability of late toxicity (e.g., secondary malignancies). Variables that correlate with survival in Hodgkin's lymphoma are often nonspecific, such as age at diagnosis and gender.

## RELATIONS AMONG FACTORS

For a variable to qualify as a useful prognostic factor, it must be significant, independent, and clinically important.[10] Many, if not all, variables are potentially of prognostic significance and many proved to be so in univariate analysis. However, variables are likely to be highly interrelated and some may be partial substitutes for one another, and few present with independent prognostic value. Moreover, factors exist that predict for a given therapy only; some for a given stage and some in the context of the presence of other factors. The use of multivariate statistical analyses is needed to assess which factors are independently significant and which only correlate with known prognostic factors but are without independent prognostic significance. This last point dramatically highlights the limits of prognostic studies, either retrospective or prospective, since the results highly depend on the variables available for all cases enrolled and the statistical model used.

## PROGNOSTIC FACTORS

### FIXED COVARIATES

As previously mentioned, agreed prognostic factors have been assessed in various settings. Table 70.1 summarizes

---

**Table 70.1  Prognostic factors shown to be independently significant**

| | |
|---|---|
| **In pathological stage I–II patients treated with radiotherapy alone** <br>   – Number of involved regions <br>   – Large tumor mass, *in particular mediastinal* <br>   – Tumor burden, i.e., combination of number of involved regions and tumor size in each region <br>   – B symptoms <br>   – Histologic subtype <br>   – Age <br>   – Gender | **In advanced disease** <br>   – Stage IV disease <br>   – Tumor burden <br>   – Very large mediastinal mass <br>   – Inguinal involvement <br>   – B symptoms <br>   – Erythrocyte sedimentation rate <br>   – Anemia <br>   – Serum albumin <br>   – Serum alkaline phosphatase <br>   – Leukocytosis <br>   – Lymphocytopenia <br>   – Serum LDH <br>   – Serum $\beta_2$-microglobulin <br>   – Histologic subtype <br>   – Age <br>   – Gender |
| **In clinical stage I–II patients treated with radiotherapy alone** <br>   – Number of involved regions <br>   – Disease confined to upper cervical nodes <br>   – Large mediastinal mass <br>   – B symptoms <br>   – Erythrocyte sedimentation rate <br>   – Anemia <br>   – Serum albumin <br>   – Histologic subtype <br>   – Age <br>   – Gender | |
| **In clinical stage I–II patients treated with combined-modality therapy** <br>   – Number of involved regions above the diaphragm <br>   – Large mediastinal mass <br>   – B symptoms <br>   – Erythrocyte sedimentation rate <br>   – Age <br>   – Gender | **Prognostic factors for laparotomy findings in supradiaphragmatic clinical stage I–II** <br>   – Number of involved regions above the diaphragm <br>   – Disease confined to upper cervical nodes <br>   – Mediastinal involvement <br>   – B symptoms <br>   – Erythrocyte sedimentation rate <br>   – Histologic subtype <br>   – Age <br>   – Gender |
| **In clinical stage I–II patients treated with chemotherapy alone**[a] <br>   – Number of involved regions <br>   – Tumor bulk <br>   – Age | |

[a]From one series only.[11]

factors shown to be independently significant on event-free survival (with event being relapse or treatment failure) in pathological stage I-II patients treated with radiotherapy alone, clinical stage I-II patients treated with radiotherapy alone, clinical stage I-II patients treated with combined-modality therapy, in those treated with chemotherapy alone (in one series only),[11] or in patients with advanced disease. Some of these factors have also proved to predict for laparotomy findings in supradiaphragmatic clinical stage I-II patients. Beside age and gender always mentioned, the number of involved regions, mediastinal involvement (more often bulky) or tumor burden, histologic subtype, B symptoms, and erythrocyte sedimentation rate are commonly reported over all settings. However, this data mostly concerns adult patients; very few are known in pediatric patients, thanks to the success obtained with combined-modality therapies since the late 70s.

### TIME-DEPENDENT COVARIATES

Similarly, prognostic factors for outcome after relapse have been reported according to initial treatment type or to the treatment given for relapse or refractory disease. In relapsing patients after initial treatment with radiotherapy alone who are given chemotherapy, the extent of disease at relapse, the type of relapse (nodal or extranodal), histologic subtype, and older age at relapse have been shown of prognostic value. In contrast, time to relapse usually does not correlate with outcome. In relapsing patients after initial chemotherapy alone or combined-modality therapy, two factors have consistently been associated with poor outcome: the response to initial treatment (complete remission, partial remission, no remission) and the duration of initial remission. These factors were independent of the type of second-line treatment. Other factors reported are the extent of disease at relapse, extranodal relapse, B symptoms at relapse, histologic subtype, stage IV at original diagnosis, and age and performance status. In relapsing patients undergoing high-dose chemotherapy and stem cell transplantation for relapse or refractory disease, several factors have shown to influence the prognosis: the response to initial treatment, the duration of initial remission, the number of failed treatments before the given relapse, and response to high-dose chemotherapy before transplantation. Other factors also reported are the extent of disease before transplantation, extranodal relapse, pleural involvement or multiple pulmonary nodules at relapse, B symptoms at relapse, increased serum lactic dehydrogenase (LDH) before transplantation, and poor performance status.

## PROGNOSTIC INDICES OR SCORES

As soon as factors have been identified to correlate with clinical outcome, investigators have combined all or part of these factors with the aim of obtaining a score that can predict for outcome: the higher the score, the lower the probability of remission, relapse or treatment failure-free survival, or overall survival. Scores were built from data accumulated in early or advanced stage patient series, enrolled or not in randomized clinical trials, or were based on individual data from randomized clinical trials analyzed using the meta-analysis approach. Only prognostic scores based on large series of patients or derived from adequate statistical analysis are reviewed next.

### PROGNOSTIC SCORES IN EARLY STAGES
#### British National Lymphoma Investigation (BNLI) index

In 1985, Haybittle and coworkers reported that age, gender, mediastinal involvement, pathologic grade based on histologic subtype, and erythrocyte sedimentation rate were independent prognostic factors on cause-specific survival in clinical stage I-IIA patients.[12] Using these factors, they derived a quantitative prognostic index based on the results of multivariate regression analysis performed on data from 743 patients. This index was expressed as follows:
I = 0.05 (age in years) + 1.0 (mediastinal involvement, coded 1 for uninvolved mediastinum, 2 for involved mediastinum) + 2.0 (pathologic grade, coded 1 if lymphocyte predominant or nodular sclerosing type 1, or 2 if nodular sclerosing type 2 or mixed cellularity) + 1.0 (erythrocyte sedimentation rate, coded 1 if below 10 mm/1st hour, 2 if between 10 and 39 mm/1st hour, and 3 if 40 mm/1st hour or above) − 1.2 (gender, coded 1 for male, 2 for female).

The index ranged from 2.5 for a young girl aged 15 without adverse factors to 11.5 for a man aged 70 with all adverse factors. In the BNLI series, the value of the index was I < 5.0 in 32% of patients, 5.0 ≤ I < 7.5 in 52%, and I ≥ 7.5 in 16%. A high index value (I ≥ 7.5) corresponded to high-risk patients, while patients with I < 7.5 had a low risk of cause-specific death whatever the level of the index.

#### German Hodgkin Study Group (GHSG) approach

The aim of the GHSG study was to adapt treatment in supradiaphragmatic clinical stage I-II patients according to their risk of occult infradiaphragmatic involvement. A retrospective multivariate analysis (logistic regression) was performed on pretherapeutic clinical characteristics of 391 laparotomized patients.[13] Twenty one percent had subdiaphragmatic disease. Of the factors (clinical including nodal presentation and biologic) tested, four independently correlated with infradiaphragmatic disease: left cervical involvement, mediastinal involvement, Karnofsky performance status less than 10, and histologic subtype (mixed cellularity or lymphocytic depletion). The regression coefficients were then used to derive a quantitative estimate of the probability of infradiaphragmatic disease for individual patients. It ended in defining two groups of patients at low or high risk. The low-risk group was composed of patients with no left cervical involvement, mediastinal involvement, and Karnofsky index equal to 10 (19% of patients), or with no left cervical involvement, mediastinal involvement, and lymphocyte predominant or nodular sclerosing histologic subtype (19% of patients), or with mediastinal involvement, Karnofsky index equal to 10 and lymphocyte predominant or nodular sclerosing histologic subtype (19% of patients). The high-risk group comprised of patients with left cervical involvement and mediastinal involvement (25% of patients), or with no mediastinal involvement and mixed cellularity or lymphocytic depletion histologic subtype (29% of patients). All other patients were considered with intermediate risk. The probability of infradiaphragmatic disease was 8% in patients at low risk and more than 35% in patients at high risk.

### European Organization for Research and Treatment of Cancer (EORTC) scoring system

Based on 25-year experience of the management of supradiaphragmatic early stage Hodgkin's lymphoma, the EORTC Lymphoma Group has defined treatment strategies based on prognostic factors with the objective of adapting the treatment aggressiveness (i.e., combined-modality therapy) to patients at high risk of treatment failure in order to avoid most treatment-related complications. In 1989, Tubiana and coworkers published the results of a multivariate analysis based on a total of 1579 patients enrolled into four successive randomized clinical trials over the 1964–1987 period.[14] Six factors were proven to independently correlate with either disease-free survival or overall survival: age (<40, 40–49, ≥50 years), gender, number of nodal areas involved (1, 2 or 3, 4 or 5), histologic type (lymphocyte predominant or nodular sclerosing), B symptoms, and erythrocyte sedimentation rate (<30, 30–49, ≥50 mm/1st hour). The originality of the publication consisted in the discussion on the balance that exists between two types of risk—the risk of treatment failure because of too light treatment and that of long-term complications following extended field irradiation or combined-modality therapy using aggressive chemotherapy. After multivariate analysis, three prognostic groups were defined. The very favorable group included females aged 39 years or less, with stage I disease, lymphocyte predominant or nodular sclerosing histologic subtype, no B symptoms, and erythrocyte sedimentation rate less than 30 mm/1st hour. They represented 6% of all patients. A simulation was performed to help in defining the unfavorable group of patients. Three options were discussed. Option A concerned patients aged 50 years or more, or with three or more nodal areas involved, or with no B symptoms and erythrocyte sedimentation rate more than or equal to 50 mm/1st hour, or with B symptoms and erythrocyte sedimentation rate more than or equal to 30 mm/1st hour. Forty-nine percent of patients were option A. Option B

had the same definition as option A except that only patients with four or five nodal areas involved were considered. Option B would include 38% of all patients. In option C, patients aged 50 years or more, or with four or five nodal areas involved, or patients aged 40–49 years with no B symptoms and erythrocyte sedimentation rate more than or equal to 50 mm/1st hour, or those with B symptoms and erythrocyte sedimentation rate more than or equal to 30 mm/1st hour were considered. Option C concerned 19% of patients. All other patients not fitting with very favorable or unfavorable definitions were considered in the favorable group, i.e., 45, 56, or 75% of all patients according to option A, B, or C, respectively. Based on the projected probability of disease-free survival and overall survival, option B was selected in the design of the H7 trial.[15] However, in this trial the presence of bulky mediastinal involvement qualified patients as an unfavorable prognostic group, although this factor was not included in the overall prognostic study performed because it was not recorded.[16] The EORTC scoring system, still in use since the H7 trial start, in particular in the two following trials H8 and H9, is presented in Table 70.2.[17–19]

Investigators who have defined a prognostic score they trust in are prone to use it in the design of the next study; they may also wait before its prognostic value is confirmed based on independent series. The design of the EORTC H7 trial was based on the newly defined EORTC scoring system; it also included an experimental strategy to test its validity. In the favorable group, patients were randomized to receive subtotal lymphoid and splenic irradiation (standard treatment) or six courses of EBVP (epirubicin, bleomycin, vinblastine, prednisone) followed by involved–field irradiation. In the unfavorable group, patients were randomized to receive six courses of MOPP/ABV (mechlorethamine, vincristine, procarbazine, prednisone, doxorubicin, bleomycin, vinblastine) hybrid and involved-field irradiation (standard treatment) or six courses of EBVP and involved-field irradiation. Beside the treatment comparison within each prognostic group, the trial design tested the prognostic value of the scoring system by comparing the two groups of patients treated with EBVP and involved-field irradiation. It is the only example of an experimental prospective design made to assess the value of a prognostic score.

## PROGNOSTIC SCORES IN ADVANCED STAGES
### St. Bartholomew's Hospital and Christie Hospital experience

Two series of patients with stage IIIB–IV were combined for a total of 301.[20] At both hospitals, patients were treated with combined-modality therapy. The end point was overall survival. Four factors emerged from multivariate analysis: age ≥45 years, male gender, absolute lymphocyte count less than 0.75 × 10⁹/L, and stage IV. Three prognostic groups could be defined. The low risk group was composed of patients aged less than

**Table 70.2** The European Organization for Research and Treatment of Cancer scoring system in supradiaphragmatic clinical stage I–II

| Factor | Score according to code |
|---|---|
| Age[a] | $< 40 = 0$, $40–49 = 1$, $\geq 50 = 9$ |
| Gender | Female = 0, male = 1 |
| Clinical stage[b] | I = 0, $II_{2-3} = 1$, $II_{4-5} = 9$ |
| B symptoms and ESR[c] | A and ESR $< 50 = 0$, B and ESR $< 30 = 1$ |
|  | A and ESR $\geq 50 = 9$ or B and ESR $\geq 30 = 9$ |
| Mediastinum[d] | Uninvolved or not bulky = 0, bulky involvement = 9 |
| Histologic subtype | Lymphocyte predominant or nodular sclerosing = 0 |
|  | Mixed cellularity or lymphocytic depletion = 1 |
| Total score | 0–38 |
| 0 | Patient belongs to the *very favorable* prognostic group |
| 1–4 | Patient belongs to the *favorable* prognostic group |
| $\geq 9$ | Patient belongs to the *unfavorable* prognostic group |

[a]In years.

[b]Five major nodal areas were defined as follows: the whole neck including the supraclavicular area (left and right); the axilla including the infraclavicular area (left and right); the whole mediastinum including the hilar nodes on both sides (one area) $II_{2-3}$, stage II with two or three nodal areas involved $II_{4-5}$, stage II with four or five nodal areas involved

[c]Erythrocyte sedimentation rate, in mm/first hour.

[d]Bulky mediastinal involvement if M/R ratio $\geq 0.35$ where M/T ratio is defined as the largest diameter of the mediastinum/ thoracic diameter at the T5-T6 level, in standing position.[16]

45 years with lymphocyte count more than $0.75 \times 10^9$ /L or female with stage IIIB (59% of patients). The high-risk group comprised male patients with stage IV disease, aged more than 45 years, or with lymphocyte count less than $0.75 \times 10^9$ /L (26% of patients). All other patients were included in the intermediate prognostic group (15% of patients). The difference in survival probability was highly significant ($P < 0.001$).

## Memorial Sloan-Kettering Cancer Center (MSKCC) experience

The series concerned 161 patients with stage IIB, IIIB, or IV disease who were treated between 1975 and 1984 according to two successive protocols.[21] All patients received combined-modality therapy. The main end point was overall survival. With multivariate analysis, five factors were shown to have independent prognostic value: age $\geq 45$ years, serum LDH $> 400$ UI/L, low (abnormal) hematocrit, inguinal involvement, and bulky mediastinal mass $\geq 0.45$ of the thoracic aperture. Since the regression coefficients corresponding to the five factors were of the same magnitude (range 1.49–2.99), each of them was considered with equal significance. Therefore, the prognostic score was derived from the sum of adverse factors present, theoretically ranging 0–5. Patients who expressed none or only one adverse factor (60% of all patients) were considered at low risk of death, while those with two or more (40% of patients) were considered at high risk of death. The same five factors plus one, bone marrow involvement, were used to predict for disease progression. Again, patients who expressed none or only one adverse factor displayed significantly better progres-sion-free survival rate at 4 years than those who expressed two or more factors.

## Italian experience

Gobbi and coworkers attempted to predict expected median survival time (EMST) including deaths from all causes.[22] Factors retained in the model were age, gender, clinical stage, histologic subtype, erythrocyte sedimentation rate, and serum albumin. A proposed equation was as follows: EMST = [326.9 − 64.6 erythrocyte sedimentation rate − 70.6 clinical stage − 60.2 histologic type − 40.4 age −29.9 serum albumin − 24.3 gender] × 0.693, that predicts a survival duration in months for a given individual.

## European bone marrow transplantation (EBMT) experience

In 1996, Federico and coworkers reported the predictive value of an index based on the MSKCC scoring system applied to stage III-IV disease with overall survival as endpoint.[23] Patients were considered at high risk of death if they presented with at least two of the following factors: mediastinal mass $\geq 0.45$, stage IV E+, high serum LDH, inguinal nodal involvement, low hematocrit, or bone marrow involvement.

## International Prognostic Index (IPI)

The International Prognostic Factors Project for Advanced Hodgkin's lymphoma was initiated by the GHSG to propose a score that could predict for both freedom from progression of disease and overall survival.[24] Twenty-five cooperative groups or institutions participated and a total of 5141 cases treated with combination chemotherapy for advanced Hogkin's disease, with or without radiotherapy, were collected. The IPI score was calculated from the set of patients with complete data (31% of all patients) and partially validated on an additional 2643 patients (51%) with not all data available. Seven factors displayed independent prognostic value on progression-free survival: serum albumin less than 4.0 g/dL, hemoglobin less than 10.5 g/dL, male gender, stage IV disease, age more than or equal to 45 years, white-cell count more than or equal to 15,000/mm$^3$, and lymphocyte count less than 600/mm$^3$ or 8% of white-cell count. All seven factors were associated with coefficients of risk that were similar (range 1.26–1.49). Therefore, the IPI score was calculated as the sum of the factors present, ranging from 0 to 7. Among the "working" patient group (N = 1618), the score was equal to 0 in 7%, 1 in 22%, 2 in 29%, 3 in 23%, 4 in 12%, and more than or equal to 5 in 7%. In the validation patient group (N = 2643), these figures were 7, 25, 31, 22, 11, and 4%, respectively. The score highly predicted for progression-free survival, and a proposal was made that patients be subgrouped in those presenting with 0–2 factors and those presenting with more than or equal to three factors. The IPI score also predicted for overall survival: the higher the score, the lower the survival rate. Later, Bierman and coworkers reported that the IPI score predicts for both event-free survival and overall survival in patients with advanced Hodgkin's lymphoma treated with autologous hematopoietic stem cell transplantation.[25] The IPI score could be calculated for 579 of the 739 advanced-stage patients enrolled into the EORTC H34 trial.[26] Forty percent of patients had 0–2 factors and 60% three factors or more. The 5-year progression-free survival rates were 84% and 74% in the two groups, respectively (P = 0.002), while the 8-year overall survival rates were 85% and 64% (P < 0.001) (unpublished data). The applicability of the IPI score to early stage disease (I-II-IIIA) was tested by the GHSG.[27] The IPI score was applied to patients enrolled into two consecutive trials and could be calculated in 961 (70%) of all patients. In patients with unfavorable early stage disease (clinical stage I–II with one or more GHSG risk factors, or IIA without any risk factor), the IPI score (0–2 vs ≥ 3) predicted for disease-free survival while it was found of no prognostic value in favorable early stage disease patients.

### PROGNOSTIC SCORES IN ALL STAGES
### Experience of the Scotland and Newcastle Lymphoma Group (SNLG) therapy working party
From 1979 to 1986, 723 Hodgkin's lymphoma patients were registered and detailed clinical and laboratory data were collected by the SNLG.[28] Sufficient information was available for 547 (76%) patients. Of these, 92 were used to develop a prognostic index and 455 for index validation. Almost half of the patients had stage III–IV disease. The end point used was overall survival.

Five factors were independently associated with a high risk of death with multivariate analysis: age, clinical stage, hemoglobin level, absolute lymphocyte count, and tumor bulk more than 10 cm. A prognostic index, I, was calculated as follows: I = 1.5858 − 0.0363 age + 0.0005 (age)$^2$ + 0.0683 clinical stage − 0.086 lymphocyte count − 0.0587 hemoglobin [+ 0.3 if bulky disease present], in which age is entered as an absolute figure, clinical stage is coded according to Ann Arbor classification (IA, IIA, IIIA coded 1, IB or IIB coded 2, IIIB coded 3, IV coded 4), absolute lymphocyte count is entered as a score (< 1.0 × 10$^9$/L coded 1, 1.0 – 1.5 × 10$^9$/L coded 2, > 1.5 – 2.0 x 10$^9$/L coded 3, > 2 × 10$^9$/L coded 4), and hemoglobin in g/dL is entered as an absolute figure. Bulky disease, if available, corresponds to the presence of a single node more than or equal to 5 cm or mediastinal to thoracic ratio more than 0.30. Applied to the patients in the validation group, the index demonstrated its ability to discriminate patients at high risk of death if I > 0.5. It was also able to discriminate patients with classical Ann Arbor stage IA and IIA disease with poor prognosis. Later, the SNLG index was used to select poor risk patients to receive intensive multiagent chemotherapy with or without autotransplant.[29]

### International Database on Hodgkin's lymphoma (IDHD) experience
In 1989, more than 14,000 cases were collected from 20 cooperative groups or institutions.[30] Data was used by Gobbi and coworkers to confirm the predictive equation that estimates for a given individual his/her EMST including deaths from all causes.[22,31] Factors selected were roughly similar to those previously published (see earlier section): age, gender, clinical stage, histologic subtype, B symptoms, serum albumin, and distribution of involved areas. An equation was derived: EMST = Exp [3.75 + 1.25 clinical stage I + 0.77 clinical stage II + 0.46 clinical stage III − 0.00046 age$^2$ + 0.85 histologic type + 0.42 B symptoms − ln (serum albumin in percentile) − 0.25 gender + 0.25 involved area distribution], with EMST expressed in months.

### EORTC Lymphoma Group experience
Of the nine randomized trials that the EORTC Lymphoma Group has conducted since 1964, five were selected that have tested modern therapies and provided similar results in term of event-free survival with treatment failure, progression, relapse, and death considered as events.[15-17,26,32] Overall, 3141 cases were available including 347 (11%) cases with advanced stage disease and low IPI score (0–2 adverse factors present). The distributions of the clinical and biological patient characteristics were similar within the five series except for bulky disease and the number of nodal areas involved that were significantly more often present among stage III-IV cases. Factors considered in the multivariate analysis included age, gender,

topography, clinical stage, mediastinal involvement, bulky disease, B symptoms, erythrocyte sedimentation rate, leukocyte count, neutrophil count, hemoglobin, and histologic subtype. In the final model performed on 2775 cases with all information available, four factors remained significant after stratification on treatment type: age more than or equal to 50 years, male gender, B symptoms, and neutrophil count more than or equal to 8000/mm$^3$. The corresponding coefficients ranged between 1.30 and 1.52, and a score was derived that considered the number of adverse factors present, i.e., 0–4. There were 23% of cases with no adverse factor, 45% with one factor, 25% with two factors, and 7% with three or four factors. The proportion of cases with three to four adverse factors was less than 1% in cases with early stage favorable prognostic features (1090 cases) according to the EORTC scoring system (Table 70.2), 12% in cases with early stage unfavorable prognostic features (1366 cases), and 11% in those with advanced stage and low IPI score (319 cases). While the progression-free survival curves of cases with zero, one, or two adverse factors did not significantly differ, that of cases with three to four factors was significantly lower. The 8-year progression-free survival rates were 86, 83, 80, and 68% in the four groups, respectively ($P < 0.001$) (unpublished data).

### PROGNOSTIC SCORES IN CHILDREN

In the last years, three groups have reported results of trials from which prognostic scoring systems have been issued. The French Society of Pediatric Oncology reported that female gender, B symptoms, nodular sclerosing histologic subtype, low hemoglobin ($< 10.5$ g/dL), and the presence of two of the following biologic factors—erythrocyte sedimentation rate more than 40 mm/1st hour, leukocytes more than $12 \times 10^9$/L, fibrinogen more than 5 g/L, $\alpha_2$–globulin less than 10 g/L, or albumin less than 35 g/L—significantly correlated (univariate analysis) with clinical outcome in 202 children with low-stage disease.[33] Patients were found at high risk if they presented with hemoglobin less than 10.5 g/dL and nodular sclerosing histologic subtype and at least two of the other five biologic factors (prognostic scale derived from multivariate analysis).

Smith and coworkers have reported the results of a prognostic factor analysis based on three series of patients treated with combined-modality therapy at three institutions.[34] Overall, the data of 328 pediatric patients was analyzed. Five factors were found of prognostic value on disease-free survival: male gender, stage IIB-IIIB-IV, bulky mediastinal disease, leukocytes more than $13.5 \times 10^3$/mm$^3$, and hemoglobin less than 11 g/dL. Because the coefficients of all five factors ranged from 1.92 to 2.08, the score proposed was equal to the sum of the factors expressed by the patient. Patients were divided into four groups with significantly different prognosis. The disease-free survival rate was 94% in patients with zero to one factor present

(50% of all patients), 85% in those with two factors (23% of patients), 71% with three factors (16% of patients), and 49% with four or five factors (11% of patients). The overall survival rate ranged from 99% to 92% for patients with less than or equal to three factors present while it was only 72% for those with four to five factors.

The German-Austrian Pediatric Hodgkin's lymphoma Study Group reported the results of a retrospective study on factors that could predict for event-free surviva.[35] Data from 552 children treated according to the HD-90 multicenter study was used. In this study, treatment was adapted to disease presentation, i.e., stage I–IIA, IIB–IIIA, and IIIB–IV. Significant univariate predictive factors were nodular sclerosing histologic subtype, B symptoms, number of involved regions and treatment. Using a multivariate regression model, only nodular sclerosing histologic subtype and B symptoms remained independent prognostic factors.

## LIMITS OF PROGNOSTIC FACTORS

Several limits can be listed that mainly depend on the kind of a given prognostic factor. One can distinguish prognostic factors whether they are objective or not, a situation that interferes with their definition.

### PROGNOSTIC FACTOR DEFINITION

Objective prognostic factors such as age, gender, height, weight, or biologic data can be estimated and their measure is generally not subjected to discussion. Automatic or validated instruments when available are very helpful. In biologic data measurement, knowledge of normal values according to either age or gender is required. However, nonobjective factors are more frequent than objective ones in the clinical research area. Histologic subtype and tumor bulk among many others can be selected as examples.

Assessment of histologic subtype depends on the experience of the pathologist and classification used. When a central review is organized involving senior experienced pathologists, very few discrepancies are noticed between diagnoses for a given case as well as few variations are observed in the distribution of various subtypes with time, i.e., within cohort of patients or studies. However, even when a central review exists, the prognostic value of pathology per se is controversial especially since the use of modern combined-modality therapy.

Tumor bulk is a recognized prognostic factor in Hodgkin's lymphoma. The way used in its evaluation, however, can very much influence the result. The Ann Arbor classification considers the number of lymph node regions involved, and their definition may vary from one study to the other. Some investigators include lung hilar nodes in the mediastinum, while others do not. In estimating mediastinal bulk, two ways of calculation have been proposed that provide different estimations.[16,36] Specht and colleagues have tried to precisely measure tumor burden and have demonstrated its prognostic value in early as well as advanced stages disease.[37–39] They used both the number of involved regions and the tumor size in each region. This approach may, however, be much difficult to apply in daily practice and sensitive to clinician attention. A more direct method of estimation of tumor burden was assessed by Gobbi and colleagues.[40] It consists of using images of the lesions obtained through computed tomography for all deep sites of involvement and those obtained by ultrasonography for superficial lesions. The sum of the volumes of the lesions is used as an estimation of the absolute tumor burden. Its ratio to the patient's body surface area represents the relative tumor burden. The latter parameter was demonstrated to be the most prognostic among all classical factors tested. Again, this approach depends highly on the radiologists' experience and their attention paid in measuring the volume of the lesions.

## ASSESSMENT OF PROGNOSTIC VALUE

While adequate statistical methods are now applied by most investigators, the material used varies from one series to the other. Prognostic factors were never assessed from a population-based series that are available from cancer registries only. The main reason is that data would be incomplete and heterogeneous and highly dependent upon the institution where the patients have been treated. Hospital-based series are biased and very often limited in number since Hodgkin's lymphoma is a rare disease. When a large single institution series is used, it generally includes patients treated over a long period of time during which treatments may have changed dramatically, leading to the loss of predictive power for most factors tested.[41] To overcome this difficulty, large homogeneous series are needed that may come from cooperative groups; alternatively, the combination of data from clinical trials with the same objectives (i.e., meta-analysis approach) has proved to be effective.

The prognostic value of scoring systems should be confirmed using independent series of patients. This approach can be applied within series when the analysis is made using a random sample of patients and the validation made using the remaining.[24] Another possibility is to apply and/or compare various scoring systems using an independent series.[42–44] Only factors or scoring systems that are consistently found of independent prognostic value in independent series should then be used.

## APPLYING PROGNOSTIC SCORES

Prognostic scores previously described can be grouped into two categories. The first category includes those that are easy to calculate, i.e., without the help of a calculator. A simple adding of adverse factors present is generally sufficient to select patients at low or high risk.

Among these are the scores proposed by the GHSG, the EORTC Lymphoma Group, the St Bartholomew's Hospital & Christie Hospital team, the MSKCC, the EBMT, and the IPI, and all scores derived from pediatric data.[13,15,20,21,23,24,33–35] The second category includes scores that necessitate more or less sophisticated calculation. It concerns the scores proposed by the BNLI, the SNLG, and by Gobbi et al.[12,22,28,31] Prognostic scores belonging to the second category have probably no chance to be used by others in contrast to the IPI score, for example, that has been adopted by most groups involved in the management of advanced stage disease.

## USE OF PROGNOSTIC FACTORS

### IN CLINICAL TRIALS

The use of prognostic factors in clinical trials usually corresponds to three purposes: study definition, stratification before randomization, and analysis of the trial results. In the definition of the study, prognostic factors are used as entry or exclusion criteria. This attitude is often based on ethical considerations since eligible patients are those for whom the benefits and risks of treatments are uncertain enough to justify randomization. It is the case in deescalation trials or in those in which better results are expected from more aggressive therapy. However, the use of prognostic factors in selecting patients may bias the trial recruitment since patient inclusion lies with the responsible local investigator who could decide to exclude borderline cases from the trial. Even central randomization does not prevent such a bias. Therefore, prognostic factors must be simple, clearly defined, easy to assess, and well accepted by all investigators participating in the trial.

Randomization is the only method to ensure comparability of the treatment groups concerning known and unknown factors. Currently randomization techniques provide adequate distribution between treatment groups especially when large numbers of patients are included. In small randomized trials, stratified randomization is designed to balance treatment allocation within predefined subgroups. However, the number of strata should be limited to avoid overstratification.

Prognostic factors not only serve in the description of the study population, they also play a role in analysis of the trial results. The omission of important known or unknown prognostic factors may bias the estimate of the treatment effect or reduce the statistical power.[45] The analysis of the results of a trial should include both univariate and multivariate tests for treatment effect. Consistent results will make the conclusion more convincing.

### IN DECISION ANALYSIS

Improvements achieved in the management and treatment of Hodgkin's lymphoma have been so important in the last 10–15 years that very few are expected in the near future. The proportion of patients cured of the disease is 90% or more in early stages and 80% or more in advanced stages. As a consequence, hematologists progressively change their objectives from better survival alone, to better survival and less late treatment-related toxicity. This concept forms the basis of most treatment strategies worldwide. Treatment strategies are usually based on the combination of known prognostic factors. In order to help investigators in selecting patients who should be offered a given treatment or to participate in a given controlled clinical trial, other approaches have been developed. Among these, decision analysis represents a tool that has been applied since the late 70s.[46–48] It is based on the use of definitions of patient risk groups (based on combinations of various prognostic factors) and on data derived from the literature. Applications have been made taking into consideration exploratory laparotomy and splenectomy, the use of stem cell transplantation, or the probability of late complications such as secondary malignancy, cardiac mortality, etc.[49–55]

## CONCLUSIONS

A large number of parameters are of prognostic significance in Hodgkin's lymphoma. A majority are more or less linked to the tumor mass itself. This is true not only for earlier mentioned factors but also for other biologic markers considered as putative prognostic factors, their prognostic significance having not yet been assessed using multivariate analysis applied to large series of cases.[56,57] Currently prevailing wisdom is to adapt treatment strategy to the a priori patient's prognosis, limiting treatment aggressiveness in patients with "favorable" prognostic factors (i.e., patients at low risk of progression/relapse) to reduce late toxicity, and increasing treatment intensity in patients with "unfavorable" prognostic factors to increase their chance of cure.

In the absence of a general consensus, factors currently used by investigators at various centers or cooperative groups are likely to differ for historical, educational, or economic reasons. This makes comparisons difficult between series, and almost impossible large-scale analysis. Adding new biologic parameters in the panoply will make it even more complicated. However, as measurable events such as treatment failure and death become rare, a huge number of patients should be prospectively followed to allow the emergence of new prognostic factors including biologic markers.[57] A general consensus on what factors should be systematically used in clinical research and on what are still a matter of debate would certainly be highly valuable.

## REFERENCES

1. Carbone PP, Kaplan HS, Musshoff K, et al.: Report of the Committee on Hodgkin's Disease Staging Classification. *Cancer Res* 31:1860, 1971.
2. Henry-Amar M, Aeppli DM, Anderson J, et al.: Workshop statistical report. In: Somers R, Henry-Amar M, Meerwaldt JH, Carde P (eds.) *Treatment Strategy in Hodgkin's Disease.* Colloque Inserm n° 196. London, Paris: Les Editions Inserm/John Libbey Eurotext; 1990: 169.
3. Lister TA, Crowther D, Sutcliffe SB, et al.: Report of a committee convened to discuss the evaluation and staging of patients with Hodgkin's disease: Cotswolds meeting. *J Clin Oncol* 7:1630, 1989. Erratum in *J Clin Oncol* 8: 1602, 1990.
4. Specht LK, Hasenclever D: Prognostic factors of Hodgkin's disease. In Mauch P, Armitage JO, Diehl V, Hoppe RT, Weiss L (eds.) *Hodgkin's Disease.* Philadelphia, PA: Lippincott Williams & Wilkins; 1999:295.
5. George SL: Identification and assessment of prognostic factors. *Semin Oncol* 15:462, 1988.
6. Byar DP: Identification of prognostic factors. In Buyse ME, Staquet MJ, Sylvester RL (eds.) *Cancer Clinical Trials: Methods and Practice.* Oxford: Oxford University Press; 1984:423.
7. Simon R: Importance of prognostic factors in cancer clinical trials. *Cancer Treat Rep* 68:185, 1984.
8. Byar DP: Problems with using observational databases to compare treatments. *Stat Med* 10:663, 1991.
9. Dixon DO, McLaughlin P, Hagemeister FB, et al.: Reporting outcomes in Hodgkin's disease and lymphoma. *J Clin Oncol* 5:1670, 1987.
10. Burke HB, Henson DE: Criteria for prognostic factors and for an enhanced prognostic system. *Cancer* 72:3131, 1993.
11. Pavlovsky S, Maschio M, Santarelli MT, et al.: Randomized trial of chemotherapy versus chemotherapy plus radiotherapy for stage I–II Hodgkin's disease. *J Natl Cancer Inst* 80:1466, 1988.
12. Haybittle JL, Hayhoe FGJ, Easterling MJ, et al.: Review of British National Lymphoma Investigation studies of Hodgkin's disease and development of prognostic index. *Lancet* I:967, 1985.
13. Rueffer U, Sieber M, Josting A, et al.: Prognostic factors for subdiaphragmatic involvement in clinical stage I-II supradiaphragmatic Hodgkin's disease: a retrospective analysis of the GHSG. *Ann Oncol* 10:1343, 1999.
14. Tubiana M, Henry-Amar M, Carde P, et al.: Towards comprehensive management tailored to prognosis factors of patients with clinical stages I and II in Hodgkin's disease. The EORTC Lymphoma Group controlled clinical trials: 1964–1987. *Blood* 73:47, 1989.
15. Noordijk EM, Carde P, Dupouy N, et al.: Combined-modality therapy for clinical stage I or II Hodgkin's lymphoma: long-term results of the European Organization for Research and Treatment of Cancer H7 randomized controlled trials. *J Clin Oncol* 24:3128, 2006.
16. Lee CKK, Bloomfield CD, Goldman AI, et al. Prognostic significance of mediastinal involvement in Hodgkin's

disease treated with curative radiotherapy. *Cancer* 46:2403, 1980.

17. Hagenbeek A, Eghbali H, Fermé C, et al.: Three cycles of MOPP/ABV hybrid and involved-field irradiation is more effective than subtotal nodal irradiation in favorable supradiaphragmatic clinical stages I-II Hodgkin's disease: Preliminary results of the EORTC–GELA H8-F randomized trial in 543 patients. *Blood* 96:575a, 2000. Abstract 2472.

18. Fermé C, Eghbali H, Hagenbeek A, et al.: MOPP/ABV hybrid and irradiation in unfavorable supradiaphragmatic clinical stages I–II Hodgkin's disease: Comparison of three treatment modalities. Preliminary results of the EORTC–GELA H8-U randomized trial in 995 patients. *Blood* 96:576a, 2000. Abstract 2473.

19. Noordijk EM, Thomas J, Fermé C, et al.: First results of the EORTC-GELA randomized trials: The H9-F trial (comparing 3 radiation dose levels) and H9-U trial (comparing 3 different chemotherapy schemes) in patients with favorable or unfavorable early stage Hodgkin's lymphoma. *J Clin Oncol* 23:561s, 2005. Abstract 6505.

20. Wagstaff J, Gregory WM, Swindell R, et al.: Prognostic factors for survival in stage IIIB and IV Hodgkin's disease: a multivariate analysis comparing two specialist centres. *Br J Cancer* 58:487, 1988.

21. Straus DJ, Gaynor JJ, Myers J, et al.: Prognostic factors among 185 adults with newly diagnosed advanced Hodgkin's disease treated with alternating potentially noncross-resistant chemotherapy and intermediate-dose radiation therapy. *J Clin Oncol* 8:1173, 1990.

22. Gobbi PG, Gobbi PG, Mazza P, et al.: Multivariate analysis of Hodgkin's disease prognosis. Fitness and use of a directly predictive equation. *Haematologica* 74:29, 1989.

23. Federico M, Clo V, Carella AM: High-dose therapy autologous stem cell transplantation vs. conventional therapy: analysis of clinical characteristics of 51 patients enrolled in the HD01 protocol. EBMT/ANZLG/Intergroup HD01 Trial. *Leukemia* 10(suppl. 2):s69, 1996.

24. Hasenclever D, Diehl V: A prognostic score for advanced Hodgkin's disease. International Prognostics Factors Project on advanced Hodgkin's disease. *N Engl J Med* 339:1506, 1998.

25. Bierman PJ, Lynch JC, Bociek RG, et al.: The International Prognostic Factors Project score for advanced Hodgkin's disease is useful for predicting outcome of autologous hematopoietic stem cell transplantation. *Ann Oncol* 13:1370, 2002

26. Aleman BMP, Raemaekers JMM, Tirelli U, et al.: Involved field radiotherapy for advanced Hodgkin's lymphoma. *N Engl J Med* 348:2396, 2003.

27. Franklin J, Paulus U, Lieberz D, et al.: Is the international prognostic score for advanced stage Hodgkin's disease applicable to early stage patients? German Hodgkin Lymphoma Study Group. *Ann Oncol* 11:617, 2000.

28. Proctor SJ, Taylor P, Donnan P, et al.: A numerical prognostic index for clinical use in identification of poor risk patients with Hodgkin's disease at diagnosis. Scotland and Newcastle Lymphoma Group (SNLG) Therapy Working Party. *Eur J Cancer* 27:624, 1991.

29. Proctor SJ, Mackie M, Dawson A, et al.: A population-based study of intensive multi-agent chemotherapy with or without autotransplant for the highest risk Hodgkin's disease patients identified by the Scotland and Newcastle Lymphoma Group (SNLG) prognostic index. A Scotland and Newcastle Lymphoma Group study (SNLG HD III). *Eur J Cancer* 38:795, 2002.

30. Somers R, Henry-Amar M, Meerwaldt JH, et al.: *Treatment Strategy in Hodgkin's Disease*. Colloque Inserm n° 196. London, Paris: Les Editions Inserm/John Libbey Eurotext; 1990.

31. Gobbi PG, Comelli M, Grignani GE, et al.: Estimate of expected survival at diagnosis in Hodgkin's disease: a means of weighting prognostic factors and a tool for treatment choice and clinical research. A report from the International Database on Hodgkin's Disease (IDHD). *Haematologica* 79:241, 1994.

32. Carde P, Hagenbeek A, Hayat M, et al.: Clinical staging versus laparotomy and combined modality with MOPP versus ABVD in early stages Hodgkin's disease : The H6 twin randomized trials from the EORTC Lymphoma Cooperative Group. *J Clin Oncol* 11:2258, 1993.

33. Landman-Parker J, Pacquement H, Leblanc T, et al.: Localized childhood Hodgkin's disease: response adapted chemotherapy with etoposide, bleomycin, vinblastine, and prednisone before low-dose radiation therapy. Results of the French Society of Pediatric Oncology study MDH90. *J Clin Oncol* 18:1500, 2000.

34. Smith RS, Chen Q, Hudson MM: Prognostic factors for children with Hodgkin's disease treated with combined-modality therapy. *J Clin Oncol* 21:2026, 2003.

35. Dieckmann K, Potter R, Hoffman J, et al.: Does bulky disease at diagnosis influence outcome in childhood Hodgkin's disease and require higher radiation doses? Results from the German-Austrian Pediatric Multicenter Trial DAL-HD90. *Int J Radiat Oncol Biol Phys* 56:644, 2003.

36. Piro AJ, Weiss DR, Hellman S: Mediastinal Hodgkin's disease: a possible danger for intubation anesthesia. Intubation danger in Hodgkin's disease. *Int J Radiat Oncol Biol Phys* 1:415, 1976.

37. Specht L, Nordentoft AM, Cold S, et al.: Tumour burden in early stage Hodgkin's disease: the single most important prognostic factor for outcome after radiotherapy. *Br J Cancer* 55:535, 1987.

38. Specht L, Nordentoft AM, Cold S, et al.: Tumor burden as the most important prognostic factor in early stage Hodgkin's disease. Relations to other prognostic factors and implications for choice of treatment. *Cancer* 61:1719, 1988.

39. Specht L, Nissen NI: Prognostic factors in Hodgkin's disease stage III with special reference to tumour burden. *Eur J Haematol* 41:80, 1988.

40. Gobbi PG, Ghirardelli ML, Solcia M, et al.: Image-aided estimate of tumor burden in Hodgkin's disease: evidence of its primary prognostic importance. *J Clin Oncol* 19:1388, 2001.

41. Hasenclever D: The disappearance of prognostic factors in Hodgkin's disease. *Ann Oncol* 13(suppl. 1):75, 2002.

42. Fermé C, Bastion Y, Brice P: Prognosis of patients with advanced Hodgkin's disease. Evaluation of four prognostic models using 344 patients included in the Groupe d'Études des Lymphomes de l'Adulte study. *Cancer* 80:1124, 1997.

43. Bettini R, Tonolini M, Maccianti E: Verification and comparison of two different predictive equations in Hodgkin's disease. *Hematologica* 82:324, 1997.

44. Gobbi PG, Zinzani PL, Broglia C, et al.: Comparison of prognostic models in patients with advanced Hodgkin's disease. Promising results from integration of the best three systems. *Cancer* 91:1467, 2001.

45. Schmoor C, Shumacher M: Effects of covariate omission and categorization when analyzing randomized trials with the Cox model. *Stat Med* 16:225, 1997.

46. Safran C, Tsichlis PN, Bluming AZ, et al.: Diagnostic planning using computer assisted decision-making for patients with Hodgkin's disease. *Cancer* 39:2426, 1977.

47. Fineberg HV: Decision trees: construction, uses, and limits. *Bull Cancer* 67:395, 1980.

48. Desforges JF: Diagnostic planning using computer assisted decision-making for the patient with Hodgkin's disease. *Bull Cancer* 67:418, 1980.

49. Corder MP, Ellwein LB: A decision-analysis methodology for consideration of morbidity factors in clinical decision-making. *Am J Clin Oncol* 7:19, 1984.

50. Corder MP, Ellwein LB: Comparison of treatments for symptomatic Hodgkin's lymphoma employing decision analysis. *Am J Clin Oncol* 7:33, 1984.

51. Desch CE, Lasala MR, Smith TJ, et al.: The optimal timing of autologous bone marrow transplantation in Hodgkin's disease patients after a chemotherapy relapse. *J Clin Oncol* 10:200, 1992.

52. Hess CF, Kortmann RD, Schmidberger H, et al.: How relevant is secondary leukaemia for initial treatment selection in Hodgkin's disease? *Eur J Cancer* 30A:1441, 1994.

53. Ng AK, Weeks JC, Mauch PM, et al.: Laparotomy versus no laparotomy in the management of early-stage, favorable-prognosis Hodgkin's disease: a decision analysis. *J Clin Oncol* 17:241, 1999.

54. Ng AK, Weeks JC, Mauch PM, et al.: Decision analysis on alternative treatment strategies for favorable-prognosis, early-stage Hodgkin's disease. *J Clin Oncol* 17:3577, 1999.

55. Ng AK, Kuntz KM, Mauch PM, et al.: Costs and effectiveness of staging and treatment options in early-stage Hodgkin's disease. *Int J Radiat Oncol Biol Phys* 50:979, 2001.

56. Axdorph U, Sjöberg J, Grimfors G, et al.: Biological markers may add to prediction of outcome achieved by the international prognostic score in Hodgkin's disease. *Ann Oncol* 11:1405, 2000.

57. Zander T, Wiedenmann S, Wolf J: Prognostic factors in Hodgkin's lymphoma. *Ann Oncol* 13(suppl. 1):67, 2002.

# Chapter 71

# CLASSIFICATION, PATHOLOGY, AND MOLECULAR GENETICS OF HODGKIN'S LYMPHOMA

*James R. Cook and Eric D. Hsi*

## CELL OF ORIGIN AND EVIDENCE OF DISRUPTED B-CELL TRANSCRIPTION FACTOR EXPRESSION

The nature and cell of origin of Hodgkin's disease (HD) has been the subject of debate since the initial description of HD in 1830.[1] Not until the mid-1990s was it recognized that the Reed-Sternberg was derived from B-cells and was in most cases a monoclonal proliferation.[2–5] These studies utilized single-cell polymerase chain reaction (PCR) from Reed-Sternberg cells to demonstrate monoclonal *IGH* rearrangements. In the pivotal study, Marafioti and colleagues examined 25 cases of HD by single-cell PCR with amplification of *IGH* or *IGK* genes. Twenty-four cases revealed gene rearrangements. Comparison of the PCR products showed that all cases were clonal and 75% of the cases had the capacity for productive rearrangements.[5] Furthermore, while the immunoglobulin (*Ig*) genes were theoretically functional, there was no transcription of *Ig* genes due to defects in the Ig gene regulatory elements.[5]

Analysis of the *IGH* sequences of Reed-Sternberg cells showed a high load of somatic mutations. The presence of these mutations, which occurs in the germinal center in normal B-cells sets the germinal center B-cell as the stage of B-cell maturation for most Reed-Sternberg cells. This concept is supported by studies of composite Hodgkin's lymphoma (HL) and non-Hodgkin's lymphoma in which a common precursor to the two lymphomas can be traced by *IGH* sequence to a germinal center type B-cell.[5,6] The results of these studies firmly establish HD as HL, a monoclonal B-cell proliferation of cells derived from germinal center or postgerminal center B-cells in the vast majority of cases.

More recent studies provide insight into the mechanisms for a disrupted B-cell transcriptional program.

Oct-2, Bob-1, and Pu.1 are important B-cell transcription factors that have all been shown to be down regulated in classical Hodgkin's lymphoma (cHL).[7–10] While they are seen in nodular lymphocyte predominant HL (nLPHL) and other B-cell lymphomas, the absence of these transcription factors serves both as an explanation for lack of Ig transcription and expression in cHL lymphoma as well as a diagnostic marker for this lymphoma. This lack of Ig expression is somewhat problematic since in normal B-cell development, the lack of Ig expression leads to apoptosis. Therefore, other genetic mechanisms must be operative to protect the cell from this fate. One explanation is overexpression of NFκB. This ubiquitous transcription factor has numerous functions in promoting cell survival and proliferation. Recent studies demonstrate the constitutive expression of activated (nuclear) NFκB in HL and that defective IkBα (an inhibitor of NFκB) is a mechanism responsible for this.[11–13] With this as background, we proceed with the pathology and classification of HL.

## CLASSIFICATION OF HODGKIN'S LYMPHOMA

The classification of HL has undergone substantial changes over the last decade, reflecting an improved understanding of the underlying biology of this neoplasm.[14] In 1966, the Rye conference modified the earlier Lukes and Butler classification system to produce four histologic subtypes of HD: Lymphocyte predominance, nodular sclerosis, mixed cellularity, and lymphocyte depletion.[15,16] This scheme was widely used for the next 30 years. The Rye classification was popular among pathologists for its simplicity and ease of use and was equally popular among clinicians because the individual subtypes were associated with prognostic differences when treated with then-current therapy.[17]

| Table 71.1 | Classification of Hodgkin's Lymphoma | |
| --- | --- | --- |
| Rye (1966) | REAL (1996) | WHO (2001) |
| Lymphocyte predominance | Lymphocyte predominance | Nodular lymphocyte predominance |
| Nodular sclerosis | Classical Hodgkin's Disease | Classical Hodgkin Lymphoma |
| Mixed cellularity | – Nodular sclerosis | – Nodular sclerosis |
| Lymphocyte depleted | – Mixed cellularity<br>– Lymphocyte depleted | – Mixed cellularity<br>– Lymphocyte depleted |

As immunophenotypic studies became part of the standard practice of hematopathology, however, it became clear that many of the cases diagnosed as lymphocyte predominance HD displayed biologic and clinical features that separated these cases from all of the other forms of HD. In addition, with improvements in standard therapy, the earlier prognostic differences between the other subtypes of HD essentially vanished. To reflect these advances, the classification of HD was modified in the revised European-American lymphoma (REAL) classification of 1994 into two large categories: lymphocyte predominance HD and classical HD.[18] The remaining histologic subtypes of the Rye classification were retained under the heading of classical HD. In addition, the term "lymphocyte-rich classical HD" was introduced to identify cases containing a lymphoid rich background, but an immunophenotype that was identical to the other forms of classical HD and to separate such cases from lymphocyte predominance HD (Table 71.1). The WHO classification of 2001 retained the overall organization of the REAL classification. However, the term "Hodgkin's disease" was replaced by "Hodgkin's lymphoma" to represent the now-definitive lymphoid histogenesis of this malignancy, and the characteristic nodular growth pattern of cases of lymphocyte predominant HL was explicitly acknowledged.[19]

## CLASSICAL HODGKIN'S LYMPHOMA

In the WHO classification, four histologic subtypes of cHL are recognized.[19] While each of these subtypes display similar immunophenotypes and molecular genetic features, there are characteristic differences in morphology and in association with the Epstein-Barr virus. The next section will first discuss the general features of cHL common to each of the subtypes, followed by descriptions of each of the subtypes that will discuss their more specific associations.

### COMMON FEATURES IN ALL SUBTYPES
#### General
Classical Hodgkin's lymphoma is a neoplasm of B-cell origin that is histologically composed of multinucleate Reed-Sternberg cells and mononuclear variants, known as Hodgkin cells.[19] Cases of otherwise typical cHL have been described that appear to be of T-cell origin, but such cases are very rare, and their most appropriate classification is a subject of controversy.[20–22] cHL is much more common than nLPHL, with cHL representing about 95% of all HL. There is a bimodal age distribution, with the first peak around 15–35 years of age, and a second peak in elderly populations. Patients typically present with nodal disease, most often involving the cervical region. Secondary involvement of extranodal sites may occur, but primary presentation at extranodal locations is unusual.

### Pathology
The lymph nodes are effaced by a proliferation of Reed-Sternberg cells and mononuclear Hodgkin variants that is accompanied by an often extensive benign, inflammatory infiltrate. Reed-Sternberg cells are defined as large cells with abundant cytoplasm, and at least two distinct nuclear lobes, each of which contain a prominent eosinophilic nucleolus. The mononuclear Hodgkin variants are large cells with a usually round nucleus and prominent nucleolus. The Reed-Sternberg and Hodgkin cells generally constitute only a small minority of the cells present in histologic sections, and in some cases the malignant cells may be quite rare. In modern practice, a definitive diagnosis of HL cannot be established by morphologic features alone, but requires confirmation by immunohistochemistry.

### Immunophenotype
The neoplastic cells in cHL are almost always positive for CD30,[23,24] and a large percentage of cases coexpress CD15 (70–80%)[24,25] and PAX5 (up to 90%) (Figure 71.1).[26,27] cHL is usually negative for CD45 and J-chain. CD20 may be found in a subset of cases but is usually present on only a minority of the neoplastic cells and expressed with variable intensity. The finding of strong CD20 expression on a large percentage of Reed-Sternberg-like cells suggests the diagnosis of a B-cell lymphoma, such as T-cell rich large B-cell lymphoma.[19] The B-cell transcription factors OCT-2 and/or BOB.1 are characteristically absent.[9] Occasionally, other B-cell antigens such as CD79a may be present. Some cases may show aberrant expression of T-cell antigens, but the finding of multiple T-cell antigens should raise the possibility of a T-cell neoplasm, such as anaplastic large cell lymphoma.

### Molecular genetics
Classical cytogenetic studies of cHL are often unsuccessful, or demonstrate only a normal karyotype. The failure of such studies to characterize the malignant cells likely is secondary to the difficulty in isolating the neoplastic cells, which typically represent only a small percentage of the cells present, combined with poor growth of the neoplastic cells in culture. When abnor-

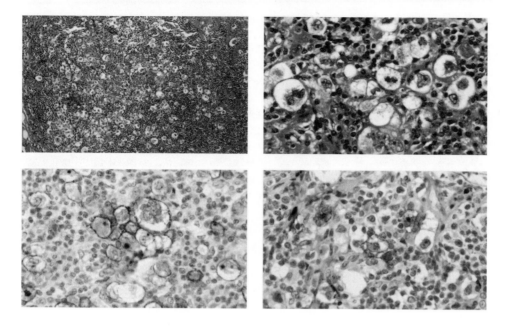

**Figure 71.1** *Nodular sclerosis Hodgkin's lymphoma. The lymph node is effaced by a lymphoid proliferation that is separated into nodules by dense collagenous bands of fibrosis (upper left). The nodules contain numerous Reed-Sternberg cells and mononuclear variants (upper right). The neoplastic cells are positive for CD30 (lower left) and CD15 (lower right)*

malities are identified, karyotypes are typically quite complex and hypertetraploidy is common.[28,29] Specific recurrent abnormalities, however, have not been identified. Clonal rearrangements of the Ig heavy chain are present in the vast majority of cases, although highly specialized, nonstandard laboratory techniques such as microdissection or single-cell PCR studies may be required to demonstrate this finding as noted earlier in this chapter. Cases with clonal T-cell receptor rearrangements appear to be very rare, and the nature of such cases is a matter of controversy.[19] In EBV positive cases, clonality of the epstein-barr virus (EBV) genome may also be identified.[30]

### NODULAR SCLEROSIS HODGKIN'S LYMPHOMA
#### General
Nodular sclerosis Hodgkin's lymphoma (NSHL) is defined as cHL where nodules of tumor cells are surrounded by bands of collagenous fibrosis. NSHL represents the most common subtype of cHL.[19]

#### Pathology
The malignant cells in NSHL include lacunar Reed-Sternberg cells, large neoplastic cells with abundant cytoplasm and characteristic retraction artifact when fixed in formalin. Bands of collagenous fibrosis surround a proliferation of Reed-Sternberg and Hodgkin cells admixed with small lymphocytes, large transformed cells, eosinophils, plasma cells, and other inflammatory cells (Figure 71.1). Some of the neoplastic cells demonstrate a shrunken, hyperchromatic appearance that has been described as "mummified" cells. When sheets of Reed-Sternberg and Hodgkin cells are present, the term "syncytial variant NHSL" has been employed.

Several grading systems have been proposed for NHSL based upon the number of Reed-Sternberg/Hodgkin

cells present. The most commonly used of these is the BNLI system, which divides cases into two grades.[31] In grade 2 NSHL, sheets of Reed-Sternberg/Hodgkin cells are present in at least 25% of the nodules. Grade 1 cases, in contrast, contain fewer neoplastic cells. Although frequently used in research protocols, this grading scheme has not gained acceptance in routine clinical practice in the United States.

#### EBV association
The incidence of EBV positivity varies with the ethnic groups studied, but is approximately 20–40% in NSHL.[30,32,33]

### MIXED CELLULARITY HODGKIN'S LYMPHOMA
#### General
The mixed cellularity Hodgkin's lymphoma (MCHL) subtype is defined by the WHO as containing scattered classical Reed-Sternberg and Hodgkin cells in a diffuse or vaguely nodular mixed inflammatory background without nodular fibrosis. MCHL is the second most common type of cHL and represents approximately 20–25% of cases.[19]

#### Pathology
Histologic sections of MCHL demonstrate effacement of the lymph node architecture by scattered Reed-Sternberg cells and variants in a diffuse or vaguely nodular mixed inflammatory proliferation (Figure 71.2). Often, there are numerous small lymphocytes, plasma cells, eosinophils, histiocytes, or neutrophils, although the relative numbers of each of these cell types varies from case to case.

#### EBV association
Approximately 75% of cases are positive for EBV.[30,32,33]

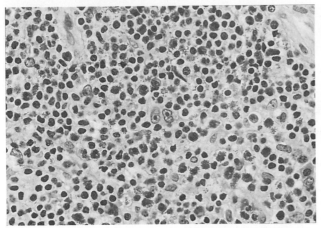

**Figure 71.2** *Mixed cellularity Hodgkin's lymphoma. A binucleate Reed-Sternberg cell is seen surrounded by small lymphocytes, eosinophils, and plasma cells*

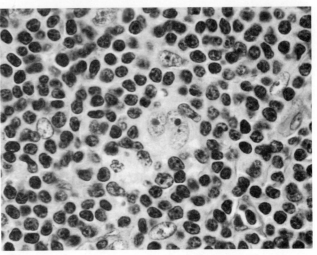

**Figure 71.4** *Lymphocyte-rich classical Hodgkin's lymphoma. At high power, a binucleate Reed-Sternberg cell is present surrounded by numerous small lymphocytes*

## LYMPHOCYTE-RICH CLASSICAL HODGKIN'S LYMPHOMA

### General

Lymphocyte-rich cHL (LRCHL) is defined as cHL containing Reed-Sternberg cells and variants in a nodular or diffuse background of numerous lymphocytes without prominent neutrophils and eosinophils.[19] Establishing a diagnosis of LRCHL, and in particular, distinguishing such cases from nLPHL, requires immunohistochemical studies. LRCHL accounts for approximately 5% of HL overall.

### Pathology

Cases of LRCHL typically display a nodular growth pattern with some of the nodules containing germinal centers. There are scattered Reed-Sternberg cells and variants, usually within the mantle zones surrounding germinal centers (Figures 71.3 and 71.4). Some of the

**Figure 71.3** *Lymphocyte-rich classical Hodgkin's lymphoma. At low power, there is a lymphoid-rich infiltrate with a predominantly diffuse growth pattern. A residual germinal center is seen (center right)*

malignant cells may show multiple folded nuclear lobes ("popcorn cells"), reminiscent of those seen in nLPHL. There is no nodular sclerosis. Although rare scattered eosinophils and neutrophils may be present, they are not a prominent feature.

### EBV association

Most cases are EBV negative.[30,32,33]

## LYMPHOCYTE-DEPLETED CLASSICAL HODGKIN'S LYMPHOMA

### General

The definition of lymphocyte-depleted classical Hodgkin's lymphoma (LDCHL) has changed dramatically over the years. Using WHO criteria, LDCHL is now defined as a diffuse proliferation of numerous Reed-Sternberg cells and variants (with an appropriate immunophenotype) without accompanying lymphocytes. Many of the cases that in the past were classified as lymphocyte depletion based upon hematoxylin and eosin morphology alone would currently be categorized as either non-Hodgkin's lymphomas (especially anaplastic large cell lymphomas) or so-called "syncytial variant" nodular sclerosis cHL. As currently defined, LDCHL is a rare entity, and there is little reliable data in the literature regarding such cases. In Western countries, this subtype appears to be somewhat more common in patients with HIV or other types of immunosuppression.

### Pathology

LDCHL typically displays numerous Reed-Sternberg cells and variants, often present in sheets, raising a differential diagnosis that includes non-Hodgkin's lymphomas. In some cases, the neoplastic cells may be scattered in a background of diffuse fibrosis. In all cases, there are very few accompanying small lymphocytes.

**EBV association**

Most of the HIV-associated cases will be positive for EBV.[34,35]

## NODULAR LYMPHOCYTE PREDOMINANT HODGKIN'S LYMPHOMA

### GENERAL

Nodular lymphocyte predominant HL is a neoplasm of germinal center B-cells that displays a growth pattern that is at least partially nodular. Whether an entirely diffuse form of LPHL exists has been controversial, and most cases formerly reported as diffuse LPHL are currently thought to represent either T-cell rich large B-cell lymphomas or LRCHL.[19] Overall, nLPHL represents approximately 5% of all cases of HL.

An intriguing association between nLPHL and a form of benign hyperplasia known as progressive transformation of germinal centers (PTGC) has led to the suggestion that PTGC may represent a precursor lesion for nLPHL.[36] PTGC may be seen within the same lymph node containing nLPHL, or PTGC may be found in biopsies without evidence of malignancy obtained either before or after the diagnosis of nLPHL. It should be noted, however, that most patients with PTGC do not go on to develop nLPHL.[37]

A small subset of patients, approximately 3–5%,[19] will go on to develop a large B-cell lymphoma. Many of these cases display the morphologic features of T-cell rich large B-cell lymphoma (TCRLBL). In fact, although the clinical features of nLPHL and TCRLBL are quite distinct, it can be difficult in some cases to distinguish between these two entities based on morphologic and immunophenotypic findings.

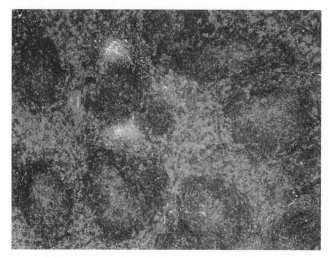

**Figure 71.5** *Nodular lymphocyte predominant Hodgkin's lymphoma. A nodular proliferation of lymphocytes and histiocytes is present*

Recognition of such cases with features overlapping nLPHL and TCRLBL has led to the suggestion that these two neoplasms may be biologically related.[38,39]

### PATHOLOGY

The neoplastic cells of nLPHL are large cells with vesicular chromatin, scant cytoplasm, and folded nuclear contours. Due to the characteristically extreme nuclear lobation, these cells are frequently described as "popcorn cells." These cells are also known as "L&H cells," a holdover of terminology from the Lukes and Butler classification that defined such cases as "lymphocytic and histiocytic Hodgkin disease."[16] Prototypical cases of nLPHL show effacement of the lymph node architecture by a nodular lymphoid proliferation. The nod-

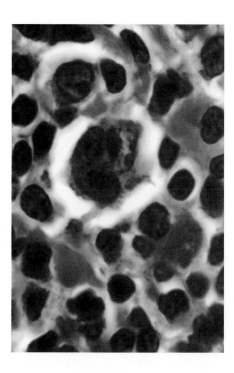

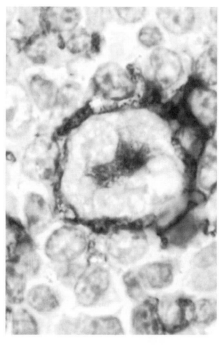

**Figure 71.6** *Nodular lymphocyte predominant Hodgkin's lymphoma. The neoplastic cells in nLPHL show multiple nuclear lobes with vesicular chromatin and prominent nucleoli (left). There is strong expression of CD20 (right)*

ules consist of many small B-cells, with scattered L&H cells (Figures 71.5 and 71.6).[17,40,41] Similar appearing diffuse areas may also be present. When diffuse areas are extensive, distinguishing nLPHL from TCRLBL may be quite difficult, especially in small biopsy specimens.

### IMMUNOPHENOTYPE

Establishing a definitive diagnosis of nLPHL, and distinguishing such cases from cHL, requires immunophenotypic studies. The neoplastic cells are positive for CD20 (Figure 71.6) and CD45 (LCA) and are characteristically negative for CD15 and CD30.[18,19,40] The L&H cells are also positive for the B-cell transcription factors, Oct-2 and BOB.1,[9] and are typically positive for the Ig-joining segment known as J-chain.[42] Approximately half of cases

are positive for epithelial membrane antigen (EMA).[19,40] Another helpful phenotypic feature of nLPHL is that the neoplastic cells are typically ringed by small T-cells that often coexpress CD57.[43,44] The presence of nodules of CD21 positive follicular dendritic cells also assists in the differential diagnosis with TCRLBL.[41]

### MOLECULAR GENETICS

Functional, clonal Ig rearrangements are generally present in the neoplastic cells. However, clonal rearrangements are rarely detected by PCR or Southern blot studies of intact tissue and have usually been identified only after single-cell microdissection.[19] Characteristic recurrent cytogenetic abnormalities have not been described.

### REFERENCES

1. Hodgkin T: On some morbid appearances of the absorbent glands and spleen. *Med Chir Trans* 17:69–97, 1832.
2. Kuppers R, Rajewsky K, Zhao M, et al.: Hodgkin disease: Hodgkin and Reed-Sternberg cells picked from histological sections show clonal immunoglobulin gene rearrangements and appear to be derived from B cells at various stages of development. *Proc Natl Acad Sci USA* 91:10962–10966, 1994.
3. Kanzler H, Kuppers R, Hansmann ML, Rajewsky K: Hodgkin and Reed-Sternberg cells in Hodgkin's disease represent the outgrowth of a dominant tumor clone derived from (crippled) germinal center B cells. *J Exp Med* 184:1495–1505, 1996.
4. Hummel M, Ziemann K, Lammert H, Pileri S, Sabattini E, Stein H: Hodgkin's disease with monoclonal and polyclonal populations of Reed-Sternberg cells. *N Engl J Med* 333:901–906, 1995.
5. Marafioti T, Hummel M, Foss HD, et al.: Hodgkin and Reed-Sternberg cells represent an expansion of a single clone originating from a germinal center B-cell with functional immunoglobulin gene rearrangements but defective immunoglobulin transcription. *Blood* 95:1443–1450, 2000.
6. Marafioti T, Hummel M, Anagnostopoulos I, Foss HD, Huhn D, Stein H: Classical Hodgkin's disease and follicular lymphoma originating from the same germinal center B cell. *J Clin Oncol* 17:3804–3809, 1999.
7. Laumen H, Nielsen PJ, Wirth T: The BOB.1 / OBF.1 coactivator is essential for octamer-dependent transcription in B cells. *Eur J Immunol* 30:458–469, 2000.
8. Re D, Muschen M, Ahmadi T, et al.: Oct-2 and Bob-1 deficiency in Hodgkin and Reed Sternberg cells. *Cancer Res* 61:2080–2084, 2001.
9. Stein H, Marafioti T, Foss HD, et al.: Down-regulation of BOB.1/OBF.1 and Oct2 in classical Hodgkin disease but not in lymphocyte predominant Hodgkin disease correlates with immunoglobulin transcription. *Blood* 97:496–501, 2001.
10. Torlakovic E, Tierens A, Dang HD, Delabie J: The transcription factor PU.1, necessary for B-cell development is expressed in lymphocyte predominance, but not classical Hodgkin's disease. *Am J Pathol* 159:1807–1814, 2001.
11. Bargou RC, Emmerich F, Krappmann D, et al.: Constitutive nuclear factor-kappaB-RelA activation is required for proliferation and survival of Hodgkin's disease tumor cells. *J Clin Invest* 100:2961–2969, 1997.
12. Krappmann D, Emmerich F, Kordes U, Scharschmidt E, Dorken B, Scheidereit C: Molecular mechanisms of constitutive NF-kappaB/Rel activation in Hodgkin/Reed-Sternberg cells. *Oncogene* 18:943–953, 1999.
13. Wood KM, Roff M, Hay RT: Defective IkappaBalpha in Hodgkin cell lines with constitutively active NF-kappaB. *Oncogene* 16:2131–2139, 1998.
14. Harris NL: Hodgkin's lymphomas: classification, diagnosis, and grading. *Semin Hematol* 36;220–232, 1999.
15. Lukes RJ, Craver L, Hall T, Rappapart H, Ruben P: Report of the Nomenclature Committee. *Cancer Res* 26:1311, 1966.
16. Lukes RJ, Butler JJ: The pathology and nomenclature of Hodgkin's disease. *Cancer Res* 26:1063–1083, 1966.
17. Butler JJ: Relationship of histological findings to survival in Hodgkin's disease. *Cancer Res* 31:1770–1775, 1971.
18. Harris NL, Jaffe ES, Stein H, et al.: A revised European-American classification of lymphoid neoplasms: a proposal from the International Lymphoma Study Group. *Blood* 84:1361–1392, 1994.
19. Stein H, Delsol G, Pileri S, et al.: Classical Hodgkin lymphoma. *Tumours of Haematopoietic and Lymphoid Tissues.* Lyon, France: IARC Press; 2001:244–253.
20. Kadin ME, Drews R, Samel A, Gilchrist A, Kocher O: Hodgkin's lymphoma of T-cell type: clonal association with a CD30+ cutaneous lymphoma. *Hum Pathol* 32:1269–1272, 2001.
21. Muschen M, Rajewsky K, Brauninger A, et al.: Rare occurrence of classical Hodgkin's disease as a T cell lymphoma. *J Exp Med* 191:387–394, 2000.
22. Seitz V, Hummel M, Marafioti T, Anagnostopoulos I, Assaf C, Stein H: Detection of clonal T-cell receptor gamma-chain gene rearrangements in Reed-Sternberg cells of classic Hodgkin diseases. *Blood* 95:3020–3024, 2000.
23. Stein H, Gerdes J, Kirchner H, Schaadt M, Diehl V: Hodgkin and Sternberg-Reed cell antigen(s) detected by an antiserum to a cell line (L428) derived from Hodgkin's disease. *Int J Cancer* 28:425–429, 1981.

24. Stein H, Mason DY, Gerdes J, et al.: The expression of the Hodgkin's disease associated antigen Ki-1 in reactive and neoplastic lymphoid tissue: evidence that Reed-Sternberg cells and histiocytic malignancies are derived from activated lymphoid cells. *Blood* 66:848–858, 1985.

25. Stein H, Uchanska-Ziegler B, Gerdes J, Ziegler A, Wernet P: Hodgkin and Sternberg-Reed cells contain antigens specific to late cells of granulopoiesis. *Int J Cancer* 29:283–290, 1982.

26. Foss HD, Reusch R, Demel G, et al.: Frequent expression of the B-cell-specific activator protein in Reed-Sternberg cells of classical Hodgkin's disease provides further evidence for its B-cell origin. *Blood* 94:3108–3113, 1999.

27. Torlakovic E, Torlakovic G, Nguyen PL, Brunning RD, Delabie J: The value of anti-pax-5 immunostaining in routinely fixed and paraffin-embedded sections: a novel pan pre-B and B-cell marker. *Am J Surg Pathol* 26:1343–1350, 2002.

28. Atkin NB: Cytogenetics of Hodgkin's disease. *Cytogenet Cell Genet* 80:23–27, 1998.

29. Deerberg-Wittram J, Weber-Matthiesen K, Schlegelberger B: Cytogenetics and molecular cytogenetics in Hodgkin's disease. *Ann Oncol* 7(suppl 4):49–53, 1996.

30. Gulley ML, Eagan PA, Quintanilla-Martinez L, et al.: Epstein-Barr virus DNA is abundant and monoclonal in the Reed-Sternberg cells of Hodgkin's disease: association with mixed cellularity subtype and Hispanic American ethnicity. *Blood* 83:1595–1602, 1994.

31. Bennett MH, MacLennan KA, Easterling MJ, Vaughan HB, Jelliffe AM, Vaughan HG: The prognostic significance of cellular subtypes in nodular sclerosing Hodgkin's disease: an analysis of 271 non-laparotomised cases (BNLI report no. 22). *Clin Radiol* 34:497–501, 1983.

32. Jarrett AF, Armstrong AA, Alexander E: Epidemiology of EBV and Hodgkin's lymphoma. *Ann Oncol* 7(suppl 4):5–10, 1996.

33. Khan G, Norton AJ, Slavin G: Epstein-Barr virus in Hodgkin disease. Relation to age and subtype. *Cancer* 71:3124–3129, 1993.

34. Uccini S, Monardo F, Ruco LP, et al.: High frequency of Epstein-Barr virus genome in HIV-positive patients with Hodgkin's disease. *Lancet* 1:1458, 1989.

35. Uccini S, Monardo F, Stoppacciaro A, et al.: High frequency of Epstein-Barr virus genome detection in Hodgkin's disease of HIV-positive patients. *Int J Cancer* 46:581–585, 1990.

36. Poppema S, Kaiserling E, Lennert K: Hodgkin's disease with lymphocytic predominance, nodular type (nodular paragranuloma) and progressively transformed germinal centres—a cytohistological study. *Histopathology* 3:295–308, 1979.

37. Ferry JA, Zukerberg LR, Harris NL: Florid progressive transformation of germinal centers. A syndrome affecting young men, without early progression to nodular lymphocyte predominance Hodgkin's disease. *Am J Surg Pathol* 16:252–258, 1992.

38. Rudiger T, Jaffe ES, Delsol G et al.: Workshop report on Hodgkin's disease and related diseases ('grey zone' lymphoma). *Ann Oncol* 9(suppl 5):S31–S38, 1998.

39. Rudiger T, Gascoyne RD, Jaffe ES, et al.: Workshop on the relationship between nodular lymphocyte predominant Hodgkin's lymphoma and T cell/histiocyte-rich B cell lymphoma. *Ann Oncol* 13(suppl 1):44–51, 2002.

40. Anagnostopoulos I, Hansmann ML, Franssila K, et al.: European Task Force on Lymphoma project on lymphocyte predominance Hodgkin disease: histologic and immunohistologic analysis of submitted cases reveals 2 types of Hodgkin disease with a nodular growth pattern and abundant lymphocytes. *Blood* 96:1889–1899, 2000.

41. Fan Z, Natkunam Y, Bair E, Tibshirani R, Warnke RA: Characterization of variant patterns of nodular lymphocyte predominant hodgkin lymphoma with immunohistologic and clinical correlation. *Am J Surg Pathol* 27:1346–1356, 2003.

42. Stein H, Hansmann ML, Lennert K, Brandtzaeg P, Gatter KC, Mason DY: Reed-Sternberg and Hodgkin cells in lymphocyte-predominant Hodgkin's disease of nodular subtype contain J chain. *Am J Clin Pathol* 86:292–297, 1986.

43. Kamel OW, Gelb AB, Shibuya RB, Warnke RA: Leu 7 (CD57) reactivity distinguishes nodular lymphocyte predominance Hodgkin's disease from nodular sclerosing Hodgkin's disease, T-cell-rich B-cell lymphoma and follicular lymphoma. *Am J Pathol* 142:541–546, 1993.

44. Poppema S: The nature of the lymphocytes surrounding Reed-Sternberg cells in nodular lymphocyte predominance and in other types of Hodgkin's disease. *Am J Pathol* 135:351–357, 1989.

# Chapter 72

# CLINICAL FEATURES AND MAKING THE DIAGNOSIS

*Kristie A. Blum and Pierluigi Porcu*

On the basis of differing morphologic, biologic, and clinical features described over the last 20 years, the currently accepted World Health Organization (WHO) Classification of Lymphoid Neoplasms recognizes two distinct clinical subtypes of Hodgkin's lymphoma (HL): classical HL and nodular lymphocyte-predominant HL.[1] Classical HL is a monoclonal lymphoid neoplasm composed of malignant Reed–Sternberg cells, which are multinucleated B cells that are CD30 and CD15 positive, surrounded by a mixed inflammatory infiltrate consisting of nonneoplastic lymphocytes, eosinophils, histiocytes, plasma cells, and fibroblasts. Four histologic subtypes of classical HL that differ in the morphology of Reed–Sternberg cells and composition of the reactive infiltrate have been identified: nodular sclerosis HL (NS HL), lymphocyte-rich HL (LR HL), mixed cellularity HL (MC HL), and lymphocyte-depleted HL (LD HL). While there is considerable overlap among these subtypes, unique clinical features have been noted with each.

Recognized as a separate entity in the WHO classification,[1] nodular lymphocyte-predominant HL is a monoclonal B-cell neoplasm characterized by a diffuse proliferation of large neoplastic cells [popcorn or lymphocytic and histiocytic (L&H) cells] that are CD20, CD79a, and CD45 positive and CD15 and CD30 negative, differing from Reed–Sternberg cells in classical HL.[2] These cells are frequently surrounded by a background infiltrate of nonmalignant small lymphocytes. This subtype comprises 3–8% of all HL,[3,4] and has distinct clinical features and patterns of relapse in several different trials and case series.[5-9]

## CLASSICAL HODGKIN'S LYMPHOMA

### EPIDEMIOLOGY

On the basis of data gathered by the Surveillance, Epidemiology, and End Results (SEER) program of the National Cancer Institute from 1975 to 2001, 7880 new cases of HL were expected in the United States in 2004, with 4330 cases in men and 3550 cases in women. From 1997 to 2001, the age-adjusted incidence rate reached 3.0/100,000 person-years, or 2.9/100,000 person-years in patients under the age of 65, and 4.3/100,000 person-years in patients 65 and older. The incidence is highest in Caucasian males, although females are commonly affected with the nodular sclerosing subtype. The median age at diagnosis is 36 years; however, as first described by MacMahon, a bimodal distribution of HL exists, with one peak in young adults (ages 15–34) and a second in patients older than 50.[10] For patients aged 15–34, age-adjusted rates of HL range from 3.1 to 4.6 per 100,000 person-years and for patients older than 50, age-adjusted rates range from 2.8 to 3.8. Fortunately, the majority of patients with HL survive, with 5-year survival rates of 85% (88% in patients younger than 65, and 52% in patients 65 and older).

### CLINICAL FEATURES

Classical Hodgkin's disease (HD) frequently presents with asymptomatic lymphadenopathy involving the cervical, supraclavicular, or mediastinal regions. Isolated subdiaphragmatic involvement is much less common, representing 3–10% of all HL cases.[11] Painful or tender lymphadenopathy is quite uncommon in HL and suggests an infectious etiology for the lymphadenopathy rather than HL. However, some patients will report pain induced by alcohol ingestion that localizes to the site of lymphomatous involvement. As the disease progresses and the nodal masses enlarge, some patients may develop dysphagia, tracheal compression, cough, hiccups, discomfort with movements of the shoulders, arms, or the neck, and skin irritation with redness or, rarely, ulceration.

While patients with cervical or supraclavicular lymphadenopathy frequently palpate an enlarged mass, patients with mediastinal presentations may complain of a persistent cough, dyspnea, or chest pain, which ultimately leads to further imaging and subsequent identification. Occasionally, patients with bulky mediastinal masses may demonstrate direct invasion of the chest wall, pleural or pericardial effusions, or superior vena caval syndrome. The pleural and pericardial effusions may not necessarily be malignant, as documented by cytology, but may result from lymphatic or venous obstruction.

In the 1960s, Rosenberg et al. described a contiguous, predictable pattern of lymphatic involvement in patients with HD.[12] Specifically, in 100 consecutive surgically staged patients with newly diagnosed HD, the sites of involvement appeared to follow specific lymphatic channels, with patients presenting with cervical involvement frequently having additional involvement of the mediastinum, hilum, or axilla, with rare involvement of the abdomen unless mediastinal structures were also involved. It is unusual to find a patient with classical HD who has involvement of the neck and lower abdomen/inguinal nodes, without contiguous involvement of the mediastinum and upper abdomen. Also, involvement of the liver or bone marrow is unusual without involvement of the spleen. Occasional patients may have neck and upper abdomen involvement, bypassing the mediastinum, which may implicate direct spread via the thoracic duct. For patients with relapsed or primary refractory HL, the orderly progression of disease along contiguous lymphatic chains does not occur, and virtually any organ including the bone marrow may be involved at relapse.

Primary extranodal/organ involvement is uncommon in HL, unless related to direct extension. For example, while primary pulmonary presentations are rare, direct extension into the lung parenchyma is frequently observed, usually in the presence of adjacent mediastinal or hilar nodes. The lung is probably one of the most common nonlymphoid organs to be involved by HL, and such involvement may be manifested by linear infiltrates, pleural effusions, or nodular infiltrates demonstrated on chest X-ray or computed tomography (CT) scan. A rare patient may present with cough, wheezing, and endobronchial extension from an area of hilar lymphadenopathy. However, determination of pulmonary involvement can be quite problematic, as HL patients are predisposed to infectious complications including bacterial, viral, and atypical pneumonias. In addition, a history of granulomatous disease or fungal infection may be responsible for pulmonary scarring or nodules. The clinical setting, response to chemotherapy, and occasionally functional imaging techniques [positron emission tomography (PET) or gallium scanning] may help differentiate these abnormalities. Splenic involvement occurs frequently in HL, in approximately 30% of patients, and, as discussed later in this chapter, cannot be reliably detected with conventional imaging techniques. Splenic size alone is not adequate to determine involvement. Bone marrow involvement is quite unusual in HL and, when present, rarely results in cytopenias. Involvement is usually focal, and detection requires adequate bone marrow biopsy specimens. It should be remembered that flow cytometric analysis of bone marrow aspirates is usually not helpful in classical HL, because Reed–Sternberg cells are infrequent and do not express surface immunoglobulins. Clonality cannot be established, and results generally reflect the background cell population. Diagnosis of bone marrow involvement, therefore, relies primarily on histopathologic analysis of an adequate core biopsy.

In addition to symptoms directly related to lymphadenopathy, patients may also complain of fevers, weight loss, night sweats, fatigue, or pruritus. B symptoms, defined as fever (>38°C or 100.4°F), unexplained weight loss (>10% body weight), or night sweats, are present in approximately 40% of patients. Since the presenting symptoms of classical HL are often nonspecific, including fatigue, cough, B symptoms, or pruritus, patients may describe these symptoms weeks to months prior to their diagnosis, and occasionally, only after persistent follow-up for these symptoms will a diagnosis be made. The Pel–Ebstein fever, an intermittent fever that recurs at variable intervals, has been associated with HL, although it is quite uncommon. The pruritus of HD can often be severe, leading to excoriations and hyperpigmentation from scratching, and may precede the diagnosis by months to years. A rare patient (typically an older male with a mixed cellularity type) will present with occult disease and fever of unknown origin. Systemic symptoms including weight loss, night sweats, and fevers may sometimes predominate, with minimal palpable adenopathy. Often only after extensive work-up, including imaging with CT scan, PET, or gallium scintigraphy, and/or bone marrow biopsy, will evidence of HL be detected. Other unusual presentations include pain related to bony involvement or nerve root compression from an epidural mass. Paraneoplastic syndromes including nephrotic syndrome, neurologic symptoms, or idiopathic thrombocytopenia purpura have also been reported and will be discussed later in this chapter.

Although the histologic subtype of HL does not appear to influence prognosis and does not alter therapeutic recommendations, each subtype is characterized by unique clinical characteristics that may guide the diagnostic evaluation as described below.

### Nodular sclerosis Hodgkin's lymphoma

The nodular sclerosis subtype accounts for 70% of classical HL.[13] This subtype is morphologically characterized by collagen bands that surround Hodgkin's or Reed–Sternberg cells. NS HL equally affects males and females and the median age at diagnosis is 28 years. At diagnosis, most patients present with stage II disease, with mediastinal involvement noted in 80% of patients, bulky disease (see Diagnostic Evaluation section for definition of bulky disease) in 54%, and splenic or lung involvement in only 10%.[4,13]

## Mixed cellularity Hodgkin's lymphoma

The mixed cellularity subtype is observed more frequently in patients with HIV disease, or in developing countries. It comprises 20–25% of classical HL cases, and is characterized by scattered Hodgkin's or Reed–Sternberg cells within a diffuse mixed inflammatory infiltrate without fibrosis.[13] In contrast to NS HL, patients with MC HL are older (median age 37), predominantly male, and often with advanced-stage disease and B symptoms. Splenic involvement is reported in 30% of patients, bone marrow involvement in 10%, and liver involvement in 3%. Mediastinal presentations are uncommon.[13]

## Lymphocyte-rich Hodgkin's lymphoma

This subtype comprises only 5% of classical HL, and again is seen most frequently in older males. Similar to MC HL, LR HL is pathologically characterized by Hodgkin's or Reed–Sternberg cells surrounded by an inflammatory infiltrate; however, these cells are primarily small lymphocytes with a notable absence of neutrophils and eosinophils.[13] Most patients present with early-stage disease, in general with peripheral node involvement. Mediastinal involvement and B symptoms are uncommon.[13]

## Lymphocyte-depleted Hodgkin's lymphoma

LD HL is the least common subtype of classical HL, often associated with HIV infection, composed of multiple, bizarre, large and small Hodgkin's or Reed–Sternberg cells in a fibrillary matrix with limited nonneoplastic inflammatory lymphocytes.[13] Abdominal organs, retroperitoneal lymph nodes, and bone marrow involvement are favored, with relative sparing of peripheral nodes. Most patients with disease are male, with advanced-stage disease and B symptoms.[13]

## Paraneoplastic syndromes

Classical HL is associated with the overexpression of a variety of cytokines and their receptors on Hodgkin's or Reed–Sternberg cells and in the surrounding inflammatory infiltrate. These cytokines, including interleukin 2 (IL-2), IL-5, IL-6, IL-7, IL-9, IL-10, IL-13, transforming growth factor β (TGFβ), and lymphotoxin A (LT-A), may be responsible for the systemic symptoms of HL and for the rare paraneoplastic syndromes associated with HL. Nephrotic syndrome, idiopathic thrombocytopenia purpura, autoimmune hemolytic anemia, and cerebellar degeneration/ataxia have all been reported in patients with HL.[14–18] Typically, nephrotic syndrome or neurologic symptoms precede a diagnosis of HL or herald a relapse, although occasionally high-dose steroids used to treat many of these syndromes may contribute to a delay in diagnosis.[14,16] Idiopathic thrombocytopenia has been described in patients preceding the diagnosis of HL, at the time of relapse, and in patients in clinical remission for HL.[17,18] Life-threatening complications of HL, including fulminant hepatic failure and lactic acidosis, have also been described,[19,20] although these situations are quite rare.

## DIAGNOSTIC EVALUATION

Initial diagnostic evaluation of HL is aimed at pathological confirmation, followed by additional evaluations to fully stage the patient. These assessments not only guide the patient's therapeutic management, but also impact prognosis. Patients with palpable lymphadenopathy should undergo an excisional biopsy in order to obtain an adequate diagnostic specimen. Fine needle aspirations are not sufficient to distinguish between classical HD and other CD30+ lymphomas including anaplastic T-cell lymphoma and diffuse large cell lymphoma. In addition, information regarding the subtype of HL (nodular sclerosing, mixed cellularity, lymphocyte rich, or lymphocyte depleted) may provide some guidance to expected clinical features.

The currently recommended diagnostic/staging work-up for patients with newly diagnosed HL is outlined in Table 72.1. The initial history and physical examination should address the presence or absence of B symptoms (defined as drenching night sweats, fever exceeding 38°C/100.4°F, or unexplained weight loss of

### Table 72.1 Recommended diagnostic work-up for patients with HL

History and physical examination
B symptoms (The absence or presence of fever (>38°C), unexplained weight loss (>10% body weight), or night sweats)
EtOH intolerance
Pruritis
Fatigue
Performance status
Examination of nodes, Waldeyer's ring, liver, and spleen

Laboratory
CBC, differential, platelets
Erthrocyte sedimentation rate (ESR)
Lactate dehydrogenase (LDH)
Liver function tests (ALT, AST, bilirubin, alkaline phosphatase)
Albumin
BUN, creatinine
Serum/urine pregnancy test (in women of childbearing age)
HIV (if risk factors or unusual clinical presentation)

Imaging studies
Chest X-ray
CT chest/abdomen/pelvis (neck, in selected cases)
PET/gallium scanning (in selected cases)

Additional procedures
Bone marrow biopsy (bilateral, preferred)
Semen/oocyte cryopreservation

EtOH, ethanol; CBC, complete blood count; ALT, alanine transaminase; AST, aspartate transaminase; BUN, blood urea nitrogen, CT, computed tomography; PET, positron emission tomography.

at least 10% of the total body weight within the last 6 months), alcohol intolerance, pruritus, fatigue, performance status, and an examination of nodes, spleen, liver, and Waldeyer's ring. On physical examination, involved lymph nodes typically are nontender, rubbery, or firm. Large lymph nodes may coalesce, forming fixed, matted masses.

Initial laboratory testing should include a complete blood count with differential, erythrocyte sedimentation rate (ESR), lactate dehydrogenase (LDH), liver function tests, albumin, blood urea nitrogen (BUN), and creatinine. Elevated white blood cell count, lymphopenia, anemia, hypoalbuminemia, and an elevated ESR all have prognostic value in the treatment of HL (Table 72.2).[21,22] In selected patients, HIV and pregnancy testing may also be indicated. Chest X-ray and CT scanning of the chest/abdomen/pelvis should be used to assess both the bulk and sites of disease at initial presentation. Patients presenting with signs or symptoms of naso-oropharyngeal involvement, such as the Waldeyer's ring, may require CT or magnetic resonance imaging (MRI) scans of the head and neck, to appropriately evaluate response. Bulky disease, usually defined as a mediastinal mass ratio (maximum width of the tumor mass divided by maximum intrathoracic diameter) exceeding 1/3 or any single nodal/tumor mass exceeding 10 cm, is also an unfavorable prognostic factor. Other imaging techniques including PET or gallium scanning may be helpful, particularly in patients with large mediastinal masses or in the setting of indeterminant lesions on CT. These modalities will be discussed later in this chapter. Finally, bone marrow biopsy should be performed to complete the staging work-up. Bone marrow involvement has been reported in 5–15% of patients at diagnosis, and is frequently associated with the presence of B symptoms.[23,24]

All patients should also be counseled regarding the risks of tobacco use during and after therapy, and fertility issues should be addressed. Specifically, with adriamycin, bleomycin, vinblastine, dacarbazine (ABVD) and Stanford V chemotherapy, there appears to be little effect on fertility, although this has not been studied exhaustively.[25,26] However, intensive regimens including bleomycin, etoposide, adriamycin, cyclophosphamide, prednisone, procarbazine (BEACOPP) or other combination salvage therapies (including, but not limited to, ifostamide, carboplatin, etoposide (ICE), dexamethasone, cytarabine, cisplatin (DHAP), and etoposide, methylpreduisolone, cytarabine, cisplatin (ESHAP)), followed by hematopoietic stem cell transplantation (SCT) for those patients who relapse, frequently affect fertility, and semen/oocyte cryopreservation is advised for those patients contemplating future parenthood. Finally, due to the high risk of second malignancies reported after combination chemotherapy and/or radiotherapy for classical HL,[27,28] all patients should be advised about the need for continual follow-up and screening mammograms in the posttreatment period.

### STAGING

Historically, staging of HL has followed the Ann Arbor staging system[29] (Table 72.3), although updated versions of this system incorporating a variety of prognostic factors exist (Table 72.4).[30] Overall, 55% of patients present with localized disease (Ann Arbor stage I–II).

The staging work-up for HD has evolved. Historically, lymphangiography, CT imaging, bone marrow biopsy, and staging laparotomy have been extensively used. Staging laparotomy evolved in an era where treatment for limited-stage (Ann Arbor stage I and II) HL consisted primarily of extended radiation therapy fields, and precise pathological staging was required to include all areas of involvement. With the detection of occult splenic or high retroperitoneal disease at the time of laparotomy in 20–30% of patients with clinical stage IA-IIA disease and 35% of patients with clinical stage IB–IIB disease,[31,32] clinical staging alone was not accurate enough to predict which patients with early-stage HL were likely to attain a prolonged disease-free survival

| Table 72.2 | Prognostic factors in HL[21,22] |
|---|---|
| **Early-stage HL[22]** | **Advanced-stage HL[21]** |
| *EORTC criteria* | Albumin <4 g/dL |
| Large mediastinal mass | Hemoglobin <10.5 g/dL |
|   Mediastinal mass ratio | Male |
|   (MMR) >1/3 | Age ≥45 years |
|   Tumor/nodal mass >10 cm | Leukocytosis |
| Age ≥50 | (WBC≥15,000/mm³) |
| ESR ≥50 without B symptoms | Lymphopenia |
| or ≥30 with B-symptoms | (Lymphocyte count |
| ≥4 sites of involvement | <8% of WBC, or |
| *GHSG criteria* | <600/mm³) |
| Large mediastinal mass | Stage IV disease |
|   Mediastinal mass ratio | |
|   (MMR) >1/3 | |
|   Tumor/nodal mass >10 cm | |
| Extranodal disease | |
| ESR ≥50 without B symptoms | |
| or ≥30 with B symptoms | |
| ≥3 sites of involvement | |
| *CCTG or ECOG criteria* | |
| Low risk disease: LPHL or NS HL, age <40, ESR <50, ≤3 regions of involvement | |
| High risk disease: All other histologies excluding LPHL or NS HL, bulky disease >10 cm, ESR ≥50, age ≥40, >3 regions of involvement | |

EORTC, European Organization for Research and Treatment of Cancer; GHSG, German Hodgkin Lymphoma Study Group; CCTG, Canadian Clinical Trials Group; ECOG, Eastern Co-Operative Oncology Group; LP HL, lymphocyte-predominant Hodgkin's lymphoma; NS HL, nodular sclerosing Hodgkin's lymphoma.

| Table 72.3 | Ann Arbor staging system for Hodgkin's lymphoma[29] |
|---|---|
| Stage I | Involvement of a single lymph node region or lymphoid structure, or involvement of a single extralymphatic site ($I_E$) |
| Stage II | Involvement of two or more lymph node regions on the same side of the diaphragm, which may be accompanied by localized contiguous involvement of an extralymphatic site or organ ($II_E$). |
| Stage III | Involvement of lymph node regions on both sides of the diaphragm, which may also be accompanied by involvement of the spleen ($III_S$) or by localized contiguous involvement of an extralymphatic site or organ ($III_E$) |
| Stage IV | Diffuse or disseminated involvement of one or more extralymphatic organs or tissues, with or without lymph node involvement. |

*Note:* The absence or presence of fever (>38°C), unexplained weight loss (>10% body weight), or night sweats should be denoted by the suffix letters A or B, respectively.

| Table 72.4 | Cotswolds update of the Ann Arbor staging system[30] |
|---|---|
| **Stage** | **Description** |
| Stage I | Involvement of a single lymph node region or lymphoid structure (e.g., spleen, thymus, Waldeyer's ring) or involvement of a single extralymphatic site ($I_E$) |
| Stage II | Involvement of two or more lymph node regions on the same side of the diaphragm (the mediastinum is a single site; hilar nodes, when involved on both sides, constitute stage II disease); localized contiguous involvement of only one extranodal organ or site and lymph node region on the same side of the diaphragm ($II_E$). The number of anatomic regions involved should be designated by a subscript (e.g., $II_3$) |
| Stage III | Involvement of lymph node regions on both sides of the diaphragm, which may also be accompanied by involvement of the spleen ($III_S$) or by localized contiguous involvement of only one extranodal organ ($III_E$) or both ($IIIS_E$) |
| III1 | With or without involvement of splenic, hilar, celiac, or portal nodes |
| III2 | With involvement of para-aortic, iliac, and mesenteric nodes |
| Stage IV | Diffuse or disseminated involvement of one or more extranodal organs or tissues, with or without associated lymph node involvement |
| Designations applicable to any disease stage | |
| A | No symptoms |
| B | Fever (temperature >38°C), drenching night sweats, unexplained weight loss of more than 10% of body weight in the preceding 6 months |
| X | Bulky disease (>1/3 widening of the mediastinum or the presence of a nodal mass >10 cm) |
| E | Involvement of single extranodal site that is contiguous or proximal to known nodal site of disease |

with radiation therapy alone. Furthermore, even for patients with pathologically confirmed stage I and II disease, the recurrence rate after extended-field radiotherapy was approximately 20%. This led to the gradual abandonment of staging laparotomy for early-stage HL, in favor of a combined modality therapeutic approach. The addition of chemotherapy to the radiation regimen minimized the importance of detection of microscopic splenic involvement, and allowed the adoption of smaller radiation therapy portals (involved field), with significant improvements in toxicity and similar, if not better, outcomes. The elimination of staging laparotomy as part of routine staging also minimized the risk of postsplenectomy sepsis in patients with compromised immune function, and prevented prolonged treatment days associated with the hospitalization for surgical staging.

**Gallium scintigraphy/positron emission tomography**
[67]Gallium scintigraphy and PET are often used to both accurately stage HL and assess response to treatment. Conventional CT scanning has not proven to be very sensitive for occult abdominal disease during the staging evaluation of HL. In addition, assessment of a residual mediastinal mass at the completion of therapy can be problematic with this modality. [67]Ga scintigraphy has proven to be more sensitive than CT in the posttreatment evaluation of HL, provided that the patient has a gallium-avid tumor at diagnosis.[33–35] The positive and negative predictive values of [67]Ga scintigraphy following treatment range from 92 to 100% and from 83 to 90%, respectively,[36,37] compared to 48% and 83% with CT.[36] PET scan using the glucose analog 2-([18]F)-fluoro-2-deoxy-D-glucose ([18]F-FDG) has emerged as a very useful tool in the evaluation and

monitoring of response in HL. In terms of diagnostic evaluation, in a small study of 11 patients undergoing staging laparotomy, the sensitivity and specificity of [18]F-FDG PET were both 100%, compared to 20% and 83%, respectively, with CT scans.[38] In a larger study of 45 patients with Hodgkin's and non-Hodgkin's lymphoma (NHL), PET scanning altered the staging in 16% of patients, although it understaged 7% of patients.[39] Even more data exist regarding the impact of PET imaging on response assessment. In 54 patients with HL (19 patients) or NHL (35 patients), all 6 patients with a positive [18]F-FDG PET relapsed—a positive predictive value of 100%, compared to 42% with conventional CT.[40] The negative predictive value of [18]F-FDG PET in this trial was 83%, with eight patients relapsing despite a negative study. In a second study in 48 patients previously treated for HL, the positive and negative predictive values of [18]F-FDG PET were both equal to 92%.[41] However, while [67]Ga scintigraphy and

$^{18}$F-FDG PET may both guide staging and treatment decisions, false positives do occur. For example, in patients younger than 25 years, a regenerating thymus can be gallium- or $^{18}$F-FDG avid, following completion of treatment of HL.[42,43] Therefore, these noninvasive radiographic modalities do have utility in the diagnostic and response evaluation of HL; however, the results need to be interpreted in conjunction with the clinical circumstances, other laboratory evaluations, and CT results. In situations where PET or $^{67}$Ga scintigraphy results contradict the clinical picture or are inconclusive, biopsy may be warranted.

## LYMPHOCYTE-PREDOMINANT HODGKIN'S LYMPHOMA

### EPIDEMIOLOGY

Classified as a distinct subtype of HL by the WHO classification,[1] LP HL is a monoclonal B-cell neoplasm characterized by a nodular polymorphic infiltrate composed of small lymphocytes, histiocytes, and large neoplastic cells, referred to as popcorn and L&H cells, that differ morphologically and immunohistochemically from Reed–Sternberg cells. L&H cells usually have one large multilobated nucleus with limited cytoplasm. These cells, unlike Hodgkin's Reed–Sternberg cells, are frequently positive for CD20 and CD79a, while negative for CD30 and CD15. Several series have also described unique clinical features for this subtype of HL.[5–9,44] LP HL represents 3–5% of all HLs and typically afflicts 30- to 50-year-old males.[4]

### CLINICAL FEATURES

In a retrospective review of 219 LP HL cases, the majority of affected patients were male (74%) and most patients presented with stage I–II disease (81%).[5,44] These patients typically present with isolated cervical, axillary, or inguinal node involvement, while mediastinal, splenic, or bone marrow involvement is uncommon.[45] Likewise, bulky disease and B symptoms are infrequent. In the same series, only 7% of patients presented with mediastinal involvement, and only 10–13% of patients had bulky disease or bone marrow involvement.[5,44]

Patients with LP HL often experience multiple relapses, although the disease progresses slowly and is usually quite responsive to therapy at the time of relapse, leading to little impact on overall survival.[44,45] The European Task Force on Lymphoma reported a 10-year overall survival exceeding 90% for patients with LP HL, compared to a 10-year progression-free survival of approximately 75%.[5,44] In a second retrospective review of 50 cases of LP HL, 78% of patients presented with early-stage disease, and overall survival at 4 years reached 92%.[8] Similar results were reported in a Stanford series of 59 patients with LP HL.[9] Interestingly, some case series have reported a high rate of second malignancies, ranging from 12 to 14%,[5,8] in patients with LP-HL, possibly attributable to either extended radiation fields or chemotherapy historically used in the treatment of this disease. In addition, transformation to diffuse large B-cell lymphoma has also been described.[46–48]

### DIAGNOSTIC EVALUATION/STAGING

The diagnostic and staging evaluation of LP HL is similar to that previously described for classical HL. Diagnosis should be confirmed by an excisional or core needle biopsy, as fine needle aspirations frequently do not yield enough tissue to visualize the typical L&H cells surrounded by the polymorphic, nodular (or nodular and diffuse) infiltrate of reactive lymphocytes and histiocytes. CD20, CD57, CD15, CD30, and CD3 staining should be performed on all specimens of LP HL. The clinical history and physical examination should again focus on the presence of B symptoms, fatigue, evaluation of performance status, and examination of nodal sites. CBC with differential, LDH, BUN, creatinine, liver function tests, and staging imaging studies should also be performed. Staging according to the Ann Arbor system (Tables 72.3 and 72.4) is again recommended. CT scan of the chest/abdomen/pelvis (neck in selected cases) and bone marrow biopsy should be performed for staging purposes. $^{18}$F-FDG PET and $^{67}$Ga scintigraphy have not been extensively evaluated for patients with LP HL, but may prove to be useful for patients with equivocal CT scans. Finally, patients should again be counseled regarding fertility, smoking cessation, and risk of second malignancies, as therapy often consists of combination chemotherapy and/or radiotherapy as has been used in classical HL.

## REFERENCES

1. Harris N, Jaffe E, Diebold J, et al.: World Health Organization Classification of neoplastic diseases of the hematopoeitic and lymphoid tissues: report of the clinical advisory committee meeting—Airlie House, Virgina, November 1997. *J Clin Oncol* 17:3835–3849, 1999.
2. Hansmann ML, Stein H, Dallenbach F, Fellbaum C: Diffuse lymphocyte-predominant Hodgkin's disease (diffuse paragranuloma). A variant of the B-cell-derived nodular type. *Am J Pathol* 138:29–36, 1991.
3. Lukes R, Butler J, Hicks E: Natural history of Hodgkin's disease as related to its pathologic picture. *Cancer* 19:317–344, 1966.
4. Colby TV, Hoppe RT, Warnke R: Hodgkin's disease: a clinicopathologic study of 659 cases. *Cancer* 49:1848–1858, 1981.
5. Diehl V, Sextro M, Franklin J, et al.: Clinical presentation, course, and prognostic factors in lymphocyte-predominant Hodgkin's disease and lymphocyte-rich

classical Hodgkin's disease: report from the European Task Force on Lymphoma Project on Lymphocyte-Predominant Hodgkin's disease. *J Clin Oncol* 17:776–783, 1999.

6. Bodis S, Kraus MD, Pinkus G, et al.: Clinical presentation and outcome in lymphocyte-predominant Hodgkin's disease. *J Clin Oncol* 15:3060–3066, 1997.

7. Franklin J, Tesch H, Hansmann ML, Diehl V: Lymphocyte predominant Hodgkin's disease: pathology and clinical implication. *Ann Oncol* 9(suppl 5):S39–S44, 1998.

8. Pappa VI, Norton AJ, Gupta RK, Wilson AM, Rohatiner AZ, Lister TA: Nodular type of lymphocyte predominant Hodgkin's disease. A clinical study of 50 cases. *Ann Oncol* 6:559–565, 1995.

9. Russell KJ, Hoppe RT, Colby TV, Burns BF, Cox RS, Kaplan HS: Lymphocyte predominant Hodgkin's disease: clinical presentation and results of treatment. *Radiother Oncol* 1:197–205, 1984.

10. MacMahon B: Epidemiological evidence on the nature of Hodgkin's disease. *Cancer* 10:1045–1054, 1957.

11. Leibenhaut M, Hoppe RT, Varghese A, Rosenberg S: Subdiaphragmatic Hodgkin's disease: laparotomy and treatment results in 49 patients. *J Clin Oncol* 5:1050–1055, 1987.

12. Rosenberg SA, Kaplan HS: Evidence for an orderly progression in the spread of Hodgkin's disease. *Cancer Res* 26:1225–1231, 1966.

13. Stein H, Delsol G, Pileri S, et al.: Classical Hodgkin lymphoma. In: Jaffe E, Harris N, Stein H, Vardiman J (eds.) *World Health Organization Classification of Tumors: Pathology and Genetics of Tumors of Haematopoietic and Lymphoid Tissues.* Lyon, France: IARC Press; 2001: 244–253.

14. Spyridonidis A, Fischer K, Glocker F, Fetscher S, Klisch J, Behringer D: Paraneoplastic cerebellar degeneration and nephrotic syndrome preceding Hodgkin's disease: case report and review of the literature. *Eur J Haematol* 68:318–321, 2002.

15. Emir S, Kutluk M, Gogus S, Buyukpamukeu M: Paraneoplastic cerebellar degeneration and Horner syndrome: association of two uncommon findings in a child with Hodgkin disease. *J Pediatr Hematol Oncol* 22:158–161, 2000.

16. Smitt P, Kinoshita A, De Leeuw B, et al.: Paraneoplastic cerebellar ataxia due to autoantibodies against a glutamate receptor. *N Engl J Med* 342:21–27, 2000.

17. Martinelli G, Zinzani P, Magagnoli M, Vianelli N, Tura S: Incidence and prognostic significance of idiopathic thrombocytopenic purpura in patients with Hodgkin's disease in complete hematological remission. *Haematologica* 83:669–670, 1998.

18. Xiros N, Binder T, Anger B, Bohlke J, Heimpel H: Idiopathic thrombocytopenic purpura and autoimmune hemolytic anemia in Hodgkin's disease. *Eur J Haematol* 40:437–441, 1998.

19. Dourakis S, Tzemanakis E, Deutsch M, Kafiri G, Hadziyannis S: Fulminant hepatic failure as a presenting paraneoplastic manifestation of Hodgkin's disease. *Eur J Gastroenterol Hepatol* 11:1055–1058, 1999.

20. Nadiminti Y, Wang JC, Chou SY, Pineles E, Tobin MS: Lactic acidosis associated with Hodgkin's disease: response to chemotherapy. *N Engl J Med* 303:15–17, 1980.

21. Hasenclever D, Diehl V: A prognostic score for advanced Hodgkin's disease. International Prognostic Factors Project on Advanced Hodgkin's Disease. *N Engl J Med* 339:1506–1514, 1998.

22. Diehl V, Stein H, Hummel M, Zollinger R, Connors JM: Hodgkin's lymphoma: biology and treatment strategies for primary, refractory, and relapsed disease. *Hematology (Am Soc Hematol Educ Program)* 225–247, 2003.

23. Munker R, Hasenclever D, Brosteanu O, Hiller E, Diehl V: Bone marrow involvement in Hodgkin's disease: an analysis of 135 consecutive cases. *J Clin Oncol* 13:403–409, 1995.

24. Bartl R, Frisch B, Burkhardt R, Huhn D, Pappenberger R: Assessment of bone marrow histology in Hodgkin's disease: correlation with clinical factors. *Br J Haematol* 51:345–360, 1982.

25. Horning SJ, Hoppe RT, Breslin S, Bartlett N, Brown W, Rosenberg S: Stanford V and radiotherapy for locally extensive and advanced Hodgkin's disease: mature results of a prospective clinical trial. *J Clin Oncol* 20:630–637, 2002.

26. Hudson MM, Greenwald C, Thompson E, et al.: Efficacy and toxicity of multiagent chemotherapy and low-dose involved-field radiotherapy in children and adolescents with Hodgkin's disease. *J Clin Oncol* 11:100–108, 1993.

27. Aleman B, van den Belt-Dusebout A, Klokman W, van't Veer M, Bartelink H, van Leeuwen F: Long-term cause-specific mortality of patients treated for Hodgkin's disease. *J Clin Oncol* 21:3431–3439, 2003.

28. Ng A, Bernardo M, Weller E, et al.: Second malignancy after Hodgkin disease treated with radiation therapy with or without chemotherapy: long-term risks and risk factors. *Blood* 100:1989–1996, 2002.

29. Carbone PP, Kaplan HS, Musshoff K, Smithers DW, Tubiana M: Report of the Committee on Hodgkin's Disease Staging Classification. *Cancer Res* 31:1860–1861, 1971.

30. Lister TA, Crowther D, Sutcliffe SB, et al.: Report of a committee convened to discuss the evaluation and staging of patients with Hodgkin's disease: Cotswolds meeting. *J Clin Oncol* 7:1630–1636, 1989.

31. Leibenhaut MH, Hoppe RT, Efron B, Halpern J, Nelsen T, Rosenberg SA: Prognostic indicators of laparotomy findings in clinical stage I–II supradiaphragmatic Hodgkin's disease. *J Clin Oncol* 7:81–91, 1989.

32. Mauch P, Larson D, Osteen R, et al.: Prognostic factors for positive surgical staging in patients with Hodgkin's disease. *J Clin Oncol* 8:257–265, 1990.

33. Zinzani PL, Zompatori M, Bendandi M, et al.: Monitoring bulky mediastinal disease with gallium-67, CT-scan and magnetic resonance imaging in Hodgkin's disease and high-grade non-Hodgkin's lymphoma. *Leuk Lymphoma* 22:131–135, 1996.

34. Front D, Israel O: The role of Ga-67 scintigraphy in evaluating the results of therapy of lymphoma patients. *Semin Nucl Med* 25:60–71, 1995.

35. Abrahamsen AF, Lien HH, Aas M, et al.: Magnetic resonance imaging and 67gallium scan in mediastinal malignant lymphoma: a prospective pilot study. *Ann Oncol* 5:433–436, 1994.

36. King SC, Reiman RJ, Prosnitz LR: Prognostic importance of restaging gallium scans following induction

chemotherapy for advanced Hodgkin's disease. *J Clin Oncol* 12:306–311, 1994.

37. Salloum E, Brandt DS, Caride VJ, et al.: Gallium scans in the management of patients with Hodgkin's disease: a study of 101 patients. *J Clin Oncol* 15:518–527, 1997.

38. Young CS, Young BL, Smith SM: Staging Hodgkin's disease with 18-FDG PET. Comparison with CT and surgery. *Clin Positron Imaging* 1:161–164, 1998.

39. Delbeke D, Martin WH, Morgan DS, et al.: 2-deoxy-2-[F-18]fluoro-D-glucose imaging with positron emission tomography for initial staging of Hodgkin's disease and lymphoma. *Mol Imaging Biol* 4:105–114, 2002.

40. Jerusalem G, Beguin Y, Fassotte MF, et al.: Whole-body positron emission tomography using 18F-fluorodeoxyglucose for posttreatment evaluation in Hodgkin's disease and non-Hodgkin's lymphoma has higher diagnostic and prognostic value than classical computed tomography scan imaging. *Blood* 94:429–433, 1999.

41. Guay C, Lepine M, Verreault J, Benard F: Prognostic value of PET using 18F-FDG in Hodgkin's disease for posttreatment evaluation. *J Nucl Med* 44:1225–1231, 2003.

42. Peylan-Ramu N, Haddy TB, Jones E, Horvath K, Adde MA, Magrath IT: High frequency of benign mediastinal uptake of gallium-67 after completion of chemotherapy in children with high-grade non-Hodgkin's lymphoma. *J Clin Oncol* 7:1800–1806, 1989.

43. Weinblatt ME, Zanzi I, Belakhlef A, Babchyck B, Kochen J: False-positive FDG-PET imaging of the thymus of a child with Hodgkin's disease. *J Nucl Med* 38:888–890, 1997.

44. Anagnostopoulos I, Hansmann ML, Franssila K, et al.: European Task Force on lymphoma project on lymphocyte predominance Hodgkin's disease: histologic and immunohistologic analysis of submitted cases reveals 2 types of Hodgkin disease with a nodular growth pattern and abundant lymphocytes. *Blood* 96:1889, 2000.

45. Stein H, Delsol G, Pileri S, et al.: Nodular lymphocyte predominant Hodgkin lymphoma. In: Jaffe E, Harris N, Stein H, Vardiman J (eds.) *World Health Organization Classification of Tumors: Pathology and Genetics of Tumors of Haematopoietic and Lymphoid Tissues.* Lyon, France: IARC Press; 2001:240–243.

46. Miettinen M, Franssila K, Saxen E: Hodgkin's disease, lymphocytic predominance nodular. Increased risk for subsequent non-Hodgkin's lymphoma. *Cancer* 51: 2293–2300, 1993.

47. Hansmann ML, Stein H, Fellbaum C, Hui P, Parwaresch M, Lennert K: Nodular paragranuloma can transform into high-grade malignant lymphoma of B type. *Hum Pathol* 20:1169–1175, 1989.

48. Greiner TC, Gascoyne RD, Anderson ME, et al.: Nodular lymphocyte-predominant Hodgkin's disease associated with large-cell lymphoma: analysis of Ig gene rearrangements by V-J polymerase chain reaction. *Blood* 87: 4302–4310, 1996.

# Chapter 73

# TREATMENT APPROACH TO CLASSICAL HODGKIN'S LYMPHOMA

*Brian J. Bolwell and Toni K. Choueiri*

## INTRODUCTION

The treatment of Hodgkin's Lymphoma (HL) has significant historical importance in the field of medical oncology. Despite being a rare malignancy, HL has represented a model for oncologic advances. HL was one of the first oncologic illnesses proved to be potentially medically cured. Radiation therapy has long been known to be curative for the majority of patients with limited stage HL. Additionally, the concept of dose intensity was demonstrated to have clinical validity in patients with HL, as a clear dose response curve in radiation therapy dose has been demonstrated. Combination chemotherapy is potentially curative for patients with advanced stage HL and represents a paradigm for combining different effective chemotherapeutic agents in a single regimen. More recently, long-term toxicities and complications of therapy, including secondary cancers, significant organ damage, and other toxicities, have been demonstrated in patients presumably cured from their HL as a result of therapy. Late toxicities have generated a spirited debate in recent years of the optimal way to treat classical HL. This chapter will present the "standard" recommendations for the treatment of HL and will also present a contrarian viewpoint.

## CLINICAL STAGE I AND II HL: "STANDARD" PRINCIPLES OF THERAPY

### INTRODUCTION

Historically, treatment algorithms were designed to determine which patients could be cured with radiation therapy alone and which patients had a poor prognosis with radiation therapy and required combination chemotherapy. This is why staging laparotomies evolved: if one could prove that a patient had no pathologic evidence of disease below the diaphram, then one might save the patient from the toxicity of combination chemotherapy and successfully treat the patient with radiation alone. There were many reasons for this treatment strategy. Extended field radiation therapy was successful, with the majority of patients with stage I and II HL being cured. In the 1970s and 1980s, acute toxicities from combination chemotherapy were significant. Antiemetic therapy was poor; the use of MOPP (mechlorethamine, oncovin (vincristine), procarbazine, and prednisone) combination chemotherapy had a known leukemogenic risk; issues of sterility were a genuine concern; and the risk of neutropenic fever and serious infections were clinically important, especially in the era prior to the availability of hematopoietic growth factors. Additionally, it was commonly felt that if patients progressed after radiation therapy, the majority could be successfully salvaged at a later date with combination chemotherapy. Thus, a 25–30% incidence of relapse after radiation therapy was deemed to be less significant because of later successful salvage with combination chemotherapy. As a result, radiation therapy continues to this day to be a primary treatment modality for limited stage HL.

### RADIATION THERAPY

A detailed description of various radiotherapy techniques is beyond the scope of this chapter. Briefly, when radiation therapy is used alone for limited stage HL, tumor doses of 150–200 cGy are generally given 5 days/week, with a total dose of 3,600–4,000 cGy delivered over approximately 5 weeks. "Boosts" of radiation therapy may be given to bulky disease sites. Given that limited stage HL is usually above the diaphram, the most common field incorporated is the *mantle field*. The mantle field encompasses the mediastinal, hilar, subcarinal, axillary, infraclavicular, supraclavicular, cervical, and submandibular lymph nodes. The para-aortic field encompasses the para-aortic nodes to approximately the L5 vertebral body. Frequently, para-aortic radiation therapy also encompasses the splenic pedicle, where the spleen is still intact. The combination of mantle, para-aortic, and pelvic radiation therapy is known as total lymphoid irradiation; the para-aortic region and pelvic region is known as an *inverted Y*.

## Radiation therapy alone

Staging laparotomy was part of the standard work up of patients with HL in the 1960s and 1970s, in part due to a lack of effective radiological techniques to evaluate abdominal and pelvic lymphadenopathy. Most patients therefore underwent pathologic staging. In contrast, at the present time few patients undergo pathologic staging. Computerized tomography and positron emission tomography (PET scanning) have lead to the common practice of clinical staging. With this evolution, some of the data concerning radiation therapy in the treatment of HL is dated.

There are several studies comparing limited field radiation therapy with broader radiation fields as the sole form of therapy in patients with limited stage HL. These studies are summarized in Table 73.1. The EORTCH 5 Trial included patients of age 40 or younger with nonbulky pathologic stage I and II, who and were considered a favorable risk group. Patients received mantle and periaortic radiation therapy versus mantle radiation therapy alone; no differences in disease-free survival (DFS) were seen between the two treatment groups.[4] Regional radiation therapy was compared to involved-field radiation therapy (IFRT) in a BLNI Trial for pathologic stage IA and IIA patients; again, there were no difference in freedom from relapse (FFR).[1]

These data contrast two other studies that reported inferior outcome in pathologically staged patients when comparing limited field radiation therapy to broader fields. The Stanford trial compared subtotal lymphoid radiation therapy with IFRT in pathologically staged IA and IIA patients; FFR was significantly different (80% vs 32%), respectively.[3] Significant differences in FFR was also found in the Collaborative clinical trial, favoring mantle/periaortic radiation therapy with IFRT.[2] The Collaborative clinical trial also found an advantage to subtotal lymphoid irradiation versus involved-field radiation for clinical stage I and II patients, in which FFR was 59% versus 32%, which was a statistically significant difference.

The utility of clinical staging in the treatment of patients with HL without a staging laparotomy was documented by the EORTCH 6 Trial.[5] In this study, favorable patients (defined as no more than two nodal sites; no B symptoms; no bulky disease; and an erythrocyte sedimentation rate <30 mm) were studied. These "favorable" patients (which constituted only 45% of patients with clinical stage I and II disease) were randomized to either subtotal nodal radiation therapy plus splenic radiation therapy versus staging laparotomy with treatment modified by the results of surgery and histology. If laparotomy was positive, patients received chemotherapy. Patients with a negative staging laparotomy, and lymphocyte predominant or nodular sclerosing histology, were treated with mantle radiation therapy alone, and other histologies received subtotal nodal radiation therapy plus splenic radiation therapy. In this study, DFS was not statistically different in the surgically staged group versus the clinically staged group. Note that 30% of patients had a positive staging laparotomy. Overall survival (OS), paradoxically, was slightly worse in the laparotomy arm (93% vs 89%). This may or may not have reflected acute or later complications as a result of surgery.

As clinical staging has become increasingly common, a majority of programs specializing in the care of lymphoma patients generally use subtotal lymphoid radiation therapy, or other modifications of extended field radiation therapy, when treating favorable stage I and II patients. Mantle radiation therapy alone is rarely used at the present time.

## Radiation therapy versus radiation therapy plus chemotherapy

Clinical trials of limited stage HL have more recently focused on the use of radiation therapy versus combined radiation therapy and chemotherapy. Decades ago, the specific chemotherapy regimen usually employed was MOPP. Given that MOPP has been replaced in the treatment of HL by ABVD (adriamycin, bleomycin, vinblastine, and dacarbazine), these pioneering studies are of only moderate relevance to today's practice. As a general statement, these studies included both pathologically staged and clinically staged patients, and generally compared subtotal lymphoid radiation therapy or total lymphoid radiation therapy versus MOPP (or a variant of MOPP) combined with limited or extended field radiation therapy. Table 73.2 shows a summary of these studies. Two studies found an advantage (FFR) in combined modality therapy (CMT), whereas the others did not. There was no difference in OS in any study. Other findings of studies of this era are important. Multiple sites of disease were associated with less favorable outcome.[8] Several studies

| Table 73.1 | Limited versus extended radiation therapy for early stage HL | | |
|---|---|---|---|
| Author | Ref. | Year | Comment |
| Hope-Stone | 1 | 1981 | Regional vs IF for PS I-IIA; regional vs IF for CSI-IIA; no difference in PFS or OS |
| Fuller | 2 | 1982 | PS I-II: extended field XRT better DFS than IF (66% vs 51%, P = 0.05) CS I-II: EF better DFS than IF (52% vs 35%, P = 0.02) |
| Rosenberg | 3 | 1985 | PS IA and IIA: STLI/TLI vs IF FFP 80% vs 32%, P = 0.0001; OS identical |
| Carde | 4 | 1988 | PS I-II STLI vs M: no difference in FFP |

XRT, radiation therapy; IF, involved field; PS, pathologic stage; CS, clinical stage; EF, extended field; STLI, subtotal lymphoid irradiation; TLI, total lymphoid irradiation; FFP, freedom from progression; M, mantle field.

**Table 73.2** Selected early trials of extended radiation therapy versus extended radiation therapy + chemotherapy in early stage HL

| Author | Ref. | Year | Comment |
|---|---|---|---|
| Jones | 6 | 1982 | PS I-II involved field XRT + MOPP vs extended field XRT—trend toward improved RFS with combined therapy ($P = 0.12$). No difference in OS. Predominant RFS effect on those patients with B symptoms ($P < 0.03$) |
| Nissen | 7 | 1982 | PS I-II randomized to extended field XRT or mantle XRT + MOPP. RFS better with combined therapy ($P < 0.05$). No difference in OS |
| Rosenberg | 3 | 1985 | PS IA—IIB Randomized to IF XRT + MOPP vs extended field XRT. Combined better RFS but no difference in OS. PS IB- IIB TLI + MOPP vs TLI. No difference in RFS or OS |
| Tubiana | 8 | 1989 | PS I-II Randomized to MOPP + extended field XRT vs TLI DFS better in combined therapy, but no difference in OS |

PS, pathologic stage; XRT, radiation therapy; IF, involved field; TLI, total lymphoid irradiation.

also concluded that large mediastinal masses (LMMs) were an adverse prognostic sign. In particular, patients with bulky mediastinal masses treated with radiation therapy alone had a high incidence of disease relapse, and most of these studies recommended CMT for this group of patients.[9–14]

An additional early trial used a different approach, as patients with limited stage HL were randomized to chemotherapy with cyclophosphamide, vinblastine, procabazine, and prednisone (CVPP) alone or CVPP plus IFRT. The study found no differences in relapse-free survival (RFS) or OS. Additional prognostic factors were age more than 45 years and more than two lymph node areas involved with HL, as well as bulky disease.[15]

A meta-analysis of 3500 patients treated on randomized trials of more versus less extensive radiation therapy and trials comparing radiation therapy plus chemotherapy to radiation therapy alone was published in 1998.[16] Adding chemotherapy reduced the risk of recurrence by 50% but did not improve OS. This was felt to be a result of an ability to salvage radiation therapy failures with subsequent chemotherapy.

### Recent trials of CMT

A sample of the recently reported randomized trials of limited stage HL is shown in Table 73.3. The usual design of the studies is a comparison of extended field radiation therapy versus abbreviated chemotherapy, combined with either limited or extended field radiation therapy. In three studies, the control group was extended field radiation therapy and abbreviated courses of chemotherapy were given with either extended-field radiation therapy or IFRT. Freedom from progression was improved in the combined modality group in all three trials; OS was identical. Bonadonna et al. investigated the use of four full cycles of ABVD chemotherapy followed by either IFRT or extended-field radiation therapy. No differences in 12-year freedom from progression or OS were noted.

All of this data has lead to the National Comprehensive Cancer Network (NCCN) practice guidelines for limited stage HL to focus on the use of extended field radiation therapy alone or CMT.[21] For clinically staged patients with supradiaphramatic presentation, the most common presentation of limited stage HL, the NCCN practice guidelines focused on three patient groups: those with no unfavorable factors, those with bulky disease, and those with nonbulky disease with an erythrocyte sedimentation rate (ESR) greater than 70 or three sites involved. The recommendations for

**Table 73.3** Recent limited stage HL randomized trials

| Author | Ref. | Year | Design | Comment |
|---|---|---|---|---|
| Hagenbeek | 17 | 2000 | 543 pts. supradiaphragmatic CS I-II, age < 50 nonbulky, randomized to MOPP/ABV hybrid × 3 + IF XRT vs STLI | 4y FFS better in combined arm: 99% vs 77% ($P < 0.0001$). OS 99% vs 95% ($P = 0.019$) |
| Press | 18 | 2001 | 326 pts. supradiaphragmatic CS I-II randomized to STLI or 3 cycles ROXO + vlb + STLI | 3y FFS better in combo arm: 94% vs 81% ($P < 0.001$). OS > 95% no difference |
| Sieber | 19 | 2002 | 571 favorable CS I-II pts. randomized to ABVD × 2 + EF vs EF alone | 2y FFP better in combo arm: 96% vs 84%, ($P < 0.05$). 2y OS 98% vs 98% |
| Bonadonna | 20 | 2004 | 136 limited stage randomized to ABVD × 4 + IF XRT or STLI | No difference in FFP or OS |

FFP, freedom from progression; CS, clinical stage; IF, involved field; EF, extended field; XRT, radiation therapy; STLI, subtotal lymphoid irradiation.

these three groups are as follows: for the favorable group, the recommendation is for subtotal lymphoid irradiation alone or CMT; for the group with bulky disease, CMT is recommended; for the nonbulky group with other high risk factors, either CMT (preferred) or subtotal lymphoid irradiation therapy is recommended. None of these recommendations for limited stage HL include chemotherapy alone.

Two recent studies have explored the use of ABVD alone for limited stage HL. A Canadian trial randomized 399 patients with nonbulky stage I-IIA disease, comparing four to six cycles of ABVD chemotherapy with extended field radiation therapy (in a high-risk group), or to two cycles of ABVD plus extended field radiation therapy (in a low-risk group). Five-year freedom from progression was slightly inferior in the ABVD group (87% vs 93%, $P = 0.006$). OS was the same, 96% (ABVD) versus 94% (standard therapy).[22] Strauss et al. studied 152 untreated clinical stage I-IIIA non-

bulky HL, comparing outcome to either six cycles of ABVD, or six cycles of ABVD followed by radiation therapy (involved-field or extended-field).[23] With five years follow-up, there was no difference in freedom from progression, or OS, in the two arms. Much smaller series have also described the clinical utility of ABVD alone in limited stage HL.[24,25]

## LATE EFFECTS AFTER PRIMARY THERAPY FOR HL

It is now known that secondary malignancies are a serious and potentially lethal consequence of primary HLe therapy. The combination of death from secondary malignancies and posttreatment cardiac mortality may result in more deaths for patients with favorable limited stage HL than does the HL itself.

Table 73.4 shows a summary of recently reported large studies examining the risk of secondary malignancies in patients who received therapy for HL. The vast majority of patients described in these studies received

| Table 73.4 | Secondary malignancy after HL therapy | | | | |
|---|---|---|---|---|---|
| Author | Ref. | Year | N | Follow-up | Findings |
| Bhatia | 26 | 1996 | 1380 | 11.4 (median) | 18-fold risk of all cancers. 7% absolute incidence at 15y. Breast cancer risk more than five times general population. BC risk associated with higher dose of radiation therapy. 46/47 solid tumor pts. received XRT ± chemotherapy. |
| Aisenberg | 27 | 1997 | 111 women stage I-II HL treated with mantle XRT | 18 y (median) | 34% of pts. aged less than 20y developed breast cancer; 22% of those aged 20–29. No plateau in incidence with time. |
| van Leeuwen, | 28 | 2000 | 1253 | 14y (median) | 25y acturioral risk of malignancy 28%; risk of solid tumors higher for younger patients; no plateau in incidence with time; 27/27 breast cancer pts. received XRT ± chemo; 48/49 other solid tumor pts. received XRT ± chemotherapy. |
| Swerdlow | 29 | 2000 | 5519 | 8.5y (mean) | 20y cumulative risk of secondary malignancy 15%; 8% solid tumors. Relative risk of solid tumors (10y, 61, breast) greater for younger pts. |
| Metayer | 30 | 2000 | 5925 | 10.5 (mean) | Sevenfold-increased risk of solid tumors, 27-fold risk of acute leukemia. 20y HL survivors have the following fold risk of developing cancers: breast—8; thyroid—38; cervix—11; GI—11. No secondary leukemic reported after 20 years, while risk of solid tumors continue. Vast majority of pts. in this cohort received XRT. |
| Ng | 31 | 2002 | 1319 | 12 (median) | Fivefold-increased risk of secondary malignancy. Risk increased with increasing radiation field size. No plateau in risk after 20 years. |
| Dores | 32 | 2002 | 32,591 | 8 (mean) | 25y after HL therapy risk of developing a solid tumor 22%; no plateau in incidence; younger age has a higher relative risk of developing a solid tumor. |

XTR, radiation therapy.

radiation therapy alone or radiation therapy in combination with chemotherapy. Several themes are apparent. Female patients receiving radiation therapy at a young age have a tremendously increased risk of developing breast cancer.[26–28] Indeed, the relative risk of developing any solid tumor is higher if the patient is treated at a younger age.[29,32] The risk of developing a solid tumor is increased if radiation therapy alone was used as opposed to chemotherapy alone.[26,28,32] The risk of solid tumors continues with time; there is no plateau in the incidence of secondary solid tumors.[32] As an example, with 25 years of follow-up, the risk of developing a secondary solid tumor is as high as 28%.[28] The risk of developing a hematologic malignancy is highest 5–10 years after therapy; there is no increased risk of hematologic malignancy after 20 years of therapy.[32] The size of the radiation therapy field is associated with an increased risk of developing secondary solid tumors.[33] Additional studies have determined that the risk of breast cancer is associated with radiation therapy dose. The risk with radiation therapy dose appears to increase linearly, from at least 4–40 Gy.[33]

A meta-analysis of over 8000 females diagnosed with HL between 1973 and 1999 was recently reported.[34] The purpose was to examine the influence of radiation therapy on the time interval to the development of breast cancer. Out of 8,036 women, 183 (2.3%) were subsequently diagnosed with breast carcinoma. The use of radiation therapy in the treatment of HL resulted in an increased risk of the development of breast carcinoma ($P < 0.01$). A regression model revealed that the use of radiotherapy had an adverse effect on long-term survival (relative risk = 1.84, $P = 0.01$).

Radiation therapy to the chest is also associated with an increased risk of ischemic coronary artery disease, involving the carotid and/or subclavian arteries, and valvular cardiac disease. A sampling of recent studies examining the relationship of radiation therapy with the development of cardiac disease is shown in Table 73.5. Some common themes to these studies are given next. The risk of ischemic coronary artery disease increases with time: there is approximately a 5–7% risk at 10 years and a 10–20% risk at 20 years.[36,39] The risk of death from ischemic heart disease is five times that of controls. The risk of ischemic death is 2–6% at 10 years and 10–12% at 20 years.[36,38] There is an eightfold risk of developing symptomatic valvular heart disease, most commonly involving the aortic valve.[39] All of these risks are associated with higher doses of radiation therapy and larger radiation therapy fields.[35,38,39] The addition of chemotherapy does not contribute to increased risk of any form of cardiac disease.[36,39] The risk of developing cardiac disease in conjunction with mantle radiation therapy seems to be particularly observed in patients who have other known cardiac risk factors, such as hypertension and elevated lipid levels.

In summary, the risk of developing coronary artery disease is dramatically increased with the use of radiation therapy to the chest. The risk of the development of solid tumors is increased with radiation therapy as well. Both of these risks continue with time and show no evidence of a plateau in their incidence with follow-up beyond 20 years.

An important but sometimes neglected article was published years ago examining the incidence of second neoplasms after ABVD in HL.[40] Over 1000 consecutive patients with HL were studied. In contrast to MOPP chemotherapy, there is no increased incidence of secondary malignancy seen in patients treated with ABVD chemotherapy.

| Table 73.5 | Recent trials of treated HL and cardiovascular disease | | | | |
|---|---|---|---|---|---|
| Author | Ref. | Year | N | Follow-uP | Comment |
| Hancock | 35 | 1993 | 2232 | 9.5 (mean) | 4% died of heart disease, 63% from CAD. Mediastinal XRT dose > 30 Gy associated with increased risk of death from MI increases with time. |
| Reinders | 36 | 2000 | 258 treated with mantle XTR | 14.2 (median) | 12% developed ischemic heart disease. Actuarial risk at 25 years of cardiac death 10%. |
| Lee | 37 | 2000 | 210 treated with mantle XTR | 15-16 (median) | 27% incidence of cardiovascular complication. Median time to cardiac event was 15 years. |
| Erikson | 38 | 2000 | 157 mantle XTR | 16 (median) | 8% died from ischemic heart disease. Greater risk with larger volume fraction and higher XRT dose. |
| Hull | 39 | 2003 | 415 chest XTR | 11 (median) | 10% developed ischemic heart disease at a median 9 years after treatment. 7% developed carotid and/or valvular dysfunction at a median of 22 years, most commonly aortic stenosis. Risk associated with higher XRT dose. Chemotherapy not associated with higher risk. |

XRT, radiation therapy; MI, myocardial infarction; CAD, coronary artery disease.

## THE CONTRARIAN APPROACH TO LIMITED STAGE HL

Virtually every textbook echoes the NCCN practice guidelines for HL in recommending radiation therapy in one form or another for limited stage disease. The radiation therapy is frequently coupled with chemotherapy, resulting in the now accepted combined modality approach. This approach has evolved for many reasons. First, it works fairly well; most patients with early stage HL are cured with this approach. Second, it builds on historical data. Initially, radiation therapy was much easier to administer to patients than was chemotherapy and resulted in generally good outcomes. Thirty years ago chemotherapy was something to avoid if at all possible. Additionally, when successful therapy for HL began there was no knowledge of long-term late effects of radiation therapy, because there was no long-term follow-up of successfully treated patients.

However, we now know that radiation therapy contributes to an increased risk of second malignancies, which continues to rise as the length of follow-up increases. Radiation therapy is also associated with cardiac toxicities that increase the risk of cardiac death in "successfully" treated patients. We also know that ABVD neither have a significant risk of secondary malignancies nor long-term cardiac toxicities (assuming that patients are monitored appropriately during the delivery of doxorubicin-based chemotherapy). Additionally, as described previously, we now have data on two recent studies examining the use of ABVD alone for limited stage HL, in which the clinical outcomes are outstanding.[23–25] A logical question to ask is why should we give radiation therapy at all. The contrarian viewpoint in the treatment of early stage HL would answer this question as follows: given our current knowledge base, there is no reason to give radiation therapy in early stage HL; simply give everyone ABVD.

Dr. Dan Longo was a pioneer in the treatment of HL. He has written several editorials recently on this subject. In 2002 he wrote,

My fear is that we have ample evidence that radiation therapy is harmful and that it is no longer needed to treat most patients with Hodgkin's lymphoma. The safest and most effective way to manage patients with Hodgkin's lymphoma is to use clinical staging followed by six cycles of combination therapy. ABVD is probably the most effective available chemotherapy regimen . . . . . . . we should be using radiation therapy more judiciously, rather than finding excuses to use it in every patient. The next generation and our patients will judge us harshly for failing to heed the obvious signs.[41]

In 2003 Dr. Longo wrote

The prevailing thinking seems to be as follows: if we give combined modality therapy we can cut back a little on the radiation dose and cut back a little on the chemotherapy cycles and that should preserve the anti tumor effects and minimize the toxicity. Au contraire. No dose of radiation therapy is without life threatening late sequelae, and six cycles of ABVD chemotherapy alone appears to be extremely effective in all stages of Hodgkin's lymphoma without any reported life threatening toxicities.[42]

Finally, in December 2004, Dr. Longo wrote an editorial and stated

Large cohorts of patients treated with radiation therapy have now been followed for many years and groups have reported that deaths related to radiation therapy treatment outnumbered deaths related to Hodgkin's lymphoma. Mediastinal radiation therapy is associated with a three fold increased risk of fatal myocardial infarction from accelerated coronary arthrosclerosis. Furthermore, patients treated with radiation therapy have a risk of developing a secondary malignancy of about 25% in 25 years with no evidence that that risk is decreasing with time . . . . . . . it is time to adopt a new approach to Hodgkin's lymphoma treatment: clinical staging followed by ABVD chemotherapy in all stages of disease. No life is without risk but such an approach removes the imminent threat posed by radiation exposure for the majority of patients.[43]

Radiation therapy has significant late toxicities that seem to be largely ignored by the oncologic community. ABVD is an extremely effective treatment of HL and not associated with long-term toxicities. The vast majority of early stage HL patients should receive ABVD alone. The possible exceptions are those with LMMs who have a positive PET scan at the end of completion of chemotherapy. Such patients might benefit from radiation therapy, although this point has not been definitively proven.

## CLINICAL STAGE III AND IV (ADVANCED) CLASSICAL HL: TREATMENT PRINCIPLES

### INTRODUCTION

Many patients present with advanced stage HL.[44] In the 1960s, DeVita and colleagues from the National Cancer Institute (NCI) introduced a multiagent chemotherapy regimen known as MOPP that established cure in over 50% of patients with advanced disease.[45] Before this era, 5-year survival from advanced HL barely reached 5%. However, MOPP had significant short- and long-term toxicities. Investigators subsequently examined other regimens, such as ABVD. ABVD yields similar survival rates as MOPP but has fewer short- and long-term toxicities. What follows is a brief review of the historical development of chemotherapy regimens for advanced HL, a discussion of the "new" regimens used for higher-risk patients, and an examination of the role of radiation therapy as part of CMT in the advanced disease setting.

## CHEMOTHERAPY REGIMENS
### MOPP and MOPP derivatives

The dosage, schedule, and frequency of MOPP chemotherapy are described in Table 73.6. Patients receive four drugs over a 2-week interval followed by a 2-week recovery period. A total of 4 weeks constitutes one cycle of treatment. Most patients receive six cycles. Historically, the dose of vincristine used in MOPP frequently exceeded the currently recognized dosage limit of 2 mg. Two updated mature studies with 10[45] and 14 years[46] follow-up, respectively, showed that 66% of patients have remained disease-free more than 10 years from the end of treatment. Forty-eight percent of advanced HL patients have survived between 9 and 21 years (median, 14 years) from the end of treatment. Nineteen percent of the complete remission cases have died of intercurrent illnesses, free of HL.[45,46]

Unfortunately, acute and long-term toxicities of MOPP regimen were significant. These toxicities ranged from nausea to death. Overall mortality approached 2.5% in the NCI series and 1.5% in smaller studies.[47] Hematologic toxicities, although reversible, were sometimes fatal, as hematopoietic growth factor compounds were not available at that time. Vincristine-associated neuropathy was clinically relevant with doses more than 2 mg. Procarbazine was associated with severe emesis, and a type I allergic reaction in rare cases.

Long-term toxicities were of even more serious concern. Most patients experienced infertility after treatment with MOPP. Males had at least an 80% risk of permanent azospermia after MOPP, while 50% of females experienced gonadal failure.[47,48] The risk appeared lower with patients younger than 25 years of age; however, accelerated early menopause seemed to be the case in every female who did recover her menses after treatment.[46] At a time when sperm banking and oocyte cryopreservation were in their early stages, many young patients, though cured, experienced significant psychological repercussions due to their infertility.

Another major problem with MOPP was the observation of myelodysplastic syndrome (MDS) and acute leukemia in up to 6% of patients. These hematologic malignancies started 2 years after treatment, with a

| Regimen | Dosage (mg/m$^2$) | Route | Schedule | Cycle duration |
|---|---|---|---|---|
| **MOPP** | | | | **28 days** |
| Mechlorethamine | 6 | IV | Days 1, 8 | |
| Vincristine[a] | 1.4 | IV | Days 1, 8 | |
| Procarbazine | 100 | PO | Days 1–14 | |
| Prednisone | 40 | PO | Days 1–14 | |
| **ABVD** | | | | **28 days** |
| Adriamycin | 25 | IV | Days 1, 15 | |
| Bleomycin | 10 | IV | Days 1, 15 | |
| Vinblastine | 6 | IV | Days 1, 15 | |
| Dacarbazine | 375 | IV | Days 1, 15 | |
| **MOPP/ABV Hybrid** | | | | **28 days** |
| Mechlorethamine | 6 | IV | Day 1 | |
| Vincristine[a] | 1.4 | IV | Day 1 | |
| Procarbazine | 100 | PO | Days 1–7 | |
| Prednisone | 40 | PO | Days 1–14 | |
| Adriamycin | 35 | IV | Day 8 | |
| Bleomycin | 10 | IV | Day 8 | |
| Vinblastine | 6 | IV | Day 8 | |
| **Stanford V** | | | | **28 days (total of three cycles)** |
| Adriamycin | 25 | IV | Day 1, 15 | |
| Vinblastine | 6 | IV | Day 1, 15 | |
| Mechlorethamine | 6 | IV | Day 1 | |
| Vincristine | 1.4 | IV | Day 8, 22 | |
| Bleomycin | 5 | IV | Day 8, 22 | |
| Etoposide | 60 | IV | Day 15, 16 | |
| Prednisone | 40 | PO | Every other day | |

Table 73.6 Main chemotherapy regimens used in advanced HL

[a]Vincristine dose capped at 2 mg.

peak around the fifth year, and were associated with an extremely poor prognosis, with a median survival of 6 months.[49] Although the risk of leukemia was mostly attributed to concomitant radiation, patients with MOPP therapy alone were at increased risk of leukemic transformation.[49,50]

MOPP derivatives were introduced in the mid 1970s with the goal of similar efficacy with less toxicity. A prospective randomized trial by the Cancer and Leukemia Group B (CALGB) examined a new combination, BOPP (BCNU (carmustine), vincristine, procarbazine, and prednisone), derived from substitution of BCNU for nitrogen mustard in the MOPP regimen. BOPP was compared to MOPP and to 2 three-drug regimens, derived by removing the procarbazine in BOPP (BOP) or removing the alkylating agent (OPP). The four-drug programs resulted in significantly higher frequency of complete remissions (BOPP 67%, MOPP 63%) than the three-drug regimens (BOP 40%, OPP 42%), and a significantly longer duration of remission and survival. In addition, BOPP had less toxicity.[51] Bakemeier et al. prospectively compared BCVPP (carmustine, cyclophosphamide, vinblastine, procarbazine, and prednisone) to MOPP. Two hundred ninety-three patients were evaluable in the induction phase of this study. The complete remission rates of BCVPP and MOPP were similar. The duration of complete remissions for previously untreated patients given BCVPP was significantly longer than that for previously untreated patients given MOPP ($P = 0.02$). Although hematologic toxicities were similar, BCVPP caused less gastrointestinal ($P = 0.0001$) and neurological toxicity ($P = 0.01$) than MOPP. More importantly, previously untreated patients achieving complete remission with BCVPP had a better OS than those receiving MOPP ($P = 0.03$).[52]

In other studies, alkylating agents such as cyclophosphamide or chlorambucil were used instead of the nitrogen mustard, resulting in similar efficacy but less treatment-related leukemia.[53,54]

### ABVD

In 1975, the ABVD regimen was introduced by Bonadonna et al. in an attempt to find a salvage treatment for MOPP failure. The dosage and schedule of this regimen are described in Table 73.6. The study involved a small number of patients (65 patients) and showed that ABVD was safe and could be used in cases of MOPP resistance. Moreover, it was well tolerated, with more than 85% of the intended dosage being delivered.[55]

The same European group published a randomized trial in a larger cohort of 237 patients comparing the "new" ABVD regimen to the standard MOPP therapy. Three cycles of either combination chemotherapy preceded and then followed subtotal or total nodal radiation. The 7-year results indicated that ABVD was statistically superior to MOPP in terms of freedom from progression (80.8% vs 62.8%), RFS (87.7% vs 77.2%),

and OS (77.4% vs 67.9%). Gonadal toxicities and leukemia were only seen in patients receiving MOPP therapy.[56] Even with the clear benefits of AVBD over MOPP in this study, it was largely criticized due to the difficulty delivering the planned MOPP dosage after receiving extensive radiation.

A landmark US study from the CALGB in 1992 randomized 361 patients with advanced HL to receive MOPP, ABVD, or a combination of MOPP alternating with ABVD. Patients not achieving a complete response or who relapsed with either MOPP alone or ABVD alone were switched to the opposite regimen. Overall survival at 5 years was 66% for MOPP, 73% for ABVD, and 75% for MOPP-ABVD ($P = 0.28$ for the comparison of MOPP, with the anthracycline-containing regimens). While an improvement in OS did not occur, ABVD regimens did have a higher rate of complete response (82% vs 67%), less hematologic toxicity, and a higher rate of failure-free survival (FFS) at 5 years (61% vs 50%), when compared to MOPP. Patients with recurrent disease after ABVD subsequently received MOPP, with 61% achieving a second remission. In comparison, only 35% of those who suffered relapse after MOPP responded to ABVD. The alternating regimen (MOPP-ABVD) was not superior to ABVD and had more hematologic toxicity.[57] Patients did not receive radiation in this study, thus allowing a direct comparison of the three chemotherapy regimens. A long-term follow-up of this study over 15 years has recently been published, demonstrating a 45% to 50% progression-free survival (PFS) and a 65% OS rate for ABVD and MOPP/ABVD.[58]

Due to the favorable outcomes associated with ABVD, it started to replace MOPP in most cases of advanced HL. Most patients were able to receive all of the planned treatments.[57] In addition, acute toxicities, such as bone marrow depression and neurotoxicities seen with MOPP, were much less frequent with ABVD. Long-term toxicities, including gonadal dysfunction, were encountered less frequently with ABVD than with MOPP, with reversibility in most of the cases.[59] In the European trial mentioned earlier,[56] no cases of therapy-related leukemia were seen with ABVD as compared with 6.5% with MOPP therapy, even with the use of radiation in both arms.

Anthracycline inclusion in the ABVD regimen were of concern initially, as doxorubicin is known to be associated with cardiomyopathy. However, six cycles of ABVD provide a total of 300 mg/m$^2$ of doxorubicin, which is well under the doses (450–500 mg/m$^2$) usually associated with cardiac toxicities.[60] Although patients who receive mantle field radiation therapy have a threefold-increased risk of fatal myocardial infarction,[35] evidence is lacking to support an additive toxicity from concomitant anthracycline use.[56]

Short-and long-term effects of bleomycin include pulmonary toxicity. In one trial, ABVD chemotherapy induced acute pulmonary toxicity that required bleomycin dose modification in 37% of patients.[61] The addition of radiation therapy resulted in a further decrease in vital capacity; however, this did not significantly affect normal daily activities. High-risk groups for bleomycin toxicity include children, patients with compromised respiratory status, or concomitant use of bleomycin and gemcitabine.[62,63]

### MOPP/ABV hybrid

This "hybrid' regimen is described in Table 73.6. Patients receive parts of a MOPP cycle combined with components of an ABVD cycle, over a 1-month period. An Eastern Cooperative Oncology Group (ECOG) trial showed a high response rate for this regimen coupled with an OS advantage when compared with sequential MOPP followed by ABVD regimen.[64] However, two other trials failed to show any FFS or OS benefit from the MOPP/ABV hybrid, when compared to an alternating regimen of MOPP/ABVD.[65,66] These mixed results prompted the initiation of an intergroup trial comparing the hybrid regimen with the standard ABVD chemotherapy. Results from this trial showed no statistical difference in FFS and 5-year OS between the two arms.[67] However, the MOPP/ABV hybrid was associated with significant treatment-related deaths, secondary malignancies, and infections.[67] As ABVD has the same overall efficacy with less toxicity than the MOPP/ABV hybrid, it continues to be the "standard treatment" in advanced HL.

### Stanford V

This regimen was introduced in 1995 with an objective of improving cure rate and limiting toxicities. Table 73.6 describes the schedule dosing of this regimen. Essentially, it is similar to the MOPP/ABV hybrid regimen but adds modest doses of Etoposide. Radiation therapy is an integral component of this regimen with 36 Gy radiation given to sites of bulky disease more than 5 cm in diameter. An initial report, followed recently by more mature data, showed an FFS of 86% with a 95% OS after 6.9 years of follow-up.[68,69] These numbers remained consistent in patients with bulky mediastinal disease.[70] Secondary malignancies and infertility were reported to be less than 10%. This favorable toxicity profile, coupled with excellent efficacy, prompted interest in this regimen as a substitute for ABVD.[71] However, a recent study from Italy showed an FFS inferiority for the Stanford regimen as compared to ABVD.[72] This study compared three chemotherapy regimens: Stanford V, ABVD, and MOPP-EBV-CAD (MEC) (a combination regimen using mechlorethamine, CCNU, vindesine, alkeran, prednisone, epidoxorubicin, vincristine, procarbazine, vinblastine, and bleomycin). Although OS was not statically different, FFS, at 56 months follow-up, was 83% for ABVD, compared to 67% for Stanford V. However, an important point is that Stanford V is a combined modality regimen, with radiation therapy routinely given in up to

85% of the patients. The Italian trial used radiation therapy in only two-thirds of patients, and frequently at suboptimal dosages. Stanford V, with or without radiation therapy, is currently being compared to ABVD in advanced HL in an intergroup trial.[71]

### BEACOPP regimen

The majority of patients with advanced HL are cured with standard anthracycline-based treatments. Approximately one-third of such patients fails to achieve a long-term remission and therefore may benefit from a more intensified initial regimen. An accurate prognostic algorithm is necessary to identify patients in whom standard treatment is likely to fail.

In 1998, a seven-factor prognostic scoring system that focused on 5-year rates of freedom from progression of disease was developed. This system, known as the international prognosis index (IPI), uses seven independent prognostic factors: serum albumin level of less than 4 g/dL; hemoglobin level of less than 10.5 g/dL; male sex; age of 45 years or older; stage IV disease (according to the Ann Arbor classification); leukocytosis (a white-cell count of at least 15,000/mm³); and lymphopenia (a lymphocyte count of less than 600/mm³, a count that was less than 8% of the white-cell count, or both). The score predicted the rate of freedom from disease progression with higher scores associated with increased risk of disease progression.[73] The IPI was incorporated in a major German trial where two "intense" regimens, known as BEACOPP (bleomycin, etoposide, adriamycin, cyclophosphamide, vincristine, procarbazine, and prednisone) were tested against COPP-ABVD, a combination that many experts find equivalent to ABVD.[74] A description of these two BEACOPP regimens (baseline and escalated) and COPP-ABVD is outlined in Table 73.7. The BEACOPP regimen was developed in an attempt to improve treatment results in advanced HL by dose and time intensification and addition of etoposide. It employs a schedule permitting a shortened 3-week cycle. With growth factor support, the dosages of cyclophosphamide, etoposide, and adriamycin were moderately escalated. The trial, known as the HL-9 trial, included more than 1000 patients with advanced disease. After a follow-up of more than 50 months, the rate of freedom from treatment failure at 5 years was 69% in the COPP-ABVD arm, 76% in the BEACOPP-baseline arm, and 87% in the escalated-arm BEACOPP arm ($P = 0.04$) for the comparison of the COPP-ABVD arm with the BEACOPP arms (both the baseline and escalated arms). The 5-year rates of OS were 83% with COPP-ABVD, 88% with BEACOPP-baseline, and 91% with BEACOPP-escalated. Only the comparison of BEACOPP-escalated and COPP-ABVD was statistically significant for OS. Taking into account the IPI, patients with poor risk factors (≥ four adverse factors) had a much more pronounced benefit from BEACOPP regimens compared to COPP-ABVD, with 5-year OS

**Table 73.7** BEACOPP (baseline), BEACOPP escalated, and COPP/ABVD regimens

| Regimen | Dosage (mg/m²) | Route | Schedule | Cycle duration |
|---|---|---|---|---|
| **BEACOPP (baseline)** | | | | **21 days** |
| Bleomycin | 10 | IV | Day 8 | |
| Etoposide | 100 | IV | Day 1–3 | |
| Adriamycin | 25 | IV | Day 1 | |
| Cyclophosphamide | 650 | IV | Day 1 | |
| Oncovin (Vincristine)[a] | 1.4 | IV | Day 8 | |
| Procarbazine | 100 | PO | Day 1–7 | |
| Prednisone | 40 | PO | Day 1–14 | |
| **BEACOPP intensified** | | | | **21 days** |
| Bleomycin | 10 | IV | Day 8 | |
| Etoposide | 200 | IV | Day 1–3 | |
| Adriamycin | 35 | IV | Day 1 | |
| Cyclophosphamide | 1250 | IV | Day 1 | |
| Oncovin (Vincristine)[a] | 1.4 | IV | Day 8 | |
| Procarbazine | 100 | PO | Day 1–7 | |
| Prednisone | 40 | PO | Day 1–14 | |
| G-CSF[b] | | SC | | |
| **COPP/ABVD** | | | | **56 days** |
| Cyclophosphamide | 650 | IV | Day 1, 8 | |
| Oncovin (Vincristine)[a] | 1.4 | IV | Day 1, 8 | |
| Procarbazine | 100 | PO | Day 1–14 | |
| Prednisone | 40 | PO | Day 1–14 | |
| Adriamycin | 25 | IV | Day 29, 43 | |
| Bleomycin | 10 | IV | Day 29, 43 | |
| Vinblastine | 6 | IV | Day 29, 43 | |
| Dacarbazine | 375 | IV | Day 29, 43 | |

[a]Vincristine dose capped at 2 mg.
[b]Granulocyte colony-stimulating factor.

exceeding 80%, as compared to 67% in the COPP-ABVD arm.[74] On the other hand, in the group of patients with zero to one adverse prognostic factors, OS did not differ among the three arms. Unfortunately, this intensification in chemotherapy resulted in a higher incidence of side effects: bone marrow toxicity, including grade 3 and 4 anemia, thrombocytopenia, infections, azospermia, and mucositis. At a median follow-up of 7 years, secondary hematologic malignancies were 2.4% in the escalated BEACOPP arm, 1% in the BEACOPP-baseline group, and 0.4% in the COPP-ABVD arm.[75] Toxicities seemed to be more significant with advanced age, as a 21% mortality was noted in patients between 66 and 75 years old.[76] Studies are currently evaluating a shorter duration of the BEACOPP regimen (14 days) in addition to growth factors.[77] Another study is evaluating a "hybrid" regimen of escalated and standard BEACOPP, where patients get four cycles of each chemotherapy regimen in an attempt to reduce toxicity and maintain same cure rates.[75] These studies are ongoing.

### ROLE OF RADIATION THERAPY IN ADVANCED HL

In addition to chemotherapy, radiation therapy presents a potentially attractive tool against advanced HL. Early observations showed that the majority of relapses occurred in previously involved, nonirradiated sites. Retrospective studies from the early 1990s showed a 10-year DFS of 89% in-patients with advanced HL who received radiation, compared to 68% in-patients without radiation.[78] Similar results were reproduced in another retrospective study.[79] These encouraging results from CMT provided the basis for randomized controlled trials, summarized in Table 73.8.

A Southwest Oncology Group (SWOG) trial randomized 278 patients with stage III and IV HL to receive additional radiation therapy or observation after achieving complete remission (CR) with MOPP-based chemotherapy.[80] In an intention-to-treat analysis, RFS and OS at 8 years of follow-up were not statistically different. Another trial from a German group randomized patients in CR after six cycles of combined COPP-ABVD to receive one additional cycle of chemotherapy with COPP-ABVD versus radiation therapy to initially involved sites. Again, DFS and OS were not different in both groups.[81] In a multicenter randomized French study, 559 patients with advanced HL were randomized to two regimens of anthracycline-based chemotherapy. Patients with an excellent response were then randomized to receive

**Table 73.8** Trials of CMT for advanced HL

| Author | Ref. | Year | N | Study | Median follow-up (months) | Comment |
|---|---|---|---|---|---|---|
| Fabian | 80 | 1994 | 278 | RCT | 96 | Based on an "intention to treat" analysis: No difference in OS or DFS between CMT and CT alone |
| Diehl | 81 | 1995 | 288 | RCT | 72 | After CR, randomized to one cycle of COPP-ABVD or 20 Gy of IFRT: No DFS or OS benefit |
| Ferme | 82 | 2000 | 559 | RCT | 48 | After CR, randomized to two cycles of the same CT or STNI: No OS or DFS difference |
| Brice | 83 | 2001 | 82 | RCT | 48 | Exclusively in LMM. After CR, randomized to two cycles of CT or STNI: RR superior in CMT but no difference in DFS or OS. |
| Loeffler | 84 | 1998 | 1740 | Meta-analysis | 120 | After CR, RT vs observation: RRTF reduced by 40% but no OS advantage, even in bulky disease. After CR, CT vs CMT: OS better in CT alone ($P = 0.045$) |
| Aleman | 85 | 2003 | 739 | RCT | 79 | After CR, two cycles of additional CT (hybrid) vs IFRT: no difference in EFS or OS |
| Laskar | 86 | 2004 | 179 | RCT | 63 | After CR with six cycles of ABVD, EFS and OS better with CMT than CT alone ($P = 0.01$ and 0.002, respectively) *Caveats:* Less than 50% of patients have advanced HL or older than 15 years. |
| Diehl | 87 | 2003 (Abstract) | 1076 | RCT | 24 | Third interim analysis: No difference in FFTF or OS between CMT and CT alone. |

RCT, randomized controlled trial; CT, chemotherapy; RT, radiation therapy; STNI, subtotal nodal irradiation; RRTF, relative risk of treatment failure; EFS, event-free survival; FFTF, freedom from treatment failure.

either "consolidation" with extensive field radiation or an additional two cycles of the same chemotherapy. Five-year DFS and OS were not different for either consolidative regimen.[82] The same authors published a subset study from the French trial that looked exclusively at patients with an LMM, a group believed by many experts to benefit from additional radiation. In this study, in patients with LMM who achieved a major response of at least 75% after six cycles of chemotherapy, consolidation radiotherapy did not add any survival benefit compared to two additional cycles of chemotherapy.[83]

A meta-analysis tried to overcome the potential false-negative outcomes from smaller studies and involved 1700 patients with advanced HL from 14 different trials.[84] Additional radiation compared to observation decreased the relapse rate by 40% without affecting the 10-year OS. On the other hand, patients who had consolidative chemotherapy had an 8% better OS compared to those with consolidative radiation therapy. Although radiation seems to delay disease recurrence, its long-term toxicities (such as AML/MDS, other secondary solid tumors, and heart disease) appear to dampen any possible long-term OS benefit. This meta-analysis was largely criticized for two reasons: the chemotherapy used was primarily MOPP-based and IFRT was used in only 50% of cases. Patients with bulky disease features, a group who could potentially benefit from radiation, were not carefully addressed in this meta-analysis.[84]

Recently, two randomized studies were published, with mixed results. The first study from Europe randomized patients with advanced HL to receive two cycles of MOPP/ABV hybrid or IFRT to involved areas after six cycles of effective chemotherapy. IFRT did not add any DFS or OS benefit compared to the two additional cycles of MOPP/ABV. IFRT was of benefit in patients achieving only a partial response after chemotherapy, and resulted in a 5-year OS similar to patients in CR.[85]

The second study, from India, explored the role of additional radiotherapy in patients achieving a CR after six cycles of ABVD. A significant difference in 8-year event-free-survival and OS was found when radiation was added to chemotherapy.[86] This was the first large, randomized study to show a survival advantage with consolidation radiation. However, this study is not widely accepted due to many limitations. More than 50% of patients had early-stage disease and were younger than 15 years. In addition, histology was in most of the cases a mixed-cellularity type, as compared to the nodular sclerosis type seen in most of the European and North American trials.

Currently, an ongoing German study (HL12) is using intensive regimens, such as like BEACOPP-type with or without IFRT, in patients with advanced HL. An interim analysis is supporting the hypothesis that radiation can further be reduced substantially after effective chemotherapy.[87]

### CONCLUSIONS OF ADVANCED HL TREATMENT

Six to eight cycles of ABVD remains the treatment of choice for advanced stage HL at this time. Both the NCCN and NCI guidelines recognize ABVD as the gold standard regimen with a high level of evidence.[88,89] Stanford V has a favorable toxicity profile, but it is not clear at this time whether it is as efficacious as ABVD. An intergroup trial is underway and will hopefully answer this question. BEACOPP regimens are gaining popularity, especially in high-risk disease; however, its toxicity profile is significant. The role of additional radiation after effective chemotherapy is at best conjec-tural, even in the bulky disease setting. Some patients with an LMM often receive additional radiation as part of initial therapy, although evidence supporting this practice is sparse. The conclusions from the current lit-erature of the role of radiation added to chemotherapy in advanced HL is that it may have a beneficial impact when the preceding drug regimen is inadequate for effective tumor control, as occurs with patients who have a partial response. However, such patients have an inherently poor prognosis, and may be appropriate candidates for autologous stem cell transplant.

Future directions using new imaging techniques such as PET scan and gene expression profiling studies will hopefully identify accurate prognostic parameters to guide therapeutic decisions.

### REFERENCES

1. Hope-Stone HF: The Place of radiotherapy in the man-agement of localised Hodgkin's disease (Report No 11). *Clin Rad* 32:519–522, 1981.
2. Fuller LM, Hutchison GB: Collaborative clinical trial for stage I and II Hodgkin's disease: significance of mediasti-nal and nonmediastinal disease in laparotomy and non-laparotomy-staged patients. *Cancer Treat Rep* 66:775–787, 1982.
3. Rosenberg SA, Kaplan HS: The Evolution and summary results of the Stanford randomized clinical trials of the management of Hodgkin's disease: 1962–1984. *Int J Radiat Oncol Biol Phys* 11:5–22, 1985.
4. Carde P, Burgers J, Henry-Amar M, et al.: Clinical stages I and II Hodgkin's Disease: a specifically tailored therapy according to prognostic factors. *J Clin Oncol* 6:239–252, 1988.
5. Carde P, Hagenbeek A, Hayat M, et al.: Clinical staging versus laparotomy and combined modality with MOPP versus ABVD in early-stage Hodgkin's disease: The H6 twin randomized trials from the European Organization for Research and Treatment of Cancer Lymphoma Cooperative Group. *J Clin Oncol* 11:2258–2272, 1993.
6. Jones SE, Coltman CA, grozea PN, DePersio EJ, Dixon DO: Conclusions from clinical trials of the Southwest Oncology Group. *Cancer Treat Rep* 66:847–853, 1982.
7. Nissen NI, Nordentoft AM: Radiotherapy versus com-bined modality treatment of stage I and II Hodgkin's dis-ease. *Cancer Treat Rep* 66:799–803, 1982.
8. Tubiana M, Henry-Amar M, Carde P, et al.: Toward com-prehensive management tailored to prognostic factors of patients with clinical stage I–II in Hodgkin's Disease. The EORTC lymphoma group controlled clinical trials: 1964–1987. *Blood* 73:47–56, 1989.
9. Crnkovich MJ, Leopold K, Hoppe RT, Mauch PM: Stage I to IIB Hodgkin's Disease: The combined experience at Stanford University and the Joint Center for Radiation Therapy. *J Clin Oncol* 5:1041–1049, 1987.
10. Mauch P, Tarbell N, Vwinstein H, et al.: Stage IA and IIA supradiaphargmatic Hodgkin's disease: prognostic factors in surgically staged patients treated with mantle and paraaortic irradiation. *J Clin Oncol* 6:1576–1583, 1988.
11. Ferrant A, Hamoir V, Binon J, Michaux J, Sokal G: Combined modality therapy for Mediastinal Hodgkin's disease: Prognostic significance of constitutional symptoms and size of disease. *Cancer* 55:317–322, 1985.
12. Longo D, Glatstein E, Duffey P, et al.: Alternating MOPP and ABVD chemotherapy plus mantle-field radiation therapy in patients with massive Mediastinal Hodgkin's disease. *J Clin Oncol* 15:3338–3346, 1997.
13. Mauch P, Goodman R, Hellman S: The Significance of mediastinal involvement in early stage Hodgkin's dis-ease. *Cancer* 42:1039–1045, 1978.
14. Liew K, Easton D, Horwich A, Barrett A, Peckham MJ: bulky mediastinal hodgkin's disease management and prognosis. *Hematol Oncol* 2:45–59, 1984.
15. Pavlovsky S, Maschio M, Santarelli T, et al.: Randomized trial of chemotherapy versus chemotherapy plus radio-therapy for stage I-II Hodgkin's Disease. *J Natl Cancer Inst* 80:1466–1473, 1988.
16. Specht L, Gray RG, Clarke MJ, Peto R: Influence of more extensive radiotherapy and adjuvant chemotherapy on long-term outcome of early-stage Hodgkin's disease: A meta-analysis of 23 randomized trials involving 3,888 patients. *J Clin Oncol* 16:830–843, 1998.
17. Hagenbeek H, Eghbali C, Fermé JH, et al.: Three cycles of MOPP/ABV (M/A) hybrid and involved-field irradiation is more effective than subtotal nodal irradiation (STNI) in favorable supradiaphragmatic clinical stages (CS) I-II Hodgkin's disease (HD): Preliminary results of the EORTC-GELA H8F randomized trial in 543 patients. *Blood* 96:5759, 2000.
18. Press OW, LeBlanc M, Lichter AS, et al.: Phase III ran-domized intergroup trial of subtotal lymphoid irradia-tion versus Doxorubicin, Vinblastine, and subtotal lym-phoid irradiation for stage IA to IIA Hodgkin's disease. *J Clin Oncol* 19:4238–4244, 2001.
19. Sieber M, Franklin J, Tesch H, et al.: Two cycles of ABVD plus extended field radiotherapy is superior to radiother-apy alone in early stage Hodgkin's Disease: Results of the German Hodgkin's Lymphoma Study Group (GHSG) Trial HD7. *Blood* 100:939, 2002.
20. Bonadona G, Bonfante V, Viviani S, Di Russo A, Villani F, Valagussa P: ABVD plus subtotal nodal versus involved-field

radiotherapy in early-stage Hodgkin's disease: long term results. *J Clin Oncol* 22:2835–2841, 2004.

21. NCCN Practice Guidelines for Hodgkin's Disease. *Oncology* 13:5A, 1999.

22. Meyer R, Gospodarowica M, Connors J, et al.: A randomized Phase III comparison of single-modality ABVD with a strategy that includes radiation therapy in patients with early-stage Hodgkin's disease: the HD-6 Trial of the National Cancer Institute of Canada Clinical Trials Group (Eastern Cooperative Oncology Group Trial JHD06). *Blood* 102:269, 2003.

23. Straus DJ, Portlock CS, Qin J, et al.: Results of a prospective randomized clinical trial of doxorubicin, bleomycin, vinblastine, and dacarbazine (ABVD) followed by radiation therapy (RT) versus ABVD alone for stages I, II, and IIIA nonbulky Hodgkin Disease. *Blood* 104:3483–3489, 2004.

24. Provencio M, España P, Millán I, Sánchez A, Cantos B, Bonilla F: the management of stage I-II supradiaphragmatic Hodgkin's disease with chemotherapy alone. *Leuk Lymphoma* 44:263–268, 2003.

25. Rueda A, Alba E, Ribelles N, Sevilla I, Ruiz I, Miramón J: Six cycles of ABVD in the treatment of stage I and II Hodgkin's lymphoma: A pilot study. *J Clin Oncol* 15:1118–1122, 1997.

26. Bhatia S, Robison L, Oberlin O, et al.: Breast Cancer and other second neoplasms after childhood hodgkin's Disease. *NEJM* 334:745–751, 1996.

27. Aisenberg A, Finkelstein D, Doppke K, Koerner F, Boivin J, Willett C: High risk of breast carcinoma after irradiation of young women with Hodgkin's disease. *Cancer* 79:1203–1210, 1997.

28. van Leeuwen F, Klokman W, van't Veer M, et al.: Long-term risk of second malignancy in survivors of hodgkin's disease treated during adolescence or young adulthood. *J Clin Oncol* 18:487–497, 2000.

29. Swerdlow AJ, Barber JA, Hudson GV, et al.: Risk of second malignancy after Hodgkin's disease in a collaborative British cohort: The relation to age at treatment. *J Clin Oncol* 18:498–509, 2000.

30. Metayer C, Lynch C, Clarke EA, et al.: Second cancers among long-term survivors of Hodgkin's disease diagnosed in childhood and adolescence. *J Clin Oncol* 18:2435–2443, 2000.

31. Ng A, Bernardo MV, Weller E, et al.: Second malignancy after Hodgkin disease treated with radiation therapy with or without chemotherapy: long-term risks and risk factors. *Blood* 100:1989–1996, 2002.

32. Dores GM, Metayer C, Curtis RE, et al.: Second malignant neoplasms among long-term survivors of Hodgkin's disease: A population-based evaluation over 25 years. *J Clin Oncol* 20:3484–3494, 2002.

33. Boice JD: Radiation and breast carcinogenesis. *Med Pediatr Oncol* 36:508–513, 2001.

34. Wendland M, Tsodikov A, Glenn MJ, Gaffney: Time interval to the development of breast carcinoma after treatment for Hodgkin disease. *Cancer* 101:1275–1282, 2004.

35. Hancock SL, Tucker MA, Hoppe RT: Factors affecting late mortality from heart disease after treatment of Hodgkin's disease. *JAMA* 1993:270:1949–1955.

36. Reinders JG, Heijmen B, Olofsen-vvan Acht M, van Putten W, Levendag PC: Ischemic heart disease after

mantle field irradiation for Hodgkin's disease in long-term follow-up. *Radiother Oncol* 51:35–42, 1999.

37. Lee CK, Aeppli D, Nierengarten ME: The need for long-term surveillance for patients treated with curative radiotherapy for Hodgkin's disease: University of Minnesota experience. *Int J Radiat Oncol Biol Phys* 48:169–179, 2000.

38. Eriksson F, Gagliardi G, Liedberg A, et al.: Long-term cardiac mortality following radiation therapy for Hodgkin's disease: analysis with the relative seriality model. *Radiother Oncol* 55:153–162, 2000.

39. Hull MC, Morris CG, Pepine CJ, Mendenhall N: Valvular dysfunction and carotid, subclavian, and coronary artery disease in survivors of Hodgkin lymphoma treated with radiation therapy. *JAMA* 290:2831–2837, 2003.

40. Valagussa P, Santoro A, Fossati Bellani F, Banfi A, Bonadonna G: Absence of treatment-induced second neoplasms after ABVD in Hodgkin's disease. *Blood* 59:488–494, 1982.

41. Longo D: The Ng/Mauch article reviewed. *Oncology* 16:610–612, 2002.

42. Longo D: Radiation therapy in the treatment of Hodgkin's Disease—Do you see what I see? *J Natl Cancer Inst* 95:928–929, 2003.

43. Longo D: Hodgkin disease: the sword of Damocles resheathed. *Blood* 104:3418, 2004.

44. Rosenberg SA, Canellos GP: Hodgkin's disease. In: Canellos GP, Lister TA, Sklar JL (eds.): *The Lymphomas*, 1st ed. Philadelphia, PA: W.B. Saunders Company; 1998:309.

45. DeVita VT Jr, Simon RM, Hubbard SM, et al.: Curability of advanced Hodgkin's disease with chemotherapy. Long-term follow-up of MOPP-treated patients at the National Cancer Institute. *Ann Intern Med* 92:587–595, 1980.

46. Longo DL, Young RC, Wesley M, et al.: Twenty years of MOPP therapy for Hodgkin's disease. *J Clin Oncol* 4:1295–1306, 1986.

47. Bonadonna G, Valagussa P, Santoro A: Alternating non-cross-resistant combination chemotherapy or MOPP in stage IV Hodgkin's disease. A report of 8-year results. *Ann Intern Med* 104:739–746, 1986.

48. Viviani S, Ragni G, Santoro A, et al.: Testicular dysfunction in Hodgkin's disease before and after treatment. *Eur J Cancer* 27:1389–1392, 1991.

49. Blayney DW, Longo DL, Young RC, et al.: Decreasing risk of leukemia with prolonged follow-up after chemotherapy and radiotherapy for Hodgkin's disease. *N Engl J Med* 16:710–714, 1987.

50. Abrahamsen JF, Andersen A, Hannisdal E, et al.: Second malignancies after treatment of Hodgkin's disease: The influence of treatment, follow-up time, and age. *J Clin Oncol* 11:255–261, 1993.

51. Nissen NI, Pajak TF, Glidewell O, et al.: A comparative study of a BCNU containing 4-drug program versus MOPP versus 3-drug combinations in advanced Hodgkin's disease: a cooperative study by the Cancer and Leukemia Group B. *Cancer* 43:31–40, 1979.

52. Bakemeier RF, Anderson JR, Costello W, et al.: BCVPP chemotherapy for advanced Hodgkin's disease: evidence for greater duration of complete remission, greater survival, and less toxicity than with a MOPP regimen.

Results of the Eastern Cooperative Oncology Group study. *Ann Intern Med* 101:447–456, 1984.

53. Bloomfield CD, Weiss RB, Fortuny I, et al.: Combined chemotherapy with cyclophosphamide, vinblastine, procarbazine, and prednisone (CVPP) for patients with advanced Hodgkin's disease. An alternative program to MOPP. *Cancer* 38:42–48, 1976.

54. Selby P, Patel P, Milan S, et al.: ChlVPP combination chemotherapy for Hodgkin's disease: long-term results. *Br J Cancer* 62:279–285, 1990.

55. Bonadonna G, Zucali R, Monfardini S, et al.: Combination chemotherapy of Hodgkin's disease with adriamycin, bleomycin, vinblastine, and imidazole carboxamide versus MOPP. *Cancer* 36:252–259, 1975.

56. Santoro A, Bonadonna G, Valagussa P, et al.: Long-term results of combined chemotherapy-radiotherapy approach in Hodgkin's disease: superiority of ABVD plus radiotherapy versus MOPP plus radiotherapy. *J Clin Oncol* 5:27–37, 1987.

57. Canellos GP, Anderson JR, Propert KJ, et al.: Chemotherapy of advanced Hodgkin's disease with MOPP, ABVD, or MOPP alternating with ABVD. *N Engl J Med* 327:1478–1484, 1992.

58. Canellos GP, Niedzwiecki D: Long-term follow-up of Hodgkin's disease trial. *N Engl J Med* 346:1417-1418, 2002.

59. Viviani S, Santoro A, Ragni G, et al.: Gonadal toxicity after combination chemotherapy for Hodgkin's disease. Comparative results of MOPP vs ABVD. *Eur J Cancer Clin Oncol* 21:601–605, 1985.

60. Lahtinen R, Kuikka J, Nousiainen T, et al.: Cardiotoxicity of epirubicin and doxorubicin: a double-blind randomized study. *Eur J Haematol* 46:301–305, 1991.

61. Hirsch A, Vander Els N, Straus DJ, et al.: Effect of ABVD chemotherapy with and without mantle or mediastinal irradiation on pulmonary function and symptoms in early-stage Hodgkin's disease. *J Clin Oncol* 14:1297–1305, 1996.

62. Mefferd JM, Donaldson SS, Link MP: Pediatric Hodgkin's disease: Pulmonary, cardiac, and thyroid function following combined modality therapy. *Int J Radiat Oncol Biol Phys* 16:679–685, 1989.

63. Bredenfeld H, Franklin J, Nogova L, et al.: Severe pulmonary toxicity in patients with advanced-stage Hodgkin's disease treated with a modified bleomycin, doxorubicin, cyclophosphamide, vincristine, procarbazine, prednisone, and gemcitabine (BEACOPP) regimen is probably related to the combination of gemcitabine and bleomycin: a report of the German Hodgkin's Lymphoma Study Group. *J Clin Oncol* 22: 2424–2429, 2004.

64. Glick JH, Young ML, Harrington D, et al.: MOPP/ABV hybrid chemotherapy for advanced Hodgkin's disease significantly improves failure-free and overall survival: the 8-year results of the intergroup trial. *J Clin Oncol* 16:19–26, 1998.

65. Viviani S, Bonadonna G, Santoro A, et al.: Alternating versus hybrid MOPP and ABVD combinations in advanced Hodgkin's disease: ten-year results. *J Clin Oncol* 14:1421–1430, 1996.

66. Connors JM, Klimo P, Adams G, et al.: Treatment of advanced Hodgkin's disease with chemotherapy–comparison of MOPP/ABV hybrid regimen with alternating courses of MOPP and ABVD: a report from the National Cancer Institute of Canada clinical trials group. *J Clin Oncol* 15:1638–1645, 1997.

67. Duggan DB, Petroni GR, Johnson JL, et al.: Randomized comparison of ABVD and MOPP/ABV hybrid for the treatment of advanced Hodgkin's disease: Report of an intergroup trial. *J Clin Oncol* 21:607–614, 2003.

68. Bartlett NL, Rosenberg SA, Hoppe RT, et al.: Brief chemotherapy, Stanford V, and adjuvant radiotherapy for bulky or advanced-stage Hodgkin's disease: a preliminary report. *J Clin Oncol* 13:1080–1088, 1995.

69. Horning SJ, Hoppe RT, Advani R, et al.: Efficacy and late effects of Stanford V chemotherapy and radiotherapy in untreated Hodgkin's disease: Mature data in early and advanced stage patients. *Blood* 104:Abstract 92, 2004.

70. Horning SJ, Williams J, Bartlett NL, et al.: Assessment of the Stanford V regimen and consolidative radiotherapy for bulky and advanced Hodgkin's disease: Eastern Cooperative Oncology Group pilot study E1492. *J Clin Oncol* 18:972–980, 2000.

71. Horning SJ, Hoppe RT, Breslin S, et al.: Stanford V and radiotherapy for locally extensive and advanced Hodgkin's disease: mature results of a prospective clinical trial. *J Clin Oncol* 20:630–637, 2002.

72. Federico M, Levis A, Luminari S, et al.: ABVD vs. Stanford V (SV) vs. MOPP-EBV-CAD (MEC) in advanced Hodgkin's lymphoma. Final results of the IIL HD9601 randomized trial. *Proc ASCO* 23:Abstract 557, 2004.

73. Hasenclever D, Diehl V: A prognostic score for advanced Hodgkin's disease. *N Engl J Med* 339:1506–1514, 1998.

74. Diehl V, Franklin J, Pfreundschuh M, et al.: Standard and increased-dose BEACOPP chemotherapy compared with COPP-ABVD for advanced Hodgkin's disease. *N Engl J Med* 348:2386–2395, 2003.

75. Diehl V, Brillant C, Franklin J, et al.: BEACOPP chemotherapy for advanced Hodgkin's disease: Further analyses of the HD0- and HD12- trials of the German Hodgkin Study Group (GHSG). *Blood* 104:Abstract 91, 2004.

76. Ballova V, Ruffer JU, Haverkamp H, et al.: A prospectively randomized trial carried out by the German Hodgkin Study Group (GHSG) for elderly patients with advanced Hodgkin's disease comparing BEACOPP baseline and COPP-ABVD (study HD9elderly). *Ann Oncol* 16:124–131, 2005.

77. Sieber M, Bredenfeld H, Josting A, et al.: 14-Day Variant of the Bleomycin, Etoposide, Doxorubicin, Cyclophosphamide, Vincristine, Procarbazine, and Prednisone regimen in advanced-stage Hodgkin's lymphoma: Results of a pilot study of the German Hodgkin's Lymphoma Study Group. *J Clin Oncol* 21: 1734–1739, 2003.

78. Yahalom J, Ryu J, Straus DJ, et al.: Impact of adjuvant radiation on the patterns and rate of relapse in advanced-stage Hodgkin's disease treated with alternating chemotherapy combinations. *J Clin Oncol* 9: 2193–2201, 1991.

79. Brizel DM, Winer EP, Prosnitz LR, et al.: Improved survival in advanced Hodgkin's disease with the use of combined modality therapy. *Int J Radiat Oncol Biol Phys* 19:535–542, 1990.

80. Fabian CJ, Mansfield CM, Dahlberg S, et al.: Low-dose involved field radiation after chemotherapy in advanced

Hodgkin disease. A Southwest Oncology Group randomized study. *Ann Intern Med* 120:903–912, 1994.

81. Diehl V, Loeffler M, Pfreundschuh M, et al.: Further chemotherapy versus low-dose involved-field radiotherapy as consolidation of complete remission after six cycles of alternating chemotherapy in patients with advance Hodgkin's disease. German Hodgkin's' Study Group (GHSG). *Ann Oncol* 6:901–910, 1995.

82. Ferme C, Sebban C, Hennequin C, et al.: Comparison of chemotherapy to radiotherapy as consolidation of complete or good partial response after six cycles of chemotherapy for patients with advanced Hodgkin's disease: results of the groupe d'etudes des lymphomes de l'Adulte H89 trial. *Blood* 95:2246–2252, 2000.

83. Brice P, Colin P, Berger F, et al.: Advanced Hodgkin's disease with large mediastinal involvement can be treated with eight cycles of chemotherapy alone after a major response to six cycles of chemotherapy. *Cancer* 92:453–459, 2001.

84. Loeffler M, Brosteanu O, Hasenclever D, et al.: Meta-analysis of chemotherapy versus combined modality treatment trials in Hodgkin's disease. International data-base on Hodgkin's Disease Overview Study Group. *J Clin Oncol* 16:818–829, 1998.

85. Aleman BM, Raemaekers JM, Tirelli U, et al.: Involved-field radiotherapy for advanced Hodgkin's lymphoma. *N Engl J Med* 348:2396–2406, 2003.

86. Laskar S, Gupta T, Vimal S, et al.: Consolidation radiation after complete remission in Hodgkin's disease following six cycles of Doxorubicin, Bleomycin, Vinblastine, and Dacarbazine chemotherapy: is there a need? *J Clin Oncol* 22:62–68, 2004.

87. Diehl V, Schiller P, Engert A, et al.: Results of the third interim analysis of the HD12 trial of the GHSG: 8 courses of BEACOPP with or without additive radiotherapy for advanced stage Hodgkin's lymphoma. *Blood* 102: Abstract 85, 2003.

88. National comprehensive Cancer network (NCCN) guidelines. Available at: www.nccn.org/professionals/physician_gls/default.asp. Accessed April 22, 2005.

89. National Cancer Institute (NCI) guidelines. Available at: www.nci.nih.gov/cancertopics/pdq/treatment/adulthodgkins/healthprofessional. Accessed April 22, 2005.

# Chapter 74

# TREATMENT APPROACH TO NODULAR LYMPHOCYTE-PREDOMINANT HODGKIN'S LYMPHOMA

*Brad Pohlman*

## INTRODUCTION AND PATHOLOGY

Nodular lymphocyte-predominant Hodgkin's Lymphoma (NLPHL) is a unique subtype of Hodgkin's lymphoma (HL), which accounts for approximately 5% of cases and has a morphology, immunophenotype, clinical presentation, natural history, and prognosis that are distinct from classical HL (CHL). This variant of HL was first described in the 1930s and recognized not only for its unique morphology but also its more indolent clinical behavior. Jackson and Parker coined the term "paragranuloma"—a term that is sometimes still seen in the literature.[1] Lukes and Butler used the term lymphocytic and histiocytic (L&H) and further divided this type into nodular and diffuse subtypes.[2] At the 1966 Rye conference, four types of HL were recognized: nodular sclerosis, mixed cellularity, lymphocyte depletion, and lymphocyte predominance (LP).[3] Although the Rye classification combined the nodular and diffuse subtypes of LPHL, subsequent studies continued to analyze the pathological and clinical differences between these two variants.[4–6] With advances in pathology and, in particular, immunohistochemistry, hematopathologists appreciated that a purely morphologic classification system was inadequate. In fact, the morphologic classifications of LPHL actually included at least two biologically distinct types of HL. This distinction was recognized in the 1994 Revised European–American Lymphoma (REAL) classification, which separated "lymphocyte predominance (paragranuloma)" from the other types of HL and added a provisional subtype of CHL, "lymphocyte-rich classical" (LRCHL).[7] More recently, the World Health Organization (WHO) classification separated HL into two broad, pathologically and clinically distinct categories: NLPHL and CHL.[8,9] The pathologic characteristics are detailed in Chapter 71. Briefly, NLPHL is a monoclonal B-cell neoplasm characterized by a nodular, or a nodular and diffuse, polymorphous proliferation of scattered large neoplastic cells known as "popcorn" or "L&H" cells.[9] Unlike the Reed–Sternberg cells of CHL, the L&H cell of NLPHL express the B-cell marker, CD20, but not CD15 or CD30. When the REAL/WHO criteria were applied to LPHL cases previously diagnosed by expert hematopathologists based on morphology alone, only three-quarters of the cases were still classified as LPHL.[10,11] Most of the other cases were reclassified as CHL and, in particular, LRCHL.

## CLINICAL FEATURES AND PROGNOSIS

### PRE-REAL/WHO SERIES

Most publications prior to the combined morphologic and immunophenotypic classification included patients with both NLPHL and CHL. Both LPHL and CHL patients were eligible for the same clinical trials. Only a small minority had LPHL and many of them were undoubtedly misdiagnosed and actually had LRCHL. Even retrospective studies as recent as 1995, which purported to analyze the specific subset of patients with LPHL, still relied on now outdated and imprecise diagnostic criteria and, therefore, must have included a significant number of LRCHL patients.

Nevertheless, many large historical series of patients with LPHL (which predated the REAL/WHO criteria and clearly included patients with CHL and, in particular, LRCHL) recognized their distinct presentation and course.[4–6,12–16] The patients were predominantly male, generally young, and frequently had asymptomatic, nonbulky, stage I or limited stage II disease involving peripheral lymph nodes. Although some series observed a pattern of frequent and sometimes late relapses, virtually all series recognized the excellent overall survival. Many of these studies observed a disturbing pattern of deaths due to other, often treatment-related, malignancies and cardiovascular disease. Some of these series appreciated differences in long-term outcome between this subtype compared to other subtypes of HL.

The development of non-Hodgkin's lymphoma (NHL) in patients with CHL or LPHL has been well documented.[12,17–24] A review from the International Data Base on Hodgkin's Disease appreciated a higher risk of NHL in patients with LPHL compared to those with CHL.[25] The NHL, primarily diffuse large B-cell lymphoma (DLBCL) and frequently the T-cell/histiocyte rich variant of DLBCL (TC/HR DLBCL), may occur simultaneously with, or sometimes years after, the diagnosis of LPHL even without any treatment.[23,24] In many of these cases, a clonal progression from HL to NHL has been documented.[24,26,27] Given the difficulty in sometimes distinguishing NLPHL and TC/HR DLBCL, some patients who actually had TC/HR DLBCL may have been initially misdiagnosed with NLPHL.[11,24,27,28] Consequently, the risk of developing NHL may actually be overestimated. While the risk of NHL after HL may be higher in NLPHL compared to CHL patients, the absolute risk is still very low—probably less than 5%.

### POST-REAL/WHO SERIES

Much of the available clinical information regarding NLPHL as currently defined is derived from the European Task Force on Lymphoma (ETFL) Project, which was initiated in 1994 and published in 1999.[29] In this large retrospective study, biopsies from cases diagnosed initially as LPHL at 17 European and American institutions were reviewed and reclassified using morphologic and immunhistochemical criteria according to a modified REAL classification. In addition, four other, relatively large, retrospective studies identified patients with NLPHL based on the REAL and/or WHO criteria.[30–33] A summary of these five studies follows. Several other recent, relatively large, retrospective series were not included in this chapter because they included only children, included patients that were reported in a subsequent publication, and/or included immunohistochemistry for diagnosis in only some of the cases.[10,34–38]

Patients with NLPHL in these five series accounted for 3–8% of all HL patients.[29–33] The presenting characteristics of these patients are shown in Table 74.1. Like the historical publications, the patients in these series were primarily young males with early stage disease. Indeed, 51–63% of patients presented with stage I disease. Frequently, these patients presented with isolated peripheral adenopathy; mediastinal involvement was appreciated in only 0–15% of the patients. A significant minority (18–20%) of patients had clinical stage (CS) I–II infradiaphragmatic disease. Stage IV was rare and accounted for only 3–12% of patients. Less than 10% of

patients had B symptoms, and bulky disease was very uncommon. A concurrent diagnosis of DLBCL was documented in only one patient.[31] The use of staging laparotomy in these retrospective series varied considerably (ranging from 0 to 88%), but results of staging laparotomy were provided in only one study.[30] In this study, only 4% of patients with CS I but 28% of patients with CS II were upstaged. Interestingly, six of eight patients with CS IIIA in this series were downstaged. The patients in these studies were diagnosed and treated over a period of many years. In general, they were treated no differently than patients with CHL of similar stage and risk factors according to standards of care at the time. Some of the patients were enrolled on clinical trials. The vast majority of patients received radiation therapy (RT) either alone or combined with chemotherapy. Some patients received radiation only to involved sites. Most received mantle or subtotal nodal irradiation (STNI). A few received total nodal irradiation. The specific chemotherapy regimens, sequence, and number of cycles varied considerably. With primary therapy, 93–98% of patients achieved a complete remission. The median follow-up in these five series ranged from 6.3 to 10.8 years. The freedom from relapse, freedom from progression, failure-free survival, or relapse-free survival ranged from 45 to 80% at 8–15 years. The HL-specific failure-free survival for the 219 NLPHL patients in the ETFL Project is shown in Figure 74.1.[29] In this series, failure-free survival was much worse for the minority of patients with stage IV disease (i.e., 24% at 8 years).[29] Relapses often occurred late; the median time to relapse was 39–53 months and ranged from 4 to 155 months. Three of these studies

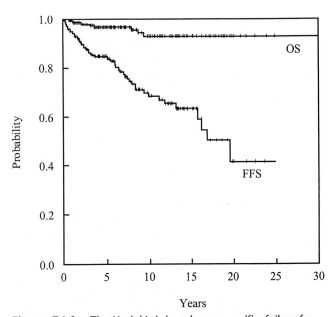

**Figure 74.1**  *The Hodgkin's-lymphoma-specific, failure-free survival and overall survival of 219 patients with nodular lymphocyte-predominant Hodgkin's lymphoma in the European Task Force Lymphoma Project. (Adapted from Ref. 29)*

**Table 74.1** Patient characteristics, treatment, and outcome in morphologically and immunophenotypically diagnosed nodular lymphocyte-predominant Hodgkin's lymphoma

| Reference | No. | Male (%) | Age (years) | Stage I/II (%) | Initial Treatment | | | | Follow-up (years) Median (range) | FFR/FFP/FFS/RFS 10 year (%) | OS 10 year (%) |
| | | | | | RT (%) | CT (%) | CMT (%) | CR (%) | | | |
|---|---|---|---|---|---|---|---|---|---|---|---|
| Bodis et al.[30] | 75 | 80 | 31% <15 77% <40 | 88 | 86 | 8 | 6 | NA | 10.8 (0.5–23.7) | FFR 80 | 93 |
| Orlandi et al.[31] | 68 | 68 | Median 35 Range 14–86 | 75 | 38 | 34 | 28 | 93 | 6.3 (1.5–20.0) | FFP 45 | 71 |
| Diehl et al.[29,39] | 219 | 74 | Median 35 72% ≦ 50 | 81 | 63 | 13 | 24 | 95 | 6.8 (NA) | 8-year FFS 74 | 8 year 94 |
| Wilder et al.[32] | 48 | 81 | Median 28 Range 16–49 87% <40 | 100[a] | 77 | 0 | 23 | NA | 9.3 (2.7–34.4) | RFS 75 | 92 |
| Feugier et al.[33] | 42 | 74 | Range 18–65 70% <40 | 100[a] | 0 | 0 | 100 | 98 | NA (6.1–22.3) | 15-year FFP 80 | 15 year 86 |

RT, radiation therapy; CT, chemotherapy; CMT, combined modality therapy; FFR, freedom from relapse; FFP, freedom from progression; FFS, failure-free survival; RFS, relapse-free survival; OS, overall survival; NA, not available.
[a]Only included stage I and II patients.

**Table 74.2** Cause of death in morphologically and immunophenotypically diagnosed nodular lymphocyte-predominant Hodgkin's lymphoma

| Reference | Total patients | Number Dead | Cause of death | | | | | |
|---|---|---|---|---|---|---|---|---|
| | | | Hodgkin's lymphoma | Non-Hodgkin's lymphoma | MDS/ AML | Solid tumors | Cardiovascular disease | Other |
| Bodis et al.[30] | 75 | 9 | 1 | – | 5 | 2 | 1 | – |
| Orlandi et al.[31] | 68 | 15 | 8 | 3 | 1 | 2 | 1 | – |
| Diehl et al.[29] | 219 | 31 | 8 | 2 | 2 | 3 | 4 | – |
| Feugier et al.[33] | 42 | 4 | 1 | 0 | 0 | 2 | 0 | 1 |

NLPHL, nodular lymphocyte-predominant Hodgkin lymphoma; MDS, myelodysplastic syndrome; AML, acute myelogenous leukemia.

suggested a continuous pattern of relapse up to 10 years or more after diagnosis and treatment.[29-31] Many patients had multiple relapses. One study suggested that patients with localized disease were less likely to relapse.[31] Another found that relapses occurred more commonly outside the initial radiation field.[32] In four of these series, subsequent NHL was documented in 0 of 71, 4 of 68, 6 of 219, and 1 of 42 patients.[29-31,33] Despite the risk of relapse, the overall survival was extraordinarily good and ranged from 71 to 94% at 8–15 years. The HL-specific overall survival for the 219 NLPHL patients in the ETFL project is shown in Figure 74.1.[29] In this series, survival was worse for patients with stage IV disease (i.e., 41% at 8 years). Of 95 deaths reported in four of these series, only 16 were attributable to HL; most of the remaining patients were in remission at the time of death.[29-31,33] Second malignancies and cardiovascular disease were the most common cause of death (Table 74.2).

## TREATMENT OF EARLY STAGE DISEASE

### PROSPECTIVE, CONTROLLED, RANDOMIZED, CLINICAL TRIALS

Several studies have defined the standard of care for patients with early stage CHL (see Chapter 73). Most, if not all, of these studies included patients with NLPHL. The German Hodgkin Lymphoma Study Group (GHSG) trial enrolled 1204 informative and eligible CS I or II patients with one or more risk factors or CS III without any risk factors.[40] A risk factor was defined as any of the following: large mediastinal mass (at least one-third of maximal thorax diameter), extranodal disease, massive splenic involvement (diffuse infiltrations or more than five focal lesions), erythrocyte sedimentation rate (ESR) ≥50 mm/h in patients without B symptoms, ≥30 mm/h in patients with B symptoms, or more than two lymph node areas of involvement. Patients with CS IIB were included on this study if they had an elevated ESR or more than two involved lymph node areas and none of the other risk factors. Patients were randomized to received four cycles of COPP (cyclophosphamide, vincristine, procarbazine, and prednisone) alternating with ABVD (doxorubicin, bleomycin, vinblastine, and dacarbazine) followed by 30-Gy extended field (EF) plus 10 Gy to bulky disease or four cycles of COPP alternating with ABVD followed by 30-Gy involved field (IF) plus 10 Gy to bulky disease. Only 8% of patients had stage I disease and 1.4% had LPHL. The National Tumor Institute of Italy enrolled 136 eligible and assessable patients with "unfavorable" stage I or any stage IIA HL. Unfavorable was defined as having any of the following characteristics: bulky disease (mediastinal mass greater than one-third of the thoracic diameter and/or nodal disease >10 cm), pulmonary hilus involvement, or contiguous extranodal extent.[41] Patients were randomized to receive either four cycles of ABVD followed by involved-field radiation therapy (IFRT) or four cycles of ABVD followed by STNI. Total radiation dose to previously involved sites was 36 Gy (in patients with confirmed complete remission following ABVD) and 40 Gy (in patients with unconfirmed complete remission or partial remission following ABVD). In patients randomized to receive STNI, the radiation dose to uninvolved sites was 30.6 Gy. Nodular sclerosis subtype accounted for 76% of the patients; the number of patients with NLPHL was not noted. Only 11% of the patients had stage I disease. In both the German and Italian studies, four cycles of chemotherapy followed by IFRT was equivalent to four cycles of chemotherapy followed by extended-field radiation therapy (EFRT). In a retrospective study of the HD1 and HD5 trials, the GHSG analyzed the outcome of CS or pathologic stage (PS) I–IIIA HL patients, who received four cycles of COPP alternating with ABVD followed by 40 Gy to areas of initially bulky disease and either 20, 30, or 40-Gy EFRT.[42] LPHL accounted for only 1–5% of the patients in these two studies. They found no significant difference in complete response rate, freedom from treatment failure, or overall survival based on the administered RT and concluded that four cycles of chemotherapy followed by 20-Gy IF/EF is sufficient treatment for most patients with early stage, nonbulky HL.

Most studies of early stage HL have included RT (either with or without chemotherapy). Only five prospective, randomized studies have evaluated chemotherapy alone for the treatment of patients with early stage HL. Two older studies in patients with early stage HL compared MOPP (mechlorethamine, vincristine, procarbazine, and prednisone) chemotherapy to STNI and obtained conflicting results.[43–45] LPHL patients accounted for only 6–7% of the patients randomized to receive chemotherapy. Recently the National Cancer Institute of Canada Clinical Trials Group and the Eastern Cooperative Oncology Group reported the preliminary results of a phase III study, which randomized 399 eligible patients with nonbulky, CS I–IIA HL to receive "standard therapy that includes RT" or chemotherapy alone.[46] Patients were stratified as either "low risk" or "high risk." Low-risk patients were younger than 40 years and had nodular sclerosis or LPHL, ESR <50 mm/h, and involvement of three or fewer disease-site regions; all other patients were high risk. Patients randomized to the "standard" arm received STNI alone (if low risk) or two cycles of ABVD followed by STNI (if high risk). Patients randomized to the chemotherapy-only arm received four cycles of ABVD (if in complete remission after two cycles) or six cycles of ABVD (if not in complete remission after two cycles). Compared to "standard" therapy, patients that received chemotherapy alone had an inferior progression-free survival (P = .006, HR = 2.6, 5-year estimates 87% vs 93%) but the same overall survival (96% vs 94%). The number of patients with NLPHL was not provided. The Grupo Argentino de Tratamiento de la Leucemia Aguda randomized 277 untreated, CS I–II HL patients (including only 33 with LPHL) to receive six cycles of CVPP (cyclophosphamide, vinblastine, procarbazine, and prednisone) or six cycles of CVPP sandwiched with 30-Gy IFRT.[47] The prospective analysis showed an improved disease-free survival in favor of combined modality therapy but similar overall survival. In favorable patients with no risk factors (defined retrospectively by Cox multivariable analysis), the disease-free survival (75% vs 70%) and overall survival (92% vs 91%) at 84 months were similar. In unfavorable patients with one or more risk factors (age greater than 45 years, more than two lymph node area involved, or bulky disease), however, the combined modality patients had an improved disease-free survival (75% vs 34%, P = 0.001) but not a statistically significant different overall survival (84% vs 66%). Finally, Memorial Sloan Kettering Cancer Center randomized patients with nonbulky, CS or, in a small minority, PS I–IIA/B or IIIA HL to receive six cycles of ABVD chemotherapy with or without 36-Gy EFRT or, in a minority, IFRT.[48] The complete response duration, freedom from progression, and overall survival were the same in both groups. Fourteen (9%) of 152 enrolled patients had LPHL; six were randomized to receive chemotherapy only. Subset analysis of the entire group according to histology failed to detect significant differences in complete response duration (P = .93), freedom from progression (P = .99), or overall survival (P = .51).

On the basis of the results of these (as well as other) studies, most patients with early stage CHL are treated with four to six cycles of combination chemotherapy (e.g., ABVD) usually followed by 20–40-Gy IFRT. But NLPHL patients comprised only a small minority of the patients in these studies and many of the patients probably had LRCHL. Furthermore, many NLPHL patients were not eligible for these studies because they lacked the necessary risk factors. Therefore, it is unclear if the results from these studies are applicable to the "typical" NLPHL patient.

### RETROSPECTIVE STUDIES OF LIMITED TREATMENT

In a recent review, Conners wrote, ". . . there is no definite evidence that LPHL is less curable than CHL . . ."[49] In another review, Diehl concluded, "there is no rationale for a less intensive treatment" of LPHL compared with CHL.[39] Yet he suggested that these "treatment strategies might be too intensive, particularly when late effects such as secondary malignancies and cardiac and pulmonary complications are taken into account." Several authors have suggested that the management of these patients should try to minimize therapy-related complications.[30,38,39,49] On the other hand, Diehl noted that the subsequent development of disease-related, rather than treatment-related, NHL in some patients suggests the need to retain (rather than reduce) currently effective primary therapy.[39] In fact, retrospective analyses support less intensive treatment at least for some patients.

Several groups have reviewed the outcome of LPHL patients treated with limited RT. In 1995, the Harvard Collaborative Oncology Group published the preliminary results of a combined prospective and retrospective analysis of 46 patients with PS I–IIA HL treated with mantle field RT alone between 1970 and 1993.[50] The prospective study was limited to patients with nodular sclerosis or LPHL and no risk factors (i.e., B symptoms, mediastinal mass greater than 1/3 of the thoracic diameter on a standing posteroanterior chest radiograph, and no subcarinal or hilar adenopathy). With a median follow-up of 32 (range 13–58) and 113 (range 56–296) months in the prospectively and retrospectively studied patients, respectively, none of the 16 LPHL patients had relapsed. The prospective study was recently updated.[51] Between October 1988 and June 2000, 87 patients with PS IA-IIA HL received 30.6–44 Gy mantle field RT. After 1995, patients with PS IA mixed cellularity, CS IA LPHL, and females with CS IA nodular sclerosis HL were also enrolled. Of the 77 pathologically staged patients, 37 had PS IA and 40 had PS IIA disease. Six patients had CS IA disease. With a median follow-up of 61 (range 13–127) months, none of the 15 LPHL patients had relapsed. Wirth et al. retrospectively studied 261 Australian patients with CS I–II HL treated with 30–40 Gy mantle field RT alone between 1969 and 1994.[52] With a median follow-up for surviving patients of 8.4 (range 1.8–27.4) years, the

10-year overall survival was 73%. On mulitvariable analysis for overall survival, age was the only important prognostic factor. The 10-year progression-free survival was 58%. On multivariable analysis, the progression-free survival was significantly better for patients with LP histology, nonmediastinal bulk less than 10 cm, three or fewer involved sites, no B symptoms, stage I, and performance status 0. The 10-year progression-free survival for 56 LPHL patients was 81% for stage I and 78% for stage II with no relapse or deaths beyond 10 years.

Patients with supradiaphragmatic CS IA LPHL have a very low probability of having disease detected below the diaphragm at staging laparotomy.[53,54] And, as noted earlier, mediastinal involvement in NLPHL is very uncommon. These data suggest that patients with CS IA NLPHL might be candidates for very limited RT. Surprisingly, little data are available on the outcome of patients with LPHL (or NLPHL as defined by the REAL/WHO criteria), who were clinically staged with modern imaging studies and treated with limited RT. Early studies showed that IFRT alone was not adequate for unselected patients with early stage HL.[55,56] Several studies, however, recognized the excellent outcome of young LPHL patients with PS or CS IA limited to suprahyoid cervical lymph node(s). Relapse following IFRT in this subset of patients is rare.[14,57–59] Recently, Schlembach et al. reported the outcome of 36 NLPHL patients (retrospectively diagnosed according to the REAL/WHO criteria) with nonbulky, stage IA ($n = 27$) or IIA ($n = 9$) involving three or less nodal regions above ($n = 27$) or below the diaphragm ($n = 9$), who received a median of 40-Gy RT alone at the MD Anderson Cancer Center between 1963 and 1996.[60] The majority of patients received "limited-field," i.e., IF ($n = 3$), regional ($n = 18$), mantle or inverted Y +/− spleen ($n = 7$); the rest of the patients received EF, i.e., subtotal or total nodal irradiation ($n = 8$). For the 24 patients with PS IA ($n = 8$) or CS IA ($n = 16$) NLPHL who received IF or regional radiotherapy, the 5-year relapse-free and overall survival were 96% and 100%, respectively. The GHSG recently presented the preliminary findings from a study in which 89 patients with CS IA NLPHL and no risk factors were treated with IFRT ($n = 44$), two to four cycles of ABVD followed by 20–30 Gy IFRT ($n = 25$), ABVD chemotherapy alone ($n = 2$), or an unknown therapy ($n = 1$).[61] Ninety-seven percent of the patients achieved a complete or unconfirmed complete remission. Two patients have relapsed and no patients have died. Follow-up, however, is relatively short.

Because of the excellent overall survival (regardless of the specific treatment) and the risk associated with treatment as well as the observations from a few reports, some authors have considered a "watch and wait" approach.[13,29,62] In one study, 31 minimally staged patients, who were initially considered to have benign lymphadenopathy but were subsequently diagnosed with LPHL, received no treatment following excision of the involved lymph node(s).[12] With median follow-up of 7 years, seven patients died 1–11 years after surgery—only one from HL and three from NHL, two from carcinoma, and two from other causes. In another study of 145 cases of LPHL, 24 stage I patients received no therapy following excision of the involved lymph node(s).[13] Fifteen of these 24 patients relapsed but 9 remained free of disease for 7–14 years. In 1988, the French Society of Pediatric Oncology (FSOP) initiated a prospective, non-randomized study.[38] At the physician's discretion, 27 children with NLPHL were either observed following lymph node excision ($n = 13$) or received (according to FSOP protocols) chemotherapy with or without 20-Gy RT. Nine of 13 observed patients had no evidence of disease following lymphadenectomy. Seven of 13 observed patients progressed a median of 24 (range 4–120) months after surgery. With a median follow-up of 70 months, 12 of 13 patients are in first ($n = 7$), second ($n = 3$), third ($n = 1$), or fifth ($n = 1$) remission and all of the patients are alive.

## TREATMENT OF ADVANCED-STAGE DISEASE

Several studies have defined the standards of care for patients with advanced-stage CHL and are discussed in Chapter 73. Based on the results of these studies, most patients in the United States are treated with ABVD, Stanford V (doxorubicin, vinblastine, vincristine, bleomycin, mechlorethamine, etoposide, and prednisone), or, less often, BEACOPP (bleomycin, etoposide, doxorubicin, cyclophosphamide, vincristine, procarbazine, and prednisone) with or without RT to sites of initially bulky disease.[63–65] LPHL accounted for only 1–5% cases so the conclusions from these studies are not necessarily applicable to NLPHL patients.

On the basis of limited data and primarily individual institutional preferences, the National Comprehensive Cancer Network (NCCN) guidelines suggest that patients with advanced (as well as early) stage NLPHL requiring chemotherapy should receive "alkylator-based" regimens.[62] Actually, very little published data are available on the most appropriate chemotherapy regimen in patients with NLPHL. In one retrospective study, 8 of 12 LPHL patients treated initially or at first relapse with MOPP or a MOPP-like regimen achieved a durable first or second complete remission, but only 2 of 6 patients treated initially or at first relapse with ABVD or EVA (etoposide, vinblastine, and doxorubicin) achieved a durable first or second complete remission.[30] A recently published study from the same institution retrospectively compared outcome of MOPP versus ABVD as salvage therapy in 100 HL patients who relapsed between 1980 and 1997 following primary RT.[66] Ninety-seven of the patients were stage I–II, and 10 had NLPHL. They observed no difference in freedom from second relapse or survival between the two groups of patients and no difference in outcome based on histology.

The results from two recent publications suggest that rituximab, an anti-CD20 monoclonal antibody with activity in B-cell NHL, may have a role in the management of patients with NLPHL. These two prospective, phase II trials evaluated the potential efficacy of a standard 4-week course of rituximab in patients with NLPHL. Between May 1999 and March 2002, GHSG enrolled 10 patients (median age 41, range 23–49 years) with NLPHL in first ($n = 5$), second ($n = 2$), or third ($n = 2$) relapse, and a median of 8.5 (range 0.5–21) years after initial diagnosis.[67] Five patients had a complete response, four patients had a partial response, and one patient (who had relapsed 6 months after initial diagnosis and soon after completing BEACOPP) progressed. Two of the nine responding patients progressed at 12 months. The other seven patients remained in remission at 9+ to 26+ months. The other study enrolled 22 NLPHL patients (median age 45, range 18–63), who were previously untreated ($n = 12$) or were in first ($n = 6$), second ($n = 3$), or fourth ($n = 1$) relapse, and a median of 11.9 (range 1–33) years after initial diagnosis and a median of 9 (range 0.4–27) years after the prior treatment.[68] The complete and partial response rates were 46% and 54%, respectively. The response duration was relatively short. Six of 12 previously untreated and 3 of 10 previously treated patients relapsed a median of 9 months after the first rituximab infusion. Eight of the nine patients relapsed exclusively at the sites of prior disease. Five of these nine patients had a repeat biopsy. Two of the five patients (including one, who was previously untreated) relapsed with DLBCL.

## GUIDELINES AND RECOMMENDATIONS

The optimal management of patients with NLPHL is uncertain and controversial. The NCCN guidelines for patients with NLPHL are complex and distinctly different than for patients with CHL; these recommendations are based on "lower-level" evidence including clinical experience, and are not always with uniform agreement among the panel members.[62] For patients with CS IA NLPHL confined to the high neck (above the hyoid bone), the NCCN guidelines recommend IF or regional RT. For patients with CS I–IIA disease at other locations, the guidelines generally recommend IF or regional RT (with or without initial chemotherapy), while for patients with more advanced disease, the guidelines recommend chemotherapy with or without RT. For patients with CS III–IVA, observation is also offered as a management option. The National Cancer Institute/Physician's data query (NCI/PDQ) website suggests that patients with nonbulky, stage I LPHL presenting in a unilateral high neck (above the thyroid notch), epitrochlear, inguinal, or femoral locations require only IF or

"regional" RT; for all other patients, it recommends the same treatment for NLPHL and CHL patients.[69] The European Organization for Research and Treatment of Cancer (EORTC) and GHSG generally treat patients with CS I–II NLPHL and no risk factors with IFRT, while they treat patients with more advanced-stage disease (i.e., CS I–II with one or more risk factors or CS III–IV) the same as patients with CHL.[70]

Based on the literature review in this chapter and the recommendations from European and American lymphoma experts, I offer the following guidelines. For patients with nonbulky, peripheral, stage IA or relatively limited, stage IIA disease, I recommend IF or regional RT. The optimal radiation dose is unknown; I recommend 30–36 Gy. For patients with bulky stage I or more advanced, stage II disease, I recommend four cycles of ABVD followed by 30 (if in complete remission) or 36-Gy (if in unconfirmed complete or partial remission) IFRT. Recent, and as yet unpublished, data from GHSG may allow some of these patients to receive as little as two cycles of ABVD and 20-Gy IFRT.[70] For patients with stage III or IV disease, I recommend six to eight cycles of combination chemotherapy (e.g., ABVD or BEACOPP). Given the poor failure-free and overall survival of stage IV NLPHL patients, standard or dose-escalated BEACOPP are particular attractive options. Recently presented, unpublished results from an Italian study, which enrolled patients with advanced-stage HL, suggested that Stanford V is inferior to ABVD.[71] The current US intergroup study is comparing ABVD to Stanford V although enrollment is limited to advanced-stage CHL patients.

## SUMMARY

NLPHL has a characteristic morphology, immunophenotype, presentation, and natural history. The clinician must recognize both its pathological and clinical characteristics and question the diagnosis if the two are discordant. Most of these patients have an excellent prognosis although long-term follow-up (i.e., greater than 10 years) in morphologically and immunophenotypically defined patients is limited. Based on the excellent 10-year survival and the relatively high risk of death from causes other than HL, therapy must not only adequately control, if not cure, the HL and ideally prevent the evolution to NHL, but also minimize both short- and long-term toxicities. This goal is perhaps even more important with NLPHL than with CHL. Future treatment strategies may incorporate anti-CD20 monoclonal antibodies, (e.g., rituximab). When relapse is suspected, a biopsy is mandatory to distinguish recurrent NLPHL from DLBCL and progressively transformed germinal centers (a benign lymphadenopathy that may occur before, after, or concurrently with NLPHL and is not necessarily indicative of disease relapse). Finally, these patients require indefinite follow-up since late relapses are possible.

## REFERENCES

1. Jackson H, Parker F: Hodgkin's disease. II: Pathology. *N Engl J Med* 231:35, 1944.
2. Lukes RJ, Butler JJ: The pathology and nomenclature of Hodgkin's disease. *Cancer Res* 26:1063, 1966.
3. Lukes RJ, Butler JJ, Hicks EB: Natural history of Hodgkin's disease as related to its pathologic picture. *Cancer* 19:317, 1966.
4. Regula DP, Hoppe RT, Weiss LM: Nodular and diffuse types of lymphocyte predominance Hodgkin's disease. *N Engl J Med* 318:214, 1988.
5. Borg-Grech A, Radford JA, Crowther D, et al.: A comparative study of the nodular and diffuse variants of lymphocyte-predominant Hodgkin's disease. *J Clin Oncol* 7:1303, 1989.
6. Pappa VI, Norton AJ, Gupta RK: Nodular type of lymphocyte predominance Hodgkin's disease. A clinical study of 50 cases. *Ann Oncol* 6:559, 1995.
7. Harris NL, Jaffe ES, Stein H, et al.: A revised European–American classification of lymphoid neoplasms: a proposal from the International Lymphoma Study Group. *Blood* 84:1361, 1994.
8. Harris NL, Jaffe ES, Diebold J, et al.: The World Health Organization classification of the neoplastic disease of the hematopoietic and lymphoid tissues. *Ann Oncol* 10:1419, 1999.
9. Stein H, Delsol G, Pileri S, et al.: Nodular lymphocyte predominant Hodgkin lymphoma. In: Jaffe ES, Harris NL, Stein H, Vardiman JW (eds.): *World Health Organization classification of tumours. Pathology and genetics of haematopoietic and lymphoid tissues.* Lyon, France: IARC Press; 2001:240.
10. Von Wasielewski R, Werner M, Fischer R, et al.: Lymphocyte-predominant Hodgkin's disease. An immunohistochemical analysis of 208 reviewed Hodgkin's disease cases from the German Hodgkin study group. *Am J Pathol* 150:793, 1997.
11. Anagnostopoulos I, Hansmann M-L, Franssila K, et al.: European task force on lymphoma project on lymphocyte predominance Hodgkin disease: histologic and immunohistologic analysis of submitted cases reveals 2 types of Hodgkin disease with a nodular growth pattern and abundant lymphocytes. *Blood* 96:1889, 2000.
12. Miettinen M, Franssila KO, Saxen E: Hodgkin's disease, lymphocyte predominance nodular-increased risk for subsequent non-Hodgkin's lymphoma. *Cancer* 54:2293, 1983.
13. Hansmann ML, Zwingers T, Boeske A, et al.: Clinical features of nodular paragranuloma (Hodgkin's disease, lymphocyte predominate type, nodular). *J Cancer Res Clin Oncol* 108:321, 1984.
14. Russell KJ, Hoppe RT, Colby TV, et al.: Lymphocyte predominant Hodgkin's disease: clinical presentation and results of treatment. *Radiother Oncol* 1:197, 1984.
15. Trudel MA, Krikorian JG, Neiman RS: Lymphocyte predominance Hodgkin's disease. A clinicopathologic reassessment. *Cancer* 59:99, 1987.
16. Tefferi A, Zellers RA, Banks PM, et al.: Clinical correlates of distinct immunophenotypic and histologic subcategories of lymphocyte-predominance Hodgkin's disease. *J Clin Oncol* 8:1959, 1990.
17. Krikorian JB, Burke JS, Rosenberg SA, Kaplan HS: Occurrence of non-Hodgkin's lymphoma after therapy for Hodgkin's disease. *N Engl J Med* 300:452, 1979.
18. Hansmann ML, Stein H, Fellbaum C, et al.: Nodular paragranuloma can transform into high-grade malignant lymphoma of T type. *Hum Pathol* 20:1169, 1989.
19. Van Leeuwen FE, Somers R, Taal BG, et al.: Increased risk of lung cancer, non-Hodgkin's lymphoma and leukemia following Hodgkin's disease. *J Clin Oncol* 7:1046, 1989.
20. Bennett MH, MacLennan KA, Vaughan Hudson G, et al.: Non-Hodgkin's lymphoma arising in patients treated for Hodgkin's disease in the BNLI: a 20-year experience. British National Lymphoma Investigation. *Ann Oncol* 2(suppl 2):83,1991.
21. Grossman DM, Hanson CA, Schnitzer B: Simultaneous lymphocyte predominant Hodgkin's disease and large-cell lymphoma. *Am J Surg Pathol* 15:668, 1991.
22. Enrici RM, Anselmo AP, Iacari V, et al.: The risk of non-Hodgkin's lymphoma after Hodgkin's disease, with special reference to splenic treatment. *Haematologica* 83:636, 1998.
23. Rueffer U, Josting A, Franklin J, et al.: Non-Hodgkin's lymphoma after primary Hodgkin's disease in the German Hodgkin's Lymphoma Study Group: incidence, treatment, and prognosis. *J Clin Oncol* 19:2026, 2001.
24. Rudiger T, Gascoyne RD, Jaffe ES, et al.: Workshop on the relationship between nodular lymphocyte predominant Hodgkin's lymphoma and T cell histiocyte-rich B cell lymphoma. *Ann Oncol* 13 (suppl 1):44, 2002.
25. Henry-Amar M: Second cancer after the treatment of Hodgkin's disease: a report from the International Database on Hodgkin's disease. *Ann Oncol* 3(suppl 4): 117, 1992.
26. Wickert RS, Weisenburger DD, Tierens A, et al.: Clonal relationship between lymphocytic predominance Hodgkin's disease and concurrent or subsequent large-cell lymphoma of B lineage. *Blood* 86:2312, 1995.
27. Greiner T, Gascoyne RD, Anderson ME: Nodular lymphocyte-predominant Hodgkin's disease associated with large-cell lymphoma: analysis of Ig Gene rearrangements by V-J polymerase chain reaction. *Blood* 88:657, 1996.
28. Boudova L, Torlakovic E, Delabie J: Nodular lymphocyte-predominant Hodgkin lymphoma with nodules resembling Tcell/histiocyte-rich B-cell lymphoma: differential diagnosis between nodular lymphocyte-predominant Hodgkin lymphoma and T-cell/histiocyte-rich B-cell lymphoma. *Blood* 102:3753, 2003.
29. Diehl V, Sextro M, Franklin J, et al.: Clinical presentation, course, and prognostic factors in lymphocyte-predominant Hodgkin's disease and lymphocyte-rich classical Hodgkin's disease: report from the European task force on lymphoma project on lymphocyte-predominant Hodgkin's disease. *J Clin Oncol* 17:776, 1999.
30. Bodis S, Kraus M, Pinkus G, et al.: Clinical presentation and outcome in lymphocyte-predominant Hodgkin's disease. *J Clin Oncol* 15:3060, 1997.
31. Orlandi E, Lazzarion M, Brusamolino E, et al.: Nodular lymphocyte predominance Hodgkin's disease: long-term observation reveals a continuous pattern of recurrence. *Leuk Lymphoma* 26:3359, 1997.
32. Wilder RB, Schlembach PJ, Jones D, et al.: European Organization for Research and Treatment of Cancer and Group d-Etude des Lymphomes de l'Adulte very favorable and favorable, lymphocyte-predominant Hodgkin disease. *Cancer* 94:1731, 2002.

33. Feugier P, Labouyre E, Djeridane M, et al.: Comparison of initial characteristics and long-term outcome of lymphocyte-predominant Hodgkin's lymphoma and classical Hodgkin's lymphoma patients at clinical stages IA and IIA prospectively treated by brief anthracycline-based chemotherapy plus extended high dose irradiation. *Blood* 104:2675, 2004.

34. Crennan E, C'Costa I, Hoe Liew K, et al.: Lymphocyte predominant Hodgkin's disease: a clinicopathologic comparative study of histologic and immunophenotypic subtypes. *Int J Radiat Oncol Biol Phys* 31:333, 1995.

35. Karayalcin G, Behm F, Gieser P, et al.: Lymphocyte predominant Hodgkin disease: clinico-pathologic features and results of treatment—the Pediatric Oncology Group experience. *Med Pediatr Oncol* 29:519, 1997.

36. Ha CS, Kavadi V, Dimopoulos M, et al.: Hodgkin's disease with lymphocyte predominance: long-term results based on current histopathologic criteria. *Int J Radiat Oncol Biol Phys* 43:329, 1999.

37. Sandoval C, Venkates L, Billups C, et al.: Lymphocyte-predominant Hodgkin disease in children. *J Pediatr Hematol Oncol* 24:269, 2002.

38. Pellegrino B, Terrier-Lacombe MJ, Oberlin O, et al.: Lymphocyte-predominant Hodgkin's lymphoma in children: therapeutic abstention after initial lymph node resection—a study of the French Society of Pediatric Oncology. *J Clin Oncol* 21:2948, 2003.

39. Diehl V, Franklin J, Sextro M, et al.: Clinical presentation and treatment of lymphocyte predominance Hodgkin's disease. In: Mauch PM, Armitage JO, Diehl V, Hoppe RT, Weiss LM (eds.) *Hodgkin's disease*. Philadelphia, PA: Lippincott; 1999:563.

40. Engert A, Schiller P, Josting A, et al.: Involved-field radiotherapy is equally effective and less toxic compared with extended-field radiotherapy after four cycles of chemotherapy in patients with early-stage unfavorable Hodgkin's lymphoma: results of the HD8 trial of the German Hodgkin's Lymphoma Study Group. *J Clin Oncol* 21:3601, 2003.

41. Bonadonna G, Bonfante V, Vivani S, et al.: ABVD plus subtotal nodal versus involved-field radiotherapy in early-stage Hodgkin's disease: long-term results. *J Clin Oncol* 22:2835, 2004.

42. Loeffler M, Diehl V, Pfreundschuh M, et al.: Dose-response relationship of complementary radiotherapy following four cycles of combination chemotherapy in intermediate-stage Hodgkin's disease. *J Clin Oncol* 15:2275, 1997.

43. Cimino G, Biti GP, Anselmo AP, et al.: MOPP chemotherapy versus extended-field radiotherapy in the management of pathological stages I-IIA Hodgkin's disease. *J Clin Oncol* 7:732, 1989.

44. Biti GP, Cimino G, Cartoni C, et al.: Extended-field radiotherapy is superior to MOPP chemotherapy for the treatment of pathologic stage I-IIA Hodgkin's disease: eight-year update of an Italian prospective randomized study. *J Clin Oncol* 10:378, 1992.

45. Longo DL, Glatstein E, Duffy PL, et al.: Radiation therapy versus combination chemotherapy in the treatment of early-stage Hodgkin's disease: seven-year results of a prospective randomized trial. *J Clin Oncol* 9:906, 1991.

46. Meyer R, Gospodarowicz M, Connors J, et al.: A randomized phase III comparison of single-modality ABVD with a strategy that includes radiation therapy in patients with early-stage Hodgkin's disease: the HD-6 trial of the National Cancer Institute of Canada Clinical Trials Group (Eastern Cooperative Oncology Group Trial JHD-6). *Blood* 102(suppl 1):Abstract 81, 2003.

47. Pavlovsky S, Mascio M, Santarelli MT, et al.: Randomized trial of chemotherapy versus chemotherapy plus radiotherapy for stage I-II Hodgkin's disease. *J Natl Cancer Inst* 890:1466, 1988.

48. Straus DJ, Portlock CS, Qin J, et al.: Results of a prospective randomized clinical trial of doxorubicin, bleomycin, vinblastine, and dacarbazine (ABVD) followed by radiation therapy (RT) vs. ABVD alone for stages I, II and IIIA non-bulky Hodgkin disease. *Blood* 194:3483, 2004.

49. Conners JM, Noordijk EV, Horning SJ: Hodgkin's lymphoma: basing the treatment on the evidence. In: Schechter GP, Broudy VC, Williams ME (eds.) *Hematology*. Washington, DC: American Society of Hematology; 2001:178.

50. Mauch PM, Canellos GP, Shulman LN, et al.: Mantle irradiation alone for selected patients with laparotomy-staged IA to IIA Hodgkin's disease: preliminary results of a prospective trial. *J Clin Oncol* 13:947, 1995.

51. Backstrand KH, Ng AK, Takvorian RW, et al.: Results of a prospective trial of mantle irradiation alone for selected patients with early-stage Hodgkin's disease. *J Clin Oncol* 19:736, 2001.

52. Wirth A, Chao M, Corry J, et al.: Mantle irradiation alone for clinical stage I-II Hodgkin's disease: long-term follow-up and analysis of prognostic factors in 261 patients. *J Clin Oncol* 17:230, 1999.

53. Leibenhaut MK, Hoppe RT, Efron B, et al.: Prognostic indicators of laparotomy findings in clinical stage I-II supradiaphragmatic Hodgkin's disease. *J Clin Oncol* 7:81, 1989.

54. Mauch P, Larson D, Osteen R, et al.: Prognostic factors for positive surgical staging in patients with Hodgkin's disease. *J Clin Oncol* 8:257, 1990.

55. Fuller L, Hutchison G: Collaborative clinical trial for stage I and II Hodgkin's disease: significance of mediastinal and nonmediastinal disease in laparotomy- and non-laparotomy-staged patients. *Cancer Treatment Rep* 66:775, 1982.

56. Rosenberg SA, Kaplan HS: The evolution and summary results of the Stanford randomized clinical trials of the management of Hodgkin's disease: 1962–1984. *Int J Radiat Oncol Biol Phys* 11:5, 1985.

57. Sutcliffe SB, Gospodarowicz MK, Bergsagel DE, et al.: Prognostic groups for management of localized Hodgkin's disease. *J Clin Oncol* 3:393, 1985.

58. Bessell EM, MacLennan KA, Toghill IO, et al.: Suprahoid Hodgkin's disease stage IA. *Radiother Oncol* 22:190, 1991.

59. Gospodarowicz MK, Sutcliffe SB, Clark RM, et al.: Analysis of supradiaphragmatic clinical stage I and II Hodgkin's disease treated with radiation alone. *Int J Radiat Oncol Biol Phys* 22:859, 1992.

60. Schlembach P, Wilder R, Jones D: Radiotherapy alone for lymphocyte-predominant Hodgkin's disease. *Cancer J* 8:377, 2002.

61. Nogova L, Reineke T, Josting A: Lymphocyte-predominant Hodgkin's disease in clinical stage IA: interim analysis of treatment options in three study generations of the German Hodgkin Study Group (GHSG). *Blood*, 102(suppl 1):Abstract 82, 2003.

62. Hoppe RT, Abrams RA, Alan AR, et al.: Hodgkin's Disease. In: *NCCN^R Practice Guidelines in Oncology—*

v.1.2004. Available at: http://www.nccn.org/professionals/physician_gls/PDF/hodgkins.pdf. Accessed October 1, 2004.

63. Canellos GP, Anders JR, Propert KJ, et al.: Chemotherapy of advanced Hodgkin's disease with MOPP, ABVD, or MOPP alternating with ABVD. *N Engl J Med* 327:1478, 1992.

64. Diehl V, Franklin J, Pfreundschuh M, et al.: Standard and increased-dose BEACOPP chemotherapy compared with COPP-ABVD for advanced Hodgkin's disease. *N Engl J Med* 348:2386, 2003.

65. Horning SJ, Hoppe RT, Breslin H, et al.: Stanford V and radiotherapy for locally extensive and advanced Hodgkin's disease: mature results of a prospective clinical trial. *J Clin Oncol* 29:630, 2002.

66. Ng AK, Li S, Neuberg D, et al.: Comparison of MOPP versus ABVD as salvage therapy in patients who relapse after radiation therapy alone for Hodgkin's disease. *Ann Oncol* 15:270, 2004.

67. Rehwald U, Schulz H, Reiser M, et al.: Treatment of relapsed CD20+ Hodgkin lymphoma with the monoclonal antibody rituximab is effective and well tolerated: results of a phase 2 trial of the German Hodgkin Lymphoma Study Group. *Blood* 101:420, 2003.

68. Ekstrand B, Lucas J, Horwitz S, et al.: Rituximab in lymphocyte-predominant Hodgkin disease: results of a phase 2 trial. *Blood* 101:4285, 2003.

69. Anonymous: Adult Hodgkin's lymphoma (PDQ®): treatment. Available at: http://cancer.gov/cancerinfo/pdq/treatment/adulthodgkins/healthprofessional. Accessed October 1, 2004.

70. Diehl V, Stein H, Hemmel M, et al.: Hodgkin's lymphoma: biology and treatment strategies for primary, refractory, and relapsed disease. In: Broudy VC, Prchal JT, Tricot GJ (eds.) *Hematology.* Washington, DC: American Society of Hematology;2003:225.

71. Federico M, Levis A, Luminari S, et al.: ABVD vs. STANFORD V vs. MOPP-EBV-CAD (MEC) in advanced Hodgkin's lymphoma. Final results of the IIL HD9601 randomized trial [abstract]. *J Clin Oncol* 22:559s, 2004. Abstract 6507.

# Chapter 75

# AUTOLOGOUS STEM CELL TRANSPLANTATION FOR HODGKIN'S LYMPHOMA

*Craig Moskowitz and Daniel Persky*

The majority of patients with Hodgkin's lymphoma (HL) are cured with radiation therapy (RT) and/or combination chemotherapy. However, patients who relapse or those with primary refractory disease have a poor outcome with conventional-dose salvage regimens. Treatment results with these salvage regimens produce a low complete remission rate and minimal survival benefit. Long-term survival is poor when either MOPP or MOPP/ABVD is administered with curative intent in the salvage setting.[1,2] Over the past two decades, results of many prospective clinical trials utilizing high-dose chemotherapy or chemoradiotherapy (HDT) with autologous stem cell transplantation (ASCT) in the salvage setting are reported, and approximately 40% of patients appear to be cured using this approach.[3]

Most early transplant studies included heavily pretreated patients receiving autologous bone marrow as the stem cell source, both of which influenced the morbidity and mortality of HDT.[4–6] With the introduction of granulocyte colony-stimulating factor (G-CSF), peripheral blood progenitor cells, better transfusion practices, more effective antibiotics, and the omission of patients with disease progression pre-ASCT, the transplant-related mortality has decreased from 15% to less than 3% in most series. Despite these strides in supportive care, long-term freedom from treatment failure (FFTF) for the patients receiving HDT/ASCT has improved by less than 10% in recent series. There are a number of pretreatment and treatment-related prognostic factors that predict for outcome.[7]

## CHEMOSENSITIVE DISEASE IS REQUIRED TO ACHIEVE BENEFIT FROM HDT/ASCT

Two randomized studies comparing full-course salvage chemotherapy (SC) administered alone with curative intent with short-course SC followed by HDT and ASCT are reported. The British National Lymphoma Investigation (BNLI) randomly assigned relapsed and primary refractory patients to either carmustine, etoposide, cytarabine, and melphalan (BEAM) HDT followed by ASCT or up to three cycles of mini-BEAM with standard support.[8] The German Hodgkin's Lymphoma Study Group (GHSG) randomly assigned patients with relapsed HL to either two cycles of dexa-BEAM (dexamethasone-BEAM) and BEAM and ASCT versus four cycles of dexa-BEAM.[9] Each study demonstrated a statistically significant improvement in FFTF for the patients treated on the HDT arms, but neither was powered to show an overall survival (OS) advantage.

The importance of pretransplant cytoreduction with SC is demonstrated in numerous previous reports.[10–13] In 1993, the lymphoma service at Memorial Sloan Kettering Cancer Center (MSKCC) published results using high-dose chemoradiotherapy in patients with biopsy-confirmed relapsed and primary refractory HL in first-generation clinical trials (MSKCC protocols 85-97 and 86-86).[14,15] The program utilized accelerated fractionation radiotherapy either as total lymphoid irradiation (TLI) or as involved field radiation (IFRT), followed by high-dose chemotherapy and ASCT. One hundred and fifty-six patients with relapsed or primary refractory disease were treated; chemosensitive disease to SC was not a requirement for subsequent HDT. At a median follow-up of 11 years, the FFTF was 45%. After the introduction of G-CSF, overall mortality of the program decreased from 18 to 6%. In this study, patients with chemosensitive disease to SC had a marked OS advantage: 61% versus 14%. These results demonstrated the feasibility of incorporating dose-intensive radiotherapy into HDT for HL and most importantly determined that patients with chemosensitive disease to SC had a marked improvement in FFTF compared to patients with refractory disease at the time of HDT.

As with aggressive non-Hodgkin's lymphoma (NHL), chemosensitive disease to SC is now suggested for transplant eligibility in the United States.[16] There is limited information regarding the optimal SC regimen. The requirements for an SC regimen are adequate cytoreduction in at least 75% of patients without extramedullary toxicity or severe bone marrow suppression, with subsequent ability to collect an adequate stem cell harvest.[17] Specifically, in the phase III randomized German study described above, of the 161 patients enrolled, 13 could not be randomized secondary to dexa-BEAM-related mortality (eight patients) or severe infection.

In 2001, we reported the results of a comprehensive program for the treatment of 82 patients with relapsed and primary refractory HL (MSKCC protocol 94-68).[18] All patients received SC with ifosfamide, carboplatin, and etoposide (ICE) and only responders were subsequently offered HDT and ASCT. All patients in this trial had biopsy-proven relapsed or refractory disease, and our data were analyzed by intent to treat. The response rate to ICE was 90%; there was no severe ICE-related extramedullary (nonhematologic) toxicity. The median number of CD34[+] cells/kg collected was $7 \times 10^6$/kg. FFTF, at a median follow-up for surviving patients of 6 years, is 55%. In the subset of patients who received HDT/ASCT (75 of 82 patients), the FFTF is 61%.

Recently, two additional SC regimens were reported to have promising, although preliminary, results. Seventy-six patients with relapsed or refractory HL were treated on a phase I/II study with gemcitabine (G), vinorelbine (N, Vinorelbine), and liposomal doxorubicin (D) (GND). The objectives were to determine the maximally tolerated dose (MTD), response rates, and toxicity of this combination; 28 patients had a prior ASCT. At a planned interim analysis of the phase II portion of the study, the overall response rate was 58% [95% exact CI (0.34, 0.80)] for the first 19 patients without prior transplant [8 partial response (PR) 3 complete response (CR)] and 68% [95% exact CI (0.44, 0.87)] for the 19 patients with prior transplant (12 PR, 1 CR). The regimen was well tolerated and, importantly, is administered in the outpatient setting.[19] IGEV consists of ifosfamide 2000 mg/m² i.v. days 1–4; gemcitabine 800 mg/m² i.v. days 1 and 4; vinorelbine 20 mg/m² i.v. day 1; prednisolone 100 mg/m² i.v. days 1–4, and G-CSF 300 μg s.c. days 7–12 or up to peripheral blood progenitor cell (PBPC) harvest. Therapy consisted of four IGEV cycles at 3-week intervals followed by HDT in responding patients. The overall response rate was 84%, and all patients but one mobilized an adequate amount of PBPC. Grade III–IV neutropenia occurred in 34% of all IGEV courses, and was dose limiting. Nonhematologic side effects were negligible.[20]

## DO PATIENTS WITH PRIMARY REFRACTORY DISEASE HAVE A SUBOPTIMAL OUTCOME WITH ASCT?

While response to SC is the major selection criteria to proceed to ASCT, other prognostic factors also predict for long-term FFTF in patients with relapsed and refractory HL. Some groups have suggested that patients with primary refractory disease do less well than those patients who achieve an initial remission to front-line therapy. There are conflicting registry data in this regard.

The North American Autologous Blood and Bone Marrow Transplant Registry (ABMTR) reported on a series of 122 primary refractory patients having 3-year progression-free survival (PFS) and OS rates of 38 and 50%, respectively, using a variety of HDT regimens. Although chemosensitivity status was unknown in less than one-third of patients, it was concluded that only B symptoms at diagnosis and a poor performance status at the time of ASCT predicted for a poor outcome.

The Groupe d'Etudes des Lymphoma de l'Adulte (GELA) reported on a group of primary refractory patients defined as progression of disease on therapy, less than 50% response to front-line therapy, or persistent bone marrow involvement after four cycles of initial chemotherapy. These patients had poor outcomes with HDT and ASCT, with 5-year freedom from second failure of 23%, even though most patients (62%) had chemosensitive disease to SC.

The GHSG evaluated 206 patients with primary refractory disease defined as progression of disease on front-line therapy, or biopsy confirmation of active disease within 90 days posttherapy. While only 70 of these 206 patients actually received HDT and ASCT, the authors concluded that HDT was no better than standard chemoradiotherapy when the data were analyzed by intent to treat.[21–24]

An underlying problem with these published refractory disease series is the lack of a uniform definition of this entity. Definitions range from progression of disease on upfront therapy to a partial response 3 months posttreatment. Moreover, the inclusion of patients with unconfirmed pathology may result in treatment of patients with aggressive NHL, with a nonmalignant disorder (infection, or sarcoid-like reactions), or with residual radiologic abnormalities but no active HL with an HDT program. These non-HL entities are often strongly positive on gallium or positron emission tomography imaging, thereby making histologic confirmation even more imperative.[25–28]

We recently reported our data in primary refractory HL, which has longer median follow-up than any of the other reported series. This report is distinguished by a repeat biopsy confirming active HL in all patients. Among the 91 patients with primary refractory HL identified for this analysis, eight (9%) were found to have diffuse large B-cell lymphoma on the repeat biopsy. In these cases, the initial diagnosis of HL was confirmed by pathology review. The presence of an aggressive NHL has both prognostic significance and affects the choice of second-line therapy; for example, the use of anti-CD20-based therapy in patients with aggressive NHL may have a critical role (i.e., rituximab or high-dose radiolabeled anti-B1).[29] With a median follow-up of

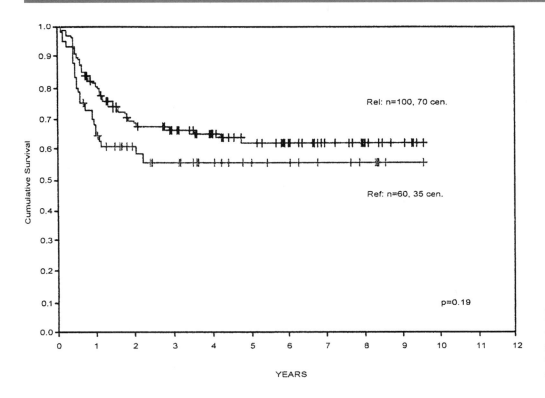

**Figure 75.1** *Overall survival of transplanted patients with relapsed or primary refractory disease*

10 years, results at many centers including data at memorial Sloar Kettering Cancer center indicate that HDT/ASCT should be considered as standard treatment for patients with primary refractory HL if chemosensitive disease to SC is established. This is summarized in Table 75.1.[30–34] We found no difference in FFTF for patients with chemosensitive primary refractory versus chemosensitive relapsed disease[35] (Figure 75.1).

## MULTIPLE FACTORS PREDICT SURVIVAL IN RELAPSED AND PRIMARY REFRACTORY HL

Many groups have reported that prognostic factors other than refractory disease can predict survival. In general these factors can be divided into four categories: (1) extent of disease (advanced stage or extranodal involvement); (2) B symptoms [or surrogate marker such as elevated erythrocyte sedimentation rate or interleukin 10 (IL-10)]; (3) remission duration of less than 1 year; (4) significant disease burden after SC. In our study of ICE SC followed by HDT and ASCT discussed above, Cox regression analysis determined that there are three factors associated with a poor outcome pre-ICE: extranodal sites of disease (ENS) ($P < 0.001$), initial remission duration $<1$ year ($P = 0.001$), and B symptoms ($P < 0.001$). Using this three-factor model, we identified three groups of patients with highly significant differences in outcome with this treatment approach. A favorable risk group having zero to one of these risk factors (56% of the patients) had FFTF of 80% measured from initiation of ICE therapy. Patients with two or three risk factors faired less well with an event-free survival (EFS) of 40%. (Figure 75.2)

This three-factor model was the basis of our third-generation risk-adapted comprehensive study. In this, study patients with no risk factor or one risk factor (ENS, initial response duration $<1$ year, or B symptoms

| Table 75.1 | Outcome of patients with primary refractory disease based upon response to salvage therapy | | | | | | |
|---|---|---|---|---|---|---|---|
| Series | PTS | Median follow-up (months) | Biopsy proven (%) | PFS (%) | OS (%) | TD (%) | Chemosensitivity |
| Vancouver | 30 | 42 | 55 | 42 | 30 | 18 | NA |
| ABMTR | 122 | 28 | NA | 38 | 50 | 12 | NS |
| GELA | 157 | 50 | 36 | 23–66 | 30–76 | 12 | $P = 0.05$ |
| GHSG | 70 | 52 | 57 | 31 | 43 | 9 | $P = 0.0001$ |
| SFGM | 86 | 29 | None | 25 | 35 | 8 | $P = 0.0001$ |
| MSKCC | 75 | 120 | 100 | 49 | 48 | 9 | $P < 0.0001$ |

TD, toxic death; SFGM, French national registry.

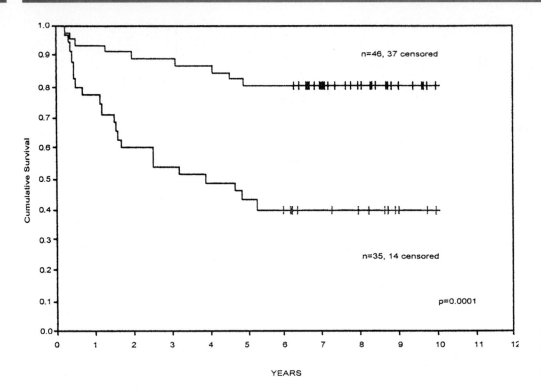

**Figure 75.2** *Overall survival of transplanted patients with relapsed or primary refractory disease*

at time of study enrollment), group A, were treated exactly the same as in the second-generation program; in that study FFTF was 80%. Patients with two risk factors, group B, received one dose of standard-dose ICE followed by a dose of augmented ICE second-line therapy as well as a more dose-intense transplant-conditioning regimen. Finally, patients with all three risk factors, group C, received a completely different regimen. Cytoreduction was done with transplant doses of ICE followed by stem cell support, which was followed by a second autotransplant. This three-arm study, however, uses one universal theme: patients must have chemosensitive disease to their "ICE" therapy—group A to standard doses of ICE, group B to augmented ICE, and group C to transplant doses of ICE. The median follow-up of the patients is now 30 months and patients with multiple risk factors have improved FFTF as compared to our previous report (unpublished data).

## RATIONALE FOR USING RADIATION THERAPY IN THE SETTING OF HDT/ASCT

RT administered with curative intent in the salvage setting has been used alone or in combination with chemotherapy. Small single-institution series of highly selected patients report a significant local control rate and 5-year FFTF of approximately 30%. The strategy of incorporating RT into HDT is based on the premise that the pattern of relapse post-HDT is similar to relapse following front-line chemotherapy; i.e., it most commonly occurs at sites of initial nodal involvement and is therefore amenable to treatment with RT. Considering the excellent local control afforded by RT,

many institutions successfully incorporated RT into their second-line therapeutic approaches; however, there remains no random assignment data that support this strategy.

RT is most commonly given in two fashions: post-transplant consolidation or as part of pretransplant cytoreduction (Table 75.2).

## CONSOLIDATIVE RADIOTHERAPY

The advantages of using RT in the post-ASCT setting include converting a CT-determined partial response to a complete response and reducing the size of the radiation field in patients with bulky disease by high-dose chemotherapy. It does not have the drawback of delaying the administration of high-dose chemotherapy or of overlapping pneumonitis, which can be seen with the combination of RT and carmustine-based HDT.[36–40] Consolidative RT may, however, produce significant myelosuppression. This has largely been avoided by waiting for proper hematologic recovery and initiating RT within 3 months of ASCT. However, due to this selection bias, patients with early disease progression post-ASCT will not be eligible to receive consolidative RT with curative intent.

One of the earlier studies by Jagannath et al. at MD Anderson Cancer Center involved treatment of 61 patients with HDT/ASCT. Of 18 patients achieving a partial response, six were converted to a CR with local RT.[41] Subsequently, Mundt et al. reported the experience at the University of Chicago with IFRT in 54 patients with relapsed/refractory HL. Forty-six percent of patients relapsed, two-thirds at sites of prior nodal

**Table 75.2** Role of involved field radiotherapy as part of management in relapsed/refractory HL

| Authors | Number of patients | Pre-ASCT | Post-ASCT | EFS/DFS/PFS | OS | Comments |
|---|---|---|---|---|---|---|
| Poen et al. | 100 | 18 | 6 | 3 year EFS: 63% vs 55%, P = 0.59 | 3 year: 70% vs 61%, P = 0.41 | Survival benefit in stages I–III |
| Pezner et al. | 86 | 26 | 3 | 2 year DFS: 44% | 2 year: 38% | IFRT impact not evaluated |
| Dawson et al. | 13 | 13 | 0 | 2 year PFS: 50% | 2 year: 84% | Prospective, phase I |
| Mundt et al. | 54 | 7 | 13 | 5 year PFS: 38.9% | 5 year (cause-specific): 46.5% | IFRT post-ASCT converted PR to CR in 10/10 |
| Lancet et al. | 70 | 0 | 27 | 5 year EFS: 44% vs 26%, P = 0.0056 | 5 year: 81% (not stratified) | |

involvement. Of 13 patients receiving IFRT after ASCT, 10 were treated at sites of persistent disease and three for CR consolidation. IFRT significantly reduced the relapse at these sites (26.3% vs 42.8%, P < 0.05) and significantly improved local control. Most importantly, all 10 patients who received IFRT at sites of persistent disease, as defined by CT criteria, were converted to a CR and had improved FFTF (40% vs 12.1%, P = 0.04) that was comparable to patients achieving CR with ASCT alone (40% vs 60.0%, P = 0.38).[42]

Lancet et al. described the experience at the University of Rochester with 27 of 70 patients who underwent ASCT receiving IFRT. Patients in CR, as defined by CT criteria, received 20 Gy to previous sites of disease while those achieving a PR posttransplant received 30 Gy within 4–8 weeks of ASCT. Five-year FFTF was significantly better in the consolidative IFRT group (44% vs 26%, P = 0.006). Consolidative RT has thus shown promise in its ability to convert some patients in PR, as defined by CT criteria, to CR with apparent long-term benefits.[43]

## PRE-ASCT CYTOREDUCTIVE RADIATION THERAPY

One of the main advantages of using RT as a part of cytoreductive therapy is maximizing response prior to HDT/ASCT, which, some groups have reported, is associated with a better outcome.[17] It also eliminates any delay in RT administration, a modality that increasingly has been left out of front-line therapy for HL. In addition, hematologic toxicity secondary to RT in the post-ASCT setting is of little clinical importance when administered pre-ASCT. Conversely it contributes to mucositis and pneumonitis, particularly if mediastinal radiation is administered.

A Stanford series by Poen et al. included 100 consecutive patients of which 24 received IFRT, 18 as part of cytoreductive therapy and six in consolidative setting. In the 39 radiation-naïve patients in this study, IFRT improved OS (93% vs 55%, P = 0.02) with a trend toward improved FFTF. For the group as a whole, FFTF and OS did not improve survival, most likely due to the selection of patients eligible to receive IFRT.[44]

In a series from the University of Toronto, Crump et al. treated 40 of 73 patients with extended-field RT to bulky sites of disease pre-ASCT. Univariate analysis determined that RT improved outcome, but this was not significant in multivariate analysis. Only disease status at transplant and relapse at irradiated sites was prognostic.[45] The same group later determined that treatment-related mortality in their series was worse in patients receiving thoracic RT, particularly if significant lung volume was irradiated or if given within 50 days of ASCT.[46]

Pezner et al. published the City of Hope experience with cytoreductive IFRT in 29 of 86 patients, 17 of whom subsequently received conditioning regimens with total body irradiation. In-field recurrences developed in 7% of the patients. Two-year disease-free survival (DFS) was 44%. Interstitial pneumonitis occurred in only three patients. However, the utility of IFRT in this program was difficult to evaluate.[47]

At MSKCC, we have used accelerated fractionated IFRT as part of cytoreduction for the past 20 years with or without total lymphoid radiation. Patients receive up to 36 Gy over a 10-day period administered in twice-daily fractions. Initially, in the pregrowth factor era, mortality with the entire program was excessive, but decreased to 6% after the introduction of G-CSF and now is 1% with the use of PBPC and more aggressive transfusion practices. Although univariate analysis supports the use of IFRT, in multivariate analysis the use of IFRT is not significant because patients with widespread extranodal disease, a worse group of patients prognostically, rarely benefit from IFRT. Interestingly <15% of failures occurred at irradiated sites.[14,18]

Recently, a small prospective study of IFRT administered pre-ASCT was reported by Dawson et al. from University of Michigan. Thirteen patients with HL received 20–36 Gy with excellent local control and a respectable 2-year FFTF of 50%, but there was a lack of association to dose or time interval pre-ASCT .[48]

Cytoreductive RT continues to be frequently employed in HDT/ASCT regimens, based mostly on retrospective institutional series. Significant toxicity, primarily pulmonary, has limited most protocols to IFRT, with the addition of more extensive RT to RT-naïve patients.

Variability of RT doses and parameters, timing of administration, and study populations have limited the ability to compare the studies. Prospective studies will be needed to address these questions as well as concerns about late toxicity, including secondary myelodysplasia and acute leukemia.

## SUMMARY

In conclusion, HDT with ASCT is standard therapy for patients with relapsed and primary refractory HL, provided chemosensitive disease to salvage chemotherapy is established. Future studies need to evaluate functional imaging in the transplant setting, standardize SC, and prospectively evaluate RT in a randomized fashion.[42,49,50]

## REFERENCES

1. Longo DL, Duffey PL, Young RC, et al.: Conventional-dose salvage combination chemotherapy in patients relapsing with Hodgkin's disease after combination chemotherapy: the low probability for cure. *J Clin Oncol* 10(2):210–218, 1992.
2. Bonfante V, Santoro A, Viviani S, et al.: Outcome of patients with Hodgkin's disease failing after primary MOPP–ABVD. *J Clin Oncol* 15(2):528–534, 1997.
3. Linch DC, Goldstone AH: High-dose therapy for Hodgkin's disease. *Br J Haematol* 107(4):685–690, 1999.
4. Bierman PJ, Bagin RG, Jagannath S, et al.: High dose chemotherapy followed by autologous hematopoietic rescue in Hodgkin's disease: long-term follow-up in 128 patients. *Ann Oncol* 4(9):767–773, 1993.
5. Chopra R, Linch DC, McMillan AK, et al.: Mini-BEAM followed by BEAM and ABMT for very poor risk Hodgkin's disease. *Br J Haematol* 81(2):197–202, 1992.
6. Gribben JG, Linch DC, Singer CR, McMillan AK, Jarrett M, Goldstone AH: Successful treatment of refractory Hodgkin's disease by high-dose combination chemotherapy and autologous bone marrow transplantation. *Blood* 73(1):340–344, 1989.
7. Moskowitz C: An update on the management of relapsed and primary refractory Hodgkin's disease. *Semin Oncol* 31(2, suppl 4):54–59, 2004.
8. Linch DC, Winfield D, Goldstone AH, et al.: Dose intensification with autologous bone-marrow transplantation in relapsed and resistant Hodgkin's disease: results of a BNLI randomised trial. *Lancet* 341(8852):1051–1054, 1993.
9. Schmitz N, Pfistner B, Sextro M, et al.: Aggressive conventional chemotherapy compared with high-dose chemotherapy with autologous haemopoietic stem-cell transplantation for relapsed chemosensitive Hodgkin's disease: a randomised trial. *Lancet* 359(9323):2065–2071, 2003.
10. Baetz T, Belch A, Couban S, et al.: Gemcitabine, dexamethasone and cisplatin is an active and non-toxic chemotherapy regimen in relapsed or refractory Hodgkin's disease: a phase II study by the National

Cancer Institute of Canada Clinical Trials Group. *Ann Oncol* 14(12):1762–1767, 2003.
11. Brice P, Bouabdallah R, Moreau P, et al.: Prognostic factors for survival after high-dose therapy and autologous stem cell transplantation for patients with relapsing Hodgkin's disease: analysis of 280 patients from the French registry. Societe Francaise de Greffe de Moelle. *Bone Marrow Transplant* 20(1):21–26, 1997.
12. Ferme C, Bastion Y, Lepage E, et al.: The MINE regimen as intensive salvage chemotherapy for relapsed and refractory Hodgkin's disease. *Ann Oncol* 6(6):543–549, 1995.
13. Gisselbrecht C, Mounier N, Ferme C, Brice P: Ifosfamide salvage treatment before autologous stem cell transplantation in patients with refractory and relapsed Hodgkin's lymphoma: a GELA experience. *Ann Oncol* 14(suppl 1): i39–i41, 2003.
14. Yahalom J, Gulati SC, Toia M, et al.: Accelerated hyperfractionated total-lymphoid irradiation, high-dose chemotherapy, and autologous bone marrow transplantation for refractory and relapsing patients with Hodgkin's disease. *J Clin Oncol* 11(6):1062–1070, 1993.
15. Yahalom J: Integrating radiotherapy into bone marrow transplantation programs for Hodgkin's disease. *Int J Radiat Oncol Biol Phys* 33(2):525–528, 1995.
16. Philip T, Guglielmi C, Hagenbeek A, et al.: Autologous bone marrow transplantation as compared with salvage chemotherapy in relapses of chemotherapy-sensitive non-Hodgkin's lymphoma. *N Engl J Med* 333(23): 1540–1545, 1995.
17. Zelenetz AD, Hamlin P, Kewalramani T, Yahalom J, Nimer S, Moskowitz CH: Ifosfamide, carboplatin, etoposide (ICE)-based second-line chemotherapy for the management of relapsed and refractory aggressive non-Hodgkin's lymphoma. *Ann Oncol* 14(suppl 1):i5–i10, 2003.
18. Moskowitz CH, Nimer SD, Zelenetz AD, et al.: A 2-step comprehensive high-dose chemoradiotherapy second-line program for relapsed and refractory Hodgkin disease:

analysis by intent to treat and development of a prognostic model. *Blood* 97(3):616–623, 2001.

19. Bartlett N, Niedzwiecki D, Johnson J, et al.: A phase I/II study of gemcitabine, vinorelbine, and liposomal doxorubicin for relapsed Hodgkin's disease: preliminary results of CALGB 59804. *Proc Am Soc Clin Oncol* 2003.

20. Balzarotti M, Magagnoli M, Spina M, et al.: IGEV regimen and high dose chemotherapy (HDT) consolidation with peripheral blood stem cell (PBSC) support for refractory-relapsed Hodgkin's disease. *Blood* 106: Abstract 2091, 2005.

21. Sweetenham JW, Carella AM, Taghipour G, et al.: High-dose therapy and autologous stem-cell transplantation for adult patients with Hodgkin's disease who do not enter remission after induction chemotherapy: results in 175 patients reported to the European Group for Blood and Marrow Transplantation. Lymphoma Working Party. *J Clin Oncol* 17(10):3101–3109, 1999.

22. Josting A, Reiser M, Rueffer U, Salzberger B, Diehl V, Engert A: Treatment of primary progressive Hodgkin's and aggressive non-Hodgkin's lymphoma: is there a chance for cure? *J Clin Oncol* 18(2):332–339, 2000.

23. Ferme C, Mounier N, Divine M, et al.: Intensive salvage therapy with high-dose chemotherapy for patients with advanced Hodgkin's disease in relapse or failure after initial chemotherapy: results of the Groupe d'Etudes des Lymphomes de l'Adulte H89 Trial. *J Clin Oncol* 20(2):467–475, 2002.

24. Lazarus HM, Rowlings PA, Zhang MJ, et al.: Autotransplants for Hodgkin's disease in patients never achieving remission: a report from the Autologous Blood and Marrow Transplant Registry. *J Clin Oncol* 17(2):534–545, 1999.

25. Bakheet SM, Powe J, Ezzat A, Rostom A: F-18-FDG uptake in tuberculosis. *Clin Nucl Med* 23(11):739–742, 1998.

26. Epelbaum R, Ben-Arie Y, Bar-Shalom R, et al.: Benign proliferative lesions mimicking recurrence of Hodgkin's disease. *Med Pediatr Oncol* 28(3):187–190, 1997.

27. Gargot D, Algayres JP, Brunet C, et al.: [Sarcoidosis and sarcoid reaction associated with Hodgkin's disease]. *Rev Med Intern* 11(2):157–160, 1990.

28. Simsek S, van Leuven F, Bronsveld W, Ooms GH, Groeneveld AB, de Graaff CS: Unusual association of Hodgkin's disease and sarcoidosis. *Neth J Med* 60(11):438–440, 2002.

29. Kewalramani T, Zelenetz AD, Nimer SD, et al.: Rituximab and ICE as second-line therapy before autologous stem cell transplantation for relapsed or primary refractory diffuse large B-cell lymphoma. *Blood* 103(10):3684–3688, 2004.

30. Wheeler C, Eickhoff C, Elias A, et al.: High-dose cyclophosphamide, carmustine, and etoposide with autologous transplantation in Hodgkin's disease: a prognostic model for treatment outcomes. *Biol Blood Marrow Transplant* 3(2):98–106, 1997.

31. Bierman PJ, Lynch JC, Bociek RG, et al.: The International Prognostic Factors Project score for advanced Hodgkin's disease is useful for predicting outcome of autologous hematopoietic stem cell transplantation. *Ann Oncol* 13(9):1370–1377, 2002.

32. Horning SJ, Chao NJ, Negrin RS, et al.: High-dose therapy and autologous hematopoietic progenitor cell transplantation for recurrent or refractory Hodgkin's disease: analysis of the Stanford University results and prognostic indices. *Blood* 89(3):801–813, 1997.

33. Reece DE, Barnett MJ, Shepherd JD, et al.: High-dose cyclophosphamide, carmustine (BCNU), and etoposide (VP16−213) with or without cisplatin (CBV +/− P) and autologous transplantation for patients with Hodgkin's disease who fail to enter a complete remission after combination chemotherapy. *Blood* 86(2):451–456, 1995.

34. Josting A, Franklin J, May M, et al.: New prognostic score based on treatment outcome of patients with relapsed Hodgkin's lymphoma registered in the database of the German Hodgkin's lymphoma study group. *J Clin Oncol* 20(1):221–230, 2002.

35. Moskowitz CH, Kewalramani T, Nimer SD, Gonzalez M, Zelenetz AD, Yahalom J: Effectiveness of high dose chemoradiotherapy and autologous stem cell transplantation for patients with biopsy-proven primary refractory Hodgkin's disease. *Br J Haematol* 124(5):645–652, 2004.

36. Alessandrino EP, Bernasconi P, Colombo A, et al.: Pulmonary toxicity following carmustine-based preparative regimens and autologous peripheral blood progenitor cell transplantation in hematological malignancies. *Bone Marrow Transplant* 25(3):309–313, 2000.

37. Dreger P, Marquardt P, Haferlach T, et al.: Effective mobilisation of peripheral blood progenitor cells with 'Dexa-BEAM' and G-CSF: timing of harvesting and composition of the leukapheresis product. *Br J Cancer* 68(5):950–957, 1993.

38. Jones RB, Matthes S, Shpall EJ, et al.: Acute lung injury following treatment with high-dose cyclophosphamide, cisplatin, and carmustine: pharmacodynamic evaluation of carmustine. *J Natl Cancer Inst* 85(8):640–647, 1993.

39. Real E, Roca MJ, Vinuales A, Pastor E, Grau E: Life threatening lung toxicity induced by low doses of bleomycin in a patient with Hodgkin's disease. *Haematologica* 84(7):667–668, 1999.

40. Reece DE, Nevill TJ, Sayegh A, et al.: Regimen-related toxicity and non-relapse mortality with high-dose cyclophosphamide, carmustine (BCNU) and etoposide (VP16-213) (CBV) and CBV plus cisplatin (CBVP) followed by autologous stem cell transplantation in patients with Hodgkin's disease. *Bone Marrow Transplant* 23(11):1131–1138, 1999.

41. Jagannath S, Armitage JO, Dicke KA, et al.: Prognostic factors for response and survival after high-dose cyclophosphamide, carmustine, and etoposide with autologous bone marrow transplantation for relapsed Hodgkin's disease. *J Clin Oncol* 7(2):179–185, 1989.

42. Mundt AJ, Sibley G, Williams S, Hallahan D, Nautiyal J, Weichselbaum RR: Patterns of failure following high-dose chemotherapy and autologous bone marrow transplantation with involved field radiotherapy for relapsed/refractory Hodgkin's disease. *Int J Radiat Oncol Biol Phys* 33(2):261–270, 1995.

43. Lancet JE, Rapoport AP, Brasacchio R, et al.: Autotransplantation for relapsed or refractory Hodgkin's disease: long-term follow-up and analysis of prognostic factors. *Bone Marrow Transplant* 22(3):265–271, 1998.

44. Poen JC, Hoppe RT, Horning SJ: High-dose therapy and autologous bone marrow transplantation for relapsed/refractory Hodgkin's disease: the impact of involved field radiotherapy on patterns of failure and survival. *Int J Radiat Oncol Biol Phys* 36(1):3–12, 1996.

45. Crump M, Smith AM, Brandwein J, et al.: High-dose etoposide and melphalan, and autologous bone marrow transplantation for patients with advanced Hodgkin's disease: importance of disease status at transplant. *J Clin Oncol* 11(4):704–711, 1993.

46. Tsang RW, Gospodarowicz MK, Sutcliffe SB, Crump M, Keating A: Thoracic radiation therapy before autologous bone marrow transplantation in relapsed or refractory Hodgkin's disease. PMH Lymphoma Group, and the Toronto Autologous BMT Group. *Eur J Cancer* 35(1): 73–78, 1999.

47. Pezner RD, Nademanee A, Niland JC, Vora N, Forman SJ: Involved field radiation therapy for Hodgkin's disease autologous bone marrow transplantation regimens. *Radiother Oncol* 34(1):23–29, 1995.

48. Dawson LA, Saito NG, Ratanatharathorn V, et al.: Phase I study of involved-field radiotherapy preceding autologous stem cell transplantation for patients with high-risk lymphoma or Hodgkin's disease. *Int J Radiat Oncol Biol Phys* 59(1):208–218, 2004.

49. Wadhwa P, Shina DC, Schenkein D, Lazarus HM: Should involved-field radiation therapy be used as an adjunct to lymphoma autotransplantation? *Bone Marrow Transplant* 29(3):183–189, 2002.

50. Yahalom J: Changing role and decreasing size: current trends in radiotherapy for Hodgkin's disease. *Curr Oncol Rep* 4(5):415–423, 2002.

# Chapter 76
# HODGKIN'S LYMPHOMA: FOLLOW-UP CARE

*Omer N. Koç*

## INTRODUCTION

The remarkable success in treatment of Hodgkin's Lymphoma (HL) creates the challenge of long-term management of patients who are, unfortunately, at risk for premature death. Despite excellent control of the disease, long-term outcome remains inferior to that of the general population. Excess mortality is, in general, due to HL itself during the first 5–10 years after diagnosis, but treatment-related complications affect survival 25–30 years after therapy. HL patients should be followed life long, and the schedule and the nature of this surveillance should be tailored to the temporal patterns of complications (Figure 76.1). While detection of recurrence may be most important during the first 5 years, detection and prevention of cardiac, thyroid, and pulmonary disease should be ongoing and screening for secondary malignancies should be employed when possible.

## PATTERNS OF RELAPSE AFTER INITIAL TREATMENT OF HODGKIN'S LYMPHOMA

Although late relapses occur, most relapses are seen within the first 5 years of treatment. Relapse risk and location are significantly affected by stage at presentation, prognostic factors, and therapy given. Long-term follow-up for patients with Hodgkin's disease reveals that approximately 70% of the disease-related deaths occur during the first 5 years and virtually no disease-related deaths are seen after 10 years. There are no data to suggest that early detection of recurrences can necessarily improve survival. However, clinical trials suggest that salvage treatment for HL is more effective when patients have minimal disease than when they have bulky disease at recurrence. However, no trial has demonstrated an advantage for treatment when disease is detected by routine screening studies versus symptomatic relapse.[1,2]

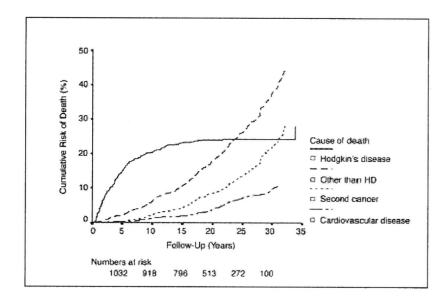

**Figure 76.1** *The actuarial risks of death from major disease categories. HD = Hodgkin's disease (From Ref. 1. Reprinted with permission from the American Society of Clinical Oncology)*

**Table 76.1** Suggested follow-up schedule for patients with Hodgkin's Lymphoma

|  | Years 0–2 | Years 3–5 | Years 5–10 |
| --- | --- | --- | --- |
| Physical examination | Every 3–4 months | Every 6 months | Once a year |
| Routine blood work[a] | Every 3–4 months | Every 6 months | Once a year |
| TFT[b], lipid profile | Once a year | Once a year | Once a year |
| Chest film | – | – | Once a year |
| CT scan | Every 3–4 months | Every 6 months | – |
| PET scan | Alternate CT/PET | Alternate CT/PET | |
| Breast cancer screen[c] | Treatment age ,17: 17–35: | Start at age 25 Start 8 years later | |

[a] Routine blood work: Complete blood count, erythrocyte sedimentation rate, and liver function tests.
[b] Patients who had neck radiotherapy.
[c] For women who had supradiaphragmatic irradiation. Annual breast MRI or ultrasound ages 25–29; annual mammogram ages 30 and above.

Despite lack of data showing a positive impact on outcome with aggressive posttreatment follow-up, many physicians utilize physical examination, blood work, and imaging studies fairly frequently during the first 2 years after therapy. This is usually followed by a less intensive schedule (Table 76.1). Typical follow-up consists of visits every 3–4 months during the first 2 years and every 6 months until year 5, and annually thereafter. These visits are generally used for physical examination, blood work, chest radiograph, and selected imaging studies. Despite such an intensive follow-up schedule, most of the relapses are detected in symptomatic patients. A study of 210 HL patients in complete remission after therapy revealed that 30 of 37 relapsed patients had symptoms of disease.[3] Only four asymptomatic relapses were detected by routine evaluation. Widespread use of sensitive imaging methods such as FDG-PET ([18]F-fluorodeoxyglucose positron emission tomography) is likely to improve the early detection rate, although it is difficult to project whether such early detection will result in improved outcome. Imaging studies such as PET scanning, with or without computed tomography (CT) scanning, are used three to four times a year during the first 2 years of follow-up despite a lack of prospective studies evaluating their impact on outcome and their cost–benefit ratio.

## FOLLOW-UP FOR LONG-TERM COMPLICATIONS OF HL TREATMENT

### SECONDARY MALIGNANCIES

Numerous studies have demonstrated that the malignancy rate is significantly higher in survivors of HL than in the general population and these malignancies have poor prognosis. Solid tumors comprise the most common type of secondary malignancy, accounting for 60–80% of cases. The risk of developing a solid tumor is increased in patients receiving radiation therapy, compared to those receiving chemotherapy alone. Secondary leukemia and non-Hodgkin's Lymphoma cases are fewer, but their relative risks are higher, since they are uncommon in the general population.[4,5] The cumulative risk of solid tumors continuously increases until at least 25 years of follow-up. In contrast, the risk of acute leukemia is mostly confined to the first 10 years.

In a German Hodgkin's Lymphoma Study Group report from 2004, 127 patients out of a cohort of 5367 developed secondary cancers (2.4%) after a median follow-up of 72 months, with overall relative risk of 2.4.[6] Of these, 24% were lung, 20% colorectal, and 10% were breast cancer. More than 50% of the patients with secondary cancers were treated with combined modality, including extended field radiotherapy. In a report from Royal Marsden Hospital, 77 second malignancies were detected out of 1039 patients (7.4%).[7] The standardized incidence ratios (SIR) were as follows: 4 for stomach, 3.8 for lung, 26.5 for bone, 16.9 for soft tissue, and 3.9 for nonmelanoma skin cancers, 4.6 for non-Hodgkin's Lymphoma, and 31.3 for acute myeloid leukemia. Patients who received radiotherapy only had an SIR of 2.6, chemotherapy only 2.1, and combined modality therapy had an SIR of 3.1. Leukemia risk was related to chemotherapy exposure alone or with radiation. Unfortunately, the relative risk of solid tumors was greater in patients who were treated at the age of 25 or younger, compared to those treated at age 55 years or older. In the Dutch series, 1253 patients with HL treated before the age of 40 were analyzed. One hundred thirty-seven secondary cancers were detected in these patients compared to 19.4 cases expected in the general population.[8] The 25-year actuarial risk of secondary cancer was 28%, and the relative risk of solid tumors increased in patients who were at a younger age during their first treatment. Most of the patients aged 20 years or younger developed second cancers before reaching 40 years and the risk appeared to decrease after 10 years. An updated Dutch series reported on 1261 patients with a median follow-up of 17.8 years[1] (Figure 76.1). There were 534 deaths, 55% due to HL. Relative risk of death from all causes was 6.8 times greater than the risk observed in general population, and this risk remained high even 30 years after treatment due to secondary tumors and cardiovascular disease (relative risk of 6.6 and 6.3, respectively). The relative risks were significantly higher for patients treated before age 20, 14.8, and 13.6, respectively, for malignancy and cardiovascular deaths. As these patients grew older however, the secondary causes of mortality declined.

Except for breast cancer, there are no guidelines for screening HL survivors for secondary malignancy. The cumulative risk of developing breast cancer is estimated to be as high as one in three by 40 years of age for those receiving supradiaphragmatic irradiation in childhood (< 16 years) and one in five by age 50 years for those treated at age 20–29 years.[9] The relative risk is increased mainly in those under the age of 30 years at the time of irradiation and is highest for those treated between the ages of 10 and 16 years. The relative risk is much lower in women aged 30–35 years (1–3.7). In comparison, the estimated risk for development of breast cancer by age 50 in the general population is one in 50. The median time to development of breast cancer after supradiaphragmatic irradiation was found to be about 15 years (range 4–20), although considerably shorter in those treated during childhood. There are no prospective trials of mammography or other screening methods in women at increased risk of breast cancer after supradiaphragmatic irradiation. In the absence of such data, clinicians have to tailor screening methods and frequency to the risk and the age of the patient at the time of treatment and the density of the breast tissue at the time of screening. Magnetic resonance imaging (MRI) scans may be more sensitive in younger women. Any method of screening should begin at a younger age than population screening for sporadic breast cancer. For those treated under the age of 17 years, screening from age 25 years is recommended; for those treated between 17 and 35 years, screening should begin 8 years after the completion of irradiation[9] (Table 76.1).

The German Hodgkin's Lymphoma Study Group also investigated secondary myeloid leukemia and myelodysplastic syndromes in patients treated for HL.[10] Forty-six patients out of a cohort of 5411 developed secondary acute myeloid leukemia/myelodysplastic syndromes (AML/MDS) after a median observation time of 55 months (1% incidence). Among these 46 patients, 30 had received cyclophosphamide, vincristine, prednisone, procarbazine/doxorubicin, bleomycin, vinblastine, dacarbazine (COPP/ABVD) or a similar regimen. There was only one patient who received ABVD alone. There were 11 patients who received Bleomycin, Etoposide, Doxorubicin, and COPP at standard or escalated doses. AML and MDS can be readily detected with a routine blood count in most patients. There may be an advantage to detect MDS early to maximize the possibility of using allogeneic transplantation for this otherwise lethal complication. Discovery of cytopenia in an HL survivor should trigger an aggressive investigation with early examination of bone marrow morphology and cytogenetics.

## CARDIAC COMPLICATIONS OF THERAPY

Cardiovascular mortality is the third main cause of death in patients with HL, after deaths due to HL and secondary malignancies. The relative risk of cardiac death is greatest in irradiated children and adolescents but the absolute risk increases with age at the time of irradiation. Cardiovascular deaths are mainly due to coronary artery disease accelerated by radiotherapy. Increased risks of cardiac events are particularly observed in patients who have known cardiac risk factors such as hypertension and hyperlipidemia. The addition of chemotherapy to radiation treatment does not appear to increase the coronary disease risk. Other late cardiac toxicities of radiation and chemotherapy include pericardial disease, cardiomyopathy, valvular defects, and conduction abnormalities.

The actuarial risk of developing symptomatic coronary artery disease is estimated to be 6% at 10 years and 10–20% at 20 years.[11,12] The actuarial risk of death from cardiac ischemia is 2–6% at 10 years and 10–12% at 15–25 years. These rates are approximately five times the rates seen in the general population. In a single-center experience, 5.5% of 475 patients treated with mantle radiotherapy had a morbid cardiac event directly related to coronary artery disease.[13] The mean interval from therapy to cardiac event was 13.1 years (range 4.4–27), and the mean age at the time of the event was 39.4 years (range 24–65). The relative risk of cardiac death was 2.8 (3.1 for males and 1.8 for females). Interestingly, in this group of patients, cardiovascular risk factors were, on average, higher than in the general population. Aggressive modification of cardiovascular risk factors should be an integral part of the follow-up management of HL survivors who had chest irradiation. The actuarial risk of other vascular events (e.g., carotid) reaches 7% at 20 years. The actuarial risk of valvular heart disease is about 5–6% with 20 years of follow-up, and the clinicians must stay alert to these complications.

## THYROID AND GONADAL DYSFUNCTION

Subclinical and clinical thyroid disease is common after treatment of HL. In a series of 151 patients, 26 cases of subclinical, 12 cases of manifest clinical hypothyroidism, and 2 cases of hyperthyroidism were documented.[14] Thyroid dysfunction was more frequent in patients who underwent mantle or neck radiotherapy. Hypothyroidism was often revealed after the sixth year of follow-up. A high incidence of thyroiditis was also reported in this group of patients. Annual monitoring of thyroid function should be incorporated in follow-up patients with HL, particularly in those treated with radiation involving neck.

The impact of therapy on fertility appears to be diminishing with judicious use of less gonadotoxic chemotherapeutics.[15] In general, patients are advised to use an effective contraception for 6–12 months after chemotherapy. After this initial period, there is no reason to discourage pregnancy in female HL survivors, since there is no documented negative impact of pregnancy on their outcome.[16,17] In addition, there appears to be no increase in the rates of stillbirths, low birth weight, congenital malformations, or early cancer development in the offspring of HL survivors.[18]

### QUALITY OF LIFE

A number of studies investigated the health-related quality of life in long-term survivors of HL. In a study from Sweden, 121 survivors were compared to a control group of 236 individuals after a median of 14 years following therapy.[19] Although their physical health was diminished, the overall quality of life was not inferior in HL patients. The German Hodgkin's Lymphoma Study Group obtained a quality-of-life questionnaire from 1981 patients at a median of 5.3 years after treatment completion.[20] Fatigue levels were much higher compared to the control population, even several years after completion of therapy. In an early-stage HL study comparing subtotal nodal radiation to combined modality therapy (CMT), there was a greater degree of symptom distress, fatigue, and poor quality of life with CMT at 6 months but the differences were not significant at 1 and 2 year time points.[21] Again, fatigue was significantly higher before therapy and persisted after therapy in these patients compared to the general population. The recognition and acknowledgment of this excess fatigue may be reassuring to the patients and may motivate them to enter in fatigue reduction programs.

### PATIENT EDUCATION

Probably the most important role of the physicians following patients with HL is the education they provide regarding recognition of potential medical problems that may arise. A well-informed patient is more likely to seek medical attention with new symptoms. However, patient teaching must be done without causing excessive alarm or anxiety in the patient and their family members, and special attention must be paid to their psychosocial state. Routine physician visits by HL survivors are probably more valuable for the sense of comfort they provide to the patients than the detection of recurrent HL or treatment complications. During these visits, it is important to review and explain potential late complications of HL treatment, discuss the psychosocial impact of their disease, and promote health maintenance, including smoking cessation, cardiovascular risk reduction, and self-examination of skin and breast tissue. Although an occasional patient will present with asymptomatic physical or laboratory findings suspicious for recurrence or treatment-related complication, most of these will be detected in symptomatic patients who return for unscheduled visits.

## CONCLUSIONS

Follow-up care of HL survivors is as important as their initial care, since they are under a constant threat of competing causes of morbidity and mortality. Although we know a great deal about relapse patterns and long-term complications of this disease, it is important to remember that there are no prospective data regarding utility of screening methods commonly used in follow-up. Therefore, all follow-up recommendations are based on clinical judgment and experience and the care paths of large cancer centers and must be tailored based on patient characteristics and the treatment given. Ongoing patient education remains an integral part of long-term follow-up of HL. Trends toward using minimally toxic and yet very effective therapy for HL are expected to reduce both recurrences and treatment complications and make follow-up simpler but not obsolete.

### REFERENCES

1. Aleman B, van den Belt-Dusebout A, Klokman W, van't Veer M, Bartelink H, van Leeuwen F: Long-term cause-specific mortality of patients treated for Hodgkin's disease. *J Clin Oncol* 21:3431, 2003.
2. Ng A, Bernardo M, Weller E, et al.: Long-term survival and competing causes of death in patients with early-stage Hodgkin's disease treated at age 50 or younger. *J Clin Oncol* 20:2101, 2002.
3. Radford J, Eardley A, Woodman C, Crowther D: Routine outpatient review following treatment for Hodgkin's disease and a efficient way of detecting relapse. *Proc Am Soc Clin Oncol* 14:86, 1995.
4. Dores G, Metayer C, Curtis R, et al.: Second malignant neoplasms among long-term survivors of Hodgkin's disease: a population-based evaluation over 25 years. *J Clin Oncol* 20:3484–3494, 2002.
5. Swerdlow A, Barber J, Hudson G, et al.: Risk of second malignancy after Hodgkin's disease in a collaborative British cohort: the relation to age at treatment. *J Clin Oncol* 18:498–509, 2000.
6. Behringer K, Josting A, Schiller P, et al.: Solid tumors in patients treated for Hodgkin's disease: a report from the German Hodgkin's Lymphoma Study Group. *Ann Oncol* 15:1079, 2004.
7. Swerdlow A, Barber J, Horwich A, Cunningham D, Milan S, Omar R: Second malignancy in patients with Hodgkin's disease treated at the Royal Marsden Hospital. *Br J Cancer* 75:116, 1997.
8. van Leeuwen F, Klokman W, van't Veer M, et al.: Long-term risk of second malignancy in survivors of Hodgkin's disease treated during adolescence or young adulthood. *J Clin Oncol* 18:487, 2000.

9. Ralleigha G, Given-Wilsonb R: Breast cancer risk and possible screening strategies for young women following supradiaphragmatic irradiation for Hodgkin's disease. *Clin Radiol* 59:647–650, 2004.

10. Josting A, Wiedenmann S, Franklin J, et al.: Secondary myeloid leukemia and myelodysplastic syndromes in patients treated for Hodgkin's disease: a report from the German Hodgkin's Lymphoma Study Group. *J Clin Oncol* 21:3440, 2003.

11. Hull M, Morris C, Pepine C, Mendenhall N: Valvular dysfunction and carotid, subclavian, and coronary artery disease in survivors of Hodgkin's Lymphoma treated with radiation therapy. *JAMA* 290:2831–2837, 2003.

12. Reinders J, Heijmen B, Olofsen-van Acht M, van Putten W, Levendag P: Ischemic heart disease after mantlefield irradiation for Hodgkin's disease in long-term follow-up. *Radiother Oncol* 51:35–42, 1999.

13. King V, Constine L, Clark D, et al.: Symptomatic coronary artery disease after mantle irradiation for Hodgkin's disease. *Int J Ratiat Oncol Biol Phys* 36:971, 1996.

14. Illes A, Biro E, Miltenyi Z, et al.: Hypothyroidism and thyroiditis after therapy for Hodgkin's disease. *Acta Haematol* 109:11, 2003.

15. Grigg A: The impact of conventional and high-dose therapy for lymph fertility. *Clin Lymphoma* 5:84, 2004.

16. Lambe M, Hsieh C, Tsaih S, Adami J, Glimelius B, Adami H: Childbearing and the risk of Hodgkin's disease. *Cancer Epidemiol Biomarkers Prev* 7:831, 1998.

17. Zwitter M, Zakelj M, Kosmelj K: A case-control study of Hodgkin's disease and pregnancy. *Br J Cancer* 73:246, 1996.

18. Swerdlow A, Jacobs P, Marks A, et al.: Fertility, reproductive outcomes, and health of offspring, of patients treated for Hodgkin's disease: an investigation including chromosome examinations. *Br J Cancer* 74:291, 1996.

19. Wettergren L, Bjorkholm M, Axforph U, Langius-Eklof A: Determinants of health-related quality of life in long-term survivors of Hodgkin's Lymphoma. *Qual Life Res* 13:1369, 2004.

20. Ruffer J, Flechtner H, Tralls P, et al.: Fatigue in long-term survivors of Hodgkin's Lymphoma; a report from the German Hodgkin's Lymphoma Study Group (GHSG). *Eur J Cancer* 39:2179, 2003.

21. Ganz P, Moinpour C, Pauler D, et al.: Health status and quality of life in patients with early-stage Hodgkin's disease treated on Southwest Oncology Group Study 9133. *J Clin Oncol* 21:3512, 2003.

# Chapter 77

# TREATMENT OF RELAPSED OR REFRACTORY HODGKIN'S LYMPHOMA AND NEW FRONTIERS IN HODGKIN'S LYMPHOMA THERAPY

*Angelo M. Carella, Angela Congiu, Sandro Nati, and Ercole Brusamolino*

## INTRODUCTION

Hodgkin's lymphoma can now be cured in more than 80% of patients, irrespective of the anatomical stage of disease and of its histologic type. In spite of this great clinical success, some patients continue to experience either resistant disease or an early or late relapse. The need for an effective salvage strategy for these patients has been one of the most important problems to be addressed in this last decade. High-dose therapy followed by the autologous stem cell transplantation (ASCT) has proved to be the most effective therapy of resistant or relapsing patients.[1-22] High-dose chemotherapy, utilized as conditioning before ASCT, is generally preceded by the use of conventional-dose salvage chemotherapy regimens aimed at debulking the disease before high-dose therapy: such salvage chemotherapy is also used for patients who are not candidates for ASCT (advanced age, poor performance status (PA), and/or comorbidities).

As a general measure, a complete clinical restaging should be done in all cases at relapse; a new biopsy for tissue diagnosis should be done, when appropriate, in cases experiencing an early relapse, but it is mandatory in patients with a late relapse. Early relapses or relapses involving extranodal sites are associated with a worse outcome compared to late relapses or to recurrences in a single nodal station.

Several factors must be taken into account in the choice of a conventional salvage therapy. Because most of the patients with Hodgkin's lymphoma receive as first-line therapy anthracyline-based regimens (ABVD or ABVD-like regimens), subsequent chemotherapy should avoid these agents due to the risk of cumulative cardiac toxicity. In general, drugs with known cross-resistance with those used in first-line therapy should

be avoided. Lastly, in order to mobilize hematopoietic progenitor cells, an effective regimen should avoid drugs that may compromise stem cell mobilization, such as nitrosourea derivatives or selected alkylating agents (melphalan, busulphan, and mechlorethamine), and possibly should include drugs with high mobilizing capacity, such as cytarabine or gemcitabine.

What follows is a critical review of what has been achieved, so far, in the salvage therapy of Hodgkin's lymphoma, with a brief account of new perspectives in the therapy of resistant/relapsing patients.

## RELAPSES AFTER RADIATION THERAPY ALONE

The prognosis of patients with Hodgkin's lymphoma, who relapse after being treated with radiotherapy alone, is generally very good. A number of studies have reviewed the outcome of conventional-dose salvage therapy in these patients.[23-31] These studies have evaluated potential prognostic factors, including disease characteristics at diagnosis and at relapse, time to relapse, and type of salvage chemotherapy. In the studies conducted in the 1980s, most of the patients relapsing after radiation therapy (RT) alone were treated with MOPP (mechlorethamine, vincristine, procarbazine, and prednisone) or similar chemotherapies.[24] A study from the Dana-Farber Cancer Institute indicated a 10-year freedom from progression (FFP) of 58% and an overall survival (OS) rate of 62%.[28] A similar analysis at Stanford University showed that the 10-year FFP and OS were both 57%[25]; the International Database on Hodgkin's lymphoma reported a 10-year OS of 58% for clinical stage I–II and of 50% for pathological stage I–II patients.[29]

The ABVD (adriamycin, bleomycin, vinblastine, and dacarbazine) regimen was initially introduced as second-line therapy for patients who had a poor response to, or relapsed after, irradiation and MOPP.[31] ABVD has subsequently proved to be superior to MOPP for both early and advanced stage Hodgkin's lymphoma and to be less toxic in term of lower risk of sterility and of subsequent leukemia.[32] A study from the National Cancer Institute of Milan demonstrated the superiority of ABVD over MOPP, with a significantly higher FFP (73% vs 42%), relapse-free survival (RFS) (81% versus 54%), and OS (80% vs 44%).[32] At variance, a study recently published from the Dana-Farber Cancer Institute has shown that the two regimens, MOPP and ABVD, had similar efficacy in patients with predominantly early-stage disease at initial RT.[33] The median follow-up was 12 years, and the 10-year FFP and OS were 70% and 89%, respectively; the type of salvage chemotherapy did not significantly influence FFP or OS; the only significant predictor for inferior FFP and OS was age greater than 50 years. The discrepancy between these two studies can be ascribed to the differences in the initial disease presentation. The results of salvage chemotherapy in more recent cohorts of patients are notably better[33] than those obtained in the earlier patients; this may be because patients who were treated in the earlier era were more likely to have presented with advanced disease or large mediastinal bulk that by current standards would have precluded the use of RT alone.[34,35]

Given the risk of leukemogenesis and of irreversible gonadal toxicity associated with MOPP chemotherapy, ABVD should be considered the salvage regimen of choice after radiation therapy failure[36]; this particularly applies to the patients given RT alone for prognostically unfavourable early-stage disease.

## RECURRENT/RESISTANT DISEASE AFTER INITIAL CHEMOTHERAPY

The therapeutic options for patients with Hodgkin's lymphoma relapsed or refractory to first-line therapy include conventional-dose salvage chemotherapy, high-dose therapy followed by ASCT, and/or allogeneic stem cell transplant.[37–39]

The need to find a second-line effective treatment for Hodgkin's lymphoma is confined almost entirely to patients presenting with advanced stage lymphoma; among these patients, however, the failure to cure is not evenly distributed across all prognostic subgroups. The landmark study by the International Prognostic Factors Project on advanced Hodgkin's lymphoma has shown that the risk of resistant/relapsing disease is less than 20% for patients with a prognostic score 0–1 (30% of total), but that it exceeds 50% for those with four or more adverse prognostic factors (19% of total).[40]

The choice of the best salvage approach should rely on the evaluation of prognostic factors and clinical characteristics of patients with recurrent or resistant disease. Since 1979, it has been observed that the length of remission after first-line therapy has a significant effect on the success of subsequent salvage treatment; thus, failures to chemotherapy can be classified as *primary resistant disease* [complete remission (CR) never achieved], as *early relapse* (within 12 months since remission), or as *late relapse* (beyond 12 months since remission). In a recent retrospective analysis of the German Hodgkin's Lymphoma Study Group on 513 patients, no patient with primary progressive disease, treated with conventional-dose chemotherapy survived more than 8 years; by contrast, the projected 20-year survival for patients with early or late relapse is 11% and 22%, respectively; thus, conventional-dose therapy has virtually no curative potential in resistant Hodgkin's lymphoma.[41]

In relapsing disease (either early or late), the most compelling evidence for the superiority of high-dose therapy over conventional-dose salvage therapy is derived from the British National Lymphoma Investigational (BNLI) and the European Blood and Marrow Transplantation (EBMT) groups.[42,43] In the first trial, patients were treated with conventional-dose mini-BEAM (carmustine, etoposide, cytarabine, and melphalan) or high-dose BEAM with autologous stem cell transplant; the actuarial 3-year event-free survival (EFS) was significantly better in patients who received high-dose therapy (53% vs 10%).[42] In the EBMT trial, patients who relapsed after chemotherapy were randomly assigned to four cycles of mini-BEAM + dexamethasone (dexa-mini-BEAM) or two cycles of dexa-mini-BEAM followed by BEAM and ASCT; the final analysis showed an FFP significantly higher in the BEAM + ASCT group (55% vs 34%).[43] Subsequently, recent studies with high-dose therapy followed by ASCT have shown 30–65% long-term disease-free survival in selected patients with refractory and relapsed disease.[10,19,39,44–49] In addition, the reduction of early transplant-related mortality from 10–15%, as reported in earlier studies, to less than 5% in more recent studies, has led to the widespread acceptance of this procedure. Therefore, there is now a general consensus that high-dose therapy and ASCT is the treatment of choice for relapsing or resistant Hodgkin's lymphoma.[39]

The role of conventional-dose salvage therapy consists of achieving the maximum tumor reduction (debulking) prior to high-dose therapy. In nearly all reported series of ASCT in relapsed Hodgkin's lymphoma, patients received some cytoreductive therapy before high-dose therapy/ASCT. Patients who relapse after chemotherapy but not respond to standard-dose salvage chemotherapy constitute the bulk of long-term survivors in transplantation studies.[6,45] Unfortunately, the design of these studies does not allow an accurate assessment of the role of cytoreduction, since many teams use a uniform standard-dose salvage chemotherapy followed by high-dose therapy and ASCT. The ability to mobilize peripheral blood progenitor cells (PBPCs) is a critical requirement for a pre-ASCT cytoreductive chemotherapy regimen. The optimal number of $CD34^+$ cells/kg needed for marrow reconstitution is undetermined but many studies have shown that $(2-3) \times 10^6$ $CD34^+$ cells/kg are enough to achieve neutrophil and platelet engraftment and to shorten the length of hospital stay.[46]

The choice of conventional salvage regimen should be also based on the evaluation of the potential cumulative risk of cardiac or pulmonary toxicity deriving from prior exposure to anthracyclines or bleomycin and on the absence of cross-resistance between the second-line drugs and those of first-line regimens (MOPP and MOPP-like, ABVD or ABVD-like regimens).

Historically, the ABVD regimen was developed when MOPP chemotherapy represented the standard first-line therapy for advanced Hodgkin's lymphoma; the ABVD combination cured about one fourth of the patients relapsing or refractory to MOPP.[50]

In the last two decades, ABVD has been the standard first-line therapy in advanced Hodgkin's lymphoma; this has led to a search of new salvage regimens incorporating new drugs (Table 77.1). Many second-line standard-dose therapy regimens have been developed,[52,62–65] several of which include platinum compounds such as cisplatin or carboplatin. While these regimens produce a fairly good overall response rate (from 50 to 80%), they are associated with substantial hematologic and nonhematologic toxicity, and hospitalization may be required either to administer the therapy or to manage complications. Overall response rates higher than 50% have been reported with the association of carmustine, etoposide, cytarabine, and melphalan (mini-BEAM)[64] and dexamethasone-BEAM (dexa-BEAM).[63] Unfortunately, both these regimens contain a nitrosourea and are poor mobi-

lizers of hematopoietic stem cells. Therefore, new drug combinations have been evaluated in order to provide sufficient disease control combined with moderate toxicity, and to allow a good PBPC mobilization for subsequent rescue after high-dose therapy. Either the combination of dexamethasone, cisplatin, and high-dose cytarabine (DHAP)[66] or that of etoposide, high-dose cytarabine, and cisplatin (ASHAP)[62] has proved to have both characteristics (good efficacy and excellent PBPC-mobilizing capacity). Other salvage regimens consist of a backbone of ifosfamide and etoposide, in association with a platinum derivative. The mitoguazone, ifosfamide, vinorelbine, and etoposide (MINE) regimen[51] was derived from the initial mitoguazone, ifosfamide, methotrexate, and etoposide (MIME) regimen.[67] In the group d'etude lymphoma (GELA) experience, among 100 patients with untreated relapses or induction failures, the MINE regimen produced an overall response rate of 75% (35% of CR); the CR response rate was 92% in patients with untreated relapses and 53% in those with induction failures; MINE was myelotoxic but was given on time at the calculated dose in 80% of patients and allowed an efficient harvest of PBPC.[51]

Recently, several variants of the ifosfamide–etoposide combination have been utilized and all these studies have confirmed that these drugs are able to produce good responses and can effectively mobilize hematopoietic progenitor cells into the peripheral blood. Two courses of VIP (etoposide, ifosfamide, and cisplatin) protocol[52] produced an overall response rate of 67%, while a combination of etoposide, prednisolone, ifosfamide, and carboplatin (EPIC)[53] produced a response rate of 70%. Sixty-five consecutive patients, 22 with primary refractory and 43 with relapsed Hodgkin's lymphoma, were treated with two biweekly cycles of ifosfamide, carboplatin, and etoposide (ICE).[54] The response rate was 88% and the

| Table 77.1 | Results of conventional salvage chemotherapy for Hodgkin's lymphoma | | | | | |
|---|---|---|---|---|---|---|
| Regimen | Reference | No. of patients | CR (%) | PR (%) | PD (%) | TRM (%) |
| MINE | 51 | 100 | 35 | 25 | 25 | 2 |
| VIP | 52 | 42 | 38 | 29 | NA | 0 |
| EPIC | 53 | 10 | 70 | NA | NA | 3 |
| ICE | 54 | 65 | 26 | 32 | 3 | 0 |
| IV | 55 | 47 | 45 | 38 | NA | 0 |
| IEV | 56 | 11 | 45 | 36 | NA | 0 |
| IEV | 57 | 18 | 50 | NA | 50 | 5 |
| GENC | 58 | 14 | 14 | 15 | NA | 0 |
| GENC | 59 | 23 | 9 | 30 | 56 | 0 |
| GDP | 60 | 23 | 17 | 21 | 31 | 0 |
| IGEV | 61 | 17 | 59 | 29 | 12 | 0 |
| ASHAP | 62 | 56 | 34 | 36 | 16 | 0 |

CR, complete remission; PR, partial remission; PD, progressive disease; TRM, therapy-related death; NA: not available.

EFS rate for patients who underwent transplantation was 68%. Predictors for outcome included B symptoms, extranodal disease, and CR duration of ≤1 year. High-dose ifosfamide and vinorelbine produced an overall response rate of 83%, with 45% complete and 38% partial responses after a median of two cycles[55]; the main toxic effect of these regimens was grade III–IV neutropenia, documented in 65% of cycles, with a median duration of 4–7 days. Almost all these standard-dose regimens were followed by PBPC collection and high-dose therapy with autologous stem cell rescue; after engraftment many patients received radiotherapy for residual disease. Of particular interest is the IEV (ifosfamide, epirubicin, and etoposide) combination[57]; this regimen was highly effective in patients relapsing after first second-line chemotherapy. Responsive patients were subsequently treated with radiotherapy. In these advanced patients, IEV was able to induce OS, RFS, and FFP of 18, 44, and 22%, respectively.

More recently, gemcitabine, a new pyrimidine antimetabolite was shown to have remarkable activity against solid tumors such as those of pancreas, lung, and bladder and to be active in vitro against leukemia and lymphoma cell lines.[68] When used as a single agent, gemcitabine is active in Hodgkin's lymphoma[58,59] and in a variety of histologic subtypes of non-Hodgkin's lymphoma, with a favorable toxicity profile compared with other cytotoxic agents.[56,69] In phase II studies in relapsed/refractory Hodgkin's lymphoma the drug was given on days 1, 8, and 15 at a dose of 1200 mg/m$^2$, with a schedule every 28 days, for a total of six cycles.[59] The overall response rate was 39%, with 9% CRs. In another study,[58] the overall response rate was 43%, with 14% CR; the patients who relapsed after a remission longer than 12 months had a better OS rate than those who relapsed earlier (67% vs 25%). In both studies the major toxicity was hematologic, with a minority of patients experiencing a grade IV toxicity. In no study did treatment-related deaths occur. According to these results this drug has been included in several salvage regimens for resistant/relapsing Hodgkin's lymphoma.

The addition of cisplatin to gemcitabine has demonstrated synergistic activity in vitro and this combination has become the standard in the treatment of advanced bladder and non-small cell lung cancer.[70] Given the moderate toxicity observed with these drugs when used at conventional doses, both have been incorporated with dexamethasone into the gemcitabine, dexamethasone, cisplatin (GDP) regimen.[71] The overall response rate achieved after the GDP regimen is 70%, (17% CRs); hematologic toxicity was mild (grade III neutropenia: 9%; grade III thrombocytopenia: 13%) and all patients successfully mobilized PBPC, with a median 10.6 × 10$^6$ CD34$^+$ cells/kg.[60]

Gemcitabine has also been associated with ifosfamide and vinorelbine in the IGEV combination. In the original experience in 17 heavily pretreated patients (chemo + radiotherapy), the overall response rate was 94%[61] and the median number of CD34$^+$ cells collected was 10.9 × 10$^6$/kg; in about 60% of patients, a single leukapheretic procedure was able to reach the number of CD34$^+$ cells necessary for the transplantation procedure. No treatment-related death was observed. The experience with the IGEV regimen has been widely confirmed also for its acceptable toxicity.

## FUTURE RESEARCH

Among the different experimental strategies in the treatment of Hodgkin's lymphoma, antibody-based constructs have given the most promising results in experimental Hodgkin's lymphoma models. Early clinical trials using immunotoxins and, more recently, monoclonal antibodies (MoAb) have demonstrated some clinical efficacy in patients with refractory Hodgkin's lymphoma.

Hodgkin's lymphoma can be a suitable candidate for MoAb-based therapy because Reed–Sternberg and Hodgkin's cells express specific surface antigens such as CD15, CD25, and CD30. So far, different approaches to eradicate tumor cells have been utilized using antibodies, including "naked" MoAb, and bispecific constructs that activate effectors cells of immune system against the target cell, immunotoxins that deliver a toxin linked to a specific antibody into the target cell, and different radioimmunoconjugates.

## MONOCLONAL ANTIBODIES FOR TREATMENT OF THE LYMPHOCYTE-PREDOMINANT HISTOLOGY

The anti-CD20 monoclonal antibody rituximab has demonstrated clinical efficacy in lymphocyte-predominant Hodgkin's lymphoma (LPHL) where Hodgkin's cells express B-cell antigens such as CD20.[72] Several multicenter phase II trials testing rituximab on refractory patients with LPHL are ongoing. In one study, 11 patients with CD20$^+$ Hodgkin's lymphoma were treated with rituximab at the standard dose of 375 mg/m$^2$, weekly for 4 weeks; nine patients (82%) achieved a complete response for which median duration was 14 months.[60] Similar results have been obtained in a trial involving 22 patients with recurrent LPHL, with an overall response rate of 100%.[73]

Treatment with rituximab was less successful in a series of 22 patients with classical Hodgkin's lymphoma, with an overall response rate of 23% and a median duration of response shorter than 8 months.[74]

## MONOCLONAL ANTIBODIES FOR TREATMENT OF CLASSICAL HODGKIN'S LYMPHOMA

Among the different target antigens on Reed–Sternberg cells, CD30 seems to be the most promising, since it is expressed at very high levels.[75] So far, two anti-CD30 MoAbs have been developed, the humanized SGN-30[76] and the fully human MDX-60.[77] The SGN-30 chimeric anti-CD30 antibody has demonstrated antitumor activity in preclinical models of Hodgkin's lymphoma and anaplastic large cell lymphoma. In a phase I single-dose trial, SGN-30 MoAb showed minimal toxicity with doses from 1 to 15 mg/kg, and antitumor activity was documented in 15% of patients (2 of 13). In a phase I/II dose-escalation study of 6 weekly infusions of SGN-30 at doses of 2, 4, 8, and 12 mg/kg, the MOAb was very well tolerated up to 8 mg/kg, and it was associated with a moderate activity.[78]

MDX-060 is a fully human IgG MoAb that recognizes CD30 and mediates killing of Reed–Sternberg cells in vitro and in xenograft tumor models. In a phase I/II dose-escalation study in patients with relapsed or refractory Hodgkin's lymphoma and other CD30+ lymphomas, MDX-060 was administered intravenously at dose levels of 0.1, 1, 5, 10, or 15 mg/kg, weekly for 4 weeks, with no dose-limiting toxicity. While the efficacy assessment has not been completed yet in all patients, preliminary results indicate that MDX-060 is well tolerated and has a clinical activity.[79]

Currently, humanized as well as fully human anti-CD30 MoAbs are being tested in clinical phase I/II studies. These MoAbs could engage the human immune system against Hodgkin's lymphoma and are capable of inducing apoptosis of Hodgkin's and Reed–Sternberg cells. In addition, these MoAbs could be combined with conventional chemotherapy and further improve the therapy of Hodgkin's lymphoma.

## SUMMARY

It is more and more difficult to test new agents since Hodgkin's lymphoma is often cured by conventional and/or high-dose therapy.[80] Nevertheless patients experiencing tumor refractoriness or early/late relapse must be able to receive effective procedures for a second remission of the disease. Clinical investigators must continue to work together to harness the objective to cure all patients with Hodgkin's lymphoma.

## REFERENCES

1. Carella A, Santini G, Santoro A,et al.: Massive chemotherapy with non-frozen autologous bone marrow transplantation in 13 cases of refractory Hodgkin's disease. *Eur J Cancer* 21:607, 1985.
2. Josting A, Reiser M, Rueffer U, Salzberger B, Diehil V, Engert A: Treatment of primary progressive Hodgkin's and aggressive non-Hodgkin's lymphoma: is there a chance for cure? *J Clin Oncol* 18:332, 2000.
3. Sureda A, Arranz R, Iriondo A, et al.: Autologous stem-cell transplantation for Hodgkin's disease: results and prognostic factors in 494 patients from the Grupo Espanol de Linfomas/Transplante Autologo de Medula Osea Spanish Cooperative Group. *J Clin Oncol* 19:1395, 2001.
4. Lazarus HM, Rowlings PA, Zhang MJ, et al.: Autotransplants for Hodgkin's disease in patients never achieving remission: a report from the Autologous Blood and Marrow Transplant Registry. *J Clin Oncol* 17:534, 1999.
5. Sweetenham JW, Carella AM, Taghipour G, et al.: High-dose therapy and autologous stem-cell transplantation for adult patients with Hodgkin's disease who do not enter remission after induction chemotherapy: results in 175 patients reported to the European Group for Blood and Marrow Transplantation Lymphoma Working Party. *J Clin Oncol* 17:3101, 1999.
6. Crump M, Smith AM, Brandwein J, et al.: High-dose etoposide and melphalan and autologous bone marrow transplantation for patients with advanced Hodgkin's disease: importance of disease status at transplant. *J Clin Oncol* 11:704, 1993.
7. Constant M: Autologous stem cell transplantation for primary refractory Hodgkin's disease: results and clinical variables affecting outcome. *Ann Oncol* 14:648, 2003.
8. Yahalom J, Gulati SC, Toia M, et al.: Accelerated hyperfractionated total-lymphoid irradiation, high-dose chemotherapy and autologous bone marrow transplantation for refractory and relapsing patients with Hodgkin's disease. *J Clin Oncol* 11: 1062, 1993.
9. Rapoport AP, Rowe JM, Kouides PA, et al.: One hundred autotransplants for relapsed or refractory Hodgkin's disease and lymphoma: value of pretransplant disease status for predicting outcome. *J Clin Oncol* 11:2351, 1993.
10. Reece DE, Connors JM, Spinelli JJ, et al.: Intensive therapy with cyclophosphamide, carmustine, etoposide ± cisplatin, and autologous bone marrow transplantation for Hodgkin's disease in first relapse after combination chemotherapy. *Blood* 83:1193, 1994.
11. Chopra R, McMillan AK, Linch DC, et al.: The place of high-dose BEAM therapy and autologous bone marrow transplantation in poor-risk Hodgkin's disease. A single-center eight-year study of 155 patients. *Blood* 81:1137, 1993.
12. Bierman PJ, Bagin RG, Jagannath S, et al.: High dose chemotherapy followed by autologous hematopoietic rescue in Hodgkin's disease: long-term follow-up in 128 patients. *Ann Oncol* 4:767, 1993.
13. Nademanee A, O'Donnell MR, Snyder DS, et al.: High-dose chemotherapy with or without total body irradiation followed by autologous bone marrow and/or peripheral blood stem cell transplantation for patients with relapsed and refractory Hodgkin's disease: results in 85 patients with analysis of prognostic factors. *Blood* 85:1381, 1995.
14. Burns LJ, Daniels KA, McGlave PB, et al.: Autologous stem cell transplantation for refractory and relapsed Hodgkin's disease: factors predictive of prolonged survival. *Bone Marrow Transplant* 16:13, 1995.
15. Lumley MA, Milligan DW, Knechtli CJ, Long SG, Billingham LJ, McDonald DF: High lactate dehydrogenase level is associated with an adverse outlook in

autografting for Hodgkin's disease. *Bone Marrow Transplant* 17:383, 1996.

16. Horning SJ, Chao NJ, Negrin RS, et al.: High-dose therapy and autologous hematopoietic progenitor cell transplantation for recurrent or refractory Hodgkin's disease: analysis of the Stanford University results and prognostic indices. *Blood* 89:801, 1997.

17. Wheeler C, Eichhoff C, Elias A, et al.: High-dose cyclophosphamide, carmustine and etoposide with autologous transplantation in Hodgkin's disease: a prognostic model for treatment outcome. *Biol Blood Marrow Transplant* 3:98, 1997.

18. Brice P, Bastion Y, Divine M: Analysis of prognostic factors after the first relapse of Hodgkin's disease in 187 patients. *Cancer* 78:1293, 1996.

19. Fermé C, Mounier N, Diviné M, et al.: Intensive salvage therapy with high-dose chemotherapy for patients with advanced Hodgkin's disease in relapsed or failure after initial chemotherapy: results of the Groupe d'Etudes des Lymphomes de l'Adulte H89 trial. *J Clin Oncol* 20:467, 2002.

20. Carella AM, Congiu AM, Gazza E, et al.: High-dose chemotherapy with autologous bone marrow transplantation in 50 advanced resistant Hodgkin's disease patients: an Italian Study Group report. *J Clin Oncol* 6:1411, 1988.

21. Yuen AR, Rosenberg SA, Hoppe RT, Halpern JD, Sandra J: Comparison between conventional salvage therapy and high-dose therapy with autografting for recurrent or refractory Hodgkin's disease. *Blood* 89:814, 1997.

22. Kessinger A, Bierman PJ, Vose JM, Armitage JO: High-dose cyclophosphamide, carmustine and etoposide followed by autologous peripheral stem cell transplantation for patients with relapsed Hodgkin's disease. *Blood* 77:2322, 1991.

23. Olver IN Wolf MM, Cruickshank D, et al.: Nitrogen mustard, vincristine, procarbazine, and prednisolone for relapse after radiation in Hodgkin's disease. An analysis of long-term follow-up. *Cancer* 62:233, 1988.

24. Longo DL, Young RC, Wesley M, et al.: Twenty years of MOPP therapy for Hodgkin's disease. *J Clin Oncol* 4:1295, 1986.

25. Roach M, Brophy N, Cox R, Varghese A, Hoppe RT: Prognostic factors for patients relapsing after radiotherapy for early-stage Hodgkin's disease. *J Clin Oncol* 8:623, 1990.

26. Mauch P, Somers R: International database on Hodgkin's disease: a cooperative effort to determine treatment outcome. *Ann Oncol* 4:59, 1992.

27. Hoppe RT: The management of Hodgkin's disease in relapse after primary radiation therapy. *Eur J Cancer* 28A:1920, 1992.

28. Healey EA, Tarbell NJ, Kalish LA, et al.: Prognostic factors for patients with Hodgkin's disease in first relapse. *Cancer* 71:2613, 1993.

29. Specht L, Horwich A, Asheley S: Salvage of relapse of patients with Hodgkin's disease in clinical stages I or II who were staged with laparotomy and initially treated with radiotherapy alone. A report from the international database on Hodgkin's disease. *Int J Radiat Oncol Biol Phys* 30:805, 1994.

30. Horwich A, Specht L, Asheley S: Survival analysis of patients with clinical stages I or II Hodgkin's disease who have relapsed after initial treatment with radiotherapy alone. *Eur J Cancer* 33:848, 1997.

31. Santoro A, Bonfante V, Bonadonna G: Salvage chemotherapy with ABVD in MOPP resistant Hodgkin's disease. *Ann Intern Med* 96:139, 1982.

32. Santoro A, Viviani S, Villareal CJ, et al.: Salvage chemotherapy in Hodgkin's disease irradiation failure: superiority of doxorubicin-containing regimens over MOPP. *Cancer Treat Rep* 70:343, 1986.

33. Ng AK, Li S, Neuberg D, et al.: Comparison of MOPP versus ABVD as salvage therapy in patients who relapse after radiation therapy alone for Hodgkin's disease. *Ann Oncol* 15:270, 2004.

34. Mauch P, Goodman R, Hellman S: The significance of mediastinal involvement in early stage Hodgkin's disease. *Cancer* 42:1039, 1978.

35. Lee CK, Bloomfield CD, Goldman AI, et al.: Prognostic significance of mediastinal involvement in Hodgkin's disease treated with curative radiotherapy. *Cancer* 46:2403, 1980.

36. Viviani S, Santoro A, Ragni G, Bonfante V, Bestetti O, Bonadonna G: Gonadal toxicity after combination chemotherapy for Hodgkin's disease. Comparative results of MOPP vs ABVD. *Eur J Cancer Clin Oncol* 21:601, 1985.

37. Diehl V, Thomas RK, Re D: Hodgkin's lymphoma—diagnosis and Therapy. *Lancet Oncol* 5:19, 2004.

38. Josting A, Raemakers JM, Diehl V, Engert A: New concepts for relapsed Hodgkin's disease. *Ann Oncol* 13(suppl 1):117, 2002.

39. Carella AM: Stem cell transplantation for Hodgkin's disease: a review of the literature. *Clin Lymphoma* 2:212, 2002.

40. Hasenclever D, Diehl V, Armitage JO, et al.: A prognostic score for advanced Hodgkin's disease. International Prognostic Factors Project on Advanced Hodgkin's Disease. *N Engl J Med* 339:1506, 1998.

41. Josting A, Franklin J, May M, et al.: New prognostic score based on treatment outcome of patients with relapsed Hodgkin's lymphoma registered in the database of the German Hodgkin's Lymphoma Study Group. *J Clin Oncol* 20:221, 2002.

42. Linch DC, Winfield D, Goldstone AH, et al.: Dose intensification with autologous bone marrow transplantation in relapsed and resistant Hodgkin's disease. *Lancet* 341:1051, 1993.

43. Schmitz N, Pfistner B, Sextro M, et al.: Aggressive conventional chemotherapy compared with high-dose chemotherapy with autologous haematopoietic stem-cell transplantation for relapsed chemosensitive Hodgkin's disease: a randomised trial. *Lancet* 359:2065, 2002.

44. Josting A, Katay L, Rueffer U, et al.: Favorable outcome of patients with relapsed or refractory Hodgkin's disease treated with-dose chemotherapy and stem cell rescue at the time of maximal response to conventional salvage therapy (dexa-BEAM). *Ann Oncol* 9:289, 1998.

45. Sweetenham JW, Taghipour G, Milligan D, et al.: High-dose therapy and ASCT for patients with HD in first relapse after chemotherapy. Results from EBMT. *Bone Marrow Transplant* 20:745, 1997.

46. Schmitz N, Linch DC, Dreger P, et al.: Randomized trial of filgrastim-mobilized PBPCT vs ABMT in lymphoma patients. *Lancet* 347:353, 1996.

47. Biermann PJ, Bagin RG, Jagannath S, et al.: High dose chemotherapy followed by autologous hematopoietic rescue in Hodgkin's disease: long-term follow-up in 128 patients. *Ann Oncol* 4:767, 1993.

48. Armitage JO, Bierman PJ, Vose JM, et al.: Autologous bone marrow transplantation for patients with relapsed Hodgkin's disease. *Am J Med* 91:605, 1991.

49. Gribben JG, Linch DC, Singer CR, McMillan AK, Jarrett M, Goldstone AH: Successful treatment of refractory Hodgkin' disease by high-dose combination chemotherapy and autologous bone marrow transplantation. *Blood* 73:340, 1989.

50. Santoro A, Bonadonna G: Prolonged disease-free survival in MOPP-resistant Hodgkin's disease after treatment with adriamycin, bleomycin, vinblastine and dacarbazine (ABVD). *Cancer Chemother Pharmacol* 2:101, 1979.

51. Ferme C, Bastion Y, Lepage E, et al.: The MINE regimen as intensive salvage chemotherapy for relapsed and refractory Hodgkin's disease. *Ann Oncol* 6:543, 1995.

52. Ribrag V, Nasr F, Bouhris JH, et al.: VIP (etoposide, ifosfamide and *cis*-platinum) as salvage intensification program in relapsed or refractory Hodgkin's disease. *Bone Marrow Transplant* 21:969, 1998.

53. Mc Bride NC, Ward MC, Mills MJ, et al.: Epic as an effective, low toxicity salvage therapy for patients with poor risk lymphoma prior to Beam high dose chemotherapy and peripheral blood progenitor cell transplantation. *Leuk Lymphoma* 33:339, 1999.

54. Moskowitz CH, Nimer SD, Zelenetz AD, et al.: A 2-step comprehensive high-dose chemoradiotherapy second-line program for relapsed and refractory Hodgkin disease: analysis by intent to treat and development of a prognostic model. *Blood* 97:616, 2001.

55. Bonfante V, Viviani S Devizzi L, et al.: High-dose ifosfamide and vinorelbine as salvage therapy for relapsed or refractory Hodgkin's disease. *Eur J Haematol* 64:51, 2001.

56. Zinzani PL, Tani M, Molinari AL, et al.: Ifosfamide, epirubicin and etoposide regimen as salvage and mobilizing therapy for relapsed/refractory lymphoma patients. *Haematologica* 87:816, 2002.

57. Anselmo AP, Meloni G, Cavalieri E, et al.: Conventional salvage chemotherapy vs high-dose therapy with autografting for recurrent or refractory Hodgkin's disease patients. *Ann Haematol* 79:79, 2000.

58. Zinzani PL, Bendandi M, Stefoni V, et al.: Value of gemcitabine treatment in heavily pretreated Hodgkin's disease patients. *Haematologica* 85:926, 2000.

59. Santoro A, Bredenfeld H, Devizzi L, et al.: Gemcitabine in the treatment of refractory Hodgkin's disease: results of a multicenter phase II study. *J Clin Oncol* 18:2615, 2000.

60. Baetz T, Belch A, Couban S, et al.: Gemcitabine, dexamethasone and cisplatin is an active and non-toxic chemotherapy regimen in relapsed or refractory Hodgkin's disease: a phase II study by the National Cancer Institute of Canada Clinical Trials Group. *Ann Oncol* 14:1762, 2003.

61. Magagnoli M, Sarina B, Balzarotti M, et al.: Mobilizing potential of ifosfamide/ vinorelbine-based chemotherapy in pretreated malignant lymphoma. *Bone Marrow Transplant* 28:923, 2001.

62. Rodriguez J, Rodriguez MA, Fayad L, et al.: ASHAP: a regimen for cytoreduction of refractory or recurrent Hodgkin's disease. *Blood* 93:3632, 1999.

63. Pfreundschuh MG, Rueffer U, Lathan B, et al.: Dexa-BEAM in patients with Hodgkin's disease refractory to multidrug chemotherapy regimens: a trial of the German Hodgkin's Disease Study Group. *J Clin Oncol* 12:580, 1994.

64. Colwill R, Crump M, Couture F, et al.: Mini-BEAM as salvage therapy for relapsed or refractory Hodgkin's disease before intensive therapy and autologous bone marrow transplantation. *J Clin Oncol* 13:396, 1995.

65. Josting A, Rudolph C, Reiser M, et al.: Time-intensified dexamethasone/cisplatin/ cytarabine. An effective salvage therapy with low toxicity in patients with relapsed and refractory Hodgkin's disease. *Ann Oncol* 13:1628, 2002.

66. Rapoport AP, Rowe JM, Kouides PA, et al.: One hundred autotransplants for relapsed or refractory Hodgkin's disease and lymphoma: value of pretransplant disease status for predicting outcome. *J Clin Oncol* 11:2351, 1993.

67. Hagemeister FB, Tannir N, McLaughlin P, et al.: MIME chemotherapy (methyl GAG, ifosfamide, methotrexate, etoposide) as treatment for recurrent Hodgkin's disease. *J Clin Oncol* 5:556, 1987.

68. Plunkett W, Huang P, Searcy CE, Gandhi V: Gemcitabine: Preclinical pharmacology and mechanisms of action. *Semin Oncol* 23:3, 1996.

69. Fosså A, Santoro A, Hiddemann W, et al.: Gemcitabine as single agent in the treatment or relapsed or refractory aggressive non-Hodgkin's lymphoma. *J Clin Oncol* 17:3786, 1999.

70. Peters GJ, Bergman AM, Ruizvan H, et al.: Interaction between cisplatin and gemcitabine *in vitro* and *in vivo*. *Semin Oncol* 22:72, 1995.

71. Josting A, Rudolpf C, Reiser M, et al.: Time-intensified dexamethasone/cisplatin/ cytarabine: an effective salvage therapy with low toxicity in patients with relapsed and refractory Hodgkin's disease. *Ann Oncol* 13:1628, 2002.

72. Rehwald U, Schulz H, Reiser M, et al.: Treatment of relapsed CD20+ Hodgkin's lymphoma with the monoclonal antibody rituximab is effective and well tolerated: results of a phase 2 trial of the German Hodgkin Lymphoma Study Group. *Blood* 101:420, 2003.

73. Ekstrand BC, Lucas JB, Horwitz SM, et al.: Rituximab in lymphocyte-predominance Hodgkin's disease: results of a phase 2 trial. *Blood* 101:4285, 2003.

74. Younes A, Romaguera J, Hagemeister F, et al.: A pilot study of rituximab in patients with recurrent classic Hodgkin's disease. *Cancer* 98:310, 2003.

75. Schwab U, Stein H, Gerdes J, et al.: Production of a monoclonal antibody specific for Hodgkin and Sternberg–Reed cells of Hodgkin's disease and a subset of normal lymphoid cells. *Nature* 299:65, 1982.

76. Wahl AF, Klussman K, Thompson JD, et al.: The anti-CD30 monoclonal antibody SGN-30 promotes growth arrest and DANN fragmentation in vitro and affects anti-tumor activity in models of Hodgkin's disease. *Cancer Res* 62:3736, 2002.

77. Borchmann P, Treml JF, Hansen H, et al.: The human anti-CD30 antibody 5F11 shows in vitro and in vivo activity against lymphoma. *Blood* 102:3737, 2003.

78. Bartlett NL, Bernstein SH, Leonard JP, et al.: Safety, anti-tumor activity and pharmacokinetics of six weekly doses

of SGN-30 (anti-CD30 monoclonal antibody) in patients with refractory or recurrent CD30+ hematologic malignancies. *Blood* 102: 647,2003. Abstract 2390.

79. Ansell S, Byrd J, Horwitz S, et al.: Phase I/II study of a fully human anti-CD30 monoclonal antibody (MDX-060) in Hodgkin's disease (HD) and anaplastic large cell lymphoma (ALCL). *Blood* 102:181, 2003. Abstract 632.

80. Connors JM: Treatment of resistant and relapsed Hodgkin's lymphoma. In: *Hematology 2003*, ASH Educational Program, San Diego, CA, Dec 6–9, 2003: 238–242.

# Section 3

# SPECIAL TOPICS IN LYMPHOMA

## Chapter 78

# EPIDEMIOLOGY OF SECOND MALIGNANCIES FOLLOWING LYMPHOMA THERAPY AND SCREENING RECOMMENDATIONS

*Jonathan W. Friedberg and Andrea K. Ng*

## INTRODUCTION

Patients with Hodgkin's lymphoma and aggressive non-Hodgkin's lymphoma (NHL) have a relatively high cure rate compared with patients with other hematologic malignancies. Despite these cures, lymphoma survivors continue to have a higher mortality rate than age- and gender-matched peers who have not had the disease. Much of this excess mortality is from second malignancies, which are now recognized as a direct consequence of curative chemotherapy and radiation therapy, and frequently have a poor prognosis. Figure 78.1 shows the cumulative incidence of observed second tumors in a cohort of survivors of Hodgkin's disease and expected tumors in a matched population. Even more than 30 years after diagnosis, patients cured of Hodgkin's lymphoma experience elevated risks of second cancers. In one study, the relative risk of death from second malignancy was 5.1 compared with age-matched controls.[1] The recent appreciation of these often-fatal late effects of treatment has focused efforts in both screening and prevention.

## SOLID TUMORS: INCIDENCE AND RISK FACTORS

The risk of solid tumors after treatment of lymphoma is most established in Hodgkin's lymphoma. However, as therapies for NHL improve and result in more survivors, it is expected that risks and risk factors for the development of solid tumors in this setting will be similar to those in Hodgkin's lymphoma. In the modern Hodgkin's lymphoma therapeutic era (post-mechlorethamine), lung and breast cancer, often appearing 15 or more years after completion of lymphoma therapy, have emerged as the most significant subtypes of second malignancy, accounting for the majority of cases.[2] Table 78.1 shows the types of solid tumors observed in a cohort of patients treated for Hodgkin's lymphoma at a single institution, representative of published experiences.

A recent study analyzed data from 32,591 patients with Hodgkin's lymphoma reported to 16 registries in North America and Europe.[3] Importantly, this included 1111 25-year survivors. In this series, there were 1726 solid tumors, with cancers of the lung, digestive tract, and

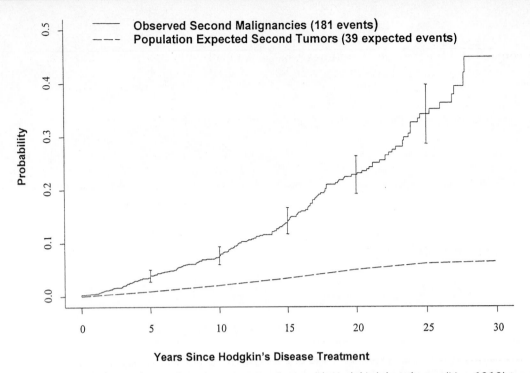

**Figure 78.1** *Cumulative incidence of second tumors among patients with Hodgkin's lymphoma (N = 1319) treated at the Joint Center for Radiation Therapy, and the expected cumulative incidence of tumors among a matched population*

breast the most common. After a progressive rise in relative risk of all solid tumors over time, there was an apparent downturn in risk at 25 years, emphasizing the importance of long-term surveillance in this population.

Radiation therapy is the most significant risk factor for developing solid tumors after lymphoma, with the majority of second cancers arising either within or at the edges of radiation fields. In the aforementioned series, temporal trends and treatment group distribution for cancers of the esophagus, stomach, rectum, breast, bladder, and thyroid all suggested a radiogenic effect. Three case–control studies have carefully evaluated the dose–response relationship between exposure to radiation therapies and the development of breast cancer and lung cancer, and demonstrated a significant trend of increasing risk of tumor development with increasing radiation dose.[4–6]

The contribution of chemotherapy alone to the risk of solid tumor development is less clear. In a cohort of patients with Hodgkin's lymphoma from the British Lymphoma Investigation Group, 31% of the population was treated with chemotherapy alone (predominantly with alkylating agents), and the relative risks of developing lung cancer after radiation therapy alone or chemotherapy alone were both significantly increased at 2.9 and 3.3, respectively.[7] A nested case–control study of lung cancer after Hodgkin's lymphoma was subsequently performed, comparing 88 cases of lung cancer with 176 matched controls.[8] Patients with a history of mechlorethamine treatment were at a significantly higher risk of developing lung cancer (RR = 1.69).

Two case-control studies on breast cancer after Hodgkin's lymphoma, however, showed a significantly decreased risk of breast cancer after alkylating chemotherapy exposure.[4,5] The relationship was dose related, with decreasing breast cancer risk with additional cycles of chemotherapy. Other data suggest the risk of breast cancer is significantly reduced in women who had premature menopause: the younger the age at menopause, the lower the risk of breast cancer.[4] These studies do report that the radiation-related risk of breast cancer, however, does not diminish in the longest follow-up, again suggesting a need for lifetime surveillance and programs of patient and physician awareness.

**Table 78.1** Tumor-type distribution of the 142 solid tumors observed in 1319 patients treated for Hodgkin's disease at the Joint Center for Radiation Therapy at a median of 12 years of follow-up

| Solid tumor type (N = 142) | N | (%) |
|---|---|---|
| Breast | 39 | (27) |
| Lung | 27 | (19) |
| Gastrointestinal | 25 | (18) |
| Sarcoma | 12 | (8) |
| Genitourinary | 12 | (8) |
| Head and neck | 9 | (6) |
| Melanoma | 8 | (6) |
| Thyroid | 5 | (4) |
| Gynecologic | 4 | (3) |
| Central nervous system | 1 | (1) |

Reports on the relationship between age at diagnosis and treatment of lymphoma and risk of second malignancy are conflicting. One consistent finding, however, is the increased risk of breast cancer for females treated for Hodgkin's lymphoma at a young age.[2,4] The cutoff age ranges from 25 to 35, beyond which the risk of breast cancer appeared to be no longer significantly increased. A cohort of 1380 children with Hodgkin's lymphoma (median age of diagnosis was 11) was followed for a median of 17 years by the Late Effects Study Group.[9] Two hundred twelve second cancers occurred in this group of patients, with breast cancer the most common malignancy. The cumulative incidence of second malignancy was 26% at 20 years. Risk factors for solid tumors clearly included young age at lymphoma diagnosis, and radiation-based therapy.

Several case–control studies have evaluated tobacco use as an additional risk factor for developing secondary neoplasms after therapy for lymphoma.[6,8] In one study, in which the smoking history was known in 90% of the patient population, patients who smoked more than 10 pack-years after the diagnosis of Hodgkin's lymphoma were at a sixfold increased risk for lung cancer compared to those with a less than one pack-year history of smoking.[10] The multiplicative effect between smoking and lymphoma therapy exposure is well described: patients who received both radiation therapy and alkylating agents were at a sevenfold increased risk of lung cancer; this risk increased to 49-fold in the setting of a greater than 10-year history of tobacco use.[6]

## MYELODYSPLASTIC SYNDROME (MDS) AND ACUTE MYELOID LEUKEMIA (AML): INCIDENCE AND RISK FACTORS

Historically, myelodysplastic syndrome (MDS) and secondary acute myelogenous leukemia have been recognized as significant complications of alkylating-agent-based chemotherapy for both indolent NHL and Hodgkin's lymphoma.[11,12] Topoisomerase inhibitors[13] and purine analogs[14] also clearly contribute to the risk of AML and MDS. With the recent introduction of alternative chemotherapy and immunotherapeutic modalities, autologous stem cell transplantation (ASCT) and radioimmunotherapy represent the lymphoma treatment modalities with the highest risk of developing MDS. In fact, MDS and AML have emerged as the major late complications of ASCT in patients with lymphoma.[15] In this setting, these disorders have an exceedingly poor prognosis, and represent the leading cause of non-disease-related death in survivors of ASCT for lymphoma.

The true incidence of MDS after nonmyeloablative radioimmunotherapy with either iodine-131 tositumomab[16] (Bexxar, GlaxoSmithKline, Philadelphia, and Corixa, Seattle) or Y-90 ibritumomab tiuxetan[17] (Zevalin, BiogenIdec, Cambridge) remains to be defined. In an analysis of 773 patients treated with I-131 tositumomab, 21 patients have developed MDS thus far, with an annualized incidence of 1.45%/year, which compares favorably to patients treated with alkylating agent chemotherapy.[18] The incidence of MDS after Y-90 ibritumomab tiuxetan appears to be similar. However, long-term follow-up of large cohorts of patients is clearly required to definitively determine the incidence of this fatal complication in the modern treatment era of indolent lymphoma, and the degree to which radioimmunotherapy contributes to this risk.

There is a substantially greater understanding of clinical risk factors for subsequent development of MDS after ASCT for lymphoma. It is expected that these risk factors may be similar in patients treated with radioimmunotherapy. Acknowledging differences in methods used to identify cases and to estimate the cumulative incidence over time, up to 10% of NHL patients treated with ASCT may develop secondary MDS within 10 years of primary therapy.[19] The majority of published studies are single-institution experiences. Important considerations in the interpretation of these studies are length and quality of patient follow-up, definition of MDS, and uniformity of treatment regimens. As expected, risk factors may differ between studies; however, the incidence over time in most studies is strikingly similar. Unlike secondary MDS from chemotherapy alone, the incidence post-ASCT appears to remain stable over time, without evidence of a plateau on the Kaplan–Meier curve.[20]

A representative series from the Dana-Farber Cancer Institute evaluated the risks and outcome of MDS in 552 patients with NHL receiving a standard conditioning regimen of 1200–1400 cGy total body irradiation (TBI) and cyclophosphamide, followed by monoclonal-antibody-purged ASCT with marrow as graft source. In this series, 41 patients developed MDS, strictly defined, a median of 47 months (range 12–129) from ASCT.[21] At the time of diagnosis of MDS, 29 patients were in remission and 12 patients had relapsed with NHL; the majority of these patients had not received further cytotoxic therapy since transplant. The absolute risk of developing MDS after ASCT for NHL was 7.4%. The cumulative risk of development of MDS was 14.5% at 10 years posttransplant.[22] In a logistic regression model, low number of stem cells infused per kilogram and prior localized irradiation were the only significant predictors of developing MDS.

The specific role of TBI conditioning in the development of MDS has been assessed by several other studies. Almost 5000 patients with lymphoma have undergone ASCT in the European Bone Marrow Transplant Registry, with 68 patients developing MDS.[23] This incidence is lower than other series, perhaps as a consequence of underreporting of this complication. The median follow-up from the date of transplant was 6.7 years for patients who developed MDS, but only 2.9 years for the patients without MDS. Multivariate analysis revealed age at transplant, exposure to TBI in conditioning, long interval between diagnosis of lymphoma and transplant, and indolent histology as independent variables predicting for subsequent MDS. For patients with Hodgkin's lymphoma, female gender was identified as a risk factor. The amount of previous chemotherapy, including cumulative alkylating agent exposure, was not found to be a significant factor.

In a case–control study of 56 patients with MDS/AML after ASCT for lymphoma, and 168 matched controls who also underwent ASCT for lymphoma but did not develop MDS/AML, the separate contributions of pretransplantation and transplantation-related therapy were assessed.[24] The intensity of pretransplant therapy did contribute to the risk of developing MDS. Transplant factors, including high-dose TBI, and peripheral blood stem cells as graft source also appeared to contribute to the risk of MDS.

It is therefore not possible to establish whether the increased risk of MDS in patients with lymphoma is truly a disease-related phenomenon, or secondary to other factors such as a tendency to use more TBI for conditioning, or exposure to high doses of alkylating agents pretransplant. The risk of MDS following ASCT for multiple myeloma[25], breast cancer,[26,27] and germ cell tumors[28] appears to be less than that in similar populations of patients with NHL following ASCT. Reported risks of developing MDS after autotransplantation for Hodgkin's lymphoma are varied, with some studies suggesting a lower risk than in similar patients with NHL following ASCT,[29–31] and others reporting a similarly high risk.[32] Confounding most of the studies of Hodgkin's lymphoma is the use of mechlorethamine prior to transplantation, which may have a more profound effect on the development of MDS than the transplant itself has.[24,31] Standard, modern regimens for Hodgkin's lymphoma clearly have significantly less risk. Between 1981 and 1998, the German Hodgkin Study Group treated 5411 patients,[33] of whom only 46 patients developed MDS/AML at a median follow-up of 55 months. Similar

**Table 78.2:    MDS/AML after ASCT for NHL and HL**

| Institution | Diagnosis | Incidence | Median follow-up[a] | Risk factors |
|---|---|---|---|---|
| Dana-Farber[21] | NHL | 41/552 | 75 months | Prior XRT<br>Low no. of cells infused |
| St. Bartholomew's[34] | NHL | 27/330 | 72 months | Older patient age<br>Prior fludarabine |
| City of Hope[13] | NHL and HL | 22/612 | Not reported | Etoposide mobilization<br>Prior XRT |
| Minnesota[35] | NHL and HL | 10/258 | 37 months | PBSCT<br>Age > 35 |
| Nebraska[36] | NHL and HL | 12/511 | Not reported | Age > 40<br>TBI conditioning |
| MD Anderson[37] | NHL | 22/493 | 21 months | TBI conditioning<br>Prior fludarabine |
| Beth Israel/Brigham[38] | NHL and HL | 6/300 | 47 months | Prior XRT<br>Number of prior relapses |
| Copenhagen[32] | NHL and HL | 6/76 | Not reported | Prior chemotherapy |
| *Registry studies* | | | | |
| EBMT[23] | NHL and HL | 66/4998 | 80 months (MDS)<br>34 months (non-MDS) | Older patient age<br>TBI conditioning<br>Indolent histology<br>Prolonged interval pre-ASCT |
| Spanish Cooperative Group[39] | HL | 12/494 | 30 months | Prior XRT<br>TBI conditioning<br>Age > 40 |
| French Cooperative Group[30] | HL | 8/467 | 21 months | Splenectomy<br>PBSCT |

*Abbreviations:* XRT: localized radiotherapy; PBSCT: peripheral blood stem cell transplantation; TBI: total body irradiation; NHL: non-Hodgkin's lymphoma; HL, Hodgkin's lymphoma; EBMT. European Group for Blood and Marrow Transplantation.

to transplant patients, the prognosis of these patients was poor, with only four patients surviving.

Table 78.2 summarizes several experiences of MDS/AML after ASCT. In summary, the reported cumulative risk of MDS exceeds 10% in several series of patients undergoing autotransplantation for NHL, and is somewhat lower after transplantation for other histologies. Older patients with extensive prior chemotherapy, patients receiving localized radiotherapy, and those receiving TBI conditioning appear to be at the highest risk for this complication.

## DETECTION OF SECOND MALIGNANCIES: STRATEGIES FOR SCREENING

The only screening test for early detection of secondary malignancies that has demonstrated benefit is mammography to detect breast cancer. In one study, 81% of 37 women with breast cancer after Hodgkin's lymphoma had mammographic abnormalities of a mass and/or microcalcifications.[41] Diller et al. reported a high frequency of mammographically detected abnormalities, supporting the value of mammographic screening in 90 patients prospectively evaluated following treatment for Hodgkin's lymphoma.[42] During the study period, 10 women developed 12 breast cancers, all of which were evident on mammogram. The role of other breast imaging modalities, including magnetic resonance imaging[43,44] and FDG-PET,[45] have not been prospectively evaluated in women following treatment for lymphoma. Moreover, the effectiveness of tamoxifen or raloxifene as chemoprevention, although demonstrated in other high-risk patients,[46] is unclear in patients treated for lymphoma. It is probably reasonable to avoid estrogen replacement therapy in these women. At the present time, we recommend annual mammography beginning 7 years after completion of radiation therapy (in a field that includes the breast) for lymphoma. For women treated before age 20, screening should probably not begin until the patient reaches age 25.[47] We anticipate, however, that additional recommendations for chemoprevention or more elaborate screening algorithms may evolve over the next few years, as current trials mature.

Despite the prevalence of lung cancer after lymphoma therapy, there is no clear role for prospective imaging as screening. The role of chest CT as screening is currently being studied in a prospective randomized trial in other high-risk groups,[48] but survivors of lymphoma are not included in the study. There are no clear data suggesting a benefit to regular imaging. However, there should be a low threshold to image the chest for any signs or symptoms that could represent a thoracic malignancy. Given the clear increased risk of secondary malignancies in patients who smoke, we recommend counseling against tobacco use.

## PREVENTION: TREATMENT REDUCTION

As outlined, the risk of both MDS/AML and solid tumors after lymphoma therapy is directly related to the cumulative treatment exposure, of both chemotherapy and radiation. A number of ongoing multi-institutional randomized trials are investigating different ways to reduce treatment for favorable prognosis Hodgkin's lymphoma, including the omission of radiation therapy, and the adoption of response-based therapy. However, longer follow-up time of these prospective randomized trials is needed to confirm to what degree the treatment reductions will translate into lower risk of second malignancy, and whether there is any trade-off with respect to failure-free survival. Even outside of a clinical trial, exposure to known stem cell toxins, including prolonged exposure to alkylating agents, purine analogs, and topoisomerase-II inhibitors, should be limited as much as possible in patients in whom ASCT or radioimmunotherapy may be considered as a treatment option. The introduction of novel biological treatment options for lymphoma, including monoclonal antibody therapy, proteosome inhibitors, and antisense therapy, may allow future minimization of such toxic therapies in many circumstances.

Clonal hematopoiesis pretransplant appears to increase the risk of subsequent MDS. There are at least five methods for assessing this risk, based on the presence of clonal abnormalities in hematopoietic cells, including standard cytogenetics, interphase fluorescence in situ hybridization, analysis for loss of heterozygosity, polymerase chain reaction for point mutations, and X-inactivation-based clonality assays.[49] Abnormalities in one of these assessments pretransplant, or before radioimmunotherapy, may represent relative contraindications to transplant. However, since no single mutation or gene rearrangement is sufficient for the development of MDS after transplant, and not all patients with cytogenetic abnormalities develop clinical MDS, these are imperfect assessments. The optimal "screening" modality has yet to be determined, and prospective studies are ongoing. However, most advocate serious consideration to deferring both radioimmunotherapy and autologous transplant in patients with clonal cytogenetic abnormalities.

Finally, to minimize the development of MDS after ASCT, chemotherapy-only conditioning regimens have similar response rates to TBI-containing regimens in most subtypes of NHL,[38,50] and may decrease risk of MDS, particularly for those patients treated with localized radiotherapy.[51,52]

## CONCLUSIONS

Second malignancies have clearly evolved to be important causes of mortality in patients with curable lymphomas. As cure rates increase, and the cohort of patients treated with aggressive autologous transplantation and novel radioimmunotherapy approaches grows, it is anticipated that the incidence of second cancers will increase significantly. Perhaps most concerning is the lack of an apparent plateau in the incidence curve, even 20–30 years after diagnosis of lymphoma.[53] For this reason, we feel it is critical that patients cured of lymphoma remain under care of medical and radiation oncologists attuned to these risks, and undergo at least annual history and physical examinations, with appropriate screening tests for second cancers. Future emphasis needs to continue on minimizing toxic therapy to prevent this devastating cost of cure.

## Acknowledgment

Dr Friedberg is supported in part by a grant from the National Cancer Institute (CA102216).

## REFERENCES

1. Aleman BM, van den Belt-Dusebout AW, Klokman WJ, et al.: Long-term cause-specific mortality of patients treated for Hodgkin's disease. *J Clin Oncol* 21:3431–3439, 2003.

2. Ng AK, Bernardo MV, Weller E, et al.: Second malignancy after Hodgkin disease treated with radiation therapy with or without chemotherapy: long-term risks and risk factors. *Blood* 100:1989–1996, 2002.

3. Dores GM, Metayer C, Curtis RE, et al.: Second malignant neoplasms among long-term survivors of Hodgkin's disease: a population-based evaluation over 25 years. *J Clin Oncol* 20:3484–3494, 2002.

4. Travis LB, Hill DA, Dores GM, et al.: Breast cancer following radiotherapy and chemotherapy among young women with Hodgkin disease. *JAMA* 290:465–475, 2003.

5. van Leeuwen FE, Klokman WJ, Stovall M, et al.: Roles of radiation dose, chemotherapy, and hormonal factors in breast cancer following Hodgkin's disease. *J Natl Cancer Inst* 95:971–980, 2003.

6. Travis LB, Gospodarowicz M, Curtis RE, et al.: Lung cancer following chemotherapy and radiotherapy for Hodgkin's disease. *J Natl Cancer Inst* 94:182–192, 2002.

7. Swerdlow AJ, Barber JA, Hudson GV, et al.: Risk of second malignancy after Hodgkin's disease in a collaborative British cohort: the relation to age at treatment. *J Clin Oncol* 18:498–509, 2000.

8. Swerdlow AJ, Schoemaker MJ, Allerton R, et al.: Lung cancer after Hodgkin's disease: a nested case-control study of the relation to treatment. *J Clin Oncol* 19:1610–1618, 2001.

9. Bhatia S, Yasui Y, Robison LL, et al.: High risk of subsequent neoplasms continues with extended follow-up of childhood Hodgkin's disease: report from the Late Effects Study Group. *J Clin Oncol* 21:4386–4394, 2003.

10. van Leeuwen FE, Klokman WJ, Stovall M, et al.: Roles of radiotherapy and smoking in lung cancer following Hodgkin's disease. *J Natl Cancer Inst* 87:1530–1537, 1995.

11. O'Donnell JF, Brereton HD, Greco FA, et al.: Acute non-lymphocytic leukemia and acute myeloproliferative syndrome following radiation therapy for non-Hodgkin's lymphoma and chronic lymphocytic leukemia: clinical studies. *Cancer* 44:1930–1938, 1979.

12. Whang-Peng J, Knutsen T, O'Donnell JF, et al.: Acute non-lymphocytic leukemia and acute myeloproliferative syndrome following radiation therapy for non-Hodgkin's lymphoma and chronic lymphocytic leukemia: cytogenetic studies. *Cancer* 44:1592–1600, 1979.

13. Krishnan A, Bhatia S, Slovak ML, et al.: Predictors of therapy-related leukemia and myelodysplasia following autologous transplantation for lymphoma: an assessment of risk factors. *Blood* 95:1588–1593, 2000.

14. Misgeld E, Germing U, Aul C, et al.: Secondary myelodysplastic syndrome after fludarabine therapy of a low-grade non-Hodgkin's lymphoma. *Leuk Res* 25:95–98, 2001.

15. Pedersen-Bjergaard J, Andersen MK, Christiansen DH: Therapy-related acute myeloid leukemia and myelodysplasia after high-dose chemotherapy and autologous stem cell transplantation. *Blood* 95:3273–3279, 2000.

16. Friedberg JW, Fisher RI: Iodine-131 tositumomab (Bexxar(R)): radioimmunoconjugate therapy for indolent and transformed B-cell non-Hodgkin's lymphoma. *Expert Rev Anticancer Ther* 4:18–26, 2004.

17. Cheson BD: Radioimmunotherapy of non-Hodgkin lymphomas. *Blood* 101:391–398, 2003.

18. Bennett JM, Zelenetz AD, Press OW, et al.: Incidence of myelodysplastic syndromes (tMDS) and acute myeloid leukemia (tAML) in patients with low-grade non-Hodgkin's lymphoma (LG-NHL) treated with Bexxar™. *Blood* 98, 2001.

19. Armitage JO, Carbone PP, Connors JM, et al.: Treatment-related myelodysplasia and acute leukemia in non-Hodgkin's lymphoma patients. *J Clin Oncol* 21:897–906, 2003.

20. Akpek G, Ambinder RF, Piantadosi S, et al.: Long-term results of blood and marrow transplantation for Hodgkin's lymphoma. *J Clin Oncol* 19:4314–4321, 2001.

21. Friedberg JW, Neuberg D, Stone RM, et al.: Outcome in patients with myelodysplastic syndrome after autologous bone marrow transplantation for non-Hodgkin's lymphoma. *J Clin Oncol* 17:3128–3135, 1999.

22. Friedberg J, Neuberg D, Freedman AS: Myelodysplasia after autotransplantation. *J Clin Oncol* 18:3446–3447, 2000.

23. Milligan DW, Ruiz De Elvira MC, Kolb HJ, et al.: Secondary leukaemia and myelodysplasia after autografting for lymphoma: results from the EBMT. EBMT Lymphoma and Late Effects Working Parties. European Group for Blood and Marrow Transplantation. *Br J Haematol* 106:1020–1026, 1999.

24. Metayer C, Curtis RE, Vose J, et al.: Myelodysplastic syndrome and acute myeloid leukemia after autotransplantation for lymphoma: a multicenter case-control study. *Blood* 101:2015–2023, 2003.

25. Govindarajan R, Jagannath S, Flick JT, et al.: Preceding standard therapy is the likely cause of MDS after autotransplants for multiple myeloma. *Br J Haematol* 95:349–353, 1996.

26. Roman-Unfer S, Bitran JD, Hanauer S, et al.: Acute myeloid leukemia and myelodysplasia following intensive chemotherapy for breast cancer. *Bone Marrow Transplant* 16:163–168, 1995.

27. Laughlin MJ, McGaughey DS, Crews JR, et al.: Secondary myelodysplasia and acute leukemia in breast cancer patients after autologous bone marrow transplant. *J Clin Oncol* 16:1008–1012, 1998.

28. Kollmannsberger C, Beyer J, Droz JP, et al.: Secondary leukemia following high cumulative doses of etoposide in patients treated for advanced germ cell tumors. *J Clin Oncol* 16:3386–3391, 1998.

29. Taylor PR, Jackson GH, Lennard AL, et al.: Low incidence of myelodysplastic syndrome following transplantation using autologous non-cryopreserved bone marrow. *Leukemia* 11:1650–1653, 1997.

30. Andre M, Henry-Amar M, Blaise D, et al.: Treatment-related deaths and second cancer risk after autologous stem-cell transplantation for Hodgkin's disease. *Blood* 92:1933–1940, 1998.

31. Harrison CN, Gregory W, Hudson GV, et al.: High-dose BEAM chemotherapy with autologous haemopoietic stem cell transplantation for Hodgkin's disease is unlikely to be associated with a major increased risk of secondary MDS/AML. *Br J Cancer* 81:476–483, 1999.

32. Pedersen-Bjergaard J, Pedersen M, Myhre J, et al.: High risk of therapy-related leukemia after BEAM chemotherapy and autologous stem cell transplantation for previously treated lymphomas is mainly related to primary chemotherapy and not to the BEAM-transplantation procedure. *Leukemia* 11:1654–1660, 1997.

33. Josting A, Wiedenmann S, Franklin J, et al.: Secondary myeloid leukemia and myelodysplastic syndromes in patients treated for Hodgkin's disease: a report from the German Hodgkin's Lymphoma Study Group. *J Clin Oncol* 21:3440–3446, 2003.

34. Micallef IN, Lillington DM, Apostolidis J, et al.: Therapy-related myelodysplasia and secondary acute myelogenous leukemia after high-dose therapy with autologous hematopoietic progenitor-cell support for lymphoid malignancies. *J Clin Oncol* 18:947, 2000.

35. Bhatia S, Ramsay NK, Steinbuch M, et al.: Malignant neoplasms following bone marrow transplantation. *Blood* 87:3633–3639, 1996.

36. Darrington DL, Vose JM, Anderson JR, et al.: Incidence and characterization of secondary myelodysplastic syndrome and acute myelogenous leukemia following high-dose chemoradiotherapy and autologous stem-cell transplantation for lymphoid malignancies. *J Clin Oncol* 12:2527–2534, 1994.

37. Hosing C, Munsell M, Yazji S, et al.: Risk of therapy-related myelodysplastic syndrome/acute leukemia following high-dose therapy and autologous bone marrow transplantation for non-Hodgkin's lymphoma. *Ann Oncol* 13:450–459, 2002.

38. Wheeler C, Khurshid A, Ibrahim J, et al.: Incidence of post transplant myelodysplasia/acute leukemia in non-Hodgkin's lymphoma patients compared with Hodgkin's disease patients undergoing autologous transplantation following cyclophosphamide, carmustine and etoposide (CBV). *Leuk Lymphoma* 40:499–509, 2001.

39. Sureda A, Arranz R, Iriondo A, et al.: Autologous stem-cell transplantation for Hodgkin's disease: results and prognostic factors in 494 patients from the Grupo Espanol de Linfomas/Transplante Autologo de Medula Osea Spanish Cooperative Group. *J Clin Oncol* 19:1395–1404, 2001.

40. Friedberg JW: Myelodysplasia after autologous stem cell transplantation. In: Atkinson K, Champlin R, Ritz J, et al. (eds.) *Clinical Bone Marrow and Stem Cell Transplantation.* Boston: Cambridge University Press, 2004.

41. Yahalom J, Petrek JA, Biddinger PW, et al.: Breast cancer in patients irradiated for Hodgkin's disease: a clinical and pathologic analysis of 45 events in 37 patients. *J Clin Oncol* 10:1674–1681, 1992.

42. Diller L, Medeiros Nancarrow C, Shaffer K, et al.: Breast cancer screening in women previously treated for Hodgkin's disease: a prospective cohort study. *J Clin Oncol* 20:2085–2091, 2002.

43. Liberman L: Breast cancer screening with MRI-what are the data for patients at high risk? *N Engl J Med* 351:497–500, 2004.

44. Kriege M, Brekelmans CT, Boetes C, et al.: Efficacy of MRI and mammography for breast-cancer screening in women with a familial or genetic predisposition. *N Engl J Med* 351:427–437, 2004.

45. Wu D, Gambhir SS: Positron emission tomography in diagnosis and management of invasive breast cancer: current status and future perspectives. *Clin Breast Cancer* 4(suppl 1):S55–S63, 2003.

46. Vogel VG, Costantino JP, Wickerham DL, et al.: The study of tamoxifen and raloxifene: preliminary enrollment data from a randomized breast cancer risk reduction trial. *Clin Breast Cancer* 3:153–159, 2002.

47. Horwich A, Swerdlow AJ: Second primary breast cancer after Hodgkin's disease. *Br J Cancer* 90:294–298, 2004.

48. MacRedmond R, Logan PM, Lee M, et al.: Screening for lung cancer using low dose CT scanning. *Thorax* 59:237–241, 2004.

49. Gilliland DG, Gribben JG: Evaluation of the risk of therapy-related MDS/AML after autologous stem cell transplantation. *Biol Blood Marrow Transplant* 8:9–16, 2002.

50. Berglund A, Enblad G, Carlson K, et al.: Long-term follow-up of autologous stem-cell transplantation for follicular and transformed follicular lymphoma. *Eur J Haematol* 65:17–22, 2000.

51. Mounier N, Gisselbrecht C: Conditioning regimens before transplantation in patients with aggressive non-Hodgkin's lymphoma. *Ann Oncol* 9:S15–S21, 1998.

52. Armitage JO: Myelodysplasia and acute leukemia after autologous bone marrow transplantation. *J Clin Oncol* 18:945, 2000.

53. Foss Abrahamsen A, Andersen A, Nome O, et al.: Long-term risk of second malignancy after treatment of Hodgkin's disease: the influence of treatment, age and follow-up time. *Ann Oncol* 13:1786–1791, 2002.

# Chapter 79

# THE APPROPRIATE USE OF PET AND GALLIUM SCANS IN LYMPHOMA

## Rebecca Elstrom

## INRODUCTION

Radiologic imaging plays a critical role in the staging and follow-up of patients with lymphoma. The initial stage of disease helps to define appropriate therapeutic interventions, and the extent and location of disease have traditionally been established through the use of anatomic imaging, in addition to physical examination and bone marrow biopsy. Furthermore, as different patients show varying degrees of responsiveness to standard chemotherapy, imaging studies can help determine whether an individual patient is responding appropriately to therapy, and therefore whether continuation of that therapy is warranted. Finally, after completion of treatment, patients are followed for evidence of relapse or progression of disease through a combination of imaging and clinical follow-up. These studies help to establish the status of disease and therefore the appropriate intervention or observation.

Anatomic imaging, such as computed tomography (CT) and magnetic resonance imaging (MRI) have been used extensively in patients with lymphoma. However, these modalities are limited by their dependence on size abnormalities in defining areas of tumor involvement. This limitation renders anatomic imaging suboptimal for detecting small foci of disease or for differentiation of viable tumor from fibrosis in a residual mass following treatment.

Functional imaging modalities, in contrast to anatomic imaging, take advantage of cellular processes to identify tissues of interest. Two such functional imaging modalities, Gallium-67 (Ga-67) scintigraphy and positron emission tomography using 18-fluoro-2-deoxyglucose (FDG-PET), utilize tracers that are taken up via metabolic pathways, therefore resulting in enhancement of highly metabolic tissues, such as tumor foci. This characteristic allows identification of tumor sites based on cellular metabolic activity rather than anatomic abnormalities, permitting detection of small foci of disease or differentiation of tumor from fibrosis. Both Ga-67 scintigraphy and FDG-PET have shown advantages in defining active lymphoma over classical imaging alone. However, the greater technical ease and apparent improved accuracy of FDG-PET imaging are contributing to its increasing acceptance as the functional imaging modality of choice in the care of lymphoma patients.

## GALLIUM-67 SCINTIGRAPHY

Gallium-67 citrate has been used since the 1970s for imaging of lymphoma and other tumors. Many malignant cells, including some lymphomas, take up large amounts of iron for use as a cofactor for ribonucleotide reductase, a key enzyme in DNA synthesis. Many malignant cells overexpress the transferrin receptor,[1-3] facilitating uptake of iron bound to transferrin. Gallium-bound transferrin binds the transferrin receptor and is therefore taken up into cells in a manner similar to iron. Ga-67 is administered intravenously and, following a distribution period of 1–2 days, can be imaged, with the best sensitivity and accuracy demonstrated by single photon emission computed tomography (SPECT).[4,5]

Using Ga-67 SPECT and higher doses of tracer, Ga-67 scintigraphy has been studied in staging and in follow-up of patients with lymphoma. It was found to be beneficial following treatment for restaging and detection of recurrence.[6,7] Different lymphoma grades and histologies have variable rates of detection, however. For example, while Ga-67 was sensitive and accurate in restaging of aggressive lymphomas, it was inadequate for detection of indolent lymphomas, and did not predict Richter's transformation in chronic lymphocytic leukemia (CLL).[8] Baseline scanning is therefore critical to establish the utility of this modality in individual tumors.

In recent years, the emergence of FDG-PET has led investigators to compare the utility of these two imaging modalities in the evaluation of lymphoma. In both Hodgkin's lymphoma (HL) and non-Hodgkin's lymphoma (NHL), FDG-PET shows higher sensitivity for staging and follow-up after treatment.[9–11] In addition, FDG-PET detects indolent lymphomas with better accuracy than does Ga-67 scintigraphy. These findings, combined with a shorter half-life of FDG and more convenient imaging characteristics, have led to FDG-PET largely replacing Ga-67 scintigraphy where FDG-PET is available.

## 18-FLUORO-2-DEOXYGLUCOSE POSITRON EMISSION TOMOGRAPHY (FDG-PET)

It has been known for decades that cancer cells have altered metabolism relative to normal cells. In the 1920s, Warburg first described the fact that cancer cells take up large amounts of glucose, performing glycolysis at an elevated rate even in the presence of oxygen.[12] Warburg hypothesized that this high rate of aerobic glycolysis was a result of dysfunctional mitochondrial electron transport, decreased production of ATP via oxidative metabolism, and a compensatory increase in ATP production by glycolysis. Others have proposed that the increased glucose uptake and glycolysis seen in cancer cells may be a primary effect, with subsequent suppression of oxidative phosphorylation. Whatever the mechanism, many cancer cells, including most lymphomas, take up excess amounts of glucose. It is this increased glucose uptake that targets FDG to cancer cells and is the basis of FDG-PET imaging of cancer.

18-Fluoro-2-deoxyglucose is a labeled glucose analog that is taken up by cells in a manner and at a rate similar to glucose. Upon entry into the cell, the molecule is phosphorylated by hexokinase, therefore trapping it inside the cell. While glucose is subsequently metabolized via glycolysis, the 2-deoxyglucose analog cannot be further metabolized, resulting in accumulation of the labeled, phosphorylated molecule within highly metabolic tissues. The label can then be detected by PET.

While FDG-PET is increasingly used in the care of patients with cancer, the optimal role for this imaging modality is still under investigation. The following sections review the status of FDG-PET imaging in detection and initial staging, response assessment, and follow-up of patients with lymphoma.

### DETECTION

The ability of FDG-PET to image lymphomas depends on the tumor's characteristic of high glucose uptake. However, the mechanisms by which this excess glucose uptake occurs, though currently under investigation, are still not completely understood. While this increased glucose uptake could act as a compensatory mechanism for highly anabolic cells to obtain building blocks for growth and proliferation, an alternative possibility is that high glucose uptake is a fundamental property of malignant cells. In the former case, one would expect that FDG avidity would depend on tumor grade, while in the latter case, the avidity may be independent of grade. Several groups have investigated different subtypes of lymphoma in an attempt to define which of these may be reliably imaged by FDG-PET.

Varying results have been reported regarding the utility of FDG-PET in imaging indolent tumors. Leskinen-Kallio and colleagues, in an early study examining FDG uptake in NHL, found poor uptake in indolent tumors.[13] In contrast, Newman et al. described comparable FDG uptake by both low- and intermediate-grade tumors.[14]

To evaluate this issue more decisively, investigators have studied the utility of FDG-PET in specific histologic subtypes of lymphoma. Elstrom and colleagues systematically evaluated specific World Health Organization (WHO) subtypes for their detectability by FDG-PET.[15] While 93% of lymphoma patients overall had tumor detectable by PET, those tumors that were not reliably detected fell within specific WHO subtypes, including marginal zone lymphoma (MZL), peripheral T-cell lymphoma (PTCL), and cutaneous B-cell lymphoma (CBCL). One limitation of this study was poor representation of some histologic subtypes, such as small lymphocytic lymphoma (SLL). Jerusalem et al. investigated FDG-PET in indolent lymphomas and found that it has poor sensitivity in imaging SLL.[16] Follicular lymphoma (FL), in contrast, including grade 1 tumors, was nearly uniformly detected in both of the above studies. These results suggest that tumor grade is not the most important predictor of FDG avidity, but rather that this avidity is based on other, as yet poorly defined, biological characteristics of the tumor.

Hoffmann and colleagues have further explored the situations in which FDG-PET imaging is useful in lymphoma. In one study they showed that, while 5 of 6 nodal MZLs were detected by FDG-PET, none of 14 extranodal MZL evaluated showed FDG avidity.[17] In another study, an evaluation of eight cases of duodenal FL, a rare manifestation of this tumor, showed that none of these lymphomas could be imaged by FDG-PET.[18] Of note, the one FL not detected by FDG-PET in the study by Elstrom et al. was an intestinal tumor. This raises the possibility that, even within broad WHO subtypes, subtle biological differences may define different imaging characteristics.

In summary, FDG-PET reliably detects most lymphomas. In the case of the most common aggressive NHL and HL, FDG-PET imaging represents an accurate assessment of disease activity. In these cases, FDG-PET can likely be used in follow-up of patients even without a baseline scan to document utility. However, in some tumors, particularly SLL, extranodal MZL, and intestinal FL, FDG avidity should be documented prior to therapy if the clinician plans to use this imaging modality for follow-up. Further studies of these issues will further clarify the generalizability of these findings.

### STAGING

Initial staging of disease presents a critical issue in the care of lymphoma patients, affecting prognosis and choice of therapy. Studies investigating the utility of FDG-PET in lymphoma have shown promising results for improving the accuracy of staging in these patients. Several groups have compared FDG-PET with traditional staging studies, such as CT, MRI, and bone marrow biopsy, in detecting specific sites of disease. In general, these investigators report improved sensitivity and specificity using FDG-PET as compared to anatomic imaging studies in both NHL and HL. The results of selected studies are presented in Table 79.1.

In addition to anatomic imaging, evaluation of bone marrow involvement represents a critical issue in staging of lymphoma. Investigations of the ability of FDG-PET to accurately stage bone marrow involvement by lymphoma have yielded conflicting results. Some have shown improved detection of bone marrow disease by PET, particularly in cases of patchy bone marrow involvement.[25] Others, however, demonstrate poor sensitivity and specificity, with a significant incidence of both false-negative FDG-PET, especially in indolent lymphomas, and false-positive FDG-PET, often in the setting of B symptoms and benign bone marrow hyperplasia.[15,26,27] At this point, FDG-PET is

---

**Table 79.1**   FDG-PET versus conventional imaging modalities (CIM) in staging lymphoma

| Studies | Histology | Patients | Major findings | Comments |
|---|---|---|---|---|
| Naumann et al.[19] | HL | 88 | PET<br>Stage change in 20%<br>Intensification of treatment in 10% | PET is especially useful in early stage |
| Partridge et al.[20] | HL | 44 | PET<br>41% upstaged<br>7% downstaged<br>Treatment modification in 25% | |
| Jerusalem et al.[21] | HL | 33 | PET<br>12% downstaged<br>1 false negative<br>9% upstaged | No changes in treatment based on PET |
| Moog et al.[22] | HL, NHL extranodal | 81 | PET<br>Identified 24 lesions not identified by CIM<br>1 false positive<br>Change of stage in 13 | |
| Hueltenschmidt et al.[23] | HL | 25 | PET<br>28% downstaged<br>12% upstaged<br>Accuracy<br>96% PET<br>56% CIM | |
| Delbeke et al.[24] | HL, NHL | 45 | PET<br>16% stage change<br>13% Treatment change<br>CIM<br>7% stage change<br>Accuracy<br>91% PET<br>84% CIM | PET and CIM are complementary |

best used as a complementary study in evaluating bone marrow involvement, ideally with follow-up biopsy of any focal areas of uptake in the setting of a negative iliac crest biopsy.

A recurring difficulty in addressing the question of FDG-PET accuracy in staging is the lack of a clear gold standard. In most cases, systematic biopsy of questionable lesions is impractical, and therefore the true result is often defined by the clinical scenario or follow-up. In spite of this limitation, however, studies have repeatedly shown improved staging information with the addition of FDG-PET.

In summary, FDG-PET scanning at initial staging can add valuable information for the clinician. First, a pretreatment FDG-PET scan documents the FDG avidity of a patient's lymphoma, confirming the utility of this modality in follow-up. In addition, PET can refine staging results of anatomic imaging by upstaging through detection of small lesions or diffuse organ involvement. Alternatively, PET may identify patients with a lower stage than suggested by anatomic imaging. However, it is clear that FDG-PET can in some cases show both false-positive and false-negative results. Therefore, discrepancies in staging must be interpreted carefully. In cases of uncertainty, questionable lesions should be biopsied if possible, particularly in cases in which treatment would be altered.

### RESPONSE ASSESSMENT

Response assessment following treatment for lymphoma provides an assessment of the adequacy of response to therapy and can help determine prognosis and the need for further therapy. Since patients who have not achieved a complete response to treatment have a poorer overall prognosis, identification of these patients early in the course of therapy may allow rapid institution of second-line therapy and, ideally, improve outcome. Unfortunately, traditional restaging modalities present pitfalls which can make accurate assessment of disease status difficult. For example, many patients retain residual anatomic abnormalities at sites of initial disease following treatment. These abnormalities may represent active lymphoma, but alternatively might represent fibrotic or necrotic tissue, in the absence of active disease. Distinguishing between these two scenarios is critical for deciding on further therapy in those patients for whom it is required, without subjecting patients for whom it is unnecessary to the toxicity of further therapy.

Potentially FDG-PET may accurately assess tumor response to therapy and therefore guide appropriate follow-up. Several investigators have studied the prognostic implications of FDG-PET following therapy, and these studies have provided promising data regarding the utility Lyf PET in this setting. Zinzani and colleagues showed that of 44 NHL and HL patients evaluated, all 13 patients with residual abnormality on FDG-PET relapsed, whereas only 1 of 24 with complete resolution of abnormal FDG uptake relapsed.[28] Similar results were found by Mikhaeel et al.,[29] who also studied a combined group of NHL and HL patients. Of 32 patients included in the study, nine had residual FDG uptake abnormalities following therapy, of which eight had relapsed at a median follow-up of 38 months. In contrast, only two of 23 patients without FDG-PET abnormalities relapsed in the same amount of time. Similarly, Jerusalem and colleagues studied a combined group of 54 NHL and HL patients,[30] showing that all patients with positive FDG-PET scan following first-line treatment relapsed within 1 year, whereas 86% of those with negative scans remained disease free at 1 year.

The utility of FDG-PET in predicting outcome following therapy in HL specifically has been investigated in several studies. Guay et al. studied 48 patients with HL following chemotherapy.[31] Of 12 patients with residual abnormality on FDG-PET, 11 relapsed, with a median progression-free interval (PFS) of 79 days. In contrast, of 36 patients with negative scans, only three relapsed with a follow-up of 5 years. Spaepen et al. also studied patients with HL who were followed for a minimum of 1 year, and showed that all five with positive posttherapy scans relapsed, while only five of 55 with negative scans relapsed.[32] In this study, the 2-year PFS was 91% in patients with a negative follow-up PET scan and 0% in those with a positive scan. Similar results were shown in a study by Dittman et al.[33] In contrast, the positive predictive value of FDG-PET was found to be only 46% in a study by de Wit and colleagues,[34] with 10 of 22 patients with positive scans relapsing.

For NHL, FDG-PET has shown similar predictive capability. Spaepen and colleagues studied a group of 93 patients with NHL with FDG-PET scans following first-line chemotherapy.[35] All 26 patients with a positive posttherapy PET scan relapsed, with a median PFS of only 73 days. In contrast, only 11 of 67 patients with a negative scan relapsed, with a much longer median PFS of 404 days. Mikhaeel et al. also showed high predictive power in a group of patients with aggressive NHL.[36] In this group of 45 patients, all nine with a positive posttreatment FDG-PET scan relapsed, whereas only six of 36 with negative scans relapsed at a median follow-up of 30 months. A third study, by Filmont and colleagues, also demonstrated the predictive power of FDG-PET in the posttreatment setting.[37] In this group of patients, the positive predictive power for relapse following a positive PET scan was 95%, whereas the negative predictive power was 83%. This study included a heterogeneous group of patients, including those undergoing first-line therapy as well as patients with relapsed disease.

In summary, FDG-PET scanning following therapy for HL and NHL contributes valuable information regarding prognosis. It appears to be most useful in prediction of early relapse. This is consistent with the idea that PET scanning reveals residual active disease and therefore more accurately defines remission status than traditional restaging techniques. FDG-PET must be interpreted with caution, however, as nonmalignant processes may also lead to abnormal uptake. On this note, it is clear that benign thymic uptake may occur after therapy, particularly in younger patients with HL. Other inflammatory or infectious processes may also cause false-positive scans. Because of these issues, positive FDG-PET scans following treatment should not be used in isolation to justify further therapy, but rather should be supplemented by clinical information and further investigation, such as biopsy, to document residual active disease. Abnormal FDG uptake in an area not previously known to be involved by lymphoma should raise particular caution. In contrast, a negative FDG-PET scan following therapy in a patient with known FDG-avid disease provides strong evidence for a meaningful complete response and good prognosis.

### EARLY RESPONSE EVALUATION

While it is clearly important to accurately assess response following treatment, an alternative approach of early evaluation during treatment could potentially identify patients who are destined to have a poor outcome with first-line therapy, allowing a change to more effective therapy while avoiding the toxicity of an ineffective chemotherapy regimen. Furthermore, an inadequate early response might predict for those patients who would benefit from immediate intensification of therapy.

The potential of FDG-PET scanning early in treatment to predict the ultimate outcome of that treatment has been investigated in several studies. Jerusalem et al. studied a group of 28 NHL patients, performing PET scans during treatment prior to completion of therapy.[38] They found that all patients with residual FDG uptake either failed to enter complete remission (CR) or relapsed, while all evaluable patients with negative scans entered CR. One third of those with negative scans subsequently relapsed during follow-up. A drawback to this study was inclusion of a heterogeneous group of patients, including multiple histologies as well as both front-line and salvage therapies. Furthermore, scans were performed at inconsistent times during treatment, after anywhere from two to five cycles of therapy. Zijlstra and colleagues evaluated the ability of PET to predict outcome in patients with aggressive NHL, when performed after 1–2 cycles of chemotherapy and found that, at 16 months follow-up, 64% of those with negative early PET remained free of disease, whereas only 25% of those with positive scans were disease free at the end of the study.[39] Kostakoglu and colleagues evaluated a mixed group of patients with either HL or NHL who had FDG-PET scans performed after one cycle of chemotherapy.[40]

Thirteen of 15 patients with positive scans either did not enter CR or relapsed following treatment. In contrast, only two of 15 with negative scans relapsed. When compared to posttreatment scans, early FDG-PET scans showed improved power to predict outcome, suggesting that early scans could be a more useful approach to response monitoring.

Several caveats to these data must be mentioned. These studies included heterogeneous groups of patients with scans performed at varying times during therapy. Before these findings can be generalized, studies must be performed in a systematic fashion, using defined groups of patients and defined imaging protocols. Furthermore, we do not yet know how to apply this information. Although patients with a positive early treatment scan appear to have a poorer prognosis than those with a negative scan, it is unclear whether changing or intensifying therapy, for example by instituting early high-dose therapy with stem cell transplant, will improve these patients' long-term outcome. At this time, therefore, the use of FDG-PET early in treatment must be considered investigational.

### PROGNOSIS IN STEM CELL TRANSPLANTATION

Autologous stem cell transplantation provides an opportunity for improved long-term survival or cure in many patients with relapsed lymphoma. However, it remains difficult to accurately predict which patients will benefit from this intensive and toxic therapy. Several groups have investigated the potential for FDG-PET performed in the peritransplant setting to predict ultimate outcome.[41–44] In general, these studies have shown that a negative FDG-PET scan during or after salvage chemotherapy strongly predicts improved PFS after transplant, while those patients with a positive FDG-PET scan prior to transplant are significantly more likely to relapse early. While the data do not definitively rule out the benefit of transplantation for those patients who retain FDG-PET-positive lesions, it may be useful in overall discussions of potential risk and benefit. As more information becomes available regarding this issue, the role of FDG-PET in pretransplantation evaluation will become clearer.

### LIMITATIONS OF FDG-PET

FDG-PET can add valuable information at several stages of care of lymphoma patients. However, this modality also has limitations which must be recognized in order to benefit optimally from its use. First, while the majority of lymphomas are detectable by FDG-PET scanning, some tumors fail to accumulate FDG, rendering them silent by this modality. While the likelihood of FDG avidity can be predicted by histology, exceptions do exist. For example, although the vast majority of FLs show FDG avidity, intestinal FLs are much less likely to take up the tracer.[18] Because of these exceptions, at this point, a baseline scan should

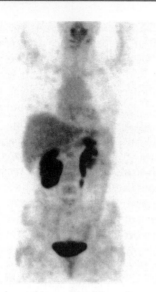

**Figure 79.1**  *Relapsed large B-cell lymphoma obscured by ureteral obstruction. A patient with a history of large B-cell lymphoma underwent FDG-PET scanning in follow-up. The intense uptake demonstrated in the right abdomen was interpreted as ureteral obstruction with no evidence of tumor. A CT scan demonstrated a mass compressing the ureter, and biopsy confirmed relapse of lymphoma*

be done in patients for whom FDG-PET will be used in follow-up.

A second limitation of FDG-PET involves difficulties of interpretation in areas of high physiologic tracer accumulation. One major example of this issue is seen in the urinary tract, as FDG is excreted via the kidneys. Tumor localized near the kidney, ureter, or bladder may not be visualized due to masking of FDG accumulation by urinary collecting structures (Figure 79.1). Alternatively, abnormal accumulations of urine may be interpreted as tumor mass, for example in the case of ureter obstruction from a cause unrelated to tumor. Another anatomic area that may present difficulty in imaging and interpretation is the cardiac region. Patients fast for several hours prior to FDG administration, therefore suppressing insulin levels. This leads to a conversion from glucose metabolism to fatty acid metabolism in adaptable tissues such as cardiac muscle, reducing FDG uptake in these tissues. In up to a third of cases, however, the heart may still take up significant amounts of FDG. While the radiologist can usually identify this uptake as cardiac, it may mask areas of malignancy in the paracardiac mediastinum. These issues emphasize the importance of concurrent anatomic imaging for optimal interpretation of FDG-PET.

Inflammatory lesions can on occasion mimic tumor on FDG-PET. Under most circumstances, inflammation can be differentiated from malignancy by intensity of uptake and spatial characteristics. In some cases, however, inflammatory lesions may masquerade as malignancy. Cases of suspected residual or recurrent tumor

visualized by FDG-PET have been documented to be infection in multiple instances.[45,46] Furthermore, postradiation inflammation may cause significant FDG accumulation. While the characteristics of uptake usually identify the process, the localization to a former site of tumor involvement can be misleading. Zhuang and colleagues have suggested that changes in FDG intensity over time may accurately differentiate tumor from inflammation, with tumor tissue continuing to increase in intensity and inflammatory lesions decreasing in intensity over the course of several hours.[47] These findings have yet to be confirmed in clinical practice.

Thymic uptake following chemotherapy, particularly in young patients with HL, is increasingly recognized as a possible cause of false-positive FDG-PET scans after therapy (Figure 79.2).[48] In an appropriate clinical setting, the clinician can recognize this phenomenon of thymic rebound as a benign event unrelated to residual tumor. However, the location of the thymus in the mediastinum, an area of frequent lymphomatous involvement, may at times make this interpretation problematic. Similarly, bone marrow may show increased uptake during or following chemotherapy due to recovery of normal hematopoiesis (Figure 79.3). Again, the clinical scenario should in most cases make interpretation of this phenomenon clear-cut.

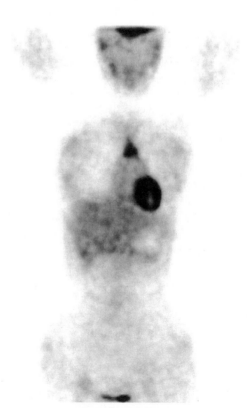

**Figure 79.2**  *Thymic rebound. An FDG-PET scan was performed 9 weeks following completion of therapy in a patient with Hodgkin's lymphoma. The mediastinal uptake is typical of benign thymic hyperplasia, and the patient remains in a complete remission*

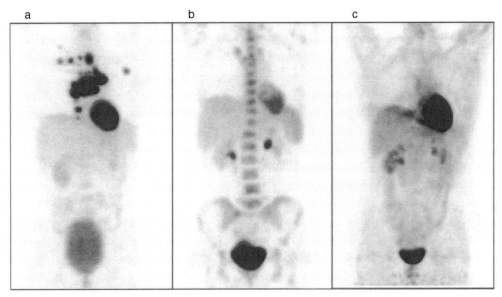

**Figure 79.3** *Physiologic uptake of FDG in a patient with large B-cell lymphoma. A patient with large B-cell lymphoma underwent baseline FDG-PET demonstrating uptake in mediastinal tumor (a). A scan performed during treatment to evaluate disease response showed resolution of FDG uptake in malignant tissues but an increase in uptake of the tracer in bone marrow, reflecting hematopoietic recovery (b). Following completion of therapy, no tracer uptake is detected in tumor or bone marrow, but physiologic cardiac uptake is demonstrated (c)*

## FUTURE DIRECTIONS

The field of functional imaging in the care of lymphoma patients is evolving rapidly. FDG-PET scanning has the potential to contribute to care of lymphoma patients in many new ways. We must, however, carefully and systematically evaluate how best to incorporate this modality in order to use it optimally. Several areas of investigation must be pursued for this aim to be realized.

Many studies have investigated the prognostic importance and treatment implications for patients with specific stages of lymphoma. However, these studies were done using conventional staging techniques. While it is reasonable to imagine that improved staging would refine our ability to predict prognosis and appropriately choose treatment, we do not at this time know how disease detected by FDG-PET will impact on these factors. For example, will low-volume disease detected only by PET, changing a patient's stage from 2 to 3, portend a worse prognosis?

A critical question for investigation is the appropriate use of FDG-PET scanning in prediction of treatment outcome. Although a positive FDG-PET scan after therapy completion would appropriately lead to investigation of the positive lesion and further treatment if confirmed to be active disease, the use of scanning during treatment is less clear. More systematic studies evaluating the outcome of patients undergoing FDG-PET scans early in treatment must be performed to define the role of this strategy in guiding treatment. Patients with specific histologies should be evaluated under defined circumstances, at a defined time during treatment, in order to clarify whether this strategy can predict outcome with high enough accuracy to guide treatment changes. Furthermore, we do not know at this time what constitutes an appropriate treatment change. It is unclear if switching to another, possibly more intensive, treatment regimen will improve outcome in these patients, or instead whether a positive scan portends a poor prognosis whatever the treatment strategy. These questions can be answered only through well-designed, prospective clinical trials.

## CONCLUSION

Functional imaging modalities have become valuable tools in the care of lymphoma patients. While Ga-67 scanning provided early benefits, the improved technical ease and greater accuracy of FDG-PET render Ga-67 scintigraphy less relevant in situations in which FDG-PET is available. FDG-PET provides important information in both initial staging of lymphoma and restaging following treatment, but its contribution appears to be dependent on tumor histology and location. Care must be taken in analysis of FDG-PET images, with the clinical scenario and characteristics of uptake guiding interpretation. Currently, FDG-PET should play a complementary role with other studies such as anatomic imaging, with biopsy and pathological confirmation of questionable lesions performed when possible. In the future, FDG-PET will provide increasingly more guidance in evaluation of prognosis and treatment effectiveness.

## REFERENCES

1. Das Gupta A, Shah VI: Correlation of transferrin receptor expression with histologic grade and immunophenotype in chronic lymphocytic leukemia and non-Hodgkin's lymphoma. *Hematol Pathol* 4:37–41, 1990.

2. Sciot R, Paterson AC, van Eyken P, Callea F, Kew MC, Desmet VJ: Transferrin receptor expression in human hepatocellular carcinoma: an immunohistochemical study of 34 cases. *Histopathology* 12:53–63, 1988.

3. Tsuchiya Y, Nakao A, Komatsu T, Yamamoto M, Shimokata K: Relationship between gallium 67 citrate scanning and transferrin receptor expression in lung diseases. *Chest* 102:530–534, 1992.

4. Front D, Israel O, Epelbaum R, et al.: Ga-67 SPECT before and after treatment of lymphoma. *Radiology* 175:515–519, 1990.

5. Tumeh SS, Rosenthal DS, Kaplan WD, English RJ, Holman BL: Lymphoma: evaluation with Ga-67 SPECT. *Radiology* 164:111–114, 1987.

6. Zinzani PL, Martelli M, Magagnoli M, et al.: Treatment and clinical management of primary mediastinal large B-cell lymphoma with sclerosis: MACOP-B regimen and mediastinal radiotherapy monitored by (67)Gallium scan in 50 patients. *Blood* 94:3289–3293, 1999.

7. Vose JM, Bierman PJ, Anderson JR, et al.: Single-photon emission computed tomography gallium imaging versus computed tomography: predictive value in patients undergoing high-dose chemotherapy and autologous stem-cell transplantation for non-Hodgkin's lymphoma. *J Clin Oncol* 14:2473–2479, 1996.

8. Cobo F, Rosinol L, Martinez A, et al.: Limitations of Gallium-67 SPECT in histological transformation of chronic lymphocytic leukaemia: an analysis of 13 patients with clinically suspected Richter's syndrome. *Br J Haematol* 119:484–487, 2002.

9. Kostakoglu L, Leonard JP, Kuji I, Coleman M, Vallabhajosula S, Goldsmith SJ: Comparison of fluorine-18 fluorodeoxyglucose positron emission tomography and Ga-67 scintigraphy in evaluation of lymphoma. *Cancer* 94:879–888, 2002.

10. Rini JN, Manalili EY, Hoffman MA, et al.: F-18 FDG versus Ga-67 for detecting splenic involvement in Hodgkin's disease. *Clin Nucl Med* 27:572–577, 2002.

11. Bar-Shalom R, Yefremov N, Haim N, et al.: Camera-based FDG PET and 67Ga SPECT in evaluation of lymphoma: comparative study. *Radiology* 227:353–360, 2003.

12. Warburg O: On the origin of cancer cells. *Science* 123:309–314, 1956.

13. Leskinen-Kallio S, Ruotsalainen U, Nagren K, Teras M, Joensuu H: Uptake of carbon-11-methionine and fluorodeoxyglucose in non-Hodgkin's lymphoma: a PET study. *J Nucl Med* 32:1211–1218, 1991.

14. Newman JS, Francis IR, Kaminski MS, Wahl RL: Imaging of lymphoma with PET with 2-[F-18]-fluoro-2-deoxy-D-glucose: correlation with CT. *Radiology* 190:111–116, 1994.

15. Elstrom R, Guan L, Baker G, et al.: Utility of FDG-PET scanning in lymphoma by WHO classification. *Blood* 101:3875–3876, 2003.

16. Jerusalem G, Beguin Y, Najjar F, et al.: Positron emission tomography (PET) with 18F-fluorodeoxyglucose (18F-FDG) for the staging of low-grade non-Hodgkin's lymphoma (NHL). *Ann Oncol* 12:825–830, 2001.

17. Hoffmann M, Kletter K, Becherer A, Jager U, Chott A, Raderer M: 18F-fluorodeoxyglucose positron emission tomography (18F-FDG-PET) for staging and follow-up of marginal zone B-cell lymphoma. *Oncology* 64:336–340, 2003.

18. Hoffmann M, Chott A, Puspok A, Jager U, Kletter K, Raderer M: 18F-fluorodeoxyglucose positron emission tomography (18F-FDG-PET) does not visualize follicular lymphoma of the duodenum. *Ann Hematol* 83:276–278, 2004.

19. Naumann R, Beuthien-Baumann B, Reiss A, et al.: Substantial impact of FDG PET imaging on the therapy decision in patients with early-stage Hodgkin's lymphoma. *Br J Cancer* 90:620–625, 2004.

20. Partridge S, Timothy A, O'Doherty MJ, Hain SF, Rankin S, Mikhaeel G: 2-Fluorine-18-fluoro-2-deoxy-D glucose positron emission tomography in the pretreatment staging of Hodgkin's disease: influence on patient management in a single institution. *Ann Oncol* 11:1273–1279, 2000.

21. Jerusalem G, Beguin Y, Fassotte MF, et al.: Whole-body positron emission tomography using 18F-fluorodeoxyglucose compared to standard procedures for staging patients with Hodgkin's disease. *Haematologica* 86:266–273, 2001.

22. Moog F, Bangerter M, Diederichs CG, et al.: Extranodal malignant lymphoma: detection with FDG PET versus CT. *Radiology* 206:475–481, 1998.

23. Hueltenschmidt B, Sautter-Bihl ML, Lang O, et al.: Whole body positron emission tomography in the treatment of Hodgkin disease. *Cancer* 91:302–310, 2001.

24. Delbeke D, Martin WH, Morgan DS, et al.: 2-deoxy-2-[F-18]fluoro-D-glucose imaging with positron emission tomography for initial staging of Hodgkin's disease and lymphoma. *Mol Imaging Biol* 4:105–114, 2002.

25. Carr R, Barrington SF, Madan B, et al.: Detection of lymphoma in bone marrow by whole-body positron emission tomography. *Blood* 91:3340–3346, 1998.

26. Chiang SB, Rebenstock A, Guan L, Alavi A, Zhuang H: Diffuse bone marrow involvement of Hodgkin lymphoma mimics hematopoietic cytokine-mediated FDG uptake on FDG PET imaging. *Clin Nucl Med* 28:674–676, 2003.

27. Najjar F, Hustinx R, Jerusalem G, Fillet G, Rigo P: Positron emission tomography (PET) for staging low-grade non-Hodgkin's lymphomas (NHL). *Cancer Biother Radiopharm* 16:297–304, 2001.

28. Zinzani PL, Magagnoli M, Chierichetti F, et al.: The role of positron emission tomography (PET) in the management of lymphoma patients. *Ann Oncol* 10:1181–1184, 1999.

29. Mikhaeel NG, Timothy AR, Hain SF, O'Doherty MJ: 18-FDG-PET for the assessment of residual masses on CT following treatment of lymphomas. *Ann Oncol* 11(suppl 1): 147–150, 2000.

30. Jerusalem G, Beguin Y, Fassotte MF, et al.: Whole-body positron emission tomography using 18F-fluorodeoxyglucose for posttreatment evaluation in Hodgkin's disease and non-Hodgkin's lymphoma has

higher diagnostic and prognostic value than classical computed tomography scan imaging. *Blood* 94: 429–433, 1999.

31. Guay C, Lepine M, Verreault J, Benard F: Prognostic value of PET using 18F-FDG in Hodgkin's disease for posttreatment evaluation. *J Nucl Med* 44:1225–1231, 2003.

32. Spaepen K, Stroobants S, Dupont P, et al.: Can positron emission tomography with [(18)F]-fluorodeoxyglucose after first-line treatment distinguish Hodgkin's disease patients who need additional therapy from others in whom additional therapy would mean avoidable toxicity? *Br J Haematol* 115:272–278, 2001.

33. Dittmann H, Sokler M, Kollmannsberger C, et al.: Comparison of 18FDG-PET with CT scans in the evaluation of patients with residual and recurrent Hodgkin's lymphoma. *Oncol Rep* 8:1393–1399, 2001.

34. de Wit M, Bohuslavizki KH, Buchert R, Bumann D, Clausen M, Hossfeld DK: 18FDG-PET following treatment as valid predictor for disease-free survival in Hodgkin's lymphoma. *Ann Oncol* 12:29–37, 2001.

35. Spaepen K, Stroobants S, Dupont P, et al.: Prognostic value of positron emission tomography (PET) with fluorine-18 fluorodeoxyglucose ([18F]FDG) after first-line chemotherapy in non-Hodgkin's lymphoma: is [18F]FDG-PET a valid alternative to conventional diagnostic methods? *J Clin Oncol* 19:414–419, 2001.

36. Mikhaeel NG, Timothy AR, O'Doherty MJ, Hain S, Maisey MN: 18-FDG-PET as a prognostic indicator in the treatment of aggressive non-Hodgkin's lymphoma-comparison with CT. *Leuk Lymphoma* 39:543–553, 2000.

37. Filmont JE, Vranjesevic D, Quon A, et al.: Conventional imaging and 2-deoxy-2-[18F]fluoro-D-glucose positron emission tomography for predicting the clinical outcome of previously treated non-Hodgkin's lymphoma patients. *Mol Imaging Biol* 5:232–239, 2003.

38. Jerusalem G, Beguin Y, Fassotte MF, et al.: Persistent tumor 18F-FDG uptake after a few cycles of polychemotherapy is predictive of treatment failure in non-Hodgkin's lymphoma. *Haematologica* 85:613–618, 2000.

39. Zijlstra JM, Hoekstra OS, Raijmakers PG, et al.: 18FDG positron emission tomography versus 67Ga scintigraphy as prognostic test during chemotherapy for non-Hodgkin's lymphoma. *Br J Haematol* 123:454–462, 2003.

40. Kostakoglu L, Coleman M, Leonard JP, Kuji I, Zoe H, Goldsmith SJ: PET predicts prognosis after 1 cycle of chemotherapy in aggressive lymphoma and Hodgkin's disease. *J Nucl Med* 43:1018–1027, 2002.

41. Filmont JE, Czernin J, Yap C, et al.: Value of F-18 fluorodeoxyglucose positron emission tomography for predicting the clinical outcome of patients with aggressive lymphoma prior to and after autologous stem-cell transplantation. *Chest*, 124:608–613, 2003.

42. Schot B, van Imhoff G, Pruim J, Sluiter W, Vaalburg W, Vellenga E: Predictive value of early 18F-fluoro-deoxyglucose positron emission tomography in chemosensitive relapsed lymphoma. *Br J Haematol* 123:282–287, 2003.

43. Spaepen K, Stroobants S, Dupont P, et al.: Prognostic value of pretransplantation positron emission tomography using fluorine 18-fluorodeoxyglucose in patients with aggressive lymphoma treated with high-dose chemotherapy and stem cell transplantation. *Blood* 102:53–59, 2003.

44. Becherer A, Mitterbauer M, Jaeger U, et al.: Positron emission tomography with [18F]2-fluoro-D-2-deoxyglucose (FDG-PET) predicts relapse of malignant lymphoma after high-dose therapy with stem cell transplantation. *Leukemia* 16:260–267, 2002.

45. Sandherr M, von Schilling C, Link T, et al.: Pitfalls in imaging Hodgkin's disease with computed tomography and positron emission tomography using fluorine-18-fluorodeoxyglucose. *Ann Oncol* 12:719–722, 2001.

46. Garrison MA, Glanton C, Rasnke M, Smith ME, Ornstein DL: Challenging cases and diagnostic dilemmas: case 1. Tracheal compression in Hodgkin's disease. *J Clin Oncol* 20:3344–3347, 2002.

47. Zhuang H, Pourdehnad M, Lambright ES, et al.: Dual time point 18F-FDG PET imaging for differentiating malignant from inflammatory processes. *J Nucl Med* 42:1412–1417, 2001.

48. Brink I, Reinhardt MJ, Hoegerle S, Altehoefer C, Moser E, Nitzsche EU: Increased metabolic activity in the thymus gland studied with 18F-FDG PET: age dependency and frequency after chemotherapy. *J Nucl Med* 42:591–595, 2001.

# Section 1
# MULTIPLE MYELOMA

## Chapter 80

# EPIDEMIOLOGY AND RISK FACTORS OF MULTIPLE MYELOMA: INSIGHTS INTO INCIDENCE AND ETIOLOGY

*Ashraf Badros*

Multiple myeloma (MM) is characterized by proliferation of malignant plasma cells in the bone marrow, bone destruction, extramedullary plasmacytoma, renal failure, and, late in the disease course, marrow failure manifested as anemia, leukopenia, and thrombocytopenia.[1] MM is customarily portrayed as an uncommon cancer. Nevertheless, MM accounts for 10% of all hematologic malignancies and 1% of all cancers. There are an estimated 74,000 new cases of MM worldwide each year with a worldwide prevalence of over 200,000 cases. MM is responsible for 2% of all cancer deaths yearly, with an estimated 57,370 deaths worldwide.[2] In the United States, there were an estimated 15,270 new MM cases in 2004 and over 11,070 yearly deaths due to MM.[3] The biology of MM suggests a multistep process as illustrated by the clinical progression from monoclonal gammopathy of unknown significance (MGUS) to the symptomatic phase of the disease. A B-cell precursor cell, after immunoglobulin gene rearrangement, is presumed to be the origin of the malignant clone in MM. The events that determine the susceptibility of B cells to undergo such malignant transformation are at best speculative.[4] The racial differences in the disease, the increased risk of developing MM with certain human leukocyte antigen

(HLA) types, and the clustering of MM in certain families suggest that genetic susceptibility may predispose certain populations to develop MM. In this chapter, the biological, environmental, chemical, and familial factors and their contributions to the pathogenesis of MM are discussed.

## DESCRIPTIVE EPIDEMIOLOGY

### TIME TRENDS

The incidence and mortality rates for MM were not available until 1950, when the disease was removed from the category of "lymphoreticular malignancies" and assigned a unique ICD code.[5] The international trends in MM rates vary significantly from country to country. There was an overall increased incidence between 1970 and 1990 with a plateau in the last decade. The incidence and prevalence of MM in selected world population is shown in Table 80.1.[2,6] This increase was attributed to underreporting in the earlier years and to improved diagnosis and more intensive surveys, especially in the elderly, in the later years (diagnostic phenomenon) rather than an actual increase in incidence.[7]

**Table 80.1**    Multiple myeloma incidence, mortality, and prevalence worldwide

| | Male | | | | Female | | | |
|---|---|---|---|---|---|---|---|---|
| | Cases[a] | ASR[b] | Deaths | Prevalence[c] | Cases[a] | ASR[b] | Death | Prevalence[c] |
| World | 39,480 | 1.5 | 30,392 | 74,315 | 34,463 | 1.12 | 26,978 | 69,262 |
| Eastern Africa | 523 | 0.43 | 414 | 761 | 341 | 0.58 | 285 | 357 |
| Middle Africa | 286 | 1.52 | 241 | 419 | 520 | 2.16 | 442 | 642 |
| Northern Africa | 381 | 0.76 | 322 | 309 | 404 | 0.67 | 328 | 516 |
| Southern Africa | 192 | 1.56 | 159 | 297 | 167 | 1.02 | 139 | 248 |
| Western Africa | 541 | 0.91 | 440 | 822 | 207 | 0.26 | 154 | 221 |
| Caribbean | 446 | 2.68 | 357 | 491 | 323 | 1.75 | 278 | 345 |
| Central America | 885 | 2.15 | 626 | 1,002 | 689 | 1.47 | 570 | 842 |
| South America | 2,381 | 1.89 | 1,889 | 2,673 | 2,196 | 1.46 | 1,846 | 2,878 |
| Northern America | 8,230 | 4.02 | 6,262 | 17,178 | 7,757 | 2.94 | 5,759 | 16,841 |
| Eastern Asia | 5,811 | 0.78 | 4,436 | 9,205 | 4,462 | 0.55 | 3,319 | 7,860 |
| South Eastern Asia | 1,537 | 0.83 | 1,241 | 1,937 | 1,001 | 0.50 | 785 | 1,226 |
| South Central Asia | 4,424 | 0.85 | 3,391 | 5,212 | 2,918 | 0.54 | 2,226 | 3,510 |
| Western Asia | 928 | 1.47 | 774 | 947 | 712 | 1.07 | 600 | 882 |
| Eastern Europe | 2,619 | 1.45 | 1,960 | 5,778 | 2,806 | 1.00 | 2,186 | 7,392 |
| Northern Europe | 2,424 | 3.19 | 2,059 | 4,987 | 2,338 | 2.36 | 1,985 | 5,212 |
| Southern Europe | 3,319 | 2.79 | 2,376 | 8,401 | 3,204 | 2.05 | 2,392 | 8,239 |
| Western Europe | 4,566 | 3.20 | 3,460 | 12,277 | 4,428 | 2.28 | 3,697 | 10,752 |
| Australia/New Zealand | 647 | 4.16 | 391 | 1,613 | 529 | 2.91 | 350 | 1,280 |
| More developed | 23,247 | 2.73 | 17,836 | 54,720 | 22,705 | 1.93 | 17,598 | 54,582 |
| Less developed | 16,223 | 0.91 | 12,550 | 19,595 | 11,754 | 0.61 | 9,379 | 14,680 |

[a]Cases: number of MM cases observed during a specific time.
[b]ASR: an age standard rate is a summary measure of the rate that a population would have if it had a standard age structure. Standardization helps to overcome the age difference between populations, as age significantly affects the incidence of MM. It is expressed per 100,000.
[c]Five-year prevalence.
Modified from Ref. 2.

## GENDER EFFECTS

The age-adjusted incidence rates for MM are higher in men (in the United States, 8090 cases were diagnosed in men versus 7180 cases in women, in the year 2004). This gender-related difference is noted across all age groups and is maintained worldwide in all reported age-specific incidence rates. This is despite the fact that MM is a disease of the elderly, and that women in general live longer than men. This gender-related difference is not only limited to the incidence of MM. There are indications that women may be more resistant than men to carcinogen exposure from occupation, radiation exposure, or smoking. In some studies, women have a better prognosis after therapy than do men.[8–12]

## RACIAL DIFFERENCE IN MM INCIDENCE

While many cancers (namely, those of the esophagus, cervix, stomach, pancreas, larynx, and prostate) have a higher rate among blacks than whites, within the hematopoietic system, MM is the only malignancy with a higher incidence among blacks. Asians have the lowest incidence rate of MM (less than 1/100,000). Table 80.2 and Figure 80.1 describe MM incidence in the US white and black males and females categorized by age at diagnosis.[3] This difference in MM incidence is also reported in Jamaica and South Africa, where blacks are reported to have a higher incidence than that reported for US blacks.[13,14] There is no definitive data to suggest that the higher incidence of MM in blacks is associated with biologically different disease. In some studies, black MM patients were, on average, 10 years younger than white patients and had higher incidence of fractures, paraplegia, and infections.[15]

Many explanations for the difference in incidence of MM between blacks and white have been proposed. Socioeconomic data showed that MM risk was significantly higher in the lowest categories of occupation, education, and income. In a population-based case–control study including 573 cases (206 blacks and 367 whites), low socioeconomic status was noted for 37% of MM in blacks and 17% in whites, and accounted for 49% of the excess incidence of MM in blacks.[16]

Differences in lifestyle between blacks and whites failed to show significant risks associated with cigarettes

**Table 80.2** Multiple myeloma incidence in the United States: white and black males and females categorized by age at diagnosis

|  | Age category at diagnosis | | | | |
|---|---|---|---|---|---|
|  | 30–39 | 40–49 | 50–59 | 60–69 | 70+ |
| White male | 0.4 | 1.8 | 7.3 | 16.3 | 35.6 |
| Black male | 1.4 | 6.4 | 18.9 | 36.8 | 66.8 |
| White female | 0.2 | 1.4 | 4.9 | 12.1 | 22.9 |
| Black female | 0.4 | 4.8 | 13.6 | 27.8 | 45.1 |

*Note:* The incidence rates were compared for males and females of all races diagnosed between 1973 and 1980 split by the age at diagnosis (30–39, 40–49, 50–59, 60–69, 70+). The *P*-value is zero to four decimal places, meaning that the trend is highly significant. The incidence rate of myeloma increases with aging across all groups. There is a higher incidence rate among male population than among females and is more in blacks than in whites.
*Source:* From Ref. 3. Rates are per 100,000 and age-adjusted to the 2000 US (19 age groups) standard.

or alcoholic beverages, and no consistent patterns with either intensity or duration of use of either were seen. These data are consistent with several studies indicating that smoking and drinking are not associated with MM.[17] Another area of controversy is the difference of dietary

habits across different racial groups and its relation to the incidence of MM. The use of vitamin C supplements by whites and the higher frequency of obesity among blacks may explain part of the higher incidence of MM among blacks. However such conjecture cannot explain the noted worldwide racial disparity of MM.[18]

Whether genetic factors contribute to the high incidence of MM among blacks is another area of controversy. Serologic typing of HLAs was conducted for blacks (46 patients and 88 controls) and whites (85 patients and 122 controls). Black patients had significantly higher frequencies than black controls for Bw65, Cw2, and DRw14. White patients had higher frequencies than white controls for A3 and Cw2. Cw2 allele had a relative MM risk of 5.7 (95% CI 1.5–26.6) and 2.6 (95% CI 1.0–7.2) for blacks and whites, respectively.[19] Some studies had reported a lower survival rate for blacks than for whites, though others did not find such a difference.[20] In a Southwest Oncology Group (SWOG) randomized trial, the survival for black patients was similar to that for white patients, both overall and adjusted for prognostic factors such as stage.[21] Not all blacks have a high incidence rate of MM; the incidence of MM in blacks living in Caribbean island is the lowest compared to other countries. Again, the younger age and aggressive presentation were noted with overall poor survival.[22]

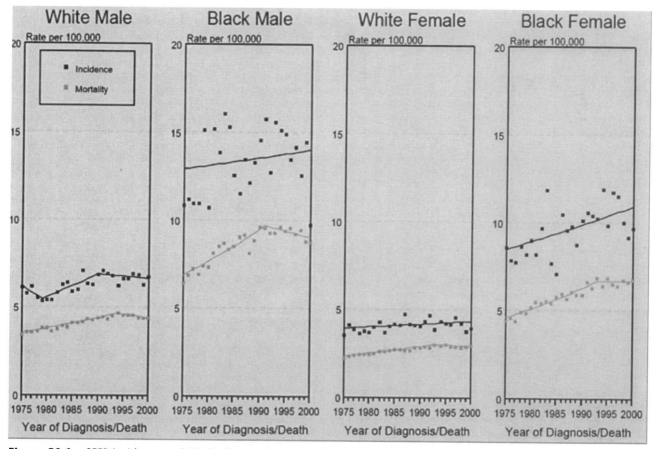

**Figure 80.1** *SEER incidence and US death rates due to myeloma, by race and sex. (Source: SEER nine areas and NCHS public use data file. Rates are age-adjusted to the 2000 US standard million population by 5-year age groups. Regression lines are calculated using the Join Point Regression Program)*

# ETIOLOGY OF MULTIPLE MYELOMA

Although the etiology of MM remains unknown, several environmental, occupational, and genetic factors have been associated with increased risk of developing MM. Although these risk factors are discussed disjointedly, it must be recognized that many factors contribute to the risk of each single case. In the search for factors that cause cancer, epidemiologists have used cohort and case–control studies. A defined population's "cohort" exposed to factors suspected of increasing the incidence of a cancer and a control "matched" group are followed for incidence of cancer. These factors are then investigated further if high incidence of a cancer is seen. Case-control studies begin with a cluster of cancer cases that are followed by investigating the exposure to various agents. Case–control studies are conducted quickly with fewer subjects. However, they are biased by selection and the ability of subjects to remember exposures.

## *MONOCLONAL GAMMOPATHY OF UNKNOWN SIGNIFICANCE*
### Incidence
MGUS indicates the presence of a monoclonal protein (M-protein) in persons without evidence of MM, macroglobulinemia, amyloidosis (AL), or related plasma cell disorders. MGUS can be associated with other disorders, including lymphoproliferative diseases, leukemia, connective tissue disorders, dermatologic diseases, and neurologic disorders.[23] MGUS is found in approximately 3% of persons older than 70 years and in about 1% of those older than 50 years. In the largest series of MGUS patients published to date that included 1384 patients from Mayo Clinic from 1960 through 1994, the risk of progression to MM was 1% per year. Patients were at risk of progression even after more than 25 years of a stable monoclonal gammopathy. The risk of developing MM was 25-fold higher when compared with a similar population (from SEER database). The concentration of the serum M-protein was the major independent predictor of progression. Patients with an immunoglobulin M (IgM) or an IgA monoclonal gammopathy had a higher risk of progression than those with an IgG monoclonal gammopathy. The presence of a urine M-protein or the reduction of one or more uninvolved immunoglobulins was not a risk factor for progression.[24] An early study that included 398 patients (270 whites and 128 blacks) showed that blacks had a two times (14.8%) higher incidence of MGUS than did whites (7.8%); this difference was statistically significant, and was noted across all age subgroups.[25] In a community-based study from the Duke Established Populations, of 1732 patients over age 70, 106 subjects (6.1%) had MGUS. There was a twofold difference in prevalence between blacks (8.4%) and whites (3.8%), $P < .001$. This biological racial difference is associated with susceptibility to an early event in the carcinogenic process leading to MM.[26] In a study from Zaragoza, Spain, the yearly incidence of monoclonal gammopathy remained stable up to 1985; from that time on, a 30–40% yearly increase was noticed, which was mainly related to MGUS and is a reflection of improved diagnosis and more vigorous application of testing to the elderly.[27] The increased rate is also noted for patients diagnosed between 1976 and 1997 in Iceland. There was an increased incidence noted between 1976 and 1980 from 5.8 (men) and 4.9 (women) to 14.7 (men) and 12.5 (women) during 1992–1997. Incidence rates were very low under 50 years of age and increased with age from 11 and 17/100,000 at age 50–54, to 169 and 119/100,000 at age 80–84, for men and women, respectively.[28]

### Risk factors
A retrospective study of 285 cases of MGUS matched with 570 controls assessed risk factors for MGUS. MGUS was significantly increased in farmers ($P < 0.005$) and industry workers ($P < 0.025$), and in those with occupational exposure to asbestos, fertilizers, mineral oils and petroleum, paints and related products, and pesticides ($P < 0.05$). Chronic immune-stimulating conditions, when considered as a group, presented a significant ($P < 0.025$) risk of MGUS, but no specific disease has been significantly associated.[29] A retrospective study from the Nurses' Health Study showed that MGUS is not increased in women with breast implants.[30] Among 6737 atomic bomb survivors, 112 developed MGUS between 1985 and 2001. The crude incidence rate was 164/100,000 person-years in the overall study population, with a sharp increase in incidence after age 60. Among 75 patients with MGUS detected in 1985, 50 patients (67%) had died by 2001, and 16 (21%) of these deaths were due to MM. Transformation from MGUS to MM was faster in exposed persons than in non-exposed persons, though that was not statistically significant.[31]

## *IMMUNE STIMULATION AND MYELOMA*
### Chronic infections and eczema
Many medical conditions associated with chronic stimulation of the immune system, such as repeated infections, allergic conditions, or autoimmune disease, have been reported to increase the risk of MM. In a case-control study, past history was abstracted from medical records for leukemia, $n = 299$; non-Hodgkin's lymphoma (NHL), $n = 100$; and MM, $n = 175$ patients, and matched with 787 controls. Prior histories of eczema and musculoskeletal conditions were associated with higher risk for MM with no role identified for chronic antigenic stimulation in the etiology of leukemia or NHL.[32] Another case–control study of 100 MM cases in whites showed no associations between MM and history of medical conditions that cause prolonged stimulation of the immune system, like

chronic infections, autoimmune disorders, allergy-related disorders, or lymphoid tissue surgery.[33]

### Gaucher's disease

Several case reports have long suspected an association between Gaucher's disease and gammopathy.[34–39] There is a reported incidence of 20% polyclonal gammopathy in this disease with an unclear percentage of monoclonal abnormalities. It is suspected that lipid deposition in Gaucher's disease results in chronic stimulation of the humoral immune system with production of polyclonal immunoglobulins that under unclear circumstances become monoclonal with development of MGUS and/or MM.[40] The use of enzyme therapy to control Gaucher's disease decreased polyclonal immunoglobulin levels but had no effect on monoclonal gammopathy. The lack of correlation between disease activity and immunoglobulin levels means that the enzyme-sensitive process affecting lipid metabolism is not directly linked to immunoglobulin deregulation.[41]

### Rheumatoid arthritis

MM has presented in patients with rheumatoid arthritis concurrently and in many cases masking the symptoms of arthritis.[42–46] IgA isotype MM is more frequently reported in rheumatoid arthritis patients.[47] Several cytokines and inflammatory molecules like interleukin 6, C–reactive protein, and the adhesion molecules ICAM-1, VCAM-1, and CD44 theoretically link MM and autoimmune disorders.[48] A report from Sweden blamed the number of X-rays in arthritis patients for the increased risk of MM.[49]

### VIRAL INFECTIONS

### Kaposi's sarcoma-associated herpesvirus

Human herpesvirus 8 (KSHV/HHV-8) was detected in the bone marrow dendritic cells of MM patients. This was considered an etiologic pathogen for MM, as it was not detected in normal individuals.[50] Unfortunately, subsequent confirmatory studies failed to establish a role of HHV-8 in the etiology of MM.[51–56] Also several clinical studies from the United States and South Africa failed to establish a link between MM and KSHV.[52,57]

### Acquired immunodeficiency syndrome

AIDS has been associated with increased incidence of high-grade B-cell lymphoma and leukemia. Several reports have described MM in HIV-infected patients.[58–68] These reports suggest that MM occurrence in AIDS patients is more than a coincidental event. Several authors suggested that MM should be considered another AIDS-associated neoplasm. In most of the reported cases, MM occurred in younger patients and had a fairly aggressive course with development of extramedullary disease, factors that may prompt physicians to publish their cases. The diagnosis of MM may be difficult in an AIDS population as renal failure, bone marrow plasmacytosis, and hypergammaglobulinemia are attributed to HIV. The challenge in diagnosis and lack of a uniform reporting system for these patients probably underestimate the true incidence of MM in AIDS patients. Biologically, it is plausible that the antigen-driven response to the viral infection and the associated increased levels of cytokines (e.g., interleukin 6) and many angiogenic factors (e.g., vascular endothelial growth factor and basic fibroblastic growth factor) can sustain the malignant clone in MM.

### Hepatitis C virus

Infection with hepatitis C virus (HCV), an RNA virus that can modulate the immune system, is associated with type II mixed cryoglobulinemia. Recently, a large case-controlled study confirmed that HCV-infected patients have a higher risk of B-cell NHL (OR = 3.7, 95% CI 1.9–7.4, $P = 0.0001$) and MM (OR = 4.5, 95% CI 1.9–10.7, $P = 0.0004$).[69] Other studies link HCV infection to Waldenstrom's macroglobulinemia and MGUS.[70,71] However, the data remain speculative and when the incidence of MM is evaluated in the context of HCV, the association is less clear.[72–74]

### Human T-cell lymphotropic virus type 1

A recent report of increased cases of MM in West Indies with incidences similar to what is reported for Afro-Americans in the United States entertained a possible link between the endemic human T-cell lymphotropic virus type 1 (HTLV-1) infection and MM, though this correlation has not been confirmed.[75]

### RADIATION EXPOSURE

Ionizing radiation is the most recognized risk factor for hematologic malignancies. Detailed prospective and retrospective studies analyzed the risk of environmental, military, occupational, and medically related sources of radiation. The issue is described in more detail below.

### Occupational exposure

The effects of low-grade protracted exposure to radiation in older age as seen in nuclear workers and individuals living in high-risk areas are at least intriguing. Several case-controlled studies reported an increased risk of MM among nuclear workers exposed to external penetrating ionizing radiation. In the international combined analyses of mortality data on 95,673 workers, more than 85.4% men, employed for at least 6 months in the nuclear industry in the United States, United Kingdom, and Canada, were monitored for external exposure to ionizing radiation. The analyses covered a total of 2,124,526 person-years at risk and 15,825 deaths, 3976 of which were due to cancer. Among the 31 specific types of cancers studied, a significant association was observed only for MM ($P = 0.037$; 44 deaths).[76] In the Sellafield British nuclear plant the cancer mortality and incidence among 14,282 workers employed between 1947 and 1975 were studied up to 1988.

Overall cancer mortality and incidence were 4% and 10%, respectively, less than that of the England and Wales populations. Among radiation workers there were significant positive correlations between accumulated radiation dose and mortality from cancers of ill-defined and secondary sites and for leukemia, but the association with MM was quite weak.[77] A study of workers at US Department of Energy facilities identified 98 MM cases/deaths and compared them to 391 age-matched controls selected from 115,143 workers at three sites. Cases were disproportionately African-American males; all were hired prior to 1948. Lifetime cumulative whole body ionizing radiation dose was not associated with MM; however, there was a positive association between MM risk and doses received at an older age.[78] The French Atomic Energy reviewed the cancer death for all workers between 1950 and 1968, after several deaths from cancer were reported in the mid 1980s. The cohort was followed up to 1990. The numbers of deaths from all causes and from all cancer sites were 44 and 21, respectively. No excess of cancer deaths was reported for the study period. The risk of death from all cancer sites increased with the duration of exposure to chemicals. The authors conclude, "the results do not justify the impression of an excess of cancer in workers of atomic facilities."[79]

### Residential exposure

In a report of all hematologic cancer cases in 489 towns within 30-km radius of Spain's seven nuclear power plants and five nuclear fuel facilities, cases of leukemia ($n = 610$), lymphoma ($n = 198$), and myeloma ($n = 122$) were matched to 477 control towns lying within a 50–100-km radius of each installation. Statistical testing revealed that with the exception of MM, none of the tumors studied showed evidence of a rise in risk with proximity to a nuclear installation.80 Taking all these data together, it appears that high-grade exposures were associated with risk of leukemia and possibly NHL, while prolonged low-grade exposure as seen in factory workers and in those living near nuclear facilities increases the risk of MM.

### *OCCUPATIONAL HAZARDS*

Many occupational exposures have been associated with MM; these include metals, rubber, wood, leather, paint, and petroleum. Several excellent reviews have discussed each occupation and its associated risks. The following is a brief summary of published studies for pertinent occupations.

### Agriculture

Agricultural work (predominantly farming) is an occupation that has been most frequently associated with MM.[81] Early reports from Iowa farmers in the 1970s showed a significantly higher mortality rate for MM and leukemia.[82] A recent update of these data suggest that association between farmers and MM is weaker than initially reported.[9,83,84] Similar results were reported from Sweden. There were 568 MM cases among 254,417 men working in agriculture, with an estimated RR of 1.20 (95% CI 1.09–1.33).[85] Meta-analyses of peer-reviewed studies of MM and farming including 32 studies published between 1981 and 1996 confirmed a low risk of MM.[86] Other studies evaluated the work environment in agriculture and risk of MM. Farming has many potential carcinogenic exposures, such as animals and zoophilic viruses, grains, dust, fertilizers, pesticides, or benzene and engine fumes. In Italy, a case-controlled study for 71 cases of leukemia, lymphoma, and myeloma estimated the risk of hematologic malignancies for agricultural workers at 1.63 (95% CI 0.69–4.34) in males and 6.00 (95% CI 1.21–25.52) in females, with significantly increased risks after DDT exposure (OR = 4.11; 95% CI 1.16–14.55).[87] In another case-control study from Italy, MM risk was not increased among workers in agriculture as a whole (OR = 1.31, 95% CI 0.62–2.74), but was increased among workers cultivating apples and pears and with exposure to chlorinated insecticides.[88] In a large cohort of 120,000 male and 85,000 female farmers in Finland, 17,000 cancer cases were observed. Compared with the incidence of cancer in the Finnish population, both genders experienced a 17–18% decreased risk of cancer. The risks were low in smoking-related cancers. Cancers with higher incidence were lip cancer and Hodgkin's disease in males. Risk of Hodgkin's disease was highest in farms without animals (RR = 1.74, CI 1.12–2.59). MM was found in excess among farmers working in pig or poultry farms.[89] Others studies failed to link farm animals to MM.[90]

### Rubber

Excess death from MM was noted in rubber workers from Akron, Ohio.[91] Similar findings were reported in a large study including 1352 white and 438 nonwhite male workers in rubber-manufacturing industry in the United States with excess bladder cancer (RR of 2.1), esophageal cancer (2.7), and MM (4.5).[92] Exposure to butadiene was associated with an increased risk of leukemia and Hodgkin's disease, while MM and lymphomas are associated with exposure to styrene.[93] However, three large studies did not find MM to be one of the cancers affecting rubber workers.[94–96]

### Benzene and related exposures

Prior case series and epidemiologic studies linked industrial exposure to benzene to development of MM.[97–100] It is accepted now that benzene exposure by itself in not a risk nor a causal factor for development of MM. This was recently reviewed in two excellent papers and is confirmed in several meta-analyses.[101–105]

### Other occupations

A recent review of 70 occupational cohort studies that addressed B-cell cancer risks in nine major industrial categories explain the limitation and inconsistency in these studies.[106] The exposure of painters to chemical compounds is complex, for there are various dyes, pigments, and solvents, which are known to be mutagenic in paint. The specific agent(s), if any, associated with the increased risk of MM in painters has not been identified. Exposure to asbestos has been linked to an increased risk of myeloma in at least two case-control studies.[33,105,107] In contrast, other case–control studies have not detected this association.[108] It will take further work to determine whether asbestos plays a role in the etiology of MM. An increased risk of MM in workers in wood, leather, and textile industries has been found in some studies, but the results are inconsistent and not universally confirmed by other investigators.[109–116] Statistical associations have been made between employment as sheet metal workers and an increased risk of MM.[113,117,118] The small numbers of cases and the lack of information on actual type and duration of exposures make it difficult to determine which occupational exposures are responsible for the elevated risks observed.

### LIFESTYLE FACTORS
#### Socioeconomic status
Socioeconomic status has been debated as an important prognostic factor in MM patients. A low socioeconomic status has been described in association with shorter survival, advanced clinical stage, and less response to chemotherapy in MM.[119–121] This is probably related to limited access to health care rather than an epidemiologic phenomenon.

#### Diet
As diet differs significantly in various racial groups, its contribution to MM has been suspected though not confirmed. The use of vitamin C supplements was reported to reduce MM risks in whites.[18] The consumption of yogurt increased the risk of developing MM while vegetables decreased that risk.[122]

#### Obesity
Recent data suggest that obesity increases the risk of MM. Excess body weight has been shown to increase the risk of death from various cancers and MM in a prospective studied population of more than 900,000 US adults. Some studies attributed the higher risk of MM in blacks to obesity, which is more common in blacks. However, recent studies showed that MM risk appears equal among black and white obese male veterans. As the prevalence of obesity and overweight worldwide increases, it is important to define its impact on cancer and to elucidate the mechanisms involved.[123,124]

#### Smoking
Several studies have proven that smoking is not linked to an excessive risk of MM for both blacks and whites

of both gender, and no consistent patterns with either intensity or duration of use have been found.[17,125–131]

#### Hair dyes
Use of permanent hair dye, especially dark dyes, contributes to death rates from MM, however the risk is small and unlikely to be a major contributor to MM.[132–139]

## GENETIC AND MOLECULAR FACTORS IN MULTIPLE MYELOMA

### FAMILIAL PREDISPOSITION
Reports of familial cluster of MM suggest that genetic factors may play a role in the etiology of MM. As previously discussed, neither specific genetic factors nor environmental exposures have been clearly implicated.[140–145] From these cases and other reviews, several observations have been made. First, there is no difference between familial and non-familial MM with regard to clinical presentation, laboratory data, and prognosis. Second, the earlier age of diagnosis in successive generations is a reflection of the genetic phenomenon of anticipation.[146] Third, individuals with familial MM appear to have a higher incidence of other hematologic malignancies. There is also a higher incidence of MGUS in many relatives of MM patients that puts them at a higher risk of developing MM.[147,148] One report of HLA typing disclosed identical haplotypes (AW24, A26, B13, and BW55) in two sisters 58 and 56 years old, diagnosed 22 months apart.[149] Other studies of familial MM in twins showed identical isotypes and in some cases similar karyotypic abnormalities.[150–152] A comprehensive family cancer database from several Swedish registries included 6 million persons. There were more than 30,000 cancers reported, and an increased cancer risk in offspring (1.1 times) was noted when the father had cancer. If both parents had cancer, the risk for sons was 1.4 and for daughters 1.3. MM was among the cancers with higher risks.[153] A population-based case-control interview study of 565 MM patients (361 whites and 204 blacks) and 2104 controls (1150 whites and 954 blacks) showed that family history of any cancer contributes to the risk of MM. The risk of MM was significantly elevated for patients who reported that a first-degree relative had MM (OR = 3.7, 95% CI 1.2–12.0) or any lymphoproliferative cancer (OR = 1.7, 95% CI 1.0–2.8), especially a sibling (OR = 2.3, 95% CI 1.1–4.5). The risk associated with familial occurrence of hematologic cancer was higher for blacks than for whites.[154] However, to date the question of genetic predisposition to MM remains unanswered.[155–159]

### POLYMORPHISM
Factors that regulate the metabolism of environmental and occupational carcinogens may be critical in

modifying MM risks in different individuals. The human xenobiotic metabolizing system is responsible for completing the detoxification of procarcinogens. The system comprises two classes of enzymes: phase 1 cytochrome P450 and phase 2 enzymes, including glutathione S-transferases (GST M1 and GST T1), paraoxonase 1 (PON1), and N-acetyltransferases (NAT) 1 and 2. Interindividual variability in the xenobiotic enzyme system can predispose certain racial groups to the carcinogenic effects of certain chemicals. In a case–control study using peripheral blood or bone marrow biopsy specimens from 90 Caucasian individuals and a control group consisting of 205 healthy Caucasian volunteer bone marrow donors, there was a significant increase in incidences of the GST T1 null; PON1 BB and NAT2 slow acetylation genotypes in MM cases compared with controls. Multivariate analysis revealed that GST T1 null was the most significant risk factor for MM. Interestingly the GST T1 enzyme has been identified as essential for benzene biodegradation. African Americans have an increased frequency of GST T1 null genotypes; this may explain the high incidence of MM. The study presents the evidence that inherited polymorphisms in genes are responsible for metabolizing carcinogens that can affect the individual risk for developing hematologic diseases.[160]

### GENE ARRAY DATA

The recent development of gene expression profiling has highlighted the sequential genetic change from normal plasma cell to a malignant one. The transformation of MGUS to MM provides an opportunity to better understand the genes involved and correlates these molecular changes with various environmental events. Recently, microarray analysis of plasma cells from 5 healthy donors, 7 patients with MGUS, and 24 MM patients established 380 genes differentially expressed between normal and MM, but a much smaller difference of only 74 genes that were differentially expressed between MGUS and MM samples. Differentially expressed genes included oncogenes/tumor-suppressor genes (LAF4, RB1, and disabled homolog 2), cell-signaling genes (RAS family members, B-cell signaling, and NF-κB genes), DNA-binding and transcription-factor genes (XBP1, zinc-finger proteins, forkhead box, and ring-finger proteins), and developmental genes (WNT and SHH pathways).[161] In a twin experiment, gene profiling of MM cells allows us to overcome the individual genetic heterogeneity. A recent study compared the gene expression profile of MM cells from a patient's bone marrow with his genetically identical healthy twin. Two hundred and ninety-six genes were upregulated and 103 genes were downregulated at least twofold in MM cells versus the normal twin plasma cells (PCs). Highly expressed genes in MM cells included cell survival pathway genes such as mcl-1, dad-1, caspase 8, and FADD-like apoptosis regulator (FLIP); oncogenes/transcriptional factors such as Jun-D, Xbp-1, calmodulin, Calnexin, and FGFR-3; stress response and ubiquitin/proteasome pathway-related genes, and various ribosomal genes reflecting increased metabolic and translational activity. Several genes were downregulated in MM cells versus healthy twin PCs including RAD51, killer cell immunoglobulin-like receptor protein, and apoptotic protease activating factor. This study provides insights into the mechanisms involved in malignant transformation in MM.[162] These new developments of the molecular mechanisms of MM will help us understand what causes the disease and develop effective preventive and treatment strategies.

## SUMMARY

The increased incidence of MM in the last 50 years is indicative of improved diagnosis of the disease and the vigorous evaluation of the increasingly aging population rather than an actual increase in incidence. MM clinical presentations range from a benign disease requiring no therapy to an aggressive malignancy reflecting the complex processes involved in initiation and propagation of the malignant clone. Genetic abnormalities possibly represent initial events that are acquired or inherited and remain dormant until environmental factors promote the proliferation of the malignant clone. Then the clone is sustained through a network of cytokines and cellular elements in the bone marrow microenvironment. The contributions of race, sex, infection, various chemicals, and hereditary factors to this process remain under investigation. Despite extensive studies, the etiology of the disease remains elusive. The studies of the genetic background, using gene array and related technologies, have provided a new opportunity to correlate specific genes with the progress of the disease.

### REFERENCES

1. Sirohi B, Powles R: Multiple myeloma. *Lancet* 363:875–887, 2004.
2. IARC: GLOBOCAN 2000: *Cancer Incidence, Mortality and Prevalence Worldwide.* Version 1.0. Lyon, France: IARC Press; 2001:No.5.
3. SEER: *SEER*Stat Database: Incidence—SEER 9 Regs Public-Use.* Nov 2003 Sub (1973–2001). Bethesda, MD: National Cancer Institute, DCCPS, Surveillance Research Program, Cancer Statistics Branch, 2004.
4. Kuehl WM, Bergsagel PL: Multiple myeloma: evolving genetic events and host interactions. *Nat Rev Cancer* 2:175–187, 2002.
5. Clark DW, Macmahon B: The incidence of multiple myeloma. *J Chronic Dis* 4:508–515, 1956.

6. Levi F, La Vecchia C, Lucchini F, Negri E: Trends in cancer mortality sex ratios in Europe, 1950–1989. *World Health Stat* Q 45:117–164, 1992.

7. Vineis P: Incidence and time trends for lymphomas, leukemias and myelomas: hypothesis generation. Working Group on the Epidemiology of Hematolymphopoietic Malignancies in Italy. *Leuk Res* 20:285–290, 1996.

8. Reizenstein P: Female superiority. *Biomed Pharmacother* 36:275–276, 1982.

9. Blair A, Dosemeci M, Heineman EF: Cancer and other causes of death among male and female farmers from twenty-three states. 23:729–742, 1993.

10. Kristensen P, Andersen A, Irgens LM, Laake P, Bye AS: Incidence and risk factors of cancer among men and women in Norwegian agriculture. *Scand J Work Environ Health* 22:14–26, 1996.

11. McDuffie HH: Women at work: agriculture. *J Occup Med* 36:1240–1246, 1994.

12. Petralia SA, Dosemeci M, Adams EE, Zahm SH: Cancer mortality among women employed in health care in 24 U.S. states, 1984–1993. *Am J Ind Med* 36:159–165, 1999.

13. Benjamin M, Reddy S, Brawley OW: Myeloma and race: a review of the literature. *Cancer Metastasis Rev* 22: 87–93, 2003.

14. Blattner WA, Jacobson RJ, Shulman G: Multiple myeloma in South African blacks. *Lancet* 1:928–929, 1979.

15. Shulman G, Jacobson RJ: Immunocytoma in black and white South Africans. *Trop Geogr Med* 32:112–117, 1980.

16. Baris D, Brown LM, Silverman DT, et al.: Socioeconomic status and multiple myeloma among US blacks and whites. *Am J Public Health* 90:1277–1281, 2000.

17. Brown LM, Pottern LM, Silverman DT, et al.: Multiple myeloma among Blacks and Whites in the United States: role of cigarettes and alcoholic beverages. *Cancer Causes Control* 8:610–614, 1997.

18. Brown LM, Gridley G, Pottern LM, et al.: Diet and nutrition as risk factors for multiple myeloma among blacks and whites in the US. *Cancer Causes Control* 12:117–125, 2001.

19. Pottern LM, Gart JJ, Nam JM, et al.: HLA and multiple myeloma among black and white men: evidence of a genetic association. *Cancer Epidemiol Biomarkers Prev* 1:177–182, 1992.

20. Garfinkel L: The epidemiology of cancer in black Americans. *Stat Bull Metrop Insur Co* 72:11–17, 1991.

21. Modiano MR, Villar-Werstler P, Crowley J, Salmon SE: Evaluation of race as a prognostic factor in multiple myeloma. An ancillary of Southwest Oncology Group Study 8229. *J Clin Oncol* 14:974–977, 1996.

22. Nossent JC, Winkel CN, van Leeuwen JC: Multiple myeloma in the Afro-Caribbean population of Curacao. *Neth J Med* 43:210–214, 1993.

23. Kyle RA, Rajkumar SV: Monoclonal gammopathies of undetermined significance: a review. *Immunol Rev* 194:112–139, 2003.

24. Kyle RA, Therneau TM, Rajkumar SV, et al.: A long-term study of prognosis in monoclonal gammopathy of undetermined significance. *N Engl J Med* 346:564–569, 2002.

25. Singh J, Dudley AW Jr, Kulig KA: Increased incidence of monoclonal gammopathy of undetermined significance in blacks and its age-related differences with whites on the basis of a study of 397 men and one woman in a hospital setting. *J Lab Clin Med* 116:785–789, 1990.

26. Cohen HJ, Crawford J, Rao MK, Pieper CF, Currie MS: Racial differences in the prevalence of monoclonal gammopathy in a community-based sample of the elderly. *Am J Med* 104:439–444, 1998.

27. Giraldo P, Rubio-Felix D, Cortes T, et al.: [Incidence, clinico-biological characteristics, and clinical course of 1,203 monoclonal gammopathies (1971–1992)]. *Sangre (Barc)* 39:343–350, 1994.

28. Ogmundsdottir HM, Haraldsdottir V, Johammesson G, et al.: Monoclonal gammopathy in Iceland: a population-based registry and follow-up. *Br J Haematol* 118: 166–173, 2002.

29. Pasqualetti P, Collacciani A, Casale R: Risk of monoclonal gammopathy of undetermined significance: a case-referent study. *Am J Hematol* 52:217–220, 1996.

30. Karlson EW, Tanasijevic M, Hankinson SE, et al.: Monoclonal gammopathy of undetermined significance exposure to breast implants. *Arch Intern Med* 161:864–867, 2001.

31. Neriishi K, Nakashima E, Suzuki G: Monoclonal gammopathy of undetermined significance in atomic bomb survivors: incidence and transformation to multiple myeloma. *Br J Haematol* 121:405–410, 2003.

32. Doody MM, Linet MS, Glass AG, et al.: Leukemia, lymphoma, and multiple myeloma following selected medical conditions. *Cancer Causes Control* 3:449–456, 1992.

33. Linet MS, Harlow SD, McLaughlin JK: A case–control study of multiple myeloma in whites: chronic antigenic stimulation, occupation, and drug use. *Cancer Res* 47:2978–2981, 1987.

34. Pinkhas J, Djaldetti M, Yaron M: Coincidence of multiple myeloma with Gaucher's disease. *Isr J Med Sci* 1:537–540, 1965.

35. Moneret-Vautrin DA, Grilliat JP, Gaucher P, et al.: [Gastric plasmacytosarcoma with IgA dysglobulinemia]. *Nouv Presse Med* 4:2799–2803, 1975.

36. Benjamin D, Joshua H, Djaldetti M, Hazaz B, Pinkhas J: Nonsecretory IgD-kappa multiple myeloma in a patient with Gaucher's disease. *Scand J Haematol* 22:179–184, 1979.

37. Shoenfeld Y, Berliner S, Pinkhas J, Beutler E: The association of Gaucher's disease and dysproteinemias. *Acta Haematol* 64:241–243, 1980.

38. Ruestow PC, Levinson DJ, Catchatourian R, Sreekanth S, Cohen H, Rosenfeld S: Coexistence of IgA myeloma and Gaucher's disease. *Arch Intern Med* 140:1115–1116, 1980.

39. Brady K, Corash L, Bhargava V: Multiple myeloma arising from monoclonal gammopathy of undetermined significance in a patient with Gaucher's disease. *Arch Pathol Lab Med* 121:1108–1111, 1997.

40. Shoenfeld Y, Gallant LA, Shaklai M, Livni E, Djaldetti M, Pinkhas J: Gaucher's disease: a disease with chronic stimulation of the immune system. *Arch Pathol Lab Med* 106:388–391, 1982.

41. Brautbar A, Elstein D, Pines G, Abrahamov A, Zimran A: Effect of enzyme replacement therapy on gammopathies

in Gaucher disease. *Blood Cells Mol Dis* 32:214–217, 2004.

42. Toth J, Kiss T, Varga S: [Multiple myeloma associated with rheumatoid arthritis]. *Orv Hetil* 113:2414–2415, 1972.

43. Perl AF: Multiple myeloma simulating rheumatoid arthritis. *Can Med Assoc J* 79:122–123, 1958.

44. Davis JS Jr, Weber FC, Bartfeld H: Conditions involving the hemopoietic system resulting in a pseudorheumatoid arthritis; similarity of multiple myeloma and rheumatoid arthritis. *Ann Intern Med* 47:10–17, 1957.

45. Buskila D, Sukenik S: [Multiple myeloma complicating rheumatoid arthritis]. *Harefuah* 115:319–321, 1988.

46. Hamano T, Ishikawa T, Yabe H, Nagai K, Nakayama S: [Rheumatoid arthritis terminating in multiple myeloma-a case report]. *Rinsho Ketsueki* 28:408–412, 1987.

47. Matsumori A, Nishiya K, Chijiwa T, et al.: [Two cases of rheumatoid arthritis associated with IgA-type multiple myeloma]. *Ryumachi* 40:26–31, 2000.

48. Usnarska-Zubkiewicz L, Czarnecka M, Wlodarczyk S, Nowak E: [Rheumatoid arthritis as a risk factor for development of multiple myeloma]. *Pol Arch Med Wewn* 97:253–259, 1997.

49. Eriksson M. Rheumatoid arthritis as a risk factor for multiple myeloma: a case–control study. *Eur J Cancer* 29A:259–263, 1993.

50. Rettig MB, Ma HJ, Vescio RA, et al.: Kaposi's sarcoma-associated herpesvirus infection of bone marrow dendritic cells from multiple myeloma patients. *Science* 276:1851–1854, 1997.

51. Tisdale JF, Stewart AK, Dickstein B, et al.: Molecular and serological examination of the relationship of human herpesvirus 8 to multiple myeloma: orf 26 sequences in bone marrow stroma are not restricted to myeloma patients and other regions of the genome are not detected. *Blood* 92:2681–2687, 1998.

52. Patel M, Mahlangu J, Patel J, et al.: Kaposi sarcoma-associated herpesvirus/human herpesvirus 8 and multiple myeloma in South Africa. *Diagn Mol Pathol* 10: 95–99, 2001.

53. Bouscary D, Dupin N, Fichelson S, et al.: Lack of evidence of an association between HHV-8 and multiple myeloma. *Leukemia* 12:1840–1841, 1998.

54. Rask C, Kelsen J, Olesen G, Nielsen JL, Obel N, Abildgaard N: Danish patients with untreated multiple myeloma do not harbour human herpesvirus 8. *Br J Haematol* 108:96–98, 2000.

55. MacKenzie J, Sheldon J, Morgan G, Cook G, Schulz TF, Jarrett RF: HHV-8 and multiple myeloma in the UK. *Lancet* 350:1144–1145, 1997.

56. Marcelin AG, Dupin N, Bouscary D, et al.: HHV-8 and multiple myeloma in France. *Lancet* 350:1144, 1997.

57. Cannon MJ, Flanders WD, Pellett PE: Occurrence of primary cancers in association with multiple myeloma and Kaposi's sarcoma in the United States, 1973–1995. *Int J Cancer* 85:453–456, 2000.

58. Voelkerding KV, Sandhaus LM, Kim HC, et al.: Plasma cell malignancy in the acquired immune deficiency syndrome. Association with Epstein-Barr virus. *Am J Clin Pathol* 92:222–228, 1989.

59. Karnad AB, Martin AW, Koh HK, Brauer MJ, Novich M, Wright J: Nonsecretory multiple myeloma in a 26-year-old man with acquired immunodeficiency syndrome, presenting with multiple extramedullary plasmacy-

tomas and osteolytic bone disease. *Am J Hematol* 32:305–310, 1989.

60. Barbanera M, Menicagli V: [Multiple myeloma in HIV infection]. *Recenti Prog Med* 81:663–665, 1990.

61. Konrad RJ, Kricka LJ, Goodman DB, Goldman J, Silberstein LE: Brief report: myeloma-associated paraprotein directed against the HIV-1 p24 antigen in an HIV-1-seropositive patient. *N Engl J Med* 328:1817–1819, 1993.

62. Kumar S, Kumar D, Schnadig VJ, Selvanayagam P, Slaughter DP: Plasma cell myeloma in patients who are HIV-positive. *Am J Clin Pathol* 102:633–639, 1994.

63. Yee TT, Murphy K, Johnson M, et al.: Multiple myeloma and human immunodeficiency virus-1 (HIV-1) infection. *Am J Hematol* 66:123–125, 2001.

64. Pouli A, Lemessiou H, Rontogianni D, et al.: Multiple myeloma as the first manifestation of acquired immunodeficiency syndrome: a case report and review of the literature. *Ann Hematol* 80:557–560, 2001.

65. Lallemand F, Fritsch L, Cywiner-Golenzer C, Rozenbaum W: Multiple myeloma in an HIV-positive man presenting with primary cutaneous plasmacytomas and spinal cord compression. *J Am Acad Dermatol* 39:506–508, 1998.

66. Talib SH, Singh J, Ranga S, Talib VH: Multiple myeloma complicating HIV-infection. A case report. *Indian J Pathol Microbiol* 40:413–416, 1997.

67. Faure I, Viallard JF, Mercie P, Bonnefoy M, Pellegrin JL, Leng B: Multiple myeloma in two HIV-infected patients. *AIDS* 13:1797–1799, 1999.

68. Elira Dokekias A, Moutschen M, Purhuence MF, Malanda F, Moyikoua A: [Multiples's myeloma and HIV infection: report of 3 cases]. *Rev Med Liege* 59:95–97, 2004.

69. Montella M, Crispo A, Frigeri F, et al.: HCV and tumors correlated with immune system: a case–control study in an area of hyperendemicity. *Leuk Res* 2001;25:775–781.

70. Silvestri F, Barillari G, Fanin R, et al.: Risk of hepatitis C virus infection, Waldenstrom's macroglobulinemia, and monoclonal gammopathies. *Blood* 88:1125–1126, 1996.

71. Gharagozloo S, Khoshnoodi J, Shokri F: Hepatitis C virus infection in patients with essential mixed cryoglobulinemia, multiple myeloma and chronic lymphocytic leukemia. *Pathol Oncol Res* 7:135–139, 2001.

72. Rabkin CS, Tess BH, Christianson RE, et al.: Prospective study of hepatitis C viral infection as a risk factor for subsequent B-cell neoplasia. *Blood* 99:4240–4242, 2002.

73. Bianco E, Marcucci F, Mele A, et al.: Prevalence of hepatitis C virus infection in lymphoproliferative diseases other than B-cell non-Hodgkin's lymphoma, and in myeloproliferative diseases: an Italian multi-center case-control study. *Haematologica* 89:70–76, 2004.

74. Hausfater P, Cacoub P, Sterkers Y, et al.: Hepatitis C virus infection and lymphoproliferative diseases: prospective study on 1,576 patients in France. *Am J Hematol* 67:168–171, 2001.

75. Besson C, Gonin C, Brebion A, Delaunay C, Panelatti G, Plumelle Y: Incidence of hematological malignancies in Martinique, French West Indies, overrepresentation of multiple myeloma and adult T cell leukemia/lymphoma. *Leukemia* 15:828–831, 2001.

76. Cardis E, Gilbert ES, Carpenter L, et al.: Effects of low doses and low dose rates of external ionizing radiation:

cancer mortality among nuclear industry workers in three countries. *Radiat Res* 142:117–132, 1995.

77. Douglas AJ, Omar RZ, Smith PG: Cancer mortality and morbidity among workers at the Sellafield plant of British Nuclear Fuels. *Br J Cancer* 70:1232–1243, 1994.

78. Wing S, Richardson D, Wolf S, Mihlan G, Crawford-Brown D, Wood J: A case control study of multiple myeloma at four nuclear facilities. *Ann Epidemiol* 10:144–153, 2000.

79. Baysson H, Laurier D, Tirmarche M, Valenty M, Giraud JM: Epidemiological response to a suspected excess of cancer among a group of workers exposed to multiple radiological and chemical hazards. *Occup Environ Med* 57:188–194, 2000.

80. Lopez-Abente G, Aragones N, Pollan M, Ruiz M, Gandarillas A: Leukemia, lymphomas, and myeloma mortality in the vicinity of nuclear power plants and nuclear fuel facilities in Spain. *Cancer Epidemiol Biomarkers Prev* 8:925–934, 1999.

81. Agu VU, Christensen BL, Buffler PA: Geographic patterns of multiple myeloma: racial and industrial correlates, State of Texas, 1969–71. *J Natl Cancer Inst* 65:735–738, 1980.

82. Burmeister LF: Cancer mortality in Iowa farmers, 1971–78. *J Natl Cancer Inst* 66:461–464, 1981.

83. Cerhan JR, Cantor KP, Williamson K, Lynch CF, Torner JC, Burmeister LF: Cancer mortality among Iowa farmers: recent results, time trends, and lifestyle factors (United States). *Cancer Causes Control* 9:311–319, 1998.

84. Blair A: Cancer risks associated with agriculture: epidemiologic evidence. *Basic Life Sci* 21:93–111, 1982.

85. Steineck G, Wiklund K: Multiple myeloma in Swedish agricultural workers. *Int J Epidemiol* 15:321–325, 1986.

86. Khuder SA, Mutgi AB: Meta-analyses of multiple myeloma and farming. *Am J Ind Med* 32:510–516, 1997.

87. Assennato G, Ferri GM, Tria G, Porro A, Macinagrossa L, Ruggieri M: [Tumors of the hemolymphopoietic tract and employment in agriculture: a case–control study carried out in an epidemiologic area in southern Italy]. *G Ital Med Lav* 17:91–97, 1995.

88. Nanni O, Falcini F, Buiatti E, et al.: Multiple myeloma and work in agriculture: results of a case–control study in Forli, Italy. *Cancer Causes Control* 9:277–283, 1998.

89. Pukkala E, Notkola V: Cancer incidence among Finnish farmers, 1979–93. *Cancer Causes Control* 8:25–33, 1997.

90. Pahwa P, McDuffie HH, Dosman JA, et al.: Exposure to animals and selected risk factors among Canadian farm residents with Hodgkin's disease, multiple myeloma, or soft tissue sarcoma. *J Occup Environ Med* 45:857–868, 2003.

91. Monson RR, Nakano KK: Mortality among rubber workers. II: Other employees. *Am J Epidemiol* 103:297–303, 1976.

92. Delzell E, Monson RR: Mortality among rubber workers. X: Reclaim workers. *Am J Ind Med* 7:307–313, 1985.

93. Matanoski G, Elliott E, Tao X, Francis M, Correa-Villasenor A, Santos-Burgoa C: Lymphohematopoietic cancers and butadiene and styrene exposure in synthetic rubber manufacture. *Ann N Y Acad Sci* 837:157–169, 1997.

94. Sorahan T, Parkes HG, Veys CA, Waterhouse JA, Straughan JK, Nutt A: Mortality in the British rubber industry 1946–85. *Br J Ind Med* 46:1–10, 1989.

95. Kogevinas M, Sala M, Boffetta P, Kazerouni N, Kromhout H, Hoar-Zahm S: Cancer risk in the rubber industry: a review of the recent epidemiological evidence. *Occup Environ Med* 55:1–12, 1998.

96. Sathiakumar N, Delzell E, Hovinga M, et al.: Mortality from cancer and other causes of death among synthetic rubber workers. *Occup Environ Med* 55:230–235, 1998.

97. Torres A, Giralt M, Raichs A: [Coexistence of chronic benzol contacts and multiple plasmacytoma. Presentation of 2 cases]. *Sangre (Barc)* 15:275–279, 1970.

98. Aksoy M: Malignancies due to occupational exposure to benzene. *Haematologica* 65:370–373, 1980.

99. Heineman EF, Olsen JH, Pottern LM, Gomez M, Raffn E, Blair A: Occupational risk factors for multiple myeloma among Danish men. *Cancer Causes Control* 3:555–568, 1992.

100. Pottern LM, Heineman EF, Olsen JH, Raffn E, Blair A: Multiple myeloma among Danish women: employment history and workplace exposures. *Cancer Causes Control* 3:427–432, 1992.

101. Bezabeh S, Engel A, Morris CB, Lamm SH: Does benzene cause multiple myeloma? An analysis of the published case–control literature. *Environ Health Perspect* 104(suppl 6):1393–1398, 1996.

102. Bergsagel DE, Wong O, Bergsagel PL, et al.: Benzene and multiple myeloma: appraisal of the scientific evidence. *Blood* 94:1174–1182, 1999.

103. Wong O, Raabe GK: Multiple myeloma and benzene exposure in a multinational cohort of more than 250,000 petroleum workers. *Regul Toxicol Pharmacol* 26:188–199, 1997.

104. Sonoda T, Nagata Y, Mori M, Ishida T, Imai K: Meta-analysis of multiple myeloma and benzene exposure. *J Epidemiol* 11:249–254, 2001.

105. Lee WJ, Baris D, Jarvholm B, Silverman DT, Bergdahl IA, Blair A: Multiple myeloma and diesel and other occupational exposures in Swedish construction workers. *Int J Cancer* 107:134–138, 2003.

106. Bukowski JA, Huebner WW, Schnatter AR, Wojcik NC: An analysis of the risk of B-lymphocyte malignancies in industrial cohorts. *J Toxicol Environ Health A* 66:581–597, 2003.

107. Golden AL, Markowitz SB, Landrigan PJ: The risk of cancer in firefighters. *Occup Med* 10:803–820, 1995.

108. Eriksson M, Karlsson M: Occupational and other environmental factors and multiple myeloma: a population based case–control study. *Br J Ind Med* 49:95–103, 1992.

109. Nandakumar A, Armstrong BK, de Klerk NH: Multiple myeloma in Western Australia: a case–control study in relation to occupation, father's occupation, socioeconomic status and country of birth. *Int J Cancer* 37:223–226, 1986.

110. Flodin U, Fredriksson M, Persson B: Multiple myeloma and engine exhausts, fresh wood, and creosote: a case–referent study. *Am J Ind Med* 12:519–529, 1987.

111. La Vecchia C, Negri E, D'Avanzo B, Franceschi S: Occupation and lymphoid neoplasms. *Br J Cancer* 60:385–388, 1989.

112. Demers PA, Boffetta P, Kogevinas M, et al.: Pooled reanalysis of cancer mortality among five cohorts of workers in wood-related industries. *Scand J Work Environ Health* 21:179–190, 1995.

113. Fritschi L, Siemiatycki J: Lymphoma, myeloma and occupation: results of a case–control *study. Int J Cancer* 67:498–503, 1996.

114. Fu H, Demers PA, Costantini AS, et al.: Cancer mortality among shoe manufacturing workers: an analysis of two cohorts. *Occup Environ Med* 53:394–398, 1996.

115. Wartenberg D, Reyner D, Scott CS: Trichloroethylene and cancer: epidemiologic evidence. *Environ Health Perspect* 108(suppl 2):161–176, 2000.

116. Costantini AS, Miligi L, Kriebel D, et al.: A multicenter case–control study in Italy on hematolymphopoietic neoplasms and occupation. *Epidemiology* 12:78–87, 2001.

117. Gallagher RP, Threlfall WJ: Cancer mortality in metal workers. *Can Med Assoc J* 129:1191–1194, 1983.

118. Morris PD, Koepsell TD, Daling JR, et al.: Toxic substance exposure and multiple myeloma: a case–control study. *J Natl Cancer Inst* 76:987–994, 1986.

119. McWhorter WP, Schatzkin AG, Horm JW, Brown CC: Contribution of socioeconomic status to black/white differences in cancer incidence. *Cancer* 63:982–987, 1989.

120. Davey Smith G, Neaton JD, Wentworth D, Stamler R, Stamler J: Mortality differences between black and white men in the USA: contribution of income and other risk factors among men screened for the MRFIT. MRFIT Research Group. Multiple Risk Factor Intervention Trial. *Lancet* 351:934–939, 1998.

121. Clayton LA, Byrd WM: The African-American cancer crisis. Part I: The problem. *J Health Care Poor Underserved* 4:83–101, 1993.

122. Vlajinac HD, Pekmezovic TD, Adanja BJ, et al.: case–control study of multiple myeloma with special reference to diet as risk factor. *Neoplasma* 50:79–83, 2003.

123. Samanic C, Gridley G, Chow WH, Lubin J, Hoover RN, Fraumeni JF Jr: Obesity and cancer risk among white and black United States veterans. *Cancer Causes Control* 15:35–43, 2004.

124. Calle EE, Rodriguez C, Walker-Thurmond K, Thun MJ: Overweight, obesity, and mortality from cancer in a prospectively studied cohort of U.S. adults. *N Engl J Med* 348:1625–1638, 2003.

125. Mills PK, Newell GR, Beeson WL, Fraser GE, Phillips RL: History of cigarette smoking and risk of leukemia and myeloma: results from the Adventist health study. *J Natl Cancer Inst* 82:1832–1836, 1990.

126. Heineman EF, Zahm SH, McLaughlin JK, Vaught JB, Hrubec Z: A prospective study of tobacco use and multiple myeloma: evidence against an association. *Cancer Causes Control* 3:31–36, 1992.

127. Brownson RC: Cigarette smoking and risk of myeloma. *J Natl Cancer Inst* 83:1036–1037, 1991.

128. Brown LM, Everett GD, Gibson R, Burmeister LF, Schuman LM, Blair A: Smoking and risk of non-Hodgkin's lymphoma and multiple myeloma. *Cancer Causes Control* 3:49–55, 1992.

129. Friedman GD: Cigarette smoking, leukemia, and multiple myeloma. *Ann Epidemiol* 3:425–428, 1993.

130. Adami J, Nyren O, Bergstrom R, et al.: Smoking and the risk of leukemia, lymphoma, and multiple myeloma (Sweden). *Cancer Causes Control* 9:49–56, 1998.

131. Stagnaro E, Ramazzotti V, Crosignani P, et al.: Smoking and hematolymphopoietic malignancies. *Cancer Causes Control* 12:325–334, 2001.

132. Brown LM, Everett GD, Burmeister LF, Blair A: Hair dye use and multiple myeloma in white men. *Am J Public Health* 82:1673–1674, 1992.

133. Zahm SH, Weisenburger DD, Babbitt PA, Saal RC, Vaught JB, Blair A: Use of hair coloring products and the risk of lymphoma, multiple myeloma, and chronic lymphocytic leukemia. *Am J Public Health* 82:990–997, 1992.

134. Herrinton LJ, Weiss NS, Koepsell TD, et al.: Exposure to hair-coloring products and the risk of multiple myeloma. *Am J Public Health* 84:1142–1144, 1994.

135. Thun MJ, Altekruse SF, Namboodiri MM, Calle EE, Myers DG, Heath CW Jr: Hair dye use and risk of fatal cancers in U.S. women. *J Natl Cancer Inst* 86:210–215, 1994.

136. Colditz GA: Hair dye and cancer: reassuring evidence of no association. *J Natl Cancer Inst* 86:164–165, 1994.

137. Grodstein F, Hennekens CH, Colditz GA, Hunter DJ, Stampfer MJ: A prospective study of permanent hair dye use and hematopoietic cancer. *J Natl Cancer Inst* 86:1466–1470, 1994.

138. Altekruse SF, Henley SJ, Thun MJ: Deaths from hematopoietic and other cancers in relation to permanent hair dye use in a large prospective study (United States). *Cancer Causes Control* 10:617–625, 1999.

139. Hartge P: Hair dyes, cancer, and epidemiology. *Cancer Invest* 18:408, 2000.

140. Berlin SO, Odeberg H, Weingart L: Familial occurrence of M-components. *Acta Med Scand* 183:347–350, 1968.

141. Boga M, Jako J, Doman J, Magyar E, Konyar E: Familial myeloma. Folia *Haematol Int Mag Klin Morphol Blutforsch* 100:201–212, 1973.

142. Maldonado JE, Kyle RA: Familial myeloma. Report of eight families and a study of serum proteins in their relatives. *Am J Med* 57:875–884, 1974.

143. Law MI: Familial occurrence of multiple myeloma. *South Med J* 69:46–48, 1976.

144. Zawadzki ZA, Aizawa Y, Kraj MA, Haradin AR, Fisher B: Familial immunopathies: report of nine families and survey of literature. *Cancer* 40:2094–2101, 1977.

145. Youinou P, le Goff P, Saleun JP, et al.: Familial occurrence of monoclonal gammapathies. *Biomedicine* 28:226–232, 1978.

146. Deshpande HA, Hu XP, Marino P, Jan NA, Wiernik PH: Anticipation in familial plasma cell dyscrasias. *Br J Haematol* 103:696–703, 1998.

147. Shoenfeld Y, Berliner S, Shaklai M, Gallant LA, Pinkhas J: Familial multiple myeloma. A review of thirty-seven families. *Postgrad Med J* 58:12–16, 1982.

148. Bourguet CC, Grufferman S, Delzell E, DeLong ER, Cohen HJ: Multiple myeloma and family history of cancer. A case–control study. *Cancer* 56:2133–2139, 1985.

149. Loth TS, Perrotta AL, Lima J, Whiteaker RS, Robinson A: Genetic aspects of familial multiple myeloma. *Mil Med* 156:430–433, 1991.

150. Ogawa M, Wurster DH, McIntyre OR: Multiple myeloma in one of a pair of monozygotic twins. *Acta Haematol* 44:295–304, 1970.

151. Snowden JA, Greaves M: IgA lambda myeloma presenting concurrently in identical twins with subsequent transformation to 'aggressive phase' in one. *Clin Lab Haematol* 17:95–96, 1995.

152. Judson IR, Wiltshaw E, Newland AC: Multiple myeloma in a pair of monozygotic twins: the first reported case. *Br J Haematol* 60:551–554, 1985.

153. Hemminki K, Vaittinen P: National database of familial cancer in Sweden. *Genet Epidemiol* 15:225–236, 1998.

154. Brown LM, Linet MS, Greenberg RS, et al.: Multiple myeloma and family history of cancer among blacks and whites in the U.S. *Cancer* 85:2385–2390, 1999.

155. Grosbois B, Jego P, Attal M, et al.: Familial multiple myeloma: report of fifteen families. *Br J Haematol* 105:768–770, 1999.

156. Lynch HT, Sanger WG, Pirruccello S, Quinn-Laquer B, Weisenburger DD: Familial MM: a family study and review of the literature. *J Natl Cancer Inst* 93:1479–1483, 2001.

157. Hemminki K: Re: familial multiple myeloma: a family study and review of the literature. *J Natl Cancer Inst* 94:462–463, 2002; author reply: 463.

158. Sobol H, Vey N, Sauvan R, Philip N, Noguchi T, Eisinger F: Re: familial multiple myeloma: a family study and review of the literature. *J Natl Cancer Inst* 94:461–462, 2002; author reply: 463.

159. Nakayama S, Kitajima K, Ueno K, Hoshino T: [Multiple myeloma in spouses-with special reference to BHC as a possible cause (author's trans)]. *Rinsho Ketsueki* 21:73–79, 1980.

160. Lincz LF, Kerridge I, Scorgie FE, Bailey M, Enno A, Spencer A: Xenobiotic gene polymorphisms and susceptibility to multiple myeloma. *Haematologica* 89:628–629, 2004.

161. Davies FE, Dring AM, Li C, et al.: Insights into the multi-step transformation of MGUS to myeloma using microarray expression analysis. *Blood* 102:4504–4511, 2003.

162. Munshi NC, Hideshima T, Carrasco D, et al.: Identification of genes modulated in multiple myeloma using genetically identical twin samples. *Blood* 103:1799–1806, 2004.

# Chapter 81

# MOLECULAR BIOLOGY, PATHOLOGY, AND CYTOGENETICS

*Silvia Ling, Lynda Campbell, Phoebe Joy Ho, John Gibson, and Douglas E. Joshua*

## INTRODUCTION

Although traditional morphology has played a secondary role to the rapid developments in molecular biology, cytogenetics, and new areas of therapy for patients with multiple myeloma, its importance cannot be underestimated. Furthermore, new cytogenetic and molecular data, which relate morphologic appearances to chromosomal translocations (i.e., the association of CD20 expression, t(11;14) translocations, and small mature plasma cell morphology),[1] have the potential to play considerable therapeutic roles in decision making about appropriate treatment for patients with myeloma.

## MORPHOLOGY

### NORMAL AND MALIGNANT PLASMA CELLS

Plasma cells are part of the normal cell population of the bone marrow. They comprise approximately 1% of the nucleated cells of normal marrow aspirates, and are equally distributed throughout the red marrow. Bone marrow findings of increased plasma cells, characteristic of myeloma, must always be taken together with other features before definite conclusions can be drawn, as high plasma cell numbers are seen in some reactive states, especially in HIV infection, autoimmune states, and liver disease. Aggregations of normal plasma cells usually occur in a perivascular distribution, with fewer than four or six cells clumped together. Normal plasma cells are of two major morphologic types. The classical "Marschalko" plasma cells are the predominant plasma cells in normal marrow. Such cells have abundant basophilic cytoplasm, paranuclear hof, and are usually devoid of nucleoli. The second appearance is of the lymphoplasmacytoid plasma cells, which are usually IgM secreting and are the predominant cells in Waldenstrom's macroglobulinemia. These cells are smaller than "Marschalko" plasma cells, with less eccentricity of the nucleus, and are more dispersed in the bone marrow without perivascular cuffing. Malignant plasma cells can be differentiated by aggregation along endosteal surfaces, large clumps, and the presence of nucleated plasmablasts or proplasmablasts. Binucleated plasma cells are occasionally seen in normal reactive marrow, and do not per se define malignancy. Electron microscopic appearances of normal plasma cells reveal peripheral chromatin condensation in an eccentric nucleus with well-developed paranuclear Golgi apparatus and cytoplasmic endoplasmic reticulum. Normal plasma cells have an even distribution of kappa and lambda staining, whereas malignant clones are light-chain restricted. Morphologic abnormalities, such as crystal formation, Russell bodies, and "flame" cells are not usually seen in normal marrows, but are by no means pathognomonic of malignancy, as they can occasionally be seen in reactive states.

### THE MORPHOLOGIC DIAGNOSIS OF MULTIPLE MYELOMA

The morphologic diagnosis of multiple myeloma and its distinction from reactive plasmacytosis relies on both the quantity of plasma cells seen and the qualitative plasma cell abnormalities, as previously mentioned. In general terms, more than 30% of plasma cells in a marrow aspirate smears constitute a major diagnostic criterion for multiple myeloma, although such a percentage may occur in other conditions, such as rheumatic disorders, inflammatory reactions of the bone marrow, and in particular, HIV infection. The demonstration of light-chain isotype restriction has become a major criterion for distinguishing malignant from reactive cases. Nuclear-cytoplasmic asynchrony is more evident in malignant plasma cells. Recently, the international myeloma working group has suggested criteria for the distinction of monoclonal gammopathy of unknown significance (MGUS), smoldering myeloma, and symptomatic myeloma. These criteria do not rely on strict morphologic criteria, but stress the clonal or light-chain isotype restriction of plasma cells.[2]

Despite attempts to define morphologic and or cytochemical features that distinguish neoplastic plasma cells from normal plasma cells, no morphologic criteria appear to be pathognomonic. Spindle-shaped crystal deposits and other cellular inclusions (see Figures 81.1 and 81.2) typical of myeloma can occasionally be seen in normal plasma cells. The diffuse eosinophilic pink staining at the cell periphery, the so-called "flame" cells (see Figure 81.3) seen mostly in IgA myeloma, can occur in other variants, as can Russell bodies which, while initially thought to be organisms, are now known to be immunoglobulin (Ig), have been seen in normal plasma cells. Variations in cell size, in multiple nucleolarity, and even cytochemical staining are not pathognomonic (see Figure 81.4). Most plasma cells stain positively for acid phosphatase, nonspecific esterase, and periodic acid–Schiff, but these are not specific for myeloma. The presence of plasmablasts (see Figure 81.5), nucleolated plasma cells often with less eccentricity and less intense staining of cytoplasm, is classical of myeloma. The number of plasmablasts has also been shown to correlate with prognosis. The presence of a large number of plasmablasts per se is probably the most important morphologic feature that distinguishes myeloma from reactive plasmacytosis, and a population of plasmablasts greater than 2% of plasma cells have been shown by the Mayo Clinic to be an adverse prognostic factor.[3]

In early myeloma, plasma cells distribute in an interstitial pattern. At a later stage, they form dense aggregates on endosteal surface, followed by nodules and sheets in advanced disease. These patterns correlate with

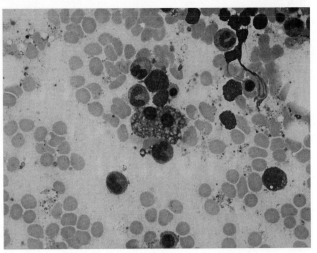

**Figure 81.2**  *Bone marrow aspirate of a patient with myeloma. Mott cells are plasma cells with multiple bluish cytoplasmic inclusion bodies*

survival, as do other major prognostic factors: plasma cell labeling index and serum $\beta_2$-microglobulin.[4–6]

The growth pattern of myeloma on trephine is also predictive of the type of skeletal defects and correlates strongly with magnetic resonance imaging findings. Nodules of plasma cells are associated with osteolytic lesions, whereas interstitial and "sarcomatous" types are associated with osteoporosis.[7]

The percentage of plasma cells on bone marrow aspirates is used as a diagnostic criterion for myeloma. According to the World Health Organization classification, major diagnostic criteria require 30% plasmacytosis, while minor criteria require 10–30% for the diagnosis of myeloma. For MGUS, marrow plasmacytosis is defined as <10%.

Monoclonality of myeloma can be demonstrated on trephine by kappa or lambda light-chain restriction by immunohistochemical stain. CD138/syndecan-1 is a useful immunohistochemical marker of normal and neoplastic plasma cells on bone marrow trephine.

### IMMUNOPHENOTYPING OF PLASMA CELLS

Immunophenotyping is a valuable technique for differentiating myeloma and normal plasma cells, and the distinction is based on the presence of phenotypic aberrations in myeloma plasma cells (MPCs) that are absent in normal plasma cells.

Normal plasma cells meet the following criteria on phenotyping: high-intensity CD38 positive, CD138 positive, CD 56 negative, CD19 positive, CD20 negative, CD28 negative, CD33 negative, and CD117 negative. Plasma cells in patients with myeloma may demonstrate other abnormalities; for example, positive CD20, CD40, and CD56, and negative CD19.[8–11]

Thus, although plasma cells are usually defined by high-intensity florescent CD38 and are CD45 negative, CD45[+] populations of plasma cells have also been studied, and these correlate with plasma cell matrixity

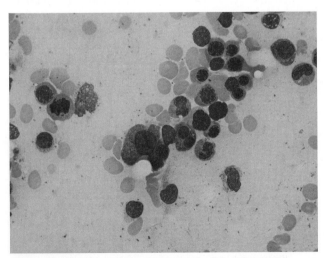

**Figure 81.1**  *Bone marrow aspirate of a patient with myeloma. Needle-shaped, azurophilic crystalline inclusions in cytoplasm of plasma cells representing Ig inclusion material*

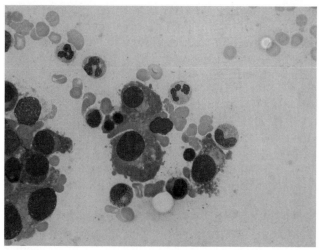

**Figure 81.3** *Bone marrow aspirate of a patient with IgA myeloma. "Flame" cells are typically associated with IgA myeloma. They are plasma cells which stain eosinophilic pink in the periphery of the cytoplasm due to the accumulation of Ig*

and proliferative capacity. Immature plasma cells are CD38$^{++}$, CD45$^{++}$, have high labeling indices, and correlate with the clinical behavior of the disease.[12] Mature malignant plasma cells are CD45 negative, have lower labeling indices, a lower incidence of P-glycoprotein expression, and oncoprotein abnormalities.[13]

## DEVELOPMENT OF PLASMA CELLS

### CELLULAR DEVELOPMENT

Lymphoid cells are derived from a common lymphoid progenitor which has the capacity to develop into a T, B, or natural killer cell.[1] The first recognizable B-cell type is a pro-B cell, which develops under the influence of transcription factors essential for B-cell commitment. The pro-B cell expresses the characteristic B-

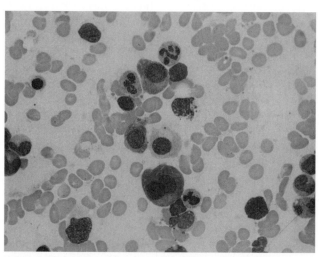

**Figure 81.4** *Binucleated plasma cell in a patient with myeloma*

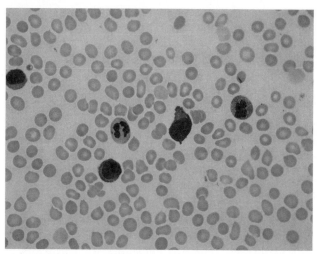

**Figure 81.5** *Plasmablasts with prominent nucleoli in a patient with plasma cell leukemia*

cell surface marker CD19, but not cytoplasmic μ immunoglobulin. It undergoes rearrangement of the Ig heavy-chain (IgH) genes, the product of which associates with that of the variable pre-beta and lambda 5 genes, which encode proteins forming the surrogate light chain. Subsequent rearrangement of true light-chain genes enables expression of surface IgM. The immature B cell thus expresses CD19, as well as cell surface IgM associated with kappa or lambda light chains, i.e., the B-cell receptor. A virgin B cell is an IgM$^+$, IgD$^+$ cell that circulates in the peripheral blood in the $G_0$ phase of cell cycle. It may be activated to proliferate and produce plasma cells and memory B cells. Such activation requires contact with T cells.

B cells with high-affinity receptors receive survival signals from antigen stimulation on dendritic cells and differentiate into memory B cells or plasmablasts, which subsequently migrate to the bone marrow and develop into plasma cells. These bone marrow plasma cells have a long life span and produce the majority of secreted Ig in the plasma. They are considered to be the normal, nonmalignant counterpart of the MPC.

### MOLECULAR ASPECTS OF PLASMA CELL DEVELOPMENT

#### IgH gene rearrangements and V gene usage in myeloma

Maturation of normal B-cell precursors to mature plasma cells involves rearrangement of the Ig genes with subsequent somatic mutation of the variable (V) region. The variable region of the Ig heavy chain is derived from three distinct gene segments encoded by the variable (V), diversity (D), and joining (J) region sequences. For the light chain, the variable region is composed of variable kappa or lambda gene segments linked to the joining segments. V gene rearrangement is dependent on the protein products of recombinase activating genes. Within the variable regions of both the Ig heavy- and light-chain genes, there are three hypervariable or complementary determining regions (CDR). These unique segments can be used as markers to detect minimal residual disease in B-cell tumors. CDR3 is the most variable portion of the Ig molecule, and is the principal site for somatic mutation and antibody affinity maturation of the Ig molecule.[14]

After variable region recombination, the isotypes of the heavy chains are determined by a process known as isotype switching. Many of the chromosomal translocations seen in multiple myeloma occur in these switch regions. The process of VDJ rearrangement and class switching allows a single B-cell clone to produce antibodies of different heavy-chain classes to the same antigenic epitope. The rearrangement of Ig genes during B-cell development is sequential, occurring at distinct stages of development. Heavy-chain genes undergo rearrangement before the light-chain genes. The product of successful heavy-chain VDJ joining activates rearrangements of the kappa locus, which precedes lambda rearrangement.

In myeloma, the malignant plasma cells have already undergone somatic mutation within the germinal center, and no ongoing mutation occurs with progressive disease. Thus, the mutation mechanism is no longer active in the malignant clone.[15,16] Analysis of the variable genes has indicated that the majority of the malignant population is derived from a post-antigen-selected plasma cell. However, less mature, minor B-cell populations of identical variable gene sequences may coexist in the circulation, both in the postswitch and preswitch populations.[17]

## ORIGIN OF THE MALIGNANT PLASMA CELL

Myeloma is characterized by proliferation of a monoclonal population of plasma cells. It is a tumor of a postgerminal center, mature B cell that has undergone antigen selection, and somatic hypermutation.[15,16,18] However, the origin of the MPC remains controversial.

Molecular studies have cast some insights into the stage of differentiation and the clonal nature of myeloma. Polymerase chain reaction and sequence analysis of the $IgV_H$ genes have shown that clonal proliferation occurs in a cell that has undergone somatic hypermutation.[15] Consequently, the unique IgH VDJ rearrangement, somatic hypermutation in the CDR regions (in particular, the hypervariable CDR3 region), becomes the signature of the malignant clone. This malignant population is intraclonally homogeneous and stable in spite of disease progression.[16,19]

Phenotypic characterization of myeloma "stem cells" has recently being proposed,[20] suggesting they are CD138+ B cells that self-replicate and differentiate into malignant CD138+ plasma cells. These subsets are small (<5%), highly clonogenic, and express CD20+ and surface IgM. They are inhibited by anti-CD20 monoclonal antibody. It was suggested that the therapeutic effect of CD20 antibodies will not be immediate and cannot be measured by standard response criteria, because they target the precursor and not the mature plasma cells that produce the clinical effects.[20]

## CYTOGENETIC ABNORMALITIES IN MYELOMA

Chromosome studies in multiple myeloma have become an important part of the management of myeloma patients. Early investigations were based on conventional karyotype analysis, with the detection of recurrent abnormalities, such as monosomy 13 and t(11;14). In recent years, developments in molecular cytogenetics ranging from metaphase and interphase fluorescent in situ hybridization (FISH) to multicolor spectral karyotyping (M-FISH) and comparative genomic hybridization (CGH) have greatly increased the range and number of detectable cytogenetic abnormalities (Figure 81.6). These techniques have overcome some limitations of conventional cytogenetics (CC) in myeloma, including (1) low mitotic index of myeloma cells; (2) multiple complex chromosomal abnormalities of myeloma complicating the identification of specific chromosomes; and (3) telomeric locations of translocational breakpoints and deletional sites, especially in 14q23.

### DELETION OF CHROMOSOME 13Q

Deletion of chromosome 13q is the most common recurrent chromosomal abnormality in myeloma. It is detected in 15–20% of myeloma by CC,[21] 50% of cases by interphase FISH in newly diagnosed myeloma patients,[22] and 30–45% of cases of MGUS.[23,24] The prognostic significance of loss of 13q identified by FISH alone has been the subject of considerable debate. Several studies based on molecular cytogenetics have shown that this abnormality is strongly associated with an unfavorable prognosis.[23,25–32] It correlates with advanced stage, elevated $\beta_2$-microglobulin, increased percentage of plasma cells, increased proliferative rate, and reduced overall survival. However, a multivariate analysis identified t(4;14), t(14;16), and the deletion of 17p13 as independent predictors of survival, while loss of 13q was found to be of only borderline significance.[33]

Chromosome 13 abnormalities are frequently associated with other chromosomal aberrations. It was observed that, while all patients carrying translocations involving the IgH locus, such as t(4;14) and t(14;16), also had loss of chromosome 13, del(13q), the reverse was not true.[24,34] This suggests the possibility that del(13q) occurred before the IgH translocation events, perhaps as an early oncogenic change. A role for monosomy 13 in the transformation of MGUS to myeloma has also been proposed, supported by a higher incidence of monosomy 13 in myeloma cases

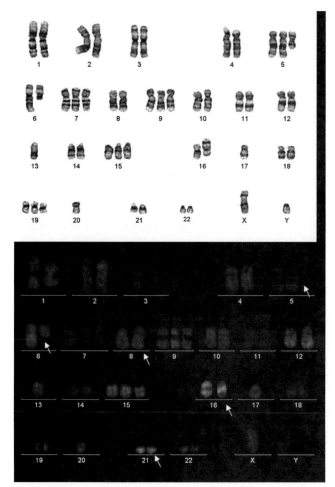

**Figure 81.6**  *Multiple myeloma karyotype: Top panel shows G-banded karyotype with extra copies of chromosomes 5, 7, 9, 15, and 19, loss of the Y chromosome, monosomy 13, and complex unbalanced rearrangements involving chromosomes 16, 17, and 20. The complex der(16) and cryptic t(8;21) were identified only on M-FISH (shown in the bottom panel). The t(8;21) breakpoint on 8q is at the site of the MYC gene*

with preexisting MGUS (70%) compared with those cases without such a history (31%).[35] Moreover, in 18 asymptomatic, untreated patients with MGUS studied serially with both CC and FISH over 6–72 months (median 30 months), del(13q14) was identified in 5 patients over the course of the study, but in only 1 of these patients was the del(13q) detected at diagnosis. All five patients proceeded to develop multiple myeloma (MM) 6–12 months after 13q deletion identification, whereas only 2/13 patients without evidence of del(13q) transformed to MM.

The majority of chromosome 13 abnormalities (92%) are complete monosomies,[22] with the remaining being partial deletions.

### IGH SWITCH TRANSLOCATION

The most common structural chromosomal abnormality in myeloma is IgH switch translocation, involving the IgH gene locus on chromosome 14q32. Using interphase FISH, its incidence is 50% in MGUS, 60–75% in multiple myeloma, and more than 80% in plasma cell leukemia.[35–38] There is a large array of non-immunoglobulin translocation partners, with the most common ones being 11q13, 4p16.3, 16q23, and 6q23. Cloning of the breakpoints of these genes has shown that they contain candidate oncogenes. As the oncogenes are translocated to der(14), they may be activated while under the control of IgH enhancers.

### Chromosome *11q13*

t(11;14) is observed in 15–20% of myeloma by FISH.[39,40] In particular, it is much more common in IgM, IgE, and nonsecretory myeloma. The breakpoints are widely scattered over a region 100–330 kb centromeric to *cyclin D1*, in contrast to mantle cell lymphoma, where the breakpoints are tightly clustered within 110 kb upstream of *cyclin D1*.[41] Cyclin D is likely to be a candidate oncogene, as supported by its being overexpressed in myeloma patients and cell lines with t(11;14).

Early studies suggested that t(11;14) was associated with a poor prognosis.[24,25,40,42] However, subsequent studies by interphase FISH have not confirmed the prognostic relationship.[40] A t(11;14) has been associated with a specific plasma cell morphology. Robillard et al. described an association between CD20 positivity, small mature plasma cell morphology, and t(11;14).[1] Another study showed an association between t(11;14) and a lymphoplasmacytoid morphology.[43] There also appeared to be a link between this morphologic subtype of MM, the t(11;14), and nonsecretory MM.[43]

### Chromosome 4p

t(4;14)(p16;q32) is present in about 15% of myeloma patients and 2–6% of patients with MGUS.[44,45] It is detectable only by molecular cytogenetics due to its extreme telomeric position. Consequent to this translocation, *FGFR3* (fibroblast growth factor receptor 3) from der(14) and *MMSET* from der(4) localized in the breakpoint regions are overexpressed.[46,47] *FGFR3* is a member of fibroblast growth factor receptor tyrosine kinases. Its mutation is shown to cause constitutive activation of the receptor in neonatal thanatropic dysplasia.[48] Similarly, in myeloma with t(4;14), it is constitutively activated.[47]

The second putative oncogene in t(4;14) is *MMSET/WHSC1*. It is a candidate gene for a multiple malformation syndrome known as Wolf–Hirschhorn syndrome. Among myeloma patients with t(4;14), approximately 32% lack *FGFR3* expression, yet express *MMSET*, supporting its role in oncogenesis.[49,50]

The t(4;14) has been shown to confer a poor prognosis. Fonseca et al.[33] reported that patients in whom this translocation had been identified, using cIg-FISH, had a significantly shorter survival (26 months vs 45 months). However, Rasmussen et al. did not find any correlation between outcome and FGFR3 overexpression,[51] and FGFR3 overexpression was identified in only 74% of patients with t(4;14) by Keats et al.[50] In the latter study, t(4;14) predicted poor survival, irrespective of FGFR3 expression.

### Chromosome 16p

t(14;16)(q32;23) occurs in about 5% of myeloma.[52,53] Its breakpoint is dispersed in a region centromeric and telomeric to the candidate oncogene *c-maf*, which is shown to be overexpressed in myeloma cell lines with this particular translocation.[54]

### Chromosome 6p

The t(6;14)(p25;q32) is present in 18% of myeloma cell lines and 5% of primary myeloma tumors.[55] This translocation places the IgH locus close to the MUM1 (multiple myeloma oncogene 1)/interferon regulatory factor 4 (IRF4) gene, which is overexpressed in myeloma cell lines. MUM1/IRF4 belongs to the family of interferon regulatory factors (IRF) that regulate B-cell proliferation and differentiation, and have in vitro oncogenic activity.

### Other chromosomal partners

Other recurrent chromosome partners in switch translocation include chromosome 8q24, 1q, and 9p13, with their corresponding potential candidate oncogene *c-myc*, IRA1 and 2, and *Pax 5*. *Pax 5* acts as a transcriptional activator and repressor, and is essential in B-cell development.[56]

### Switch translocations—implication for pathogenesis

Thirty to fifty percent of multiple myeloma is preceded by MGUS. As indicated earlier, the incidence of the chromosome 14q23 translocation increases from 47% in MGUS, to 60% in intramedullary myeloma and 70–80% in plasma cell leukemia.[35,38] It occurs in the premalignant stage (MGUS) and is stable within the myeloma population of each tumor. It is proposed to be the primary translocation that initiates oncogenesis.[57] Conversely, changes such as complex *c-myc* translocations that do not occur in MGUS and tend to be heterogeneous within tumors are probably secondary/late events that contribute to disease progression.

### NUMERICAL CHANGES

Numerical changes are common in myeloma, occurring in 89–90% of cases using conventional and molecular cytogenetics.[26] They are divided into "hypodipoid/pseudodiploid" and "hyperdiploid" changes. "Hypodiploidy" is associated with a poor prognosis, and the common ones are loss of chromosomes 8, 13, 14, and X, with the most prevalent one being monosomy 13. The common "hyperdiploidy" identified by both CC and FISH includes trisomies 1, 3, 5, 7, 9 , 11 ,15 ,19, and 21.[21,58,59] Hyperdiploidy is associated with a good prognosis.

### C-myc REARRANGEMENT

*C-myc* rearrangement has been found in about 15% of myeloma and primary plasma cell leukemia in a large cohort of patients examined by interphase FISH,[60] in 50% of advanced myeloma,[61] and in 55–95% of myeloma cell lines.[60,61] Those that involve the Ig loci, i.e., t(8;14) and t(8;22), account for only 25%, with the remaining being highly complex and heterogeneous rearrangements with nonreciprocal translocations, multiple deletions, and duplications. *C-myc* rearrangements correlate with elevated $\beta_2$-microglobulin, which is a poor prognostic indicator. Its incidence in MGUS (3%) and smoldering myeloma (4%) is much lower than in active disease.[60] For these reasons, it is reasonable to suggest that the *c-myc* rearrangement is a secondary/late oncogenic event.

### OTHER MOLECULAR ABERRATIONS NOT AFFECTING THE Ig LOCI

These include chromosomes 11q and 8 rearrangements; duplication of 1q21-31; reciprocal translocation of 1q with 15p, 16p, and 5q; *p53*, N-*ras*, and K-*ras* mutation; complex translocations involving three or more chromosomes, and whole arm translocations.

Aberrations of p53, the tumor suppressor gene on chromosome 17p13, have been postulated to play a role in myeloma pathogenesis, with p53 deletions found to be a predictor of poor survival.[62] The p53 tumor suppressor gene is involved in the control of normal cellular proliferation, differentiation, and apoptosis, as well as DNA replication and repair. Although previous CC studies indicated a low frequency of p53 mutations and deletions in myeloma, 3–9%,[62] molecular cytogenetic studies have demonstrated a much higher incidence. Monoallelic deletions of chromosome 17p involving p53 have been detected by FISH in approximately one-third of newly diagnosed myeloma patients, and were also associated with reduced survival.[63] Many of these abnormalities are small interstitial deletions that are detectable only by FISH.[63] The higher frequency of p53 mutations in plasma cell leukemia and relapsed disease, as compared with myeloma at diagnosis, may indicate their role as a late molecular aberration in myeloma progression.[64]

N-*ras* and K-*ras* mutation are rare in MGUS, indolent disease, and solitary plasmacytomas, but have been reported to occur in 10–40% of patients with active disease, and even higher in advance disease. With the more sensitive allele-specific amplification method, the frequencies are higher: 55% at diagnosis and 81% at relapse.

### PROGNOSTIC SIGNIFICANCE—AN OVERVIEW

Even early CC studies demonstrated the adverse prognostic significance of abnormal karyotypes in myeloma.[65] Patients with abnormal karyotypes are more likely to have features of aggressive disease: lower hemoglobin, higher $\beta_2$-microglobulin, higher labeling index, and higher percentage of plasma cells in the marrow ($P < .0001$)[66] and, in long-term follow-up, patients with the best outcome are those with no evidence of cytogenetic abnormalities at either diagnosis or relapse.[31]

By CC, the most consistent chromosomal abnormality associated with poor prognosis is del(13q), including both complete and partial deletions.[25,27] This finding has since been confirmed in most molecular cytogenetics series.[23,29,31,33] Conventional karyotyping has also demonstrated the poor prognostic significance associated with chromosome 11q translocations, including t(11;14) translocation and reciprocal translocations with chromosomes 8, 9, and 12.[25,42] However, this was not confirmed by molecular cytogenetics.[40] The combination of aberrations of both chromosomes 11 and 13 results in a dismal outcome.[25]

The hyperdiploid group, comprising 30–40%, is usually considered to carry a favorable prognosis, whereas hypodiploidy is associated with a poor prognosis.

### EPIGENETIC EVENTS

An epigenetic event is defined as a genetic modification without alterations of DNA nucleotide sequences. Hypermethylation is an epigenetic event that is frequently associated with myeloma. It leads to the inactivation of genes, including death-associated protein kinase (*DAPK*), *SOCS1*, *p15*, and *p16*.

Hypermethylation of *p15* and *p16* was observed in 75 and 67% of one group of myeloma patients, respectively.[67] Hypermethylation of *p15* and *p16* was associated with blastic disease in myeloma, and may be causally related to plasmacytoma development.[67] Hypermethylation of *p16* was also shown to correlate with an increased proliferative rate of plasma cells, shorter survival, and poor outcome, albeit not as an independent prognostic factor.[68] In MGUS, the frequencies of *p15* and *p16* hypermethylation were similar to myeloma patients, suggesting an early genetic change rather than a late transformation event.[69]

### GENE EXPRESSION PROFILING

The unique gene expression profile of myeloma has allowed the identification of multitudes of genes that could be involved in the pathogenesis of myeloma, and that might become potential therapeutic targets. Myeloma can be distinguished accurately from normal plasma cells based on gene expression profiling of 120 genes; however, it is indistinguishable from MGUS by this approach. Myeloma can be subdivided molecularly into four groups (MM1–MM4) by an unsupervised hierarchical clustering, with the MM4 group being the highly proliferative myeloma cell lines and the MM1 group consisting of MGUS and normal plasma cells. The main difference lies in the high expression of genes involved in cell cycling and DNA metabolism in the MM4 subgroup,[70,71] and correlates

with a high incidence of karyotypic abnormalities, increased $\beta_2$-microglobulin, and increased creatinine, all of which are features of high-risk disease.

## MYELOMA MICROENVIRONMENT

Cytogenetics and molecular studies have indicated that multiple genetic events are implicated in the pathogenesis of myeloma. In particular, IgH switch translocations are proposed to be the primary event in MGUS, with additional events contributing to transformation of the malignant clone to intramedullary myeloma. During this phase, myeloma cells produce factors that create a bone marrow microenvironment that is essential for survival, growth, and differentiation. Subsequently, secondary translocations or dysregulation of oncogenes lead to growth independent of the bone marrow milieu and a clinical course that is aggressive with frequent extramedullary manifestation.

### INTERLEUKIN 6

Interleukin 6 (IL-6) is involved in the proliferation and differentiation of plasmablastic cells[72–74] into Ig-secreting mature plasma cells.[75–77] This process is also dependent on the interaction between fibronectin, produced by bone marrow stromal cells (BMCLs), and receptor VLA-4 and VLA-5 on bone marrow Ig-secreting plasma cells.[77]

In multiple myeloma, IL-6 is a major autocrine and paracrine growth factor.[78–82] This is based on in vitro and in vivo studies, which have shown that anti-IL-6 antibody almost completely inhibits proliferation of myeloma cells. Bone marrow stroma is the predominant source of IL-6 and its secretion is upregulated by transforming growth factor β, IL-1β, and IL-10, which is produced by BMCLs and myeloma cells.[83] IL-6 correlates with disease activity in plasma cell dyscrasia.[84,85] Higher levels of serum IL-6 and soluble IL-6 receptors are associated with disease progression and poor prognosis.[84–86] Soluble IL-6 receptor/IL-6 complex activates gp130 and increases the IL-6 sensitivity of myeloma cell lines.[87]

Activation of the gp130 IL-6 transducer is a key signal for myeloma proliferation. It mediates the IL-6 as well as other myeloma growth factors/cytokines including leukocyte inhibitory factor, OSM, IL-11, and CNTF.

Other cytokines interact with IL-6 and influence myeloma growth. IL-1α, IL-2, IL-4, and IL-10 induce partial differentiation of B cells to normal plasmablastic cells. Interferon alpha has differing effects on myeloma, depending on the surface receptors on myeloma cells. It stimulates IL-6-dependent proliferation in some myeloma cell lines, but prolongs the plateau phase in patients responsive to therapy. Interferon gamma is a potent inhibitor of myeloma proliferation via downregulation of IL-6 receptor complex.

## TUMOR NECROSIS FACTOR ALPHA

The major effect of tumor necrosis factor alpha (TNF-α) is stimulation of IL-6 production in BMSCs. It upregulates the adhesion molecules on myeloma and BMSCs, and hence triggers IL-6 secretion from BMSCs via activation of NF-κB.[88,89] TNF-α induces modest proliferation of myeloma cells via mitogen-activated protein kinase (MAPK)/ERK activation and not Stat3. It is possibly through the inhibition of the TNF-α pathway that proteosome inhibitors and thalidomide have their therapeutic effects. It also protects myeloma cells against drug-induced apoptosis.[90]

## VASCULAR ENDOTHELIAL GROWTH FACTOR

Neovascularization is an important pathogenetic factor of myeloma. Increased bone marrow angiogensis correlates with disease progression.[18,91–98] Vascular endothelial growth factor (VEGF) plays an important role in neovascularization of myeloma. It regulates endothelial cell function, vessel budding, and tube formation. In particular, it stimulates migration and proliferation of myeloma cells in an autocrine and paracrine loop.[99]

VEGF is produced by myeloma cells and BMCLs that are adhered to myeloma cells. It also augments the secretion of IL-6 by BMCLs.

## INSULIN GROWTH FACTOR-I

Insulin growth factor is an autocrine growth factor and migratory factor of myeloma cells. It activates predominantly the phosphoinositol 3-kinase (PI-3K) signaling pathway, with some contribution to the MAPK pathway. It stimulates proliferation, inhibits apoptosis, and enhances migration through endothelial cells and BMCLs.[100–102]

## MACROPHAGE INFLAMMATORY PROTEIN-1 ALPHA

Macrophage inflammatory protein-1 alpha (MIP-1α) is a chemokine that belongs to the RANTES (regulated on activation, normal T expressed and secreted) family of chemokines. Its role in myeloma lytic lesions is well described. More recently, it is shown that it has been correlated with tumor burden and survival in myeloma patients.[103,104]

## REFERENCE

1. Robillard N, et al.: CD20 is associated with a small mature plasma cell morphology and t(11;14) in multiple myeloma. *Blood* 102(3):1070–1071, 2003.
2. International Myeloma Working Group: Criteria for the classification of monoclonal gammopathies, multiple myeloma and related disorders: a report of the International Myeloma Working Group. *Br J Haematol* 121(5):749–757, 2003.
3. Greipp PR, et al.: Plasmablastic morphology—an independent prognostic factor with clinical and laboratory correlates: Eastern Cooperative Oncology Group (ECOG) myeloma trial E9486 report by the ECOG Myeloma Laboratory Group. *Blood* 91(7):2501–2507, 1998.
4. Bartl R, et al.: Bone marrow histology and serum beta 2 microglobulin in multiple myeloma—a new prognostic strategy. *Eur J Haematol Suppl* 51:88–98, 1989.
5. Schambeck CM, et al.: Characterization of myeloma cells by means of labeling index, bone marrow histology, and serum beta 2-microglobulin. *Am J Clin Pathol* 106(1):64–68, 1996.
6. Peest D, et al.: Prognostic value of clinical, laboratory, and histological characteristics in multiple myeloma: improved definition of risk groups. *Eur J Cancer* 29A(7):978–983, 1993.
7. Bartl R, Frisch B: Bone marrow histology in multiple myeloma: prognostic relevance of histologic characteristics. *Hematol Rev* 3:87–108, 1989.
8. San Miguel JF, et al.: Immunophenotypic evaluation of the plasma cell compartment in multiple myeloma: a tool for comparing the efficacy of different treatment strategies and predicting outcome. *Blood* 99(5): 1853–1856, 2002.
9. Ocqueteau M, et al.: Immunophenotypic characterization of plasma cells from monoclonal gammopathy of undetermined significance patients. Implications for the differential diagnosis between MGUS and multiple myeloma. *Am J Pathol* 152(6):1655–1665, 1998.
10. Ocqueteau M, et al.: Expression of the CD117 antigen (c-Kit) on normal and myelomatous plasma cells. *Br J Haematol* 95(3):489–493, 1996.
11. Rawstron AC, et al.: Circulating plasma cells in multiple myeloma: characterization and correlation with disease stage [see comment]. *Br J Haematol* 97(1):46–55, 1997.
12. Joshua D, et al.: The labelling index of primitive plasma cells determines the clinical behaviour of patients with myelomatosis [see comment]. *Br J Haematol* 94(1):76–81, 1996.
13. Pope B, et al.: The functional phenotype of the primitive plasma cell in patients with multiple myeloma correlates with the clinical state. *Leuk Lymphoma* 27(1–2): 83–91, 1997.
14. Bakkus MH, et al.: The clonogenic precursor cell in multiple myeloma. *Leuk Lymphoma* 18(3–4):221–229, 1995.
15. Bakkus MH, et al.: Evidence that multiple myeloma Ig heavy chain VDJ genes contain somatic mutations but show no intraclonal variation. *Blood* 80(9):2326–2335, 1992.
16. Ralph QM, et al.: Advancement of multiple myeloma from diagnosis through plateau phase to progression does not involve a new B-cell clone: evidence from the Ig heavy chain gene. *Blood* 82(1):202–206, 1993.
17. Bakkus MH, et al.: Evidence that the clonogenic cell in multiple myeloma originates from a pre-switched but somatically mutated B cell. *Br J Haematol* 87(1):68–74, 1994.
18. Vescio RA, et al.: Myeloma Ig heavy chain V region sequences reveal prior antigenic selection and marked

somatic mutation but no intraclonal diversity. *J Immunol* 155(5):2487–2497, 1995.

19. Taylor BJ, et al.: Intraclonal homogeneity of clonotypic immunoglobulin M and diversity of nonclinical post-switch isotypes in multiple myeloma: insights into the evolution of the myeloma clone. *Clin Cancer Res* 8(2):502–513, 2002.

20. Matsui W, et al.: Characterization of clonogenic multiple myeloma cells. *Blood* 103(6):2332–2336, 2004.

21. Lai JL, et al.: Improved cytogenetics in multiple myeloma: a study of 151 patients including 117 patients at diagnosis. *Blood* 85(9):2490–2497, 1995.

22. Avet-Louseau H, et al.: Chromosome 13 abnormalities in multiple myeloma are mostly monosomy 13. *Br J Haematol* 111(4):1116–1117, 2000.

23. Konigsberg R, et al.: Predictive role of interphase cytogenetics for survival of patients with multiple myeloma. *J Clin Oncol* 18(4):804–812, 2000.

24. Fonseca R, et al.: The t(4;14)(p16.3;q32) is strongly associated with chromosome 13 abnormalities in both multiple myeloma and monoclonal gammopathy of undetermined significance [see comment]. *Blood* 98(4):1271–1272, 2001.

25. Tricot G, et al.: Poor prognosis in multiple myeloma is associated only with partial or complete deletions of chromosome 13 or abnormalities involving 11q and not with other karyotype abnormalities. *Blood* 86(11):4250–4256, 1995.

26. Perez-Simon JA, et al.: Prognostic value of numerical chromosome aberrations in multiple myeloma: a FISH analysis of 15 different chromosomes. *Blood* 91(9):3366–3371, 1998.

27. Zojer N, et al.: Deletion of 13q14 remains an independent adverse prognostic variable in multiple myeloma despite its frequent detection by interphase fluorescence in situ hybridization. *Blood* 95(6):1925–1930, 2000.

28. Fonseca R, et al.: Deletions of chromosome 13 in multiple myeloma identified by interphase FISH usually denote large deletions of the q arm or monosomy. *Leukemia* 15(6):981–986, 2001.

29. Facon T, et al.: Chromosome 13 abnormalities identified by FISH analysis and serum beta2-microglobulin produce a powerful myeloma staging system for patients receiving high-dose therapy. *Blood* 97(6):1566–1571, 2001.

30. Fassas AB, et al.: Both hypodiploidy and deletion of chromosome 13 independently confer poor prognosis in multiple myeloma. *Br J Haematol* 118(4):1041–1047, 2002.

31. Shaughnessy J Jr, et al.: Prognostic impact of cytogenetic and interphase fluorescence in situ hybridization-defined chromosome 13 deletion in multiple myeloma: early results of total therapy II. *Br J Haematol* 120(1):44–52, 2003.

32. Kaufmann H, et al.: Both chromosome 13 abnormalities by metaphase cytogenetics and deletion of 13q by interphase FISH only are prognostically relevant in multiple myeloma. *Eur J Haematol* 71(3):179–183, 2003.

33. Fonseca R, et al.: Clinical and biologic implications of recurrent genomic aberrations in myeloma. *Blood* 101(11):4569–4575, 2003.

34. Sawyer JR, et al.: Identification of new nonrandom translocations in multiple myeloma with multicolor spectral karyotyping. *Blood* 92(11):4269–4278, 1998.

35. Avet-Loiseau H, et al.: 14q32 translocations and monosomy 13 observed in monoclonal gammopathy of undetermined significance delineate a multistep process for the oncogenesis of multiple myeloma. Intergroupe Francophone du Myelome. *Cancer Res* 59(18):4546–4550, 1999.

36. Fonseca R, et al.: Genomic abnormalities in monoclonal gammopathy of undetermined significance [see comment]. *Blood* 100(4):1417–1424, 2002.

37. Moreau P, et al.: Recurrent 14q32 translocations determine the prognosis of multiple myeloma, especially in patients receiving intensive chemotherapy. *Blood* 100(5):1579–1583, 2002.

38. Avet-Loiseau H, et al.: Cytogenetic, interphase, and multicolor fluorescence in situ hybridization analyses in primary plasma cell leukemia: a study of 40 patients at diagnosis, on behalf of the Intergroupe Francophone du Myelome and the Groupe Francais de Cytogenetique Hematologique. *Blood* 97(3):822–825, 2001.

39. Avet-Loiseau H, et al.: Oncogenesis of multiple myeloma: 14q32 and 13q chromosomal abnormalities are not randomly distributed, but correlate with natural history, immunological features, and clinical presentation. *Blood* 99(6):2185–2191, 2002.

40. Avet-Loiseau H, et al.: High incidence of translocations t(11;14)(q13;q32) and t(4;14)(p16;q32) in patients with plasma cell malignancies. *Cancer Res* 58(24):5640–5645, 1998.

41. Ronchetti D, et al.: Molecular analysis of 11q13 breakpoints in multiple myeloma. *Blood* 93(4):1330–1337, 1999.

42. Fonseca R, et al.: Multiple myeloma and the translocation t(11;14)(q13;q32): a report on 13 cases. *Br J Haematol* 101(2):296–301, 1998.

43. Garand R, et al.: t(11;14) and t(4;14) translocations correlated with mature lymphoplasmacytoid and immature morphology, respectively, in multiple myeloma [see comment]. *Leukemia* 17(10):2032–2035, 2003.

44. Avet-Loiseau H, et al.: Monosomy 13 is associated with the transition of monoclonal gammopathy of undetermined significance to multiple myeloma. Intergroupe Francophone du Myelome. *Blood* 94(8):2583–2589, 1999.

45. Malgeri U, et al.: Detection of t(4;14)(p16.3;q32) chromosomal translocation in multiple myeloma by reverse transcription-polymerase chain reaction analysis of IGH-MMSET fusion transcripts. *Cancer Res* 60(15):4058–4061, 2000.

46. Richelda R, et al.: A novel chromosomal translocation t(4; 14)(p16.3; q32) in multiple myeloma involves the fibroblast growth-factor receptor 3 gene [see comment]. *Blood* 90(10):4062–4070, 1997.

47. Chesi M, et al.: Frequent translocation t(4;14)(p16.3;q32.3) in multiple myeloma is associated with increased expression and activating mutations of fibroblast growth factor receptor 3. *Nat Genet* 16(3):260–264, 1997.

48. Webster MK, et al.: Profound ligand-independent kinase activation of fibroblast growth factor receptor 3

by the activation loop mutation responsible for a lethal skeletal dysplasia, thanatophoric dysplasia type II. *Mol Cell Biol* 16(8):4081–4087, 1996.

49. Santra M, et al.: A subset of multiple myeloma harboring the t(4;14)(p16;q32) translocation lacks FGFR3 expression but maintains an IGH/MMSET fusion transcript. *Blood* 101(6):2374–2376, 2003.

50. Keats JJ, et al.: In multiple myeloma, t(4;14)(p16;q32) is an adverse prognostic factor irrespective of FGFR3 expression. *Blood* 101(4):1520–1529, 2003.

51. Rasmussen T, et al.: FGFR3 dysregulation and clinical outcome in myeloma [see comment]. *Br J Haematol* 120(1):166, 2003.

52. Sawyer JR, et al.: Multicolour spectral karyotyping identifies new translocations and a recurring pathway for chromosome loss in multiple myeloma. *Br J Haematol* 112(1):167–174, 2001.

53. Sawyer JR, et al.: Jumping translocations of chromosome 1q in multiple myeloma: evidence for a mechanism involving decondensation of pericentromeric heterochromatin. *Blood* 91(5):1732–1741, 1998.

54. Chesi M, et al.: Frequent dysregulation of the c-maf proto-oncogene at 16q23 by translocation to an Ig locus in multiple myeloma. *Blood* 91(12):4457–4463, 1998.

55. Shaughnessy J Jr, et al.: Cyclin D3 at 6p21 is dysregulated by recurrent chromosomal translocations to immunoglobulin loci in multiple myeloma. *Blood* 98(1):217–223, 2001.

56. Emelyanov AV, et al.: The interaction of Pax5 (BSAP) with Daxx can result in transcriptional activation in B cells. *J Biol Chem* 277(13):11156–11164, 2002.

57. Bergsagel PL, Kuehl WM: Chromosome translocations in multiple myeloma. *Oncogene* 20(40):5611–5622, 2001.

58. Calasanz MJ, et al.: Cytogenetic analysis of 280 patients with multiple myeloma and related disorders: primary breakpoints and clinical correlations. *Genes Chromosomes Cancer* 18(2):84–93, 1997.

59. Sawyer JR, et al.: Cytogenetic findings in 200 patients with multiple myeloma. *Cancer Genet Cytogenet* 82(1):41–49, 1995.

60. Avet-Loiseau H, et al.: Rearrangements of the *c-myc* oncogene are present in 15% of primary human multiple myeloma tumors. *Blood* 98(10):3082–3086, 2001.

61. Shou Y MM, Gabrea A, et al.: Diverse karyotypic abnormalities of the c-myc locus associated with c-myc dysregulation and tumour progression in multiple myeloma. *Proc Natl Acad Sci USA* 97:228–233, 2000.

62. Preudhomme C, et al.: Rare occurrence of P53 gene mutations in multiple myeloma. *Br J Haematol* 81(3):440–443, 1992.

63. Drach J, et al.: Presence of a p53 gene deletion in patients with multiple myeloma predicts for short survival after conventional-dose chemotherapy. *Blood* 92(3):802–809, 1998.

64. Neri A, et al.: p53 gene mutations in multiple myeloma are associated with advanced forms of malignancy. *Blood* 81(1):128–135, 1993.

65. Seong C, et al.: Prognostic value of cytogenetics in multiple myeloma. *Br J Haematol* 101(1):189–194, 1998.

66. Debes-Marun CS, et al.: Chromosome abnormalities clustering and its implications for pathogenesis and prognosis in myeloma [see comment]. *Leukemia* 17(2):427–436, 2003.

67. Ng MH, et al.: Frequent hypermethylation of p16 and p15 genes in multiple myeloma. *Blood* 89(7):2500–2506, 1997.

68. Mateos MV, et al.: Methylation is an inactivating mechanism of the p16 gene in multiple myeloma associated with high plasma cell proliferation and short survival. *Br J Haematol* 118(4):1034–1040, 2002.

69. Guillerm G, et al.: p16(INK4a) and p15(INK4b) gene methylations in plasma cells from monoclonal gammopathy of undetermined significance. *Blood* 98(1):244–246, 2001.

70. Zhan F, et al.: Global gene expression profiling of multiple myeloma, monoclonal gammopathy of undetermined significance, and normal bone marrow plasma cells [see comment]. *Blood* 99(5):1745–1757, 2002.

71. Tarte K, et al.: Gene expression profiling of plasma cells and plasmablasts: toward a better understanding of the late stages of B-cell differentiation. *Blood* 102(2):592–600, 2003.

72. Jourdan M, et al.: Constitutive production of interleukin-6 and immunologic features in cardiac myxomas. *Arthritis Rheum* 33(3):398–402, 1990.

73. Suematsu S, et al.: IgG1 plasmacytosis in interleukin 6 transgenic mice. *Proc Natl Acad Sci USA* 86(19):7547–7551, 1989.

74. Suematsu S, et al.: Generation of plasmacytomas with the chromosomal translocation t(12;15) in interleukin 6 transgenic mice. *Proc Natl Acad Sci U S A* 89(1):232–235, 1992.

75. Vernino L, et al.: Generation of nondividing high rate Ig-secreting plasma cells in cultures of human B cells stimulated with anti-CD3-activated T cells. *J Immunol* 148(2):404–410, 1992.

76. Roldan E, et al.: Cytokine network regulating terminal maturation of human bone marrow B cells capable of spontaneous and high rate Ig secretion in vitro. *J Immunol* 149(7):2367–2371, 1992.

77. Roldan E, Garcia-Pardo A, Brieva JA: VLA-4-fibronectin interaction is required for the terminal differentiation of human bone marrow cells capable of spontaneous and high rate immunoglobulin secretion. *J Exp Med* 175(6):1739–1747, 1992.

78. Sonneveld P, Schoester M, de Leeuw K: In vitro Ig-synthesis and proliferative activity in multiple myeloma are stimulated by different growth factors. *Br J Haematol* 79(4):589–594, 1991.

79. Tanabe O, et al.: BSF-2/IL-6 does not augment Ig secretion but stimulates proliferation in myeloma cells. *Am J Hematol* 31(4):258–262, 1989.

80. Zhang XG, Klein B, Bataille R: Interleukin-6 is a potent myeloma-cell growth factor in patients with aggressive multiple myeloma. *Blood* 74(1):11–13, 1989.

81. Klein B, et al.: Paracrine rather than autocrine regulation of myeloma-cell growth and differentiation by interleukin-6. *Blood* 73(2):517–526, 1989.

82. Herrmann F, et al.: Interleukin-4 inhibits growth of multiple myelomas by suppressing interleukin-6 expression [retraction in *Blood* 93(10):3573, 1999 May 15]. *Blood* 78(8):2070–2074, 1991.

83. Urashima M, et al.: Transforming growth factor-beta1: differential effects on multiple myeloma versus normal B cells. *Blood* 87(5):1928–1938, 1996.

84. Bataille R, et al.: Serum levels of interleukin 6, a potent myeloma cell growth factor, as a reflect of disease severity in plasma cell dyscrasias. *J Clin Invest* 84(6): 2008–2011, 1989.

85. Reibnegger G, et al.: Predictive value of interleukin-6 and neopterin in patients with multiple myeloma. *Cancer Res* 51(23 pt 1):6250–6253, 1991.

86. Griepp PR, G.J., Kalish LA, Oken MM, Miller AM, Kyle RA, Klein B: Independent prognostic value for serum soluble interleukin-6 receptor (sIL-6R) in Eastern Cooperative Oncology Group (ECOG) myeloma trial E9487. *Proc Am Soc Clin Oncol* 12:404, 1993.

87. Gaillard JP, et al.: Increased and highly stable levels of functional soluble interleukin-6 receptor in sera of patients with monoclonal gammopathy. *Eur J Immunol* 23(4):820–824, 1993.

88. Chauhan D, et al.: Multiple myeloma cell adhesion-induced interleukin-6 expression in bone marrow stromal cells involves activation of NF-kappa B. *Blood* 87(3):1104–1112, 1996.

89. Hideshima T, et al.: The role of tumor necrosis factor alpha in the pathophysiology of human multiple myeloma: therapeutic applications. *Oncogene* 20(33):4519–4527, 2001.

90. Damiano JS, et al.: Cell adhesion mediated drug resistance (CAM-DR): role of integrins and resistance to apoptosis in human myeloma cell lines. *Blood* 93(5):1658–1667, 1999.

91. Vacca A, et al.: Bone marrow angiogenesis and progression in multiple myeloma. *Br J Haematol* 87(3):503–508, 1994.

92. Vacca A, et al.: Bone marrow neovascularization, plasma cell angiogenic potential, and matrix metalloproteinase-2 secretion parallel progression of human multiple myeloma. *Blood* 93(9):3064–3073, 1999.

93. Ribatti D, et al.: Bone marrow angiogenesis and mast cell density increase simultaneously with progression of human multiple myeloma. *Br J Cancer* 79(3–4): 451–455, 1999.

94. Xu JL, et al.: Proliferation, apoptosis, and intratumoral vascularity in multiple myeloma: correlation with the clinical stage and cytological grade. *J Clin Pathol* 55(7): 530–534, 2002.

95. Rajkumar SV, et al.: Prognostic value of bone marrow angiogenesis in multiple myeloma. *Clin Cancer Res* 6(8):3111–3116, 2000.

96. Rajkumar SV, Kyle RA: Angiogenesis in multiple myeloma. *Semin Oncol* 28(6):560–564, 2001.

97. Pruneri G, et al.: Microvessel density, a surrogate marker of angiogenesis, is significantly related to survival in multiple myeloma patients. *Br J Haematol* 118(3):817–820, 2002.

98. Moehler TM, et al.: Angiogenesis in hematologic malignancies. *Ann Hematol* 80(12):695–705, 2001.

99. Podar K, et al.: Vascular endothelial growth factor triggers signaling cascades mediating multiple myeloma cell growth and migration. *Blood* 98(2):428–435, 2001.

100. Qiang YW, Kopantzev E, Rudikoff S: Insulinlike growth factor-I signaling in multiple myeloma: downstream elements, functional correlates, and pathway cross-talk. *Blood* 99(11):4138–4146, 2002.

101. Qiang YW, et al.: Insulin-like growth factor I induces migration and invasion of human multiple myeloma cells. *Blood* 103(1):301–308, 2004.

102. Georgii-Hemming P, et al.: Insulin-like growth factor I is a growth and survival factor in human multiple myeloma cell lines. *Blood* 88(6):2250–2258, 1996.

103. Choi SJ, et al.: Macrophage inflammatory protein 1-alpha is a potential osteoclast stimulatory factor in multiple myeloma. *Blood* 96(2):671–675, 2000.

104. Terpos E, et al.: Serum levels of macrophage inflammatory protein-1 alpha (MIP-1alpha) correlate with the extent of bone disease and survival in patients with multiple myeloma. *Br J Haematol* 123(1):106–109, 2003.

# Chapter 82

# CLINICAL FEATURES AND MAKING THE DIAGNOSIS OF MULTIPLE MYELOMA

## Yi-Hsiang Chen

Multiple myeloma is, with rare exceptions, a systemic disease. The neoplastic plasma cells cause various organ dysfunctions through tumor cell invasion and, more importantly, through the pathologic effects of the monoclonal immunoglobulins (Ig) and/or free Ig light chains. In addition, myeloma cells secrete, and stimulate normal stromal cells in the bone marrow microenvironment to secrete, a host of cytokines that mediate various biologic effects. Thus, patients with multiple myeloma may exhibit an array of clinical manifestations.

## PRESENTING FEATURES

Despite increasing awareness of this disease entity and advances in the diagnostic technology that have led to early diagnosis, the major presenting features in most patients remain remarkably consistent. Table 82.1 summarizes the initial findings in groups of patients seen at various periods of time in the last three to four decades.[1-3] The findings in a small group of young and older patients are also included for comparison.[4,5] The most frequent presentations are symptoms arising from myeloma involvement of bone and the bone marrow.

### BONE PAIN

Bone pain is the most frequent presenting symptom. It may precede the diagnosis for months. It most commonly begins in the back and lower chest, less often in the ribs or extremities. Back pain is usually insidious, and is aggravated by weight bearing and movement. Acute exacerbation of back pain often occurs with compression fractures of the vertebrae. The chest pain from rib lesions is generally mild, aggravated by movement and position, but may be pleuritic and associated with dyspnea, particularly when rib fracture or pleural effusion develops. Bone pain may become severe when pathologic fracture occurs spontaneously or with trivial trauma. Physical examination may illicit bone tenderness of the affected regions. Radicular pain

and paresthesia along the dermatome distribution may precede the onset of motor weakness or loss of sphincter control from spinal cord or nerve root compression, and are important warning signs to look for clinically.

### SYSTEMIC SYMPTOMS AND SIGNS

Weakness, fatigue, anorexia, palpitation, and dyspnea on exertion are common symptoms of anemia. The onset is insidious. The symptoms are generally mild, but worsen with the development of renal insufficiency. Symptoms of renal failure may supervene, including periorbital and dependent edema. In *hypercalcemic* patients, nausea, vomiting, constipation, polyuria, polydipsia, headache, and lethargy may develop.

### FEVER AND INFECTION

Fever from myeloma occurs in <1% of patients.[1,2] Its presence demands workup for infection. Infection occurs in about 10% of patients, but the incidence almost doubles in those older than 75 years.[5] Recurrent pneumonia, sinusitis, and urinary tract infections may precede the diagnosis. In untreated patients with infection, Gram-positive organisms predominate.

### RENAL FAILURE

Renal insufficiency (serum creatinine >2 mg/dL) is present in 20–30% of patients at diagnosis.[1-7] This may be an underestimation. In a study of more than 1300 newly diagnosed patients, the frequency of renal failure increased from 31 to 49%, when the creatinine clearance was also measured.[6] Renal failure affected 24% of patients with IgG, 31% with IgA, 100% with IgD, and 52% with light-chain myeloma. Advanced age, late disease stage, heavy light-chain proteinuria, and hypercalcemia were identified as risk factors.[6] Occasionally, severe acute renal failure is the first manifestation of myeloma. This is often precipitated by confounding events, such as dehydration, infection, and hypercalcemia.[8-10] Over the course of the disease,

| Table 82.1 | Changing presenting features in multiple myeloma | | | | | |
| --- | --- | --- | --- | --- | --- | --- |
| Clinical features | 1960–71 (1)[a] | 1985–98 (2) | 1972–86 (3) | 1987–90 (3) | Age <40 (4) | Age >75 (5) |
| *Symptoms* | | | | | | |
| Bone pain | 68% | 58 | 60 | 37 | 66 | 62 |
| Weakness, fatigue | – | 32 | 65 | 42 | 33 | – |
| Infection | 12 | – | 10 | 12 | 11 | 20 |
| Hemorrhage | 7 | – | 4 | 2 | – | – |
| *Signs* | | | | | | |
| Hepatomegaly | 21 | 4 | 30 | 32 | <5 | – |
| Splenomegaly | 5 | 1 | 3 | 2 | <5 | – |
| Lymphadenopathy | 4 | 1 | 4 | 1 | <5 | – |
| *Laboratory findings* | | | | | | |
| Anemia (Hb <12 g/dL) | 62 | 73 | 61 | 39 | 60 | 32 (≤10 g/dL) |
| Leukopenia (<4000/μL) | 16 | 20 | 5 | 7 | 18 | 28 (<2, 500/mL) |
| Thrombocytopenia (<100,000/μL) | 13 | 5 | 11 | 3 | 4 | 5 |
| Hypercalcemia | 30 | 28 | 20 | 18 | 30 | 17 |
| Creatinine >2mg/dL | 30 | 19 | 14 | 10 | 29 | 35 |
| *Previous MGUS* | – | 20 | – | – | – | – |
| *Incidental diagnosis* | – | – | 14 | 34 | – | – |

[a]Numbers in parentheses in the first row indicate references.

over 50% of patients will develop renal failure from myeloma. Renal failure may also be due to hypertension, diabetes, or other comorbid conditions in older patients. Detailed urinalysis is required to differentiate various forms of myeloma renal diseases. Myeloma cells may be detected in the urine sediment.[11]

### LESS COMMON PRESENTATIONS

Bleeding manifestations and symptoms related to polyneuropathy, hyperviscosity, and amyloidosis are present occasionally at diagnosis.

## CLINICAL MANIFESTATIONS AND PATHOPHYSIOLOGY

Multiple myeloma may involve practically every organ system. Myeloma cells, originating from postgerminal center B lymphocytes (see Chapter 81), proliferate primarily in the bone marrow microenvironment. Thus, hematopoietic tissues and the skeletal system are uniformly affected at the earliest stage of disease.

### BLOOD AND BONE MARROW CHANGES

Anemia is present in 60–80% of patients at presentation.[1–5] It is usually mild to moderate in severity and is normocytic, normochromic in morphology. The anemia has the characteristics of anemia of chronic inflammation (formerly anemia of chronic disease) with low serum iron, decreased transferrin saturation, and elevated ferritin. The reticulocyte count is low, reflecting a hypoproliferative state. A bone marrow examination commonly reveals erythroid hypoplasia and a varying

degree of myeloma cell infiltration. The pathogenetic mechanisms of anemia in myeloma are beginning to be elucidated. Inflammatory cytokines, including interleukin-1 (IL-1), tumor necrosis factors (TNFs), and IL-6, often elevated in myeloma patients, suppress hematopoiesis.[12] Within the bone marrow microenvironment, myeloma cells, expressing high levels of cell surface Fas-L and TNF-related apoptosis-including ligand (TRAIL), induce apoptosis of the surrounding immature erythroblasts by binding to the respective death receptors on erythroblasts.[13] The increased level of IL-6 induces excessive hepatic production of hepcidin, which inhibits the intestinal iron absorption and release of iron from reticuloendothelial cells, thus interfering with the iron use.[14] In addition, inappropriate erythropoietin response, seen in 25% of patients (and more often as the disease progresses), contributes to the development of anemia, which frequently responds to erythropoietin treatment.[15,16] In addition to inflammatory cytokines, hyperviscosity may be a cause of the blunted erythropoietin response.[12,17] Finally, in some patients, the degree of anemia is accentuated because of an expanded plasma volume,[18] which in turn is likely a consequence of an increased level of IL-6.[19]

Severe anemia can occur particularly in patients who have renal failure. Macrocytic anemia with an elevated mean corpuscular volume is seen in up to 20% of patients.[20] A few patients may have concomitant folate or vitamin $B_{12}$ deficiencies, but most have macrocytosis of unknown cause.[20] On the other hand, microcytic, iron-deficiency anemia can develop from gastrointestinal (GI) bleeding in patients who have amyloid involvement of the GI tract. RBC rouleaux formation and high erythrocyte sedimentation rate are characteristically seen in patients with high monoclonal protein. Rarely, Howell–Jolly bodies may be present in patients with massive amyloid infiltration of the spleen.

Leukopenia and thrombocytopenia occur in 10–15% of patients at diagnosis. In some, thrombocytosis develops, presumably from the thrombopoietic effect of IL-6.[1,2,21] This occurs more often in patients with osteosclerotic myeloma. Occasional plasma cells or plasmacytoid lymphocytes can be seen in the peripheral blood smear. A marked increase in plasma cells, 20% of leukocytes or ≥2000/μL, is seen in rare cases of primary plasma cell leukemia and more commonly in the terminal phase of myeloma.[22]

The bone marrow shows myeloma cell infiltration that varies from 10% to total replacement. Myeloma cells are morphologically monomorphic with large, round nuclei and an open chromatin pattern. This is in contrast to reactive plasmacytosis, in which a heterogeneous population of plasma/plasmacytoid cells with variously sized nuclei and condensed chromatin is seen. In some cases, plasmablastic morphology may predominate and predicts a poorer outcome.[23] On the bone marrow section, the pattern of myeloma cell infiltration may be diffuse, interstitial, or focal. These patterns appear to be of prognostic significance.[24] Some degree of fibrosis, unaccompanied by characteristic features of myeloid metaplasia, is found in up to 10% of patients but has no apparent effect on the clinical course of disease.[24,25] With special staining, increased microvascular density can be seen in patients with advanced disease and is a poor prognostic factor.[26]

### BLOOD CHEMISTRIES

Abnormalities in blood chemistries reflect various organ dysfunctions and metabolic derangements and include elevated blood urea nitrogen, serum creatinine, calcium, and hepatic enzymes. Serum albumin level is often depressed consequent to specific transcriptional down-regulation of the albumin gene by IL-6 and other inflammatory cytokines.[27,28] The severity of hypoalbuminemia, correlated with the stage of disease, is an important prognostic factor.[29] C-reactive protein, a surrogate marker for IL-6, and β$_2$-microglobulin, a marker for myeloma tumor load, are increased in some patients.[30] Elevated levels of serum lactic dehydrogenase, seen in 11% of untreated patients and more frequently in patients with high tumor mass, predict for chemoresistance and a shorter survival.[31] A large amount of paraprotein in the serum causes reduced anion gap, "spurious" hyponatremia, and rarely, "spurious" hypercalcemia due to the binding of calcium by paraproteins.[32]

### HEMOSTATIC DEFECTS

Prothrombin time and partial thromboplastin time are generally normal. A prolonged thrombin time, however, is the most frequent abnormal coagulation finding in patients with myeloma.[33] It is occasionally associated with bleeding diathesis, manifested as epistaxis, ecchymosis, hematoma, or postsurgical bleeding, but more often it is asymptomatic. The underlying cause is the interference of fibrin monomer polymerization by paraproteins.[34,35] A heparin-like anticoagulant, unrelated to monoclonal protein, was also reported in some patients.[36] Rarely, specific inhibitors to coagulation factors, such as factor VIII, and reduced plasma concentration of fibrinogen, factors II, V, VII, VIII, X, and XI were reported.[33,37] Acquired factor X deficiency, due to absorption and rapid clearance of factor X by the amyloid fibrils, was seen in a few patients with amyloid light chain (AL) amyloidosis.[38] Bleeding time may be prolonged, and platelet aggregation, adhesion, and platelet factor III activity may be reduced, possibly from the coating of paraprotein on platelet surface. This abnormality is clinically significant in patients with paraprotein concentration in excess of 5 g/dL.[39] Rarely, an acquired von Willebrand syndrome may develop. Monoclonal proteins either bind to von Willebrand factor itself, or interfere with its binding to platelet glycoprotein, or inhibit the binding of fibrinogen to platelets.[40,41]

### MYELOMA BONE DISEASE AND HYPERCALCEMIA

Hypercalcemia occurs in 20–30% of patients at diagnosis, often in association with skeletal system involvement. In a recent large series, radiographs at diagnosis were abnormal in 79% of patients, with discrete lytic lesions in 66% and diffuse osteoporosis in 22%. Osteosclerotic lesions occurred in about 0.5% of patients and are associated with POEMS syndrome in some patients.[2,42]

### MYELOMA RENAL DISEASES

The renal failure in myeloma may take one of several forms (Table 82.2) and is often multifactorial in an individual patient. Specific myeloma-related processes affect renal tubular and/or glomerular functions. Direct invasion of renal parenchyma by myeloma cells occurs rarely and mostly in the terminal phase of the disease.

### TUBULAR DYSFUNCTION

Free light chains (Bence Jones protein) play a crucial role in causing renal damage in myeloma patients. The nephrotoxicity of certain light chains has previously been demonstrated. Incubation of light chain with renal cortical tissue slides inhibited organic ion trans-

| Table 82.2 | Renal dysfunctions |
| --- | --- |
| Reversible | Irreversible (mostly) |
| Volume depletion | Myeloma cast nephropathy |
| Hypercalcemia | Renal amyloidosis |
| Hyperuricemia | Immunoglobulin deposition |
| Renal tubular acidosis | diseases |
| Hyperviscosity syndrome | Myeloma cell infiltration |
| Pyelonephritis | |

port, gluconeogenesis, and ammonia formation,[43] while microperfusion of nephrons with light chain isolated from myeloma patients with renal failure, but not those with normal renal function, led to obstruction of the distal tubules and cast formation.[44] Furthermore, intraperitoneal injection of light chains from myeloma patients with a variety of renal lesions reproduced similar lesions in mice in 22 of 27 cases. Light chains from patients without renal disease were much less likely (4/13) to induce renal lesions.[45] Thus, the properties of any particular light chain dictate the nature of renal damage in myeloma renal diseases.

### Myeloma cast nephropathy

Myeloma cast nephropathy (MCN) is the most common form of myeloma renal disease and frequently progresses to chronic renal failure. It is often precipitated by dehydration, hypercalcemia, and use of diuretics or nonsteroidal anti-inflammatory drugs, all causing a reduction in glomerular filtration. Renal failure is reversible in about 50% of patients.[8–10,46] The physical basis for light-chain nephrotoxicity has not been elucidated. The initial finding that the isoelectric point of light chain was the determinant for its nephrotoxicity has not been confirmed.[45,47] Nevertheless, coprecipitation of light chain and Tamm-Horsfall protein in distal tubules leads to obstructing cast formation, tubular atrophy, disruption of the basement membrane, interstitial inflammation and fibrosis and eventually nephrosclerosis, all features characteristic of "myeloma kidney".[46,48]

### Acquired Fanconi syndrome

Acquired Fanconi syndrome occurs rarely. It may precede overt myeloma for years.[46,49] Patients may have azotemia and various degrees of proteinuria, glycosuria, aminoaciduria, and phosphaturia. On renal biopsy, the damaged proximal tubular cells show atrophic changes and contain crystalline cytoplasmic inclusions without overt lesions of cast nephropathy. This syndrome is almost always associated with κ light-chain proteinuria. Recent analysis of light chains in these patients showed a preferential involvement of Vκ1 subgroup of limited germline origin. This light-chain V domain contains unusual hydrophobic sequences that are resistant to proteolysis by lysosomal cathepsin B. The accumulation of indigestible nephrotoxic light chains in proximal tubular cells provides a plausible explanation for the functional impairment.[50]

### Distal tubular dysfunction

Distal tubular dysfunction with impairment in urinary acidification and concentration may occur as a part of renal failure or rarely as an isolated defect.[46,49]

## GLOMERULAR DYSFUNCTION

### Monoclonal immunoglobulin deposition disease

Direct deposition of monoclonal light chain and/or, more rarely, fragments of heavy chain may lead to renal failure in myeloma patients.[51–53] Renal biopsy reveals nodular sclerosing glomerulopathy. Glomeruli are enlarged with a diffuse and nodular expansion of the mesangial matrix, with little thickening in glomerular basement membrane (GBM). Variable degrees of tubular basement membrane (TBM) thickening, tubular atrophy, and interstitial fibrosis are also present. Immunofluorescent staining shows linear monoclonal light-chain deposit in GBM and TBM in light-chain deposition disease (LCDD). In heavy-chain deposition disease (HCDD) or mixed light/heavy-chain disease (LHCDD), heavy-chain fragment and complement deposits are also present. In about 80% of LCDD, the light chain is of κ isotype.[54] Both κ and λ are seen in HCDD, while CH1 constant domain appears to be deleted in the deposits of heavy-chain fragment.[55] Commonly, a mixed picture of LCDD and MCN is present. Compared with MCN, monoclonal immunoglobulin deposition disease (MIDD) is more likely to lead to nephrotic syndrome, and may precede the diagnosis of myeloma. Systemic light-chain deposition in other organs may occur in some patients.[51] The incidence of LCDD appears low. However, in a series of 118 myeloma patients with renal failure who underwent renal biopsy, LCDD was found in 19%.[53]

### Renal amyloidosis (see also Chapter 90)

Amyloidosis occurs in 7–10% of patients with myeloma.[1] The most common renal manifestation is nonspecific proteinuria, although microscopic hematuria may occur. About 25% of patients with AL amyloidosis have serum creatinine values >2 mg/dL. The glomerular filtration rate may be reduced in 50% of patients. About 15% of patients show clinical nephrotic syndrome.[56] Among 118 myeloma patients with renal failure and a renal biopsy, renal amyloidosis was found in 25%.[53] The kidney size is usually normal or slightly enlarged on imaging studies, but small, contracted kidneys can be seen. Renal biopsy shows amyloid deposition in glomerular mesangium and GBM. Amyloid material stains with Congo red and exhibits apple-green birefringence on polarized light. Electron micrographs reveal characteristic nonbranching fibrils with a distinct diameter of 7.5–10 nm.[57]

## NEUROLOGIC MANIFESTATIONS

Neurologic dysfunctions in patients with myeloma may result directly from tumor invasion or indirectly from the effects of myeloma proteins. In addition, metabolic derangements, hypercalcemia, hyperviscosity, and uremia affect neurologic functions (Table 82.3).

## SPINAL CORD COMPRESSION AND RADICULOPATHY

Extension of vertebral body plasmacytoma and collapse of bony structures lead to compression of the spinal cord or dorsal roots by epidural tumors. Occasionally, paravertebral tumor invades the spinal canal through intervertebral foramina. The incidence

| Table 82.3 | Neurologic complications |
|---|

Metabolic encephalopathies: hypercalcemia, hyperviscosity syndrome, uremia
Cord compression, radiculopathy
Meningeal plasmacytosis/CNS plasmacytoma
Cryoglobulinemia (vasculitis)
Peripheral polyneuropathies
    POEMS syndrome/osteosclerotic myeloma
    Amyloid neuropathy
    Polyneuropathy associated with myeloma
    Polyneuropathy associated with cryoglobulinemia

of this complication is about 15%.[58,59] The thoracic spine is more commonly involved. IgA myeloma and extensive cortical bone involvement appear to pose a greater risk.[59] Plain radiographs of the spine may reveal vertebral collapse and/or vertebral or paravertebral masses. Uncommon neurologic manifestations may occur with cranial plasmacytoma, either as a part of multiple myeloma or as a solitary lesion.

### MENINGEAL INVOLVEMENT

Meningeal myelomatosis occurs rarely. Limited reports have recently been reviewed.[60] Patients may experience headache, mentation changes, multiple cranial nerve palsies, and speech and gait disturbances.[61] IgD and IgA myelomas appear to be overrepresented in these cases. Advanced stage with high tumor-labeling index, and, in particular, plasma cell leukemia (19%) are common causes of central nervous system (CNS) disease. Specific laboratory findings include the presence of myeloma cells[62] and paraprotein in the cerebrospinal fluid (CSF).[63]

### PERIPHERAL NEUROPATHIES

Peripheral polyneuropathy develops in 1–8% of patients with myeloma.[64,65] The true incidence may be higher because of a high proportion of subclinical disease as suggested by electrodiagnostic studies.[66] The neuropathy may be sensory, motor, or sensorimotor, and consists of a heterogeneous group of disorders detailed below.

### Osteosclerotic myeloma and POEMS syndrome

Osteosclerotic bone lesions are seen in about 3% of patients with multiple myeloma.[67,68] Patients with *osteosclerotic myeloma* are on average about 10 years younger than those with classic myeloma, with a mean age at diagnosis of 55 years. Male gender predominates. The incidence of anemia, renal failure, hypercalcemia, and bone pain is lower than in classic myeloma. Monoclonal protein concentration is usually low. Osteosclerotic bone lesions are often limited in number, and bone marrow plasmacytosis is mild or absent. Peripheral polyneuropathy, however, occurs in 40–50% of patients and may precede other symptoms of myeloma.[65,68] Similarly, multiple myeloma that is

associated with polyneuropathies occurs at a younger age with a male predominance. In about 50% of cases, pure osteosclerotic or mixed sclerotic/lytic bone lesions are seen, although pure lytic lesions occur in about 25% of patients.[42,69] In both groups, the monoclonal IgG or IgA are almost exclusively associated with λ light-chain isotype. Clearly, these two groups of patients exhibit similar and overlapping features. Other unusual clinical manifestations, variably expressed in these patients, include organomegaly, endocrinopathy, and skin lesions. This constellation of clinical features is emphasized by the designation of an acronym, POEMS (plasma cell dyscrasia with polyneuropathy, organomegaly, endocrinopathy, M protein, and skin changes) syndrome.[70,71] For uniform diagnosis, it was recently proposed that a diagnosis of POEMS be made when a patient meets two major criteria—polyneuropathy and monoclonal plasmaproliferative disorder—and one of the minor criteria—sclerotic bone lesions, Castleman's disease, organomegaly (liver, spleen, lymph nodes), endocrinopathy (adrenal, thyroid, pituitary, gonads, parathyroid, pancreas), skin changes (hyperpigmentation, hypertrichosis, plethora, hemangiomata, white nails), and papilledema.[72] The POEMS syndrome is associated with various plasma cell dyscrasias. The incidence was 1.4% in 2714 patients with plasma cell dyscrasias, excluding myeloma.[73] Five to 20% of POEMS syndrome occurs in patients with typical myeloma with significant bone marrow plasmacytosis. Osteosclerotic or mixed sclerotic/lytic bone lesions occur in 90%. In about 45% of patients, the bone lesion is solitary.[74] The neuropathy in POEMS syndrome, form extensive demyelination with various degree of axonal degeneration, resembles chronic inflammatory demyelinating polyneuropathy. In the great majority, it is a chronic, distal sensorimotor neuropathy with symmetrical numbness and dysesthesia of legs, progressively extending proximally, accompanied by ascending weakness. Reflexes are severely depressed. Cranial nerves are spared, and autonomic involvement is very rare.[75,76]

### Osteolytic myeloma

Peripheral polyneuropathy also occurs in typical myeloma and resembles paraneoplastic neuropathy associated with other neoplasia. It is mostly a mild sensorimotor neuropathy from axonal degeneration, with some degree of segmental demyelination.[76] Distal numbness, tingling, and weakness affect the legs more than the arms. The autonomic system is not involved.

### Amyloid neuropathy

Systemic amyloidosis complicates the course of myeloma in 7–10% of patients. Amyloid neuropathy occurs in about 15% of patients with systemic AL amyloidosis.[56,77] In the nervous system, amyloid may be deposited, often focally, in epineurial and endoneurial connective tissues and vessel walls of peripheral nerves, dorsal ganglia, and autonomic ganglia.[78] Sural nerve biopsy reveals axonal degeneration with a lesser degree of demyelination, affecting mostly unmyelinated or lightly myelinated fibers.[79] The absence of blood–nerve barrier in dorsal root and sympathetic ganglia may predispose these sites to amyloid deposition.[80] Electrodiagnostic studies show decreased action potential amplitude, reduced sensory responses, and normal or mildly reduced conduction velocity.[81] The neuropathy is progressive, sensory dominant, with prominent pain and temperature sense loss. The most common initial presentation is burning or painful paresthesia with mild weakness of lower extremities. Symptoms of autonomic dysfunction include orthostatic hypotension, impotence, and urinary retention.

### Carpal tunnel syndrome

The deposition of amyloid in the flexor retinaculum entraps the median nerve. Carpel tunnel syndrome is the most common neurologic finding in systemic amyloidosis. Electrodiagnostic studies show diminished sensory action potential, prolonged distal latency, and denervation of abductor pollicis brevis. Hand and wrist pain and numbness and paresthesia of the middle and radial fingers are common. Thenar muscle atrophy may occur in severe, chronic case.

### Cryoglobulinemia

About 6% of myeloma proteins are cryoglobulins.[82] Cryoglobulins, especially type II and III, have been associated with neuropathy. *Mononeuropathy* or *mononeuropathy multiplex* may occur as a consequence of vasculitis. *Polyneuropathy*, possibly due to ischemic demyelination, has also been reported.[83,84] In eight cases of myeloma with cryoglobulinemia, one patient was reported to have polyneuropathy, which improved transiently with plasmapheresis and chemotherapy.[82]

### *SYSTEMIC AMYLOIDOSIS (SEE ALSO CHAPTER 90)*

AL amyloidosis complicates the course of myeloma in 7–10% of patients.[1,85] It is more commonly associated with myeloma of λ light-chain type. Amyloidogenic light chains preferentially involve certain Vκ and VΛ germline genes. The specific *V* gene is often associated with a propensity for a specific pattern of organ infiltration, suggesting an organ tropism of amyloidogenic light chain.[86,87] Amyloid protein may deposit in many organs in the body.[88] Serious organ dysfunctions develop when the kidneys, peripheral nervous system, and heart are involved. Cardiac amyloidosis results in arrhythmia, conduction defect, and restrictive cardiomyopathy. Involvement of the GI tract may produce mobility disorders and malabsorption. Pulmonary amyloidosis precipitates respiratory failure. Amyloid angiopathy causes spontaneous skin and mucosal bleeding. Amyloid may also deposit in the skin, endocrine organs, joints, and other tissues, occa-sionally producing a pressure effect. Rarely, cortical bone involvement by amyloid results in pathologic fracture.

### *IMMUNE DYSFUNCTION*

The susceptibility to bacterial infections in patients with myeloma has long been recognized.[89] Infection may be the presenting feature in 10% of patients. Patients at the initiation of treatment and at relapse are at higher risk for infection.[90–92] Other risk factors are decreased polyclonal Ig and renal failure. Gram-positive infections are common before chemotherapy, while Gram-negative organisms predominate after chemotherapy.[92]

Multiple defects in the immune system have been identified. The deficiencies of the uninvolved polyclonal Ig correlate with higher infection risks and are likely to be the major cause of infection.[93] This *secondary antibody deficiency (or functional hypogammaglobulinemic state)* is mainly due to defective antibody production in the immune responses to antigenic stimulation, particularly in the primary immune responses,[90,94] though the accelerated concentration-dependent catabolism of IgG may also be a factor.[95] The underlying mechanism has been extensively studied in patients and in a murine plasmacytoma model. In human disease, lower numbers of peripheral blood and bone marrow B lymphocytes and plasma cell precursors, repeatedly observed in myeloma patients, indicate a suppression of B-cell proliferation and maturation. This suppression appears reversible when myeloma is effectively treated.[96,97]

### *HYPERVISCOSITY SYNDROME*

Hyperviscosity syndrome occurs in fewer than 5% of IgG and in 5–10% of IgA myeloma patients.[98,99] The type of monoclonal immunoglobulin and the plasma concentration are the main determinants for the development of hyperviscosity. In one study of IgG myeloma, hyperviscosity occurred in 4.2% of 238 patients, and in 22% of 46 patients with serum IgG level above 5.0 g/dL.[98] The IgG$_3$ subtype, with a tendency for aggregation, and unusually asymmetrical IgG molecules with a high axial ratio, pose higher risks.[100,101] Similarly, myeloma patients with polymeric IgA are much more likely to develop hyperviscosity syndrome than those with the monomeric form.[99,102] Hyperviscosity has also been reported in unusual cases of light-chain myeloma.[103]

The circulatory disturbances resulting from hyperviscosity lead to various clinical manifestations. Headache, blurred vision, reduced visual acuity, and drowsiness are common. Occasionally, patients may present with dementia or psychosis.[104] Progressive, severe CNS dysfunction results in obtundation, vertigo, seizure, gait ataxia, and coma. Dyspnea may precede overt congestive heart failure. Bleeding occurs most commonly as epistaxis, ecchymosis, and sometimes GI bleeding. Fundoscopic examination, revealing characteristic retinal flame-shaped hemorrhages, engorged, tortuous, segmented retinal veins ("box-caring"), and papilledema, should be performed initially and repeatedly during the course of treatment.

### EXTRAMEDULLARY PLASMACYTOMA

*Primary extramedullary plasmacytoma* occurs rarely and involves most commonly the upper air passages and paranasal sinuses (90%), though a variety of organ involvement has been reported.[105] The clinical manifestations depend on the sites of involvement. In the head and neck region, painless or painful mass may be the first sign. Nasal obstruction, discharge, epistaxis, hoarseness, or hemoptysis may occur. Less commonly involved sites include lung, GI tract, lymph nodes, and the thyroid gland. Only about 20% of patients will have serum monoclonal proteins, and the bone marrow is not involved. Diagnosis is made by histologic or cytologic demonstration of myeloma cells in the biopsied specimen. Establishment of monoclonality, by specific antibody staining for cytoplasmic immunoglobulin to show light-chain restriction or immunoglobulin gene rearrangement, is sometimes necessary to differentiate this entity from reactive plasmacytosis. A bone survey is necessary to exclude bone involvement, and magnetic resonance imaging (MRI) or $^{18}$F-fluorodeoxyglucose positron emission tomography ($^{18}$F-FDG PET) may be used to detect other soft tissue involvement.[106]

More commonly, extramedullary plasmacytomas develop at the terminal phase of myeloma. A wide variety of organs have been shown to be invaded in postmortem examination.[85] With increasingly effective chemotherapy, more patients develop extramedullary plasmacytoma during the late phase of their disease.

### SOLITARY PLASMACYTOMA OF BONE

Solitary plasmacytoma of bone occurs in 3–5% of myeloma patients. It is more common in men (male-to-female ratio 2:1) and at a younger age (50 vs 65 years). It involves mainly the axial bones, particularly vertebrae. Local bone pain and occasionally pathologic fracture may be the presenting feature. Anemia, hypercalcemia, and renal impairment are absent. A serum monoclonal immunoglobulin, usually of low concentration, is detected in about 50% of patients. The bone marrow is not involved, by definition. A bone survey should be done to exclude more extensive disease.

The diagnostic criteria for solitary plasmacytoma of the bone and solitary extramedullary plasmacytoma are not well defined. Because a fraction of these patients, presumably those with truly localized disease, appear curable with radical radiotherapy,[107] stringent criteria that allow precise diagnosis of a potentially curable disease are needed. Questions have been raised as to the need for using sensitive molecular techniques to assess marrow involvement and for advanced imaging methods, such as MRI or PET, to exclude disseminated diseases. Guidelines on the diagnosis and treatment have recently been proposed.[107]

### UNCOMMON MYELOMA: IgD AND IgE MYELOMA

Patients with IgD myeloma have a higher rate of renal failure, extramedullary lesions, amyloidosis, and leukemic manifestation. Serum paraprotein is low, often difficult to detect, and is associated with λ light chain in more than 80% of patients. Rare IgE myeloma also shows a tendency for developing into plasma cell leukemia.[108]

## CLINICAL EVALUATION

The diagnosis of myeloma may not be obvious even in a "typical" case, as the presenting symptoms are not specific. Increasingly, patients are referred for evaluation after seeking medical attention for unexplained anemia, neuropathy, or renal failure. Incidental finding of a monoclonal serum protein is also becoming more frequent. A comprehensive evaluation of patients suspicious for a diagnosis of myeloma starts with thorough history and physical examination. The clinical findings help to direct further investigations for the precise diagnosis and quantification of the extent of disease.

### LABORATORY INVESTIGATION

Laboratory investigations are directed at defining various organ dysfunctions due to myeloma, and a number of studies, required for establishing a diagnosis and staging, should be routinely included.[109]

### HEMATOLOGIC EVALUATION

A complete blood count with differential is required. Optional determinations for serum iron, transferrin saturation, and ferritin are done for patients with microcytic indices, while serum folate and vitamin $B_{12}$ level are evaluated for those with macrocytic indices.

### BIOCHEMICAL EVALUATION

Serum blood urea nitrogen, creatinine, electrolytes, and serum calcium are required tests. Serum albumin, lactate dehydrogenase, $β_2$-microglobulin, and C-reactive protein (CRP) are useful prognostic markers.

### IMMUNOGLOBULIN MEASUREMENTS

Serum protein electrophoresis is required for detecting monoclonal Ig. Cellulose acetate or agarose gel electrophoresis is commonly used. The latter was shown to be more sensitive.[110] A monoclonal immunoglobulin (M spike) is identified as a discrete, homogeneous band on electrophoresis or as spikes in the γ, β, or $α_2$ region of the densitometer tracing. Two M proteins may occur rarely (biclonal gammopathy). Immunofixation is then used to determine the isotype of the paraprotein, using specific antibodies to $\gamma$, $\alpha$, $\mu$, $\delta$, and/or $\varepsilon$ heavy-chain isotypes and to $\kappa$ and $\lambda$ light-chain isotypes. Typing for IgD and IgE is not routinely done and should be requested when IgD or IgE myeloma is suspected.

Urinary protein electrophoresis should be performed on an 80–100 × concentrated random sample. Immunofixation electrophoresis more sensitive for detecting proteins in low concentration, should also be performed. If monoclonal free light chain is identified, a 24-h urine collection should be sent for quantifying daily excretion of light chain and other proteins, especially albumin. The urine dipstick is not sensitive to Bence Jones protein. Urinary light chains that occasionally form multiple, equally spaced bands ("ladder pattern") are generally polyclonal.[111]

### BONE MARROW EXAMINATION (SEE ALSO CHAPTER 81)

A bone marrow aspiration and core biopsy are required for determining the extent and the histologic pattern of myeloma cell infiltration. The percent myeloma cells in the marrow should be enumerated. In selected cases, immunocytological studies, most commonly using immunoperoxidase staining, are performed for demonstrating light-chain restriction in monoclonal plasma cells. Other markers, such as Ki-67,[112] can be assessed. Optional flow cytometric study of the bone marrow is helpful in detailed characterization of the malignant myeloma cells. The nuclear ploidy, S-phase fraction, the expression of B-cell differentiation antigens, adhesion molecules, and occasionally the myeloid markers are of some prognostic interest. If available, a plasma cell labeling index, usually by bromodeoxyuridine labeling, should be obtained for its prognostic importance.[30] Cytogenetic and fluorescence in situ hybridization analyses for numeric and structural abnormalities and for specific rearrangement of chromosomes should be requested whenever possible. The cytogenetic analysis of myeloma cells has significant prognostic value and provides a basis for a molecularly based classification of myeloma (Chapters 80 and 81). Abnormalities in chromosome 13 are particularly ominous.[113]

### IMAGING STUDIES
#### Plain X-ray

A skeletal survey is required and should include lateral and anteroposterior views of the skull, cervical, thoracic, and lumbar spines, chest, pelvis, femurs, and humeri. Radiographs of focal lesions are needed when clinically indicated. Myeloma involves most frequently the axial bones, the sites of red marrow. On X-ray, multiple, osteolytic lesions may be present, and are characteristically "punched out." Extensive erosion of the cortex in weight-bearing bones needs to be identified and may require urgent preventive measures to avoid pathologic fracture.

### Radionuclide scans
**Diphosphonate** Conventional diphosphonate radionuclide bone scans, depending on the osteoblastic activity of the lesion, have a sensitivity of only 40–60% and thus are of limited use.[114,115]

#### Tc 99m MIBI
Scanning with Tc 99m 2-methoxyisobutylisonitrile, a lipophilic, cationic agent accumulated in metabolically active tissues and extruded from the cells through MDR-1 p-glycoprotein, has recently been shown to have a higher sensitivity. Diffuse bone marrow uptake or focal enhanced bone lesions may be detected. The latter lesions are concordant with radiographic bone lesions in about 70% of the cases. It was suggested that the lesions detected by Tc 99m MIBI represented active disease sites, and the intensity of radionuclide uptake correlated with the disease activity, as reflected by high levels of disease markers, such as $\beta$2-microglobulin and CRP.[116–118] Its clinical utility is still experimental.

#### 18F-FDG PET
Whole-body $^{18}$F-FDG-PET also detects diffuse and/or focal increased uptake of radionuclide in myeloma patients. In a study of 66 patients, a positive scan was obtained in all 16 untreated patients with active myeloma, including four (25%) who had a negative radiographic bone survey.[106] Extramedullary plasmacytoma was detected and verified by histologic examination. Importantly, tests for MGUS were negative, and new lesions were found in relapsed patients. A comparative study with Tc 99m MIBI and FDG-PET suggests the former reflects more the extent of disease, while the latter is more sensitive to active proliferative lesions.[119] The validity of FDG-PET has yet to be determined.

### COMPUTED TOMOGRAPHY
Computed tomography (CT) detects bone destruction similar to plain radiographs, but with higher sensitivity.

### MAGNETIC RESONANCE IMAGING
MRI is useful in detecting myelomatous involvement of the bone marrow. The patterns of infiltration can be focal, diffuse, or mixed.[120] In a study of 77 patients examined with MRIs of the thoracic and lumbar spines, three stages of bone disease could be graded: stage I, no focal or diffuse infiltration; stage II, ≤10 foci or mild diffuse infiltration; and stage III, >10 foci or strong diffuse infiltration. This MRI staging correlates strongly with survival and can be used as a bone lesion scale in Durie–Salmon staging system.[121] MRI is also useful in following bone lesions after treatment, as plain radiographs may not show significant changes,

**Table 82.4** Diagnostic criteria for (symptomatic) multiple myeloma

(1) Tumor criteria:
  Monoclonal plasma cells in the bone marrow >10% and/or
  Biopsy-documented plasmacytoma
  Monoclonal protein in serum and/or urine

(2) End organ damages, one or more of the following
  **C**alcium elevation in the blood (serum calcium >10.5 mg/dl or upper limit of normal)
  **R**enal insufficiency (serum creatinine >2 mg/dl)
  **A**nemia (hemoglobin <10 g/dl or 2 g/dl < normal)
  **B**one disease: lytic lesions or osteoporosis
  Others: symptomatic hyperviscosity, amyloidosis, recurrent bacterial infections (>2 episodes in 12 months)

For patients with a solitary bone lesion or osteoporosis without fracture as the sole defining criteria, ≥30% bone marrow plasmacytosis is required for the diagnosis of systemic myeloma. For monoclonal protein, no specific level is required and it is absent in non-secretory myeloma.

even in responsive disease.[122] MRI is the current imaging of choice in evaluating spinal cord compression.

Imaging studies, other than plain radiography, are not routinely used. MRI and PET appear promising, and further investigations may find them useful in detecting focal or residual disease and in better quantifying the extent of disease.[123]

## DIFFERENTIAL DIAGNOSIS

The required investigations detailed above assure the gathering of sufficient information for making the diagnosis. In most patients with symptomatic, progressive myeloma, the diagnosis is readily made by the presence of marked bone marrow plasmacytosis, monoclonal protein in serum and/or urine, and osteolytic bone lesions, all the major criteria for myeloma. Minor criteria, including anemia, hypercalcemia, renal insufficiency, and suppression of nonparaproteins, help establish the diagnosis in cases where bone disease is not obvious.[124] The myeloma-related disorders, however, are a heterogeneous group, including multiple myeloma, smoldering myeloma, indolent myeloma, MGUS, solitary plasmacytoma of the bone, extramedullary plasmacytoma, and plasma cell leukemia. In addition, systemic AL amyloidosis, Waldenstrom's macroglobulinemia, and heavy-chain diseases also share the features of the neoplasia of Ig-secreting cells (see Chapters 88 and 90). The distinction among some of these disorders is not precise, and the diagnostic criteria used vary among experts. A number of classification systems are often used, including that by Durie–Salmon,[125] by the Mayo group,[2,126] the Southwest Oncology Group (SWOG),[127] and by the British Columbia Cancer Agency.[128] A comparison of these classification systems in 157 patients with plasma cell dyscrasias showed that 80% of the cases could be classified by all systems, and in 64%, the diagnosis was concordant. Not unexpectedly, the discrepancies occurred primarily among the smoldering myeloma, indolent myeloma, and multiple myeloma stage I groups.[124] Thus, currently, the selection of a particular diagnosis and classification system makes relatively little difference in treatment approach.

Recent efforts by international groups aim at simplifying the classification for uniform application.[123,129] Recognizing that myeloma-related disorders have a wide spectrum of overlapping features, the proposed classification emphasizes the importance of myeloma-related organ or tissue impairment (end-organ damage) in the clinical course of patients and in decision making for systemic therapy. The proposed diagnostic criteria, not greatly different from current classifications, have greater clarity.[123,129] Tables 82.4–82.6 list the criteria for (symptomatic) multiple myeloma, MGUS, smoldering (indolent or asymptomatic) myeloma, nonsecretory myeloma, solitary plasmacytoma of the bone, and extramedullary plasmacytoma. In addition, plasma cell leukemia is defined by the presence of monoclonal plasma cells of ≥2000/μL in the peripheral blood and ≥20% plasma cells in WBC differential count.

The biological basis for various classifications of myeloma-related disorders is unclear. Molecular studies have shown that similar genetic alterations occur in all variants of myeloma,[130] and in gene expression profiling, MGUS is not distinguishable from early

**Table 82.5** Diagnostic criteria for monoclonal gammopathy of undetermined significance (MGUS), smoldering or indolent or asymptomatic myeloma (SM), and non-secretory myeloma (NSMM)

| | MGUS | SM | NSMM |
|---|---|---|---|
| (1) Monoclonal plasma cells in the bone marrow | <10% | ≥10% | ≥10% |
| (2) M-spike: | | | |
| serum IgG or | <3.0 g/dl | ≥3.0 g/dl | absent[a] |
| serum IgA or | <2.0 g/dl; | ≥2.0 g/dl | absent[a] |
| urine Bence Jones protein | <1.0 g/24 h | ≥1.0 g/24 h | absent[a] |
| (3) End organ damage | absent | absent | presnet |

[a]by immunofixation.
Presence of all three criteria are required for diagnosis, except in SM where only one of (1) and (2) criteria is sufficient.

| Table 82.6 | Solitary plasmacytoma of the bone, solitary extramedullary plasmacytoma | |
| --- | --- | --- |
| | Solitary plasmacytoma of the bone | Solitary extramedullary plasmacytoma |
| Biopsy-documented plasmacytoma | Bone, single site[a] | Extraosseous, single site[a] |
| Monoclonal plasma cells in the bone marrow | <10% | Normal bone marrow |
| M protein in serum and/or urine | Absent[b] | Absent[b] |
| End-organ damage | Absent | Absent |

[a]X-ray and MRI and/or FDG-PET imaging (if performed) should be negative outside of the primary site.
[b]Low concentration of M protein may be present in some patients (and may decrease after local treatment).

myeloma.[131,132] Nevertheless, the classification provides a useful framework for clinical approach to patients with these disorders.

## CONCLUDING REMARKS

Past investigations in myeloma and its related diseases have been fruitful in delineating the pathophysiologic processes of these disorders, and in elucidating the basic biology of the immune system. Continued research in this area promises to refine our understanding of these disorders and, more importantly, will identify molecular targets for the next generation of effective therapeutics.

### Acknowledgment
The help of my wife, Yu-His Chen, MD, in preparing this manuscript is acknowledged with gratitude and affection.

## REFERENCES

1. Kyle RA: Multiple myeloma. Review of 869 cases. *Mayo Clin Proc* 50:29, 1975.
2. Kyle RA, Gertz MA, Witzig TE, et al.: Review of 1027 patients with newly diagnosed multiple myeloma. *Mayo Clin Proc* 78:21, 2003.
3. Riccardi A, Gobbi PG, Ucci G, et al.: Changing clinical presentation of multiple myeloma. *Eur J Cancer* 27:1401, 1991.
4. Blade J, Kyle RA, Greipp PR: Presenting features and prognosis in 72 patients with multiple myeloma who were younger than 40 years. *Br J Haematol* 93:345, 1996.
5. Rodon P, Linassier C, Gauvain J-B, et al.: Multiple myeloma in elderly patients: presenting features and outcome. *Eur J Haematol* 66:11, 2001.
6. Knudsen LM, Hippe E, Hjorth M, et al.: Renal function in newly diagnosed multiple myeloma—a demographic study of 1353 patients. The Nordic Myeloma Study Group. *Eur J Haematol* 53:207, 1994.
7. Blade J, Fernandez-Llama P, Bosch F, et al.: Renal failure in multiple myeloma: presenting features and predictors of outcome in 94 patients from a single institution. *Arch Intern Med* 158:1889, 1998.
8. DeFronzo RA, Humphrey RL, Wright JE, et al.: Acute renal failure in multiple myeloma. *Medicine* 54:209, 1975.
9. DeFronzo RA, Cooke CR, Wright JR, et al.: Renal function in patients with multiple myeloma. *Medicine* 57:151, 1978.
10. Cohen DJ, Sherman WH, Osserman EF, et al.: Acute renal failure in patients with multiple myeloma. *Am J Med* 76:247, 1984.
11. Pringle JP, Graham RC, Bernier GM: Detection of myeloma cells in the urine sediment. *Blood* 43:137, 1974.
12. Means RT Jr: Pathogenesis of the anemia of chronic disease: a cytokine-mediated anemia. *Stem cell* 13:32, 1995.
13. Silvestris F, Cafforio P, Tucci M, et al.: Negative regulation of erythroblast maturation by Fas-L+/TRAIL+ highly malignant plasma cells: a major pathogenetic mechanism of anemia in multiple myeloma. *Blood* 99:1305, 2002.
14. Nemeth E, Rivera S, Gabayan V, et al.: Il-6 mediates hypoferremia of inflammation by inducing the synthesis of the iron regulatory hormone hepcidin. *J Clin Invest* 113:1271, 2004.
15. Beguin Y, Yerna M, Loo M, et al.: Erythropoiesis in multiple myeloma: defective red cell production due to inappropriate erythropoietin production. *Br J Haematol* 82:648, 1992.
16. Ludwig H, Fritz E, Kotzmann H, et al.: Erythropoietin treatment of anemia associated with multiple myeloma. *N Engl J Med* 322:1693, 1990.
17. Singh A, Eckardt KU, Zimmermann A, et al.: Increased plasma viscosity as a reason for inappropriate erythropoietin formation. *J Clin Invest* 91:251, 1993.
18. Alexanian R: Blood volume in monoclonal gammopathy. *Blood* 49:301, 1977.
19. Atkins MB, Kappler K, Mier JW, et al.: Interleukin-6-associated anemia: determination of the underlying mechanism. *Blood* 86:1288, 1995.
20. Hoffbrand AV, Hobbs JR, Kremenchuzky S, et al.: Incidence and pathogenesis of megaloblastic erythropoiesis in multiple myeloma. *J Clin Pathol* 20:699, 1967.
21. Baatout S: Interleukin-6 and megakaryocytopoiesis: an update. *Ann Hematol* 73:157, 1996.
22. Kosmo MA, Gale RP: Plasma cell leukemia. *Semin Hematol* 24:202, 1987.
23. Greipp PR, Raymond NM, Kyle RA, et al.: Multiple myeloma: significance of plasmablastic subtype in morphological classification. *Blood* 65:305, 1985.

24. Bartl R, Frisch B, Burkhardt T, et al.: Bone marrow histology in myeloma: its importance in diagnosis, prognosis, classification and staging. *Br J Haematol* 51:361, 1982.

25. Krzyzaniak RL, Buss DH, Cooper MR, et al.: Marrow fibrosis and multiple myeloma. *Am J Clin Pathol* 89:63, 1988.

26. Vacca A, Ribatti D, Roncali L, et al.: Bone marrow angiogenesis and progression in multiple myeloma. *Br J Haematol* 87:503, 1994.

27. Castell JV, Gomez-Lechon MJ, David M, et al.: Interleukin-6 is the major regulator of acute phase protein synthesis in adult human hepatocytes. *FEBS Lett* 242:237, 1989.

28. Moshage HJ, Kleter BE, van Pelt JF, et al.: Fibrinogen and albumin synthesis are regulated at the transcriptional level during the acute phase response. *Biochim Biophys Acta* 950:450, 1988.

29. Chen Y, Magalhaes MC: Hypoalbuminemia in patients with multiple myeloma. *Arch Intern Med* 150:605, 1990.

30. Greipp PR, Lust JA, O'Fallon WM, et al.: Plasma cell labeling index and beta 2-microglobulin predict survival independent of thymidine kinase and C-reactive protein in multiple myeloma. *Blood* 81:3382, 1993.

31. Dimopoulos MA, Barlogie B, Smith TL, et al.: High serum lactate dehydrogenase level as a marker for drug resistance and short survival in multiple myeloma. *Ann Intern Med* 115:931, 1991.

32. Merlini G, Fitzpatrick LA, Siris ES, et al.: A human myeloma immunoglobulin G binding four moles of calcium associated with asymptomatic hypercalcemia. *J Clin Immunol* 4:185, 1984.

33. Perkins HA, MacKenzie HR, Fundenberg HH: Hemostatic defects in dysproteinemias. *Blood* 35:695, 1970.

34. Coleman M, Vigliano EM, Weksler ME, et al.: Inhibition of fibrin monomer polymerization by lambda myeloma globulins. *Blood* 39:210, 1972.

35. Cohen I, Amir J, Ben-Shaul Y, et al.: Plasma cell myeloma associated with an unusual myeloma protein causing impairment of fibrin aggregation and platelet function in a patient with multiple malignancies. *Am J Med* 48:766, 1970.

36. Khoory MS, Nesheim ME, Bowie EJW, et al.: Circulating heparin sulfate proteoglycan anticoagulant from a patient with a plasma cell disorder. *J Clin Invest* 65:666, 1980.

37. Lackner H: Hemostatic abnormalities associated with dysproteinemias. *Semin Hematol* 10:125, 1973.

38. Furie B, Greene E, Furie BC: Syndrome of acquired factor X deficiency and systemic amyloidosis. *N Engl J Med* 297:81, 1977.

39. Penny R, Castaldi PA, Whitsed HM: Inflammation and haemostasis in paraproteinaemias. *Br J Haematol* 20:35, 1971.

40. DiMinno G, Coraggio F, Cerbone AM, et al.: A myeloma paraprotein with specificity for platelet glycoprotein IIIa in a patient with a fatal bleeding disorder. *J Clin Invest* 77:157, 1986.

41. Tefferi A, Nichols WL: Acquired von Willebrand's disease: concise review of occurrence, diagnosis, pathogenesis, and treatment. *Am J Med* 103:536, 1997.

42. Driedger H, Pruzanski W: Plasma cell neoplasia with peripheral polyneuropathy. A study of five cases and a review of the literature. *Medicine (Baltimore)* 59:301, 1980.

43. Preuss HG, Weiss FR, Iammarino RM, et al.: Effect on rat kidney slice function in vitro of proteins from the urine of patients with myelomatosis and nephrosis. *Clin Sci Mol Med* 46:283, 1974.

44. Sanders PW, Booker BB: Pathobiology of cast nephropathy form human Bence Jones proteins. *J Clin Invest* 89:630, 1991.

45. Solomon A, Weiss DT, Kattine AA: Nephrotoxic potential of Bence Jones proteins. *N Engl J Med* 324:1845, 1991.

46. Kyle RA: Monoclonal gammopathy and the kidney. *Ann Rev Med* 40:53, 1989.

47. Clyne DH, Pera AJ, Thompson RE: Nephrotoxicity of Bence Jones proteins: the importance of the isoelectric point. *Kidney Int* 16:345, 1979.

48. Huang ZQ, Kirk AA, Connelly KG, et al.: Bence Jones proteins bind to a common peptide segment of Tamm-Horsfall glycoprotein to promote heterotypic aggregation. *J Clin Invest* 92:2975,1993.

49. Maldonado JE, Velosa JA, Kyle RA, et al.: Fanconi syndrome in adults: a manifestation of a latent form of myeloma. *Am J Med* 58:354, 1975.

50. Messiaen T, Deret S, Mougenot B, et al.: Adult Fanconi syndrome secondary to light chain gammopathy. Clinicopathologic heterogeneity and unusual features in 11 patients. *Medicine (Baltimore)* 79:135, 2000.

51. Buxbaum JN, Chuba JV, Hellman GC, et al.: Monoclonal immunoglobulin deposition disease: light chain and light and heavy chain deposition diseases and their relation to light chain amyloidosis. *Ann Intern Med* 112:455, 1990.

52. Lin J, Markowitz GS, Valeri AM, et al.: Renal monoclonal immunoglobulin deposition disease: the disease spectrum. *J Am Soc Nephrol* 12:1482, 2001.

53. Montseny J-J, Kleinknecht D, Meyrier A, et al.: Long-term outcome according to renal histological lesions in 118 patients with monoclonal gammopathies. *Nephrol Dial Transplant* 13:1438, 1998.

54. Heilman RL, Velosa JA, Holley KE, et al.: Long-term follow-up and response to chemotherapy in patients with light-chain deposition disease. *Am J Kidney Dis* 20:34, 1992.

55. Moulin B, Deret S, Mariette X, et al.: Nodular glomerulosclerosis with deposition of monoclonal immunoglobulin heavy chains lacking CH1. *J Am Soc Nephrol* 10:519, 1999.

56. Kyle RA, Greipp PR: Amyloidosis (AL). Clinical and laboratory features in 229 cases. *Mayo Clin Proc* 58:665, 1983.

57. Merlini G, Bellotti V: Molecular mechanisms of amyloidosis. *N Engl J Med* 349:583, 2003.

58. Brenner B, Carter A, Tatarsky I, et al.: Incidence, prognostic significance and therapeutic modalities of central nervous system involvement in multiple myeloma. *Acta Haematol* 68:77, 1982.

59. Woo E, Yu YL, Ng M, et al.: Spinal cord compression in multiple myeloma: who gets it? *Aust N Z J Med* 16:671, 1986.

60. Petersen SL, Wagner A, Gimsing P: Cerebral and meningeal multiple myeloma after autologous stem cell transplantation. A case report and review of the literature. *Am J Hematol* 62:228, 1999.

61. Woodruff RK, Ireton HJC: Multiple cranial nerve palsies as the presenting feature of meningeal myelomatosis. *Cancer* 49:1710, 1982.

62. Afifi AM: Myeloma cells in the cerebrospinal fluid in plasma cell neoplasia. *J Neurol Neurosurg Psychiatry* 37:1162, 1974.

63. Hansotia P, Gani K, Friedenberg W: Cerebrospinal fluid monoclonal gammopathy in multiple myeloma and Waldenstrom's macroglobulinemia. *Neurology* 33:1411, 1983.

64. Kelly JJ, Kyle RA, Miles JM, et al.: The spectrum of peripheral neuropathies in myeloma. *Neurology* 31:24, 1981.

65. Reitan JB, Pape E, Fossa SD, et al.: Osteosclerotic myeloma with polyneuropathy. *Acta Med Scand* 208:137, 1980.

66. Walsh JC: The neuropathy of multiple myeloma: an electrophysiological and histological study. *Arch Neurol* 25:404, 1971.

67. Evison G, Evans KT: Bone sclerosis in multiple myeloma. *Br J Radiol* 40:81, 1967.

68. Driedger H, Pruzanski W: Plasma cell neoplasia with osteosclerotic lesions. *Arch Intern Med* 139:892, 1979.

69. Kelly JJ Jr, Kyle RA, Miles JM, et al.: Osteosclerotic myeloma and peripheral neuropathy. *Neurology* 33:202, 1983.

70. Nakanishi T, Sobue I, Toyokura Y, et al.: The Crow–Fukase syndrome: a study of 102 cases in Japan. *Neurology* 34:712, 1984.

71. Bardwick PA, Zvaifler NJ, Gill GN, et al.: Plasma cell dyscrasia with polyneuropathy, organomegaly, endocrinopathy, M protein, and skin changes: the POEMS syndrome. *Medicine* 59:311, 1980.

72. Dispenzieri A, Kyle RA, Lacy MQ, et al.: POEMS syndrome: definitions and long-term outcome. *Blood* 101:2496, 2003.

73. Diego Miralles G, O'Fallon JR, Talley NJ: Plasma-cell dyscrasia with polyneuropathy. The spectrum of POEMS syndrome. *N Engl J Med* 327:1919, 1992.

74. Soubrier MJ, Dubost J-J, Sauvezie BJM: POEMS syndrome: a study of 25 cases and a review of the literature. *Am J Med* 97:543, 1994.

75. Ropper AH, Gorson KC: Neuropathies associated with paraproteinemia. *N Engl J Med* 338:1601, 1998.

76. Kelly JJ Jr: Peripheral neuropathies associated with monoclonal proteins. A clinical review. *Muscle Nerve* 8:138, 1985.

77. Kyle RA, Dyck PJ: Amyloidosis and neuropathy. In: Dyck PJ, Thomas PK, Griffin JW, eds. *Peripheral Neuropathy*. Philadelphia: WB Saunders; 1993: 1294–1309.

78. Davies-Jones GA, Esiri MM: Neuropathy due to amyloid in myelomatosis. *Br Med J* 2:444, 1971.

79. Thomas PK, King RH: Peripheral nerve changes in amyloid neuropathy in myeloma. *Brain* 97:395, 1974.

80. Verghese JP, Bradley WG, Nemni R, et al.: Amyloid neuropathy in multiple myeloma and other plasma cell dyscrasias. *J Neurol Sci* 59:237, 1983.

81. Kelly JJ Jr: The electrodiagnostic findings in peripheral neuropathy associated with monoclonal gammopathy. *Muscle Nerve* 6:504, 1983.

82. Brouet J-C, Clauvel J-P, Danon F, et al.: Biologic and clinical significance of cryoglobulins. *Am J Med* 57:775, 1974.

83. Gemignani F, Pavesi F, Fiocchi A, et al.: Peripheral neuropathy in essential mixed cryoglobulinaemia. *J Neurol Neurosurg Psychiatry* 55:116, 1992.

84. Nemni R, Corbo M, Fazio R, et al.: Cryoglobulinaemic neuropathy. A clinical, morphological and immunocytochemical study of 8 cases. *Brain* 111:541, 1988.

85. Kapadia SB: Multiple myeloma: a clinicopathologic study of 62 consecutively autopsied cases. *Medicine (Baltimore)* 59:380, 1980.

86. Comenzo RL, Zhang Y, Martinez C, et al.: The tropism of organ involvement in primary systemic amyloidosis: contributions of Ig V(L) germ line gene use and clonal plasma cell burden. *Blood* 98:714, 2001.

87. Abraham RS, Geyer SM, Price-Troska TL, et al.: Immunoglobulin light chain variable (V) region genes influence clinical presentation and outcome in light chain-associated amyloidosis (AL). *Blood* 101:3801, 2003.

88. Kyle RA, Gertz MA: Primary systemic amyloidosis: clinical and laboratory features in 474 cases. *Semin Hematol* 32:45, 1995.

89. Glenchur H, Zinneman HH, Hall WH: A review of 51 cases of multiple myeloma: emphasis on pneumonia and other infections as complications. *Arch Intern Med* 103:173, 1959.

90. Hargreaves RM, Lea JR, Griffiths H, et al.: Immunological factors and risk of infection in plateau phase myeloma. *J Clin Pathol* 48:260, 1995.

91. Perri RT, Hebbel RP, Oken MM: Influence of treatment and response status on infection risk in multiple myeloma. *Am J Med* 71:935, 1981.

92. Savage DG, Lindenbaum J, Garrett TJ: Biphasic pattern of bacterial infection in multiple myeloma. *Ann Intern Med* 96:47, 1982.

93. Cwynarski MT, Cohen S: Polyclonal immunoglobulin deficiency in myelomatosis and macroglobulinaemia. *Clin Exp Immunol* 8:237, 1971.

94. Fahey JL, Scoggins R, Utz JP, et al.: Infection, antibody response, and gamma globulin components in multiple myeloma and macroglobulinemia. *Am J Med* 35:689, 1963.

95. Waldmann TA, Strober W: Metabolism of immunoglobulins. *Prog Allergy* 13:1, 1969.

96. Pilarski LM, Mant MJ, Ruether BA, et al.: Severe deficiency of B lymphocytes in peripheral blood from multiple myeloma patients. *J Clin Invest* 74:1301, 1984.

97. Rawstron AC, Davies FE, Owen RG, et al.: B-lymphocyte suppression in multiple myeloma is a reversible phenomenon specific to normal B-cell progenitors and plasma cell precursors. *Br J Haematol* 100:176, 1998.

98. Pruzanski W, Watt JG: Serum viscosity and hyperviscosity syndrome in IgG multiple myeloma. *Ann Intern Med* 77:853, 1972.

99. Roberts-Thomson PJ, Mason DY, MacLennan IC: Relationship between paraprotein polymerization and clinical features in IgA myeloma. *Br J Haematol* 33:117, 1976.

100. Capra JD, Kunkel HG: Aggregation of γG3 proteins. Relevance to the hyperviscosity syndrome. *J Clin Invest* 49:610, 1970.

101. MacKenzie MR, Fudenberg HH, O'Reilly RA: The hyperviscosity syndrome. I. In IgG myeloma. The role of protein concentration and molecular shape. *J Clin Invest* 49:15, 1970.

102. Chandy KG, Stockley RA, Leonard RC, et al.: Relationship between serum viscosity and intravascular IgA polymer concentration in IgA myeloma. *Clin Exp Immunol* 46:653, 1981.

103. Carter PW, Cohen HJ, Crawford J: Hyperviscosity syndrome in association with kappa light chain myeloma. *Am J Med* 86:591, 1989.

104. Mueller J, Hotson JR, Langston JW: Hyperviscosity induced dementia. *Neurology* 33:101, 1983.

105. Malpas JS, Cavenagh JD: Plasmacytoma. In Malpas JS, Bergsagel DE, Kyle RA, Anderson KC, eds. *Myeloma. Biology and Management.* 3rd ed. Philadelphia: WB Saunders; 2004: 353–360.

106. Durie BGM, Waxman AD, D'Agnolo A, et al.: Whole-body $^{18}$F-FDG PET identifies high-risk myeloma. *J Nucl Med* 43:1457, 2002.

107. Soutar F, Lucraft H, Jackson G, et al.: Guidelines on the diagnosis and treatment of solitary plasmacytoma of bone and solitary extramedullary plasmacytoma. *Br J Haematol* 124:717, 2004.

108. Bergsagel DE, Pruzanski W: Syndromes and special presentations associated with plasma cell myeloma. In Wiernik PH, Goldman JM, Dutcher JP, Kyle RA, eds. *Neoplastic Diseases of the Blood.* 4th ed. Cambridge, UK: Cambridge University Press; 200:547.

109. Smith A, Wisloff F, Samson D: Guidelines on the diagnosis and management of multiple myeloma 2005. *Br J Haematol* 132:410, 2005.

110. Katzmann JA, Clark R, Wiegert E, et al.: Identification of monoclonal proteins in serum: a quantitative comparison of acetate, agarose gel, and capillary electrophoresis. *Electrophoresis* 18:1775, 1997.

111. Harrison HH: "Ladder light chain" or "pseudo-oligoclonal" pattern in urinary immunofixation electrophoresis (IFE) studies: a distinctive IFE pattern and an explanatory hypothesis relating it to free polyclonal light chains. *Clin Chem* 37:1559, 1991.

112. Alexandrakis MG, Passam F, Kyriakou D, et al.: Ki-67 proliferation index: correlation with prognostic parameters and outcome in multiple myeloma. *Am J Clin Oncol* 27:8, 2004.

113. Shaughnessy J Jr, Tian E, Sawyer J, et al.: Prognostic impact of cytogenetic and interphase fluorescence in situ hybridization-defined chromosome 13 deletion in multiple myeloma: early results of total therapy II. *Br J Haematol* 120:44, 2003.

114. Wahner HW, Kyle RA, Beabout JW: Scintigraphic evaluation of the skeleton in multiple myeloma. *Mayo Clinic Proc* 55:739, 1980.

115. Bataille R, Chevalier J, Rossi M, et al.: Bone scintigraphy in plasma-cell myeloma: a prospective study of 70 patients. *Radiology* 145:801, 1982.

116. Adams BK, Fataar A, Nizami MA: Technetium-99m-sestaMIBI uptake in myeloma. *J Nucl Med* 37:1001, 1996.

117. Pace L, Catalano L, Pinto AM, et al.: Different patterns of technetium-99m sestamibi uptake in multiple myeloma. *Eur J Nucl Med* 25:714, 1998.

118. Alexandrakis MG, Kyriakou DS, Passam F, et al.: Value of Tc-99m sestamibi scintigraphy in the detection of bone lesions in multiple myeloma: comparison with Tc-99m methylene diphosphonate. *Ann Hematol* 80:349, 2001.

119. El-Shirbiny AM, Yeung H, Imbriaco M, et al.: Technetium-99m-MIBI versus fluorine-18-FDG in diffuse multiple myeloma. *J Nucl Med* 38:1208, 1997.

120. Moulopoulos LA, Varma DGK, Dimopoulos MA, et al.: Multiple myeloma: spinal MR imaging in patients with untreated, newly diagnosed disease. *Radiology* 185:833, 1992.

121. Baur A, Staebler A, Nagel D, et al.: Magnetic resonance imaging as a supplement for the clinical staging system of Durie and Salmon? *Cancer* 95:1334, 2002.

122. Rahmouni A, Divine M, Mathieu D, et al.: MR appearance of multiple myeloma before and after treatment. *Am J Roentgenol* 160:1053, 1993.

123. Durie BGM, Kyle RA, Belch A, et al.: Myeloma management guidelines: a consensus report from the scientific advisors of the international myeloma foundation. *Hematol J* 4:379, 2003.

124. Ong F, Hermans J, Noordijk EM, et al.: Is the Durie and Salmon diagnostic classification system for plasma cell dyscrasias still the best choice? *Ann Hematol* 70:19, 1995.

125. Durie BGM: Staging and kinetics of multiple myeloma. *Semin Oncol* 13:300, 1986.

126. Greipp PR: Monoclonal gammopathies: new approaches to clinical problems in diagnosis and prognosis. *Blood Rev* 3:222, 1992.

127. Jacobson JL, Hussein MA, Barlogie B, et al.: A new staging system for multiple myeloma patients based on the Southwest Oncology Group (SWOG) experience. *Br J Haematol* 122:441, 2003.

128. Lymphoma Tumor Group. Plasma cell disorders. In: *Cancer Treatment Policies.* Vancouver: British Columbia Cancer Agency; 1992:4–6.

129. Kyle RA, Child JA, Anderson K: Criteria for the classification of monoclonal gammopathies, multiple myeloma and related disorders: a report of the international myeloma working group. *Br J Haematol* 121:749, 2003.

130. Kuehl WM, Bergsagel PL: Multiple myeloma: evolving genetic events and host interactions. *Nature Rev Cancer* 2:175, 2002.

131. Zhan F, Hardin J, Kordsmeier B, et al.: Global gene expression profiling of multiple myeloma, monoclonal gammopathy of undetermined significance, and normal bone marrow plasma cells. *Blood* 99:1745, 2002.

132. Davies FE, Dring AM, Li C, et al.: Insights into the multistep transformation of MGUS to myeloma using microarray expression analysis. *Blood* 102:4504, 2003.

# Chapter 83

# INITIAL TREATMENT APPROACH TO MULTIPLE MYELOMA

*Jeffrey A. Zonder*

## INTRODUCTION

Most of the 15,000 people per year in the United States who develop multiple myeloma (MM)[1] require some form of treatment at the time of diagnosis. Combination regimens incorporating alkylating agents, corticosteroids, and/or anthracyclines have been used for decades, with little overall progress during that time in terms of survival or cure rate.[2, 3] High-dose chemotherapy with autologous stem cell support (HDC/ASCS), shown in some studies to offer a modest survival benefit, is nonetheless noncurative (summarized below, and in greater detail in Chapter 90). Thalidomide plus dexamethasone (TD) has recently emerged as the most widely used front-line regimens in the United States, and other thalidomide-containing combinations, as well as ones incorporating bortezomib (Velcade; PS-341) or lenalidomide (Revlimid; CC-5013), are currently being studied. New regimens are often difficult to compare to more established therapies for a variety of reasons. The most important endpoint of therapy, survival, is not known for many newer regimens. Additionally, with the exception of Melpahlan-Prednisone-Thalidomide (MPT), newer combinations have not been compared in a randomized fashion to standards like Melphalan-Prednisone (MP) or Vincristine-Doxorubicin (Adriamycin)-Dexamethasone (VAD) (described in detail below, Tables 83.1 and 83.2). Increasingly, surrogate endpoints are being used to assess new agents and combinations, with some debate as to the best indicator of clinical efficacy. Though it is widely held that complete response (CR) rate is the best predictor of long-term survival,[4, 5] some investigators have shown other endpoints such as time to disease progression may correlate more strongly.[6] There is the least amount of data to support the use of partial reduction in serum or urine M-protein concentration as a surrogate efficacy endpoint, but it is often used in Phase II studies where the goal is often to determine if a regimen has enough "promise" to warrant larger-scale Phase III trials. For further discussion regarding response assessment, please refer to Chapter 91.

When treatment for a patient with newly diagnosed MM is being considered, the first question the clinician must ask is, "Does the patient require *any* treatment right now?" Definite indications for therapy include bone pain or the presence of multiple lytic skeletal lesions, cytopenias or renal dysfunction without other identifiable causes, hypercalcemia, or a high serum or urine M-protein level. Less common manifestations, such as amyloidosis or paraprotein-related hyperviscosity, also represent indications to initiate systemic therapy. Recently published management guidelines emphasize that asymptomatic newly diagnosed myeloma (formerly termed indolent or smoldering myeloma) should *not* be treated with cytotoxic therapy.[7] It is clear that many of these patients can be followed for an extended period of time without intervention or complications.[8] At least two randomized studies have addressed this point. In the first, a group of Swedish investigators randomized 50 patients with asymptomatic MM to either immediate or deferred therapy with MP.[9] There were no differences in response rate, response duration, or survival, despite the fact that therapy was started on average a year later in the deferred-therapy arm. Riccardi et al. also found no differences in response rate or overall survival (OS) amongst 145 patients enrolled on a prospective study with a similar design.[10] In contrast to the Swedish experience, patients treated at the time of disease progression had a shorter duration of response. Thalidomide, 200–800 mg/day, has been investigated as treatment of asymptomatic MM in a group of 29 patients at the Mayo Clinic.[11] Although the majority of patients exhibited reduction in M-protein levels, 37% of patients progressed to symptomatic myeloma by 2 years, and 28% experienced grade 3-4 drug toxicity. It is thus premature to recommend the use of thalidomide in this setting outside of a clinical trial designed to assess whether it retards the time to progression to overt disease compared to observation alone. Initiation of bisphosphonates in patients with asymptomatic MM in an effort to prevent the development of symptomatic skeletal disease is also being

**Table 83.1**   Combination chemotherapy regimens for multiple myeloma

| Regimen | Drugs | Doses | Frequency |
|---------|-------|-------|-----------|
| MP | Melphalan | 8–9 mg/m² PO, days 1–4 | q 28 days |
| | Prednisone | 60 mg/m² (or 100 mg) PO, days 1–4 | |
| M2 (VBMCP)[31] | Vincristine | 0.03 mg/kg IVP, day 1 | q 28 days |
| | Carmustine (BCNU) | 1 mg/kg IVPB, day 1 | |
| | Melphalan | 0.1 mg/kg PO, days 1–7 | |
| | Cyclophosphamide | 1 mg/kg IVPB, day 1 | |
| | Prednisone | 1 mg/kg PO, days 1–7 | |
| VMCP/VBAP[34] | Vincristine | 1 mg IVP, day 1 | q 28 days |
| | Melphalan | 5–6 mg/m² PO, days 1–4 | |
| | Cyclophosphamide | 100–125 mg/m² PO, days 1–4 | |
| | Prednisone | 60 mg/m² PO, days 1–4 | |
| | (alternating with) | | |
| | Vincristine | 1 mg IVP, day 1 | |
| | Carmustine (BCNU) | 30 mg/m² IVPB, day 1 | |
| | Doxorubicin | 30 mg/m² IVP, day 1 | |
| | Prednisone | 60 mg/m² PO, days 1–4 | |
| ABCM[77] | Doxorubicin | 30 mg/m² IVP, day 1 | q 5–6 weeks |
| | Carmustine (BCNU) | 30 mg/m² IVPB, day 1 | |
| | Cyclophosphamide | 100 mg/m² PO, days 22–25 | |
| | Melphalan | 6 mg/m² PO, days 22–25 | |
| EDAP[44] | Etoposide | 100 mg/m²/day, CIV, days 1–4 | q 28 days |
| | Dexamethasone | 40 mg/day IV / PO, days 1–4 | |
| | Cytarabine (Ara-C) | 1 g/m² IVPB, day 5 | |
| | Cisplatin | 25 mg/m²/day, CIV, days 1–4 | |
| DCEP[111,162] | Dexamethasone | 40 mg/day, IV / PO, days 1–4 | q 28 days |
| | Cyclophosphamide | 400 mg/m²/day, CIV, days 1–4 | |
| | Etoposide | 40 mg/m²/day, CIV, days 1–4 | |
| | Cisplatin | 10 mg/m²/day, CIV, days 1–4 | |
| MOCCA[163] | Methylprednisolone | 0.8 mg/kg PO, days 1–7 | q 35 days |
| | Vincristine | 0.03 mg/kg IVP, day 1 | |
| | Lomustine (CCNU) | 40 mg PO, day 1 | |
| | Cyclophosphamide | 10 mg/kg IVPB, day 1 | |
| | Melphalan | 0.25 mg/kg PO, days 1–4 | |

explored,[12] but there is insufficient data to support routine use at present,[13] particularly in light of the recently recognized association between long-term bisphosphonate use and the uncommon but potentially serious problem of osteonecrosis of the jaw (ONJ).[14, 15]

## CONVENTIONAL REGIMENS FOR INITIAL THERAPY OF MULTIPLE MYELOMA

### MELPHALAN AND OTHER ALKYLATING AGENTS

Melphalan, usually in combination with prednisone (the "MP" regimen, Table 83.1), has been used to treat MM since the 1960s. A small randomized study comparing different schedules of melphalan, with or without prednisone, showed a distinct advantage in favor of intermittent ("pulse") melphalan with prednisone as compared to either pulse or daily melphalan alone,[16] though not all subsequent studies have con-

firmed superiority of this schedule.[17, 18] In the MP regimen, the initial dose of oral melphalan is 8–9 mg/m² daily along with prednisone 100 mg/day (or 60 mg/m²/day) for four consecutive days, approximately every 4 weeks. While the oral administration of melphalan is convenient, absorption can sometimes be unpredictable,[19] and therefore the dose may need to be titrated upward in subsequent cycles, until modest myelosuppression (i.e., absolute neutrophil count ~1000/MM³ weeks after the start of the cycle) is seen. Also, in patients with renal insufficiency, pronounced cytopenias can develop with full melphalan dosing, and a starting dose of 4–6 mg/m²/day for 4 days is recommended, with careful monitoring of hematologic toxicity. Objective responses, usually occurring within the first two to three cycles of MP, can be expected in 50–60% of patients and last on average 1.5–2 years.[20] Because of the low toxicity and ease of administration of oral MP, it is often selected as the initial therapy in

**Table 83.2**    Dosage schedules for VAD and related regimens

| Regimen | Drugs | Doses | Frequency |
|---|---|---|---|
| VAD[37] | Vincristine<br>Doxorubicin<br>Dexamethasone | 0.4 mg/day, CIV, days 1–4<br>9 mg/m$^2$/day, CIV, days 1–4<br>40 mg/d, days 1–4, 9–12, 17–20 (odd cycles)<br>days 1–4, 14–18 (even cycles)<br>(alternatively, DEX on days<br>1–4 and 14–18 *every* cycle, using a<br>q 28 day schedule) | q 28–35 d |
| Bolus VAD[164] | Vincristine<br>Doxorubicin<br>Dexamethasone | 0.4 mg/day, CIV, days 1–4<br>9 mg/m$^2$/day, CIV, days 1–4<br>40 mg/day, days 1–4, 9–12, 17–20 (odd cycles)<br>days 1–4, 14–18 (even cycles) | q 28–35 d |
| DVd[49] | Liposomal Doxorubicin (Doxil)<br>Vincristine<br>Dexamethasone | 40 mg/m$^2$, IVPB, day 1<br>2 mg IVP, day 1<br>40 mg/day, PO/IV, days 1–4 | q 28 days |
| VAMP[42]<br><br>(C-VAMP) | Vincristine<br>Doxorubicin<br>Methylprednisolone<br>(add Cyclophosphamide) | 0.4 mg/day, CIV, days 1–4<br>9 mg/m$^2$/day, CIV, days 1–4<br>1 g, IV/PO, days 1–5<br>(500 mg/m$^2$ IVPB, days 1, 8, 15) | q 28 days |
| MOD[41] | Mitoxantrone<br>Vincristine<br>Dexamethasone | 9 mg/m$^2$/day, CIV, days 1–4<br>0.4 mg/day, CIV, days 1–4<br>40 mg/day, days 1–4, 9–12, 17–20 | q 35 days |
| VND[43] | Vincristine<br>Mitoxantrone<br>Dexamethasone | 0.4 mg/day, CIV, days 1–4<br>3 mg/m$^2$/day, CIV, days 1–4<br>40 mg/day, days 1–4 | q 28 days |
| VECD[50] | Vincristine<br>Epirubicin<br>Cyclophosphamide<br>Dexamethasone | 1.5 mg IVP, day 1<br>20 mg/m$^2$ IVP, days 2, 3<br>200 mg/m$^2$ IVPB, days 1–3<br>20 mg/m$^2$ PO/IV, days 1–5 | q 28 days |
| VID[54] | Vincristine<br>Idarubicin (oral)<br>Dexamethasone | 1.6 mg/m$^2$ IVP (max: 2 mg), day 1<br>10 mg/m$^2$ PO, days 1–4<br>40 mg/d PO/IV, days 1–4, 9–12, 17–20 | q 28 days |
| Z-Dex[53] | Idarubicin (oral)<br>Dexamethasone | 10 mg/m$^2$ PO, days 1–4<br>40 mg/d PO/IV, d 1–4 | q 28 days |

elderly patients and other patients not going on to HDC/ASCS (see discussion below).

Oral cyclophosphamide (Cytoxan), with or without steroids, has been shown to be equally effective as oral melphalan.[21, 22] Intravenous (IV) cyclophosphamide, 600–1200 mg/m$^2$ every 3–6 weeks, is effective therapy and is also a viable alternative to oral melphalan.[23, 24] More intensive IV cyclophosphamide dosing, such as 600 mg/m$^2$/day for four consecutive days, is feasible[25] but not typically considered because of the effectiveness of less-toxic lower doses. Very high-dose IV cyclophosphamide (i.e., 4–7 g/m$^2$ followed by G-CSF or GM-CSF) is often used after induction to mobilize stem cells for collection prior to HDC/ASCS.[26–28] It is likely that high-dose cyclophosphamide priming provides additional antimyeloma effect beyond that achieved by prior induction therapy,[29] though there is no evidence that this results in any benefit over priming with growth factors alone in terms of transplant outcome.[30]

Many alkylator-based combination chemotherapy regimens have been evaluated and compared to MP. A meta-analysis showed no difference in response duration or OS in more than 6600 patients participating in 27 randomized trials,[20] but two particular regimens warrant comment. The M2 regimen (see Table 83.1) generated interest in the United States after an Eastern Cooperative Oncology Group (ECOG) randomized trial demonstrated modest superiority over MP.[31] Objective responses occurred in more than 70% of patients receiving M2, but 5-year OS was an unimpressive 26%. In contrast, a European study comparing VAD and M2 did not demonstrate superior response rate or OS for the 46 patients treated with M2.[32] Interest in this regimen may be revived somewhat by the recent report of the US Intergroup study comparing VAD followed by two cycles of M2 versus VAD followed by HDC/ASCS in more than 800 patients, discussed in detail below, in which patients treated with

M2, had equivalent overall outcomes to those getting HDC/ASCS.[33] VMCP alternating with VBAP (VMCP/VBAP, Table 83.1) was used in the positive IFM 90 HDC/ASCS study.[34] All patients received VMCP/VBAP induction, and then patients randomized to conventional therapy received additional cycles of the same regimen. In a SWOG study comparing VMCP/VBAP to MP, the alternating regimen demonstrated a superior response rate (53% vs 32%) and median OS (43 months vs 23 months).[35] Another randomized study comparing these regimens, however, did not demonstrate either a response rate or survival advantage for VMCP/VBAP.[36]

### VAD AND RELATED REGIMENS

With no overall improvement in outcome seen with the alkylator-based combination regimens developed in the 1970s and 1980s, regimens utilizing anthracyclines administered by continuous infusion were developed, with the rationale that continuous drug exposure would more effectively target slowly cycling plasma cells. One such regimen is VAD: vincristine 0.4 mg/day and doxorubicin (Adriamycin) 9 mg/m$^2$/day as a continuous infusion, with pulses of dexamethasone (orally or IV intravenously) 40 mg/day on days 1–4, 9–11, 17–20 in repeating 28- to 35-day cycles.[37] Approximately two-thirds of previously untreated patients will respond to VAD, usually within two to three cycles.[38-40] Unfortunately, despite the continuous infusion of chemotherapy in VAD and other regimens[41-43] (see Table 83.2), the majority of these responses are partial,[38-40, 42, 44] as seen with earlier bolus regimens. Also, long-term survival of nontransplanted myeloma patients treated with VAD is not significantly better than that seen with MP.[3, 20] VAD is a reasonable option in patients with renal insufficiency because, in contrast to melphalan, neither vincristine nor doxorubicin requires dosage adjustment for impaired creatinine clearance. The widespread popularity of VAD since its advent in the 1980s until the last few years is accounted for by another factor as well: the dramatic increase in the use of HDC/ASCS. Several groups have reported a clear negative impact on stem cell mobilization and subsequent engraftment (particularly platelets) from prior melphalan therapy.[45-47] Accordingly, VAD (two to four cycles) was often the initial regimen used in patients for whom HDC/ASCS was planned. More recently, TD has supplanted VAD as the most widely used regimen in such patients.

Central line placement and use of an ambulatory pump for regimens like VAD are inconvenient and are associated with infections and thrombotic complications. This, and the recognition that infusional regimens have not changed the overall course of MM compared to MP, has led to interest in more convenient bolus or oral variations on VAD (see Table 83.2). Randomized studies have shown that both "bolus VAD," with the standard doses of each drug given as an IV injection on days 1–4, and also the DVd regimen have similar efficacy to traditional VAD.[48, 49] DVd consists of pegylated doxorubicin (Doxil™) 40 mg/m$^2$ IVPB on day 1, Vincristine 2 mg IVP on day 1, and dexamethasone 40 mg/day on days 1–4. In a Phase II study, DVd induced major responses in 88% of newly diagnosed patients and was well tolerated overall.[49] It is noteworthy that grade 3-4 palmar-plantar erythrodysesthesia, a Doxil-related toxicity not seen with traditional VAD, occurred in approximately 20% of patients. The VECD protocol, using bolus injections of vincristine 1.5 mg day 1 and epirubicin 20 mg/m$^2$ days 2 and 3 with 1-hour infusions of cyclophosphamide 200 mg/m$^2$ days 1–3 and oral dexamethasone 20 mg/m$^2$ days 1–5, is yet another regimen with comparable efficacy to VAD.[50] Bolus VAD or VECD are less expensive than either standard infusional VAD[51] or DVd. In a preliminary cost analysis, DVd was shown to be less costly than VAD if the latter was administered on an inpatient basis.[52] Given the significantly higher drug costs associated with DVd,[52] this might not hold true at centers where both regimens are given in the outpatient setting.

Oral VAD variants have also been developed, and these are likely to have similar efficacy to traditional VAD.[53, 54] The lack of availability of oral anthracyclines in the United States at present makes these less relevant for standard practice, however.

### HIGH-DOSE DEXAMETHASONE MONOTHERAPY

Dexamethasone, 20 mg/m$^2$/day on days 1–4, 9–12, and 17–20, induces responses in previously untreated patients with MM 40–50% of the time,[55, 56] suggesting that dexamethasone accounts for most of the benefit derived from VAD and TD (described below). Dexamethasone monotherapy may be preferred for frail patients, since the toxicity is generally less than that seen with VAD or TD. Still, primary pulse dexamethasone treatment is somewhat more toxic than MP,[57] and patients should be monitored closely for specific side effects, including hyperglycemia, gastrointestinal bleeding, mood disorder, insomnia, weight gain, increased susceptibility to infections, and rarely pancreatitis.[58]

### THALIDOMIDE AND DEXAMETHASONE

Thalidomide has activity against relapsed and refractory myeloma as a single agent[59-65] and in combination with pulse dexamethasone,[66, 67] with responses noted in 25–55% of patients in various trials. In two large Phase II studies of TD in previously *untreated* patients, response rates of 64% and 72% were reported.[68, 69] Investigators from the Mayo Clinic treated 50 patients with 200 mg of thalidomide daily with dexamethasone 40 mg/day on days 1–4, 9–12, and 17–20.[68] In the other study, 40 patients at M.D. Anderson Cancer Center (MDACC) were started on thalidomide 100–200 mg daily with dose increase to 400 mg/day allowed (median maximum dose achieved was 200 mg/day), and dexamethasone 20 mg/m$^2$ on the same schedule as in the Mayo trial.[69] As would be predicted from trials involving patients with relapsed/ refractory MM,[65, 66] thalidomide therapy caused neuropathy, sedation, and constipation. Thrombotic complications occurred in 12% and 15% of patients treated in these two induction trials. In the MDACC study, a 25% thrombosis rate was observed in the first 24 patients treated, despite prophylaxis with 1 mg of coumadin daily. The next 16 patients received therapeutic doses of coumadin or low-molecular-weight heparin and no thrombotic events occurred.[69] Based on the results of these Phase II trials, a randomized study comparing TD to dexamethasone alone was undertaken by ECOG. In this study, after four cycles of randomized therapy, patients with at least stable disease were given the option of proceeding to HDC/ ASCS. Although a statistically higher response rate was observed in the patients treated with TD (63% vs 41%), they also experienced more toxicity (including thrombotic complications), without any difference in survival.[70] TD induction has no negative effect on stem cell collection and quality of subsequent engraftment in patients treated with going on to HDC/ASCS.[68, 70, 71] Conclusions regarding the long-term outcome for patients treated with TD *without* subsequent HDC/ ASCS on this ECOG study are limited because almost all patients went on to high-dose therapy. The overall duration of response and survival for the 21 patients continuing TD beyond four cycles were 18 and 21 months, respectively,[72] similar to the rates noted in the initial report of a large randomized trial of dexamethasone ± thalidomide without HDC/ASCS (TTP: 17 months, OS: 25 months).[73] These results are very similar to what one can expect from traditional cytotoxic regimens such as VAD. This, plus the fact that this convenient oral regimen can be used safely prior to HDC/ASCS or in the setting of renal insufficiency,[74] has made TD the most widely used induction regimen in the United States.

## HIGH-DOSE CHEMOTHERAPY AND AUTOLOGOUS STEM CELL SUPPORT

The role of HDC/ASCS is somewhat controversial at present. Many clinicians consider HDC/ASCS to be the "standard of care" for suitable candidates early in the course of their treatment, typically after two to four cycles of induction therapy. The data available from published studies has recently been summarized in overviews and management guidelines,[7, 55, 75] and will be reviewed here briefly (also, refer to Chapter 90).

A randomized trial from the Intergroupe Francophone du Myélome (IFM) comparing HDC/ASCS to nonmyeloablative therapy (VMCP/VBAP) demonstrated a superior outcome for those patients treated with intensive therapy.[34] In this trial involving 200 patients aged 65 years or less, the myeloablative preparative regimen consisted of melphalan 140 mg/m$^2$ plus 8 Gy total body irradiation. The response rate, 5-year event-free survival (EFS) and 5-year OS were all higher in the transplant arm of the trial (81% vs 55%, 28% vs 10%, and 52% vs 12%, respectively). The median OS for the HDC/ASCS arm was just over 1 year longer (57 months vs 44 months). A similar 1-year OS advantage (54 months vs 42 months) was also demonstrated in the more recent Medical Research Council (MRC) VII trial,[76] which involved 401 patients randomized to either HDC/ASCS or a conventional chemotherapy ("ABCM,"[77] Table 83.1). The fact that the transplanted patients in the MRC study did not do any better than those in the IFM trial is disappointing, since the patients in the MRC study received stem cells instead of bone marrow, and generally received a transplant preparative regimen (melphalan 200 mg/m$^2$ (MEL 200)) proven to be superior to that used in the IFM study.[78]

Two nonrandomized studies comparing the outcome of HDC/ASCS to historical controls also suggest survival benefit from transplant. The Arkansas group compared outcome for 123 patients treated with the "Total Therapy I (TTI)" tandem transplant regimen with that of matched historical controls treated on prior Southwest Oncology Group (SWOG) with conventional chemotherapy.[79] Median EFS and OS were 49 and 62 months in the TTI group versus 22 and 48 months in the conventionally treated group. The Nordic Myeloma Study Group compared the results of therapy in 274 patients treated with HDC/ASCS and 274 matched historical controls who would have met current criteria for HDC/ASCS.[80] The intensive therapy group had a 3-year OS of approximately 70% versus 55% in the nontransplant group. Log-rank comparison of the survival curves showed a difference that was highly statistically significant. Based on the preceding data, several experts in the field of MM have concluded that HDC/ASCS offers some benefit over standard regimens and it should be considered standard therapy for suitable patients.[7, 55]

In contrast to the results of the above-mentioned studies, a preliminary report from the PETHEMA investigators of a randomized trial comparing continued conventional chemotherapy to HDC/ASCS (MEL 200) in more than 200 patients who responded to initial conventional chemotherapy showed a similar median OS of approximately 5.5 years for both groups.[81] It is possible that the exclusion of patients who did not respond to initial chemotherapy influenced the outcome of this study, making the results difficult to compare with those of the IFM and MRC studies. The Dutch–Belgian Hemato-Oncology Cooperative Study Group (HOVON) also conducted a randomized study in which patients received either HDC/ASCS or "intermediate dose melphalan" (140 mg/m²). EFS and OS were the same for each arm (21 vs 22 months, and 50 vs 47 months, respectively).[82]

More recently, the preliminary results of a US Intergroup randomized study were reported, and as in the PETHEMA trial, no survival benefit was observed.[83] Following VAD induction and high-dose cyclophosphamide with stem cell collection, patients received either HDC/ASCS (MEL 140 + 12 Gy TBI) or two cycles of the M2 regimen. Eight hundred and four patients started VAD, but only 510 were randomized after induction. For nearly all of the almost 300 patients who did not proceed with randomization, the reason was failure to respond to induction therapy. Thirty-nine patients on this trial with matched sibling donors underwent allogeneic stem cell transplant before this arm of the study was closed due to a high (but not surprising) treatment-related mortality of 39% in the first year. In the other two arms, there was no difference in the response rate, 7-year progression free survival (17% for HDC/ASCS vs 16% for chemotherapy), or 7-year OS (37% vs 42%). Interestingly, despite the early mortality seen in the small group of patients who underwent allogeneic transplantation, there was a 7-year OS of approximately 40% (very similar to that for the other groups), with an apparent survival curve plateau suggesting possible cures in some cases.[33] Reasons offered by the investigators for the lack of benefit with HDC/ASCS include unexpectedly good outcome in the conventional therapy arm compared to prior experience and the fact that over half of the patients progressing after M2 went on to be treated with HDC/ASCS.[33] A previously published French randomized study demonstrated equivalent survival for patients randomized to treatment with HDC/ASCS as rescue therapy upon progression, versus immediately following conventional therapy,[84] lending some credence to the latter assertion. It is possible that improved supportive measures and postprogression use of newer antimyeloma agents such as thalidomide or bortzeomib could have contributed to the longer-than-expected survival seen in this study, as well. Regardless of the reason(s), the equivalent results with nonmyeloablative therapy and HDC/ASCS in this large, well-conducted study will likely complicate decision making for patients and clinicians.

It has become evident that the subset of MM patients with deletion of all or part of chromosome 13 (Δ13), detected by either standard cytogenetic techniques or by fluorescence in situ hybridization (FISH), have inferior outcome compared to patients lacking Δ13.[85–87] Even with tandem melphalan-based autologous transplants, the 5-year OS for patients with Δ13 is only 16%,[85] slightly *inferior* to the 22% observed for similar patients treated in another trial with the non-myeloablative VBMCP regimen.[88] With poor outcome despite HDC/ASCS consistently demonstrated, other treatment options ought to be explored. At our center,

we have offered patients under age 60 with Δ13 HDC/ASCS followed by a nonmyeloablative ("mini") allogeneic transplant. The rationale for this is to try and gain "graft-versus-myeloma" benefit[89, 90] without the excessive early mortality seen with standard allogeneic transplantation.[91, 92] There is published anecdotal evidence that patients with Δ13 can enjoy extended benefit after such treatment.[93, 94] Variations on this approach have been described in several published reports.[94–96] Large studies more formally evaluating the strategy of HDC/ASCS "conditioning" followed by nonmyeloablative allogeneic stem cell transplant are currently underway.

All of the randomized trials of HDC/ASCS exclude patients with markedly impaired renal function, as well as patients older than 65–70 years. The available data suggests HDC/ASCS is possible in these groups,[97–102] though the potential for increased treatment-related toxicity should be recognized. For example, a preparative regimen of melphalan 140 mg/m² may be optimal for patients with impaired renal function.[103] It may also be desirable to use less intensive IV melphalan (i.e., 60–140 mg/m²) in older patients with MM to reduce toxicity.[97] Such regimens in older patients may be able to achieve results comparable to those seen with more intensive transplant regimens.[104]

New issues related to HDC continue to emerge. Tandem autologous transplant has been shown in one randomized trial to yield superior outcome to single transplant,[5] but there is evidence to suggest that the subset of patients actually benefiting from a second transplant are those not attaining a CR or nCR with the first one and who are able to undergo the second procedure within 6–12 months.[5, 105] Given the mixed data on single HDC/ASCS, the role of tandem transplant in *any* patient group remains ambiguous. As allogeneic stem cell transplant techniques become increasingly refined, the potential role of this modality will need to be explored further. Finally, the rapid expansion of novel antimyeloma agents in recent years has led to vigorous debate as to how these agents should be incorporated into both transplant and nontransplant treatment paradigms.

## NEWER REGIMENS AND NOVEL AGENTS

### MELPHALAN-PREDNISONE-THALIDOMIDE

The results of two large randomized studies comparing MP to MPT, undertaken after an Italian Phase II of MP plus low-dose thalidomide (MPT) in patients with previously untreated MM demonstrated a remarkable 93% overall response rate (45% CR/nCR),[106] have recently reported. Palumbo et al. randomized 255 patients between the ages of 60 and 85 with newly diagnosed MM to either MP or MPT. All patients received six 4-week cycles of MP, and patients randomized to the MPT arm also received thalidomide 100 mg daily until either disease progression or unacceptable toxicity.[107] Patients receiving MPT had a superior overall response rate (76% vs 48%), CR/nCR rate (28% vs 7%), and 2-year EFS rate (54% vs 27%; $p$ = 0.0006). Three-year OS was also higher—80% for MPT versus 64% for MP—although this difference did not reach statistical significance. The increased efficacy of MPT came at the price of increased toxicity, particularly infectious and thrombotic complications. The incidence of grade 3-4 nonhematologic adverse events was 48% in the MPT arm, compared to 25% in the MP arm ($p$ = 0.0002). Prior to the introduction of prophylactic enoxaparin, 20% of patients receiving MPT developed deep vein thromboses (DVTs). After enoxaparin 40 mg subcutaneously once daily was added, the incidence of DVTs dropped to 3%, resulting in an overall incidence of 12% on this trial. The IFM compared MP (12 cycles), MPT (thalidomide ≤ 400 mg/day through the end of MP), and a high-dose melphalan-based regimen (VAD × 2, then cyclophosphamide 3 g/m² to mobilize stem cells, then MEL(100) with ASCS × 2) in 476 patients between the ages of 65–75 with previously untreated MM.[108] The median progression-free survival for MPT was 29 months (compared to 17 months for MP ($p$ < 0.0001) and 19 months for MEL(100) ($p$ = 0.0001)). Median OS, which was 30 months for MP and 39 months for MEL(100), was not reached in the MPT arm after 56 months median follow-up ($p$ = 0.0008 for MPT vs MP, $p$ = 0.014 for MPT vs MEL(100)).

## COMBINATION CHEMOTHERAPY WITH CONCURRENT THALIDOMIDE

The addition of daily thalidomide (50 mg/day initially, escalated to a maximum of 400 mg/day) to the DVd regimen (described above) appears to result in greatly enhanced antimyeloma activity in both the relapsed/refractory and up-front settings.[109] After a median of six cycles of therapy, 46% of newly diagnosed patients had either a CR or nCR, a rate comparable to that seen with HDC/ASCS.[34] It remains to be seen whether the time to disease progression will be as long as that typically expected from HDC/ASCS. The regimen is clearly more toxic than DVd alone, requiring prophylactic antibiotics because of high rates of infection, particularly pneumonia, and also daily aspirin because of a high rate of DVTs.[109] The latter complication is not wholly unexpected, given the higher rate of thrombotic complications seen with TD.[68, 69] Investigators at the University of Arkansas have published their extensive experience using combination chemotherapy with thalidomide in both the up-front and relapsed setting (Table 83.3).[110-112] As in the other trials discussed, an increased rate of DVT was observed with these combinations, particularly during concomitant anthracycline and thalidomide administration.[111, 112]

Based on the results of the two randomized studies discussed above, some clinicians have adopted MPT as the preferred regimen for newly diagnosed MM patients who are not going on to get HDC/ASCS and who are judged likely to be able to tolerate the added toxicity of the regimen compared to MP. Incorporation of thalidomide into other combination chemotherapy induction regimens will ultimately only be justified if there is proven, meaningful clinical benefit that outweighs increases in toxicity.

## BORTEZOMIB (VELCADE)

Bortezomib is the first proteasome inhibitor approved by the FDA for treatment of relapsed–refractory MM. In Phase II trials involving heavily pretreated patients, including several with markedly impaired renal function, Bortezomib 1.3 mg/m² as an IV push twice weekly for 2 weeks followed by a week break demonstrated a 35% overall response rate, including 10% CR/nCR.[113] Two Phase II studies in newly diagnosed

| Table 83.3 | Combination regimens containing thalidomide | | |
|---|---|---|---|
| Regimen | Drugs | Doses | Frequency |
| TD[68,69] | Dexamethasone | 40 mg/day PO/IV, days 1–4, 9–12, 17–20 | q 28–35 days |
| | Thalidomide | 200–600 mg/day PO (start 100–200) | |
| TD-PACE[110] | Dexamethasone | 40 mg/day PO/IV, days 1–4 | q 28 days |
| | Thalidomide | 400 mg/day PO | |
| | Cisplatin | 10 mg/m²/day, CIV, days 1–4 | |
| | Doxorubicin | 10 mg/m²/day, CIV, days 1–4 | |
| | Cyclophosphamide | 400 mg/m²/day, CIV, days 1–4 | |
| | Etoposide | 40 mg/m²/day, CIV, days 1–4 | |
| DVd-T[109] | Liposomal Doxorubicin (Doxil) | 40 mg/m², IVPB, day 1 | q 28 days |
| | Vincristine | 2 mg IVP, day 1 | |
| | Dexamethasone | 40 mg/day, PO/IV, days 1–4 | |
| | Thalidomide | 200–400 mg/day PO (start 50–100) | |
| MP-T[106] | Melphalan | 4 mg/m² PO, days 1–7 | q 28–35 d |
| | Prednisone | 40 mg/m² PO, days 1–7 | |
| | Thalidomide | 100 mg/day PO | |

myeloma suggest that the response rate may be much higher when the drug is used in combination with dexamethasone earlier in the disease course. Jagannath et al. treated 32 patients with newly diagnosed MM with standard dose bortezomib and added pulse dexamethasone for patients who did not achieve at least a partial response after two cycles or a CR after four cycles.[114] The response rate to bortezomib alone was 40% after two cycles, partial responses in almost all cases. Dexamethasone was added for 22 patients, leading to improved responses in 15 cases. The overall response rate for the study was ultimately 88%, with 25% attaining CR/nCR. An IFM study involving 52 newly diagnosed patients treated with bortezomib plus dexamethasone showed similarly impressive results: 66% overall response rate and 21% CR rate.[115] In this study, subsequent stem cell collection was successful in 44 out of 44 patients in whom this was attempted, demonstrating that bortezomib can be used as initial therapy for patients planning to undergo HDC/ASCS. Peripheral sensory neuropathy occurred in just under a third of the patients enrolled on each of these two studies, and 14% of the enrollees in the French study had grade 2-3 neuropathy.[114, 115] Bortezomib dose reduction results in improvement of treatment-related neuropathy in half or more of cases.[114] Other investigators have explored adding bortezomib to cytotoxic chemotherapeutic combination regimens. The PAD regimen, which combines bortezomib (1.3 mg/m$^2$ days 1,4,8,11), infusional adriamycin (9 mg/m$^2$/day CIV), and dexamethasone (40 mg/d days 1-4 every cycle, and days 8-11, 15-18 cycle 1 only), has been shown in a large Phase II study to be both feasible and exceptionally active, with an overall response rate of 95% (CR rate 24%).[116] Based on the very high overall and complete response rates seen with the PAD regimen, some clinicians (including the author) are already using the PAD regimen rather than VAD for the initial treatment of MM patients presenting with renal failure. Similarly impressive response rates were noted in a Phase I-II study of MP plus bortezomib in previously untreated MM patients.[117] For further discussion regarding bortezomib as treatment for relapsed–refractory MM, please refer to Chapter 92. If larger studies validate the promising results seen thus far, it is probable that in the future bortezomib will become widely used early in the course of disease management.

### LENALIDOMIDE (CC-5013; REVLIMID)

Lenalidomide is a member of a class of thalidomide analogues called immunmodulatory drugs, or IMiDs. In vitro, lenalidomide modulates cytokine production and T-lymphocyte stimulation at least 100 times more potently than thalidomide.[118, 119] Phase I trials in relapsed–refractory patients using doses ranging from 5 mg/day to 50 mg/day have shown response rates of 40–71%, even in patients previously treated with thalidomide.[120, 121] The toxicity profile of lenalidomide is very different than that of thalidomide, with thrombocytopenia and neutropenia predominating, and essentially no sedation, constipation, or neuropathy. The response rate among 34 patients with newly diagnosed MM treated with lenalidomide 25 mg daily for 21 out of every 28 days with pulse dexamethasone (40 mg/day on days 1–4, 9–12, 17–20) was 91% (CR 6%).[122] ECOG has completed accrual to a large randomized study of lenalidomide with two different doses of dexamethasone, and the Southwest Oncology Group is currently conducting a 500-person randomized, double-blinded study comparing dexamethasone to dexamethasone plus lenalidomide (LD). The results of these two studies will establish whether LD could be an appropriate front-line regimen for patients with MM.

## DURATION OF THERAPY

The risk of some chemotherapy-associated complications is related to cumulative lifetime dose of a given agent. Relevant examples include cardiomyopathy and anthracyclines,[123] neuropathy and vinca alkyloids or thalidomide,[124] and stem cell injury from melphalan.[45-47] Thus, the benefit of ongoing treatment must be continuously weighed against the risk of developing potentially irreversible toxicities. In patients not undergoing HDC/ASCS, initial therapy is typically continued for at least two to four cycles beyond maximal response, unless concern over toxicity mandates stopping sooner. Indefinite "maintenance" with ongoing chemotherapy is not beneficial in the case of MP[125] and is not feasible with VAD. There is insufficient data to make a recommendation at this time on the optimal duration of TD therapy (NCCN Guidelines v.1 2006; www.nccn.org/professionals/physician_gls/PDF/myeloma.pdf), but most clinicians continue therapy until there is evidence of either disease progression or unacceptable toxicity. There is data to support benefit from ongoing corticosteroids as a form of maintenance. A SWOG trial showed that 50 mg of prednisone every other day after achievement of maximal response to chemotherapy extends median duration of both remission and survival by 9 months,[126] a modest benefit which must be weighed against the potential adverse effects of chronic steroid use in certain patients (e.g., diabetics). The preliminary findings of a trial comparing dexamethasone maintenance (40 mg/day for four consecutive days every month) to observation following induction therapy confirm a 9-month improvement in time to disease progression, but no survival advantage was found.[127] Maintenance therapy with Interferon-α (IFN) has been explored in a multitude of trials, the results of which are summarized in two published meta-analyses.[128, 129] IFN maintenance prolongs both response duration and OS by only 4–6 months in a minority of patients with significant toxicity and cost, making it difficult for most clinicians to recommend with enthusiasm.

## SUPPORTIVE CARE

Adjunctive measures addressing three complications of MM—skeletal disease, anemia, and thrombosis—deserve mention. For a more general discussion of palliative care issues in hematologic malignancies, please refer to Chapter 115.

### MANAGEMENT OF SKELETAL DISEASE

Bone disease in the form of lytic lesions, pathological fractures, or osteoporosis are present at diagnosis over three-quarters of the time,[130] ultimately leading to significant morbidity in many patients with MM. While external beam radiation therapy is remarkably effective palliation for pain relief from existing lesions, it is the localized therapy without the potential to reduce the risk of skeletal complications outside of the radiation port.

Bone resorption in MM results occurs due to stimulation of osteoclasts, which in turn results predominantly from receptor activator of NF-κB (RANK) signaling by RANK-ligand.[131, 132] Bisphosphonates are synthetic pyrophosphate analogues that inhibit osteoclast function directly though disruption of intracellular biochemical pathways[133, 134] or induction of apoptosis,[135] or indirectly by stimulating production of the inhibitory RANK decoy molecule, osteoprotegerin.[136] The two bisphosphonates currently approved for use in treating MM-related bone disease are pamidronate (Aredia) and zoledronic acid (Zometa). Pamidronate, 90 mg intravenously over 4 hours every 4 weeks, has been shown in randomized trials to significantly reduce the rate of skeletal complications associated with MM compared to placebo, 28% versus 44% at 12 months, as well as delaying the median time to first skeletal complication from 12 months to 21 months.[137] This effect persisted with treatment extended out to almost 2 years.[138] It should be noted that this dose of pamidronate can be given safely over 60–90 minutes. Zoledronic acid is a newer bisphosphonate with 1000 times the potency of pamidronate and an even shorter infusional time of 15 minutes. In a randomized trial with extended follow-up, comparing zoledronic acid 4 mg every 3–4 weeks to pamidronate 90 mg, comparable efficacy in preventing skeletal complications was observed.[139, 140] As a result of these trials, the American Society of Clinical Oncology has released clinical guidelines recommending the routine use of either pamidronate or zoledronic acid for MM patients with lytic bone lesions or myeloma-related osteopenia.[13] There is no consensus on the optimal duration of bisphosphonate therapy, but the widespread practice of indefinite monthly administration of these agents has recently come under scrutiny with the recognition of ONJ as an uncommon toxicity associated with prolonged bisphosphonate use.[14] Patients with ONJ develop exposed areas of chronic, nonhealing necrotic bone in their mouths, in many cases after tooth extraction. While much work remains to be done in terms of fully characterizing this problem, some groups have developed treatment guidelines which reflect the currently available information on ONJ and bisphosphonates.[15] Newer approaches to treating myeloma-related bone disease include percutaneous kyphoplasty or vertebroplasty of vertebral compression fractures related to lytic lesions[141, 142] or osteoporosis[143]; utilization of radioactive Strontium-89[144]; and recombinant osteoprotegerin or the soluble RANK-ligand receptor, RANK-Fc, to block the osteoclast-activating effects of endogenous RANK-ligand in the marrow microenvironment.[145, 146]

### MANAGEMENT OF ANEMIA

Several studies have been performed to assess the efficacy of recombinant erythropoietin (rHuEPO; Epogen, Procrit) administered subcutaneously to patients with MM with a hemoglobin value of less than 10 g/dL.[147–150] Although there were methodological flaws making interpretation of the results of individual trials problematic, taken together they suggest that half or more of such patients may benefit in terms of increase in hemoglobin concentration[147–150] and reduction in transfusion requirements.[147, 150] Based on these results, the American Society of Clinical Oncology and the American Society of Hematology guidelines recommend consideration of rHuEPO use for myeloma patients with anemia that does not improve after initiation of therapy with chemotherapy or glucocorticoids.[151] Concurrent use of rHuEPO with either thalidomide or lenalidomide may be associated with an increased risk of DVTs, and therefore caution is recommended when considering its use in this setting.[152] The starting dose of rHuEPO should be 150 units/kg thrice weekly for a minimum of 4 weeks, with consideration of an increase to 300 units/kg/dose for an additional 4–8 weeks if there has been less than a 1–2 g/dL increase in hemoglobin. Forty-thousand units subcutaneously once weekly, with an increase to 60,000 units as needed, is an accepted and widely used alternative. A randomized study comparing an alternative erythropoietic agent, weekly darbepoetin alfa (Aranesp; dose: 2.25 μg/kg/wk), to placebo was published after the release of these guidelines, and the results demonstrate comparable efficacy.[153] Studies evaluating administration of higher doses of darbepoetin every 2 to 3 weeks in patients with other cancers receiving chemotherapy suggest that less-frequent dosing is feasible,[154, 155] but at present, there is insufficient data in patients with myeloma or other hematologic malignancies.

### THROMBOSIS

Patients with MM have a high baseline incidence of thrombotic complications—perhaps as high as 10%.[156] Treatment with either thalidomide or lenalidomide in combination with either glucocorticoids[69, 70, 157, 158] or chemotherapy[111, 112, 159] appears to increase this risk.

All MM patients receiving these IMiD-containing combinations should receive some form of thromboprophylaxis. There is evidence to support the use of full-dose warfarin,[69] prophylactic dose enoxaparin,[107] and aspirin (ASA) 81–325 mg daily.[122, 159, 158] These preventative agents have not been compared head-to-head. The favorable cost- and toxicity-profile of ASA has made this the most attractive option for patients and clinicians, though some experts have advocated full-dose warfarin or enoxaparin as preferred options.[160]

## SUMMARY

As our understanding of MM expands, treatment paradigms are changing. It is becoming increasingly apparent that tumor-specific biologic features, such as the presence of chromosome 13 abnormalities, or patient-specific clinical factors, such as renal failure or advanced age, result in biologically or functionally distinct disease states, likely requiring "tailoring" of treatment. Although cure remains an elusive goal, it appears that for some subsets of patients, emerging therapies may finally be starting to have an impact on survival. For example, the addition of thalidomide to MP clearly improves survival in older patients who are not candidates for HDC/ASCS. Once optimal strategies for combining thalidomide and other new agents such as bortezomib and lenalidomide with traditional cytotoxic drugs are established, better quality (i.e., more complete) responses may be able to be obtained without having to use HDC/ASCS. The benefits of HDC/ASCS have recently been questioned with the negative results of a large randomized US intergroup trial, but high-dose therapy will likely remain a part of MM therapy for the foreseeable future, particularly as allogeneic transplant techniques evolve.

## REFERENCES

1. Jemal A, Tiwari RC, Murray T, et al.: Cancer statistics, 2004. *CA Cancer J Clin* 54(1):8–29, 2004.
2. Alexanian R, Dimopoulos M: The treatment of multiple myeloma. *N Engl J Med* 330(7):484–489, 1994.
3. Crowley J, Jacobson J, Alexanian R: Standard-dose therapy for multiple myeloma: the Southwest Oncology Group experience. *Semin Hematol* 38(3): 203–208, 2001.
4. Blade J, Vesole DH, Gertz M: High-dose therapy in multiple myeloma. *Blood* 102(10):3469–3470, 2003.
5. Attal M, Harousseau JL, Facon T, et al.: Single versus double autologous stem-cell transplantation for multiple myeloma. *N Engl J Med* 349(26):2495–2502, 2003.
6. Durie BG, Jacobson J, Barlogie B, Crowley J: Magnitude of response with myeloma frontline therapy does not predict outcome: importance of time to progression in southwest oncology group chemotherapy trials. *J Clin Oncol* 22(10):1857–1863, 2004.
7. Durie BG, Kyle RA, Belch A, et al.: Myeloma management guidelines: a consensus report from the scientific advisors of the International Myeloma Foundation. *Hematol J* 4(6):379–398, 2003.
8. Kyle RA, Greipp PR: Smoldering multiple myeloma. *N Engl J Med* 302(24):1347–1349, 1980.
9. Hjorth M, Hellquist L, Holmberg E, Magnusson B, Rodjer S, Westin J: Initial versus deferred melphalan-prednisone therapy for asymptomatic multiple myeloma stage I—a randomized study. Myeloma Group of Western Sweden. *Eur J Haematol* 50(2):95–102, 1993.
10. Riccardi A, Mora O, Tinelli C, et al.: Long-term survival of stage I multiple myeloma given chemotherapy just after diagnosis or at progression of the disease: a multi-centre randomized study. Cooperative Group of Study and Treatment of Multiple Myeloma. *Br J Cancer* 82(7):1254–1260, 2000.
11. Rajkumar SV, Gertz MA, Lacy MQ, et al.: Thalidomide as initial therapy for early-stage myeloma. *Leukemia* 17(4):775–779, 2003.
12. Musto P, Falcone A, Sanpaolo G, Bodenizza C, LaSala A, Carella AM: Zoledronate for early-stage, untreated myeloma: an interim report of a randomized study [abstract]. *Proc Am Soc Clin Oncol* 23, 600. 2004.
13. Berenson JR, Hillner BE, Kyle RA, et al.: American Society of Clinical Oncology clinical practice guidelines: the role of bisphosphonates in multiple myeloma. *J Clin Oncol* 20(17):3719–3736, 2002.
14. Ruggiero SL, Mehrotra B, Rosenberg TJ, Engroff SL: Osteonecrosis of the jaws associated with the use of bisphosphonates: a review of 63 cases. *J Oral Maxillofac Surg* 62(5):527–534, 2004.
15. Lacy MQ, Dispenzieri A, Gertz MA, et al.: Mayo clinic consensus statement for the use of bisphosphonates in multiple myeloma. *Mayo Clin Proc* 81(8):1047–1053, 2006.
16. Alexanian R, Haut A, Khan AU, et al.: Treatment for multiple myeloma. Combination chemotherapy with different melphalan dose regimens. *JAMA* 208(9): 1680–1685, 1969.
17. Report on the second myelomatosis trial after five years of follow-up. Medical Research Council's Working Party on Leukaemia in Adults. *Br J Cancer* 42(6): 813–822, 1980.
18. McArthur JR, Athens JW, Wintrobe MM, Cartwright GE: Melphalan and myeloma. Experience with a low-dose continuous regimen. *Ann Intern Med* 72(5):665–670, 1970.
19. Alberts DS, Chang SY, Chen HS, Evans TL, Moon TE: Oral melphalan kinetics. *Clin Pharmacol Ther* 26(6): 737–745, 1979.
20. Combination chemotherapy versus melphalan plus prednisone as treatment for multiple myeloma: an overview of 6,633 patients from 27 randomized trials. Myeloma Trialists' Collaborative Group. *J Clin Oncol* 16(12):3832–3842, 1998.
21. Medical Research Council's Working Party on Leukaemia in Adults: Myelomatosis: comparison of

melphalan and cyclophosphamide therapy. *Br Med J* 1(750):640–641, 1971.

22. Rivers SL, Patno ME: Cyclophosphamide vs melphalan in treatment of plasma cell myeloma. *JAMA* 207(7): 1328–1334, 1969.

23. Kyle RA, Seligman BR, Wallace HJ Jr, Silver RT, Glidewell O, Holland JF: Mutiple myeloma resistant to melphalan (NSC-8806) treated with cyclophosphamide (NSC-26271), prednisone (NSC-10023), and chloroquine (NSC-187208). *Cancer Chemother Rep* 59(3):557–562, 1975.

24. Aitchison R, Williams A, Schey S, Newland AC: A randomised trial of cyclophosphamide with and without low dose alpha-interferon in the treatment of newly diagnosed myeloma. *Leuk Lymphoma* 9(3):243–246, 1993.

25. Lenhard RE, Daniels MJ, Oken MM, et al.: An aggressive high dose cyclophosphamide and prednisone regimen for advanced multiple myeloma. *Leuk Lymphoma* 13(5–6):485–489, 1994.

26. Goldschmidt H, Hegenbart U, Haas R, Hunstein W: Mobilization of peripheral blood progenitor cells with high-dose cyclophosphamide (4 or 7 g/m2) and granulocyte colony-stimulating factor in patients with multiple myeloma. *Bone Marrow Transplant* 17(5):691–697, 1996.

27. Martinez E, Sureda A, Dalmases CD, et al.: Mobilization of peripheral blood progenitor cells by cyclophosphamide and rhGM-CSF in multiple myeloma. *Bone Marrow Transplant* 18(1):1–7, 1996.

28. Fitoussi O, Perreau V, Boiron JM, et al.: A comparison of toxicity following two different doses of cyclophosphamide for mobilization of peripheral blood progenitor cells in 116 multiple myeloma patients. *Bone Marrow Transplant* 27(8):837–842, 2001.

29. Cremer FW, Kiel K, Wallmeier M, Haas R, Goldschmidt H, Moos M: Leukapheresis products in multiple myeloma: lower tumor load after mobilization with cyclophosphamide plus granulocyte colony-stimulating factor (G-CSF) compared with G-CSF alone. *Exp Hematol* 26(10):969–975, 1998.

30. Alegre A, Tomas JF, Martinez-Chamorro C, et al.: Comparison of peripheral blood progenitor cell mobilization in patients with multiple myeloma: high-dose cyclophosphamide plus GM-CSF vs G-CSF alone. *Bone Marrow Transplant* 20(3):211–217, 1997.

31. Oken MM, Harrington DP, Abramson N, Kyle RA, Knospe W, Glick JH: Comparison of melphalan and prednisone with vincristine, carmustine, melphalan, cyclophosphamide, and prednisone in the treatment of multiple myeloma: results of Eastern Cooperative Oncology Group Study E2479. *Cancer* 79(8):1561–1567, 1997.

32. Monconduit M, Menard JF, Michaux JL, et al.: VAD or VMBCP in severe multiple myeloma. The Groupe d'Etudes et de Recherche sur le Myelome (GERM). *Br J Haematol* 80(2):199–204, 1992.

33. Barlogie B, Kyle RA, Anderson KC, et al.: Comparable survival in multiple myeloma (MM) with high dose therapy (HDT) employing MEL 140 mg/m2 + TBI 12 Gy autotransplants versus standard dose therapy with VBMCP and no benefit from interferon (IFN) maintenance: results of intergroup trial S9321. Session type: oral session [abstract]. *Blood* 102(11):42a. 2004.

34. Attal M, Harousseau JL, Stoppa AM, et al.: A prospective, randomized trial of autologous bone marrow transplantation and chemotherapy in multiple myeloma. Intergroupe Francais du Myelome. *N Engl J Med* 335(2):91–97, 1996.

35. Salmon SE, Haut A, Bonnet JD, et al.: Alternating combination chemotherapy and levamisole improves survival in multiple myeloma: a Southwest Oncology Group Study. *J Clin Oncol* 1(8):453–461, 1983.

36. Boccadoro M, Marmont F, Tribalto M, et al.: Multiple myeloma: VMCP/VBAP alternating combination chemotherapy is not superior to melphalan and prednisone even in high-risk patients. *J Clin Oncol* 9(3): 444–448, 1991.

37. Barlogie B, Smith L, Alexanian R: Effective treatment of advanced multiple myeloma refractory to alkylating agents. *N Engl J Med* 310(21):1353–1356, 1984.

38. Alexanian R, Barlogie B, Tucker S: VAD-based regimens as primary treatment for multiple myeloma. *Am J Hematol* 33(2):86–89, 1990.

39. Samson D, Gaminara E, Newland A, et al.: Infusion of vincristine and doxorubicin with oral dexamethasone as first-line therapy for multiple myeloma. *Lancet* 2(8668):882–885, 1989.

40. Anderson H, Scarffe JH, Ranson M, et al.: VAD chemotherapy as remission induction for multiple myeloma. *Br J Cancer* 71(2):326–330, 1995.

41. Phillips JK, Sherlaw-Johnson C, Pearce R, et al.: A randomized study of MOD versus VAD in the treatment of relapsed and resistant multiple myeloma. *Leuk Lymphoma* 17(5–6):465–472, 1995.

42. Raje N, Powles R, Kulkarni S, et al.: A comparison of vincristine and doxorubicin infusional chemotherapy with methylprednisolone (VAMP) with the addition of weekly cyclophosphamide (C-VAMP) as induction treatment followed by autografting in previously untreated myeloma. *Br J Haematol* 97(1):153–160, 1997.

43. Cavo M, Benni M, Ronconi S, et al.: Melphalan-prednisone versus alternating combination VAD/MP or VND/MP as primary therapy for multiple myeloma: final analysis of a randomized clinical study. *Haematologica* 87(9):934–942, 2002.

44. Barlogie B, Jagannath S, Desikan KR, et al.: Total therapy with tandem transplants for newly diagnosed multiple myeloma. *Blood* 93(1):55–65, 1999.

45. Gertz MA, Lacy MQ, Inwards DJ, et al.: Factors influencing platelet recovery after blood cell transplantation in multiple myeloma. *Bone Marrow Transplant* 20(5):375–380, 1997.

46. Prince HM, Imrie K, Sutherland DR, et al.: Peripheral blood progenitor cell collections in multiple myeloma: predictors and management of inadequate collections. *Br J Haematol* 93(1):142–145, 1996.

47. Tricot G, Jagannath S, Vesole D, et al.: Peripheral blood stem cell transplants for multiple myeloma: identification of favorable variables for rapid engraftment in 225 patients. *Blood* 85(2):588–596, 1995.

48. Dimopoulos MA, Pouli A, Zervas K, et al.: Prospective randomized comparison of vincristine, doxorubicin and dexamethasone (VAD) administered as intravenous bolus injection and VAD with liposomal doxorubicin as first-line treatment in multiple myeloma. *Ann Oncol* 14(7):1039–1044, 2003.

49. Hussein MA, Wood L, Hsi E, et al.: A phase II trial of pegylated liposomal doxorubicin, vincristine, and reduced-dose dexamethasone combination therapy in newly diagnosed multiple myeloma patients. *Cancer* 95(10):2160–2168, 2002.

50. Fossa A, Muer M, Kasper C, Welt A, Seeber S, Nowrousian MR: Bolus vincristine and epirubicin with cyclophosphamide and dexamethasone (VECD) as induction and salvage treatment in multiple myeloma. *Leukemia* 12(3):422–426, 1998.

51. Al-Zoubi A, Emmons R, Walsh W, O'Donnell J, Stewart M, Jani CR: The efficacy and cost of bolus VAD (vincristine, doxorubicin, and dexamethasone) administered as a rapid intravenous infusion for untreated multiple myeloma—a phase II study [abstract]. *Proc Am Soc Clin Oncol* 22:614, 2003.

52. Hussein MA, Wildgust M, Fastenau J, Piech CT: Cost effectiveness of DVd vs VAd in newly diagnosed multiple myeloma [abstract]. *Proc Am Soc Clin Oncol* 23:567, 2004.

53. Cook G, Sharp RA, Tansey P, Franklin IM: A phase I/II trial of Z-Dex (oral idarubicin and dexamethasone), an oral equivalent of VAD, as initial therapy at diagnosis or progression in multiple myeloma. *Br J Haematol* 93(4):931–934, 1996.

54. Glasmacher A, Haferlach T, Gorschluter M, et al.: Oral idarubicin, dexamethasone and vincristine (VID) in the treatment of multiple myeloma. *Leukemia* 11(suppl 5):S22–S26, 1997.

55. Kumar A, Loughran T, Alsina M, Durie BG, Djulbegovic B: Management of multiple myeloma: a systematic review and critical appraisal of published studies. *Lancet Oncol* 4(5):293–304, 2003.

56. Alexanian R, Dimopoulos MA, Delasalle K, Barlogie B: Primary dexamethasone treatment of multiple myeloma. *Blood* 80(4):887–890, 1992.

57. Facon T, Mary JY, Pegourie B, et al.: Dexamethasone-based regimens versus melphalan-prednisone for elderly multiple myeloma patients ineligible for high-dose therapy. *Blood* 107(4):1292–1298, 2006.

58. Levine RA, McGuire RF: Corticosteroid-induced pancreatitis: a case report demonstrating recurrence with rechallenge. *Am J Gastroenterol* 83(10):1161–1164, 1988.

59. Kneller A, Raanani P, Hardan I, et al.: Therapy with thalidomide in refractory multiple myeloma patients—the revival of an old drug. *Br J Haematol* 108(2):391–393, 2000.

60. Juliusson G, Celsing F, Turesson I, Lenhoff S, Adriansson M, Malm C: Frequent good partial remissions from thalidomide including best response ever in patients with advanced refractory and relapsed myeloma. *Br J Haematol* 109(1):89–96, 2000.

61. Rajkumar SV, Fonseca R, Dispenzieri A, et al.: Thalidomide in the treatment of relapsed multiple myeloma. *Mayo Clin Proc* 75(9):897–901, 2000.

62. Hus M, Dmoszynska A, Soroka-Wojtaszko M, et al.: Thalidomide treatment of resistant or relapsed multiple myeloma patients. *Haematologica* 86(4):404–408, 2001.

63. Tosi P, Ronconi S, Zamagni E, et al.: Salvage therapy with thalidomide in multiple myeloma patients relapsing after autologous peripheral blood stem cell transplantation. *Haematologica* 86(4):409–413, 2001.

64. Yakoub-Agha I, Attal M, Dumontet C, et al.: Thalidomide in patients with advanced multiple myeloma: a study of 83 patients—report of the Intergroupe Francophone du Myelome (IFM). *Hematol J* 3(4):185–192, 2002.

65. Barlogie B, Desikan R, Eddlemon P, et al.: Extended survival in advanced and refractory multiple myeloma after single-agent thalidomide: identification of prognostic factors in a phase 2 study of 169 patients. *Blood* 98(2):492–494, 2001.

66. Dimopoulos MA, Zervas K, Kouvatseas G, et al.: Thalidomide and dexamethasone combination for refractory multiple myeloma. *Ann Oncol* 12(7):991–995, 2001.

67. Palumbo A, Giaccone L, Bertola A, et al.: Low-dose thalidomide plus dexamethasone is an effective salvage therapy for advanced myeloma. *Haematologica* 86(4):399–403, 2001.

68. Rajkumar SV, Hayman S, Gertz MA, et al.: Combination therapy with thalidomide plus dexamethasone for newly diagnosed myeloma. *J Clin Oncol* 20(21):4319–4323, 2002.

69. Weber D, Rankin K, Gavino M, Delasalle K, Alexanian R: Thalidomide alone or with dexamethasone for previously untreated multiple myeloma. *J Clin Oncol* 21(1):16–19, 2003.

70. Rajkumar SV, Blood E, Vesole D, Fonseca R, Greipp PR: Phase III clinical trial of thalidomide plus dexamethasone compared with dexamethasone alone in newly diagnosed multiple myeloma: a clinical trial coordinated by the Eastern Cooperative Oncology Group. *J Clin Oncol* 24(3):431–436, 2006.

71. Ghobrial IM, Dispenzieri A, Bundy KL, et al.: Effect of thalidomide on stem cell collection and engraftment in patients with multiple myeloma. *Bone Marrow Transplant* 32(6):587–592, 2003.

72. Dingli D, Rajkumar SV, Nowakowski GS, et al.: Combination therapy with thalidomide and dexamethasone in patients with newly diagnosed multiple myeloma not undergoing upfront autologous stem cell transplantation: a phase II trial. *Haematologica* 90(12):1650–1654, 2005.

73. Rajkumar SV, Hussein MA, Catalano L, et al.: A multicenter, randomized, double-blind, placebo-controlled trial of thalidomide plus dexamethasone versus dexamethasone alone as initial therapy for newly diagnosed multiple myeloma [abstract]. *J Clin Oncol* 24(suppl 18S):426S, 2006.

74. Tosi P, Zamagni E, Cellini C, et al.: Thalidomide alone or in combination with dexamethasone in patients with advanced, relapsed or refractory multiple myeloma and renal failure. *Eur J Haematol* 73(2):98–103, 2004.

75. Barlogie B, Shaughnessy J, Tricot G, et al.: Treatment of multiple myeloma. *Blood* 103(1):20–32, 2004.

76. Child JA, Morgan GJ, Davies FE, et al.: High-dose chemotherapy with hematopoietic stem-cell rescue for multiple myeloma. *N Engl J Med* 348(19):1875–1883, 2003.

77. MacLennan IC, Chapman C, Dunn J, Kelly K: Combined chemotherapy with ABCM versus melphalan for treatment of myelomatosis. The Medical Research Council Working Party for Leukaemia in Adults. *Lancet* 339(8787):200–205, 1992.

78. Moreau P, Facon T, Attal M, et al.: Comparison of 200 mg/m(2) melphalan and 8 Gy total body irradiation plus 140 mg/m(2) melphalan as conditioning regimens for peripheral blood stem cell transplantation in patients with newly diagnosed multiple myeloma: final analysis of the Intergroupe Francophone du Myelome 9502 randomized trial. *Blood* 99(3):731–735, 2002.

79. Barlogie B, Jagannath S, Vesole DH, et al.: Superiority of tandem autologous transplantation over standard therapy for previously untreated multiple myeloma. *Blood* 89(3):789–793, 1997.

80. Lenhoff S, Hjorth M, Holmberg E, et al.: Impact on survival of high-dose therapy with autologous stem cell support in patients younger than 60 years with newly diagnosed multiple myeloma: a population-based study. Nordic Myeloma Study Group. *Blood* 95(1):7–11, 2000.

81. Blade J, Sureda A, Ribera J: High-dose therapy auto-transplantation vs continued conventional chemotherapy in multiple myeloma patients responding to initial treatment chemotherapy. Results of a prospective randomized trial from the Spanish Cooperative Group [abstract]. *Blood* 98:815a, 2001.

82. Segeren CM, Sonneveld P, van der HB, et al.: Overall and event-free survival are not improved by the use of myeloablative therapy following intensified chemotherapy in previously untreated patients with multiple myeloma: a prospective randomized phase 3 study. *Blood* 101(6):2144–2151, 2003.

83. Barlogie B, Kyle RA, Anderson KC, et al.: Standard chemotherapy compared with high-dose chemoradiotherapy for multiple myeloma: final results of phase III US Intergroup Trial S9321. *J Clin Oncol* 24(6):929–936, 2006.

84. Fermand JP, Ravaud P, Chevret S, et al.: High-dose therapy and autologous peripheral blood stem cell transplantation in multiple myeloma: up-front or rescue treatment? Results of a multicenter sequential randomized clinical trial. *Blood* 92(9):3131–3136, 1998.

85. Desikan R, Barlogie B, Sawyer J, et al.: Results of high-dose therapy for 1000 patients with multiple myeloma: durable complete remissions and superior survival in the absence of chromosome 13 abnormalities. *Blood* 95(12):4008–4010, 2000.

86. Facon T, Avet-Loiseau H, Guillerm G, et al.: Chromosome 13 abnormalities identified by FISH analysis and serum beta2-microglobulin produce a powerful myeloma staging system for patients receiving high-dose therapy. *Blood* 97(6):1566–1571, 2001.

87. Worel N, Greinix H, Ackermann J, et al.: Deletion of chromosome 13q14 detected by fluorescence in situ hybridization has prognostic impact on survival after high-dose therapy in patients with multiple myeloma. *Ann Hematol* 80(6):345–348, 2001.

88. Fonseca R, Harrington D, Oken MM, et al.: Biological and prognostic significance of interphase fluorescence in situ hybridization detection of chromosome 13 abnormalities (delta13) in multiple myeloma: an eastern cooperative oncology group study. *Cancer Res* 62(3):715–720, 2002.

89. Tricot G, Vesole DH, Jagannath S, Hilton J, Munshi N, Barlogie B: Graft-versus-myeloma effect: proof of principle. *Blood* 87(3):1196–1198, 1996.

90. Libura J, Hoffmann T, Passweg J, et al.: Graft-versus-myeloma after withdrawal of immunosuppression following allogeneic peripheral stem cell transplantation. *Bone Marrow Transplant* 24(8):925–927, 1999.

91. Alyea E, Weller E, Schlossman R, et al.: Outcome after autologous and allogeneic stem cell transplantation for patients with multiple myeloma: impact of graft-versus-myeloma effect. *Bone Marrow Transplant* 32(12):1145–1151, 2003.

92. Bjorkstrand BB, Ljungman P, Svensson H, et al.: Allogeneic bone marrow transplantation versus autologous stem cell transplantation in multiple myeloma: a retrospective case-matched study from the European Group for Blood and Marrow Transplantation. *Blood* 88(12):4711–4718, 1996.

93. Laterveer L, Verdonck LF, Peeters T, Borst E, Bloem AC, Lokhorst HM: Graft versus myeloma may overcome the unfavorable effect of deletion of chromosome 13 in multiple myeloma. *Blood* 101(3):1201–1202, 2003.

94. Badros A, Barlogie B, Siegel E, et al.: Improved outcome of allogeneic transplantation in high-risk multiple myeloma patients after nonmyeloablative conditioning. *J Clin Oncol* 20(5):1295–1303, 2002.

95. Maloney DG, Molina AJ, Sahebi F, et al.: Allografting with nonmyeloablative conditioning following cytoreductive autografts for the treatment of patients with multiple myeloma. *Blood* 102(9):3447–3454, 2003.

96. Singhal S, Safdar A, Chiang KY, et al.: Non-myeloablative allogeneic transplantation ('microallograft') for refractory myeloma after two preceding autografts: feasibility and efficacy in a patient with active aspergillosis. *Bone Marrow Transplant* 26(11):1231–1233, 2000.

97. Palumbo A, Triolo S, Argentino C, et al.: Dose-intensive melphalan with stem cell support (MEL100) is superior to standard treatment in elderly myeloma patients. *Blood* 94(4):1248–1253, 1999.

98. Reece DE, Bredeson C, Perez WS, et al.: Autologous stem cell transplantation in multiple myeloma patients <60 vs >/=60 years of age. *Bone Marrow Transplant* 32(12):1135–1143, 2003.

99. Siegel DS, Desikan KR, Mehta J, et al.: Age is not a prognostic variable with autotransplants for multiple myeloma. *Blood* 93(1):51–54, 1999.

100. Sirohi B, Powles R, Mehta J, et al.: The implication of compromised renal function at presentation in myeloma: similar outcome in patients who receive high-dose therapy: a single-center study of 251 previously untreated patients. *Med Oncol* 18(1):39–50, 2001.

101. Badros A, Barlogie B, Siegel E, et al.: Results of autologous stem cell transplant in multiple myeloma patients with renal failure. *Br J Haematol* 114(4):822–829, 2001.

102. Lee CK, Zangari M, Barlogie B, et al.: Dialysis-dependent renal failure in patients with myeloma can be reversed by high-dose myeloablative therapy and autotransplant. *Bone Marrow Transplant* 33(8):823–828, 2004.

103. Fassas A, Tricot G: Results of high-dose treatment with autologous stem cell support in patients with multiple myeloma. *Semin Hematol* 38(3):231–242, 2001.

104. Palumbo A, Bringhen S, Bertola A, et al.: Multiple myeloma: comparison of two dose-intensive melphalan regimens (100 vs 200 mg/m(2)). *Leukemia* 18(1):133–138, 2004.

105. Morris C, Iacobelli S, Brand R, et al.: Benefit and timing of second transplantations in multiple myeloma: clinical findings and methodological limitations in a European Group for Blood and Marrow Transplantation registry study. *J Clin Oncol* 22(9):1674–1681, 2004.

106. Palumbo A, Bertola A, Musto P, et al.: Oral melphalan, prednisone, and thalidomide for newly diagnosed myeloma patients [abstract]. *Proc Am Soc Clin Oncol* 23:567, 2004.

107. Palumbo A, Bringhen S, Caravita T, et al.: Oral melphalan and prednisone chemotherapy plus thalidomide compared with melphalan and prednisone alone in elderly patients with multiple myeloma: randomised controlled trial. *Lancet* 367(9513):825–831, 2006.

108. Facon T, Mary JY, Harousseau JL, et al.: Superiority of melphalan-prednisone (MP) + thalidomide (THAL) over MP and autologous stem cell transplantation in the treatment of newly diagnosed elderly patients with multiple myeloma. *J Clin Oncol* 24(suppl 18S):1S, 2006.

109. Agrawal NR, Hussein M, Elson P, Karam M, Reed J, Srkalovic G: Pegylated doxorubicin (DOX), vincristine (V), reduced frequency dexamethasone (d), and thalidomide (T) (DVd-T) in newly diagnosed (nmm) and relapsed refractory (rmm) multiple myeloma patients [abstract]. *Blood* 102(11):237a, 2004.

110. Lee CK, Barlogie B, Munshi N, et al.: DTPACE: an effective, novel combination chemotherapy with thalidomide for previously treated patients with myeloma. *J Clin Oncol* 21(14):2732–2739, 2003.

111. Zangari M, Siegel E, Barlogie B, et al.: Thrombogenic activity of doxorubicin in myeloma patients receiving thalidomide: implications for therapy. *Blood* 100(4):1168–1171, 2002.

112. Zangari M, Anaissie E, Barlogie B, et al.: Increased risk of deep-vein thrombosis in patients with multiple myeloma receiving thalidomide and chemotherapy. *Blood* 98(5):1614–1615, 2001.

113. Richardson PG, Barlogie B, Berenson J, et al.: A phase 2 study of bortezomib in relapsed, refractory myeloma. *N Engl J Med* 348(26):2609–2617, 2003.

114. Jagannath S, Durie BG, Wolf J, et al.: Bortezomib therapy alone and in combination with dexamethasone for previously untreated symptomatic multiple myeloma. *Br J Haematol* 129(6):776–783, 2005.

115. Harousseau JL, Attal M, Leleu X, et al.: Bortezomib plus dexamethasone as induction treatment prior to autologous stem cell transplantation in patients with newly diagnosed multiple myeloma: results of an IFM phase II study. *Haematologica* 91(11):1498–1505, 2006.

116. Oakervee HE, Popat R, Curry N, et al.: PAD combination therapy (PS-341/bortezomib, doxorubicin and dexamethasone) for previously untreated patients with multiple myeloma. *Br J Haematol* 129(6):755–762, 2005.

117. Mateos MV, Hernandez JM, Hernandez MT, et al.: Bortezomib plus melphalan and prednisone in elderly untreated patients with multiple myeloma: results of a multicenter phase 1/2 study. *Blood* 108(7):2165–2172, 2006.

118. Muller GW, Chen R, Huang SY, et al.: Amino-substituted thalidomide analogs: potent inhibitors of TNF-alpha production. *Bioorg Med Chem Lett* 9(11):1625–1630, 1999.

119. Corral LG, Haslett PA, Muller GW, et al.: Differential cytokine modulation and T cell activation by two distinct classes of thalidomide analogues that are potent inhibitors of TNF-alpha. *J Immunol* 163(1):380–386, 1999.

120. Richardson PG, Schlossman RL, Weller E, et al.: Immunomodulatory drug CC-5013 overcomes drug resistance and is well tolerated in patients with relapsed multiple myeloma. *Blood* 100(9):3063–3067, 2002.

121. Barlogie B: Thalidomide and CC-5013 in multiple myeloma: the University of Arkansas experience. *Semin Hematol* 40(suppl 4):33–38, 2003.

122. Rajkumar SV, Hayman SR, Lacy MQ, et al.: Combination therapy with lenalidomide plus dexamethasone (Rev/Dex) for newly diagnosed myeloma. *Blood* 106(13):4050–4053, 2005.

123. Singal PK, Iliskovic N: Doxorubicin-induced cardiomyopathy. *N Engl J Med* 339(13):900–905, 1998.

124. Gottschalk PG, Dyck PJ, Kiely JM: Vinca alkaloid neuropathy: nerve biopsy studies in rats and in man. *Neurology* 18(9):875–882, 1968.

125. Alexanian R, Gehan E, Haut A, Saiki J, Weick J: Unmaintained remissions in multiple myeloma. *Blood* 51(6):1005–1011, 1978.

126. Berenson JR, Crowley JJ, Grogan TM, et al.: Maintenance therapy with alternate-day prednisone improves survival in multiple myeloma patients. *Blood* 99(9):3163–3168, 2002.

127. Shustik C, Belch A, Robinson S, et al.: Dexamethasone (dex) maintenance versus observation (obs) in patients with previously untreated multiple myeloma: a National Cancer Institute of Canada Clinical Trials Group Study: MY.7 [abstract]. *Proc Am Soc Clin Oncol* 23:558, 2004.

128. Fritz E, Ludwig H: Interferon-alpha treatment in multiple myeloma: meta-analysis of 30 randomised trials among 3948 patients. *Ann Oncol* 11(11):1427–1436, 2000.

129. The Myeloma Trialists' Collaborative Group: Interferon as therapy for multiple myeloma: an individual patient data overview of 24 randomized trials and 4012 patients. *Br J Haematol* 113(4):1020–1034, 2001.

130. Kyle RA: Multiple myeloma: review of 869 cases. *Mayo Clin Proc* 50(1):29–40, 1975.

131. Sezer O, Heider U, Zavrski I, Kuhne CA, Hofbauer LC: RANK ligand and osteoprotegerin in myeloma bone disease. *Blood* 101(6):2094–2098, 2003.

132. Yaccoby S, Pearse RN, Johnson CL, Barlogie B, Choi Y, Epstein J: Myeloma interacts with the bone marrow microenvironment to induce osteoclastogenesis and is dependent on osteoclast activity. *Br J Haematol* 116(2):278–290, 2002.

133. Luckman SP, Coxon FP, Ebetino FH, Russell RG, Rogers MJ: Heterocycle-containing bisphosphonates cause apoptosis and inhibit bone resorption by preventing protein prenylation: evidence from structure-activity relationships in J774 macrophages. *J Bone Miner Res* 13(11):1668–1678, 1998.

134. Luckman SP, Hughes DE, Coxon FP, Graham R, Russell G, Rogers MJ: Nitrogen-containing bisphosphonates inhibit the mevalonate pathway and prevent post-translational prenylation of GTP-binding proteins, including Ras. *J Bone Miner Res* 13(4):581–589, 1998.

135. Frith JC, Monkkonen J, Auriola S, Monkkonen H, Rogers MJ: The molecular mechanism of action of the antiresorptive and antiinflammatory drug clodronate: evidence for the formation in vivo of a metabolite that inhibits bone resorption and causes osteoclast and macrophage apoptosis. *Arthritis Rheum* 44(9):2201–2210, 2001.

136. Viereck V, Emons G, Lauck V, et al.: Bisphosphonates pamidronate and zoledronic acid stimulate osteoprotegerin production by primary human osteoblasts. *Biochem Biophys Res Commun* 291(3):680–686, 2002.

137. Berenson JR, Lichtenstein A, Porter L, et al.: Efficacy of pamidronate in reducing skeletal events in patients with advanced multiple myeloma. Myeloma Aredia Study Group. *N Engl J Med* 334(8):488–493, 1996.

138. Berenson JR, Lichtenstein A, Porter L, et al.: Long-term pamidronate treatment of advanced multiple myeloma patients reduces skeletal events. Myeloma Aredia Study Group. *J Clin Oncol* 16(2):593–602, 1998.

139. Rosen LS, Gordon D, Kaminski M, et al.: Zoledronic acid versus pamidronate in the treatment of skeletal metastases in patients with breast cancer or osteolytic lesions of multiple myeloma: a phase III, double-blind, comparative trial. *Cancer J* 7(5):377–387, 2001.

140. Rosen LS, Gordon D, Kaminski M, et al.: Long-term efficacy and safety of zoledronic acid compared with pamidronate disodium in the treatment of skeletal complications in patients with advanced multiple myeloma or breast carcinoma: a randomized, double-blind, multicenter, comparative trial. *Cancer* 98(8):1735–1744, 2003.

141. Fourney DR, Schomer DF, Nader R, et al.: Percutaneous vertebroplasty and kyphoplasty for painful vertebral body fractures in cancer patients. *J Neurosurg* 98(suppl 1):21–30, 2003.

142. Lieberman I, Reinhardt MK: Vertebroplasty and kyphoplasty for osteolytic vertebral collapse. *Clin Orthop* (suppl 415):S176–S186, 2003.

143. Peters KR, Guiot BH, Martin PA, Fessler RG: Vertebroplasty for osteoporotic compression fractures: current practice and evolving techniques. *Neurosurgery* 51(suppl 5):96–103, 2002.

144. Hayek D, Ritschard J, Zwahlen A, Courvoisier B, Donath A: [Use of strontium-89 in the analgesic treatment of bone metastases]. *Schweiz Med Wochenschr* 110(31–32):1154–1159, 1980.

145. Pearse RN, Sordillo EM, Yaccoby S, et al.: Multiple myeloma disrupts the TRANCE/osteoprotegerin cytokine axis to trigger bone destruction and promote tumor progression. *Proc Natl Acad Sci U S A* 98(20):11581–11586, 2001.

146. Body JJ, Greipp P, Coleman RE, et al.: A phase I study of AMGN-0007, a recombinant osteoprotegerin construct, in patients with multiple myeloma or breast carcinoma related bone metastases. *Cancer* 97(suppl 3):887–892, 2003.

147. Cazzola M, Messinger D, Battistel V, et al.: Recombinant human erythropoietin in the anemia associated with multiple myeloma or non-Hodgkin's lymphoma: dose finding and identification of predictors of response. *Blood* 86(12):4446–4453, 1995.

148. Dammacco F, Silvestris F, Castoldi GL, et al.: The effectiveness and tolerability of epoetin alfa in patients with multiple myeloma refractory to chemotherapy. *Int J Clin Lab Res* 28(2):127–134, 1998.

149. Garton JP, Gertz MA, Witzig TE, et al.: Epoetin alfa for the treatment of the anemia of multiple myeloma. A prospective, randomized, placebo-controlled, double-blind trial. *Arch Intern Med* 155(19):2069–2074, 1995.

150. Osterborg A, Boogaerts MA, Cimino R, et al.: Recombinant human erythropoietin in transfusion-dependent anemic patients with multiple myeloma and non-Hodgkin's lymphoma—a randomized multicenter study. The European Study Group of Erythropoietin (Epoetin Beta) Treatment in Multiple Myeloma and Non-Hodgkin's Lymphoma. *Blood* 87(7):2675–2682, 1996.

151. Rizzo JD, Lichtin AE, Woolf SH, et al.: Use of epoetin in patients with cancer: evidence-based clinical practice guidelines of the American Society of Clinical Oncology and the American Society of Hematology. *J Clin Oncol* 20(19):4083–4107, 2002.

152. Knight R, DeLap RJ, Zeldis JB: Lenalidomide and venous thrombosis in multiple myeloma. *N Engl J Med* 354(19):2079–2080, 2006.

153. Hedenus M, Adriansson M, San Miguel J, et al.: Efficacy and safety of darbepoetin alfa in anaemic patients with lymphoproliferative malignancies: a randomized, double-blind, placebo-controlled study. *Br J Haematol* 122(3):394–403, 2003.

154. Kotasek D, Steger G, Faught W, et al.: Darbepoetin alfa administered every 3 weeks alleviates anaemia in patients with solid tumours receiving chemotherapy; results of a double-blind, placebo-controlled, randomised study. *Eur J Cancer* 39(14):2026–2034, 2003.

155. Mirtsching B, Charu V, Vadhan-Raj S, et al.: Every-2-week darbepoetin alfa is comparable to rHuEPO in treating chemotherapy-induced anemia. Results of a combined analysis. *Oncology* (Huntingt) 16(suppl 11):31–36, 2002.

156. Srkalovic G, Cameron MG, Rybicki L, Deitcher SR, Kattke-Marchant K, Hussein MA: Monoclonal gammopathy of undetermined significance and multiple myeloma are associated with an increased incidence of venothromboembolic disease. *Cancer* 101(3):558–566, 2004.

157. Rajkumar SV, Blood E: Lenalidomide and venous thrombosis in multiple myeloma. *N Engl J Med* 354(19):2079–2080, 2006.

158. Zonder JA, Barlogie B, Durie BG, McCoy J, Crowley J, Hussein MA: Thrombotic complications in patients with newly diagnosed multiple myeloma treated with lenalidomide and dexamethasone: benefit of aspirin prophylaxis. *Blood* 108(1):403, 2006.

159. Baz R, Li L, Kottke-Marchant K, et al.: The role of aspirin in the prevention of thrombotic complications of thalidomide and anthracycline-based chemotherapy for multiple myeloma. *Mayo Clin Proc* 80(12):1568–1574, 2005.

160. Zonder JA, Barlogie B, Durie BG, McCoy J, Crowley J, Hussein MA: Thrombotic complications in patients with newly diagnosed multiple myeloma treated with lenalidomide and dexamethasone: benefit of aspirin prophylaxis. *Blood* 108(1):403, 2006.

161. Rajkumar SV: Thalidomide therapy and deep venous thrombosis in multiple myeloma. *Mayo Clin Proc* 80(12):1549–1551, 2005.

162. Corso A, Arcaini L, Caberlon S, et al.: A combination of dexamethasone, cyclophosphamide, etoposide, and cisplatin is less toxic and more effective than high-dose cyclophosphamide for peripheral stem cell mobilization in multiple myeloma. *Haematologica* 87(10): 1041–1045, 2002.

163. Palva IP, Ahrenberg P, Ala-Harja K, et al.: Treatment of multiple myeloma with an intensive 5-drug combination or intermittent melphalan and prednisone; a randomised multicentre trial. Finnish Leukaemia Group. *Eur J Haematol* 38(1):50–54, 1987.

164. Segeren CM, Sonneveld P, van der HB, et al.: Vincristine, doxorubicin and dexamethasone (VAD) administered as rapid intravenous infusion for first-line treatment in untreated multiple myeloma. *Br J Haematol* 105(1):127–130, 1999.

# Chapter 84

# VARIANTS OF MULTIPLE MYELOMA

*Robert A. Kyle and S. Vincent Rajkumar*

Variants of multiple myeloma consist of solitary plasmacytoma of bone, extramedullary plasmacytoma, multiple solitary plasmacytomas, plasma cell leukemia, smoldering multiple myeloma, nonsecretory myeloma, immunoglobulin (Ig) D myeloma, and POEMS syndrome (osteosclerotic myeloma).

## SOLITARY PLASMACYTOMA OF BONE

Solitary plasmacytoma of bone is characterized by the presence of a tumor consisting of monoclonal plasma cells, identical to those in myeloma, and no other features of multiple myeloma.[1]

### CLINICAL FEATURES

Solitary plasmacytoma of bone is uncommon and occurs in 3–5% of patients with plasma cell neoplasms. It occurs more commonly in men than in women. The median age at diagnosis is approximately 55 years, which is a decade younger than that for multiple myeloma.

The most common symptom initially is pain at the site of the skeletal lesion. Severe back pain or cord compression may be the presenting feature. Pathologic fractures or a soft tissue extension of a solitary plasmacytoma, such as in a rib, may result in a palpable mass.

The axial skeleton is more commonly involved than is the appendicular skeleton.[2] Thoracic vertebrae are more often involved than are lumbar, sacral, or cervical vertebrae. Involvement of the distal axial skeleton below the knees or elbows is extremely rare. The recommended laboratory tests for identifying this entity are listed in Table 84.1.

### DIAGNOSIS

The diagnosis is based on histologic evidence of a tumor consisting of monoclonal plasma cells and the absence of multiple myeloma on the basis of bone marrow, radiographic, and appropriate studies of blood and urine. Complete skeletal radiographs must show no other lesions of multiple myeloma (Table 84.2). If magnetic resonance imaging of the spine and pelvis reveals skeletal lesions, the condition should be classified as smoldering multiple myeloma. Approximately one–fourth to one–third of patients with an apparently solitary plasmacytoma will have abnormalities on magnetic resonance imaging.[5–7] These patients are at greater risk for progression to multiple myeloma. Immunofixation of serum and concentrated urine ideally should have no monoclonal (M) protein, but approximately half of the patients do have a small amount of M protein in the serum or urine. This often disappears after tumoricidal radiation. Most patients with solitary plasmacytoma of bone have normal, uninvolved immunoglobulin levels.[1] There is no anemia, hypercalcemia, or renal insufficiency that is related to the plasmacytoma. Although the bone marrow aspirate and biopsy must contain no evidence of multiple myeloma, a few plasma cells may be seen.

### TREATMENT

Tumoricidal radiation is the treatment of choice. The patient should receive 4000–5000 cGy over approximately 4 weeks. Even if the plasmacytoma has been excised for diagnostic purposes, radiotherapy should also be given. The local response rate exceeds 80–90%.[8] In one series, all solitary plasmacytomas less than 5 cm in size were controlled by radiotherapy.[9]

There is no convincing evidence that adjuvant or prophylactic chemotherapy will prevent the development of multiple myeloma.[10–12] However, in an uncontrolled study, adjuvant chemotherapy delayed the time to progression to 59 months, compared with 29 months for patients treated with only radiation, but did not affect the rate of conversion.[8] In another report of 53 patients with solitary plasmacytomas randomized to receive either radiotherapy plus melphalan and prednisone for 3 years or radiotherapy alone, disease–free survival and overall survival improved in the chemotherapy group. After a median follow-up of 8.9 years, 22 of 25 patients were alive and free of disease in the chemotherapy group, compared with 13 of 28 patients in the radiotherapy-only group ($P < .01$).[13]

| Table 84.1   Laboratory tests recommended for solitary plasmacytoma |
|---|
| History and physical examination |
| Hemoglobin, leukocytes with differential and platelets |
| Serum calcium and creatinine |
| Serum protein electrophoresis and immunofixation, quantitative serum immunoglobulins |
| Electrophoresis of aliquot from 24-h urine specimen followed by immunofixation |
| $\beta_2$-Microglobulin, C-reactive protein, and lactate dehydrogenase |
| Skeletal survey including humeri and femurs |
| Bone marrow aspirate and biopsy |
| Peripheral blood plasma cell count and labeling index, if available |
| Magnetic resonance imaging or computed tomography |

From Ref. 3, with permission from Elsevier.

However, on the basis of all available data, adjuvant therapy should not be given to patients with solitary plasmacytoma of bone.[1] The use of systemic chemotherapy may obscure recognition of patients cured by radiotherapy. In addition, early exposure to systemic treatment may increase the number of resistant subclones and restrict later therapeutic approaches. In one report, secondary leukemia developed in four of seven patients with solitary plasmacytoma of bone who had received adjuvant melphalan-based chemotherapy after completion of radiotherapy.[14]

## NATURAL HISTORY

Overt multiple myeloma develops in at least 50% of patients with solitary plasmacytoma of bone.[2,8,9,15] In our report of 46 patients, 77% of those who progressed did so within 4 years.[2] Dimopoulos et al.[16] found that two–thirds of patients who progressed did so within 3 years.

The patterns of failure in our series included development of multiple myeloma in 54%, failure local recurrence in 11%, and development of new solitary bone lesions without evidence of myeloma in 2%. Four of the five local failures in our series occurred in the spine, and all the patients had received less than 45 Gy to the initial lesion.

The overall survival rate in a series of 46 patients was 74% at 5 years and 45% at 10 years. The 5- and 10-year disease-free survival rates were 43% and 25%, respectively. In a series of 12 patients with solitary plasmacytoma of the vertebral column, multiple myeloma developed in 50%.[17] Fifty-eight percent patients were alive at 5 years and 25% at 10 years. An additional 72 patients with solitary plasmacytoma of the spine were identified in the English literature. The mean disease-free duration of survival for the 84 patients was 76 months. The average overall duration of survival was 92 months. The 5-year disease-free survival rate was 60%, and the 10-year disease-free survival rate was 16%.[17]

In one series, conversion to myeloma occurred in 9 of 11 patients (82%) who had lesions 5 cm or larger, whereas only 5 to 18 patients (28%) who remained stable had lesions that were 5 cm or larger (7).

## PROGNOSTIC FACTORS

Relapse rates are higher in older patients[9] and in patients presenting with axial lesions.[18] The persistence of an M protein after radiation therapy is a predictor of subsequent development of multiple myeloma in several studies.[8,16] In one series, persistence of the M protein for more than 1 year after radiation therapy was the only independent adverse prognostic factor for myeloma-free survival and cause-specific survival with multivariate analysis when included variables were resolution vs persistence of the M protein after radiation therapy, presence or

| Table 84.2   Classification of plasma cell disorders | |
|---|---|
| Category | Criteria |
| Solitary plasmacytoma (bone or extramedullary) | Absent or small monoclonal protein in serum or urine<br>Single area of destruction<br>Bone marrow not consistent with myeloma<br>Normal skeletal survey |
| Multiple solitary plasmacytomas | Absent or small monoclonal protein in serum or urine<br>More than one localized area of destruction<br>Normal bone marrow |
| Monoclonal gammopathy of undetermined significance (MGUS) | Monoclonal protein <3 g/dL<br>Bone marrow plasma cells < 10%<br>No end-organ damage[a] |
| Smoldering (asymptomatic) multiple myeloma (SMM) | Monoclonal protein ≥3 g/dL or bone marrow plasma cells ≥ 10%<br>No end-organ damage[a] |
| Symptomatic multiple myeloma (MM) | Monoclonal protein in serum or urine<br>Clonal bone marrow plasma cells or plasmacytoma<br>Presence of end-organ damage[a] |

[a]End-organ damage: anemia, lytic bone lesions, renal failure, or hypercalcemia thought to be related to plasma cell proliferative disorder.
From Ref. 4, with permission from Mayo Foundation.

absence of an M protein at diagnosis, presence or absence of an associated soft tissue mass on computed tomography or magnetic resonance imaging, size of serum M protein at diagnosis, age, spinal vs nonspinal location, Karnofsky performance score, total radiation dose, and tumor size. In patients with an M protein persisting for more than 1 year, multiple myeloma developed within 2.2 years of therapy.[5] Of the 60 patients in that series, 75% had an M protein at diagnosis. The 10-year myeloma-free survival rate was 91% in patients whose M protein disappeared, and 29% in those whose M protein did not disappear at 1 year after radiation therapy.

In contrast, we found no difference in the 5-year disease-free survival rate among patients with or without an M protein at diagnosis.[2] The failure rate was 75% in patients with a persistent M protein after radiation and 71% in those in whom the M protein disappeared. The median time to failure was 40 months for the patients with a persistent M protein and 36 months for those in whom the M protein disappeared with therapy.

We studied angiogenesis in 25 patients with solitary plasmacytoma of bone. High-grade angiogenesis was present in 64% of the plasmacytomas, whereas angiogenesis was low in the bone marrow of all 25 patients. The median vascular density was 26 (range 20–50) in the high-grade group ($n = 16$) and 11 (range 2–16) in the low-grade group ($n = 9$). Progression to myeloma occurred in 9 of the 16 patients in the high-grade angiogenesis group and in only 1 of the 9 patients with low-grade angiogenesis. The progression-free survival rate was significantly shorter in those with high-grade angiogenesis. There was no correlation between median vascular density and age, M-protein level, urinary light chain, $\beta_2$-microglobulin level, or tumor location. In a multivariate Cox, analysis, persistence of M protein, angiogenesis grade, and spinal vs nonspinal tumor location were independently prognostic for progression. Patients who had both a persistent M-protein spike and high-grade angiogenesis (six patients) were five times more likely to have progression than did the rest of the group ($P = .01$).[19]

### FOLLOW-UP

After radiation therapy, patients should have a complete blood count, serum calcium and creatinine determinations, and serum and urine immunofixation every 4–6 months for 1 year and annually thereafter. A metastatic bone survey or magnetic resonance imaging should be performed every year or sooner if an M protein develops, if a persistent M protein increases in size, or if any features suggestive of multiple myeloma occur.

## EXTRAMEDULLARY PLASMACYTOMA

Extramedullary plasmacytoma is a plasma cell tumor that arises outside the bone marrow. Extramedullary plasmacytoma accounts for up to 3% of plasma cell malignancies.[15] The median age of patients is about 60

years, and the majority of patients are male.[15] Approximately 80% of tumors involve the upper respiratory tract, including the sinuses and nasal cavity, larynx, and nasopharynx. Epistaxis, rhinorrhea, and nasal obstruction are the most frequent symptoms.

In a review of 714 cases of extramedullary plasmacytoma, 82% involved the upper respiratory tract. Seventy-four percent of plasmacytomas involving the upper aerodigestive tract occurred in male patients. Extramedullary plasmacytomas in the 155 cases not involving the upper aerodigestive region were in the gastrointestinal tract (40%), urogenital region (25%), skin (17%), lung (10%), breast (4%,) conjunctiva (2%), and retroperitoneum (1%).[20]

In a review of the literature, Anghel et al.[21] described 17 patients with a primary solitary testicular plasmacytoma at diagnosis. The median age was 53.5 years. Nine patients died of progressive disease, six were alive without evidence of disease, and two were alive with disease. Twenty-five patients with plasmacytoma localized to the lymph nodes were reported.[22] Cervical nodes were involved in 56%, abdominal in 16%, and mediastinal in 12%. Bone marrow examinations and metastatic bone surveys showed no evidence of multiple myeloma. Ten patients had localized disease, and none had development of multiple myeloma.

Pulmonary involvement may occur. Koss et al.[23] reported two patients with extramedullary plasmacytoma involving the mediastinal lymph nodes and three with parenchymal involvement. When the authors considered their 5 cases in combination with 14 others from the literature, the overall 2-year survival rate was 66%, and the 5-year survival rate was 40%.[23]

### DIAGNOSIS

Extramedullary plasmacytoma is diagnosed on the basis of finding a monoclonal plasma cell tumor in an extramedullary site, in the absence of multiple myeloma in the bone marrow and on radiographic tests, without protein spikes using appropriate studies of blood and urine (Table 84.2). Poorly differentiated neoplasms and lymphoma may be difficult to differentiate from plasmacytomas. In this situation, immunohistochemistry and flow cytometry are helpful in making the diagnosis. There is a higher incidence of IgA M-protein subtype in extramedullary plasmacytoma.

### TREATMENT

The treatment of choice for extramedullary plasmacytoma is tumoricidal radiation at a dosage of 4000 cGy over 4 weeks.

### COURSE

Tsang et al.[9] reported local recurrence in 7% of patients receiving tumoricidal radiation. All local failures were in patients with bulky tumors 5 cm or more in diameter. Progression to multiple myeloma occurs in 10–15% of patients, which is much less common than in patients with solitary plasmacytoma of bone.[9,20,24,25]

In one review, the overall 5-year survival rate with pulmonary plasmacytoma was 40%,[23] whereas it was 60–82% in three separate series of patients with plasmacytoma mainly in the head and neck region.[24–26] A detailed literature search found that there were more than 400 publications between 1905 and 1997.[20] The median overall duration of survival was more than 25 years for patients who received a combination of radiation and surgery. Median duration of survival for patients receiving surgical intervention only was 13 years, whereas it was 12 years for those receiving radiation therapy alone. Overall, 61% had no recurrence or development of multiple myeloma; 22% had recurrence of extramedullary plasmacytoma; and 16% had conversion to multiple myeloma.

Extramedullary plasmacytoma may be classified as low-, intermediate-, or high-grade, depending on histologic grading. In one study, local control after radiation therapy was achieved in 15 of 18 patients (83%) with low-grade disease and in only 1 of 6 patients (17%) with intermediate- to high-grade tumors.[24]

## MULTIPLE SOLITARY PLASMACYTOMAS

The condition termed *multiple solitary plasmacytomas* is characterized by the simultaneous or sequential occurrence of discrete lesions in either bone or soft tissue (extramedullary). In contrast to multiple myeloma, the bone marrow is normal and radiography and magnetic resonance imaging show no evidence of diffuse skeletal involvement (Table 84.2). There is no end-organ damage other than the localized bone lesions. Multiple plasmacytomas may be treated with tumoricidal radiation, when recurrent, if there is no evidence of multiple myeloma. Large numbers of solitary plasmacytomas or recurrent lesions at short intervals are an indication for systemic therapy similar to that for multiple myeloma, such as autologous stem cell transplantation.

## PLASMA CELL LEUKEMIA

Plasma cell leukemia (PCL) is a rare form of plasma cell dyscrasia characterized by the presence of at least $2.0 \times 10^9/L$ and more than 20% plasma cells in the peripheral blood differential leukocyte count. PCL may be classified as primary, when it presents in the leukemic phase, or secondary, when there is leukemic transformation of a previously recognized multiple myeloma. Approximately 60% of patients with PCL have the primary type.[27,28] Secondary PCL occurs in about 1% of patients with multiple myeloma.

### PATHOPHYSIOLOGY
The reason that some patients present with PCL and others have evolvement to it is unclear. Primary PCL is a distinct entity because its presenting features, response

to chemotherapy, and survival are different from those in multiple myeloma. In patients with primary PCL who respond to chemotherapy, PCL almost always reappears at relapse, whereas only 1% of patients with multiple myeloma evolve to a secondary PCL.[30]

Primary PCL cells have a higher expression of CD20 antigen than do cells from multiple myeloma.[28] Plasma cells from both primary and secondary PCL usually lack CD56 antigen, which is important in anchoring plasma cells to the bone marrow stroma.[31] One study showed that the expression of CD28 appears to differentiate primary from secondary PCL.[31]

In one report, more than 80% of patients with PCL were diploid or hypodiploid compared with 40% of patients with multiple myeloma, and 60% of patients with multiple myeloma were hyperdiploid (33). In another series, 17 of 20 (85%) patients were nonhyperdiploid, 2 were equivocal, and 1 was hyperdiploid.[29]

Cytogenetic studies show a complex karyotype with multiple structural and numeric abnormalities in most cases. Fluorescence in situ hybridization showed monosomy of chromosome 13 in 12 of 13 patients.[28] In contrast, cytogenetic findings associated with a favorable outcome such as trisomy of chromosomes 6, 9, and 17 are absent in primary PCL.[28] In a report of 20 patients with PCL (13 primary and 7 secondary), 15 had IgH translocations. Two-thirds of the translocations were t(11;14)(q13;q32), which is an unfavorable prognostic feature. Fourteen patients (70%) had deletion of chromosome 13, whereas 10 had t(17;p13.1) (p53 locus), which are both unfavorable prognostic features.

Mutations of N- and K-*ras* oncogenes have been reported in up to 58% of patients with PCL.[32,33] Amplification of the c-*myc* oncogene at the DNA level with concomitant overexpression has been reported.[34] In two series, 4 of 12 (33%) and 3 of 10 (30%) patients with PCL had p53 mutations.[33,35] Hypomethylation of p16 has been reported in PCL.[36]

Interleukin 6 (IL–6) is the major plasma cell growth factor in vitro and in vivo in patients with multiple myeloma.[37] In a series of 13 patients with PCL, all had significant spontaneous cell growth after 5 days in culture and all had significant growth when stimulated with exogenous IL–6.[38] The role of IL–6 is supported by blockage of plasma cell proliferation when treated with anti–IL–6 monoclonal antibody.[39]

### CLINICAL FEATURES
PCL is uncommon. Most reports consist of single cases or small series, with the exception of three reviews reporting at least 25 cases each. The main clinical and laboratory features, the response to therapy, and the duration of survival of patients with primary PCL in the three reviews are summarized in Table 84.3. Noel and Kyle[27] included patients with PCL diagnosed between 1960 and 1985, while another two series[28,40] included patients with a more recent diagnosis of PCL.

**Table 84.3**   Primary plasma cell leukemia: clinical and laboratory features in three series including at least 25 patients each

| Feature | Noel and Kyle[27] | Dimopoulos et al.[40] | Garcia-Sanz et al.[28] |
|---|---|---|---|
| No. of patients | 25 | 27 | 26 |
| Median age, years | 53 | 57 | 55 |
| Sex (M/F) | 15/10 | NR | 12/14 |
| Extramedullary involvement (%) | >50 | 37 | 23 |
| Lytic bone lesions (%) | 44 | NR | 48 |
| Hemoglobin <10 g/dL (%) | >50 | 82 | 54 |
| Platelet count <100 × 10⁹/L (%) | >50 | 67 | 48 |
| Calcium ≥11 mg/dL (%) | >50 | 44 | 48 |
| Creatinine ≥2 mg/dL (%) | NR | 37 | 44 |
| Monoclonal protein type (%) | | | |
| IgG | 12.5 (2/16) | 52 | 54 |
| IgA | 25 (4/16)[a] | 15 | 4 |
| IgD | 6 (1/16) | 0 | 8 |
| Light-chain | 44 (7/16) | 28 | 31 |
| Nonsecretory | 12.5 (2/16) | 7 | 4 |
| Response to treatment (%) | 47 | 37 | 38 |
| Median survival (months) | 6.8 | 12 | 8 |

IgA, immunoglobulin A; IgD, immunoglobulin D; IgG, immunoglobulin G; NR, not reported.
[a]One case was biclonal (IgAλ, IgEλ).
From Ref. 41, with permission from Elsevier.

The median age ranged between 53 and 57 years, which is a decade younger than that in a large recent myeloma cohort.[42] Patients with primary PCL are younger and have a higher incidence of hepatosplenomegaly and lymphadenopathy, a higher platelet count, fewer lytic lesions, a lower serum M-protein level, and longer survival than do patients with secondary PCL.[27,28] It is obvious from these series that primary PCL has a more aggressive clinical presentation than does multiple myeloma with a higher frequency of extramedullary involvement, anemia, thrombocytopenia, hypercalcemia, and renal impairment. The presence of lytic bone lesions is lower than that observed in multiple myeloma.

### THERAPY AND SURVIVAL

In general, therapeutic options are similar to treatment of multiple myeloma, except that more intensive therapy is needed, and outcomes are significantly inferior.

The outcome of 68 patients from the literature with well-documented primary PCL treated before 1986 has been described.[27] Fifty-two of the patients received a single alkylating agent, mainly melphalan with or without prednisone, as initial therapy. A complete or partial response was documented in 28 patients (54%). The median duration of survival was slightly more than 1 year in patients who responded to therapy, but less than 1 month for nonresponding patients. The other 16 patients were treated with combination chemotherapy, which resulted in a response rate of 75% and a median duration of survival for all 16 patients of 9.5 months. In the Mayo Clinic series of 25 patients with primary PCL, 7 of 15 patients responded to melphalan with or without prednisone. Despite the response rate of 47%, the median time to progression or death in these 15

patients was 8.7 months. The median duration of survival for all 25 patients with PCL was 6.8 months, and only 4 patients survived for more than 2 years.

The overall response rate in the series by Dimopoulos et al.[40] was 37%. They noted that failure to achieve 50% clearing of peripheral blood plasma cells within 10 days after initiation of treatment was a predictor of no response. The median duration of survival was 12 months. A short survival was caused mainly by the large number of patients dying of disease complications during the first 2 months of treatment. In that series, patients treated with vincristine, doxorubicin (adriamycin), and dexamethasone (VAD) or with cyclophosphamide and etoposide had a response rate of 59% and a median duration of survival of 20 months. These improved results are probably due to a decrease in early mortality as a result of a rapid reduction of tumor mass, and due to improved supportive therapy. Garcia-Sanz et al.[28] reported an overall response rate of 38%. The response rate and survival were lower in patients treated with melphalan and prednisone than in those given alternating courses of vincristine, cyclophosphamide, melphalan, and prednisone (VCMP) or vincristine, 1,3-bis(2-chlorethyl)-1-nitrosourea (BCNU), doxorubicin (adriamycin), and prednisone (VBAP).

Treatment with a single alkylating agent plus prednisone is not adequate for patients with primary PCL. Combination chemotherapy with VAD, cyclophosphamide, and etoposide or alternating VCMP and VBAP yields better responses. High-dose therapy followed by autologous stem cell transplantation should be offered to responding patients if age and clinical condition do not preclude transplantation.[43] Thalidomide also may be a useful agent.[44]

Secondary PCL usually is a terminal event in patients with relapsed or refractory myeloma. Unfortunately, the median duration of survival in these patients is about 1 month.[27] Thalidomide may be of some benefit in this situation.[45]

## SMOLDERING (ASYMPTOMATIC) MULTIPLE MYELOMA

The point of transition from monoclonal gammopathy of undetermined significance (MGUS) to smoldering multiple myeloma is not sharply defined biologically. By definition, MGUS consists of an M-protein value less than 3 g/dL, bone marrow plasma cell value less than 10%, and absence of anemia, renal insufficiency, hypercalcemia, or skeletal lesions attributable to the neoplastic plasma cell proliferation (Table 84.2). However, if the M-protein value is 3 g/dL or more or the bone marrow contains 10% or more plasma cells, the term *smoldering (asymptomatic) multiple myeloma* is used (Table 84.2).[4] Frequently, a reduction of uninvolved immunoglobulins in the serum and a small amount of M protein in the urine are found. These findings are consistent with multiple myeloma, but anemia, renal insufficiency, and skeletal lesions are not present. That is, there is no evidence of end-organ damage. In addition, the plasma cell labeling index is low.

Smoldering multiple myeloma occurs in approximately 15% of all cases of newly diagnosed multiple myeloma.[1] The prevalence estimates of smoldering multiple myeloma are variable because many reports include asymptomatic patients with lytic lesions on skeletal survey. Some exclude skeletal lesions but include patients who have lytic lesions on magnetic resonance imaging. A true prevalence derived from strict criteria for smoldering multiple myeloma is not available. Most patients with smoldering multiple myeloma eventually have progression to symptomatic myeloma, and the risk of progression is higher than with MGUS.[1] Some patients may remain stable for many years.[46] The median time for progression to symptomatic disease is 1–3 years. One study found only a 20% risk of progression at 6 years, but patients were considered to have smoldering multiple myeloma only if they had no disease progression after 1 year of follow-up.[47]

### PREDICTORS OF PROGRESSION
Assessment of predictors of progression in smoldering multiple myeloma is hampered by varying diagnostic criteria used to define the condition. Several studies include patients with asymptomatic lytic lesions as well. Future studies of smoldering multiple myeloma will need to use more uniformly accepted criteria so that results can be compared.

Patients with an increase in the number of circulating peripheral blood monoclonal plasma cells are at higher risk for progression to myeloma. An increased plasma cell labeling index of the bone marrow indicates that symptomatic multiple myeloma is present or will develop in the near future.

The three most important prognostic factors for progression in one series included a serum monoclonal protein concentration more than 3.0 g/dL, IgA subtype, and urinary M-protein excretion of more than 50 mg/day. Patients with more than two of these features had a median time to progression of 17 months; those with two factors had a median time to progression of 40 months; and patients who had none of these features had a median time to progression of 95 months.[48]

Other studies have found that abnormalities on magnetic resonance imaging can predict disease progression in patients with smoldering multiple myeloma.[1] Whether patients who have abnormalities on magnetic resonance imaging should be considered as having smoldering multiple myeloma is debatable. Nevertheless, these patients can be considered to have low-grade multiple myeloma and can be observed without therapy, similar to those with smoldering multiple myeloma.

### MANAGEMENT
The current standard of care in smoldering multiple myeloma is close follow-up every few months without any chemotherapy. This recommendation results from trials that found no significant improvement in overall survival in patients who received immediate treatment with melphalan plus prednisone for stage I or asymptomatic myeloma, compared with those who received treatment at progression. Hjorth and colleagues[49] assigned 50 patients with asymptomatic stage I myeloma to observation versus melphalan plus prednisone chemotherapy. No differences were found in overall survival between the two groups. In another series of 44 patients with asymptomatic myeloma, survival times were similar with immediate or deferred therapy.[50]

Investigational approaches may be considered for selected patients in appropriate trials. Thalidomide is being studied as a single agent, and a partial response rate of approximately 35% has been noted. However, a phase III randomized study comparing no therapy with thalidomide or other agents such as bisphosphonates, IL-1β inhibitors, clarithromycin, or dehydroepiandrosterone is required before making any recommendations concerning therapy of smoldering multiple myeloma.

## POEMS SYNDROME (OSTEOSCLEROTIC MYELOMA)

POEMS (*p*olyneuropathy, *o*rganomegaly, *e*ndocrinopathy, *M* protein, and *s*kin changes) syndrome, or osteosclerotic myeloma, is characterized by chronic sensorimotor peripheral neuropathy with predominating motor disability.[51] Additional features include sclerotic bone lesions, Castleman's disease, papilledema, edema, ascites, pleural effusion, erythrocytosis, and thrombocytosis.

### CLINICAL FEATURES

Peripheral neuropathy was present in all of our 99 patients and usually dominates the clinical picture.[52] Symptoms usually begin in the feet and consist of tingling or paresthesias. Motor involvement follows the sensory symptoms. Both begin distally and are symmetric and progress proximally. More than half of the patients have severe weakness and may have difficulty in climbing stairs, rising from a chair, or gripping objects firmly. In contrast to the neuropathy associated with primary amyloidosis (AL), autonomic symptoms are not a feature. Bone pain and pathologic fractures are major findings in symptomatic myeloma, but occur rarely in POEMS syndrome.

Physical examination reveals a symmetric, sensorimotor neuropathy involving the extremities. Muscle weakness is usually more marked than sensory loss. Touch, pressure, vibratory, and joint position senses are often involved, whereas loss of temperature discrimination and nociception occur less frequently. Papilledema was present in almost one-third of our patients. However, other cranial nerves are not affected.

Hepatomegaly, splenomegaly, and lymphadenopathy were present in about one-fourth of patients. Hyperpigmentation was present in almost one-half of patients, but it was easily overlooked. Hypertrichosis, manifested by coarse black hair, appeared on the extremities in one-fourth of our patients, and telangiectasia and hemangiomas were present in 10%. Peripheral edema was found in one-fourth of our patients, but ascites and pleural effusion were uncommon. Clubbing of the fingers has been noted but was infrequent in our series.

### LABORATORY FEATURES

Almost 20% of our patients had polycythemia. Anemia was not a feature of the syndrome. Thrombocytosis was noted in more than half of our patients. Hypercalcemia and renal insufficiency were rare.

All of our patients had evidence of a monoclonal plasma cell proliferative process. Eighty-five percent had an M protein in the serum, but the level was modest and the median value was 1.1 g/dL. This is similar to the 75% reported by Nakanishi et al.[53] in a review of 102 patients with the syndrome. Forty patients had an M protein in the urine, but the amount was small and the median value was 100 mg/24 h.

All of our patients had a monoclonal λ-proliferative process. IgAλ was found in 44 patients, and IgGλ was found in 40. Only one patient had an IgMλ protein. A clonal λ plasma cell proliferative process was shown by immunohistochemical staining in all 12 patients who did not have an M protein in their serum or urine.

The bone marrow was most often nondiagnostic. Only 14% of patients had a bone marrow plasmacytosis of more than 10%, which is similar to the findings of Soubrier et al.[54] Only four of our patients had more than 20% plasma cells, but none of them had lytic bone lesions or anemia.

Endocrine abnormalities were found in two-thirds of our patients at presentation. Hypogonadism was the most common abnormality, and 71% of males had erectile dysfunction. Twenty-four of 28 patients who had serum testosterone levels measured had a reduction. Gynecomastia was found in 17 men. Prolactin levels were not increased. Hypothyroidism was found in 14% of patients. An additional 12% had a mild increase in the thyroid-stimulating hormone level but had normal thyroxin levels. Abnormalities of the adrenal-pituitary axis were present in 16%. In five additional patients, adrenal insufficiency developed during follow-up.

### SCLEROTIC BONE LESIONS

Conventional radiographs showed osteosclerotic lesions in 95% of our patients. Lytic lesions without evidence of sclerosis are rare. Approximately half of our patients had mixed sclerotic and lytic lesions. Forty-seven percent of our patients had only sclerotic lesions. A single solitary lesion was found in 45%, and the remainder had multiple lesions. The pelvis, spine, ribs, and proximal extremities are most often involved. In rare instances, multiple myeloma is associated with diffuse osteosclerotic bone lesions, and affected patients must be differentiated from those with POEMS syndrome.

### PATHOPHYSIOLOGY

The cause of POEMS syndrome is unknown. Patients frequently have higher levels of IL–1β, tumor necrosis factor α, and IL–6 than do patients with multiple myeloma.[55] Levels of vascular endothelial growth factor are also frequently increased.[56] Antibodies to human herpesvirus 8 were reported in seven of nine patients with POEMS syndrome and Castleman's disease. Six of seven patients had human herpesvirus 8 DNA sequences.[57]

Electromyography shows slowing of nerve conduction and severe attenuation of compound muscle action potentials.[58] Distal fibrillation potentials are found on needle electromyography. Both axonal degeneration and demyelination are found in sural nerve biopsy specimens. Ono et al.[59] reported a loss of demyelinated fibers and an increased frequency of axonal degeneration in teased fibers. Cerebrospinal fluid protein levels are increased in almost all patients. More than half of our patients had a cerebrospinal fluid protein value more than 100 mg/dL.[60]

Castleman's disease (giant cell lymph node hyperplasia, angiofollicular lymph node hyperplasia) has also been associated with POEMS syndrome.[61] In our experience, about 15% of patients with POEMS syndrome also have Castleman's disease.

Renal involvement may be a feature of POEMS syndrome. Nakamoto et al.[62] reviewed 52 cases of POEMS syndrome with renal abnormalities. Approximately half of the patients had creatinine levels more than 1.5 mg/dL, and 10% required dialysis.

Pulmonary hypertension also has been noted in POEMS syndrome.[63] Pulmonary hypertension developed in 5 of 20 patients with POEMS syndrome, and increased levels of IL–1β, IL–6, tumor necrosis factor α, and vascular endothelial growth factor were found in all cases.[64] Five of our patients had pulmonary hypertension and restrictive lung disease; respiratory failure developed in four of them. Respiratory disease was responsible for death in 17% of our patients.

Hyperpigmentation, hypertrichosis, and hemangiomas were the major dermatologic findings in our series.[52] Four patients have been described with POEMS syndrome and a violaceous skin patch overlying a solitary plasmacytoma of bone, along with enlarged regional lymph nodes. One patient had POEMS syndrome, whereas in another, POEMS syndrome developed after excision of the plasmacytoma. The authors suggested the term *AESOP syndrome* for *a*denopathy and *e*xtensive *s*kin patch *o*verlying a *p*lasmacytoma.[65]

Forty-one thrombotic events occurred in 18 of our patients. These consisted of stroke, myocardial infarction, or Budd-Chiari syndrome. Four patients with POEMS syndrome have been reported with acute arterial thrombotic events.[66]

### DIAGNOSIS AND COURSE

POEMS syndrome must be considered in the differential diagnosis of a patient presenting with a sensorimotor peripheral neuropathy. A metastatic bone survey must be done in search for osteosclerotic lesions. These lesions can be subtle and easily confused with fibrous dysplasia or a vertebral hemangioma. The M-protein level in the serum and urine is low and may be easily overlooked. The diagnosis depends on the demonstration of increased numbers of monoclonal plasma cells and a biopsy specimen from the osteosclerotic lesion.

The natural history is one of progressive peripheral neuropathy over a period of years until the patient is bedridden. Death usually occurs from inanition or terminal pneumonia. The median overall duration of survival in our 99 patients was 13.7 years.

### THERAPY

Radiation in a dose of 40–50 cGy is indicated for patients with single or multiple osteosclerotic lesions in a limited area. More than half of the patients show substantial improvement of neuropathy. Of our 13 patients who did not respond to radiation, 9 received less than 4000 cGy. The improvement may be slow and may not be apparent for 6 months or longer. Some patients continue to improve for 2–3 years after radiation therapy.

Systemic therapy is necessary if the patient has widespread osteosclerotic lesions. Melphalan and prednisone were given to 48 of our patients, and improvement was noted in 44%. Combination chemotherapy induced responses in 27% of 15 treated patients. Prednisone or dexamethasone as a single agent was given to 41 of our patients, and there was an apparent improvement in only 15%. Plasma exchange, intravenous immunoglobulin, cyclosporine, and azathioprine were ineffective.

Autologous stem cell transplantation after high-dose melphalan should be seriously considered for patients younger than 70 years with widespread osteosclerotic lesions. The stem cells should be collected before the patient is exposed to alkylating agents because they will damage the hematopoietic stem cells. The mortality associated with the procedure is only 1–2%.[67–70]

## NONSECRETORY MYELOMA

Patients with nonsecretory myeloma have no M protein in either the serum or urine with immunofixation. This finding occurs in 1–5% of all patients with multiple myeloma.[42,71–74] In 1027 patients with newly diagnosed myeloma, we found no M protein in the serum and urine with immunofixation in 29 (2.8%).[42]

Immunoperoxidase and immunofluorescence studies on plasma cells should be performed in all patients with nonsecretory myeloma. A cytoplasmic M protein is identified in about 85% of patients; no M protein can be found in the remaining, and these patients are considered to have "nonproducer" nonsecretory myeloma.[75–78]

Ultrastructural study of plasma cells shows the typical features observed in plasma cells of patients who have an M protein in the serum and urine.[79,80] In contrast, in some cases of nonproducer or truly nonsecretory myeloma, ultrastructural studies show highly undifferentiated plasma cells.[77,81] The lack of M protein in the serum and urine of patients with nonsecretory myeloma may be from (1) the inability of plasma cells to excrete the immunoglobulin, (2) the low synthetic capacity of immunoglobulin production, (3) increased intracellular degradation, or (4) rapid extracellular degradation of abnormal immunoglobulins. Interestingly, the light chain is of κ type in about 75% of patients with nonsecretory myeloma.

### CLINICAL FEATURES

The main presenting features in four series of nonsecretory myeloma with at least seven patients are shown in Table 84.4. In the largest series, consisting of 29 patients, the median age was a decade younger than that of a usual patient with myeloma. In that series, almost 70% of patients had low tumor mass. No patient had a hemoglobin level less than 11 g/dL or renal failure, and only two patients had hypercalcemia. In the other series, the presenting features of nonsecretory myeloma were similar to those in patients with M

**Table 84.4** Nonsecretory myeloma: presenting features in four series including at least seven patients

| Feature | Azar et al.[71] | Dreicer and Alexanian[73] | Cavo et al.[72] | Bourantas[82] |
|---|---|---|---|---|
| No. of patients | 7 | 29 | 7 | 9 |
| Median age (years) | 62 | 54 | 55 | 53 |
| Sex (M/F) | 4/3 | 16/13 | 2/5 | 4/5 |
| Hemoglobin <11 g/dL, no. of patients | 6 | 0 | 5 | 6 |
| Calcium ≥11.5 mg/dL, no. of patients | NR | 2 | 0 | 4 |
| Creatinine ≥2 mg/dL, no. of patients | NR | 0 | 0 | 1 |
| High tumor mass (stage III disease), no. of patients | NR | 2[a] | 6 | 8 |
| Lytic bone lesions, no. of patients | 6 | 29 | 5 | 9 |

NR, not reported.
[a] Stage not including skeletal involvement.
From Ref. 41, with permission from Elsevier.

protein, except for the absence of renal insufficiency. Most patients had stage III disease, and the majority had a marked reduction of normal polyclonal immunoglobulins. Almost all patients had lytic lesions.

In the series of 29 patients, the condition remained nonsecretory throughout in 22 patients (76%). During follow-up, M protein developed in the serum in five patients (two with monoclonal heavy chain and three with monoclonal light chain). In two others, a monoclonal light chain developed in the urine. The uninvolved immunoglobulins were reduced in 92%. None of the patients with nonsecretory myeloma had a serum creatinine value more than 2 mg/dL. In contrast, the serum creatinine value was increased in 35% of the patients with light-chain myeloma. Median duration of survival was 38 months for patients with nonsecretory myeloma, 34 months for those with light-chain myeloma, and 33 months for the entire cohort of 1027 patients.[42]

### RESPONSE TO THERAPY AND SURVIVAL

Therapy is similar to that for multiple myeloma. The lack of a measurable M protein makes evaluation of response to therapy difficult. Evaluation of response is based on improvement in the symptoms of bone pain, correction of anemia and hypercalcemia if initially present, reduction of extramedullary plasmacytomas, no increase in lytic bone lesions, and decrease in the proportion of bone marrow plasma cells. The advent of free light-chain assays is useful for monitoring the progress of patients with nonsecretory myeloma. Drayson et al.[94] reported abnormal free light chains in 68% of patients with nonsecretory myeloma. Dreicer and Alexanian[73] reported that 80% of patients responded to initial chemotherapy.

In several series, survival of patients with nonsecretory myeloma was similar to that of patients with a measurable M protein.[71,72,79,80] Dreicer and Alexanian[73] reported a median duration of survival of 39 months, whereas Bourantas[82] noted 45 months. The median of 38 months in our study was not statistically different from that in patients with a measurable M protein.[42]

## IMMUNOGLOBULIN D MYELOMA

IgD myeloma accounts for about 2% of all cases of multiple myeloma.[83,84] Although the presence of an IgD M protein is almost always indicative of a malignant plasma cell disorder such as multiple myeloma or primary amyloidosis, two well-documented cases of MGUS of the IgD type have been reported.[85,86] Thus, the presence of a serum IgD M protein is not always associated with a malignant plasma cell proliferative process.

### CLINICAL FEATURES

The data on IgD myeloma come from reports on a few cases and small series, two large reviews of the reported cases in the literature,[87,88] and single-institution experience in 53 cases.[89,90]

The main clinical and laboratory features reported in four series of IgD myeloma including at least 20 patients are summarized in Table 84.5.[87,88,89,90,91] The median age at presentation was 55–60 years, which is slightly younger than that in a general myeloma population. The initial presenting symptoms were not different from those reported in usual myeloma cases. In two series, a moderate lymph node enlargement, a rare finding in multiple myeloma, was present in about 10% of patients.[88,90] Although one series had a low incidence of extramedullary plasmacytoma,[91] the reported incidence of extraosseous spread in IgD myeloma ranges from 19 to 63%.[84,88,90] In one of the studies, 7 of 53 patients (13%) had extradural plasmacytomas at diagnosis.[90] Amyloidosis was reported in 44% of patients at autopsy.[87] In a single-institution series, however, the frequency of associated amyloidosis was 19%.[90] IgD myeloma has been associated with a higher frequency of PCL.[87,88,92] The incidence of renal failure is higher in IgD myeloma.[87,88,90,91]

The serum protein electrophoretic pattern differs in that only 60% of patients with IgD myeloma have an M-protein spike. Furthermore, the amount of the M protein rarely exceeds 2 g/dL.[90] Almost all patients

**Table 84.5    Immunoglobulin D myeloma: clinical and laboratory features in four series including at least 20 patients[a]**

| Feature | Jancelewicz et al.[87] | Fibbe and Jansen[91] | Shimamoto et al.[88] | Bladé et al.[90] |
|---|---|---|---|---|
| No. of patients | 133 | 21 | 165 | 53 |
| Median age (years) | 56 | 59 | 55 | 60 |
| Sex (M/F) | 98/31 | 15/6 | 125/40 | 33/20 |
| Extramedullary involvement (%) | >23 | NR | 27 | 19 |
| Lytic bone lesions (%) | 79 | 43 | NR | 72 |
| Hemoglobin <10 g/dL (%) | 29 | 33 | NR | 29 |
| Calcium ≥11 mg/dL (%) | 30 | 33 | 34 | 22 |
| Creatinine ≥2 mg/dL (%) | 31[b] | 38 | 43 | 33 |
| κ/λ ratio | 115/13 | 19/2 | 133/29 | 32/20 |
| Median survival (months) | 13.7 | 17 | 12 | 21 |

NR, not reported.
[a] In some series, data were not available in all cases.
[b] Blood urea nitrogen ≥75 mg/dL.
From Ref. 41, with permission from Elsevier.

with IgD myeloma have light-chain proteinuria, and more than half have more than 1 g/24 h.[90] In most series of IgD myeloma, increased λ light chain has been reported,[87,88,91,93] but in a large single-institution series the frequency of λ light chain was 60%.[90] IgD myeloma should always be excluded in patients with a discrete M-protein spike on serum protein electrophoresis and only a monoclonal κ or λ light chain on immunofixation.

In summary, patients with IgD myeloma often present with a small band or no spike on serum protein electrophoresis and light-chain proteinuria. Almost one-fifth have associated amyloidosis. Because these features are also typical of light-chain myeloma, IgD can be considered a variant. The presence of IgD M protein and the predominance of the λ light chain are the major distinctive findings.

## THERAPY AND SURVIVAL

Treatment and response to therapy in patients with IgD myeloma is similar to that in patients with myeloma of other immunologic types.[87,90,95] In several series, the median duration of survival of patients with IgD myeloma ranged from 12 to 17 months.[84,87,88,91] Fahey et al.[95] reported a median duration of 2 years in 15 patients. In the Mayo Clinic series of 53 patients, the median duration of survival was 21 months, but for the 26 patients in whom the diagnosis was made after 1980 the median survival was 31 months.[90] Three patients in that series survived for more than 10 years, and one of them was considered to have been cured.[96]

### Acknowledgment

This work is supported in part by research grant no. CA62242 from the National Institutes of Health.

## REFERENCES

1. Dimopoulos MA, Moulopoulos LA, Maniatis A, et al.: Solitary plasmacytoma of bone and asymptomatic multiple myeloma. *Blood* 96:2037, 2000.
2. Frassica DA, Frassica FJ, Schray MF, et al.: Solitary plasmacytoma of bone: Mayo Clinic experience. *Int J Radiat Oncol Biol Phys* 16:43, 1989.
3. Kyle RA: Monoclonal gammopathy of undetermined significance and solitary plasmacytoma: implications for progression to overt multiple myeloma. *Hematol Oncol Clin North Am* 11:71–87, 1997.
4. International Myeloma Working Group: Criteria for the classification of monoclonal gammopathies, multiple myeloma and related disorders: a report of the International Myeloma Working Group. *Br J Haematol* 121:749, 2003.
5. Wilder RB, Ha CS, Cox JD, et al.: Persistence of myeloma protein for more than one year after radiotherapy is an adverse prognostic factor in solitary plasmacytoma of bone. *Cancer* 94:1532, 2002.
6. Moulopoulos LA, Dimopoulos MA, Weber D, et al.: Magnetic resonance imaging in the staging of solitary plasmacytoma of bone. *J Clin Oncol* 11:1311, 1993.
7. Pertuiset E, Bellaiche L, Liote F, et al.: Magnetic resonance imaging of the spine in plasma cell dyscrasias: a review. *Rev Rhum Engl Ed* 63:837, 1996.
8. Holland J, Trenkner DA, Wasserman TH, et al.: Plasmacytoma: treatment results and conversion to myeloma. *Cancer* 69:1513, 1992.
9. Tsang RW, Gospodarowicz MK, Pintilie M, et al.: Solitary plasmacytoma treated with radiotherapy: impact of tumor size on outcome. *Int J Radiat Oncol Biol Phys* 50:113, 2001.
10. Bolek TW, Marcus RB, Mendenhall NP: Solitary plasmacytoma of bone and soft tissue. *Int J Radiat Oncol Biol Phys* 36:329, 1996.
11. Shih LY, Dunn P, Leung WM, et al.: Localised plasmacytomas in Taiwan: comparison between extramedullary plasmacytoma and solitary plasmacytoma of bone. *Br J Cancer* 71:128, 1995.
12. Galieni P, Cavo M, Avvisati G, et al.: Solitary plasmacytoma of bone and extramedullary plasmacytoma: two different entities? *Ann Oncol* 6:687, 1995.
13. Aviles A, Huerta-Guzman J, Delgado S, et al.: Improved outcome in solitary bone plasmacytomata with combined therapy. *Hematol Oncol* 14:111, 1996.
14. Delauche-Cavallier MC, Laredo JD, Wybier M, et al.: Solitary plasmacytoma of the spine: long-term clinical course. *Cancer* 61:1707, 1988.
15. Knowling MA, Harwood AR, Bergsagel DE: Comparison of extramedullary plasmacytomas with solitary and

multiple plasma cell tumors of bone. *J Clin Oncol* 1:255, 1983.

16. Dimopoulos MA, Goldstein J, Fuller L, et al.: Curability of solitary bone plasmacytoma. *J Clin Oncol* 10:587, 1992.

17. McLain RF, Weinstein JN: Solitary plasmacytomas of the spine: a review of 84 cases. *J Spinal Disord* 2:69, 1989.

18. Bataille R, Sany J: Solitary myeloma: clinical and prognostic features of a review of 114 cases. *Cancer* 48:845, 1981.

19. Kumar S, Fonseca R, Dispenzieri A, et al.: Prognostic value of angiogenesis in solitary bone plasmacytoma. *Blood* 101:1715, 2003.

20. Alexiou C, Kau RJ, Dietzfelbinger H, et al.: Extramedullary plasmacytoma: tumor occurrence and therapeutic concepts. *Cancer* 85:2305, 1999.

21. Anghel G, Petti N, Remotti D, et al.: Testicular plasmacytoma: report of a case and review of the literature. *Am J Hematol* 71:98, 2002.

22. Menke DM, Horny HP, Griesser H, et al.: Primary lymph node plasmacytomas (plasmacytic lymphomas). *Am J Clin Pathol* 115:119, 2001.

23. Koss MN, Hochholzer L, Moran CA, et al.: Pulmonary plasmacytomas: a clinicopathologic and immunohistochemical study of five cases. *Ann Diagn Pathol* 2:1, 1998.

24. Susnerwala SS, Shanks JH, Banerjee SS, et al.: Extramedullary plasmacytoma of the head and neck region: clinicopathological correlation in 25 cases. *Br J Cancer* 75:921, 1997.

25. Miller FR, Lavertu P, Wanamaker JR, et al.: Plasmacytomas of the head and neck. *Otolaryngol Head Neck Surg* 119:614, 1998.

26. Strojan P, Soba E, Lamovec J, et al.: Extramedullary plasmacytoma: clinical and histopathologic study. *Int J Radiat Oncol Biol Phys* 53:692, 2002.

27. Noel P, Kyle RA: Plasma cell leukemia: an evaluation of response to therapy. *Am J Med* 83:1062, 1987.

28. Garcia-Sanz R, Orfao A, Gonzalez M, et al.: Primary plasma cell leukemia: clinical, immunophenotypic, DNA ploidy, and cytogenetic characteristics. *Blood* 93:1032, 1999.

29. Santana-Davila R, Rajkumar SV, Ahmann GJ, et al.: High incidence of p 53 deletion in plasma cell leukemia (PCL), and multiple myeloma (mm) with leukemic transformation (MMLT) [abstract]. *Blood* 102:680a, 2003.

30. Woodruff RK, Malpas JS, Paxton AM, et al.: Plasma cell leukemia (PCL): a report on 15 patients. *Blood* 52:839, 1978.

31. Pellat-Deceunynck C, Barille S, Jego G, et al.: The absence of CD56 (NCAM) on malignant plasma cells is a hallmark of plasma cell leukemia and of a special subset of multiple myeloma. *Leukemia* 12:1977, 1998.

32. Corradini P, Ladetto M, Voena C, et al.: Mutational activation of N- and K-*ras* oncogenes in plasma cell dyscrasias. *Blood* 81:2708, 1993.

33. Portier M, Moles JP, Mazars GR, et al.: *p53* and *RAS* gene mutations in multiple myeloma. *Oncogene* 7:2539, 1992.

34. Sumegi J, Hedberg T, Bjorkholm M, et al.: Amplification of the c-*myc* oncogene in human plasma-cell leukemia. *Int J Cancer* 36:367, 1985.

35. Neri A, Baldini L, Trecca D, et al.: *p53* gene mutations in multiple myeloma are associated with advanced forms of malignancy. *Blood* 81:128, 1993.

36. Urashima M, Teoh G, Ogata A, et al.: Characterization of p16 (INK4A) expression in multiple myeloma and plasma cell leukemia. *Clin Cancer Res* 3:2173, 1997.

37. Zhang XG, Klein B, Bataille R: Interleukin-6 is a potent myeloma-cell growth factor in patients with aggressive multiple myeloma. *Blood* 74:11, 1989.

38. Zhang XG, Bataille R, Widjenes J, et al.: Interleukin-6 dependence of advanced malignant plasma cell dyscrasias. *Cancer* 69:1373, 1992.

39. Klein B, Wijdenes J, Zhang XG, et al.: Murine anti-interleukin-6 monoclonal antibody therapy for a patient with plasma cell leukemia. *Blood* 78:1198, 1991.

40. Dimopoulos MA, Palumbo A, Delasalle KB, et al.: Primary plasma cell leukaemia. *Br J Haematol* 88:754, 1994.

41. Bladé J, Kyle RA: Nonsecretory myeloma, immunoglobulin D myeloma, and plasma cell leukemia. *Hematol Oncol Clin North Am* 13:1259, 1999.

42. Kyle RA, Gertz MA, Witzig TE, et al.: Review of 1027 patients with newly diagnosed multiple myeloma. *Mayo Clin Proc* 78:21, 2003.

43. Hovenga S, de Wolf JT, Klip H, et al.: Consolidation therapy with autologous stem cell transplantation in plasma cell leukemia after VAD, high-dose cyclophosphamide and EDAP courses: a report of three cases and a review of the literature. *Bone Marrow Transplant* 20:901, 1997.

44. Johnston RE, Abdalla SH: Thalidomide in low doses is effective for the treatment of resistant or relapsed multiple myeloma and for plasma cell leukaemia. *Leuk Lymphoma* 43:351, 2002.

45. Tsiara S, Chidos A, Kapsali H, et al.: Thalidomide administration for the treatment of resistant plasma cell leukemia. *Acta Haematol* 109:153, 2003.

46. Kyle RA, Greipp PR: Smoldering multiple myeloma. *N Engl J Med* 302:1347, 1980.

47. Cesana C, Klersy C, Barbarano L, et al.: Prognostic factors for malignant transformation in monoclonal gammopathy of undetermined significance and smoldering multiple myeloma. *J Clin Oncol* 20:1625, 2002.

48. Weber DM, Dimopoulos MA, Moulopoulos LA, et al.: Prognostic features of asymptomatic multiple myeloma. *Br J Haematol* 97:810, 1997.

49. Hjorth M, Hellquist L, Holmberg E, et al., for the Myeloma Group of Western Sweden: Initial versus deferred melphalan—prednisone therapy for asymptomatic multiple myeloma stage I: a randomized study. *Eur J Haematol* 50:95, 1993.

50. Grignani G, Gobbi PG, Formisano R, et al.: A prognostic index for multiple myeloma. *Br J Cancer* 73:1101, 1996.

51. Bardwick PA, Zvaifler NJ, Gill GN, et al.: Plasma cell dyscrasia with polyneuropathy, organomegaly, endocrinopathy, M protein, and skin changes: the POEMS syndrome. Report on two cases and a review of the literature. *Medicine (Baltimore)* 59:311, 1980.

52. Dispenzieri A, Kyle RA, Lacy MQ, et al.: POEMS syndrome: definitions and long-term outcome. *Blood* 101:2496, 2003.

53. Nakanishi T, Sobue I, Toyokura Y, et al.: The Crow-Fukase syndrome: a study of 102 cases in Japan. *Neurology* 34:712, 1984.

54. Soubrier MJ, Dubost JJ, Sauvezie BJ, and the French Study Group on POEMS Syndrome: POEMS syndrome: a study of 25 cases and a review of the literature. *Am J Med* 97:543, 1994.

55. Gherardi RK, Belec L, Soubrier M, et al.: Overproduction of proinflammatory cytokines imbalanced by their antagonists in POEMS syndrome. *Blood* 87:1458, 1996.

56. Watanabe O, Maruyama I, Arimura K, et al.: Overproduction of vascular endothelial growth factor/vascular permeability factor is causative in Crow–Fukase (POEMS) syndrome. *Muscle Nerve* 21:1390, 1998.

57. Pelec L, Mohamed AS, Authier FJ, et al.: Human herpesvirus 8 infection in patients with POEMS syndrome-associated multicentric Castleman's disease. *Blood* 93:3643, 1999.

58. Sung JY, Kuwabara S, Ogawara K, et al.: Patterns of nerve conduction abnormalities in POEMS syndrome. *Muscle Nerve* 26:189, 2002.

59. Ono K, Ito M, Hotchi M, et al.: Polyclonal plasma cell proliferation with systemic capillary hemangiomatosis, endocrine disturbance, and peripheral neuropathy. *Acta Pathol Jpn* 35:251, 1985.

60. Kelly JJ Jr, Kyle RA, Miles JM, et al.: Osteosclerotic myeloma and peripheral neuropathy. *Neurology* 33:202, 1983.

61. Bitter MA, Komaiko W, Franklin WA: Giant lymph node hyperplasia with osteoblastic bone lesions and the POEMS (Takatsuki's) syndrome. *Cancer* 56:188, 1985.

62. Nakamoto Y, Imai H, Yasuda T, et al.: A spectrum of clinicopathological features of nephropathy associated with POEMS syndrome. *Nephrol Dial Transplant* 14:2370, 1999.

63. Ribadeau-Dumas S, Tillie-Leblond I, Rose C, et al.: Pulmonary hypertension associated with POEMS syndrome. *Eur Respir J* 9:1760, 1996.

64. Lesprit P, Godeau B, Authier FJ, et al.: Pulmonary hypertension in POEMS syndrome: a new feature mediated by cytokines. *Am J Respir Crit Care Med* 157:907, 1998.

65. Lipsker D, Rondeau M, Massard G, et al.: The AESOP (adenopathy and extensive skin patch overlying a plasmacytoma) syndrome: report of 4 cases of a new syndrome revealing POEMS (polyneuropathy, organomegaly, endocrinopathy, monoclonal protein, and skin changes) syndrome at a curable stage. *Medicine (Baltimore)* 82:51, 2003.

66. Lesprit P, Authier FJ, Gherardi R, et al.: Acute arterial obliteration: a new feature of the POEMS syndrome? *Medicine (Baltimore)* 75:226, 1996.

67. Jaccard A, Royer B, Bordessoule D, et al.: High-dose therapy and autologous blood stem cell transplantation in POEMS syndrome. *Blood* 99:3057, 2002.

68. Rovira M, Carreras E, Bladé J, et al.: Dramatic improvement of POEMS syndrome following autologous haematopoietic cell transplantation. *Br J Haematol* 115:373, 2001.

69. Dispenzieri A, Lacy MQ, Litzow MR, et al.: Peripheral blood stem cell transplant (PBSCT) in patients with POEMS syndrome [abstract]. *Blood* 98:391b, 2001.

70. Peggs KS, Paneesha S, Kottaridis PD, et al.: Peripheral blood stem cell transplantation for POEMS syndrome. *Bone Marrow Transplant* 30:401, 2002.

71. Azar HA, Zaino EC, Pham TD, et al.: "Nonsecretory" plasma cell myeloma: observations on seven cases with electron microscopic studies. *Am J Clin Pathol* 58:618, 1972.

72. Cavo M, Galieni P, Gobbi M, et al.: Nonsecretory multiple myeloma: presenting findings, clinical course and prognosis. *Acta Haematol* 74:27, 1985.

73. Dreicer R, Alexanian R: Nonsecretory multiple myeloma. *Am J Hematol* 13:313, 1982.

74. Turesson I, Grubb A: Non-secretory or low-secretory myeloma with intracellular kappa chains: report of six cases and review of the literature. *Acta Med Scand* 204:445, 1978.

75. Franchi F, Seminara P, Teodori L, et al.: The non-producer plasma cell myeloma: report of a case and review of the literature. *Blut* 52:281, 1986.

76. Indiveri F, Barabino A, Santolini ME, et al.: "Nonsecretory" multiple myeloma: report of a case. *Acta Haematol* 51:302, 1974.

77. Mancilla R, Davis GL: Nonsecretory multiple myeloma: immunohistologic and ultrastructural observations on two patients. *Am J Med* 63:1015, 1977.

78. Stavem P, Froland SS, Haugen HF, et al.: Nonsecretory myelomatosis without intracellular immunoglobulin: immunofluorescent and ultramicroscopic studies. *Scand J Haematol* 17:89, 1976.

79. Joyner MV, Cassuto JP, Dujardin P, et al.: Non-excretory multiple myeloma. *Br J Haematol* 43:559, 1979.

80. Rubio-Felix D, Giralt M, Giraldo MP, et al.: Nonsecretory multiple myeloma. *Cancer* 59:1847, 1987.

81. Gach J, Simar L, Salmon J: Multiple myeloma without M-type proteinemia: report of a case with immunologic and ultrastructure studies. *Am J Med* 50:835, 1971.

82. Bourantas K: Nonsecretory multiple myeloma. *Eur J Haematol* 56:109, 1996.

83. Ameis A, Ko HS, Pruzanski W: M components: a review of 1242 cases. *Can Med Assoc* 114:889, 1976.

84. Hobbs JR: Immunochemical classes of myelomatosis: including data from a therapeutic trial conducted by a Medical Research Council working party. *Br J Haematol* 16:599, 1969.

85. Bladé J, Kyle RA: IgD monoclonal gammopathy with long-term follow-up. *Br J Haematol* 88:395, 1994.

86. O'Connor ML, Rice DT, Buss DH, et al.: Immunoglobulin D benign monoclonal gammopathy: a case report. *Cancer* 68:611, 1991.

87. Jancelewicz Z, Takatsuki K, Sugai S, et al.: IgD multiple myeloma: review of 133 cases. *Arch Intern Med* 135:87, 1975.

88. Shimamoto Y, Anami Y, Yamaguchi M: A new risk grouping for IgD myeloma based on analysis of 165 Japanese patients. *Eur J Haematol* 47:262, 1991.

89. Sinclasr D: IgD myeloma: clinical, biological and laboratory features. *Clin Lab* 48:617, 2002.

90. Bladé J, Lust JA, Kyle RA: Immunoglobulin D multiple myeloma: presenting features, response to therapy, and survival in a series of 53 cases. *J Clin Oncol* 12:2398, 1994.

91. Fibbe WE, Jansen J: Prognostic factors in IgD myeloma: a study of 21 cases. *Scand J Haematol* 33:471, 1984.

92. Pruzanski W, Rother I: IgD plasma cell neoplasia: clinical manifestations and characteristic features. *Can Med Assoc J* 102:1061, 1970.

93. Chernokhvostova EV, Batalova TN, German GP, et al.: Immunodiagnosis of IgD multiple myeloma: a report of 17 cases. *Folia Haematol Int Mag Klin Morphol Blutforsch* 108:539, 1981.

94. Drayson M, Tang LX, Drew R, et al.: Serum free light-chain measurements for identifying and monitoring patients with nonsecretory multiple myeloma. *Blood* 97:2900, 2001.

95. Fahey JL, Carbone PP, Rowe DS, et al.: Plasma cell myeloma with D-myeloma protein (IgD myeloma). *Am J Med* 45:373, 1968.

96. Kyle RA: IgD multiple myeloma: a cure at 21 years. *Am J Hematol* 29:41, 1988.

# Chapter 85

# ALLOGENEIC STEM CELL TRANSPLANTATION FOR MULTIPLE MYELOMA

*Edwin P. Alyea*

## INTRODUCTION

Multiple myeloma is a clonal neoplasm of terminally differentiated B cells which accounts for about 1% of new cancers.[1] Despite an increased understanding of the biology of the malignant plasma cell, myeloma remains incurable with current chemotherapy. Although multiple myeloma is highly sensitive to chemotherapy, combination chemotherapy regimens have not achieved better outcomes than achieved by melphalan and prednisone therapy.[2] Large comparative studies have demonstrated superior response rates, overall survival, and event-free survival using high-dose therapy and autologous Stem cell transplant (SCT) compared with conventional therapy.[3] Despite the improved outcome after autologous transplantation, long-term disease-free survival remains disappointingly low at 15–20%, with disease relapse being the primary reason for treatment failure.[4] Myeloablative allogeneic stem cell transplantation achieves long-term disease-free survival in 15–20% patients with myeloma. The curative potential of allografting is based upon two principles. First, high-dose myeloablative therapy may eradicate disease, and hematopoiesis is restored using a tumor-free stem cell allograft. Second, donor cells mediate an immunologic antitumor effect that eradicates minimal residual disease (MRD) posttransplant. This immunologic effect has been termed the "graft-versus-leukemia (GvL) effect" or, in multiple myeloma, the graft-versus-myeloma (GvM) effect. For allogeneic SCT to achieve its full potential in the treatment of patients with myeloma, efforts are now being directed toward both reducing the attendant toxicity of allogeneic SCT and enhancing the GvM effect after transplant. Identification of the mediators and targets of the GvM effect may allow for more directed immunotherapy for myeloma in the future.

## STANDARD THERAPY AND AUTOLOGOUS STEM CELL TRANSPLANT IN MULTIPLE MYELOMA

Alkylating agents administered with corticosteroids have been the mainstay of therapy for patients with multiple myeloma over the last three decades. Most commonly, melphalan is combined with prednisone, and patients are treated every 6 weeks. Many attempts have been made to increase the intensity of standard therapy, but combination chemotherapy regimens have not led to an improvement in survival. Specifically, a meta-analysis of 6633 patients treated in comparative trials of melphalan and prednisone versus combination chemotherapy showed these treatments to be equivalent.[5] Currently, the response rate to conventional chemotherapy is 40–60%, with a median survival of 3 years from diagnosis. Unfortunately, this disease remains incurable with conventional chemotherapy.

The demonstration that high-dose melphalan can induce higher remission rates in patients who are otherwise refractory to conventional-dose melphalan has provided the framework for multiple trials of autologous stem cell transplantation in this disease.[3,6–8] A randomized trial of 200 newly diagnosed patients in France demonstrated an improved response rate (81% vs 57%) and 5-year probability of event-free survival (28% vs 10%) for patients undergoing high-dose therapy and autologous SCT, compared with standard-dose chemotherapy.[3] A second randomized trial of 401 previously untreated patients demonstrated both an improved overall survival and progression-free survival for patients receiving intensive therapy, including an autologous transplant, compared with standard therapy.[9] Other randomized studies have not demonstrated an improved overall survival or event-free survival, but have demonstrated a prolonged time to treatment failure and improved quality of life.[10]

Although response rates are high following autologous transplantation, long-term follow up demonstrates that few patients are cured using this approach.

Efforts continue to improve the results of autologous transplantation for patients with myeloma. A recent randomized trial demonstrated that sequential autologous transplantation resulted in a superior overall survival compared with a single autologous transplantation.[11] While results of autologous transplant in myeloma appear encouraging, relapse of disease is the principal reason for the failure of this approach. Reinfusion of tumor cells at the time of transplant may contribute to disease relapse in some patients, as has been demonstrated in other types of autologous transplantation.[12] In an effort to reduce relapse rates, attention has focused on allogeneic transplant as a method to provide a tumor-free stem cell source for patients. In addition, the recognition of the existence of a potent GvM effect has renewed interest in allogeneic transplantation for myeloma.

## MONITORING OF PATIENTS AFTER TRANSPLANTATION

Criteria for defining a complete response (CR) in patients with myeloma undergoing transplantation have evolved over time and may account in some cases for the differing CR rates observed in clinical trials. Early trials from the European Stem cell Transplant Registry (EBMTR) defined CR as the disappearance of immunoglobulin in serum and light chains in the urine using conventional electrophoresis or immunofixation, as well as the absence of myeloma cells in the marrow.[13,14] Using a more strict definition, investigators at Dana-Farber Cancer Institute (DFCI) and Fred Hutchinson Cancer Research Center (FHCRC) have required the absence of detectable monoclonal protein by immunofixation to define a CR. In an effort to establish uniform criteria for response, transplant registries have proposed criteria based upon immunofixation for defining CR, PR, relapse, and progressive disease in patients with multiple myeloma treated with high-dose therapy.[15]

Polymerase chain reaction (PCR) based techniques have also been used to evaluate MRD in patients with myeloma after high-dose therapy. PCR for MRD in multiple myeloma involves the amplification of the $V_H$ family of primers to identify the patient-specific immunoglobulin complementarity-determining region (CDRIII) sequences. Patient-specific primers can then be used to follow patients over time. Using the $V_H$ family primers alone, one myeloma cell in $10^3$–$10^4$ normal cells can be detected. Increased sensitivity can be obtained using patient specific primers, to the degree that one myeloma cell in a background of $10^5$–$10^6$ normal cells can be identified. Investigators are now using PCR to assess patients after transplantation and have reported in one study that molecular CR, defined as PCR negativity, occurs more frequently after allografting (7 of 14 patients) than after autografting (2 of 15 patients).[16] Quantitative PCR using "Real-Time" technology can now also be used to follow patients with myeloma and provide a better estimate of the burden of disease.[17]

## CLINICAL TRIAL RESULTS OF MYELOABLATIVE ALLOGENEIC TRANSPLANTATION

Results from several large trials of myeloablative allogeneic SCT in patients with myeloma are available both from cooperative groups and several single institutions (Table 85.1). The EBMTR has reported the results of 162 patients receiving allogeneic Stem cell transplant for multiple myeloma at over 40 centers in Europe and South Africa.[13,18,23] The median age was 43 years, and 52% of the patients had evidence of chemotherapy-sensitive disease at the time of transplant. Although the ablative regimens differed between centers, the majority (72%) of patients received high-dose chemotherapy, most commonly cyclophosphamide and melphalan, combined with total body irradiation (TBI). Graft-versus-host disease (GvHD) prophylaxis also varied by center. Cyclosporine was combined either with methotrexate (48%) or with other agents (20%). T-cell depletion, either alone or in combination with other agents, was used in 33% of patients. The overall treatment-related mortality (TRM) was 25%, with most patients succumbing to complications of infection, interstitial pneumonitis, or GvHD. The overall CR rate was 44%, and the overall actuarial survival rates at 4 years and 9 years after were 32 and 18%, respectively. Relapse-free survival was 34% at 6 years for those patients who attained a CR after transplant.

Similar results have been reported from several large single institutions. In the FHCRC experience, 80 patients underwent myeloablative allogeneic

**Table 85.1  Results of allogeneic transplantation in multiple myeloma**

| | N | Treatment-Related mortality (%) | Complete remission rate following stem cell transplant (%) | References |
|---|---|---|---|---|
| EBMTR | 162 | 25 | 44 | 13,18 |
| Royal Marsden | 33 | 54 | 36 | 19 |
| Seattle | 80 | 56 | 36 | 20 |
| Dana-Farber | 61 | 10 | 23 | 21 |
| Vancouver | 19 | 16 | 58 | 22 |

transplantation for multiple myeloma.[20] Sixty patients received marrow from HLA-identical sibling donors, and 20 patients from mismatched or unrelated donors. The majority of patients had chemotherapy-refractory disease. Ablative therapy consisted of busulfan and cyclophosphamide in 57 patients, and cyclophosphamide and TBI in 23 patients. The majority of patients (56%) received cyclosporine with methotrexate as GvHD prophylaxis and the remaining received cyclosporine and prednisone (37%). The TRM was 56%, with infection, veno-occlusive disease, and complications of GvHD being the most common causes of treatment failure. Despite the increased TRM, the CR rate was 36% in this highly refractory group of patients. Overall and progression-free survival was 20 and 16%, respectively, at 5 years after transplant.

Sixty-one patients with multiple myeloma have undergone allogeneic SCT at DFCI.[21,24] The majority of patients had advanced Durie–Salmon stage II–III disease at diagnosis, and all patients had chemotherapy-sensitive disease at the time of transplant. The ablative regimen included cyclophosphamide and TBI in 80% of patients, and busulfan and cyclophosphamide in the remaining 20% of patients in whom prior radiation therapy precluded the use of TBI. All patients received marrow allografts from HLA-matched sibling donors which were T-cell depleted using anti-CD6 monoclonal antibody and complement lysis as the only form of GvHD prophylaxis. The overall TRM was low (10%), primarily due to the fact that only 17% of patients developed grade II or greater GvHD. The CR rate was 22%, and 60% of patients achieved PR. The median and progression-free survival was 22 months and 12 months, respectively.

Recently, Martinelli et al. reported the results of 68 patients receiving allogeneic transplantation. The majority (56) received bone marrow, while the remaining 16 patients received peripheral blood stem cells (PBSCs). Conditioning regimens included cyclophosphamide and TBI in 48 patients, and busulfan and cyclophosphamide in 20 patients. GvHD prophylaxis consisted of cyclosporine with or without methotrexate in 31 patients and T-cell depletion in 37 patients. Thirty-eight patients achieved a CR at a median of 36 months.[25] Twelve patients achieving a CR were evaluated by PCR and 9 (75%) were PCR negative. Only 1 of 4 patients who were PCR positive relapsed during the follow-up period.[26]

Overall, the results of allogeneic SCT in patients with multiple myeloma demonstrate CR rates ranging from 22 to 50%. In many trials the treatment-related toxicity was high (25–56%), primarily related to complications of GvHD, infection, and disease relapse. To improve outcome, efforts have focused on methods to reduce both complications of GvHD and disease relapse.

## TREATMENT-RELATED TOXICITY AND GvHD FOLLOWING MYELOABLATIVE ALLOGENEIC TRANSPLANTATION

While allogeneic transplantation following myeloablative therapy is associated with potent antitumor activity in patients with myeloma, most clinical trials have reported significant TRM, limiting the effectiveness of this approach. Acute and chronic GvHD contribute to the high TRM. The incidence of grade II–IV acute GvHD in patients receiving cyclosporine and methotrexate ranges as high as 78% in some studies, with an incidence of grade III–IV GvHD of 14–19%. In the EBMTR registry, patients with grades III and IV GvHD had an extremely poor survival.[14,23]

Using selective T-cell depletion with anti-CD6 monoclonal antibody and complement lysis, investigators at DFCI have reduced the incidence of significant GvHD after transplant in patients with multiple myeloma. When T-cell depletion is used as the only means of GvHD prophylaxis, the incidence of severe grade III or IV acute GvHD is less than 7%, with no deaths attributable to GvHD.[21] No evidence of GvHD was identified in 47% of patients, while 36% and 12% patients had grades I and II GvHD, respectively. Chronic GvHD was noted in only 20% of patients. Using an in vivo T-cell depletion approach, Kroger et al. reported a similar low incidence of severe GvHD and an overall 6-year progression-free survival of 31%.[27] Unfortunately, this reduction in toxicity related to GvHD has not been associated with an increased overall survival rate. As an example, a recent study using a partial T-cell depletion approach after myeloablative transplantation was associated with a low complete response rate (6%) after transplanation.[28] The EBMTR has reported that patients receiving T-cell depletion had a similar survival in comparison to patients receiving other methods of GvHD prophylaxis.[14,23]

## MYELOABLATIVE CONDITIONING REGIMENS

A variety of conditioning regimens have been explored using allogeneic transplantation for multiple myeloma. Cyclophosphamide, in combination with TBI or busulfan, has been used most commonly. No particular regimen has been identified to be superior in terms of CR rates, toxicity, or long-term outcome. As an example, EBMTR studies using a variety of conditioning regimens did not demonstrate any difference in response rates between regimens with or without TBI.[13,14] Data from FHCRC support this finding: modified TBI added to busulfan and cyclophosphamide did not result in improvement of either relapse or survival of patients transplanted in the setting of advanced disease.[20]

Melphalan has also been included in the conditioning regimen for allogeneic transplantation. A small study of 14 patients treated with melphalan in addition to busulfan and cyclophosphamide demonstrated a low TRM.[22] In another study, 10 of 13 patients receiving melphalan 110–120 mg/m$^2$ in combination with TBI achieved a CR, and 9 patients remained disease free at 7–70 months after transplantation.[29] The overall disease-free survival with short follow-up in this study approached 70%.

## PROGNOSTIC FACTORS AND OUTCOME AFTER MYELOABLATIVE ALLOGENEIC TRANSPLANTATION

Prognostic factors influencing outcome have been analyzed in patients with multiple myeloma receiving allogeneic SCT. The EBMTR analysis demonstrated improved survival associated with female gender (41% at 4 years), stage I disease at diagnosis (52% at 4 years), treatment with one regimen prior to ablative therapy (42% at 4 years), and achieving CR prior to SCT (64% at 3 years).[13,14,23] IgA subtype and a low serum $\beta_2$-microglobulin also conferred a favorable prognosis. Ability to achieve a CR following transplantation was the most favorable prognostic factor associated with prolonged survival.

In 80 patients receiving transplantation at FHCRC, time from diagnosis to transplant was found to be a significant prognostic factor.[20] Patients undergoing transplant more than 1–3 years after diagnosis had a 2.5 times greater 100-day mortality, compared with patients transplanted in the first year after diagnosis. Patients receiving transplantation beyond the first year after diagnosis or those with Durie–Salmon stage III disease had a 1.8 and 2.0 times greater risk of dying from any cause, respectively. Adverse factors predicting relapse or disease progression included female patients receiving marrow grafts from male donors, as well as extensive chemotherapy (greater than eight cycles) prior to transplant. Only Durie–Salmon stage at the time of transplant influenced relapse or progression-free survival, with stage III patients at increased risk, compared with stage I or stage II patients.

Analyzing the outcome of 62 patients undergoing allogeneic transplantation at DFCI, advanced disease was the factor associated with inferior progression-free survival and overall survival. Other factors, such as age less than 40, donor/patient sex, Ig isotype, or time from diagnosis to transplant, were not found to be significant.[24]

These analyses demonstrate that advanced-stage disease is associated with inferior outcomes after transplant. Data from FHCRC suggest that transplant is more successful if performed early after diagnosis and prior to extensive therapy. Unfortunately, the TRM associated with myeloablative allogeneic transplantation at present is high in patients with myeloma, and use of this modality in patients earlier in their disease course must, therefore, be considered carefully.

## SYNGENEIC TRANSPLANTATION

The FHCRC and the EBMTR have reported long-term follow-up of patients receiving syngeneic transplants. Five of the nine evaluable patients treated at the FHCRC achieved a CR after transplant, three a PR, and one patient had no response. Of the five patients who achieved a CR, three relapsed and one died of myelodysplastic syndromes; one patient remains in remission with a small monoclonal spike at 15 years after transplant. Two patients died of treatment-related complications early after transplant.[30]

The EBMTR has reported on 24 patients who received syngeneic transplant.[31] Sixty-eight percent entered a CR. Three of 17 patients relapsed, and 2 died of transplant-related complications. The overall survival and progression-free survival are 73 months and 72 months, respectively. These data were compared with EBMTR results for autologous and allogeneic transplants. The relapse rate was lower after syngeneic than autologous transplant, but similar to that observed after allogeneic transplant. These results suggest that the higher relapse rate seen after autologous transplant compared to syngeneic transplant is related either to reinfusion of malignant cells in the autograft or to the presence of a GvM effect in the setting of syngeneic transplantation.

## MYELOABLATIVE PERIPHERAL BLOOD STEM CELL TRANSPLANTATION

Use of allogeneic PBSCs has increased over the last several years. PBSC transplantation results in more rapid engraftment and requires shorter hospital stays than does SCT.[32] Relatively few myeloablative allogeneic PBSC transplants have been performed to date in patients with multiple myeloma. In one small study, 10 patients received granulocyte colony-stimulating factor mobilized PBSCs (median of $9.7 \times 10^8$ mononuclear cells/kg and $14.3 \times 10^6$ CD34$^+$ cells/kg) from HLA-identical siblings.[33] Engraftment was rapid, with a median time to both neutrophil and platelet engraftment of only 13 days. Four patients developed grade II or greater GvHD; two patients died, one of multiorgan toxicity. While follow-up is limited, the CR rate was 71%.

## COMPARISON OF MYELOABLATIVE ALLOGENEIC AND AUTOLOGOUS STEM CELL TRANSPLANTATION

The results of myeloablative allogeneic and autologous transplant for patients with multiple myeloma have

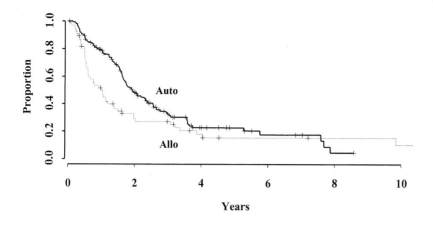

**Figure 85.1** *Progression-free survival: comparison of patients receiving either autologous or myeloablative allogeneic transplantation for multiple myeloma*

been compared.[23,24,34–36] The EBMTR performed a retrospective case-matched analysis comparing 189 patients treated with allogeneic transplantation with an equal number of patients undergoing autologous transplant.[23] The groups were comparable, except that the median age of patients receiving autologous transplants was 49 years, significantly greater than the median age of 43 years in patients undergoing allogeneic transplant. The CR rate was similar for both groups; however, the TRM was significantly higher for allogeneic transplant recipients (41% vs 13%). This difference in TRM resulted in a significantly improved median survival for patients treated with autologous transplant (34 months) versus allogeneic transplant (18 months). After 4 years of follow-up, the survival curves for the allogeneic and autologous patient cohorts come together, and thereafter the long-term survival rates in both groups were comparable.

Sixty-two patients receiving a myeloablative allogeneic transplantation were compared with 162 patients receiving autologous transplantation at DFCI.[24] The groups were comparable, with the exception that patients receiving autologous transplantation had a higher median age, 50 years versus 45 years; received

transplantation earlier after diagnosis; and had received fewer regimens prior to transplantation. Patients receiving autologous transplantation had a superior overall and progression-free survival at 2 years after transplantation, 74 and 48% respectively, compared with patients receiving allogeneic transplantation, 58 and 28%, respectively. By 4 years after transplantation, overall survival and progression-free survival were similar—41 and 23% for autologous recipients and 39 and 18% for allogeneic transplant recipients, respectively (Figure 85.1). The 4-year cumulative TRM was significantly higher for the allogeneic transplant patients, 24% versus 13% for autologous transplant patients. Relapse of disease was the most common cause of treatment failure for both transplant procedures, but was higher for patients receiving autologous transplantation, 56%, compared with 46% for those receiving allogeneic transplantation (Figure 85.2). Therefore, despite the lower incidence of relapse following allogeneic transplantation, the high TRM following allogeneic transplantation results in an inferior overall survival when compared with autologous transplantation. The lower relapse rate is in part related to the potent GvM effect mediated by the allogeneic immune system. Efforts are

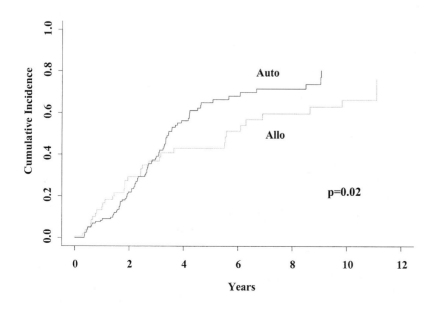

**Figure 85.2** *Comparison of risk of relapse after myeloablative allogeneic transplantation and autologous transplantation*

currently focused on reducing the treatment-related toxicity of transplantation using nonmyeloablative conditioning regimens while preserving the GvM effect.

## GRAFT-VERSUS-MYELOMA EFFECT AND DONOR LYMPHOCYTE INFUSION

Similar to chronic myelogenous leukemia, there are several lines of indirect evidence supporting the existence of an alloimmune antimyeloma response, or GvM effect. This evidence includes the observation that molecular remissions are more common after allogeneic transplantation than after autologous transplantation in patients with myeloma.[16] In addition, the relapse rates are lower after allogeneic transplant compared with autologous transplantation. Some patients with persistent evidence of disease after allogeneic transplantation gradually achieve complete remission without further therapy. Finally, it has been shown that vaccination of the allogeneic donor against the patient's idiotypic protein can facilitate transfer of donor immunity to myeloma at the time of transplantation.[37]

Studies of donor lymphocyte infusion (DLI) provide direct evidence of the existence of a GvM effect[38–41] (Table 85.2). The overall response rate to DLI in patients with myeloma approaches 45%, with complete responses noted in about 25% of patients. Durable complete responses are noted in half of the patients who obtain a complete remission, with follow-up over 7 years in some patients. Interestingly, extramedullary recurrence has been noted in some patients.[45]

DLI in patients with myeloma is associated with a high incidence of GvHD. In one study of 13 patients treated with DLI, 66% developed evidence of acute GvHD and 56% chronic GvHD.[38] Quantitative PCR has been used to follow patients after DLI and demonstrates the close correlation between the onset of GvHD and GvM.[46] Strategies explored to reduce GvHD following DLI include the infusion of lower numbers of donor cells, infusion of selective donor cell populations such as CD4$^+$ cells,[40,47] or use of T cells transduced with thymidine kinase, which allows for systemic treatment of the recipient with ganciclovir in the event that severe GvHD develops.[48–50] Lokhorst and colleagues reported responses in some patients with doses as low as $1 \times 10^7$ CD3$^+$ cells/kg.[51]

There is a strong association between GvHD and a GvM effect, and whether GvHD and GvM are distinct remains unclear. A review of DLI studies in patients with multiple myeloma reported that 18 of 22 patients who developed GvHD responded to the infusion, while only 2 of 7 patients who did not develop GvHD responded.[41] A second study of 54 patients demonstrated an overall response rate of 52%, with 73% of patients who developed evidence of chronic GvHD responding to DLI.[52] Responses to DLI have occurred in the absence of clinical GvHD, and several patients remain in durable remission without evidence of GvHD, suggesting that GvM may indeed be separable from GvHD in some patients. In an attempt to prevent relapse and to induce a GvM effect in the minimal disease setting, prophylactic DLI after myeloablative transplantation has been explored.

## INDUCTION OF GvM AFTER MYELOABLATIVE TRANSPLANT

Improvement in outcome of myeloablative allogeneic transplantation requires reducing TRM and maximizing the GvM effect. One strategy involves combining a myeloablative T-cell-depleted transplantation with DLI in hopes of reducing the TRM associated with the transplant procedure while augmenting the GvM effect. Twenty-four patients at DFCI were enrolled in a trial combining a T-cell-depleted myeloablative transplant with prophylactic DLI, 6 months after transplantation.[53] Twenty-one patients received cyclophosphamide and TBI ablative therapy; busulfan and cylophosphamide were used in those three patients in whom prior radiation precluded TBI. The bone marrow was purged of T cells with anti-CD6 monoclonal antibody as the sole means of GvHD prophylaxis. Despite the use of T-cell depletion, just over half of the 24 patients were eligible to receive DLI. Reasons for not receiving DLI included rapid relapse, transplant-related complications such as interstitial pneumonitis, and GvHD. Nine of the 11 patients who were eligible to receive DLI at 6 months demonstrated a response,

| Table 85.2 | Results of Patients with Multiple Myeloma treated with DLI | | | | |
|---|---|---|---|---|---|
| Studies | N | Prior chemotherapy | CR (%) | PR (%) | Overall RR (%) |
| Salama et al.[42] | 25 | 3 | 7 (33) | 2 (8) | 9 (36) |
| Lokhorst et al.[38] | 27 | 13 | 6 (22) | 8 (29) | 14 (52) |
| DFCI[40,53] | 21 | 0 | 9 (43) | 6 (29) | 15/21 (71) |
| Huff et al.[43] | 16 | 0 | 6 (38) | 2 (13) | 8/15 (50) |
| Peggs et al.[44] | 19 | 0 | 1 (5) | 8 (42) | 9/19 (47) |

**Table 85.3** Results of nonmyeloablative allogeneic transplantation in multiple myeloma

| References | N | Donor | Prior auto | Conditioning regimen for NST | Treatment-related mortality | Event-free survival |
|---|---|---|---|---|---|---|
| Arkansas[54] | 31 | MRD 25 URD 6 | | Melphalan based | 10% at 100 days | 1 year 55% 2 year 31% |
| MD Anderson[55] | 22 | MRD 13 URD 9 | | Fludarabine Melphalan | 19% at 100 days 40% at 1 year | 2 year 19% |
| Hamburg[56] | 21 | URD 21 | | Fludarbine Melphalan ATG | 10% at 100 days 26% at 1 year | 2 year 53% |
| Hamburg[57] | 17 | MRD 7 MMRD 2 URD 8 | Yes | Fludarbine Melphalan ATG | 11% at 100 days | 1 year 71% |
| Seattle[58] | 54 | MRD 54 | Yes | TBI | 0% at 100 days | 2 year 55% |

MRD, matched related donor; MMRD, mismatched related donor; URD: unrelated donor; TBI, total body irridiation; ATG, antithymocyte globulin

with 6 complete responses and 3 partial responses. Six patients developed acute GvHD after DLI, and four patients progressed to chronic GvHD. This approach demonstrates that a significant GvM effect can be induced by the administration of DLI after transplant; however, its effect on overall outcome will require further follow-up. Ultimately, identifying the T cells mediating GvM and their target antigens will allow DLI with antigen-specific T cells to both enhance efficacy and avoid toxicity.

## NONMYELOABLATIVE STEM CELL TRANSPLANTATION FOR MYELOMA

Nonmyeloablative stem cell transplantation (NST) has been explored as an alternative to myeloablative transplantation for patients with myeloma. A variety of conditioning regimens and GvHD prophylactic regimens have been employed[54–58] (Table 85.3). Several of these studies have combined an autologous transplant procedure with a nonmyeloablative transplantation in order to achieve better disease control and greater host immune suppression prior to proceeding to nonmyeloablative transplantation. Overall, these studies report TRM at 100 days ranging from 0 to 19% and event-free survival rates at 2 years ranging from 19 to 55%. While initial results are encouraging, data are not yet available on the durability of these responses. Early attempts to reduce GvHD complications after nonmyeloablative transplantation using a T-cell depletion followed by DLI approach have not been encouraging.[59]

Prognostic features associated with an improved outcome after nonmyeloablative transplantation include chemotherapy-sensitive disease, good performance status, complete remission after transplantation, and evidence of chronic GvHD.[60] Patients with deletions of 13q were at increased risk of relapse after NST, compared with patients without this abnormality.[61] These results demonstrate that induction of the GvM effect may lead to significant remissions in patients with myeloma. Identifying the targets of the GvM reaction may help make this therapy more efficacious and specific.

## TARGETS OF GvM EFFECT

Several potential targets of the GvM effect have been proposed (Table 85.4). Previous studies have focused on targeting the immunoglobulin idiotype (Id) as a tumor antigen in myeloma, an approach that has also been used in B-cell non-Hodgkin's lymphoma.[66,67] Investigators have generated specific anti-Id T-cell responses in patients with myeloma after high-dose chemotherapy or autologous transplantation. Demonstrating that this approach can be adoptively transferred, immunization of the donor against the patient's Id protein has resulted in the development of Id-specific T-cell responses in recipients after allogeneic transplantation.[37] Studies are attempting to use this strategy in nonmyeloablative transplantation as well.

**Table 85.4** Potential target antigens of the graft-versus-myeloma effect

| Potential targets | References |
|---|---|
| **Targets identified by T cells** | |
| Idiotype | 37 |
| MUC-1 | 62 |
| MAGE family | 63 |
| hTERT | 64 |
| **Targets identified by SEREX** | |
| BCMA | 65 |
| ROCK-1 | |
| KIAA0053 | |
| HOMER 3B | |

Other candidates targeted by T cells include MUC-1 and members of the MAGE family of genes. MUC-1 is an immunogenic epithelial mucin present in several solid tumors and has also been identified on malignant plasma cells.[62,68] MUC-1-specific cytotoxic T-cell lymphocytes have been isolated in the bone marrow of patients with myeloma.[62,69] Vaccination trials in myeloma are underway, targeting the MUC-1 antigen.[70,71] Genes of the MAGE family are expressed in myeloma and anti-MAGE CTL clones are identified and were able to kill myeloma cell lines in vitro.[63]

Distinct populations of T cells may mediate GvHD and GvM. Specifically, clonal populations of T cells emerged in three of four patients after CD4[+] DLI.[72] The clones that were detected early after DLI correlated with GvM effect, while those clones appearing later were associated with the onset of GvHD. Interestingly, clones associated with GvM were often detectable prior to DLI and expanded up to 10-fold after DLI. In contrast, clones associated with GvHD were undetectable prior to DLI. These findings suggest that DLI may mediate GvM via an indirect effect on preexisting T-cell populations, while GvHD post-DLI is mediated by new T-cell populations that develop after DLI.

While much attention has focused on T cells, evidence is emerging that B cells and humoral immunity may also play an important role in the GvM effect. Animal studies have emphasized the importance of interactions between humoral responses and T-cell responses, both CD4[+] and CD8[+].[73,74] Using SEREX, a technique in which the patient's serum is used to screen recombinant cDNA expression libraries, a large number of serologically defined tumor-associated antigens have been identified.[75–78] Ten gene products have been identified in myeloma patients responding to CD4[+] DLI using this tool.[65] Two of the genes identified were also weakly recognized in a patient with chronic GvHD, perhaps suggesting a link between GvM and chronic GvHD. Two antigens identified, BCMA and ROCK-1, are highly expressed in primary myeloma cells as well as in myeloma cell lines, and further characterization of these myeloma antigens is being pursued to determine if they may serve as rational therapeutic targets.

## FUTURE DIRECTIONS

### ADOPTIVE IMMUNOTHERAPY

Data demonstrate that DLI mediates a significant GvM effect, and this offers the potential to effectively and selectively treat MRD after transplantation.[38,40] Defining the role and timing of DLI after nonmyeloablative transplantation is currently underway. Efforts to identify the mediators of GvM and their target antigens are in progress, and hopefully it will be possible to expand antigen-specific DLI ex vivo to treat patients while at the same time reducing the complications related to GvHD.

Strategies are also available for increasing the antigen-presenting capacity of myeloma cells and their ability to stimulate donor T cells targeting myeloma. CD40 activation of myeloma cells upregulates Class I and Class II HLA and costimulatory molecules,[79] and CD40-activated myeloma cells trigger a brisk allogeneic, as well as autologous, T-cell response.[80,81] In preclinical studies, histocompatible donor cells can be expanded ex vivo using CD40-activated patient myeloma cells as stimuli.

Another strategy for ex vivo expansion of T cells for adoptive immunotherapy is directed toward a novel, widely expressed tumor antigen derived from the telomerase catalytic subunit (hTERT).[64] hTERT is a ribonucleoprotein expressed in high levels in more than 85% of human cancers, including multiple myeloma, but is expressed in few normal tissues. In preliminary studies using donor cells, this expansion strategy has been used to generate MHC Class I restricted CTL that are specific for an hTERT peptide and kill hTERT-bearing myeloma cells. These studies will establish the conditions for testing the efficacy and safety of allogeneic, as well as autologous, hTERT CTL immunotherapy, and may provide the framework for a subsequent clinical treatment protocol in myeloma.

### VACCINATION

Vaccination is another promising area for inducing antimyeloma immunity. T-cell recognition of myeloma is suggested by the restricted usage of Vα and Vβ segments in the peripheral blood[82]; the presence of activated Id-reactive CD8[+] cells[83] as well as CD4[+] cells[84]; the growth of T-cell clones by stimulation with IL-2 and F(ab')2 fragments derived from autologous Id[85]; as well as the production of cytokines such as interferon γ(IFN-γ), interleukin 2 (IL-2), and IL-4 after stimulation with autologous Id.[86,87] The Id-reactive population includes T cells that are not MHC restricted and that recognize conformational epitopes on Ig, as well as CD4[+] and CD8[+] cells, which recognize Id-derived peptides in association with MHC Class I and Class II molecules.[88] The Id-reactive T-cell expansion has been correlated with tumor load,[83,87] and a shift from type I to type II T-cell response has been correlated with disease progression.[85] It has been shown that vaccination with Id[67,89] or the use of Id-pulsed dendritic cells[90] can trigger Id-specific humoral and T-cell response in some patients with myeloma, even after high-dose therapy and autologous transplantation.

As discussed previously, it is possible to vaccinate the donor against the patient's idiotypic protein prior to transplant and transfer specific donor immunity at the time of allografting.[37,91] This strategy is under active investigation, coupling donor immunization pretransplant with patient vaccination following transplantation to boost antitumor immunity. Activated tumor cells, such as CD40-activated myeloma cells, or possibly tumor-associated antigens, such as MUC-1, or BMCA, may be used to vaccinate donors prior to transplantation.

## CONCLUSIONS

Allogeneic transplantation in patients with multiple myeloma can achieve high response rates, and long-term remission in some patients. Unfortunately, the toxicity associated with myeloablative transplantation has limited the success of this approach. The recogni-tion of the existence of the GvM myeloma effect has renewed interest in allogeneic transplantation in patients with myeloma, now using a nonmyeloablative approach in hopes of reducing toxicity related to the transplant procedure. DLI remains an effective method for inducing a GvM effect, and the role of DLI after non-myeloablative transplant is being defined. Efforts to identify the targets, mechanism of action of the GvM effect, as well as methods to enhance the GvM effect are underway. Identification of targets and an understand-ing of the mechanism of action may lead to more spe-cific allogeneic immune therapies in the future.

## REFERENCES

1. Landis S, Murray T, Bolden S, Wingo P: Cancer statistics. *CA Cancer J Clin* 49:8–31, 1999.
2. Gregory WM, Richards MA, Malpas JS: Combination chemotherapy versus melphalan and prednisolone in the treatment of multiple myeloma: an overview of published trials [see comments]. *J Clin Oncol* 10:334–342, 1992.
3. Attal M, Harousseau JL, Stoppa AM, et al.: A prospective, randomized trial of autologous Stem cell transplantation and chemotherapy in multiple myeloma. Intergroupe Francais du Myelome [see comments]. *N Engl J Med* 335:91–97, 1996.
4. Desikan R, Barlogie B, Sawyer J, et al.: Results of high-dose therapy for 1000 patients with multiple myeloma: durable complete remissions and superior survival in the absence of chromosome 13 abnormalities. *Blood* 95:4008–4010, 2000.
5. Combination chemotherapy versus melphalan plus prednisone as treatment for multiple myeloma: an overview of 6,633 patients from 27 randomized trials. Myeloma Trialists' Collaborative Group. *J Clin Oncol* 16:3832–3842, 1998.
6. Anderson K: Who benefits from high-dose therapy for mulitple myeloma? *J Clin Oncol* 13:1291–1296, 1995.
7. Barlogie B, Jagannath S, Desikan KR, et al.: Total therapy with tandem transplants for newly diagnosed multiple myeloma. *Blood* 93:55–65, 1999.
8. Schlossman RL, Anderson KC: Stem cell transplantation in multiple myeloma. *Curr Opin Oncol* 11:102–108, 1999.
9. Child JA, Morgan GJ, Davies FE, et al.: High-dose chemotherapy with hematopoietic stem-cell rescue for multiple myeloma. *N Engl J Med* 348:1875–1883, 2003.
10. Segeren CM, Sonneveld P, van der Holt B, et al.: Overall and event-free survival are not improved by the use of myeloablative therapy following intensified chemother-apy in previously untreated patients with multiple myeloma: a prospective randomized phase 3 study. *Blood* 101:2144–2151, 2003.
11. Attal M, Harousseau JL, Facon T, et al.: Single versus double autologous stem-cell transplantation for multiple myeloma. *N Engl J Med* 349:2495–2502, 2003.
12. Rill DR, Santana VM, Roberts WM, et al.: Direct demon-stration that autologous stem cell transplantation for solid tumors can return a multiplicity of tumorigenic cells. *Blood* 84:380–383, 1994.

13. Gahrton G, Tura S, Ljungman P, et al.: Allogeneic Stem cell transplantation in multiple myeloma. *N Engl J Med* 325:1267–1273, 1991.
14. Gahrton G, Tura S, Ljungman P, et al.: Prognostic factors in allogeneic Stem cell transplantation for multiple myeloma [see comments]. *J Clin Oncol* 13:1312–1322, 1995.
15. Blade J, Samson D, Reece D, et al.: Criteria for evaluating disease response and progression in patients with multi-ple myeloma treated by high-dose therapy and haemopoietic stem cell transplantation. Myeloma Subcommittee of the EBMT. European Group for Blood and Marrow Transplant. *Br J Haematol* 102:1115–1123, 1998.
16. Corradini P, Voena C, Tarella C, et al.: Molecular and clinical remissions in multiple myeloma: role of autolo-gous and allogeneic transplantation of hematopoietic cells. *J Clin Oncol* 17:208–215, 1999.
17. Ladetto M, Donovan JW, Harig S, et al.: Real-time poly-merase chain reaction of immunoglobulin rearrange-ments for quantitative evaluation of minimal residual disease in multiple myeloma. *Biol Blood Marrow Transplant* 6:241–253, 2000.
18. Gahrton G, Tura S, Flesch M, et al.: Stem cell transplan-tation in multiple myeloma: report from the European Cooperative Group for Stem cell Transplantation. *Blood* 69:1262, 1987.
19. Kulkarni S, Powles RL, Treleaven JG, et al.: Impact of previous high-dose therapy on outcome after allograft-ing for multiple myeloma. *Stem cell Transplant* 23:675–680, 1999.
20. Bensinger WI, Buckner CD, Anasetti C, et al.: Allogeneic marrow transplantation for multiple myeloma: an analysis of risk factors on outcome. *Blood* 88:2787–2793, 1996.
21. Schlossman R, Alyea E, Orsini E, Anderson K: Immune based strategies to improve hematopoietic stem cell transplantation in mulitple myeloma. In: Dicke K, Keating A, eds. *Autologous Marrow and Blood Transplantation.* Charlottesville, VA: Carden, Jennings Publishing; 1999:207–221.
22. Reece DE, Shepherd JD, Klingemann HG, et al.: Treatment of myeloma using intensive therapy and allo-geneic Stem cell transplantation. *Stem cell Transplant* 15:117–123, 1995.

23. Bjorkstrand B, Ljungman P, Svensson H, et al.: Allogeneic Stem cell transplantation versus autologous stem cell transplantation in multiple myeloma: a retrospective case-matched study from the European Group for Blood and Marrow Transplantation. *Blood* 88:4711–4718, 1996.

24. Alyea E, Weller E, Schlossman R, et al.: Outcome after autologous and allogeneic stem cell transplantation for patients with multiple myeloma: impact of graft-versus-myeloma effect. *Stem cell Transplant* 32:1145–1151, 2003.

25. Martinelli G, Terragna C, Zamagni E, et al.: Molecular remission after allogeneic or autologous transplantation of hematopoietic stem cells for multiple myeloma. *J Clin Oncol* 18:2273–2281, 2000.

26. Cavo M, Terragna C, Martinelli G, et al.: Molecular monitoring of minimal residual disease in patients in long-term complete remission after allogeneic stem cell transplantation for multiple myeloma. *Blood* 96:355–357, 2000.

27. Kroger N, Einsele H, Wolff D, et al.: Myeloablative intensified conditioning regimen with in vivo T-cell depletion (ATG) followed by allografting in patients with advanced multiple myeloma. A phase I/II study of the German Study Group Multiple Myeloma (DSMM). *Stem cell Transplant* 31:973–979, 2003.

28. Lokhorst HM, Segeren CM, Verdonck LF, et al.: Partially T-cell-depleted allogeneic stem-cell transplantation for first-line treatment of multiple myeloma: a prospective evaluation of patients treated in the phase III study HOVON 24 MM. *J Clin Oncol* 21:1728–1733, 2003.

29. Russell NH, Miflin G, Stainer C, et al.: Allogeneic Stem cell transplant for multiple myeloma [letter]. *Blood* 89:2610–2611, 1997.

30. Bensinger WI, Demirer T, Buckner CD, et al.: Syngeneic marrow transplantation in patients with multiple myeloma. *Stem cell Transplant* 18:527–531, 1996.

31. Gahrton G, Svensson H, Bjorkstrand B, et al.: Syngeneic transplantation in multiple myeloma—a case-matched comparison with autologous and allogeneic transplantation. European Group for Blood and Marrow Transplantation. *Stem cell Transplant* 24:741–745, 1999.

32. Bensinger WI, Weaver CH, Appelbaum FR, et al.: Transplantation of allogeneic peripheral blood stem cells mobilized by recombinant granulocyte colony-stimulating factor. *Blood* 85:1655–1658, 1995.

33. Majolino I, Corradini P, Scime R, et al.: Allogeneic transplantation of unmanipulated peripheral blood stem cells in patients with multiple myeloma. *Stem cell Transplant* 22:449–455, 1998.

34. Mehta J, Tricot G, Jagannath S, et al.: Salvage autologous or allogeneic transplantation for multiple myeloma refractory to or relapsing after a first-line autograft? *Stem cell Transplant* 21:887–892, 1998.

35. Couban S, Stewart AK, Loach D, Panzarella T, Meharchand J: Autologous and allogeneic transplantation for multiple myeloma at a single centre. *Stem cell Transplant* 19:783–789, 1997.

36. Reynolds C, Ratanatharathorn V, Adams P, et al.: Allogeneic stem cell transplantation reduces disease progression compared to autologous transplantation in patients with multiple myeloma. *Stem cell Transplant* 27:801–807, 2001.

37. Kwak LW, Taub DD, Duffey PL, et al.: Transfer of myeloma idiotype-specific immunity from an actively immunised marrow donor. *Lancet* 345:1016–1020, 1995.

38. Lokhorst HM, Schattenberg A, Cornelissen JJ, Thomas LL, Verdonck LF: Donor leukocyte infusions are effective in relapsed multiple myeloma after allogeneic Stem cell transplantation. *Blood* 90:4206–4211, 1997.

39. Tricot G, Vesole DH, Jagannath S, Hilton J, Munshi N, Barlogie B: Graft-versus-myeloma effect: proof of principle. *Blood* 87:1196–1198, 1996.

40. Alyea EP, Soiffer RJ, Canning C, et al.: Toxicity and efficacy of defined doses of CD4(+) donor lymphocytes for treatment of relapse after allogeneic Stem cell transplant. *Blood* 91:3671–3680, 1998.

41. Mehta J, Singhal S: Graft-versus-myeloma. *Stem cell Transplant* 22:835–843, 1998.

42. Salama M, Nevill T, Marcellus D, et al.: Donor leukocyte infusions for multiple myeloma. *Stem cell Transplant* 26:1179–1184, 2000.

43. Huff CA, Fuchs EJ, Noga SJ, et al.: Long-term follow-up of T cell-depleted allogeneic Stem cell transplantation in refractory multiple myeloma: importance of allogeneic T cells. *Biol Blood Marrow Transplant* 9:312–319, 2003.

44. Peggs KS, Thomson K, Hart DP, et al.: Dose-escalated donor lymphocyte infusions following reduced intensity transplantation: toxicity, chimerism, and disease responses. *Blood* 103:1548–1556, 2004.

45. Byrne JL, Fairbairn J, Davy B, Carter IG, Bessell EM, Russell NH: Allogeneic transplantation for multiple myeloma: late relapse may occur as localised lytic lesion/plasmacytoma despite ongoing molecular remission. *Stem cell Transplant* 31:157–161, 2003.

46. Voena C, Malnati M, Majolino I, et al.: Detection of minimal residual disease by real-time PCR can be used as a surrogate marker to evaluate the graft-versus-myeloma effect after allogeneic stem cell transplantation. *Stem cell Transplant* 32:791–793, 2003.

47. Giralt S, Hester J, Huh Y, et al.: CD8-depleted donor lymphocyte infusion as treatment for relapsed chronic myelogenous leukemia after allogeneic Stem cell transplantation. *Blood* 86:4337–4343, 1995.

48. Bonini C, Verzeletti S, Servida P, et al.: Transfer of the HSV-TK gene into donor peripheral blood lymphocytes for in vivo immunomodulation of donor antitumor immunity after ALLO- SCT (meeting abstract). *Blood* 84:110a, 1994.

49. Bonini C, Ferrari G, Verzeletti S, et al.: HSV-TK gene transfer into donor lymphocytes for control of allogeneic graft-versus-leukemia [see comments]. *Science* 276:1719–1724, 1997.

50. Link CJ Jr, Traynor A, Seregina T, Burt RK: Adoptive immunotherapy for leukemia: donor lymphocytes transduced with the herpes simplex thymidine kinase gene. *Cancer Treat Res* 101:369–375, 1999.

51. Lokhorst HM, Schattenberg A, Cornelissen JJ, et al.: Donor lymphocyte infusions for relapsed multiple myeloma after allogeneic stem-cell transplantation: predictive factors for response and long-term outcome. *J Clin Oncol* 18:3031–3037, 2000.

52. Lokhorst HM, Wu K, Verdonck LF, et al.: The occurrence of graft-versus-host disease is the major predictive factor for response to donor lymphocyte infusions in multiple myeloma. *Blood* 103:4362–4364, 2004.

53. Alyea E, Schossman R, Canning C, et al.: CD6 T cell depleted allogeneic Stem cell transplant followed by CD4+ donor lymphocyte infusion for patients with multiple myeloma. *Blood* 94:609a, 1999.

54. Badros A, Barlogie B, Siegel E, et al.: Improved outcome of allogeneic transplantation in high-risk multiple myeloma patients after nonmyeloablative conditioning. *J Clin Oncol* 20:1295–1303, 2002.

55. Giralt S, Weber D, Cohen A, et al.: *Non Myeloablative Conditioning with Fludarabine and Melphalan for Patients with Multiple Myeloma*. Keystone, CO: ASBMT; 1999:43.

56. Kroger N, Sayer HG, Schwerdtfeger R, et al.: Unrelated stem cell transplantation in multiple myeloma after a reduced-intensity conditioning with pretransplantation antithymocyte globulin is highly effective with low transplantation-related mortality. *Blood* 100:3919–3924, 2002.

57. Kroger N, Schwerdfeger R, Kiehl M, et al.: Autologous stem cell transplantation followed by a dose-reduced allograft induces high complete remission rate in mutiple myeloma. *Blood* 100(3):755–760, 2002.

58. Maloney DG, Molina AJ, Sahebi F, et al.: Allografting with nonmyeloablative conditioning following cytoreductive autografts for the treatment of patients with multiple myeloma. *Blood* 102:3447–3454, 2003.

59. Peggs KS, Mackinnon S, Williams CD, et al.: Reduced-intensity transplantation with in vivo T-cell depletion and adjuvant dose-escalating donor lymphocyte infusions for chemotherapy-sensitive myeloma: limited efficacy of graft-versus-tumor activity. *Biol Blood Marrow Transplant* 9:257–265, 2003.

60. Lee CK, Badros A, Barlogie B, et al.: Prognostic factors in allogeneic transplantation for patients with high-risk multiple myeloma after reduced intensity conditioning. *Exp Hematol* 31:73–80, 2003.

61. Kroger N, Schilling G, Einsele H, et al.: Deletion of chromosome band 13q14 as detected by fluorescence in situ hybridization is a prognostic factor in patients with multiple myeloma who are receiving allogeneic dose-reduced stem cell transplantation. *Blood* 103:4056–4061, 2004.

62. Takahashi T, Makiguchi Y, Hinoda Y, et al.: Expression of MUC1 on myeloma cells and induction of HLA-unrestricted CTL against MUC1 from a multiple myeloma patient. *J Immunol* 153:2102–2109, 1994.

63. van Baren N, Brasseur F, Godelaine D, et al.: Genes encoding tumor-specific antigens are expressed in human myeloma cells. *Blood* 94:1156–1164, 1999.

64. Vonderheide RH, Hahn WC, Schultze JL, Nadler LM: The telomerase catalytic subunit is a widely expressed tumor-associated antigen recognized by cytotoxic T lymphocytes. *Immunity* 10:673–679, 1999.

65. Bellucci R, Wu CJ, Chiaretti S, et al.: Complete response to donor lymphocyte infusion in multiple myeloma is associated with antibody responses to highly expressed antigens. *Blood* 103:656–663, 2004.

66. Osterborg A, Yi Q, Henriksson L, et al.: Idiotype immunization combined with granulocyte-macrophage colony-stimulating factor in myeloma patients induced type I, major histocompatibility complex-restricted, CD8- and CD4-specific T-cell responses. *Blood* 91:2459–2466, 1998.

67. Massaia M, Borrione P, Battaglio S, et al.: Idiotype vaccination in human myeloma: generation of tumor-specific immune responses after high-dose chemotherapy. *Blood* 94:673–683, 1999.

68. Barratt-Boyes SM: Making the most of mucin: a novel target for tumor immunotherapy. *Cancer Immunol Immunother* 43:142–151, 1996.

69. Noto H, Takahashi T, Makiguchi Y, Hayashi T, Hinoda Y, Imai K: Cytotoxic T lymphocytes derived from bone marrow mononuclear cells of multiple myeloma patients recognize an underglycosylated form of MUC1 mucin. *Int Immunol* 9:791–798, 1997.

70. Tanaka Y, Koido S, Chen D, Gendler SJ, Kufe D, Gong J: Vaccination with allogeneic dendritic cells fused to carcinoma cells induces antitumor immunity in MUC1 transgenic mice. *Clin Immunol* 101:192–200, 2001.

71. Brossart P, Heinrich KS, Stuhler G, et al.: Identification of HLA-A2-restricted T-cell epitopes derived from the MUC1 tumor antigen for broadly applicable vaccine therapies. *Blood* 93:4309–4317, 1999.

72. Orsini E, Alyea EP, Schlossman R, et al.: Changes in T cell receptor repertoire associated with graft-versus-tumor effect and graft-versus-host disease in patients with relapsed multiple myeloma after donor lymphocyte infusion. *Stem cell Transplant* 25:623–632, 2000.

73. Dhodapkar KM, Krasovsky J, Williamson B, Dhodapkar MV: Antitumor monoclonal antibodies enhance cross-presentation of Cellular antigens and the generation of myeloma-specific killer T cells by dendritic cells. *J Exp Med* 195:125–133, 2002.

74. Nishikawa H, Tanida K, Ikeda H, et al.: Role of SEREX-defined immunogenic wild-type cellular molecules in the development of tumor-specific immunity. *Proc Natl Acad Sci U S A* 98:14571–14576, 2001.

75. Sahin U, Tureci O, Schmitt H, et al.: Human neoplasms elicit multiple specific immune responses in the autologous host. *Proc Natl Acad Sci U S A* 92:11810–11813, 1995.

76. Old LJ, Chen YT: New paths in human cancer serology. *J Exp Med* 187:1163–1167, 1998.

77. Wu CJ, Yang XF, McLaughlin S, et al.: Detection of a potent humoral response associated with immune-induced remission of chronic myelogenous leukemia. *J Clin Invest* 106:705–714, 2000.

78. Sahin U, Tureci O, Pfreundschuh M: Serological identification of human tumor antigens. *Curr Opin Immunol* 9:709–716, 1997.

79. Urashima M, Chauhan D, Uchiyama H, Freeman GJ, Anderson KC: CD40 ligand triggered interleukin-6 secretion in multiple myeloma. *Blood* 85:1903–1912, 1995.

80. Schultze JL, Cardoso AA, Freeman GJ, et al.: Follicular lymphomas can be induced to present alloantigen efficiently: a conceptual model to improve their tumor immunogenicity [published erratum appears in *Proc Natl Acad Sci U S A* 92(23):10818, 1995 Nov 7]. *Proc Natl Acad Sci U S A* 92:8200–8204, 1995.

81. Teoh G, Tai Y-T, Greenfield E, Anderson K: Tumor rejection antigen 1 (GRP94) expression is induced by CD40 ligand activation of multiple myeloma cells and mediates allogeneic T cell reactivity [abstract]. *Blood*. In press.

82. Janson CH, Grunewald J, Osterborg A, et al.: Predominant T cell receptor V gene usage in patients with abnormal clones of B cells. *Blood* 77:1776–1780, 1991.

83. Dianzani U, Pileri A, Boccadoro M, et al.: Activated idiotype-reactive cells in suppressor/cytotoxic subpopulations of monoclonal gammopathies: correlation with diagnosis and disease status. *Blood* 72:1064–1068, 1988.

84. Moss P, Gillespie G, Frodsham P, Bell J, Reyburn H: Clonal populations of CD4+ and CD8+ T cells in patients with multiple myeloma and paraproteinemia. *Blood* 87:3297–3306, 1996.

85. Osterborg A, Masucci M, Bergenbrant S, Holm G, Lefvert AK, Mellstedt H: Generation of T cell clones binding F(ab′)2 fragments of the idiotypic immunoglobulin in patients with monoclonal gammopathy. *Cancer Immunol Immunother* 34:157–162, 1991.

86. Yi Q, Osterborg A, Bergenbrant S, Mellstedt H, Holm G, Lefvert AK: Idiotype-reactive T-cell subsets and tumor load in monoclonal gammopathies. *Blood* 86:3043–3049, 1995.

87. Osterborg A, Yi Q, Bergenbrant S, Holm G, Lefvert AK, Mellstedt H: Idiotype-specific T cells in multiple myeloma stage I: an evaluation by four different functional tests. *Br J Haematol* 89:110–116, 1995.

88. Yi Q, Holm G, Lefvert AK: Idiotype-induced T cell stimulation requires antigen presentation in association with HLA-DR molecules. *Clin Exp Immunol* 104:359–365, 1996.

89. Bergenbrant S, Yi Q, Osterborg A, et al.: Modulation of anti-idiotypic immune response by immunization with the autologous M-component protein in multiple myeloma patients. *Br J Haematol* 92:840–846, 1996.

90. Reichardt VL, Okada CY, Liso A, et al.: Idiotype vaccination using dendritic cells after autologous peripheral blood stem cell transplantation for multiple myeloma—a feasibility study. *Blood* 93:2411–2419, 1999.

91. Kwak LW, Pennington R, Longo DL: Active immunization of murine allogeneic Stem cell transplant donors with B-cell tumor-derived idiotype: a strategy for enhancing the specific antitumor effect of marrow grafts. *Blood* 87:3053–3060, 1996.

# Chapter 86

# DEFINITION OF REMISSION, PROGNOSIS, AND FOLLOW-UP

## S. Vincent Rajkumar and Angela Dispenzieri

## INTRODUCTION

Multiple myeloma is typically incurable, with a median survival of 3–4 years.[1–3] Conventional chemotherapy with melphalan and prednisone (MP) produces a response rate of approximately 50%, with complete responses (CRs) in less than 10% of patients.[4] Combination chemotherapy with additional cytotoxic agents improves response rates (60–70%), but without significant survival benefit compared to MP.[4–6]

The careful evaluation of the efficacy of the various therapeutic options and their impact on patient outcome has implications for both practice and research. In this chapter, we review the current criteria for evaluating response to therapy in myeloma, summarize established and novel prognostic factors for the disease, and briefly outline the recommended follow-up for patients.

## DEFINITION OF REMISSION (RESPONSE) CRITERIA

Strict remission (response) criteria are required to monitor effectiveness of therapy in patients and to evaluate new drugs and interventions. Response criteria are also required to compare various therapeutic alternatives, both in clinical practice and in prospective trials. In some, but not all instances, response to therapy also serves as a marker for a good clinical outcome. In addition to response rates, other estimates of successful therapy in myeloma include measurements such as progression-free (PFS) and overall survival (OS).

### BASIC PRINCIPLES

The goals of assessing response differ between clinical practice and clinical trials. In practice, clinicians use various parameters to make an informed judgment about whether a given therapy is effective in a patient with myeloma, and to adjust therapy as needed. This includes assessment of M-protein levels on the basis of published response criteria, as well as other clinical variables. There is room for discretion when certain results are not available or are deemed clinically unnecessary. In clinical trials, however, there is a need to adhere to strict criteria to ensure that reported results are reliable and reproducible, as well as to ensure that results can be compared across clinical trials.

Several well-established response and survival criteria have been developed for myeloma over the years, primarily for use in clinical trials, though they have also been used to guide clinical practice. These criteria define various categories of response. They also define progressive disease, which is important in calculating PFS and event-free survival (EFS). The four most commonly used response criteria are those of the Chronic Leukemia-Myeloma Task Force,[7] Southwest Oncology Group (SWOG),[8,9] Eastern Cooperative Oncology Group (ECOG),[10] and the European Group for Blood and Bone Marrow Transplant/International Bone Marrow Transplant Registry/American Bone Marrow Transplant Registry (EBMT/IBMTR/ABMTR).[11] Recently the International Myeloma Working Group has published uniform response criteria.[11a]

### CRITERIA FOR RESPONSE AND PROGRESSION

Serum and urine M-protein levels should be determined by electrophoresis rather than by quantitative immunoglobulin measurement. Exceptions are made in cases in which the M-protein value may be unreliable. In these cases, quantitative immunoglobulins should be used. To assess response and progression, however, serum protein electrophoresis (SPEP) values should be compared only to SPEP values and quantitative immunoglobulin values only to quantitative immunoglobulin values.

The international uniform response criteria[11a] are the standard criteria for clinical trials and have been adopted recently by cooperative groups such as ECOG. These criteria partially take into account hemoglobin, calcium, bone changes, and bone marrow plasmacytosis for assessment of response, but rely heavily on measurement of serum and urine M protein.

For clinical trial purposes certain arbitrary levels of serum and urine M-protein values are considered "measurable," to ensure that a decrease in the M protein meeting requirements for response would be of sufficient magnitude to not be considered a laboratory variation. A "measurable" serum M protein is typically defined as ≥1 g/dL and a "measurable" urine M spike is defined as ≥200 mg/24 h. Responses cannot be reliably ascertained using M-protein measurements if the baseline values are below the "measurable" threshold.

### Standard definition of response and progression

By definition, the criteria require that M-protein reductions be confirmed by consecutive determinations. Responding patients should also have no evidence of progressive disease.

Bone marrow biopsies are not required to confirm PR or MR, but are required for the definition of CR and to evaluate response in patients with nonsecretory myeloma. Skeletal radiographs are not required to confirm response, but should not show evidence of progression if performed. A summary of the criteria listed below is provided in Table 86.1.

***Complete response*** Patients who have complete disappearance of M protein (negative immunofixation on the serum and urine) and 5% or fewer bone marrow plasmacytosis are considered to have achieved a CR. In addition, any soft-tissue plasmacytomas should disappear, and there should be no known increase in the size or number of lytic bone lesions. Patients meeting criteria for CR who have no clonal cells in the bone marrow and have a normal free light chain ratio are categorized as "stringent CR."

***Very good partial response*** The VGPR category is a useful measure of response that has gained clinical signifi-cance, as patients who achieve at least a VGPR with the first autologous stem cell transplant do not benefit from a second (tandem) transplant. For practical purposes, it distinguishes patients who have had near disappearance in their M spike but are still immunofixation positive from those who merely have a 50% reduction in their serum M spike. To be considered VGPR, patients must meet all of the following criteria:

■ greater than or equal to 90% reduction of M protein from serum (also includes achievement of a detectable but not quantifiable monoclonal protein by SPEP or by immunofixation only);
■ urine M spike to be ≤100 mg/24 h (also includes achievement of a detectable but not quantifiable monoclonal protein by urine protein electrophoresis or by immunofixation only);
■ no increase in size or number of lytic bone lesions.

***Partial response*** To be considered a PR, patients should have a ≥50% reduction in the level of the serum monoclonal protein and a reduction in 24-h urinary light-chain excretion either by ≥90% or to <200 mg/24 h. If present at baseline, there should also be a ≥50% reduction in the size of any soft-tissue plasmacytomas (by radiography or clinical examination), and there should be no increase in the number or size of lytic bone lesions. (Development of a compression fracture does not exclude response.) FLC criteria are used in patients without measurable disease.

In patients with nonsecretory myeloma, a ≥50% reduction in plasma cells in a bone marrow aspirate and on trephine biopsy must be documented in place of the M-protein and FLC requirements provided baseline bone marrow plasma cell percentage is 30% or

| Table 86.1 | Response criteria for myeloma | |
|---|---|---|
| Response category[a] | Monoclonal protein/plasmacytoma | Bone marrow |
| Complete response (CR) | ■ Negative immunofixation on the serum and urine and <br> ■ Disappearance of any soft-tissue plasmacytomas | ≤5% plasma cells |
| Very good partial response[b] | ■ ≥90% reduction of serum M protein and <br> ■ Serum and urine M protein detectable on immunofixation but not on electrophoresis, or <br> ■ Urine M protein <100 mg/24 h and <br> ■ Disappearance of any soft-tissue plasmacytomas | |
| Partial response | ■ ≥50% reduction of serum M protein and <br> ■ Reduction in 24-h urinary M protein by ≥90% or to <200 mg/24 h <br> ■ If present at baseline, a ≥50% reduction in size of soft-tissue plasmacytomas <br> ■ If serum and urine M protein unmeasurable, a ≥50% decrease in the difference between involved and uninvolved free light-chain (FLC) levels is required in place of the M-protein criteria[b] | Not a response requirement except in nonsecretory myeloma where a ≥50% reduction in plasma cells is required in place of M protein |

[a]The criteria for response require M-protein reductions to be confirmed by consecutive determinations and that there be no known increase in the size or number of lytic bone lesions on skeletal imaging.
[b]Should not be used to assess response if serum and/or urine M protein are measurable. Baseline involved FLC level must be 10 mg/dL (100 mg/L) or higher and serum FLC ratio must be abnormal for FLC criteria to be used to assess response.

higher. At Mayo Clinic, these bone marrow criteria are also used for patients in whom neither the serum nor the urine M-protein levels are "measurable" at baseline, i.e., patients with oligosecretory myeloma.

*Stable disease* Failure to meet response criteria for CR, VGPR, PR, or progressive disease is considered as stable disease.

*Relapse from CR* Patients in CR are considered to have "relapse from CR" if there is reappearance of serum or urine M protein by immunofixation or electrophoresis, development of $\geq$5% plasma cells in the bone marrow, or appearance of any other sign of progression (i.e., new plasmacytoma, lytic bone lesion, or hypercalcemia). Relapse from CR is used only to calculate disease free survival (DFS).

*Progressive disease* Progressive disease for patients not in CR is defined by the presence of one or more of the following features, and is used to calculate time to progression (TTP) and progression free survival (PFS):

■ increase in serum M protein to >25% above the lowest response level, which must also be an absolute increase of at least 0.5 g/dL;
■ increase in 24-h urine M protein to >25% above the lowest remission value, which must also be an absolute increase of at least 200 mg/24 h of urine M protein;
■ increase in bone marrow plasmacytosis by >25% above the lowest remission value, which must also be an absolute increase of at least 10% bone marrow plasma cells;
■ development of new soft-tissue plasmacytomas or bone lesions. Compression fracture does not exclude continued response and may not indicate progression;
■ definite increase in size of existing plasmacytomas or bone lesions. At Mayo Clinic, a definite increase is defined as a 50% (and at least 1 cm) increase as measured serially by the sum of the products of the cross diameters of the measurable lesion; and
■ development of hypercalcemia as defined by serum calcium >11.5 mg/dL (not attributable to any other cause);
■ progression based on FLC criteria (see below).

The Bladé criteria require that M-protein levels for relapse from CR and progression listed above be confirmed by at least one repeat investigation.

### Definitions for response using the free light-chain assay

The serum *free* light-chain (FLC) assay is of particular use in monitoring response to therapy in patients who have oligosecretory or nonsecretory myeloma, in whom serial bone marrow biopsies are often impractical and cumbersome.

The test is highly sensitive and consists of two separate assays: one to detect free kappa (normal range 0.33–1.94 mg/dL) and the other to detect free lambda (normal range 0.57–2.63 mg/dL) light chains.[12] In addition to measuring the levels of free-light chain, the test also allows assessment of clonality based on the ratio of kappa/lambda light-chain levels (normal reference range 0.26–1.65).[13] Patients with a kappa/lambda FLC ratio <0.26 are typically defined as having monoclonal lambda FLC, and those with ratios >1.65 are defined as having a monoclonal kappa FLC. The monoclonal light-chain isotype is referred to as the "involved" FLC isotype, and the opposite light-chain type is the "uninvolved" FLC type. Thus, a patient with a ratio of >1.65 on the FLC ratio has a monoclonal kappa FLC isotype, where the kappa is the "involved" FLC and the lambda is the "uninvolved" FLC.

When using the FLC assay, the FLC levels vary considerably with changes in renal function and do not solely represent monoclonal elevations. Thus, both the level of the involved and the uninvolved FLC isotype (i.e., the involved/uninvolved ratio or involved/uninvolved difference) should be considered in assessing response. The criteria listed below take this factor into account.

Until further validation, the serum FLC assay criteria should be used in assessing response and progression only if the baseline serum and/or urine M proteins are not "measurable" by the traditional criteria discussed earlier. In addition, the baseline level of the involved FLC should be at least $\geq$10 mg/dL and the FLC assay should have an abnormal ratio (clonal).

*Complete response* To be considered a CR, normalization of the FLC ratio and negative serum and urine immunofixation are required. In addition, patients should meet other nonparaprotein requirements for CR.

*Partial response* To be considered a PR, a 50% decrease in the difference between involved and uninvolved FLC levels, is required in place of the M-protein criteria. Other requirements of PR must also be met.

*Progressive disease* The following change qualifies as progression:

■ a 50% increase in the difference between involved and uninvolved FLC levels from the lowest response level, which must also be an absolute increase of at least 10 mg/dL.

### ESTIMATES OF SURVIVAL

Several estimates of survival have been developed to assess the efficacy of therapy and to describe prognosis in clinical cancer research. These include OS, disease-free survival (DFS), PFS, and EFS. OS is the gold standard for comparing therapeutic strategies, but has limitations because even in randomized trials patients often cross over to treatment offered in the opposing arm when discontinuing assigned therapy.

PFS, usually defined as time from start of therapy to disease progression or death,[14] can serve as a surrogate for OS. EFS, which is the duration from start of therapy to predefined events such as disease progression or relapse, death, or serious toxicity, can also be used as an important endpoint. When EFS is defined from start of therapy to death from any cause or progression (whichever occurs earlier),[15,16] it is the same as PFS. On the other hand, time to progression (TTP)[17] is usually measured from start of therapy to disease progression, with deaths due to causes other than progression not counted as an event, but censored at that time point.

Response duration, which is measured only in responding patients, also provides an estimate of drug efficacy. In myeloma, often only a subset of patients respond to a specific drug, and although TTP or PFS for the entire cohort may appear small, the benefit in responders may be substantial.[17,18]

DFS applies only to patients achieving a CR, and refers to the duration from onset of CR to first evidence of relapse. Since it applies to only a small subset of patients with myeloma, it is probably not a good endpoint in this disease.

### COMPARING RESPONSE RATES AND SURVIVAL

A comparison of response and survival between patients receiving different therapeutic strategies can be reliably made only in the context of a randomized (phase III) trial. As a general rule, response rates and estimates of survival should not be compared between trials, e.g., comparing two separate phase II (nonrandomized, single-arm) trials, except as a hypothesis generating exercise, even if the same response and survival criteria are used in the trials being compared.

## PROGNOSTIC FACTORS

There is significant variation in survival of patients with myeloma; though median survival is 3 years,[1] some patients can live longer than 7–10 years.[19–22] Several prognostic factors that identify groups of patients with significantly different survival probabilities have been identified, and have become indispensable for patient care and counseling (Table 86.2). These factors are also increasingly used for risk stratification in clinical trials to ensure that treatment arms are truly comparable.

Age, stage, hemoglobin concentration, creatinine, calcium, albumin, immunoglobulin class subtype, and extent of bone marrow involvement are all significant predictors of survival.[23–25] However, they add minimal additional prognostic value, once the major independent prognostic factors are known.[26,27] These include serum $\beta_2$-microglobulin ($\beta_2$M), bone marrow plasma cell labeling index (PCLI), karyotypic chromosome 13 deletion or hypodiploidy, plasmablastic morphology, lactate dehydrogenase (LDH), and C-reactive protein (CRP).[24,28]

| Table 86.2 Prognostic factors in myeloma |
| --- |
| **Clinically useful, major prognostic factors** |
| Performance status |
| Stage (by the ISS staging system) |
| Cytogenetic studies (conventional cytogenetics and/or interphase FISH) |
| ■ Deletion 13 |
| ■ Hypodiploidy |
| ■ t (4;14), t(14;16), or deletion 17p |
| Lactate dehydrogenase |
| Plasmablastic morphology |
| Plasma cell labeling index (limited availability) |
| Circulating plasma cells (limited availability) |
| **Biologically relevant prognostic factors, with limited clinical utility** |
| Microvessel density |
| Ras and p53 mutations |
| Immunophenotyping |
| Serum IL-6 and soluble IL-6 Receptors |

### STANDARD CLINICAL AND LABORATORY FACTORS

#### Age

As expected, age has an influence on the outcome of patients with myeloma.[26,27] In particular, patients younger than 40 years of age have a median survival that exceeds 50 months.[29] In a recent cohort study, OS was 41 months in patients less than 70 years of age, compared to 26 months in older patients.[1] However, age does not seem to add major prognostic information once the $\beta_2$M and PCLI are known.[27] Age also does not appear to be a significant variable for predicting survival after autotransplantation for myeloma, though age restrictions in the larger randomized transplant trials have been to 60 or 65 years.[15,16] Retrospective analyses of subsets of older patients transplanted at other large transplant centers suggest that a specific age limit need not be imposed in selecting patients for autologous stem cell transplantation.[30]

#### Performance status

Performance status is probably the single most powerful predictor of outcome in myeloma, but its value has not been highlighted in the literature. Kyle and colleagues reported on a study of 1027 consecutive patients with newly diagnosed myeloma seen at the Mayo Clinic, in which performance status of 3–4 (using the ECOG scoring system) had a more adverse impact on outcome than any other single variable including PCLI and $\beta_2$M.[1] One of the reasons performance status is not on the list of many studies evaluating prognosis is that most of these studies use cohorts of patients from clinical trials. Most clinical trials automatically exclude those with performance status 3–4 from participating. In contrast, the study by Kyle et al. included all patients with myeloma seen at the Mayo Clinic between 1985 and 1998, not just patients enrolling in clinical trials. The relative risk of a performance status of 3–4 was 1.9 [95% confidence interval (CI) 1.6–2.4], compared to 1.5 for PCLI (95% CI 1.3–1.7) and $\beta_2M$ (95% CI 1.3–1.8). In that study, which predated the era of new active agents against myeloma, patients with good performance status had a median survival of 36 months, compared to 11 months for those with performance status of 3–4.

## Stage

Since 1975, the Durie–Salmon staging system (Table 86.3) has been used to stage multiple myeloma. The median survival is about 5 years for those with stage IA disease and 15 months for those with stage IIIB disease using this system. The Durie–Salmon staging essentially measures tumor burden and is limited in the categorization of bone lesions.[24,31] Some studies have also failed to confirm the prognostic value of the Durie–Salmon stage.[26,31] The Durie–Salmon staging largely loses prognostic value once the PCLI and $\beta_2M$ are known.[27]

**Table 86.3** Durie-Salmon staging for multiple myeloma

| Stage I |
| --- |
| All of the following: |
| Hemoglobin >10 g/dL<br>Serum calcium <12 mg/dL |
| On radiograph, normal bone structure or solitary bone plasmacytoma only |
| Low M-component production rates |
| IgG <5 g/dL |
| IgA <3 g/dL |
| Urine light-chain M-component on electrophoresis <4 g/24 h |
| **Stage II** |
| Fitting neither Stage I nor III |
| **Stage III** |
| One or more of the following: |
| Hemoglobin <8.5 g/dL |
| Serum calcium >12 mg/ dL |
| Advanced lytic bone lesions |
| High M-component rates |
| IgG >7 g/dL |
| IgA >5 g/dL |
| Urine light-chain M-component on electrophoresis >12 g/24 h |
| **Subclassification** |
| A: Serum creatinine <2 mg/dL |
| B: Serum creatinine ≥2 mg/dL |

Modified from Durie BG, Salmon SE: A clinical staging system for multiple myeloma. Correlation of measured myeloma cell mass with presenting clinical features, response to treatment, and survival. *Cancer* 36:842–854,1975; with permission of John Wiley & Sons , Inc.

**Table 86.4** International staging system for multiple myeloma

| Stage | Median survival (months) |
| --- | --- |
| **Stage I**<br>$\beta_2M$ <3.5 and albumin ≥3.5 | 62 |
| **Stage II**<br>Not meeting criteria for Stage I or III | 44 |
| **Stage III**<br>$\beta_2M$ >5.5 | 29 |

Adapted from Greipp PR, San Miguel JF, Durie BG, et al.: A new International staging system (ISS) for multiple myeloma (MM) from the International Myeloma Working Group. *J Clin Oncol* 23(15): 3412–3420, 2005; with permission of the American Society of Clinical Oncology.

Recently, Greipp et al. have developed a new staging for myeloma built with international consensus as a replacement to the Durie–Salmon staging. The new International Staging System (ISS) was a collaborative effort by investigators from 17 institutions worldwide and involved data from 11,171 patients. It overcomes some of the drawbacks of the Durie–Salmon staging and is extremely simple to use. The ISS divides patients into three distinct stages and prognostic groups based solely on the $\beta_2M$ and albumin levels in the serum (Table 86.4).

### C-reactive protein

The CRP is an acute-phase reactant. It is produced by hepatic cells in response to interleukin 6 (IL-6). The serum CRP is a widely available, inexpensive assay, and has been proposed as a surrogate for measurement of IL-6 levels.

Several studies have shown that the CRP has prognostic value in myeloma. [32,33] However, Mayo Clinic and ECOG studies have failed to confirm the value of CRP as an independent prognostic factor.[26,27]

### Other miscellaneous clinical and laboratory parameters

Several readily available clinical and laboratory parameters, such as hemoglobin concentration, creatinine, calcium, albumin, immunoglobulin class subtype, and extent of bone marrow involvement, are also predictors of survival.[23–25,34] Some, such as hemoglobin, albumin, and creatinine, are already incorporated into staging systems. When independent factors are known, they do not add significant additional prognostic information.[26,27]

### MAJOR INDEPENDENT PROGNOSTIC FACTORS
### Plasma cell labeling index and measures of plasma cell proliferation

PCLI is a measurement of the proliferative activity of the neoplastic plasma cells in myeloma.[27,35] The assay is done on the bone marrow aspirate, using a slide-based immunofluorescence method. The principle underlying the PCLI is that cells in the S phase of the cell cycle incorporate bromodeoxyuridine, which is then recognized by a specific monoclonal antibody (BU-1) directed against it.

Several studies have demonstrated the prognostic value of PCLI in myeloma. A high PCLI predicts both poor OS and PFS. On multivariate analysis, PCLI has consistently demonstrated independent prognostic value.[33,36–42] Most investigators use a cutoff value of 1 or 2% to identify those with a poor prognosis. At the Mayo Clinic, a cutoff of 1% or higher has been defined as a high value. In one study, Greipp et al. found the median survival of patients with a PCLI $\geq$1% to be 17 months, compared to 42 months in those with a PCLI <1%.[27] In another study, the median survival was 21 and 43 months in patients with a PCLI <2% versus those with values $\geq$2%, respectively.[43]

One of the limitations of the PCLI is that only a few laboratories in the United States are presently performing the test. To overcome this limitation, flow cytometric methods of estimating the proportion of plasma cells in S phase have been developed. San Miguel and colleagues analyzed the cell cycle distribution of plasma cells in 120 untreated multiple myeloma patients, using simultaneous CD38 and DNA staining.[44] A high percentage (>3%) of plasma cells in the S phase was an independent prognostic factor for poor survival.

### β2-microglobulin

$\beta_2 M$ is a small protein that forms the light chain of the human leukocyte antigen, and has a molecular weight of 11,800.[45] It is normally excreted by the kidney, and its serum concentration is elevated in renal failure. There is an excellent correlation between serum $\beta_2 M$ levels and myeloma tumor burden in the absence of renal failure.[46]

A high serum $\beta_2 M$ level is an established predictor of poor survival in patients treated with conventional chemotherapy for myeloma.[27,47,48] $\beta_2 M$ is also an independent predictor of CR, OS, and EFS after transplantation for myeloma.[22,49–51] As discussed earlier, it has been incorporated into the ISS, and hence does not need to be considered independent of the staging in the future.[52] The utility of serial $\beta_2 M$ is undefined, and it should not be used as a marker for evaluating disease course or response to therapy.

### Cytogenetic abnormalities

Cytogenetic abnormalities are of major prognostic significance in acute leukemias and myelodysplastic syndromes. Among myeloma patients treated with standard-dose or high-dose chemotherapy, the presence of cytogenetic abnormalities has significant prognostic value.[24,53,54] Cytogenetic abnormalities are usually complex (>3 abnormalities) in myeloma.[53,55] Approximately 20% of patients with newly diagnosed disease have abnormalities on conventional karyotypic analysis.[53] In contrast, the incidence of such abnormalities in relapsed myeloma increases to 40% or higher.[53,56–58] Recent studies show that cytogenetic abnormalities are present in most, if not all, patients with myeloma if sensitive interphase fluorescent in situ hybridization techniques (FISH) are used.[59–61] The most common cytogenetic changes include deletion of chromosome 13 (30–55% of patients), deletion of 17p13.1 (10%), t(11;14)(q13;q32) (15–20%), t(4;14)(p16.3;q32) (15%), and t (14;16) (q32;q23) (5%).[54] The discrepancy is due to the low proliferative activity of neoplastic plasma cells and the resulting lack of metaphases, which are essential for karyotypic analysis but not for interphase FISH, which does not require dividing cells.[54,62]

Several groups have reported on the prognostic value of cytogenetic abnormalities detected by karyotyping in myeloma.[49,58,63] Tricot and colleagues studied 427 patients undergoing transplantation and found that patients with chromosomal abnormalities had a significantly worse outcome compared to those with normal cytogenetics: OS 29 months versus 55 months, and EFS 19 months versus 36 months, respectively. Similar results are seen in patients with relapsed and refractory myeloma as well.[58]

There is a significant correlation between the presence of cytogenetic abnormalities and a high PCLI.[55,64] Since the two variables are correlated, the PCLI may not add significant predictive value to a model that already contains cytogenetics, and vice versa. However, there are trends that suggest that the two variables may achieve independent prognostic significance if studies are done with a larger sample size.

*Deletion of chromosome 13*  Several studies show that deletion of chromosome 13 [Figure 86.1(a) and 86.1(b)] has a particularly adverse prognostic effect.[21,22,65–67] The abnormality is monosomy for the chromosome in approximately 85% of cases, while in 15% it represents interstitial deletions involving mainly 13q14.[68,69]

When present, the prognostic effect of deletion 13 detected by conventional karyotypic analysis is highly significant. In a study of 1000 patients with myeloma who received autologous stem cell transplantation, the 5-year survival rate was 16% in those with karyotypic deletion 13 (163 patients), compared to 44% in those without the abnormality (830 patients) ($P < 0.001$). Five-year EFS was 0% versus 28% ($P < 0.001$), respectively.[22]

The adverse prognostic effect is also demonstrable (although to a slightly lesser extent) when deletion 13 is recognized using interphase FISH studies.[70–73] In four different studies, median OS ranged from 15 to 35 months among patients with deletion 13 by interphase FISH, compared to 50–65 months in those without the abnormality.[70,72–74] Importantly, in contrast to karyotypic deletion 13, which is detected in only 15% of patients, approximately 35–55% of patients have abnormalities that can be detected by interphase FISH.[54]

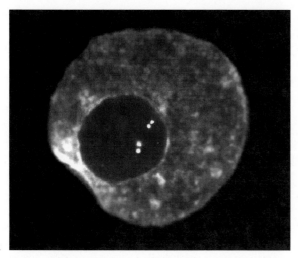
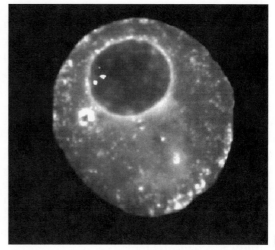

a                                                                                          b

**Figure 86.1** *FISH showing (a) normal plasma cell with two copies of chromosome 13 (two probes for each copy), and (b) plasma cell in myeloma with deletion of one copy of chromosome 13*

The abnormality may also have therapeutic implications, since patients who demonstrate the presence of deletion 13 by karyotypic analysis appear to receive minimal benefit from single or tandem autologous stem cell transplantation.[22,73] Unfortunately, nonmyeloablative transplantation does not appear to overcome the poor prognostic effect either.[75,76]

***Other cytogenetic changes*** The presence of t(4;14) (p16.3;q32), t(14;16)(q32q23), and 17p13, which are usually detected by molecular genetic studies such as interphase FISH or metaphase spectral karyotype imaging, are associated with a markedly adverse prognosis.[71,77–79]

### Plasmablastic morphology

Based on well-defined morphologic criteria, it is possible to identify a subgroup of patients with myeloma who have plasmablastic features on bone marrow examination.[80]

Plasmablastic morphology is considered to be present (plasmablastic myeloma) when ≥2% plasmablasts comprise the bone marrow plasma cell population.[26]

Using the above criteria, a large study of 453 newly diagnosed patients by the ECOG demonstrated that plasmablastic morphology is a powerful, independent adverse prognostic factor for survival.[26] In this study, median OS was 1.9 years in patients with plasmablastic myeloma, compared to 3.7 years in those with nonplasmablastic morphology.

One limitation of using plasmablastic morphology as a prognostic factor is that the interpretation is subjective, and significant interobserver variation may be present.

### Circulating plasma cells and peripheral blood labeling index

Circulating myeloma cells are difficult to find in routinely stained peripheral blood slides in most patients with myeloma. However, with the use of multiparameter flow cytometry, or by using the slide-based immunofluorescence method (similar to that described for the PCLI), these cells can be easily detected and quantified (Figure 86.2).[81–84] Witzig and colleagues have shown that the presence of large numbers of circulating plasma cells is associated with poor prognosis.[85] In a study of 254 patients with myeloma, OS was poorer among those with a high level of circulating peripheral blood plasma cells: median survival, 2.4 years (high levels) versus 4.4 years (low or undetectable levels), and $P < 0.001$.[85]

Circulating plasma cells also predict for patients with smoldering multiple myeloma (SMM) that are likely to progress sooner to active disease.[83] In a study of 57 patients with SMM, the median TTP for patients with abnormal circulating plasma cells was 0.75 years, compared to 2.5 years for the rest ($P < 0.01$).

Although powerful prognostic factors, circulating plasma cells, and peripheral blood labeling index are limited by their availability. Flow cytometric methods to detect circulating plasma cells are being studied and can be readily incorporated into clinical practice once well validated.

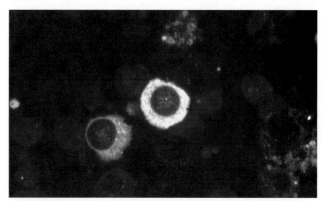

**Figure 86.2** *Circulating plasma cells as seen on florescent microscopy after staining for cytoplasmic immunoglobulin light chains*

### Lactate dehydrogenase

LDH is a powerful, independent prognostic factor in myeloma.[64,86,87] One limitation of the LDH is that only a small proportion of patients with myeloma (5–11%) have an elevated level.[88] Nevertheless, when elevated, it predicts for a markedly adverse prognosis.

### OTHER PROGNOSTIC MARKERS WITH BIOLOGICAL IMPORTANCE

Numerous other prognostic factors have been identified, many of which are of major biological importance, as they shed light on the mechanisms of disease progression in myeloma. However, their impact on outcome is minimal once the major independent factors described above are known, thus limiting their clinical utility as prognostic tools.

### Microvessel density

Studies in myeloma indicate that bone marrow angiogenesis is increased in myeloma (Figure 86.3).[89–92] There is also evidence that bone marrow angiogenesis correlates with the proliferation of neoplastic plasma cells and may be important in disease progression and activity.[89,90] Several studies now show that increased angiogenesis measured by microvessel density is a significant adverse prognostic factor in myeloma.[93–96] In the ECOG study, OS was significantly longer in patients with low-grade angiogenesis (53 months), compared to those with high-grade (24 months) or intermediate-grade angiogenesis (48 months) ($P = 0.18$).[97]

### Interleukin 6

Although IL-6 is an important growth factor in the differentiation of normal B lymphocytes to plasma cells,[98,99] it does not generally induce proliferation of normal B lymphocytes or plasma cells.[100] In contrast, IL-6 can induce a significant proliferative response in myeloma cells.[98] It appears to have both an autocrine and paracrine role in the growth and proliferation of myeloma cells.[98,101] The proliferative response of myeloma cells to IL-6 is a major factor that distinguishes malignant proliferating from normal nonproliferating plasma cells.[100]

Serum IL-6 levels are elevated in about one-third of myeloma patients, and are more frequently elevated in plasma cell leukemia. IL-6 levels correlate with bone marrow plasmacytosis, serum LDH, $\beta_2M$, and calcium.[102,103]

### Soluble IL-6 receptors

The activity of IL-6 in myeloma appears to be modulated by the expression of soluble IL-6 receptors (sIL-6R).[100,104,105] In the presence of IL-6, sIL-6R associates with glycoprotein 130 (gp130), and leads to signal transduction and augmentation of the IL-6 proliferation effect.[106] sIL-6R potentiates the proliferative effect of IL-6 on myeloma cells up to 10-fold.[104,105]

An elevated sIL-6R level has independent poor prognostic value in myeloma.[28,33] A multivariate analysis of 388 patients showed independent prognostic significance for a sIL-6R >300.[33] The sIL-6R level did not correlate with PCLI or other prognostic variables. Adding sIL-6R to PCLI and $\beta_2M$ allowed improved prognostic classification, doubling the proportion identified as high risk.

### Immunophenotyping

Certain immunophenotypic features have been suggested to have prognostic value. CD20+ plasma cells in myeloma have been associated with a more aggressive course of disease.[107] Initial reports suggested that the presence or coexpression of CD10 or surface immunoglobulin may represent poor prognostic features in myeloma. However, the prognostic value of CD10 in myeloma is unclear, as others have reported conflicting results.[107–109] Further, only 15% of myeloma cells are positive for CD10, limiting its role as a prognostic factor. The presence of surface immunoglobulin may be indicative of more immature plasma cell clone. It does not appear that any of these immunophenotypic characteristics of plasma cells have independent prognostic value in myeloma.

### Oncogenes and tumor suppressor genes

Mutations in the *ras* oncogene have been noted in plasma cells of myeloma, more commonly in the advanced phase of the disease.[110,111] Liu and colleagues examined the mutational status of the N- and K-*ras* genes in 160 newly diagnosed multiple myeloma patients enrolled on the ECOG phase III clinical trial E9486.[112] The incidence of *ras* mutations was 39%. Patients with K-*ras*, but not N-*ras*, mutations had a significantly shorter median survival, 2.0 years versus 3.7 years, $P < 0.02$.[112]

Mutations of the tumor suppressor gene p53 have also been studied. The incidence of p53 point mutations

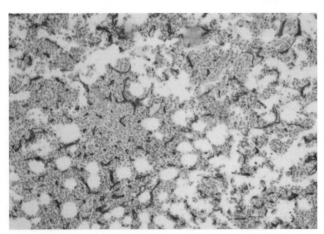

**Figure 86.3** *Increased bone marrow microvessels in myeloma bone marrow as visualized by immunohistochemical staining for CD34*

in myeloma in one study was 13%.[113] Mutations were more common (43%) in the more advanced and clinically aggressive forms of the myeloma.

### Alternative measures of plasma cell proliferation

Besides the PCLI and S-phase estimations, other methods are available to evaluate the proliferative activity of the plasma cells. Immunohistochemical staining of bone marrow using the Ki-67 antibody has been proposed as a surrogate marker for the PCLI, because it identifies plasma cells undergoing active cell division.[114] The correlation between the results of this assay and disease activity is good, but comparisons suggest a wider variation of results and lack of correlation with the PCLI.[115]

Similarly, the use of the proliferating cell nuclear antigen (PCNA) monoclonal antibody has been proposed as a surrogate marker of cell proliferation.[116] The results of PCNA correlate more closely with PCLI than with the Ki-67 assay.

### T- and B-cell levels

Several studies have shown that baseline and posttreatment levels of T and B lymphocytes may be important to outcome in myeloma. San Miguel and colleagues demonstrated that loss of $CD4^+$ T cells is associated with a worse prognosis in myeloma patients.[117] Similarly, an elevated level of T cells with activation markers or plasma cell markers has been associated with an unfavorable outcome.[118] Kay and colleagues showed that approximately 20% of patients with myeloma have increased levels of circulating $CD19^+$ B cells.[119] Low numbers of circulating $CD19^+$ B-cell level (<125 μL) were associated with more advanced disease (clinical stage III, $P = 0.033$). Survival was better in patients with higher levels of circulating CD19 cells (≥125 μL, $P < 0.0001$). CD19 was found to be an independent prognostic factor.

Recently, Kay and colleagues have confirmed the above findings in an ECOG phase III trial involving 504 newly diagnosed patients with myeloma treated with standard-dose chemotherapy.[120] Higher baseline levels of CD3(+), CD4(+), CD8(+), and CD19(+) cells were each associated with improved survival. Porrata and colleagues have demonstrated that early lymphocyte recovery is important for survival, postautologous transplanatation in myeloma.[121]

### Other novel factors

An association between high serum levels of the carboxy terminal of telopeptide of type I collagen (ICTP) and survival has been suggested in newly diagnosed myeloma patients.[122] In one study, patients with high serum level of ICTP had poorer OS compared to those with low levels with a median survival of 3.5 years versus 4.1 years, respectively ($P = 0.001$).[123]

Serum levels of thymidine kinase also have prognostic value in myeloma.[124] Thymidine kinase may identify a small subset of patients with a high PCLI. An elevated IL-2 level is associated with a better prognosis.[125]

### COMBINING INDEPENDENT PROGNOSTIC FACTORS TO PREDICT OUTCOME

A combination of independent prognostic factors provides greater prognostic information than any one prognostic factor alone. Table 86.5 provides two other models in which readily available prognostic factors have been combined to provide powerful prognostic information.

| Table 86.5 | Combining major prognostic factors to predict outcome in myeloma | | | | |
|---|---|---|---|---|---|
| Series | Prognostic factors | Combination | No. of patients | Overall survival (OS) | Event-free survival (EFS) |
| Facon et al.[73] | Deletion 13 by FISH | None high | 110 | Median not reached at 111 month | Median 37 months |
| | β₂-microglobulin | One high | | Median 47 months | Median 27 months |
| | | Both high | | Median 25 months | Median 15 months |
| Desikan et al.[22] | β₂-microglobulin | None abnormal | 1000 | 62% at 5 years | 41% at 5 years |
| | Karyotypic deletion 13 | Any 1–3 abnormal with exception of deletion 13 | | 20–52% at 5 years | 12–34% at 5 years |
| | More than 12 months therapy prior to transplant | Deletion 13 present | | 5–35% at 5 years | 0% at 5 years |
| | C-reactive protein | All 4 factors abnormal | | 5% at 5 years | 0% at 5 years |
| Greipp et al.[126] | Plasma cell labeling index | None high | 493 | 46% at 5 years | Not available |
| | β₂-microglobulin | Either one high | | 31% at 5 years | Not available |
| | | Both high | | 9% at 5 years | Not available |

## FOLLOW-UP

The follow-up of patients with multiple myeloma is dependent on a number of factors, including phase of disease (early untreated vs relapsed refractory), the stage, presence or absence of ongoing therapy, mode of therapy, and comorbidity. Patients are typically evaluated every 4–6 weeks during active therapy, and every 3–4 months when in the plateau phase of disease on no therapy or only maintenance therapy. Patients with active treatment or disease-related complications may need more frequent monitoring.

The suggested clinical and laboratory evaluations to be performed at follow-up are given in Table 86.6. These are guidelines and need to be modified according to clinical need.

### Acknowledgments

This work is supported by grants CA 107476, 62242, 100080, and 93842 from the National Cancer Institute, National Institutes of Health, Bethesda, MD.

**Table 86.6** Standard tests for follow-up

**Routine tests to be done at each follow-up**
- Complete blood counts
- Serum chemistries (include serum creatinine, electrolytes, and calcium)
- Serum protein electrophoresis
- Urine protein electrophoresis

**Every 6–12 months**
- Skeletal survey

**Based on clinical situation**
- Serum and urine protein immunofixation (at baseline and to document complete response)
- Bone marrow biopsy (at baseline, as needed to clarify clinical state, and if needed to confirm Progression/response)
- $\beta_2$ microglobulin, plasma cell labeling index, cytogenetics, circulating plasma cells, LDH, CRP (at base line, and as needed to clarify clinical state)

## REFERENCES

1. Kyle RA, Gertz MA, Witzig TE, et al.: Review of 1,027 patients with newly diagnosed multiple myeloma. *Mayo Clin Proc* 78:21–33, 2003.
2. Kyle RA: Multiple myeloma: review of 869 cases. *Mayo Clin Proc* 50:29–40, 1975.
3. Rajkumar SV, Gertz MA, Kyle RA, Greipp PR: Current therapy for multiple myeloma. *Mayo Clin Proc* 77:813–822, 2002.
4. Myeloma Trialists' Collaborative Group: Combination chemotherapy versus melphalan plus prednisone as treatment for multiple myeloma: an overview of 6,633 patients from 27 randomized trials. *J Clin Oncol* 16:3832–3842, 1998.
5. Alexanian R, Dimopoulos M: The treatment of multiple myeloma. *N Engl J Med* 330:484–489, 1994.
6. Oken MM, Harrington DP, Abramson N, Kyle RA, Knospe W, Glick JH: Comparison of melphalan and prednisone with vincristine, carmustine, melphalan, cyclophosphamide, and prednisone in the treatment of multiple myeloma: results of Eastern Cooperative Oncology Group Study E2479. *Cancer* 79:1561–1567, 1997.
7. Anonymous: Proposed guidelines for protocol studies. I: Introduction. II: Plasma cell myeloma. III: Chronic lymphocytic leukemia. IV: Chronic granulocytic leukemia. *Cancer Chemother Rep* 34:141–173, 1973.
8. Alexanian R, Bonnet J, Gehan E, et al.: Combination chemotherapy for multiple myeloma. *Cancer* 30:382–389, 1972.
9. McLaughlin P, Alexanian R: Myeloma protein kinetics following chemotherapy. *Blood* 60:851–855, 1982.
10. Oken MM, Kyle RA, Greipp PR, et al.: Complete remission induction with combined VBMCP chemotherapy and interferon (rIFN alpha 2b) in patients with multiple myeloma. *Leuk Lymphoma* 20:447–452, 1996.

11. Blade J, Samson D, Reece D, et al.: Criteria for evaluating disease response and progression in patients with multiple myeloma treated by high-dose therapy and haemopoietic stem cell transplantation. Myeloma Subcommittee of the EBMT. European Group for Blood and Marrow Transplant. *Br J Haematol* 102:1115–1123, 1998.
11a. Durie BGM, Harousseau J-L, Miguel JS, et al.: International uniform response criteria for multiple myeloma. *Leukemia* 20(9):1467–1473, 2006.
12. Abraham RS, Clark RJ, Bryant SC, et al.: Correlation of serum immunoglobulin free light chain quantification with urinary Bence Jones protein in light chain myeloma. *Clin Chem* 48:655–657, 2002.
13. Katzmann JA, Clark RJ, Abraham RS, et al.: Serum reference intervals and diagnostic ranges for free kappa and free lambda immunoglobulin light chains: relative sensitivity for detection of monoclonal light chains. *Clin Chem* 48:1437–1444, 2002.
14. Child JA, Morgan GJ, Davies FE, et al.: High-dose chemotherapy with hematopoietic stem-cell rescue for multiple myeloma. *N Engl J Med* 348:1875–1883, 2003.
15. Attal M, Harousseau JL, Stoppa AM, et al.: A prospective, randomized trial of autologous bone marrow transplantation and chemotherapy in multiple myeloma. Intergroupe Francais du Myelome. *N Engl J Med* 335:91–97, 1996.
16. Attal M, Harousseau JL, Facon T, et al.: Single versus double autologous stem-cell transplantation for multiple myeloma. *N Engl J Med* 349:2495–2502, 2003.
17. Richardson PG, Barlogie B, Berenson J, et al.: A phase 2 study of bortezomib in relapsed, refractory myeloma. *N Engl J Med* 348:2609–2617, 2003.

18. Kumar S, Gertz MA, Dispenzieri A, et al.: Response rate, durability of response, and survival after thalidomide therapy for relapsed multiple myeloma. *Mayo Clin Proc* 78:34–39, 2003.

19. Kyle RA: Long-term survival in multiple myeloma. *N Engl J Med* 308:314–316, 1983.

20. Attal M, Harousseau JL, Facon T, et al.: Single versus double autologous stem-cell transplantation for multiple myeloma. *N Engl J Med* 26:2495–2502, 2003.

21. Barlogie B, Jagannath S, Desikan KR, et al.: Total therapy with tandem transplants for newly diagnosed multiple myeloma. *Blood* 93:55–65, 1999.

22. Desikan R, Barlogie B, Sawyer J, et al.: Results of high-dose therapy for 1000 patients with multiple myeloma: durable complete remissions and superior survival in the absence of chromosome 13 abnormalities. *Blood* 95:4008–4010, 2000.

23. Greipp PR: Prognosis in myeloma. *Mayo Clin Proc* 69:895–902, 1994.

24. Kyle RA: Prognostic factors in multiple myeloma. *Stem Cells* 2:56–63, 1995.

25. Greipp PR, Gaillard JP, Klein B, et al.: Independent prognostic value for plasma cell labeling index (PCLI), immunofluorescence microscopy plasma cell percent (IMPCP), beta 2-microglobulin (B2M), soluble interleukin-6 receptor (sIL-6R), and c-reactive protein (CRP) in myeloma trial E9487 [meeting abstract]. *Blood* 84:385a, 1994.

26. Greipp PR, Leong T, Bennett JM, et al.: Plasmablastic morphology—an independent prognostic factor with clinical and laboratory correlates: Eastern Cooperative Oncology Group (ECOG) myeloma trial E9486 report by the ECOG Myeloma Laboratory Group. *Blood* 91:2501–2507, 1998.

27. Greipp PR, Lust JA, O'Fallon WM, Katzmann JA, Witzig TE, Kyle RA: Plasma cell labeling index and beta 2-microglobulin predict survival independent of thymidine kinase and C-reactive protein in multiple myeloma. *Blood* 81:3382–3387, 1993.

28. Greipp PR: Prognosis in myeloma. *Mayo Clin Proc* 69:895–902, 1994.

29. Blade J, Kyle RA, Greipp PR: Presenting features and prognosis in 72 patients with multiple myeloma who were younger than 40 years. *Br J Haematol* 93:345–351, 1996.

30. Siegel DS, Desikan KR, Mehta J, et al.: Age is not a prognostic variable with autotransplants for multiple myeloma. *Blood* 93:51–54, 1999.

31. Rapoport BL, Falkson HC, Falkson G: Prognostic factors affecting the survival of patients with multiple myeloma. A retrospective analysis of 86 patients. *Afr Med J* 79:65–67, 1990.

32. Bataille R, Boccadoro M, Klein B, Durie B, Pileri A: C-reactive protein and beta-2 microglobulin produce a simple and powerful myeloma staging system. *Blood* 80:733–737, 1992.

33. Greipp PR, Gaillard JP, Kalish LA, et al.: Independent prognostic value for serum soluble interleukin-6 receptor (sIL-6R) in Eastern Cooperative Oncology Group (ECOG) Myeloma Trial E9487 [meeting abstract]. *Proc Annu Meet Am Soc Clin Oncol* 12:404, 1993.

34. Bartl R, Frisch B, Fateh-Moghadam A, Kettner G, Jaeger K, Sommerfeld W: Histologic classification and staging of multiple myeloma. A retrospective and prospective study of 674 cases. *Am J Clin Pathol* 87:342–355, 1987.

35. Greipp PR, Witzig TE, Gonchoroff NJ: Immunofluorescent plasma cell labeling indices (Li) using a monoclonal antibody (Bu-1). *Am J Hematol* 20:289–292, 1985.

36. Greipp PR, Katzmann JA, O'Fallon WM, Kyle RA: Value of beta 2-microglobulin level and plasma cell labeling indices as prognostic factors in patients with newly diagnosed myeloma. *Blood* 72:219–223, 1988.

37. Greipp PR, Witzig TE, Gertz MA, et al.: Clinical application of cell kinetics to patients with monoclonal gammopathy and multiple myeloma. *Cell Tissue Kinet* 23:348, 1990.

38. Boccadoro M, Marmont F, Tribalto M, et al.: Early responder myeloma: kinetic studies identify a patient subgroup characterized by very poor prognosis. *J Clin Oncol* 7:119–125, 1989.

39. Boccadoro M, Marmont F, Tribalto M, et al.: Multiple myeloma: VMCP/VBAP alternating combination chemotherapy is not superior to melphalan and prednisone even in high-risk patients. *J Clin Oncol* 9:444–448, 1991.

40. Latreille J, Barlogie B, Johnston D, Drewinko B, Alexanian R: Ploidy and proliferative characteristics in monoclonal gammopathies. *Blood* 59:43–51, 1982.

41. Cornelissen JJ, Sonneveld P, Schoester M, et al.: MDR-1 expression and response to vincristine, doxorubicin, and dexamethasone chemotherapy in multiple myeloma refractory to alkylating agents. *J Clin Oncol* 12:115–119, 1994.

42. Montecucco C, Riccardi A, Ucci G, et al.: Analysis of human myeloma cell population kinetics. *Acta Haematol (Basel)* 75:153–156, 1986.

43. Greipp PR, Oken MM, Kalish LA, Miller AM, Kyle RA: Independent prognostic value for plasma cell labeling index (PCLI) and beta 2-microglobulin (B2M) in Eastern Cooperative Oncology Group (ECOG) Myeloma Trial E9487 [meeting abstract]. *Proc Annu Meet Am Soc Clin Oncol* 11, 1992.

44. San Miguel JF, Garcia-Sanz R, Gonzalez M, et al.: A new staging system for multiple myeloma based on the number of S-phase plasma cells. *Blood* 85:448–455, 1995.

45. Katzmann JA, Greipp PR, O'Fallon WM, Kyle RA: Serum beta 2-microglobulin. *Mayo Clin Proc* 61:752–753, 1986.

46. Garewal H, Durie BG, Kyle RA, Finley P, Bower B, Serokman R: Serum beta 2-microglobulin in the initial staging and subsequent monitoring of monoclonal plasma cell disorders. *J Clin Oncol* 2:51–57, 1984.

47. Bataille R, Durie BG, Grenier J: Serum beta2 microglobulin and survival duration in multiple myeloma: a simple reliable marker for staging. *Br J Haematol* 55:439–447, 1983.

48. Bataille R, Vincent C, Revillard JP, Sany J: Serum beta-2-microglobulin binding activity in monoclonal gammopathy: correlative study and clinical significance. *Eur J Cancer Clin Oncol* 19:1075–1080, 1983.

49. Tricot G, Sawyer JR, Jagannath S, et al.: Unique role of cytogenetics in the prognosis of patients with myeloma receiving high-dose therapy and autotransplants. *J Clin Oncol* 15:2659–2666, 1997.

50. Rajkumar SV, Fonseca R, Lacy MQ, et al.: Beta 2-microglobulin and bone marrow plasma cell involvement predict complete responders among patients undergoing blood cell transplantation for myeloma. *Bone Marrow Transplant* 23:1261–1266, 1999.

51. Harousseau JL, Attal M: The role of stem cell transplantation in multiple myeloma. *Blood Rev* 16:245–253, 2002.

52. Greipp PR, San Miguel JF, Durie BG, et al.: A new International Staging System (ISS) for multiple myeloma (MM) from the International Myeloma Working Group. *Blood* 102:190a, 2003. Abstract 664.

53. Dewald GW, Kyle RA, Hicks GA, Greipp PR: The clinical significance of cytogenetic studies in 100 patients with multiple myeloma, plasma cell leukemia, or amyloidosis. *Blood* 66:380–390, 1985.

54. Fonseca R, Barlogie B, Bataille R, et al.: Genetics and cytogenetics of multiple myeloma: a workshop report. *Cancer Res* 64:1546–1558, 2004.

55. Rajkumar SV, Fonseca R, Dewald DW, et al.: Cytogenetic abnormalities correlate with the plasma cell labeling index and extent of bone marrow involvement in myeloma. *Cancer Genet Cytogenet* 113:73–77, 1999.

56. Lai JL, Zandecki M, Mary JY, et al.: Improved cytogenetics in multiple myeloma: a study of 151 patients including 117 patients at diagnosis. *Blood* 85:2490–2497, 1995.

57. Sawyer JR, Waldron JA, Jagannath S, Barlogie B: Cytogenetic findings in 200 patients with multiple myeloma. *Cancer Genet Cytogenet* 82:41–49, 1995.

58. Rajkumar SV, Fonseca R, Lacy MQ, et al.: Abnormal cytogenetics predict for poor survival after high-dose therapy and autologous blood cell transplantation in multiple myeloma. *Bone Marrow Transplant* 1999.

59. Drach J, Schuster J, Nowotny H, et al.: Multiple myeloma: high incidence of chromosomal aneuploidy as detected by interphase fluorescence in situ hybridization. *Cancer Res* 55:3854–3859, 1995.

60. Drach J, Angerler J, Schuster J, et al.: Interphase fluorescence in situ hybridization identifies chromosomal abnormalities in plasma cells from patients with monoclonal gammopathy of undetermined significance. *Blood* 86:3915–3921, 1995.

61. Zandecki M: Multiple myeloma-almost all patients are cytogenetically abnormal. *Br J Haematol* 94:217–227, 1996.

62. Brigaudeau C, Trimoreau F, Gachard N, et al.: Cytogenetic study of 30 patients with multiple myeloma: comparison of 3 and 6 day bone marrow cultures stimulated or not with cytokines by using a miniaturized karyotypic method. *Br J Haematol* 96:594–600, 1997.

63. Simpson DR, Berkahn LC, Squire J, et al.: Prognostic significance of cytogenetics in patients with multiple myeloma referred for autologous stem cell transplant (ABMT). *Blood* 90(suppl 1):527a, 1997.

64. Rajkumar SV, Fonseca R, Lacy MQ, et al.: Abnormal cytogenetics predict poor survival after high-dose therapy and autologous blood cell transplantation in multiple myeloma. *Bone Marrow Transplant* 24:497–503, 1999.

65. Seong C, Delasalle K, Hayes K, et al.: Prognostic value of cytogenetics in multiple myeloma. *Br J Haematol* 101:189–194, 1998.

66. Tricot G, Barlogie B, Jagannath S, et al.: Poor prognosis in multiple myeloma is associated only with partial or complete deletions of chromosome 13 or abnormalities involving 11q and not with other karyotype abnormalities. *Blood* 86:4250–4256, 1995.

67. Shaughnessy J Jr, Tian E, Sawyer J, et al.: Prognostic impact of cytogenetic and interphase fluorescence in situ hybridization-defined chromosome 13 deletion in multiple myeloma: early results of total therapy II. *Br J Haematol* 120:44–52, 2003.

68. Fonseca R, Oken MM, Harrington D, et al.: Deletions of chromosome 13 in multiple myeloma identified by interphase FISH usually denote large deletions of the q arm or monosomy. *Leukemia* 15:981–986, 2001.

69. Avet-Louseau H, Daviet A, Sauner S, Bataille R, Intergroupe Francophone du M: Chromosome 13 abnormalities in multiple myeloma are mostly monosomy 13. *Br J Haematol* 111:1116–1117, 2000.

70. Fonseca R, Harrington D, Oken MM, et al.: Biological and prognostic significance of interphase fluorescence is situ hybridization detection of chromosome 13 abnormalities in multiple myeloma: an Eastern Cooperative Oncology Group study. *Cancer Res* 62:715–720, 2002.

71. Fonseca R, Blood E, Rue M, et al.: Clinical and biologic implications of recurrent genomic aberrations in myeloma. *Blood* 101:4569–4575, 2003.

72. Zojer N, Konigsberg R, Ackermann J, et al.: Deletion of 13q14 remains an independent adverse prognostic variable in multiple myeloma despite its frequent detection by interphase fluorescence in situ hybridization. *Blood* 95:1925–1930, 2000.

73. Facon T, Avet-Loiseau H, Guillerm G, et al.: Chromosome 13 abnormalities identified by FISH analysis and serum beta2-microglobulin produce a powerful myeloma staging system for patients receiving high-dose therapy. *Blood* 97:1566–1571, 2001.

74. Perez-Simon JA, Garcia-Sanz R, Tabernero MD, et al.: Prognostic value of numerical chromosome aberrations in multiple myeloma: a FISH analysis of 15 different chromosomes. *Blood* 91:3366–3371, 1998.

75. Moreau P, Garban F, Facon T, et al.: Preliminary Results of the IFM9903 and IFM9904 protocols comparing autologous followed by miniallogeneic transplantation and double autologous transplant in high-risk de novo multiple myeloma. *Blood* 102:43a, 2003.

76. Kroger N, Schilling G, Einsele H, et al.: Deletion of chromosome band 13q14 as detected by fluorescence in situ hybridization is a prognostic factor in patients with multiple myeloma who are receiving allogeneic dose-reduced stem cell transplantation. *Blood* 103:4056–4061, 2004.

77. Moreau P, Facon T, Leleu X, et al.: Recurrent 14q32 translocations determine the prognosis of multiple myeloma, especially in patients receiving intensive chemotherapy. *Blood* 100:1579–1583, 2002.

78. Keats JJ, Reiman T, Maxwell CA, et al.: In multiple myeloma, t(4;14)(p16;q32) is an adverse prognostic factor irrespective of FGFR3 expression. *Blood* 101:1520–1529, 2003.

79. Drach J, Ackermann J, Fritz E, et al.: Presence of a P53 gene deletion in patients with multiple myeloma predicts for short survival after conventional-dose chemotherapy. *Blood* 92:802–809, 1998.

80. Greipp PR, Raymond NM, Kyle RA, O'Fallon WM: Multiple myeloma: significance of plasmablastic subtype in morphological classification. *Blood* 65:305–310, 1985.

81. Witzig TE, Gonchoroff NJ, Katzmann JA, Therneau TM, Kyle RA, Greipp PR: Peripheral blood b cell labeling indices are a measure of disease activity in patients with monoclonal gammopathies. *J Clin Oncol* 6:1041–1046, 1988.

82. Witzig TE, Dhodapkar MV, Kyle RA, Greipp PR: Quantitation of circulating peripheral blood plasma cells and their relationship to disease activity in patients with multiple myeloma. *Cancer* 72:108–113, 1993.

83. Witzig TE, Kyle RA, O'Fallon WM, Greipp PR: Detection of peripheral blood plasma cells as a predictor of disease course in patients with smoldering multiple myeloma. *Br J Haematol* 87:266–272, 1994.

84. Witzig TE: Detection of malignant cells in the peripheral blood of patients with multiple myeloma: clinical implications and research applications. *Mayo Clin Proc* 69:903–907, 1994.

85. Witzig TE, Gertz MA, Lust JA, Kyle RA, O'Fallon WM, Greipp PR: Peripheral blood monoclonal plasma cells as a predictor of survival in patients with multiple myeloma. *Blood* 88:1780–1787, 1996.

86. Rajkumar SV, Fonseca R, Lacy MQ, et al.: Plasmablastic morphology is an independent predictor of poor survival after autologous stem cell transplantation for multiple myeloma. *J Clin Oncol* 17:1551–1557, 1999.

87. Dimopoulos MA, Barlogie B, Smith TL, Alexanian R: High serum lactate dehydrogenase level as a marker for drug resistance and short survival in multiple myeloma. *Ann Intern Med* 115:931–935, 1991.

88. Dimopoulos MA, Moulopoulos A, Smith T, Delasalle KB, Alexanian R: Risk of disease progression in asymptomatic multiple myeloma. *Am J Med* 94:57–61, 1993.

89. Vacca A, Ribatti D, Roncali L, et al.: Bone marrow angiogenesis and progression in multiple myeloma. *Br J Haematol* 87:503–508, 1994.

90. Vacca A, Ribatti D, Roncali L, Dammacco F: Angiogenesis in B cell lymphoproliferative diseases. Biological and clinical studies. *Leuk Lymphoma* 20:27–38, 1995.

91. Rajkumar SV, Fonseca R, Witzig TE, Gertz MA, Greipp PR: Bone marrow angiogenesis in patients achieving complete response after stem cell transplantation for multiple myeloma. *Leukemia* 13:469–472, 1999.

92. Munshi N, Wilson CS, Penn J, et al.: Angiogenesis in newly diagnosed multiple myeloma: poor prognosis with increased microvessel density (MVD) in bone marrow biopsies. *Blood* 92:98a, 1998. Abstract 400.

93. Rajkumar SV, Leong T, Roche PC, et al.: Prognostic value of bone marrow angiogenesis in multiple myeloma. *Clin Cancer Res* 6:3111–3116, 2000.

94. Rajkumar SV, Mesa RA, Fonseca R, et al.: Bone marrow angiogenesis in 400 patients with monoclonal gammopathy of undetermined significance, multiple myeloma, and primary amyloidosis. *Clin Cancer Res* 8:2210–2216, 2002.

95. Sezer O, Niemoller K, Eucker J, et al.: Bone marrow microvessel density is a prognostic factor for survival in patients with multiple myeloma. *Ann Hematol* 79:574–577, 2000.

96. Munshi NC, Wilson C: Increased bone marrow microvessel density in newly diagnosed multiple myeloma carries a poor prognosis. *Semin Oncol* 28:565–569, 2001.

97. Rajkumar SV, Leong T, Fonseca R, et al.: Bone marrow angiogenesis has prognostic value in multiple myeloma. An Eastern Cooperative Oncology Group study. *Proc Am Soc Clin Oncol* 18:19a, 1999. Abstract 68.

98. Kishimoto T: The biology of interleukin-6. *Blood* 74:1–10, 1989.

99. Klein B, Zhang XG, Lu ZY, Bataille R: Interleukin-6 in human multiple myeloma. *Blood* 85:863–872, 1995.

100. Lust JA, Donovan KA: Biology and transition of monoclonal gammopathy of undetermined significance (MGUS) to multiple myeloma. *Cancer Control* 5:209–217, 1998.

101. Donovan KA, Lacy MQ, Kline MP, et al.: Contrast in cytokine expression between patients with monoclonal gammopathy of undetermined significance or multiple myeloma. *Leukemia* 12:593–600, 1998.

102. Nachbaur DM, Herold M, Maneschg A, Huber H: Serum levels of interleukin-6 in multiple myeloma and other hematological disorders: correlation with disease activity and other prognostic parameters. *Ann Hematol* 62:54–58, 1991.

103. Solary E, Guiguet M, Zeller V, et al.: Radioimmunoassay for the measurement of serum IL-6 and its correlation with tumour cell mass parameters in multiple myeloma. *Am J Hematol* 39:163–171, 1992.

104. Gaillard JP, Bataille R, Brailly H, et al.: Increased and highly stable levels of functional soluble interleukin-6 receptor in sera of patients with monoclonal gammopathy. *Eur J Immunol* 23:820–824, 1993.

105. Gaillard JP, Liautard J, Klein B, Brochier J: Major role of the soluble interleukin-6/interleukin-6 receptor complex for the proliferation of interleukin-6-dependent human myeloma cell lines. *Eur J Immunol* 27:3332–3340, 1997.

106. Lust JA, Donovan KA, Kline MP, Greipp PR, Kyle RA, Maihle NJ: Isolation of an mRNA encoding a soluble form of the human interleukin-6 receptor. *Cytokine* 4:96–100, 1992.

107. San Miguel JF, Gonzalez M, Gascon A, et al.: Immunophenotypic heterogeneity of multiple myeloma: influence on the biology and clinical course of the disease. Castellano-Leones (Spain) Cooperative Group for the study of monoclonal gammopathies. *Br J Haematol* 77:185–190, 1991.

108. Durie BG, Grogan TM: CALLA-positive myeloma: an aggressive subtype with poor survival. *Blood* 66:229–232, 1985.

109. Epstein J, Xiao HQ, He XY: Markers of multiple hematopoietic-cell lineages in multiple myeloma. *N Engl J Med* 322:664–668, 1990.

110. Neri A, Murphy JP, Cro L, et al.: Ras oncogene mutation in multiple myeloma. *J Exp Med* 170:1715–1725, 1989.

111. Matozaki S, Nakagawa T, Nakao Y, Fujita T: RAS gene mutations in multiple myeloma and related monoclonal gammopathies. *Kobe J Med Sci* 37:35–45, 1991.

112. Liu P, Leong T, Quam L, et al.: Activating mutations of N- and K-ras in multiple myeloma show different clinical associations: analysis of the Eastern Cooperative Oncology Group Phase III Trial. *Blood* 88:2699–2706, 1996.

113. Neri A, Baldini L, Trecca D, Cro L, Polli E, Maiolo AT: p53 gene mutations in multiple myeloma are associated with advanced forms of malignancy. *Blood* 81:128–135, 1993.

114. Drach J, Gattringer C, Glassl H, Drach D, Huber H: The biological and clinical significance of the KI-67 growth fraction in multiple myeloma. *Hematol Oncol* 10:125–134, 1992.

115. Girino M, Riccardi A, Luoni R, Ucci G, Cuomo A: Monoclonal antibody Ki-67 as a marker of proliferative activity in monoclonal gammopathies. *Acta Haematol* 85:26–30, 1991.

116. Ide K, Ahmann GJ, Roche PC, Greipp PR: Evaluation of a PCNA labeling index in multiple myeloma (MM). *Blood* 80:486a, 1992.

117. San Miguel JF, Gonzalez M, Gascon A, et al.: Lymphoid subsets and prognostic factors in multiple myeloma. Cooperative Group for the Study of Monoclonal Gammopathies. *Br J Haematol* 80: 305–309, 1992.

118. Oritani K, Katagiri S, Tominaga N, et al.: Aberrant expression of immunoglobulin light chain isotype in B lymphocytes from patients with monoclonal gammopathies: isotypic discordance and clonal B-cell excess. *Br J Haematol* 75:10–15, 1990.

119. Kay NE, Oken MM, Bone N, et al.: Circulating CD19+ blood cell levels in myeloma. ECOG Myeloma Clinical Trials Laboratory Study Group. *Blood* 86:4000–4001, 1995.

120. Kay NE, Leong TL, Bone N, et al.: Blood levels of immune cells predict survival in myeloma patients: results of an Eastern Cooperative Oncology Group phase 3 trial for newly diagnosed multiple myeloma patients. *Blood* 98:23–28, 2001.

121. Porrata LF, Gertz MA, Inwards DJ, et al.: Early lymphocyte recovery predicts superior survival after autologous hematopoietic stem cell transplantation in multiple myeloma or non-Hodgkin lymphoma. *Blood* 98:579–585, 2001.

122. Elomaa I, Virkkunen P, Risteli L, Risteli J: Serum concentration of the cross-linked carboxyterminal telopeptide of type I collagen (ICTP) is a useful prognostic indicator in multiple myeloma. *Br J Cancer* 66:337–341, 1992.

123. Trendle MC, Leong T, Kyle RA, et al.: Measurements of serum markers of bone metabolism in patients with newly diagnosed multiple myeloma: a study from the ECOG myeloma clinical trials group [meeting abstract]. *Proc Annu Meet Am Assoc Cancer Res* 38:446, 1997.

124. Brown RD, Joshua DE, Ioannidis RA, Kronenberg H: Serum thymidine kinase as a marker of disease activity in patients with multiple myeloma. *Aust N Z J Med* 19:226–232, 1989.

125. Cimino G, Avvisati G, Amadori S, et al.: High serum IL-2 levels are predictive of prolonged survival in multiple myeloma. *Br J Haematol* 75:373–377, 1990.

126. Greipp PR, Leong TL, Kay NE, Van Ness BG, Oken MM, Kyle RA: From ECOG myeloma trial E9486: a prognostic index based on tumor burden, proliferation and host immune status. *Blood* 90(suppl 1): Abstract 1561, 1997.

# Chapter 87

# TREATMENT OF RELAPSED OR REFRACTORY MULTIPLE MYELOMA AND NEW FRONTIERS IN MULTIPLE MYELOMA THERAPY

*Manmeet Ahluwalia and Mohamad A. Hussein*

## INTRODUCTION

Despite several recent therapeutic advances, multiple myeloma (MM) remains incurable, and unfortunately most patients experience relapse after responding to initial therapies, including high-dose chemotherapy and stem cell transplantation (SCT). Long-term remissions are rare. With conventional chemotherapy, the 5-year median survival rate is approximately 25%, and approximately 10% of patients live longer than 10 years.[1] Multiple regulatory pathways involving cytokines, adhesion molecules, angiogenesis, and resistance mechanisms contribute to the development and progression of the disease. The complex pathophysiology of MM makes it difficult to manage the disease successfully. Over the past 5 years, remarkable improvement in the understanding of the disease biology has resulted in the development of targeted therapy interrupting single or multiple survival pathways for the disease. Newer agents have been developed that have provided hope for better management of relapsed and refractory MM. Further research is ongoing to target multiple pathways of the disease simultaneously for more efficient and durable treatment of the disease.

## THE BIOLOGY OF MULTIPLE MYELOMA

The bone marrow microenvironment consists of extracellular matrix proteins, stromal cells, monoclonal myeloma cells, vascular endothelial cells, osteoblasts, osteoclasts, and lymphocytes. The interactions among the myeloma cells, stromal cells, adhesion molecules, cytokines, and the factors involved in angiogenesis play a key role in the pathogenesis of MM and in the refractoriness of the disease.

Multiple regulatory pathways are involved in the development and progression of MM. Interleukin 6 (IL-6) is an important cytokine in myeloma cell growth and proliferation.[2] Close cell-to-cell contact between myeloma cells and the bone marrow stromal cells triggers a large amount of IL-6 production that supports the growth of these cells and protects them from apoptosis induced by dexamethasone or other chemotherapeutic agents.[3] In addition, IL-6 can enhance the effect of other osteoclastogenic factors, such as receptor activator of nuclear factor (RANK) ligand (RANKL), parathyroid-hormone-related peptide (PTHrP), macrophage inflammatory protein 1α (MIP-1α), IL-1, and tumor necrosis factor α (TNFα).

Nuclear factor kappa B (NF-κB) is a protein that is believed to be central to the pathophysiology of MM. The Rel/NF-κB family of proteins includes inducible dimeric transcription factors that recognize and bind a common sequence motif in nuclear DNA.[4–7] NF-κB, the major transcription factor in this family, is a p50/RelA heterodimer (p50/p65) present in the cytoplasm of almost all cells.[7,8] NF-κB regulates cell growth and apoptosis, as well as the expression of various cytokines, adhesion molecules, and their receptors.[9] NF-κB is normally bound in the cytoplasm to its inhibitor I-κB.[7] Stimulation of cells by cytokines, stress, or chemotherapy can trigger signaling cascades that lead to activation of I-κB kinase (a heterodimeric protein kinase that catalyzes I-κB phosphorylation). I-κB is then degraded by the proteasome pathway, releasing free active NF-κB. After release from I-κB, activated NF-κB translocates to the nucleus and binds to the promoter regions of several target genes, thereby triggering their transcription. This in turn leads to increased expression of various cytokines and chemokines, adhesion molecules, and cyclin D, which promote cell growth and survival.[6] NF-κB activation also leads to increased expression of adhesion molecules, such as ICAM-1 and VCAM-1 by MM cells, thus facilitating the binding of the myeloma cells to stroma, in turn causing NF-κB-mediated upregulation of IL-6 secretion by the stromal cells and contributing to drug resistance.[10,11] Therefore, treatment strategies targeting NF-κB, the malignant cell–stroma interaction, and the complex cytokine network could result in regulation of the growth and development of the MM cells.

## DRUG RESISTANCE MECHANISMS

MM cells, unlike the cells of most other hematologic malignancies, are highly resistant to chemotherapy. The membrane cell survival proteins, Bcl-2 and Bcl-X$_L$, are overexpressed in most MM cells through interaction with the environment and are associated with inhibition of apoptosis. Upregulation of these antiapoptotic members of Bcl-2 contribute to the drug resistance seen in MM cells.[12,13] In a study by Tu et al., Bcl-X$_L$ overexpression in bone marrow biopsy samples strongly correlated with decreased patient response to melphalan, vincristine, doxorubicin, and dexamethasone.[13] Response rates were 83–87% in non-Bcl-X$_L$-expressing patients, compared to 20–31% in Bcl-X$_L$-expressing patients.[13]

Drug resistance continues to pose considerable challenge to successful treatment of MM patients.[14] Tumor cells develop resistance to cytotoxic agents due to several mechanisms, including those mediated by drug transporter proteins, such as P-glycoprotein (P-gp),[15] increased activity of the transcription factor, NF-κB,[16] or lung-resistance-related protein (LRP; a major vault protein).[17] Acquired drug resistance in MM cells usually manifests as a multidrug-resistant phenotype.[15,18]

The expression of P-gp has not been shown to be elevated in patients who have not received any chemotherapy or who have been treated only with melphalan.[19] P-gp expression may be elevated in approximately 75% of patients treated with vincristine, doxorubicin, and dexamethasone (VAD).[19,20] The degree of P-gp expression in myeloma cells correlates with the cumulative dose of doxorubicin and vincristine given to the patient.

LRP is a major nuclear vault protein that blocks the transport of drugs from the cytoplasm to the nucleus by forming central plugs of the nuclear pore complexes. Its spectrum of cross-resistance is wide, covering not only the classical multi-drug resistance (MDR) phenotype, but also the platinol- and melphalan-resistant phenotypes.[17,21] P-gp can be expressed in up to half of patients with MM, and is associated with a poor response to melphalan-based induction chemotherapy and shorter overall survival duration.[22] The response rate was lower in patients expressing LRP (54%) compared to those lacking it (87%). Thus, LRP has been proposed as an important genetic marker for predicting poor therapeutic response and outcome.[22] There is increased expression of LRP in patients with p53 deletion and P-gp. LRP and P-gp might share a similar regulatory mechanism

mediated by p53, and further research exploring the role of these genes is underway.[22]

## PROTEASOME INHIBITOR: BORTEZOMIB

Bortezomib (N-pyrazine carbonyl-L-phenylalanine-L-leucine boronic acid, previously known as PS-341 or MLN-341), a boronic acid dipeptide, is a specific inhibitor of the proteasome pathway.[23,24] Bortezomib inhibits the proteasome pathway in a rapid and reversible manner by binding directly with the 20S proteasome complex and blocking its enzymatic activity. The proteasome pathway regulates the degradation of the NF-κB inhibitor, I-κB.[25,26] Several effects of bortezomib, including the induction of apoptosis in the malignant plasma cell, appear to be mediated through inhibition of NF-κB. Bortezomib prevents the degradation of I-κB and thereby inhibits NF-κB activation.[5]

In view of encouraging in vitro data, a phase I study using bortezomib was initiated in patients with refractory hematologic malignancies (MM, lymphoma) to determine the maximum tolerated dose (MTD), dose-limiting toxicity (DLT), and pharmacodynamics of the molecule.[27] Bortezomib was administered at doses ranging from 0.4 to 1.38 mg/m$^2$, twice weekly for 4 weeks, followed by a 2-week rest. DLTs, including grade III hyponatremia, fatigue and malaise, and hypokalemia, were observed at the highest dose levels (1.38 mg/m$^2$ and 1.20 mg/m$^2$); 1.04 mg/m$^2$ was considered the MTD. Although grade IV events did occur, none was felt to be related to bortezomib. Evidence of antineoplastic activity was observed in patients with MM and non-Hodgkin's lymphoma. Of the nine evaluable patients with plasma cell dyscrasias, a complete response was observed in one patient, and the remaining eight showed evidence of decreased paraprotein levels or bone marrow plasmacytosis. In another phase I trial, DLTs were nonhematologic and included diarrhea and painful sensory neuropathy. Grade III sensory neuropathy was experienced by two of 12 patients treated at the highest dose level (1.56 mg/m$^2$).[28] Based on the preclinical and phase I activity in MM, a phase II study (SUMMIT) was initiated in patients with relapsed and refractory MM.[24] The dose established for bortezomib in the treatment of relapsed/refractory myeloma was 1.3 mg/m$^2$ given twice weekly on days 1, 4, 8, and 11 every 21 days.[24] This schedule of at least 72 h between the dosages of bortezomib allows for the recovery of the inhibited proteasome, thus minimizing the incidence of significant and severe side effects. Dexamethasone (20 mg the day of and after each bortezomib dose) was permitted if progressive disease was observed after two cycles, or in the presence of stable disease after four cycles. A total of 202 heavily pretreated patients were enrolled. Of the 202 patients entered, 193 were evaluable for response. The overall response rate [complete remission (CR) + partial response (PR) + minimal response (MR)] was 35% (67 of

193 patients). Seven patients (4%) had a CR, and 12 (6%) had a near-CR (NCR) (myeloma protein undetectable by electrophoresis but immunofixation positive). An additional 34 patients (18%) achieved a PR, and 14 (7%) others an MR.[24] The median time to disease progression for bortezomib as a single agent was 7 months, compared with 3 months that was reported for the patients' previous therapy ($P = 0.01$). In a landmark analysis, patients who achieved a CR or PR by the end of the second cycle survived significantly longer than those achieving other types of responses. Additional clinical benefits observed in these patients included increases in hemoglobin levels and platelet counts, resulting in a reduction in transfusion requirements. Moreover, levels of unaffected immunoglobulins improved. The factors that predicted poor response to bortezomib were older age ($\geq 65$ years) and $\geq 50\%$ plasma cells in the bone marrow. In this bortezomib trial, serum $\beta_2$-microglobulin level, number or type of previous therapies, and chromosomal abnormalities, including chromosome 13 deletions, did not predict for poor response. This observation might be important for future development of bortezomib therapy in combination with other agents or strategies, especially in patients with poor prognosticators.[24,29,30]

Drug-related adverse events of any grade occurring in >25% of patients included nausea (55%), diarrhea (44%), fatigue (41%), thrombocytopenia (40%), peripheral neuropathy (31%), vomiting (27%), and anorexia (25%). The most common grade III adverse events included thrombocytopenia (28%), fatigue (12%), peripheral neuropathy (12%), and neutropenia (11%). The most common grade IV events included thrombocytopenia (3%) and neutropenia (3%). Peripheral neuropathy was more likely to occur in patients who suffered from neuropathy at baseline (80%). Among the 33 patients who did not have evidence of peripheral neuropathy on study entrance, 17 developed peripheral neuropathy during the course of therapy. Most of the adverse events reported during the trial were manageable with standard supportive symptomatic therapy.

Bortezomib is an active agent in the management of relapsed/refractory MM, with responses occurring relatively quickly (within 6 weeks of the initiation of therapy). In view of its ability to sensitize myeloma cells to other biologics and chemotherapeutic agents,[22,31,32] further development using the agent in combination with other agents at low dosages is in progress. A maintenance strategy is being investigated as part of the phase III, APEX (Assessment of Proteasome Inhibition for Extending Remissions) trial. Studies defining the dose and the frequency are urgently needed to maximize the benefits of this drug's mechanisms of action.

## THALIDOMIDE

Thalidomide is unique in that it is the only anticancer agent in the treatment of MM that maintains the same high response rate in newly diagnosed as well as in the relapsed and refractory MM patients.[33,34] Thalidomide, also known as alpha-(N-phthalimido) glutarimide, consists of a two-ringed structure with an asymmetric carbon in the glutarimide ring that exists as an equal mixture of S- (−) and R- (+) enantiomers that interconvert rapidly under physiologic conditions. This makes attempts at isolation of the dextro form, in an effort to eliminate teratogenicity, unsuccessful. As it is sparingly soluble in water and ethanol, there is no intravenous formulation.[35] Thalidomide undergoes rapid pH-dependent hydrolysis in aqueous solution. Mean terminal half-lives for a 200-mg dose range from 4 to 9 h, whereas higher doses of 800 mg have a substantially longer terminal half-life of approximately 8 h.[36] Pharmacokinetics in renal and hepatic dysfunction is not well established; in patients with renal failure secondary to MM, however, similar dose levels to those for patients with non-impaired renal function are used.

Thalidomide inhibits angiogenesis and induces apoptosis of established neovasculature in experimental models.[37,38] The bone marrows of MM patients show prominent vascularization, which correlates positively with high plasma cell labeling index disease activity and independently confers a poor prognosis.[39–42] Moreover, the plasma levels of various angiogenic cytokines, such as basic fibroblast growth factor and vascular endothelial growth factor (VEGF), are elevated in patients with active myeloma.[40–42]

The first study of thalidomide in MM by Singhal et al.[43] consisted of 84 previously treated patients with refractory myeloma, 76 of whom had relapsed after high-dose chemotherapy. Oral thalidomide was administered as a single agent for a median of 80 days (range 2–465). The starting dose was 200 mg daily, and this was increased by 200 mg every 2 weeks to a maximum of 800 mg/day. The response was assessed based on a reduction of myeloma protein in serum or urine that lasted for at least 6 weeks. The serum or urine levels of paraprotein were reduced by at least 90% in eight patients, two had a complete remission (CR), six patients had a 75% reduction of paraprotein, seven patients had a 50% reduction, while six had a 25% reduction, accounting for a total rate of response of 32%. Reductions in the paraprotein levels were apparent within 2 months in 78% of the patients who responded to therapy. This was associated with increased hemoglobin levels and decreased numbers of plasma cells in the bone marrow. The microvascular density of bone marrow, however, did not significantly change in responding patients. After 12 months of follow-up, Kaplan–Meier estimates of the mean ($\pm$SE) rates of event-free survival and overall survival for all patients were $22 \pm 5\%$ and $58 \pm 5\%$, respectively.[43] A more recent follow-up included 169 patients with advanced myeloma, in whom 67% had abnormal cytogenetics (CG) and 76% a prior autotransplant.[44] A 25% reduction in the M protein was noted in 37% of

| | | | Partial | EFS | | OS | |
|---|---|---|---|---|---|---|---|
| References | No. of patients | Thalidomide dose (mg) | response or better (%) | % of patients | Duration of follow-up | % of patients | Duration of follow-up |
| Yakoub-Agha et al.[45] | 83 | 400 | 48 | 50 | 1 year | 57 | 1 year |
| Mileshkin et al.[45] | 75 | 600 | 28 | 50 | 5.5 months | 50 | 15 months |
| Neben et al.[47] | 83 | 400 | 20 | 45 | 1 year | 86 | 1 year |

**Table 87.1**    Thalidomide in relapsed/refractory multiple myeloma

EFS, event-free survival; OS, overall survival.

the patients, and $\geq 50\%$ reduction in 30% of the patients; NCR or CR occurred in 14%, more frequently in patients with low plasma cell labeling index and normal CG. Two-year event-free and overall survival rates were $20 \pm 6\%$ and $48 \pm 6\%$, respectively. Superior 2-year event-free and overall survival was seen in patients with normal CG, normal plasma cell labeling index, and $\beta_2$-microglobulin of 3 mg/L or less. The therapy was well tolerated considering that most of the patients were previously heavily treated for their advanced disease. At least one third of patients had mild or moderate constipation, weakness or fatigue, or somnolence. More severe adverse effects were infrequent (occurring in fewer than 10% of patients), and hematologic effects were rare.[43] Similar findings have been reported by other study groups (Table 87.1).

### COMBINATION THERAPY

Pegylated doxorubicin (Doxil), vincristine, and dexamethasone (DVd) is an active combination used in the management of newly diagnosed MM with equivalent response rates and quality of responses to those of VAD therapy.[48,49] Moreover, in the relapsed/refractory setting, the response rates are modest and durable only when patients achieve a NCR or better, which is a rare occurrence (overall response rate is 22% and NCR is <5%).[50] DVd significantly reduces the amount of abnormal angiogenic activity in treated patients; however, this finding does not impact progression-free survival.[48] Thalidomide has a direct antimyeloma effect in addition to its ability to modulate integrins, rendering the myeloma cell vulnerable and sensitized to different chemotherapeutic agents. It was combined with DVd in newly diagnosed active MM as well as in advanced progressing relapsed/refractory disease, with the primary objective of improving the response rate, quality of response, and of maintaining the antiangiogenic activity achieved with the DVd regimen. The overall CR/NCR rate was 47% in relapsed/refractory patients, compared to 46% in newly diagnosed disease.[50] Time to best response was similar for both groups. Stable disease or improvement occurred in 89% of the patients with relapsed/refractory disease.

Early studies from the University of Arkansas have shown that patients with $\beta_2$-microglobulin of 3gm/dL or less, normal CG, and normal plasma cell labeling index were the most sensitive to thalidomide therapy.[44] A phase II study evaluated the role and efficacy of thalidomide in combination with interferon alpha-2B.[46] In this trial, a multivariate analysis for overall survival demonstrated that age greater than 65 years (median, 9.2 months vs longer than 26 months; $P = 0.011$), raised serum lactate dehydrogenase levels ($P = 0.002$), and raised serum creatinine ($P = 0.007$) predicted inferior outcomes. Those factors could have been influenced by the addition of interferon to the therapy.

Overall, thalidomide as a single agent or in combination is well tolerated. Tolerability depends on the starting dose of therapy, the maximal target dose, the cumulative dose, and the type of agents with which thalidomide is combined and the intensity of the schedule for those agents. The most critical side effect that is noted is the increased incidence of deep venous thrombosis. Plasma cell dyscrasia appears to be associated with a high incidence of thrombotic events.[51] This finding is supported by the increased incidence of thrombotic events in patients with monoclonal gammopathy who are not receiving any active therapy. Of interest is the absence of any significant increase in the incidence of those events with the use of thalidomide in combination with dexamethasone, when the latter was used in a less intense schedule compared to the more frequent, intense steroid timetable.[33,34,52] When used in combination with chemotherapy, particularly anthracyclines, the incidence of deep venous thrombosis is significantly increased and can be reduced to baseline by the use of low-dose aspirin or low-molecular-weight heparin.[50,52] In summary, when thalidomide is used as a single agent or in combination with a nonintense steroid schedule (dexamethasone at 40 mg/day for 4 days with 10 days off), prophylactic anticoagulation is not warranted. When used in combination with anthracycline-based regimens, low-dose aspirin prevents deep venous thrombosis with no side effects.

In patients with relapsed or refractory disease who are slowly progressing, it is reasonable to consider the use of thalidomide as a single agent, starting with a low dose of 50 mg daily and incrementing this dose by 50 mg a week to a maximum of 400 mg/day. This dose strategy allows patients to develop tolerance to the side effects, especially somnolence, and capitalizes on the data suggesting that the cumulative dose in the first 3 months of therapy could influence the outcome of therapy.[45,47] If patients do respond to monotherapy, then progress at a later time, the addition of steroids provides another chance at a response that could be as high as 50%.[53] In patients with more advanced disease or with quickly progressing MM, the use of thalidomide in combination with steroids or chemotherapy is reasonable. In this population, the time to achieve a response is approximately 0.7 months, and the response rates are around 70%.[53] The use of thalidomide in combination with DVd improves the response rate and the quality of response. The progression-free survival at 14 months is significantly improved when compared to DVd alone, and the results appear to be better than what was noted with thalidomide and dexamethasone alone.[50,53] A phase III trial is in progress to compare dexamethasone and thalidomide to DVd-T.

## IMMUNOMODULATORY ANALOGS OF THALIDOMIDE

The efficacy of thalidomide has been limited by adverse effects, which include sedation, neuropathy, constipation, and deep vein thrombosis. This spurred the development of thalidomide-derived immunomodulatory analogs, known as immunomodulatory drugs (ImiDs). Like thalidomide, IMiDs inhibit angiogenesis and act directly on MM cells to induce both apoptosis and growth arrest in resistant cells. They also block the adhesion of myeloma cells to bone marrow stromal cells and the associated protection against apoptosis, and thus affect myeloma cell growth, survival, and migratory factors such as IL-6, tumor necrosis factor $\alpha$ (TNF$\alpha$), and VEGF. In addition, they expand natural killer cell and T-cell numbers, and improve function against human myeloma cells and enhance their susceptibility to antibody-dependent cell-mediated cytotoxicity in vivo.[54–56] The addition of an amino group at position 4 of the phthaloyl ring in thalidomide structure led to the generation of CC-4047, and with the further removal of a carbonyl on the ring CC-5013 (lenalidomide) was created. ImiDs are up to 50,000 times more potent at inhibiting TNF$\alpha$ than is the thalidomide parent compound in vitro, and are markedly more stable.[57]

Promising preclinical data led to the first phase I study of thalidomide analog CC-5013 in 2001, when 25 patients with relapsed and refractory MM were treated with 5–50 mg/day of CC-5013. Patients enrolled in this study had received a median of three prior regimens, including autologous SCT and prior thalidomide in approximately two thirds of the patients. Grade III myelosuppression developed after 28 days in all 13 patients treated at the highest dose level of 50 mg/day. In 12 of these patients, dose reduction to 25 mg/day was well tolerated and was considered the maximum-tolerated dose.[58] No significant constipation or neuropathy was seen in any cohort, and encouragingly, responses were seen in 17 (71%) of 24 assessable patients, including 11 patients (46%) who had received prior thalidomide.[58] Further studies evaluating CC-5013, either alone or in combination with dexamethasone, have shown encouraging results in patients with MM at first relapse, or for relapsed/refractory MM.[59] Further studies, including a phase III trial, are ongoing in evaluating the efficacy of CC-5013 (with and without dexamethasone) in patients with relapsed or refractory disease.[60]

In a recently published phase I trial of 24 patients with relapsed or refractory disease treated with CC-4047, Schey et al. reported encouraging results. Sixty-seven percent of patients achieved greater than 25% reduction in paraprotein, 13 patients (54%) had greater than 50% reduction in paraprotein, and four (17%) of 24 patients entered a CR.[61]

## ARSENIC TRIOXIDE

Arsenic trioxide is an antitumor agent with a multifaceted mechanism of action that induces apoptosis in vitro in MM cell lines and freshly isolated cells from MM patients. In preliminary studies, it has demonstrated good clinical activity in patients with late-stage MM. Arsenic trioxide affects myeloma cell survival, possibly through the inhibition of glutathione peroxidase, inducing apoptosis and inhibiting the proliferation of MM cell lines and primary MM cells in a dose-dependent manner.[62,63] Unlike the antitumor activity of dexamethasone, which is inhibited by IL-6, arsenic-trioxide-induced apoptosis is not prevented by IL-6.[63] Arsenic trioxide induces apoptosis through activation of caspases 8 and 10 in mutated p53 myeloma cells, while it does so by activation of caspase 9 in the mitochondrial apoptotic pathway in myeloma cells with functional p53.[64] In addition, it inhibits TNF$\alpha$-induced cell adhesion, inhibits secretion of IL-6 and VEGF, and increases dexamethasone-induced apoptosis.[65,66] The cytotoxic action of arsenic trioxide is increased when administered with ascorbic acid in vitro.[67]

Cross-resistance to other chemotherapeutic agents is less likely with arsenic trioxide because it can induce dose-dependent apoptosis in drug-resistant MM cell lines.[68] Antiangiogenic properties, such as inhibition of VEGF production and capillary formation, also promote the antitumor efficacy of arsenic trioxide.[68] In addition, treatment with arsenic trioxide increases lymphokine-activated killer cell activity and upregulates CD38 ligand and CD38 on immune effector cells and myeloma cells, indicating that immunomodulation may contribute to its antitumor activity.[69] A recent phase II, multicenter, open-label study of arsenic trioxide (ATO) was conducted in 24 MM patients (eight with relapsed disease and 16 refractory to prior therapy).[68]

Patients received ATO 0.25 mg/kg/day for 5 days/week during the first 2 weeks of each 4-week cycle. Sixteen patients had grade III or IV neutropenia and one required antibiotics. Eight of 24 (33%) patients had reductions in serum M-protein levels in excess of 25%, while an additional 6 (25%) patients had stable disease.[68] The median time to response was 67.5 days, with a median duration of response of 130 days.[68] Arsenic trioxide therapy lowered serum creatinine levels in two patients with high baseline values. These data show that ATO is active and reasonably well tolerated as a single-agent salvage therapy, even in patients with late-stage, relapsed and refractory MM.

## TRANSPLANTATION

The role of the autologous hematopoietic progenitor cell transplant in the management of relapsed MM evolved in the late 1980s and early 1990s. This is covered in greater detail in Chapter 83.

## NOVEL AGENTS

### FARNESYLTRANSFERASE INHIBITORS

Farnesylation is the first and most important step in the posttranslational modification of Ras proteins, which are mutated in up to 30–40% of patients with MM.[70] Mutated Ras activates Ras-dependent pathways, including the MAPK (mitogen-activated protein kinase) and the PK13 cascades, to form cross-linked complexes that favor cell survival. In preclinical trials, R115777 inhibited the growth and survival of MM cells even in the presence of IL-6.[71] In a phase II trial, R115777 was used to treat 43 patients who had previously received treatment for MM. Disease stabilization (defined as 0–25% decrease in the level of paraprotein) occurred in 64% of patients. Fatigue was the most common side effect.[72]

### HISTONE DEACETYLASE INHIBITORS

Histone deacytylase (HDAC) inhibitors are a new class of chemotherapeutic reagents that cause growth arrest and apoptosis of neoplastic cells. In a recent study, depsipeptide, a new member of the HDAC inhibitors, induced apoptosis in myeloma cell lines in a time- and dose-dependent fashion, and in primary patient myeloma cells.[73] Another HDAC inhibitor, suberoylanilide hydroxamic acid (SAHA), potently induced apoptosis of human MM cells.[74] SAHA treatment has been shown to suppress the activity of the proteasome and expression of its subunits, thereby enhancing MM cell sensitivity to proteasome inhibition by bortezomib (PS-341).[74] SAHA also enhances the anti-MM activity of other proapoptotic agents, including dexamethasone, cytotoxic chemotherapy, and thalidomide analogs.[74] This agent has shown encouraging results in a phase I trial.[75]

### INHIBITORS OF VEGF RECEPTOR

VEGF stimulates autocrine and paracrine growth of MM cells. VEGF achieves its action through its binding to three tyrosine kinase receptors—VEGF receptor 1(also called FMS-like tyrosine kinase receptor 1), VEGF receptor 2 (also called kinase insert domain containing receptor), and VEGF receptor 3 (also called FMS-like tyrosine kinase receptor 4).[76] VEGF receptor 1 is the most commonly expressed VEGF in MM patients. In a phase II study, no objective response was seen in patients with refractory MM when treated with VEGF receptor 2 (SU5416).[77] However, antiangiogenic properties of SU5416 can be used in combination with other agents in treating relapsed/refractory MM.

### BISPHOSPHONATES

Bisphosphonates have a widely recognized antiosteoclastic activity and have been shown to decrease skeletal events in patients with MM.[78] There is growing evidence of direct antitumor action of bisphosphonates on MM cells. Bisphosphonates act through inhibition of the ubiquitous mevalonate pathway, inducing apoptosis of tumor cells, suppressing proliferation and migration of endothelial cells, and by inhibiting angiogenesis.[76] In addition, bisphosphonates decrease IL-6 production and induce apoptosis of osteoclasts through inhibition of farnesyl and gernanyl transferase activity. Bisphosphonates increase $\gamma\delta$ T cells, which cause increased apoptosis of the MM cells.[79] Immunomodulatory effects of bisphosphonates are further being explored.

### OTHER AGENTS

Other agents that are under investigation for their role in the treatment of MM include those that act by interrupting intracellular signaling pathways, including the inhibitors of insulin-like growth factor 1 (IGF-1) receptor, inhibitors of the heat-shock protein 90, and the soluble RANKL antagonist, which decreases bone resorption. Inhibitors of lysophosphatidic acid acyltransferase $\beta$ (CT-32176, CT-32458, and CT-32615) in combination with HDAC inhibitors are under study for their role in MM treatment.[76] Table 87.2 lists new agents now under study for treatment of relapsed or refractory MM.

## SALVAGE THERAPIES

Traditionally, salvage therapies included combination chemotherapy, such as vincristine, doxorubicin, and dexamethasone (VAD). VAD was the first effective treatment for melphalan-resistant myeloma.[80] Other agents that have shown efficacy in relapsed or refractory myeloma, especially myeloma with high proliferative activity, include combinations such as DCEP (dexamethasone pulsing and 4-day continuous infusion

| Table 87.2   Novel agents under study in treatment of relapsed/refractory multiple myeloma |
| --- |
| Proteasome inhibitor (PS-341, bortezomib) |
| Thalidomide |
| Immunomodulatory derivatives (ImiDs) |
| Arsenic trioxide |
| Heat-shock proteins |
| Anti-VEGF antibodies |
| Farnesyltransferase inhibitors |
| Histone deacetylase inhibitors |
| Bcl-2 antisense molecules |
| 2-Methoxyestradiol |
| Bisphosphonates |
| IGF-1 receptor inhibitors |
| RANKL antagonist |
| Lysophosphatidic acid acyltransferase β inhibitors |
| Vaccines |

of cyclophosphamide, etoposide, and cisplatin) or DT-PACE, in which thalidomide and doxorubicin are added to DCEP.[81]

## SUMMARY

Disease progression in MM is associated with complex biologic pathways and processes, making it difficult to manage the disease successfully, and increasing the probability of relapse. The pathophysiology of MM contributes to the development of resistance to standard therapy. Over the past 2–3 years, there has been a remarkable expansion in drug development for MM that will probably result in a positive impact on survival. This has included development of bortezomib, lenalidomide, and "rediscovering" thalidomide and arsenic trioxide, agents that have shown promise in treatment of relapsed and refractory myeloma.

Novel treatment strategies are further needed to target the underlying pathogenic mechanisms, but they must be safe for a predominantly older patient population. Nontraditional therapeutic agents having novel mechanisms of action are under investigation. The current approach is to target the progression of myeloma at multiple different pathways simultaneously. It is probably time to proceed on two simultaneous developmental tracks: one, the continuation of the current strategy to develop targeted therapy; the other, to properly define the dose, frequency, and combination strategies of the available new agents. Combination of novel agents with established therapy may fill an unmet need in the management of relapsed/refractory MM.

## REFERENCES

1. Pandit S, Vesole DH: Relapsed multiple myeloma. *Curr Treat Options Oncol* 2:261–269, 2001.
2. Anderson KC, Lust JA: Role of cytokines in multiple myeloma. *Semin Hematol* 36:14–20, 1999.
3. Grigorieva I, Thomas X, Epstein J: The bone marrow stromal environment is a major factor in myeloma cell resistance to dexamethasone. *Exp Hematol* 26:597–603, 1998.
4. Gilmore TD, Koedood M, Piffat KA, White DW: Rel/NF-kappaB/IkappaB proteins and cancer. *Oncogene* 13:1367–1378, 1996.
5. Hideshima T, Chauhan D, Richardson P, et al.: NF-kappa B as a therapeutic target in multiple myeloma. *J Biol Chem* 277:16639–16647, 2002.
6. Karin M, Ben-Neriah Y: Phosphorylation meets ubiquitination: the control of NF-[kappa]B activity. *Annu Rev Immunol* 18:621–663, 2000.
7. Karin M: How NF-kappaB is activated: the role of the IkappaB kinase (IKK) complex. *Oncogene* 18(49):6867–6874, 1999.
8. Mitsiades N, Mitsiades CS, Poulaki V, et al.: Biologic sequelae of nuclear factor-kappaB blockade in multiple myeloma: therapeutic applications. *Blood* 99:4079–4086, 2002.
9. Almond J, Cohen GM: The proteasome: a novel target for cancer chemotherapy. *Leukemia* 16:433–443, 2002.
10. Chauhan D, Uchiyama H, Akbarali Y, et al.: Multiple myeloma cell adhesion-induced interleukin-6 expression in bone marrow stromal cells involves activation of NF-kappa B. *Blood* 87:1104–1112, 1996.
11. Hazlehurst LA, Damiano JS, Buyuksal I, Pledger WJ, Dalton WS: Adhesion to fibronectin via beta1 integrins regulates p27kip1 levels and contributes to cell adhesion mediated drug resistance (CAM-DR). *Oncogene* 19:4319–4327, 2000.
12. Hallek M, Bergsagel PL, Anderson KC: Multiple myeloma: increasing evidence for a multistep transformation process. *Blood* 91:3–21, 1998.
13. Tu Y, Renner S, Xu F, et al.: BCL-X expression in multiple myeloma: possible indicator of chemoresistance. *Cancer Res* 58:256–262, 1998.
14. Dalton WS: Mechanisms of drug resistance in hematologic malignancies. *Semin Hematol* 34:3–8, 1997.
15. Gottesman MM, Pastan I: Biochemistry of multidrug resistance mediated by the multidrug transporter. *Annu Rev Biochem* 62:385–427, 1993.
16. Wang CY, Cusack JC Jr, Liu R, Baldwin AS Jr: Control of inducible chemoresistance: enhanced anti-tumor therapy through increased apoptosis by inhibition of NF-B. *Nat Med* 5:412–417, 1999.
17. Scheffer GL, Schroeijers AB, Izquierdo MA, Wiemer EA, Scheper RJ: Lung resistance-related protein/major vault protein and vaults in multidrug-resistant cancer. *Curr Opin Oncol* 12:550–556, 2000.
18. Dalton WS, Jove R: Drug resistance in multiple myeloma: approaches to circumvention. *Semin Oncol* 26:23–27, 1999.

19. Grogan TM, Spier CM, Salmon SE, et al.: P-glycoprotein expression in human plasma cell myeloma: correlation with prior chemotherapy. *Blood* 81:490–495, 1993.

20. Cornelissen JJ, Sonneveld P, Schoester M, et al.: MDR-1 expression and response to vincristine, doxorubicin, and dexamethasone chemotherapy in multiple myeloma refractory to alkylating agents. *J Clin Oncol* 12:115–119, 1994.

21. Kitazono M, Sumizawa T, Takebayashi Y, et al.: Multidrug resistance and the lung resistance-related protein in human colon carcinoma SW-620 cells. *J Natl Cancer Inst* 91:1647–1653, 1999.

22. Yang HH, Ma MH, Vescio RA, Berenson JR: Overcoming drug resistance in multiple myeloma: the emergence of therapeutic approaches to induce apoptosis. *J Clin Oncol* 21:4239–4247, 2003.

23. Adams J, Palombella VJ, Sausville EA, et al.: Proteasome inhibitors: a novel class of potent and effective antitumor agents. *Cancer Res* 59:2615–2622, 1999.

24. Richardson PG, Barlogie B, Berenson J, et al.: A phase 2 study of bortezomib in relapsed, refractory myeloma. *N Engl J Med* 348:2609–2617, 2003.

25. Palombella VJ, Rando OJ, Goldberg AL, Maniatis T: The ubiquitin-proteasome pathway is required for processing the NF-kappa B1 precursor protein and the activation of NF-kappa B. *Cell* 78:773–785, 1994.

26. Palombella VJ, Conner EM, Fuseler JW, et al.: Role of the proteasome and NF-kappaB in streptococcal cell wall-induced polyarthritis. *Proc Natl Acad Sci U S A* 95:15671–15676, 1998.

27. Orlowski RZ, Stinchcombe TE, Mitchell BS, et al.: Phase I trial of the proteasome inhibitor PS-341 in patients with refractory hematologic malignancies. *J Clin Oncol* 20:4420–4427, 2002.

28. Aghajanian C, Soignet S, Dizon DS, et al.: A phase I trial of the novel proteasome inhibitor PS341 in advanced solid tumor malignancies. *Clin Cancer Res* 8:2505–2511, 2002.

29. Barlogie B, Desikan R, Eddlemon P, et al.: Extended survival in advanced and refractory multiple myeloma after single-agent thalidomide: identification of prognostic factors in a phase 2 study of 169 patients. *Blood* 98:492–494, 2001.

30. Desikan R, Barlogie B, Sawyer J, et al.: Results of high-dose therapy for 1000 patients with multiple myeloma: durable complete remissions and superior survival in the absence of chromosome 13 abnormalities. *Blood* 95:4008–4010, 2000.

31. Ma MH, Yang HH, Parker K, et al.: The proteasome inhibitor PS-341 markedly enhances sensitivity of multiple myeloma tumor cells to chemotherapeutic agents. *Clin Cancer Res* 9:1136–1144, 2003.

32. Yang HH, Vescio R, Schenkein D, Berenson JR: A prospective, open-label safety and efficacy study of combination treatment with bortezomib (PS-341), velcade and melphalan in patients with relapsed or refractory multiple myeloma. *Clin Lymphoma* 4:119–122, 2003.

33. Rajkumar SV, Hayman S, Gertz MA, et al.: Combination therapy with thalidomide plus dexamethasone for newly diagnosed myeloma. *J Clin Oncol* 20:4319–4323, 2002.

34. Weber D, Rankin K, Gavino M, Delasalle K, Alexanian R: Thalidomide alone or with dexamethasone for previously untreated multiple myeloma. *J Clin Oncol* 21:16–19, 2003.

35. Warren NJ and Celgene Corp: Thalomid capsules (thalidomide) prescription product insert; 1998.

36. Chen TL, Vogelsang GB, Petty BG, et al.: Plasma pharmacokinetics and urinary excretion of thalidomide after oral dosing in healthy male volunteers. *Drug Metab Dispos* 17:402–405, 1989.

37. D'Amato RJ, Loughnan MS, Flynn E, Folkman J: Thalidomide is an inhibitor of angiogenesis. *Proc Natl Acad Sci U S A* 91:4082–4085, 1994.

38. Kenyon BM, Browne F, D'Amato RJ: Effects of thalidomide and related metabolites in a mouse corneal model of neovascularization. *Exp Eye Res* 64:971–978, 1997.

39. Rajkumar SV, Fonseca R, Witzig TE, Gertz MA, Greipp PR: Bone marrow angiogenesis in patients achieving complete response after stem cell transplantation for multiple myeloma. *Leukemia* 13:469–472, 1999.

40. Vacca A, Ribatti D, Roncali L, et al.: Bone marrow angiogenesis and progression in multiple myeloma. *Br J Haematol* 87:503–508, 1994.

41. Vacca A, Ribatti D, Roncali L, Dammacco F: Angiogenesis in B cell lymphoproliferative diseases. Biological and clinical studies. *Leuk Lymphoma* 20:27–38, 1995.

42. Vacca A, Di LM, Ribatti D, et al.: Bone marrow of patients with active multiple myeloma: angiogenesis and plasma cell adhesion molecules LFA-1, VLA-4, LAM-1, and CD44. *Am J Hematol* 50:9–14, 1995.

43. Singhal S, Mehta J, Desikan R, et al.: Antitumor activity of thalidomide in refractory multiple myeloma. *N Engl J Med* 341:1565–1571, 1999.

44. Barlogie B, Desikan R, Eddlemon P, et al.: Extended survival in advanced and refractory multiple myeloma after single-agent thalidomide: identification of prognostic factors in a phase 2 study of 169 patients. *Blood* 98:492–494, 2001.

45. Yakoub-Agha I, Attal M, Dumontet C, et al.: Thalidomide in patients with advanced multiple myeloma: a study of 83 patients—report of the Intergroupe Francophone du Myelome (IFM). *Hematol J* 3:185–192, 2002.

46. Mileshkin L, Biagi JJ, Mitchell P, et al.: Multicenter phase 2 trial of thalidomide in relapsed/refractory multiple myeloma: adverse prognostic impact of advanced age. *Blood* 102:69–77, 2003.

47. Neben K, Moehler T, Benner A, et al.: Dose-dependent effect of thalidomide on overall survival in relapsed multiple myeloma. *Clin Cancer Res* 8:3377–3382, 2002.

48. Hussein MA, Wood L, Hsi E, et al.: A Phase II trial of pegylated liposomal doxorubicin, vincristine, and reduced-dose dexamethasone combination therapy in newly diagnosed multiple myeloma patients. *Cancer* 95:2160–2168, 2002.

49. Rifkin RM, Gregory SA, Mohrbacher A, et al.: Pegylated liposomal doxorubicin, vincristine, and dexamethasone provide significant reduction intoxicity compared with doxorubicin, vincristine, and dexamethasone in patients with newly diagnosed multiple myeloma: a Phase III multicenter, randomized trial. *Cancer* 106(4):848–858, 2006.

50. Hussein MA, Baz R, Srkaloviz G, et al.: Phase II study of pegylated doxorubicin, vincristine, decreased-frequency dexamethasone, and thalidomide in newly diagnosed and relapsed multiple myeloma. *Mayo Clin Proc* 81(7):889–895, 2006.

51. Srkalovic G, Cameron MG, Rybicki L, et al.: Monoclonal gammopathy of undetermined significance and multiple myeloma are associated with an increased incidence of venothromboembolic disease. *Cancer* 101:558–566, 2004.

52. Zangari M, Barlogie B, Anaissie E, et al.: Deep vein thrombosis in patients with multiple myeloma treated with thalidomide and chemotherapy: effects of prophylactic and therapeutic anticoagulation. *Br J Haematol* 126:715–721, 2004.

53. Anagnostopoulos A, Weber D, Rankin K, Delasalle K, Alexanian R: Thalidomide and dexamethasone for resistant multiple myeloma. *Br J Haematol* 121:768–771, 2003.

54. Davies FE, Raje N, Hideshima T, et al.: Thalidomide and immunomodulatory derivatives augment natural killer cell cytotoxicity in multiple myeloma. *Blood* 98: 210–216, 2001.

55. Hideshima T, Chauhan D, Shima Y, et al.: Thalidomide and its analogs overcome drug resistance of human multiple myeloma cells to conventional therapy. *Blood* 96: 2943–2950, 2000.

56. Lentzsch S, LeBlanc R, Podar K, et al.: Immunomodulatory analogs of thalidomide inhibit growth of Hs Sultan cells and angiogenesis in vivo. *Leukemia* 17:41–44, 2003.

57. Bartlett JB, Dredge K, Dalgleish AG: The evolution of thalidomide and its IMiD derivatives as anticancer agents. *Nat Rev Cancer* 4:314–322, 2004.

58. Richardson PG, Schlossman RL, Weller E, et al.: Immunomodulatory drug CC-5013 overcomes drug resistance and is well tolerated in patients with relapsed multiple myeloma. *Blood* 100:3063–3067, 2002.

59. Richardson P, Schlossman R, Jagannath S, et al.: Thalidomide for patients with relapsed multiple myeloma after high-dose chemotherapy and stem cell transplantation: results of an open-label multicenter phase 2 study of efficacy, toxicity, and biological activity. *Mayo Clin Proc* 79:875–882, 2004.

60. Richardson P, Anderson K: Immunomodulatory analogs of thalidomide: an emerging new therapy in myeloma. *J Clin Oncol* 22:3212–3214, 2004.

61. Schey SA, Fields P, Bartlett JB, et al.: Phase I study of an immunomodulatory thalidomide analog, CC-4047, in relapsed or refractory multiple myeloma. *J Clin Oncol* 22:3269–3276, 2004.

62. Park WH, Seol JG, Kim ES, et al.: Arsenic trioxide-mediated growth inhibition in MC/CAR myeloma cells via cell cycle arrest in association with induction of cyclin-dependent kinase inhibitor, p21, and apoptosis. *Cancer Res* 60:3065–3071, 2000.

63. Rousselot P, Labaume S, Marolleau JP, et al.: Arsenic trioxide and melarsoprol induce apoptosis in plasma cell lines and in plasma cells from myeloma patients. *Cancer Res* 59:1041–1048, 1999.

64. Liu Q, Hilsenbeck S, Gazitt Y: Arsenic trioxide-induced apoptosis in myeloma cells: p53-dependent G1 or G2/M cell cycle arrest, activation of caspase-8 or caspase-9, and synergy with APO2/TRAIL. *Blood* 101:4078–4087, 2003.

65. Hayashi T, Hideshima T, Akiyama M, et al.: Arsenic trioxide inhibits growth of human multiple myeloma cells in the bone marrow microenvironment. *Mol Cancer Ther* 1:851–860, 2002.

66. Hussein MA: Trials of arsenic trioxide in multiple myeloma. *Cancer Control* 10:370–374, 2003.

67. Grad JM, Bahlis NJ, Reis I, et al.: Ascorbic acid enhances arsenic trioxide-induced cytotoxicity in multiple myeloma cells. *Blood* 98:805–813, 2001.

68. Hussein MA, Saleh M, Ravandi F, et al.: Phase 2 study of arsenic trioxide in patients with relapsed or refractory multiple myeloma. *Br J Haematol* 125:470–476, 2004.

69. Hussein MA: Arsenic trioxide: a new immunomodulatory agent in the management of multiple myeloma. *Med Oncol* 18:239–242, 2001.

70. End DW: Farnesyl protein transferase inhibitors and other therapies targeting the Ras signal transduction pathway. *Invest New Drugs* 17:241–258, 1999.

71. Le GS, Pellat-Deceunynck C, Harousseau JL, et al.: Farnesyl transferase inhibitor R115777 induces apoptosis of human myeloma cells. *Leukemia* 16:1664–1667, 2002.

72. Alsina M, Fonseca R, Wilson EF, et al.: Farnesyltransferase inhibitor tipifarnib is well tolerated, induces stabilization of disease, and inhibits farnesylation and oncogenic/tumor survival pathways in patients with advanced multiple myeloma. *Blood* 103:3271–3277, 2004.

73. Khan SB, Maududi T, Barton K, Ayers J, Alkan S: Analysis of histone deacetylase inhibitor, depsipeptide (FR901228), effect on multiple myeloma. *Br J Haematol* 125:156–161, 2004.

74. Mitsiades CS, Mitsiades NS, McMullan CJ, et al.: Transcriptional signature of histone deacetylase inhibition in multiple myeloma: biological and clinical implications. *Proc Natl Acad Sci U S A* 101:540–545, 2004.

75. Kelly WK, Richon VM, O'Connor O, et al.: Phase I clinical trial of histone deacetylase inhibitor: suberoylanilide hydroxamic acid administered intravenously. *Clin Cancer Res* 9:3578–3588, 2003.

76. Bruno B, Rotta M, Giaccone L, et al.: New drugs for treatment of multiple myeloma. *Lancet Oncol* 5:430–442, 2004.

77. Zangari M, Anaissie E, Stopeck A, et al.: Phase II study of SU5416, a small molecule vascular endothelial growth factor tyrosine kinase receptor inhibitor, in patients with refractory multiple myeloma. *Clin Cancer Res* 10:88–95, 2004.

78. Ashcroft AJ, Davies FE, Morgan GJ: Aetiology of bone disease and the role of bisphosphonates in multiple myeloma. *Lancet Oncol* 4:284–292, 2003.

79. Kunzmann V, Bauer E, Feurle J, et al.: Stimulation of gammadelta T cells by aminobisphosphonates and induction of antiplasma cell activity in multiple myeloma. *Blood* 96:384–392, 2000.

80. Barlogie B, Smith L, Alexanian R: Effective treatment of advanced multiple myeloma refractory to alkylating agents. *N Engl J Med* 310:1353–1356, 1984.

81. Lee CK, Barlogie B, Munshi N, et al.: DTPACE: an effective, novel combination chemotherapy with thalidomide for previously treated patients with myeloma. *J Clin Oncol* 21:2732–2739, 2003.

# Section 2

# SPECIAL TOPICS IN MULTIPLE MYELOMA

## Chapter 88

# HYPERVISCOSITY SYNDROME

*Marcel N. Menke and Steve P. Treon*

## INTRODUCTION

Hyperviscosity syndrome (HVS) can be caused by various clinical conditions. It can be observed in conditions where the hematocrit is raised, such as polycythemia vera and pseudopolycythemia, or where serum proteins are increased or their composition is altered, such as in paraproteinemias, hyperfibrinogenemia, or hypoalbuminemia, as well as in inflammatory syndromes, hypothermia, increased red blood cell aggregability, and reduced red cell deformability due to various congenital and acquired conditions, such as sickle cell anemia, hyperlipoproteinemia, thrombosis, or diabetes.[1-8]

The most common cause of HVS encountered by hematologists is monoclonal and occasional polyclonal paraproteinemias, particularly those characterized by large molecular compounds with a high intrinsic viscosity, such as immunoglobulin M (IgM). Therefore, among cases of HVS caused by paraproteinemias the most frequent diagnosis is Waldenström's macroglobulinemia (WM), a B-cell disorder characterized by overproduction of monoclonal IgM. Approximately 17% of all WM patients show clinical symptoms related to hyperviscosity (HV).[9] HVS can also occur in patients with multiple myeloma, malignant lymphoproliferative diseases, lymphoma, monoclonal gammopathy of undetermined significance (MGUS), and primary amyloidosis.[2,10-12] These diseases can occur as a result of a monoclonal paraproteinemia of either IgM, IgG, or IgA.

## PATHOPHYSIOLOGY OF HVS

### IMMUNOGLOBULINS

Paraproteinemias due to excess concentrations of immunoglobulin molecules represent the main disorder of blood that primarily contribute to HVS. Excess concentrations of immunoglobulins are primarily present in the plasma. There are five immunoglobulin classes: IgG, IgA, IgM, IgD, and IgE.

Immunoglobulin M, with which HVS is most commonly observed, is a large molecular compound that is secreted in a pentamer form and weighs approximately one million daltons. IgM may bind water through its carbohydrate component and can also form aggregates. Due to its large size, 70–95% of the IgM produced is found in the intravascular compartment.[13,14] As a result of its osmotic draw, IgM leads to expanded blood volume, and can surreptitiously lead to a factitious anemia. Paraproteinemias due to smaller sized immunoglobulins, such as IgG and IgA, can also cause HVS, but usually at much higher serum levels than IgM due to their capacity to diffuse across blood barriers. Immunoglobulins, which are cationic, can also lower the repulsive forces between normally anionic erythrocytes and further contribute to HVS through rouleaux formation.[15]

### SYMPTOMATIC THRESHOLD OF VISCOSITY

Serum viscosity is often measured in centipoises (cp), which is a measure of viscosity relative to water. The normal range of serum viscosity is between 1.2 and 1.8 cp. Patients with nonmalignant inflammatory disorders can display elevated serum viscosities above 1.8 cp, but generally are under the symptomatic threshold leading to HVS. Fahey et al.[16] first reported on the "symptomatic threshold" of viscosity in 1965 in patients with monoclonal gammopathies. While acknowledging in their studies that the serum viscosity at which symptoms occurred varied between patients, no patient exhibited symptoms at a serum viscosity of less than 4 cp. Similarly, Crawford et al. reported in a series of 126 patients with monoclonal gammopathies that patients usually became symptomatic at serum viscosity levels of >4 cp, whereas, none of the patients in this series who had a serum viscosity of <3 cp exhibited HVS.[17] In a study of 56 patients with malignant paraproteinemias, retinopathy was always associated with serum viscosities ≥3.8 cp, though in some patients with serum viscosity levels between 2 and 3 cp, bleeding and neurologic symptoms were observed.[18] Numerous additional studies have also confirmed the appearance of symptoms at serum viscosity levels of 4–5 cp.[19–22]

While many investigators have focused on the use of serum viscosity levels to evaluate HVS, others have emphasized the use of whole blood viscosity wherein both immunoglobulin and hematocrit levels are taken into account.[23] However, in follow-up studies, MacKenzie et al. demonstrated that serum viscosity levels were as reliable as whole blood viscosity levels in identifying HVS in patients with monoclonal gammopathies.[24] This is probably due to the high concentration of immunoglobulins present in serum. However, HVS was reported in a patient with low immunoglobulin levels, in whom a high whole blood viscosity level was detected, which likely was due to extensive red cell paraprotein interactions. It therefore appears that evaluation of the whole blood viscosity may reveal in certain individuals the presence of HVS.

## CLINICAL FINDINGS

The clinical findings for HVS are summarized in Table 88.1. Symptoms due to HV can be categorized into (1) general symptoms, such as tiredness, fatigue, weight loss, and anorexia, (2) neurologic symptoms, such as headaches, nausea, vertigo, dizziness, ataxia, paresthesia, decreased hearing, and rarely coma, and (3) vascular disturbances, such as epistaxis, gingival and gastrointestinal hemorrhages or menorrhagia, congestive heart failure, retinopathy (including retinal hemorrhages), papilledema, dilated retinal veins and visual disturbances, and perfusion-related renal problems. The typical opthalmologic changes in a WM patient with HVS are depicted in Figure 88.1.

### ASSOCIATED MANIFESTATIONS OF HVS
#### Retinal findings
Circulatory disturbances due to HV can be best appreciated by ophthalmoscopy. Approximately 10% of

| Table 88.1 | Clinical symptoms of hyperviscosity |
| --- | --- |

(1) General symptoms
- Tiredness/fatigue
- Loss of weight
- Anorexia

(2) Neurologic symptoms
- Headache
- Nausea
- Vertigo
- Dizziness that can rarely lead to coma
- Ataxia
- Paresthesia
- Decreased hearing

(3) Vascular disturbance
- Epistaxis
- Gingival and gastrointestinal hemorrhages or menorrhagia
- Congestive heart failure
- HV-related retinopathy
- HV-related kidney problems

patients with HV due to WM have symptoms of visual disturbance, and up to 50% of these patients will demonstrate ocular changes.[25–27] The percentage of retinal involvement in patients with HV due to other paraproteinemias is unknown, but such cases have been reported.[28,29] In a recent study, Menke et al. examined 46 patients with WM by indirect ophthalmoscopy and the laser Doppler blood flow technique, which assessed retinal vessel diameter and blood flow.[30] These studies showed a relationship between retinal vessel caliber, particularly retinal veins, and serum viscosity, with increases in the caliber of vessels accompanying increases in serum viscosity.[28,30] Fluorescein angiography has also been used to investigate retinal microcirculation, with finding of increased arteriovenous passage times and vessel diameters in WM patients with increased serum viscosities.[28,29]

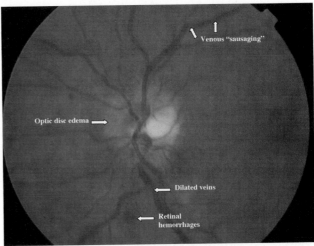

**Figure 88.1** *Ocular exam of a patient with Waldenström's macroglobulinemia depicting typical findings of hyperviscosity*

Among the first clinical signs of HV is the appearance of peripheral and mid-peripheral dot- and blot-like hemorrhages in the retina, which are best appreciated with indirect ophthalmoscopy and scleral depression.[30,31] In more severe cases of HVS, dot, blot, and flame-shaped hemorrhages can appear in the macular area, and may be accompanied by retinal edema and visual disturbance. Although visual acuity usually improves with plasmapheresis treatment, irreversible visual loss has been reported.[32] Some patients with HVS show papilledema and markedly dilated and tortuous veins with focal constrictions, predominantly at the arterio-venous junctions (i.e., venous sausaging). Other clinical findings associated with HVS can include intraretinal exudates resulting from more severe leakage from retinal vessels and retinal detachments.[33] Fluorescein angiography may be helpful in cases of intraretinal exudates in identifying areas of leakage.

### Corneal and conjunctival findings

Slitlamp examination frequently reveals sludging of red blood cells in the conjunctival vessels. Keratoconjunctivitis associated with HV in patients with WM has also been reported. In some cases, corneal and conjunctival crystals consisting of immunoglobulin deposits can be found in patients with paraproteinemia.[34]

### Neurologic findings

Common neurologic symptoms of HVS include headaches, nausea, vertigo, and dizziness, which rarely can progress to coma.[1,14,35,36] Some patients with HVS can show sensorineural hearing loss.[37] In most cases, neurologic symptoms usually appear at higher viscosity levels (i.e., >4 cp), though early appearance before retinal findings at lower serum viscosity levels (i.e., 2–3 cp) has also been reported.[18]

Several animal models have been used to investigate the neurologic consequences of HVS. The effects of blood hyperviscosity on functional integrity in the brain stem have been investigated using brain stem auditory evoked potentials.[38] Animals with elevated blood hyperviscosity showed either a total lack of any waveforms, or a prolongation of waves, indicating a severe disturbance in functional brain stem integrity, which could be improved partially with hemodilution therapy. In a study investigating the cerebral cortical blood flow and oxygen metabolism in newborn piglets with hyperviscosity, cerebral cortical blood flow and oxygen delivery were found to be decreased.[39] Moreover, in studies of the cerebral microcirculation in macroglobulinemic mice, decreased plasma velocities in the presence of increased serum viscosities were observed, whereas red blood cell velocities were within normal limits or even elevated. These findings suggest that alterations of viscosity can lead to disturbances in the microcirculation of the cerebral cortex, and are likely to account at least in part for the neurologic manifestations of HVS.[40]

### Kidney findings

Renal failure is an uncommon manifestation of HVS, and may result from perturbations in renal perfusion, leading to ischemic injury of the kidney. In experimental animal models, the influence of blood rheology on glomerular hemodynamics has been investigated. Elevation of either serum or whole blood viscosity resulted in renal vasodilation and decreased renal blood flow.[41,42] Ischemic acute tubular necrosis as a result of HVS has also been reported in a patient with WM.[43] In HVS-related renal dysfunction, decreased urine output, defects in concentrating and diluting urine, and increased serum creatinine may be observed.[43] In such cases, a kidney biopsy can be considered. Increased mesangial matrix, cytoplasmatic vacuolation of the epithelial cells lining the proximal tubules, foci of atypical lymphoplasmacytoid infiltration in the interstitium, and mitosis in the tubules as a sign of regenerative activity may be observed in biopsy specimens from a patient with HVS-induced renal injury.

## TREATMENT OF HYPERVISCOSITY SYNDROME

### PLASMA EXCHANGE/PLASMAPHERESIS

Plasmapheresis can be successfully used as an emergent therapy for patients with immunoglobulin-related HVS. Typically, two to four courses of plasmapheresis are required to achieve symptomatic control. However, marked improvement in HVS can occur even after the first course of plasmapheresis. The benefit of plasmapheresis usually lasts 4–6 weeks in patients with immunoglobulin-related HVS, and should be considered a temporizing measure until definitive therapy can be initiated to control disease.[44] Plasmapheresis can also be effective in reverting HV-associated retinopathy.[28,30,45,46] Improvements in renal function after plasmapheresis have also been reported in patients with hyperviscosity-related renal failure.[43]

In general, the response of patients to plasmapheresis depends on three main factors: (1) the intravascular component of the protein; (2) the volume exchanged; and (3) the synthesis rate of the protein being removed. The IgM molecule is large, with 70–95% localized in the intravascular compartment. A single plasma exchange can result in a reduction in serum IgM by 35%, with a concomitant decrease of 50–60% in serum viscosity.[47] In contrast to IgM, only 40% of IgG and IgA immunoglobulins are intravascular. Therefore, plasmapheresis is more likely to be successful in patients with WM, as opposed to multiple myeloma. There is no evidence that regular removal of monoclonal proteins accelerates or reduces their rate of synthesis. Concurrent systemic chemotherapy is therefore required for long-term management. However, plasmapheresis may be rarely indicated on a long-term basis in patients with hyperviscosity who are drug resistant or whose only clinical problem is due to the paraprotein (e.g., immunoglobulin-related neuropathy) rather than tumor burden.[14]

## REFERENCES

1. Gertz MA, Kyle RA: Hyperviscosity syndrome. *J Intens Care Med* 10(3):128–141, 1995 May–Jun.
2. Kyle RA, Garton JP: The spectrum of IgM monoclonal gammopathy in 430 cases. *Mayo Clin Proc* 62(8): 719–731, 1987 Aug.
3. Pickart LR, Thaler MM: Fatty acids, fibrinogen and blood flow: a general mechanism for hyperfibrinogenemia and its pathologic consequences. *Med Hypotheses* 6(5): 545–557, 1980 May.
4. Richardson SG, Matthews KB, Cruickshank JK, Geddes AM, Stuart J: Coagulation activation and hyperviscosity in infection. *Br J Haematol* 42(3):469–480, 1979 Jul.
5. Eckmann DM, Bowers S, Strecker M, Cheung AT: Hematocrit, volume expander, temperature, and shear rate effects on blood viscosity. *Anesth Analg* 91(3): 539–545, 2000 Sep.
6. Koppensteiner R: Blood rheology in emergency medicine. *Semin Thromb Hemost* 22(1):89–91, 1996.
7. Somer T, Meiselman HJ: Disorders of blood viscosity. *Ann Med* 25(1):31–39, 1993 Feb.
8. Gordge MP, Patel A, Faint RW, Rylance PB, Neild GH: Blood hyperviscosity and its relationship to progressive renal failure in patients with diabetic nephropathy. *Diabet Med* 7(10):880–886, 1990 Dec.
9. Merlini G, Baldini L, Broglia C, et al.: Prognostic factors in symptomatic Waldenstrom's macroglobulinemia. *Semin Oncol* 30(2):211–215, 2003 Apr.
10. Kopp WL, Beirne GJ, Burns RO: Hyperviscosity syndrome in multiple myeloma. *Am J Med* 43(1):141–146, 1967 Jul.
11. Lindsley M, Teller D, Noonan B, Peterson M, Mannik M: Hyperviscosity syndrome in multiple myeloma. A reversible, concentration-dependent aggregation of the myeloma protein. *Am J Med* 54(4):682–688, 1973 May.
12. Tuddenham EGD, Whittaker JA, Bradley JS, Lilleyman JS, James DR: Hyperviscosity syndrome in IgA multiple myeloma. *Br J Haematol* 27:65–76, 1974.
13. Jensen KB: Metabolism of human γ-macroglobulin (IGM) in normal man. *Scand J Clin Lab Invest* 24:205, 1969.
14. Johnson SA: Waldenström's macroglobulinemia. *Rev Clin Hematol* 6(4):421–434, 2002 Dec.
15. Ballas SK: The erythrocyte sedimentation rate, rouleaux formation and hyperviscosity syndrome. Theory and fact. *Am J Clin Pathol* 63(1):45–48, 1975 Jan.
16. Fahey JL, Barth WF, Solomon A: Serum hyperviscosity syndrome. *JAMA* 192:464–467, 1965.
17. Crawford J, Cox EB, Cohen HJ: Evaluation of hyperviscosity in monoclonal gammopathies. *Am J Med* 79(1): 13–22, 1985 Jul.
18. Russel JA, Powles RL: The relationship between serum viscosity, hypervolemia and clinical manifestations associated with circulating paraprotein. *Br J Haematol* 39(2): 163–175, 1978 Jun.
19. Capra JD, Kunkel HG: Aggregation of gamma-G3 proteins: relevance to the hyperviscosity syndrome. *J Clin Invest* 49(3):610–621, 1970 Mar.
20. Castleman B, Scully RE, McNeely BU: Case records of the Massachusetts General Hospital. Weekly clinicopathological exercises. *N Engl J Med* 34:213, 1972.
21. Dine ME, Guay AT, Snyder LM: Hyperviscosity syndrome with IgA myeloma. *Am J Med Sci* 264(2):111–115, 1972 Aug.
22. Wolf RE, Alperin JB, Ritzmann SE, Levin WC: IgG-K-multiple myeloma with hyperviscosity syndrome—response to plasmapheresis. *Arch Intern Med* 129(1): 114–117, 1972 Jan.
23. Mannik M: Blood viscosity in Waldenström's macroglobulinemia. *Blood* 44(1):87–98, 1974 Jul.
24. MacKenzie MR, Lee TK: Blood viscosity in Waldenström macroglobulinemia. *Blood* 49(4):507–510, 1977 Apr.
25. Deuel TF, Davis P, Avioli LV: Waldenstrom's macroglobulinemia. *Arch Intern Med* 143(5):986–988, 1983 May.
26. McCallister BD, Bayrd ED, Harrison EG, Mc Guckin WF: Primary macroglobulinemia: review with a report of thirty-one cases and notes on the value of continous chlorambucil therapy. *Am J Med* 43:394–434, 1967.
27. Martin NH: Macroglobulinemia. A clinical and pathological study. *Q J Med* 29:179–197, 1960 Apr.
28. Luxenberg MN, Mausolf FA: Retinal circulation in the hyperviscosity syndrome. *Am J Ophthalmol* 70(4): 588–598, 1970 Oct.
29. Dobberstein H, Solbach U, Weinberger A, Wolf S: Correlation between retinal microcirculation and blood viscosity in patients with hyperviscosity syndrome. *Clin Hemorheol Microcirc* 20:31–35, 1999.
30. Menke MN, Feke GT, McMeel JW, Branagan A, Hunter Z, Treon SP: Hyperviscosity-related retinopathy in Waldenström's macroglobulinemia. *Arch Ophthalmol* In press.
31. Goen TM, Terry JE: Mid-peripheral hemorrhages secondary to Waldenström's macroglobulinemia. *J Am Optom Assoc* 57(2):109–112, 1986 Feb.
32. Thomas EL, Olk RJ, Markman M, Braine H, Patz A: Irreversible visual loss in Waldenstrom's macroglobulinemia. *Br J Ophthalmol* 67(2): 102–106, 1983 Feb.
33. Grindle CF, Buskard NA, Newman DL: Hyperviscosity retinopathy. A scientific approach to therapy. *Trans Ophthalmol Soc U K* 96(2):216–219, 1976 Jul.
34. Orellana J, Friedman AH: Ocular manifestations of multiple myeloma, Waldenstrom's macroglobulinemia and benign monoclonal gammopathy. *Surv Ophthalmol* 26(3):157–169, 1981 Nov–Dec.
35. Gertz MA, Fonseca R, Rajkumar SV: Waldenström's macroglobulinemia. *Oncologist* 5(1):63–67, 2000.
36. Blumenthal DT, Glenn MJ: Neurologic manifestations of hematologic disorders. *Neurol Clin* 20(1):265–281, 2002 Feb.
37. Syms MJ, Arcila ME, Holtel MR: Waldenstrom's macroglobulinemia and sensorineural hearing loss. *Am J Otolaryngol* 22(5):349–353, 2001 Sep–Oct.
38. Bernath I, Bernat I, Pongracz E, Koves P, Szakacs Z, Horvath A: Effects of blood hyperviscosity on functional

intergrity in the brain stem: a brain stem evoked auditory potential study. *Clin Hemorheol Microcirc* 31(2): 123–128, 2004.

39. Goldstein M, Stonestreet BS, Brann BS IV, Oh W: Cerebral cortical blood flow and oxygen metabolism in normocythemic hyperviscous newborn piglets. *Pediatr Res* 24(4):486–489, 1988 Oct.

40. Rosenblum WI: Erythrocyte velocity and fluorescein transit time in the cerebral microcirculation of macroglobulinemic mice: differential effect of a hyperviscosity syndrome on the passage time of erythrocytes and plasma. *Microvasc Res* 3(3):288–296, 1971 Jul.

41. Simchon S, Chen RY, Carlin RD, Fan FC, Jan KM, Chien S: Effects of blood viscosity on plasma renin activity and renal hemodynamics. *Am J Physiol* 250:F40–F46, 1986 Jan.

42. McDonald KM: Influence of blood rheology on intrarenal blood flow distribution. *Am J Physiol* 230(5):1448–1454, 1976 May.

43. Wong PN, Mak SK, Lo KY, Tong GM, Wong AK: Acute tubular necrosis in a patient with Waldenstrom's macroglobulinemia and hyperviscosity syndrome. *Nephrol Dial Transplant* 15(10):1684–1687, 2000 Oct.

44. Gertz MA, Anagnostopoulos A, Anderson K, et al.: Treatment recommendations in Waldenstrom's macroglobulinemia: consensus panel recommendations from the Second International Workshop on Waldenstrom's Macroglobulinemia. *Semin Oncol* 30(2):121–126, 2003 Apr.

45. Feman SS, Stein RS: Waldenstrom's macroglobulinemia, a hyperviscosity manifestation of venous stasis retinopathy. *Int Ophthalmol* 4(1–2):107–112, 1981 Aug.

46. Freidman AH, Marchevsky A, Odel JG, Gerber MA, Thung SN: Immunofluorescent studies of the eye in Waldenstrom's macroglobulinemia. *Arch Ophthalmol* 98(4):743–746, 1980 Apr.

47. Reinhart WH, Lutolf O, Nydegger UR, Mahler F, Straub PW: Plasmapheresis for hyperviscosity syndrome in macroglobulinemia Waldenstrom and multiple myeloma: influence on blood rheology and the microcirculation. *J Lab Clin Med* 119(1):69–76, 1992 Jan.

# Chapter 89

# MONOCLONAL GAMMOPATHY OF UNDETERMINED SIGNIFICANCE

*Shaji Kumar, Philip R. Greipp*

## BACKGROUND AND DEFINITIONS

Presence of small amounts of monoclonal protein in the serum detected by protein electrophoresis, in the absence of clinical or laboratory evidence of multiple myeloma (MM), Waldenström macroglobulinemia, light chain amyloidosis, or related disorders, was described over half a century ago. Since Waldenström's initial description of "essential hyperglobulinemia," this entity has been described by multiple terms, including idiopathic paraproteinemia and idiopathic, asymptomatic, benign, or nonmyelomatous, monoclonal gammopathy. The common theme to all these early descriptions was the presumed "benign" nature of the abnormality and the relatively stable levels of paraprotein in these patients. However, long-term follow-up of these patients has proven that "benign monoclonal gammopathy" is a misnomer. These patients have a definite risk of progression to MM, macroglobulinemia, or amyloidosis, and at the time of diagnosis it is impossible to predict with any degree of confidence as to who will have disease progression. This led to coining of the term monoclonal gammopathy of undetermined significance (MGUS), highlighting the uncertain nature of the abnormality at the time of initial detection.

The hallmark of MGUS is the presence of monoclonal protein (M protein) in individuals with no clinical or laboratory evidence of MM, macroglobulinemia, light chain amyloidosis, or related plasma cell disorders. It is characterized by M protein less than 3 gm/dL in the serum with an absence or small amounts of M protein in the urine; fewer than 10% clonal plasma cells in the bone marrow; absence of bony lytic lesions, anemia, hypercalcemia, or renal insufficiency related to the paraproteinemia. While some of the abnormalities, such as anemia and renal insufficiency, are common in this patient population, it is imperative that an alternate cause for the abnormality be identified prior to making the diagnosis of MGUS. The stability of the paraprotein over time and lack of development of additional abnormalities are important for the definition of MGUS, though at the time of initial detection of the M protein these factors are indeterminate. Some studies that followed these patients for long term have required demonstrated stability of the M protein for at least 1 year for inclusion in the study.

## EPIDEMIOLOGY

There appear to be some variation in the prevalence of this disease, based on geography and race. In a study from a small southeastern Minnesota community, M protein was found in 15 of the 1200 adults (1.25%) aged 50 years or older.[1] In a study from Sweden, of 6995 adult patients aged 25 years or older, Axelsson reported presence of an M protein in 1%.[2] Saleun et al. detected a monoclonal protein in the sera of 334 persons, from among 30,279 French adults studied, translating to a prevalence of 1.1%.[3] In a study from Greece, a paraprotein was detected in 75 of the 1564 patients (aged 50–95 years) studied, of whom 60 were classified as having MGUS.[4] Among Japanese patients older than 50 years, Kurihara reported the presence of M protein in 71 of 2007 samples (3.5%).[5] In a convenience sample of community-dwelling elderly subjects aged 63–95 years seen for health screening examinations, Bowden found an M protein in 2.7% of Japanese, compared to 10% of Americans.[6] African Americans have been reported to have a higher prevalence of M proteins compared to that reported in Caucasians.[7] In a study of 1732 elderly subjects (>70 years) selected by stratified random household sampling, Cohen found 106 (6.1%) with a monoclonal gammopathy.[8] African Americans (8.4%) had a greater than twofold prevalence of monoclonal gammopathy compared to whites (3.8%).

The prevalence of monoclonal gammopathy increases with age, and is greater in men than women.[9] In the Japanese study, 11% of those from 80 to 89 years had detectable paraprotein in the sera.[5] In the study by

Cohen, the incidence of MGUS among those older than 70 years was 3.6%.[8] In a study of residents from a retirement home, the prevalence of monoclonal gammopathies was 6% in those younger than 80 years, compared to 14% in those older than 90 years.[10] Ligthart et al. reported the presence of M protein among 23% of 439 patients aged 75–84, compared to a control group aged 25–34 years, of whom none had a detectable paraprotein.[11] There is a slight preponderance of male gender among MGUS patient populations (Male:Female ratio of 1.1 to 1.2).[8,12–14] A familial occurrence of monoclonal gammopathies has been reported.[15]

## DIAGNOSIS

The detection of a paraprotein in the serum is often an incidental finding in a healthy individual undergoing routine testing, or in someone undergoing evaluation for an unrelated disorder. An agarose gel electrophoresis is the preferred method for evaluation of M protein in the serum, and is more sensitive than cellulose acetate. The monoclonal protein appears as a localized band on the agarose gel electrophoresis, and when converted to a densitometric tracing appears as a tall spike or peak (Figure 89.1). The M spike is usually seen in the $\beta$ or $\gamma$ region of the densitometer tracing, though occa-

sionally it can occupy the $\alpha_2$-globulin region. In contrast, a polyclonal increase in the gamma globulin is manifested as a broad peak in the $\gamma$ region. Once an electrophoretic abnormality suggestive of M protein is seen on the electrophoresis, immunofixation should be performed to confirm the presence of the monoclonal protein as well as to characterize the heavy-chain class (G, A, M, E, or D) and the type of light chain ($\kappa$ or $\lambda$). In addition to identifying the presence of the monoclonal protein, the protein can be quantitated by rate nephelometry, which is important for the follow-up of these patients. Nephelometry results may be higher than those expected on the basis of the densitometry tracing from serum protein electrophoresis, especially in the case of IgM.

An M protein may also be present in the urine, which should be examined in patients with monoclonal gammopathies. Similar techniques are used for urine protein electrophoresis, and should be performed on 24-h collections. The percentage of M protein on the densitometer tracing, and the total protein excretion over a 24-hour period, will allow calculation of the M protein excreted during this time period.

Once an M protein is identified, the next step is to rule out the presence of another plasma cell disorder, such as MM, amyloidosis, or macroglobulinemia (see differential diagnosis, below). A compete blood count

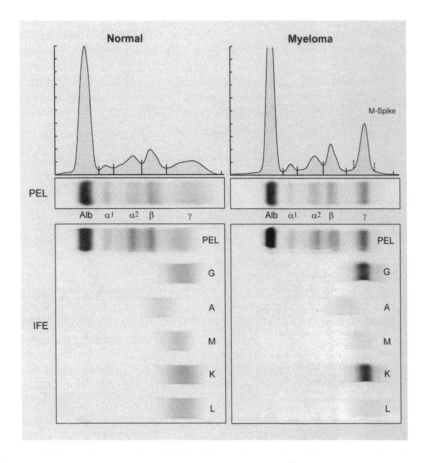

**Figure 89.1** *Serum protein electrophoresis and immunofixation. The left side panels show the protein electrophoresis and immunofixation pattern from a normal serum sample. On the right is a patient with myeloma and IgG kappa monoclonal protein. The monoclonal protein appears as an abnormal band on the agarose gel electrophoresis that is converted to an M-spike in the gamma region on the densitometric tracing. The immunofixation demonstrates the type pf M-protein as an IgG kappa*

and chemistry panel, including calcium and creatinine, should be obtained in all individuals. C-reactive protein and $\beta_2$-microglobulin levels should be obtained as well. The presence of anemia or renal insufficiency points toward a more advanced plasma cell proliferative disorder, unless another explanation is found. A bone marrow biopsy to estimate the plasma cell percentage is not necessary for the diagnosis of MGUS, and should be reserved for those with higher amounts of M protein ($>1.5$ gm/dL) or if there is a strong clinical suspicion for another plasma cell disorder. A skeletal survey that includes films of the long bones and skull should be obtained, especially in those with larger M-protein levels and in those whom clinical suspicion for MM is high.

## CLINICAL AND LABORATORY FEATURES

The majority of patients with MGUS are asymptomatic. Exceptions are the patients in whom associated disorders develop, the strongest association being neuropathy, as described below (Associated Disorders). The median age at diagnosis of MGUS was 72 years in the Mayo Clinic series and 63 years (24–91 years) in the Italian series.[12,13] Laboratory findings include the M protein in serum, which is less than 3 gm/dL by definition. The median M-protein concentration in the 1384 patients reported by Kyle et al. was 1.3 gm/dL (range: unmeasurable to 3 gm/dL). The M protein was an IgG subtype in nearly two-third of the patients, IgA in 12%, and IgM in 15%.[13] IgD MGUS is rare, and isolated case reports can be seen in the literature.[16,17] Given the rarity of this class of immunoglobulins among MGUS patients, finding an IgD spike should raise suspicion of MM, amyloidosis, or plasma cell leukemia. A biclonal gammopathy (presence of two distinct monoclonal proteins) was seen in about 3% of patients. The light chain was kappa in nearly 60% and lambda in the remaining 40%. The levels of the polyclonal uninvolved immunoglobulins were decreased in nearly a third of the patients in this study. Other studies have reported lesser proportions of patients with reductions in the polyclonal immunoglobulins.[12] Light chains were detectable in 31% of patients with MGUS, with only 17% having 24-h light chain excretions of over 150 mg. The bone marrow plasma cell percentage, when evaluated, varies between 0 and 10%, with median values of 3–5% in different studies.[12,13] The plasma cell labeling index (PCLI), a measure of the plasma cell proliferative rate, is characteristically low. Anemia may be present in some of the patients, and is usually related to iron deficiency, renal insufficiency, or myelodysplasia, which are common in this population. Nearly 23% of patients in the Mayo study had hemoglobin values of less than 12 gm/dL.

Conventional cytogenetics fail to demonstrate any significant chromosomal abnormalities in the plasma cells in MGUS, which is likely a reflection of the low proliferative rate of these cells. More recently, several authors have reported the presence of chromosomal abnormalities in MGUS, similar to that seen in myeloma, using interphase fluorescence in situ hybridization techniques.[18–21] Fonseca et al. studied 59 patients with MGUS in whom 27 (46%) had IgH translocations. A t(11;14)(q13;q32) was found in 15 (25%) of 59 patients, a t(4;14)(p16.3;q32) in 9% of the patients, and a t(14;16)(q32;q23) in 5% of the patients. Deletion 13 was noted in nearly half of the patients with MGUS who were studied. Patients with a chromosome 13 deletion may be at a higher risk of progression to myeloma.[19]

Long-term follow-up studies have provided valuable information about the outcome of these patients. It is not clear if the life expectancy of this population as a group is changed compared to those without MGUS. Blade et al., in his study of 128 persons with MGUS, did not find any significant difference in the survival probability of persons with MGUS compared to a control population, even though progression to malignancy was clearly associated with a shorter survival.[22] In the initial Mayo Clinic series of 241 patients, the overall survival was shorter among those with MGUS compared to an age- and sex-adjusted population.[23] Among the 1384 patients from southeastern Minnesota, evaluated at Mayo Clinic between 1960 and 1994, the median survival among those with MGUS was clearly shorter (8.1 years) compared to the expected survival (11.8) for an age- and sex-matched population.[13] Among the 1324 cases of MGUS identified between 1978 and 1993 in North Jutland County, Denmark, a twofold higher mortality rate was observed compared to the expected rate for that population.[24] Malignant transformation explained only 20% of the excess mortality in this group. The rest was likely due to other coexisting medical conditions in this patient population, especially during the period immediately following diagnosis.

Patients with MGUS can go on to develop other plasma cell proliferative disorders, such as MM, amyloidosis, Waldenström's macroglobulinemia, or a lymphoproliferative disorder. Direct progression to plasma cell leukemia also has been reported.[25] The risk of progression persists throughout the course of the disease. Among the 1384 patients seen at Mayo Clinic since 1970 and followed for a total of 11,009 person-years (median 15.4 years; range 0–35 years), 115 patients (8%) developed one of the above-mentioned disorders.[13] These included 75 patients with myeloma, 19 with lymphoma, 10 with primary amyloidosis, 7 with macroglobulinemia, 3 with chronic lymphocytic leukemia (CLL), and 1 with a plasmacytoma. The cumulative risk of progression was 10% at 10 years, 21% at 20 years, and 26% at 25 years, translating to a 1% annual risk. In addition, there were 32 patients in whom the M-protein level rose to over 3 gm/dL or the bone marrow plasma cell percentage increased to >10% without development of overt symptomatic myeloma. The risk of development of MM was calculated to be over 25 fold among these patients, and that of macroglobulinemia and amyloidosis 46 and 8.4 fold, respectively. The risk of developing lymphoma or CLL, though higher, was not as dramatic as that for the plasma cell disorders. The majority of patients with MGUS (70%) died of unrelated causes during the follow-up period, with no evidence of progression. The risk of progression is remarkably similar across multiple studies. Among the 1104 patients with MGUS reported by Cesana et al., at a median follow-up of 65 months, the M protein remained stable in 907 patients (82%); 111 patients (10%) died from unrelated causes and 64 patients (5.8%) had a malignant transformation.[12] This included myeloma (43 patients), macroglobulinemia (12), lymphoma (6), plasmacytoma (1), and CLL (1). Baldini et al. reported a 6.8% rate of malignant transformation among the 335 patients who were followed for a median of 70 months.[26] Among the 128 patients with MGUS studied by Blade et al., progression was seen in 10.2% at a median follow up of 56 months.[22] Carter reported a 6.2% rate of transformation among 64 patients studied for over 3 years.[27] Among the 313 patients reported by Paladini et al., 14% of the patients followed for 5–8 years and 18% of those with more than 8 years of follow-up developed a malignant B-cell dyscrasia.[28] The mean duration to progression was 63 months (27–138 months) from initial recognition of the paraprotein. Similar results have been reported by others.[29,30] In a study of 1229 patients from the Danish Cancer Registry, the relative risk of developing MM, Waldenström's macroglobulinemia, and non-Hodgkin's lymphoma was significantly increased, and the increase was independent of the time from diagnosis.[31] However, the relative risk of CLL was not significantly increased.

Spontaneous disappearance of the M protein has been reported, and was seen in 27 patients (2%) in the Mayo Clinic study. Most of these patients had low levels of M protein at the time of diagnosis. In the Italian study, spontaneous disappearance was noted in 19 patients (1.7%).[12] Similar rates of spontaneous disappearance have been reported in other series, as well.[27]

## RISK FACTORS FOR PROGRESSION

Identifying patients with MGUS who are at high risk of progression is important; both from the standpoint of prognostication as well as for design and implementation of trials aimed at preventing progression. At the time of diagnosis, it is difficult to predict the disease

**Table 89.1    Factors associated with increased risk of progression**

1. Higher M-protein levels at diagnosis
2. IgA or IgM
3. Higher percentage of plasma cells in bone marrow
4. Suppression of un-involved immunoglobulins
5. Presence of circulating plasma cells or clonal B cells
6. Bone density abnormalities
7. Advanced age
8. Bence Jones Proteinuria
9. Elevated ESR
10. Abnormal free light chain ratio

ESR, erythrocyte sedimentation rate.

course for an individual, even though several clinical and laboratory markers have been suggested based on results from large groups of prospectively followed patients with MGUS (Table 89.1). In the Mayo Clinic study of 1384 patients with MGUS, factors associated with a higher risk of progression included higher M-protein levels and non-IgG (IgA or IgM) subgroups.[13] The risk of progression to MM or a related disorder at 10 years after diagnosis of MGUS was 6% for an initial M-protein level of 0.5 g/dL or less, 7% for a level of 1 g/dL, 11% for 1.5 g/dL, 20% for 2 g/dL, 24% for 2.5 g/dL, and 34% for 3.0 g/dL. The initial concentration of the M protein appears to be one of the most important risk factors, and similar results have been observed in other large studies. In the Italian series reported by Cesana et al., patients with MGUS who had more than 1.9 g/dL of M protein had twice the rate of progression compared to those with less than 0.95 g/dL.[12] In a Danish study reported by Gregersen et al., the risk of progression increased with increasing M-protein concentration.[14] The type of immunoglobulin also appears to have predictive value, with those having an IgG paraprotein being at lower risk of progression compared to those with an IgA or IgM M protein. In the Italian study, patients with an IgA or IgM M protein had nearly twice the rate of progression compared to those with IgG. In a series of 128 persons with MGUS reported by Blade et al., the IgA type of MGUS was the only variable associated with a higher probability of progression.[22] In the Danish study, the relative risk of progression for IgA and IgM were 1.8 and 1.1, respectively, compared to IgG type paraprotein.[14] The proportion of plasma cells in the bone marrow may help predict the risk of progression. Cesana et al. noted an event rate of 0.64/100 person-years among those with 0–5% plasma cells in the marrow, compared to 1.35 and 5.96/100 person-years for those with 6–9% and ≥10% plasma cells, respectively.[12] Baldini et al. reported a transformation rate of 6.8% among those with a plasma cell percentage of <10%, which increased to over 30% in those with 10–30% plasma cells in their marrow. Similar results have been seen in other studies.[32] Suppression of uninvolved immunoglobulins (immunoglobulin classes other than the M protein), characteristically seen in myeloma, can also be seen in patients with MGUS. In the Mayo study, nearly 38% of the patients with MGUS had reduction in the uninvolved immunoglobulin.[13] Baldini et al. reported a 3.6 fold elevated risk of progression with suppression of one uninvolved immunoglobulin and a 13.1 fold increased risk when two of the polyclonal immunoglobulins were decreased.[26] Cesana et al. reported a relative risk of 1.6 for reduction in one normal immunoglobulin, and 7.6 for reduction in two normal immunoglobulins. Similar predictive values for suppression of polyclonal immunoglobulins have been reported by others.[14] Clonal plasma cells can be detected in the peripheral blood in up to 20% of the patients with MGUS using immunofluorescence microscopy. Presence of circulating clonal plasma cells in these patients appears to predict for an increased risk of progression. In one study, patients who had circulating plasma cells were twice as likely (relative risk of 2.2) to progress, most commonly to myeloma, compared to those without circulating plasma cells.[33] Increased numbers of clonal B cells in the circulation has also been associated with a higher risk of progression.[34] Quantification of free light chains (FLCs) in the serum offers a new method for disease assessment in patients with paraproteinemias. The presence of an abnormal kappa/lambda FLC ratio (kappa/lambda ratio <0.26 or >1.65) in the serum may help identify those at a higher risk of progression of their underlying MGUS.[35] In a study of 1384 patients with MGUS, an abnormal ratio was detected in 379 patients (33%). The risk of progression in these patients was significantly higher (hazard ratio 3.5, 95% CI 2.3–5.5; $p < 0.001$) compared to those with a normal ratio. The presence of Bence Jones proteinuria nearly tripled the rate of progression in two large studies, and may help predict risk of progression.[12,26] Increased rates of bone resorption have been reported in MGUS patients who are at high risk of progression.[36] Modern imaging techniques, such as whole-body positron emission tomography ([18]F-FDG PET), may predict patients with stable disease, though further studies are needed to validate these findings.[37] Increased age has been reported as a risk factor in a few studies. Baldini et al. reported a 3.6 fold higher risk of progression for

those older than 70 years.[26] In one study, a low sCD16 (soluble Fc gamma receptor type III) level in patients with MGUS indicated a high likelihood of rapid progression to MM.[38]

## DIFFERENTIAL DIAGNOSIS

Once the presence of an M protein is detected on protein electrophoresis or immunofixation, it is important to consider and rule out other plasma cell proliferative disorders, including MM, amyloidosis, and macroglobulinemia. The presence of anemia without another explanation, hypercalcemia, lytic bone lesions, renal insufficiency that cannot be attributed to another cause, M protein > 3 gm/dL, large amounts of paraprotein in the urine, bone marrow plasma cells of over 10%, or a high bone marrow PCLI should all raise the suspicion of MM, rather than MGUS. However, no one clinical feature distinguishes one from the other with certainty, and differentiation of myeloma from MGUS may be difficult (Table 89.2) There is a distinct group of patients with features consistent with MGUS except for an M-protein concentration of ≥3gm/dL and ≥10% plasma cells in the marrow, for whom the term smoldering (asymptomatic) multiple myeloma (SMM) has been coined.[39,40] This group of patients has also been referred to as having monoclonal gammopathy of borderline significance (MGBS).[26] These patients often have small amounts of M protein in the urine and a reduction of uninvolved immunoglobulins, as well as a low labeling index. At the time of diagnosis, it is often difficult to predict the course of these patients, and this condition is difficult to distinguish from symptomatic myeloma and needs to be closely followed. Patients with SMM are at a higher risk of progression to another plasma cell disorder compared to those with MGUS. In the group of patients reported by Baldini et al., the risk of malignant transformation for the MGBS group was 37% at a median follow-up of 53 months, compared to 6.8% for those with MGUS. Cesana et al. reported a higher risk of progression for patients with SMM (19.7%), compared to 5.8% among those with MGUS, at a median follow-up of 65–72

| Table 89.2 | Diagnostic features of MGUS, SMM, and MM |
|---|---|
| **Disease stage** | **Diagnostic Features** |
| Monoclonal gammopathy of Undetermined significance (MGUS) | ■ Serum monoclonal protein <3 g/dL<br>■ Bone marrow plasma cells <10%<br>■ Absence of anemia, renal failure, hypercalcemia, and lytic bone lesions |
| Smoldering multiple myeloma (SMM) | ■ Serum monoclonal protein ≥3 g/dL or bone marrow plasma cells ≥10%<br>■ Absence of anemia, renal failure, hypercalcemia, and lytic bone lesions |
| Symptomatic multiple myeloma (MM) | ■ Presence of a serum or urine monoclonal protein<br>■ Bone marrow plasmacytosis<br>■ Anemia, renal failure, hypercalcemia, or lytic bone lesions |

months. This group of patients may need immediate treatment for their disease, though many have a relatively stable course for several years.

While high serum levels of M protein and large amounts of M protein in the urine increases the likelihood of myeloma, MGUS patients can occasionally have high levels of Bence Jones protein in their urine, and there is no cutoff value that can be reliably used for discrimination. As many as 17% of patients with MGUS can have urinary monoclonal proteins of more than 150 mg/24 h.[13] While reduction of uninvolved immunoglobulin points toward myeloma, these findings can be seen in as many as 38% of the patients with MGUS.[13] While >10% plasma cells in the bone marrow points toward myeloma, some of these patients can have a stable clinical course, as previously mentioned. Atypical plasma cells, especially those with a plasmablastic morphology, point toward myeloma, even though they may occasionally be seen in patients with MGUS or SMM. In a study of 566 patients enrolled in a multicenter trial (MGUS = 295; myeloma = 266), consistent differences were observed in the bone marrow histology between patients with MGUS and MM.[41] Changes in bone marrow composition from MGUS to early MM and to advanced MM followed a precise pattern which, in addition to increasing plasma cell percentage, included a shift from plasmocytic to plasmablastic cytology, an increase in bone marrow cellularity and fibrosis, a change in bone marrow infiltration (becoming diffuse rather than interstitial), a decrease in residual hematopoiesis, and an increase in osteoclasts. Patients with MGUS generally have plasma cell labeling index values close to 0, which may be a valuable discriminator when other features are equivocal.[42] A value of over 0.4% raises the likelihood of myeloma or impending transformation to one. However, nearly a third of patients with symptomatic myeloma can have normal labeling index values. The value of the labeling index in differentiating benign monoclonal gammopathy from myeloma has been reported by others.[43,44] The ratio of the plasma cell cytoplasmic light chains has been suggested as a useful differentiating feature, with a ratio of 8 or below pointing toward MGUS.[45] Circulating clonal plasma cells can be detected using immunofluorescence microscopy, flow cytometry, or more sensitive techniques, such as allele specific oligonucleotide-polymerase chain reaction (ASO-PCR) in patients with monoclonal gammopathies, and are seen in higher numbers in patients with myeloma compared to those with MGUS.[46] In patients with MGUS and SMM, the presence of these cells predicts for a higher risk of progression.

While the presence of lytic bone lesions in the setting of a monoclonal protein points to myeloma, this patient population is at risk for other malignancies, and the bone lesions may be related to metastatic disease. Occasional patients have one or more sclerotic bone lesions, M protein in the serum or urine (typically lambda), endocrine and skin abnormalities, and often debilitating neuropathy—a syndrome referred to as osteosclerotic myeloma or POEMS syndrome. More sensitive imaging of the bone using techniques such as MRI or whole body PET imaging may help distinguish patients with MGUS from those with other disorders. Bellaiche et al. performed MRIs of the thoracolumbar spine in 24 patients with MGUS comparing the results to those in 44 patients with myeloma.[47] All findings on magnetic resonance examination were normal in those with MGUS, whereas findings on 38 patients (86%) with MM were abnormal. CT evaluations of the thoracolumbar spine, iliac crests, and sacrum showing lacunae larger than 5 mm with trabecular disruption have been reported in myeloma—a finding not observed in any of the patients with MGUS.[48] Durie et al. found that a normal whole-body $^{18}$F-FDG PET reliably identified patients with stable MGUS.[37] Others have reported that markers of increased bone turnover, such as carboxy-terminal telopeptide of type I collagen (ICTP) and deoxypyridinoline (Dpd), may help distinguish patients with MGUS.[49] Bataille et al., using histomorphometric parameters of bone resorption, demonstrated decreased levels of bone resorption in MGUS compared to active MM.[36]

Levels of cytokines either in the serum or those demonstrated in the plasma cells have been suggested as having diagnostic value. Interleukin (IL)-1β is produced by plasma cells from patients with MM, whereas those from patients with MGUS rarely do.[50] IL-1β is thought to be an important player in the osteoclast-mediated bone destruction seen in myeloma. Serum levels of IL-6 have been reported to be higher in patients with myeloma compared to in those with MGUS. In one study, significant serum IL-6 levels were detected in only 3% of the MGUS/SMM group, compared to 35% of the overt MM group and 100% of those with plasma cell leukemia.[51] Serum levels of IL-2 have been reported to be higher in MGUS patients compared to those with myeloma.[52] Serum β$_2$ microglobulin, while increased in myeloma compared to MGUS, does not have enough discriminatory power to be of clinical value in differentiating between MGUS and myeloma.[53–55]

Increased bone marrow angiogenesis is a prominent feature of MM and is a prognostic factor for overall survival. Patients with MGUS do not have any significant increase in the bone marrow microvessel density, though the clinical applicability of this test is low given that many patients with myeloma can have normal findings.[56] Presence of cytoplasmic 5'nucleotidase (c5NT) in plasma cells has been reported to discriminate between MGUS and myeloma.[57]

An M-protein can be detected in the presence of many lymphoproliferative disorders, including non-Hodgkin's lymphoma and CLL, and should be kept in mind when evaluating these patients. Over a ten year period, Malacrida et al. performed protein electrophoresis on

102,000 samples, detecting 730 cases of M-protein, of whom 114 could be classified as B cell malignancies and 261 as monoclonal gammopathy of undefined significance.[58]

## DISEASE ASSOCIATIONS

Several hematological and non-hematological conditions have been associated with monoclonal gammopathies. Many of these conditions are likely to occur with increased frequency in this older patient group, making it difficult to identify true associations.

Various lymphoproliferative disorders have been described in the context of monoclonal gammopathies. In a long-term study of 430 patients with a monoclonal IgM in the serum, Kyle et al. found 28 patients (7%) with lymphoma, 21 (5%) with CLL, and 62 (14%) with other malignant lymphoproliferative diseases. Among those with an apparently benign monoclonal gammopathy, nearly a fifth subsequently progressed to have a lymphoid malignancy.[59] In a study of 1144 patients, using serum protein electrophoresis, Alexanian et al. found an M-protein (IgG) in 2.3% of the 400 patients with CLL and lymphocytic lymphoma.[60] IgM peaks were seen in 4.5% of patients with lymphomas. Noel et al. reported on 100 patients with CLL seen over a fourteen year period, all of whom had an M-protein in the serum or urine. IgG (51%) was noted most often, followed by IgM (38%) and IgA (1%), with light chains alone in the remainder.[61] Monoclonal gammopathy has also been reported in association with hairy cell leukemia, adult T-cell leukemia, and chronic myeloid leukemia, though the strength of the association remains indeterminate.

Acquired von-Willebrand disease has been described in association with monoclonal gammopathies as well as other malignant disorders.[62,63] Bleeding time is prolonged in most patients, and is associated with marked reductions in plasma von Willebrand factor antigen and ristocetin cofactor activity, and a type 2 pattern of von Willebrand multimer distribution. Other hematological disorders that have been associated with monoclonal gammopathies include polycythemia vera, myelofibrosis, myelodysplastic syndrome, and pernicious anemia. Lupus-like anti-coagulant activity has been associated with the monoclonal protein in patients with monoclonal gammopathies.[64]

Another common association that has been seen with monoclonal gammopathies is peripheral neuropathy.[65–68] Nearly 10% of patients with idiopathic peripheral neuropathy have a monoclonal protein detectable in their serum or urine, a prevalence rate nearly five times of that seen in general population.[69] The frequency of the neuropathy in different series varies widely, likely a reflection of the criteria used to identify it as well as the thoroughness of the search for a monoclonal protein and the clinical or electrophysiologic criteria used to diagnosis neuropathy.[70] The neuropathy seen in association with MGUS is typically a peripheral neuropathy, and autonomic nerve or cranial nerve involvement is not usually seen. The association appears to be the strongest with IgM monoclonal gammopathies.[71,72] In one study, the prevalence of peripheral neuropathy among patients with IgM monoclonal gammopathies was as high as 32%.[73] The monoclonal protein binds to myelin associated glycoprotein (MAG) in nearly half of the patients with an IgM-MGUS associated neuropathy.[70] Among the 65 patients with MGUS and sensorimotor peripheral neuropathy seen at Mayo Clinic, 31 patients had IgM, 24 had IgG, and 10 had IgA.[65] IgM-MGUS associated neuropathies were characterized by a higher frequency of sensory loss and ataxia, higher frequency of nerve conduction abnormalities, and a higher frequency of dispersion of the compound muscle action potential. Neither the amount of IgM nor the estimated size of the monoclonal peak was associated with the severity of neuropathy. The type and severity of IgM-MGUS neuropathies associated with anti-MAG antibodies were not significantly different from those without anti-myelin-associated glycoprotein antibodies. Patients with IgM-associated neuropathy had more severe demyelination on nerve conduction studies compared to IgG associated neuropathy in one small study, though clinical feature were indistinguishable.[74] Patients with IgM associated neuropathy may have a more progressive course, with significantly more weakness and sensory signs.[75]

Patients with MGUS associated neuropathy often present with a clinical picture resembling chronic inflammatory demyelinating polyneuropathy (CIDP). Simmons et al. compared a group of 77 patients with idiopathic CIDP with 26 patients in whom CIDP was associated with MGUS.[76] Patients with CIDP and MGUS had, on average, a more indolent course and less severe weakness, despite similar findings on electrophysiological studies. These patients also demonstrated less functional impairment, more frequent sensory loss, and more abnormal sensory conduction studies. However, given the greater improvement of idiopathic CIDP patients with treatment, both groups had similar outcomes from their initial episodes of weakness. However, nerve conduction studies may not always be helpful in distinguishing between demyelinating neuropathies associated with a paraprotein and idiopathic demyelinating polyneuropathy.[77] Diagnostic criteria for demyelinating neuropathy associated with monoclonal proteins have been proposed.[78] Even though the neuropathy associated with MGUS is typically a predominantly demyelinating process which can have additional features of axonal degeneration, pure or predominant axonal degeneration also has been reported.[79] Axonal neuropathy in this setting presents as a mild, symmetric, slowly progressive, predominantly sensory, neuropathy usually limited to the legs. When compared with

MGUS neuropathy of demyelinating type, the axonal process was associated with less vibration and proprioceptive loss, did not include leg ataxia, less often had generalized areflexia, had less prevalence of IgM gammopathy and anti-MAG antibodies, and had lower CSF protein concentrations. Even though fewer patients with axonal neuropathy improved with therapy, the illness was generally milder with less disability.

The treatment of MGUS associated neuropathy is difficult. Plasmapheresis has been studied by many, with variable benefit. In a double blind trial from Mayo Clinic, significant benefit was seen with plasma exchange, especially among those with IgG or IgA MGUS.[80] Intermittent cyclophosphamide and prednisone has been reported to produce improvements or stabilization of the neuropathy in a small study.[81] Fludarabine has been used with some benefit in patients with IgM associated peripheral neuropathy.[82] There are scattered reports of benefit from high dose therapy in patients with debilitating peripheral neuropathy.[83]

The association of neuropathy and monoclonal gammopathy in the presence of osteosclerotic bone lesions is a distinct entity. The constellation of *Polyneuropathy*, *Organomegaly*, *Endocrinopathy*, *M* protein and *Skin* changes or POEMS syndrome, also known as osteosclerotic myeloma, Crow Fukase syndrome, or Takasuki syndrome is a poorly understood phenomenon.[84] These patients usually have sclerotic bone lesions on skeletal survey. Other clinical findings include papilledema, pedal edema, hyperpigmentation, hypertrichosis, gynecomastia, hepatosplenomegaly, and lymphadenopathy. Laboratory testing may reveal abnormalities of multiple endocrine glands, including the thyroid, parathyroid, and adrenals, as well as polycythemia and thrombocytosis. Almost all patients have small amounts of M-protein in the serum, and the associated light chain is lambda in virtually every patient. Patients with single osteosclerotic lesion can often be treated with radiation therapy to the lesion with significant benefit. Patients with multiple lesions often need systemic therapy, and autologous stem cell transplantation has been successful in selected patients.[85]

Motor neuron disease has been associated with MGUS. In a study of 56 patients with motor neuron disease, 6 (10.7%) were found to have a monoclonal protein (4 with IgG and 2 with IgA), compared to a control group of 121 age-matched patients with other neurological disorders, in whom only 5 patients (4.1%) had a monoclonal protein.[86] Presence of gammopathy in this study appeared to correlate with the absence of marked upper motor neuron involvement and with elevated CSF protein concentration.

Autoimmune disorders such as rheumatoid arthritis,[87] lupus erythematosus,[88] and polymyositis[89] have been reported in association with monoclonal gammopathies. Paraproteins with activity against rheumatoid factor, as well monoclonal anti-nuclear antibodies, have been reported.[90] A higher prevalence of anti-phospholipid antibodies have been reported in association with monoclonal gammopathy.[91]

## DISEASE VARIANTS

*Biclonal gammopathies:* The simultaneous presence of more than one type of M-protein can be seen in as many as 5% of patients with monoclonal gammopathies. This likely represents the proliferation of two separates clones of plasma cells, producing M-proteins of different immunoglobulin classes. Patients with three different types of M-proteins also have been reported. Most of these were associated with malignant lymphoproliferative disorders, though a few were of undetermined significance. Kyle et al. reported on 57 patients with biclonal gammopathy, of whom 37 had a biclonal gammopathy of undetermined significance.[92] These patients had clinical features indistinguishable from those with monoclonal gammopathies. The remaining patients with a biclonal gammopathy had myeloma, macroglobulinemia, or another lymphoproliferative disorder. Nilsson et al. found 20 patients (2%) from among 1034 patients with monoclonal gammopathy, who had two distinct monoclonal spikes; 3 were associated with lymphoma, 7 with myelomatosis, 9 with monoclonal gammopathy of undetermined significance (MGUS), and 1 with lupus erythematosus disseminatus.[93]

*Idiopathic Bence Jones Proteinuria:* Patients may present with isolated monoclonal FLCs in the urine, or Bence Jones proteinuria. Several patients have been reported with Bence Jones proteinuria, with disease that has remained stable over long periods of follow up. Kyle reported nine patients with Bence Jones proteinuria of over 1 g/24 hours with no serum M-protein and no evidence of another plasma cell proliferative disorder.[94,95] While symptomatic myeloma developed in three of these patients at 8–21 years of follow up, two were followed for 12 years with no evidence of progression. Similar outcomes have been reported by others.[96] While patients with idiopathic Bence Jones proteinuria can stay stable over long periods, some studies have suggested an increased risk of progression in patients with light chain proteinuria, and they need to be followed closely.

## MANAGEMENT

The cornerstone of the management is regular follow up, so that any disease progression can be detected and appropriate therapy can be instituted. At the time of initial diagnosis, other plasma cell disorders should be ruled out, as mentioned before. Patients with small amounts of M-protein in their serum (< 0.5 g/dL) may not require a bone marrow examination or skeletal survey, given the low risk of progression seen in this group. However, the choice of tests should be dictated by the clinical assessment, and if suspicion is high, a complete workup, including bone marrow examination, skeletal survey, and urine protein electrophoresis, should be performed. The serum protein electrophoresis should be repeated at least annually to demonstrate stability of the M-protein. Patients with higher levels of M-protein, especially those with over 2 gm/dL, should have metastatic bone survey, quantitation of immunoglobulins, 24 hour urine examination for monoclonal protein, and a bone marrow aspirate and biopsy. A bone marrow PCLI, if available, should be performed, as this will provide valuable prognostic information. Serum $\beta_2$ microglobulin and C-reactive protein should be obtained. If these tests are consistent with the diagnosis of MGUS, serum protein electrophoresis should be performed in three months. If results do not indicate any progression, they should be repeated every 6–12 months. Patients who, at diagnosis, have factors predicting higher risk of progression, will need closer follow up. They should be re-evaluated for progression in the interval period if clinical symptoms or signs raise suspicion for progression. The risk of progression never disappears, and patients need lifelong follow up.

## REFERENCES

1. Kyle RA, Finkelstein S, Elveback LR, et al.: Incidence of monoclonal proteins in a Minnesota community with a cluster of multiple myeloma. *Blood* 40:719–724, 1972.
2. Axelsson U, Bachmann R, Hallen J: Frequency of pathological proteins (M-components) in 6,995 sera from an adult population. *Acta Med Scand* 179:235–247, 1966.
3. Saleun JP, Vicariot M, Deroff P, et al.: Monoclonal gammopathies in the adult population of Finistere, France. *J Clin Pathol* 35:63–68, 1982.
4. Anagnostopoulos A, Evangelopoulou A, Sotou D, et al.: Incidence and evolution of monoclonal gammopathy of undetermined significance (MGUS) in Greece. *Ann Hematol* 81:357–361, 2002.
5. Kurihara Y, Shiba K, Fukumura Y, et al.: Occurrence of serum M-protein species in Japanese patients older than 50 years based on relative mobility in cellulose acetate membrane electrophoresis. *J Clin Lab Anal* 14:64–69, 2000.
6. Bowden M, Crawford J, Cohen HJ, et al.: A comparative study of monoclonal gammopathies and immunoglobulin levels in Japanese and United States elderly. *J Am Geriatr Soc* 41:11–14, 1993.
7. Singh J, Dudley AW Jr, Kulig KA: Increased incidence of monoclonal gammopathy of undetermined significance in blacks and its age-related differences with whites on the basis of a study of 397 men and one woman in a hospital setting. *J Lab Clin Med* 116: 785–789, 1990.
8. Cohen HJ, Crawford J, Rao MK, et al.: Racial differences in the prevalence of monoclonal gammopathy in a community-based sample of the elderly. *Am J Med* 104:439–444, 1998.
9. Ogmundsdottir HM, Haraldsdottir V, Johannesson GM, et al.: Monoclonal gammopathy in Iceland: a population-based registry and follow-up. *Br J Haematol* 118:166–173, 2002.
10. Crawford J, Eye MK, Cohen HJ: Evaluation of monoclonal gammopathies in the "well" elderly. *Am J Med* 82:39–45, 1987.
11. Ligthart GJ, Radl J, Corberand JX, et al.: Monoclonal gammopathies in human aging: increased occurrence with age and correlation with health status. *Mech Ageing Dev* 52:235–243, 1990.
12. Cesana C, Klersy C, Barbarano L, et al.: Prognostic factors for malignant transformation in monoclonal gammopathy of undetermined significance and smoldering multiple myeloma. *J Clin Oncol* 20:1625–1634, 2002.
13. Kyle RA, Therneau TM, Rajkumar SV, et al.: A long-term study of prognosis in monoclonal gammopathy of undetermined significance. *N Engl J Med* 346:564–569, 2002.
14. Gregersen H, Mellemkjaer L, Ibsen JS, et al.: The impact of M-component type and immunoglobulin concentration on the risk of malignant transformation in patients with monoclonal gammopathy of undetermined significance. *Haematologica* 86:1172–1179, 2001.
15. Bizzaro N, Pasini P: Familial occurrence of multiple myeloma and monoclonal gammopathy of undetermined significance in 5 siblings. *Haematologica* 75:58–63, 1990.
16. Blade J, Kyle RA: IgD monoclonal gammopathy with long-term follow-up. *Br J Haematol* 88:395–396, 1994.
17. Kinoshita T, Nagai H, Murate T, et al.: IgD monoclonal gammopathy of undetermined significance. *Int J Hematol* 65:169–172, 1997.
18. Fonseca R, Bailey RJ, Ahmann GJ, et al.: Genomic abnormalities in monoclonal gammopathy of undetermined significance. *Blood* 100:1417–1424, 2002.
19. Avet-Loiseau H, Li JY, Morineau N, et al.: Monosomy 13 is associated with the transition of monoclonal gammopathy of undetermined significance to multiple myeloma. Intergroupe Francophone du Myelome. *Blood* 94:2583–2589, 1999.
20. Avet-Loiseau H, Facon T, Daviet A, et al.: 14q32 translocations and monosomy 13 observed in monoclonal gammopathy of undetermined significance delineate a multistep process for the oncogenesis of multiple myeloma. Intergroupe Francophone du Myelome. *Cancer Res* 59:4546–4550, 1999.
21. Bernasconi P, Cavigliano PM, Boni M, et al.: Long-term follow-up with conventional cytogenetics and band 13q14 interphase/metaphase in situ hybridization monitoring in monoclonal gammopathies of undetermined significance. *Br J Haematol* 118:545–549, 2000.
22. Blade J, Lopez-Guillermo A, Rozman C, et al.: Malignant transformation and life expectancy in monoclonal gammopathy of undetermined significance. *Br J Haematol* 81:391–394, 1992.
23. Kyle RA: Monoclonal gammopathy of undetermined significance. Natural history in 241 cases. *Am J Med* 64:814–826, 1978.

24. Gregersen H, Ibsen J, Mellemkjoer L, et al.: Mortality and causes of death in patients with monoclonal gammopathy of undetermined significance. *Br J Haematol* 112:353–357, 2001.

25. Pasqualetti P, Casale R: Monoclonal gammopathy of undetermined significance evolving directly in primary plasma cell leukemia. *Biomed Pharmacother* 51:284–285, 1997.

26. Baldini L, Guffanti A, Cesana BM, et al: Role of different hematologic variables in defining the risk of malignant transformation in monoclonal gammopathy. *Blood* 87:912–918, 1996.

27. Carter A, Tatarsky I: The physiopathological significance of benign monoclonal gammopathy: a study of 64 cases. *Br J Haematol* 46:565–574, 1980.

28. Paladini G, Fogher M, Mazzanti G, et al: Idiopathic monoclonal gammopathy. Long-term study of 313 cases. *Recenti Prog Med* 80:123–132, 1989.

29. van de Poel MH, Coebergh JW, Hillen HF: Malignant transformation of monoclonal gammopathy of undetermined significance among out-patients of a community hospital in southeastern Netherlands. *Br J Haematol* 91:121–125, 1995.

30. Carrell RW, Colls BM, Murray JT: The significance of monoclonal gammopathy in a normal population. *Aust N Z J Med* 1:398–401, 1971.

31. Gregersen H, Mellemkjaer L, Salling Ibsen J, et al.: Cancer risk in patients with monoclonal gammopathy of undetermined significance. *Am J Hematol* 63:1–6, 2000.

32. Ucci G, Riccardi A, Luoni R, et al.: Presenting features of monoclonal gammopathies: an analysis of 684 newly diagnosed cases. Cooperative group for the study and treatment of multiple myeloma. *J Intern Med* 234:165–173, 1993.

33. Kumar S, Rajkumar SV, Kyle RA, et al.: Prognostic value of circulating plasma cells in monoclonal gammopathy of undetermined significance. *Blood* 103:3494, 2003.

34. Isaksson E, Bjorkholm M, Holm G, et al.: Blood clonal B-cell excess in patients with monoclonal gammopathy of undetermined significance (MGUS): association with malignant transformation. *Br J Haematol* 92:71–76, 1996.

35. Rajkumar SV, Kyle RA, Therneau T, et al.: presence of an abnormal serum free light ratio is an independent risk factor for progression in Monoclonal Gammopathy of Undetermined Significance (MGUS). *Blood* 104, 2004.

36. Bataille R, Chappard D, Basle MF: Quantifiable excess of bone resorption in monoclonal gammopathy is an early symptom of malignancy: a prospective study of 87 bone biopsies. *Blood* 87:4762–4769, 1996.

37. Durie BG, Waxman AD, D'Agnolo A, et al.: Whole-body (18)F-FDG PET identifies high-risk myeloma. *J Nucl Med* 43:1457–1463, 2002.

38. Mathiot C, Mary JY, Tartour E, et al.: Soluble CD16 (sCD16), a marker of malignancy in individuals with monoclonal gammopathy of undetermined significance (MGUS). *Br J Haematol* 95:660–665, 1996.

39. Durie BG: Staging and kinetics of multiple myeloma. *Semin Oncol* 13:300–309, 1986.

40. Kyle RA, Greipp PR: Smoldering multiple myeloma. *N Engl J Med* 302:1347–1349, 1980.

41. Riccardi A, Ucci G, Luoni R, et al.: Bone marrow biopsy in monoclonal gammopathies: correlations between pathological findings and clinical data. The Cooperative Group for Study and Treatment of Multiple Myeloma. *J Clin Pathol* 43:469–475, 1990.

42. Greipp PR, Kyle RA: Clinical, morphological, and cell kinetic differences among multiple myeloma, monoclonal gammopathy of undetermined significance, and smoldering multiple myeloma. *Blood* 62:166–171, 1983.

43. Boccadoro M, Gavarotti P, Fossati G, et al.: Low plasma cell 3(H) thymidine incorporation in monoclonal gammopathy of undetermined significance (MGUS), smouldering myeloma and remission phase myeloma: a reliable indicator of patients not requiring therapy. *Br J Haematol* 58:689–696, 1984.

44. Lokhorst HM, Boom SE, Terpstra W, et al.: Determination of the growth fraction in monoclonal gammopathy with the monoclonal antibody Ki-67. *Br J Haematol* 69:477–481, 1988.

45. Majumdar G, Grace RJ, Singh AK, et al.: The value of the bone marrow plasma cell cytoplasmic light chain ratio in differentiating between multiple myeloma and monoclonal gammopathy of undetermined significance. *Leuk Lymphoma* 8:491–493, 1992.

46. Billadeau D, Van Ness B, Kimlinger T, et al.: Clonal circulating cells are common in plasma cell proliferative disorders: a comparison of monoclonal gammopathy of undetermined significance, smoldering multiple myeloma, and active myeloma. *Blood* 88:289–296, 1996.

47. Bellaiche L, Laredo JD, Liote F, et al.: Magnetic resonance appearance of monoclonal gammopathies of unknown significance and multiple myeloma. The GRI Study Group. *Spine* 22:2551–2557, 1997.

48. Laroche M, Assoun J, Sixou L, et al.: Comparison of MRI and computed tomography in the various stages of plasma cell disorders: correlations with biological and histological findings. Myelome-Midi-Pyrenees Group. *Clin Exp Rheumatol* 14:171–176, 1996.

49. Jakob C, Zavrski I, Heider U, et al.: Bone resorption parameters [carboxy-terminal telopeptide of type-I collagen (ICTP), amino-terminal collagen type-I telopeptide (NTx), and deoxypyridinoline (Dpd)] in MGUS and multiple myeloma. *Eur J Haematol* 69:37–42, 2002.

50. Lacy MQ, Donovan KA, Heimbach JK, et al.: Comparison of interleukin-1 beta expression by in situ hybridization in monoclonal gammopathy of undetermined significance and multiple myeloma. *Blood* 93:300–305, 1999.

51. Bataille R, Jourdan M, Zhang XG, et al.: Serum levels of interleukin 6, a potent myeloma cell growth factor, as a reflect of disease severity in plasma cell dyscrasias. *J Clin Invest* 84:2008–2011, 1989.

52. Cimino G, Avvisati G, Amadori S, et al.: High serum interleukin-2 levels in patients with monoclonal gammopathy of undetermined significance (MGUS) and multiple myeloma. *Nouv Rev Fr Hematol* 31:329–332, 1989.

53. Bataille R, Grenier J, Sany J: Beta-2-microglobulin in myeloma: optimal use for staging, prognosis, and treatment—a prospective study of 160 patients. *Blood* 63:468–476, 1984.

54. Chelazzi G, Senaldi G: Serum beta 2-microglobulin levels in multiple myeloma and monoclonal gammapathy of undetermined significance: a clinical study of 55 patients. *Ric Clin Lab* 16:53–58, 1986.

55. Elias J, Dauth J, Senekal JC, et al.: Serum beta-2-microglobulin in the differential diagnosis of monoclonal gammopathies. *S Afr Med J* 79:650–653, 1991.

56. Rajkumar SV, Mesa RA, Fonseca R, et al.: Bone marrow angiogenesis in 400 patients with monoclonal gammopathy of undetermined significance, multiple myeloma, and primary amyloidosis. *Clin Cancer Res* 8:2210–2216, 2002.

57. Majumdar G, Heard SE, Singh AK: Use of cytoplasmic 5'nucleotidase for differentiating malignant from benign monoclonal gammopathies. *J Clin Pathol* 43:891–892, 1990.

58. Malacrida V, De Francesco D, Banfi G, et al.: Laboratory investigation of monoclonal gammopathy during 10 years of screening in a general hospital. *J Clin Pathol* 40:793–797, 1987.

59. Kyle RA, Garton JP: The spectrum of IgM monoclonal gammopathy in 430 cases. *Mayo Clin Proc* 62:719–731, 1987.

60. Alexanian R: Monoclonal gammopathy in lymphoma. *Arch Intern Med* 135:62–66, 1975.

61. Noel P, Kyle RA: Monoclonal proteins in chronic lymphocytic leukemia. *Am J Clin Pathol* 87:385–388, 1987.

62. Kumar S, Pruthi RK, Nichols WL: Acquired von Willebrand's syndrome: a single institution experience. *Am J Hematol* 72:243–247, 2003.

63. Lamboley V, Zabraniecki L, Sie P, et al.: Myeloma and monoclonal gammopathy of uncertain significance associated with acquired von Willebrand's syndrome. Seven new cases with a literature review. *Joint Bone Spine* 69:62–67, 2002.

64. Bellotti V, Gamba G, Merlini G, et al.: Study of three patients with monoclonal gammopathies and 'lupus-like' anticoagulants. *Br J Haematol* 73:221–227, 1989.

65. Gosselin S, Kyle RA, Dyck PJ: Neuropathy associated with monoclonal gammopathies of undetermined significance. *Ann Neurol* 30:54–61, 1991.

66. Kyle RA: Monoclonal proteins in neuropathy. *Neurol Clin* 10:713–734, 1992.

67. Kelly JJ: Neuropathies of monoclonal gammopathies of undetermined significance. *Hematol Oncol Clin North Am* 13:1203–1210, 1999.

68. Gorson KC: Clinical features, evaluation, and treatment of patients with polyneuropathy associated with monoclonal gammopathy of undetermined significance (MGUS). *J Clin Apheresis* 14:149–153, 1999.

69. Kissel JT, Mendell JR: Neuropathies associated with monoclonal gammopathies. *Neuromuscul Disord* 6:3–18, 1996.

70. Nobile-Orazio E, Barbieri S, Baldini L, et al.: Peripheral neuropathy in monoclonal gammopathy of undetermined significance: prevalence and immunopathogenetic studies. *Acta Neurol Scand* 85:383–390, 1992.

71. Suarez GA, Kelly JJ Jr: Polyneuropathy associated with monoclonal gammopathy of undetermined significance: further evidence that IgM-MGUS neuropathies are different than IgG-MGUS. *Neurology* 43:1304–1308, 1993.

72. Vallat JM, Jauberteau MO, Bordessoule D, et al.: Link between peripheral neuropathy and monoclonal dysglobulinemia: a study of 66 cases. *J Neurol Sci* 137:124–130, 1996.

73. Baldini L, Nobile-Orazio E, Guffanti A, et al.: Peripheral neuropathy in IgM monoclonal gammopathy and Waldenstrom's macroglobulinemia: a frequent complication in elderly males with low MAG-reactive serum monoclonal component. *Am J Hematol*.45:25–31, 1994.

74. Simovic D, Gorson KC, Ropper AH: Comparison of IgM-MGUS and IgG-MGUS polyneuropathy. *Acta Neurol Scand* 97:194–200, 1998.

75. Notermans NC, Wokke JH, Lokhorst HM, et al.: Polyneuropathy associated with monoclonal gammopathy of undetermined significance. A prospective study of the prognostic value of clinical and laboratory abnormalities. *Brain* 117(Pt 6):1385–1393, 1994.

76. Simmons Z, Albers JW, Bromberg MB, et al.: Presentation and initial clinical course in patients with chronic inflammatory demyelinating polyradiculoneuropathy: comparison of patients without and with monoclonal gammopathy. *Neurology* 43:2202–2209, 1993.

77. Bromberg MB, Feldman EL, Albers JW: Chronic inflammatory demyelinating polyradiculoneuropathy: comparison of patients with and without an associated monoclonal gammopathy. *Neurology* 42:1157–1163, 1992.

78. Notermans NC, Franssen H, Eurelings M, et al.: Diagnostic criteria for demyelinating polyneuropathy associated with monoclonal gammopathy. *Muscle Nerve* 23:73–79, 2000.

79. Gorson KC, Ropper AH: Axonal neuropathy associated with monoclonal gammopathy of undetermined significance. *J Neurol Neurosurg Psychiatry* 63:163–168, 1997.

80. Dyck PJ, Low PA, Windebank AJ, et al.: Plasma exchange in polyneuropathy associated with monoclonal gammopathy of undetermined significance. *N Engl J Med* 325:1482–1486, 1991.

81. Notermans NC, Lokhorst HM, Franssen H, et al.: Intermittent cyclophosphamide and prednisone treatment of polyneuropathy associated with monoclonal gammopathy of undetermined significance. *Neurology* 47:1227–1233, 1996.

82. Wilson HC, Lunn MP, Schey S, et al.: Successful treatment of IgM paraproteinaemic neuropathy with fludarabine. *J Neurol Neurosurg Psychiatry* 66:575–580, 1999.

83. Lee YC, Came N, Schwarer A, et al.: Autologous peripheral blood stem cell transplantation for peripheral neuropathy secondary to monoclonal gammopathy of unknown significance. *Bone Marrow Transplant* 30:53–56, 2002.

84. Dispenzieri A, Kyle RA, Lacy MQ, et al.: POEMS syndrome: definitions and long-term outcome. *Blood* 101:2496–2506, 2003.

85. Dispenzieri A, Moreno-Aspitia A, Suarez GA, et al.: Peripheral blood stem cell transplantation in 16 patients with POEMS syndrome, and a review of the literature. *Blood* 104:3400–3407, 2004.

86. Lavrnic D, Vidakovic A, Miletic V, et al.: Motor neuron disease and monoclonal gammopathy. *Eur Neurol* 35:104–107, 1995.

87. Zawadzki ZA, Benedek TG: Rheumatoid arthritis, dysproteinemic arthropathy, and paraproteinemia. *Arthritis Rheum* 12:555–568, 1969.

88. Michaux JL, Heremans JF: Thirty cases of monoclonal immunoglobulin disorders other than myeloma or macroglobulinemia. A classification of diseases associated with the production of monoclonal-type immunoglobulins. *Am J Med* 46:562–579, 1969.

89. Kiprov DD, Miller RG: Polymyositis associated with monoclonal gammopathy. *Lancet* 2:1183–1186, 1984.

90. Hardiman KL, Horn S, Manoharan A, et al.: Rheumatic autoantibodies in the sera of patients with paraproteins. *Clin Exp Rheumatol* 12:363–368, 1994.

91. Stern JJ, Ng RH, Triplett DA, et al.: Incidence of antiphospholipid antibodies in patients with monoclonal gammopathy of undetermined significance. *Am J Clin Pathol* 101:471–474, 1994.

92. Kyle RA, Robinson RA, Katzmann JA: The clinical aspects of biclonal gammopathies. Review of 57 cases. *Am J Med* 71:999–1008, 1981.

93. Nilsson T, Norberg B, Rudolphi O, et al.: Double gammopathies: incidence and clinical course of 20 patients. *Scand J Haematol* 36:103–106, 1986.

94. Kyle RA, Greipp PR: "Idiopathic" Bence Jones proteinuria: long-term follow-up in seven patients. *N Engl J Med* 306:564–567, 1982.

95. Kyle RA, Maldonado JE, Bayrd ED: Idiopathic Bence Jones proteinuria—a distinct entity? *Am J Med* 55:222–226, 1973.

96. Kanoh T, Ohnaka T, Uchino H, et al.: The outcome of idiopathic Bence Jones proteinuria. *Tohoku J Exp Med* 151:121–126, 1987.

# Chapter **90**
# AMYLOIDOSIS

## *Madhav V. Dhodapkar*

## DEFINITION

The term *amyloidosis* is used to describe a heterogeneous group of protein deposition diseases in which misfolding of proteins plays a prominent role.[1,2] This process generates insoluble toxic fibrillar protein aggregates that are deposited in tissues in a characteristic β-pleated structure. These deposits are identified based on their apple-green birefringence under a polarizing light microscope after staining with Congo red dye, and by the presence of rigid nonbranching fibrils 7–10 nm in diameter on electron microscopy. Historically, the amyloidoses were classified as "primary" when no apparent etiology was evident, and "secondary" when resulting from chronic infectious or inflammatory states.[3] In 1971, Glenner demonstrated the presence of immunoglobulin (Ig) light chains in primary amyloid fibrils.[4] Since then, several other proteins have been characterized, and the chemical nature of the amyloidogenic protein forms the basis of the current classification (Table 90.1).[5]

Pathologically, all amyloid deposits share some common constituents, such as amyloid P component and glycosaminoglycans, but differ in the nature of the precursor protein. Clinically, the amyloidoses are still classified as localized to a single organ, or systemic.[6] The most common localized form is Alzheimer's disease, which affects more than 12 million people worldwide.[7] In the western world, the two most common forms of systemic amyloidosis are AL (or Ig light chain) amyloidosis and reactive amyloidosis due to chronic inflammatory diseases (e.g., rheumatoid arthritis). Hereditary amyloidosis is an ever expanding group of disorders that pose difficult diagnostic problems.[8] In this chapter, we will largely focus on AL amyloidosis as it is associated with hematologic diseases.

## MOLECULAR PATHOGENESIS

### PROPERTIES OF AMYLOIDOGENIC PROTEINS

To date, at least 21 different proteins have been recognized as causative agents of amyloid diseases.[5] Despite heterogeneous structure and function, all these proteins generate morphologically indistinguishable amyloid fibrils. The current nomenclature for amyloidosis is based on this diversity of precursor proteins. For example, amyloidosis involving Ig light chains (L) or transthyretrin (TTR) is classified as AL or ATTR, respectively. The conversion of the native protein into a β-sheet structure is a pathologic process closely linked to physiologic protein folding. The pathogenically misfolded proteins may form in several ways. The protein may have an intrinsic property to assume a pathologic conformation that becomes evident with ageing (e.g., normal transthyretin in patients with senile systemic amyloidosis),[9] or with persistently high concentrations in the serum (e.g., β-2 microglobulin in patients undergoing long-term hemodialysis).[10] Other mechanisms include mutations in the protein, as in many hereditary amyloidoses, or proteolytic remodeling of the precursors, as in β-amyloid precursors in Alzheimer's disease. The mechanisms can act independently or together. Other environmental influences, such as proteolysis, pH, and oxidation states, also seem to play important roles in the formation of amyloid fibrils.[11]

### AMYLOIDOGENICITY OF IG LIGHT CHAINS

Only a small proportion of Ig light chains are amyloidogenic. For example, AL amyloidosis occurs in only about 12–15% of patients with myeloma.[12] Certain structural features are related to amyloiodogenicity: the λ isotype and the Vλ6 variability subgroup.[13] Two Vλ gene segments, 6a and 3r, seem to contribute to nearly 40% of the amyloidogenic λ light chains.[14,15] There is some evidence that some of the amyloidogenic light chains undergo antigen-driven selection and mutations.[14] Development of mutations in these proteins can then lead to destabilization of key structural domains and generation of an aggregation prone state.[16] Improved understanding of the mechanisms of amyloidogenicity of the Ig light chains may allow the development of targeted therapies.

### MECHANISMS OF TISSUE DAMAGE AND SPECIFICITY

A remarkable aspect of amyloidoses is the diversity of organ distribution. Specific proteins aggregate

**Table 90.1    Major types of amyloidosis: Classification and clinical presentation**

| Type | Precursor | Distribution | Syndrome |
|------|-----------|--------------|----------|
| AL | Ig light chain | Systemic or localized | Primary amyloidosis |
| AA | Serum amyloid A | Systemic | Secondary amyloidosis reactive to chronic infections or inflammation, including periodic fever syndromes |
| ATTR | Transthyretin | Systemic | Prototypic familial amyloid polyneuropathy |
|  |  | Localized | Senile cardiac amyloidosis |
| Aβ | Aβ precursor | Localized | Alzheimers; ageing |
| APrP | Prion protein | Localized | Prion associated disorders |
| ACys | Cystatin C | Localized | Icelandic amyloid angiopathy |
| AFib | Fibrinogen Aα chain | Systemic | Hereditary, renal |
| Aβ2M | β-2 microglobulin | Systemic | Chronic hemodialysis |
| AApoA1 | Apolipoprotein AI | Systemic | Liver, kidney, heart |
| AApoAII | Apolipoprotein AII | Systemic | Liver, kidney, heart |
| A Lys | Lysozyme | Systemic | Kidney, liver, spleen |
| A Gel | Gelsolin | Systemic | Finnish hereditary amyloidosis |
| AIAPP | Islet-associated peptide | Localized | Amyloid of the islets; Type II diabetes |

predominantly in defined target organs: β-2 microglobulin in the joints, fibrinogen Aα in the kidney, and the transthyretin Met30 variant in the peripheral nerves.[17] In AL amyloid, virtually every organ may be involved, most commonly the heart, kidneys, nerves, and liver. Importantly, the pattern of organ involvement may differ greatly between patients and seems to determine outcome. The reasons behind differences in organ tropism in different patients is not clear, but may be due to properties of the light chains themselves, or to their interactions with specific tissue glycosaminoglycans or cell-surface receptors, such as the receptor for advanced glycation end products (RAGE).[18]

An equally important, but poorly understood aspect of this disease is the mechanism by which the deposited amyloid fibrils cause tissue damage or organ dysfunction. For example, amyloid deposition in the heart due to either light chain or transthyretin-related amyloid leads to different clinical outcomes.[19] Several possible explanations for the mechanism of tissue injury have been put forth. These include interactions with RAGE receptors,[18] inflammatory response due to fibrillar intermediates, or direct cytoxicity of oligomeric precursors.[20] Several clinical clues suggest that some of these mechanisms may be operative in AL amyloid as well. For example, significant improvement in organ function may occur after chemotherapy has halted the production of amyloidogenic light chains, but before the expected resolution of the amyloid deposits in the involved tissues.[11,21] Improved understanding of the mechanism of amyloid-associated tissue injury may allow novel approaches to

preserve organ function and prolong survival in these patients.

## CLINICAL FEATURES

Clinical features in this group of diseases is highly diverse and depends on the nature of the organs involved. The nature of the amyloid (e.g., AL, ATTR) is a key determinant of pattern of organ involvement and dysfunction. Clinically, it is still useful to think in terms of localized or systemic forms of amyloidosis.[6]

### LOCALIZED AMYLOIDOSES

Localized deposits of amyloidosis in the genitourinary tract (e.g., bladder, ureter) or tracheobronchial tree (e.g., vocal cords) are nearly always localized, even though the fibrils themselves are often AL.[22,23] Skin amyloid is often localized and can be classified into lichen, macular, or nodular. The lichen and macular forms are easily treated with surgical resection. A common presentation of localized soft-tissue amyloid is carpal tunnel syndrome, which is generally treated with surgical release. These patients do not have systemic plasma cell dyscrasia and do not require systemic therapy.

### SYSTEMIC AMYLOIDOSIS
#### Immunoglobulin light chain-associated amyloidosis (AL)

AL is derived from Ig light chains, and most patients have plasma cell dyscrasia.[24,25] Patients regularly have free light chains detectable in the serum or the urine.

The clonal burden of plasma cells, however, is low and most patients have less than 10% plasma cells. Presence of lytic bone lesions and significant marrow plasmacytosis (more than 30%) should lead to a diagnosis of associated myeloma. However, in most instances, the clonal plasma cell burden in AL amyloidosis is nonprogressive, analogous to monoclonal gammopathy of undetermined significance or smoldering myeloma. It is the unique biologic properties of the light chain that leads to organ dysfunction and shortened survival.

Patients with AL generally present with one of the following seven syndromes:

1. Cardiomyopathy, with or without congestive heart failure,
2. Nephrotic range proteinuria, with or without renal insufficiency,
3. Hepatomegaly with elevated serum alkaline phosphatase,
4. Axonal peripheral neuropathy,
5. Autonomic neuropathy manifest as orthostatic hypotension,
6. Small intestinal involvement leading to pseudo-obstruction and alternating constipation and diarrhea, and
7. Soft-tissue involvement leading to arthropathy, macroglossia, and jaw or limb claudication.

These clinical features are consistent with AL, but there is significant overlap with other forms of amyloid, including AA, AF, or dialysis-associated amyloid.[24,25] It is therefore critical to establish the correct type of amyloid before initiation of therapy.

The dominant organs/systems involved in AL are cardiac, renal, neurologic, and gastrointestinal. Symptomatic cardiac involvement occurs in up to 25–50% of patients.[6] Cardiac manifestations mainly reflect myocardial involvement, and patients present with restrictive cardiomyopathy and diastolic dysfunction. Echocardiography is the most important tool in the diagnosis of cardiac involvement. The major echocardiographic features are increased left ventricular wall thickness, left atrial enlargement, and diastolic dysfunction, though these are not specific for AL amyloidosis.[26] Serum levels of troponins and brain natriuretic peptide appear to correlate with cardiac involvement and prognosis in early studies.[27,28] Renal involvement is generally manifest as nephrosis or renal insufficiency, and present in over half of the patients at diagnosis.[29] Sensorimotor peripheral neuropathy is present at diagnosis in about 15–30% of patients.[30] Autonomic neuropathy often co-exists with peripheral neuropathy and may present as orthostasis, or gut/bladder motility disturbances.

### Secondary amyloidosis (AA)

The most common manifestations of secondary (AA) amyloidosis are nephrotic range proteinuria and bowel involvement with diarrhea. AA may therefore be difficult to distinguish from AL.[31] In the west, AA mostly occurs in the setting of chronic inflammatory conditions (such as poorly controlled rheumatoid arthritis or ankylosing spondylitis), or chronic infections (e.g., osteomyelitis).[25] In the developing countries, AA is much more common as a complication of tuberculosis, leprosy, or malaria. In the Middle East, familial Mediterranean fever (FMF) is a common cause of AA. Although most patients do have an antecedent history of attacks of polyserositis, rash, or arthritis, there are genetic pedigrees of FMF, wherein AA can develop without antecedent symptoms.[32]

### Familial amyloidosis (AF)

Familial forms of amyloid are more common than AA. The most common presentation is progressive axonal peripheral and autonomic neuropathy.[17] However, patients can present with cardiomyopathy or with hepatic or renal amyloid. The most common forms of familial amyloidoses are due to mutations in the transthyretin (TTR) molecule.[9] To date, more than 60 mutations in the *TTR* gene have been described and associated with amyloid neuropathy. Nearly half of these patients do not have a family history. Therefore, an absence of family history does not exclude the diagnosis of AF. A distinct type of AF is seen in African American men. An allele of TTR called isoleucine 122 (*ILE122*) is carried by 3.9% of African-Americans.[19] The inheritance of this allele is a major cause of cardiac amyloidosis in elderly African American men. Cardiac amyloidosis can also occur from the deposition of wild type, as opposed to mutant, TTR. This form, referred to as "senile cardiac amyloidosis," occurs in 10–25% of people older than 80 years. Inherited forms of renal amyloid also occur, generally manifest as nephrosis. The amyloid in these instances may be a mutant fibrinogen-A-α chain, mutant lysozyme, apolipoprotein-A-I, or A-II. The distinction between AF and AL is critical and of more than academic importance. For example, liver transplantation done before the development of severe neuropathy or cardiomyopathy can produce durable regressions in patients with transthyretin-related amyloidosis.[33]

## DIAGNOSTIC WORKUP

The diagnosis of amyloidosis depends on the pathologic demonstration of typical congophilic deposits. The most common strategy is to take the biopsy from the most easily available tissue. Small amyloid deposits often occur in subcutaneous tissue of most people with AL or AA amyloidosis. For this reason, an abdominal fat aspirate is often used as an initial screen. However, a negative result does not exclude a diagnosis of AL, and other sites, such as rectal mucosa, marrow, and particularly the involved organ may need to be sampled.

The most important element of the diagnosis is typing of the amyloid deposit, as several amyloid states can have overlapping features. The presence of serum or urine monoclonal protein strongly supports AL amyloid. However, monoclonal proteins can be incidental in 3% of elderly patients.[34] Therefore, there would be a small false positive rate if this were the only criterion used. Most amyloid treatment centers recommend typing of the tissue with commercial antisera for AA, TTR, and κ and λ light chains. Antisera are also available for other proteins such as fibrinogen, lysozyme, or apolipoprotein, but are reserved for more complex cases.

Once the diagnosis and type of amyloid have been established, the next step is to determine the extent of organ dysfunction. In AL amyloidosis, evaluation of renal function (e.g., 24-hour urine collection for immunofixation and total protein) and cardiac involvement (e.g., echocardiogram, holter monitor, serum troponin, and brain natriuretic peptide) should be undertaken even in the absence of symptoms. Studies to evaluate the underlying clone in AL amyloid should include bone marrow biopsy, studies to quantify monoclonal Ig in the serum and urine, serum-free light chains, serum β-2 microglobulin, and a skeletal survey to exclude lytic bone disease. Other evaluations, such as electromyogram and stool studies for malabsorption, are based on the nature of disease-related symptoms. Rabiolabeled serum amyloid P component (SAP) has been used to image amyloid involvement, but this test has limited availability.[35] Approaches to visualize AL deposits in a noninvasive fashion are an area of active research.

## PROGNOSTIC FACTORS

The heterogeneity of clinical features and outcome in AL amyloidosis have inspired attempts to identify key determinants of prognosis in these patients. Presence of congestive heart failure and the total number of organs/systems involved are predictive of adverse outcome in several studies.[25] However, these features are quite subjective and may depend on the extent of evaluation of organ involvement. More recent studies have begun to test more objective criteria based on laboratory tests that have predictive value in other plasma cell diseases. These studies have identified serum level of β-2 microglobulin and markers of cardiac involvement (brain natriuretic peptide and troponins) as dominant predictors of outcome.[27,28,36,37] Assessment of prognostic factors is likely to assume major importance in the therapy of AL, as patient selection has a major effect on the outcome with some newer approaches (such as high-dose chemotherapy). Ongoing research will help clarify the impact of light chain variable region (VL) usage and other features of the amyloidogenic protein as predictors of outcome in AL.[38]

## EVALUATION OF RESPONSE

Evaluation of response to therapy in AL amyloidosis is largely based on surrogate measures that assess improvement in the underlying plasma cell clone and in AL-related organ dysfunction.[39] The hematologic response definition is quite comparable to that used in multiple myeloma, though the level of the monoclonal Ig in AL is quite low compared to myeloma. Most AL treatment centers also follow serum levels of free light chains as surrogate markers,[40] although this assay has not yet been fully incorporated or compared with the traditional response criteria used in most published studies with AL amyloid. Currently, improvement in AL-related organ dysfunction remains the gold standard by which the clinical efficacy of therapies against AL amyloid is judged. Although a consensus is beginning to emerge, these criteria are somewhat arbitrary. It is notable that histologic evidence of regression of AL deposits has not been documented in most studies. Indeed, improved organ function can occur without actual regression of amyloid deposits.[21]

## PRINCIPLES OF THERAPY

Most of the current therapies in AL and other amyloidoses are targeted toward the amyloidogenic precursor. The underlying principle is that deposition/resorption of amyloid is a dynamic process. Reduction in precursors or inhibition of amyloid formation will therefore shift the balance toward regression of deposits. A greater degree of reduction in precursors may lead to more durable responses. As the precursors themselves may be responsible for organ dysfunction, this approach may also help preserve organ function.

For example, therapies targeted to the underlying plasma cell clone may lead to reduction in amyloidogenic light chains, and thereby improved organ function.[1] Improvement in dialysis-related Aβ-2 microglobulin can occur with renal transplantation to reduce the levels of serum β-2 microglobulin. In patients with ATTR, liver transplantation has been pursued to provide a source of normal TTR from the transplanted liver. Durable regressions have been observed in several patients in whom liver transplantation was done before the development of severe neuropathy or cardiomyopathy.[33] Patients who receive such transplants late in the disease course, however, can show disease progression due to the deposition of wild type TTR in the heart that already has a nidus of mutant TTR.

## SUPPORTIVE CARE

Another important advance has been the improvements in supportive measures for AL-related organ dysfunction.[6] Careful attention to intravascular volume and cardiac function is essential. Many patients with renal involvement require assistance in the form of dialysis, although renal transplants have also been performed in some patients with otherwise good risk disease. Amyloidosis can develop in the graft if the precursor protein is not well controlled. Orthostasis can be treated with elastic stockings, fluorocortisone, and midodrine. Refractory diarrhea has been treated with antidiarrheals, somatostatin analogs, and even diverting colostomies.

## SPECIFIC THERAPY FOR AL AMYLOIDOSIS

### MELPHALAN AND PREDNISONE

The use of melphalan and prednisone (MP) to treat AL amyloidosis followed their establishment as effective therapy for multiple myeloma. A three-arm trial randomized 219 patients to colchicine alone, oral melphalan (0.15 mg/kg per day for 7 days) and prednisone (0.8 mg/kg per day for 7 days) every 6 weeks, or a combination of melphalan, prednisone, and colchicine (MPC).[41] The median survival for patients receiving MP was 17 months, compared to 8.5 months for colchicine alone. Another trial comparing MPC to MP found improved survival with MP-based therapy.[42] These studies have helped establish MP as one of the standard approaches to treat AL. However, most patients do not respond to this therapy, with objective responses seen in only 15–20% of patients. Most of these responses are limited to the patients with renal-only disease with preserved renal function. The median time to response is long (12 months), which necessitates prolonged therapy. This, however, has other consequences, such as the development of myelodysplasia or acute leukemia (actuarial risk of 21% at 3.5 years).[43] In spite of these limitations, MP is used frequently in the therapy of AL, particularly in older patients, as it is relatively well tolerated.

### DEXAMETHASONE BASED THERAPIES

In 1997, Dhodapkar et al. first described the clinical activity of dexamethasone (DEX) in AL amyloidosis.[44] Several studies have since confirmed this finding.[45–48] In a recent US Intergroup trial, 93 patients were treated with induction therapy with pulsed DEX, followed by DEX and alpha interferon as maintenance.[37] Complete hematologic remissions (CHR) were observed in 24 %. Improvement in AL-related organ function was seen in 45% of patients. Overall survival in the entire cohort was 31 months. The presence of congestive heart failure (CHF) and elevated serum β-2 microglobulin were dominant adverse prognostic factors. Patients with both of these features do poorly with DEX and should not be treated with this regimen. DEX has also been administered as a part of regimens that include melphalan[49] or doxorubicin-vincristine,[45] with promising results. However, whether the addition of these agents adds significantly to DEX alone remains unclear. The use of melphalan may have an impact on stem cell collection in patients eligible for stem cell transplantation, and should therefore be avoided before stem cell collection.

The tolerance to DEX in AL amyloid is lower than that in myeloma. This has prompted investigators to use reduced doses at the initiation of therapy, with dose escalation based on tolerance. Controlled studies are needed to compare DEX-based regimens to MP and to stem cell transplantation. Recent studies have identified the activity of several new drugs, such as thalidomide and bortezomib in combination with DEX in myeloma.[50,51] These regimens are currently undergoing active evaluation in the therapy of AL amyloidosis.

### STEM CELL TRANSPLANTATION IN AL AMYLOIDOSIS

The utility of high-dose melphalan and autologous stem cell transplantation in myeloma has been demonstrated through controlled studies. This has prompted several investigators to pursue this form of therapy in AL amyloidosis. Most of the published data are from a few amyloid centers.[52–54] The largest experience is from Boston University Medical Center. In the last update, 394 of 701 patients evaluated were eligible for this form of therapy.[21] Hematologic complete remissions (HCR) were observed in 40% of patients. Improvement in at least one organ was seen in 66% of patients with HCR and 30% of those without HCR. Median survival of the entire cohort was 4.6 years, but the early mortality was 13%. These data suggest that durable improvements in AL-related organ function can be achieved in AL amyloid using high-dose chemotherapy. Due to the higher transplantation-related mortality, some investigators are now pursuing risk-adapted approaches to melphalan dosing.[55]

Although the data with autologous stem cell transplant (ASCT) are promising, the degree to which they are impacted by patient selection factors remains unclear. Survival of patients eligible for transplantation, but treated with other approaches, is comparable to that reported in the ASCT experience in at least two, but not all studies.[37,56,57] These data underscore the need for controlled trials to address the value of high-dose melphalan and ASCT in AL amyloid. We recommend that the application of high-dose chemotherapy and stem cell transplantation in AL amyloidosis be carried out only in the context of clinical trials, or by groups experienced in this approach.[55]

### NEWER INVESTIGATIONAL APPROACHES

In view of the activity of several new agents in myeloma, these agents are now also being tested in patients with AL amyloidosis. However, the tolerance to drugs such as thalidomide is lower in this patient population.[58] Based on its binding to amyloid fibrils in vivo, iododeoxydoxorubicin was tested in a phase I/II trial, but yielded a low (15%) response rate as a single agent.[59] Hrncic et al. reported on an experimental model in which injection of antibody directed against amyloidogenic light chains led to regression of amyloid deposits.[60] This has not yet been tested in humans. Another approach in early clinical testing involves targeted pharmacologic depletion of serum amyloid P component, which may have broad utility in several amyloid states.[61]

## CONCLUSIONS

The amyloidoses are a diverse group of disorders characterized by pathologic protein folding, conformation, and deposition.[1,2] These disorders exhibit considerable clinical heterogeneity but share many pathogenic mechanisms. Current therapies are directed mostly toward reducing the supply of precursor proteins. Improved understanding of the pathogenic mechanisms is likely to yield novel approaches to therapy of these diseases.

## REFERENCES

1. Dhodapkar MV, Merlini G, Solomon A: Biology and therapy of immunoglobulin deposition diseases. *Hematol Oncol Clin North Am* 11:89–110, 1997.
2. Merlini G, Bellotti V: Molecular mechanisms of amyloidosis. *N Engl J Med* 349:583–596, 2003.
3. Bennhold H: Ein spezifishe amyloidfarbung mit kongoroot. *Muenchner Medizinische* 69:1537–1547, 1922.
4. Glenner G, Terry W, Harada M: Amyloid fibril proteins: proof of homology with immunoglobulin light chains by sequence analysis. *Science* 172:1150–1154, 1971.
5. Westermark P, Benson MD, Buxbaum JN: Amyloid fibril protein nomenclature. *Amyloid* 9:197–200, 2002.
6. Falk R, Comenzo R, Skinner M: The systemic amyloidoses. *N Engl J Med* 337:898–909, 1997.
7. Hardy J, Selkoe DJ: The amyloid hypothesis of Alzheimer's disease: progress and problems on the road to therapeutics. *Science* 297:353–356, 2002.
8. Lachmann HJ, Booth DR, Booth SE: Misdiagnosis of hereditary amyloidosis as AL amyloidosis. *N Engl J Med* 346:1786–1791, 2002.
9. Saraiva MJ: Transthyretin amyloidosis: a tale of weak interactions. *FEBS Lett* 498:201–203, 2001.
10. Drueke TB: Beta-2 microglobulin and amyloidosis. *Nephrol Dial Transplant* 15:17–24, 2000.
11. Merlini G, Westermark P: The systemic amyloidoses: clearer understanding of the molecular mechanisms offers hope for more effective therapies. *J Intern Med* 255:159–178, 2004.
12. Kyle RA, Gertz MA: Primary systemic amyloidosis: clinical and laboratory features in 474 cases. *Semin Hematol* 32:45–59, 1995.
13. Ozaki S, Abe M, Wolfenbarger D, Weiss DT, Solomon A: Preferential expression of human lambda light chain variable region subgroups in multiple myeloma, AL amyloidosis, and Waldentrom's macroglobulinemia. *Clin Immunol Immunopathol* 71:183–189, 1994.
14. Perfetti V, Ubbiali P, Vignarelli MC, et al.: Evidence that amyloidogenic light chains undergo antigen-driven selection. *Blood* 91:2948–2954, 1998.
15. Perfetti V, Casarini S, Palladini G, et al.: Analysis of V(lambda)-J(lambda) expression in plasma cells from primary (AL) amyloidosis and normal bone marrow identifies 3r (lambdaIII) as a new amyloid-associated germline gene segment. *Blood* 100:948–953, 2002.
16. Hurle MR, Helms LR, Li L, Chan W, Wetzel R: A role for destabilizing amino acid replacements in light chain amyloidosis. *Proc Natl Acad Sci USA* 91:5446–5450, 1994.
17. Buxbaum JN, Tagoe CE: The genetics of amyloidoses. *Ann Rev Med* 51:543–569, 2000.
18. Yan SD, Zhu H, Zhu A, et al.: Receptor-dependent cell stress and amyloid accumulation in systemic amyloidosis. *Nat Med* 6:643–651, 2000.
19. Jacobson DR, Pastore RD, Yaghoubian R, et al.: Variant-sequence transthyretin (isoleucine 122) in late-onset cardiac amyloidosis in black Americans. *N Engl J Med* 336:466–473, 1997.
20. Walsh DM, Klyubin I, Fadeeva JV, et al.: Naturally secreted oligomers of amyloid beta protein potently inhibit hippocampal long-term potentiation in vivo. *Nature* 416:535–539, 2002.
21. Skinner M, Sanchorawala V, Seldin DC, et al.: High-dose melphalan and autologous stem-cell transplantation in patients with AL amyloidosis: an 8-year study. *Ann Intern Med* 140:85–93, 2004.
22. Crocitto LE, Eastham JA, Zien L, Skinner EC, Huffman JL: Management and evaluation of localized amyloidosis of the bladder: two case reports. *Urology* 44:282–284, 1994.
23. O'Regan A, Fenlon HM, Beamis JF Jr, Steele MP, Skinner M, Berk JL: Tracheobronchial amyloidosis. The Boston University experience from 1984 to 1999. *Medicine (Baltimore)* 79:69–79, 2000.
24. Gertz MA, Lacy MQ, Dispenzieri A: Amyloidosis. *Hematol Oncol Clin North Am* 13:1211–1233, ix, 1999.
25. Gertz MA, Lacy MQ, Dispenzieri A: Amyloidosis: recognition, confirmation, prognosis, and therapy. *Mayo Clin Proc* 74:490–494, 1999.
26. Dubrey SW, Cha K, Skinner M, LaValley M, Falk RH: Familial and primary (AL) cardiac amyloidosis: echocardiographically similar diseases with distinctly different clinical outcomes. *Heart* 78:74–82, 1997.
27. Dispenzieri A, Kyle RA, Gertz MA, et al.: Survival in patients with primary systemic amyloidosis and raised serum cardiac troponins. *Lancet* 361:1787–1789, 2003.
28. Palladini G, Campana C, Klersy C, et al.: Serum N-terminal pro-brain natriuretic peptide is a sensitive marker of myocardial dysfunction in AL amyloidosis. *Circulation* 107:2440–2445, 2003.
29. Gertz MA, Lacy MQ, Dispenzieri A: Immunoglobulin light chain amyloidosis and the kidney. *Kidney Int* 61:1–9, 2002.
30. Rajkumar SV, Gertz MA, Kyle RA: Prognosis of patients with primary systemic amyloidosis who present with dominant neuropathy. *Am J Med* 104:232–237, 1998.

31. Perfetti V, Garini P, Vignarelli MC, Marinone MG, Zorzoli I, Merlini G: Diagnostic approach to and follow-up of difficult cases of AL amyloidosis. *Haematologica* 80:409–415, 1995.

32. Grateau G: The relationship between familial Mediterranean fever and amyloidosis. *Curr Opin Rheumatol* 12:61–64, 2000.

33. Bergethon PR, Sabin TD, Lewis D, Simms RW, Cohen AS, Skinner M: Improvement in the polyneuropathy associated with familial amyloid polyneuropathy after liver transplantation. *Neurology* 47:944–951, 1996.

34. Kyle RA, Rajkumar SV: Monoclonal gammopathies of undetermined significance. *Hematol Oncol Clin North Am* 13:1181–1202, 1999.

35. Hawkins PN, Aprile C, Capri G, et al.: Scintigraphic imaging and turnover studies with iodine-131 labelled serum amyloid P component in systemic amyloidosis. *Eur J Nucl Med* 25:701–708, 1998.

36. Pardanani A, Witzig TE, Schroeder G, et al.: Circulating peripheral blood plasma cells as a prognostic indicator in patients with primary systemic amyloidosis. *Blood* 101:827–830, 2003.

37. Dhodapkar MV, Hussein MA, Rasmussen E, et al.: Clinical efficacy of high dose dexamethasone with maintenance dexamethasone/alpha interferon in patients with primary systemic amyloidosis: results of United States Intergroup trial Southwest Oncology Group SWOG 9628. *Blood* 104: 3520–3526, 2004.

38. Comenzo RL, Wally J, Kica G, et al.: Clonal immunoglobulin light chain variable region germline gene use in AL amyloidosis: association with dominant amyloid-related organ involvement and survival after stem cell transplantation. *Br J Haematol* 106:744–751, 1999.

39. Gertz MA, Kyle RA, Greipp PR: Response rates and survival in primary systemic amyloidosis. *Blood* 77:257–262, 1991.

40. Abraham RS, Katzmann JA, Clark RJ, Bradwell AR, Kyle RA, Gertz MA: Quantitative analysis of serum free light chains. A new marker for the diagnostic evaluation of primary systemic amyloidosis. *Am J Clin Pathol* 119:274–278, 2003.

41. Kyle RA, Gertz MA, Greipp PR, et al.: A trial of three regimens for primary amyloidosis: colchicine alone, melphalan and prednisone, and melphalan, prednisone, and colchicine. *N Engl J Med* 336:1202–1207, 1997.

42. Skinner M, Anderson J, Simms R, et al.: Treatment of 100 patients with primary amyloidosis: a randomized trial of melphalan, prednisone, and colchicine versus colchicine only. *Am J Med* 100:290–298, 1996.

43. Gertz MA, Kyle RA: Acute leukemia and cytogenetic abnormalities complicating melphalan treatment of primary systemic amyloidosis. *Arch Intern Med* 150:629–633, 1990.

44. Dhodapkar MV, Jagannath S, Vesole D, et al.: Treatment of AL-amyloidosis with dexamethasone plus alpha interferon. *Leuk Lymphoma* 27:351–356, 1997.

45. Lachmann HJ, Gallimore R, Gillmore JD, et al.: Outcome in systemic AL amyloidosis in relation to changes in concentration of circulating free immunoglobulin light chains following chemotherapy. *Br J Haematol* 122: 78–84, 2003.

46. Gertz MA, Lacy MQ, Lust JA, Greipp PR, Witzig TE, Kyle RA: Phase II trial of high-dose dexamethasone for previously treated immunoglobulin light-chain amyloidosis. *Am J Hematol* 61:115–119, 1999.

47. Gertz MA, Lacy MQ, Lust JA, Greipp PR, Witzig TE, Kyle RA: Phase II trial of high-dose dexamethasone for untreated patients with primary systemic amyloidosis. *Med Oncol* 16:104–109, 1999.

48. Palladini G, Anesi E, Perfetti V, et al.: A modified high-dose dexamethasone regimen for primary systemic (AL) amyloidosis. *Br J Haematol* 113:1044–1046, 2001.

49. Palladini G, Perfetti V, Obici L, et al.: The association of melphalan and high-dose dexamethasone is effective and well tolerated in patients with AL (primary) amyloidosis ineligible for stem cell transplantation. *Blood* 103:2936–2938, 2004.

50. Singhal S, Mehta J, Desikan R, et al.: Antitumor activity of thalidomide in refractory multiple myeloma. *N Engl J Med* 341:1565–1571, 1999.

51. Richardson PG, Barlogie B, Berenson J, et al.: A phase 2 study of bortezomib in relapsed, refractory myeloma. *N Engl J Med* 348:2609–2617, 2003.

52. Gertz MA, Lacy MQ, Dispenzieri A, et al.: Stem cell transplantation for the management of primary systemic amyloidosis. *Am J Med* 113:549–555, 2002.

53. Comenzo RL, Gertz MA: Autologous stem cell transplantation for primary systemic amyloidosis. *Blood* 99:4276–4282, 2002.

54. Moreau P, Leblond V, Bourquelot P, et al.: Prognostic factors for survival and response after high-dose therapy and autologous stem cell transplantation in systemic AL amyloidosis: a report on 21 patients. *Br J Haematol* 101:766–769, 1998.

55. Gertz MA, Lacy MQ, Dispenzieri A: Therapy for immunoglobulin light chain amyloidosis: the new and the old. *Blood Rev* 18:17–37, 2004.

56. Dispenzieri A, Lacy MQ, Kyle RA, et al.: Eligibility for hematopoietic stem-cell transplantation for primary systemic amyloidosis is a favorable prognostic factor for survival. *J Clin Oncol* 19:3350–3356, 2001.

57. Dispenzieri A, Kyle RA, Lacy MQ, et al.: Superior survival in primary systemic amyloidosis patients undergoing peripheral blood stem cell transplant : a case control study. *Blood* 103: 3960–3963, 2004.

58. Dispenzieri A, Lacy MQ, Rajkumar SV, et al.: Poor tolerance to high doses of thalidomide in patients with primary systemic amyloidosis. *Amyloid* 10: 257–261, 2003.

59. Gertz MA, Lacy MQ, Dispenzieri A, et al.: A multicenter phase II trial of 4'-iodo-4'deoxydoxorubicin (IDOX) in primary amyloidosis (AL). *Amyloid* 9:24–30, 2002.

60. Hrncic R, Wall J, Wolfenbarger DA, et al.: Antibody-mediated resolution of light chain-associated amyloid deposits. *Am J Pathol* 157:1239–1246, 2000.

61. Pepys MB, Herbert J, Hutchinson WL, et al.: Targeted pharmacological depletion of serum amyloid P component for treatment of human amyloidosis. *Nature* 417:254–259, 2002.

# Chapter 91
# TREATMENT OF COMPLICATIONS IN MULTIPLE MYELOMA

*Paul Masci*

Although multiple myeloma (MM) is classified under the heading of indolent non-Hodgkin's lymphomas, the pathophysiologic mechanisms of this disease often cause significant morbidity. Long-term survival rates for patients with MM have consistently improved over the last 30 years.[1] Thus, managing the acute and chronic complications of this disease can be challenging. This chapter will review the basic mechanisms of target organ complications of MM and provide a summary of literature-based recommendations for managing such complications.

## ANEMIA

Anemia in the patient with MM is defined by a hemoglobin value 2 gm/dL below the institutional limits of normal or a hemoglobin concentration less than 10 gm/dL.[2] It is present in approximately two-thirds of newly diagnosed patients and will eventually occur in nearly all patients.[2] The causes are multifactorial and include the replacement of normal hematopoietic cells by the expanding plasma cell burden, myelosuppression related to chemotherapy, and an increase of plasma volume secondary to high serum M-protein levels, which may lead to spurious declines in hemoglobin concentration.[3] Importantly, overproduction of interleukin-6 (IL-6) in the bone marrow microenvironment can cause an attenuated response to erythropoietin.[4] This process may be exacerbated in patients who have compromised renal function and lower endogenous erythropoietin levels.

The use of exogenous recombinant erythropoietin has been studied in patients with MM. Small, single institution studies suggested benefit in those patients with low endogenous levels.[5,6] Subsequent randomized trials have confirmed this benefit.[7,8] In a double-blinded study, 25 patients were randomized to receive placebo or erythropoietin 150 U/kg three times per week for 6 weeks.[7] The dose was doubled in nonresponders after 6 weeks in the erythropoietin group; patients in the placebo arm were crossed over to receive erythropoietin in an open label fashion if no response was observed after 12 weeks on study. Although the number of evaluable patients was small ($n = 20$), the results were significant. Sixty percent of the patients receiving erythropoietin had a complete response, whereas no responses occurred in the placebo group. Thirty percent of these patients did have a complete response when crossed over to receive erythropoietin. The median dose for the responding group was 120 U/kg. The type of chemotherapy and pretreatment serum erythropoietin levels did not predict response to exogenous erythropoietin.[7]

A second trial included 120 transfusion-dependent patients with either MM or low-grade non-Hodgkin's lymphoma. Patients were randomly assigned to receive either a fixed dose or an escalating dose of erythropoietin, or placebo.[8] Response, defined by elimination of transfusion need and an increase in hemoglobin by at least 2 gm/dL, occurred in 60% of those patients receiving erythropoietin. No difference in response was found for the fixed versus escalating dose of erythropoietin.[8] Multivariate analysis did suggest that endogenous erythropoietin level was the most important predictor of response.[8]

As these trials included small numbers of patients, the current consensus guidelines do not recommend the routine use of erythropoietin in MM patients not receiving chemotherapy. For those MM patients receiving chemotherapy, or with no improvement in hemoglobin following control of disease, erythropoietin use is recommended if a hemoglobin level $\leq 10$ gm/dL is observed.[9] Guidelines for recombinant erythropoietin use are presented in Table 91.1.

A large retrospective study suggested that approximately 14% of newly diagnosed plasma cell dyscrasia patients have serologic evidence of $B_{12}$ deficiency.[10] Newly diagnosed MM patients should be screened for $B_{12}$ deficiency by use of serum $B_{12}$ and methylmalonic acid (MMA) levels. In the absence of renal insufficiency, a serum $B_{12}$ level < 200 pg/mL or a serum $B_{12}$ level 200–300 pg/mL with an elevated MMA are diagnostic

**Table 91.1**    Recommendations for erythropoietin use in multiple myeloma

■ Consider for all MM patients receiving chemotherapy with a hemoglobin level ≤10 g/dL. There is no satisfactory data to support routine erythropoietin use in MM patients in the absence of chemotherapy.

■ Most trials have studied multiple doses per week. The recommended starting dose is 150 U/kg three times per week for a minimum of 4 weeks. The dose may be escalated to 300 U/μg three times weekly for up to 4–8 more weeks if no response to initial dose. The evidence for once weekly dosing, i.e., 40,000 units, is less strong, but acceptable clinically.

■ The dose can be titrated to maintain hemoglobin levels at or near 12 g/dL. Erythropoietin may also be held and restarted once hemoglobin levels decline 10 g/dL. Patients who do not respond to optimized doses by 6–8 weeks are unlikely to do so and erythropoietin should be discontinued.

■ The use of erythropoietin in patients with isolated plasmacytoma, or other plasma cell dyscrasia is not recommended. Anemia in these patients should prompt further work-up for underlying MM.

Adapted from Ref. 9

of B[12] deficiency.[10] Such patients should receive vitamin B[12] replacement therapy.

## HYPERCALCEMIA

Hypercalcemia may be observed in approximately 15–30% of newly diagnosed patients with MM.[11,12] The mechanism of hypercalcemia is likely due to increased osteoclastic resorptive activity.[13] Calcium levels should be corrected for serum albumin. Furthermore, some patients may have spurious elevations of serum calcium because of increased binding by paraproteins. Therefore, ionized serum calcium levels should be measured to aid in the diagnosis of hypercalcemia for patients with high monoclonal protein levels.[3]

Clinically, hypercalcemia is associated with lethargy, confusion, polydypsia, polyuria, constipation, and nausea.[11] Untreated hypercalcemia will lead to renal insufficiency, a problem to which patients with MM are already prone. Therefore, prompt treatment once recognized is essential.

Urgent treatment of hypercalcemia is accomplished through increased urinary calcium excretion by volume expansion with intravenous saline. The addition of diuretics to aid in maintaining adequate urine output and calciuresis may cause other electrolyte abnormalities and exacerbate volume depletion. Therefore, diuretics are probably best avoided in the initial management of hypercalcemia. Some investigators recommend corticosteroids, i.e., prednisone 25 mg daily as an adjunctive treatment.[12]

Bisphosphonates inhibit the resorptive action of osteoclasts (see the next section on skeletal complications) and can be effective in the management of hypercalcemia in the patient with MM.[14,15] Two bisphosphonates, pamidronate (Aredia; Novartis Pharmaceuticals, East Hanover, NJ) and zoledronate (Zometa; Novartis Pharmaceuticals, East Hanover, NJ) have been studied for the treatment of hypercalcemia of malignancy.[16] One large randomized trial suggested that zoledronate (4 mg or 8 mg) may be superior to pamidronate (90 mg) in achieving corrected serum calcium levels to less than 10.8 mg/dL, time to response, and duration of response.[16] However, this study, which included 275 eligible patients with hypercalcemia of malignancy, enrolled only 23 (8.4%) with MM.[16] Therefore, it is reasonable to treat MM patients with hypercalcemia with either agent.

## RENAL COMPLICATIONS

Renal insufficiency is found in up to 20% of patients with MM at the time of diagnosis and about 10% of all patients will eventually develop severe renal failure.[2,17] The morbidity and mortality of this complication is significant; MM patients account for approximately 0.9% of the dialysis patients in the United States and up to 2% of dialysis patients in Great Britain.[17,18] A review of the United States Renal Data System reveals that the 2-year all-cause mortality for dialysis patients with MM/light chain disease is higher than for all other dialysis patients (58% vs 31%; $P < 0.01$ by log-rank test).[18]

Several independent mechanisms are responsible for the acute and chronic renal insufficiency observed in patients with MM: direct tubulointerstitial damage and cast nephropathy caused by filtered fee light-chain proteins (Bence-Jones proteins), light chain deposition disease, primary amyloidosis, hypercalcemia, and, rarely, type I myeloma associated cryoglobulinemia.

Filtered light-chain proteins (both κ and λ) can cause an acute or chronic renal insufficiency by two pathophysiologic mechanisms.[19,20] In vitro studies suggest that human-derived light-chains are directly toxic to proximal tubular cells in rat nephrons causing both altered function and morphology in a perfusion, time-dependent fashion.[19] This mechanism is believed to underlie the tubulointerstitial nephropathy found in patients with MM.[19] Light-chain proteins may also form intraluminal proteinacious casts through noncovalent binding with the normally present Tamm-Horsfall glycoproteins.[21] These casts can obstruct the distal tubules, leading to an obstructive cast nephropathy ("myeloma kidney").[20] Increasing calcium, sodium, and chloride concentrations in the tubule fluid can augment the aggregation of light-chains and Tamm-Horsfall protein.[22] Dehydration can cause both decreased filtrate flow and increased light-chain concentration, further accelerating cast formation.[23] Therefore, obstructive cast nephropathy usually manifests as acute renal insufficiency with nonnephrotic clinical features.

Multiple myeloma patients with acute renal insufficiency may benefit from plasma exchange or plasmapheresis. A small randomized trial was conducted in which patients with MM and Bence-Jones proteinuria (> 1 g/day) were randomly assigned to receive plasma exchange or control.[24] Twenty-nine patients were enrolled, 24 of whom initially required dialysis; the five not requiring dialysis had serum creatinine levels in excess of 5 mg/dL. All patients received concurrent therapy with cytotoxic drugs and corticosteroids. Those in the plasma exchange group underwent a 3–4 L exchange per day for five consecutive days. Patients in the plasma exchange group had a significant reduction in proteinuria ($P < 0.01$) associated with a significant increase in urine output ($P < 0.001$) compared to the control group.[24] Thirteen of the 15 patients (87%) allocated to plasma exchange no longer required dialysis at the end of the study period, with an average serum creatinine recovery of 2.6 mg/dL, while only two of the 14 patients (14%) in the control group improved with cytotoxic treatment alone.[24] Importantly, a significant improvement in 1 year overall survival was observed when compared to the control group (66% vs 28%; $P < 0.01$).[24]

The importance of the tubular cast burden in a similar population of patients was described in a trial of plasmapheresis.[25] Twenty-one patients with overt MM all received cytotoxic therapy, corticosteroids, and forced diuresis. Eleven were randomly assigned to receive plasmapheresis three times per week for 1 to 4 weeks. Renal biopsies were performed on nine of the patients in the plasmapheresis group and seven of the patients in the control group. The patients in the two groups had similar outcomes, with no differences observed between groups for improved serum creatinine value, need for long-term hemodialysis, or overall median survival (approximately 18 months for both).[25] However, blinded evaluation of renal biopsy specimens (available from 16 patients on trial) for myeloma cast formation and tubulointerstitial changes consisting of inflammation, atrophic loss, and fibrosis was performed. Five out of seven patients (71%) with 2–3+ cast formation went on to require hemodialysis, while only two of nine (22%) with ≤ 1+ cast formation became dialysis dependent.[25]

The results of these two small studies may seem conflicting. However, they differed in choice of pheresis technique and cytotoxic regimen. Also, patients in the second study had an average time from recognition of renal impairment to study entry of 1.21 months.[25] This suggests that patients with acute renal insufficiency caused by myeloma kidney with low disease burden may benefit from plasma exchange if it is instituted with cytotoxic chemotherapy soon after recognition of impaired renal function. Indeed, an empiric trial of plasmapheresis in any MM patient with acute renal failure not initially responsive to volume replacement is warranted as renal biopsy is logistically impractical in all patients.[12]

Light-chain (rarely heavy chain) deposition disease and primary amyloidosis are pathophysiologically similar. Both are histologically characterized by the deposition of immunoglobulin (Ig) light or heavy chains within various body tissues. Amyloid protein (usually λ light chain) deposition is histologically and molecularly unique in the formation of characteristic β-pleated fibrils identified by an apple-green color when stained with Congo red dye. Light-chain (usually κ light chain) and the rare heavy-chain deposition diseases lead to a nonfibrillary accumulation of light (or heavy) chains. In the kidney, light chain deposition is detected by immunohistochemical staining and found in a linear distribution within the glomerular and/or tubular basement membranes.[26] Electron microscopy may reveal granular electron dense deposits in the same places.[26]

Generally, the clinical manifestation of renal light chain or amyloid deposition is nephrotic range proteinuria with a nonoliguric, chronically progressive renal insufficiency. Treatment of patients with advanced renal disease from amyloid or light-chain deposition disease is often unsatisfactory. However, a multicenter trial including 64 patients with renal impairment from amyloidosis treated with a pulse dose strategy of dexamethasone demonstrated improved renal function in 39% at a median of 4 months.[27]

In summary, patients with acute renal insufficiency caused by cast nephropathy may have improvement with hydration, plasma exchange, and treatment of the underlying MM. Those with amyloid or light-chain deposition disease may benefit from dexamethasone treatment. All patients with MM should be encouraged to drink liberal amounts of water and avoid the use of non-steroidal anti-inflammatory drugs (NSAIDs). Clinicians should use intravenous contrast judiciously in patients with MM, especially in those with volume depletion and heavy urine ligh- chain excretion, as the risk of precipitating acute renal insufficiency is increased in these patients.[28] Hypercalcemia should be corrected promptly in these patients, as they may be especially prone to exacerbations of underlying chronic renal insufficiency.

## INFECTIOUS COMPLICATIONS

Infectious complications are frequent in patients with MM and an important cause of mortality in this disease.[29] Data suggest that approximately 25% of newly diagnosed patients initially seek care because of recurrent infections, especially of the respiratory and urinary tracts.[30,31] The underlying mechanisms leading to compromised immune function in patients with MM are incompletely understood, but are likely related to defects in both primary and secondary immune responses. Low serum levels of normal Ig in patients with MM have long been recognized, and an imbalance in the proportion of Th1 to Th2 cells has recently been described.[32,33] Patients receiving cytotoxic chemotherapy and corticosteroids may be further immunocompromised due to myelosuppression.

Hypogammaglobulinemia may account for the increased susceptibility to polysaccharide encapsulated organisms, particularly at the time of diagnosis and following initial treatment (see next).[34,35] However, infections with gram negative bacilli and *Staphylococcus aureus* appear to be more common causes of serious and lethal infections in those patients undergoing chemotherapy within the first 2 months after diagnosis.[36–38] In addition, such infections frequently necessitate delaying chemotherapy. Efforts to reduce the occurrence of infection in those patients undergoing initial treatment are warranted.

Trimethoprim-sulfamethoxazole (TMP-SMX) has been investigated as a prophylactic agent in a small, randomized, multicenter trial of newly diagnosed patients undergoing chemotherapy for MM.[35] This antibiotic was chosen based on low expense, tolerability, and previous experience in other patients with other causes of immunocompromise.[35] Fifty-seven patients with MM were randomized to receive prophylaxis consisting of two TMP-SMX 80/400 mg tablets every 12 hours for 2 months, or to a control group that received no prophylaxis. Chemotherapy was administered to all patients; 50% received melphalan plus prednisone, while all others received more intensive combination chemotherapy. The two groups were well balanced with respect to age, gender, and stage of disease. Data collection continued for 3 months after the start of chemotherapy for patients in both groups. Fifty-four patients of the 57 entered were evaluable. Overall, 12 (46%) of the patients assigned to the control group and five (18%) of the patients who received TMP-SMX experienced any infection during the 3 month observation period ($P = 0.04$).[35] Bacterial infections were significantly more frequent during the first 2 months in the control group compared to the prophylactic group (35% vs 4%; $P = 0.004$).[35] Although not statistically significant, four deaths occurred in the control group while only one occurred in the prophylactic group.[35] TMP-SMX caused skin rash requiring cessation of treatment in six (21%) patients. One patient developed exfoliative dermatitis.[35]

Although reactions to TMP-SMX were observed, this study demonstrated that prophylactic administration of antibiotics is feasible and may confer clinical benefit. The practice of administering a prophylactic antibiotic is not routinely followed, but some centers do recommend prophylaxis for all patients undergoing initial chemotherapy.[39] The choice of agent is not settled, and an National Cancer Institute

(NCI)-sponsored trial is currently ongoing comparing TMP-SMX, a fluoroquinolone, or placebo in a similar patient population.

Hypogammaglobulinemia has been suggested to be the cause of susceptibility to infections with polysaccharide encapsulated organisms in patients with MM, similar to infections in patients with primary Ig deficiency.[34] Moreover, myeloma patients appear to be more prone to pathogens such as *Streptococcus pneumoniae* or *Haemophilus influenzae* in the time period following initial chemotherapy. Efforts to enhance secondary immune function with passive immunization by administration of intravenous immunoglobulin (IVIG) have been evaluated.

Results from a phase I trial demonstrated that IVIG could be safely given to patients with MM.[40] Seventeen patients were given doses of IVIG ranging from 150 mg/kg to 500 mg/kg. The infusions were well tolerated, with no significant toxicities. The investigators measured functional antibody to hepatitis B surface antigen and found a range in the half-life from 7 to 20 days for the entire group.[40] The kinetics of the antibody did not appear to be related to the M-protein subtype or baseline native immunoglobulin G (IgG) levels.[40]

To assess the prophylactic role of IVIG in preventing serious infections, a prospective, randomized, double-blinded, placebo-controlled, multicenter trial including patients with stable phase MM was conducted.[41] Patients were not eligible if they had early, progressive, or terminal MM or received any prophylactic antibiotics within the 2 weeks preceding study entry.[41] Eighty-three patients were enrolled and randomized to receive IVIG 0.4 g/kg or placebo (0.4% albumin) every 4 weeks for 1 year. Patients were stratified by baseline Ig levels. Severity of infection was prospectively defined; major infections included culture positive sepsis or clinical sepsis syndrome without documented organism, meningitis, and pneumonia requiring hospitalization. Moderate infections consisted of acute bronchitis, upper respiratory or urinary tract infections, skin cellulitis or abscess, and localized zoster. Serious infections included all those considered major or moderate, whereas infections were considered minor if antibiotics were not clinically indicated. Patients were well balanced with respect to age, stage, and performance status. Thirty-two of the 42 (76%) patients randomized to IVIG and 26 of the 41 (63%) patients in the placebo group had baseline Ig levels below normal.[41] No episodes of sepsis or pneumonia occurred in the IVIG treatment group, whereas 10 episodes occurred in the placebo group ($P = 0.002$).[41] Respiratory infections other than pneumonia were also significantly less frequent in the IVIG group (6 episodes vs 18; $P = 0.0097$).[41] Three patients withdrew from the IVIG group because of infusion reactions. No comment was made as to how baseline Ig levels affected outcome. However, analysis of 54 patients who had received Pneumovax 1 month prior to study entry showed that those with poor response to the vaccine (i.e., less than twofold increase or final specific IgG < 40 U/mL) who also received IVIG had six episodes of infection compared with 16 episodes in poor responders in the placebo arm during 128 patient-month follow ups ($P = 0.033$).[41] The short follow-up did not allow for survival analysis.[41] The implication is that those patients who are unable to mount an immune response may benefit from IVIG during stable phase MM. Until further studies exploring risk of infusion reactions, overall survival, quality of life (QOL), and cost effectiveness are available, the routine use IVIG in stable phase MM patients is not routinely recommended. Similarly, there are no prospective data to suggest benefit from IVIG in MM patients with acute bacterial infections.

Patients with hematologic malignancies often inquire about yearly influenza vaccination, and physicians differ on their recommendations. Data is available to guide decision making. Thirty-four consecutive patients with either a chronic lymphoproliferative disorder ($n = 28$) or MM ($n = 6$) were given a virosomal influenza vaccine preparation.[42] The MM patients had a mean time from diagnosis to study entry of 3 years (range 1–11). A hemagglutinin inhibition assay (HAI) to assess antibody response to three strains of influenza was performed on all patients at baseline and 1 month after vaccination. Seroconversion (HAI titre ≥ 1:20 in previously seronegative subjects, or a fourfold or greater increase of the titre in previously positive subjects) to all three strains occurred in three of the six (50%) MM patients; seroconversion to at least two of the three strains was documented in two (33%) MM patients, and no response occurred in one patient.[42] Two mild injection site reactions were reported for the entire 34 patient study population, and none of the MM patients in this study developed influenza in the ensuing 3-month follow-up.

A separate study evaluated the response of MM patients to immunization with pneumococcal (Pneumovax II) and *H. influenzae* type b (Hib) vaccination. Fifty-two MM patients, of whom seven patients had undergone high-dose therapy with autologous stem cell transplantation within the preceding 6 months, were offered vaccination.[43] At baseline, 94% of the patients had *S. pneumoniae* antibody titers below the protective level. Postvaccination, 39% achieved protective levels. Similarly, 54% of patients had nonprotective titers of *H. influenzae* antibodies, whereas 75% developed protective titers following vaccination.[43] High-dose therapy followed by autologous transplant predicted for poor response to Hib vaccine ($P = 0.04$).[43] These results suggest that routine measurement of antibodies in patients with MM to both *S. pneumoniae* and *H. influenzae* should be performed and, if found to be low, vaccination should be offered.

## SKELETAL COMPLICATIONS

The skeletal complications of MM are the most distressing of all the end-organ complications encountered in this disease. Osteopenia and lytic bone lesions are a cause of disabling pain and pathologic fractures. Spinal cord compression may result as well. Thirty percent of patients will present with nonvertebral fractures and more than 50% will present with back pain or vertebral fractures.[44,45] Approximately 80% of patients will have radiographic evidence of osteoporosis, lytic lesions, or fractures at the time of diagnosis.[2]

Osteoporosis, focal lysis, and hypercalcemia all result from increased osteoclastic activity. The molecular mechanism causing this enhanced activity is incompletely understood, but continues to be an area of intense investigation. The current paradigm proposes that an imbalance in osteoprotegerin (OPG) and osteoprotegerin ligand (OPGL) are central to bone resorption.[46] OPGL is known to activate osteoclastic cells via the receptor activator of NF-κB (RANK).[46] Ex vivo coculture studies suggest that plasma cells derived from patients with MM modulate osteoblast and bone marrow stromal cell production of OPGL and its decoy receptor OPG in such a way that OPG is downregulated while OPGL itself is upregulated.[46] Recombinant OPG is currently in clinical development and the results of a phase I trial have been published.[47]

### BISPHOSPHONATES

Bisphosphonates are a class of drugs that are structural analogs of endogenous pyrophosphate.[15] Carbon substitution for the central oxygen atom makes the molecule resistant to hydrolysis and allows for the addition of two side chains necessary for calcium crystal and bone mineral affinity.[15] Bisphosphonates are selectively deposited to sites of increased bone turnover and are ingested by osteoclasts, causing inhibition their resorptive capacity.[48,49] Currently, two bisphosphonates, pamidronate (Aredia; Novartis Pharmaceuticals, East Hanover, NJ) and zoledronate (Zometa; Novartis Pharmaceuticals, East Hanover, NJ), are Food and Drug Administration (FDA) approved in the United States for use in MM patients with lytic bone disease.

Bisphosphonates have been extensively studied in patients with MM (see Table 91.2). In general, no overall survival benefit has been observed with their use; rather, significant reductions in clinically measurable skeletal related events (SREs) can be achieved.[15] In larger trials, an SRE is defined as pathologic fracture, spinal cord compression, or need for radiation or surgical intervention.[50,51] In addition to these clinical endpoints, some studies have included hypercalcemia as an SRE.[52,53]

When given to MM patients undergoing chemotherapy, pamidronate 90 mg IV over 4 hours monthly can significantly reduce serum and urinary markers of bone

| Table 91.2 | Randomized trials of bisphosphonate therapy in multiple myeloma | |
| --- | --- | --- |
| | Pamidronate 90 mg IV over 4 hours every 4 weeks | Zoledronate 4 or 8 mg IV every 3–4 weeks for 12 months |
| References | 48,53 | 51 |
| Study design | Randomized double-blind, placebo-controlled trial | Randomized, double-blind, comparative trial |
| Efficacy evaluation | Pamidronate vs placebo | Noninferiority study zoledronate vs pamidronate |
| Primary endpoint | Combined SREs at 9 months | Combined SREs |
| Sample size, n | 392 (all MM) | 1,648 (513 MM, 1,130 breast cancer) |
| Treatment course | First vs second or greater chemotherapy | First treatment |
| Percent patients with osteolytic bone lesions at entry | 100 | 100 |
| **Results** | | |
| Pain score decline | Yes | Yes, equal to pamidronate |
| Time to first SRE | ~12 vs 21 months | Median 12.3 months zoledronate vs 12.0 months pamidronate (P = NS) |
| SREs per year | 28% vs 44% at 12 months; 38% vs 51% at 21 months | 47–49% zoledronate vs 49% pamidronate |
| Nonvertebral fractures | 15% vs 10% | NR |
| Vertebral fractures | NR | NR |
| Radiotherapy needed | 25% vs 34% | 0.47 vs 0.71 per year (P = 0.018) |
| NNT to a avoid one event | 6.2 at 12 months; 7.7 at 21 months | N/A |

NNT, Number needed to treat; NR, Not reported; N/A, Non applicable; NS, Not significant.
Adapted from Ref. 14.

resorption (cross-linked N-telopeptides of type-I collagen), IL-6, CRP, and β2-microglobulin, which may lead to a significant reduction of pain.[54]

A large randomized international multicenter placebo-controlled trial led to the FDA approval of pamidronate in MM patients with lytic bone lesions.[50] Patients with stage III MM and at least one lytic skeletal lesion undergoing chemotherapy were randomly assigned to receive placebo or pamidronate 90 mg IV over 4 hours monthly for a planned 21 months. Patients were stratified into those receiving first-line chemotherapy or second-line and beyond. The primary end point was number of SREs after nine doses, in which an SRE was defined as pathologic fracture, need for radiation or surgery, and spinal cord compression.[50] Three hundred ninety-two patients were included in the safety and survival analysis, while only eligible patients were included in the efficacy analysis (n = 196 in pamidronate group vs n = 181 in placebo group). The time to first skeletal event was significantly less in the pamidronate group (P = 0.001 by the log-rank test).[50] The mean number of SREs per year was observed to be reduced from 2.1 in the placebo group to 1.1 in the pamidronate group at the planned primary time end point (P = 0.0006).[50] Two patients were withdrawn from the pamidronate treatment secondary to an allergic reaction and hypocalcemia. Renal insufficiency was not reported in any patients. Follow-up analysis at 21 months continued to show effect as the proportion of patients treated with

pamidronate developing any skeletal event was less than the placebo group (P = 0.015).[55] Subset analysis identified longer survival in the patients treated with pamidronate who were also receiving second-line or beyond chemotherapy when compared to patients in the placebo arm (21 months vs 14 months; P = 0.041).[55] Objective measures of QOL showed declines in the placebo-treated patients.[15]

Zoledronate at doses of 4 mg and 8 mg IV over 5 minutes were shown to be superior to pamidronate 90 mg IV over 2 hours in the treatment of hypercalcemia of malignancy.[16] Additionally, a trial comparing two doses of zoledronate (2 mg and 4 mg) to pamidronate 90 mg in patients with MM or bone metastases from breast cancer suggested equivalent efficacy in reduction of SREs.[52] These studies provided a rationale for a direct efficacy comparison of pamidronate and zoledronate in a multicenter, double-blind trial.[53] The trial included 1648 eligible patients with either stage III MM (n = 510) or metastatic breast cancer (n = 1138). Patients were randomly assigned to receive pamidronate at 90 mg or zoledronate at either 4 or 8 mg. Doses in all arms were given every 3–4 weeks. Patients in the 8 mg treatment arm were later reassigned to receive 4 mg because of renal safety concerns with high-dose zoledronate. The primary endpoint was an analysis of the proportion of patients experiencing at least one SRE over a 13 month period.[53] Median time to first SRE and the proportion of patients with any SRE calculated on an intent-to-treat basis were similar among all patient groups, with no statistically significant differences noted.[53] Percentages of adverse renal events were similar in patients receiving pamidronate and zoledronate at 4 mg (0.2% and 0.5%, respectively).[53] This study led to the FDA approval of zoledronate 4 mg IV infused over at least 15 minutes monthly for the treatment of osteolytic bone lesions in patients with MM.[15]

Clodronate (Bonefos; Roche Pharmaceuticals, Nutley, NJ) is available in oral and parenteral formulations and was the first bisphosphonate to demonstrate efficacy for MM patients in earlier European trials. Three hundred fifty patients undergoing their first systemic treatment for MM with oral melphalan and prednisolone were randomly assigned to receive clodronate 2.4 g orally daily or placebo for up to 2 years.[45] Significantly fewer patients in the treatment group had progression of osteolytic lesions by 24 months (12% vs 24%; $P = 0.026$).[45] However, clodronate has less potency than pamidronate or zoledronate and must be taken daily.[15] Additionally, clodronate is not yet FDA approved in the United States; clinical trials are in progress.

Ibandronate (Bondronat; Rhone-Poulenc Rorer, Collegeville, PA) is a newer bisphosphonate with an approximate 2-log greater potency than pamidronate.[15,56] A recent phase III, placebo-controlled trial of 198 evaluable MM patients demonstrated that a monthly 2 mg IV bolus of ibandronate did not lead to a significant improvement in the number of SREs per patient-year (2.13 for ibandronate vs 2.05 for placebo).[57] Post hoc analysis suggested that ibandronate-treated patients with reductions in bone formation markers (alkaline phosphatase, osteocalcin, and urinary C-terminal telopeptide of type-I collagen) did have fewer SREs compared to placebo patients.[57] However, a recently published comparison trial showed pamidronate 90 mg monthly caused greater reductions in markers of bone resorption and disease activity (paraprotein, CRP, and β2-microglobulin) than ibandronate 4 mg monthly.[58]

Osteonecrosis of the mandible is a recently described potential complication of long-term bisphosphonate therapy.[59] A retrospective review describes 56 patients who received IV bisphosphonate therapy for more or equal to 1 year presenting with lesions typical of non-healing tooth extraction sockets or exposed mandibular bone not amenable to conservative debridement or antibiotic therapy.[59] Other risk factors in the development of osteonecrosis in these patients included chemotherapy, corticosteroids, and poor oral hygiene.[59] Based on these findings, the pharmaceutical manufacturer has issued a warning recommending dental examinations along with any indicated preventative dentistry prior to placing patients with risk factors (those receiving chemotherapy, corticosteroids, or who have poor oral hygiene) on chronic bisphosphonate therapy. Furthermore, invasive dental procedures should be avoided during treatment.

A consensus panel of the American Society of Clinical Oncology (ASCO) has developed evidence-based guidelines for the use of bisphosphonates in patients with MM.[15] As previously summarized, level II evidence (i.e., evidence from at least one well-designed experimental study) supports the use of pamidronate 90 mg IV infused over at least 2 hours or zoledronate 4 mg IV infused over at least 15 minutes every 3–4 weeks for MM patients who have plain film radiograph evidence of a lytic bone lesion(s).[15] Bisphosphonate therapy is not routinely recommended for patients with monoclonal gammopathy of undetermined significance, smoldering myeloma, solitary plasmacytomas without evidence of other lytic lesions, or MM patients with osteopenia on bone mineral density measurements and no other evidence of lytic lesions.[15] The duration of bisphosphonate therapy has not been studied, and no clear recommendations on stopping treatment exist.[15] The consensus panel recommends discontinuing treatment if the benefit is no longer exceeding the inconvenience of monthly infusions or significant side effects develop.[15] Additionally, judicious use of longer term therapy is prudent in light of the newly described complication of mandibular osteonecrosis.

## PATHOLOGIC FRACTURES

Once pathologic fractures occur, they can cause severe pain and structural instability, leading to postural deformities and possibly spinal cord compression. Clinically useful adjuncts include radiation, analgesia, and surgical intervention.

## RADIATION

External beam radiation therapy is used in the majority of patients with fractures and isolated plasmacytomas. It can be useful for urgent pain control and relief of neurologic compromise. The typical dose is 30 Gy delivered in 10 fractions; however no standard dose is defined.

## SURGICAL INTERVENTIONS

### Vertebroplasty

Vertebroplasty has been used to relieve pain in patients with pathologic vertebral or osteoporotic compression fractures.[60] It is accomplished by the injection of low-viscosity bone cement into a damaged vertebral body.[61] Two drawbacks to the procedure have been suggested: the technique is not able to restore normal structure of the spine, and cement leakage may occur.[60]

### Kyphoplasty

Kyphoplasty is another surgical technique designed to restore height to collapsed vertebral bodies in order to decrease pain and improve function and mobility. The method involves the insertion of a deflated balloon into the potential space between the upper and lower end-plates of the collapsed vertebrae and inflating the balloon to push the vertebral end-plates apart, thus restoring height. The expanded cavity is then filled with a viscous, partially cured cement, thus supporting the expanded endplates and minimizing the potential for leak.[60] A prospective cohort study of 55 kyphoplasty procedures in 18 MM patients with osteolytic vertebral compression fractures demonstrated an average gain of 34% of lost height with no major procedure-related complications.[60] Patients also experienced a significant improvement in objective scores of bodily pain, physical function, vitality, and social function.[60] Importantly, patients in this study had a mean duration of symptoms prior to procedure of 11 months (range 0.5–24 months), suggesting that patients with "old" fractures should be evaluated by an orthopedic surgeon skilled in this technique to assess potential benefit.

## THROMBOEMBOLIC EVENTS

Patients with MM have a higher risk of developing a deep venous thrombosis (DVT) when compared to the general population.[62,63] A retrospective study using univariate analysis has identified a personal or family history of DVT, immobility, a low serum albumin level, and a high leukocyte count to be associated with risk of DVT in patients with MM or other plasma cell dyscrasias.[63] Newly diagnosed MM patients or those with a chromosome 11 abnormality appear to have an increased risk as well.[64] Currently, however, there is no role for the routine prophylaxis of DVT in such patients.

Thalidomide has been identified as an active drug in both newly diagnosed and relapsed or refractory MM patients.[65] The incidence of DVT in patients receiving single-agent thalidomide appears to be low.[63] In a large phase II trial of 169 patients with advanced and refractory MM given single-agent thalidomide, DVT was observed in 2% of the patients.[66] However, thalidomide is thrombogenic when given in combination with either dexamethasone or chemotherapy; results of published and unpublished studies report an incidence of 11–28%.[67–70] The thrombogenic potential of thalidomide is particularly high when combined with doxorubicin-containing regimens.[68,70,71] Although the full mechanisms of thrombosis is unclear, data from a small cohort of patients treated with thalidomide and dexamethasone for relapsed or refractory MM demonstrated a significant decrease in thrombomodulin within the first month of treatment.[72] The temporal risk of thalidomide-associated DVT in MM patients appears to be highest during induction regimens early in the course of disease.[73] The immunomodulatory thalidomide derivative, CC-5013 (lenalidomide; Celgene, Warren, NJ), does not appear to have the same thrombogenic risk as thalidomide.[74]

Prophylactic strategies with both anticoagulants and antiplatelet agents are being explored; no evidence-based guidelines are yet available. A study reporting the results of MM patients who received high-dose chemotherapy with or without thalidomide prior to autologous stem cell transplantation has recently been published.[73] Patients randomized to receive chemotherapy with thalidomide were also randomized, in sequential cohorts, to receive either warfarin 1 mg per day or low molecular weight heparin (LMWH; enoxaparin 40 mg s.c. qd). Patients who received chemotherapy alone in this trial had a 14% incidence of DVT. Those who received chemotherapy and thalidomide with or without warfarin had no difference in the incidence of DVT (34% vs 31%), suggesting no efficacy for low-dose warfarin prophylaxis.[73] However, patients who received chemotherapy, thalidomide, and LMWH had the same incidence of DVT when compared to matched controls who received chemotherapy alone (15% vs 15%).[73] Therefore, LMWH seems to attenuate the added thrombogenic risk conferred by thalidomide in patients receiving thalidomide and high dose chemotherapy.

In a phase II study of pegylated, liposomal doxorubicin, vincristine, reduced frequency dexamethasone, and thalidomide (DVd-T) for patients with relapsed or refractory MM, a 25% incidence of DVT was observed in the first 20 patients treated.[70] Low-dose aspirin 81 mg daily was administered to subsequent patients and the incidence of DVT decreased to 13%, a rate comparable to those patients receiving chemotherapy without thalidomide.[70]

## SUMMARY

Caring for patients with MM is very challenging. The availability and activity of modern chemotherapy regimens as well as newer classes of drugs with novel mechanisms of action in addition to aggressive transplant regimens has collectively changed the course of MM to that of a chronic disease for a sizeable number of patients. Hence, patients will potentially be receiving several courses of therapy and proper supportive care can enhance QOL and delay or prevent serious complications. Finally, oncology practitioners need to realize that progressive renal insufficiency, anemia, or infection may all herald disease relapse. Therefore, it is reasonable to reassess all parameters of renal and hepatic function in addition to requantification of marrow plasma cell burden and paraproteins in a previously stable patient with new or progressive symptoms.

# REFERENCES

1. Jemal A, Tiwari RC, Murray T, et al.: Cancer statistics, 2004. CA Cancer J Clin 54:8–29, 2004.
2. Criteria for the classification of monoclonal gammopathies, multiple myeloma and related disorders: a report of the International Myeloma Working Group. Br J Haematol 121:749–57, 2003.
3. Tricot G: Multiple myeloma and other plasma cell disorders. In: Hoffman R, Benz EJ, Shattil SJ, et al. (eds.): Hematology Basic Principles and Practice, 3rd ed. New York: Churchill Livingstone; 2000:1398–1416.
4. Beguin Y: Erythropoiesis and erythropoietin in multiple myeloma. Leuk Lymphoma 18:413–421, 1995.
5. Ludwig H, Fritz E, Kotzmann H, et al.: Erythropoietin treatment of anemia associated with multiple myeloma. N Engl J Med 322:1693–1699, 1990.
6. Barlogie B, Beck T: Recombinant human erythropoietin and the anemia of multiple myeloma. Stem Cells 11:88–94, 1993.
7. Garton JP, Gertz MA, Witzig TE, et al.: Epoetin alfa for the treatment of the anemia of multiple myeloma. A prospective, randomized, placebo-controlled, double-blind trial. Arch Intern Med 155:2069–2074, 1995.
8. Osterborg A, Boogaerts MA, Cimino R, et al.: Recombinant human erythropoietin in transfusion-dependent anemic patients with multiple myeloma and non-Hodgkin's lymphoma—a randomized multicenter study. The European Study Group of Erythropoietin (Epoetin Beta) Treatment in Multiple Myeloma and Non-Hodgkin's Lymphoma. Blood 87:2675–2682, 1996.
9. Rizzo JD, Lichtin AE, Woolf SH, et al.: Use of epoetin in patients with cancer: evidence-based clinical practice guidelines of the American Society of Clinical Oncology and the American Society of Hematology. J Clin Oncol 20:4083–4107, 2002.
10. Baz R, Alemany C, Green R, et al.: Prevalence of vitamin B12 deficiency in patients with plasma cell dyscrasias: a retrospective review. Cancer 101:790–795, 2004.
11. Niesvizky R, Warrell RP, Jr.: Pathophysiology and management of bone disease in multiple myeloma. Cancer Invest 15:85–90, 1997.
12. Kyle RA: Update on the treatment of multiple myeloma. Oncologist 6:119–124, 2001.
13. Body JJ, Bartl R, Burckhardt P, et al.: Current use of bisphosphonates in oncology. International Bone and Cancer Study Group. J Clin Oncol 16:3890–3899, 1998.
14. Bataille R, Harousseau JL: Multiple myeloma. N Engl J Med 336:1657–1664, 1997.
15. Berenson JR, Hillner BE, Kyle RA, et al.: American Society of Clinical Oncology clinical practice guidelines: the role of bisphosphonates in multiple myeloma. J Clin Oncol 20:3719–3736, 2002.
16. Major P, Lortholary A, Hon J, et al.: Zoledronic acid is superior to pamidronate in the treatment of hypercalcemia of malignancy: a pooled analysis of two randomized, controlled clinical trials. J Clin Oncol 19:558–567, 2001
17. Iggo N, Winearls CG, Davies DR: The development of cast nephropathy in multiple myeloma. QJM 90:653–656, 1997.
18. Abbott KC, Agodoa LY: Multiple myeloma and light chain-associated nephropathy at end-stage renal disease in the United States: patient characteristics and survival. Clin Nephrol 56:207–210, 2001.
19. Sanders PW, Herrera GA, Galla JH: Human Bence Jones protein toxicity in rat proximal tubule epithelium in vivo. Kidney Int 32:851–861, 1987.
20. Sanders PW, Booker BB: Pathobiology of cast nephropathy from human Bence Jones proteins. J Clin Invest 89:630–639, 1992.
21. Huang ZQ, Kirk KA, Connelly KG, et al.: Bence Jones proteins bind to a common peptide segment of Tamm-Horsfall glycoprotein to promote heterotypic aggregation. J Clin Invest 92:2975–2983, 1993.
22. Sanders PW, Booker BB, Bishop JB, et al.: Mechanisms of intranephronal proteinaceous cast formation by low molecular weight proteins. J Clin Invest 85:570–576, 1990.
23. Myatt EA, Westholm FA, Weiss DT, et al.: Pathogenic potential of human monoclonal immunoglobulin light chains: relationship of in vitro aggregation to in vivo organ deposition. Proc Natl Acad Sci U S A 91:3034–3038, 1994.
24. Zucchelli P, Pasquali S, Cagnoli L, et al.: Controlled plasma exchange trial in acute renal failure due to multiple myeloma. Kidney Int 33:1175–1180, 1988.
25. Johnson WJ, Kyle RA, Pineda AA, et al.: Treatment of renal failure associated with multiple myeloma. Plasmapheresis, hemodialysis, and chemotherapy. Arch Intern Med 150:863–869, 1990.
26. Pozzi C, D'Amico M, Fogazzi GB, et al.: Light chain deposition disease with renal involvement: clinical characteristics and prognostic factors. Am J Kidney Dis 42:1154–1163, 2003.
27. Dhodapkar MV, Hussein MA, Rasmussen E, et al.: Clinical efficacy of high dose dexamethasone with maintenance dexamethasone/alpha interferon in patients with primary systemic amyloidosis: results of United States intergroup trial southwest oncology group (SWOG) S9628. Blood 12:3520–3526, 2004.
28. McCarthy CS, Becker JA: Multiple myeloma and contrast media. Radiology 183:519–521, 1992.
29. Kyle RA: Multiple myeloma: review of 869 cases. Mayo Clin Proc 50:29–40, 1975.
30. Longo DL: Plasma cell disorders. In: Braunwald E, Fauci AS, Isselbacher KJ, et al. (eds.): Harrison's Principles of Internal Medicine, 16th ed. New York: McGraw-Hill; 2005.
31. Salonen J, Nikoskelainen J: Lethal infections in patients with hematological malignancies. Eur J Haematol 51:102–108, 1993.
32. McKelvey EM, Fahey JL: Immunoglobulin changes in disease: quantitation on the basis of heavy polypeptide chains, IgG (gammaG), IgA (gammaA), and IgM (gammaM), and of light polypeptide chains, type K (I) and type L (II). J Clin Invest 44:1778–1787, 1965.
33. Murakami H, Ogawara H, Hiroshi H: Th1/Th2 cells in patients with multiple myeloma. Hematology 9:41–45, 2004.
34. Hargreaves RM, Lea JR, Griffiths H, et al.: Immunological factors and risk of infection in plateau phase myeloma. J Clin Pathol 48:260–266, 1995.
35. Oken MM, Pomeroy C, Weisdorf D, et al.: Prophylactic antibiotics for the prevention of early infection in multiple myeloma. Am J Med 100:624–628, 1996.

36. Perri RT, Hebbel RP, Oken MM: Influence of treatment and response status on infection risk in multiple myeloma. *Am J Med* 71:935–940, 1981.

37. Savage DG, Lindenbaum J, Garrett TJ: Biphasic pattern of bacterial infection in multiple myeloma. *Ann Intern Med* 96:47–50, 1982.

38. Rayner HC, Haynes AP, Thompson JR, et al.: Perspectives in multiple myeloma: survival, prognostic factors and disease complications in a single centre between 1975 and 1988. *Q J Med* 79:517–525, 1991.

39. Kyle RA: Multiple Myeloma. Diagnostic challenges and standard therapy. *Semin Hematol* 38:11–14, 2001.

40. Gordon DS, Hearn EB, Spira TJ, et al.: Phase I study of intravenous gamma globulin in multiple myeloma. *Am J Med* 76:111–116, 1984.

41. Chapel HM, Lee M, Hargreaves R, et al.: Randomised trial of intravenous immunoglobulin as prophylaxis against infection in plateau-phase multiple myeloma. The UK Group for Immunoglobulin Replacement Therapy in Multiple Myeloma. *Lancet* 343:1059–1063, 1994.

42. Rapezzi D, Sticchi L, Racchi O, et al.: Influenza vaccine in chronic lymphoproliferative disorders and multiple myeloma. *Eur J Haematol* 70:225–230, 2003.

43. Robertson JD, Nagesh K, Jowitt SN, et al.: Immunogenicity of vaccination against influenza, Streptococcus pneumoniae and Haemophilus influenzae type B in patients with multiple myeloma. *Br J Cancer* 82:1261–1265, 2000.

44. Croucher PI, Apperley JF: Bone disease in multiple myeloma. *Br J Haematol* 103:902–910, 1998.

45. Lahtinen R, Laakso M, Palva I, et al.: Randomised, placebo-controlled multicentre trial of clodronate in multiple myeloma. Finnish Leukaemia Group. *Lancet* 340:1049–1052, 1992.

46. Giuliani N, Bataille R, Mancini C, et al.: Myeloma cells induce imbalance in the osteoprotegerin/osteoprotegerin ligand system in the human bone marrow environment. *Blood* 98:3527–3533, 2001.

47. Body JJ, Greipp P, Coleman RE, et al.: A phase I study of AMGN-0007, a recombinant osteoprotegerin construct, in patients with multiple myeloma or breast carcinoma related bone metastases. *Cancer* 97:887–892, 2003.

48. Body JJ: Bisphosphonates. *Eur J Cancer* 34:263–269, 1998.

49. Fleisch H: Bisphosphonates: mechanisms of action. *Endocr Rev* 19:80–100, 1998.

50. Berenson JR, Lichtenstein A, Porter L, et al.: Efficacy of pamidronate in reducing skeletal events in patients with advanced multiple myeloma. Myeloma Aredia Study Group. *N Engl J Med* 334:488–493, 1996.

51. Rosen LS, Gordon D, Kaminski M, et al.: Long-term efficacy and safety of zoledronic acid compared with pamidronate disodium in the treatment of skeletal complications in patients with advanced multiple myeloma or breast carcinoma: a randomized, double-blind, multicenter, comparative trial. *Cancer* 98:1735–1744, 2003.

52. Berenson JR, Rosen LS, Howell A, et al.: Zoledronic acid reduces skeletal-related events in patients with osteolytic metastases. *Cancer* 91:1191–1200, 2001.

53. Rosen LS, Gordon D, Kaminski M, et al.: Zoledronic acid versus pamidronate in the treatment of skeletal metastases in patients with breast cancer or osteolytic lesions

54. Terpos E, Palermos J, Tsionos K, et al.: Effect of pamidronate administration on markers of bone turnover and disease activity in multiple myeloma. *Eur J Haematol* 65:331–336, 2000.

55. Berenson JR, Lichtenstein A, Porter L, et al.: Long-term pamidronate treatment of advanced multiple myeloma patients reduces skeletal events. Myeloma Aredia Study Group. *J Clin Oncol* 16:593–602, 1998.

56. Muhlbauer RC, Bauss F, Schenk R, et al.: BM 21.0955, a potent new bisphosphonate to inhibit bone resorption. *J Bone Miner Res* 6:1003–1011, 1991.

57. Menssen HD, Sakalova A, Fontana A, et al.: Effects of long-term intravenous ibandronate therapy on skeletal-related events, survival, and bone resorption markers in patients with advanced multiple myeloma. *J Clin Oncol* 20:2353–2359, 2002.

58. Terpos E, Viniou N, de la Fuente J, et al.: Pamidronate is superior to ibandronate in decreasing bone resorption, interleukin-6 and beta 2-microglobulin in multiple myeloma. *Eur J Haematol* 70:34–42, 2003.

59. Ruggiero SL, Mehrotra B, Rosenberg TJ, et al.: Osteonecrosis of the jaws associated with the use of bisphosphonates: a review of 63 cases. *J Oral Maxillofac Surg* 62:527–534, 2004.

60. Dudeney S, Lieberman IH, Reinhardt MK, et al.: Kyphoplasty in the treatment of osteolytic vertebral compression fractures as a result of multiple myeloma. *J Clin Oncol* 20:2382–2387, 2002.

61. Deramond H, Depriester C, Galibert P, et al.: Percutaneous vertebroplasty with polymethylmethacrylate. Technique, indications, and results. *Radiol Clin North Am* 36:533–546, 1998.

62. Barlogie B, Jagannath S, Desikan KR, et al.: Total therapy ith tandem transplants for newly diagnosed multiple myeloma. *Blood* 93:55–65, 1999.

63. Srkalovic G, Cameron MG, Rybicki L, et al.: Monoclonal gammopathy of undetermined significance and multiple myeloma are associated with an increased incidence of venothromboembolic disease. *Cancer* 101:558–566, 2004.

64. Zangari M, Barlogie B, Thertulien R, et al.: Thalidomide and deep vein thrombosis in multiple myeloma: risk factors and effect on survival. *Clin Lymphoma* 4:32–435, 2003.

65. Hussein MA: Nontraditional cytotoxic therapies for relapsed/refractory multiple myeloma. *Oncologist* 7(suppl 1):20–29, 2002.

66. Barlogie B, Desikan R, Eddlemon P, et al.: Extended survival in advanced and refractory multiple myeloma after single-agent thalidomide: identification of prognostic factors in a phase 2 study of 169 patients. *Blood* 98:492–494, 2001.

67. Offidani M, Corvatta L, Marconi M, et al.: Thalidomide plus oral melphalan compared with thalidomide alone for advanced multiple myeloma. *Hematol J* 5:312–317, 2004.

68. Zangari M, Siegel E, Barlogie B, et al.: Thrombogenic activity of doxorubicin in myeloma patients receiving thalidomide: implications for therapy. *Blood* 100:1168–1171, 2002.

69. Zangari M, Anaissie E, Barlogie B, et al.: Increased risk of deep-vein thrombosis in patients with multiple

myeloma receiving thalidomide and chemotherapy. *Blood* 98:1614–1615, 2001.

70. Hussein M, Elson P, Tso E, et al.: Doxil (D), Vincristine (V), Decadron (d) and Thalidomide (T) (DVd-T)for Relpased/Refractory Multiple Myeloma (RMM). *Blood* 100(suppl): 2002.

71. Comenzo R, Hassoun H, Reich L, et al.: *Doxorubicin and Dexamethasone followed by Thalidomide and Dexamethasone as Initial Therapy for Symptomatic Patients with Multiple Myeloma.* Washington, DC: American Society of Hematology; 2003.

72. Corso A, Lorenzi A, Terulla V, et al.: Modification of thrombomodulin plasma levels in refractory myeloma patients during treatment with thalidomide and dexamethasone. *Ann Hematol* 83:588–591, 2004.

73. Zangari M, Barlogie B, Anaissie E, et al.: Deep vein thrombosis in patients with multiple myeloma treated with thalidomide and chemotherapy: effects of prophylactic and therapeutic anticoagulation. *Br J Haematol* 126:715–721, 2004.

74. Richardson PG, Schlossman RL, Weller E, et al.: Immunomodulatory drug CC-5013 overcomes drug resistance and is well tolerated in patients with relapsed multiple myeloma. *Blood* 100:3063–3067, 2002.

Chapter **92**

# PRINCIPLES OF HEMATOPOIETIC STEM CELL TRANSPLANTATION TO TREAT HEMATOLOGIC MALIGNANCIES

*Michael R. Bishop*

## INTRODUCTION

Hematopoietic stem cell transplantation (HSCT) is the process of infusing hematopoietic stem and progenitor cells, which are used primarily to restore normal hematopoiesis or to treat malignancy.[1–3] The term HSCT has replaced the relatively archaic term *bone marrow transplantation* for two specific reasons. First, the stem and progenitor cells used in HSCT can be obtained from a variety of sources other than the bone marrow, including the peripheral blood and umbilical cord blood.[4] It is more important to characterize HSCT according to where the stem cells used for transplantation are derived. The use of hematopoietic stem cells derived from patients themselves is referred to as autologous HSCT.[1,3] Transplantation of hematopoietic stem cells derived from an identical twin is referred to as syngeneic HSCT, and transplantation of hematopoietic stem cells from stem cells other than the patient or an identical twin is referred to as allogeneic HSCT. The stem cells used for HSCT are of hematopoietic origin, as more primitive stem cells are of interest for regenerative therapy, highlighting their plasticity and unique biologic characteristics.[5]

### HISTORY OF HEMATOPOIETIC STEM CELL TRANSPLANTATION

The clinical application of HSCT is less than 50 years old, and its origins are related to identification of the severe myelosuppressive effects of radiation that were observed among nuclear bomb survivors at Hiroshima and Nagasaki.[6] Intense research began at that time to develop methods to reverse the myelosuppressive effects of radiation, including the infusion of bone marrow.[7–10] In 1949, Jacobson reported on the effects of shielding the spleen of mice from lethal doses of irradiation.[7] Shielding of the spleen protected nearly all mice at a total body irradiation dose of 700 cGy, while unshielded mice all died from marrow aplasia. As the dose of radiation was raised to 1050 cGy, approximately one-third of the shielded mice survived, and a dose of 1200 cGy was lethal to all mice. At autopsy, these latter radiation groups were found to have died from fibrosis of the lungs, liver, and kidneys. The authors erroneously concluded that shielding the spleen was protecting a humoral factor that affected hematopoiesis; however, it would subsequently be determined that early hematopoietic progenitors were actually protected from the effects of radiation. From these early studies, theories evolved that radiation and chemotherapy could be administered at controlled, yet highly myelosuppressive doses, which were capable of eliminating malignant hematopoietic clones, and that normal hematopoiesis could be reestablished by the infusion of normal bone marrow. Early animal studies of HSCT were thwarted by incompatibility between bone marrow recipients and donors leading to a high degree of graft rejection.[10] Among animals that did not reject their marrow grafts, a syndrome of weight loss, alopecia, diarrhea, and eventually death was commonly observed.[11] This syndrome was referred to as "runting" disease, which we now refer to clinically as graft-versus-host disease (GVHD), and is discussed in more detail next. The most significant breakthrough for HSCT in particular and for all forms of organ transplantation in general was the recognition that the major histocompatibility complex (MHC) and human leukocyte antigens (HLA) were the major determinants of graft rejection.[12] After the development of clinical methods to determine HLA, which permitted the "matching" of bone marrow donors and recipients, the first successful clinical stem cell transplantation trials among patients with severe combined immunodeficiency disorders and advanced acute leukemias were reported in the late 1960s and early 1970s.[1,10] Today, HSCT is a standard treatment for many immunodeficiency states, metabolic disorders (e.g., Hurler's syndrome), defective hematopoietic states (e.g., severe aplastic anemia, thalassemia), and a variety of malignancies. It is currently being investigated in nonmalignant diseases, including autoimmune diseases (e.g., rheumatoid arthritis and multiple sclerosis) and the emerging field of regenerative medicine, which takes advantage of the plasticity of stem cells, to repair defective or damaged tissues (e.g., cardiac muscle after a myocardial infarction).[13,14] This chapter will focus primarily on the rationale for the application of HSCT in the treatment of hematologic malignancies.

## CLINICAL DECISION-MAKING IN HEMATOPOIETIC STEM CELL TRANSPLANTATION

Hematologic malignancies are particularly amenable to the beneficial effects of HSCT due to their relative sensitivity to cytotoxic chemotherapy and radiation, as well as their susceptibility to immunologic effects that are associated with allogeneic HSCT. The intent of HSCT for the treatment of malignancy is to have a significant impact on survival and to potentially cure the disease. The curative intent of HSCT is imperative, as the procedure is associated with a significant degree of morbidity and mortality as compared to other forms of therapy. As such, the decision to employ HSCT is based primarily on the inherent risk of the disease itself versus the potential benefit and inherent risks of the various forms of HSCT being considered. This decision takes into careful consideration many factors, including the specific disease, the available alternative treatment options, the disease state (remission, sensitivity to chemotherapy), patient age and performance status, and availability of a stem cell source. Once it is determined that a patient could potentially benefit from HSCT, the decisions as to what type of transplant (allogeneic vs autologous vs syngeneic), what type of conditioning regimen, and the timing of the transplant (first complete remission vs first relapse) need to be made. These decisions are primarily based upon the aforementioned factors and supplemented by the amount of risk that the patient (and physician) is willing to accept.

## TYPES OF HEMATOPOIETIC STEM CELL TRANSPLANTATION

### ALLOGENEIC HEMATOPOIETIC STEM CELL TRANSPLANTATION
#### Histocompatibility
The choice of a syngeneic, autologous, or allogeneic HSCT is relatively predetermined for most patients, as few patients have an identical twin and the availability of an allogeneic donor is limited. In allogeneic HSCT,

stem cells are obtained from someone (i.e., the donor) other than the patient (i.e., the recipient). Donor and recipient are generally identical or "matched" for HLA, which are derived from the MHC located on chromosome 6.[15] A single set of MHC alleles, described as a haplotype, is inherited from each parent, resulting in HLA pairs. The most important HLA include HLA-A, HLA-B, HLA-C, DR, and DQ loci. Among siblings, the genes that encode for HLA-B and C are located so close to each other in the MHC that one is rarely inherited without the other. As a result, an HLA match among siblings is referred to a "6 of 6," as they are matched for HLA-A, B, and DR; however, in actuality they are matched for all of the HLA antigens.[3] The other antigens, such as HLA-C, become more important when alternative sources of hematopoietic stem cells are used, such as those from unrelated donors and cord blood, which are described in more detail next and in Chapter 98.[16]

### Graft-versus-leukemia effect
The distinctive characteristics of allogeneic HSCT are that the stem cell graft is free of contamination by malignant cells and contains T-cells that are capable of mediating an immunologic reaction against foreign antigens. This latter characteristic can be a major advantage if the immunologic response is directed against malignant cells, referred to as the graft-versus-leukemia (GVL) or graft-versus-tumor effect, thus potentially eradicating disease and reducing the chance of disease relapse. However, if the immunologic response is directed against antigens present on normal tissues, it can lead to the destruction of normal organs, described clinically as GVHD. The risk of both graft rejection (host-versus-graft reaction) and GVHD rises with HLA-disparity.

The GVL effect was initially recognized in animal models and subsequently noted among patients undergoing allogeneic HSCT for acute and chronic leukemias.[17-20] The clinical importance of the interactions between immunocompetent donor T cells and tumor cells in mediating GVL effect is supported by an increased rate of relapse in allogeneic stem cell grafts from which T cells have been removed (T cell depletion), an inverse correlation between relapse and severity of GVHD, and an increased rate of relapse after syngeneic or autologous HSCT using the same myeloablative conditioning regimen.[20,21] These data suggested that T cells within the allograft were directly involved in eradicating leukemia. Finally, the most compelling evidence for a T cell-mediated GVL effect originates from the observation that infusion of allogeneic lymphocytes, a donor lymphocyte infusion (DLI), at a time remote from the transplant conditioning regimen, can successfully treat leukemia relapse after allogeneic HSCT.[22-25] In an initial report, DLI therapy was given to three patients with chronic myelogenous leukemia (CML) whose disease had recurred after an allogeneic HSCT.[22] The DLI, without any additional cytotoxic therapy, resulted in sustained cytogenetic and molecular remissions. Evidence of a GVL effect similarly has been observed against other hematologic malignancies, including multiple myeloma and lymphomas.[26,27] Over time, it became increasingly apparent that a significant part of the curative potential of allogeneic HSCT could be directly attributed to the GVL effect. However, there is tremendous variability relative to the clinical effectiveness of the GVL effect against different hematologic malignancies after allogeneic HSCT. Factors that affect the GVL effect after allogeneic HSCT include the presence of mixed T cell chimerism, the development of tolerance between donor and host, the relative susceptibility of the hematologic malignancy to the GVL effect, and suboptimal GVL reactivity.[28]

The expression of surface or intracellular molecules on malignant cells is essential for recognition or elimination by effector T cells. Malignant cells may directly down-regulate effector cells through secretion of inhibitory factors such as transforming growth factor-beta (TGF-β).[29] Malignant cells may also down-regulate HLA class I and class II molecules, may have low- or missing expression of costimulatory molecules, such as CD80, CD83, CD86, CD40, and intercellular adhesion molecule, or alter the presentation antigenic peptide sequences.[30–33] The cytotoxic effects of effector cells are primarily mediated through the Fas-ligand pathway or tumor necrosis factor (TNF) receptors, or through direct binding of perforin and activation of granzyme B.[34] Decreased Fas ligand expression or reduced perforin binding can impair the potency of the GVL effect.[35–37]

It has long been recognized that an optimal GVL effect requires efficient antigen presentation by antigen presenting cells, such as dendritic cells, and appropriate costimulatory signals to T cells.[38–40] In HLA-mismatched allogeneic HSCT, natural killer (NK) cells have been found to exert strong alloimmune response that contributes to a potent clinical GVL effect.[41] The interaction of killer-cell immunoglobulin-like receptors (KIR), expressed on NK cells, with MHC inhibits the cytotoxic activity of NK cells.[42–44] In allogeneic HSCT where donors and recipients are mismatched for HLA (HLA-mismatched or haploidentical HSCT), a lack of appropriate HLA class I ligands in the recipient can inhibit the KIR of donor NK cells, facilitating a strong GVL effect.[42] Although a beneficial effect of NK cell alloreactivity has been observed in haploidentical HSCT, there has been conflicting data relative to any benefit in the setting allogeneic HSCT from unrelated donors.[45,46]

The failure to detect clinical evidence of a GVL effect after allogeneic HSCT can be partially attributed to the biologic characteristics of the disease, such as histology and chemotherapy sensitivity.[47] There are significant differences in the susceptibility of various hematologic malignancies to the GVL effect, and there can be significant differences in the susceptibility of particular hematologic malignancies relative to their histologies.[21,48] Evidence of a GVL effect and the efficacy of DLI in non-Hodgkin's lymphoma (NHL) have been primarily limited to follicular or "low-grade" histologies, with only anecdotal cases in patients with diffuse large B-cell or more aggressive NHL histologies.[48,49] This may reflect the biologic characteristics, such as growth rate or antigen expression, of the respective histologies. In some cases, a clinical GVL effect is not possible, as certain hematologic malignancies can be localized in immunologically "privileged" sites, such as the central nervous system.[50]

An extremely important clinical factor relative to the susceptibility of hematologic malignancies to the GVL effect is chemotherapy sensitivity.[48,51] In extremely chemotherapy-refractory patients, the GVL effect may be insufficiently potent to be clinically detectable, because the tumor growth rate exceeds the ability of the immune effect to eliminate disease. Patients with chemotherapy-sensitive disease also tend to have less of a disease burden, and the greatest efficacy of the GVL effect has been observed in minimal residual disease states.[24] Specifically, relapse is higher among patients who are not in remission at the time of allogeneic HSCT or DLI.[52] In chronic phase CML, the efficacy of DLI is inversely related to the disease burden; the highest response rates to DLI have been observed among CML patients with disease detectable only by polymerase chain reaction methods, and the lowest efficacy is observed among patients with hematologic relapses.[53]

### Selection of allogeneic stem donor

The choice of donor for an allogeneic HSCT takes into account several factors, including the patient's disease, disease state, and urgency in obtaining a donor. When allogeneic HSCT is being considered for a patient, a fully HLA-matched sibling is the preferred donor, as the risk of graft rejection and GVHD are the least with this source of allogeneic stem cells.[3] For patients who lack a fully HLA-matched sibling donor, the preferred alternative sources for allogeneic stem cells include an unrelated fully HLA-matched donor, a partially HLA-matched cord blood unit, or a partially HLA-matched family member.[54–56] A major disadvantage of an unrelated donor is that the average time required to identify and procure an HLA-matched unrelated donor is approximately 2–4 months, which may be inadequate for patients with rapidly progressive malignancies.[57] The alternative stem cell source to an unrelated bone marrow donor for allogeneic HSCT is umbilical cord blood.[55,57,58] The major advantages of umbilical cord stem cells is that they can be obtained in fewer than 4 weeks and cord blood units mismatched for up to 3 of 6 HLA may be used for allogeneic HSCT. This degree of HLA mismatching is acceptable, as the overwhelming percentage of T cells within the cord blood unit are naive, and the incidence of GVHD is comparable or less than that associated with an HLA-matched unrelated bone marrow donor. The major disadvantage of umbilical cord blood units is that they are associated with a high degree of graft rejection, especially in adults. Engraftment- and treatment-related mortality appears to be directly related to umbilical cord cell dose.[55,57,58] The other significant disadvantage is that once the cord blood unit is used, there is no way to go back and get additional cells for a DLI or in the event of graft failure.

### SYNGENEIC HEMATOPOIETIC STEM CELL TRANSPLANTATION

Syngeneic HSCT uses stem cells from an identical twin.[59,60] As the stem cells are genetically identical with the recipient, the major advantages of a syngeneic HSCT are that they are not associated with GVHD or graft rejection. Another significant advantage of syngeneic HSCT, which is shared with allogeneic HSCT, is that there is no risk of contamination by malignant cells. The major disadvantage is that the syngeneic HSCT does not provide a GVL effect that is associated with allogeneic HSCT; conversely, however, syngeneic HSCT is not associated with GVHD or graft rejection. This results in a relatively low risk of treatment-related morbidity and mortality. The greatest disadvantage is that far less than 1% of patients have an identical twin, making this an unavailable option for the overwhelming majority of patients. However, when an identical twin is available, syngeneic HSCT is considered the preferred type of HSCT in almost all clinical situations, due to the aforementioned advantages.

### AUTOLOGOUS HEMATOPOIETIC STEM CELL TRANSPLANTATION

Autologous HSCT uses stem cells from patients themselves. The principle behind both syngeneic and autologous HSCT is that certain malignancies, such as leukemias, have a steep dose-response curve to chemotherapy and, to a relative degree, radiation.[61-63] The major limitation to the administration of higher doses of chemotherapy or radiation, in order to obtain a maximal response, are the myelosuppressive effects of these therapies. Autologous, allogeneic, and syngeneic hematopoietic stem cells are primarily used as a "rescue" product to restore hematopoiesis after patients have received high-dose chemotherapy and/or radiation. The amount of chemotherapy and radiation that can be administered prior to transplant, referred to as the conditioning or preparative regimen, is limited due to associated toxicities to other organs. This limitation in the amount of therapy that can be delivered may permit the survival of resistant tumor cells, which accounts for the relapses that are observed after HSCT.[64,65] Relapse rates are lower after allogeneic HSCT, as this form of transplant provides a potential GVL effect at the expense of increased treatment-related morbidity and mortality, primarily through GVHD.[19-21]

### Tumor contamination and "purging"

The major advantages of autologous hematopoietic stem cells are that almost every patient can serve as his/her own donor and there is no graft rejection or GVHD, although attempts have been made to induce autologous GVHD and GVL, as discussed next. Thus, autologous HSCT is also associated with a relatively low treatment-related mortality rate, which varies with disease, disease state, and age. The major disadvantages are that the autologous stem cell graft may be contaminated with tumor cells and, similar to syngeneic HSCT, is not associated with a GVL effect. The contribution of autograft contamination by tumor cells to relapse has varying clinical significance.[66-68] Attempts have been made to remove or "purge" tumor cells from the autograft using various methods prior to autologous HSCT.[69-71] However, there is only retrospective and anecdotal evidence that autograft purging results in an improved clinical outcome.[48,72]

### Autologous graft-versus-host disease

Although the high rate of relapse after autologous HSCT has in part been attributed to tumor contamination of the autograft, a similar relapse rate has also been observed with syngeneic HSCT, which is free of tumor contamination.[21] It is more likely that relapses are due to endogenous tumor cells that survived the cytotoxic effects of the conditioning regimen. It has been hypothesized that these high relapse rates with either syngeneic or autologous HSCT are due to the absence of a GVL effect. Attempts have been made to induce GVHD and an associated GVL effect in the autologous HSCT setting. Murine studies indicated that administration of the immunosuppressive drug cyclosporine after autologous HSCT elicited an autoimmune syndrome with pathology virtually identical to GVHD.[73] The GVHD observed after autologous and syngeneic HSCT in murine models was associated with the development of a highly restricted repertoire of CD8+ autoreactive T cells that recognized a peptide from the invariant chain, termed CLIP, presented by MHC class II molecules.[74] These autoreactive T cells produced type 1 cytokines, including interferon-gamma, interleukin-2 (IL-2), and TNF-α. These studies led to clinical trials in patients with lymphoma and acute leukemia.[75,76] Although clinical and histologic evidence of GVHD was demonstrated in these trials, there was no clear evidence of a clinical benefit in terms of a reduction in relapse rates.

### Sources of hematopoietic stem cells

Hematopoietic stem cells may be obtained from the bone marrow, the peripheral blood, and from umbilical cord blood. Hematopoietic stem cells from bone marrow are used in both autologous and allogeneic stem cell transplantation, although far less frequently than in the past. Peripheral blood hematopoietic stem cells are used in approximately 90% of autologous HSCT and in approximately 70% of allogeneic HSCT.[77] The predominance of this stem cell source is related to the relative ease in attainment and moderate improvement in the rate of hematopoietic recovery after infusion, as compared to hematopoietic stem cells derived from bone marrow. Hematopoietic stem cells from cord blood are collected immediately after delivery of a baby. A minimally acceptable cord blood unit dose is $1.7 \times 10^5$ CD34$^+$ cells per the patient's weight in kilograms, to assure engraftment in the allogeneic HSCT setting.[78] This criterion is a significant problem for adult patients, where the application of cord blood transplantation has been associated with delayed hematopoietic recovery, especially platelets; graft failure; and a relatively high treatment-related mortality compared to other sources of allogeneic hematopoietic stem cells.

## CONDITIONING REGIMENS FOR HEMATOPOIETIC STEM CELL TRANSPLANTATION

As described previously, prior to the infusion of hematopoietic stem cells, patients receive regimens with the intent of "conditioning" or "preparing" the patient for the infusion of hematopoietic stem cells.[1,3] Most conditioning or preparative regimens consist of chemotherapy alone or combined with radiation, radioimmunoconjugates, and/or monoclonal antibodies that target T cells (e.g., alemtuzumab).[1,3,79,80] The choice of conditioning regimen is dependent upon the type of transplant (allogeneic vs autologous vs syngeneic) and the specific disease being treated.

### MYELOABLATIVE CONDITIONING REGIMENS
The earliest conditioning regimens were designed for the treatment of acute leukemias with syngeneic and allogeneic HSCT.[81] As previously discussed, these early conditioning regimens allowed the administration of maximum doses (i.e., "high-dose") of chemotherapy and/or radiation for the eradication of disease. In the case of an allogeneic HSCT, the conditioning regimen also had to be adequately immunosuppressive to prevent graft rejection, as the recipient's immune system is capable of recognizing the donor hematopoietic stem cells as foreign. The most commonly used chemotherapy agents are alkylating agents (e.g., cyclophosphamide) with or without total lymphoid or total body irradiation at doses varying between 800 and 1440 cGy. The doses of chemotherapy and radiation used in these regimens are referred to as myeloablative, as they result in a degree of myelosuppression and immunosuppression that is nearly universally fatal

without the infusion of hematopoietic stem cells as a rescue product.[82]

### NON-MYELOABLATIVE AND REDUCED-INTENSITY CONDITIONING REGIMENS
The demonstration that an immune-mediated GVL effect plays a central role in the therapeutic efficacy of allogeneic HSCT led to the hypothesis that myeloablative conditioning regimens were not essential for tumor eradication.[83] This subsequently led investigators to develop less intense conditioning regimens that were adequately immunosuppressive to permit the engraftment of donor hematopoietic stem cells, and could serve as a platform for the administration of donor T cells as adoptive cellular therapy.[84] A variety of nonmyeloablative, also referred to as reduced-intensity, conditioning regimens have been reported.[85–88] All share the similar goal of providing sufficient immunosuppression to achieve donor engraftment of an allogeneic hematopoietic stem cell graft while attempting to minimize toxicity. The most important clinical question is whether this reduction in toxicity comes at the cost of a loss of antitumor activity within the conditioning regimen.

## CLINICAL EFFICACY OF HEMATOPOIETIC STEM CELL TRANSPLANTATION IN HEMATOLOGIC MALIGNANCIES

There is clinical evidence that syngeneic, autologous, and allogeneic HSCT all provide benefit, defined as response, freedom of progression, or overall survival, for the majority of hematologic malignancies.[3] However, the beneficial effects of these various forms of HSCT vary greatly with each hematologic malignancy. Myeloablative conditioning regimens with syngeneic, autologous, or allogeneic HSCT result in higher response rates than conventional cytotoxic agents for almost all hematologic malignancies. However, the durability of these responses and their effect on survival varies from disease to disease. Similarly, there is evidence of a clinical GVL effect in almost every hematologic disease; however, the potency and clinical relevance is highly variable. This section will briefly cover the susceptibility of hematologic malignancies to the different forms and effects of HSCT.

### CHRONIC MYELOGENOUS LEUKEMIA
Chronic myelogenous leukemia is highly susceptible to the GVL effect, as evidenced by the response of CML to DLI, and that long-term, leukemia-free survival rates exceed 70% for patients who were transplanted in early chronic phase.[89,90] GVL effect against CML clearly exists, as the greatest efficacy of DLI has been demonstrated in CML. Several studies have implicated peptides associated with the product of *bcr-abl*, but a specific antigen has yet to be identified.[91] However,

studies in CML provide several important insights on the efficacy of DLI in specific, and GVL in general, relative to disease status and lymphocyte dose.[22,52,53,92] Chronic phase CML is particularly responsive to DLI, with remission rates of 50–80%.[53,92] In contrast, response rates of accelerated and acute ("blast") phase CML varies between 10% and 30%; the more advanced states of the CML are inversely correlated to the response to DLI. These variable response rates reflect the biology of disease relative to antigen and MHC presentation, as well as growth rate. In patients with more advanced CML, the GVL effect may be insufficiently potent to be clinically detectable, because the leukemic growth rate exceeds the ability of the immune effect to eliminate disease. There is also considerable variability of response to DLI among CML patients in chronic phase. For CML patients with cytogenetic or molecular relapses, the response rates are approximately 60–70% and 80–90%, respectively.[53,92] In contrast, the response to DLI among patients with chronic phase CML with morphologic or hematologic relapses is approximately 50–60%. Increased lymphocyte dose appears to improve DLI efficacy against relapse, but it is also associated with increased toxicity in the form of GVHD.[92] However, lower DLI doses are as effective as higher doses in patients with a low disease burden. These variations in response suggest that tumor bulk plays an important role in the efficacy of DLI in CML. All of these factors, including disease biology, disease state, and tumor bulk, appear to play significant roles relative to the susceptibility of hematologic malignancies to a GVL effect. Autologous HSCT has limited efficacy in CML due to the relative lack of sensitivity of CML cells to cytotoxic therapy, and more importantly due to difficulty in obtaining a relatively tumor-free autograft.[93] Due to the tremendous clinical success of imatinib (STI-571, Gleevec), the emerging predominant strategy is to use allogeneic HSCT in patients with more advanced CML, and for patients who have failed or progressed on Gleevec.[94]

### ACUTE LEUKEMIAS AND MYELODYSPLASTIC SYNDROMES

Acute myelogenous leukemia (AML), along with acute lymphocytic leukemia (ALL), were some of the first malignancies in which HSCT was demonstrated to have efficacy.[19,21,81] Initial studies of myeloablative allogeneic HSCT demonstrated that this treatment was capable of resulting in long-term survival for a minority of patients with refractory and relapsed AML.[81] Subsequent studies suggested that a GVL effect contributed to the success of allogeneic HSCT in AML.[19,21] The evidence for a GVL effect in ALL is less convincing.[95] In contrast to data in CML, the clinical responses of relapsed AML and ALL to DLI are generally less than 50%, with particularly disappointing results for ALL.[25,52,95] A number of antigens have been identified as potential targets in AML, explaining the efficacy of

allogeneic HSCT in this disease. These antigens are expressed only on a minority of AML cells, and on normal tissues.[96–98] Similarly, the response of myelodysplastic syndrome to DLI is relatively poor, although allogeneic HSCT is the only known curative therapy for patients with MDS.[99]

### MULTIPLE MYELOMA

The efficacy of high-dose chemotherapy in multiple myeloma has led to inclusion of autologous HSCT as part of its initial therapy.[100,101] Due to unique biologic characteristics, there are clinical data demonstrating that the inclusion of more than one cycle of high-dose chemotherapy with autologous HSCT may improve upon the results of a single transplant.[102] Although there is clear evidence of a GVL effect against multiple myeloma, a tumor-specific antigen has not been identified. The use of myeloablative allogeneic HSCT is controversial, as they have been associated with a high mortality rate.[103] Results of allogeneic HSCT in multiple myeloma have been improved with the use of nonmyeloablative conditioning regimens.[104]

### LYMPHOMA

Due its relative sensitivity to chemotherapy, there is substantial evidence that autologous HSCT is efficacious for patients with primary refractory or chemotherapy-sensitive recurrent malignant lymphomas of specific histologies, including "intermediate-grade" (e.g., disease diffuse large B-cell), NHL, and Hodgkin's lymphomas.[105–108] The demonstration of a potent GVL effect against lymphomas is less clear, and the efficacy of DLI in lymphoma is anecdotal at best.[47–49] When specific comparisons were made between syngeneic, autologous, and allogeneic HSCT in different types of lymphoma, a clear GVL effect was not demonstrated.[48] Thus, the specific role of allogeneic HSCT has not been defined; however, there is evidence that nonmyeloablative allogeneic HSCT may provide benefit for patients with recurrent follicular and advanced non-Hodgkin's lymphoma, as well as for Hodgkin's lymphoma.[51,109]

### SUMMARY

Hematopoietic stem cell transplantation represents a treatment option that can result in significant improvements, and in many cases cures, for a variety of hematologic malignancies. In the autologous and syngeneic HSCT settings, the efficacy is attributed almost solely to the ability of high-dose chemotherapy and radiotherapy to overcome resistant mechanisms within malignant cells; however, relapse of disease remains the primary reason for treatment failure. Relapse is significantly less in the allogeneic HSCT setting. This reduction in relapse rates is attributed to a T cell-mediated GVL effect, but it comes at the expense of GVHD, resulting in high treatment-related morbidity and mortality. Advances in the understanding of T cell biology and tumor immunology, which includes identification of immunogenic cancer antigens and an increased ability to identify and expand T cells with tumor reactivity, will lead to the translation of the GVL effect into the syngeneic and autologous HSCT settings. Current studies of adoptive cellular therapy in solid tumors, particularly melanoma, suggest that this is highly possible.[110] In the allogeneic HSCT setting, the situation is somewhat reversed, as clinical applications and success at treating malignancy leads the scientific understanding of the biology of these tumor regressions. To this extent, efforts are underway to elucidate the mechanism(s) of curative allogeneic GVL effects. This understanding is of significant importance, as it may allow one to identify mechanisms of GVL mediation that are distinct from GVHD, resulting in an improved therapeutic ratio. It is apparent that the fields of autologous and allogeneic HSCT therapy conceptually overlap, with each application attempting to achieve a maximal response against cancer cells with relatively reduced toxicity, specifically reduced GVHD in allogeneic HSCT and a reasonable degree of tumor-specific autoimmunity in autologous HSCT.

## REFERENCES

1. Thomas E, Storb R, Clift RA, et al.: Bone-marrow transplantation (two parts). *N Engl J Med* 292:832, 895, 1975.
2. Quesenberry P, Levitt L: Hematopoietic stem cells (third of three parts). *N Engl J Med* 301:868, 1979.
3. Armitage JO: Bone marrow transplantation. *N Engl J Med* 330:827,1994.
4. Weissman IL: Translating stem and progenitor cell biology to the clinic: barriers and opportunities. *Science* 287:1442, 2000.
5. Rafii S, Lyden D: Therapeutic stem and progenitor cell transplantation for organ vascularization and regeneration. *Nat Med* 9:702, 2003.
6. Clark ML, Lynch FX: Clinical symptoms of radiation sickness, time to onset and duration of symptoms among Hiroshima survivors in the lethal and median lethal ranges of radiation. *Mil Surg* 111:360, 1952.
7. Jacobson LO, Marks EK, Robson MJ, et al.: Effect of spleen protection on mortality following X-irradiation. *J Lab Clin Med* 34:1538, 1949.
8. Rekers PE, Coulter MP, Warren S: Effects of transplantation of bone marrow into irradiated animals. *Arch Surg* 60:635, 1950.
9. Dameshek W: Bone marrow transplantation; a present-day challenge. *Blood* 12:321, 1957.
10. Groth CG, Brent LB, Calne RY, et al.: Historic landmarks in clinical transplantation: conclusions from the consensus conference at the University of California, Los Angeles. *World J Surg* 24:834, 2000.
11. Siskind GW, Thomas L: Studies on the runting syndrome in newborn mice. *J Exp Med* 110:511, 1959.
12. Wilson RE, Henry L, Merrill JP: A model system for determining histocompatibility in man. *J Clin Invest* 42:1497, 1963.
13. Brenner MK: Haematopoietic stem cell transplantation for autoimmune disease: limits and future potential. *Best Pract Res Clin Haematol* 17:359, 2004.
14. Orlic D, Kajstura J, Chimenti S, et al.: Bone marrow cells regenerate infarcted myocardium. *Nature* 410:701, 2001.
15. McCluskey J, Peh CA: The human leucocyte antigens and clinical medicine: an overview. *Rev Immunogenet* 1:3, 1999.
16. Hurley CK, Wade JA, Oudshoorn M, et al.: A special report: histocompatibility testing guidelines for hematopoietic stem cell transplantation using volunteer donors. *Tissue Antigens* 53:394, 1999.
17. Barnes DHW, Loutit JF: Treatment of murine leukaemia with X-rays and homologous bone marrow. *Br J Haematol* 3:241, 1957.
18. Mathé G, Amiel JL, Schwartzenberg L, et al.: Successful allogeneic bone marrow transplantation in man: chimerism, induced specific tolerance and possible antileukemic effects. *Blood* 25:179, 1965.
19. Weiden PL, Flournoy N, Thomas ED, et al.: Antileukemic effect of graft-versus-host disease in human recipients of allogeneic-marrow grafts. *N Engl J Med* 300:1068, 1979.
20. Weiden PL, Sullivan KM, Flournoy N, et al.: Antileukemic effect of chronic graft-versus-host disease: contribution to improved survival after allogeneic marrow transplantation. *N Engl J Med* 304:1529, 1981.
21. Horowitz MM, Gale RP, Sondel PM, et al.: Graft-versus-leukemia reactions after bone marrow transplantation. *Blood* 75:555, 1990.
22. Kolb HJ, Mittermüller J, Clemm C, et al.: Donor leukocyte transfusions for treatment of recurrent chronic myelogenous leukemia in marrow transplant patients. *Blood* 76:2462, 1990.
23. Porter DL, Roth MS, McGarigle C, et al.: Induction of graft-versus-host disease as immunotherapy for relapsed chronic myeloid leukemia. *N Engl J Med* 330:100, 1994.
24. Kolb HJ, Schattenberg A, Goldman JM, et al.: Graft-versus-leukemia effect of donor lymphocyte transfusions in marrow grafted patients. European Group for Blood and Marrow Transplantation Working Party Chronic Leukemia. *Blood* 86:2041, 1995.
25. Collins RH, Jr, Shpilberg O, Drobyski WR, et al.: Donor leukocyte infusions in 140 patients with relapsed malignancy after allogeneic bone marrow transplantation. *J Clin Oncol* 15:433, 1997.
26. Jones RJ, Ambinder RF, Piantadosi S, et al: Evidence of a graft-versus-lymphoma effect associated with allogeneic bone marrow transplantation. *Blood* 77:649, 1991.
27. Tricot G, Vesole DH, Jagannath S, et al.: Graft-versus-myeloma effect: proof of principle. *Blood* 87:1196, 1996.
28. Truitt RL, Horowitz MM, Atasoylu AA, et al.: Graft-versus-leukemia effect of allogeneic bone marrow transplantation: clinical and experimental aspects of

late leukemia relapse. In: Stewart THM, Wheelock EF, (eds.): *Cellular Immune Mechanisms and Tumor Dormancy.* Boca Raton, FL: CRC Press; 1992:111.

29. Bergmann L, Schui DK, Brieger J, et al.: The inhibition of lymphokine-activated killer cells in acute myeloblastic leukemia is mediated by transforming growth factor-beta 1. *Exp Hematol* 23:1574, 1995.

30. Brouwer RE, van der HP, Schreuder GM, et al.: Loss or downregulation of HLA class I expression at the allelic level in acute leukemia is infrequent but functionally relevant, and can be restored by interferon. *Hum Immunol* 63:200, 2002.

31. Brouwer RE, Hoefnagel J, Borger van Der BB, et al.: Expression of co-stimulatory and adhesion molecules and chemokine or apoptosis receptors on acute myeloid leukaemia: high CD40 and CD11a expression correlates with poor prognosis. *Br J Haematol* 115:298, 2001.

32. Dermime S, Mavroudis D, Jiang YZ, et al.: Immune escape from a graft-versus-leukemia effect may play a role in the relapse of myeloid leukemias following allogeneic bone marrow transplantation. *Bone Marrow Transplant* 19:989, 1997.

33. Kolb HJ, Schmid C, Barrett AJ, Schendel DJ: Graft-versus-leukemia reactions in allogeneic chimeras. *Blood* 103:767, 2004.

34. Schimmer AD, Hedley DW, Penn LZ, Minden MD: Receptor- and mitochondrial-mediated apoptosis in acute leukemia: a translational view. *Blood* 98:3541, 2001.

35. Tsukada N, Kobata T, Aizawa Y, et al.: Graft-versus-leukemia effect and graft-versus-host disease can be differentiated by cytotoxic mechanisms in a murine model of allogeneic bone marrow transplantation. *Blood* 93:2738, 1999.

36. Lehmann C, Zeis M, Schmitz N, Uharek L: Impaired binding of perforin on the surface of tumor cells is a cause of target cell resistance against cytotoxic effector cells. *Blood* 96:594, 2000.

37. Hsieh MH, Korngold R: Differential use of FasL- and perforin-mediated cytolytic mechanisms by T-cell subsets involved in graft-versus-myeloid leukemia responses. *Blood* 96:1047, 2000.

38. Gimmi CD, Freeman GJ, Gribben JG, et al.: Human T-cell clonal anergy is induced by antigen presentation in the absence of B7 costimulation. *Proc Natl Acad Sci USA* 90:6586, 1993.

39. Avigan D: Dendritic cells: development, function and potential use for cancer immunotherapy. *Blood Rev* 13:51, 1999.

40. Appleman LJ, Boussiotis VA: T cell anergy and costimulation. *Immunol Rev* 192:161, 2003.

41. Ruggeri L, Capanni M, Urbani E, et al.: Effectiveness of donor natural killer cell alloreactivity in mismatched hematopoietic transplants. *Science* 295:2097, 2002.

42. Ruggeri L, Capanni M, Casucci M, et al.: Role of natural killer cell alloreactivity in HLA-mismatched hematopoietic stem cell transplantation. *Blood* 94:333, 1999.

43. Farag SS, Fehniger TA, Ruggeri L, et al.: Natural killer cell receptors: new biology and insights into the graft-versus-leukemia effect. *Blood* 100:1935, 2002.

44. Gao JX, Liu X, Wen J, et al.: Two-signal requirement for activation and effector function of natural killer cell response to allogeneic tumor cells. *Blood* 102:4456, 2003.

45. Davies SM, Ruggieri L, DeFor T, et al.: Evaluation of KIR ligand incompatibility in mismatched unrelated donor hematopoietic transplants. Killer immunoglobulin-like receptor. *Blood* 100:3825, 2002.

46. Giebel S, Locatelli F, Lamparelli T, et al.: Survival advantage with KIR ligand incompatibility in hematopoietic stem cell transplantation from unrelated donors. *Blood* 102:814, 2003.

47. Bishop MR: The graft-versus-lymphoma effect: fact, fiction, or opportunity? *J Clin Oncol* 21:3713, 2003.

48. Bierman PJ, Sweetenham JW, Loberiza FR, Jr, et al.: Lymphoma Working Committee of the International Bone Marrow Transplant Registry and the European Group for Blood and Marrow Transplantation. Syngeneic hematopoietic stem-cell transplantation for non-Hodgkin's lymphoma: a comparison with allogeneic and autologous transplantation—The Lymphoma Working Committee of the International Bone Marrow Transplant Registry and the European Group for Blood and Marrow Transplantation. *J Clin Oncol* 21:3744, 2003.

49. Grigg A, Ritchie D: Graft-versus-lymphoma effects: clinical review, policy proposals, and immunobiology. *Biol Blood Marrow Transplant* 10:579, 2004.

50. Salutari P, Sica S, Micciulli G, et al.: Extramedullary relapse after allogeneic bone marrow transplantation plus buffy-coat in two high risk patients. *Haematologica* 81:182, 1996.

51. Robinson SP, Goldstone AH, Mackinnon S, et al.: Lymphoma Working Party of the European Group for Blood and Bone Marrow Transplantation. Chemoresistant or aggressive lymphoma predicts for a poor outcome following reduced-intensity allogeneic progenitor cell transplantation: an analysis from the Lymphoma Working Party of the European Group for Blood and Bone Marrow Transplantation. *Blood* 100:4310, 2002.

52. Porter DL, Collins RH, Jr, Shpilberg O, et al.: Long-term follow-up of patients who achieved complete remission after donor leukocyte infusions. *Biol Blood Marrow Transplant* 5:253, 1999.

53. Dazzi F, Szydlo RM, Cross NC, et al.: Durability of responses following donor lymphocyte infusions for patients who relapse after allogeneic stem cell transplantation for chronic myeloid leukemia. *Blood* 96:2712, 2000.

54. Kernan NA, Bartsch G, Ash RC, et al.: Analysis of 462 transplantations from unrelated donors facilitated by the National Marrow Donor Program. *N Engl J Med* 328:593, 1993.

55. Rubinstein P, Carrier C, Scaradavou A, et al.: Outcomes among 562 recipients of placental-blood transplants from unrelated donors. *N Engl J Med* 339:1565, 1998.

56. Aversa F, Tabilio A, Velardi A, et al.: Treatment of high-risk acute leukemia with T-cell-depleted stem cells from related donors with one fully mismatched HLA haplotype. *N Engl J Med* 339:1186, 1998.

57. Grewal SS, Barker JN, Davies SM, Wagner JE: Unrelated donor hematopoietic cell transplantation: marrow or umbilical cord blood? *Blood* 101:4233, 2003.

58. Laughlin MJ, Eapen M, Rubinstein P, et al.: Outcomes after transplantation of cord blood or bone marrow from unrelated donors in adults with leukemia. *N Engl J Med* 351:2265, 2004.

59. Fefer A, Cheever MA, Greenberg PD: Identical-twin (syngeneic) marrow transplantation for hematologic cancers. *J Natl Cancer Inst* 76:1269, 1986.

60. Gale RP, Horowitz MM, Ash RC, et al.: Identical-twin bone marrow transplants for leukemia. *Ann Intern Med* 120:646, 1994.

61. Frei E, III, Canellos GP: Dose: a critical factor in cancer chemotherapy. *Am J Med* 69:585,1980.

62. Saijo N: Chemotherapy: the more the better? Overview. *Cancer Chemother Pharmacol* 40:S100, 1997.

63. Kimler BF, Park CH, Yakar D, Mies RM: Radiation response of human normal and leukemic hemopoietic cells assayed by in vitro colony formation. *Int J Radiat Oncol Biol Phys* 11:809, 1985.

64. Schabel FM, Jr, Trader MW, Laster WR, Jr, et al.: Patterns of resistance and therapeutic synergism among alkylating agents. *Antibiot Chemother* 23:200, 1978.

65. Harris AL: DNA repair: relationship to drug and radiation resistance, metastasis and growth factors. *Int J Radiat Biol Relat Stud Phys Chem Med* 48:675, 1985.

66. Brenner MK, Rill DR, Moen RC, et al.: Gene marking to trace origin of relapse after autologous bone-marrow transplantation. *Lancet* 341:85, 1993.

67. Sharp JG, Kessinger A, Mann S, et al.: Outcome of high-dose therapy and autologous transplantation in non-Hodgkin's lymphoma based on the presence of tumor in the marrow or infused hematopoietic harvest. *J Clin Oncol* 14:214, 1996.

68. Gertz MA, Witzig TE, Pineda AA, et al.: Monoclonal plasma cells in the blood stem cell harvest from patients with multiple myeloma are associated with shortened relapse-free survival after transplantation. *Bone Marrow Transplant* 19:337, 1997.

69. Yeager AM, Kaizer H, Santos GW, et al.: Autologous bone marrow transplantation in patients with acute nonlymphocytic leukemia, using ex vivo marrow treatment with 4-hydroperoxycyclophosphamide. *N Engl J Med* 315:141, 1986.

70. Gribben JG, Freedman AS, Neuberg D, et al.: Immunologic purging of marrow by PCR before autologous bone marrow transplantation for B-cell lymphoma. *N Engl J Med* 325:1525, 1991.

71. Vescio R, Schiller G, Stewart AK, et al.: Multicenter phase III trial to evaluate CD34(+) selected versus unselected autologous peripheral blood progenitor cell transplantation in multiple myeloma. *Blood* 93:1858, 1999.

72. Alvarnas JC, Forman SJ: Graft purging in autologous bone marrow transplantation: a promise not quite fulfilled. *Oncology (Huntingt)* 18:867, 2004.

73. Hess AD: Syngeneic/autologous graft-vs-host disease: mobilization of autoimmune mechanisms as antitumor immunotherapy. *Cancer Control* 1:201, 1994.

74. Hess AD, Thoburn CJ, Chen W, Horwitz LR: Complexity of effector mechanisms in cyclosporine-induced syngeneic graft-versus-host disease. *Biol Blood Marrow Transplant* 6:13, 2000.

75. Jones RJ, Vogelsang GB, Hess AD, et al.: Induction of graft-versus-host disease after autologous bone marrow transplantation. *Lancet* 1:754, 1989.

76. Yeager AM, Vogelsang GB, Jones RJ, et al.: Induction of cutaneous graft-versus-host disease by administration of cyclosporine to patients undergoing autologous bone marrow transplantation for acute myeloid leukemia. *Blood* 79:3031, 1992.

77. Goldman JM, Horowitz MM: The International Bone Marrow Transplant Registry. *Int J Hematol* 76(suppl 1):393, 2002.

78. Wagner JE, Barker JN, DeFor TE, et al.: Transplantation of unrelated donor umbilical cord blood in 102 patients with malignant and nonmalignant diseases: influence of CD34 cell dose and HLA disparity on treatment-related mortality and survival. *Blood* 100:1611, 2002.

79. Thomas ED: High-dose therapy and bone marrow transplantation. *Semin Oncol* 12(4 suppl 6):15, 1985.

80. Simpson D: T-cell depleting antibodies: new hope for induction of allograft tolerance in bone marrow transplantation? *Bio Drugs* 17:147, 2003.

81. Thomas ED, Buckner CD, Banaji M, et al.: One hundred patients with acute leukemia treated by chemotherapy, total body irradiation and allogeneic marrow transplantation. *Blood* 49:511, 1977.

82. Baranov A, Gale RP, Guskova A, et al.: Bone marrow transplantation after the Chernobyl nuclear accident. *N Engl J Med* 321:205, 1989.

83. Sullivan KM, Storb R, Buckner CD, et al.: Graft-versus-host disease as adoptive immunotherapy in patients with advanced hematologic neoplasms. *N Engl J Med* 320:828, 1989.

84. McCarthy NJ, Bishop MR: Nonmyeloablative allogeneic stem cell transplantation: early promise and limitations. *Oncologist* 5:487, 2000.

85. Giralt S, Estey E, Albitar M, et al.: Engraftment of allogeneic hematopoietic progenitor cells with purine analog-containing chemotherapy: harnessing graft-versus-leukemia without myeloablative therapy. *Blood* 89:4531, 1997.

86. Slavin S, Nagler A, Naparstek E, et al.: Nonmyeloablative stem cell transplantation and cell therapy as an alternative to conventional bone marrow transplantation with lethal cytoreduction for the treatment of malignant and nonmalignant hematologic diseases. *Blood* 91:756, 1998.

87. McSweeney PA, Niederwieser D, Shizuru JA, et al.: Hematopoietic cell transplantation in older patients with hematologic malignancies: replacing high-dose cytotoxic therapy with graft-versus-tumor effects. *Blood* 97:3390, 2001.

88. Perez-Simon JA, Kottaridis PD, Martino R, et al.: Spanish and United Kingdom Collaborative Groups for Nonmyeloablative Transplantation. Nonmyeloablative transplantation with or without alemtuzumab: comparison between 2 prospective studies in patients with lymphoproliferative disorders. *Blood* 100:3121, 2002.

89. Goldman JM, Apperley JF, Jones L, et al.: Bone marrow transplantation for patients with chronic myeloid leukemia. *N Engl J Med* 314:202, 1986.

90. Hansen JA, Gooley TA, Martin PJ, et al.: Bone marrow transplants from unrelated donors for patients with chronic myeloid leukemia. *N Engl J Med* 338:962, 1998.

91. Pinilla-Ibarz J, Cathcart K, Scheinberg DA: CML vaccines as a paradigm of the specific immunotherapy of cancer. *Blood Rev* 14:111, 2000.

92. Mackinnon S, Papadopoulos EB, Carabasi MH, et al.: Adoptive immunotherapy evaluating escalating doses of donor leukocytes for relapse of chronic myeloid

leukemia after bone marrow transplantation: separation of graft-versus-leukemia responses from graft-versus-host disease. *Blood* 86:1261, 1995.

93. Bhatia R, McGlave PB: Autologous hematopoietic cell transplantation for chronic myelogenous leukemia. *Hematol Oncol Clin North Am* 18:715, 2004.

94. Hughes TP, Kaeda J, Branford S, et al; International randomised study of interferon versus STI571 (IRIS) study group. Frequency of major molecular responses to imatinib or interferon alfa plus cytarabine in newly diagnosed chronic myeloid leukemia. *N Engl J Med* 349:1423, 2003.

95. Collins RH, Jr, Goldstein S, Giralt S, et al.: Donor leukocyte infusions in acute lymphocytic leukemia. *Bone Marrow Transplant* 26:511, 2000.

96. van der Harst D, Goulmy E, Falkenburg JH, et al.: Recognition of minor histocompatibility antigens on lymphocytic and myeloid leukemic cells by cytotoxic T-cell clones. *Blood* 83:1060, 1994.

97. Molldrem JJ, Komanduri K, Wieder E: Overexpressed differentiation antigens as targets of graft-versus-leukemia reactions. *Curr Opin Hematol* 9:503, 2002.

98. Goulmy E: Minor histocompatibility antigens: allo target molecules for tumor-specific immunotherapy. *Cancer J* 10:1, 2004.

99. Cutler CS, Lee SJ, Greenberg P, et al.: A decision analysis of allogeneic bone marrow transplantation for the myelodysplastic syndromes: delayed transplantation for low-risk myelodysplasia is associated with improved outcome. *Blood* 104:579, 2004.

100. Attal M, Harousseau JL, Stoppa AM, et al.: A prospective, randomized trial of autologous bone marrow transplantation and chemotherapy in multiple myeloma. Intergroupe Francais du Myelome. *N Engl J Med* 335:91, 1996.

101. Child JA, Morgan GJ, Davies FE, et al.: Medical Research Council Adult Leukaemia Working Party. High-dose chemotherapy with hematopoietic stem-cell rescue for multiple myeloma. *N Engl J Med* 348:1875, 2003.

102. Attal M, Harousseau JL, Facon T, et al.: InterGroupe Francophone du Myelome. Single versus double autologous stem-cell transplantation for multiple myeloma. *N Engl J Med* 349:2495, 2003. Erratum in *N Engl J Med* 350:2628, 2004.

103. Bensinger WI, Buckner CD, Anasetti C, et al.: Allogeneic marrow transplantation for multiple myeloma: an analysis of risk factors on outcome. *Blood* 88:2787, 1996.

104. Maloney DG, Molina AJ, Sahebi F, et al.: Allografting with nonmyeloablative conditioning following cytoreductive autografts for the treatment of patients with multiple myeloma. *Blood* 102:3447, 2003.

105. Vose JM, Anderson JR, Kessinger A, et al.: High-dose chemotherapy and autologous hematopoietic stem-cell transplantation for aggressive non-Hodgkin's lymphoma. *J Clin Oncol* 11:1846, 1993.

106. Philip T, Guglielmi C, Hagenbeek A, et al.: Autologous bone marrow transplantation as compared with salvage chemotherapy in relapses of chemotherapy-sensitive non-Hodgkin's lymphoma. *N Engl J Med* 333:1540, 1995.

107. Moskowitz CH, Nimer SD, Zelenetz AD, et al.: A 2-step comprehensive high-dose chemoradiotherapy second-line program for relapsed and refractory Hodgkin disease: analysis by intent to treat and development of a prognostic model. *Blood* 97:616, 2001.

108. Moskowitz CH, Kewalramani T, Nimer SD, et al.: Effectiveness of high dose chemoradiotherapy and autologous stem cell transplantation for patients with biopsy-proven primary refractory Hodgkin's disease. *Br J Haematol* 124:645, 2004.

109. Dean RM, Bishop MR: Allogeneic hematopoietic stem cell transplantation for lymphoma. *Clin Lymphoma* 4:238, 2004.

110. Dudley ME, Wunderlich JR, Robbins PF, et al.: Cancer regression and autoimmunity in patients after clonal repopulation with antitumor lymphocytes. *Science* 298:850, 2002.

# Chapter 93

# PRINCIPLES OF HLA MATCHING AND THE NATIONAL MARROW DONOR PROGRAM

*Edward J. Ball*

## INTRODUCTION

Transplantation of allogeneic hematopoietic stem cells is a potentially curative treatment for a number of hematologic malignancies and other diseases.[1] The best success of this therapy is achieved using HLA-identical sibling donors, but only 30–35% of patients have such donors. Alternate donors that have been used include partially HLA-matched related donors and unrelated donors. The use of alternate donors is generally associated with increased rates of severe complications and mortality. Efforts to reduce complications associated with alternate-donor transplantation include HLA matching and protocols designed to improve engraftment and reduce graft-*versus*-host disease (GVHD).

The HLA complex is intimately involved in human allogeneic stem cell transplantation, being critically involved in GVHD, graft failure, and graft-versus-leukemia (GVL) effects. Each of these is a reflection of the normal function of HLA molecules in immune responses to pathogenic agents. The principle functions of HLA molecules are to bind peptides and to serve as recognition elements for T lymphocyte and natural killer (NK) cell receptors.[2,3]

## HLA GENETIC ORGANIZATION

The HLA (human leukocyte antigen) complex is the name of the human major histocompatibility complex (MHC). It is located on chromosome 6 (6p21.3), covers about 3600 kilobases of DNA, and contains in excess of 120 expressed genes.[4,5] Two classes of HLA molecules are central to the control of immune responses: class I (HLA-A, -B, -C) and class II (HLA-DR, -DQ, -DP)[6,7] (Figure 93.1). Class I molecules are heterodimorphic glycoproteins whose alpha chain (~45 kD) is encoded by HLA-complex genes (*HLA-A\**, *-B\**, *C\**) and whose beta chain is $\beta_2$-microglobulin ($\beta_2$-M), encoded on chromosome 15 (15q21–22.2).[8] Class II molecules are also heterodimeric glycoproteins, but both alpha and beta chains (~28–32 kD) are encoded within the HLA complex (alpha genes *HLA-DRA1\**, *-DQA1\**, *-DPA1\** and beta genes *HLA-DRB1\**, *-DRB3\**, *-DRB4\**, *-DRB5\**, *-DQB1\**, *-DPB1\**).

### VARIATION IN HLA GENETIC ORGANIZATION

Complexity of the HLA region is manifest at several levels. As noted above, each HLA chromosomal segment or haplotype has multiple class I and class II loci. However, there is variation in the number of *HLA-DRB* genes present on commonly occurring haplotypes. There are five different prototypic haplotypes that are very commonly observed[9–11] (Figure 93.2). Thus, haplotypes expressing DR1, DR8, or DR10 typically have only the *DRB1\** gene that can be expressed, while most other haplotypes have *DRB1\** and a second gene expressed (*DRB3\**, *DRB4\**, or *DRB5\**, encoding DR52, DR53, and DR51 antigens, respectively). It should be noted that exceptions to these prototypic haplotypes are known.[12–15] These exceptional haplotypes may be difficult to match in unrelated-donor searches. Further, some reasonably frequent haplotypes do not express a second DR antigen as a result of an inactivating mutation, e.g., HLA-B57, *DRB1\*0701*, *DRB4\*01030102N*, *DQB1\*030302*[16]; *DRB1\*1502*, *DRB5\*0108N*, *DQB1\*0501*[17]; HLA-B52, *DRB1\*1502*, *DRB5\*0110N*, *DQB1\*0503*.[18]

## HLA STRUCTURE AND FUNCTION

The HLA class I[19,20] and class II[21,22] molecules were revealed by crystallographic studies to be similar in overall structure. The extracellular portion of both molecules is composed of four domains (Figure 93.3). A peptide binding structure formed by the two domains most distal to the cell membrane ($\alpha 1$, $\alpha 2$ of class I and $\alpha 1$, $\beta 1$ of class II) sits atop two membrane proximal domains ($\alpha 3$ and $\beta_2$M of class I and $\alpha 2$, $\beta 2$ of class II). The intron/exon arrangement of the class I and class II HLA

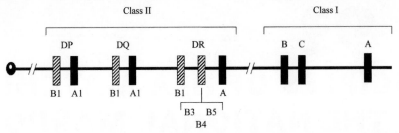

**Figure 93.1**   *HLA class I and class II genes of the HLA complex. This figure shows an abbreviated representation of the HLA region of chromosome 6. The relative locations of the genes commonly evaluated in transplant matching are shown. Solid bars represent α-chain genes and slashed bars represent β-chain genes. When present, the DRB3\*, DRB4\*, or DRB5\* genes are located between the DRA1\* and DRB1\* genes*

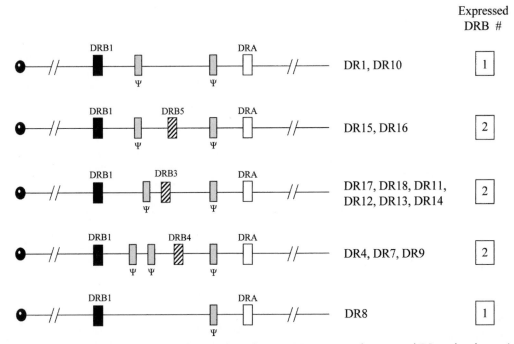

**Figure 93.2**   *Prototypic HLA-DR haplotypes. The number of HLA-DRB genes and expressed DR molecules varies with different haplotypes. In this figure five common or prototypic HLA haplotypes, the normally associated DR types, and number of expressed DR molecules are shown. ψ indicates a nonexpressed DRB pseudogene*

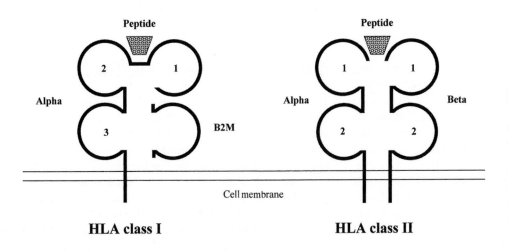

**Figure 93.3**   *Domain structure of HLA molecules. HLA class I and class II molecules are heterodimeric glycoproteins composed of four external domains. The two most external domains of each molecule form a peptide binding structure that is recognized by T-cell receptors*

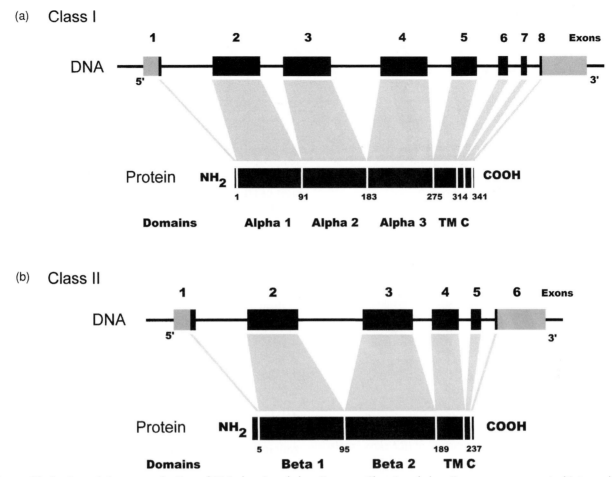

**Figure 93.4** *Exon–intron organization of HLA class I and class II genes. Class I and class II genes are segmented into multiple exons separated by noncoding introns. Each external protein domain of the mature molecules is encoded by different exons*

genes (Figure 93.4) corresponds in large part to the domain structure of the encoded molecules. Exons 2, 3, 4 of the class I alpha genes primarily encode the alpha 1, 2, 3 domains of the class I protein. In class II molecules, the alpha and beta gene products each contribute one domain to the peptide binding structure of the heterodimer. HLA class I molecules are found on nearly all nucleated cells. Class II molecules have a more restricted distribution, being found on B lymphocytes, activated T lymphocytes, macrophages, and dendritic cells.

### T-CELL RECOGNITION OF HLA

As noted previously, the principal function of HLA molecules is to acquire peptide fragments and to interact with effector T cells or NK cells. Peptide fragments bound by HLA molecules are found in a cleft whose walls are formed by more or less parallel alpha helices that sit atop a floor formed by β-pleated sheets (Figure 93.5). In class I molecules, six pockets are formed that accommodate side chains of the bound peptides.[20,25] Most of the highly polymorphic amino acid positions can be classified according to whether their side chains engage the bound peptide or the T-cell receptor (TCR) (contact residues).[26] In a similar fashion, the peptide binding[21,22] and TCR contact residues of class II mole-

cules have been addressed in crystallographic studies.[27] While any HLA molecule can bind numerous different peptides, there is a selective or preferential binding of peptides (peptide binding motif) that is determined by the polymorphic HLA pocket residues. Since the TCR engages both bound peptide and TCR contact residues of the HLA molecule, T-cell specificity is influenced by both types of residues.

In HLA-identical transplants there are no foreign HLA molecules to which the donor can respond. However, cytotoxic T cells against minor histocompatibility antigens arise and can mediate GVHD and GVL.[28,29] In these cases, peptides from the minor histocompatibility antigens are bound by host HLA molecules and are presented to donor T cells. In essence, such T cells are responding to a foreign peptide in a "self" HLA molecule.

In an allogeneic response to a mismatched HLA antigen, a large portion of T cells are activated.[30] While peptide-independent recognition of MHC has been demonstrated in some studies,[31,32] most alloreactive T cells would appear to recognize foreign MHC in a peptide-dependent or a peptide-specific fashion.[33–38] Thus, despite most peptide-binding residues being inaccessible to TCRs, they can influence the T-cell response by

(a)

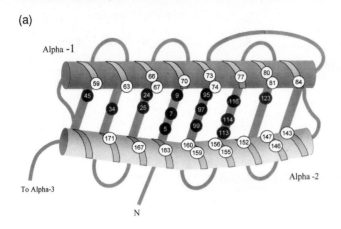

(b)

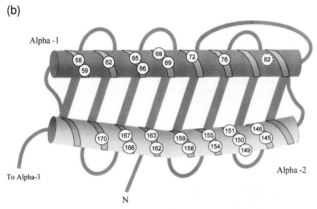

**Figure 93.5** *Peptide-binding structure of HLA class I molecules. This figure shows a representation of the peptide-binding structure formed by the α-1 and α-2 protein domains of a class I molecule. (a) Amino acid residues involved in peptide binding and (b) amino acid residues that contact the T-cell receptor. Residue positions in white are located in α-helical segments and those in black are located in β-pleated sheet segments of the molecule. The indicated residues are those designated in Ref. 23 and/or 24*

dictating which peptides are bound and their orientation by the foreign HLA molecules. Since T cells specific for foreign HLA plus peptides are not negatively selected during thymic selection, alloreactive T cells of this sort can represent a large fraction of the mature T-cell repertoire.

### NK CELL RECOGNITION OF HLA

NK cells are lymphocytes of the innate immune system that function early to control infections and have the ability to kill certain tumor cells.[3,39] Lysis by NK cells is inversely related to target cell expression of class I MHC molecules. Since a number of viruses and tumor cells down regulate expression of class I molecules to avoid killing by cytotoxic T cells, NK cells are able to counter this adaptation. At the same time, the expression of class I molecules by healthy cells prevents their killing by NK cells. The inhibition of lysis is mediated by a set of NK-cell receptors specific for class I molecules. Among these are CD94/NKG2A, which recognize a subset of HLA class I leader peptides bound by the nonclas-

sic HLA-E molecule[40] and certain killer immunoglobulin-like receptors (KIR) (Table 93.1). Inhibitory receptors KIR2DL1, KIR2DL2, KIR2DL3 recognize an HLA-Cw amino acid motif dimorphism at positions 77 and 80,[41–44] the latter having been shown to be a receptor contact residue in crystallographic studies.[43,44] KIR3DL1 is specific for the HLA-Bw4 epitope of a subset of HLA-B molecules.[45] The Bw4 epitope is determined by amino acids in the region of 77 to 83 of the HLA heavy chain. KIR3DL2 has been indicated to be specific for HLA-A3 and -A11.[46,47] Studies have indicated that KIR recognition of HLA is dependent on bound peptides, but there is little indication that the peptide contributes to the specificity of the interaction.[3]

In the normal autologous setting, all NK cells have at least one inhibitory receptor that interacts with an autologous HLA class I molecule, thus preventing attack against normal cells. In an HLA class I mismatched transplant there may be donor NK clones that are able to attack recipient cells because the class I ligands for the inhibitory receptors are not present on these cells. It has been indicated that these cells can mediate an effective GVL effect in HLA-mismatched transplants.[48–50]

### ANTIBODY RECOGNITION OF HLA

Alloantibodies directed against determinants of allogeneic HLA molecules can arise as a result of pregnancy, blood transfusion, and transplantation. Such antibodies are well known to cause rejection of solid organ transplants.[51] The presence of patient antibodies against mismatched donor HLA antigens and a positive lymphocyte crossmatch is strongly associated with engraftment failure or graft rejection.[52,53] For patients lacking an HLA-matched donor, recognizing the presence of HLA antibodies and defining the specificity(ies) can be very important in finding compatible donors. Antibody reactivity and specificity can be determined by testing against panels of HLA-typed cells or purified HLA antigens.

| Table 93.1 | HLA ligands for inhibitory KIR | | |
|---|---|---|---|
| **Inhibitory KIR** | | | **HLA ligand** |
| KIR2DL1 | HLA-C Group 2 | Lys-80 | Cw2, Cw4, Cw5, Cw6, etc. |
| KIR2DL2, KIR2DL3 | HLA-C Group 1 | Asn-80 | Cw1, Cw3, Cw7, Cw8, etc. |
| KIR3DL1 | HLA-B Bw4 alleles | Residues 77-83 | B51, B27, B38, B63, etc. |
| KIR3DL2 | HLA-A3, -A11 | | |

The commonly considered inhibitory killer immunoglobulin-like receptors (KIR) and associated HLA class I ligands are shown. HLA-C group specificity is associated with amino acids at residue position 80; Lysine (Lys, K) or Asparagine (Asn, N). Representative HLA-C group and Bw4 antigens are shown

## POLYMORPHISM OF HLA GENES AND PRODUCTS

### HLA NOMENCLATURE

Two nomenclature systems exist for the HLA system. The HLA system was originally described using alloantisera reactive with antigenic determinants of HLA molecules expressed at the cell surface and a nomenclature developed around that typing system. With the advent of DNA-based methods in the mid-1980s a dramatic increase in the level of polymorphism was revealed and required an additional nomenclature system. Alleles identified by DNA typing were grouped according to nucleotide sequence homology, but to the degree possible the allele names retained a relation to the serologic or antigen-level names.

Figure 93.6 outlines the basics of the DNA-based nomenclature. HLA allele names indicate the locus (e.g., *HLA-A**) followed by up to eight digits that refer to a unique nucleotide sequence. With the exception of *HLA-DPBI**, the first two digits of an HLA allele name can be referred to as a family or group designation that signifies a high level of sequence homology. *DPBI** allele names are not grouped into homology-related families in general. This group or family in many, but not all, cases correlates with the serologic or antigen-level typing of the allele product. The third and fourth digits relate to the encoded protein product of the allele. The fifth and sixth digits, when present, indicate nucleotide sequence variant alleles that encode the same protein product due to codon redundancy (synonymous alleles). The seventh and eighth digits refer to allele nucleotide polymorphism outside of the coding portions (exons) of the allele. In some cases, these noncoding variations cause important functional characteristics of the allele, such as null or low expression. These expression variants can also be shown with an appended letter suggestive of the expression variation (e.g., N = null, L = low, S = soluble). The most current listing of HLA alleles can be found at http://www.ebi.ac.uk/imgt/hla/index.html.[54]

In the laboratory, HLA alleles or molecules can be defined at different levels. Serologic HLA typing defines HLA products based on the pattern of reactivity with selected antibodies. DNA typing systems generally test for particular sequence motifs using sequence-specific oligonucleotide primer amplification (PCR-SSP) and/or oligonucleotide probe hybridization (PCR-SSOP) or direct sequencing (SBT) of amplified gene segments. Low-to-intermediate level resolution DNA test systems identify group or family level types (two digit nomenclature) that correlate in large part to antigen- or serologic-level typing. High-resolution DNA systems indicate specific alleles or a very limited set of allele possibilities. Aside from expression variant alleles, the first four digits of an allele name can be considered to fully define the expressed HLA product (four digit nomenclature).

In many cases, the first two digits of the HLA allele name correspond to the serologic or antigen name of the encoded product. For example, *A*01*, *A*02*, *B*07*, *B*08* alleles serologically type as A1, A2, B7, and B8 for all of the characterized alleles. In other cases, the allele group and serologic antigen name do not have this mnemonic similarity. For example, the *B*40* group of alleles encode B60 (e.g., *B*4001*) and B61 (e.g., *B*4002*) antigens by serology. In these cases, the alleles are clearly related based on sequence homology, but are distinct in key residues that are involved in formation of epitopes recognized by antibodies (and T cells). The best source that correlates serologic antigen names with HLA alleles is that of Schreuder and colleagues.[55] Since many new HLA alleles discovered in DNA-based testing are not serologically characterized, the antigen-level assignment is not formally known. In many cases the probable antigen-level assignment can be surmised by a knowledge of which amino acid sequence motifs are important in antigen definition. A useful resource for this can be found at http://tpis.upmc.edu/tpis/HLAMatchmaker/.[56]

### HLA ALLELES

The genes of the HLA complex include the most polymorphic human genes with known function. For class I and class II loci that may be considered for matching in transplantation, there are more than 1700 alleles described (Table 93.2) (http://www.ebi.ac.uk/imgt/hla/index.html).[54] Considering the number of loci present per haplotype and the number of alleles at each locus, there is the formal possibility of an incredibly large number of distinct HLA haplotypes (>9 × 10[9] for

HLA-A*020101

HLA-**A**\*020101       A locus

HLA-A***02**0101       Group / Family

HLA-A*02**0101**       Allele identifier

HLA-A*0201**01**  ⎤
                  ⎥  Distinct bases    Synonymous
HLA-A*0201**02**  ⎦  Same protein      alleles

HLA-DRB4*010301**01**  ⎤ Intron & regulatory
HLA-DRB4*010301**02N** ⎦       variants

HLA-DRB4*01030102**N**     Null allele

HLA-A*24020102**L**      Low-expression allele

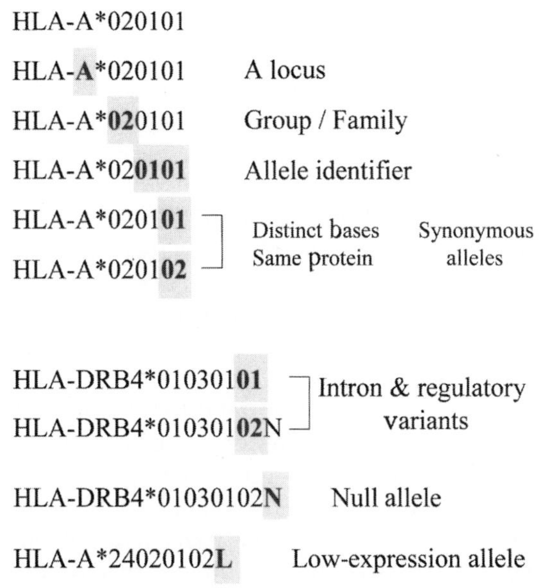

**Figure 93.6**   *HLA nomenclature. HLA DNA-based nomenclature consists of the HLA complex name followed by the locus identifier and a multidigit allele identifier with or without a qualifying letter designation. The significance of various positions is indicated in this figure*

| Table 93.2 | Polymorphism of HLA genes | | | | | | | |
| --- | --- | --- | --- | --- | --- | --- | --- | --- |
| **HLA class I** | | | | | | **HLA class II** | | |
| Locus | Alleles | Expression variants | | | | Locus | Alleles | Null Variants |
| | | Null | Low | Soluble | | | | |
| HLA-A | 313 | 20 | 2 | 0 | | HLA-DRB1 | 377 | 0 |
| HLA-B | 587 | 15 | 0 | 1 | | HLA-DRB3 | 41 | 0 |
| HLA-C | 139 | 2 | 0 | 0 | | HLA-DRB4 | 13 | 3 |
| | | | | | | HLA-DRB5 | 18 | 2 |
| | | | | | | HLA-DQA1 | 28 | 1 |
| | | | | | | HLA-DQB1 | 56 | 0 |
| | | | | | | HLA-DPA1 | 20 | 0 |
| | | | | | | HLA-DPB1 | 110 | 2 |

The number of alleles described for each of the indicated HLA loci is shown in the middle column. The number of expression variant alleles is indicated in adjacent columns. Data represent WHO listed alleles as of July 2004.[52]

HLA-A, -B, -C, -DRB1) and tissue types. However, the practical numbers encountered are much smaller on two accounts. First, many of the described alleles occur at very low frequency in most or all populations. Thus, the majority of individuals in a population can be accounted for by a relatively limited number of alleles at the commonly typed loci.[57,58] Second, alleles at different loci appear together more frequently than expected by chance due to linkage disequilibrium.[6,59,60] As an example, *HLA-A*0101,B*0801, Cw*0701,DRB1*0301,DQB1*0201* may represent ~5% of the haplotypes in Northern European populations despite an expectation of about 0.007% based on the product of the individual gene frequencies. Patients with common or linkage HLA haplotypes more often find well-matched donors in unrelated-donor registries than do those with uncommon associations.[61–63]

The level of polymorphism of the HLA genes is not equally distributed among the coding exons. For class I HLA genes, exons 2 and 3 are more polymorphic than other exons. For class II genes, exon 2 is the most polymorphic exon. As noted earlier, these exons encode the protein domains that form the peptide binding structure and interface for the T-cell[22,26,27] and NK-cell receptors.[43,44,64] Most of the highly polymorphic positions of these domains are involved in peptide-binding or TCR contact[26] (Figure 93.5). It may be that matching for these residues is more important than others in reducing adverse transplant outcome, although data supporting this are lacking as of yet.

### ETHNIC DIFFERENCES IN HLA ALLELE AND HAPLOTYPE FREQUENCIES

Certain alleles and allele combinations (haplotypes) have very different frequencies in different ethnic or racial groups.[58,65–67] Further, a greater complexity due to the variety of alleles and haplotypes is also seen in some groups. The probability of finding an HLA-matched unrelated donor is affected both by this complexity and by the number of individuals of that group represented in the various registries.[66,68–70] These considerations are the basis for unrelated donor registry recruitment efforts among minority groups.

### HLA EXPRESSION VARIANTS (NULL, SOLUBLE, AND LOW-EXPRESSION ALLELES)

A number of HLA class I and class II genes have been described with mutations that prevent cell surface expression ("null" or "soluble") or cause reduced expression ("low")[54,71] (Table 93.2). The greatest number of these expression variant alleles have been described for *HLA-A** and *-B**, but have been observed for most, if not all, HLA loci. While most of these variants are rare, some are not and may often appear as part of extended haplotypes (e.g., *DRB4*01030102N*,[16] *DRB5*0108N*,[17] *DRB5*0110N*,[18] *A*24020102L*,[72] *Cw*0409N*[73]). Known expression variants can be typed by DNA methods, but serologic typing is useful for generic exclusion of such alleles.

The consequences of mismatches for null expression variants have not been reported. However, since the null alleles are generally considered not to produce surface HLA molecules, mismatching between an expressed and nonexpressed allele could result in allostimulation and an adverse transplant outcome.

The *A*24020102L* allele produces surface antigen sufficient to stimulate a T-cell response even though not detected by anti-A24 antibodies in serologic typing.[74] Severe acute GVHD in an *A*24020102L* patient transplanted with an *A*24*-negative donor was reported by Zanone-Ramseier and colleagues.[75]

## HLA MATCHING IN STEM CELL TRANSPLANTATION RELATED DONORS

### HLA-IDENTICAL SIBLING DONORS

HLA-identical related donors (typically siblings) are generally considered to produce superior transplant outcome results compared to HLA-matched unrelated donors.[76,77] It is against this subset of donors that all other alternate donor types are compared with regard to transplant outcome.

Since there is a 50% chance of two siblings inheriting the same HLA haplotype from a parent, there is a 25% chance that they will inherit the same chromosome from each parent. Overall, about 30–35% of patients find an HLA-matched sibling donor for transplantation. Serologic typing and low-resolution DNA typing for HLA-A, -B, -C, -DR may be sufficient to identify an HLA-identical sibling when enough family members have been studied to demonstrate that the same haplotypes were inherited (identity by descent). If not initially typed, HLA-DP typing may also be performed to exclude the possibility of a crossover in the interval between DR/DQ and DP. If two siblings have not been shown to be HLA identical by descent, there is the possibility that they have not inherited the same HLA haplotypes, but rather different haplotypes that are only similar at the tested loci. In such cases, additional study of untested loci and DNA testing at high resolution are warranted. If not initially studied, the inclusion of HLA-C and -DP testing is often useful to identify distinct haplotypes. Although HLA-identical relatives are generally siblings, more distant relatives are sometimes found to be HLA identical. This may be suggested by the architecture of the family and should be addressed when HLA-identical siblings are not identified.

### HLA-MATCHED RELATED DONORS

While HLA-identical siblings have inherited the same haplotypes from each parent, other HLA-matched family members may be identified. These may include siblings, parents, and more distantly related individuals. Such individuals have typically inherited one HLA haplotype in common with the patient and a second, matched haplotype of independent origin. Since one haplotype is of independent origin, a higher level of HLA testing is needed to determine the level of similarity of the nonshared haplotype. Both the patient and the prospective donor should be tested for all relevant HLA loci at high resolution. Even when the nonshared haplotype is found to be identical at each tested locus, identity cannot be assumed for untested loci or DNA segments that may be relevant to transplant outcome (e.g., minor histocompatibility antigens, cytokine genes). Thus, donors HLA identical by descent may be preferred to over matched, but haplotype distinct related donors.

An HLA-matched, but haplotype distinct related donor may be favored over a matched unrelated donor on at least three counts. First, the shared haplotype is identical (within the boundaries marked by the tested loci), including any additional genes that may be important to transplant outcome. Second, a related donor is expected to share more minor histocompatibility genes with the patient than an unrelated donor. Third, a related donor is generally more accessible and may result in a more timely transplant.

When an HLA-identical sibling is not identified in the immediate family, the possibility that a more distant relative might be matched should be considered.[78] This may be particularly relevant when the patient has a rare HLA allele or haplotype paired with a haplotype that is frequent in the general population. The probability of finding a more distant matched relative is a function of the number of relatives available and the frequency of the more common haplotype in the general population or the ethnic group of the family. Allele and haplotype frequencies in various populations are available.[57,58,65–70] The typical approach is to first determine which branch of the family carries the rare HLA allele or haplotype (e.g., maternal or paternal) and then to trace the rare haplotype by typing additional key relatives.

### PARTIAL HLA-MATCHED RELATED DONORS

Partial HLA-matched related donors (PMRD) have been utilized as alternative donors for patients without an HLA-identical or phenotypically matched related donor.[48–50,79–85] These cases nearly always involve a shared HLA haplotype between the patient and donor. The nature and number of mismatched HLA antigens or alleles can have an important effect on transplant outcome.

With partially matched related donors, the possibility of patient antibodies reactive with the mismatched HLA antigens should be addressed to avoid the associated risk of graft failure. Identification of patient antibodies against mismatched HLA antigens and a positive lymphocyte crossmatch against the donor strongly correlates with increased risk of graft failure.[52,53,86]

#### Single-antigen-mismatched related donors

For patients without an HLA-matched related donor, a single-antigen- or allele-mismatched sibling donor is available in less than 5% of cases. Such cases may represent a recombinant HLA haplotype in the patient or donor, which can be demonstrated by family study. Other cases may represent two similar, but entirely unrelated haplotypes being present in the family. For unproven cases and unrelated haplotypes, high-resolution DNA typing and additional locus testing (e.g., Cw, DP) are needed.

Compared to HLA-identical sibling transplants, related single HLA-mismatched transplants have been reported to have equivalent[84,85] or reduced[76,87,88] overall survival. Increased risk of severe acute GVHD has been reported with both class I and class II (DRB1*) mismatches, although it may be higher with DRB1* mismatches.[85,87] Increased risk of graft failure and GVHD is associated with single-antigen PMRD donor transplants, but may be offset in part by lower relapse rates due to GVL effect observed in some studies. The stage of disease when the patient is transplanted is an important variable in transplant outcome. In some[76,87] but not all[85,88] reports, the negative overall survival effect of mismatch was observed in low- or standard-risk patients but not or less in high-risk patients where relapse may be a more imminent factor. When compared to unrelated donor transplants, single HLA-mismatched PMRD transplants have been reported to have comparable[76,85,87,89] overall survival.

### Haploidentical HLA-mismatched related donors

Related donors sharing one HLA haplotype, but with a greater level of HLA disparity have also been used.[48–50,79,81,83,84,90] The greater level of disparity is associated with increased engraftment failure, GVHD, and transplant-related mortality (TRM).[76,87,91] Drobyski and colleagues[83] found that matched, unrelated-donor transplants had better outcomes than related donors, with more than one HLA mismatch for class I (A,B) or class II (DRB1*,DQB1*). Improved results may be obtained with more extensive GVHD prophylaxis, rigorous donor T cell depletion, and high stem cell doses.[48–50,79] Ruggeri and colleagues[48,49] found that NK cells can have a profound effect in patients receiving rigorously T-cell-depleted stem cells from single haplotype matched donors. In patients who lacked an HLA ligand for an inhibitory KIR present in the stem cell donor (see Table 93.1), donor NK cells capable of killing patient lymphoblasts were found. In patients with myeloid disease, especially AML, KIR epitope mismatched transplants had increased engraftment and lower relapse rates than did KIR epitope matched cases. Leung and colleagues,[50] in a study of pediatric patients, reported a stronger correlation by testing donor cells for KIR expression and extended the observation to ALL patients. The authors suggest that when inhibitory KIR receptors of donor NK cells are not engaged by recipient ligands they are able to mediate a strong GVL effect and may also promote engraftment. Whether a similar benefit may apply in unrelated stem cell transplants is not established since conflicting studies have been reported.[92–95]

## UNRELATED DONORS

Since only about 30–35% of patients needing a stem cell transplant have a suitably HLA-matched relative able to donate, the majority of patients need alternate donors. As indicated earlier, some additional patients can be transplanted with partially matched related donors with acceptable outcomes. Nevertheless, many patients do not have suitable related donors and seek unrelated donors. Over the years, a number of national and international donor registries have been set up to facilitate unrelated-donor transplants. There are currently more than 9 million prospective donors registered along with a significant number of stored cord blood units (CBU).

### HLA-MATCHED UNRELATED DONORS

While HLA-identical sibling donors produce the best transplant outcomes,[84] closely matched unrelated donors (MUD) can also produce acceptable results.[96,97] Sources of stem cells for unrelated donor transplants include bone marrow[97] peripheral blood stem cells (PBSC),[98] and umbilical cord blood cells.[99–103]

In sibling donor transplants, serologic or low resolution HLA testing sufficient to prove haplotype identity is adequate, but this is not the case when unrelated donors are being considered. With the advent of DNA-based HLA testing, it was quickly apparent that serologically defined HLA antigens represent multiple distinct alleles in most cases.[55] The available literature on the role of HLA matching in stem cell transplant outcome varies both with regard to the number of HLA loci tested and the resolution level of the testing performed.

### Which HLA loci should be matched?

As shown in Table 93.3, matching for many of the HLA loci has been reported to be important in affecting transplant outcome, and there has been general consensus that mismatches for HLA-A, -B, and -DR loci are important. Studies using DNA typing methods have demonstrated the importance of matching for HLA-C in MUD transplants.[104–106,108,109,123] Thus, matching for HLA-A, -B, -Cw, and DRB1* is supported by numerous studies. Conflicting results have been reported regarding the importance of matching for HLA-DQ and -DP (Table 93.3). In some cases, the effect of mismatch was observed when coupled with mismatches at other loci but not in isolation. The effect of mismatches at DRB3*, DRB4*, and DRB5* (secondary DRB) has not been evaluated. It can be argued that all of these loci should be matched between patient and donor if possible since products of all of these alleles can elicit T-cell responses.[124,125] Because of strong linkage disequilibrium between DRB1* and DQ and the secondary DRB loci, matching can generally be accomplished. However, since linkage disequilibrium between DRB1* and DP is much lower, otherwise very well matched donors are frequently mismatched at DP. If included in a matching algorithm, some centers may use HLA-DP matching to distinguish among otherwise matched donors.

**Table 93.3** Effect of HLA matching on unrelated donor transplant outcome

| HLA Locus | Matching benefit | Literature citation | |
| --- | --- | --- | --- |
| | | Match benefit | Lack of benefit |
| A | Yes | 104–107 | |
| B | Yes | 104–107 | |
| C | Yes | 104–111 | |
| DRB1 | Yes | 105, 106, 112 113, 114 | 104 |
| DRA | No | | |
| DRB3, DRB4, DRB5 | Unknown | | |
| DQA1 | No | | 106 |
| DQB1 | Variable reports | 110, 115, 116 | 106, 113 |
| DPA1 | Variable reports | 117 | 106, 118 |
| DPB1 | Variable reports | 118–121 | 104, 106, 113, 128 |

### What level of matching is appropriate?

Initially, the importance of matching for HLA-A, -B, and -DR was established by serologic or antigen-level assignment.[126,127] With DNA-based typing it was subsequently shown that allele- or high-resolution-level matching for DRB1* was associated with lower GVHD and TRM,[112–114,128,129] being most evident when donors were otherwise matched for class I antigens. Since the mid-1990s most centers have matched unrelated donors for DRB1* at the allele- or high-resolution-typing level whenever possible, and often with preference over matching for class I.

Until the later 1990s, most studies of HLA matching involved antigen- or low-resolution-level HLA class I typing and may not have considered HLA-C.

A number of recent large studies have investigated the role of class I matching using allele-level DNA typing. Petersdorf and colleagues[23,107] found that single-antigen-level or multiple-allele-level class I (A, B, C), but not class II, mismatches in the HVG (host *versus* graft) vector were associated with graft failure in CML patients. The risk of graft failure was particularly high when the mismatch was only in the HVG direction (donor is mismatched at a locus for which the patient is homozygous). In a subsequent study,[110] allele- or antigen-level HLA-A, -B, -C mismatches were associated with increased mortality in low risk, but not higher risk CML patients. Two large registry studies of transplants performed at multiple centers and in multiple disease types have also been reported. Morishima and colleagues[104,105] found that single

HLA-A, -B, -C, and -DRB1* antigen- or allele-level mismatches were associated with increased acute GVHD, and class I mismatches were risk factors for failed engraftment. Flomenberg and colleagues[106] found that antigen or low-resolution mismatching at HLA-A, -B, or -Cw was significantly associated with increased mortality. No significant mortality risk was found for single locus mismatches found only at the allele level (i.e., antigen level matched), although a trend was shown for HLA-A allele mismatches. For severe acute GVHD, only HLA-A antigen-level mismatches were significantly associated although trends for association for HLA-B and -C were present. In sum, these studies show that HLA-A, -B, -C antigen or low-resolution mismatches are clearly associated with reduced overall survival. The effect is at least similar to mismatches for HLA-DRB1* and has called into question the common practice of giving matching preference to DRB1* when choosing partially mismatched unrelated donors. With regard to allele-level versus antigen-level class I mismatches, it would appear that single-antigen-level mismatches are more strongly associated with severe consequences than are allele-level mismatches. However, trends toward allele mismatch effect and indications of cumulative or synergistic effects of multiple allele mismatches suggest that allele-level matching for at least HLA-A, -B, -C, and -DRB1* should be utilized when possible. Similar high-resolution matching for HLA-DQ and -DP is also supported by reports by individual centers.

### WHAT IF HLA-MATCHED DONORS ARE NOT AVAILABLE?

If related donors and matched unrelated donors are not available, one may choose to consider partially matched unrelated donors. As discussed earlier, mismatched unrelated donors have increased risk of severe complications and increased mortality. However, despite the increased risk, successful outcomes are observed. Transplantation in these cases may benefit from alternate donor sources, protocols designed to minimize the risk of increased complication rates, or selection of donors whose mismatches may elicit less severe immune responses.

### ALTERNATE DONOR SOURCES
#### Unrelated cord blood stem cells

Unrelated cord blood (UCB) cell transplantation has been used successfully to treat pediatric and smaller adult patients.[99,101–103] Patients receiving HLA mismatched related and UCB transplants have a lower rate of severe acute GVHD and mortality than is observed in marrow transplants with a similar level of HLA mismatch.[101] Stem cell or nucleated cell dose is critical to successful engraftment and is the most important factor affecting patient survival in cord transplants.[99,101–103] However, minimizing HLA mismatches is still important in cord transplants. Rubinstein and

Stevens[103] reported that risk of severe acute GVHD correlated with HLA mismatch. Considering HLA-A, -B (antigen level) and -DRB1* matching, severe GVHD was seen in 8, 19, and 28% for 6/6, 5/6, and ≤4/6 HLA mismatches, respectively.

### T-cell depleted stem cell products

T-cell depletion of stem cell products can effectively reduce GVHD, but was found to be associated with an increased relapse rate due to the loss of a GVL effect.[79,80] However, as noted previously, rigorous T-cell depletion/CD34⁺ enrichment has been successful in related, haplotype mismatched donor transplants, particularly when the HLA mismatch prevents KIR inhibition of donor NK cells.[48,49,50] This might also apply to unrelated donors, but conflicting indications have so far been reported.[92–95] Another approach may be to transplant T-depleted donor stem cells and then at a later date infuse reserved donor T cells when the patient hematopoietic system has been replaced.[130] The intent being to avoid the massive initial stimulation of donor T cells by patient hematopoietic cells ("cytokine storm") that may promote GVHD, but recovering a GVL effect at a later point.

### CAN ACCEPTABLE HLA MISMATCHES BE PREDICTED?

Even with the large number of prospective donors listed by the various registries around the world, many patients do not find a matched donor even for HLA-A, -B, -C, -DRB1*. Despite the increased risk associated with HLA-mismatched transplants, acceptable results are achieved for many patients despite an imperfectly matched donor. The question raised is whether certain HLA mismatches are better tolerated than others and if so, whether this can be applied to donor selection to improve outcome.

Comparing different prospective allele mismatches simply on the basis of the number of mismatched amino acids is unlikely to be helpful. More likely to be useful would be a qualitative analysis of the mismatched residues. As discussed previously, most alloreactive T cells recognize foreign MHC in a peptide-dependent or a peptide-specific fashion,[33–38] leading to the speculation that HLA amino acids involved in peptide binding and TCR interaction may be more important to matching than other positions (see Figure 93.5). Antigen-level class I mismatches pose a greater risk than allele-level mismatches for graft failure[112] and increased mortality.[106] Petersdorf and colleagues[23] observed that there were a greater number of differences in peptide binding and especially TCR contact residues in the antigen-mismatched donor/recipient pairs rather than in allele-level mismatched donor/recipient pairs. Ferrara and colleagues[131] found that transplanted patients whose donors were mismatched at residue 116 of HLA class I molecules (A, B, or Cw) were at higher risk of severe GVHD and increased

mortality than those with mismatches at other residues.[131] This residue is in the floor of the cleft and is expected to contribute to peptide-binding specificity.[19] In addition to the molecular position of the mismatched residue, the nature of the mismatched amino acid may relate to the impact of the change. Substitution with amino acids of similar character may have less effect than that with dissimilar amino acids.

The ability to associate particular HLA allele mismatches with different levels of complication risk would be useful to distinguish among mismatched prospective donors. Elsner and colleagues[24,132] have developed an online tool that compares HLA alleles based on quantitative, positional, and qualitative evaluation of the mismatched amino acids and produces a dissimilarity score (http://histocheck.de./). Shaw and colleagues[133] studied 26 HLA-A allele level mismatched transplants but did not find a correlation of the dissimilarity scores and transplant outcome. That HLA allele pairs can be compared with regard to probability of T-cell stimulation is a logical premise. However, further large studies of HLA allele level typed transplant pairs will be needed to determine clinical validity of this approach.

## UNRELATED DONOR REGISTRIES

For patients without a suitable related donor, searching unrelated donor registries may provide a suitable donor.[134] The National Marrow Donor Program (NMDP) is the largest of the registries with over 5 million prospective marrow/PBSC donors and 31,000 CBU[135–137] (http://www.nmdpresearch.org/index.html). NMDP searches include donors from Bone Marrow Donors Worldwide, representing registries from 39 countries and bringing the total number of prospective donors to over 9 million (http://www.bmdw.org/database/donors.htm). As discussed previously, the prospect of finding a match for a patient with uncommon or rare HLA alleles may be different in various populations. Thus, a search of different registries may be more likely to provide a matched donor. In the NMDP registry, five major groups are represented: Caucasian (67.4%), Hispanic (10.6%), African American (9.9%), Asian/Pacific Islander (7.8%), American Indian/Alaska Native (1.6%).[136] The CBU Registry has about 30% minority representation. Of the registrants, approximately two-thirds have at least serologic or antigen-level typing for HLA-A, -B, -DR.

When a search is requested a list of potentially matched registrants or CBU is generated. NMDP search reports indicate prospective marrow/PBSC donors with potential for 5/6 and 6/6 (A, B, DR) matches and 4/6, 5/6, and 6/6 for CBU. From among those likely to be matched, a sample for confirmatory and additional HLA testing can be requested. This typing can be performed by the transplant center laboratory or an NMDP reference laboratory. The NMDP requires that both patient and donor be HLA typed at high resolution or allele level for HLA-A*, -B*, and -C* (minimal exons 2 and 3) and DRB1* before donation can occur. This does not indicate that patient and donor must be matched at high resolution for these loci. The intent is to allow analysis of the effect of allele-level matching on transplant outcome.

The prospect of finding a preliminary HLA-A, -B, -DR matched registry donor (i.e. serologic level typing) is 87% for Caucasians, 75% for Asian/Pacific Islander, 85% for Hispanic and 60% for African Americans according to NMDP statistics.[135] However, when allele-level matching and other loci are considered, the probability of a full match drops markedly. Tiercy and colleagues[138,139] indicated that half or less of their patients with preliminary matches (A, B, DR antigen level) were able to find allele-level matched donors for HLA-A, -B, -Cw, -DRB1, -DRB3, -DRB5, -DQB1. Finding highly matched donors for patients of ethnic minorities is especially difficult.[62,70]

### STRATEGIES FOR UNRELATED DONOR SEARCHES

Identification of a prospective unrelated stem cell donor is based principally on HLA matching. The patient should be initially typed for all relevant loci at allele/high resolution even though registry-matching algorithms are currently based on A, B, DR. This information can be used to indicate the probability that a matched donor will be found and may suggest the number of donors from a preliminary search that should be recruited for confirmatory or higher resolution testing. Since an increasing proportion of registry donors have been typed at high resolution and for more loci, the preliminary search results may already indicate well-matched donors that can be requested for confirmatory typing. Patients that have common HLA alleles and haplotypes more often find matched unrelated donors[61–63] and one can expect that only a few donors need to be typed to find a well-matched donor over the HLA-A through DQ interval. In contrast, rare alleles or haplotypes may indicate that a greater number of donors need to be considered.

In some searches, a large number of donors are possible matches by low resolution typing, and the problem becomes identifying those that may be more likely to match the patient. These can sometimes be prioritized on the basis of additional loci that have been tested. As mentioned previously, the HLA complex displays a high level of linkage disequilibrium between loci. Thus, one may selectively perform confirmatory testing on donors who are listed as DRB1*13, DQB1*0604 or DRB1*13, DRB3*0301 for a patient who is DRB1*1302, since these are the most common associations for this allele. Another example would be typing B44, Cw5 prospective donors to enrich for the

B*4402 subtype as opposed to the other common B44 subtype of B*4403.

Some HLA alleles or haplotypes may be rare in the general population but more common in particular ethnic or racial groups. This information can be used to focus a donor search in those groups' registries that are more likely to have individuals that match the patient. Thus, for a patient who is DRB1*1503 one may focus confirmatory testing mainly on African American donors listed as DRB1*15 rather than DRB1*15 Caucasians since the frequency of this allele differs markedly in the two groups (>80% vs <5%, respectively). A number of references regarding HLA antigen or allele frequencies in different populations are available.[57,58,140] In some cases, donors may be matched for a patient but have been incorrectly typed or listed on the registry. This problem is most apparent for donors who only have serologic-based typing as is more often seen for antigens that are difficult to assign by serologic typing.[141] If no matches are indicated for a patient with one of these difficult antigens, one should consider repeating the registry search using a surrogate antigen that the proper antigen may have been mistyped as (e.g., A26 to replace A66). Some problem antigens may have been missed entirely in serologic typing and running a second registry search without that antigen may pick up a matched donor (e.g., A74, particularly when paired with another A19 group antigen).

Patients with null or expression variant alleles may be difficult to match in registry searches, although the indications that the more common variants may appear as part of extended haplotypes may be somewhat encouraging.[16–18,72,73] Donors with expression variants mismatched to patients can be excluded on the basis of serologic- or DNA-based typing.

### SEARCHES FOR HLA-MISMATCHED UNRELATED DONORS

For a significant fraction of patients a fully matched donor may not be obtained. Tiercy and colleagues[138] indicated that their patients for whom full HLA-matched donors were not found fell into four categories (1) a rare allele in the patient, (2) an unusual B-DR or DR-DQ haplotype in the patient, (3) an antigen that is split into more than two alleles with greater than 10% frequency (e.g., DRB1*04), (4) a B antigen that has multiple Cw associations (e.g., B*51). Since some patients can do well with mismatched donors, the issue may become finding prospective donors that represent minimal mismatches to the patient, as discussed previously. Given the high level of linkage disequilibrium, especially between HLA-B and -Cw and between DR and DQ, mismatches at B or DR are very often also found to be mismatched at Cw or DQ, respectively. This may affect the choice of prospective donors on whom to perform additional testing to avoid multilocus mismatches.

## SUMMARY

HLA matching between patient and donor is a critical component in determining the success of allogeneic stem cell transplantation. High-level matching is associated with improved engraftment, reduced severe GVHD, and improved patient survival. Mismatching at most HLA loci has been correlated with adverse outcome in at least some reports, and there is essential consensus that matching for HLA-A, -B, -Cw, and -DRB1* is important for improved outcome.

It is important to develop consensus on the effect of mismatching for other HLA loci that have not been well studied or for which there are conflicting indications. Since a significant fraction of patients do not have fully matched donors (related or unrelated), it is important to determine if certain HLA mismatches may be better tolerated than others and produce less risk of adverse outcome. This will require the study of large numbers of patient/donor pairs that have been HLA typed at allele level for each of the polymorphic loci.

## REFERENCES

1. Buchner T: Treatment of adult acute leukemia. *Curr Opin Oncol* 9:18, 1997.
2. Germain R: Antigen processing and presentation. In: Paul W (ed.) *Fundamental Immunology*. 2nd ed. Philadelphia, PA: Lippincott-Raven;1999:287.
3. Lanier LL: NK cell receptors. *Annu Rev Immunol* 16:359, 1998.
4. The MHC sequencing consortium: Complete sequence and gene map of a human major histocompatibility complex. *Nature* 401:921, 1999.
5. Mungall AJ, Palmer SA, Sims SK, et al.: The DNA sequence and analysis of human chromosome 6. *Nature* 425:805, 2003.
6. Klein J, Sato A: The HLA system. First of two parts. *N Engl J Med* 343:702, 2000.
7. Margulies D: The major histocompatibility complex. In: Paul W (ed.) *Fundamental Immunology*. 4th ed. Philadelphia, PA: Lippincott-Raven;1999:263.
8. Goodfellow P, Jones E, Van Heyningen V, et al.: The beta2-microglobulin gene is on chromosome 15 and not in the HL-A region. *Nature* 254:267, 1975.
9. Andersson G, Larhammar D, Widmark E, et al.: Class II genes of the human major histocompatibility complex. Organization and evolutionary relationship of the DR beta genes. *J Biol Chem* 262:8748, 1987.
10. Gorski J, Rollini P, Mach B: Structural comparison of the genes of two HLA-DR supertypic groups: the loci encoding DRw52 and DRw53 are not truly allelic. *Immunogenetics* 25:397, 1987.
11. Kawai J, Ando A, Sato T, et al.: Analysis of gene structure and antigen determinants of DR2 antigens using DR gene transfer into mouse L cells. *J Immunol* 142:312, 1989.
12. Tautz C, Marsh DG, Baur X: A novel HLA-haplotype containing a DRB5 gene not associated with DRB1*15 or DRB1*16 alleles. *Tissue Antigens* 39:91, 1992.
13. Nesci S, Talevi N, Andreani M, et al.: An unusual DRB1*1503 haplotype without a detectable DRB5 locus in a black African family. *Tissue Antigens* 49:53, 1997.
14. Robbins F, Hurley CK, Tang T, et al.: Diversity associated with the second expressed HLA-DRB locus in the human population. *Immunogenetics* 46:104, 1997.
15. Wade JA, Hurley CK, Hastings A, et al.: Combinatorial diversity in DR2 haplotypes. *Tissue Antigens* 41:113, 1993.
16. Sutton VR, Kienzle BK, Knowles RW: An altered splice site is found in the DRB4 gene that is not expressed in HLA-DR7, Dw11 individuals. *Immunogenetics* 29:317, 1989.
17. Voorter CE, Roeffaers HE, du Toit ED, et al.: The absence of DR51 in a DRB5-positive individual DR2ES is caused by a null allele (DRB5*0108N). *Tissue Antigens* 50:326, 1997.
18. Balas A, Ocon P, Vicario JL, et al.: HLA-DR51 expression failure caused by a two-base deletion at exon 2 of a DRB5 null allele (DRB5*0110N) in a Spanish gypsy family. *Tissue Antigens* 55:467, 2000.
19. Saper MA, Bjorkman PJ, Wiley DC: Refined structure of the human histocompatibility antigen HLA-A2 at 2.6 A resolution. *J Mol Biol* 219:277, 1991.
20. Bjorkman PJ, Saper MA, Samraoui B, et al.: Structure of the human class I histocompatibility antigen, HLA-A2. *Nature* 329:506, 1987.
21. Brown JH, Jardetzky TS, Gorga JC, et al.: Three-dimensional structure of the human class II histocompatibility antigen HLA-DR1. *Nature* 364:33, 1993.
22. Stern LJ, Brown JH, Jardetzky TS, et al.: Crystal structure of the human class II MHC protein HLA-DR1 complexed with an influenza virus peptide. *Nature* 368:215, 1994.
23. Petersdorf EW, Hansen JA, Martin PJ, et al.: Major-histocompatibility-complex class I alleles and antigens in hematopoietic-cell transplantation. *N Engl J Med* 345: 1794, 2001.
24. Elsner HA, DeLuca D, Strub J, et al.: HistoCheck: rating of HLA class I and II mismatches by an internet-based software tool. *Bone Marrow Transplant* 33:165, 2004.
25. Garrett TP, Saper MA, Bjorkman PJ, et al.: Specificity pockets for the side chains of peptide antigens in HLA-Aw68. *Nature* 342:692, 1989.
26. Bjorkman PJ, Saper MA, Samraoui B, et al.: The foreign antigen binding site and T cell recognition regions of class I histocompatibility antigens. *Nature* 329:512, 1987.
27. Hennecke J, Carfi A, Wiley DC: Structure of a covalently stabilized complex of a human alphabeta T-cell receptor, influenza HA peptide and MHC class II molecule, HLA-DR1. *Embo J* 19:5611, 2000.
28. Goulmy E, Schipper R, Pool J, et al.: Mismatches of minor histocompatibility antigens between HLA-

identical donors and recipients and the development of graft-versus-host disease after bone marrow transplantation. *N Engl J Med* 334:281, 1996.

29. Goulmy E: Human minor histocompatibility antigens: new concepts for marrow transplantation and adoptive immunotherapy. *Immunol Rev* 157:125, 1997.

30. Sherman LA, Chattopadhyay S: The molecular basis of allorecognition. *Annu Rev Immunol* 11:385, 1993.

31. Elliott TJ, Eisen HN: Cytotoxic T lymphocytes recognize a reconstituted class I histocompatibility antigen (HLA-A2) as an allogeneic target molecule. *Proc Natl Acad Sci USA* 87:5213, 1990.

32. Smith PA, Brunmark A, Jackson MR, et al.: Peptide-independent recognition by alloreactive cytotoxic T lymphocytes (CTL). *J Exp Med* 185:1023, 1997.

33. Wang W, Man S, Gulden PH, et al.: Class I-restricted alloreactive cytotoxic T lymphocytes recognize a complex array of specific MHC-associated peptides. *J Immunol* 160:1091, 1998.

34. Kovalik JP, Singh N, Mendiratta SK, et al.: The alloreactive and self-restricted CD4+ T cell response directed against a single MHC class II/peptide combination. *J Immunol* 165:1285, 2000.

35. Rotzschke O, Falk K, Faath S, et al.: On the nature of peptides involved in T cell alloreactivity. *J Exp Med* 174:1059, 1991.

36. Chattopadhyay S, Theobald M, Biggs J, et al.: Conformational differences in major histocompatibility complex-peptide complexes can result in alloreactivity. *J Exp Med* 179:213, 1994.

37. Weber DA, Terrell NK, Zhang Y, et al.: Requirement for peptide in alloreactive CD4+ T cell recognition of class II MHC molecules. *J Immunol* 154:5153, 1995.

38. Munz C, Obst R, Osen W, et al.: Alloreactivity as a source of high avidity peptide-specific human CTL. *J Immunol* 162:25, 1999.

39. Parham P, McQueen KL: Alloreactive killer cells: hindrance and help for haematopoietic transplants. *Nat Rev Immunol* 3:108, 2003.

40. Borrego F, Ulbrecht M, Weiss EH, et al.: Recognition of human histocompatibility leukocyte antigen (HLA)-E complexed with HLA class I signal sequence-derived peptides by CD94/NKG2 confers protection from natural killer cell-mediated lysis. *J Exp Med* 187:813, 1998.

41. Colonna M, Borsellino G, Falco M, et al.: HLA-C is the inhibitory ligand that determines dominant resistance to lysis by NK1- and NK2-specific natural killer cells. *Proc Natl Acad Sci USA* 90:12000, 1993.

42. Moretta A, Sivori S, Vitale M, et al.: Existence of both inhibitory (p58) and activatory (p50) receptors for HLA-C molecules in human natural killer cells. *J Exp Med* 182:875, 1995.

43. Boyington JC, Motyka SA, Schuck P, et al.: Crystal structure of an NK cell immunoglobulin-like receptor in complex with its class I MHC ligand. *Nature* 405:537, 2000.

44. Fan QR, Long EO, Wiley DC: Crystal structure of the human natural killer cell inhibitory receptor KIR2DL1-HLA-Cw4 complex. *Nat Immunol* 2:452, 2001.

45. Gumperz JE, Litwin V, Phillips JH, et al.: The Bw4 public epitope of HLA-B molecules confers reactivity with natural killer cell clones that express NKB1, a putative HLA receptor. *J Exp Med* 181:1133, 1995.

46. Dohring C, Scheidegger D, Samaridis J, et al.: A human killer inhibitory receptor specific for HLA-A1,2. *J Immunol* 156:3098, 1996.

47. Pende D, Biassoni R, Cantoni C, et al.: The natural killer cell receptor specific for HLA-A allotypes: a novel member of the p58/p70 family of inhibitory receptors that is characterized by three immunoglobulin-like domains and is expressed as a 140-kD disulphide-linked dimer. *J Exp Med* 184:505, 1996.

48. Ruggeri L, Capanni M, Casucci M, et al.: Role of natural killer cell alloreactivity in HLA-mismatched hematopoietic stem cell transplantation. *Blood* 94:333, 1999.

49. Ruggeri L, Capanni M, Urbani E, et al.: Effectiveness of donor natural killer cell alloreactivity in mismatched hematopoietic transplants. *Science* 295:2097, 2002.

50. Leung W, Iyengar R, Turner V, et al.: Determinants of antileukemia effects of allogeneic NK cells. *J Immunol* 172:644, 2004.

51. Terasaki PI: Humoral theory of transplantation. *Am J Transplant* 3:665, 2003.

52. Anasetti C, Amos D, Beatty PG, et al.: Effect of HLA compatibility on engraftment of bone marrow transplants in patients with leukemia or lymphoma. *N Engl J Med* 320:197, 1989.

53. Mickelson EM, Petersdorf E, Anasetti C, et al.: HLA matching in hematopoietic cell transplantation. *Hum Immunol* 61:92, 2000.

54. Robinson J, Waller MJ, Parham P, et al.: IMGT/HLA and IMGT/MHC: sequence databases for the study of the major histocompatibility complex. *Nucleic Acids Res* 31:311, 2003.

55. Schreuder GM, Hurley CK, Marsh SG, et al.: The HLA dictionary 2004: a summary of HLA-A, -B, -C, -DRB1/3/4/5, -DQB1 alleles and their association with serologically defined HLA-A, -B, -C, -DR, and -DQ antigens. *Hum Immunol* 66:170, 2005.

56. Duquesnoy RJ, Marrari M: HLAMatchmaker: a molecularly based algorithm for histocompatibility determination. II: Verification of the algorithm and determination of the relative immunogenicity of amino acid triplet-defined epitopes. *Hum Immunol* 63:353, 2002.

57. Klitz W, Maiers M, Spellman S, et al.: New HLA haplotype frequency reference standards: high-resolution and large sample typing of HLA DR-DQ haplotypes in a sample of European Americans. *Tissue Antigens* 62:296, 2003.

58. Cao K, Hollenbach J, Shi X, et al.: Analysis of the frequencies of HLA-A, B, and C alleles and haplotypes in the five major ethnic groups of the United States reveals high levels of diversity in these loci and contrasting distribution patterns in these populations. *Hum Immunol* 62:1009, 2001.

59. Begovich AB, McClure GR, Suraj VC, et al.: Polymorphism, recombination, and linkage disequilibrium within the HLA class II region. *J Immunol* 148:249, 1992.

60. Bugawan TL, Klitz W, Blair A, et al.: High-resolution HLA class I typing in the CEPH families: analysis of linkage disequilibrium among HLA loci. *Tissue Antigens* 56:392, 2000.

61. Pedron B, Duval M, Elbou OM, et al.: Common genomic HLA haplotypes contributing to successful donor search in unrelated hematopoietic transplantation. *Bone Marrow Transplant* 31:423, 2003.

62. Oudshoorn M, Cornelissen JJ, Fibbe WE, et al.: Problems and possible solutions in finding an unrelated bone marrow donor. Results of consecutive searches for 240 Dutch patients. *Bone Marrow Transplant* 20:1011, 1997.

63. Tron de Bouchony E, Leberre C, Dauriac C, et al.: Relevance of 10 Caucasian HLA haplotypes in searches for unrelated bone marrow donors for 100 patients from a single center. Bone *Marrow Transplant* 15:845, 1995.

64. Boyington JC, Brooks AG, Sun PD: Structure of killer cell immunoglobulin-like receptors and their recognition of the class I MHC molecules. *Immunol Rev* 181:66, 2001.

65. Imanishi T, Akaza T, Kimura A, et al.: Allele and haplotype frequencies for HLA and complement loci in various ethnic groups. In: Tsuji K, Aizawa M, Sasazuki T (eds.) *HLA 1991.* Oxford:Oxford University Press;1992: 1065.

66. Mori M, Beatty PG, Graves M, et al.: HLA gene and haplotype frequencies in the North American population: the National Marrow Donor Program Donor Registry. *Transplantation* 64:1017, 1997.

67. Schipper RF, D'Amaro J, Bakker JT, et al.: HLA gene haplotype frequencies in bone marrow donors worldwide registries. *Hum Immunol* 52:54, 1997.

68. Beatty PG, Boucher KM, Mori M, et al.: Probability of finding HLA-mismatched related or unrelated marrow or cord blood donors. *Hum Immunol* 61:834, 2000.

69. Mori M, Graves M, Milford EL, et al.: Computer program to predict likelihood of finding an HLA-matched donor: methodology, validation, and application. Biol *Blood Marrow Transplant* 2:134, 1996.

70. Beatty PG, Mori M, Milford E: Impact of racial genetic polymorphism on the probability of finding an HLA-matched donor. *Transplantation* 60:778, 1995.

71. Parham P: Filling in the blanks. *Tissue Antigens* 50:318, 1997.

72. Dunn PP, Turton JR, Downing J, et al.: HLA-A*24020102L in the UK blood donor population. *Tissue Antigens* 63: 589, 2004.

73. Pinto C, Smith AG, Larsen CE, et al.: HLA-Cw*0409N is associated with HLA-A*2301 and HLA-B*4403-carrying haplotypes. *Hum Immunol* 65:181, 2004.

74. Magor KE, Taylor EJ, Shen SY, et al.: Natural inactivation of a common HLA allele (A*2402) has occurred on at least three separate occasions. *J Immunol* 158:5242, 1997.

75. Zanone-Ramseier R, Gratwohl A, Gmur J, et al.: Sequencing of two HLA-A blank alleles: implications in unrelated bone marrow donor matching. *Transplantation* 67:1336, 1999.

76. Szydlo R, Goldman JM, Klein JP, et al.: Results of allogeneic bone marrow transplants for leukemia using donors other than HLA-identical siblings. *J Clin Oncol* 15:1767, 1997.

77. Weisdorf DJ, Anasetti C, Antin JH, et al.: Allogeneic bone marrow transplantation for chronic myelogenous leukemia: comparative analysis of unrelated versus matched sibling donor transplantation. *Blood* 99:1971, 2002.

78. Schipper RF, D'Amaro J, Oudshoorn M: The probability of finding a suitable related donor for bone marrow transplantation in extended families. *Blood* 87:800, 1996.

79. Aversa F, Tabilio A, Velardi A, et al.: Treatment of high-risk acute leukemia with T-cell-depleted stem cells from related donors with one fully mismatched HLA haplotype. *N Engl J Med* 339:1186, 1998.

80. Henslee-Downey PJ, Abhyankar SH, Parrish RS, et al.: Use of partially mismatched related donors extends access to allogeneic marrow transplant. *Blood* 89:3864, 1997.

81. Aversa F, Tabilio A, Terenzi A, et al.: Successful engraftment of T-cell-depleted haploidentical "three-loci" incompatible transplants in leukemia patients by addition of recombinant human granulocyte colony-stimulating factor-mobilized peripheral blood progenitor cells to bone marrow inoculum. *Blood* 84:3948, 1994.

82. Godder KT, Hazlett LJ, Abhyankar SH, et al.: Partially mismatched related-donor bone marrow transplantation for pediatric patients with acute leukemia: younger donors and absence of peripheral blasts improve outcome. *J Clin Oncol* 18:1856, 2000.

83. Drobyski WR, Klein J, Flomenberg N, et al.: Superior survival associated with transplantation of matched unrelated versus one-antigen-mismatched unrelated or highly human leukocyte antigen-disparate haploidentical family donor marrow grafts for the treatment of hematologic malignancies: establishing a treatment algorithm for recipients of alternative donor grafts. *Blood* 99:806, 2002.

84. Beatty PG, Clift RA, Mickelson EM, et al.: Marrow transplantation from related donors other than HLA-identical siblings. *N Engl J Med* 313:765, 1985.

85. Ottinger HD, Ferencik S, Beelen DW, et al.: Hematopoietic stem cell transplantation: contrasting the outcome of transplantations from HLA-identical siblings, partially HLA-mismatched related donors, and HLA-matched unrelated donors. *Blood* 102:1131, 2003.

86. Anasetti C: The role of the immunogenetics laboratory in marrow transplantation. *Arch Pathol Lab Med* 115:288, 1991.

87. Kanda Y, Chiba S, Hirai H, et al.: Allogeneic hematopoietic stem cell transplantation from family members other than HLA-identical siblings over the last decade (1991–2000). *Blood* 102:1541, 2003.

88. Hasegawa W, Lipton JH, Messner HA, et al.: Influence of one human leukocyte antigen mismatch on outcome of allogeneic bone marrow transplantation from related donors. *Hematology* 8:27, 2003.

89. Leung WH, Turner V, Richardson SL, et al.: Effect of HLA class I or class II incompatibility in pediatric marrow transplantation from unrelated and related donors. *Hum Immunol* 62:399, 2001.

90. Mehta J, Singhal S, Gee AP, et al.: Bone marrow transplantation from partially HLA-mismatched family donors for acute leukemia: single-center experience of 201 patients. *Bone Marrow Transplant* 33:389, 2004.

91. Beatty PG: Marrow transplantation using volunteer unrelated donors in a comparison of mismatched family donor transplants: a Seattle perspective. *Bone Marrow Transplant* 14(suppl 4):S39, 1994.

92. Giebel S, Locatelli F, Lamparelli T, et al.: Survival advantage with KIR ligand incompatibility in hematopoietic stem cell transplantation from unrelated donors. *Blood* 102:814, 2003.

93. Davies SM, Ruggieri L, DeFor T, et al.: Evaluation of KIR ligand incompatibility in mismatched unrelated donor hematopoietic transplants. Killer immunoglobulin-like receptor. *Blood* 100:3825, 2002.

94. Bornhauser M, Schwerdtfeger R, Martin H, et al.: Role of KIR ligand incompatibility in hematopoietic stem cell transplantation using unrelated donors. *Blood* 103:2860, 2004.

95. Gagne K, Brizard G, Gueglio B, et al.: Relevance of KIR gene polymorphisms in bone marrow transplantation outcome. *Hum Immunol* 63:271, 2002.

96. Stroncek DF: Results of bone marrow transplants from unrelated donors. *Transfusion* 32:180, 1992.

97. Kernan NA, Bartsch G, Ash RC, et al.: Analysis of 462 transplantations from unrelated donors facilitated by the National Marrow Donor Program. *N Engl J Med* 328:593, 1993.

98. Stroncek DF, Confer DL, Leitman SF: Peripheral blood progenitor cells for HPC transplants involving unrelated donors. *Transfusion* 40:731, 2000.

99. Rubinstein P, Carrier C, Scaradavou A, et al.: Outcomes among 562 recipients of placental-blood transplants from unrelated donors. *N Engl J Med* 339:1565, 1998.

100. Gluckman E, Rocha V, Boyer-Chammard A, et al.: Outcome of cord-blood transplantation from related and unrelated donors. Eurocord Transplant Group and the European Blood and Marrow Transplantation Group. *N Engl J Med* 337:373, 1997.

101. Barker JN, Wagner JE: Umbilical cord blood transplantation: current practice and future innovations. *Crit Rev Oncol Hematol* 48:35, 2003.

102. Rocha V, Cornish J, Sievers EL, et al.: Comparison of outcomes of unrelated bone marrow and umbilical cord blood transplants in children with acute leukemia. *Blood* 97:2962, 2001.

103. Rubinstein P, Stevens CE: Placental blood for bone marrow replacement: the New York Blood Center's program and clinical results. *Baillieres Best Pract Res Clin Haematol* 13:565, 2000.

104. Sasazuki T, Juji T, Morishima Y, et al.: Effect of matching of class I HLA alleles on clinical outcome after transplantation of hematopoietic stem cells from an unrelated donor. Japan Marrow Donor Program. *N Engl J Med* 339:1177, 1998.

105. Morishima Y, Sasazuki T, Inoko H, et al.: The clinical significance of human leukocyte antigen (HLA) allele compatibility in patients receiving a marrow transplant from serologically HLA-A, HLA-B, and HLA-DR matched unrelated donors. *Blood* 99:4200, 2002.

106. Flomenberg N, Baxter-Lowe LA, Confer D, et al.: Impact of HLA class I and class II high resolution matching on outcomes of unrelated donor bone marrow transplantation: HLA-C mismatching is associated with a strong adverse effect on transplant outcome. *Blood*, 104:1923, 2004.

107. Petersdorf EW, Gooley TA, Anasetti C, et al.: Optimizing outcome after unrelated marrow transplantation by comprehensive matching of HLA class I and II alleles in the donor and recipient. *Blood* 92:3515, 1998.

108. Tiercy JM, Passweg J, Van Biezen A, et al.: Isolated HLA-C mismatches in unrelated donor transplantation for CML. *Bone Marrow Transplant* 34:249, 2004.

109. Petersdorf EW, Longton GM, Anasetti C, et al.: Association of HLA-C disparity with graft failure after marrow transplantation from unrelated donors. *Blood* 89:1818, 1997.

110. Petersdorf EW, Anasetti C, Martin PJ, et al.: Limits of HLA mismatching in unrelated hematopoietic cell transplantation. *Blood* 104:2976, 2004.

111. El Kassar N, Legouvello S, Joseph CM, et al.: High resolution HLA class I and II typing and CTLp frequency in unrelated donor transplantation: a single-institution retrospective study of 69 BMTs. *Bone Marrow Transplant* 27:35, 2001.

112. Petersdorf EW, Longton GM, Anasetti C, et al.: The significance of HLA-DRB1 matching on clinical outcome after HLA-A, B, DR identical unrelated donor marrow transplantation. *Blood* 86:1606, 1995.

113. Petersdorf EW, Kollman C, Hurley CK, et al.: Effect of HLA class II gene disparity on clinical outcome in unrelated donor hematopoietic cell transplantation for chronic myeloid leukemia: the US National Marrow Donor Program Experience. *Blood* 98:2922, 2001.

114. Devergie A, Apperley JF, Labopin M, et al.: European results of matched unrelated donor bone marrow transplantation for chronic myeloid leukemia. Impact of HLA class II matching. Chronic Leukemia Working Party of the European Group for Blood and Marrow Transplantation. *Bone Marrow Transplant* 20:11, 1997.

115. Gajewski J, Gjertson D, Cecka M, et al.: The impact of T-cell depletion on the effects of HLA DR beta 1 and DQ beta allele matching in HLA serologically identical unrelated donor bone marrow transplantation. *Biol Blood Marrow Transplant* 3:76, 1997.

116. Petersdorf EW, Longton GM, Anasetti C, et al.: Definition of HLA-DQ as a transplantation antigen. *Proc Natl Acad Sci USA* 93:15358, 1996.

117. Schaffer M, Aldener-Cannava A, Remberger M, et al.: Roles of HLA-B, HLA-C and HLA-DPA1 incompatibilities in the outcome of unrelated stem-cell transplantation. *Tissue Antigens* 62:243, 2003.

118. Varney MD, Lester S, McCluskey J, et al.: Matching for HLA DPA1 and DPB1 alleles in unrelated bone marrow transplantation. *Hum Immunol* 60:532, 1999.

119. Loiseau P, Esperou H, Busson M, et al.: DPB1 disparities contribute to severe GVHD and reduced patient survival after unrelated donor bone marrow transplantation. *Bone Marrow Transplant* 30:497, 2002.

120. Shaw BE, Potter MN, Mayor NP, et al.: The degree of matching at HLA-DPB1 predicts for acute graft-versus-host disease and disease relapse following haematopoietic stem cell transplantation. *Bone Marrow Transplant* 31:1001, 2003.

121. Petersdorf EW, Gooley T, Malkki M, et al.: The biological significance of HLA-DP gene variation in haematopoietic cell transplantation. *Br J Haematol* 112: 988, 2001.

122. Petersdorf EW, Smith AG, Mickelson EM, et al.: The role of HLA-DPB1 disparity in the development of acute graft-versus-host disease following unrelated donor marrow transplantation. *Blood* 81:1923, 1993.

123. Nagler A, Brautbar C, Slavin S, et al.: Bone marrow transplantation using unrelated and family related donors: the impact of HLA-C disparity. *Bone Marrow Transplant* 18:891, 1996.

124. Ottenhoff TH, Elferink DG, Termijtelen A, et al.: HLA class II restriction repertoire of antigen-specific T cells. II: Evidence for a new restriction determinant associated with DRw52 and LB-Q1. *Hum Immunol* 13:117, 1985.

125. Berle EJ Jr, Thorsby E: Both DR and MT class II HLA molecules may restrict proliferative T-lymphocyte responses to antigen. *Scand J Immunol* 16:543, 1982.

126. Beatty PG, Anasetti C, Hansen JA, et al.: Marrow transplantation from unrelated donors for treatment of hematologic malignancies: effect of mismatching for one HLA locus. *Blood* 81:249, 1993.

127. Davies SM, Shu XO, Blazar BR, et al.: Unrelated donor bone marrow transplantation: influence of HLA A and B incompatibility on outcome. *Blood* 86:1636, 1995.

128. Tiercy JM, Morel C, Freidel AC, et al.: Selection of unrelated donors for bone marrow transplantation is improved by HLA class II genotyping with oligonucleotide hybridization. *Proc Natl Acad Sci USA* 88:7121, 1991.

129. Speiser DE, Tiercy JM, Rufer N, et al.: High resolution HLA matching associated with decreased mortality after unrelated bone marrow transplantation. *Blood* 87:4455, 1996.

130. Kolb HJ, Schmid C, Barrett AJ, et al.: Graft-versus-leukemia reactions in allogeneic chimeras. *Blood* 103:767, 2004.

131. Ferrara GB, Bacigalupo A, Lamparelli T, et al.: Bone marrow transplantation from unrelated donors: the impact of mismatches with substitutions at position 116 of the human leukocyte antigen class I heavy chain. *Blood* 98:3150, 2001.

132. Elsner HA, Blasczyk R: Sequence similarity matching: proposal of a structure-based rating system for bone marrow transplantation. *Eur J Immunogenet* 29:229, 2002.

133. Shaw BE, Barber LD, Madrigal JA, et al.: Scoring for HLA matching? A clinical test of HistoCheck. *Bone Marrow Transplant* 34:367, 2004.

134. Hurley CK, Fernandez Vina M, Setterholm M: Maximizing optimal hematopoietic stem cell donor selection from registries of unrelated adult volunteers. *Tissue Antigens* 61:415, 2003.

135. Kollman C, Abella E, Baitty RL, et al.: Assessment of optimal size and composition of the U.S. national registry of hematopoietic stem cell donors. *Transplantation* 78:89, 2004.

136. Karanes C: Unrelated donor stem cell transplant: donor selection and search process. *Pediatr Transplant* 7(suppl 3): 59, 2003.

137. Karanes C, Confer D, Walker T, et al.: Unrelated donor stem cell transplantation: the role of the National Marrow Donor Program. *Oncology* 17:1036, 2003.

138. Tiercy JM, Villard J, Roosnek E: Selection of unrelated bone marrow donors by serology, molecular typing and cellular assays. *Transpl Immunol* 10:215, 2002.

139. Tiercy J, Bujan-Lose M, Chapuis B, et al.: Bone marrow transplantation with unrelated donors: what is the probability of identifying an HLA-A/B/Cw/DRB1/B3/B5/DQB1-matched donor? *Bone Marrow Transplant* 26:437, 2000.

140. Zachary AA, Bias WB, Johnson A, et al.: Antigen, allele, and haplotype frequencies report of the ASHI minority antigens workshops: part 1, African–Americans. *Hum Immunol* 62:1127, 2001.

141. Noreen HJ, Yu N, Setterholm M, et al.: Validation of DNA-based HLA-A and HLA-B testing of volunteers for a bone marrow registry through parallel testing with serology. *Tissue Antigens* 57:221, 2001.

# Chapter 94

# STEM CELL MOBILIZATION

## Auayporn Nademanee

Hematopoietic progenitors cells (HPC) were first demonstrated in human peripheral blood (PB) in 1971.[1] In normal individuals small amounts of peripheral blood stem cells (PBSC) are present in the PB during steady state hematopoiesis and many aphereses are required to obtain adequate PBSC for transplant. In the mid 1980s, autologous PBSC transplantations (PBSCT) were performed successfully as an alternative to bone marrow transplantation (BMT) in patients with malignant lymphoma, breast cancer, and acute leukemia.[2–4] These studies showed that hematopoietic engraftment can be achieved with stem cells collected from the circulating blood rather than from the bone marrow (BM) and hematopoietic reconstitution using stem cells collected during steady-state was similar to BM. However, while most patients experienced a complete and stable hematopoietic reconstitution, some patients had slow platelet recovery or experienced a subsequent fall in PB count with nonmobilized PBSCT. This raises some concerns about the ability of circulating stem cells collected during steady state to sustain life-long hematopoiesis. Some investigators added PBSC to autologous BM grafts in an attempt to shorten the duration of neutropenia and enhance hematopoietic recovery. However, only the addition of PBSC collected after prior myelosuppressive therapy,[5] not during the steady state,[6] were found to accelerate hematopoietic recovery and prompt engraftment.

Blood progenitor cell mobilization in humans was initially noted during recovery from myelosuppressive chemotherapy.[7] The advances in knowledge in stem cell biology, the availability of hematopoietic growth factors, the availability of large-scale, continuous-flow leukopheresis, and an improved technique for progenitor cells assay, have increased the use of mobilized PBSC for transplantation. PBSC have several advantages when compared to BM grafts, including the fact that it is an outpatient procedure and no general anesthesia is required. In addition, results from randomized studies have shown that the hematopoietic recovery following myeloablative therapy was much more rapid with mobilized PBSC autografts than with BM autografts followed by growth factor.[8] This has lead to the widespread use of mobilized PBSC in all autologous transplant settings and in many allogeneic transplant settings.

## MECHANISM OF STEM CELL MOBILIZATION

Despite the success of PBSCT, the exact mechanism involved in PBSC mobilization and homing is not well understood. There is evidence that cytotoxic agents disrupt normal marrow endothelial cell barriers and thus facilitate homing and release of hematopoietic stem cells (HSC). A number of different cytokines are also known to up- or downregulate specific adhesion molecules on both progenitor cells and endothelium and may mediate both the binding and release of HSC and progenitor cells.

A significant number of studies in the past few years have revealed insights into regulation of HSC release, migration, and homing as well as the mechanism of different mobilization pathways. Under steady-state conditions, most of the stem cells are maintained in the $G_0$ phase of the cell cycle by interaction with stromal cells in the BM, while there is only a small proportion of stem cells in the S or $G_2/M$ phase of the cell cycle. Adhesive interaction between the $CD34^+$ hematopoietic stem cell with cellular and matrix components of the BM environment are involved in stem cell mobilization.[9] Primitive HSC express a wide range of cell adhesion molecules (CAM), including members of the integrin, selectin, immunoglobulin superfamily, and CD 44 families of adhesion molecules. The mobilization process is initiated by stress-induced activation of neutrophils and osteoclasts by chemotherapy and repeated stimulation with cytokines, resulting in shedding and release of membrane-bound stem cell factor (SCF), proliferation of progenitor cells, as well as activation and/or degradation of adhesion molecules such as very late antigen (VLA-4) and L-selectin. Recent studies suggest the interaction between CXCR4 and its ligand stromal-derived factor-1 (SDF-1) plays a key role in stem cell mobilization.[10] Active signaling through SDF-1/CXCR4 and upregulation of adhesion molecules are required for homing, whereas downregulation of adhesion molecules and

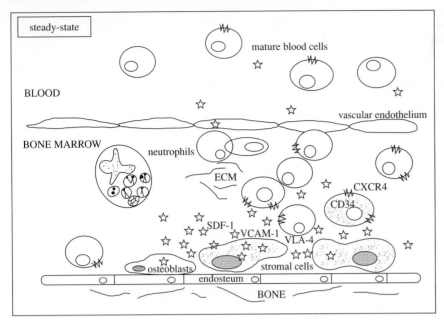

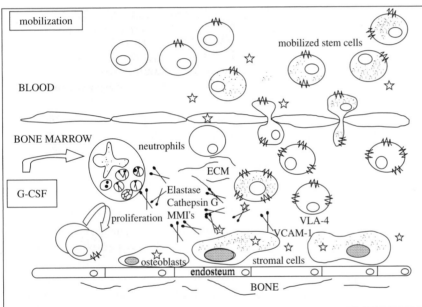

**Figure 94.1** *A model for stem cell mobilization by G-CSF. In steady state (upper panel), stem cells are localized in close proximity to stromal cells. Retention is mediated by adhesion molecules such as VCAM-1/VLA-4 and through SDF-1/CXCR4 interactions. During mobilization (lower panel), G-CSF induces both cell proliferation and release of neutrophil proteases (elastase, cathepsin G, and MMPs), which participate in cell egress by degrading retention signals (VCAM-1 and SDF-1) and by remodeling the extracellular matrix. Upregulation of CXCR-4 on BM cells during G-CSF-induced mobilization suggests active participation of SDF-1/CXCR4 interactions in the migration of cells toward the blood. (From Lapidot and Petit[10], used with Permission.)*

disruption of SDF-1/CXCR4 signaling are required for mobilization of HSC. Lapidot and Petit have recently suggested a model wherein granulocyte colony-stimulating factor (G-CSF) stimulation induces proteases such as neutrophil elastase and other matrix metalloproteases that markedly reduce local BM of SDF-1, resulting in the egress of HSC and progenitor cells from BM into PB.[10] Mobilized CD34+ cells have lower levels of VLA-4, c-kit expression, and CXCR4 expression compared with steady-state BM and PB. The release of CD34+ cells from the marrow is contingent upon an extensive decrease in L-selectin and moderate decrease in VLA-4 expression on CD34+ cells, and therefore, VLA-4 might have a role in facilitation of extravasation and release of CD34+ cells from the marrow into blood stream. The reduced c-kit expression before the egress of HSC in the circulation is inversely correlated with stem cell yield. The activation

of the metalloproteinase (MMP)-9 leading to the release of c-kit-L is a decisive checkpoint for the mobilization of HSC as it promotes the recruitment of stem cells into PB. The proposed mechanism of stem cell mobilization is shown in Figure 94.1.

## PARAMETERS USED FOR MEASUREMENT OF PBSC

HSC are clonogenic cells capable of self-renewal and multilineage differentiation. Progenitor cells are oligolineage cells that are already more restricted in their differentiation potential and are not able to self-renew. The expression of the antigen CD34 and lineage negativity are often used as surrogate markers for HSC and progenitor cells. The percentage of CD34+ cells in PB under steady-state conditions is about 0.06% and about 1.1% in BM.[11]

Other parameters used to measure the quantity of PBSC include nucleated and mononuclear cell number (MNC) and colony-forming unit granulocyte-macrophage (CFU-GM). Several studies have shown that the number of MNC count correlates poorly with engraftment kinetics, thus it is no longer used for PBSC enumeration. Both the CFU-GM and CD34+ assays are the two most commonly used indicators which have been shown to predict the time to engraftment. Numerous studies have shown a relationship between the dose of CD34+ cells, the concentration of CFU-GM, and the time to engraftment.[12,13] However, CFU-GM assays require significant laboratory skill, and methodology in different laboratories varies greatly. Therefore, quantifying CD34+ cells by flow cytometry is now the method of choice for determining graft adequacy. Moreover, the CD34+ cell count has been shown to be a good predictor for engraftment kinetics, especially for platelets.

## METHODS OF STEM CELL MOBILIZATION

### MYELOSUPPRESSIVE CHEMOTHERAPY

Several methods to mobilize PBSC from an extra vascular location into circulation have been described. Myelosuppressive chemotherapy was the first method described for stem cell mobilization.[14] During the recovery phase after myelosuppressive chemotherapy, there was a 14- to 100-fold increase in peripheral blood CFU-GM above the baseline. The extent of this increase is proportional to the severity and duration of the cytopenia. High-dose cyclophosphamide (CY) is the most commonly used regimen since it is active against most tumors. However, there are several disadvantages to chemotherapy mobilization, including the length of time required, toxicity, neutropenic fever and/or sepsis, bleeding diathesis, and the unpredictable timing of apheresis. In addition, little or no increase in peripheral blood CFU-GM was observed in some patients who had received extensive prior therapy and patients with marrow involvement with tumor.[15] With the introduction of hematopoietic growth factors, it is no longer acceptable to use myelosuppressive chemotherapy alone for stem cell mobilization.

### HEMATOPOIETIC GROWTH FACTORS ALONE

Several hematopoietic growth factors have been used to mobilize PBSC including G-CSF, granulocyte macrophage colony-stimulating factor (GM-CSF), interleukin-3 (IL-3), and SCF. Currently, G-CSF is the most commonly used agent to mobilize PBSC because of its potency and lack of serious toxicity. There are several common features observed during mobilization with hematopoietic growth factors.[16] First, mobilization kinetics are similar, with peak levels of circulating HPCs generally achieved after 5–10 days of growth factor.

Second, a broad spectrum of HPCs is mobilized, including pluripotential, and committed myeloid, megakaryocytic, and erythroid progenitors. Third, the increase in circulating HPCs is associated with decreased numbers of HPCs in BM. And finally, mobilized HPCs have characteristic phenotypic features distinct from those of HPCs that reside in the BM under steady-state conditions. Relative to BM, a higher percentage of mobilized PBSC are in the $G_0$ or $G_1$ phase of cell cycle, and the expression of VLA-4 and c-kit on their surfaces is reduced. A recent study showed that HPCs are selectively mobilized after the M phase of cell cycle thus providing a potential explanation for preponderance of HPCs in the $G_0$ or $G_1$ phase of the cell cycle in blood.

The mechanism by which growth factors mobilize PBSC is not clearly understood. Recent animal studies have provided some insight into stem cell trafficking in the BM and the role of adhesion molecules in HPC mobilization.[16–18] The model of HPC mobilization by G-CSF is shown in Figure 94.2.

### G-CSF

G-CSF stimulates neutrophil granulopoiesis in a dose-dependent manner. The level of PB progenitor cells

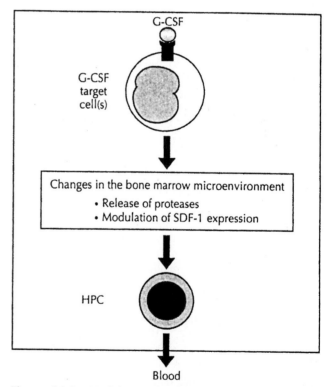

**Figure 94.2** *Model of hematopoietic progenitor cell mobilization by granulocyte colony-stimulating factor. In this model, G-CSF-induced HPC mobilization occurs in two steps. In the first step, G-CSF activates a target cell population (as yet undefined). The second step is the generation of secondary signals by these activated cells, leading in turn to HPC mobilization. Potential secondary signals include protease release by activated cells and the modulation of stromal-derived factor-1 (SDF-1) expression in the BM. (From Thomas et al.[16], used with permission.)*

increase from 40- to 80-fold after 4–5 days of G-CSF and returns to baseline value within 4–6 days after cessation of G-CSF. Sheridan et al.[19] were the first to report that hematopoietic reconstitution can be accomplished after G-CSF-mobilized PBSC following high-dose chemotherapy. The time to platelet and RBC transfusion independence was shorter with G-CSF-mobilized PBSC. Chao et al.[20] reported the results of hematopoietic recovery in 85 patients with Hodgkin's disease who received autologous PBSCT using PBSC collected during steady-state or G-CSF-mobilized PBSC, with or without BM. The use of G-CSF-mobilized PBSC resulted in a significantly accelerated time to recovery of granulocytes (10 days vs 12 days; $P < 0.01$) and platelet engraftment (13 days vs 30 days; $P < 0.001$).

Two randomized studies have also shown the benefits of G-CSF-mobilized PBSC compared to autologous BM after high-dose therapy. Fifty-eight patients with heavily pretreated Hodgkin's and non-Hodgkin's lymphoma (NHL) were randomized to receive either G-CSF-mobilized PBSC or autologous BM.[21] All patients received G-CSF after transplant. Patients who received G-CSF-mobilized PBSC had faster engraftment of both absolute neutrophit count (ANC) $> 0.5 \times 10^9$/L (11 days vs 14 days; $P = 0.005$) and platelet recovery more or equal to $20 \times 10^9$/L (16 days vs 23 days; $P = 0.02$). Similar results were reported by Hartman et al.[8] in a larger randomized study of 129 patients with solid tumor and lymphomas. In addition, a cost analysis showed that the total cost was decreased by 17% in adults and 29% in children receiving PBSC transplantation.

The doses of G-CSF used for mobilization are also important and several studies have shown that using higher doses of G-CSF results in a higher number of CD34+, or CFU-GM yield and a lesser number of collections. Nademanee et al.[22] showed a dose-response effect for G-CSF, with a sevenfold increase in the number of CD34+ cells in the PB over the baseline value for 5 μg/kg perday and 28 times for 10 μg/kg per day. Similarly, there were 10- and 17-fold increases in CFU-GM over baseline for 5μg/kg per day and 10 μg/kg per day of G-CSF, respectively. Weaver et al.[23] conducted randomized studies to evaluate different doses of G-CSF, 10, 20, 30, or 40 μg/kg per day on yields of CD 34+cells in patients with breast cancer. The median number of CD34+ cells collected after 10 μg/kg per day was $0.7 \times 10^6$/kg per apheresis (range 0.1–4.4) as compared to 1.2 (range 0.1–6.8) after 30 μg/kg per day ($P = 0.04$). Patients receiving 10 μg/kg had lower yields of CD34+ cells and had a 3.3-fold increase in the probability of not achieving more or equal to $5.0 \times 10^6$ CD34+ cells per kg as compared to patients receiving 20–40 μg/kg. These data suggest that doses of G-CSF $> 10$ μg/kg per day mobilize more CD34+ cells and may be useful when high numbers of CD34+ cells are desired.

### GM-CSF

GM-CSF is a multilineage CSF because it stimulates the proliferation and differentiation of HPCs into neutrophil, eosinophil, and monocyte colonies. GM-CSF functions in conjunction with other cytokines, erythropoietin and IL-3, to promote the proliferation and differentiation of erythroid and megakaryocytic progenitors, respectively. Administration of GM-CSF not only increases the number of monocytes but also increases the function of monocytes and macrophages including oxidative metabolism, cytotoxicity, and Fc-dependent phagocytosis. GM-CSF enhances dendritic cell maturation, proliferation, and migration.[24] The ability of GM-CSF to mobilize PBSC was first reported by Socinski et al.[25] in 13 patients with sarcoma. After 4–7 days of GM-CSF at doses of 4–64 μg/kg per day by continuous infusion, they found an 18-fold increase in peripheral blood CFU-GM and an eightfold increase in erythroid burst-colony forming units (BFU-E). Haas et al.[26] observed an 8.5-fold increase in the number of circulating CFU-GM using a continuous infusion of GM-CSF at 250 μg/m² per day. A total of six aphereses were performed and the median number of MNC and CFU-GM collected was $36 \times 10^9$ and $209 \times 10^4$, respectively.

The efficacy of GM-CSF for stem cell mobilization has been compared with G-CSF in both normal donors and in cancer patients. Peters et al.[27] suggested that GM-CSF is less efficacious than G-CSF in mobilization and found that the total numbers of CD 34+, CD 33+, and CD7+ cells collected per kg were higher in G-CSF mobilization than with GM-CSF. Weisdorf et al.[28] found no significant advantage for either drug as mobilizing agents for PBSC used for autologous transplant in lymphoma patients. Lane et al.[29] evaluated the PBSC mobilization efficacy of G-CSF at 10 μg/kg per day ($n = 8$), GM-CSF 10 μg/kg per day ($n = 5$), or GM plus G-CSF each at 5 μg/kg per day ($n = 5$) in normal donors. The median CD34+ cell yield with the combination regimen and with G-CSF was significantly higher than with GM-CSF alone. It is widely accepted that as a single agent, G-CSF mobilizes more CD34+ cells than does GM-CSF.

### G-CSF/GM-CSF

Since the two growth factors mobilize different cells, concurrent or sequential administration of these growth factors may be synergistic. Spitzer et al.[30] conducted a randomized study comparing G-CSF plus GM-CSF each at 5 μg/kg per day with G-CSF 10 μg/kg per day for stem cell mobilization in 50 patients with lymphoma and solid tumors. There were no statistically significant differences in either the CD34+ cell yield or the rate of hematopoietic recovery between the two groups. Winter et al.[31] conducted a phase I/II study of combined G-CSF and GM-CSF either sequential, G-CSF followed by GM-CSF or GM-CSF followed by G-CSF, or concurrent G-CSF/GM-CSF for mobilization of PBSC. The administration of G-CSF to patients already receiving GM-CSF results in 80-fold increase in HPC over the baseline; however, the addition of GM-CSF to G-CSF was less effective.

## G-CSF/SCF

SCF is an early acting hematopoietic factor that displays pronounced synergies with other hematopoietic growth factors such as GM-CSF, G-CSF, erythropoietin, IL-3, and IL-6 to stimulate proliferation of erythroid, megakaryocytic, granulocytic, and mast and basophil progenitor cells. The SCF receptor (c-*kit*) is present on many tissues of neuroectodermal, epithelial, and hematopoietic origin.

In patients with stage II/III breast cancer with no previous chemotherapy, Glaspy et al.[32] showed that the leukapheresis yield was 70% higher for those receiving SCF 10 μg/kg perday concomitantly with G-CSF than those receiving G-CSF alone. The combination of SCF+G-CSF has also been shown to be effective in patients with breast cancer with previous chemotherapy and those with heavily pretreated lymphoma. Moskowitz et al.[33] conducted a phase I/II randomized trial of SCF (5, 10, 15, or 20 μg/kg per day) plus G-CSF 10 μg/kg per day, or G-CSF 10 μg/kg per day alone to mobilize PBSC in NHL patients. The combination of SCF+G-CSF was better than G-CSF alone for patients who had received extensive prior therapy. Similar results were reported by Stiff et al.[34] in another randomized study using SCF 20 μg/kg per day plus G-CSF 10 μg/kg per day versus G-CSF 10 μg/kg per day in 102 heavily pretreated patients with Hodgkin's disease and NHL. Compared with the G-CSF alone group, the SCF+G-CSF group showed an increase in the proportion of patients reaching the target yield within five leukaphereses (44% vs 17%; $P = 0.002$): reduction in the number of leukaphereses required to reach the target yield, increase in the median yield of CD34$^+$ cells per leukapheresis ($0.73 \times 10^6$/kg vs $0.48 \times 10^6$/kg; $P = 0.04$), and an increase in the median total CD34$^+$ cells collected within five leukaphereses ($3.6 \times 10^6$/kg vs $2.4 \times 10^6$/kg; $P = 0.05$). These results suggest that SCF plus G-CSF was more effective than G-CSF alone for mobilizing PBSC in heavily pretreated patients. However, SCF administration can be associated with anaphylactic reactions due to mast cell-mediated reactions. Therefore, premedication with ranitidine, albuterol, and either diphenhydramine or cetirizine are required. Due to the high incidence of allergic reactions and the need for observation after administration SCF is difficult to use in standard clinical practice. SCF is not commercially available in the United States.

### G-CSF/recombinant human thrombopoietin

Thrombopoietin (TPO) is a naturally occurring glycosylated peptide growth factor and the primary regulator of megakaryocytopoiesis. In preclinical models, TPO has been shown to accelerate the reconstitution of BM CD34$^+$ cells and to increase the number of circulating PB progenitor cells after a mid-lethal dose of total body irradiation. TPO has also been shown to enhance proliferation of early progenitor cells committed to the erythroid and myelomonocytic lineage. Results from phase I studies of recombinant human TPO (rhTPO) in the myelosuppressive and myeloablative settings indicate that rhTPO, alone and combined with chemotherapy and G-CSF, increases the number of progenitor and CD34$^+$ cells in the PB.[35] Linker et al.[36] conducted a randomized, double-blind, multicenter trial in 134 patients to evaluate the efficacy of rhTPO for mobilization and reconstitution after high-dose chemotherapy and PBSCT. For the mobilization phase, patients received study drug at a dose of 0.5 μg/kg, or 15 μg/kg, or placebo given intravenously on days 1, 3. and 5 before initiation of G-CSF 10μg/kg per day on day 5 and leukapheresis starting on day 9. After high-dose chemotherapy and PBSCT, patients were randomly assigned to receive rhTPO 1.5 μg/kg on day 0, +2, +4, and +6 with either G-CSF 5 μg/kg per day or GM-CSF 250μg/m$^2$ per day, or placebo plus G-CSF 5 μg/kg per day. Administration of rhTPO followed by G-CSF produced a nearly twofold increase in median CD34$^+$ cell dose per leukapheresis with a higher CD34$^+$ cell yield when rhTPO started before day 5. Comparing rhTPO to placebo, a higher percentage of patients achieved the minimum yield of CD34$^+$ cell more or equal to $2 \times 10^6$/kg (92% vs 75%; $P = 0.050$) as well as the target yield of more or equal to $5 \times 10^6$ CD34$^+$/kg (79% vs 46%; $P = 0.011$). rhTPO also significantly reduced the median number of aphereses required to achieve both a minimum graft (one rhTPO vs two placebo) and a target graft (two rhTPO vs four placebo). However, rhTPO given after transplantation did not enhance platelet recovery. None of the patients developed neutralizing antibodies that cross-react with endogenous TPO. These results suggest that rhTPO is safe and effective in enhancing mobilization and increasing leukapheresis efficiency.

### CHEMOTHERAPY PLUS GROWTH FACTORS FOR STEM CELL MOBILIZATION

Although chemotherapy alone can produce increases in progenitors in PB, multiple phase II studies have shown that the addition of growth factors such as G-CSF and GM-CSF to myelosuppressive chemotherapy enhances mobilization and allows for more progenitors to be collected with fewer apheresis procedures while reducing myelotoxicity. Siena et al.[37] reported that after high-dose CY, an approximately 30-fold expansion of CFU-GM numbers was observed. This increase was further magnified, to over 100 times control values, when GM-CSF was given to accelerate post-CY hematopoietic recovery. These precursors were both increased in number and enriched in the more immature forms. In addition, there was an increase of the most immature CD34$^+$/CD33$^-$ progenitors to multipotent and unipotent colony-forming cells (CD34$^+$/CD33$^+$) in PB. In a randomized cross-over trial reported by Koc et al.,[38] high-dose CY plus G-CSF results in mobilization of more progenitors than GM-CSF plus G-CSF when tested in the same patient regardless of whether CY+GCSF was given as the first or second mobilizing strategy.

The magnitude of the increase in circulating stem cells is related to the intensity of myelosuppressive chemotherapy used. Cyclophosphamide at doses of 1.5, 4, or 7 g/m$^2$ and G-CSF or GM-CSF are effective in mobilizing PBSC; however higher stem-cell yields were obtained with higher doses of CY (7 g/m$^2$).[39] When G-CSF was administered from the day after CY, white blood cell (WBC) decreased reaching a nadir around day 7 or 8 followed by an abrupt increase in WBC and PB CD34$^+$ cell counts. Peak circulating CD34$^+$ cells and progenitors were seen on approximately day 9 or 10. PBSC collection usually begins on day 10 or when WBC > 1 × 10$^9$/L.

While high-dose CY followed by GM-CSF or G-CSF is the most frequently chemotherapy/growth factor mobilization regimen, it has several limitations, including potential cardiotoxicity, hemorrhagic cystitis, nausea, and vomiting. Several investigators have reported the effectiveness of high-dose etoposide (2 g/m$^2$) with GM-CSF or G-CSF as a mobilizing strategy.[40] It is associated with minimal nonhematologic toxicity and has antitumor activity. Several other combination chemotherapy regimens are also effective for stem cell mobilization. Studies suggest that the combination of CY + etoposide, or CY + Taxol or CY+ etoposide + cisplatin are more effective than CY alone.

The dose and type of growth factor utilized with chemotherapy may also be important. Although GM-CSF was the first cytokine to enhance PBSC mobilization by chemotherapy, it is now less commonly used than G-CSF, probably because of side effects such as fever and hypoxemia. The dose of G-CSF used with chemotherapy is lower than when used alone for stem cell mobilization (10–24 μg/kg per day). A higher dose of G-CSF 16 μg/kg per day rather than a lower dose of 8 μg/kg per day was more effective in patients with a variety of malignancies. In a randomized trial reported by Weaver et al.,[41] G-CSF or GM-CSF followed by G-CSF after mobilizing chemotherapy was more effective in patients with solid tumors and hematologic malignancies than GM-CSF. In contrast, for patients with NHL, GM-CSF followed by G-CSF permitted more efficient collection of a target number of CD34$^+$ cells than did GM-CSF, while G-CSF was the least efficient of the three cytokine strategies.

It is difficult to conclude which combination of chemotherapy and growth factor is the optimal regimen given the heterogeneity of patient population, the different mobilizing chemotherapy regimens, and the different cytokines used. Moreover, there is no difference in time to recovery of neutrophils and platelets among patients transplanted with PBSC mobilized by different techniques as long as a minimum number of CD34$^+$ cells/kg is given. In general, chemotherapeutic agents that are effective for underlying malignancies should be used for pretransplant cytoreduction as well as PBSC mobilization.[42] Agents that are known to damage stem cells such as melphalan should be avoided.

## NEW STRATEGY FOR PBSC MOBILIZATION

### AMD 3100

AMD 3100 is a selective antagonist of the chemokine receptor CXCR4, which is present on WBCs. AMD 3100 also reversibly blocks the binding of CXCR4 with SDF-1. In a phase I study, it was noted that AMD 3100 induced leucocytosis. Broxmeyer et al. demonstrated a 40-fold increase in the mobilization of hematopoietic progenitors within 1 h of AMD 3100 injection in mice.[43] Results from a phase-I study in 10 healthy volunteers[44] and 13 patients with multiple myeloma or NHL[45] demonstrated that AMD 3100 rapidly mobilized PBSC. The absolute CD34$^+$ cell count increased from 2.6/μL to 15.6/μL, and 16.2/μL at 4 h and 6 h, respectively, after AMD 3100 administration. Recent studies confirm that AMD 3100 and G-CSF are synergistic. Injection of AMD 3100 given on the fifth day of G-CSF resulted in a striking 50-fold increase in the number of circulating CD34$^+$ cells. In addition, PBSC mobilized by AMD 3100 have a higher repopulation potential in human-mouse xenografts than G-CSF-mobilized PBSC. Liles et al.[46] recently demonstrated that a 240 μg/kg injection of AMD 3100 followed the same day of a single large volume leukapheresis yielded a mean of 3.1 × 10$^6$ CD34$^+$ cells/kg. Based on these results, AMD 3100 may not only be effective for the rapid mobilization of CD34$^+$ cells in patients who have received chemotherapy, but also for mobilization of normal volunteer donors.

## OPTIMAL TIME FOR PBSC COLLECTION

The timing of PBSC collection is important in order to maximize the number of progenitors harvested. Using growth factor alone for mobilization, apheresis is usually performed on days 5, 6, and 7 of G-CSF administration. Progenitor cell levels start to decrease after day 8 even with continuation of G-CSF. Following chemotherapy mobilization, it is recommended to start PBSC collection at 12–14 days after chemotherapy when WBC >1 × 10$^9$/L.[47] For chemotherapy + growth factor mobilization, apheresis usually starts when the WBC reaches 2–5 × 10$^9$/L. However, some studies suggest that a delay in PBSC collection until WBC >10 × 10$^9$/L may be more optimal. A strong linear relationship between the number of CFU-GM and CD34$^+$ cells in both the leukaphresis product and PB on the day of collection has been well established. Several studies have shown that the number of circulating CD34$^+$ cells predicts the extent of PBSC collection and may be used to anticipate or delay leukapheresis, as well as to shorten or extend the duration of procedure. At present CD34$^+$cells measurement is preferable since it is a more direct measurement of progenitor cells, and it should be used to guide stem cell collection.[48]

## TARGET AND THRESHOLD

In most studies, $20 \times 10^4$ CFU-GM/kg or $2 \times 10^6$ CD34$^+$ cells/kg is generally accepted as the minimum threshold below which rapid hematopoietic reconstitution may not occur. In a study reported by Bensinger et al.,[49] patients receiving more than $2.5 \times 10^6$ CD34$^+$cells/kg had more rapid neutrophil and platelet recovery than patients who received less than that. However, comparing patients who received more than $5 \times 10^6$ CD34$^+$ cells/kg to those receiving $2.5–5 \times 10^6$ CD34$^+$ cells/kg, there was no difference in neutrophil engraftment but there was more rapid recovery of platelets. They also found that very high level of CD34$^+$ cells ($>10 \times 10^6$ CD34$^+$ cells/kg) did not result in a significant faster recovery of either neutrophils or platelets. Kiss et al.[50] showed that patients who received more or equal to $5 \times 10^6$ CD34$^+$ cells/kg were found to have statistically significantly faster neutrophil recovery (median 10 days vs 11 days; $P = 0.002$) and platelet recovery (median 9 days vs 21 days; $P = 0.004$) than those receiving less than that. Based on these studies, a minimum cell dose of $2.5 \times 10^6$ CD34$^+$ cells/kg may be sufficient to ensure rapid recovery of neutrophils and platelet; the optimal transplant cell dose of $5 \times 10^6$ CD34$^+$ cells/kg is recommended.

Previous chemotherapy is also an important factor in determining a threshold of CD34$^+$ cells for rapid engraftment. Tricot et al.[51] analyzed 225 patients receiving autologous PBSC transplants for multiple myeloma and found that the minimum CD34$^+$ cell threshold was more or equal to $2 \times 10^6$ cells/kg for patients receiving less than 6 months of melphalan, but more than $5 \times 10^6$ CD34$^+$ cells/kg were required for patients who received more than 12 months of melphalan.

## FACTORS AFFECTING PBSC COLLECTION

Several factors have been shown to be significant determinants of progenitor cell yield including the amount of previous chemotherapy, the number of cycles, the degree of BM involvement, previous wide-field radiation, the interval between previous chemotherapy and mobilization, and exposure to stem cell toxic drugs.[52,53] These factors are indicators of hematopoietic reserve. Haas et al.[54] found that previous cytotoxic chemotherapy and radiotherapy adversely affected the yield of CD34$^+$ cells with each cycle of chemotherapy associated with an average decrease of $0.2 \times 10^6$ CD34$^+$ cells/kg per apheresis in nonirradiated patients, and large field radiotherapy reduced the collection yields by an average of $1.8 \times 10^6$ CD34$^+$ cells/kg. Glaspy et al.[32] reported that frequency of previous chemotherapy, even with regimens that are not considered stem cell toxin, can decrease the number of CD34$^+$ cells harvested in patients with breast cancer. Tricot et al.[51]

found a correlation between duration of exposure to previous chemotherapy, especially alkylating agents, and mobilization yield in patients with multiple myeloma. They reported that 91% of patients with exposure of less than 6 months reach more than $5 \times 10^6$ CD34$^+$ cells/kg as compared to only 28% of patients with exposure more than 24 months. Dreger et al.[55] reported that prior exposure to stem cell toxic agents such as Carmustine (BCNU) and melphalan was associated with poor stem cell yield. Fludarabine treatment was proven to be associated with poor PBSC mobilization[56] as well as other stem cell toxic agents such as nitrogen mustard, procarbazine, or more than 7.5 g of cytarabine chemotherapy.[57]

Some investigators found that measurement of BM CFU-GM and CD34$^+$ cells during steady-state can be used to predict for PBSC mobilization. Kotasek et al.[15] reported a higher premobilization BM CFU-GM level immediately before CY mobilization predicts for successful collection of CFU-GM. Other investigators have shown that a lower CD34$^+$ cell percentage ($<2.5\%$) of the BM products before PBSC mobilization predicts for suboptimal PBSC collection.[58] Low platelet counts on the first day of stem cell collection[59] and low numbers of circulating natural killer (CD3$^-$16$^+$56$^+$) cells[60] prior to administration of mobilization therapy have predicted for poor mobilization. Gazitt et al.[61] evaluated expression of adhesion molecules on CD34$^+$ cell in PB of NHL patients and found that good mobilizers had a relatively higher percentage of CD34$^+$ cells expressing the VLA-4 antigen.

## MOBILIZATION OF TUMOR CELLS AND ITS CLINICAL SIGNIFICANCE

Several studies have shown that tumor cells could be mobilized in PB after chemotherapy and G-CSF.[62] Circulating tumor cells may be present in patients with certain malignancies regardless of marrow involvement. The presence of these cells in circulation appears to correlate with disease activity and stage. The possibility of infusing cancer cells into patients at the time of PBSC transplant is known to occur in breast cancer, lymphoma, multiple myeloma (MM), and leukemia. However, the biologic significance of infusing PBSC contaminated with tumor cells remains uncertain. Gene-marking studies and retrospective clinical trials have demonstrated that contaminating tumor cells can contribute to disease recurrence after high-dose therapy and autologous PBSCT.[63] However, other investigators found no increase in the incidence of relapse following high-dose therapy and infusing of tumor contaminated PBSCs.[64] A 3 to 5-log reduction in malignant contamination in the PBSC can be achieved by CD34$^+$ cell selection.[65] However, phase III randomized study showed no improvement in disease-free and overall survival with CD34$^+$ cell selection.[66] In addition, delay at engraftment and an increase in the incidence of infectious complications have been reported following CD34[+] enriched transplant.

## MOBILIZATION OF ALLOGENEIC STEM CELLS

Despite the rapid engraftment and the reduction in transplant-related mortality with mobilized PBSC, there are some concerns about the increased risk of acute and chronic graft-versus-host-disease (GVHD) due to the higher numbers of T cells in mobilized PBSC products. Korbling et al.[67] compared the allograft content of G-CSF mobilized PBSC to cellular contents of BM harvest and showed that there was a three- to fourfold increase in CD34[+] cells and a 10- to 20-fold increase in the number of CD3[+] T cells in PBSC products compared to BM harvest. There have been several randomized trials comparing BM and PBSC in the allogeneic transplant setting, but the results were inconclusive.[68,69] However, most studies demonstrated a significant enhancement of neutrophil and platelet recovery with allogeneic PBSCT, but a survival benefit was observed only in patients with advanced hematologic malignancies. The risk of acute GVHD was not significantly increased with allogeneic PBSCT. However, a modest increase in chronic GVHD has been reported in several studies. A meta-analysis of 15 phase II and phase III trials assessing the risk of GVHD in allogeneic PBSC and BM demonstrated a modest increased relative risk of acute GVHD (relative risk 1.2) and a significant increased risk of chronic GVHD (relative risk 1.8) in recipients of allo-

geneic PBSCT.[70] In addition, there was a significant reduction in risk of relapse after PBSC allografts.

Similar to autologous PBSC studies, the numbers of mobilized CD34[+] cells correlate well with engraftment. Allogeneic PBSC recipients who received more than $5 \times 10^6$ CD34[+] cells/kg had a 95% chance of both neutrophil and platelet recovery by day +15.[71] However, infusion of allogeneic PBSC $> 8 \times 10^6$ CD34[+] cells/kg has been shown to result in poor survival presumably due to increased rates of chronic GVHD and its complications.

## CONCLUSIONS

Currently, mobilized PBSCs are the preferable and major source of stem cells harvested for autologous, and possibly, allogeneic transplantation because of the higher cell yield, faster hematopoietic and immune reconstitution, and decreased procedural risks compared with harvested BM cells. Measurement of PB CD34[+] cells before collection is necessary for efficient and cost-effective stem cell collection. PBSC collection should be performed early in the course of disease to avoid chemotherapy-induced stem cell damage and to reduce the risk of therapy-induced myelodysplasia. Different mobilization strategies are needed for patients who are at high risk for poor mobilization. Over the last decade, significant progress has been made in understanding the mechanisms of PBSC mobilization and stem cell homing. This has led to the development of new agents that are being tested in clinical trials, which will eventually lead to development of improved mobilization protocols especially for poor mobilizers.

## REFERENCES

1. McCredie KB, Hersh EM, Freireich EJ: Cells capable of colony formation in the peripheral blood in man. *Science* 171:293–294, 1971.
2. Juttner CA, To LB, Haylock DN, et al.: Peripheral blood stem cell selection, collection and auto-transplantation. *Prog Clin Biol Res* 333:447–460, 1990.
3. Kessinger A, Armitage JO, Landmark JD, Weisenburger DD: Reconstitution of human hematopoietic function with autologous cryopreserved circulating stem cells. *Exp Hematol* 14:192–196, 1986.
4. Korbling M, Dorken B, Ho AD, et al.: Autologous transplantation of blood-derived hemopoietic stem cells after myelablative therapy in a patient with Burkitt's lymphoma. *Blood* 67:529–532, 1986.
5. Gianni AM, Bregni M, Siena S, et al.: Rapid and complete hemopoietic reconstitution following combined transplantation of autologous blood and marrow cells. A changing role for high dose chemo-radiotherapy? *Hematol Oncol* 7:139–148, 1989.
6. Lobo F, Kessinger A, Landmark JD, et al.: Addition of peripheral blood stem cells collected without mobilization techniques to transplanted autologous bone marrow did not hasten marrow recovery following mye-

loablative therapy. *Bone Marrow Transplant* 8:389–392, 1991.
7. Richman CM, Weiner RS, Yankee RA: Increase in circulating stem cells following chemotherapy in man. *Blood* 47:1031–1039, 1976.
8. Hartmann O, Corroller AGL, Blaise D, et al.: Peripheral blood stem cell and bone marrow transplantation for solid tumors and lymphomas: hematologic recovery and costs: a randomized, controlled trial. *Ann Intern Med* 126:600–607, 1997.
9. Papayannopoulou T: Current mechanistic scenarios in hematopoietic stem/progenitor cell mobilization. *Blood* 103:1580–1585, 2004.
10. Lapidot T, Petit I: Current understanding of stem cell mobilization: the roles of chemokines, proteolytic enzymes, adhesion molecules, cytokines and stromal cells. *Exp Hematol* 30:973–981, 2002.
11. Fruehauf S, Haas R, Conradt C, et al.: Peripheral blood progenitor cell (PBPC) counts during steady-state hematopoiesis allow to estimate the yield of mobilized PBPC after filgrastim (R-metHuG-CSF)-supported cytotoxic chemotherapy. *Blood* 85:2619–2626, 1995. Comments.

12. Siena S, Bregni M, Brando B, et al.: Flow cytometry for clinical estimation of circulating hematopoietic progenitors for autologous transplantation in cancer patients. *Blood* 77:400–409, 1991.

13. To LB, Haylock DN, Simmons PJ, et al.: The Biology and clinical uses of blood stem cells. *Blood* 89:2233–2258, 1997.

14. To LB, Shepperd KM, Haylock DN, et al.: Single high doses of cyclophosphamide enable the collection of high numbers of hemopoietic stem cells from the peripheral blood. *Exp Hematol* 18:442–447, 1990.

15. Kotasek D, Shepherd KM, Sage RE, et al.: Factors affecting blood stem cell collections following high-dose cyclophosphamide mobilization in lymphoma, myeloma and solid tumors. *Bone Marrow Transplant* 9:11–17, 1992.

16. Thomas J, Liu F, Link DC: Mechanisms of mobilization of hematopoietic progenitors with granulocyte colony-stimulating factor. *Curr Opin Hematol* 9:183–189, 2002.

17. Link DC: Mechanisms of granulocyte colony-stimulating factor-induced hematopoietic progenitor-cell mobilization. *Semin Hematol* 37(suppl 2):25–32, 2000.

18. Gazitt Y: Comparison between granulocyte colony-stimulating factor and granulocyte-macrophage colony-stimulating factor in the mobilization of peripheral blood stem cells. *Curr Opin Hematol* 9:190–198, 2002.

19. Sheridan WP, Begley CG, Juttner CA, et al.: Effect of peripheral-blood progenitor cells mobilized by filgrastim (G-CSF) on platelet recovery after high-dose chemotherapy. *Lancet* 339:640–644, 1992.

20. Chao NJ, Schriber JR, Grimes K, et al.: Granulocyte Colony-stimulating factor "mobilized" peripheral blood progenitor cells accelerate granulocyte and platelet recovery after high-dose chemotherapy. *Blood* 81:2031–2035, 1993.

21. Schmitz N, Linch DC, Dreger P: Filgastim-mobilised peripheral blood progenitor cell transplantation in comparison with autologous bone marrow transplantation: results of a randomised phasde III trial in lymphoma patients. *Lancet* 347:353–357, 1996.

22. Nademanee A, Sniecinski I, Schmidt GM, et al.: High-dose therapy followed by autologous perpheral blood stem cell transplantation for patients with Hodgkin's disease and non-Hodgkin's lymphoma using unprimed and granulocyte colony-stimulating factor mobilized peripheral blood stem cells. *J Clin Oncol* 12:2176–2186, 1994.

23. Weaver CH, Birch R, Greco FA, et al.: Mobilization and harvest of peripheral blood stem cells: randomized evaluations of different doses of filgastim. *Br J Haematol* 100:338–347, 1998.

24. Armitage JO: Emerging applications of recombinant human granulocyte-macrophage colony-stimulating factor. *Blood* 92:4491–4508, 1998.

25. Socinski MA, Cannistra SA, Elias A, et al.: Granulocyte-macrophage colony stimulating factor expands the circulating haemopoietic progenitor cell compartment in man. *Lancet* 1:1194–1198, 1988.

26. Haas R, Ho AD, Bredthauer U, et al.: Successful autologous transplantation of blood stem cells mobilized with recombinant human granulocyte-macrophage colony-stimulating factor. *Exp Hematol* 18: 94–98, 1990.

27. Peters WP, Rosner G, Ross M, et al.: Comparative effects of Granulocyte-macrophage colony-stimulating factor (GM-CSF) and granylocyte colony-stimulating factor (G-CSF) on priming peripheral blood progenitor cells for use with autologous bone marrow after high-dose chemotherapy. *Blood* 81:1709–1719, 1993.

28. Weisdorf D, Miller J, Verfaillie C, et al.: Cytokine-primed bone marrow stem cells vs peripheral blood stem cells for autologous transplantation: a randomized comparison of GM-CSF vs. G-CSF. *Biol Blood Bone Marrow Transplant* 3:217–233, 1997.

29. Lane TA, Law P, Maruyama M, et al.: Harvesting and enrichment of hematopoietic progenitor cells mobilized into the peripheral blood of normal donors by granulocyte-macrophage colony-stimulating factor (GM-CSF) or G-CSF: potential role in allogeneic marrow transplantation. *Blood* 85:275–282, 1995.

30. Spitzer G, Adkins D, Mathews M, et al.: Randomized comparson of G-CSF + GM-CSF vs G-CSF alone for mobilization of peripheral blood stem cells: effect on hematopoietic recovery after high-dose chemotherapy. *Bone Marrow Transplant* 20:921–930, 2004.

31. Winter JN, Lazarus HM, Rademaker A, et al.: Phase I/II study of combined granulocyte colony-stimulating factor and granulocyte-macrophage colony-stimulating factor administration for the mobilization of hematopoietic progenitor cells. *J Clin Oncol* 14:277–286, 1996.

32. Glaspy JA, Shpall EJ, LeMaistre CF, et al.: Peripheral blood progenitor cell mobilization using stem cell factor in combination with filgrastim in breast cancer patients. *Blood* 90:2939–2951, 1997.

33. Moskowitz CH, Stiff P, Gordon MS, et al.: Recombinant methionyl human stem cell factor and filgrastim for peripheral blood progenitor cell mobilization and transplantation in non-Hodgkin's lymphoma patients --áresults of a phase I/II trial. *Blood* 89:3136–3147, 1997.

34. Stiff P, Gingrich R, Luger S, et al.: A randomized phase 2 study of PBPC mobilization by stem cell factor and filgrastim in heavily pretreated patients with Hodgkin's disease or non-Hodgkin's lymphoma. *Bone Marrow Transplant* 26:471–481, 2004.

35. Somlo G, Sniecinski I, ter Veer A, et al.: Recombinant human thrombopoietin in combination with granulocyte colony-stimulating factor enhances mobilization of peripheral blood progenitor cells, increases peripheral blood platelet concentration, and accelerates hematopoietic recovery following high-dose chemotherapy. *Blood* 93:2798–2806, 1999.

36. Linker C, Anderlini P, Herzig R, et al: Recombinant human thrombopoietin augments mobilization of peripheral blood progenitor cells for autologous transplantation. *Biol Blood Marrow Transplant* 9:405–413, 2003.

37. Siena S, Bregni M, Brando B, et al.: Circulation of CD34+ hematopoietic stem cells in the peripheral blood of high-dose cyclophosphamide-treated patients: enhancement by intravenous recombinant human granulocyte-macrophage colony-stimulating factor. *Blood* 74:1905–1914, 1989.

38. Koc ON, Gerson SL, Cooper BW, et al.: Randomized cross-over trial of progenitor-cell mobilization: high-dose cyclophosphamide plus granulocyte colony-stimulating factor (G-CSF) versus granulocyte-macrophage colony-stimulating factor plus G-CSF. *J Clin Oncol* 18:1824–1830, 2000.

39. Goldschmidt H, Hegenbart U, Haas R: Mobilization of peripheral blood progenitor cells with high-dose cyclophosphamide (4 or 7 gm/m²) and granulocyte colony-stimulating factor in patients with multiple myeloma. *Bone Marrow Transplant* 17:691–687, 1996.

40. Copelan EA, Ceselski SK, Ezzone SA, et al.: Mobilization of peripheral-blood progenitor cells with high-dose etoposide and granulocyte colony-stimulating factor in patients with breast cancer, non-Hodgkin's lymphoma, and Hodgkin's disease. *J Clin Oncol* 15:759–765, 1997.

41. Weaver CH, Schulman KA, Wilson-Relyea B, et al.: Randomized trial of filgrastim, sargramostim, or sequential sargramostim and filgrastim after myelosuppressive chemotherapy for the harvesting of peripheral-blood stem cells. *J Clin Oncol* 18:43, 2000.

42. Moskowitz CH, Bertino JR, Glassman JR, et al.: Ifosfamide, carboplatin, and etoposide: a highly effective cytoreduction and peripheral-blood progenitor-cell mobilization regimen for transplant-eligible patients with non-Hodgkin's lymphoma. *J Clin Oncol* 17:3776–3785, 1999.

43. Broxmeyer HE, Hangoc G, Cooper S: AMD3100, an antagonist of CXCR4 and mobilization of myeloid progenitor cells, is a potent mobilizer of competitive repopulating long term marrow self renewing stem cells in mice. *Blood* 100(suppl):609a, 2004.

44. Liles WC, Broxmeyer HE, Rodger E, et al.: Mobilization of hematopoietic progenitor cells in healthy volunteers by AMD3100, a CXCR4 antagonist. *Blood* 102:2728–2730, 2003.

45. Devine SM, Flomenberg N, Vesole DH, et al.: Rapid mobilization of CD34+ Cells following administration of the CXCR4 antagonist AMD3100 to patients with multiple myeloma and non-Hodgkin's lymphoma. *J Clin Oncol* 22:1095–1102, 2004.

46. Liles WC, Rodger E, Broxmeyer HE: Mobilization and collection of CD34+ progenitor cells from normal human volunteers with AMD 3100, a CXCR antagonist, and G-CSF. *Blood* 100(suppl):109a, 2002.

47. Fukuda H, Kojima S, Matsumoto K, et al: Auto-transplantation of peripheral blood stem cells mobilized by chemotherapy and recombinant human granulocyte colony-stimulating factor in childhood neuroblastoma and non-Hodgkin's lymphoma. *Br J Haematol* 80:327, 1992.

48. Siena S, Schiavo R, Pedrazzoli P, et al.: Therapeutic relevance of CD34 cell dose in blood cell transplantation for cancer therapy. *J Clin Oncol* 18:1360–1377, 2000.

49. Bensinger W, Appelbaum F, Rowley S, et al.: Factors that influence collection and engraftment of autologous peripheral-blood stem cells. *J Clin Oncol* 13:2547–2555, 1995.

50. Kiss JE, Rybka WB, Winkelstein A: Relationship of CD 34+ cell dose to early and late hematopoiesis following autologous peripheral blood stem cell transplantation. *Bone Marrow Transplant* 19:303–310, 2004.

51. Tricot G, Jagannath S, Vesole D, et al.: Peripheral blood stem cell transplants for multiple myeloma: identification of favorable variables for rapid engraftment in 225 patients. *Blood* 85:588–596, 1995.

52. Goldschmidt H, Hegenbart U, Wallmeier M, et al.: Factors influencing collection of peripheral blood progenitor cells following high-dose cyclophosphamide and granulocyte colony-stimulating factor in patients with multiple myeloma. *Br J Haematol* 98:736–755, 1997.

53. Watts MJ, Sullivan AM, Jamieson E, et al.: Progenitor-cell mobilization after low-dose cyclophosphamide and granulocyte colony-stimulating factor: an analysis of progenitor-cell quantity and quality and factors predicting for these parameters in 101 pretreated patients with malignant lymphoma. *J Clin Oncol* 15:535–546, 1997.

54. Haas R, Mohle R, Fruhauf S, et al.: Patient characteristics associated with successful mobilizing and autografting of peripheral blood progenitor cells in malignant lymphoma. *Blood* 83:3787–3794, 1994.

55. Dreger P, Kloss M, Petersen B, et al.: Autologous progenitor cell transplantation: prior exposure to stem cell-toxic drugs determines yield and engraftment of peripheral blood progenitor cell but not of bone marrow grafts. *Blood* 86:3970–3978, 1995.

56. Ketterer N, Salles G, Moullet I, et al.: Factors associated with successful mobilization of peripheral blood progenitor cells in 200 patients with lymphoid malignancies. *Brit J Haematol* 103:235–241, 1998.

57. Moskowitz CH, Glassman JR, Wuest D, et al.: Factors affecting mobilization of peripheral blood progenitor cells in patients with lymphoma. *Clin Cancer Res* 4: 311–316, 1998.

58. Passos-Coelho JL, Braine HG, Davis JM, et al.: Predictive factors for peripheral-blood progenitor-cell collections using a single large-volume leukapheresis after cyclophosphamide and granulocyte-macrophage colony-stimulating factor mobilization. *J Clin Oncol* 13: 705–714, 1995.

59. Zimmerman TM, Michelson GC, Mick R, et al.: Timing of platelet recovery is associated with adequacy of leukapheresis product yield after cyclophosphamide and G-CSF in patients with lymphoma. *J Clin Apheresis* 14: 31–34, 1999.

60. Stewart DA, Guo D, Juider J, et al.: The CD 3-16+56+NK cell count independently predicts autologous blood stem cell mobilization. *Bone Marrow Transplant* 27:1237–1243, 2004.

61. Gazitt Y, Liu Q: Plasma levels of SDF-1 and expression of SDF-1 receptor on CD34+ cells in mobilized peripheral blood of non-Hodgkin's lymphoma patients. *Stem Cells* 19:37–45, 2001.

62. Brugger W, Bross KJ, Glatt M, et al.: Mobilization of tumor cells and hematopoietic progenitor cells into peripheral blood of patients with solid tumors. *Blood* 83: 636–640, 1994.

63. Brenner MK, Rill DR, Moen RC: Gene-marking to trace origin of relapse after autologous bone marrow transplantation. *Lancet* 341:85–86, 2004.

64. Cooper BW, Moss TJ, Ross AA, et al.: Occult tumor contamination of hematopoietic stem-cell products does not affect clinical outcome of autologous transplantation in patients with metastatic breast cancer. *J Clin Oncol* 16:3509–3517, 1998.

65. Brugger W, Scheding S, Bock T, et al.: Purging of peripheral blood progenito cell autografts and treatment of minimal residual disease. *Stem Cells* 15(suppl 1): 159–165, 2004. Abstract.

66. Stewart AK, Vescio R, Schiller G, et al.: Purging of autologous peripheral-blood stem cells using cd34 selection

does not improve overall or progression-free survival after high-dose chemotherapy for multiple myeloma: results of a multicenter randomized controlled trial. *J Clin Oncol* 19:3771–3779, 2001.

67. Korbling M, Anderlini P: Peripheral blood stem cell versus bone marrow allotransplantation: does the source of hematopoietic stem cells matter? *Blood* 98:2900–2908, 2001.

68. Bensinger WI, Martin PJ, Storer B, et al.: Transplantation of bone marrow as compared with peripheral-blood cells from hla-identical relatives in patients with hematologic cancers. *N Engl J Med* 344: 175–181, 2001.

69. Couban S, Simpson DR, Barnett MJ, et al.: A randomized multicenter comparison of bone marrow and peripheral blood in recipients of matched sibling allogeneic transplants for myeloid malignancies. *Blood* 100: 1525–1531, 2002.

70. Cutler C, Giri S, Jeyapalan S, et al.: Acute and chronic graft-versus-host disease after allogeneic peripheral-blood stem-cell and bone marrow transplantation: a meta-analysis. *J Clin Oncol* 19:3685–3691, 2001.

71. Brown RA, Adkins D, Goodnough LT, et al.: Factors that influence the collection and engraftment of allogeneic peripheral blood stem cells in patients with hematologic malignancies. *J Clin Oncol* 15:3067, 1997.

# Chapter 95

# STEM CELL TRANSPLANTATION FOR SOLID TUMORS AND NONMALIGNANT CONDITIONS

## E. Randolph Broun

## INTRODUCTION

The use of high-dose chemotherapy (HDC) with stem cell rescue has found utility in a number of settings. Clearly for some diseases (i.e., relapsed intermediate-grade non-Hodgkin's lymphoma) this represents the best available therapy and is the standard of care. This determination was made as a result of carefully designed clinical trials showing a clear advantage to this approach over conventional-dose chemotherapy in a randomized fashion. In other diseases (such as germ cell cancer), the incidence of the disease is such that large randomized trials are not easily performed; yet well-designed trials have demonstrated the superiority of this approach in comparison to conventional-dose chemotherapy. There are other diseases (such as breast cancer and ovarian cancer) in which early enthusiasm has been tempered by the results of randomized trials failing to show any advantage for high-dose chemotherapy. Finally, there are a number of diseases (amyloidosis, renal cell cancer, melanoma, and others) in which the value of high-dose therapy with either autologous or allogeneic stem cell transplant is undetermined. This chapter will review the state of the art in high-dose therapy with stem cell rescue for solid tumors and a variety of other disorders.

## BREAST CANCER

The prognosis of patients with advanced breast cancer, either high-risk or metastatic disease, remains poor. The majority of patients with high-risk primary breast cancer, defined by extensive axillary nodal involvement or inflammatory carcinoma, experience relapse after multimodality therapy including surgery, adjuvant chemotherapy, and radiotherapy (RT). Metastatic breast cancer (MBC) remains incurable.

Given this situation, the early enthusiasm for the use of high-dose therapy with stem cell or bone marrow (BM) rescue was not surprising.[1] Phase II studies in both high-risk and MBC yielded results that seemed superior to those obtained with standard-dose chemotherapy.

### HDC FOR MBC
#### Phase II studies

Initial trials of high-dose therapy in MBC targeted patients with refractory,[2,3] untreated,[4] and responding disease.[5–8] It soon became clear that high-dose therapy produced high complete remission (CR) rates and a consistent long-term event-free survival (EFS) rate of 10–25% in patients transplanted after response to first-line chemotherapy.[9] Outcome after tandem cycles of the same HDC regimen appears comparable to a single HDC cycle.[10–14]

Retrospective analyses identified attainment of a CR to pretransplant induction chemotherapy and low tumor burden as the two most important independent prognostic factors of favorable outcome after HDC, whereas liver involvement and extensive prior chemotherapy exerted an adverse effect.[15] This information was utilized to design a trial to test whether patients with low tumor burden might benefit from high-dose therapy. Sixty patients who were rendered disease free by local treatment, either by pretransplant surgery or posttransplant RT, were enrolled in a study of high-dose cyclophosphamide/cisplatin/BCNU (carmustine) with stem cell rescue. At a median follow-up of 5 years, the EFS and overall survival (OS) rates were 52 and 62%, respectively.[16] In conclusion, these early phase II trials demonstrated impressive results in patients for whom the outlook was otherwise quite poor.

### Randomized trials in MBC

Eight randomized trials of HDC in MBC have been reported to date. Of these, six have compared high-dose therapy to conventional-dose chemotherapy, and two have evaluated the timing of high-dose therapy: early versus late.

Stadtmauer et al.[17] compared a single cycle of high-dose therapy to maintenance conventional-dose chemotherapy in 184 patients responding to a long course of conventional-dose chemotherapy. At a median follow-up of 67 months, an intent-to-treat analysis showed no differences between the two arms in EFS (4% vs 3%) or OS (14% vs 13%). Surprisingly, the partial remission (PR) to CR conversion rate, while small, was higher in the maintenance conventional-dose chemotherapy arm than in the HDC arm (9% vs 6%). This trial has been widely criticized because of its 45% dropout rate.

Using a similar approach, a group of Canadian investigators randomized 224 patients with chemoresponsive MBC to receive either additional conventional-dose chemotherapy or a single cycle of high-dose therapy with conventional-dose chemotherapy. In its first intent-to-treat analysis at a median follow-up of 19 months, significant differences in favor of HDC were observed in EFS (38% vs 24%, $P = 0.01$), but not OS (median 2 vs 2.3 years, $P = 0.9$). This trial suffered high attrition (21%) and transplant-related mortality (TRM) (7.7%) rates in the transplant arm.[18]

In the French National PEGASE-03 study, Biron et al.[19] randomized 180 responding patients to one cycle of high-dose therapy with conventional-dose chemotherapy or observation. High-dose therapy was well tolerated, with a TRM of 1% and an increase in the CR rate from 11 to 24% ($P = 0.0002$). Interestingly, in this study with a median follow-up of 48 months, there was a significant improvement in EFS in favor of high-dose therapy (27% vs 10%, $P = 0.0005$).

Crown et al.[20] looked at initial therapy with tandem high-dose therapy compared with conventional-dose doxorubicin/docetaxel followed by maintenance chemotherapy in 110 patients with MBC. The response rate on the high-dose arm was significantly better, with overall response (71% vs 29%) and CR rates (44% vs 6%) better than the control arm. Using EFS as the primary endpoint, the high-dose arm was superior (16% vs 9%, $P = 0.01$) at a median follow-up of 42 months.

Following a similar design, Schmid et al.[21] compared two sequential cycles of high-dose therapy to six to nine cycles of another modern conventional-dose chemotherapy regimen of doxorubicin and paclitaxel in 92 untreated patients. The CR rate and EFS were significantly superior in the transplant arm, without significant differences in OS at a follow-up of 14 months.

In the other French trial, Lotz et al.[22] randomized 61 responding MBC patients to additional conventional-dose chemotherapy or one HDC cycle. The apparently large differences seen in favor of the transplant arm in EFS (median 35 months vs 20 months) and OS (median 43 months vs 20 months, with 5-year OS rates

30% vs 18%) did not reach statistical significance in this study.

Finally, investigators at Duke University conducted two small trials with a crossover design, comparing early versus late use of HDC in MBC patients in CR,[23] and with bone-only disease,[24] respectively. In those studies, patients were randomized to immediate HDC with one cycle of cyclophosphamide/cisplatin/BCNU or observation, with the same HDC offered to patients in the control arm upon relapse or progression. In both trials the immediate transplant arm had significantly superior EFS (25% vs 10%, and 17% vs 9%, respectively) with no significant benefit in OS, compared to late transplant (33% vs 38%, and 28% vs 22%, respectively).

In summary, eight randomized trials in MBC, enrolling 1020 patients, have been reported. None are particularly large with half enrolling 100 or fewer patients. EFS differences in favor of high-dose therapy were seen in seven of those eight trials,[18–24] with the only exception being the Philadelphia study.[17] Longer follow-up is needed to see if the EFS advantage translates into an OS benefit.

### HIGH-DOSE THERAPY FOR HIGH-RISK BREAST CANCER
#### Phase II studies

The use of high-dose therapy with, initially, BM and, later, Peripheral blood progenitor cell(s) (PBPC) rescue was first explored and reported by Peters et al.[25] at Duke University and by Gianni et al.[26] at Milan. Each reported results that appeared superior to outcomes after conventional-dose chemotherapy using similar patient selection criteria. Specifically, Peters et al. reported a 72% 5-year EFS in a prospective phase II trial of high-dose cyclophosphamide/cisplatin/BCNU in patients with 10 or more positive axillary nodes. These results have stood the scrutiny of time, with 61% EFS rate at 11-year follow-up.[27] Gianni et al.[26] used a sequential high-dose single-agent regimen in this patient population. At a median follow-up of 4 years, the observed EFS rate was 57%.

#### Randomized trials in high-risk breast cancer

Rodenhuis et al.[28] randomized 885 patients with four or more involved lymph nodes to receive four cycles of conventional-dose chemotherapy followed by one more cycle of conventional-dose chemotherapy or one cycle of HDC. At a median follow-up of 57 months, there was a trend for an EFS advantage in favor of high-dose therapy (65% vs 59%, $P = 0.09$), with no significant OS differences. The EFS of those patients randomized to high-dose therapy who were actually transplanted appeared superior to those in the control arm ($P = 0.03$). Prospectively planned subset analysis showed that high-dose therapy improved EFS among patients with 10 or more involved nodes (68% vs 49%, $P = 0.05$).

In the Cancer and Leukemia Group B (CALGB) 9082 trial, Peters et al.[29] randomized 785 patients with

10 or more positive nodes to receive four conventional-dose chemotherapy cycles followed by one cycle of cyclophosphamide/cisplatin/BCNU or by one additional cycle of those drugs at intermediate doses with granulocyte colony-stimulating factor support. Twenty-five patients who relapsed on the intermediate-dose arm (15%) received subsequent salvage high-dose therapy. At a median follow-up of 5 years, the intent-to-treat EFS (61% vs 60%, $P = 0.5$) and OS rates (70% vs 72%, $P = 0.2$) were similar in the high- and intermediate-dose arms. There were fewer relapses in the transplant arm (32% vs 43%), which represented a 31% relative reduction in the incidence of relapses. Unfortunately, the high 10% treatment-related mortality rate observed in the high-dose arm of this trial (versus 0% in the other arm) offset the decrease in recurrences.

The Eastern Cooperative Oncology Group (ECOG) randomized 540 patients with 10 or more involved nodes to receive six cycles of conventional-dose chemotherapy with or without consolidation with one cycle of high-dose cyclophosphamide/thiotepa with BM support and, towards the end of the study, with PBPC support. With a median follow-up of 6.1 years, there was no significant difference between the high-dose and conventional-dose chemotherapy arms in EFS (55% vs 48%, $P = 0.1$) or OS (58% vs 62%, $P = 0.3$).[30]

In the Anglo-Celtic trial, Crown et al.[31] randomized 605 patients with four or more positive nodes to receive conventional-dose chemotherapy followed by one high-dose therapy cycle or maintenance conventional-dose chemotherapy. At a median follow-up of 4 years, the first planned analysis did not reveal differences in EFS (51% vs 54%, $P = 0.6$) or OS (63% vs 62%, $P = 0.8$).

Nitz et al.[32] enrolled 403 patients with 10 or more positive nodes to receive a modern dose-dense regimen or two sequential cycles of high-dose therapy with PBPC support. At a median follow-up of 39 months, there was superiority of the transplant arm in EFS (62% vs 48%, $P = 0.001$) and OS (75.6% vs 66%, $P = 0.05$).

In a French trial, Roch et al.[33] randomized 314 patients to receive conventional-dose chemotherapy followed by one cycle of high-dose therapy or observation. At a median follow-up of 33 months, there was an EFS benefit in favor of high-dose therapy in EFS (71% vs 55%, $P = 0.002$), but not OS (84% vs 85%, $P = 0.3$).

In summary, review of these randomized studies presents a conflicting picture. A common theme is relatively short follow-up. While there are several negative trials after fairly long follow-up,[29,30,34,35] other studies have already shown superiority of transplant in their first analyses,[32,33] or suggested a nonsignificant trend in favor of transplant.[28,36] Unfortunately the situation in high-risk breast cancer is similar to that in metastatic disease, with further follow-up needed to

see if the consistent advantage in EFS translates into an improvement in OS.

## OVARIAN CARCINOMA

Major improvements are needed in the treatment of advanced ovarian cancer. While the introduction of, initially, cisplatin and, later, taxanes has improved the outcome of these patients, less than 25% of stage III patients achieve long-term disease-free survival (DFS) with current multimodal management, including debulking surgery and conventional-dose chemotherapy. For patients with relapsed disease, salvage conventional-dose chemotherapy is not curative. Stage IV patients have a 5-year survival of less than 5%.

### HDC FOR RECURRENT DISEASE

The largest single-center experience is that reported by Stiff et al. from Loyola University.[37] This group reported on 100 patients, most with heavily pretreated, platinum-refractory, bulky disease. Patients were treated with a carboplatin- or melphalan-based high-dose regimen with BM or PBPC rescue. Median EFS and OS times were 7 and 13 months, respectively. Tumor bulk and platinum sensitivity were significant prognostic factors with an important finding being that the few patients with low bulk, platinum-sensitive disease had a respectable outcome.

These results were confirmed to a retrospective analysis of 421 patients from the Autologous Blood and Marrow Transplant Registry (ABMTR), receiving high-dose therapy between 1989 and 1996, in most cases for relapsed disease. Most patients had extensive prior chemotherapy, 41% of them had platinum-resistant tumors, 38% had bulky disease, and only 8% received transplants as part of the initial therapy. In this poor-prognosis population, 2-year EFS and OS rates were 12 and 35%, respectively. Younger age, good performance status, nonclear cell histology, remission status at transplantation, and platinum sensitivity were associated with better outcomes.

A retrospective analysis of 254 patients from the European Group for Blood and Marrow Transplant (EBMT) Registry evaluated the front-line use of HDC.[38] Half of them were transplanted while having residual disease, and 40% in first CR or near CR.

Outcome was improved for those patients transplanted in remission compared to those with resistant tumors, with a median EFS of 18 months versus 9 months, and median OS of 33 months versus 14 months.

The only completed randomized trial addressing the efficacy of HDC enrolled patients with low-burden, chemosensitive disease receiving first-line therapy. One hundred and ten patients with tumors of less than 2 cm were randomized to second-look laparotomy after four to six cycles of platinum-based chemotherapy, to receive consolidation with high-dose carboplatin/cyclophosphamide with PBPC support, or three maintenance cycles of conventional carboplatin/cyclophosphamide. An intent-to-treat preliminary analysis of this study showed a significant improvement of EFS in the transplant arm (median 22 months vs 11 months, $P$ = 0.03). Unfortunately, a similar trial addressing this crucial question, the US National Cancer Institute sponsored Intergroup trial, was closed prematurely due to poor accrual.

In summary, available data from phase II trials suggest that high-dose therapy offers a potential benefit for patients with platinum-sensitive disease at the time of remission. The only randomized trial comparing HDC to conventional-dose chemotherapy has shown fairly large EFS differences in favor of transplant as consolidation therapy for high-risk patients. In contrast, patients with residual disease at second-look surgery, or who have relapsed, have a much worse outcome.

## SMALL-CELL LUNG CANCER

Most patients with small-cell lung cancer (SCLC) respond to chemotherapy, but such responses are usually of relatively short duration, and survival has not significantly increased over the past two decades, either in limited or in extensive disease. These discouraging results prompted the investigation of high-dose chemotherapy with autologous stem cell transplant (ASCT) in the early 1980s. Initial studies testing one or two high-dose chemotherapy cycles as front-line therapy showed no improvement in outcome compared to historical controls.[39–42] Subsequently, delayed high-dose chemotherapy with ASCT was tested as consolidation therapy for a response obtained with conventional-dose chemotherapy. Spitzer et al.[43] reported 4-year OS of 19% among 32 such patients with limited disease (LD). There is only one reported randomized trial of HDC in SCLC.[44] Patients responding to induction chemotherapy were randomized to one additional cycle or to high-dose cyclophosphamide/BCNU/etoposide with ASCT. Although patients received cranial irradiation, no chest RT was delivered. The transplant arm showed improved responses and EFS, but OS was not significantly different between both groups, in part due to a 17% TRM rate on the high-dose arm. All patients with extensive disease (ED) relapsed in both arms of the study.

Subsequent studies incorporated thoracic and cranial RT after transplant. Elias et al.[45] treated 36 LD patients with a sequence of induction therapy, high-dose chemotherapy with cyclophosphamide/cisplatin/BCNU, and chest and cranial RT after hematologic recovery. Median EFS was 21 months, with a 5-year OS of 41%. All seven patients transplanted in partial response to induction therapy relapsed. However, the 5-year progression-free survival (PFS) was 53% for the

29 patients transplanted in CR. Leyvraz et al.[46] from the EBMT treated 69 patients (30 with LD and 39 with ED) with three sequential courses of high-dose chemotherapy (ifosfamide, carboplatin, and etoposide) with ASCT as initial therapy. RT, not required but recommended for responders, was administered to 37 patients to the chest, and prophylactically to the brain to 24 patients. Predictably, patients with LD had better outcome than those with ED, with a median OS of 18 months vs 11 months, and 2-year OS rates of 32% vs 5%.

## MELANOMA

The prognosis of metastatic melanoma is dismal. Research of HDC for this disease dates back more than 40 years.[47] Early trials with high-dose single agents with BCNU,[48] melphalan,[49] or thiotepa[50] achieved higher response rates than those expected with conventional-dose chemotherapy, but of brief duration. Disease confined to skin or lymph nodes was more likely to respond. High-dose combinations of melphalan/BCNU,[51] cyclophosphamide/cisplatin/BCNU,[52] or DTIC (dacarbazine)/melphalan/ifosfamide[53] showed higher activity than did single-agent therapy, but no improvement in outcome.

In summary, the use of HDC in melanoma remains experimental. While HDC may provide a favorable setting for testing of immunotherapy against minimal residual melanoma,[54] it is unlikely that HDC and ASCT will play a meaningful role in the management of this disease in the foreseeable future.

## BRAIN TUMORS

Most patients with malignant brain gliomas relapse after surgery and RT, and die within 2 years of diagnosis. The addition of chemotherapy offers a modest survival advantage, especially for younger patients with anaplastic astrocytoma (AA), but virtually none to those with high-grade glioblastoma multiforme (GM). Standard salvage therapy is not curative. The poor outcome of adult patients with malignant gliomas prompted many trials in the 1980s of high-dose single-agent BCNU, a drug with good central nervous system (CNS) penetration.[55–57] Initial trials in patients with refractory tumors showed high response rates, although of brief duration. High-dose BCNU was subsequently moved up to first-line therapy, combined with surgery and RT. Johnson et al. reported their experience in 25 patients with unresectable grade III or IV gliomas. These patients were treated with BCNU 1050 mg/m$^2$ followed by autologous stem cell transplant and cranial radiotherapy. They reported a median survival of 26 months, significantly better than a group of historical controls albeit with short follow-up.[58] The largest series was reported by

Durando et al.[59] in 114 newly diagnosed patients, who were treated with surgery, high-dose BCNU, and RT. At a median follow-up of more than 7 years, the EFS and OS rates were 14 and 24%, respectively. Extent of prior surgery, histology (median OS of 12 months for GM vs 81 months for AA), and young age were predictive of outcome. These observations are consistent with those from nonconcurrent matched-pair comparisons, which did not suggest benefit from high-dose BCNU in patients with high-grade GM.[60]

In summary, available results of HDC in adult patients with high-grade GM, largely employing high-dose single-agent BCNU, do not appear to improve outcome compared to conventional therapy. Further research may identify a role of HDC, in the setting of multimodal treatment, for young patients with AA.

## ADULT SOFT-TISSUE SARCOMA

Small series of metastatic soft-tissue sarcoma patients treated with high-dose chemotherapy have been reported. When used as initial[61] or salvage therapy for refractory disease,[62] high-dose chemotherapy has not produced a clear survival benefit. However, results appeared improved when used as consolidation after induction conventional-dose chemotherapy, particularly for patients transplanted in CR. Blay et al.[63] treated 30 patients with responsive metastatic disease with high-dose ifosfamide, etoposide, and cisplatin. At a median follow-up of 94 months, the EFS and OS rates were 21 and 23%, respectively. Those patients in CR before high-dose chemotherapy had a better outcome than those in PR (5-year OS 75% vs 5%).

## ADULT SMALL ROUND-CELL TUMORS

The family of small round-cell tumors includes Ewing's sarcomas, primitive neuroectodermal tumors (PNET), rhabdomyosarcomas (RMS), and desmoplastic small round-cell tumors (DSRCT). The results reported to date from high-dose chemotherapy are generally disappointing in RMS, and uniformly dismal in DSRCT.[61,64] In contrast, results appear encouraging (25–50% long-term EFS rates) in chemotherapy-sensitive high-risk or advanced PNET/Ewing's sarcomas.[65,66] The benefit of total body irradiation in this setting, employed in most early studies, has been seriously questioned in recent years.[67] In contrast, melphalan appears to be an important agent in HDC for this disease, and there is debate as to the merits of inclusion of busulfan.[68]

## GERM CELL CANCER

Germ cell cancer (GCT) is an uncommon malignancy that occurs most often in young men, and accounts for about 1% of malignancies in men. There are groups of patients who do poorly despite the best therapeutic efforts: some of these have poor prognostic factors at diagnosis, such as far-advanced disease, choriocarcinoma, or markedly elevated serum markers; others do not achieve remission, or relapse following primary or salvage therapy; and, finally, a few patients demonstrate refractoriness to cisplatin. In each of these settings, high-dose therapy with hematopoietic stem cell rescue (HSCR) has been attempted, with varying degrees of success.

The initial study was a phase I dose-escalation study, done in collaboration with Vanderbilt University,[69] which examined the use of two courses of high-dose carboplatin and VP-16 with ABMT, in patients with GCTs that were either cisplatin refractory (defined as progression of disease within 4 weeks of previous cisplatin-based therapy) or recurrent after a minimum of two prior courses of cisplatin-based therapy. Thirty-three patients were entered on this trial: The initial 13 patients were treated with escalating doses of carboplatin, to establish a maximum-tolerated dose in combination with 1200 mg/m² VP-16; the subsequent 20 patients were treated with VP-16 1200 mg/m² and the phase II dose of carboplatin, 1500 mg/m², given in three divided doses on days −7, −5, and −3. Toxicities seen in the protocol were the expected severe myelosuppression, moderate enterocolitis, and stomatitis. Grade III hepatic toxicity (more than fivefold increase in liver enzymes), usually in association with massive infection, was observed in 8/33 patients. Significant ototoxicity, neurotoxicity, and nephrotoxicity were not seen, despite the heavy previous exposure to cisplatin in this group of patients. Treatment-related mortality was 7/33 (21%), and causes of death included infection[70] and veno-occlusive disease of the liver.[71] This was a very heavily pretreated patient population, with over one-half having received three or more prior chemotherapy (CT) regimens, and 67% were cisplatin refractory. Eight patients achieved a CR, and six a PR, for an overall response rate of 44% (95% confidence interval, 27–63%). Of these, 8/14 patients remained alive and disease free with 18 months of follow-up. CR could be achieved despite advanced disease or cisplatin refractoriness. The use of high-dose carboplatin and VP-16 can provide long-term DFS as third- or fourth-line salvage therapy in a small percentage of patients, and overt cisplatin resistance can occasionally be overcome with this approach.

A larger phase II trial was carried out through the ECOG, utilizing the same dose and schedule of agents as in the phase II portion of the initial study.[72] The same eligibility criteria were used for this study. Forty patients were entered on this multi-institution cooperative group effort between July 1988 and September 1989: 22/38 (58%) evaluable patients proceeded to the second course of high-dose therapy. Toxicity was similar to that seen in the phase I trial, with 5/38 (13%)

patients dying of treatment-related causes. Nine patients (24%) achieved a CR, including two who were rendered disease free with post-SCT surgical resection, and eight achieved a PR, for an overall response rate of 45%. Achievement of a CR was associated with testicular, rather than extragonadal, primary ($P = .12$), absence of liver metastases ($P = .08$), and embryonal cell type ($P = .11$).

A striking finding in this study was the poor outcome in patients with nonseminomatous primary mediastinal germ cell tumors. Unfortunately. this report mirrors the experience at other institutions.

A phase I trial, with further dose escalation of the combination of carboplatin and VP-16, was subsequently carried out. Thirty-two patients were enrolled on a careful dose-escalation schema of each of these agents. The maximum-tolerated dose level was carboplatin 700 mg/m$^2$ and VP-16 750 mg/ m$^2$, given daily on days $-6$, $-5$, and $-4$. Dose-limiting toxicity for this regimen was mucositis. There were five treatment deaths: four caused by sepsis and multiorgan failure, and one by CNS hemorrhage. Significant ototoxicity was also seen. These higher doses are used in the treatment of patients in first relapse, or with limited prior therapy.[73]

The overall cure rate for patients with recurrent testis cancer, treated with ifosfamide (IFX) and cisplatin-based salvage CT, is in the range of 20–25%.[74] A logical step to improve the outcome of these patients was the use of high-dose therapy at time of first relapse. The initial trial at Indiana University used two rounds of conventional-dose IFX and cisplatin, with either vinblastine or VP-16 (depending on prior treatment), followed by a single round of high-dose therapy with ABMT, using carboplatin and VP-16 in the dose and schedule used in the ECOG phase II trial. Twenty-five patients were enrolled in this study between July 1989 and January 1992. There was one early death due to sepsis during conventional-dose induction therapy, and no transplant-related deaths on this study. Eighteen of 25 patients completed the planned treatment, including high-dose therapy and ABMT. With a median follow-up of 19 months (range 4–30 months), 9/25 (36%) were alive and free of disease; three had relapsed, and were alive with disease; and six had died of progressive disease.[75] A follow-up trial examined the use of two cycles of high-dose therapy with HSCR in 25 patients in first relapse of cisplatin-sensitive testicular GCT. At a median follow-up of 26 months, 13/25 (52%) were alive and free of disease, and only one had died of treatment-related causes.[76]

A number of conclusions can be drawn from this series of studies. It is clear that a fraction (15–20%) of patients with GCT, which is either multiply relapsed or overtly cisplatin-refractory, can be cured with high-dose carboplatin and VP-16 with ABMT.[69,73,77,78] For this population of patients, ABMT is clearly not an investigational therapy, and, in fact, represents the therapy with the greatest curative potential. It is important to note that cisplatin-refractory patients are rarely cured, and new and innovative approaches are needed. Finally, the use of high-dose therapy with ABMT in patients with gonadal GCT in first relapse, who are platinum-sensitive, is quite successful, with high response rates and low toxicity.

A number of institutions in Europe have reported their experience in the treatment of GCT with high-dose therapy and HSCR.

Droz et al.[79] reported on 17 patients treated with cisplatin (200 mg/m$^2$), VP-16 (1750 mg/m$^2$), and cyclophosphamide (6400 mg/m$^2$) with BM rescue. This was a heavily pretreated group of patients, and they observed CRs in 9/17 (53%), with 4/17 patients in long-term DFS. Among the refractory patients treated on this protocol, there were no long-term survivors. This group went on to carry out a randomized trial of conventional-dose therapy [cisplatin (200 mg/m$^2$), vinblastine, and bleomycin given every 3 weeks for three to four cycles] versus high-dose therapy with BM rescue, in patients with poor-risk characteristics. One hundred fifteen patients were enrolled, of whom 114 were evaluable. The 2-year survival was 82% in the conventional-dose arm, and 60% in the high-dose arm, a statistically insignificant difference. Unfortunately, this trial suffered from some deficiencies: the dose intensity and total dose of cisplatin was actually higher on the conventional-dose arm than the transplant arm, and small number of patients precluded definite conclusions. Nonetheless, this study did not show an advantage for the use of high-dose therapy with BM rescue for the initial treatment of poor-risk GCT patients.[80]

Rosti et al.[81] published the Italian multicenter experience with high-dose carboplatin, IFX, and etoposide with BM rescue in the treatment of 28 patients. They observed that the five long-term disease-free survivors in this group were all cisplatin sensitive at the time of transplant, and concluded that cisplatin refractoriness predicted for a universally poor outcome. Two other groups have reported a significant experience with the addition of IFX to the combination of carboplatin and VP-16. The German Testicular Cancer Cooperative Study Group published their initial phase I/II experience with this regimen in 1994.[82] They reported 74 patients, 20 of whom were treated with the phase II doses of carboplatin (1500 mg/m$^2$), VP-16 (2400 mg/m$^2$), and IFX (10 g/m$^2$). IFX was again administered by prolonged infusion. Renal toxicity in this group was mild, with a median maximum serum creatinine level of 1.4 mg/dL; however, with escalating doses of carboplatin, much more severe renal toxicity was observed. Of 23 patients with cisplatin-refractory disease, only 1 was alive, free of disease, with a 7-month follow-up. This group updated their results in 1997,[83] revealing an OS of 38%, with a failure-free survival of 31% at 5 years. There were no long-term survivors among cisplatin-refractory patients. Late toxicities of renal insufficiency, paresthesias, and ototoxicity were seen in 20–30% of survivors.

Lotz et al.[84] carried out a phase I/ll trial of this regimen, using a tandem transplant schema in 39 patients, including five with metastatic trophoblastic disease. Overall, there were 13 CRs and four PRs, for an overall response rate of 46%. Thirty-three patients treated on this trial had cisplatin-refractory disease (defined as failure to respond/progression on cisplatin-based CT or relapse within 4 weeks of cisplatin-based CT). In this group there were 21 patients with gonadal GCT, nine of whom achieved a CR with a median duration of 29 months (range 2–84+ months), and no patient with refractory extragonadal GCT was a long-term survivor. The investigators concluded that cisplatin refractoriness could be overcome with dose-intense therapy. The use of high-dose therapy with HSCR has been successful and life-saving for some patients, but many questions remain. In particular, those with primary mediastinal nonseminomatous GCT in relapse, and those with cisplatin-refractory disease, are helped either rarely or not at all. The cumulative information on relapsed mediastinal GCT indicates that this group of patients should be spared the rigors of high-dose therapy and autologous stem cell transplantation. New and innovative approaches are needed for these patients. For those who have cisplatin-refractory disease, the question is more difficult. There appears to be a fraction of such patients who are long-term disease-free survivors in most large series. This is a small fraction, probably no more than 5%, and yet, it is not zero. Ideally, however, such patients should be enrolled in clinical trials to develop more effective approaches. The use of allotransplantation in these two groups has yet to be explored, and may be worthy of evaluation.

## ALLOGENEIC STEM CELL TRANSPLANTATION FOR SOLID TUMORS

Allogeneic stem cell transplantation is an effective therapy for a variety of hematologic malignancies. Early clinical observations indicate that a graft-versus-malignancy effect may be present after allogeneic transplant in advanced solid tumors.

The toxicity and TRM associated with conventional, fully ablative allografting was prohibitive in typical patients with solid tumors who might benefit from such an approach. In recent years, many transplant groups have explored the activity of reduced-intensity conditioning regimens with the aim to reduce regimen-related toxicity and TRM.[85] Different groups have used a variety of approaches to achieve the necessary immunosuppression including fludarabine-based regimens,[86-88] low-dose fractionated total-body irradiation,[89] thymic irradiation, and T-cell-depleting antibodies[90] or cytotoxic drugs in combination with monoclonal antibodies.[91]

The occurrence of a graft-versus-malignancy effect that can be exploited for the treatment of solid tumors

may be inferred from early reports of a few cases that used allogeneic, fully ablative transplantation. A graft-versus-malignancy effect was first described after allografting for breast cancer.[92] Subsequently, Ueno et al.[93] reported a small series of breast cancer patients treated with a high-dose alkylating agent regimen. In two of these cases, a disease response occurred during acute graft-versus-host disease (GvHD). More recently, Bay et al.[94] described responses attributable to a graft-versus-malignancy effect in four patients with refractory ovarian cancer. An anecdotal report identified a complete response in a patient with non-SCLC who had acute GvHD following a myeloablative allogeneic transplant for acute leukemia.[95] Thus, several tumors have been demonstrated to be susceptible to an immune-mediated graft-versus-malignancy effect after allogeneic SCT. The toxicities of fully ablative conditioning, however, precluded clinical trials to explore this more fully. The improved safety profile of non-myeloablative allogeneic SCT allowed a number of investigators to initiate pilot studies in chemotherapy-refractory diseases. Advanced renal cell cancer (RCC) and metastatic melanoma were chosen as candidates for these studies because of their poor prognosis and susceptibility to immune therapy. In 2000, Childs et al.[96] from the National Institutes of Health (NIH) reported a clear graft-versus-malignancy effect in metastatic, cytokine-refractory renal carcinoma: in their report, disease regression occurred in 53% of 19 patients, and was associated with GvHD and full donor T-cell engraftment. Three of four patients who achieved a complete response survived without evidence of disease, including the first patient who remains in remission 4.5 years after the transplant. Disease response occurred primarily in the lungs, but other sites responded as well. The NIH results have been recently updated by Igarashi et al.[97] demonstrating that 23 of the first 55 patients had regression of metastatic disease compatible with a graft-versus-malignancy effect. Five patients died from transplant-related causes, acute GvHD being the major toxicity associated with the procedure. Other investigators have since confirmed these first observations. Rini et al.[98] demonstrated 4 partial responses in 15 patients who had undergone allogeneic SCT. Nine of these patients had sustained donor engraftment, with four treatment-related deaths. Blaise et al.[99] reported their experience of reduced-intensity allografting in a variety of solid tumors; notably, their approach resulted in a rapid engraftment and a low overall TRM (9%). Renal cell cancer patients, most of whom had a progressive disease at time of treatment, had a response rate of 8%.

## AMYLOIDOSIS

The use of high-dose therapy and stem cell transplant for primary amyloidosis has gained in popularity recently.

Given the dismal outcome of patients with a diagnosis of AL amyloidosis, with or without conventional-dose therapy, a number of groups have carried out trials exploring the use of high-dose therapy in this setting. It is clear that the selection of patients with amyloidosis for high-dose therapy is of the utmost importance. The extent of organ involvement prior to high-dose therapy accounts for most of the transplant-related morbidity and mortality.[100,101] In one trial, 43 patients were transplanted; those with two or more involved organs had a 100-day survival of 33% as compared with 81% for those with more than two organs involved. The Mayo Clinic treated 66 patients with a treatment-related mortality of 14%. Multivariate analysis revealed that serum creatinine and number of organs involved were the key predictors of survival. The 30-month survival was 72% overall, but was <20% for patients with more than two organs involved. They have therefore published a risk-adapted model for the selection of these patients.[102]

There is one randomized trial reported in which patients received either high-dose therapy as initial therapy or two cycles of oral melphalan and prednisone followed by high-dose therapy. One hundred patients were enrolled and randomized (52 to arm 1 and 48 to arm 2). Nine patients in arm 1 and 16 in arm 2 did not proceed to high-dose therapy. Survival of patients on arm 1 at 1 year was 70% compared with 58% for arm 2 (*P* = 0.04), and 35% of patients in both arms who underwent high-dose therapy achieved a CR.[103]

In summary, the best treatment for AL amyloidosis has yet to be identified. The use of a risk-adapted model as proposed by the Mayo Clinic group makes high-dose therapy feasible for a larger proportion of these patients,; yet-well designed clinical trials are needed to define more effective, safer, therapy for patients with this otherwise devastating diagnosis.

## REFERENCES

1. Antman KH: High-dose chemotherapy with autologous hematopoietic stem-cell support for breast cancer in North America. *J Clin Oncol* 15:1870, 1997.
2. Eder JP: High dose combination alkylating agent chemotherapy with autologous bone marrow support for metastatic breast cancer. *J Clin Oncol* 4:646, 1986.
3. Peters WP: High-dose combination chemotherapy with autologous bone marrow support: a phase I trial. *J Clin Oncol* 4:646, 1986.
4. Peters WP: High-dose combination chemotherapy with bone marrow support as initial treatment for metastatic breast cancer. *J Clin Oncol* 6:1368, 1988.
5. Antman K: A phase II study of high-dose cyclophosphamide, thiotepa, and carboplatin with autologous bone marrow support in women with measurable advanced breast cancer responding to standard-dose therapy. *J Clin Oncol* 10:102, 1992.
6. Jones RB: AFM induction chemotherapy followed by intensive alkylating agent consolidation with autologous bone marrow support (ABMS) for advanced breast cancer: current results. *Proc Am Soc Clin Oncol* 7:121, 1990.
7. Laport GF: High-dose chemotherapy consolidation with autologous stem cell rescue in metastatic breast cancer: a 10-year experience. *Bone Marrow Transplant* 21:127, 1998.
8. Rizzieri DA: Prognostic and predictive factors for patients with metastatic breast cancer undergoing aggressive induction therapy followed by high-dose chemotherapy with autologous stem-cell support. *J Clin Oncol* 17:3064, 1999.
9. Nieto Y: Prognostic evaluation of the early lymphocyte recovery inpatients with advanced metastatic and non-metastatic breast cancer receiving high-dose chemotherapy with an autologous stem-cell transplant. *Clin Cancer Res.* 10:5076, 2004.
10. Ayash LJ: Double dose-intensive chemotherapy with autologous marrow and peripheral-blood progenitor-cell support for metastatic breast cancer: a feasibility study. *J Clin Oncol* 12:37, 1994.
11. Broun ER: Tandem autotransplantion for the treatment of metastatic breast cancer. *J Clin Oncol* 13:2050, 1994.
12. Dunphy FR: Treatment of estrogen receptor-negative or hormonally refractory breast cancer with double high-dose chemotherapy intensification and bone marrow support. *Clin Oncol* 8:1207, 1990.
13. Rodenhuis S: Feasibility of multiple courses of high-dose cyclophosphamide, thiotepa, and carboplatin for breast cancer or germ cell cancer. *J Clin Oncol* 14:1473, 1996.
14. Shapiro CL: Repetitive cycles of cyclophosphamide, thiotepa, and carboplatin intensification with peripheral-blood progenitor cells and filgrastim in advanced breast cancer patients. *J Clin Oncol* 15:674, 1997.
15. Nieto Y: Status of high-dose chemotherapy for breast cancer: a review. *Biol Blood Marrow Transplant* 6:476, 2000.
72. Bewick M: Expression of C-erbB-2/HER-2 in patients with metastatic breast cancer undergoing high-dose chemotherapy and autologous blood stem cell support. *Bone Marrow Transplant* 24:377, 1999.
16. Nieto Y: Prognostic model for relapse after high-dose chemotherapy with autologous stem-cell transplantation for stage IV oligometastatic breast cancer. *J Clin Oncol* 20:707, 2004.
17. Stadtmauer EA: Conventional-dose chemotherapy compared with high-dose chemotherapy plus autologous hematopoietic stem-cell transplantation for metastatic breast cancer. *N Engl J Med* 342:1069, 2000.
18. Crump M: A randomized trial of high-dose chemotherapy (HDC) with autologous peripheral blood stem cell support (AHPCT) compared to standard chemotherapy in women with metastatic breast cancer: a National Cancer Institute of Canada (NCIC) Clinical Trials Group study. *Proc Am Soc Clin Oncol* 20:21a, 2001. Abstract 82.

19. Biron P: High dose thiotepa (TTP), cyclophosphamide (CPM) and stem cell transplantation after 4 FEC 100 compared with 4 FEC alone allowed a better disease free survival but the same overall survival in first line chemotherapy for metastatic breast cancer. Results of the PEGASE 03 French protocol. *Proc Am Soc Clin Oncol* 21:42a, 2002. Abstract 167.

20. Crown J: Superiority of tandem high-dose chemotherapy (HDC) versus optimized conventionally-dosed chemotherapy (CDC) in patients (pts) with metastatic breast cancer (MBC): The International Breast Cancer Dose Intensity Study (IBDIS 1). *Proc Am Soc Clin Oncol* 22:23a, 2003. Abstract 88.

21. Schmid P: Randomized trial of up front tandem high-dose chemotherapy (HD) compared to standard chemotherapy with doxorubicin and paclitaxel (AT) in metastatic breast cancer (MBC). *Proc Am Soc Clin Oncol* 21:43a, 2002. Abstract 171.

22. Lotz J-P: Intensive chemotherapy and autograft of hematopoietic stem cells in the treatment of metastatic breast cancer: results of the national protocol PEGASE 04 [in French]. *Hematol Cell Ther* 41:71, 1999.

23. Peters WP: A large, prospective, randomized trial of high-dose combination alkylating agents (CPB) with autologous cellular support (ABMS) as consolidation for patients with metastatic breast cancer achieving complete remission after intensive doxorubicin-based induction therapy (AFM). *Proc Am Soc Clin Oncol* 15:121a, 1996.

24. Madan B: Improved survival with consolidation high-dose cyclophosphamide, cisplatin and carmustine (HD-CPB) compared with observation in women with metastatic breast cancer (MBC) and only bone metastases treated with induction adriamycin, 5-fluorouracil and methotrexate (AFM): a phase III prospective randomized comparative trial. *Proc Am Soc Clin Oncol* 19:48a, 2000.

25. Peters WP: High-dose chemotherapy and autologous bone marrow support as consolidation after standard-dose adjuvant therapy for high-risk primary breast cancer. *J Clin Oncol* 11:1132, 1993.

26. Gianni AM: Efficacy, toxicity and applicability of high-dose chemotherapy as adjuvant treatment in operable breast cancer with 10 or more involved axillary nodes: five year results. *J Clin Oncol* 15:2312, 1997.

27. Nikcevich DA: Ten year follow-up after high-dose chemotherapy and autologous bone marrow support as consolidation after standard-dose adjuvant therapy for high-risk primary breast cancer. *Proc Am Soc Clin Oncol* 21:415a, 2002.

28. Rodenhuis S, Bontenbal M, Beex LVAM, et al.: High-dose chemotherapy with hematopoietic stem-cell rescue for high-risk breast cancer. *N Engl J Med* 349:7, 2003.

29. Peters WP: Updated results of a prospective, randomized comparison of two doses of combination alkylating agents (AA) as consolidation after CAF in high-risk primary breast cancer involving ten or more axillary lymph nodes (LN): CALGB 9082/SWOG 9114/NCIC Ma-13. *Proc Am Soc Clin Oncol* 20:21, 2001.

30. Tallman M: Conventional adjuvant chemotherapy with or without high dose chemotherapy and autologous stem-cell transplantation in high-risk breast cancer. *N Engl J Med* 349:17, 2003.

31. Crown JP: High-dose chemotherapy (HDC) with autograft (PBP) support is not superior to cyclophosphamide (CPA), methotrexate and 5-FU (CMF) following doxorubicin (D) induction in patients (pts) with breast cancer and 4 or more involved axillary lymph nodes (4+LN): The Anglo-Celtic I study. *Proc Am Soc Clin Oncol* 21:42a, 2002. Abstract 166.

32. Nitz UA: Tandem high dose chemotherapy versus dose-dense conventional chemotherapy for patients with high risk breast cancer: interim results from a multi-center phase III trial. *Proc Am Soc Clin Oncol* 22:832a, 2003. Abstract 3344.

33. Roch HH: High dose chemotherapy (HDC) improves early outcome for high risk ($N > 7$) breast cancer patients: the PEGASE 01 trial. *Proc Am Soc Clin Oncol* 20:27a, 2001. Abstract 102.

34. Bergh J: Tailored fluoruracil, epirubicin, and cyclophosphamide compared with marrow-supported high-dose chemotherapy as adjuvant treatment for high-risk breast cancer: a randomised trial. *Lancet* 356:1384, 2000.

35. Gianni A: Five-year results of the randomized clinical trial comparing standard versus high-dose myeloablative chemotherapy in the adjuvant treatment of breast cancer with $> 3$ positive nodes (LN+). *Proc Am Soc Clin Oncol* 20:21a, 2001. Abstract 80.

36. Basser R: Randomized trial comparing up-front, multi-cycle dose-intensive chemotherapy (CT) versus standard dose CT in women with high-risk stage 2 or 3 breast cancer (BC): first results from IBCSG trial 15–95. *Proc Am Soc Clin Oncol* 22:6a, 2003. Abstract 20.

37. Stiff PJ: High-dose chemotherapy with autologous transplantation for persistent/relapsed ovarian cancer: a multivariate analysis of survival for 100 consecutively treated patients. *J Clin Oncol* 15:1309, 1997.

38. Ledermann JA: High-dose chemotherapy for ovarian carcinoma: long-term results from the Solid Tumour Registry of the European Group for Blood and Marrow Transplantation (EBMT). *Ann Oncol* 12:693, 2001.

39. Farha P: High-dose chemotherapy and autologous bone marrow transplantation for the treatment of small-cell lung carcinoma. *Cancer* 52:1351, 1983.

40. Souhami RL: High-dose cyclophosphamide with autologous bone marrow transplantation for small-cell lung carcinoma of the bronchus. *Cancer Chemother Pharmacol* 10:205, 1983.

41. Souhami RL: High-dose cyclophosphamide in small-cell carcinoma of the lung. *J Clin Oncol* 3:958, 1985.

42. Souhami RL: Intensive chemotherapy with autologous bone marrow transplantation for small-cell lung cancer. *Cancer Chemother Pharmacol* 24:321, 1989.

43. Spitzer G: High-dose intensification therapy with autologous bone marrow support for limited small-cell bronchogenic carcinoma. *J Clin Oncol* 4:4, 1986.

44. Humblet Y: Late intensification chemotherapy with autologous bone marrow transplantation in selected small-cell carcinoma of the lung: a randomized study. *J Clin Oncol* 5:1864, 1987.

45. Elias AD: Dose-intensive therapy for limited-stage small-cell lung cancer: long-term outcome. *J Clin Oncol* 17:1175, 1999.

46. Leyvraz S: Multiple courses of high-dose ifosfamide, carboplatin, and etoposide with peripheral-blood progenitor

cells and filgrastim for small-cell lung cancer: a feasibility study by the European Group for Blood and Marrow Transplantation. *J Clin Oncol* 17:3531, 1999.

47. Ariel IM: Treatment of disseminated melanoma with phenylalanine mustard (melphalan) and autogenous bone marrow transplants. *Surgery* 51:582, 1962.

48. Phillips GL: A phase I–II study; intensive BCNU (1,3-bis (2-chloroethyl)-1-nitrosourea, NSC 409962) and autologous bone marrow transplantation for refractory cancer. *Cancer* 52:1792, 1982.

49. Cornbleet MA: Treatment of advanced malignant melanoma with high-dose melphalan and autologous bone marrow transplantation. *Br J Cancer* 61:330, 1990.

50. Wolff SN: High-dose thiotepa with autologous bone marrow transplantation for metastatic malignant melanoma: results of phase I and II studies of the North American Bone Marrow Transplantation Group. *J Clin Oncol* 7:245, 1989.

51. Herzig R: Treatment of metastatic melanoma with intensive melphalan-BCNU combination chemotherapy and cryopreserved autologous bone marrow transplantation. *Proc Am Soc Clin Oncol* 3:264, 1984.

52. Shea TC: Malignant melanoma: treatment with high-dose combination alkylating agent chemotherapy and autologous bone marrow support. *Arch Dermatol* 124:878, 1988.

53. Thatcher D: High-dose double alkylating agent chemotherapy with DTIC, melphalan, or ifosfamide and marrow rescue for metastatic malignant melanoma. *Cancer* 63:1296, 1989.

54. Lister J: Autologous peripheral blood stem cell transplantation and adoptive immunotherapy with activated natural killer cells in the immediate post-transplant period. *Clin Cancer Res* 1:607, 1995.

55. Johnson DB: Prolongation of survival for high-grade malignant gliomas with adjuvant high-dose BCNU and autologous bone marrow transplantation. *J Clin Oncol* 5:783, 1987.

56. Phillips GL: Intensive BCNU chemotherapy and autologous bone marrow transplantation for malignant glioma. *J Clin Oncol* 4:639, 1986.

57. Takvorian T: Autologous bone marrow transplantation: host effects of high-dose BCNU. *J Clin Oncol* 1:610, 1983.

58. Johnson DB: Prolongation of survival for high-grade malignant gliomas with adjuvant high dose BCNU and autologous bone marrow transplantation. *J Clin Oncol* 5:783–789, 1987.

59. Durando X: High-dose BCNU followed by autologous hematopoietic stem cell transplantation in supratentorial high-grade malignant gliomas: a retrospective analysis of 114 patients. *Bone Marrow Transplant* 31:559, 2003.

60. Goodwin W: A retrospective comparison of high-dose BCNU with autologous marrow rescue plus radiotherapy vs IV BCNU plus radiation therapy in high grade gliomas. *Proc Am Soc Clin Oncol* 8:90, 1989.

61. Kessinger A: High dose therapy with autologous hematopoietic stem cell rescue for patients with metastatic soft tissue sarcoma. *Proc Am Soc Clin Oncol* 13:A1674, 1994.

62. Elias AD: Phase I study of high-dose ifosfamide, carboplatin and etoposide with autologous hematopoietic stem cell support. *Bone Marrow Transplant* 15:373, 1995.

63. Blay JY: High-dose chemotherapy with autologous hematopoietic stem-cell transplantation for advanced soft tissue sarcoma in adults. *J Clin Oncol* 18:3643, 2000.

64. Bertuzzi A: Prospective study of high-dose chemotherapy and autologous peripheral stem cell transplantation in adult patients with advanced desmoplastic small round-cell tumour. *Br J Cancer* 89:1159, 2003.

65. Bertuzzi A: High-dose chemotherapy in poor-prognosis adult small round-cell tumors: clinical and molecular results from a prospective study. *J Clin Oncol* 20:2181, 2002.

66. Burdach S: Allogeneic and autologous stem-cell transplantation in advanced Ewing tumors. An update after long-term follow-up from two centers of the European Intergroup study EICESS. *Ann Oncol* 11:1451, 2000.

67. Burdach S: High-dose therapy for patients with primary multifocal and early relapsed Ewing's tumors: results of two consecutive regimens assessing the role of total body irradiation. *J Clin Oncol* 21:3072, 2003.

68. Burdach S: High-dose chemoradiotherapy (HDC) in the Ewing family of tumors (EFT). *Crit Rev Oncol Hematol* 41:169, 2003.

69. Nichols CR: Dose-intensive chemotherapy in refractory germ cell cancers: a phase I trial of high dose carboplatin and etoposide with autologous bone marrow transplantation. *J Clin Oncol* 7:932–939, 2005.

70. Motzer RJ: The role of ifosfamide plus cisplatin-based chemotherapy as salvage therapy for patients with refractory germ cell tumors. *Cancer* 66:2476–2481, 2005.

71. Williams SW: Treatment of disseminated germ cell tumors with cisplatin, bleomycin and either vinblastine or etoposide. *N Engl J Med* 316:1435–1440, 1987.

73. Nichols CR: High-dose carboplatin and etoposide with autologous bone marrow transplantation in refractory germ cell cancer: an Eastern Cooperative Group protocol. *J Clin Oncol* 10:558–563, 1992.

74. Broun ER: Salvage therapy with high-dose chemotherapy and autologous bone marrow support in the treatment of primary nonseminomatous mediastinal germ cell tumors. *Cancer* 68:1513–1515, 1991.

75. Broun ER: High-dose carboplatin/VP-16 plus ifosfamide with autologous bone marrow support in the treatment of refractory germ cell tumors. *Bone Marrow Transplant* 7:53–56, 1991.

76. Broun ER: Tandem high-dose chemotherapy with autologous bone marrow transplantation for initial relapse of testicular germ cell cancer. *Cancer* 79:1605–1610, 1997.

77. Broun ER, Nichols CR, Mandanas R; et al.: Dose escalation study or high-dose carboplatin and etoposide with autologous bone marrow support in patients with recurrent and refractory germ cell tumors. *Bone Marrow Transplant* 16:353–358, 1995.

78. Broun ER: Long-term outcome of patients with relapsed and refractory germ cell tumors treated with high-dose chemotherapy and autologous bone marrow rescue. *Ann Intern Med* 117:124–128, 1992.

79. Droz JP: Long-term survivors after salvage high-dose chemotherapy with bone marrow rescue in refractory germ cell cancer. *Eur J Cancer* 27:831–835, 1991.

80. Chevreau C: Early intensified chemotherapy with autologous bone marrow transplantation in first line treatment of poor risk non-seminomatous germ cell tumors. Preliminary results of a French randomized trial. *Eur Urol* 23:213–218, 1993.

81. Rosti G: High-dose chemotherapy with autologous bone marrow transplantation in germ cell tumors; a phase II study. *Ann Oncol* 3:809–812, 1992.

82. Siegert W: High-dose treatment with carboplatin, etoposide and ifosfamide followed by autologous stem cell transplantation in relapsed or refractory germ cell cancer: a phase I/ll study. *J Clin Oncol* 12:1223–1231, 1994.

83. Beyer J: Long-term survival of patients with recurrent or refractory germ cell tumors after high-dose chemotherapy. *Cancer* 79:161–168, 1997.

84. Lotz JP: High-dose chemotherapy with ifosfamide, carboplatin, and etoposide combined with autologous bone marrow transplantation for the treatment of poor prognosis germ cell tumors and metastatic trophoblastic disease in adults. *Cancer* 75:874–885, 1995.

85. Barrett J: Non-myeloablative stem cell transplants. *Br J Haematol* 11:6, 2000.

86. Giralt S: Engraftment of allogeneic hematopoietic progenitor cells with purine analog-containing chemotherapy: harnessing graft-versus-leukemia without myeloablative therapy. *Blood* 89:4531, 1997.

87. Khouri IF: Transplant-lite: induction of graft-versus-malignancy using fludarabine-based nonablative chemotherapy and allogeneic blood progenitor-cell transplantation as treatment for lymphoid malignancies. *J Clin Oncol* 16:2817, 1998.

88. Slavin S: Nonmyeloablative stem cell transplantation and cell therapy as an alternative to conventional bone marrow transplantation with lethal cytoreduction for the treatment of malignant and nonmalignant hematologic diseases. *Blood* 91:756, 1998.

89. Kanda Y: Allogeneic reduced intensity stem cell transplantation for advanced pancreatic cancer. *Proc Am Soc Clin Oncol* 22:834, 2003. Abstract 3353.

90. Sykes M: Mixed lymphohaemopoietic chimerism and graft-versus-lymphoma effects after non-myeloablative therapy and HLA-mismatched bone-marrow transplantation. *Lancet* 353:1755, 1999.

91. Kottaridis PD: In vivo CAMPATH-1H prevents graft-versus-host disease following nonmyeloablative stem cell transplantation. *Blood* 96:2419, 2000.

92. Eibl B: Evidence for a graft-versus-tumor effect in a patient treated with marrow ablative chemotherapy and allogeneic bone marrow transplantation for breast cancer. *Blood* 88:1501, 1996.

93. Ueno NT: Allogeneic peripheral-blood progenitor-cell transplantation for poor-risk patients with metastatic breast cancer. *J Clin Oncol* 16:986, 1998.

94. Bay JO: Allogeneic hematopoietic stem cell transplantation in ovarian carcinoma: results of five patients. *Bone Marrow Transplant* 30:95, 2002.

95. Moscardo F: Graft-versus-tumour effect in non-small-cell lung cancer after allogeneic peripheral blood stem cell transplantation. *Br J Haematol* 111:708, 2000.

96. Childs R: Regression of metastatic renal-cell carcinoma after nonmyeloablative allogeneic peripheral-blood stem-cell transplantation. *N Engl J Med* 343:750, 2002.

97. Igarashi T, Mena O, Re F, et al.: Exploring the role of allogeneic immunotherapy for non-hematologic malignancies: proof of concept and potential immune mechanism of graft-vs-tumor effects in solid tumors. *Haematologica* 87(suppl 1):2, 2002.

98. Rini BI: Allogeneic stem-cell transplantation of renal cell cancer after nonmyeloablative chemotherapy: feasibility, engraftment and clinical results. *J Clin Oncol* 20:2017, 2002.

99. Blaise D: Reduced-intensity preparative regimen and allogeneic stem cell transplantation for advanced solid tumors. *Blood* 103:435, 2004.

100. Comenzo RL: Hematopoietic cell transplantation for primary systemic amyloidosis: what have we learned. *Leuk Lymphoma* 37:245–258.

101. Gertz MA: Blood stem cell transplantation as therapy for primary systemic amyloidosis(AL). *Bone Marrow Transplant* 26:963–969, 2000.

102. Gertz MA: Stem cell transplantation for management of primary amyloidosis. *Blood* 98:816, 2001.

103. Sanchorawala V: High dose intravenous melphalan and autologous stem cell transplantation as initial therapy or following 2 cycles of oral chemotherapy for the treatment of AL amyloidosis: results of prospective randomized trial. *Blood* 98:815, 2001.

104. Loehrer PJ Sr: Vinblastine plus ifosfamide plus cisplatin as initial salvage therapy in recurrent germ cell tumor. *J Clin Oncol* 16:2500–2504, 1998.

105. Broun ER: Early salvage therapy for germ cell cancer using high-dose chemotherapy with autologous bone marrow support. *Cancer* 73:1716–1720, 1994.

# Chapter 96

# NONMYELOABLATIVE CONDITIONING REGIMEN FOR ALLOGENEIC HEMATOPOIETIC CELL TRANSPLANTATION

*Frédéric Baron, Marie-Térèse Little, and Rainer Storb*

## INTRODUCTION

Due to regimen-related toxicities, the use of conventional allogeneic hematopoietic cell transplantation (HCT) has been restricted to younger and medically fit patients. This is unfortunate, as the median ages at diagnosis of patients with most hematologic malignancies, such as acute and chronic leukemias, lymphomas, multiple myeloma, or myelodysplastic syndromes, range from 65 to 70 years (Table 96.1).[1] The curative potential of allogeneic HCT is the result of eradication of malignant cells by high-dose chemotherapy and total body irradiation (TBI), and of immune-mediated graft-versus-tumor (GvT) effects.[2,3] The power of the GvT effects, which are mediated by lymphocytes, has led several groups of investigators to infuse donor lymphocytes (donor lymphocyte infusion, DLI) in patients who have relapsed with hematologic malignancies after allogeneic HCT.[4,5] The induction of durable remissions by DLI demonstrated that the GvT effects were capable of eradicating some hematologic malignancies by themselves, even in the absence of chemotherapy. This prompted the introduction of reduced-intensity conditioning regimens[6–8] or truly nonmyeloablative regimens for allogeneic HCT[9–11] that are mainly based on GvT effects. The lower degrees of regimen-related toxicities associated with these procedures have allowed the extension of allogeneic HCT to patients previously deemed ineligible for high-dose conventional approaches due to age or comorbidities.[9]

## AIMS OF CONDITIONING REGIMENS

### MAKING SPACE FOR DONOR CELLS

Immature progenitor cells occupy defined niches within the marrow stroma to obtain the necessary support for proliferation and differentiation.[12] To allow access for donor cells to these niches, it was commonly believed that at least some host stem cells must be eradicated by the conditioning regimen. However, there is now evidence that allogeneic grafts can create their own marrow space via subclinical graft-versus-host reactions. First, dogs conditioned only with 4.5 Gy irradiation targeted to the cervical, thoracic, and upper abdominal lymph node chains, and administered postgrafting immunosuppression with mycophenolate mofetil (MMF, a purine synthesis inhibitor) and cyclosporine (CSP) achieved long-term mixed hematopoietic chimerism, as well as in the lymph nodes and bone marrow spaces that were shielded from irradiation.[13] Secondly, HLA-identical bone marrow can stably engraft without any conditioning regimen or postgrafting immunosuppression in infants with severe combined immunodeficiency disease (SCID).[14] Thirdly, allografts have been successfully carried out with postgrafting immunosuppression with MMF and CSP, but without conditioning in some human patients with T-cell deficiencies other than SCID.[15] Finally, sustained engraftment has been accomplished in dogs after selective T-cell ablation with bismuth-213-labeled anti-TCRαβ monoclonal antibody and postgrafting MMF/CSP.[16]

### TUMOR ERADICATION

Radiation or chemotherapy dose-effect curves for tumor eradication are usually straight on a log scale: each radiation or chemotherapy dose increment kills the same fraction of malignant cells. Thus, allogeneic HCT was first used as a means to deliver otherwise supralethal doses of TBI.[17,18] The major demonstration of the antitumor efficacy of supralethal chemoradiotherapy was evidenced by the superiority of autologous HCT over conventional chemotherapy in various hematologic

| Table 96.1 | Age of patients at diagnoses and at HCT[1] | | |
|---|---|---|---|
| | Median ages patient (years) | | |
| | Recent allogeneic HCT recipients (FHCRC) | | At diagnoses (SEERS) |
| Disease | Related donor | Unrelated donor | |
| CML | 40 | 36 | 67 |
| AML | 28 | 33 | 68 |
| NHL | 33 | 35 | 65 |
| MM | 45 | 45 | 70 |
| CLL | 51 | 46 | 71 |
| HD | 29 | 28 | 34 |
| MDS | 40 | 41 | 68 |
| Overall | 40 (n = 1428) | 35 (n = 1277) | – |

HCT, hematopoietic cell transplantation; FHCRC, Fred Hutchinson Cancer Research Center; SEERS, Surveillance, Epidemiology and End Results; CML, chronic myeloid leukemia; AML, acute myeloid leukemia; NHL, non-Hodgkin's lymphoma; MM, multiple myeloma; CLL, chronic lymphocytic leukemia; HD, Hodgkin's disease; MDS, myelodysplastic syndrome.

| Table 96.2 | Effect of TBI dose and postgrafting immunosuppression on engraftment of DLA-identical marrow grafts | |
|---|---|---|
| TBI dose (Gy) | Postgrafting immunosuppression | No. of dogs with stable engraftment (%)[a]/no. of dogs transplanted |
| 9.2 | None[28] | 20/21 (95%) |
| 4.5 | None[29] | 6/17 (35%) |
| 4.5 | Cyclosporine[29] | 7/7 (100%) |
| 2.0 | Cyclosporine[30] | 0/4 (0%) |
| 2.0 | Methotrexate + cyclosporine[30] | 2/5 (40%) |
| 2.0 | Mycophenolate mofetil + cyclosporine[30] | 11/12 (92%) |
| 2.0 | Sirolimus + cyclosporine[31] | 6/7 (86%) |
| 1.0 | Mycophenolate mofetil + cyclosporine[30] | 0/6 (0%) |
| 1.0 | Cyclosporine + G-PBMC[b32] | 5/8 (63%) |

[a] Mixed or full chimerism.
[b] Granulocyte colony-stimulating factor mobilized peripheral blood mononuclear cells.

malignancies.[19] However, high-dose pretransplant therapy does not completely eradicate the malignancy in all patients. Attempts to improve disease-free survival by increasing the intensity of the conditioning regimens were usually accompanied by increases in transplant-related mortality (TRM), and overall as well as disease-free survivals remained unchanged or worsened.[20,21]

### PREVENTION OF HEMATOPOIETIC STEM CELL REJECTION

It is necessary to abolish host defenses prior to transplantation to avoid immune-mediated graft rejection caused by alloreactive cytotoxic host T lymphocytes in the major histocompatibility complex (MHC)-identical setting[16,22] and by alloreactive cytotoxic host T lymphocytes, host natural killer (NK) cells, and HLA-specific antibodies in the MHC-mismatched setting.[23,24] The risks of graft rejection increase in cases of HLA disparities or host sensitization to major and minor histocompatibility antigens via administration of multiple blood products.[25,26] Both the conditioning regimen and the donor T lymphocytes are instrumental in the destruction of the host immune system. The latter implies that T-cell depletion of the graft as a method to prevent graft-versus-host disease (GvHD) may also have deleterious effects on engraftment.[27]

### TBI DOSE DE-ESCALATION IN THE DLA-IDENTICAL DOG MODEL

In the preclinical canine dog leukocyte antigen (DLA)-identical transplant model, a dose-response relationship with respect to TBI and allogeneic marrow engraftment has been demonstrated (Table 96.2). A single TBI dose of 9.2 Gy was sufficiently immunosuppressive to allow engraftment of DLA-identical littermate marrow in 95% of dogs not given postgrafting immunosuppression.[28] When the dose was decreased to 4.5 Gy, only 41% of dogs had stable engraftment.[29] When dogs were given 4.5 Gy TBI and posttransplant prednisone, none engrafted.[29] However, the addition of postgrafting CSP for 5 weeks led to engraftment in all animals studied.[29] When the TBI dose was further decreased to 2 Gy, postgrafting immunosuppression, either with CSP alone or with a combination of CSP and methotrexate (MTX), resulted in graft rejection with autologous recovery in the majority of the dogs.[30] On the other hand, a postgrafting immunosuppressive regimen combining CSP and MMF lead to the development of stable mixed chimerism in 11 of 12 dogs studied.[30] However, when the TBI dose was further decreased to 1 Gy, stable long-term engraftment did not occur, demonstrating a delicate balance between host and donor cells.[30] More recently, the combination of rapamycin (sirolimus) and CSP was found to be as effective as MMF/CSP in dogs given DLA-identical marrow followed by 2 Gy TBI (Figure 96.1).[31] However, here again, stable long-term engraftment did not occur when the TBI dose was further decreased to 1 Gy.[31]

There is some evidence that the rejections observed after 1 Gy TBI are due to immune-mediated host antigraft reactions. First, stable mixed chimerism could be achieved after only 1 Gy TBI by reducing the intensity of host immune responsiveness before HCT with the help of the fusion peptide, CTLA4-Ig, which blocks T-cell costimulation through the B7-CD28 signal pathway.[33] Second,

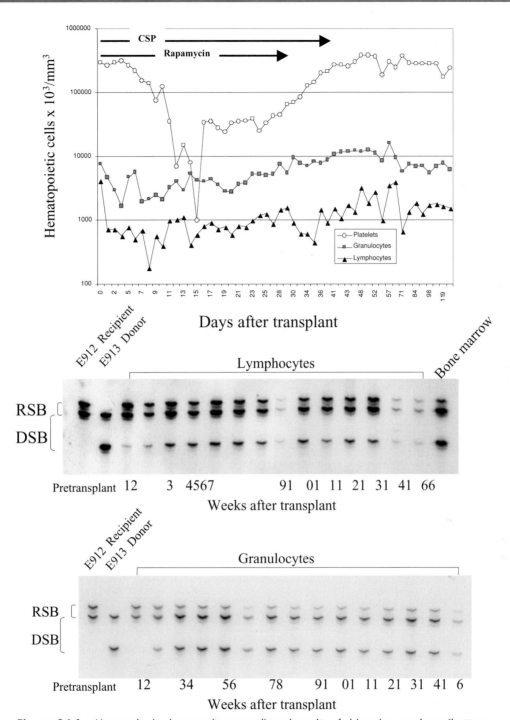

**Figure 96.1** *Hematologic changes (top panel) and results of chimerism analyses (bottom panel) in a dog conditioned with 2 Gy TBI before a DLA-identical littermate marrow graft and given a combination of rapamycin and CSP for postgrafting immunosuppression. (Reprinted from Baron F, et al.: Hematopoietic cell transplantation: five decades of progress. Arch Med Res 34:528–524, 2003; with permission from IMSS.)*

Zaucha et al. demonstrated that the addition of granulocyte colony-stimulating factor mobilized peripheral blood mononuclear cells (G-PBMC) to marrow grafts allowed for a reduction in the pretransplant TBI to 1 Gy and omission of MMF.[32] This effect was due to donor CD3 cells contained in G-PBMC, because the addition of the CD3-depleted fraction of G-PBMC resulted in graft rejection in six of seven recipients.[32]

## REDUCED-INTENSITY OR NONMYELOABLATIVE CONDITIONING REGIMENS

A number of reduced-intensity or truly nonmyeloablative conditioning regimens have been developed for clinical use (Table 96.3). Most of the reduced-intensity conditioning regimens do not meet criteria

**Table 96.3** Example of RIC or NMCR currently under investigation

| Center | Preparative regimen | Postgraft immuno-suppression | No. of patients (median age in years) | Diseases | GvHD Acute (grade II–IV) | GvHD Chronic | NRM (time after transplant) | Outcome |
|---|---|---|---|---|---|---|---|---|
| MD Anderson[34] | Fludarabine 25 mg/m²/day (or 2-CDA 12 mg/m²) × 5 days Melphalan 140–180 mg/m² | FK506 + MTX | 86 (52) | Hematologic malignancies | 49% | 68% | 37% (at 100 days) | 2-year OS 28% 2-year DFS 23% |
| United Kingdom[35] | Fludarabine 30 mg/m²/day × 5 days Melphalan 140 mg/m² Campath-1H 20 mg/day × 5 days | CSP +/– MTX | 44 (41) | Hematologic malignancies. 19 patients had a previous failed transplant | 3/44. 1 after DLI | NR | 11% (at 12 months) | 1-year OS 73% 1-year PFS 71% |
| Jerusalem[36] | Fludarabine 30 mg/m²/day × 6 days  Busulfan (p.o.) 4 mg/kg/day × 2 days ATG 5–10 mg/kg/day × 4 days | CSP +/– MTX | 24 (35) | CML in first chronic phase | 75%[a] | 55% | 3 patients (days 116, 499, and 726) | 5-year DFS 85% |
| MD Anderson[37] | Fludarabine 25 mg/m²/day × 5 days or Fludarabine 30 mg/m²/day × 3 days Cyclophosmphamide 1g/m²/day × 2 days or 750 mg/m²/day × 3 days +/– Rituximab | FK506 + MTX | 20 (51) | Lymphomas | 20% | 64% | 2 (at day 45 and before 10 months) | 2-year DFS 84% |
| National Institutes of Health[38] | Fludarabine 25 mg/m²/day × 5 days Cyclophosphamide 60 mg/kg/day × 2 days | CSP | 15 (50) | Hematologic + solid malignancies | 10/15 patients. 1 after DLI | NR | 2 patients (days 59 and 205) | 8/15 patients survived between 121 and 409 (median 200) days |
| Boston[10] | Cyclophosphamide 50 mg/kg/day × 3–4 days ATG 30 mg/kg/day × 3 days or 15 mg/kg/day × 4 days Thymic irradiation 700 cGy in patients who have not received previous mediastinal irradiation | CSP | 21 | Hematologic malignancies | 12 patients 6 after DLI | NR | 2 patients (days 77 and 180) | At a median follow-up of 445 days: 11 patients were surviving 7 patients were surviving free of progression |

table continues

**Table 96.3** continued

| Center | Preparative regimen | Postgraft immuno-suppression | No. of patients (median age in years) | Diseases | GvHD Acute (grade II–IV) | GvHD Chronic | NRM (time after transplant) | Outcome |
|---|---|---|---|---|---|---|---|---|
| **Seattle** (unrelated)[39] | Fludarabine 30 mg/m²/day × 3 days TBI 2 Gy | CSP + MMF | 89 (53) | Hematologic malignancies. 69 patients (78%) had high-risk diseases | 52% | 37% at 1 year[b] | 16% (at 12 months) | 1-year OS 52% 1-year PFS 38% |
| **Seattle** (related)[18] | TBI 2 Gy +/− Fludarabine 30 mg /m²/day × 3 days. | CSP + MMF | 212 (55) | Hematologic malignancies. | 44% | 65% | 4.7% (at 100 days) | At a median follow-up of 11.5 months 68% were surviving 52% were surviving free of progression |

[a]grade I–IV; [b] extensive chronic GvHD
NRM, nonrelapse mortality; 2-CDA, cladribine; ATG, antithymocyte globulin; CSP, cyclosporine; FK506, tacrolimus; MTX, methotrexate; BM, bone marrow; OS, overall survival; DFS, disease-free survival; PFS, progression-free survival; NR, not reported; RIC, reduced-intensity conditioning regimen; NMCR, nonmyeloablative conditioning regimen.

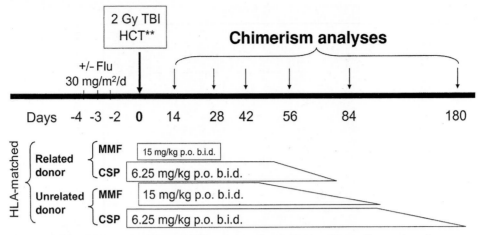

**Figure 96.2** *Nonmyeloablative HCT regimens for patients with malignancies given grafts from HLA-matched related and unrelated donors. (Reprinted from Baron F, Storb R, Little MT: Hematopoietic cell transplantation: five decades of progress.* Arch Med Res *34:528–524, 2003; with permission from IMSS.)*

of nonmyeloablative conditioning. These include (1) no eradication of host hematopoiesis; (2) prompt hematologic recovery (<4 weeks) without transplant; and (3) presence of mixed chimerism upon engraftment. Reduced-intensity conditioning regimens are aimed at eliminating host-versus-graft reactions and producing major antitumor effects. Conversely, non-myeloablative conditioning regimens rely on optimization of pre- and posttransplant immunosuppression to overcome host-versus-graft reactions to allow engraftment, and eradication of tumors depend nearly exclusively on the GvT effect. In patients with slowly progressing diseases [i.e., chronic lymphocytic leukemia (CLL), low-grade non-Hodgkin's lymphoma (NHL), and chronic myeloid leukemia (CML) in first chronic phase] or with more aggressive diseases in complete remission, a nonmyeloablative conditioning regimen might be sufficient to achieve engraftment and cure the malignant disease. However, cytoreduction might be required in patients with aggressive diseases (acute leukemia, multiple myeloma, high-grade lymphoma, Hodgkin's disease), who are not in complete remission at the time of the transplant.

### REDUCED-INTENSITY CONDITIONING REGIMENS

Most reduced-intensity conditioning regimens have combined purine analogs (fludarabine, cladribine, or pentostatin) and alkylating agents, usually cyclophosphamide, busulfan, or melphalan. In 1997, Giralt et al. reported engraftment of HLA-identical related transplants after a reduced-intensity conditioning regimen combining fludarabine 30 mg/m$^2$/day × 4 days, cytarabine zg/m$^2$/day × 4 days, and idarubicin 12 mg/m$^2$/day × 3 days.[6] Initial engraftment was greater than 90% with TRM around 20%. Giralt et al. subsequently reported a more intense regimen combining fludarabine (120–125 mg/m$^2$) and melphalan (140––180 mg/m$^2$) for patients with advanced leukemia,

multiple myeloma, or renal cell carcinoma.[34] Nonrelapse mortalities at 100 days and 1 year after the transplant were around 20 and 40%, respectively.[34] The Jerusalem group developed another protocol combining fludarabine, antithymocyte globulin (ATG), and low-dose oral busulfan.[7] This regimen allowed the achievement of full donor chimerism in the majority of the patients with a low TRM. However, most patients included in this study were younger and would be considered eligible for conventional allogeneic HCT. Kottaridis et al. used another regimen combining Campath-1H (100 mg/m$^2$), melphalan (140 mg/m$^2$), and fludarabine (150 mg/m$^2$).[35,40] This regimen allowed engraftment with low incidences of GvHD and TRM in HLA-matched related and unrelated recipients.

### NONMYELOABLATIVE CONDITIONING REGIMENS

Childs et al. developed a regimen combining cyclophosphamide (120 mg/kg) and fludarabine (125 mg/m$^2$).[11,38] TRM was 12% at 1 year in metastatic renal cell carcinoma patients. Spitzer et al. showed that mixed chimerism could be achieved with a regimen combining cyclophosphamide, thymic irradiation (in patients who had not previously received mediastinal radiation therapy), and ATG.[10] However, around 30% of the patients subsequently rejected their transplant.

Based on the canine allogeneic transplant model, we studied the induction of mixed chimerism jointly with other centers, using low-dose (2 Gy) pretransplant TBI combined with postgrafting immunosuppression consisting of MMF and CSP, initially in HLA-matched related recipients (Figure 96.2).[9] Typically, patients did not become severely pancytopenic, and more than 50% of eligible patients were treated entirely in the outpatient setting.[9] Two-year nonrelapse mortality was 7%.[9] Nonfatal graft rejection was observed in 16% of

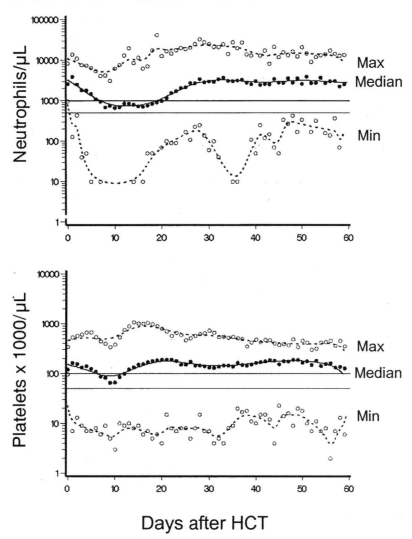

**Figure 96.3** *Neutrophil and platelet changes in 212 patients with malignancies conditioned with 2 Gy TBI +/− fludarabine (30 mg/m²/day × 3 days) and given HLA-matched related G-PBMC grafts. (Reprinted from Storb R: ASCO Educational Book 77–83, 2002; with permission from the American Society of Clinical Hematology.)*

patients.[9] Therefore, in subsequent patients, three doses of fludarabine (30 mg/m²/day) were added, and rejections decreased to 3%.[18] We studied a similar protocol that extended the duration of postgrafting immunosuppression with MMF and CSP to 96 and 180 days, respectively, to condition patients for HLA-matched unrelated donor grafts (Figure 96.2).[39,41]

## CHIMERISM EVALUATION AND ENGRAFTMENT KINETICS

### ASSESSMENT OF HEMATOPOIETIC CHIMERISM

The assessment of hematopoietic chimerism required more sensitive techniques than conventional cytogenetic analyses because of the availability of only small numbers of dividing cells. The most widely used techniques have been fluorescent in situ hybridization (FISH), with X- and Y-specific probes in case of sex-

mismatched transplant, and polymerase-chain-reaction-based assays of polymorphic mini- (variable number tandem repeats) or micro-satellite markers in case of sex-matched transplant. Other techniques based on restriction fragment length polymorphism have also been used.

### ENGRAFTMENT KINETICS

The engraftment kinetics after a nonmyeloablative conditioning regimen were first analyzed by Childs et al.[38] The authors studied chimerism evolution in 15 patients conditioned with cyclophosphamide and fludarabine. Postgrafting immunosuppression was carried out with CSP alone. The patterns of engraftment varied considerably among their patients, but most often full donor chimerism was achieved earlier in T cells than in granulocytes, and the achievement of full donor T-cell chimerism preceded GvHD and antitumor responses. The kinetics of B-cell recovery were distinct from those of myeloid and T-cell lineages, while NK-cell chimerism was closely correlated with T-cell chimerism.

Ueno et al. studied chimerism evolution in 23 patients, with metastatic tumors transplanted after a reduced-intensity conditioning regimen combining fludarabine and melphalan.[42] Postgrafting immunosuppression consisted of tacrolimus and short MTX. All patients showed 100% T-cell and granulocyte chimerisms on days 30 and 100 after the transplant.

Keil et al. analyzed the impact of day 28 chimerism on outcome after nonmyeloablative HCT in 38 patients conditioned with fludarabine followed by low-dose (2 Gy) TBI.[43] Postgrafting immunosuppression was carried out with MMF and CSP. Generally, donor T-cell chimerism lagged behind myeloid chimerism. In addition, patients with <90% donor T cells on day 28 after the transplant had significantly higher risks of graft rejection and relapse and significantly worse progression-free survival than patients with ≥90% donor T cells.

Baron et al. analyzed T-cell chimerism in 35 patients conditioned with TBI (2 Gy) alone ($n = 15$), TBI (2 Gy) and fludarabine ($n = 13$), or fludarabine and cyclophosphamide ($n = 7$). Patients received either unmanipulated ($n = 18$), CD8-depleted ($n = 11$), or CD34-selected G-PBMC ($n = 6$). Median donor T-cell contributions on days 28, 60, 100, 180, and 365 in recipients of unmanipulated G-PBMC were 75, 85, 87, 90, and 100%, respectively. Evolution of donor T-cell chimerism did not differ significantly between recipients of unmanipulated and CD8-depleted G-PBMC, while CD34 selection resulted in significantly decreased donor T-cell chimerism.[44]

We analyzed the kinetics of donor engraftment in peripheral blood hematopoietic subpopulations from 120 patients conditioned with 2 Gy TBI +/− fludarabine and postgrafting immunosuppression with MMF and CSP.[45] On day 14 posttransplant, the highest degree of donor chimerism was noted in the NK-cell fraction, followed by lymphocytes, monocytes, and granulocytes. By day 28, donor granulocyte chimerism had surpassed those in the remaining cell populations. Most patients remained mixed chimeras for at least 180 days posttransplant, with greater than 60% donor chimerism in each subpopulation except in patients with CML or MDS, who had lower percentages of donor T-cell chimerisms. Patients receiving G-PBMC had higher degrees of donor T-cell chimerism than recipients of marrow. Greater intensity of therapy before HCT was also associated with higher degrees of donor chimerisms. Low donor T-cell chimerism on day 14 (<50% CD3$^+$ T cells) was strongly associated with a higher risk of graft rejection.

Taken altogether, these results suggest that the engraftment kinetics after nonmyeloablative or reduced-intensity conditioning HCT depend on the intensity of pretransplant chemotherapy, the intensity of the preparative regimens, and whether the grafts have been depleted of T-cells or not. Moreover, monitoring mixed chimerism early after transplant may predict transplantation outcomes and/or allow early intervention to prevent graft rejection or disease progression.

## TOXICITY

There are important differences in toxicities among the various studies, in part related to the intensities of the regimens used, the ages of the patients studied, and the nature of the grafts used (sibling vs unrelated and HLA-matched vs mismatched). The 100-day TRM ranged from <5% in HLA-matched nonmyeloablative HCT recipients conditioned with low-dose TBI +/− fludarabine[18] to 37% in patients given melphalan and purine-analog-containing preparative regimens.[34] In a multicenter European Bone Marrow Transplant (EBMT) study reporting on 188 transplants for lymphoma with various reduced-intensity or nonmyeloablative conditioning regimens, the 100-day and 1-year probabilities of TRM were 13 and 26%, respectively, and those were significantly higher in older patients.[46]

Analysis of data from the first 45 patients receiving 2 Gy TBI as a conditioning regimen showed that no patients experienced regimen-related painful mucositis, pulmonary toxicity, cardiac toxicity, veno-occlusive disease of the liver, hemorrhagic cystitis, or new onset alopecia.[9] Fifty-three percent of eligible patients were treated entirely in the outpatient department, with others having relatively short hospitalizations (median 8 days). The hematologic changes were much milder than those observed after conventional HCT (Figure 96.3). Platelet and red blood cell transfusion requirements were significantly reduced in these patients compared to a concurrent group of myeloablative recipients, with 77% of patients not requiring platelet and 37% not requiring red blood cell transfusions.[47] Liver and lung toxicities were also significantly reduced after nonmyeloablative HCT. The frequency of a bilirubin >4 mg/dL was 26% at 200 days in 193 consecutive nonmyeloablative HCT recipients versus 48% at 100 days in 1419 consecutive allogeneic HCT recipients conditioned with cyclophosphamide-based myeloablative regimens.[48] The 120-day cumulative incidence of idiopathic pneumonia syndrome was 2.2% in 183 nonmyeloablative HCT recipients versus 8.4% in 917 recipients of myeloablative conditioning regimens.[49]

## GRAFT-VERSUS-HOST DISEASE

Most reports show that GvHD is a major cause of morbidity and mortality after reduced-intensity or nonmyeloablative conditioning regimens.[7,9,34,39,41] In the EBMT lymphoma study, grade II–IV acute GvHD was seen in 29% of in vivo T-cell-depleted HCT recipients, versus 58% of T-cell-replete HCT recipients ($P = 0.03$).[46] In multivariate analysis, both T-cell depletion of grafts and grafts from sibling donors were associated with lower GvHD incidences.[46] In a French study that used a conditioning regimen of fludarabine, busulfan, and ATG, the cumulative incidence of grade II–IV acute GvHD was 36%, and the 2-year cumulative incidence of chronic GvHD was 43%.[50] In multivariate analysis, a lower incidence of acute GvHD was significantly associated with higher ATG doses infused during conditioning ($P = 0.0005$), whereas the use of G-PBMC instead of marrow as the stem cell source was the only risk factor for the development of chronic GvHD ($P = 0.0007$). Not surprisingly, the relapse rates were much lower in patients who experienced GvHD than in those without it, suggesting potent GvT effects.

We recently compared GvHD in 44 nonmyeloablative and 52 age-matched conventional HCT recipients (ablative group).[51] HCT included grafts from both related and unrelated donors who were at least serologically matched for HLA-A, -B, and -C, and allele-level matched for HLA-DRB1 and -DQB1. The median patient age was 56 years in the nonmyeloablative group versus 54 years in the ablative group. Postgrafting immunosuppression was MMF and CSP in the nonmyeloablative group, and MTX plus CSP ($n = 48$) or MMF plus CSP ($n = 4$) in the ablative group. Grades II–IV and III–IV acute GvHD to day 100 were lower among unrelated recipients in the nonmyeloablative group than among those in the ablative group ($P = 0.01$ and $0.01$, respectively). Peaks of skin and gastrointestinal morbidities occurred between 6 and 12 months in the nonmyeloablative group and during the first month in the ablative group. Interestingly, 7 of 10 nonmyeloablative HCT recipients who required steroid treatment for cutaneous GvHD after day +80 had acute inflammatory changes similar to those seen in acute GvHD ("late onset acute GvHD"). These observations emphasized that a new GvHD classification that is based on criteria emphasizing the quality of target organ involvement rather than temporal presentation would be required to assess GvHD after nonmyeloablative HCT. The median time to initiation of corticosteroids was 3.0 months in the nonmyeloablative group versus 0.9 months ($P < 0.001$) in the ablative group. Significantly smaller proportions of nonmyeloablative compared to ablative recipients required steroids during each of the first 3 months after HCT (month 1, $P < 0.001$; month 2, $P < 0.001$; month 3, $P = 0.02$). However, differences in steroid requirements between the nonmyeloablative and the ablative groups were no longer significant beyond the first 3 months after HCT. The 15-month cumulative incidence of death with manifestations of GvHD under treatment was 24% in the nonmyeloablative group versus 35% not significant (NS) in the ablative group. One-year overall survival was 68% in the nonablative group versus 50% ($P = 0.04$) in the ablative group.

## IMMUNE RECONSTITUTION AND INFECTIONS

To date, few reports have analyzed immune reconstitution after nonmyeloablative HCT. Mohty et al. showed that early CD8[+] T lymphocyte and NK-cell recoveries after HCT with a reduced-intensity conditioning regimen take place, whereas naïve CD4[+]CD45RA[+] T lymphocytes remained below normal values during the first months after the transplant.[52] Similar results were reported by Baron et al.[44] We recently compared immune reconstitution after conventional and non-myeloablative transplantation.[53] During the first 6 months, absolute lymphocyte subset counts were similar, but counts of cytomegalovirus (CMV)-specific T-helper lymphocytes were higher at days 30 and 90 in the nonmyeloablative patient group. Conventional transplant recipients had higher naïve CD4 and CD8 counts 1 year after the HCT, probably reflecting lower counts of recent thymic emigrants in nonmyeloablative recipients; this finding might be related to the older age of nonmyeloablative recipients.

Mohty et al. analyzed infectious complications occurring during the first 6 months after HLA-identical sibling transplantation with an ATG-based reduced-intensity conditioning regimen.[54] The 6 month cumulative incidences of bacteremia, positive CMV antigenemia, and fungal infection were 25, 42, and 8%, respectively.

Junghanss et al. compared the incidence of post-transplant CMV infections in 56 nonmyeloablative recipients with that in 112 matched controls who were treated by conventional HCT during the same time period.[55] CMV disease occurred in neither low- and intermediate-risk CMV nonmyeloablative or control patients. The 100-day incidence of CMV disease for high-risk CMV patients (defined as recipients serologically positive for CMV) was 9% in the nonmyeloablative group versus 19% ($P = 0.08$) in the control group. However, the 1-year probability of CMV disease for high-risk CMV patients was similar in the two groups ($P = 0.87$). The onset of CMV disease was significantly delayed in the nonmyeloablative group compared to the control group (medians of 130 days vs 52 days, $P = 0.02$). These results agreed with the evolution of CMV-specific immunity after nonmyeloablative or conventional HCT, and emphasized that nonmyeloablative HCT recipients should receive CMV surveillance beyond day 100 and preemptive ganciclovir treatment similar to that routinely given to recipients of myeloablative regimens.

The same authors analyzed the incidence of bacterial infections during the first 100 days and of fungal infections during the first year posttransplantation.[56]

The 30- and 100-day incidences of bacteremia were 9 and 27% in the nonmyeloablative group versus 27% (P = 0.01) and 41% (P = 0.07) in the control group, respectively. Invasive aspergillosis occurred at a similar rate (15% in the nonmyeloablative group vs 9% in the control group, P = NS). Fukuda et al. analyzed risks and outcomes of invasive fungal infections in 163 nonmyeloablative HCT recipients. The 1-year cumulative incidence of proven or probable invasive fungal infections, invasive mold infections, invasive aspergillosis, and invasive candidiasis were 19, 15, 14, and 5%, respectively. Invasive mold infections occurred late (median 107 days) after nonmyeloablative HCT. Risks factors were GvHD and CMV disease. Nonrelapse mortality in nonmyeloablative recipients' was 22%, of which 39% were mold infection related.

## PRELIMINARY RESULTS WITH NONMYELOABLATIVE CONDITIONING

### HLA-MATCHED RELATED GRAFTS

We recently reviewed results of the first 212 patients treated by our group of collaborators.[18] Conditioning regimens consisted of 2 Gy TBI alone (n = 102), or 90 mg/m$^2$ fludarabine plus 2 Gy TBI (n = 110). Patient diagnoses included multiple myeloma (n = 66), acute leukemias or myelodysplastic syndromes (n = 58), chronic leukemias (n = 43), lymphomas (n = 41), and other hematologic malignancies (n = 4). Median patient age was 55 (range 18–73) years. The declines in blood counts after HCT were generally modest. The incidences of grade II, III, and IV acute GvHD were 29, 10, and 5%, respectively. Chronic GvHD was seen in 65% of patients. With a median follow-up of 11.5 (3–42) months, overall survival and progression-free survival were 63 and 52%, respectively. Typically, remissions occurred over extended periods of time, and some patients achieved complete remissions beyond 1 year posttransplant.

### HLA-MATCHED UNRELATED GRAFTS

Maris et al. reported the results in 89 patients given grafts from unrelated donors matched for HLA-A, -B, and -C antigens and HLA-DRB1 and -DQBI alleles.[39] The median patient age was 53 (range 5–69) years. Diagnoses included were acute leukemias (n = 17), myelodysplastic syndromes (n = 21), chronic leukemias (n = 19), multiple myeloma (n = 7), lymphomas (n = 17), or other hematologic malignancies (n = 8). Stem cell sources were marrow (n = 18) or G-PBMC (n = 71). Durable engraftment was observed in 85% of G-PBMC and 56% of marrow recipients (P = 0.007). Factors associated with increased risks of graft rejection were marrow instead of G-PBMC as stem cell source and the absence of chemotherapy preceding HCT. Cumulative probabilities of grades II, III, and IV acute GvHD were 42, 8, and 2%, respectively. Chronic

extensive GvHD was seen in 37% of patients. Grades II–IV acute GvHD (P = 0.02) and chronic GvHD (P = 0.04) were associated with decreased risks of relapse. Nonrelapse mortality at day 100 and 1 year were 11 and 16%, respectively. One-year overall and progression-free survivals were 57 and 44% for G-PBMC recipients, and 33 (P = 0.13) and 17% (P = 0.02), respectively, for marrow recipients. Risk factors favorably associated with improved overall survival in a multivariate analysis included <5% blasts in the marrow before HCT, low relapse risk disease category, transplantation from female donors, and CD3$^+$ cell doses ≥2.33 × 10$^8$ cells/kg.

## HCT WITH NONMYELOABLATIVE CONDITIONING AFTER FAILURE OF PREVIOUS HCT

Given that TRM after a second myeloablative allogeneic HCT in adults ranges from 50 to 80%,[57] several authors have investigated the use of nonmyeloablative or reduced-intensity conditioning regimens in this setting. Nagler et al. described 12 high-risk, heavily treated patients with a median age of 33 (range 8–63) years who received HLA-identical sibling (n = 9) or unrelated (n = 3) HCT[58] for acute leukemias or lymphomas. Patients were conditioned with a reduced-intensity regimen consisting of fludarabine (180 mg/m$^2$), busulfan (8 mg/kg/day), and ATG (40 mg/kg). Three-year TRM and progression-free survival rates were 10 and 50%, respectively. Branson et al. reported on 38 patients with refractory, progressive, or relapsed lymphoproliferative diseases after autologous HCT.[59] The median age was 44 (range 25–64) years. The conditioning regimen consisted of Campath-1H (100 mg), fludarabine (150 mg/m$^2$), and melphalan (140 mg/m$^2$). Fourteen-month TRM and progression-free survival rates were 20 and 50%, respectively. Feinstein et al. studied 55 patients with a median age of 43 (range 18–69) years who failed previous myeloablative autologous (n = 49), allogeneic (n = 4), or syngeneic (n = 2) HCT.[60] All patients were considered ineligible for conventional allografts because of age (older than 30 years), medical infirmity, or high-risk of TRM (prior high-dose TBI or dose-limiting organ irradiation). Twelve patients had disease that remained untreated after they failed conventional HCT, and 13 others had treatment-refractory disease at the time of the nonmyeloablative HCT. The nonmyeloablative conditioning regimen consisted of 2 Gy TBI alone (n = 7), or 2 Gy TBI and 90 mg/m$^2$ fludarabine (n = 48). Donors were HLA-identical siblings (n = 31) or HLA-matched unrelated donors (n = 24). Thirty-three patients died a median of 127 days (range 7–834 days) after HCT: 21 of relapse, 11 of TRM, and 1 of suicide. The TRM rate on day 100 was 11%, with an estimated 1-year TRM rate of 20%. One-year progression-free survival was 28%, and untreated disease at the time of the nonmyeloablative HCT increased the risk of death.

## RESULTS IN DIFFERENT DISEASE SETTINGS
### Myeloid malignancies

Or et al. reported results of a reduced-intensity conditioning regimen HCT in 24 CML patients in first chronic phase. Patients had a median age of 35 (range 3–63) years.[36] Nineteen received their HCT from HLA-matched family members (18 siblings and one father), and five patients received their HCT from HLA-matched unrelated donors. The 5-year probability of progression-free survival was 85% [95% confidence interval (CI) 70–100%], suggesting that results after a reduced-intensity conditioning regimen may be as good as after myeloablative conditioning in chronic-phase CML. Feinstein et al.[61] reported outcomes in 18 patients with de novo ($n = 13$) or secondary ($n = 5$) AML in first complete remission who received a nonmyeloablative HCT from HLA-identical sibling donors. Median age was 59 (range 36–73) years. Conditioning consisted of 2 Gy TBI alone ($n = 10$) or combined with fludarabine ($n = 8$). Two rejections were observed in patients not given fludarabine, and one of the two died with relapse. At a median follow-up of 766 days, seven patients have remained in complete remission. The 1-year estimates of TRM, overall survival, and progression-free survival were 17 (95% CI 0–35%), 54 (95% CI 31–78%), and 42% (95% CI 19–66%), respectively. For the 13 patients older than 55 years, the figures were 8 (95% CI 0–22%), 68 (95% CI 43–94%), and 59% (95% CI 31–87%), respectively. These results are promising, as the 1-year progression-free survival for AML patients older than 55 years is around 45% with conventional chemotherapy.

### Chronic lymphocytic leukemia

Dreger et al. reported results of 77 patients who received reduced-intensity conditioning regimen HCT ($n = 34$) or nonmyeloablative HCT ($n = 43$) for CLL in EBMT-affiliated centers.[62] The median age was 54 (range 30–66) years, and the median number of previous chemotherapy regimens was 3 (range 0–8). Eight patients were in complete remission, 42 in partial remission, and 27 had refractory disease at transplant. The 1-year probability of TRM was 18% (95% CI 9–37%), and the 2-year probabilities of overall survival and progression-free survival were 72 (95% CI 61–83%) and 56% (95% CI 43–69), respectively.

Sorror et al. recently reported outcomes in 14 chemotherapy-refractory CLL patients who received a nonmyeloablative HCT from HLA-matched unrelated donors.[63] The median patient age was 58 (range 48–67) years. Two patients rejected their transplants. With a median follow-up of 19 months, seven patients were in complete remission, two in partial remission, and two had stable disease. Estimated 2-year progression-free survival was 62%.

### Lymphoma

Robinson et al. reported results in 188 patients with lymphoma [low-grade NHL $n = 52$, high-grade NHL ($n = 62$), Hodgkin's disease ($n = 52$), and mantle cell lymphoma ($n = 22$)] who received various reduced-intensity conditioning regimens or nonmyeloablative HCT in EBMT-affiliated centers.[46] The median age was 40 (range 2–61) years, and the median number of prior treatment courses was 3 (range 0–6). Forty-eight percent of patients had undergone prior autologous transplantation. The 1-year probability of TRM was 25.5%. The 1-year probability of progression-free survival was 46%, and was significantly better in patients with chemosensitive disease, Hodgkin's disease, and low-grade NHL.

### Multiple myeloma

We recently reported results in 54 multiple myeloma patients who first received a cytoreductive autologous HCT followed by a planned nonmyeloablative HCT.[64] Patients were 29–71 (median 52) years old and had previously treated stage II or III multiple myeloma. Forty-eight percent had refractory (35%) or relapsed (13%) disease. Conditioning regimens for autologous and nonmyeloablative transplants were melphalan 200 mg/m[2] and 2 Gy TBI, respectively. Nonmyeloablative HCT was performed 40–229 (median 62) days after the autologous transplant. The 100-day mortalities after autologous and allogeneic HCT were 2 and 2%, respectively. With a median follow-up of 552 days after allografting, 57% of patients achieved complete remissions and 26% partial remissions. Of the 28 patients with responsive disease entering the trial (complete/partial remissions), 3 have died and 2 have had disease progression. In contrast, of the 26 patients with relapsed or refractory disease at study entry, 9 have died. Causes of death in both groups were complications related to GvHD ($n = 4$), progression ($n = 3$), pulmonary failure ($n = 2$), lung cancer ($n = 1$), CMV infection ($n = 1$), and encephalopathy ($n = 1$). The estimated 2-year overall and progression-free survivals were 78 and 55%, respectively.

## SUMMARY

Reduced-intensity conditioning and nonmyeloablative regimens allowed engraftment of allogeneic hematopoietic cells and the development of GvT effects. Remarkably, a minimally toxic regimen of 2 Gy TBI with or without fludarabine followed by postgrafting immunosuppression with MMF and CSP assured engraftment rates similar to those following myeloablative conditioning. Antitumor responses occurred after the achievement of full donor T-cell chimerism, though complete remissions required extended periods of time, with some patients achieving complete remissions more than 1 year after transplant. In patients with slowly progressing diseases such as CLL, low-grade NHL, chronic-phase CML, or with more aggressive diseases in complete remission, nonmyeloablative conditioning may be sufficient to achieve engraftment and cure. In patients with aggressive diseases such as acute leukemias, multiple myeloma, high-grade lymphomas, and Hodgkin's disease not in complete remission, cytoreduction by preceding chemotherapy or autologous HCT may be required. Remaining challenges include prevention of both severe GvHD and infections, in particular invasive fungal infections. Further progress in adoptive transfer of T-cell populations with relative tumor specificity is likely to make HCT after reduced-intensity or nonmyeloablative regimens more effective, and might even extend the use of allogeneic HCT to the therapy of nonhematopoietic malignancies.

## REFERENCES

1. Molina AJ, Storb RF: Hematopoietic stem cell transplantation in older adults. In: Rowe JM, Lazarus HM, Carella AM (eds.) *Handbook of Bone Marrow Transplantation.* 1st ed. London: Martin Dunitz Ltd; 2000:111.
2. Weiden PL, Flournoy N, Thomas ED, et al.: Antileukemic effect of graft-versus-host disease in human recipients of allogeneic-marrow grafts. *N Engl J Med* 300:1068, 1979.
3. Sullivan KM, Weiden PL, Storb R, et al.: Influence of acute and chronic graft-versus-host disease on relapse and survival after bone marrow transplantation from HLA-identical siblings as treatment of acute and chronic leukemia. *Blood* 73:1720, 1989.
4. Kolb HJ, Schattenberg A, Goldman JM, et al.: Graft-versus-leukemia effect of donor lymphocyte transfusions in marrow grafted patients. European Group for Blood and Marrow Transplantation Working Party Chronic Leukemia. *Blood* 86:2041, 1995.
5. Collins RH Jr, Goldstein S, Giralt S, et al.: Donor leukocyte infusions in acute lymphocytic leukemia. *Bone Marrow Transplant* 26:511, 2000.
6. Giralt S, Estey E, Albitar M, et al.: Engraftment of allogeneic hematopoietic progenitor cells with purine analog-containing chemotherapy: harnessing graft-versus-leukemia without myeloablative therapy. *Blood* 89:4531, 1997.
7. Slavin S, Nagler A, Naparstek E, et al.: Nonmyeloablative stem cell transplantation and cell therapy as an alternative to conventional bone marrow transplantation with lethal cytoreduction for the treatment of malignant and nonmalignant hematologic diseases. *Blood* 91:756, 1998.
8. Khouri IF, Keating M, Körbling M, et al.: Transplant-lite: induction of graft-versus-malignancy using fludarabine-based nonablative chemotherapy and allogeneic blood progenitor-cell transplantation as treatment for lymphoid malignancies. *J Clin Oncol* 16:2817, 1998.
9. McSweeney PA, Niederwieser D, Shizuru JA, et al.: Hematopoietic cell transplantation in older patients with hematologic malignancies: replacing high-dose cytotoxic therapy with graft-versus-tumor effects. *Blood* 97:3390, 2001.
10. Spitzer TR, McAfee S, Sackstein R, et al.: Intentional induction of mixed chimerism and achievement of antitumor responses after nonmyeloablative conditioning therapy and HLA-matched donor bone marrow transplantation for refractory hematologic malignancies. *Biol Blood Marrow Transplant* 6:309, 2000.
11. Childs R, Chernoff A, Contentin N, et al.: Regression of metastatic renal-cell carcinoma after nonmyeloablative allogeneic peripheral-blood stem-cell transplantation. *N Engl J Med* 343:750, 2000.
12. Simmons PJ, Przepiorka D, Thomas ED, et al.: Host origin of marrow stromal cells following allogeneic bone marrow transplantation. *Nature* 328:429, 1987.
13. Storb R, Yu C, Barnett T, et al.: Stable mixed hematopoietic chimerism in dog leukocyte antigen-identical littermate dogs given lymph node irradiation before and pharmacologic immunosuppression after marrow transplantation. *Blood* 94:1131, 1999.
14. Buckley RH, Schiff SE, Schiff RI, et al.: Hematopoietic stem-cell transplantation for the treatment of severe combined immunodeficiency. *N Engl J Med* 340:508, 1999.
15. Woolfrey AE, Nash RA, Sanders JE, et al.: A nonmyeloablative regimen for induction of multi-lineage hematopoietic mixed donor-host chimerism in nonmalignant disorders. *Blood* 98(pt 1):784a, 3390, 2000.
16. Bethge WA, Wilbur DS, Storb R, et al.: Selective T-cell ablation with bismuth-213-labeled anti-TCRαβ as nonmyeloablative conditioning for allogeneic canine marrow transplantation. *Blood* 101:5068, 2003.
17. Barnes DWH, Corp MJ, Loutit JF, et al.: Treatment of murine leukaemia with x-rays and homologous bone marrow. Preliminary communication. *Br Med J* 2:626, 1956.
18. Storb, R.: Allogeneic hematopoietic stem cell transplantation—yesterday, today, and tomorrow. *Exp Hematol* 31:1, 2003.
19. Zittoun RA, Mandelli F, Willemze R, et al.: Autologous or allogeneic bone marrow transplantation compared with intensive chemotherapy in acute myelogenous leukemia. *N Engl J Med* 332:217, 1995.
20. Clift RA, Buckner CD, Appelbaum FR, et al.: Allogeneic marrow transplantation in patients with acute myeloid leukemia in first remission: a randomized trial of two irradiation regimens. *Blood* 76:1867, 1990.
21. Clift RA, Buckner CD, Appelbaum FR, et al.: Allogeneic marrow transplantation in patients with chronic myeloid leukemia in the chronic phase: a randomized trial of two irradiation regimens. *Blood* 77:1660, 1991.
22. Barsoukov AA, Moore PF, Storb R, et al.: The use of an anti-TCRαβ monoclonal antibody to control host-versus-graft reactions in canine marrow allograft recipients conditioned with low dose total body irradiation. *Transplantation* 67:1329, 1999.
23. Raff RF, Deeg HJ, Loughran TP Jr, et al.: Characterization of host cells involved in resistance to marrow grafts in dogs transplanted from unrelated DLA-nonidentical donors. *Blood* 68:861, 1986.
24. Sandmaier BM, Storb R, Bennett KL, et al.: Epitope specificity of CD44 for monoclonal antibody dependent facilitation of marrow engraftment in a canine model. *Blood* 91:3494, 1998.

25. Anasetti C, Amos D, Beatty PG, et al.: Effect of HLA compatibility on engraftment of bone marrow transplants in patients with leukemia or lymphoma. *N Engl J Med* 320:197, 1989.

26. Martin PJ, Hansen JA, Buckner CD, et al.: Effects of in vitro depletion of T cells in HLA-identical allogeneic marrow grafts. *Blood* 66:664, 1985.

27. Maraninchi D, Gluckman E, Blaise D, et al.: Impact of T-cell depletion on outcome of allogeneic bone-marrow transplantation for standard-risk leukaemias. *Lancet* 2:175, 1987.

28. Storb R, Raff RF, Appelbaum FR, et al.: What radiation dose for DLA-identical canine marrow grafts? *Blood* 72:1300, 1988.

29. Yu C, Storb R, Mathey B, et al.: DLA-identical bone marrow grafts after low-dose total body irradiation: effects of high-dose corticosteroids and cyclosporine on engraftment. *Blood* 86:4376, 1995.

30. Storb R, Yu C, Wagner JL, et al.: Stable mixed hematopoietic chimerism in DLA-identical littermate dogs given sublethal total body irradiation before and pharmacological immunosuppression after marrow transplantation. *Blood* 89:3048, 1997.

31. Hogan WJ, Little M-T, Zellmer E, et al.: Postgrafting immunosuppression with sirolimus and cyclosporine facilitates stable mixed hematopoietic chimerism in dogs given sublethal total body irradiation before marrow transplantation from DLA-identical littermates. *Biol Blood Marrow Transplant* 9:489, 2003.

32. Zaucha JM, Zellmer E, Georges G, et al.: G-CSF-mobilized peripheral blood mononuclear cells added to marrow facilitates engraftment in nonmyeloablated canine recipients: CD3 cells are required. *Biol Blood Marrow Transplant* 7:613, 2001.

33. Storb R, Yu C, Zaucha JM, et al.: Stable mixed hematopoietic chimerism in dogs given donor antigen, CTLA4Ig, and 100 cGy total body irradiation before and pharmacologic immunosuppression after marrow transplant. *Blood* 94:2523, 1999.

34. Giralt S, Thall PF, Khouri I, et al.: Melphalan and purine analog-containing preparative regimens: reduced-intensity conditioning for patients with hematologic malignancies undergoing allogeneic progenitor cell transplantation. *Blood* 97:631, 2001.

35. Kottaridis PD, Milligan DW, Chopra R, et al.: In vivo CAMPATH-1H prevents graft-versus-host disease following nonmyeloablative stem cell transplantation. *Blood* 96:2419, 2000.

36. Or R, Shapira MY, Resnick I, et al.: Nonmyeloablative allogeneic stem cell transplantation for the treatment of chronic myeloid leukemia in first chronic phase. *Blood* 101:441, 2003.

37. Khouri IF, Saliba RM, Giralt SA, et al.: Nonablative allogeneic hematopoietic transplantation as adoptive immunotherapy for indolent lymphoma: low incidence of toxicity, acute graft-versus-host disease, and treatment-related mortality. *Blood* 98:3595, 2001.

38. Childs R, Clave E, Contentin N, et al.: Engraftment kinetics after nonmyeloablative allogeneic peripheral blood stem cell transplantation: full donor T-cell chimerism precedes alloimmune responses. *Blood* 94:3234, 1999.

39. Maris MB, Niederwieser D, Sandmaier BM, et al.: HLA-matched unrelated donor hematopoietic cell transplantation after nonmyeloablative conditioning for patients with hematologic malignancies. *Blood* 102:2021, 2003.

40. Chakraverty R, Peggs K, Chopra R, et al.: Limiting transplantation-related mortality following unrelated donor stem cell transplantation by using a nonmyeloablative conditioning regimen. *Blood* 99:1071, 2002.

41. Niederwieser D, Maris M, Shizuru JA, et al.: Low-dose total body irradiation (TBI) and fludarabine followed by hematopoietic cell transplantation (HCT) from HLA-matched or mismatched unrelated donors and postgrafting immunosuppression with cyclosporine and mycophenolate mofetil (MMF) can induce durable complete chimerism and sustained remissions in patients with hematological diseases. *Blood* 101:1620, 2003.

42. Ueno NT, Cheng YC, Rondon G, et al.: Rapid induction of complete donor chimerism by the use of a reduced-intensity conditioning regimen composed of fludarabine and melphalan in allogeneic stem cell transplantation for metastatic solid tumors. *Blood* 102:3829, 2003.

43. Keil F, Prinz E, Moser K, et al.: Rapid establishment of long-term culture-initiating cells of donor origin after nonmyeloablative allogeneic hematopoietic stem-cell transplantation, and significant prognostic impact of donor T-cell chimerism on stable engraftment and progression-free survival. *Transplantation* 76:230, 2003.

44. Baron F, Schaaf-Lafontaine N, Humblet-Baron S, et al.: T-cell reconstitution after unmanipulated, CD8-depleted or CD34-selected nonmyeloablative peripheral blood stem-cell transplantation. *Transplantation* 76:1705, 2003.

45. Baron F, Baker JE, Storb R, et al.: Kinetics of engraftment in patients with hematologic malignancies given allogeneic hematopoietic cell transplantation after nonmyeloablative conditioning. *Blood* 104(8):2254, 2004.

46. Robinson SP, Goldstone AH, Mackinnon S, et al.: Chemoresistant or aggressive lymphoma predicts for a poor outcome following reduced-intensity allogeneic progenitor cell transplantation: an analysis from the Lymphoma Working Party of the European Group for Blood and Bone Marrow Transplantation. *Blood* 100:4310, 2002.

47. Weissinger F, Sandmaier BM, Maloney DG, et al.: Decreased transfusion requirements for patients receiving nonmyeloablative compared with conventional peripheral blood stem cell transplants from HLA-identical siblings. *Blood* 98:3584, 2001.

48. Hogan WJ, Maris M, Storer B, et al.: Hepatic injury after nonmyeloablative conditioning followed by allogeneic hematopoietic cell transplantation: a study of 193 patients. *Blood* 103(1):78, 2004.

49. Fukuda T, Hackman RC, Guthrie KA, et al.: Risks and outcomes of idiopathic pneumonia syndrome after nonmyeloablative and conventional conditioning regimens for allogeneic hematopoietic stem cell transplantation. *Blood* 102:2777, 2003.

50. Mohty M, Bay JO, Faucher C, et al.: Graft-versus-host disease following allogeneic transplantation from HLA-identical sibling with antithymocyte globulin-based reduced-intensity preparative regimen. *Blood* 102:470, 2003.

51. Mielcarek M, Martin PJ, Leisenring W, et al.: Graft-versus-host disease after nonmyeloablative versus

conventional hematopoietic stem cell transplantation. *Blood* 102:756, 2003.

52. Mohty M, Gaugler B, Faucher C, et al.: Recovery of lymphocyte and dendritic cell subsets following reduced intensity allogeneic bone marrow transplantation. *Hematology* 7:157, 2002.

53. Maris M, Boeckh M, Storer B, et al.: Immunologic recovery after hematopoietic cell transplantation with nonmyeloablative conditioning. *Exp Hematol* 31:941, 2003.

54. Mohty M, Jacot W, Faucher C, et al.: Infectious complications following allogeneic HLA-identical sibling transplantation with antithymocyte globulin-based reduced intensity preparative regimen. *Leukemia* 17:2168, 2003.

55. Junghanss C, Boeckh M, Carter RA, et al.: Incidence and outcome of cytomegalovirus infections following nonmyeloablative compared with myeloablative allogeneic stem cell transplantation, a matched control study. *Blood* 99:1978, 2002.

56. Junghanss C, Marr KA, Carter RA, et al.: Incidence and outcome of bacterial and fungal infections following nonmyeloablative compared with myeloablative allogeneic hematopoietic stem cell transplantation: a matched control study. *Biol Blood Marrow Transplant* 8:512, 2002.

57. Ringdén O, Labopin M, Gorin NC, et al.: The dismal outcome in patients with acute leukaemia who relapse after an autograft is improved if a second autograft or a matched allograft is performed. *Bone Marrow Transplant* 25:1053, 2000.

58. Nagler A, Or R, Naparstek E, et al.: Second allogeneic stem cell transplantation using nonmyeloablative conditioning for patients who relapsed or developed secondary malignancies following autologous transplantation. *Exp Hematol* 28:1096, 2000.

59. Branson K, Chopra R, Kottaridis PD, et al.: Role of nonmyeloablative allogeneic stem-cell transplantation after failure of autologous transplantation in patients with lymphoproliferative malignancies. *J Clin Oncol* 20:4022, 2002.

60. Feinstein LC, Sandmaier BM, Maloney DG, et al.: Allografting after nonmyeloablative conditioning as a treatment after a failed conventional hematopoietic cell transplant. *Biol Blood Marrow Transplant* 9:266, 2003.

61. Feinstein LC, Sandmaier BM, Hegenbart U, et al.: Non-myeloablative allografting from human leucocyte antigen-identical sibling donors for treatment of acute myeloid leukaemia in first complete remission. *Br J Haematol* 120:281, 2003.

62. Dreger P, Brand R, Hansz J, et al.: Treatment-related mortality and graft-versus-leukemia activity after allogeneic stem cell transplantation for chronic lymphocytic leukemia using intensity-reduced conditioning (Review). *Leukemia* 17:841, 2003.

63. Sorror ML, Maris M, Storer B, et al.: Nonmyeloablative (NM) conditioning and allogeneic hematopoietic cell transplantation (HCT) with HLA-matched unrelated donor (URD) for patients (Pts) with chemotherapy-refractory chronic lymphocytic leukemia (CLL). *Blood* 102(pt 1):482a, 1757, 2003.

64. Maloney DG, Molina AJ, Sahebi F, et al.: Allografting with nonmyeloablative conditioning following cytoreductive autografts for the treatment of patients with multiple myeloma. *Blood* 102:3447, 2003.

# Chapter 97

# UMBILICAL CORD BLOOD TRANSPLANTATION

## Ian Horkheimer and Nelson Chao

## INTRODUCTION

Transplantation of hematopoietic stem cells (HSCs) collected from bone marrow (BM) or peripheral blood (PB) of related and unrelated donors has become a successful treatment option for several malignant and nonmalignant disorders (Table 97.1). Further success has been hampered by the limited number of suitable HLA-matched donors, the prolonged length of donor unit procurement, and significant transplant-related morbidity. Over the past 15 years, in efforts to overcome these obstacles, allogeneic transplantation using umbilical cord blood (UCB) as an alternative source of HSCs has been investigated.

The use of UCB as a source of HSCs was proposed in the early 1980s. UCB cells have been shown in vitro to demonstrate both self-renewal and hematopoietic differentiation capabilities.[1-4] Umbilical cord blood transplantation (UCBT) entered the clinical arena in 1988 when a child with severe Fanconi anemia was successfully transplanted using UCB harvested from an HLA-matched sibling.[5] The Placental Blood Project was launched in 1993 to evaluate the clinical utility of expanding UCB as a source of HSCs. Shortly thereafter, mismatched related and unrelated UCBTs in children with high-risk leukemia were performed.[6] Since 1998, more than 2500 UCBTs have been completed—75% performed in children and the remaining 25% in adults.[7] Potential advantages of UCB as an alternative source of HSCs include (1) negligible risk to donor, (2) absence of donor attrition, (3) ease of procurement and rapid allocation, (4) reduced risk of graft-versus-host disease (GVHD), and (5) less stringent HLA-matching restrictions.

## UCB BANKING

Given today's population dynamics, the estimated probability of any patient obtaining an HLA-matched related-donor HSC unit is approximately 30–40%.[8] The likelihood of securing a matched unrelated donor unit varies according to ancestry and is less likely in patients of certain racial and ethnic backgrounds. As such, approximately 50% of all patients requiring allogeneic transplantation are unable to secure an unrelated HLA-matched donor unit.[9] As an alternative source of HSC, UCB has the potential to alleviate this donor shortage. UCB banks have been developed to optimize the chances of finding a suitable donor for allogeneic transplantation. Netcord, a cooperative network of large experienced UCB banks in the United States, Europe, Japan, and Australia was founded in 1998 to establish minimum UCBT standards, reach an international agreement on aspects that protect the infant donor and mother, and facilitate the matching process. As of March 2004, over 150,000 UCB units have been banked in 36 UCB registries throughout 21 countries.[10]

### ETHICAL CONSIDERATIONS

UCB as an alternative source for allogeneic transplantation has generated several ethical concerns.[11] In 1997, a working group composed of experts in medicine, blood banking, law, ethics, anthropology, and the social sciences convened to examine these issues.[12] A consensus statement to inform public policy and raise awareness regarding UCB banking procedures was generated. This statement addressed the following dilemmas: (1) the potential promise of UCB as an investigational agent, (2) maintaining linkage of the donors and stored UCB units, (3) the uncertainty of autologous UCB banking, (4) monitoring of private-sector marketing practices, (5) assuring equitable UCB banking recruitment and use, and (6) the process of obtaining informed consent.

### INFORMED CONSENT

Informed consent is routinely a prerequisite for the procedures of UCB banking. Prenatal efforts are often directed at recruiting potential donors. Information regarding the risks and benefits of the collection, storage, and potential uses of UCB are explained to parents of prospective donors. By convention, the mother must consent by proxy as UCB is technically of fetal

**Table 97.1** Diseases treated by UCBT

| Malignant | Nonmalignant |
| --- | --- |
| Acute lymphocytic leukemia | Fanconi's anemia |
| Acute myeloid leukemia | Severe combined immunodeficiency |
| Chronic myelogenous leukemia | Severe aplastic anemia |
| Juvenile chronic myelogenous leukemia | Osteopetrosis |
| Chronic lymphocytic leukemia | Thalassemia |
| Hodgkin's lymphoma | Myelofibrosis |
| Non-Hodgkin's lymphoma | Sickle cell anemia |
| Neuroblastoma | Hurler's syndrome |
| | Myelodysplastic syndrome |
| | Wiskott–Aldrich syndrome |
| | Adrenoleukody-strophy |
| | Blackfan–Diamond Syndrome |
| | Hunter syndrome |
| | Amegakaryocytic thrombocytopenia |
| | Lesch–Nyhan Syndrome |
| | Gunther's disease |
| | Kostman syndrome |
| | X-linked lymphoproliferative disorder |

origin. At least four models of obtaining informed consent exist: before labor, during labor, after collection, and phased.[13] Before-labor consent allows the donor parent(s) to review and examine the consent documents weeks to months prior to childbirth. Donors not exposed to recruitment efforts, often as a result of inadequate prenatal care, may be excluded; potential restriction in the diversity of the global UCB bank may result. During-labor consent occurs during the early phase of labor. Consent for testing and donation may also be obtained at this time. The after-collection model does not require consent for UCB collection. Once collected, an informed consent process for testing and donation is engaged. This may be troublesome given various personal, cultural, and religious beliefs toward UCB. In light of the potential advantages and disadvantages of these consent models, a phased consent policy has been adopted by some authorities. The premise upon which this policy is based is that the decision to collect UCB is not necessarily closely linked to the decision to test or donate the unit. In the first phase, information regarding UCB is dispersed during prenatal visits. Consent for the second and third phase may be completed at this time. Omission of the first phase does not preclude progression to the second or third phases. The second phase begins during labor when a consent form is delivered and reviewed explaining the process of UCB collection. The final phase is completed after delivery when the mother may agree to the processing, storage, and potential transplantation of the collected UCB.

Policies and recommendations vary based on patient demographics and the practices of health care providers. Nearly all centers employing in vitro UCB collection methods require prelabor consent. The largest UCB bank in the world, the New York Blood Center, uses the after-collection model. The phased-consent policy has been adopted by the American Red Cross, North Central Blood Services Cord Blood Bank. The American Medical Association Working Group on Ethical Issues of Umbilical Cord Blood Banking states "In general, when UCB collection is anticipated, the norm should be to obtain written informed consent before labor and delivery, followed by an affirmation of this consent after delivery."[12]

## COLLECTION

Optimal yield of mononuclear cells remains a critical factor in UCB collection. A suitable UCB unit has been defined as a volume of at least 40 ml (excluding anticoagulant) and a total nucleated cell (TNC) count of $6 \times 10$.[8,14] Factors associated with improved UCB harvest include fewer previous births, larger infant size, greater gestational age, longer umbilical cord, and larger placenta.[15,16] Two methods of UCB collection exist in utero and ex utero. *In utero* collection is initiated within seconds of delivery of the baby but prior to expulsion of the placenta. The umbilical cord is clamped, transected, and disinfected. The umbilical vein is then punctured with a 16-gauge needle connected to a standard closed blood donor collection system (450 ml) containing approximately 20–30 ml of CPDA (citrate, phosphate, dextrose, adenine) anticoagulant, and drained by gravity. *Ex utero* UCB collection takes place immediately following placental delivery. The delivered placenta is placed in a plastic-lined absorbent cotton pad suspended from a support frame. Within minutes, the disinfected umbilical cord vein is punctured and drained into a blood donor set containing CPDA anticoagulant. The method of collection varies between UCB banks and among collection sites within UCB banks. A small, randomized single-institution trial detected a statistically significant increase in mean volume (83.26 ml vs. 48.42 ml) and mononuclear cell numbers ($3.12 \times 10^8$ vs. $1.806 \times 10^8$) with *in utero* collection.[17] This was supported by a retrospective single-institution analysis.[18] A large, retrospective multicenter analysis of five programs established by the American Red Cross Cord Program argued equivalency between *in utero* and *ex utero* methods.[19]

## PROCESSING, STORAGE, AND PREPARATION FOR USE

In 1995, the National Heart, Lung, and Blood Institute funded three UCB banks and six transplant centers to assist in establishing standard operation procedures for the collection, processing, and investigation of UCB use.[14] Several modifications of the standard procedure of UCB processing and storage have been developed to reduce unit size (and thus storage costs) and enhance red blood cell (RBC) depletion while maintaining sterility and HSC composition and activity.[20–26] Three to five milliliters of UCB is removed for HLA-typing, disease testing, microbiological cultures, progenitor cell assays, and assessment of total nucleated and CD34+ cell counts. RBC depletion and volume reduction begin with the addition of 6% hydroxyethyl starch to enhance RBC sedimentation. The mixture is centrifuged at 50$g$ for 5 minutes. The leukocyte-containing supernatant is then centrifuged at 400$g$ for 10 min yielding a sediment of white cells. The leukocyte pellet is resuspended in plasma and diluted to a final volume of 20 ml.

UCB is cryopreserved with chilled dimethyl sulfoxide to a final concentration of 10% and a total volume of 25 ml. The sample is placed in aluminum containers and frozen to −50°C in a −80°C freezer. The UCB unit is then transferred to a liquid nitrogen storage device where it may be housed for several years.[27]

Preparation of a frozen UCB unit for infusion is similar to the procedure used for PB stem cell units. The unit is placed in a sterile, sealable plastic bag, submerged, and gently agitated in a 37°C water bath. When thawed, equal volumes of 10% dextran and 5% albumin are added to a volume double of that was originally collected. The suspension is then centrifuged at 250$g$ for 10 min. The pellet is resuspended with equal volumes (50 ml) of 10% dextran and 5% albumin. Samples of the final unit are sent for bacterial and fungal cultures.

### HLA TYPING AND UCB TESTING

UCB is HLA typed and subjected to a standard battery of laboratory tests prior to storage. More specific testing for genetic diseases is guided by the donor's history. As a result of the prospective HLA typing and testing, the time required to find a UCB donor and proceed to transplantation is significantly reduced compared to that required for BM sources[28] (Table 97.2). HLA typing in preparation for allogeneic transplantation has largely focused on class I (HLA-A and HLA-B) and class II (DRB) antigens. Class I antigens are typed by serologic methods (microlymphocytotoxicity assay), while class II antigens are identified with molecular biology techniques (low- and high-resolution polymerase chain reaction (PCR)). HLA typing of UCB poses certain obstacles, particularly for the serologic assays. Available tissue is often limited due to efforts to maximize the volume of cells available for infusion. The sample size may be inadequate for either initial or repeat typing efforts. In addition, interference with serologic reagents, a high background of dead cells, and contamination of the sample with immature erythroblasts and early myeloid cells may make the results uninterpretable. Given this, recent interest in

molecular typing of class I antigens has been generated. A review of 1644 UCB units deemed 14.5% of the serologically HLA-typed class I antigens unsatisfactory due to cross-reactions, false positives, unclear split assessments, or an inability to perform the assay due to poor cell viability.[29] Of these unreliable samples 100 were analyzed using molecular biology (PCR) methods, which found that the initial serologic HLA type was incorrectly determined in 56.7% of the units. Nearly 20% could not be typed due to high cell mortality. Similar results were reported in a separate review of over 200 consecutively HLA-typed UCB units.[30]

## UCB BIOLOGIC CHARACTERIZATION AND IMMUNE RECONSTITUTION

Successful allogeneic transplantation relies on hematopoietic recovery and immune reconstitution and maturation, processes that depend in part on the cellular components of the graft. HSCs can be identified by in vitro colony assays and can be further characterized phenotypically using flow cytometric techniques. Human HSCs have been defined as either pluripotent or lineage committed. Pluripotent HSCs have the capacity for both self-renewal and sustained differentiation, whereas lineage-committed human HSCs have the potential for self-renewal but are destined to differentiate along a specific hematopoietic lineage. Pluripotent HSCs are CD34+CD38−CD90+ HLA-DR−. Lineage-committed HSCs are CD34+38+, with coexpression of either CD33 (myeloid), CD15 (late myeloid), CD64 (granulomonocytic), CD71 (erythroid), CD61 (megakaryocytic), CD7 (T cell), or CD19 (B cell) antigens. UCB contains a disproportionately higher number of phenotypically immature HSCs. UCB immune function is also thought to be immature. In vitro, UCB T cells demonstrate decreased allogeneic responses following primary antigen stimulation.[31,32]

| Table 97.2 | Tests commonly performed on UCB |
|---|---|
| ABO and Rh blood group antigens | |
| Blood group antibody screen | |
| HLA class I and II typing | |
| Hemoglobin electrophoresis | |
| G-6PD activity | |
| Osmotic fragility and spectrin/ankrin analysis | |
| VDRL/RPR | |
| Bacterial and fungal cultures | |
| Cytomegalovirus (CMV) IgM antibody | |
| Hepatitis B virus core antibody and surface antigen | |
| Hepatitis C virus antibody and PCR | |
| Human immunodeficiency virus (HIV) ELISA/Western Blot, p24 antigen, and PCR | |
| Human T-lymphocyte virus (HTLV) I, II ELISA/Western Blot | |

Following allogeneic stem cell transplant, engraftment is dependent on pluripotent and myeloid lineage-committed HSCs. B-cell reconstitution begins with differentiation of donor-derived HSCs and CD34$^+$CD38$^+$CD19$^+$CD20$^+$ B-lineage committed HSCs in the PB and BM. T-cell reconstitution is believed to occur initially by a thymic-independent pathway. Antigen stimulation drives the conversion of naïve CD45RA$^+$CD45RO$^-$ T cells present in the allograft to memory CD45RA$^-$CD45RO$^+$ T cells with resultant limited T-cell receptor (TCR) diversity.[33–35] Following this, a thymic-dependent pathway is responsible for further immune reconstitution. CD34$^+$CD38$^+$CD7$^+$CD3$^-$ T-lineage-specific HSCs repopulate in the BM and migrate to the thymus. These HSCs down-regulate CD34 antigen and eventually become CD4$^+$CD8$^+$ T-cell precursors. TCRs are up-regulated as is CD3 antigen. CD4 or CD8 antigen is then selectively lost, resulting in a more durable and diverse naïve CD45RA$^+$CD45RO$^-$ CD4$^+$ or CD8$^+$ T-cell repertoire.[33,36,37]

### BIOLOGIC CHARACTERIZATION

Comparative flow cytometry analyses of the cellular content of UCB, BM, and PB units have been performed.[38,39] The absolute number of pluripotent HSCs was significantly reduced in UCB units as compared to BM and PB units. A mean of $0.21 \times 10^6$ cells/UCB unit was approximately 1/10 that of the other sources, but these HSCs were present at a higher frequency (UCB 3.39%, BM 1.47%, PB 1.82%). UCB units also possessed a significantly lower absolute number of myeloid-committed HSCs (26–65 fold) and fewer total lymphocytes ($0.59 \times 10^9$ cells/unit) as compared to BM and PB sources. Of these lymphocytes, the frequency of B cells in UCB samples (18.5%) was similar to BM units and approximately twice that of PB units. The percentage of B-lineage-specific HSCs was greater in UCB units (3.79%) as compared to PB units, although no difference was detected in the frequency of immature CD19$^+$CD20$^-$ B cells and mature CD19$^+$CD20$^+$ B cells. The proportion of T cells in UCB samples (58%) was similar to that of BM, both of which were decreased as compared to PB samples (71.2%). T-lineage-specific HSCs were present at a three- to fourfold higher frequency in UCB units (12.1%) as compared to BM and PB units. UCB units also had a higher frequency of naïve CD45RA$^+$CD45RO$^-$ CD4$^+$ and CD8$^+$ cells. The percentage of NK cells (CD3$^-$CD16/56$^+$) was highest in UCB units as compared to that in BM and PB sources (24.8%, 15.0%, and 8.5%, respectively).

### IMMUNE RECONSTITUTION

Following UCBT, B-cell recovery is commonly regained within weeks, while T-cell competence is often not complete for 12–36 or more months. Quantitative assessment of immune reconstitution may be performed by determining lymphocyte subset counts. Qualitative determination may be undertaken by evaluation of T-cell-receptor excision circles (TRECs)—stable, nonreplicating episomal DNA by-products of the TCR rearrangement process. TRECs provide an estimate of the thymus's ability to produce new T cells.[40] Analysis of TCR Vβ-chain complimentary determining region 3 (CDR3) is a measure of TCR diversity.[41]

Quantitative immune reconstitution in children the first 100 days post-UCBT has been evaluated.[42] B-cell counts increased to normal levels 30–90 days post-transplant as did serum immunoglobulin levels. NK cell counts remained within the normal range during the first 100 days. CD4$^+$ and CD8$^+$ T-cell counts did not recover during this period. Additional pediatric patients were followed several months post-UCBT.[43] CD4$^+$ and CD8$^+$ cells recovered at medians of 12 and 9 months. Multivariate analysis of factors affecting lymphocyte subsets revealed that GVHD had an adverse affect on CD4$^+$ recovery. Recipients of unrelated-donor grafts had worse CD8$^+$ recovery. A separate analysis in children found that naïve and memory T-cell counts reached normal levels between 6 and 12 months post-UCBT in children. In adults, CD4$^+$ and CD8$^+$ T cells did not reach normal levels until 2 years post-UCBT, while naïve and memory T-cell recovery were delayed until 3 years post-UCBT.[44] TREC determination and Vβ-chain TCR CDR3 analysis following UCBT has been assessed in both children and adults.[44,45] TREC levels and Vβ-chain TCR diversity were limited in both populations in the first 2–6 months post-UCBT. In children, TCR diversity broadened as early as 9 months; TREC levels were detectable 1 year post-UCBT. In adults, development of TCR diversity was delayed until nearly 3 years post-UCBT. TREC levels were first detected at 18 months. Increasing TREC levels in both children and adults coincided with the appearance of naïve CD4$^+$ T cells. These data suggest that the antigen-driven peripheral expansion of T cells following pediatric UCBT is more short lived as a result of earlier thymic-dependent immune reconstitution. Following adult UCBT, thymic-dependent immune reconstitution is more delayed.

### CLINICAL DATA

The promising results of UCB as an alternative source of HSCs in pediatric related- and unrelated-donor transplantation generated worldwide interest. In 1992, in an attempt to more quickly learn the true risks and benefits of UCBT, the International Cord Blood Transplant Registry (ICBTR), now a part of the International Bone Marrow Transplant Registry (IBMTR), was established as a repository of clinical data on the outcomes of patients who received UCB. EuroCord, a registry and forum for the development of cooperative studies within the European community, was formed in 1995. Success in the pediatric population eventually led to UCBT for adult diseases. Analyses of UCBT clinical data have shown that the most important factor in predicting the rate and likelihood of engraftment is the number of nucleated cells infused (cell dose = TNC/kg). On the basis of the increased body mass of adults, the reduced cell dose limits the utility of UCB in this population. GVHD appears to occur less frequently following UCBT as compared to transplantation from BM and PB sources. This is thought to be a consequence of the immature immune characteristics of UCB. As a result of the reduced rates of GVHD, a greater degree of HLA disparity is allowed, further enlarging the potential-donor pool. Given the immature immune function of UCB grafts, a diminished graft-versus-leukemia (GVL) effect has been postulated but not observed. GVL effect following UCBT is believed to be the result of early $CD3^-CD16/56^+$ NK-cell recovery eventually followed by T-cell reconstitution. Transplant-related mortality (TRM) following UCBT remains a significant limitation, particularly in the adult population, and is most often a result of the conditioning regimen, failed or delayed engraftment (infection and/or hemorrhage), or GVHD.

### PEDIATRIC RELATED-DONOR UCBT

The clinical data reported on pediatric related-donor UCBT are largely based on the experiences of the ICBTR[46,47] and the EuroCord Registry[48–50] (Table 97.3). The ICBTR reported on 74 children with a median age of 4.9 years. Both malignant and nonmalignant diseases were treated. The conditioning regimen was total body irradiation (TBI) based in half of the patients. GVHD prophylaxis consisted of cyclosporine and either prednisone or methotrexate. HLA type was identical or disparate at one locus in 75% of the patients. The EuroCord Registry reported on 138 patients with a median age of 5 years, 63% of whom had a malignant disease. The conditioning regimen varied according to disease and age, but again was TBI based in approximately half of the patients. GVHD prophylaxis consisted mainly of cyclosporine. The majority of the grafts were HLA identical.

The ICBTR reported a 91% engraftment rate at day 60 with median neutrophil recovery at 22 days in closely HLA-matched patients. Platelet recovery occurred at a median of 51 days. There was no statistical correlation between engraftment and cell dose. The EuroCord Registry noted an 83% probability of engraftment with neutrophil recovery occurring at a median of 26 days. This was associated with a cell dose of $\geq 3.7 \times 10^7$/kg.

The ICBTR recorded a 3% rate of acute GVHD in patients with 0–1 HLA mismatch, followed by three cases of chronic GVHD. The EuroCord Registry reported acute grade II–IV GVHD in 20% of patients and chronic GVHD in 6%. Fifty percent of patients

| Table 97.3 Pediatric related donor UCBT | | |
|---|---|---|
| | ICBTR[46,47] | EuroCord[48–50] |
| Cell Dose (TNC/kg) | $4.7 \times 10^7$ | $4.0 \times 10^7$ |
| Engraftment %: median days to neutrophil recovery | 91%[a] <br> 22 | 83% <br> 26 |
| Acute GVHD | 3% | 20% |
| TRM | NA | NA |
| Relapse | 49% | 22% |
| Survival: <br> EFS <br> OS | 46%[b] <br> 76%[c] <br> 62%[d] | NA <br> <br> 63%[e] |

UCBT, umbilical cord blood transplantation; ICBTR, International Cord Blood Transplant Registry; TNC, total nucleated cells; GVHD, graft-versus-host disease; TRM, transplant-related mortality; EFS, event-free survival; OS, overall survival; NA, not available.
[a]Observed at 60 days.
[b]Observed in patients with malignant diseases.
[c]Observed in patients with nonmalignant diseases.
[d]Observed at 1.6 years.
[e]Observed at 1 year.

with any HLA disparity developed grade II–IV GVHD, while only 9% did so in HLA-identical transplants.

Initial reports from the ICBTR and EuroCord Registry noted relapse in 49 and 22% of patients with malignancies. The ICBTR reported a 46% event-free survival (EFS) for patients with a malignant disease compared to 78% for patients with a nonmalignant condition. The overall survival (OS) for all patients was 62%, with a median follow-up of 1.6 years. Those who were HLA matched or disparate at one loci had a higher OS of 72%. The EuroCord Registry reported an OS of 63% at 1 year. The 2-year OS varied with disease—46% in patients with malignancies, 76% with aplastic anemia, 79% with inborn errors of metabolism, and 100% with hemoglobinopathies. OS correlated with infusion of $\geq 3.7$ ($10^7$ TNC/kg, HLA identity (73% if HLA-identical and 33% with any HLA-disparity), age <6, weight <20 kg, and negative cytomegalovirus (CMV) serology.

In a multivariate analysis of data from the EuroCord Registry after related-donor HLA-matched UCBTs and SCTs, it was found that neutrophil and platelet recovery following UCBT were delayed as compared to that in SCT. Rates of acute and chronic GVHD were reduced following UCBT (RR 0.40 and 0.35, respectively). Survival was similar.[51]

### PEDIATRIC UNRELATED-DONOR UCBT

Data regarding pediatric unrelated-donor UCBT, of which nearly two-thirds were in patients with malignant diseases, have been reported by at least four sources: Minnesota/Duke,[46,52,53] New York Blood

**Table 97.4    Pediatric unrelated donor UCBT**

|  | Minnesota/Duke[46,52,53] | IMBTR[54] | EuroCord[49,50,55] | Minnesota[56] |
|---|---|---|---|---|
| Cell Dose (TNC/kg) | $4.0 \times 10^7$ | NA | $4.5 \times 10^7$ | $3.1 \times 10^7$ |
| Engraftment: median days to neutrophil recovery | %94% 24 | 91%[a] 28 | 82%[a] 29 | 88%[b] 23 |
| Acute GVHD: grade II–IV grade III–IV | 40% 10% | 44% 22% | 39% NA | 39% 11% |
| TRM | NA | NA | 34%[c] 65%[d] | 30%[e] 35%[f] |
| Relapse | NA | 14%[g] | 31%[c] 77%[d] | 37%[f] |
| Survival: EFS OS | NA 40%[f] | 54%[h] NA | 36%[f] NA | NA 58%[e] 47%[f] |

UCBT, umbilical cord blood transplantation; ICBTR, International Cord Blood Transplant Registry; TNC, total nucleated cells; GVHD, graft-versus-host disease; TRM, transplant-related mortality; EFS, event-free survival; OS, overall survival; NA, not available.
[a]Observed at 60 days.
[b]Observed at 42 days
[c]Observed in good risk malignancies.
[d]Observed in advanced malignancies.
[e]Observed at 1 year.
[f]Observed at 2 years.
[g]Observed in patients with leukemia.
[h]Observed at 100 days.

Center (NYBC) (IBMTR)[54] EuroCord Registry,[49,50,55] and Minnesota[56] (Table 97.4). The Minnesota/Duke group reported on 85 children with a median age of 5.6 years. The conditioning regimen varied, as did GVHD prophylaxis. Eleven percent were HLA identical, 35% were disparate at one locus, and the remaining grafts were mismatched at ≥2 loci. The NYBC registry (IBMTR) reported on 562 patients (460 of which were pediatric). Seven percent of the grafts were HLA identical, 39% were disparate at one locus, and 54% were mismatched at ≥2 loci. The EuroCord Registry reported on 291 patients with a median age of 5 years. The conditioning regimen varied according to disease. Seventeen percent were HLA identical with the remaining disparate at ≥1 loci. The Minnesota group reported on 102 patients (80 of which were pediatric). The median age was 7.4 years and the median weight was 25.9 kg. The conditioning regimen was mainly TBI/Cyclophosphamide(Cy). All patients received antithymocyte globulin (ATG). GVHD prophylaxis was largely cyclosporine and methylprednisolone. Fourteen percent were HLA identical, 43% were disparate at one locus, and the remaining grafts were mismatched at ≥2 loci.

The Minnesota/Duke group reported engraftment in 94% of the patients at a median of 24 days. Engraftment correlated with a cell dose $\geq 3 \times 10^7$/kg. The early use of granulocyte colony-stimulating factor and a conditioning regimen other than TBI also improved hematopoietic recovery. The IBMTR noted a median time to neutrophil recovery of 28 days. Ninety-one percent of the patients recovered their neutrophil counts by day 60. More rapid engraftment was associated with a greater number of UCB unit precryopreservation leukocytes and greater HLA identity. Platelet engraftment occurred in 58% of the patients by day 100 and 85% by day 180, with more rapid recovery in younger patients and those without infection or GVHD. The EuroCord Registry observed neutrophil recovery in 82% of the patients by day 60. The median time to recovery was 29 days. In a subgroup analysis, 79% of the patients with acute leukemia recovered neutrophil counts by 60 days. This correlated with a cell dose $\geq 3.7 \times 10^7$/kg. The Minnesota group recorded an engraftment rate of 88% by day 42. The median time to neutrophil recovery was 23 days and correlated with a CD34+ cell dose $\geq 1.7 \times 10^5$/kg. Platelet recovery occurred in 65% of the patients by six months, with a median time to recovery of 86 days. Platelet recovery was associated with younger age, higher CD34+ cell dose, and the lack of acute grade III–IV GVHD.

The Minnesota/Duke group noted acute grade II–IV GVHD in 40% of the patients and grade III–IV GVHD in 10%. No association between HLA disparity and acute GVHD was observed. The IBMTR, EuroCord Registry, and Minnesota group reported similar rates of acute grade II–IV GVHD. The IBMTR reported a trend ($p$ = 0.06) toward significance of an association between acute GVHD and HLA disparity. The observed rates of chronic GVHD from these sources ranged from 9 to 25%.

The EuroCord Registry's subgroup analysis of patients with acute leukemia noted a 1-year TRM of 34% in those with good risk disease as compared to 65% in those with advanced disease. The Minnesota group reported 1- and 2-year TRM rates of 30 and 35%. By univariate analysis, a reduction in 1-year TRM to 20% was demonstrated if the CD34$^+$ cell dose was ≥1.7 × 10$^5$/kg. Reduced TRM was also predicted by younger age, higher cell dose, and the absence of severe GVHD. By Cox regression analysis, CD34$^+$ cell dose, development of severe GVHD, and age were the only factors predictive of TRM. The IBMTR noted relapse in 14% of the patients with leukemia. Higher rates were seen in patients with advanced disease and acute myeloid leukemia (AML). The EuroCord Registry reported relapse in 31% of the patients with good risk leukemia as compared to 77% in patients with poor risk disease. The Minnesota group observed a 37% cumulative incidence of relapse at 2 years. By Cox regression analysis, this was associated with age and malignancy risk group, but not cell dose, HLA match, or prior acute/chronic GVHD.

The IBMTR reported a 54% EFS at 100 days. By multivariate analysis, correlation was noted between EFS and cell dose, HLA identity, diagnosis (CML > Fanconi anemia > severe aplastic anemia), younger age, and the location of the transplantation center. The EuroCord Registry reported a 2-year EFS of 21% in patients with aplastic anemia, 36% with malignant diseases, and 51% with inborn errors of metabolism. Of the patients with acute leukemia, the 2-year EFS was 49% in good risk patients as compared to 8% in those with advanced disease. The Minnesota/Duke group reported a 40% OS at 2 years. The Minnesota group observed an OS of 58% at 1 year and 47% at 2 years. The OS increased to 70% at 1 year in patients receiving ≥1.7 × 10$^5$ CD34$^+$ cells/kg. By univariate analysis, OS was associated with younger age, nonmalignant disease, higher cell dose, and the absence of severe GVHD. By Cox regression analysis, HLA match, CD34$^+$ cell dose, and absence of severe GVHD predicted OS.

The EuroCord Registry completed a comparative analysis of pediatric unrelated UCBTs and unmanipulated or T-cell depleted SCTs in patients with acute leukemia.[57] The majority of UCBTs were HLA mismatched. The median cell dose for those undergoing UCBT was 3.8 × 10$^7$/kg. Disease characteristics, conditioning regimens, and GVHD prophylaxis varied. A delay in neutrophil engraftment was noted in those undergoing UCBT (32 days as compared to 18 and 16 days in unmanipulated and T-cell depleted SCT, respectively). The rate of acute grade II–IV GVHD was reduced in UCBTs (35% as compared to 58 and 20%). A greater early TRM was observed in UCBTs (39%). Two-year EFS was improved in unmanipulated SCTs (43%), but was similar in T-cell depleted SCTs and UCBTs (37%, and 31%, respectively).

### PEDIATRIC UNRELATED-DONOR UCBT FOR MALIGNANT DISEASES

The EuroCord Registry reported unrelated-donor UCBT data from 95 children (median age 4.8 years) with AML.[58] Eight percent were HLA identical, 46% were disparate at one locus, and 43% were mismatched at ≥2 loci. The median cell dose was 4.4 × 10$^7$/kg. The median time to neutrophil recovery was 26 days. By multivariate analysis, neutrophil recovery correlated with the status of disease at transplantation and the use of hematopoietic growth factor immediately post-UCBT. Acute GVHD was seen in 35% of patients and was not predicted by HLA disparity. Chronic GVHD was noted in 5 of 53 patients. The 100-day TRM was 20%. Relapse occurred in 26% of the patients and was associated with weight ≥21 kg and active disease at the time of transplantation. The 2-year EFS was 42% with an OS of 49%. Disease status and major ABO incompatibility predicted EFS and OS.

### PEDIATRIC UCBT FOR NONMALIGNANT DISEASES

Data regarding pediatric UCBT for nonmalignant diseases are limited to abstract reports[59–62] and publications by Locatelli et al.[63] and Staba et al.[64] Locatelli et al. reported on 44 patients, three-quarters of whom had a hemoglobinopathy/thalassemia and one-quarter had sickle cell disease (SCD). The UCB donor was related in all transplants. Ninety-three percent of the grafts were HLA identical. Neutrophil recovery at 60 days occurred in 89% of the patients. The median time to neutrophil recovery was 23 days. Platelet recovery was reported in 90% of the patients at a median of 39 days. Acute GVHD developed in 11% of the patients. The 2-year Kaplan-Meier estimate of EFS was 79% for patients with thalassemia and 90% for those with SCD. OS was 100%.

Staba et al. reported on 20 consecutive patients with Hurler's syndrome. All UCB donors were unrelated. The median age was 11 months. One patient was HLA identical, 11 were disparate at one locus, and the remaining grafts were mismatched at ≥2 loci. The conditioning regimen was Busulfan(Bu)/Cy/ATG. GVHD prophylaxis consisted of cyclosporine and methylprednisolone. The mean cell dose was 8.34 × 10$^7$/kg

| Table 97.5    Adult unrelated donor UCBT | | | | |
|---|---|---|---|---|
| | EuroCord[50,69] | Laughlin et al.[70] | Sanz et al.[71] | Duke[72,73] |
| Median cell dose (TNC/kg) | $1.7 \times 10^7$ | $1.6 \times 10^7$ | $1.71 \times 10^7$ | $1.6 \times 10^7$ |
| Engraftment: % | 81%[a] | 100%[a] | 91%[b] | 80%[c] |
| median days to neutrophil recovery | 32 | 27 | 22 | 26 |
| Acute GVHD: | | | | |
| grade II–IV | 38% | 60% | NA | 41% |
| grade III–IV | NA | 20% | NA | 22% |
| TRM | 50%[d] | 50%[d] | 43%[d] | 56% |
| Relapse | NA | 4/54[e] | 0 | 7/25[e] |
| Survival: | | | | |
| EFS | 21%[g] | 26%[h] | 53%[g] | 15%[k] |
| OS | 27%[g] | 28%[i] | 55%[j] | 19%[k] |

UCBT, umbilical cord blood transplantation; ICBTR, International Cord Blood Transplant Registry; TNC, total nucleated cells; GVHD, graft-versus-host disease; TRM, transplant-related mortality; EFS, event-free survival; OS, overall survival; NA, not available.
[a]Observed at 60 days.
[b]Observed at 30 days.
[c]Observed at 50 days.
[d]Observed at 100 days.
[e]Observed in 4 of 54 patients with malignancies.
[f]Observed in 7 of 25 patients with malignancies that engrafted and survived 100 days.
[g]Observed at 1 year.
[h]Observed at 40 months.
[i]Observed at 22 months.
[j]Observed at 8 months.
[k]Observed at 3 years.

and the mean number of CD34[+] cells infused was $2.51 \times 10^5$/kg. The median time to neutrophil recovery was 24 days. Twenty-five percent of patients developed acute grade II–IV GVHD. Two patients developed chronic GVHD. The EFS at a median of 905 days was 85%.

### ADULT UNRELATED-DONOR UCBT

Adult unrelated-donor UCBT has been performed predominantly in relapsed hematological malignancies, with the exception of a small series of patients with de novo AML.[65] The adult UCBT data are less mature than those of the pediatric population, yet reasonable rates of engraftment have been observed. Unfortunately, high TRM rates and marginal survival limit this treatment option to a select group of adult patients. The data have been reported in abstract form[66–68] and from the following sources: EuroCord,[50,69] Laughlin et al.,[70] Sanz et al.,[71] and Duke[72,73](Table 97.5). The EuroCord Registry reported on 108 patients with a median age of 26 years and a median weight of 60 kg. GVHD prophylaxis was predominantly cyclosporine and corticosteroids. 6% of the grafts were HLA identical, 35% were disparate at one locus, and 59% were mismatched at ≥2 loci. Laughlin et al. reported on 68 patients with a median age of 31.4 years and a median weight of 69.2 kg. The conditioning regimen was largely TBI

based/ATG. GVHD prophylaxis was cyclosporine alone or cyclosporine and methylprednisolone. Two grafts were HLA identical, 26% were disparate at one locus, and 71% were mismatched at ≥2 loci. Sanz et al. reported on 22 patients with a median age of 29 years and a median weight of 69.5 kg. The conditioning regimen consisted of Bu/Cy/ATG/thiotepa. GVHD prophylaxis was cyclosporine and prednisone. One graft was HLA identical, 13 were disparate at one locus, and 8 were mismatched at ≥2 loci. The Duke group reported on 57 patients with a median age of 31 years and a median weight of 70 kg. The conditioning regimen was TBI or Bu based plus ATG. GVHD prophylaxis was cyclosporine and methylprednisolone. Two grafts were HLA identical, eight were disparate at one locus, and the remaining grafts were mismatched at ≥2 loci.

The EuroCord Registry reported engraftment in 81% of the patients at 60 days. The median time to neutrophil recovery was 32 days and was associated with a cell dose ≥$1.7 \times 10^7$/kg. Laughlin et al. reported a 90% engraftment rate at 42 days. The median time to neutrophil recovery was 27 days, while the median times to platelet and RBC recovery were 58 and 60 days, respectively. The neutrophil recovery rate was more rapid if the TNC count before freezing was ≥$1.87 \times 10^7$/kg. Sanz et al. observed engraftment in all 20 patients who survived longer than 30 days. The median time to neutrophil recovery was 22 days. The Duke group recorded a median time to neutrophil recovery of 26 days. No association was noted with cell dose. The median time to platelet recovery was 84 days and was predicted by a CD34$^+$ cell dose $\geq 1.37 \times 10^5$/kg.

The EuroCord Registry documented acute GVHD in 38% of the patients and chronic GVHD in 26%. Laughlin et al. noted acute grade II–IV GVHD in 60% of the patients and grade III–IV GVHD in 20%. Sanz et al. reported similar rates. Long et al. noted grade II–IV GVHD in 30% of the patients and grade III–IV GVHD in 16%. Eight of 25 evaluable patients developed chronic GVHD.

The EuroCord Registry experienced a TRM of 56% at 180 days. This was improved with a cell dose $\geq 2.0 \times 10^7$/kg, greater HLA identity, inactive disease, and transplantation after 1998. Laughlin et al. noted a 100-day TRM of 50%, similar to that reported by Sanz et al. and Long et al. The EuroCord Registry noted a "low" rate of relapse, as did Laughlin et al. (4 of 54 patients with a malignancy). Sanz et al. did not report any relapses. The Duke group observed relapse in 7 of 25 patients who engrafted and survived longer than 100 days.

The EFS reported by the EuroCord Registry was 21% at 1 year. Laughlin et al. noted a 26% EFS at 22 months. This correlated with a CD34$^+$ dose $\geq 1.2 \times 10^5$/kg. Long et al. recorded a 3-year EFS of 15%, improved with age $\leq 32$ years. The EuroCord Registry reported an OS of 27% at 1 year. This was improved in patients with CML in chronic phase or acute leukemia in CR1/CR2. The cell dose was also important since those patients who received $\leq 1 \times 10^7$/kg had a 75% probability of death as compared to 30% if the dose was $\geq 3 \times 10^7$/kg. Laughlin et al. noted an OS of 28% at 22 months. Sanz et al. observed an 8-month OS of 55% (five patients had CML). Long et al. reported a 3-year OS of 19%.

## CURRENT AND FUTURE DIRECTIONS

Delayed engraftment with prolonged neutropenia following UCBT may lead to life-threatening infections. Cell dose has been shown to be critical in predicting the rate of engraftment. Investigators have developed techniques to increase the number of UCB stem cells available for transplantation by ex vivo expansion, with the goal of shortening the period of neutropenia.[74–77] These preclinical advances are yet to be translated into improved clinical outcomes. Preliminary results of multidonor, pooled UCB units have been reported in a small series of adult patients.[78] TRM is a major complication of allogeneic SCT. Toxicities of the conditioning regimens often limit allogeneic transplantation to younger patients with relatively few comorbidities. In efforts to expand this therapy to older and more frail patients, nonmyeloablative conditioning regimens have been developed. These regimens have been applied in small series of adult UCBTs.[79–85] High rates of engraftment (cumulative incidence of 94% with median neutrophil recovery in 9.5 days), severe GVHD (9%), TRM (28%), and survival (EFS 31% and OS 39%) have been reported.[79]

## REFERENCES

1. Traycoff CM, Kosak ST, Grigsby S, et al.: Evaluation of ex vivo expansion potential of cord blood and bone marrow hematopoietic progenitor cells using cell tracking and limiting dilution analysis. *Blood* 85:2059–2068, 1995.

2. Cairo MS, Law P, van de Ven C, et al.: The in vitro effects of stem cell factor and PIXY321 on myeloid progenitor formation (CFU-GM) from immunomagnetic separated CD34+ cord blood. *Pediatr Res* 32:277–281, 1992.

3. van de Ven C, Ishizawa L, Law P, et al.: IL-11 in combination with SLF and G-CSF or GM-CSF significantly increases expansion of isolated CD34+ cell population from cord blood vs. adult bone marrow. *Exp Hematol* 23:1289–1295, 1995.

4. Lu L, Xiao M, Shen RN, et al.: Enrichment, characterization, and responsiveness of single primitive CD34 human umbilical cord blood hematopoietic progenitors with high proliferative and replating potential. *Blood* 81:41–48, 1993.

5. Gluckman E, Broxmeyer HA, Auerbach AD, et al.: Hematopoietic reconstitution in a patient with Fanconi's anemia by means of umbilical-cord blood from an HLA-identical sibling. *N Engl J Med* 321:1174–1178, 1989.

6. Kurtzberg J, Graham M, Casey J, et al.: The use of umbilical cord blood in mismatched related and unrelated hemopoietic stem cell transplantation. *Blood Cells* 20:275–283, 1994; discussion: 284.

7. Sanz MA, Sanz GF: Unrelated donor umbilical cord blood transplantation in adults. *Leukemia* 16:1984–1991, 2002.

8. Armitage JO: Bone marrow transplantation. *N Engl J Med* 330:827–838, 1994.

9. Confer D: Unrelated marrow donor registries. *Curr Opin Hematol* 4:408–412, 1997.

10. bmdw.org/Addresses/USA.html.

11. Burgio GR, Gluckman E, Locatelli F: Ethical reappraisal of 15 years of cord-blood transplantation. *Lancet* 361:250–252, 2003.

12. Sugarman J, Reisner EG, Kurtzberg J: Ethical aspects of banking placental blood for transplantation. *JAMA* 274:1783–1785, 1995.

13. Vawter DE, Rogers-Chrysler G, Clay M, et al.: A phased consent policy for cord blood donation. *Transfusion* 42:1268–1274, 2002.

14. Fraser JK, Cairo MS, Wagner EL, et al.: Cord Blood Transplantation Study (COBLT): cord blood bank standard operating procedures. *J Hematother* 7:521–561, 1998.

15. Nakagawa R, Watanabe T, Kawano Y, et al.: Analysis of maternal and neonatal factors that influence the nucleated and CD34+ cell yield for cord blood banking. *Transfusion* 44:262–267, 2004.

16. Ballen KK, Wilson M, Wuu J, et al.: Bigger is better: maternal and neonatal predictors of hematopoietic potential of umbilical cord blood units. *Bone Marrow Transplant* 27:7–14, 2001.

17. Surbek DV, Schonfeld B, Tichelli A, et al.: Optimizing cord blood mononuclear cell yield: a randomized comparison of collection before vs after placenta delivery. *Bone Marrow Transplant* 22:311–312, 1998.

18. Solves P, Moraga R, Saucedo E, et al.: Comparison between two strategies for umbilical cord blood collection. *Bone Marrow Transplant* 31:269–273, 2003.

19. Lasky LC, Lane TA, Miller JP, et al.: In utero or ex utero cord blood collection: which is better? *Transfusion* 42:1261–1267, 2002.

20. Bertolini F, Battaglia M, Zibera C, et al.: A new method for placental/cord blood processing in the collection bag. I: Analysis of factors involved in red blood cell removal. *Bone Marrow Transplant* 18:783–786, 1996.

21. Nagler A, Peacock M, Tantoco M, et al.: Separation of hematopoietic progenitor cells from human umbilical cord blood. *J Hematother* 2:243–245, 1993.

22. Harris DT, Schumacher MJ, Rychlik S, et al.: Collection, separation and cryopreservation of umbilical cord blood for use in transplantation. *Bone Marrow Transplant* 13:135–143, 1994.

23. Sousa T, de Sousa ME, Godinho MI, et al.: Umbilical cord blood processing: volume reduction and recovery of CD34+ cells. *Bone Marrow Transplant* 19:311–313, 1997.

24. Armitage S, Fehily D, Dickinson A, et al.: Cord blood banking: volume reduction of cord blood units using a semi-automated closed system. *Bone Marrow Transplant* 23:505–509, 1999.

25. M-Reboredo N, Diaz A, Castro A, et al.: Collection, processing and cryopreservation of umbilical cord blood for unrelated transplantation. *Bone Marrow Transplant* 26:1263–1270, 2000.

26. Rubinstein P, Dobrila L, Rosenfield RE, et al.: Processing and cryopreservation of placental/umbilical cord blood for unrelated bone marrow reconstitution. *Proc Natl Acad Sci USA* 92:10119–10122, 1995.

27. Broxmeyer HE, Cooper S: High-efficiency recovery of immature haematopoietic progenitor cells with extensive proliferative capacity from human cord blood cryopreserved for 10 years. *Clin Exp Immunol* 107(suppl 1):45–53, 1997.

28. Barker JN, Krepski TP, DeFor TE, et al.: Searching for unrelated donor hematopoietic stem cells: availability and speed of umbilical cord blood versus bone marrow. *Biol Blood Marrow Transplant* 8:257–260, 2002.

29. Poli F, Scalamogna M, Crespiatico L, et al.: Comparison of serological and molecular typing for HLA-A and -B on cord blood lymphocytes. *Tissue Antigens* 51:67–71, 1998.

30. Laurenti L, Perrone MP, Bafti MS, et al.: HLA typing strategies in a cord blood bank. *Haematologica* 87:851–854, 2002.

31. Risdon G, Gaddy J, Broxmeyer HE: Allogeneic responses of human umbilical cord blood. *Blood Cells* 20:566–570, 1994; discussion: 571–572.

32. Roncarolo MG, Bigler M, Ciuti E, et al.: Immune responses by cord blood cells. *Blood Cells* 20:573–585, 1994; discussion: 585–586.

33. Roux E, Helg C, Dumont-Girard F, et al.: Analysis of T-cell repopulation after allogeneic bone marrow transplantation: significant differences between recipients of T-cell depleted and unmanipulated grafts. *Blood* 87:3984–3992, 1996.

34. Roux E, Helg C, Chapuis B, et al.: T-cell repertoire complexity after allogeneic bone marrow transplantation. *Hum Immunol* 48:135–138, 1996.

35. Dumont-Girard F, Roux E, van Lier RA. et al.: Reconstitution of the T-cell compartment after bone marrow transplantation: restoration of the repertoire by thymic emigrants. *Blood* 92:4464–4471, 1998.

36. Roux E, Dumont-Girard F, Starobinski M, et al.: Recovery of immune reactivity after T-cell-depleted bone marrow transplantation depends on thymic activity. *Blood* 96:2299–2303, 2000.

37. Mackall CL, Granger L, Sheard MA, et al.: T-cell regeneration after bone marrow transplantation: differential CD45 isoform expression on thymic-derived versus thymic-independent progeny. *Blood* 82:2585–2594, 1993.

38. Theilgaard-Monch K, Raaschou-Jensen K, Schjodt K, et al.: Pluripotent and myeloid-committed CD34+ subsets in hematopoietic stem cell allografts. *Bone Marrow Transplant* 32:1125–1133, 2003.

39. Theilgaard-Monch K, Raaschou-Jensen K, Palm H, et al.: Flow cytometric assessment of lymphocyte subsets, lymphoid progenitors, and hematopoietic stem cells in allogeneic stem cell grafts. *Bone Marrow Transplant* 28:1073–1082, 2001.

40. Bogue M, Roth DB: Mechanism of V(D)J recombination. *Curr Opin Immunol* 8:175–180, 1996.

41. Gorski J, Yassai M, Zhu X, et al.: Circulating T cell repertoire complexity in normal individuals and bone marrow recipients analyzed by CDR3 size spectratyping. Correlation with immune status. *J Immunol* 152:5109–5119, 1994.

42. Abu-Ghosh A, Goldman S, Slone V, et al.: Immunological reconstitution and correlation of circulating serum inflammatory mediators/cytokines with the incidence of acute graft-versus-host disease during the first 100 days following unrelated umbilical cord blood transplantation. *Bone Marrow Transplant* 24:535–544, 1999.

43. Niehues T, Rocha V, Filipovich AH, et al.: Factors affecting lymphocyte subset reconstitution after either related or unrelated cord blood transplantation in children—a Eurocord analysis. *Br J Haematol* 114:42–48, 2001.

44. Klein AK, Patel DD, Gooding ME, et al.: T-cell recovery in adults and children following umbilical cord blood transplantation. *Biol Blood Marrow Transplant* 7:454–466, 2001.

45. Talvensaari K, Clave E, Douay C, et al.: A broad T-cell repertoire diversity and an efficient thymic function indicate a favorable long-term immune reconstitution after cord blood stem cell transplantation. *Blood* 99:1458–1464, 2002.

46. Wagner JE, Kurtzberg J: Cord blood stem cells. *Curr Opin Hematol* 4:413–418, 1997.

47. Wagner JE, Kernan NA, Steinbuch M, et al.: Allogeneic sibling umbilical-cord-blood transplantation in children with malignant and non-malignant disease. *Lancet* 346: 214–219, 1995.

48. Rocha V, Chastang C, Souillet G, et al.: Related cord blood transplants: the Eurocord experience from 78 transplants. Eurocord Transplant group. *Bone Marrow Transplant* 21(suppl 3):S59–S62, 1998.

49. Gluckman E, Rocha V, Boyer-Chammard A, et al.: Outcome of cord-blood transplantation from related and unrelated donors. Eurocord Transplant Group and the European Blood and Marrow Transplantation Group. *N Engl J Med* 337:373–381, 1997.

50. Gluckman E: Current status of umbilical cord blood hematopoietic stem cell transplantation. *Exp Hematol* 28:1197–1205, 2000.

51. Locatelli F, Rocha V, Chastang C, et al.: Factors associated with outcome after cord blood transplantation in children with acute leukemia. Eurocord-Cord Blood Transplant Group. *Blood* 93:3662–3671, 1999.

52. Kurtzberg J, Laughlin M, Graham ML, et al.: Placental blood as a source of hematopoietic stem cells for transplantation into unrelated recipients. *N Engl J Med* 335: 157–166, 1996.

53. Wagner JE, Rosenthal J, Sweetman R, et al.: Successful transplantation of HLA-matched and HLA-mismatched umbilical cord blood from unrelated donors: analysis of engraftment and acute graft-versus-host disease. *Blood* 88:795–802, 1996.

54. Rubinstein P, Carrier C, Scaradavou A, et al.: Outcomes among 562 recipients of placental-blood transplants from unrelated donors. *N Engl J Med* 339:1565–1577, 1998.

55. Gluckman E, Rocha V, Chastang C: European results of unrelated cord blood transplants. Eurocord Group. *Bone Marrow Transplant* 21(suppl 3):S87–S91, 1998.

56. Wagner JE, Barker JN, DeFor TE, et al.: Transplantation of unrelated donor umbilical cord blood in 102 patients with malignant and nonmalignant diseases: influence of CD34 cell dose and HLA disparity on treatment-related mortality and survival. *Blood* 100:1611–1618, 2002.

57. Rocha V, Cornish J, Sievers EL, et al.: Comparison of outcomes of unrelated bone marrow and umbilical cord blood transplants in children with acute leukemia. *Blood* 97:2962–2971, 2001.

58. Michel G, Rocha V, Chevret S, et al.: Unrelated cord blood transplantation for childhood acute myeloid leukemia: a Eurocord Group analysis. *Blood* 102: 4290–4297, 2003.

59. Rocha V, Chastang C, Pasquini R, et al.: Cord blood transplant in patients with bone marrow failure syndromes. *Blood* 92:136a, 1998.

60. Howrey R, Martin P, Ciocci G: Unrelated cord blood transplantation for correction of genetic diseases. *Blood* 92:291a, 1998.

61. Ortega J, Yaniv L, Rocha V, et al.: Unrelated cord blood transplantation for inborn errors. *Blood* 1998:291a, 1998.

62. Ortega J, Rocha V, Wall D, et al.: Unrelated cord blood transplant in children with severe primary immunodeficiencies. An Eurocord analysis. *Blood* 98:667a, 2001.

63. Locatelli F, Rocha V, Reed W, et al.: Related umbilical cord blood transplantation in patients with thalassemia and sickle cell disease. *Blood* 101:2137–2143, 2003.

64. Staba SL, Escolar ML, Poe M, et al.: Cord-blood transplants from unrelated donors in patients with Hurler's syndrome. *N Engl J Med* 350:1960–1969, 2004.

65. Ooi J, Iseki T, Takahashi S, et al.: Unrelated cord blood transplantation for adult patients with advanced myelodysplastic syndrome. *Blood* 101:4711–4713, 2003.

66. Goldberg S, Chedid S, Jennis A, et al.: Unrelated umbilical cord blood transplantation in adults: a single institution experience. *Blood* 96:208a, 2000.

67. Cornetta K, Laughlin M, Carter S, et al.: Umbilical cord blood transplantation in adults: results of a prospective, multi-institutional, NHBLI sponsored trial. *Blood* 100: 42a, 2002.

68. Iseki T, Ooi J, Tomonari A, et al.: Unrelated cord blood transplantation in adults with hematological malignancy: a single institution experience. *Blood* 98:665a, 2001.

69. Gluckman E: Hematopoietic stem-cell transplants using umbilical-cord blood. *N Engl J Med* 344:1860–1861, 2001.

70. Laughlin MJ, Barker J, Bambach B, et al.: Hematopoietic engraftment and survival in adult recipients of umbilical-cord blood from unrelated donors. *N Engl J Med* 344:1815–1822, 2001.

71. Sanz GF, Saavedra S, Planelles D, et al.: Standardized, unrelated donor cord blood transplantation in adults with hematologic malignancies. *Blood* 98:2332–2338, 2001.

72. Long GD, Laughlin M, Madan B, et al.: Unrelated umbilical cord blood transplantation in adult patients. *Biol Blood Marrow Transplant* 9:772–780, 2003.

73. Koh L, Chao NJ: Umbilical cord blood transplantation in adults using myeloablative and nonmyeloablative preparative regimens. *Biol Blood Marrow Transplant* 10(1):1–22, 2004.

74. Stiff P, Pecora A, Parthasarathy M, et al.: Umbilical cord blood transplants in adults using a combination of unexpanded and ex vivo expanded cells: preliminary clinical observations. *Blood* 92:646a, 1998.

75. Shpall E, Quinones R, Hami L, et al.: Transplantation of cancer patients receiving high dose chemotherapy with ex vivo expanded cord blood cells. *Blood* 92:646a, 1998.

76. Pecora A, Stiff P, Jennis A, et al.: Prompt and durable engraftment in two older adult patients with high risk chronic myelogenous leukemia (CML) using ex vivo expanded and unmanipulated unrelated cord blood. *Bone Marrow Transplant* 25:797–799, 2000.

77. Jaroscak J, Martin P, Waters-Pick B, et al.: A phase 1 trial of augmentation of unrelated umbilical cord blood transplantation with ex vivo expanded cells. *Blood* 92: 646a, 1998.

78. Barker J, Weisdorf D, DeFor T, et al.: Impact of multiple unit unrelated donor umbilical cord blood transplantation in adults: preliminary analysis of safety and efficacy. *Blood* 98:2791a, 2001.

79. Barker JN, Weisdorf DJ, DeFor TE, et al.: Rapid and complete donor chimerism in adult recipients of unrelated donor umbilical cord blood transplantation after reduced-intensity conditioning. *Blood* 102:1915–1919, 2003.

80. Rizzieri DA, Long GD. Vredenburgh JJ, et al.: Successful allogeneic engraftment of mismatched unrelated cord

blood following a nonmyeloablative preparative regimen. *Blood* 98:3486–3488, 2001.

81. McSweeney P: Nonmyeloablative allogeneic hematopoietic cell transplants: any role for rheumatoid arthritis? *J Rheumatol Suppl* 64:49–54, 2001.

82. McSweeney P, Bearman S, Jones R, et al.: Nonmyeloablative hematopoietic cell transplants using cord blood. *Blood* 98:2794a, 2001.

83. Hwang W, Tan P, Goh Y, et al.: Minimal toxicity of an immunosuppression-based nonmyeloablative condition-ing regimen for mismatched unrelated umbilical cord blood transplantation. *Blood* 100:5437a, 2002.

84. Cairo M, Harrison L, Del Toro G, et al.: Reduced intensity (RI) umbilical cord blood (UCB) and matched family donor (MFD) allogeneic stem cell transplantation (AlloSCT) in children and adolescents with malignant and nonmalignant disease. *Blood* 100:5432a, 2002.

85. Goggins T, Rizzieri DR: Nonmyeloablative allogeneic stem cell transplantation using alternative donors. *Cancer Control* 11:86–96, 2004.

Chapter **98**

# GRAFT-VERSUS-HOST DISEASE: NEW PERSPECTIVES ON PATHOBIOLOGY AND THERAPY

*Thomas R. Spitzer and Robert Sackstein*

## INTRODUCTION

The transplantation of healthy hematopoietic stem cells into a patient with aplastic anemia or leukemia is potentially curative therapy, but the development of graft-versus-host disease (GVHD)—which often occurs even when the donor and recipient are siblings fully matched at the HLA loci—significantly limits survival. The first descriptions of GVHD following allogeneic bone marrow transplant in humans were made in the 1960s. Significant strides in prophylaxis of GVHD have been made over the past four decades by the use of pharmacologic agents such as methotrexate and cyclosporine and by manipulation of the donor cell inoculum to limit the infusion of effector donor lymphocytes. However, given the extensive clinical observations and investigations on the nature of this complication, it is remarkable that the diagnosis of GVHD is still clinically challenging and that this complication continues to pose a formidable obstacle to successful allogeneic hematopoietic stem cell transplantation (HSCT). On the other hand, patients with GVHD have improved leukemia-free survival (the graft-versus-leukemia (GVL) effect) and this graft-versus-malignancy (GVM) effect, a beneficial by-product of the alloreactivity of the donor cells, may extend to lymphomas, myeloma, and even solid tumors.[1-4] Thus, a major question in HSCT biology is how to preserve a GVM effect while eliminating GVHD. This chapter will review some of the critical issues in the clinical manifestations and pathobiology of GVHD, including the results of recent investigations using an in vitro lymphocyte-skin adhesion assay to better define the mechanisms of GVHD. Advances during the past decade in the prevention and treatment of GVHD including recent evidence for a role of cellular modulation of GVHD will also be reviewed.

## CLINICAL PRESENTATION AND PATHOBIOLOGY OF ACUTE GVHD

GVHD occurs in two forms, "acute" and "chronic," defined separately by the timing of onset posttransplant and by differences in the clinical presentation and pathology of affected target organs. Acute GVHD, by classical definition, is GVHD that occurs within 100 days of HSCT, usually around the time of leukocyte engraftment or shortly thereafter. Though this operational term is useful in delineating GVHD occurring immediately posttransplant from the more indolent and progressive changes of chronic GVHD, it is important to note that acute GVHD can occur beyond 100 days posttransplant, particularly in the setting of donor lymphocyte infusions (DLI) used in the prevention or treatment of disease relapse. There are three principal target tissues affected in acute GVHD—the skin, liver, and gut. Although the clinical staging and the overall grading of acute GVHD is based on the relative level of involvement of these three tissues (Table 98.1), other organs, especially the lymphoid tissues and the bone marrow, are targets of the GVHD reaction.

The most common tissue affected in acute GVHD is the skin, with over 80% of patients with GVHD manifesting skin eruptions.[5] The typical skin presentation consists of a maculopapular rash that can resemble a sunburn, initially involving the ears, neck, shoulders, upper chest and back, and the palms and soles of the extremities. The extent of skin surface involved and the presence of bullae or desquamation define the different stages of skin involvement. The clinical findings of cutaneous GVHD are corroborated by histologic analysis of skin biopsy material, and, therefore, discrete pathologic criteria contribute to the diagnosis of cutaneous GVHD (Table 98.1).[6] However, the characteristic pathologic changes of acute cutaneous GVHD are not

| Table 98.1 | Histologic grading for acute cutaneous GVHD | | | |
| --- | --- | --- | --- | --- |
| Grade 0 | Grade 1 | Grade 2 | Grade 3 | Grade 4 |
| Normal skin | Perivascular mononuclear cell infiltrates | Perivascular mononuclear cell infiltrates | Grade 2 changes plus epidermolysis and bulla formation (from fusion of basilar vacuoles) | Denudation of epidermis (separation of epidermis from dermis) |
| | Vacuolar degradation of epidermal–dermal junction | Vacuolar degradation | | |
| | | Dyskeratotic cells or eosinophilic bodies in the epidermis | | |

specific for GVHD alone and can occur in a variety of other cutaneous diseases and reactions. Many skin eruptions occur posttransplant in response to the preparative regimen, hypersensitivity to drugs (e.g., antibiotics), infections, and even the recovery of leukocytes, and, therefore, there is no "gold standard" for accurate pathologic diagnosis of GVHD.[7] Moreover, there is no correlation between the numbers of infiltrating mononuclear cells or of dyskeratotic cells in skin specimens and the clinical outcome.[7] The diagnosis of cutaneous GVHD is based on exclusion of other confounding contributors such as drugs and viral exanthems, and depends upon *clinicopathologic correlation*, i.e., clinical history and manifestations supported by characteristic pathologic changes. Indeed, the timing of the clinical manifestations is an important component of the diagnosis, as some pathologists will consider GVHD in the differential only if characteristic histopathologic changes occur during or after engraftment.

Involvement of the gut and liver in GVHD is usually accompanied by skin changes, but, rarely, these tissues can be involved separately or together without skin manifestations. The primary clinical manifestation of gut GVHD is diarrhea and abdominal pain. The diarrhea is initially watery in nature but, commonly, becomes bloody requiring transfusion support with platelets and red cells. The volume of diarrhea defines the different stages of gut involvement. Rectal biopsy is helpful in the diagnosis of gut GVHD, particularly when diarrhea occurs in the absence of cutaneous eruptions. The early finding of lymphocytic infiltrates at the crypts—accompanied by necrosis and dropout of crypt cells—is characteristic of the diagnosis, but, again, is not pathognomonic for GVHD. Like the skin, different pathologic stages are recognized culminating in mucosal denudation (grade 4), and the differential includes drug reactions and infection (particularly cytomegalovirus infection). Hepatic GVHD is manifested by a rise in the conjugated bilirubin, and the level of total bilirubin elevation defines the clinical stages of liver disease. Lymphocytic infiltrates in the interlobular and marginal bile ducts are characteristic

histopathologic findings, which lead to the clinically identifiable cholestatic picture.

As mentioned above, the timing of skin, gut, and liver changes is a critical component of the diagnosis of GVHD. Although a "hyperacute" form of GVHD can occur typically in HLA-mismatched donor—recipient pairs, manifested by fever and markedly accelerating skin changes with diarrhea and hyperbilirubinemia before engraftment, most acute GVHD will initially present about the time of engraftment or thereafter. Within the past several years, characteristic clinical findings of an "engraftment syndrome" have been described in recipients of both autologous and allogeneic stem cell transplants.[8–10] This syndrome typically consists of noninfectious fever, a maculopapular skin eruption resembling GVHD, capillary leak with resultant weight gain and pulmonary infiltrates/effusions, and, not uncommonly, hyperbilirubinemia and diarrhea. The fact that these changes occur in autologous transplant recipients indicates that the pathophysiology of this entity does not depend on alloreactivity per se. Interestingly, the skin biopsy findings are consistent with GVHD.[8] Treatment of this syndrome requires prompt administration of corticosteroids to prevent complications of capillary leak, including renal dysfunction and pulmonary failure.

The pathophysiology of the engraftment syndrome may overlap with that of acute GVHD. The common feature in these entities may be primary endothelial damage as a consequence of inflammatory mediators such as IL-2, TNF-$\alpha$ and IFN-$\gamma$, released locally by infiltrating perivascular lymphocytes.[8,11–13] In GVHD, however, there is also evidence of direct cell-mediated immunologic reactivity resulting in microvascular injury.[14] One effect of combining cyclosporin A and rapamycin is to modify the migration capabilities of lymphocytes, by altering lymphocyte and/or endothelial adhesive structures mediating lymphocyte recruitment from the vasculature and into the tissue. In this regard, corticosteroids, the first-line pharmacologic agents in the treatment of acute GVHD, also profoundly affect lymphocyte migration to lymphoid and extra-lymphoid tissues,[15,16] and decreased lymphocyte infiltrates in affected tissues are a prognostic sign for steroid-responsiveness in GVHD therapy.[17]

In Billingham's classic description of the elements required for the development of GVHD,[18] three requirements were emphasized: (1) The host must be incapable of rejecting the graft; (2) The graft must contain immunocompetent cells; and (3) There must be incompatibilities in transplantation antigens between donor and host. Despite the fact that this description needs to be modified somewhat in light of evidence of GVHD occurring in the setting of blood transfusions, solid organ transplants, and in the case of cyclosporin-induced autologous GVHD (due to induction of autoreactive T cells[19]), Billingham's tenets reflect important basic principles in the biology of GVHD. However, given the data reviewed above and the pathologic evidence of lymphocytic infiltrates consistently accompanying GVHD-induced tissue injury, a fourth requirement to Billingham's criteria must be proposed: effector lymphocytes must migrate to the target tissues in GVHD.

The pathologic hallmark of acute GVHD is mononuclear cell infiltrates in the involved tissues.[20,21] The pathogenesis of acute GVHD involves the migration of both alloreactive lymphocytes and of NK cells into target tissues.[22-25] A central role for alloreactive T cells in the development of GVHD is indicated by the fact that T-cell depletion of donor marrow significantly abrogates the incidence of GVHD.[26] Indeed, the lymphocytic infiltrates of dermal GVHD are composed of donor-derived cells.[27] Infiltrating NK cells may contribute to tissue damage in GVHD by their local release of inflammatory cytokines such as TNF-$\alpha$ and IFN-$\gamma$.[28,29] The NK cell infiltrates are also donor-derived,[30] indicating that their localization in tissues is likewise due to recruitment from the circulation.

## PREVENTION OF GVHD

The central dilemma regarding the prevention of GVHD is how to preserve a potent GVM effect of the transplant while avoiding the deleterious aspects of clinical GVHD. Conventional strategies that have been attempted for the prevention of GVHD have focused on either pharmacologic intervention or ex vivo T-cell (or T-cell subset) depletion. More recently, manipulation of the host—donor cellular environment has been attempted in an effort to dissociate GVM from GVHD.

### PHARMACOLOGIC STRATEGIES

The availability of cyclosporine-based pharmacoprophylaxis in the early to mid 1980s represented a major advance in the field of clinical HSCT. Prospective randomized trials evaluating the combination of cyclosporine and methotrexate compared with cyclosporine or methotrexate alone for leukemia or severe aplastic anemia were conducted.[31,32] Significant reductions in the incidence of acute GVHD were seen in both studies. In the case of transplantation for hematologic malignancy (acute myelogenous leukemia in first complete remission or chronic phase chronic myelogenous leukemia) an overall survival benefit was realized. However, for severe aplastic anemia a survival difference did not reach statistical significance. Pharmacologic GVHD prophylaxis alone has been shown to be considerably less effective in the prevention of GVHD following HLA-mismatched donor HSCT.[33,34] For recipients of HLA-2 or -3 antigen mismatched non-T-cell-depleted transplants, acute GVHD incidence exceeds 70–80% and transplant-related mortality is very high.[33] Despite these limitations, cyclosporine-based pharmacoprophylactic strategies have had a major impact on the practice of clinical HSCT. The reduction in acute GVHD-related morbidity and mortality has allowed for the transplantation of considerably older patients and of patients without HLA genotypically identical sibling donors.

More recently, there have been several reported pharmacologic advances in the prevention of GVHD (Table 98.2). Triple drug immunoprophylaxis (cyclosporine, methotrexate, and corticosteroids) has been shown to be superior to cyclosporine and corticosteroids alone for the prevention of GVHD following HLA-matched donor HSCT for hematologic malignancies.[35] The lack of an overall survival benefit (perhaps due to an impairment of the GVM effect) and an increased infection risk associated with more intensive immunosuppressive regimens have underscored the limitations of this approach.

The introduction of tacrolimus has represented an advance in the management of GVHD. Two multicenter prospective randomized trials comparing tacrolimus and methotrexate with cyclosporine and methotrexate for GVHD prophylaxis following HSCT for hematologic malignancies have been conducted.[36,37] In the first trial involving HLA genotypically identical sibling donors, a significant reduction in the incidence of GVHD in the tacrolimus-treated patients was observed.[36] The second trial involved patients receiving transplants from HLA-matched unrelated donors. Once again, GVHD incidence was reduced in the tacrolimus-treated group.[37] In both trials, however, no significant difference in overall survival between two treatment groups was observed. The toxicity profile of tacrolimus was somewhat different than that of cyclosporine. More neurotoxicity was observed with tacrolimus. However, there was less renal impairment and hypertension in tacrolimus-treated patients.

Newer agents are presently being evaluated for GVHD prophylaxis. Rapamycin, an mTOR inhibitor that has been shown to cause G1 cell cycle arrest, has been evaluated in several GVHD prophylaxis strategies.

**Table 98.2    GVHD prophylaxis strategies**

| Pharmacologic | Result |
| --- | --- |
| Methotrexate | Limited GVHD protection |
| Methotrexate + CYA or corticosteroids | Improved prophylaxis compared with single-agent methotrexate; survival advantage in aplastic anemia |
| Methotrexate + tacrolimus | Superior prophylaxis compared with CYA/methotrexate but no survival advantage |
| Methotrexate + CYA + corticosteroids | Superior prophylaxis compared with CYA/methotrexate but no survival advantage |
| Tacrolimus + sirolimus +/− methotrexate | Promising GVHD protection in HLA-matched related and unrelated donor settings |
| CYA 1 MMF | Promising GVHD protection with less morbidity than with methotrexate combinations (mucositis, myelosuppression) |
| **Ex vivo T-cell depletion** | |
| **Pan T-cell depletion** | |
| Negative selection | Decreased GVHD but increased relapse rate, engraftment failure |
| Positive (CD34⁺ cell) selection | Decreased GVHD but increased relapse rate, engraftment failure. Possible protection from PTLD by B-cell depletion |
| **Selective T-cell depletion** | |
| CD8⁺ cell depletion (bone narrow) | Decreased GVHD, apparent preservation of GVL effect but increased engraftment failure |

GVHD, graft-versus-host disease; CYA, cyclosporine; MMF, mycophenolate mofetil; GVL, graft-versus-leukemia.

In combination with tacrolimus and methotrexate, or tacrolimus alone, a very low incidence of acute GVHD has been reported following HLA-matched unrelated donor transplantation and HLA-matched related donor transplantation, respectively.[38,39]

Mycophenolate mofetil (MMF) is a purine antagonist which in combination with cyclosporine has been effective in the prevention of GVHD in preclinical (canine) models[40] and in clinical trials following HLA-matched nonmyeloablative transplantation.[41] Recently, the combination of MMF and tacrolimus was shown to have similar GVHD protective effects as cyclosporine and methotrexate following HLA-matched myeloablative stem cell transplantation.[42] Mucositis was reportedly less frequent than with methotrexate-containing regimens and delayed engraftment was obviated.

### EX VIVO T-CELL DEPLETION

A series of experimental and clinical observations have shown that GVHD can be effectively prevented by infusing less than $1–5 \times 10^5$ T cells/kg of recipient body weight.[43,44] Early enthusiasm for the ex vivo removal of immunocompetent T cells from the marrow graft, however, was tempered by an increased risk of engraftment failure and relapse of the underlying malignancy.[45–47] This increased relapse risk was somewhat disease-specific. In chronic myelogenous leukemia (CML), for example, an increase in relapse risk from approximately 10–20% following HLA-matched donor non-T-cell-depleted transplantation to 60–80% following T-cell-depleted transplantation was observed.[47] In acute myelogenous leukemia (AML) in first remission, on the other hand, an effect of T-cell depletion on probability of relapse was not apparent.[48]

Given the limitations of ex vivo T-cell depletion, this strategy has not reached widespread acceptance for the prevention of GVHD following HLA genotypically identical donor HSCT for hematologic malignancies, particularly CML. However, given the more profound impact of GVHD on mortality risk following HLA nongenotypically identical donor transplants, T-cell-depletion strategies are being reevaluated.

In an effort to diminish the problems of engraftment failure and relapse following ex vivo T-cell depletion, recent investigations have focused on the depletion of selective T-cell subsets. Ex vivo depletion of CD8⁺ T cells has been shown to result in an apparent reduction of GVHD with no increase in relapse probability following HLA-matched sibling donor HSCT for CML.[49] An increased risk of engraftment failure, however, has further demonstrated the importance of T cells in overcoming host alloresistance to engraftment.

Recently, adoptive cellular immunotherapy via DLI has been increasingly utilized for its capacity to enhance GVH alloreactivity and to impart a potent GVM effect.[50,51] In CML, for example, a cytogenetic and molecular remission is achieved with DLI for the treatment of relapse following allogeneic HSCT in the majority of cases, demonstrating that a potent antitumor effect, with at least a several log tumor cell cytoreduction, is achievable.[50–53] In a nonrandomized comparison of non-T-cell-depleted transplants and CD6⁺ T-cell-depleted transplants for CML (followed by DLI at time of relapse), similar survival probabilities were realized.[54] Not surprisingly an increased probability of relapse occurred in the T-cell-depleted transplant recipients, but the majority of these patients achieved a second remission with DLI, which in most cases appeared to be durable. This suggests that for at least selected patients who are at high risk for transplant-related morbidity or mortality an ex vivo T-cell-depleted HSCT followed by DLI for posttransplant relapse may be a rational treatment strategy.

Given the potent antitumor potential of DLI and experimental evidence suggesting that delayed DLI may be associated with a substantially lower risk of GVHD than with early T-cell infusion(s), clinical trials evaluating ex vivo T-cell-depleted bone marrow or peripheral blood progenitor cell (PBPC) transplants followed by delayed T-cell infusions have been conducted.[55–57] Preliminary results suggest that this strategy is feasible and that delayed DLI can be performed without a prohibitive risk of GVHD.[56] The optimal dosing and timing of delayed T-cell infusion(s) remain to be determined.

## CELLULAR MODULATION OF GVHD AND THE SEPARATION OF GVHD FROM GVM

Experimental and clinical experience have suggested that host cells surviving the transplant conditioning regimen may be instrumental in the regulation of GVHD.[58–61] The availability of sensitive methods for detecting the presence of residual host cells (e.g., microsatellite analyses evaluating variable number of tandem repeat sequences) has demonstrated that at least a transient presence of host cells in many patients can be seen following HSCT.[62,63] An increased incidence of acute GVHD with increasing intensity of the preparative regimen, possibly because of the increased cytokine release and damage to host elements following these aggressive preparative regimens, has been observed.[64] A relationship between the presence of mixed lymphohematopoietic chimerism and a reduced incidence of acute GVHD has also been seen in some series.[65–67]

In several animal models the intentional induction of mixed lymphohematopoietic chimerism has been associated with a reduction in the incidence of GVHD.[40,60,68,69] These mixed chimeric states are achievable following either myeloablative preparative regimens in which a combination of mixed T-cell-depleted syngeneic and T-cell-depleted allogeneic marrow is transplanted ("mixed" marrow transplantation) or following nonablative preparative regimens with peri-transplant in vivo anti-T-cell therapy.[58,68,70,71]

Clinical trials at the Massachusetts General Hospital have been conducted utilizing similar nonmyeloablative preparative regimens for the induction of mixed chimerism followed by DLI in patients with advanced hematologic malignancies.[72–74] Mixed chimerism has been reliably achieved with regimens consisting of cyclophosphamide, anti-T-cell antibody therapy, and thymic irradiation. Sustained remissions of chemorefractory lymphoproliferative malignancies have been observed in a number of patients who achieved mixed chimerism followed by either spontaneous conversion to full donor hematopoiesis or DLI, which resulted in chimerism conversion. In several cases this chimerism conversion following DLI was not accompanied by significant clinical GVHD, providing proof of principal that GVHD is separable from GVM in mixed chimeras given delayed DLI. Sustained mixed lymphohematopoietic chimerism was also shown to be achievable following haploidentical stem cell transplantation.[72] An increased risk of GVHD in recipients of haploidentical transplants has, however, prompted a revision of the strategy in an effort to induce a GVH free state of mixed chimerism as a platform for DLI. A combination of vigorous in vivo T-cell depletion with an anti-CD2 monoclonal antibody and ex vivo T-cell depletion (using a CD34+ cell selection device) has resulted in the uniform induction of mixed chimerism following haploidentical stem cell transplantation with minimal or no GVHD. The conversion of chimerism, in some cases following delayed DLI, and in some cases with minimal or no GVHD, has provided further evidence that GVHD and GVM are separable, even in the haploidentical transplant setting.

Other cellular modulatory approaches to separate clinical GVHD from GVHD have included the administration of exogenous cytokines posttransplant to dissociate T-cell subset effector function[75–77] (Table 98.3). Early clinical trials have not substantiated a benefit of high-dose IL-2 posthaploidentical stem cell transplantation.[78] However, the optimal timing and dosing of IL-2 may not have been achievable clinically.

| Table 98.3 | Separation of GVHD from GVT |
|---|---|
| Method | Mechanism |
| Induction of mixed lymphohematopoietic chimerism, delayed DLI | ■ Initial bidirectional tolerance<br>■ Resolution of pro-inflammatory cytokine milieu prior to DLI<br>■ Confinement of the GVL alloresponse to the lymphohematopoietic space |
| Ex vivo T-cell subset (CD8+ cell) depletion | GVHD protection from CD8+ cell removal, preservation of GVT effect from CD4+ cells, other effector cell populations |
| Enrichment for CD4+, CD25+ cells | Inhibition of GVHD by T-regulatory cells |
| ATG/TLI conditioning | Increase of regulatory natural killer T cells |
| Depletion of L-selectin+ T cells | Inhibition of The capacity of T cells to home to lymph nodes |

DLI, donor lymphocyte infusion; GVL, graft-versus-leukemia; GVHD, graft-versus-host disease.

Manipulation of the cellular environment of the graft may also contribute to a separation of GVHD and GVM. As discussed above, CD8$^+$ T-cell-depleted marrow grafts may be associated with less GVHD and preservation of potent GVL effect,[49] and CD8$^+$ T-cell-depleted DLI have been shown to induce remissions in patients with hematologic malignancies in relapse after allogeneic stem cell transplantation, with less GVHD than occurs with unmanipulated DLI (with comparable numbers of CD4$^+$ cells).[79]

On the basis of preclinical murine models showing that NK1.1$^+$ TCR $\alpha\beta^+$ cells have non-major histocompatibility complex (MHC)-restricted natural suppressor activity and the percentage of these cells can be increased by the administration of total lymphoid irradiation (TLI) and antithymocyte globulin (ATG), clinical trials utilizing TLI/ATG have been initiated by Strober and colleagues in an effort to suppress GVHD and preserve a GVL effect.[80] A comparable human CD8$^+$ NK$^+$ cell population of natural suppressor cells has been shown to be increased in percentage following TLI/ATG conditioning. Impressive GVHD protection and disease-free survival probabilities have been demonstrated in early clinical trials of reduced-intensity of transplantation for advanced hematologic malignancies.[81]

Given the complexity of the cellular and cytokine interactions that affect the incidence and severity of GVHD, an only preliminary understanding of how the host—donor cellular environment might be manipulated to prevent GVHD exists. Which host or donor regulatory cells are important in the suppression of GVHD, for example, remain to be determined. Several cell populations including the NK1.1$^+$ murine cell population and the CD4$^+$ CD25$^+$ cell subset and lymphokine-activated killer cells exhibiting both veto and natural suppressor activity have been postulated as having a regulatory role in the suppression of the GVH reaction.[82,83] Given the compelling experimental and clinical evidence for a protective effect of cytokines and regulatory cell populations, future efforts should be made to define the mechanism of these effects and hopefully optimize their clinical benefits.

## TREATMENT OF GVHD

### ACUTE GVHD

The treatment of acute GVHD, particularly severe (grade III–IV) GVHD, remains inadequate. Corticosteroids are the mainstay of therapy for acute GVHD, particularly if they are not utilized as prophylaxis.[84,85] Several studies have established the response rates for treatment of GVHD with corticosteroids.[86,87] The highest response rates have been demonstrated in cutaneous GVHD (>60%). Sustained response rates of only 20–40% have been seen for visceral (gut and liver) GVHD. Long-term survival has been correlated with the grade of GVHD and response to medical therapy. Patients with grade

III or IV GVHD who do not achieve a complete remission of their GVHD with medical therapy have a less than 50% probability of long-term survival; mortality rates in excess of 90% have been reported for grade IV GVHD.[5] Most patients who receive corticosteroids for grades II–IV GVHD require long-term corticosteroid administration. Substantial morbidity which usually accompanies long-term corticosteroid administration includes heightened infection risk, hypertension, diabetes mellitus, osteoporosis and aseptic necrosis of the hip and other bones, and proximal myopathy.[85]

Given the substantial morbidity with intensive corticosteroid therapy of acute GVHD, attempts have been made to both improve the response rate of treatment and to provide a steroid sparing effect by adding additional immunosuppressive therapy (Table 98.4). In a randomized trial comparing prednisone with equine antithymocyte globulin and prednisone for the initial treatment for acute grades II–IV GVHD, response rates were the same.[88] There were more infectious complications in the combined therapy group. No difference in survival was observed between the two groups at day 100 and after 6 months and 2 years. In a comparison of upfront methylprednisolone versus methylprednisolone/daclizumab (an anti-IL-2 receptor monoclonal antibody) for acute GVHD, response rates were also similar.[89] Significantly worse 100-day and 1-year survival for the combined therapy group led to early closure of the trial. The increased mortality in the

| Table 98.4 | Treatment strategies for GVHD |
|---|---|
| **Acute GVHD** | **Chronic GVHD** |
| Pharmacologic immunosuppression | Pharmacologic immunosuppression |
|   Corticosteroids |   Corticosteroids |
|   Cyclosporine |   Cyclosporine |
|   Tacrolimus |   Tacrolimus |
|   Sirolimus |   Sirolimus |
| Mycophenolate mofetil |   Azathioprine |
| |   Mycophenolate mofetil |
| Antibody Therapy | Thalidomide |
|   Polyclonal | Clofazimine |
|   Antithymocyte globulin (equine, rabbit) | |
|   Monoclonal | T-cell modulation |
|   Anti-T-cell (anti-CD3, CD2, ect) |   Extracorporeal photopheresis |
|   Daclizumab (anti-IL-2 receptor) | |
|   Infliximab (anti-TNF-salpha) | |
|   Alemtuzumab (anti-CD52$^+$) | |
| Other biologic therapy Denileukin diftitox | |
| Gene therapy Thymidine kinase suicide gene transduction/ganciclovir | |

GVHD, graft-versus-host disease.

combination group was attributed to both relapse and GVHD-related mortality, possibly as a result of a negative impact on regulatory (CD4$^+$CD25$^+$) cells due to daclizumab.

Thus, corticosteroids alone (or in combination with a calcineurin inhibitor which is often still being administered at the onset of GVHD) remain the initial treatment of choice for grades II–IV GVHD. For patients who do not respond to methylprednisolone (or an equivalent corticosteroid) at a dose of 2 mg/kg/day, several possible strategies exist. Increasing the steroid dose to 5 mg/kg or higher has been evaluated in previous noncontrolled situations.[90] While a dose—response relationship may exist for corticosteroids, higher doses (particularly those of 10 mg/kg/day or greater) are associated with increased steroid-related complications and transplant-related mortality. Equine or rabbit antithymocyte globulin has been used most frequently as second-line therapy. While transient responses are common, particularly in cutaneous GVHD, the mortality rate in patients requiring ATG for steroid refractory acute GVHD is very high (approximately 90%) owing primarily to opportunistic infections.[87,91] Several other therapies, on the basis of their targeting of cytokines and/or effector cell populations, have been evaluated in steroid refractory GVHD. Favorable response rates have been seen with monoclonal antibodies targeting tumor necrosis factor-alpha (infliximab)[92] and the IL-2 receptor (daclizumab and basiliximab).[93,94] A fusion protein consisting of IL-2 and diphtheria toxin has shown promising activity in steroid refractory GVHD.[95] The transient nature of the responses is not surprising given the complex, multifactorial mechanisms of GVHD. The cumulative immunosuppressive effect of corticosteroids and other immunosuppressive agents to which these potent highly specific immunosuppressive agents are added is also not surprisingly notable for a very high risk of infectious complications. In an experience from the MD Anderson Cancer Center with infliximab for steroid refractory GVHD an overall response rate of 65% was seen, with most of the patients (62%) achieving a complete remission. Fungal, bacterial, and viral infections were seen in 46, 69, and 57% of the patients, respectively. Estimated overall survival probability from the time of the transplant was only 31%.[91]

In an effort to more specifically target effector T cells while avoiding the more broad immunosuppressive effects of pharmacologic immunosuppressive therapy, gene therapy approaches have been evaluated for the treatment of acute GVHD. T cells transduced with a herpes viral thymidine kinase gene have been evaluated in preclinical transplant models and in preliminary clinical trials with ganciclovir administered in the event of GVHD, resulting in death of the effector T cells and in some instances, reversal of the GVHD.[96] Improving the efficiency of gene transduction and preservation of the cells that mediate a GVM effect remain important future goals of this strategy.

### CHRONIC GVHD

The treatment of chronic GVHD has also been problematic with long-term immunosuppressive therapy required for many patients with symptomatic disease. With the routine use of PBPC, and the transplantation of older patients, the problem of extensive chronic GVHD has increased.[97,98] Treatment strategies must weigh the need to ameliorate the clinical manifestations of chronic GVHD against the risks of long-term (often lifetime) administration of immunosuppressive medications (including but not limited to infection, osteonecrosis, and secondary malignancy). Some recent series have focused on local control of chronic GVHD manifestations, such as oral cyclosporine rinses or ophthalmic cyclosporine solution for xerostomia and xerophthalmia, respectively.[99,100] Extracorporeal photopheresis has been shown to be an effective salvage strategy for patients with steroid refractory GVHD.[101] The cumulative morbidity of immunosuppressive therapy can hopefully be lessened with this approach. Long-term venous access issues can be problematic given the heightened infection risk of patients with chronic GVHD.

The optimal therapy for extensive chronic GVHD remains uncertain. An alternate-day corticosteroid and cyclosporine regimen has been shown to be effective in the management of chronic GVHD with an acceptable toxicity profile.[102] Corticosteroids as a single agent have been shown to be superior to combined corticosteroids and azathioprine for chronic GVHD.[103] For their steroid sparing effect, however, combination regimens are often employed in the treatment of chronic GVHD. Newer agents with substantial activity in chronic GVHD include MMF[104] and sirolimus[105] (Table 98.4). Thalidomide has demonstrated some activity in steroid refractory chronic GVHD.[106] Clofazimine has been shown to have efficacy in the treatment of the connective tissue variant of chronic GVHD.[107] Ursodiol may ameliorate the clinical manifestations of hepatic GVHD.[108] Other vitally important supportive care aspects of the management of chronic GVHD include immunoglobulin repletion for patients with severe hypogammaglobulinemia, antimicrobial prophylaxis (e.g., penicillin for *Streptococcus pneumoniae*, co-trimoxazole for pneumocystis carinii pneumonia (PCP) prophylaxis), physical therapy to prevent joint contractures, and frequent dental and ophthalmological evaluations to address dental hygiene and to evaluate for and treat corneal ulceration, and ocular infections, respectively.

### SUMMARY

Though significant strides in the prevention and therapy of GVHD have been made over the last two decades, a greater understanding of the molecular immunology of this complication is still needed in order to develop more effective therapies to eliminate GVH while maintaining beneficial alloreactivity against malignancy. Though there may not be a single therapeutic approach that will achieve this aim, the considerable experimental and clinical evidence indicates that modulation of tissue-specific homing, in combination with lower toxicity preparative regimens and selective enrichment or depletion of effector T cells, will yield novel and effective alternatives to minimize the risk of GVHD. These approaches, combined with judicious application(s) of immunopharmacologic agents, may prove sufficient to achieve the full curative promise of allogeneic HSCT.

## REFERENCES

1. Weiden P, Flournoy N, Sanders J, et al.: Antileukemic effect of graft-versus-host disease contributes to improved survival after allogeneic marrow transplantation. *Transplant Proc* 13:248, 1981.
2. Jones J, Ambinder R, Piantodosi S, Santos G: Evidence of a graft-versus-lymphoma effect associated with allogeneic bone marrow transplantation. *Blood* 77:649, 1996.
3. Tricot G, Vesole D, Jagannath S, et al.: Graft-versus-myeloma effect: proof of principle. *Blood* 87:1196, 1996.
4. Eibl B, Schwaighofer H, Nachbaur D, et al.: Evidence of a graft-versus-tumor effect in a patient treated with marrow ablative chemotherapy and allogeneic bone marrow transplantation for breast cancer. *Blood* 88:1501, 1996.
5. Martin P, Schoch G, Fisher L, et al.: A retrospective analysis of therapy for acute graft-versus-host disease: initial treatment. *Blood* 76:1464, 1990.
6. Lerner Kao G, Storb R: Histopathology of graft-versus-host reaction (GVHR) in human recipients of marrow from HLA matched sibling donors. *Transplant Proc* 6:367, 1974.
7. Horn TD: Acute cutaneous eruptions after marrow ablation: roses by other names? *J Cutan Pathol* 21:385, 1994.
8. Lee CK, Gingrich R, Hohl R, et al.: Engraftment syndrome in autologous bone marrow and peripheral stem cell transplantation. *Bone Marrow Transplant* 16:175, 1995.
9. Cahill RA, Spitzer TR, Mazumder A, et al.: Marrow engraftment and clinical manifestations of capillary leak syndrome. *Bone Marrow Transplant* 18:177, 1996.
10. Ravoet C, Feremans W, Husson B, et al.: Clinical evidence for an engraftment syndrome associated with early and steep neutrophil recovery after autologous blood stem cell transplantation. *Bone Marrow Transplant* 18:943, 1996.
11. Dickinson A, Sviland L, Dunn J, et al.: Demonstration of direct involvement of cytokines in graft-versus-host reaction using an in vitro human skin explant model. *Bone Marrow Transplant* 7:209, 1991.
12. Antin JH, Ferrara JLM: Cytokine dysregulation and acute graft-versus-host disease. *Blood* 80:2964, 1992.
13. Carayol G, Bourhis JH, Guillard M, et al.: Quantitative analysis of T helper 1, T helper 2, and inflammatory cytokine expression in patients after allogeneic bone marrow transplantation. *Transplantation* 63:1307, 1997.
14. Dumler J, Beschorner W, Farmer E, et al.: Endothelial-cell injury in cutaneous acute graft-versus-host disease. *Am J Pathol* 135:1097, 1989.
15. Sackstein R: Lymphocyte migration following bone marrow transplantation. *Annal New York Acad Sci* 770:177, 1995.
16. Sackstein R, Borenstein M: The effects of corticosteroids on lymphocyte recirculation in humans: analysis of the mechanism of impaired lymphocyte migration to lymph node following methylprednisolone administration. *J Invest Med* 43:68, 1995.
17. Sviland L, Pearson A, Green M, et al.: Prognostic importance of histological and immunopathological assessment of skin and rectal biopsies in patients with GVHD. *Bone Marrow Transplant* 11:215, 1993.
18. Billingham R: The biology of graft-versus-host reaction. *Harvey Lect* 62:21, 1966.
19. Fischer A, Beschorner W, Hess A: Syngeneic graft-versus-host disease: failure of autoregulation in self/non-self discrimination. *Blood* 20:493, 1988.
20. Woodruff J, Hansen J, Good R, et al.: The pathology of the graft-versus-host reaction (GVHR) in adult receiving bone marrow transplants. *Transplant Proc* 8:675, 1976.
21. Horn T, Bauer D, Vogelsang G, et al.: Reappraisal of histological features of the acute cutaneous graft-versus-host reaction based on an allogeneic rodent model. *J Invest Dermatol* 103:206, 1994.
22. Lampert I, Janossy G, Suitters A, et al.: Immunological analysis of the skin in graft-versus-host disease. *Clin Exp Immunol* 50:123, 1982.
23. Kaye V, Neumann P, Kersey J, et al.: Identity of immune cells in graft-versus-host disease of the skin. *Am J Pathol* 116:436, 1984.
24. Rhoades J, Cibull M, Thompson J, et al.: Role of natural killer cells in the pathogenesis of human acute graft-versus-host disease. *Transplantation* 56:113, 1993.
25. Takata M, Imai T, Hirone T: Immunoelectron microscopy of acute graft-versus-host disease of the skin after allogeneic bone marrow transplantation. *J Clin Pathol* 46:801, 1993.
26. Korngold R, Sprent J: Lethal graft-versus-host disease after bone marrow transplantation across minor histocompatability barriers in mice. *J Exp Med* 148:1687, 1978.
27. Thomas J, Wakeling W, Imrie S, et al.: Chimerism in skin of bone marrow transplant recipients. *Transplantation* 38:475, 1984.
28. Chong AF, Scuderi P, Grimes W, et al.: Tumor targets stimulate IL-2 activated killer cells to produce interferon-y and tumor necrosis factor. *J Immunol* 142:2133, 1989.
29. Xun C, Brown S, Jennings C, et al.: Acute graft-versus-host-like disease induced by transplantation of human

activated natural killer cells into SCID mice. *Transplantation* 56:409, 1993.

30. Ferrara J, Guillen F, van Dijken P, et al.: Evidence that large granular lymphocytes of donor origin mediate acute graft-versus-host disease. *Transplantation* 47:50, 1989.

31. Storb R, Deeg H, Farewell V, et al.: Marrow transplantation for severe aplastic anemia: methotrexate alone compared with a combination of methotrexate and cyclosporine for prevention of acute graft-versus-host disease. *Blood* 68:119, 1986.

32. Storb R, Deeg HF, Farewell V, et al.: Methotrexate and cyclosporine compared with cyclosporine alone for prophylaxis of acute graft-versus-host disease after marrow transplantation for leukemia. *N Eng J Med* 314:729, 1986.

33. Beatty PG, Clift FM, Mickelson BB, et al.: Marrow transplantation from related donors other than HLA-identical siblings. *N Engl J Med* 313:765, 1985.

34. Chan KW, Fryer CJ, Danegri JF, Buskard NA, Phillips GL: Allogeneic bone marrow transplantation using partially-matched related donor. *Bone Marrow Transplant* 2:27, 1987.

35. Chao N, Schmidt C, Nilan J, et al.: Cyclosporine, methotrexate and prednisone compare with cyclosporine and prednisone for prophylaxis of acute graft-versus-host disease. *New Engl J Med* 329:1225, 1993.

36. Ratanatharathorn V, Nash R, Przepiorka D, et al.: Phase III study comparing methotrexate and tracrolimus (Prograf FK506) with methotrexate and cyclosporine for graft-versus-host disease prophylaxis after HLA-identical sibling bone marrow transplantation. *Blood* 7:2303, 1998.

37. Nash R, Antin J, Karanes C, et al.: Phase III study comparing tacrolimus (FK506) with cyclosporine (CSP) for prophylaxis of acute graft-versus-host disease (GVHD) after marrow transplantation from unrelated donors. *Blood* 96:2062, 2000.

38. Cutler C, Kim HT, Hochberg E, et al.: Sirolimus and tacrolimus without methotrexate as graft-versus-host disease prophylaxis after matched related donor peripheral blood stem cell transplantation. *Biol Blood Marrow Transplant* 10:328, 2004.

39. Alyea EP, Neuberg D, Cutler C, et al.: Sirolimus, tacrolimus and low dose methotrexate as graft-versus-host disease prophylaxis after matched related and unrelated nonmyeloablative transplantation is well tolerated and associated with low incidence of acute GVHD. *Blood* 102:711a, 2003.

40. Storb R, Yu C, Wagner JL, et al.: Stable mixed hematopoietic chimerism in DLA-identical littermate dogs given sublethal total body irradiation before and pharmacological immunosuppression after marrow transplantation. *Blood* 89:3048, 1997.

41. McSweeney PA, Niederwieser D, Shizuru JA, Sandmaier BM: Hematopoietic cell transplantation in older patients with hematologic malignancies: replacing high-dose cytotoxic therapy with graft-versus-tumor effects. *Blood* 97:3390, 2001.

42. Nash RA, Johnson L, Parker PM, et al.: A phase I/II study of mycophenolate mofetil (MMF) in combination with cyclosporine (CSP) for prophylaxis of graft-versus-host disease (GVHD) after myeloablative conditioning and allogeneic hematopoietic cell transplantation (HCT): dose escalation of MMF. *Blood* 102:240a, 2003.

43. Verdonck L, de Gast G, van Heugten H, Dekker A: A fixed low number of T cells in HLA-identical allogeneic bone marrow transplantation. *Blood* 75:776, 1990.

44. Verdonck L, Dekker A, de Gast G, et al.: Allogeneic bone marrow transplantation with a fixed low number of T cells in the marrow graft. *Blood* 83:3090, 1994.

45. Martin P, Hansen J, Torok-Storb B, et al.: Graft failure in patients receiving T-cell-depleted HLA-identical allogeneic bone marrow transplants. *Bone Marrow Transplant* 3:445, 1988.

46. Butturini A, Gale R: T-cell depletion in bone marrow transplants for leukemia: current results and future directions. *Bone Marrow Transplant* 3:185, 1988.

47. Marmont A, Horowitz M, Gale R, et al.: T-cell depletion of HLA-identical transplants in leukemia. *Blood* 78:2120, 1991.

48. Passweg J, Tiberghien P, Cahn J, et al.: Graft-versus-leukemia effects in T lineage and B lineage acute lymphoblastic leukemia. *Bone Marrow Transplant* 21:153, 1998.

49. Champlin R, Ho W, Gajewski J, et al.: Selective depletion of CD8+ T lymphocytes for prevention of graft-versus-host disease after allogeneic bone marrow transplantation. *Blood* 76:418, 1990.

50. Porter DL, Roth MS, McGarigle C, et al.: Induction of graft-versus-host disease as immunotherapy for relapsed chronic myeloid leukemia. *N Engl J Med* 330:100, 1994.

51. Porter DL, Antin JH: The graft-versus-leukemia effects of allogeneic cell therapy. *Annu Rev Med* 50:369, 1999.

52. Collins RH Jr, Shpilberg O, Drobyski WR, et al.: Donor leukocyte infusions in 140 patients with relapsed malignancy after allogeneic bone marrow transplantation. *J Clin Oncol* 15:433, 1997.

53. Porter DL, Collins RH Jr, Hardy C, et al.: Treatment of relapsed leukemia after unrelated donor marrow transplantation with unrelated donor leukocyte infusions. *Blood* 95:1214, 2000.

54. Sehn LH, Alyea EP, Weller E, et al.: Comparative outcomes of T-cell-depleted and non-T-cell-depleted allogeneic bone marrow transplantation for chronic myelogenous leukemia: impact of donor lymphocyte infusion. *J Clin Oncol* 17:561, 1999.

55. Van Rhee F, Feng L, Cullis J, et al.: Relapse of chronic myeloid leukemia after allogeneic bone marrow transplantation: the case for giving donor leukocyte infusions before the onset of hematologic relapse. *Blood* 83:3377, 1994.

56. Barrett A, Mavroudis D, Tisdale J, et al.: T-cell-depleted bone marrow transplantation and delayed T cell add-back to control acute GVHD and conserve a graft-versus-leukemia effect. *Bone Marrow Transplant* 21:543, 1998.

57. Petz LD, Yam P, Wallace BR, et al.: Mixed hematopoietic chimerism following bone marrow transplantation for hematologic malignancies. *Blood* 70:133, 1987.

58. Sykes M, Sheard MA, Sachs DH, et al.: Graft-versus-host-related immunosuppression induced in mixed chimeras by alloresponses against either host or donor

lymphohematopoietic cells. *J Exp Med* 168:2391, 1988.

59. Sykes M, Sharabi Y, Sachs D, et al.: Achieving alloengraftment without graft-versus-host disease: approaches using mixed allogeneic bone marrow transplantation. *Bone Marrow Transplant* 3:379, 1988.

60. Sharabi Y, Abraham VS, Sykes M, et al.: Mixed allogeneic chimeras prepared by a non-myeloablative regimen: requirement for chimerism to maintain tolerance. *Bone Marrow Transplant* 9:191, 1992.

61. Huss R, Deeg JH, Gooley T, et al.: Effect of mixed chimerism on graft-versus-host disease, disease recurrence and survival after HLA-identical marrow transplantation for aplastic anemia or chronic myelogenous leukemia. *Bone Marrow Transplant* 18:767, 1996.

62. Suttorp M, Schmitz N, Dreger P, et al.: Monitoring of chimerism after allogeneic bone marrow transplantation with unmanipulated marrow by use of DNA polymophisms. *Leukemia* 7:679, 1993.

63. Socie G, Lawler M, Gluckman E, et al.: Studies on hemopoietic chimerism following allogeneic bone marrow transplantation in the molecular biology era. *Leuk Res* 19:467, 1995.

64. Hagglund L, Bostom L, Remberger M, et al.: Risk factors for acute graft-versus-host disease in 291 consecutive HLA-identical bone marrow transplant recipients. *Bone Marrow Transplant* 16:747, 1995.

65. Hill RS, Pertersen FB, Storb R, et al.: Mixed hematologic chimerism after allogeneic marrow transplantation for severe aplastic anemia is associated with a higher risk of graft rejection and a lessened incidence of acute graft-versus-host disease. *Blood* 67:811, 1986.

66. Roy DC, Tantravaho R, Murray C, et al.: Natural history of mixed chimerism after bone marrow transplantation with CD6-depleted allogeneic marrow: a stable equilibrium. *Blood* 75:296,1990.

67. Bertheas MF, Lafage P, Levy M, et al.: Influence of mixed chimerism on the results of allogeneic bone marrow transplantation for leukemia. *Blood* 78:3103, 1991.

68. Ildstad ST, Wren SM, Bluestone JA, et al.: Effect of selective T-cell depletion of host and/or donor bone marrow lymphopoietic repopulation, tolerance, and graft-versus-host disease in mixed allogeneic chimeras (B10 + B10.D2-B10). *J Immunol* 136:28,1986.

69. Kawai T, Cosimi AB, Colvin RB, et al.: Mixed allogeneic chimerism and renal allograft tolerance in cynomologous monkeys. *Transplantation* 59:256,1995.

70. Sykes M, Szot GL, Swenson K, Pearson DA: Induction of high levels of allogeneic hematopoietic reconstitution and donor specific tolerance without myelosuppressive conditioning. *Nature Med* 3:783,1997.

71. Pelot MR, Pearson DA, Swenson K, et al.: Lymphohematopoietic graft-vs.-host reactions can be induced without graft-vs.-host disease in murine mixed chimeras established with a cyclophosphamide-based nonmyeloablative conditioning regimen. *Biol Blood Marrow Transplant* 22:133, 1999.

72. Sykes M, Preffer F, Saidman SL, et al.: Mixed lymphohematopoietic chimerism is achievable following non-myeloablative therapy and HLA-mismatched donor marrow transplantation. *Lancet* 353:1755, 1999.

73. Spitzer TR, McAfee S, Sackstein R, et al.: Intentional induction of mixed chimerism and achievement of antitumor responses after nonmyeloablative conditioning therapy and HLA-matched donor bone marrow transplantation for refractory hematologic malignancies. *Biol Blood Marrow Transplant* 6:309, 2000.

74. Spitzer TR, McAfee SL, Dey BR, et al.: Nonmyeloablative haploidentical stem-cell transplantation using anti-CD2 monoclonal antibody (MEDI-507)-based conditioning for refractory hematologic malignancies. *Transplantation* 75:1748, 2003.

75. Sykes M, Harty W, Szot G, Pearson D: Interleukin-2 inhibits graft-versus-host disease promoting activity of CD4+ cells while preserving CD4 and CD8-mediated graft-versus-leukemia effects. *Blood* 83:2560,1994.

76. Sykes M, Abraham V, Harty W, Pearson D: IL-2 reduces graft-versus-host disease and preserves a graft-versus-leukemia effect by selectively inhibiting CD4+ T cell activity. *J Immunol* 150:197, 1993.

77. Sykes M, Szot GL: Nguyen P, Pearson D, et al.: Interkeukin-12 inhibits murine graft-versus-host disease. *Blood* 86:2429, 1995.

78. Champlin RE, Passweg JR, Zhang MJ, et al.: Interleukin-2 for prevention of graft-versus-host disease after haploidentical marrow transplantation. *Transplantation* 58:858, 1994.

79. Alyea EP, Canning C, Neuberg D, et al.: CD8+ cell depletion of donor lymphocyte infusions using cd8 monoclonal antibody-coated high-density microparticles (CD8-HDM) after allogeneic hematopoietic stem cell transplantation: a pilot study. *Bone Marrow Transplant* 34:123, 2004.

80. Lan F, Zeng D, Higuchi M, Higgins JP, Strober S: Host conditioning with total lymphoid irradiation and antithymocyte globulin prevents graft-versus-host disease: the role of CD1-reactive natural killer T cells. *Biol Blood Marrow Transplant* 9:355, 2003.

81. Lowsky R, Jones SD, Mitra S, et al.: Non-myeloablative conditioning with total lymphoid irradiation (TLI) and anti-thymocyte globulin (ATG) for allogeneic hematopoietic cell transplantation (HCT) results in high levels of regulatory natural killer T-cells and low incidences of acute GVHD and tumor relapse. *Blood* 102:152a, 2003.

82. Colby C, Sykes M, Sachs DH, et al.: Cellular modulation of acute graft-versus-host disease. *Biol Blood Marrow Transplant* 3:287, 1997.

83. Mehta JPR, Singhal S, Horton C, Treleaven J: Outcome of autologous rescue after failed engraftment of allogeneic marrow. *Bone Marrow Transplant* 17:213, 1996.

84. Deeg H, Henslee-Downey P: Management of acute graft-versus-host disease. *Bone Marrow Transplant* 6:1,1990.

85. Lazarus H, Vogelsang G, Rowe J, et al.: Prevention and treatment of acute graft-versus-host disease: the old and new. A report from the Eastern Cooperative Oncology Group (ECOG). *Bone Marrow Transplant* 19:577, 1997.

86. Doney K, Weiden P, Storb R, Thomas E: Treatment of graft-versus-host disease in human allogeneic marrow graft recipients: a randomized trial comparing antithymocyte globulin and corticosteroids. *Am J Hematol* 11:1, 1981.

87. Kennedy M, Deeg J, Strob R, et al.: Treatment of acute graft-versus-host disease after allogeneic marrow transplantation. *Am J Med* 78:978, 1985.

88. Cragg L, Blazar BR, Defor T, et al.: A randomized trial comparing prednisone with antithymocyte globulin/ prednisone as an initial systemic therapy for moderately severe acute graft-versus-host disease. *Biol Blood Marrow Transplant* 6:441, 2000.

89. Lee SJ, Zahrieh D, Agura E, et al.: Effect of up-front daclizumab when combined with steroids for the treatment of acute graft-vs.-host disease: results of a randomized trial. *Blood* 104(5):1559—1564, 2004.

90. Oblon D, Elfenbein G, Goedert M, et al.: Successful therapy of acute graft versus host disease (aGVHD) with high dose methyl-prednisolone (MP). *Proc Am Assoc Cancer Res* 29:82a, 1988.

91. Khoury H, Kashyap A, Adkins DR, et al.: Treatment of steroid-resistant acute graft-versus-host disease with antithymocyte globulin. *Bone Marrow Transplant* 27:1059, 2001.

92. Couriel DR, Saliba R, Hicks K, et al.: Tumor necrosis factor alpha blockade for the treatment of steroid-refractory acute GVHD. *Blood* 104(3):649-654, 2004.

93. Przepiorka D, Kerman NA, Ippoliti C, et al.: Daclizumab, a humanized anti-interleukin-2 receptor alpha chain antibody for the treatment of acute graft-versus-host disease. *Blood* 95:83, 2000.

94. Massenkeil G, Rackwitz S, Genvresse I, Rosen O, Dorken B, Arnold R: Basiliximab is well tolerated and effective in the treatment of steroid-refractory acute graft-versus-host disease after allogeneic stem cell transplantation. *Bone Marrow Transplant* 30:899, 2002.

95. Ho VT, Zahrieh D, Hochberg E, et al.: Safety and efficacy of denileukin diftitox in patients with steroid refractory graft-versus-host disease (GVHD) after allogeneic hematopoietic stem cell transplantation (HSCT). *Blood* 102:242a, 2003.

96. Tiberghien P, Reynolds CW, Keller J, et al.: Ganciclovir treatment of herpes simplex thymidine kinase-transduced primary T lymphocytes: an approach for specific in vivo donor T-cell depletion after bone marrow transplantation? *Blood* 84:1333, 1994.

97. Sorror ML, Maris MB, Storer B, et al.: Comparing morbidity and mortality of HLA-matched unrelated donor hematopoietic cell transplantation after nonmyeloablative and myeloablative conditioning: influence of pre-transplant comorbidities. *Blood* 104(5):1550—1558, 2004.

98. Couriel DR, Saliba RM, Giralt S, et al.: Acute and chronic graft-versus-host disease after ablative and nonmyeloablative conditioning for allogeneic hematopoietic transplantation. *Biol Blood Marrow Transplant* 10:178, 2004.

99. Epstein JB, Truelove EL: Topical cyclosporine in a bioadhesive for treatment of oral lichenoid mucosa; reaction: an open label clinical trial. *Oral Surg Oral Med Oral Pathol Oral Radiol Endod* 82:523, 1996.

100. Kiang E, Tesavibul N, Yee R, Kellaway J, Przepiorka D: The use of topical cyclosporine A in ocular graft-versus-host disease. *Bone Marrow Transplant* 22:147, 1998.

101. Apisarnthanarax N, Donato M, Korbling M, et al.: Extracorporeal photopheresis therapy in the management of steroid-refractory or steroid-dependent cutaneous chronic graft-versus-host disease after allogeneic stem cell transplantation: feasibility and results. *Bone Marrow Transplant* 31:459, 2003.

102. Sullivan KM, Witherspoon RP, Storb R, et al.: Alternating-day cyclosporine and prednisone for treatment of high-risk chronic graft-v-host disease. *Blood* 72:555, 1988.

103. Sullivan KM, Witherspoon RP, Storb R, et al.: Prednisone and azathioprine compared with prednisone and placebo for treatment of chronic graft-v-host disease: prognostic influence of prolonged thrombocytopenia after allogeneic marrow transplantation. *Blood* 72:546, 1988.

104. Kim JG, Sohn SK, Kim DH, et al.:Different efficacy of mycophenolate mofetil as salvage treatment for acute and chronic GVHD after allogeneic stem cell transplant. *Eur J Haematol* 73:56, 2004.

105. Benito AI, Furlong T, Martin PJ, et al.: Sirolimus (rapamycin) for the treatment of steroid-refractory acute graft-versus-host disease. *Transplantation* 72:1924, 2001.

106. Vogelsang GB, Farmer ER, Hess AD, et al.: Thalidomide for the treatment of chronic graft-versus-host disease. *N Engl J Med* 326:1055, 1992.

107. Lee SJ, Wegner SA, McGarigle C, Bierer BE, Antin JH: Treatment of chronic graft-versus-host disease with clofazimine. *Blood* 89:2298, 1997.

108. Chiba T, Yokosuka O, Kanda T, et al.: Hepatic graft-versus-host disease resembling acute hepatitis: additional treatment with ursodeoxycholic acid. *Liver* 22:514, 2002.

# Chapter 99

# INFECTIOUS COMPLICATIONS FOLLOWING STEM CELL TRANSPLANTATION

*David L. Longworth*

## INTRODUCTION

Hematopoietic stem cell transplantation (HSCT) has been increasingly used in the treatment of malignant and nonmalignant hematologic disorders, autoimmune diseases, and genetic and metabolic diseases. More than 50,000 HSCTs are performed annually worldwide.[1] Despite significant advances in defining optimal immunosuppressive regimens, in shortening the duration of neutropenia through the availability of hematopoietic growth factors, and in preventing and managing infectious and noninfectious complications, HSCTs continue to be associated with significant morbidity and mortality. Infectious and noninfectious complications such as graft-versus-host-disease (GVHD), adult respiratory distress syndrome (ARDS), and venoocclusive disease (VOD) are the major contributors to adverse outcome.

This chapter focuses on the recognition, management, and prevention of infectious complications following autologous and allogeneic HSCT. Guidelines focusing on infection prevention were recently published by the Centers for Disease Control and Prevention,[2] and include general and infection-specific strategies, as well as recommendations regarding infection control. The latter is beyond the scope of this discussion and the reader is referred to the guidelines as well as to a recent excellent review regarding infection control management in HSCT.[3]

A thorough pretransplant infectious disease evaluation is essential in HSCT candidates. Specific infectious complications following HSCT are predictable and can be anticipated based upon the sequential suppression of the various components of host defense associated with the conditioning regimen and subsequent HSCT.[4] The clinical syndromes that most commonly occur and the pathogens involved vary over time. For purposes of differential diagnosis in the HSCT recipient with suspected infection, three distinct periods of

infection risk exist, each with unique deficiencies in host immune function.[5] These include the preengraftment period (from the initiation of the conditioning regimen to engraftment), the early engraftment period (from engraftment to day 100), and the late engraftment period in allogeneic HSCT recipients (from day 100 until cessation of immunosuppressive medications). This chapter reviews the appropriate pretransplant infectious disease evaluation; the immune defects and associated infectious complications during the preengraftment, early engraftment, and late engraftment periods; and the prevention, diagnosis, and management of selected syndromes and pathogens encountered in HSCT recipients.

## PRETRANSPLANT EVALUATION

A careful pretransplant infectious disease history should be obtained in all HSCT candidates (Table 99.1). This should include a history of prior bacterial, mycobacterial, and opportunistic infections, especially invasive fungal infections produced by *Aspergillus* or *Candida* species. In those with prior invasive fungal disease, a careful clinical and radiographic evaluation should be performed to exclude residual active disease, which would require aggressive treatment prior to HSCT. Antimicrobial susceptibility profiles of recent bacterial pathogens should be noted, as patients may remain colonized with these organisms. Patients with a prior history of tuberculosis, exposure to tuberculosis, or positive skin test for tuberculosis should be evaluated clinically and with chest radiograph for evidence of active disease. A travel history should be obtained to identify potential exposure, even in the remote past, to *Strongyloides stercoralis*, which may reactivate in the face of immunosuppression. Patients with potential exposure or unexplained peripheral eosinophilia should be screened pretransplant for

**Table 99.1    Components of a pre-HSCT infectious diseases evaluation**

- Complete infectious disease history, including prior infections, antimicrobial susceptibility profiles, and their management
- In those with prior invasive fungal infection or nocardiosis, clinical evaluation and imaging studies to assess disease activity
- Travel and immunization history
  Selected screening for *Strongyloides stercoralis* and *Trypanosoma cruzi* in those at risk
- Evaluation for TB exposure, clinical, and radiographic evaluation in those at-risk
- Dental evaluation
- Serologic testing for CMV, HSV, VZV, EBV, hepatitis A,B,C, HIV 1 and 2, *Toxoplasma gondii, Treponema pallidum*

*S. stercoralis* with an enzyme-linked immunosorbent assay, which has a sensitivity exceeding 90% in detecting latent asymptomatic infection. Seropositive individuals should receive ivermectin prior to HSCT. Individuals who were born or have resided in areas of South America, Central America, or Mexico where Chagas disease is endemic, or who have received a blood transfusion while visiting those areas, should be screened for *Trypanosoma cruzi* IgG using at least two serologic tests.[2] Serologic testing should also be performed to identify prior exposure to cytomegalovirus (CMV), varicella zoster virus (VZV), herpes simplex virus (HSV), human immunodeficiency virus 1 and 2 (HIV), hepatitis A, B and C, Epstein—Barr Virus (EBV), *Toxoplasma gondii*, and *Treponema pallidum*. CMV-seronegative HSCT recipients are at-risk for acquiring CMV from seropositive donors or blood products. CMV-seronegative candidates for allogeneic HSCT with a CMV-seronegative donor should receive only CMV-seronegative or leukocyte-reduced red cells and platelets.[2]

A formal dental evaluation should be performed in all HSCT candidates and, if necessary, restorative work completed prior to transplant so as to minimize the occurrence of infection from oral mucositis associated with the conditioning regimen. This is especially important given the emergence of viridans streptococci as important pathogens in the early transplant period.[6]

## THE PREENGRAFTMENT PERIOD

The preengraftment period commences with the initiation of the preparative regimen and ends at the time of engraftment. This usually occurs by about day 20 in autologous HSCT recipients and by day 30 in allogeneic HSCT recipients, but may vary depending upon the conditioning regimen and the underlying disease. The presence of indwelling intravascular devices,

mucositis of the mouth and gastrointestinal tract, neutropenia, and lymphopenia are the major defects in host defense that occur during the preengraftment period. These are present in both autologous and allogeneic HSCT recipients, and thus the types of infectious complications seen in these respective groups are similar; however, the shorter duration of neutropenia in autologous HSCT recipients is responsible for a lower incidence of infectious complications in these individuals.

### MICROBIOLOGY

Table 99.2 summarizes the common pathogens encountered during the preengraftment period. The most common portals of entry for bacterial infection during this period include central venous catheters and mucositis of the mouth and gut arising from the preparative regimen. Thus, not surprisingly, bacterial pathogens such as viridans streptococci and Gram-negative bacilli from the mouth and gastrointestinal tract, respectively, and skin organisms such as coagulase negative staphylococci are the most common bacterial pathogens encountered in the preengraftment period. Up to 12% of infections occur prior to transplant.[4] Although Gram-negative infections were common during the 1980s, the use of prophylactic oral antibiotics such as fluoroquinolones and trimethoprim-sulfamethoxazole at the onset of neutropenia has led to a shift in the spectrum of bacterial pathogens seen in the preengraftment period. Gram-positive organisms now account for a majority of bacterial infections and for 50% of bacteremias.[7,8] Coagulase negative staphylococci

**Table 99.2    Common pathogens encountered during the preengraftment period**

| Pathogen | Site of origin/involvement |
|---|---|
| **Bacteria** | |
| *Staphylococci* | Skin, intravascular devices |
| *Streptococci* | Mouth, GI tract |
| *Gram-negative bacilli* | GI tract |
| *Clostridium difficile* | Colon |
| **Viruses** | |
| Herpes simplex 1 | Mouth, esophagus |
| Herpes simplex 2 | Genitals, anus, skin |
| Community respiratory viruses | Upper respiratory tract, pneumonia |
| **Fungi** | |
| *Candida* species | Originate from gut May involve bloodstream, mouth, esophagus, skin, intravascular devices; rarely viscera or bone marrow |
| *Aspergillus* species | Pneumonia, sinusitis; rarely CNS and skin |

and viridans streptococci have emerged as dominant pathogens, and the latter have been associated with a shock syndrome.[9] Penicillin resistance is an emerging problem in viridans streptococci.[10] Gram-negative infections are the second most common cause of bacterial infections in the preengraftment period, and now include less common and more often multiresistant organisms such as *Enterobacter, Acinetobacter, Klebsiella, Citrobacter* and *Stenotrophomonas* species. Vancomycin-resistant enterococci and *Clostridium difficile* are important emerging pathogens, although diarrhea following HSCT is infectious in fewer than 15% of cases.[11,12]

HSV and community-acquired respiratory viruses (CRV) are the most common viral pathogens encountered in the preengraftment period. Autologous and allogeneic HSCT recipients appear to be at similar risk for these viral infections. HSV infections are almost always attributable to reactivation of latent asymptomatic infection in seropositive individuals. In the absence of prophylaxis, 70–80% of seropositive individuals will reactivate HSV in the preengraftment period, with a peak incidence at 2–3 weeks posttransplant. HSV type 1 (HSV 1) accounts for 85% of episodes and produces gingivostomatitis[4]; infection in the mouth may spread to the trachea, esophagus or lungs. In the initial posttransplant period, up to half of mouth lesions may be attributable to HSV 1.[4] The remaining 15% of HSV reactivation episodes are due to HSV type 2 involving the genitals or other cutaneous sites.

Reactivation of other human herpes viruses (HHV) in the early posttransplant period, including HHV-6 and HHV-8, has been associated with the development of clinical symptoms. HHV-6 may reactivate in seropositive recipients of both autologous and allogeneic HSCTs, on average at 2–4 weeks posttransplant.[13,14] An anti-CD3 monoclonal antibody for prophylaxis against acute GVHD in allogeneic HSCT recipients appears to increase the risk of HHV-6 reactivation, which has been associated with the development of fever, rash, interstitial pneumonia, encephalitis, delayed white cell engraftment, and an increase in the severity of GVHD.[14,15] HHV-8 reactivation was recently reported to cause fever, rash, and hepatitis 2–3 weeks following autologous HSCT.[16] The pathogenetic significance of HHV-7 reactivation has been debated; HHV-7 may serve as a cofactor for the development of CMV disease following organ transplantation.[17]

CRV infections may develop in both autologous and allogeneic HSCT recipients and tend to mirror the seasonal occurrence of influenza, parainfluenza, respiratory syncytial virus (RSV), and rhinovirus infections in the community. Outbreaks of RSV and influenza have been described on stem cell transplant units.[18,19] Prevention of infection and containment of outbreaks require meticulous attention to infection control practices, cohorting of infected individuals, immunization against influenza of health care workers and at-risk HSCT candidates pretransplant, and influenza prophylaxis on HSCT units during outbreaks.[2,19] Influenza, parainfluenza, and RSV may produce lower respiratory tract infection in the early posttransplant period with significant morbidity and mortality[20,21]; tracheobronchitis and pneumonia are usually heralded by the onset of upper respiratory tract symptoms, such as rhinorrhea, sinus congestion, and sore throat. Lymphopenia appears to be a risk factor for progression to lower respiratory tract infection in HSCT recipients with influenza.[21] Other pathogens, such as *Aspergillus* species, are frequently isolated in patients with influenza involving the lower respiratory tract. Antiviral therapy in HSCT recipients with influenza with a neuraminidase inhibitor is preferred to amantidine or rimantidine, as neuraminidase inhibitors appear to shorten the duration of viral shedding.[21] Inhaled ribavirin and intravenous immunoglobulin have been advocated for those with RSV. The optimal therapy for a parainfluenza lower respiratory tract infection has not been defined; in a recent study involving allogeneic and autologous HSCT recipients with parainfluenza pneumonia, inhaled ribavirin with or without immunoglobulin did not improve survival.[22] Adenovirus infections occur in up to 6% of pediatric HSCT recipients, often following engraftment, but occasionally in the preengraftment period.[23] Hemorrhagic cystitis, hemorrhagic colitis, pneumonia, nephritis, and hepatic failure are the most common presentations; disseminated disease has been reported.

Invasive fungal infections due to molds and *Candida* species are important clinical problems in the preengraftment period. Autologous HSCT recipients have a lower incidence of these infections compared with those receiving allogeneic transplants. Prior to 1990, *Candida albicans, C. tropicalis,* and *C. parapsilosis* were the most common causes of invasive fungal infections in this setting. However, the demonstration in the early 1990s of the utility of fluconazole prophylaxis in reducing the incidence of superficial and invasive fungal infections in HSCT recipients and its subsequent widespread use[24,25] has led to a decline in the incidence of infections from these organisms. Fluconazole prophylaxis in HSCT recipients has also led to the emergence of the fluconazole-resistant yeasts *C. krusei* and *C. glabrata* as important pathogens in the preengraftment period, and to the emergence of aspergillosis as the most common invasive fungal infection following HSCT.

Candidal infections can present in the preengraftment period as superficial cutaneous infection, thrush, esophagitis, urinary tract infections, fungemia, or as disseminated infection involving the skin, viscera, and bone marrow. Although infection most often arises from organisms that colonize mucosal surfaces, infection of intravascular devices or contamination of infusates such as total parenteral nutrition (TPN) fluid are occasional causes of candidal bloodstream infections. Risk factors for invasive candidal infections include prolonged and severe neutropenia, breakdown of mucosal barriers, and the use of broad spectrum antibiotics, corticosteroids, and TPN.[26]

Invasive molds are a growing cause of morbidity and mortality in the preengraftment period, especially in allogeneic HSCT recipients.[27] Invasive aspergillosis following HSCT occurs in a bimodal distribution, with peak onsets at 16 days and 96 days following HSCT.[27] While the overall incidence of invasive aspergillosis is higher in allogeneic HSCT recipients, early onset disease is more common in autologous HSCT recipients.[27] Risk factors for early onset disease occurring within 40 days of HSCT include transplantation for hematologic malignancy without first remission, HLA-mismatched related donor, HSCT outside a laminar airflow room, and HSCT during summer months.[27] Pneumonia, often with cavitation, is the most common clinical syndrome; invasive aspergillosis can also involve the sinuses, brain, and skin. Other emerging fungal pathogens include *Fusarium* species and the *Zygomycetes*. Fusariosis typically presents as fungemia with hematogenous spread to the skin, and occurs in a trimodal distribution following allogeneic HSCT, with peak incidences prior to engraftment, at 62 days, and beyond 1 year following HSCT.[28] Survival is poor, especially in those with neutropenia. *Zygomycetes*, which present with sinopulmonary disease and for which iron overload and decompensated diabetes mellitus represent risk factors, have been increasingly seen in HSCT recipients receiving antifungal prophylaxis with voriconazole.[26,29,30]

### EVALUATION AND MANAGEMENT OF THE FEBRILE PATIENT

The differential diagnosis of fever in the HSCT recipient in the preengraftment period includes infectious and noninfectious causes, as summarized in Table 99.3. The differential diagnosis is guided by the presence or absence of localizing symptoms and physical findings and by the prior infectious disease history. Routine cultures of blood should be obtained, including through respective lumens of intravascular devices. In multilumen central venous catheters, infection may be confined to the inner surface of a single lumen. Cultures of urine, stool assays for *C. difficile* toxin, nasopharygeal specimens for direct fluorescent antibody testing for CRVs, and mouth cultures for HSV should be obtained as clinically indicated. Plain films of the chest may disclose an infiltrate even in the absence of respiratory symptoms and should be obtained. In patients with sinus symptoms, computed tomography of the sinuses is preferred to sinus plain films. In persistently febrile individuals and those at high risk for invasive aspergillosis, computed tomography of the chest should be performed in search of an occult infiltrate, even if the chest radiograph is normal. In those with a halo sign or cavitary infiltrate, both

**Table 99.3** Common causes of fever in the HSCT recipient in the preengraftment period

| Syndrome | Common pathogens |
| --- | --- |
| Bacteremia<br>    Intravascular devices<br>    Bowel<br>    Other | *Staphylococci*<br>*Viridans streptococci*<br>Gram-negative bacilli |
| Oral Mucositis, Esophagitis | Noninfectious<br>Herpes simplex virus |
| Diarrhea | Noninfectious<br>*Clostridium difficile* |
| Pneumonia | Mouth flora (aspiration)<br>Gram-negative bacilli<br>*Staphylococci*<br>Community respiratory viruses<br>*Aspergillus* species |
| Intravascular device | *Staphylococci*<br>Gram-negative bacilli<br>*Candida* species |
| Noninfectious causes<br>    Drug fever<br>    Chemical aspiration<br>    Engraftment syndrome | |

suggestive of invasive pulmonary aspergillosis, bronchoscopy is indicated to establish a microbiologic diagnosis.

The selection of an empiric antimicrobial regimen should be guided by the suspected anatomic origin of the fever, by the pathogens suspected, and by local susceptibility profiles of institutional isolates. It is imperative to prospectively monitor and report to clinicians the antimicrobial susceptibility profiles of bacterial pathogens encountered within the institution and on the stem cell transplant unit, as this may impact on the selection of empiric antibacterial regimens and identify potential outbreaks.[2] The recent change by the National Committee on Clinical Laboratory Standards in the breakpoint defining susceptibility of coagulase negative staphylococci to methicillin has led to the reclassification of >95% of coagulase negative staphylococci as methicillin-resistant. As these organisms are the most common cause of intravascular device-related bacteremia in HSCT recipients, this has resulted in increasing pressure to include vancomycin in empiric antibacterial regimens in febrile HSCT recipients. The emergence of vancomycin-resistant enterococci and vancomycin-intermediate and vancomycin-resistant *Staphylococcus aureus*[31] has led, on the other hand, to recommendations to minimize indiscriminate vancomycin use.[2] However, a recent single center study suggested that early empiric vancomycin administration with as little as two doses between days −7 and +7 dramatically reduced the incidence of viridans streptococcal bacteremia in HSCT recipients.[32] Therefore, vancomycin may be included in the initial coverage of febrile HSCT recipients pending cultures, but its long-term empiric use in the absence of a microbiologic diagnosis or strong clinical indication is discouraged. Persistent fever despite antifungal prophylaxis with fluconazole or low-dose amphotericin should heighten concern about invasive fungal infection and prompt consideration of empiric antifungal therapy with higher dose amphotericin B or voriconazole.

### PROPHYLAXIS AND THERAPY

Routine decontamination of the gut is not recommended for HSCT candidates.[2] The use of oral fluoroquinolones and an agent active against Gram-positive cocci in asymptomatic neutropenic patients reduces the occurrence of Gram-positive and Gram-negative bacteremias, but has no impact on fever-related morbidity or infection-related mortality.[33] A novel strategy to reduce the occurrence of oral mucositis after intensive chemotherapy using palifermin (recombinant human keratinocyte growth factor) has demonstrated promise. In a double-blind, placebo-controlled trial involving patients with hematologic malignancies, palifermin recipients had less severe mucositis, a shorter duration of mucositis, and a lower incidence of fever during neutropenia and bacteremia compared with placebo recipients.[34]

Acyclovir prophylaxis is indicated for all HSV-seropositive HSCT candidates and has been shown to reduce the occurrence of viral reactivation.[35] Prophylaxis should commence at the initiation of the preparative regimen and continue to engraftment or to the resolution of mucositis.[2] Valacyclovir has not been FDA-approved for this indication.

Antifungal prophylaxis is indicated during neutropenia in all allogeneic and most autologous HSCT recipients. Fluconazole has been recommended by the Centers for Disease Control and Prevention, the Infectious Disease Society of America, and the American Society of Blood and Marrow Transplantation,[2] but is not effective in the prevention of infections due to *Aspergillus* species, *C. krusei*, and *C. glabrata*. This has led some centers to use other agents for antifungal prophylaxis, including low or moderate dose amphotericin B, liposomal amphotericin B, inhaled or nasal amphotericin B, and voriconazole. Unfortunately, the efficacy of these various prophylactic strategies has not been demonstrated in well designed clinical trials. Moreover, the zygomycetes have emerged as important pathogens in patients receiving voriconazole prophylaxis or therapy.[29,30] Oral itraconazole should not be used because of its variable absorption; its interactions with other agents such as cyclosporine, methylprednisolone, rifampin, antiepileptics, and warfarin; and the prolonged time required to achieve steady state concentrations in the blood.[2] New antifungals

are in development and may have a future role in prophylaxis against fungal infections in HSCT recipients. A recent large, randomized, double-blind, multicenter, prospective phase 3 clinical trial compared fluconazole with micafungin, a new echinocandin, for prophylaxis against invasive fungal infections in neutropenic patients undergoing autologous and allogeneic HSCT.[36] Micafungin was superior to fluconazole across treatment groups and was associated with a lower incidence of aspergillosis and colonization with *C. glabrata*.

Empiric antibacterial therapy in febrile HSCT recipients should be guided by the suspected site of infection and by knowledge of antimicrobial susceptibility profiles of institutional isolates as well as by organisms previously infecting or colonizing the patient. Catheter-related infections can often be cured without device removal, except in those with tunnel, fungal, or mycobacterial infections and in those who are hemodynamically unstable. Empiric antifungal therapy in persistently febrile neutropenic patients has traditionally been amphotericin B. A recent randomized, double-blind, multicenter study compared the echinocandin caspofungin with liposomal amphotericin B for empiric therapy in 1095 persistently febrile neutropenic patients, of whom 75 were HSCT recipients.[37] Caspofungin was as effective and better tolerated than amphoterin B, with lower incidences of nephrotoxicity and infusion-related side effects.

For decades amphotericin B has been the treatment of choice for invasive aspergillosis and other filamentous fungi; however, response rates have been disappointing, and as low as 10–15% in allogeneic HSCT recipients.[38] Several alternative agents have recently become available with superior efficacy. Voriconazole is a broad-spectrum triazole with activity against most *Candida* and *Aspergillus* species. In a randomized, unblinded trial comparing high-dose amphotericin B with voriconazole for primary therapy in 277 patients with suspected or proven invasive aspergillosis, many of whom were HSCT recipients, voriconazole had superior efficacy and fewer serious side effects compared with amphotericin B. After 12 weeks, 52.8% of voriconazole recipients versus 31.6% in the amphotericin B group had responded to therapy, though transient visual disturbances occurred in nearly half of voriconazole recipients.[39]

While superior to amphotericin B, voriconazole is not uniformly effective and many patients require salvage therapy. Several recent studies have examined alternative strategies. The utility of the echinocandin caspofungin was examined in 83 patients with invasive aspergillosis who were refractory to or intolerant of conventional therapy; 79.5% had failed conventional therapy with formulations of amphotericin B and 25% were HSCT recipients.[40] Forty-five percent responded to caspofungin, including 50% with pulmonary aspergillosis and 23% with disseminated disease; however, HSCT recipients had a poorer response compared with those with hematologic malignancies. In a small, single center observational study, HSCT recipients with refractory invasive aspergillosis were treated with a combination of voriconazole and caspofungin, and compared with an earlier group treated with voriconazole alone.[41] In this nonrandomized study, patients who received combination therapy had improved survival at 3 months compared with historical controls who received voriconazole monotherapy.

## THE EARLY ENGRAFTMENT PERIOD

The early engraftment period begins with the resolution of neutropenia and continues to approximately day 100. The risk of infection in this period is substantially lower in autologous compared with allogeneic HSCT recipients. With the resolution of neutropenia, most patients quickly heal their mucositis. However, GVHD in allogeneic HSCT recipients can lead to recurrent breakdown of mucosal barriers in the gastrointestinal tract, predisposing to recurrent bacterial or fungal bloodstream infections. Nearly all allogeneic HSCT recipients require indwelling vascular devices through this period, which pose an ongoing risk for bacterial infection. Impaired cell-mediated immunity is the major risk factor for infection in this period, especially in allogeneic HSCT recipients, which may be further compromised by the immunosuppressive therapy required to prevent rejection or treat GVHD. Additional immune defects in this period include hyposplenism, diminished neutrophil opsonic and phagocytic function, and the deleterious effects of immunomodulating viruses such as CMV and HHV6.

### MICROBIOLOGY

The pathogens requiring consideration in the early postengraftment period are summarized in Table 99.4. Bacterial infections arising from indwelling intravascular devices and mucositis in the setting of GVHD continue to occur in the early postengraftment period. The microbiology of these infections is similar to that encountered in the preengraftment period. Invasive fungal infections due to resistant yeasts, *Aspergillus* species, *Fusaria* species, and zygomycetes also occur during this period. GVHD, graft failure, and corticosteroid therapy are major risk factors for invasive aspergillosis, whose peak incidence in allogeneic HSCT recipients occurs at this time.[27] Patients remain at-risk for CRV infections. Unlike children, in whom adenovirus infection is more often seen in the preengraftment period, adult patients tend to develop adenovirus infection beyond 90 days.[42] As in children, pneumonia, hemorrhagic cystitis, hemorrhagic colitis, and nephritis are the major clinical syndromes.

**Table 99.4** Pathogens encountered in the early postengraftment period

| Pathogens | Common sites of involvement, origin |
|---|---|
| **Common** | |
| **Bacteria** | |
| *Staphylococci* | Intravascular devices |
| *Streptococci* | Mouth and bowel with GVHD |
| *Enterococci* | Mouth and bowel with GVHD |
| Gram-negative bacilli | Intravascular devices, GI tract with GVHD |
| **Viruses** | |
| CMV | Viremia, pneumonia, enterocolitis; reactivation of latent infection, primary infection |
| **Fungi** | |
| *Aspergillus* species | Pneumonia, CNS |
| ***Less Common*** | |
| **Bacteria** | |
| *Legionella* species | Pneumonia, exclude nosocomial water source |
| *Listeria monocytogenes* | Meningoencephalitis, bacteremia |
| **Viruses** | |
| Adenovirus | Pneumonia, nephritis, hemorrhagic cystitis, hemorrhagic colitis, hepatitis |
| HHV6 | Fever, rash, interstitial pneumonia, encephalitis |
| Community-acquired respiratory | Upper respiratory tract infections, pneumonia viruses |
| **Fungi** | |
| Zygomycetes | Pneumonia, sinusitis |
| *Candida* species | Fungemia, hepatosplenic candidiasis, disseminated infection; intravascular devices and gut with GVHD |
| *Fusaria* species | Fungemia, cutaneous disease, pneumonia |
| *Pseudallescheria boydii* | Pneumonia |
| **Parasites** | |
| *Pneumocystis carinii* | Pneumonia |
| *Toxoplasma gondii* | CNS, pneumonia, disseminated disease; reactivation of latent infection |
| *Strongyloides stercoralis* | Enterocolitis, pneumonia, bowel perforation, Gram-negative bacteremia; accelerated autoinfection cycle |

Several pathogens require special comment. Legionellosis is uncommon but has been reported in the setting of HSCT.[43] The disease may occur in the pretransplant or preengraftment periods, but is most common in the early engraftment period.[43] A sentinel case occurring beyond day 10 of hospitalization should raise the possibility of nosocomial transmission, and an appropriate epidemiologic and environmental investigation is mandatory.[2] Unrecognized nosocomial transmission of legionellosis for over a decade in the transplant setting has been described.[44] HSCT patients with legionellosis present with fever and lobar, patchy, or nodular pulmonary infiltrates. In those with nodular infiltrates, the disease may mimic invasive pulmonary aspergillosis, the most common cause of such infiltrates in this setting. HSCT recipients with legionellosis are at increased risk for mortality and may require more prolonged courses of therapy than immunocompetent individuals.[44] *Legionella pneumophila* infections are more often fatal than those due to non-*pneumophila Legionella* strains.

Listeriosis in HSCT recipients is rare, but occurs most often in the early postengraftment period.[45] Meningoencephalitis and bacteremia are the most common clinical presentations. A history of high-risk food ingestion associated with listeriosis is typically absent.

Parasitic infections are uncommon following HSCT, but are most likely to occur in the early postengraftment period. The incidence of *Pneumocystis carinii* pneumonia has declined dramatically with the widespread use of chemoprophylaxis. The median time to onset is 9 weeks following HSCT. Patients typically present with fever, worsening dyspnea, dry cough, and interstitial pulmonary infiltrates.[46] One hundred and ten cases of toxoplasmosis have been described following HSCT[47]; 64% have occurred between days 31 and 100, likely representing reactivation of latent infection in the face of immunosuppression. Forty-eight percent of cases have been confined to the brain. Disseminated infection occurred in 48%. Fever was the most common sign, but was only present in 43%. Focal neurologic symptoms, headache, altered mentation, and respiratory complaints were present in a minority of patients. Meningitis occasionally accompanies cerebral toxoplasmosis, and the organism can been identified on cytologic examination of cerebrospinal fluid. Hyperinfection strongyloidiasis is rare following HSCT and has not been reported in autologous recipients.[2] Immunosuppression in allogeneic recipients leads to acceleration of the autoinfection cycle of *S. stercoralis* in those with unrecognized asymptomatic infection. Patients typically develop symptoms 4–6 weeks from the initiation of immunosuppressive therapy consisting of fever, diarrhea, respiratory symptoms, and occasionally intestinal perforation owing to widespread migration of larval parasites through the bowel wall and the lungs.[48] Specimens of stool, sputum, and bronchoalveolar lavage fluid typically demonstrate larvae of *S. stercoralis* on parasitologic examination.

CMV is the most important and common viral pathogen encountered in the early postengraftment period. In the era prior to prophylactic or preemptive therapy, morbidity and mortality from CMV were substantial. Among seropositive allogeneic HSCT recipients, the group at greatest risk, the incidence of CMV infection varied from 42% to 69%; symptomatic disease developed in 16–25%, with pneumonia in up to 5%.[49] The incidence in autologous HSCT recipients was lower but still substantial. Prior to the availability of antiviral therapy, mortality from CMV pneumonia following HSCT approached 50%.[50] The widespread used of targeted prophylaxis or preemptive therapy from engraftment to day 100 in allogeneic HSCT recipients has led to a significant decline in the incidence of symptomatic disease during the early engraftment period, but late disease beyond day 100 is increasingly recognized.[5,51] Risk factors for symptomatic CMV disease include advanced age, conditioning with total body irradiation, seropositive recipient status, HSCT from a matched unrelated donor, CD34+ allogeneic HSCT, acute GVHD, and high titers of circulating CMV. Symptomatic disease is uncommon in autologous HSCT recipients; patients at higher risk include seropositive recipients with underlying hematologic malignancies, those receiving intensive conditioning regimens, and recent recipients of fludarabine or 2-chlorodeoxyadenosine.[2] CMV appears to be immunomodulatory and seronegative allogeneic HSCT recipients with seropositive donors have a higher risk of death from bacterial and fungal infections.[49]

The common clinical syndromes produced by CMV include fever without localizing findings, interstitial pneumonia, enterocolitis, and bone marrow suppression. Hepatitis, retinitis, and CNS disease are less common.

### EVALUATION AND MANAGEMENT OF THE FEBRILE PATIENT

The differential diagnosis of fever in the early engraftment period is broad. Essential considerations include the patient's prior infectious disease history in the preengraftment and pretransplant periods; timing of onset of fever; the presence or absence of localizing signs and symptoms; the presence or absence of GVHD or symptoms suggestive of GVHD; risk of CMV; and current medications. The differential diagnosis for common clinical syndromes is summarized in Table 99.5 and includes both infectious and noninfectious causes.

Fever at the time of engraftment raises several special considerations, including engraftment syndrome, which is often accompanied by a diffuse maculopapular rash; acute GVHD; or flare of occult infection as leucocytes return and migrate to a site of inflammation.

Fever in the absence of localizing symptoms during the early postengraftment period has many causes. Bacteremia or fungemia from intravascular devices or from the bowel in patients with GVHD may present without localizing symptoms. Patients with pulmonary

**Table 99.5   Common causes of fever in the early engraftment period**

| Syndrome | Common sources, pathogens |
|---|---|
| Fever at engraftment | Engraftment syndrome |
| | Acute GVHD |
| | Occult focal infection |
| **Fever without localizing findings** | |
| ■ Bacteremia | Intravascular devices |
| | *Staphylococci* |
| | Gram-negative bacilli |
| | Gut GVHD |
| | Gram-negative bacilli |
| | *Enterococci* |
| ■ Fungemia | Intravascular devices |
| | *Candida* species |
| | Gut GVHD |
| | *Candida* species |
| ■ Occult pneumonia | Aspergillosis |
| | Fusariosis |
| | Zygomycosis |
| ■ Sinusitis | GVHD, bacterial infection |
| ■ Viral infections | CMV, HHV6 |
| ■ Drug fever | Penicillins, cephalosporins, trimethoprim-sulfamethoxazole, vancomycin, phenytoin |
| **Fever and a pulmonary infiltrate** | |
| ■ Fungal pneumonia | Aspergillosis, Fusariosis, Zygomycosis |
| ■ Bacterial pneumonia | *Staphylococci*, Gram-negative bacilli, Legionellosis |
| ■ Viral pneumonia | CMV, community respiratory viruses |
| ■ Noninfectious causes | Aspiration, idiopathic interstitial pneumonia, diffuse alveolar hemorrhage |
| **Fever with diarrhea** | |
| ■ GVHD | |
| ■ C. *difficile* | |
| ■ CMV | |
| ■ Community viruses | |

fungal infections such as aspergillosis, fusariosis, or zygomycosis may lack cough, dyspnea, and hemoptysis at the outset. Sinusitis from infection or GVHD may be asymptomatic except for fever. CMV infection may present only with fever and must be strongly considered in CMV seropositive allogeneic HSCT recipients and seronegative recipients with a CMV seropositive donor. HSCT recipients who are CMV D-/R- have a small risk of CMV in this period. The concern for reactivation CMV is heightened in at-risk and high-risk individuals who are being followed and monitored prospectively for viremia, rather than receiving prophylaxis from the time of engraftment. Fever without

localizing signs or symptoms may also occur as an initial manifestation of adenovirus infection or reactivation of HHV6. Noninfectious causes of fever include early GVHD and new medications. Medications which are most likely to cause drug fever include trimethoprim-sulfamethoxazole, penicillins, cephalosporins, vancomycin, and phenytoin.

The differential diagnosis of fever and a pulmonary infiltrate includes infectious and noninfectious causes. Infectious causes include bacterial pneumonia (including legionellosis), pulmonary fungal infections, and CRV infections during seasonal outbreaks. Noninfectious causes include diffuse alveolar hemorrhage (though fever may be absent), aspiration pneumonia, and idiopathic interstitial pneumonia.

In patients with fever and diarrhea, concerns include GVHD, CMV or adenovirus enterocolitis, *C. difficile*-associated diarrhea, and community-acquired viral gastroenteritis caused by rotavirus, Norwalk virus, or coxsackievirus during seasonal outbreaks. Diarrhea is infectious in origin in a minority of HSCT patients during this period.

The differential diagnosis of fever and rash depends upon the appearance of the rash. If maculopapular, concerns include engraftment syndrome, acute GVHD (especially if the rash involves the palms and soles), drug reaction, and reactivation of HHV6. A papulopustular rash consisting of only a few scattered lesions should suggest disseminated candidiasis. Nodular skin lesions may occur with disseminated aspergillosis or fusariosis, disseminated cryptococcosis, and nocardiosis. The latter two infections are rare following HSCT, especially in the early postengraftment period, and are generally encountered beyond 100 days. A vesicular rash should suggest HSV or VZV, the latter being uncommon between days 30 and 100.

The diagnostic evaluation should be tailored based upon the presence or absence of localizing signs and symptoms to suggest a source of fever. Blood cultures for bacterial pathogens are indicated in most patients. In those with clinical clues as to the cause of fever, additional cultures and imaging studies may be pursued. In those without localizing findings, blood cultures should be obtained from each lumen of indwelling vascular devices and peripherally. Fungal blood cultures should be collected if unexplained fever persists. Patients at-risk for CMV infection should be tested using the pp65 antigenemia assay, polymerase chain reaction, or hybrid capture for CMV viremia. Computed tomographic scans of the sinuses, chest, and abdomen should be considered in search of occult sinusitis, occult pulmonary infiltrates, and thickening of the bowel wall suggestive of GVHD or infectious enterocolitis. Biopsy for histopathologic examination and culture may establish a diagnosis in patients with rash; vesicular lesions should be unroofed and scraped for viral culture. In patients with fever and pulmonary infiltrates, bronchoscopy should be strongly considered.

## PROPHYLAXIS AND THERAPY

Antibacterial prophylaxis is recommended in allogeneic HSCT recipients who develop chronic GVHD and should be targeted at encapsulated organisms, including *Streptococcus pneumoniae, Hemophilus influenzae,* and *Neisseria meningitidis.*[2] Selection of a regimen should be guided by local pneumococcal susceptibility profiles. Prophylaxis against *Pneumocystis carinii* is indicated in allogeneic HSCT recipients and should commence with engraftment and extend through all periods of immunodeficiency and for at least 6 months.[2] High-risk autologous HSCT recipients are candidates for PCP prophylaxis, including those with underlying hematologic malignancies, recipients of intensive preparative regimens or graft manipulation, and recent recipients of fludarabine or 2-chlorodeoxyadenosine. Trimethoprim-sulfamethoxazole is the preferred agent. In allergic individuals, desensitization should be attempted. In those unable to tolerate trimethoprim-sulfamethoxazole, alternative agents include dapsone, atovaquone, and aerosolized pentamidine. The latter is least effective and should only be used in patients unable to tolerate other regimens.

Prophylaxis against *I. gondii* is recommended in allogeneic HSCT patients with active GVHD or with a prior history of *Toxoplasma* chorioretinitis.[2] Trimethoprim-sulfamethoxazole is preferred, though rare break-through cases have occurred.[52] In sulfa-intolerant patients, clindamycin, pyrimethamine, and leucovorin may be substituted.

Prophylaxis against yeast infections is not routinely recommended following engraftment. The utility of and optimal regimen for prophylaxis against aspergillosis in the early postengraftment period is unclear; many centers nevertheless choose to continue *Aspergillus* prophylaxis though this period, especially in high-risk individuals with GVHD.

All allogeneic HSCT recipients at-risk for CMV, including CMV seropositive recipients and seronegative recipients with seropositive donors, should either receive prophylaxis commencing at engraftment or should be monitored at least weekly for evidence of CMV viremia.[2] Several tests may be used to detect CMV viremia, including the pp65 antigenemia assay, CMV-DNA PCR, or hybrid capture DNA detection. Routine and rapid shell vial cultures are less sensitive and more time-consuming. CMV-DNA PCR is extremely sensitive, but has a low positive predictive value.[53] Patients with detectable antigenemia on 2 or more consecutive tests positive for CMV DNA should commence preemptive therapy. Ganciclovir given intravenously has been the agent of choice for prophylaxis and preemptive treatment. However, one recent multicenter, randomized study compared oral valacyclovir with intravenous ganciclovir from engraftment to day 100 in CMV seropositive allogeneic HSCT recipients and found oral valacyclovir comparably effective.[53] Once commenced, ganciclovir should be continued through day 100 or at least for 3 weeks in those receiving preemptive therapy, whichever is longer. If tests are available to detect viremia, a negative test result should be confirmed prior to discontinuing ganciclovir. A prophylactic strategy is preferred in centers unable to perform CMV antigen detection or CMV DNA detection by PCR or hybrid capture. Some centers with these capabilities nevertheless prefer a prophylactic strategy, while others advocate preemptive therapy so as to limit unnecessary ganciclovir exposure, as ganciclovir prophylaxis has been associated with more neutropenia, delayed recovery of CMV-specific immune responses, and a higher incidence of invasive fungal and bacterial infections.[2,49,54] Neutropenia arising on ganciclovir may be managed with G-CSF, or by holding the drug for several days. In those unable to tolerate ganciclovir, foscarnet may be used. The strategies of CMV prophylaxis and preventive therapy have reduced the incidence of CMV disease in the early postengraftment period. There is increasing evidence, however, of late CMV disease beyond day 100 in high-risk patients.[51] Risk factors for late disease include the presence of chronic GVHD, corticosteroid use, delayed development of high avidity anti-CMV antibody, low CD4 count, and receipt of a matched unrelated or T-cell-depleted HSCT.[2] The utility of extended prophylaxis in high-risk patients has not been proven; these individuals should be monitored for evidence of CMV viremia beyond day 100, especially during intensification of immunosuppression. If detected, 3 weeks of preemptive therapy is recommended.

Because CMV disease is rare following autologous HSCT, screening for viremia is not routinely recommended, except in high-risk patients with underlying hematologic malignancies, in those who have recently received fludarabine or 2-chlorodeoxyadenosine, or in recipients of particularly intensive preparative regimens.[2] In such individuals, monitoring to day 60 has been suggested; viremic patients should receive 3 weeks of preemptive therapy.

Patients with tissue invasive CMV disease, such as pneumonia and enterocolitis, should receive 3 weeks of therapy.[5] Ganciclovir-resistant CMV is rare and usually occurs in immunodeficient patients who have previously received multiple courses of ganciclovir. Sustained viremia through ganciclovir should suggest the presence of UL97 genotypic resistance mutations and prompt a switch to foscarnet.

## THE LATE ENGRAFTMENT PERIOD

The late engraftment period commences at day 100 and continues until the discontinuation of all immunosuppressive therapy and the absence of GVHD. Beyond day 100, autologous HSCT recipients have a more rapid return of immune function compared with allogeneic recipients, and their risk of opportunistic infection is low. Defects in humoral, cellular, and reticuloendothelial immune function persist beyond day 100 in allogeneic HSCT recipients for up to 18–36 months, especially in those with GVHD and in those who have received matched unrelated, mismatched family-related, or umbilical cord blood HSCTs. In general, the risk of opportunistic infection correlates with the severity of chronic GVHD during this period.

### MICROBIOLOGY

Allogeneic HSCT recipients who continue to require indwelling intravascular devices and who have disrupted mucosal barriers from chronic GVHD remain at-risk for bacterial infections from these sites. In addition, because of humoral immunodeficiency, these patients are at higher risk of infection with encapsulated organisms such as *S. pneumoniae* and *H. influenzae*. These typically present as bacteremia, pneumonia, or sinusitis.

Allogeneic HSCT recipients are at-risk beyond day 100 for a number of viral infections. As many will be out of hospital, CRV infections continue to pose a threat. Late-onset CMV disease is increasingly common, and in a recent study developed in 17.8% of allogeneic HSCT recipients a median of 169 days after transplantation.[55] Mortality was 46%, and 38% of survivors had a second episode a median of 79 days following the first episode. Risk factors at 3 months for late CMV disease and death included GVHD, absolute lymphopenia <100 lymphocytes/cc, CD4 T-lymphocyte count <50 cells/cc, prior CMV antigenemia, and absent CMV-specific T-cell responses. Beyond 3 months, continued antigenemia or CMV DNA detection in peripheral leucocytes or plasma predicted late disease and death.

VZV is common following HSCT and occurs in both autologous and allogeneic HSCT recipients.[56] Eighty-six percent of cases occur within the first 18 months, with a median onset at 5 months.[5,56] Risk factors include age >10, radiation as part of the conditioning regimen, and VZV seropositivity.[56] Patients with dermatomal disease are at-risk for cutaneous or visceral dissemination, especially in the setting of GVHD. Atypical presentations of VZV with few vesicles or pain in the abdomen or back can occur. Atypical generalized zoster presents with multiple vesicular lesions without a dermatomal distribution. In those with dermatomal disease, the presence of more than 10 lesions outside the dermatome defines cutaneous dissemination. Visceral dissemination may involve the lungs, liver, or CNS.

EBV infection is common following HSCT, especially in EBV seronegative patients with a seropositive donor. Symptomatic disease is less common and may include fever with a mononucleosis-like illness, aplastic anemia, meningoencephalitis, or posttransplant lymphoproliferative disorder (PTLD). PTLD is the most feared manifestation of EBV infection and arises due to polyclonal or monoclonal B-cell activation in the setting of inadequate EBV-specific T cell immune surveillance. PTLD may present as a mono-like illness, as focal mass lesions in various sites, such as the lung or brain, as intestinal bleeding or perforation, or as widespread disease involving multiple organs, mimicking lymphoma. Onset typically occurs 3–5 months following HSCT. The incidence varies from <1% in matched related allogeneic HSCT recipients to up to 18% in certain high-risk groups, including recipients of matched unrelated, mismatched or T-cell depleted allografts, and those who receive GVHD prophylaxis with T-cell specific monoclonal antibodies or antithymocyte globulin.[57,58]

Mycobacterial infections due to *M. tuberculosis* and nontuberculous mycobacteria are rare but reported following HSCT and typically present with a median onset at 4–5 months following transplantation.[59,60] Nontuberculous mycobacterial infections present as catheter-related infections, or as pulmonary, cutaneous, or disseminated disease. *M. tuberculosis* most often produces reactivation pulmonary disease, but rarely presents with pleural, nodal, cutaneous, marrow, or CNS involvement.

### EVALUATION AND MANAGEMENT OF THE FEBRILE PATIENT

The differential diagnosis of fever in the late post engraftment period is broad, as many patients will be out of hospital and at-risk for community-acquired infectious diseases. The risk of opportunistic infection is proportionate to the extent of GVHD present and the degree of residual immunodeficiency. Autologous HSCT recipients are much less likely to have an opportunistic infection compared with allogeneic patients. The diagnostic evaluation and management should be guided by the history, by the presence or absence of localizing complaints, by the presence or absence of GVHD and the degree of immunodeficiency, and by the prior infectious disease history.

The differential diagnosis of fever without localizing symptoms or signs should include bacteremia, late-onset CMV disease, and PTLD. Although patients with chronic GVHD or indwelling intravascular devices remain at-risk for bloodstream infections with staphylococci and Gram-negative bacilli, encapsulated organisms should be suspected. All patients should have blood cultures obtained. High-risk patients for late-onset CMV disease should be screened for CMV viremia. PTLD is rare, but circulating EBV may be sought by PCR and high titers correlate with a greater likelihood of PTLD. If suspected, CT scans to identify adenopathy or masses in the chest, abdomen or pelvis should be performed.

In febrile patients without an obvious source of infection, empiric antibiotic therapy should be strongly considered pending blood cultures and should include coverage of *S. pneumoniae*, *H. influenzae*, and

*N. meningitidis.* Knowledge regarding the local incidence of penicillin-resistant pneumococci is essential in selecting a regimen. Patients with proven bacteremia with an encapsulated organism should be screened for hypogammaglobulinemia. Patients with late CMV viremia or invasive disease should be treated as outlined previously; clearance of viremia should be documented at the conclusion of 3 weeks of antiviral therapy.

The differential diagnosis in patients with a pneumonia syndrome depends upon the history, the likelihood of opportunistic infection, and the radiographic pattern of the infiltrate. In patients with acute onset of fever, a productive cough and a focal infiltrate, pneumococcal or *H. influenzae* pneumonia should be suspected. The presence of a nodular or cavitary infiltrate should suggest aspergillosis, tuberculosis, nocardiosis, zygomycosis, or PTLD. Interstitial infiltrates should suggest CMV, PCP, CRV, or noninfectious causes, which may account for up to 50% of cases in this setting. Diagnostic evaluation should include blood cultures and examination of expectorated sputum for pathogens suspected from the history and radiographic findings. Bronchoscopy may be necessary to establish a diagnosis in those with nodular, cavitary or interstitial infiltrates.

Sinusitis and otitis media from encapsulated organisms occur with higher frequency in the late engraftment period; symptoms to suggest these diagnoses should be carefully sought in allogeneic HSCT recipients with fever. Patients with VZV may present with dermatomal or atypical pain that heralds the onset of rash by up to 72 h.

## PROPHYLAXIS AND THERAPY

Patients with chronic GVHD should receive prophylactic antibiotic therapy directed against encapsulated organisms as long as immunosuppressive treatment is being administered; the regimen should be selected based upon local resistance patterns of *S. pneumoniae* and *H. influenzae*.[2] The 23-valent pneumococcal polysaccharide vaccine should be administered 12–24 months after HSCT and HiB conjugate vaccine should be given at 12, 14, and 24 months as well.[2] Patients with hypogammaglobulinemia may require replacement therapy if they experience recurrent infections with encapsulated organisms, or at the time of a serious first episode.

CMV prophylaxis is not recommended beyond day 100, but high-risk patients should receive biweekly screening. Ganciclovir should be administered for at least 3 weeks if viremia is detected. EBV and VZV prophylaxis are not recommended.[2] Anecdotal reports have suggested efficacy of acyclovir and ganciclovir in patients with PTLD, but no large trials have been performed and antiviral therapy is not recommended.[2] If possible, immunosuppression should be reduced if PTLD is identified. The administration of donor-derived, EBV-specific cytotoxic T cells has demonstrated promise in the prevention of PTLD in high-risk patients.[61] Influenza immunization is indicated on an annual basis beginning 6 months after HSCT.[2]

## REFERENCES

1. Barnes RA, Stallard N: Severe infections after bone marrow transplantation. *Curr Opin Crit Care* 7:362–366, 2001.
2. Centers for Disease Control and Prevention. Guidelines for preventing opportunistic infections among hematopoietic stem cell transplant recipients. *MMWR* 49(RR-10):1–125, 2000.
3. Kusne S, Krystofiak S: Infection control issues after bone marrow transplantation. *Curr Opin Infect Dis* 14:427–431, 2001.
4. Sable CA, Donowitz GR: Infections in bone marrow transplant recipients. *Clin Infect Dis* 18:273–284, 1993.
5. van Burik JA, Weisdorf: Hematopoietic stem cell therapy: infections in recipients of blood and marrow transplantation. *Hemat/Oncol Clin North Am* 13:1065–1089, 1993.
6. Shenep JL: Viridans-group streptococcal infections in immunocompromised hosts. *Internat J Antimicrob Agents* 14:129–135, 2000.
7. Elishoov H, Or R, Strauss N, et al.: Nosocomial colonization, septicemia, and Hickman-Broviac catheter-related infections in bone marrow transplant recipients. A 5-year prospective study. *Medicine (Baltimore)* 77:83–101, 1998.
8. Mossad SB, Longworth DL, Goormastic M, et al.: Early infectious complications in autologous bone marrow transplantation: a review of 219 patients. *Bone Marrow Transplant* 18:265–271, 1996.
9. Steiner M, Villablanca J, Kersey J, et al.: Viridans streptococcal shock in bone marrow transplantation patients. *Am J Hematol* 42:354–358, 1993.
10. Alcaide F, Linares JA, Pallares R, et al.: In vitro activities of 22 beta-lactam antibiotics against penicillin-resistant and penicillin-susceptible viridans group *Streptococci* isolated from blood. *Antimicrob Agents Chemother* 39:2243–2247, 1995.
11. Kirkpatrick BD, Harrington SM, Smith D, et al.: Outbreak of vancomycin-dependent *Enterococcus faecium* in a bone marrow transplant unit. *Clin Infect Dis* 29:1268–1273, 1999.
12. Cox GJ, Matsui SM, Lo RS, et al.: Etiology and outcome of diarrhea after marrow transplantation: a prospective study. *Gastroenterology* 107:1398–1407, 1994.
13. Kadakia MP, Rybka WB, Stewart JA, et al.: Human herpes virus 6: infection and disease following autologous and allogeneic bone marrow transplantation. *Blood* 87:5341–5354, 1996.
14. Imbert-Marcille BM, Tang XW, Lepelletier D, et al.: Human herpes virus 6 infection after autologous or allogeneic stem cell transplantation: a single-center prospective longitudinal study of 92 patients. *Clin Infect Dis* 31:881–886, 2000.

15. Zerr DM, Gooley TA, Yeung L, et al.: Human herpesvirus 6 reactivation and encephalitis in allogeneic bone marrow transplant recipients. *Clin Infect Dis* 33:763–771, 2001.

16. Luppi M, Barozzi P, Schultz TF, et al.: Nonmalignant disease associated with human herpesvirus 8 reactivation in patients who have undergone autologous peripheral blood stem cell transplantation. *Blood* 96:2355–2357, 2000.

17. Yoshikawa T: Human herpesvirus-6 and 7 infections in transplantation. *Pediatr Transplant* 7:11–17, 2003.

18. Harrington RD, Hooten TM, Hackman RC, et al.: An outbreak of respiratory syncytial virus infection in a bone marrow transplant center. *J Infect Dis* 165:987–993, 1992.

19. Weinstock DM, Eagen J, Malak SA, et al.: Control of influenza A on a bone marrow transplant unit. *Infect Control Hosp Epidemiol* 21:730–732, 2000.

20. Ljunman P, Ward KN, Crooks BNA, et al.: Respiratory virus infections after stem cell transplantation: a prospective study from the infectious diseases working party of the European group for blood and marrow transplantation. *Bone Marrow Transplant* 28:479–484, 2001.

21. Nichols WG, Guthrie KA, Corey L, et al.: Influenza infections after hematopoietic stem cell transplantation: risk factors, mortality, and the effect of antiviral therapy. *Clin Infect Dis* 39:1300–1306, 2004.

22. Nichols WG, Corey L, Gooley T, et al.: Parainfluenza virus infections after hematopoietic stem cell transplantation: risk factors, response to antiviral therapy, and effect on transplant outcome. *Blood* 98:573–578, 2001.

23. Hale GA, Heslop HE, Krance RA, et al.: Adenovirus infection after pediatric bone marrow transplantation. *Bone Marrow Transplant* 23:277–282, 1999.

24. Goodman JL, Winston DJ, Greenfield RA, et al.: A controlled trial of fluconazole to prevent fungal infections in patients undergoing bone marrow transplantation. *N Engl J Med* 326:845–851, 1992.

25. Slavin MA, Osborne B, Adams R, et al.: Efficacy and safety of fluconazole prophylaxis for fungal infections after marrow transplantation—a prospective, randomized, double-blind study. *J Infect Dis* 171:1545–1552, 1995.

26. De La Rosa GR, Champlin RE, Kontoyiannis DP: Risk factors for the development of invasive fungal infections in allogeneic blood and marrow transplant recipients. *Transplant Infect Dis* 4:3–9, 2002.

27. Wald A, Leisenring, van Burik J, Bowden R: Epidemiology of *Aspergillus* infections in a large cohort of patients undergoing bone marrow transplantation. *J Infect Dis* 175:1459–1466, 1997.

28. Nucci M, Marr KA, Queiroz-Telles F, et al.: Fusarium infection in hematopoietic stem cell transplant recipients. *Clin Infect Dis* 38:1237–1242, 2004.

29. Siwek GT, Dodgson KJ, de Magalhaes-Silverman M, et al.: Invasive zygomycosis in hematopoietic stem cell transplant recipients receiving voriconazole prophylaxis. *Clin Infect Dis* 39:584–587, 2004.

30. Imhof A, Balajee A, Fredricks DN, et al.: Breakthrough fungal infections in stem cell transplant recipients receiving voriconazole. *Clin Infect Dis* 39:743–746, 2004.

31. Fridkin SK: Vancomycin-intermediate and resistant *Staphylococcus aureus*: what the infectious disease specialist needs to know. *Clin Infect Dis* 32:108–115, 2001.

32. Jaffe D, Jakubowski A, Sepkowitz K, et al.: Prevention of peritransplantation viridans streptococcal bacteremia with early vancomycin administration: a single-center observational cohort study. *Clin Infect Dis* 39:1625–1632, 2004.

33. Cruciani M, Rampazzo R, Malena M, et al.: Prophylaxis with fluoroquinolones for bacterial infections in neutropenic patients: a meta-analysis. *Clin Infect Dis* 23:795–805, 1996.

34. Spielberger R, Stiff P, Bensinger W, et al.: Palifermin for oral mucositis after intensive therapy for hematologic cancers. *N Engl J Med* 351:2590–2598, 2004.

35. Epstein JB, Ransier A, Sherlock CH, et al.: Acyclovir prophylaxis of oral herpes virus during bone marrow transplantation. *Eur J Cancer Biol Oral Oncol* 32B:158, 1996.

36. van-Burik JH, Ratanatharathorn V, Stepan DE, et al.: Micafungin versus fluconazole for prophylaxis against invasive fungal infections during neutropenia in patients undergoing hematopoietic stem cell transplantation. *Clin Infect Dis* 39:1407–1416, 2004.

37. Walsh TJ, Teppler H, Donowitz G, et al.: Caspofungin versus liposomal amphotericin B for empirical antifungal therapy in patients with persistent fever and neutropenia. *N Engl J Med* 351:1391–1402, 2004.

38. Lin S, Schranz J, Teutsch S: Aspergillosis case fatality rate: systematic review of the literature. *Clin Infect Dis* 32:358–366, 2001.

39. Herbrecht R, Denning DW, Patterson TF, et al.: Voriconazole versus amphotericin B for primary therapy of invasive aspergillosis. *N Engl J Med* 347:408–415, 2002.

40. Maertens J, Raad I, Petrikkos G, et al.: Efficacy and safety of caspofungin for treatment of invasive aspergillosis in patients refractory to or intolerant of conventional antifungal therapy. *Clin Infect Dis* 39:1563–1571, 2004.

41. Marr K, Boeckh M, Carter RA, et al.: Combination antifungal therapy for invasive aspergillosis. *Clin Infect Dis* 39:797–802, 2004.

42. Flomenberg P, Babbitt J, Dobryski W: Increasing incidence of adenovirus in bone marrow transplant recipients. *J Infect Dis* 169:775–781, 1994.

43. Harrington RD, Woolfrey AE, Bowden R, et al.: Legionellosis in a bone marrow transplant center. *Bone Marrow Transplant* 18:361–368, 1996.

44. Kool JL, Fiore AE, Kioski CM, et al.: More than 10 years of unrecognized nosocomial transmission of Legionnaires' disease among transplant patients. *Infect Control Hosp Epidemiol* 19:898–904, 1998.

45. Chang J, Powles R, Paton N, et al.: Listeriosis in bone marrow transplant recipients: incidence, clinical features, and treatment. *Clin Infect Dis* 21:1289–1290, 1995.

46. Tuan IZ, Dennison D, Weisdorf D: *Pneumocystis carinii* pneumonitis following bone marrow transplantation. *Bone Marrow Transplant* 10:267–272, 1992.

47. Mele A, Paterson PJ, Prentice HG, et al.: Toxoplasmosis in bone marrow transplantation: a report of two cases and systematic review of the literature. *Bone Marrow Transplant*;29:691–698, 2002.

48. Liu LX, Weller PF: Strongyloidiasis and other intestinal nematode infections. *Infect Dis Clin North Am* 6:655–682, 1993.

49. Nichols WG, Corey L, Gooley T, et al.: High risk of death due to bacterial and fungal infections among cytomegalovirus (CMV)-seronegative recipients of stem cell transplants from seropositive donors: evidence of indirect effects of primary CMV infection. *J Infect Dis* 185:273–282, 2002.

50. Reed EC, Bowden RA, Davidliker PS, et al.: Treatment of cytomegalovirus pneumonia with ganciclovir and intravenous cytomegalovirus immunoglobulin in patients with bone marrow transplants. *Ann Intern Med* 109:783–788, 1988.

51. Wolf D, Lurain N, Zuckerman T, et al.: Emergence of late cytomegalovirus central nervous system disease in hematopoietic stem cell transplant recipients. *Blood* 101:463–465, 2003.

52. Slavin MA, Meyers JD, Remington JS, et al.: *Toxoplasma gondii* infection in marrow transplant recipients: a 20-year experience. *Bone Marrow Transplant* 13:549–557, 1994.

53. Winston DJ, Yeager AM, Chandrasekar PH, et al.: Randomized comparison of oral valacyclovir and intravenous ganciclovir for prevention of cytomegalovirus disease after allogeneic bone marrow transplantation. *Clin Infect Dis* 36:749–758, 2003.

54. Boeckh M, Gooley TA, Myerson D, et al.: Cytomegalovirus pp65 antigenemia- guided early treatment with ganciclovir versus ganciclovir at engraftment after allogeneic marrow transplantation: a randomized double blind study. *Blood* 88:4063–4071, 1996.

55. Boeckh M, Leisenring W, Riddell S, et al.: Late cytomegalovirus disease and mortality in recipients of allogeneic hematopoietic stem cell transplants: importance of viral load and T-cell immunity. *Blood* 101:407–414, 2003.

56. Chang CS, Miller W, Haake R, et al.: Varicella zoster infection after bone marrow transplantation: incidence, risk factors and complications. *Bone Marrow Transplant* 13:277–283, 1994.

57. Zutter MM, Martin PJ, Sale GE, et al.: Epstein–Barr virus lymphoproliferation after bone marrow transplantation. *Blood* 72:520–529, 1988.

58. Gerritsen EJ, Stam ED, Hermans J, et al.: Risk factors for developing EBV-related B cell lymphoproliferative disorders (BPLD) after non-HLA-identical BMT in children. *Bone Marrow Transplant* 18:377–382, 1996.

59. Doucette K, Fishman J: Nontuberculous mycobacterial infection in hematopoietic stem cell and solid organ transplant recipients. *Clin Infect Dis* 38:1428–1439, 2004.

60. Cordonnier C, Martino R, Trabasso P, et al.: Mycobacterial infection: a difficult and late diagnosis in stem cell transplant recipients. *Clin Infect Dis* 38:1229–1236, 2004.

61. Rooney CM, Smith CA, Ng CY, et al.: Infusion of cytoxic T cells for the prevention of Epstein–Barr virus-induced lymphoma in allogeneic transplant recipients. *Blood* 92:1549–1555, 1998.

# Chapter **100**

# NONINFECTIOUS COMPLICATIONS OF STEM CELL TRANSPLANTATION

*Scott I. Bearman*

## INTRODUCTION

Blood or marrow transplantation is the standard of care for many hematologic malignancies and selected nonmalignant diseases. Whether transplantation succeeds or fails depends, in part, on the ability of the patient to tolerate the preparative treatment. This chapter will focus on the major toxicities of *myeloablative* preparative regimens. Reduced-intensity regimens are usually described as being *nonmyeloablative*. Some of these regimens are, in fact, are quite toxic. Although this is a generalization, it is safe to say that reduced-intensity regimens are associated with fewer early treatment-related deaths. Where these regimens are most appropriately used remains the subject of intense investigation. A more detailed discussion of this approach can be found elsewhere in this text.

## REGIMEN-RELATED TOXICITY

Toxicities that can be directly attributed to the preparative regimen are referred to as regimen-related toxicities (RRTs). Excluded are infection, hemorrhage, and graft-versus-host disease (GVHD). Less clear are the toxicities that are the result of GVHD prophylaxis. Although flawed, a set of criteria developed in Seattle in the late 1980s remains one of the few designed to evaluate toxicity from myeloablative therapy.[1] This system was devised in patients who were prepared for transplantation using cyclophosphamide and total body irradiation (TBI). Life-threatening or fatal RRT was more common in patients who received higher TBI doses, who were transplanted with relapsed disease, and who received allogeneic versus autologous grafts. It also demonstrated that RRT was cumulative. Patients who developed grade 2 RRT in three or more organs were more likely to die by day 100 than those who developed grade 2 RRT in fewer organs.

Preparative regimens, particularly those that are myeloablative, usually employ noncross resistant drugs with nonoverlapping, nonhematopoietic toxicities. Dose-limiting toxicities are to nonhematopoietic organs and are similar among the different regimens (Table 100.1). The spectrum of such toxicities may change as newer immunosuppressive regimens that do not include methotrexate are studied.[2–5]

### CARDIAC TOXICITY

Cardiac toxicity is the dose-limiting toxicity of the oxazophosphorine chemotherapeutic agents cyclophosphamide and ifosfamide. Pathologically, cardiac toxicity is characterized by hemorrhagic pancarditis. Patients with severe cardiac toxicity can develop severe congestive heart failure and pericardial effusions with tamponade within 24–48 h of receiving high-dose cyclophosphamide or ifosfamide.[6,7] Risk factors reported for severe cardiac toxicity include previous treatment with anthracyclines[8,9] and reduced left-ventricular function prior to transplant.[10]

Murdych and Weisdorf evaluated the incidence of serious cardiac complications over a 20-year period in more than 2800 patients transplanted at the University of Minnesota.[11] Twenty-six of 2921 (<1%) patients developed life-threatening cardiac toxicity, half of whom died. Severe cardiac toxicity remains an uncommon complication of high-dose cytoreduction. However, subclinical cardiac toxicity, manifested by asymptomatic pericardial effusions and echocardiographic evidence of left-ventricular dysfunction, is not uncommon.[8,12,13]

The pathogenesis of cardiac toxicity is unclear. Several groups have measured troponin 1 (Tn1) levels in patients receiving high-dose chemotherapy. Morandi and colleagues measured Tn1 levels in 16 breast cancer patients who received 7 g/m$^2$ of cyclophosphamide as part of a high-dose chemotherapy regimen.[14] Cyclophosphamide was given in five divided doses every 3 h

**Table 100.1**  Dose-limiting toxicities of drugs commonly used in myeloablative preparative regimens

| Drug | Organ at risk |
| --- | --- |
| Cyclophosphamide | Heart, bladder, liver |
| Busulfan | Lungs, liver |
| Etoposide | Mucosa |
| BCNU | Lungs |
| Melphalan | Mucosa |

over a 13-h period. Tn1 was measured at baseline and at 6, 12, 24, and 48 h after the first dose of cyclophosphamide. Levels never exceeded normal values in any of the patients studied and were not measurable in 12 of the 16 patients.

However, this may not be the case with anthracycline-containing high-dose regimens. Cardinale and colleagues measured Tn1 levels shortly after transplant and 1 month later. Patients were segregated into three groups: those whose levels remained normal (Tn1 −/− group), those with only an early rise in troponin (Tn1 +/− group), and those whose troponin levels were elevated at both time points (Tn1 +/+ group). Echocardiograms were performed in all patients prior to and at various times following transplant. They reported that left ventricular ejection fractions did not change in the Tn1 −/− patient group and less than 1% of patients had cardiac events. Cardiac events were much more common in patients whose Tn1 levels increased, even transiently. Patients in the Tn1 +/+ group had a significantly greater number of cardiac events (84%) than patients in the Tn1 +/− group (37%).[15] These results suggest that cardiac toxicity after high-dose anthracyclines occurs by disruption of myocardial membranes while cardiac toxicity after high-dose cyclophosphamide occurs by another mechanism, possibly affecting endothelium or interstitium.[16]

Cardiac toxicity following autologous transplantation for AL amyloidosis is common and often severe. Cardiac involvement is common in patients with AL amyloidosis and is associated with an increased risk of cardiac toxicity following transplant. Investigators at Boston University reported that 20 of 28 patients who died within 3 months of transplant had evidence of amyloid cardiomyopathy prior to transplant.[17] The Mayo Clinic group reported that five out of six patients with interventricular septal wall thickness greater than 15 mm died after transplant, none of whom had congestive heart failure or reduced left ventricular function.[18]

Life-threatening arrthymias are common in patients transplanted for AL amyloid. Moreau et al. reported that three of nine patients who died within 1 month of transplant had fatal cardiac arrthymias.[19] Cardiac complications may be more common among AL amyloid patients even after less intense preparative therapy. Comenzo and colleagues reported that 5 of 30 patients who received 100 mg/m² of melphalan rather than the standard 200 mg/m² died of transplant-related complications by day 100. Two had cardiac arrests. Their pretransplant ejection fractions were 37% and 40%.[20]

### MUCOSAL AND GASTROINTESTINAL TOXICITY

Most of the drugs or modalities used in myeloablative regimens produce mucosal injury, including etoposide, melphalan, and TBI. About 75% of patients who are prepared using myeloablative regimens develop mucositis.[1,21,22] It is the most common complaint of transplant patients.[23,24] Injury to actively dividing cells in the basal cell layer begins with the first cytoreductive treatment and lasts 10–14 days, leading to atrophy, ulceration, and local infection, which is also compounded by neutropenia. Severe mucositis is associated with an increased risk of bacteremia. Utilization of total parenteral nutrition, number of febrile days, and total charges all correlate with increasing severity of mucositis.[25]

A number of strategies to prevent mucositis have been studied. Glutamine, an essential amino acid that has been reported to protect the mucosa,[26,27] has been the subject of several randomized trials. One study found no benefit while the other two reported a benefit for patients receiving glutamine supplementation.[28–30] In the largest of these studies, Anderson randomized 193 patients to receive or not to receive oral glutamine. Autologous stem cell recipients benefited with less pain and narcotic use while allogeneic transplant patients did not. However, day 28 survival was superior for allogeneic patients who received glutamine. The authors suggested that allogeneic transplant patients did not benefit because of the use of methotrexate for GVHD prophylaxis.

Both G-CSF and GM-CSF have been studied to prevent mucositis. Patients who receive conventional dose chemotherapy appear to benefit from hematopoietic growth factors but transplant patients do not.[31,32] Interleukin-11 (IL-11) has been reported to reduce mucositis in autologous transplant recipients.[33] The benefits of IL-11 appear to be outweighed by the risks among allogeneic transplant recipients. Antin and coworkers studied IL-11 in allotransplant recipients prepared with cyclophosphamide/TBI who received cyclosporine and methotrexate as GVHD prophylaxis. The study was stopped early due to excessive toxicity.[34]

There have been several recent studies with promising new agents to prevent mucositis. Keratinocyte growth factor (KGF) is a member of the heparin-binding family of fibroblast growth factor 7 and stimulates the proliferation and differentiation of epithelial cells from several tissues, including the gastrointestinal tract.[35,36] KGF was shown to reduce mucositis in animals receiving chemotherapy and/or radiation.[37,38] Spielberger and colleagues recently reported the results of a prospective, randomized placebo-controlled study of KGF in patients prepared for autologous transplant with TBI and high-dose etoposide and cyclophosphamide.[39] Patients given KGF before and after high-dose chemoradiotherapy had less WHO grade 3 and 4 oral mucositis and required less narcotics and total parenteral nutrition. The duration of mucositis was reduced, as well.

The synthetic protegrin iseganen has also been studied to prevent mucositis in transplant patients. Protegrins are naturally occurring antibiotic peptides derived from specific granules of neutrophils, with a very broad spectrum of activity. Vesole and colleagues conducted a phase II study of iseganen in 187 transplant patients prepared with mucositis-causing regimens.[40] Mucositis was reduced by 42% in patients who took this agent for 4 or more days prior to stem cell infusion. Recently, a prospective randomized trial of iseganen was conducted and reported. Giles et al. randomized 501 patients to receive or not to receive iseganen with myeloablative therapy. In this study, the incidence and severity of mucositis was not different in the two groups.[41]

There have also been several studies of the cytoprotectant amifostine. Amifostine is an organic thiophoshate that is dephosphorylated by membrane bound alkaline phosphatase to its active metabolite WR-1065. It is a potent free radical scavenger and has been shown to be cytoprotective against radiotherapy and certain chemotherapeutic agents, such as cisplatin and nitrogen mustard.[42,43] Amifostine has been studied in the transplant setting in patients prepared with high-dose melphalan. Phillips and colleagues have reported a phase I/II study of melphalan dose escalation with amifostine. Mucositis was not greater in patients treated with escalated doses of melphalan (with amifostine) than in patients treated with the standard dose of 200 mg/m$^2$ without amifostine.[44,45]

Other gastrointestinal complaints, such as nausea and vomiting, pain, and diarrhea are common after high-dose chemotherapy and/or TBI. Patients experience nausea and vomiting due to effects on the brain's emesis center or because of direct mucosal toxicity. Treatment of mucosal pain with opiates can also cause or worsen nausea. The type 3 serotonin antagonists ondansetron, grantisetron, and tropisetron are effective in about half of patients.[46,47] Delayed nausea and vomiting remain significant problems in transplant patients.[48] Newer agents such as palonosetron, another 5-HT3 antagonist and aprepitant, a neurokinin-1 receptor antagonist, may have a role in transplant patients.[49]

## VENOOCCLUSIVE DISEASE OF THE LIVER/SINUSOIDAL OBSTRUCTION SYNDROME

Hepatic toxicity is, arguably, the most problematic RRT after ablative preparative therapy. Patients with hepatic toxicity develop painful hepatomegaly and retain fluid early in the course of the disease, which is followed by rising bilirubin and, sometimes, transaminases.[50-52] Clinical signs of portal hypertension precede those of hepatic parenchymal injury (hyperbilirubinemia, elevated transaminases). Furthermore, not all patients have hepatic venular occlusion on biopsy or autopsy material.[51] For this reason, DeLeve and colleagues have suggested that the more appropriate name for this toxicity is *sinusoidal obstruction syndrome* (SOS) rather than venoocclusive disease (VOD).

The sinusoidal endothelial cell (SEC) appears to be the primary target in this syndrome. The endothelial marker plasminogen activator inhibitor-1 increases early and specifically in patients with SOS–VOD.[53,54] Another endothelial marker, thrombomodulin, also increases after high-dose therapy.[55] Hyaluronic acid, which is metabolized by SEC, has also been reported to be elevated in patients with SOS–VOD.[56] Coculture of SEC and hepatocytes and exposure to cyclophosphamide results in greater damage to SEC compared to hepatocytes. It is believed that metabolic activation of cyclophosphamide by hepatocytes generates the toxic metabolite acrolein, which produces the injury. Supporting intracellular levels of glutathione can reverse this injury.[57] Busulfan affects cyclophosphamide metabolism by reducing glutathione levels in hepatocytes and SEC.[58,59] This is probably why SOS–VOD occurs less frequently when cyclophosphamide administration precedes busulfan than the other way around.[60] Fatal VOD can occur after IV busulfan plus cyclophosphamide although busulfan levels are far more reliable after intravenous administration.[61]

Fluid retention and painful hepatomegaly are the first signs of SOS–VOD and appear on or around the date of stem cell infusion. Hyperbilirubinemia develops about a week later. Ascites is uncommon in patients with mild or moderate disease while about half of patients with severe disease develop ascites.[50] The most common cause of death in patients with SOS–VOD is multiorgan failure rather than liver failure.[50,62] Rapid increases in weight and bilirubin characterize patients with SOS–VOD who are more likely to die.

Active hepatic parenchymal inflammation (elevated transaminases),[50] second transplants using ablative preparation,[63] and preexisting hepatic fibrosis[64,65] have been reported to be risk factors for SOS–VOD. Elevated levels of soluble thrombomodulin and von Willebrand factor prior to transplant have been reported in patients who went on to develop SOS–VOD, suggesting that endothelial injury prior to the start of preparative therapy is also a risk factor.[66]

Historically, SOS–VOD was a common complication of ablative transplant, with up to 53% of patients developing this problem and up to two thirds of affected patients dying.[50] More recent reports suggest that the incidence of SOS–VOD is much less.[67] The decrease in incidence and severity of SOS–VOD may be due to healthier patients with fewer underlying risk factors (chronic hepatitis C being largely eliminated), and the use of less intensive preparative regimens.

An association between SOS–VOD and treatment with gemtuzumab ozogamicin, a humanized anti-CD33 monoclonal antibody conjugated to the antitumor antibiotic calicheamicin, has been reported.[68–70] SOS–VOD after gemtuzumab ozogamicin has been reported in both transplant and nontransplant settings. Recently, Wadleigh et al. reported that SOS–VOD was more common in patients who received gemtuzumab ozogamicin prior to transplant than in patients who did not receive gemtuzumab ozogamicin. Furthermore, only patients who received gemtuzumab ozogamicin within 3.5 months of their transplant developed SOS–VOD.[71] Rajvanshi et al. reported on the outcome of patients who received gemtuzumab for relapsed AML *after* a previous stem cell transplant. Eleven of 23 patients developed SOS–VOD.[69] Histologic material was available from five patients. Extensive sinusoidal collagen deposition was seen, suggesting that gemtuzumab ozogamicin targets CD33$^+$ cells within the sinusoids.

Fractionated TBI results in less SOS–VOD than single fraction.[72] Shielding the liver during TBI may reduce SOS–VOD but may increase the risk of relapse.[73] Many institutions use ursodeoxycholic acid[74,75] but it is unclear whether survival is impacted by this agent. Spontaneous recovery is the usual outcome for patients with SOS–VOD who recover and treatment is supportive.

Richardson and colleagues have studied defibrotide (DF), a single-stranded polydeoxyribonucleotide with anti-ischemic, antithrombotic and thrombolytic activity and no significant anticoagulant effects, in patients with severe SOS–VOD.[76] A total of 102 patients with severe SOS–VOD, 97% of whom had multiorgan dysfunction, have now been treated.[77] Fifty-four percent of patients achieved complete responses. Median PAI-1 levels decreased and protein C increased in patients who achieved complete responses. No significant adverse events occurred. There are also anecdotal reports of using N-acetylcysteine[78] and L-glutamine[79,80] for prevention or treatment of SOS–VOD. Surgical or invasive approaches have been used for patients with severe SOS–VOD, with mixed results. Several patients have even been treated with portosystemic shunts[81] or liver transplantation.[82–84] Transplantation was successful in several patients.

## RENAL DYSFUNCTION

Renal dysfunction occurs commonly after ablative high-dose preparative therapy. The causes include tumor lysis, infusion of cryopreserved marrow or stem cells, certain chemotherapeutic agents, and nephrotoxins. Ifosfamide, melphalan, and cisplatin are the agents used in high-dose regimens most likely to cause

renal dysfunction. Renal dysfunction due to these drugs is usually mild and reversible. Severe renal dysfunction occurs most commonly in association with dysfunction of multiple organs.

The manifestations of early and late renal dysfunction after transplantation are different. About 40% of patients develop early renal dysfunction, which may require dialysis in 25–50% of the affected patients.[85] Early renal dysfunction is more likely in allotransplant recipients due to GVHD prophylaxis with cyclosporine or tacrolimus. Severe dysfunction is more common in the setting of nephrotoxic antibiotics or sepsis. Treatment of early renal dysfunction is supportive and requires delicate management of intravascular volume, diuretics, hemodialysis, or ultrafiltration. Most patients who need dialysis die.

Late renal dysfunction usually manifests as hemolytic uremic syndrome (HUS). Patients present with microangiopathic hemolytic anemia, hypertension, renal failure, and encephalopathy. Both autologous and allogeneic patients develop late renal dysfunction, which is often attributable to TBI. Partial shielding of the kidneys can reduce the incidence of HUS.[62,86] Cyclosporine, tacrolimus, and sirolimus can also cause HUS.[87–89] HUS due to cyclosporine or tacrolimus is usually not improved by switching to the other agent.[90] Several groups have studied amifostine in the transplant setting to prevent renal toxicity, with mixed results.[91,92]

The issue of whether preexisting renal dysfunction precludes patients from transplant has also been recently studied. Patients with AL amyloidosis commonly develop nephrotic syndrome and/or renal insufficiency. High-dose melphalan and autologous stem cell transplantation can improve nephrotic syndrome in many patients.[17,18,93,94] In the immediate peritransplant period renal function usually worsens and then improves.[95] Unfortunately, most patients with AL amyloidosis have progressive renal dysfunction over time. Those patients who achieve complete hematologic responses after autologous transplant preserve their renal function better than patients who have persistent disease after transplant. Renal failure does not preclude transplantation for patients with AL amyloidosis provided cardiac and pulmonary function are satisfactory. AL amyloid patients with renal failure who undergo transplant develop more toxicity than other patients but their complete remission rates and 1-year survival are comparable to patients without end-stage renal disease.[17]

San Miguel and colleagues[96] reviewed the outcomes of 566 patients with multiple myeloma in the Spanish Autologous Stem Cell Transplantation registry. Patients were categorized according to renal function (abnormal function at diagnosis but normal at transplant; abnormal at both diagnosis and transplant; normal at both diagnosis and transplant). Treatment-related mortality was significantly greater in patients who had abnormal renal function at both diagnosis and transplant. They reported that poor performance status, hemoglobin ≤9.5 mg/dL, and creatinine ≥5 mg/dL were independent risk factors for TRM. Renal function did not affect response to transplant.

Badros et al. transplanted 81 multiple myeloma patients with renal failure, including 38 on dialysis.[97] Sixty patients (including 27 on dialysis) received 200 mg/m² of melphalan while 21 received 140 mg/m². Patients on dialysis developed significantly more pulmonary complications and encephalopathy. Early treatment-related mortality was not influenced by the dose of melphalan. Only 31 of the 81 patients received a second planned cycle of high-dose melphalan. The patients in this study who received two transplants did not do any better than those who were transplanted once.

### NEUROTOXICITY

Some agents used in transplant regimens can cause central nervous system (CNS) toxicity and peripheral neuropathy. Antiseizure medications providing therapeutic levels can prevent seizures that can occur after high-dose busulfan.[98,99] CNS toxicity occurring after high-dose cytarabine can be reduced by careful attention to renal function and dose adjustment when indicated.[100,101]

Leukoencephalopathy is a progressive and often fatal form of CNS toxicity that presents with seizure, confusion, dysarthria, weakness, and coma, usually several months posttransplant.[102,103] Most patients who develop leukoencephalopathy have received radiation and/or intrathecal therapy after transplant. Cyclosporine or tacrolimus can also cause leukoencephalopathy that tends to occur earlier than leukoencephalopathy due to CNS therapy and usually improves after discontinuation of treatment.[104] Neurotoxicity as a result of cyclosporine resolves or improves in most patients after switching to tacrolimus.[90]

Some patients develop cognitive dysfunction after stem cell transplantation. Phipps and colleagues conducted a prospective study of neurocognitive function in children who underwent transplant and found that age at the time of transplant was the single predictor of late neurocognitive sequelae. Patients who were 6 years of age or older had a minimal risk of cognitive sequelae while younger patients, particularly those younger than 3 years of age, had a greater risk.[105] Some adults also experience neuropsychological impairment after transplant, characterized by slowed reaction time, difficulty with attention and concentration, and troubles with reasoning and problem solving,[106] which was correlated with TBI dose. The incorporation of taxanes in high-dose regimens has increased the incidence of peripheral neuropathy in transplant patients.[107–113] Whether taxane drug levels correlate with neurotoxicity is unclear.[107,113]

### HEMORRHAGIC CYSTITIS

Hemorrhagic cystitis after transplant may be caused by cyclophosphamide or ifosfamide. The nonenzymatic metabolite of these agents, acrolein, causes hyperemia and ulceration of the bladder mucosa, resulting in hemorrhage and focal necrosis. Previously treatment with busulfan appears to increase the risk of hemorrhagic cystitis.[114] Prophylaxis includes hyperhydration with forced diuresis, bladder irrigation, or mesna. There is no clear preferred strategy. Randomized studies comparing one prophylactic strategy to another have had mixed results.[115–119]

BK polyoma virus is another cause of hemorrhagic cystitis.[117,120–123] Several investigators have demonstrated the presence of BK viruria in patients undergoing transplant, not all of whom had hemorrhagic cystitis. Neither background viral reactivation nor urothelial damage explain the increase in BK viruria in patients with hemorrhagic cystitis. This data was corroborated by Bogdonovic and colleagues, who also found that the risk of hemorrhagic cystitis from BK virus was the viral load.[124]

Late hemorrhagic cystitis can also be caused by adenovirus. In both culture and PCR analyses, 60% and 57% of patients were positive for adenovirus, respectively. PCR was not quantitative in this study and therefore no information is available regarding the number of viral copies and extent of disease.[125]

Early microscopic hematuria usually resolves spontaneously. Late hemorrhagic cystitis can result in significant bleeding and pain and treatment can be problematic. A number of therapies have been reported, including bladder instillation with formalin,[126] prostaglandin E$_1$[127] or alum,[128] electrode fulguration,[129] suprapubic cystostomy,[130] and embolization of vesicle arteries.[131] Several patients have been treated with intravesical antibiotics.[132] Most of these reports are anecdotal, making it difficult to determine whether one is superior to another. Hemorrhagic cystitis may be more common in recipients of unrelated donor stem cells.[133]

### PULMONARY TOXICITY

Idiopathic pneumonia syndrome occurs in 10% or less of patients who undergo transplantation using myeloablative preparative regimens. It occurs in similar frequency among allogeneic and autologous transplant recipients and has a high case-fatality rate, about 75%.[134,135] IPS occurs a median of 21 days posttransplant and appears to be more common in allogeneic transplant recipients with severe acute GVHD and in patients transplanted for diagnoses other than leukemia.[134] Almost 70% of patients with IPS require mechanical ventilation a median of 2 days after the onset of radiographic changes. Ventilated patients rarely survive to be discharged from the hospital.[136,137] Patients with IPS who die usually do so as a result of respiratory failure. Steroids are usually ineffective.

The precise mechanism of IPS is unclear, although the data suggest that a number of proinflammatory events in the peritransplant period are responsible. BAL fluid of patients with lung injury contains increased amounts of TNF-α.[138,139] Schots et al. reported that serum levels of TNF-α and the inflammatory cytokines IL-6 and IL-8 are increased in patients who develop major treatment-related complications, including IPS.[140] In a small series of patients, neutralization of TNF-α with Etanercept, a soluble, dimeric TNF-α binding protein, resulted in significant improvement in pulmonary function in patients with IPS.[141]

Other investigators have studied potential markers for IPS, in the hope that they might identify patients at risk and intervene before development of clinical disease. DiNubile and colleagues measured plasma gelsolin levels in 24 patients undergoing allogeneic stem cell transplantation.[142] Gelsolin is one of several proteins found in plasma that bind actin. There was a significant association between the last measured gelsolin level and survival time posttransplant. Lower gelsolin levels were associated with a higher chance of dying. The authors postulate that the conditioning regimen produces tissue injury that depletes circulating gelsolin.[143]

## CONCLUSION

The reduction in toxicity due to ablative regimens is not likely to diminish by the development of new ablative programs. In fact, there are few examples of truly new ablative regimens. Rather, better understanding of the pathophysiology of RRTs will lead to new approaches for their prevention and treatment. Development of newer immunosuppressive regimens, such as the combination of tacrolimus or cyclosporine with mycophenolate mofetil, is likely to make a much greater impact on toxicity than changes in the ablative program itself.

### REFERENCES

1. Bearman SI, Appelbaum FR, Buckner CD, et al.: Regimen-related toxicity and early post-transplant survival in patients undergoing marrow transplantation. *J Clin Oncol* 6:1562–68, 1988.
2. McSweeney PA, Abhyankar S, Becker C, et al.: Low incidence of early transplant mortality using tacrolimus and mycophenolate mofetil for GVHD prevention after conventional allografting. *Blood* 100(suppl 1):1623, 2002.
3. McSweeney P, Abhyankar S, Petersen F, et al.: Tacrolimus and mycophenolate mofetil for GVHD prevention after unrelated donor transplants. *Blood* 102(suppl):2654, 2003.
4. Cutler C, Kim HT, Hochberg E, et al.: Sirolimus and tacrolimus without methotrexate as graft-versus-host disease prophylaxis after matched related donor peripheral blood stem cell transplantation. *Biol Blood Marrow Transplant* 10:328–336, 2004.
5. Nash RA, Johnston L, Parker PM, et al.: A phase I/II study of mycophenolate mofetil in combination with cyclosporine for prophylaxis of graft versus host disease after myeloablative conditioning and allogeneic hematopoietic cell transplantation: dose escalation of MMF. *Blood* 102(suppl 1):844, 2003.
6. Gottdeiner JS, Appelbaum FR, Ferrans VJ, et al.: Cardiotoxicity associated with high-dose cyclophosphamide therapy. *Arch Int Med* 141:758–763, 1981.
7. Angelucci E, Mariotti E, Lucarelli G, et al.: Sudden cardiac tamponade after chemotherapy for marrow transplantation in thalassaemia. *Lancet* 339:287–289, 1992.
8. Steinherz LJ, Steinherz PG, Mangiacasale D, et al.: Cardiac changes with cyclophosphamide. *Med Ped Oncol* 9:417–422, 1981.
9. Larsen RL, Barber G, Heise CT, et al.: Exercise assessment of cardiac function in children and young adults before and after bone marrow transplantation. *Pediatrics* 89:722–729, 1992.

10. Bearman SI, Petersen FB, Schor RA, et al.: Radionuclide ejection fractions in the evaluation of patients being considered for bone marrow transplantation: risk for cardiac toxicity. *Bone Marrow Transplant* 5:173–177, 1990.
11. Murdych T, Weisdorf DJ: Serious cardiac complications during bone marrow transplantation at the University of Minnesota, 1977–1997. *Bone Marrow Transplant* 28:283–287, 2001.
12. Kupari M, Volin L, Suokas A, et al.: Cardiac involvement in bone marrow transplantation: electrocardiographic changes, arrhythmias, heart failure and autopsy findings. *Bone Marrow Transplant* 5:91–98, 1990.
13. Quezado ZMN, Wilson WH, Cunnion RE, et al.: High-dose ifosfamide is associated with severe, reversible cardiac dysfunction. *Ann Int Med* 118:31–36, 1993.
14. Morandi P, Ruffini PA, Benvenuto GM, et al.: Serum cardiac troponin I levels and ECG/echo monitoring in breast cancer patients undergoing high-dose (7 g/m²) cyclophosphamide. *Bone Marrow Transplant* 28:277–282, 2001.
15. Cardinale D, Sandri MT, Colombo A, et al.: Prognostic value of troponin 1 in cardiac risk stratification of cancer patients undergoing high-dose chemotherapy. *Circulation* 109:2749–2754, 2004.
16. Morandi P, Ruffini PA, Benvenuto GM, et al.: Serum cardiac troponin I levels and ECG/echo monitoring in breast cancer patients undergoing high-dose (7 g/m²) cyclophosphamide. *Bone Marrow Transplant* 28:277–282, 2001.
17. Sanchorawala V, Wright DG, Seldin DC, et al.: An overview of the use of high-dose melphalan with autologous stem cell transplantation for the treatment of AL amyloidosis. *Bone Marrow Transplant* 28:637–642, 2001.
18. Gertz MA, Lacy MQ, Gastineau DA, et al.: Blood stem cell transplantation as therapy for primary systemic amyloidosis (AL). *Bone Marrow Transplant* 26:963–969, 2000.

19. Moreau P, Leblond V, Bourquelot P, et al.: Prognostic factors for survival and response ater high-dose therapy and autologous stem cell transplantation in systemic AL amyloidosis: a report on 21 patients. *Br J Haematol* 101:766–769, 1998.

20. Comenzo RL, Sanchorawala V, Fisher C, et al.: Intermediate-dose intravenous melphalan and blood stem cells mobilized with sequential GM + G-CSF or G-CSF alone to treat AL (amyloid light chain) amyloidosis. *Brit J Haematol* 104:553–559, 1999.

21. Woo SB, Sonis ST, Monopoli MM, et al.: A longitudinal study of oral ulcerative mucositis in bone marrow transplant recipients. *Cancer* 72:1612–1617, 1993.

22. Pico JL, Avila-Garavito A, Naccahie P: Mucositis: its occurance, consequences, and treatment in the oncology setting. *Oncologist* 3:446–451, 1998.

23. Bellm LA, Epstein JB, Rose-Ped A, et al.: Patient reports of complications of bone marrow transplantation. *Supp Care Cancer* 8:33–39, 2000.

24. Stiff P: Mucositis associated with stem cell transplantation: current status and innovative approaches to management. *Bone Marrow Transplant* 27(suppl 2):S3-S11, 2001.

25. Horowitz MM, Oster G, Fuchs H, et al.: Oral Mucositis Assessment Scale (OMAS) as a predictor of clinical and economic outcomes in bone marrow transplant patients. *Blood* 94(suppl 1):399a, 1999.

26. Fox AD, Kripke SA, De Paula J, et al.: Effect of a glutamine suppled enteral diet on methotrexate-induced enterocolitis. *J Parrenter Enteral Nutr* 12:325–331, 1988.

27. O'Dwyer ST, Scott T, Smith RJ, et al.: 5-Fluorouracil toxicity on small intestine but not white blood cells is decreased by glutamine. *Clin Res* 35:367a, 1987.

28. Anderson PM, Ramsay NK, Shu XO, et al.: Effect of low-dose oral glutamine on painful stomatitis during bone marrow transplantation. *Bone Marrow Transplant* 22:339–344, 1998.

29. Coghlin Dickson TM, Wong RM, Offrin RS, et al.: Effect of oral glutamine supplation during bone marrow transplantation. *J Parenter Enteral Nutr* 24:61–66, 2000.

30. Huang EY, Leung SW, Wang CJ, et al.: Oral glutamine to alleviate radiation-induced oral mucositis: a pilot randomized trial. *Int J Radiat Oncol Biol Phys* 46:535–539, 2000.

31. Nemunitis J, Rosenfeld CS, Ash R, et al.: Phase III randomized, double-blind placebo-controlled trial of rhGM-CSF following allogeneic bone marrow transplantation. *Bone Marrow Transplant* 15:949–954, 1995.

32. Atkinson K, Biggs JC, Downs K, et al.: GM-CSF after allogeneic bone marrow transplantation: accelerated recovery of neutrophils, monocytes, and lymphocytes. *Aust NZ J Med* 21:686–692, 1991.

33. Schwerkoske J, Schwartzberg L, Weaver C, et al.: A phase I, double-masked, placebo-controlled study to evaluate tolerability of Neumega (rh IL-11; opreleukin) to reduce mucositis in patient with solid tumor or lymphoma receiving high dose chemotherpay with autologous peripheral blood stem cell reinfusion. *Proc Am Soc Clin Oncol* 18:584a, 1999.

34. Antin JH, Lee SJ, Neuberg D, et al.: A phase I/II double-blind, placebo-controlled study of recombinant human interleukin-11 for mucositis and acute GVHD prevention in allogeneic stem cell transplantation. *Bone Marrow Transplant* 29:373–377, 2002.

35. Rubin JS, Osada H, Finch PW, et al.: Purification and characterization of a newly identified growth factor specific for epithelial cells. *Proc Nat Acad Sci USA* 86:802–806, 1989.

36. Rubin JS, Bottaro DB, Chedid M, et al.: Keratinocyte growth factor. *Cell Biol Int* 19:399–411, 1995.

37. Farrell CL, Bready JV, Rex KL, et al.: Keratinocyte growth factor protects mice from chemotherapy and radiation-induced gastrointestinal injury and mortality. *Cancer Res* 58:933–939, 1998.

38. Farrell CL, Rex KL, Kaufman SA, et al.: Effects of keratinocyte growth factor in the squamous epithelium of the upper aerodigestive tract of normal and irradiated mice. *Int J Radiat Biol* 75:609–620, 1999.

39. Spielberger R, Emmanouilides C, Stiff P, et al.: Use of recombinant human keratinocyte growth factor can reduce severe oral mucositis in patients with hematologic malignancies undergoing autologous peripheral blood progenitor cell transplantation after radiation-based conditioning—results of a phase 3 trial. *Proc Am Soc Clin Oncol* 22:3642, 2003.

40. Vesole DH, Fuchs HJ. IB-367 reduces the number of days of severe oral mucositis complicating myeloablative chemotherapy. *Blood* 94(suppl 1):154a, 1999.

41. Giles FJ, Rodriguez R, Weisdorf D, et al.: A phase III, randomized, double-blind, placebo-controlled, study of iseganen for the reduction of stomatitis in patients receiving stomatotoxic chemotherapy. *Leuk Res* 28:559–565, 2004.

42. Yuhas JM, Culo F: Selective inhibition of the nephrotoxicity of cisdichlorodiammineplatinum (II) by WR-2721 without altering its antitumor activity. *Cancer Treat Rep* 64:57–64, 1980.

43. Valeriote F, Tolen S: Protection and potentiation of nitrogen mustard cytotoxicity by WR-2721. *Cancer Res* 42:4330–4341, 1982.

44. Phillips GL, Meisenburg B, Hale GA, et al.: Amifostine cytoprotection of escalating doses of melphalan and autologous hematopoietic stem cell transplantation: final results of a phase I & II study. *Proc Am Soc Clin Oncol* 20:24, 2001.

45. Thumma S, Hari P, Bredeson C, et al.: Phase I/II trial of dose escalation of melphalan with amifostine cytoprotection supported by autologous hematopoietic stem cell transplant in multiple myeloma patients > 65 years. *Blood* 102(suppl 1);3663, 2003.

46. Fox-Geiman MP, Fisher SG, Kiley K, et al.: Double-blind comparative trial of oral ondansetron versus oral granisetron versus IV ondansetron in the prevention of nausea and vomiting associated with highly emetogenic preparative regimens prior to stem cell transplantation. *Biol Blood Marrow Transplant* 7:596–603, 2001.

47. Lacerda JF, Martins C, Carmo JA, et al.: Randomized trial of ondansetron, granisetron, and tropisetron in the prevention of acute nausea and vomiting. *Transplant Proc* 32:2680–2681, 2000.

48. Eagle DA, Gian V, Lauwers GY, et al.: Gastroparesis following bone marrow transplantation. *Bone Marrow Transplant* 28:59–62, 2001.

49. Navari RM: Pathogenesis-based treatment of chemotherapy-induced nausea and vomiting—two new agents. *J Support Oncol* 1:89–103, 2003.

50. McDonald GB, Hinds MS, Fisher LB, et al.: Venocclusive disease of the liver and multiorgan failure after bone marrow transplantation: a cohort study of 355 patients. *Ann Intern Med* 118:255–267, 1993.

51. Shulman HM, Fisher LB, Schoch HG, et al.: Venocclusive disease of the liver after marrow transplantation: histologic correlates of clinical signs and symptoms. *Hepatology* 19:1171–1180, 1994.

52. Strasser SI, McDonald GB, Schoch HG, et al.: Severe hepatocellular injury after hematopoietic cell transplant: incidence and etiology in 2136 consecutive patients. *Hepatology* 32:299, 2000.

53. Salat C, Holler E, Reinhardt B, et al.: Parameters of the fibrinolytic system in patients undergoing BMT: elevation of PAI-1 in veno-occlusive disease. *Bone Marrow Transplant* 14:747–750, 1994.

54. Salat C, Holler E, Kolb H-J, et al.: Plasminogen activator inhibitor-1 confirms the diagnosis of hepatic veno-occlusive disease in patients with hyperbilirubinemia after bone marrow transplantation. *Blood* 89:2184–2188, 1997.

55. Testa S, Manna A, Porcellini A: Increased plasma level of vascular endothelial glycoprotein thrombomodulin as an early indicator of endothelial damage in bone marrow transplantation. *Bone Marrow Transplant* 18:383-388, 1996.

56. Fried MW, Duncan A, Seroka S, et al.: Serum hyaluronic acid in patients with veno-occlusive disease following bone marrow transplantation. *Bone Marrow Transplant* 27:635–639, 2001.

57. DeLeve LD: Cellular target of cyclophosphamide toxicity in murine liver: role of glutathione and site of metabolic activation. *Hepatology* 24:830–837, 1996.

58. Slattery JT, Kalhorn TF, McDonald GB: Conditioning regimen-dependent disposition of cyclophosphamide and hydroxycyclophosphamide in human marrow transplantation patients. *J Clin Oncol* 14:1484–1494, 1996.

59. DeLeve LD, Wang X: Role of oxidative stress and glutathione in busulfan toxicity in cultured murine hepatocytes. *Pharmacology* 60:143–154, 2000.

60. Meresse V, Hartmann O, Vassal G, et al.: Risk factors of hepatic venocclusive disease after high-dose busulfan-containing regimens followed by autologous bone marrow transplantation: a study in 136 children. *Bone Marrow Transplant* 10:135–141, 1992.

61. Andersson BS, Kashyap A, Gian V, et al.: Conditioning therapy with intravenous busulfan and cyclophosphamide (IV Bu CY2) for hematologic malignancies prior to allogeneic stem cell transplantation: a phase II study. *Biol Blood Marrow Transplant* 8:145–154, 2002.

62. Zager RA: Acute renal failure in the setting of bone marrow transplantation. *Kidney Int* 46:1443–1458, 1994.

63. Radich JP, Sanders JE, Buckner CD, et al.: Second allogeneic marrow transplantation for patients with recurrent leukemia after initial transplantation with total-body irradiation-containing regimens. *J Clin Oncol* 11:304–313, 1993.

64. Tanikawa S, Mori S, Ohhashi K, et al.: Predictive markers for hepatic veno-occlusive disease after hematopoietic stem cell transplantation in adults: a prospective single center study. *Bone Marrow Transplant* 26:881–886, 2000.

65. Rio B, Bauduer F, Arrago JP: N-terminal peptide of type III procollagen: a marker for the development of hepatic veno-occlusive disease after BMT and a basis for determining the timing of prophylactic heparin. *Bone Marrow Transplant* 11:471–472, 1993.

66. Richard S, Seigneur M, Blann A, et al.: Vascular endothelial lesion in patients undergoing bone marrow transplantation. *Bone Marrow Transplant* 18:955-959, 1996.

67. Carreras E, Bertz H, Arcese W, et al.: Incidence and outcome of hepatic veno-occlusive disease after blood or marrow transplantation: a prospective cohort study of the European Group for *Blood* and Marrow Transplantation. European Group for Blood and Marrow Transplantation Chronic Leukemia Working Party. *Blood* 92:3599–3604, 1998.

68. Giles FJ, Kantarjian HM, Kornblau SM, et al.: Mylotarg™ (gemtuzumab ozogamicin) therapy is associated with hepatic venooclusive disease in patients who have not received stem cell transplantation. *Cancer* 92:406–413, 2001.

69. Sievers EL, Larson RA, Stadtmauer, et al.: Efficacy and safety of gemtuzumab ozogamicin in patients with CD33-positive acute myeloid leukemia in first relapse. *J Clin Oncol* 19:3244-3254, 2001.

70. Rajvanshi P, Shulman HM, Sievers EL, et al. Hepatic sinusoidal obstruction after gemtuzumab ozogamicin (Mylotarg) therapy. *Blood* 99:2310–2314, 2002.

71. Wadleigh M, Richardson PG, Zahrieh D, et al.: Prior gemtuzumab ozogamicin exposure significantly increases the risk of veno-occlusive disease in patients who undergo myeloablative allogeneic stem cell transplantation. *Blood* 102:1578–1582, 2003.

72. Grinsky T, Benhamou E, Bourhis J-H, et al.: Prospective randomized comparison of single-dose versus hyper-fractionated total-body irradiation in patients with hematologic malignancies. *J Clin Oncol* 18:981–986, 2000.

73. Anderson JE, Appelbaum FR, Schoch G, et al.: Relapse after allogeneic bone marrow transplantation for refractory anemia is increased by shielding lungs and liver during total body irradiation. *Biol Blood Marrow Transplant* 7:163–170, 2001.

74. Essell JH, Schroeder MT, Harman GS, et al.: Ursodiol prophylaxis against hepatic complications of allogeneic bone marrow transplantation. *Ann Intern Med* 128:975-981, 1998.

75. Ohashi K, Tanabe J, Watanabe R, et al.: The Japanese multicenter open randomized trial of ursodeoxycholic acid prophylaxis for hepatic veno-occlusive disease after stem cell transplantation. *Am J Hematol J* 64:32–38, 2000.

76. Hagglund H, Ringden O, Ericzon BG, et al.: Treatment of hepatic venocclusive disease with recombinant human tissue plasminogen activator or orthotopic liver transplantation after allogeneic bone marrow transplantation. *Transplantation* 62:1076–1080, 1996.

77. Richardson PG, Murakami C, Jin Z, et al.: Multi-institutional use of defibrotide in 88 patients after stem cell transplantation with severe veno-occlusive disease and multisystem organ failure: response without significant toxicity in a high-risk population and factors predictive of outcome. *Blood* 100:4337–4343, 2002.

78. Richardson PG, Soiffer RJ, Antin JH, et al.: Defibrotide for the treatment of severe veno-occlusive disease and multi-system organ failure post SCT. Final results of a phase II, multicenter, randomized study and preliminary analyses of surrogate markers and ultrasound findings. *Blood* 104(suppl 1):360, 2004.

79. Ringden O, Remberger M, Lehmann S, et al.: N-acetylcysteine for hepatic veno-occlusive disease after allogeneic stem cell transplantation. *Bone Marrow Transplant* 25:993–996, 2000.

80. Goringe AP, Brown S, O'Callaghan U, et al.: Glutamine and vitamin E in the treatment of hepatic veno-occlusive disease following high-dose chemotherapy. *Bone Marrow Transplant* 21: 829–832, 1998.

81. Brown SA, Goringe A, Fegan C, et al.: Parenteral glutamine protects hepatic function during bone marrow transplantation. *Bone Marrow Transplant* 22:281–284, 1998.

82. Murray JA, LaBrecque DR, Gingrich RD, et al.: Successful treatment of hepatic venocclusive disease in a bone marrow transplant patient with a side-to-side portacaval shunt. *Gastroenterol* 92:1073–1077, 1987.

83. Nimer SD, Milewicz AL, Champlin RE, et al.: Successful treatment of hepatic venocclusive disease in a bone marrow transplant patient with orthotopic liver transplantation. *Transplantation* 49:819–821, 1990.97.

84. Rapaport AP, Doyle HR, Starzl T, et al.: Orthotopic liver transplantation for life-threatening veno-occlusive disease of the liver after allogeneic bone marrow transplant. *Bone Marrow Transplant* 8:421–424, 1991.

85. Zager RA, O'Quigley J, Zager BK, et al.: Acute renal failure following bone marrow transplantation: a retrospective study of 272 patients. *Am J Kidney Dis* 13:210–216, 1989.

86. Lawton CA, Barber-Derus SW, Murray JK, et al.: Influence of renal shielding on the incidence of late renal dysfunction associated with T-lymphocyte depleted bone marrow transplantation in adult patients. *Int J Rad Oncol Biol Phys* 23:681–686, 1992.

87. Singh N, Gayowski T, Marino JR: Hemolytic uremic syndrome in solid-organ transplant recipients. *Transpl Int* 9: 68–75, 1996.

88. Woo M, Przepiorka D, Ippoliti C, et al.: Toxicities of tacrolimus and cyclosporin A after allogeneic blood stem cell transplantation. *Bone Marrow Transplant* 20:1095–1098, 1997.

89. Benito AI, Furlong T, Martin PJ, et al.: Sirolimus (rapamycin) for the treatment of steroid-refractory acute graft-versus-host disease. *Transplantation* 72:1924–1929, 2001.

90. Furlong T, Storb R, Anasetti C, et al.: Clinical outcome after conversion to FK506 (tacrolimus) therapy for acute graft-versus-host disease resistant to cyclosporine or for cyclosporine-associated toxicities. *Bone Marrow Transplant* 26:985–991, 2000.

91. Phillips GL, Meisenberg B, Hale GA, et al.: Amifostine cytoprotection of escalating doses of melphalan and autologous hematopoietic stem cell transplantation: final results of a phase I and II study. *Proc Am Soc Clin Oncol* 20:24, 2001.

92. Hartmann JT, von Vangerow A, Fels LM, et al.: A randomized trial of amifostine in patients with high-dose VIC chemotherapy plus autologous blood stem cell transplantation. *Brit J Cancer* 84:313–320, 2001.

93. San Miguel JF, Lahuerta JJ, Garcia-Sanz R, et al.: Are myeloma patients with renal failure candidates for autologous stem cell transplantation? *Hematol J* 1: 28–36, 2000.

94. Badros A, Barlogie B, Siegel E, et al.: Results of autologous stem cell transplant in multiple myeloma patients with renal failure. *Br J Haematol* 114:822–829, 2001.

95. Dember LM, Sanchorawala V, Seldin DC, et al.: Effect of dose-intensive intravenous melphalan and autologous blood stem-cell transplantation on AL amyloidosis-associated renal disease. *Ann Intern Med* 134:746–753, 2001.

96. Sezer O, Schmid P, Shweigert M, et al.: Rapid reversal of nephrotic syndrome due to primary systemic AL amyloidosis after VAD and subsequent high-dose chemotherapy with autologous stem cell support. *Bone Marrow Transplant* 23:967–969, 1999.

97. Vassal G, Deroussent A, Hartmann O, et al.: Dose-dependent neurotoxicity of high-dose busulfan in children: a clinical and pharmacological study. *Cancer Res* 50:6203–6207, 1990.

98. Grigg AP, Shepherd JD, Phillips GL: Busulphan and phenytoin. *Ann Intern Med* 111:1149–1150, 1989.

99. Damon LE, Mass R, Linker CA: The association between high-dose cytarabine neurotoxicity and renal insufficiency. *J Clin Oncol* 7:1563–1568, 1989.

100. Rubin EH, Anderson JW, Berg DT, et al.: Risk factors for high-dose cytarabine neurotoxicity: an analysis of a Cancer and Leukemia Group B trial in patients with acute myeloid leukemia. *J Clin Oncol* 10:948–953, 1992.

101. Smith GA, Damon LE, Rugo HS, et al.: High-dose cytarabine dose modification reduces the incidence of neurotoxocity in patients with renal insufficiency. *J Clin Oncol* 15:833–839, 1997.

102. Bleyer WA: Neurologic sequelae of methotrexate and ionizing radiation: a new classification. *Cancer Treat Rep* 65(suppl):89–98, 1981.

103. Thompson CB, Sander JE, Flournoy N, et al.: The risks of central nervous system relapse and leukoencephalopathy in patients receiving bone marrow transplants for acute leukemia. *Blood* 67:195–199, 1986.

104. Bechstein WO: Neurotoxicity of calcineurin inhibitors: impact and clinical management. *Transplant Int* 13:313–326, 2000.

105. Phipps S, Dunavant M, Srivastava DK, et al.: Cognitive and academic functioning in survivors of pediatric bone marrow transplantation. *J Clin Oncol* 18:1004–1011, 2000.

106. Andrykowski MA, Altmaier EM, Barnett RL, et al.: Cognitive dysfunction in adult survivors of allogeneic marrow transplantation: relationship to dose of total body irradiation. *Bone Marrow Transplant* 6:269–276, 1990.

107. Stemmer SM, Cagnoni PJ, Shpall EJ, et al.: High-dose paclitaxel, cyclophosphamide, and cisplatin with autologous hematopoietic progenitor-cell support: a phase I trial. *J Clin Oncol* 14:1463–1472, 1996.

108. Doroshow JH, Synold T, Somlo G et al.: High-dose infusional paclitaxel (P), platinum (DDP), cyclophosphamide (CY), and cyclosporine A (CSA) with peripheral blood progenitor cell rescue for high risk primary and responsive metastatic breast cancer. *Proc Am Soc Clin Oncol* 16:235, 1997.

109. Mayordomo JI, Yubero A, Cajal R, et al.: Phase I trial of high-dose paclitaxel in combination with cyclophosphamide, thiotepa and carboplatin with autologous peripheral blood stem cell rescue. *Proc Am Soc Clin Oncol* 16:102, 1997.

110. Gluck S, Arnold A, Dulude H, et al.: High-dose cyclophosphamide, mitoxantrone and paclitaxel with blood progenitor cell support for the treatment of metastatic breast cancer. *Proc Am Soc Clin Oncol* 15:137, 1996.

111. Vahdat L, Papadopoulos K, Balmaceda C, et al.: Phase I trial of sequential high-dose chemotherapy with escalating dose paclitaxel, melphalan, and cyclophosphamide, thiotepa, and carboplatin with peripheral blood progenitor support in women with responding metastatic breast cancer. *Clin Cancer Res* 4:1689–1695, 1998.

112. Nieto Y, Cagnoni PJ, Shpall EJ, et al.: Phase I trial of docetaxel (DTX) (Taxotere) with peripheral blood progenitor cell (PBPC) support, with melphalan (MEL) and carboplatin (CB), in refractory advanced cancer. *Proc Am Soc Clin Oncol* 19:217, 2000.

113. Papadopoulos KP, Egorin MJ, Huang M, et al.: The pharmacokinetics and pharmacodynamics of high-dose paclitaxel monotherapy (825 mg/m² continuous infusion over 24 h) with hematopoietic support in women with metastatic breast cancer. *Cancer Chemother Pharmacol* 47:45–50, 2001.

114. Thomas AE, Patterson J, Prentice HG, et al.: Haemorrhagic cystitis in bone marrow transplantation patients: possible increased risk associated with prior busulphan therapy. *Bone Marrow Transplant* 1:347–355, 1987.

115. Hows JW, Mehta A, Ward L, et al.: Comparison of mesna with forced diuresis to prevent cyclophosphamide induced haemorrhagic cystitis in marrow transplantation: a prospective randomized study. *Brit J Cancer* 50:753–756, 1984.

116. Vose JM, Reed EC, Pippert GC, et al.: Mesna compared with continuous bladder irrigation as uroprotection during high-dose chemotherapy and transplantation: a randomized trial. *J Clin Oncol* 11:1306–1310, 1993.

117. Bedi A, Miller CB, Hanson JL, et al.: Association of BK virus with failure of prophylaxis against hemorrhagic cystitis following bone marrow transplantation. *J Clin Oncol* 13:1103–1109, 1995.

118. Ringdén O, Ruutu, T, Remberger M, et al.: A randomized trial comparing busulfan versus total body irradiation in allogeneic marrow transplant recipients with leukemia: a report from the Nordic Bone Marrow Transplantation Group. *Blood* 83:2723–2730, 1994.

119. Ringdén O, Ruutu T, Remberger M, et al.: A randomized trial comparing busulfan versus total body irradiation in allogeneic marrow transplant recipients with hematological malignancies. *Transplant Proc* 26:1831–1832, 1994.

120. Leung AYH, Suen CKM, Lie AKW, et al.: Quantification of polyoma BK viruria in hemorrhagic cystitis complicating bone marrow transplantation. *Blood* 98:1972–1978, 2001.

121. Arthur RR, Shah KV, Baust SJ, et al.: Association of BK viruria with hemorrhagic cystitis in recipients of bone marrow transplants. *N Engl J Med* 315: 230–234, 1986.

122. Apperly JF, Rice SJ, Bishop JA, et al.: Late-onset hemorrhagic cystitis associated with urinary excretion of polyomaviruses after bone marrow transplantation. *Transplantation* 43:108–112, 1987.

123. Chan PK, Ip KW, Shiu SY, et al.: Association between polyomaviruria and microscopic haematuria in bone marrow transplant recipients. *J Infect* 29:139–146, 1994.

124. Bogdanovic G, Priftakis P, Giraud G, et al.: Association between a high BK virus load in urine samples of patients with graft-versus-host disease and development of hemorrhagic cystitis after hematopoietic stem cell transplantation. *J Clin Microbiol* 42:5394–5396, 2004.

125. Akiyama H, Kurosu T, Sakashita C, et al.: Adenovirus is a key pathogen in hemorrhagic cystitis associated with bone marrow transplantation. *Clin Infect Dis* 32:1325–1330, 2001.

126. Shrom SH, Donaldson MH, Duckett JW, et al.: Formalin treatment for intractable hemorrhagic cystitis. A review of the literature with 16 additional cases. *Cancer* 38: 1785–1789, 1976.

127. Trigg ME, O'Reilly J, Rumelhart S, et al.: Prostaglandin E₁ bladder instillations to control severe hemorrhagic cystitis. *J Urol* 143:92–94, 1990.

128. Efros MD, Ahmed T, Coombe N, et al.: Urologic complications of high-dose chemotherapy and bone marrow transplantation. *Urology* 43:355–360, 1994.

129. Lapides J: Treatment of delayed intractable hemorrhagic cystitis following radiation or chemotherapy. *J Urol* 104:707–708, 1970.

130. Baronciani D, Angelucci E, Erer B, et al.: Suprapubic cystotomy as treatment for severe hemorrhagic cystitis after bone marrow transplantation. *Bone Marrow Transplant* 16:267–270, 1995.

131. Gine E, Rovira M, Real I, et al.: Successful treatment of severe hemorrhagic cystitis after hemopoietic cell transplantation by selective embolization of the vesical arteries. *Bone Marrow Transplant* 31:923–925, 2003.

132. Fanourgiakis P, Georgala A, Vekemans M, et al.: Intravesical instillation of cidofovir in the treatment of hemorrhagic cystitis caused by adenovirus type 11 in a bone marrow transplant recipient. *Clin Infect Dis* 40: 199–201, 2005.

133. El-Zimaity M, Saliba R, Chan K, et al.: Hemorrhagic cystitis after allogeneic hematopoietic stem cell transplantation: donor type matters. *Blood* 103:4674–4680, 2004.

134. Kantrow SP, Hackman RC, Boeckh M, et al.: Idiopathic pneumonia syndrome. Changing spectrum of lung injury after marrow transplantation. *Transplantation* 63:1079–1086, 1997.

135. Wingard JR, Mellits ED, Sostrin MB, et al.: Interstitial pneumonitis after bone marrow transplantation. Nine-year experience at a single institution. *Medicine* 67: 175–186, 1988.

136. Bach PB, Schrag D, Nierman DM, et al.: Identification of poor prognostic features among patients requiring mechanical ventilation after hematopoietic stem cell transplant. *Blood* 98:3234–3240, 2001.

137. Khassawneh BY, White P, Anaissie EJ, et al.: Outcome from mechanical ventilation after autologous peripheral

blood stem cell transplantation. *Chest* 121:185–188, 2002.

138. Hauber HP, Mikkila A, Erich JM, et al.: TNF alpha, interleukin-10 and interleukin-18 expression in cells of the bronchoalveolar lavage in patients with pulmonary complications following bone marrow or peripheral stem cell transplantation: a preliminary study. *Bone Marrow Transplant* 30:485–490, 2002.

139. Clark JG, Madtes DK, Martin TR, et al.: Idiopathic pneumonia after bone marrow transplantation: cytokine activation and lipopolysaccharide amplification in the bronchoalveolar compartment. *Crit Care Med* 27:1800–1806, 1999.

140. Cooke KR, Hill GR, Gerbitz A, et al.: Tumor necrosis factor-α neutralization reduces lung injury after experimental allogeneic bone marrow transplantation. *Transplantation* 70:272–279, 2000.

141. Schots R, Kaufman L, Van Riet I, et al.: Proinflammatory cytokines and their role in the development of major transplant-related complications in the early phase after allogeneic bone marrow transplantation. *Leukemia* 17:1150–1156, 2003.

142. DiNubile MJ, Stossel TP, Ljunghusen OC, et al.: Prognostic implications of declining plasma gelsolin levels after allogeneic stem cell transplantation. *Blood* 100:4367–4371, 2002.

143. Mounzer KC, Moncure M, Smith YR, et al.: Relationship of admission gelsolin levels to clinical outcomes in patients after major trauma. *Am J Respir Crit Care Med* 160:1673–1681, 1999

Chapter **101**

# PHARMACOLOGY OF TRADITIONAL AGENTS USED TO TREAT HEMATOLOGIC MALIGNANCIES

*Jennifer L. Shamp*

## THE HISTORY OF CANCER CHEMOTHERAPY

The term *chemotherapy* refers to the treatment of cancer or other malignant diseases by using specific drugs that selectively destroy growing cells. Prior to the advent of chemotherapy, two main modalities were used in the treatment of cancer: surgery and radiation. Both options, although effective for many types of cancer, are localized forms of therapy. Chemotherapy provided the first systemic form of treatment, using the bloodstream as a means of disseminating drug to both the tumor site as well as areas of metastasis. Additionally, this provided a major breakthrough in the treatment of hematologic malignancies, such as leukemia and lymphoma, which had previously been virtually untreatable with surgery or radiation.

The advent of modern chemotherapy originated during World War I, with the observation that soldiers who had been exposed to mustard gas, or sulfur mustard, experienced significant decreases in their white blood cell counts, specifically their lymphocytes. Krumbaar first described these findings in 1919, as he noted atrophy of lymphoid and testicular tissue, as well as bone marrow depression, in soldiers who had been subject to poisonings.[1] This observation led investigators to take a closer look at nitrogen mustard, a compound closely related to sulfur mustard, as an antitumor agent. Various animal studies took place throughout the 1920s and 1930s, and advances in the use of nitrogen mustard as a topical anticancer agent were made.[1] With the start of World War II, initiatives in chemical warfare again intensified. Further study of nitrogen mustard and related compounds suggested that the basic effects on cellular mechanisms could be compared to that of X-rays. A true breakthrough occurred at Yale University in 1942, when Goodman, Gilman, Philips, and Allen discovered the systemic antitumor activity of nitrogen mustard.[2] Because of wartime secrecy, these findings were not published until 1946. Their observations in animals led to the first human study, in 1942, of a man with "x-ray resistant lymphosarcoma." After 10 days of therapy with this compound, the result was striking, as the patient's tumors had virtually melted away.[3] Although the patient relapsed one month later, a new era in the treatment of cancer had begun.

## CHEMOTHERAPEUTIC AGENTS USED IN THE TREATMENT OF HEMATOLOGIC MALIGNANCIES

### ALKYLATING AGENTS

Thousands of variants of the basic chemical structure of nitrogen mustard have been developed over the years, but few have matched the success and utility of the original compound. These variants include some of the oldest, yet most valuable of all antineoplastic drugs. Five basic types of alkylating agents are currently in use.

- Nitrogen mustard derivatives (mechlorethamine, cyclophosphamide, ifosfamide, melphalan, chlorambucil)
- Ethylenimines (triethylenemelanime, thiotepa, altremaine)
- Alkyl sulfonates (busulfan)
- Nitrosoureas (carmustine, streptozocin)
- Triazenes (dacarbazine)

The chemotherapeutic effect of alkylating agents is attributed to their highly reactive alkyl groups, which form covalent bonds with nucleophilic groups found on proteins and nucleic acids.[4] The alkylating agents by nature are strong electrophiles (electron acceptors), which react quickly with nucleophiles (electron donors) found on DNA bases, such as phosphate, amino, sulfhydryl, hydroxyl, carboxyl, and imidazole groups. Ultimately, these bonds result in cross-linking of DNA base pairs, either between two strands of DNA or within the same strand. This cross-linking prevents the DNA strand from unwinding properly for replication, ultimately leading to inhibition of DNA synthesis and cell death.[4,5] It is thought that apoptosis is stimulated by p53 pathways in response to this DNA damage. Alkylating agents can affect cells at any point in the cell cycle (cell-cycle nonspecific), but rapidly dividing cells experience the strongest insult.

### Toxicity

As Krumbhaar noted in 1919, poisoning caused by sulfur mustard is characterized by aplasia of bone marrow, dissolution of lymphoid tissue, and ulceration of the gastrointestinal tract.[1] While the alkylating agents differ somewhat in spectrum of activity and severity of adverse effects, most exhibit toxicities similar to those observed with the original agent. These compounds are typically dose-limited by suppressive effects on the bone marrow. Myelosuppression often manifests acutely, with an onset of 6–10 days and recovery within 14–21 days.[5] Some compounds, such as busulfan and carmustine, exhibit a prolonged suppression of granulocytes and platelets, and for this reason are commonly used in stem cell transplant preparative regimens. Suppression of both cellular and humoral immunity occurs frequently. The rapidly dividing cells of the intestinal mucosa are particularly sensitive to the effects of alkylating agents, evidenced by mucositis and stomatitis. Specific organ toxicities, such as pulmonary fibrosis, have been reported with all alkylating agents. In addition, this entire class of compounds is associated with a high incidence of secondary malignancies, affecting up to 5% of exposed patients[6] (Table 101.1).

### Selected alkylating agents

*Cyclophosphamide* Cyclophosphamide is a nitrogen-mustard derivative that possesses a broad spectrum of activity. Its clinical usefulness is widespread, and it remains a key component of treatment regimens for a variety of malignancies, including non-Hodgkin's lymphoma and acute lymphocytic leukemia.[5] Additionally, the immunosuppressive properties of cyclophosphamide have been found to be effective in the treatment of various nonmalignant conditions, such as Wegener's granulomatosis, rheumatoid arthritis, nephrotic syndrome, and control of organ rejection after transplantation.[5]

Cyclophosphamide is a prodrug and requires activation by hepatic cytochrome P450 2B enzymes for its therapeutic effect. It is converted to 5-hydroxyphosphamide, which exists in equilibrium with its tautomer, aldophosphamide. Further conversion to phosphoramide mustard in susceptible cells results in liberation of the active alkylating compound and subsequent cell toxicity.[17]

*Pharmacokinetics/metabolism:* Cyclophosphamide is well absorbed from the gastrointestinal tract and is available for both oral and intravenous administration. It distributes widely to tissues, and penetrates the CNS to a small extent.[18] Hepatic metabolism is required for conversion of cyclophosphamide to its active form as well as inactive metabolites. These inactive metabolites undergo renal excretion along with unchanged drug (<15%).[18]

*Toxicity:* The dose-limiting toxicity of cyclophosphamide is myelosuppression, mainly leukopenia. While white blood cells are sensitive to cyclophosphamide, platelets are less affected. Alopecia, dose-dependent nausea and vomiting, mucositis, and stomatitis are common. Cardiac dysfunction, manifesting as congestive heart failure, has occurred rarely. Cyclophosphamide may potentiate the cardiac toxicity of anthracyclines.[5] The classic toxicity associated with cyclophosphamide (as well as the structurally related ifosfamide) is hemorrhagic cystitis, which has been reported in up to 15% patients.[9] Acrolein, a toxic metabolite of both cyclophosphamide and ifosfamide, is thought to bind to crucial thiols in the bladder wall, causing mucosal damage. This creates a syndrome of hematuria, urinary frequency, and irritation.[19] In severe cases, massive hemorrhage and bladder carcinoma can occur. Aggressive hydration and therapy with the detoxifying agent mesna, which binds acrolein in the bladder and prevents mucosal attachment, can minimize the risk of this effect.[19]

*Busulfan* Busulfan is an alkyl sulfonate derivative that reacts with the N7 position of guanosine, leading to cross-linking of DNA strands and subsequent inhibition of DNA synthesis. Busulfan is unique in that it affects the cells of myeloid origin to a greater extent than those of lymphoid origin.[5] In addition, busulfan is toxic to hematopoietic stem cells and is thus frequently used in stem cell transplant preparative regimens.

*Pharmacokinetics/metabolism:* Busulfan is rapidly and completely absorbed from the gastrointestinal tract and is available for oral and intravenous administration. It distributes widely throughout the body and achieves CSF levels similar to concurrent plasma levels.[12,19] The compound undergoes extensive metabolism in the liver and is a substrate for cytochrome P450 3A3/4. Approximately 10–50% metabolites are excreted in the urine. Half-life ranges from 2 to 3 h.[19]

*Toxicity:* The most notable toxicity of busulfan is the profound suppression of the bone marrow; severe pancytopenia is also common and often indication of the compound. This is a delayed effect, with the onset of myelosuppression occurring 7–10 days after the therapy is initiated. Other common toxicities include urticaria, skin hyperpigmentation, and alopecia. At

**Table 101.1** Alkylating agents in the treatment of hematologic malignancies

| Agent | Clinical uses | Mechanism of action | Common toxicities |
|---|---|---|---|
| **Nitrogen mustard derivatives** | | | |
| Mechlorethamine | HD, NHL | Bifunctional alkylating agent with two reactive groups[5] | Acute<br>■ DLT[a] = Myelosuppression (onset 4–7 days)<br>■ Severe nausea/vomiting (onset 30 min to 2 h[7])<br>■ Extravasation (vesicant)<br>Chronic<br>■ Secondary malignancies<br>■ Sterility |
| Cyclo-phosphamide | NHL, HD, BMT, CLL, ANLL, ALL, myeloma | Activated by hepatic oxidase enzymes to reactive agent phosphoramide mustard | Acute<br>■ DLT = Myelosuppression (onset 7 days[8])<br>■ Dose-dependent nausea/vomiting (onset 8 h)<br>■ Alopecia (onset 3 weeks[8])<br>■ Hemorrhagic cystitis (onset ranges from 24 h to several weeks[9])<br>■ Nephrotoxicity<br>Chronic<br>■ Nephrotoxicity |
| Melphalan | Myeloma, BMT | L-phenylalanine mustard; classic bifunctional alkylating agent | Acute<br>■ DLT = Myelosuppression: prolonged and cumulative (onset 7 days, nadir up to 4–6 weeks after therapy[10])<br>■ Dose-dependent nausea/vomiting/mucositis<br>Chronic<br>■ Secondary malignancies, including AML and myelodysplasia |
| Chlorambucil | CLL, NHL, HD | Aromatic analog of nitrogen mustard; bifunctional alkylating agent with selective cytotoxicity for lymphocytes | Acute<br>■ DLT = Myelosuppression (onset 7 days, recovery 28 days[11])<br>Chronic<br>■ Secondary malignancies, including acute leukemias |
| **Alkyl sulfonates** | | | |
| Busulfan | BMT, CML | Bifunctional alkylating agent with greater cytotoxicity to myeloid cell lines | Acute<br>■ DLT = Myelosuppression (onset 7–10 days[12])<br>■ Mild nausea/vomiting<br>■ Hepatic VOD (with doses > 16 mg/day[12])<br>■ Skin hyperpigmentation<br>■ Generalized tonic-clonic seizures<br>Chronic<br>■ Sterility<br>■ Interstitial pulmonary fibrosis (may occur 1–10 years after therapy[12,13])<br>■ Secondary malignancies |

*table continues*

| Table 101.1 | continued | | |
|---|---|---|---|
| Agent | Clinical uses | Mechanism of action | Common toxicities |
| **Nitrosoureas** | | | |
| Carmustine | Myeloma, HD, NHL, BMT | Metabolized to active alkylating agent plus isocyanate compounds that may exert additional cytotoxic effects | Acute<br>■ DLT = Myelosuppression (onset 14 days, complete recovery may take 6–8 weeks[14])<br>■ Severe nausea/vomiting (onset 2–6 h)<br>■ Pain at injection site<br>■ Facial flushing, dizziness<br>■ Nephrotoxicity (glomerulosclerosis, tubular loss, interstitial fibrosis)<br>■ Hyperpigmentation<br>Chronic<br>■ Pulmonary toxicity; interstitial pneumonitis and fibrosis |
| **Triazenes** | | | |
| Procarbazine | HD | Atypical alkylating agent; requires hepatic activation to active compound which interferes with DNA, RNA, and protein synthesis | Acute<br>■ DLT = Myelosuppression (onset 14 days, recovery 28 days[15])<br>■ Anorexia, nausea/vomiting<br>■ Facial flushing, pain at injection site<br>Chronic<br>■ Sterility<br>■ Secondary malignancies |
| Dacarbazine | HD | Requires activation to reactive intermediates (methyl-carbonium ions) that alkylate nucleic acids; thus, DNA, RNA, and protein synthesis is inhibited | Acute<br>■ Severe nausea/vomiting (onset 1–2 h, may last up to 12 h[16])<br>■ Myelosuppression (mild); (onset 7 days, recovery 21–28 days)<br>■ Anaphylactic reactions<br>■ Photosensitivity<br>■ Flu-like syndrome (may last several days after infusion[17])<br>■ Extravasation (irritant)<br>Chronic<br>■ Hepatocellular necrosis |

[a]DLT = dose-limiting toxicity.

higher doses, such as those used in stem cell transplant regimens, adverse effects become more severe. Mild nausea and vomiting may occur. In addition, because of its ability to readily penetrate the CNS, busulfan can lower the seizure threshold, causing generalized tonic-clonic seizures.[12] For this reason, prophylactic antiepileptic medications are commonly administered. Veno-occlusive disease, or VOD, is thought to be associated with high doses of busulfan.[12] Finally, pulmonary toxicity can occur. "Busulfan lung" is characterized by pulmonary fibrosis and presenting symptoms include nonproductive cough, shortness of breath, and weight loss.[5,12,19] This complication may correlate with duration of busulfan therapy, with a higher incidence occurring in those who have received greater than 3 years of treatment. It is often fatal, with average survival of 5 months after diagnosis.[19]

### ANTIMETABOLITES
As a class, antimetabolites exhibit S-phase specific cytotoxicity. These agents chemically resemble the purine and pyrimidine nucleoside bases involved in normal cellular DNA replication (adenine, guanine, cytosine, and thymine) or impair enzymes involved in protein or DNA synthesis. These nucleoside analogs essentially "trick" cells into incorporating the toxic drug into newly synthesized DNA strands in place of normal nucleotide bases.[5,20] This leads to synthesis inhibition and chain termination. Multiple antimetabolites are currently in use (Table 101.2).

**Table 101.2** Antimetabolite compounds and selected toxicities

| Agent | Mechanism of action | Clinical uses | Common toxicities |
|---|---|---|---|
| **Purine analogs** | | | |
| Fludarabine, Fludara | Adenosine analog; incorporated into DNA resulting in chain termination; also inhibits ribonucleotide reductase, which depletes cells of deoxyribonucleotide triphosphate pools | CLL, NHL | ■ DLT[a] = Myelo-suppression (onset 10–14 days[21]) <br> ■ Neurotoxicity <br> ■ Immunosuppression (can last up to 2 years[22]) <br> ■ Mild nausea/vomiting <br> ■ Interstitial pneumonitis (onset ranges from 3 days after first cycle to 6 days after seventh cycle[23]) |
| Cladribine, 2-CDA, Leustatin | Adeosine analog; incorporated into DNA resulting in chain termination; also inhibits ribonucleotide reductase, which depletes cells of deoxyribonucleotide triphosphate pools | Hairy cell leukemia, NHL | ■ DLT = Myelo-suppression (onset 7–14 days[24]) <br> ■ Immunosuppression (onset 4–6 months; typically lasts 1 year, may last up to 40 months[24]) <br> ■ Fever |
| 6-Mercaptopurine, 6-MP | Hypoxanthine analog; interferes with purine biosynthesis; also incorporated into DNA resulting in chain termination[25] | ALL | ■ Mucositis <br> ■ Diarrhea <br> ■ Mild myelosuppression (onset 7–10 days[24]) <br> ■ Hepatotoxicity, jaundice (onset typically 2–3 months[24]) |
| 6-Thioguanine, 6-TG | Guanine analog; incorporated into DNA resulting in chain termination[25] | AML, ALL | ■ DLT = Myelo-suppression (onset 7–10 days[26]) <br> ■ Mild nausea/vomiting <br> ■ Immunosuppression[26] <br> ■ Mucositis <br> ■ Diarrhea |
| **Pyrimidine analogs** <br> Cytarabine, Cytosine arabinoside, Ara-C, Cytosar-U | Cytidine analog; incorporated into DNA resulting in chain termination; also inhibits DNA polymerase resulting in decreased DNA synthesis/repair | AML, ALL, CNS leukemia, NHL | Moderate dose <br> ■ DLT = Myelo-suppression (onset 4–7 days[27]) <br> ■ Alopecia <br> ■ Mild nausea/vomiting <br> High dose (>1 g/m$^2$) <br> ■ Cerebellar toxicity (onset typically 5 days[28]) <br> ■ Myelosuppression <br> ■ Severe nausea/vomiting (onset 1–3 h, typically lasts 3–8 h[27]) <br> ■ Conjunctivitis <br> ■ Transient hepatic dysfunction (elevation of serum transaminases) <br> ■ Pulmonary complications <br> ■ "Ara-C syndrome": allergic reaction characterized by fever, myalgias, rash, conjunctivitis (onset 12 h after infusion[28]) |

*table continues*

**Table 101.2**    continued

| Agent | Mechanism of action | Clinical uses | Common toxicities |
|---|---|---|---|
| Gemcitabine, Gemzar | Cytidine analog; incorporated into DNA resulting in chain termination;[29,30] Also inhibits ribonucleotide reductase, depleting cells of deoxyribonucleotides required for DNA synthesis | Investigational use in Hodgkin's disease, cutaneous T-cell lymphoma, mantle cell lymphoma, CLL | ■ DLT = Myelo-suppression (onset 7–10 days[31]) <br> ■ Hepatic transaminase elevations (transient) <br> ■ Proteinuria, hematuria <br> ■ Generalized rash <br> ■ Flu-like symptoms, fever (onset 6–12 hours[31]) |
| Decitabine, 2'-deoxy-5-azacytidine, Aza dC, DAC, dezocitidine | Cytidine analog; incorporated into DNA resulting in chain termination; once incorporated into DNA, inhibits DNA methyltransferase enzymes (DNMTs), preventing the transfer of a methyl group to DNA strands[32]. Formerly silenced genes are subsequently activated, altering cell differentiation and apoptosis pathways. | Investigational studies in refractory AML, CLL, Small lymphocytic lymphoma, MDS | ■ Myelosuppression (onset 14 days, may last up to 30 days) <br> ■ Nausea/vomiting <br> ■ Fatigue, lethargy <br> ■ Hepatic transaminase elevations |
| 5-azacytidine | Cytidine analog; incorporated into DNA resulting in chain termination; once incorporated into DNA, inhibits DNA methyltransferase enzymes (DNMTs), preventing the transfer of a methyl group to DNA strands[32]. Formerly silenced genes are subsequently activated, altering cell differentiation and apoptosis pathways. Also incorporated into RNA, altering tRNA methylation and inhibiting protein synthesis[32]. | CML, AML, myelodysplasia | ■ Myelosuppression <br> ■ Nausea/vomiting <br> ■ Diarrhea <br> ■ Mutagenic potential |
| Pentostatin, 2-Deoxycoformycin, Nipent | Inhibits adenosine deaminase, which metabolizes adenosine and deoxyadenosine; leads to accumulation of deoxyadenosine triphosphate (dATP), which inhibits ribonucleotide reductase and causes cell death | Hairy cell leukemia | ■ DLT = Myelo-suppression (onset 7–10 days[33]) <br> ■ Immunosuppression <br> ■ Severe nausea/vomiting (onset 12–24 h after infusion[11]) <br> ■ Transient hepatic transaminase elevations <br> ■ Nephrotoxicity and neurotoxicity (rare at current doses) <br> ■ Transient lethargy, confusion |
| Folic acid analog <br> Methotrexate | Folic acid analog; binds DHFR and inhibits conversion of folic acid to active "tetrahydro" form, which deprives cells of necessary precursor for thymidylate and purine synthesis[9] | ALL, CNS leukemia, NHL, BMT | ■ DLT = Myelo-suppression (onset 4–7 days) <br> ■ Mucositis, stomatitis (onset 3–7 days[11]) <br> ■ Hepatic transaminase elevations (onset 12–24 h, usually lasts 10 days[11]) <br> ■ Pulmonary toxicity <br> ■ Nephrotoxicity |

[a]DLT = dose-limiting toxicity.

## Antimetabolites: Selected nucleoside analogs

***Cytarabine*** Cytarabine is an antimetabolite that is currently considered the foundation of treatment for AML. It is one of the most active agents available against this disease and has been considered an integral component of induction and postremission therapy for the past two decades. In addition, cytarabine exhibits significant activity against lymphomas, meningeal leukemia, and meningeal lymphoma. It has little use in the treatment of solid tumors. Cytarabine is administered in a wide range of doses, and evidence supports a significant dose-response effect.[34]

Chemically, cytarabine is the arabinose analog of the nucleotide base cytosine. Arabinose analogs differ from human analogs by the placement of a hydroxyl group on the sugar moiety of the nucleoside. Cytarabine penetrates cells via a carrier-mediated transport process, where it must be phosphorylated by the enzyme deoxycytidine kinase (dCK) to its active form, ara-CTP. Because of its structural similarity to cytosine, ara-CTP is directly incorporated into DNA in place of cytosine, where it terminates strand elongation by inhibiting DNA replication. This antimetabolite effect is thought to be the main mechanism of cytarabine activity at moderate doses (100–200 mg/m²). In addition, cytarabine further affects DNA synthesis by direct inhibition of the enzyme DNA polymerase, which is responsible for strand elongation as well as DNA repair. The degree of activity correlates linearly with the degree of incorporation into DNA. This is heavily influenced by the plasma cytarabine concentration.[35]

*Pharmacokinetics/metabolism:* Cytarabine is degraded within the cell by cytidine deaminase to the inactive compound uracil arabinoside, or ara-U. Cytarabine is widely distributed in the body, with a volume of distribution approximating total plasma volume. It penetrates the CNS and achieves concentrations approximately 20–40% of simultaneous plasma levels.[19] Cytarabine is metabolized extensively in the liver and excreted as metabolites within 36 h; approximately 80% is excreted in the urine as ara-U. The plasma half-life is 2–6 h, while the CSF half-life is longer, ranging from 2 to11 h.[5,19]

*Toxicity:* Toxicity of cytarabine is dose-dependent; at higher doses (>1 g/m²), cytarabine is dose-limited by cerebellar toxicity. This often manifests as a syndrome of dysarthria, nystagmus, and ataxia, and may progress to generalized encephalopathy and seizures. Some degree of CNS toxicity has been documented in up to 40% of patients receiving high-dose cytarabine.[19] This is typically reversible upon discontinuation of drug, but may be permanent. It is highly correlated with older age, renal dysfunction, and elevated alkaline phosphatase levels, and dose adjustments are strongly recommended for both groups of patients.[5,19,36,37] In addition, high-dose cytarabine can cause severe conjunctivitis, maculopapular skin rash, palmar-plantar erythema, and hepatic toxicity characterized by cholestatic jaundice. At lower doses, cytarabine can cause significant myelosuppression. Alopecia and dose-related nausea and vomiting are common as well.[5]

***Gemcitabine*** Gemcitabine is a pyrimidine analog, structurally similar to cyarabine, and was initially developed as an attempt to expand upon the cytotoxic effects of the latter agent. Chemically, it differs from cytarabine by the substitution of geminal fluorines for the hydroxyl group at the 2' position.[20,38] This chemical alteration allows for greater cellular permeability and increased affinity for the enzyme dCK, which phosphorylates gemcitabine to its active gemcitabine-5'-triphosphate form.[38] This compound, upon incorporation into DNA, results in chain termination. Increased cellular transport and increased affinity for dCK allow for greater intracellular retention and accumulation of gemcitabine as compared to cytarabine. This may account for the extended spectrum of activity seen with the newer compound.[25] In addition, there is evidence that gemcitabine inhibits ribonucleotide reductase, leading to the depletion of cellular deoxyribonucleotide triphosphate pools. This not only depletes cells of active nucleotides essential for DNA synthesis, but also propagates the toxicity of gemcitabine. Cells are forced to further incorporate gemcitabine into DNA strands because of the lack of competition with normal nucleotides. Additionally, as a result of the structural conformation of gemcitabine, a normal base pair is routinely added to DNA strands just after incorporation of the toxic compound. This effectively protects gemictabine from being excised by DNA repair enzymes from the newly formed strand, and ensures cell death. This mechanism has been termed "masked chain termination." Gemcitabine has demonstrated activity in a variety of solid as well as hematologic malignancies, including Hodgkin's disease, mantle cell lymphoma, and chronic lymphocytic leukemia.[38]

*Pharmacokinetics/metabolism:* Extensive deamination of gemcitabine occurs in the gastrointestinal tract; therefore, the compound is not active orally and is available only as a solution for injection. Deamination by cytidine deaminase is the primary metabolic route, which occurs in liver, plasma, and peripheral tissues. More than 90% of drug is recovered in the urine as the difluorouridine metabolite.[5,19] Because of the dependence of half-life on infusion duration, many infusion schedules have been evaluated. A longer infusion duration (>70 min) is associated with a longer half-life (4–10 h) and increased clinical activity.[29,30]

*Toxicity:* The dose-limiting toxicity associated with gemcitabine is myelosuppression, mainly consisting of neutropenia. Nausea and vomiting are mild. Acutely (within 6–12 h of drug administration), fever and flu-like symptoms, such as headache, chills, malaise, and myalgias, are common. Elevations in hepatic transaminases may occur and caution should be used when treating patients with underlying hepatic dysfunction.[39] Mild proteinuria and hematuria have been reported frequently.[5,19] A generalized, macropapular rash occurs in approximately 25% of patients; this is typically reversible and does not usually require discontinuation of drug.[19]

*Fludarabine*    Fludarabine monophosphate is a structural analog of the purine adenine. Initially, the arabinose analog of adenine, ara-A, was developed. However, because of the rapid inactivation by adenosine deaminase enzymes, the drug exhibited less than optimal antitumor activity. The addition of a fluorine atom resulted in a compound that retained antitumor activity, while resisting inactivation by deaminase enzymes.[5] Thus, F-ara-A or fludarabine was developed. This compound is highly effective in the treatment of chronic lymphocytic leukemia; in addition, it has activity in acute leukemia and non-Hodgkin's lymphoma.[19]

Similar to cytarabine and other nucleoside analogs, fludarabine requires transport into tumor cells and activation to its triphosphate form for cytotoxic activity. The first step in this phosphorylation is performed by the enzyme dCK, which results in the active compound F-ara-ATP. This compound is active in both dividing and resting cells.[40] DNA synthesis inhibition results from competitive uptake of F-ara-ATP, rather than adenine, by dividing cells for incorporation into DNA strands. Once incorporated, chain elongation is halted, inhibiting DNA synthesis. F-ara-ATP exhibits additional activity through inhibition of specific enzymes, such as DNA polymerase α, DNA ligase, and topoisomerase II.[41] These actions are S-phase specific, and incorporation of fludarabine into DNA at this point in cell division is required for apoptosis. Unlike cytarabine, fludarabine is also incorporated into RNA, where it inhibits the RNA polymerase II enzyme. Subsequently, RNA transcription is terminated, and protein synthesis cannot be achieved. This may account for the activity of fludarabine in resting cells.[41] Finally, evidence indicates that fludarabine may activate apoptotic pathways as well, by stimulating APAF-1, which subsequently leads to activation of caspase-9 and caspase-3 pathways.[40]

*Pharmacokinetics/metabolism:* Fludarabine is inactivated by deaminase enzymes, particularly adenine deaminase. Its terminal elimination half-life is approximately 10 h and renal excretion is the primary route of elimination.[42] As excess toxicity results from accumulation of drug in renal dysfunction, dosage adjustments are recommended for patients with moderate renal dysfunction (creatinine clearance 30–70 ml/min). Fludarabine should be avoided for patients with severe renal dysfunction (creatinine clearance <30 ml/min).[43]

*Toxicity:* When fludarabine was first developed, doses were limited by neurologic toxicity. At these higher doses, a syndrome of delayed CNS toxicity was seen, characterized by paralysis and coma. It was eventually found that fludarabine could be used in lower doses, maintaining activity at less risk to the patient. For the doses used currently, severe CNS toxicity is rare.[19] A small portion of patients experience some degree of neurotoxicity, which can manifest as somnolence, paresthesias, and peripheral neuropathies. The dose-limiting toxicity of fludarabine is now considered to be myelosuppression.[5,19,42] Immunosuppression is common as well, and suppression of CD4 and CD8 cells can last up to a year before returning to normal levels. Slowly reversible, dose-dependent pulmonary toxicity consistent with interstitial pneumonitis has been reported rarely.

### Antimetabolites: Folic acid analog

*Methotrexate*    Methotrexate is a unique antimetabolite that is used in a multitude of malignancies, including solid tumors, lymphomas, and lymphocytic leukemias as well as a variety of autoimmune and inflammatory disorders. This agent is the most well characterized and widely used of all the antimetabolites.

Methotrexate differs structurally from folic acid by replacement of a hydroxyl group with an amino group on the pteridine ring, as well as an additional methyl group.[19] Access to the target site of action is achieved through specific intracellular transport systems, which are mediated by the reduced folate carrier and folate receptor protein. Methotrexate exerts its cytotoxic effect through inhibition of the enzyme dihydrofolate reductase (DHFR). This enzyme is responsible for converting dietary folates to their reduced or active "tetrahydro" form for use by cells in thymidylate and purine synthesis. Through binding of DHFR to methotrexate, intracellular pools of reduced folates are depleted and synthesis of DNA is prevented.[5] This action can be overcome by supplying the active tetrahydro form of folate to cells exogenously; this compound is known as leucovorin or folinic acid.

*Pharmacokinetics/metabolism:* Oral bioavailability is variable and incomplete. Methotrexate distributes widely to tissues, including the CNS. In moderate doses, CNS levels are low; however, at high methotrexate doses ($>1$ gm/m$^2$) therapeutic CNS levels are achieved. Methotrexate can accumulate in fluid collections, such as pleural fluid and ascites. These fluid accumulations can act as reservoirs, slowly releasing methotrexate into the bloodstream over a prolonged time course.[19] Methotrexate undergoes hepatic metabolism and enterohepatic cycling to various metabolites, which are eliminated renally (filtration and active secretion). Methotrexate solubility is pH-dependent, and methotrexate can crystallize in the renal tubules at high doses.[5] Alkalinization of the urine increases the solubility of methotrexate, minimizing the risk of this complication. Terminal half-life is approximately 8–10 h, but can be prolonged to over 20 h in patients with renal insufficiency, impaired enterohepatic cycling, or significant third-space fluids.[19]

*Toxicity:* The dose-limiting toxicity of methotrexate is myelosuppression. Granulocytes and platelets are the cell lines most affected. Mucositis, stomatitis, and mucosal ulceration can be severe. At higher doses, nephrotoxicity and acute renal failure can result from intratubular precipitation of drug. Hepatic toxicity is characterized by elevations in serum transaminases and bilirubin, portal fibrosis, and occasionally cirrhosis. Pulmonary toxicity is rare but potentially fatal. CNS toxicity can result from intravenous administration as well as direct intrathecal administration.[19]

## ANTITUMOR ANTIBIOTICS

### Antitumor antibiotics: Anthracyclines, anthracene derivatives

*Daunorubicin, doxorubicin, idarubicin* Anthracyclines are among the most effective antineoplastic agents ever developed; the various compounds have been in use for more than 20 years (Table 101.3). They possess a wide spectrum of activity against a variety of solid tumors and hematologic malignancies and are an essential component of current therapies in AML, ALL, and Hodgkin's disease, to name a few. These compounds share an aglycone or sugar moiety attached to a four-membered anthracene ring complex, known as a chromophore. It is this chromophore that gives these drugs their intense coloring. The original anthracyclines, doxorubicin and daunorubicin, were derived from the pigment-producing bacteria *Streptomyces peucetius* in the early 1960s.[58]

The anthracene derivatives are cell-cycle nonspecific; however, they exert the greatest activity against rapidly dividing cells. The mechanism of action of these agents is still being elucidated and remains somewhat controversial. There is evidence supporting a variety of mechanisms.[58,59] Traditionally, anthracyclines have been considered intercalating agents. Because of

**Table 101.3** Common properties of anthracene and anthracenedione derivatives

| Agent | Dosing information | Clinical uses | Dose adjustments |
|---|---|---|---|
| **Anthracene derivatives** | | | |
| Doxorubicin | Dose range, 40–75 mg/m² Maximum cumulative dose,[44] 550 mg/m² <br><br> * If prior RT, 450 mg/m² | All, Hodgkin's disease, NHL, sarcomas, germ cell tumors, many solid tumors (breast, stomach, head/neck, liver, bladder) | Renal impairment[45] <br> ■ CrCl<10 ml/min: give 75% dose <br> Hepatic impairment[46] <br> ■ Bilirubin 1.2–3 mg/dl: give 50% dose <br> ■ Bilirubin 3.1–5 mg/dl: give 25% dose <br> ■ Bilirubin >5 mg/dl: avoid use |
| Daunorubicin | Dose range, 45–90 mg/m² Maximum cumulative dose,[47] 550 mg/m² <br><br> * If prior RT, 400 mg/m² | ALL, AML | Renal impairment[48] <br> ■ CrCl<10 ml/min: give 75% dose <br> Hepatic impairment[48] <br> ■ Bilirubin 1.2–3 mg/dl: give 75% dose <br> ■ Bilirubin 3.1–5 mg/dl: give 50% dose <br> ■ Bilirubin >5 mg/dl: Avoid use |
| Idarubicin | Dose range, 10–12 mg/m² Maximum cumulative dose: doses of 150–290 mg/m² have resulted in 5% chance of cardio-myopathy[49] | AML, ALL | Renal impairment[50] <br> ■ Serum creatinine ≥2 mg/dl: give 75% dose <br> Hepatic impairment[50,51] <br> ■ Bilirubin 1.5–5 mg/dl: give 50% dose <br> ■ Bilirubin >5 mg/dl: avoid use |
| **Anthracene-dione derivatives** | | | |
| Mitoxantrone | Dose range, 10–15 mg/m² Maximum cumulative dose: doses exceeding 80–120 mg/m² have been associated with a higher incidence of cardio-myopathy[52–56] | AML | Renal impairment[57]: not necessary <br> Hepatic impairment: dose reduction advised; no guidelines available |

their planar structure and positively charged sugar moieties, anthracyclines are thought to "intercalate" or insert between negatively charged phosphate bridges of DNA base pairs, binding tightly and creating covalent bonds. Two types of bonds are formed: more stable drug–DNA cross-links and less stable drug–DNA adducts.[58] These bonds create torsional strain and lead to DNA deformation and uncoiling. Additionally, this intercalation interferes with several enzymes involved in DNA replication and transcription, including helicase, DNA polymerase, and RNA polymerase.[59]

Anthracyclines are also considered potent topoisomerase II poisons. Topoisomerase is an enzyme that temporarily relieves torsional strain during DNA synthesis. The topoisomerase enzymes accomplish this task by causing temporary single-strand (topoisomerase I) or double-strand (topoisomerase II) DNA breaks, and subsequently resealing these breaks after twisting of the double helix is modified. A structurally dependent function of the anthracene derivatives is to stabilize a reaction intermediate in which DNA strands are cleaved and covalently linked to topoisomerase II, impeding DNA resealing. This DNA damage is followed by growth arrest in G1 and G2 phases and programmed cell death.[58]

Generation of free radicals and subsequent lipid peroxidation occurs with anthracyclines as well, and this mechanism is thought to contribute to the efficacy as well as the cardiotoxicity of these compounds. Electron transfer and reduction of anthracyclines takes place quickly, leading to the formation of superoxide anions and hydrogen peroxide. These highly reactive compounds bind iron, generating the most toxic of the hydroxyl radicals, which can cleave DNA. The ability of various tissues to diffuse these free radicals is thought to account for the characteristic distribution of anthracycline toxicity.[5,58]

*Pharmacokinetics/metabolism:* Anthracyclines as a class distribute rapidly and widely to all body tissues except the CNS, accounting for a large distribution volume. Metabolism occurs mainly in the liver, followed by biliary excretion. Elimination is biphasic, with estimated half-lives of approximately 30 h for doxorubicin, 15–20 h for daunorubicin, and 15–20 h for idarubicin. Renal elimination accounts for <10% of total clearance with each of these compounds; however, enough drug escapes to color the urine bright red or orange.[19]

*Toxicity:* The most common short-term toxicity associated with these compounds is myelosuppression, characterized mainly by leukopenia. Other common effects include alopecia, moderately severe nausea and vomiting, and mucositis. The most notorious adverse effect associated with the anthracyclines is cardiotoxicity. This typically manifests as chronic congestive cardiomyopathy, which is cumulative and dose-dependent.[58] It is thought to result from numerous factors related to anthracycline treatment, including

free-radical accumulation in the cardiac myocytes, increased membrane lipid peroxidation, changes in adrenergic function and adenylate cyclase, irreversible decrease in mitochondrial calcium loading and ATP content, and induction of nitric oxide synthase, leading to nitric oxide activation of metalloproteinases. These effects depend on peak drug concentrations as well as cumulative dose.[58] Continuous infusion may decrease the risk of cardiotoxicity by decreasing the peak concentration; however, this results in much greater stomatitis.[19] Patients are also at risk for late onset cardiotoxicity, characterized by left ventricular dysfunction and arrhythmias.

### Antitumor antibiotics: Anthracenedione derivatives

*Mitoxantrone*   Mitoxantrone, developed in an attempt to create an anthracene derivate with an improved toxicity profile, is actually an anthracenedione. Structurally, it is composed of a three-membered anthracene complex and lacks a sugar moiety.[19] Mitoxantrone intercalates between DNA base pairs, resulting in inhibition of DNA synthesis and function, as well as inhibiting topoisomerase II. However, it is thought to have a decreased tendency for free radical formation and thus there is a lower chance of cardiotoxicity. Recent reports have challenged this assumption, however, and it is generally thought to exhibit a similar cardiotoxicity profile to the structurally similar anthracyclines.[60]

### Antitumor antibiotics: Miscellaneous compounds

*Bleomycin*   Bleomycin is a small peptide compound that is isolated from the fungus *Streptomyces verticillus*. While the drug contains 13 identifiable peptide fractions, the primary component (approximately 70% of commercial product) is bleomycin A2. Bleomycin requires the presence of iron for activity; bleomycin–iron complexes can bind directly to DNA, and upon oxidation, form free radical intermediates that lead to single and double strand breaks.[61] The DNA lesions introduced by bleomycin are similar to those seen with ionizing radiation.[62] This agent has activity in a variety of malignancies, including testicular cancer and Hodgkin's lymphoma, and is an integral component in the treatment of these diseases.

*Pharmacokinetics/metabolism:* Bleomycin is poorly absorbed orally, and is available only as a solution for injection. It distributes to intracellular and extracellular fluid, and achieves its highest concentrations in skin, kidney, lung, and heart tissues. It does not penetrate the CNS.[61] Bleomycin is degraded by the enzyme bleomycin hydrolase, which is present in tissues throughout the body. Lowest levels of this enzyme are found in the skin and lungs, which may account for the toxicity profile associated with this agent. Renal excretion is the primary route of bleomycin elimination, with 45–70% of drug excreted unchanged in the urine.[19] Dose adjustments are recommended in patients with renal dysfunction, as elimination half-life is extended from 2 to 4 h to more than 20 h in these patients.[19]

*Toxicity:* The skin and lungs are the organs most sensitive to the toxic effects of bleomycin. Mucocutaneous toxicity is common, and typically occurs 14–21 days after treatment.[5] This can present as erythema, hyperpigmentation, ulceration, skin peeling, and thickening of the nail beds. Stomatitis and alopecia are common as well. Pulmonary toxicity is dose-limiting and can occur months after completion of therapy. It has been associated with cumulative dose (>400 units) as well as advanced age, renal dysfunction, preexisting pulmonary disease, and previous chest irradiation.[19] Interstitial pneumonitis is characteristic, presenting as cough and dyspnea with nonspecific radiograph findings. This complication can be fatal or reversible. Hypersensitivity reactions, such as fever and chills, occur in up to 25% of patients treated with bleomycin. These reactions are thought to be due to direct release of pyrogens rather than histamine, and can often be managed with antipyretics.[19] Nausea and vomiting are mild, as is myelosuppression.

## VINCA ALKALOIDS

### Vincristine, vinblastine, vindesine, vinorelbine

The vincas are natural compounds originally derived from the periwinkle plant. Two of these compounds, vincristine and vinblastine, are used in the treatment of a variety of hematological malignancies, including lymphocytic leukemia, lymphoma, Hodgkin's disease, and myeloma.

Vinca alkaloids are known as "spindle poisons," because of their ability to inhibit the assembly of microtubules. This targeting of microtubules is thought to be one of the most important sites of antitumor activity discovered to date.[63] These compounds act by directly binding to the "vinca domain" on tubulin, blocking its ability to polymerize into microtubules.[64] Microtubules are cytoskeletal fibers, comprising tubulin subunits, which are responsible for a variety of cellular functions crucial to mitosis, including chromosomal segration and maintenance of cellular shape. Disruption of microtubule dynamics by vinca alkaloids results in absence of a mitotic spindle, which leads to irregular dispersion of chromosomes throughout the cytoplasm. Ultimately, cells are arrested during mitosis in the metaphase/anaphase transition, and apoptosis occurs. Microtubules are responsible for a variety of other cellular functions as well, including cellular transport and motility, phagocytosis, neurotransmission, and axonal transport.[65] Inhibition of these nonmitotic cellular functions may account for some of the adverse effects common to the vinca alkaloids.

*Pharmacokinetics/metabolism:* Vinca alkaloids, as a class, are poorly absorbed from gastrointestinal tract. They are only available for intravenous administration. Distribution occurs mainly within the blood, and the compounds bind tightly to blood components. Penetration of the CNS is poor. All four compounds are metabolized extensively by the liver and excreted in the bile. Small amounts of unchanged drug are recovered in the urine. Dosage adjustments are recommended for patients with hepatic dysfunction to avoid excessive toxicity.[19]

*Toxicity:* Although vincas are structurally similar, their spectra of activity and adverse effects differ significantly. The dose-limiting toxicity of vincristine is neurotoxicity, likely due to inhibition of microtubule effects related to neuronal transmission.[65] This can manifest as sensory and/or motor neuropathy and is characterized by paresthesias, palsies, and pain. Autonomic complications, such as abdominal pain, orthostatic hypotension, constipation, and paralytic ileus, may also occur. For this reason, vincristine doses have traditionally been limited to 2 mg, although recent protocols are challenging this maximum dose. Other adverse effects associated with vincristine include SIADH and alopecia. Fatal cases of intrathecal administration have been reported.[66] While the potential for myelosuppression exists with vincristine, it is uncommon at standard doses. Conversely, the dose-limiting toxicity for vinblastine and vinorelbine is myelosuppression. Anemia and thrombocytopenia can occur, but leukopenia is most significant.[5] Although neurotoxicity may occur, it is much less common than with vincristine. This primarily manifests as myalgias and arthralgias and occurs more commonly with vinorelbine than vinblastine.[5]

## PODOPHYLLOTOXIN DERIVATIVES

### Etoposide, teniposide

Podophyllotoxin is an extract from the mandrake plant (mayberry or podophyllum). This compound is a well-known spindle poison that binds to microtubule proteins and inhibits assembly of microtubules. The podophyllotoxin derivatives, etoposide and teniposide, while originally developed in an effort to retain the activity of podophyllotoxin, both exert their antitumor activity through a different mechanism.[5,67] Teniposide differs from etoposide by the addition of a sulfur-containing group in place of a methyl group on the sugar ring and is approximately 10-fold more potent than etoposide in vitro.[19] These agents are active against a variety of malignancies, including small cell lung cancer, testicular cancer, leukemia, and lymphoma.

Etoposide and teniposide are thought to exert their activity by binding to topoisomerase II, forming stable ternary complexes with DNA and topoisomerase II. As a result, topoisomerase II remains bound between the free end of the cleaved DNA strand and the drug, unable to reseal the broken DNA. This ultimately results in accumulation of strand breaks and subsequent cell death.[5,68] Because these compounds target the enzyme topoisomerase II, drug administration schedule is important as this enzyme is expressed only in certain phases of mitosis. Thus, continuous administration is advantageous because it maximizes the likelihood of exposing a dividing tumor cell to the drug. Indeed, one study showed this dramatic effect by comparing 1-day administration of etoposide (500 mg/m$^2$) to 5-day administration (100 mg/m$^2$/day) in SCLC patients. Although the same total dose of drug was administered, the response rate of the group receiving single-day infusion was 10%, while the consecutive treatment group had a response rate of 89%.[69] Thus, exposing cells to lower concentrations of drug for prolonged times is thought to maximize the therapeutic effect of the topoisomerase II inhibitors.

*Pharmacokinetics/metabolism:* Both drugs bind significantly to plasma proteins. Etoposide is approximately 50% absorbed from the gastrointestinal tract and is available orally. Considerable pharmacokinetic interpatient variability exists with both intravenous and oral dosing.[70] Etoposide and teniposide undergo extensive metabolism in the liver. It is estimated that 30–70% of etoposide is excreted renally, while this accounts for only 5–20% of teniposide elimination. Dose adjustments are recommended for patients with moderate renal dysfunction (estimated creatinine clearance <50 ml/min) in order to avoid excessive toxicity.[71,72] Various metabolites have been identified for both compounds, but their significance has been disputed.

*Toxicity:* Toxicities of the two agents are similar. The dose-limiting toxicity for both is myelosuppression, which mainly manifests as leukopenia. Thrombocytopenia occurs less often and is usually not as severe.[5] Reversible alopecia, mild nausea and vomiting, and stomatitis are common. Allergic reactions including anaphylaxis have been observed. These are more common with tenioposide, which is less-water soluble than etoposide. Hepatotoxicity has been reported in up to 3% of patients receiving etoposide, consisting of hyperbilirubinemia, ascites, and transaminase elevations. Secondary leukemias, including AML and APL, have been reported. Toxicity in general is enhanced in patients with low serum albumin levels because of the decreased binding of the drug and increased free levels.[19]

## MISCELLANEOUS AGENTS

### L-Asparaginase

***Erwinia asparaginase, pegaspargase,* Escherichia coli L-*asparaginase*** L-Asparaginase is a compound that is actually an enzyme, L-asparagine aminohydrolase. The original, most commonly used agent is derived from *Escherichia coli*. Other available forms include a derivative produced by *Erwinia chrysanthemi* and the longer-acting pegylated asparaginase (pegaspargase). L-asparaginase possesses activity against malignancies of lymphocytic origin and is mainly used in the treatment of ALL. L-Asparaginase acts by breaking down

L-Asparagine, a nonessential amino acid required by cells for protein and nucleic acid synthesis. Most cells are able to synthesize adequate supplies of asparagine on their own; however, certain malignant cells, particularly those of lymphocytic origin, lack the synthetase enzyme required for asparagine formation. These cells are particularly sensitive to the effects of L-asparaginase. By converting existing cellular supplies of asparagine to aspartic acid and ammonia, L-asparaginase quickly depletes cells of this amino acid, thus inhibiting protein synthesis.[73]

*Pharmacokinetics/metabolism:* L-Asparaginase is not absorbed orally and is available only for parenteral administration. Distribution volume approximates plasma volume, and L-asparaginase does not penetrate CNS significantly.[5] Metabolism of L-asparaginase occurs through systemic degradation,[74] and the drug is cleared by the reticuloendothelial system.

*Toxicity:* While toxicity to the bone marrow is minimal, L-asparaginase and related compounds are associated with a variety of adverse effects. Hypersensitivity reactions, including anaphylaxis, can occur immediately and have been reported in up to 43% of patients treated with the *E. coli*-derived compound. Because allergic reactions are more likely to occur with intravenous administration,[75] asparaginase is typically given by intramuscular or subcutaneous injection. Patients who do react to *E. coli*-derived asparaginase may be switched to another source of drug, either pegaspargase or *Erwinia asparaginase*. This is associated with a high success rate and may enable the patient to complete a prescribed course of therapy. L-Asparaginase is also associated with coagulation abnormalities. It is thought that asparaginase depletes plasma proteins involved in both coagulation and fibrinolysis, including fibrinogen, factor IX, factor XI, antithrombin III, protein C, and protein S.[76,77] Both bleeding and thrombosis have been reported.[76–78] Pancreatitis is another complication associated with asparaginase and routine monitoring of amylase or lipase is recommended.[5,79]

### Hydroxyurea

While hydroxyurea is not a nucleoside analog, it is generally considered to be an antimetabolite due to its similar mechanism of action to this class of drugs. Structurally, it is an analog of urea and inhibits the enzyme ribonucleotide reductase. As a result of this inhibition, ribonucleotides are prevented from being converted to the active deoxyribonucleotide forms necessary for DNA synthesis and repair. Subsequently, DNA synthesis cannot occur and cells are stranded in the S phase or the G1–S interface.[19]

*Pharmacokinetics/metabolism:* Hydroxyurea is well absorbed from the gastrointestinal tract and is available for oral administration. Bioavailability is approximately 80–100%. It is widely distributed throughout

| Table 101.4 | Mechanisms of resistance to traditional antineoplastic agents |
|---|---|
| **Chemotherapeutic class** | **Mechanisms of resistance** |
| Alkylating agents | ■ Mutations of p53 tumor suppressor gene<br>■ Decreased transport of drug by active transport mechanisms<br>■ Increased production of nucleophilic substances (electron donors) that bind and detoxify reactive alkyl groups<br>■ Increased activity of DNA repair enzymes<br>■ Increased metabolism of drug to inactive form[81] |
| Antimetabolites: nucleoside analogs | ■ Inefficient cellular uptake and insufficient intracellular concentration of drug due to deficient transport mechanisms<br>■ Increased degradation of active compound by enzymes (cytidine deaminase or 5′-nucleotidase)<br>■ Loss of deoxycytidine kinase (dCK) gene, which converts drug to active form[35,82] |
| Antimetabolites: folic acid analog (Methotrexate) | ■ Saturated active transport mechanisms<br>■ Increased production of DHFR (dihydrofolate reductase)<br>■ Slower rates of thymidylate synthesis<br>■ Alterations in binding affinity of DHFR and methotrexate[5] |
| L-Asparaginase | ■ Increased levels of enzyme asparagine synthetase within tumor cells[5,19] |
| Anthracene derivatives | ■ Increased drug efflux mechanisms, such as P-glycoprotein or MDR-1<br>■ Decreased expression of topoisomerase II enzyme<br>■ Mutation of topoisomerase II enzyme[81,83] |
| Vinca alkaloids | ■ Increased levels of P-glycoprotein membrane efflux pump<br>■ Altered expression of tubulin isotypes<br>■ Tubulin mutations<br>■ Altered expression of microtubule-regulatory proteins[64,84] |
| Podophyllotoxin derivatives | ■ Amplification of MDR-1 gene mutation<br>■ Decreased expression of topoisomerase II enzyme<br>■ Mutation of topoisomerase II enzyme<br>■ Mutation of p53 tumor suppressor gene[5,81] |
| Hydroxyurea | ■ Increased expression of ribonucleotide reductase5,19 |

the body, with levels detected in the CNS, fluid accumulations, and breast milk. While significant interpatient variability exists, approximately 50% of hydroxyurea is hepatically metabolized, with 50% of drug eliminated as urea and unchanged drug in urine.[5,19]

*Toxicity:* The dose-limiting toxicity of hydroxyurea is myelosuppression. This is often the desired therapeutic effect as well. Mild nausea and vomiting is common, which is more severe with higher doses. Finally, skin pigmentation and macropapular rash may occur[80] (Table 101.4).

## TREATMENT OF HEMATOLOGIC MALIGNANCIES: SUMMARY

Many valuable agents have been developed for the treatment of hematologic malignancies since the first patient with lymphoma was treated with nitrogen mustard in 1942. While these traditional agents have broad therapeutic potential and are currently considered integral components of treatment regimens for leukemias and lymphomas, they are associated with a variety of toxicities as well. Nausea and vomiting, myelosuppression, alopecia, mucositis, infertility, and carcinogenesis are just some of the adverse effects commonly associated with these compounds. This has a dramatic impact on patients' quality of life. More recently, great advances have been made in understanding the molecular biology of cancer. New therapies are being developed to specifically target only those cells exhibiting genetic mutations, thus protecting healthy cells from unnecessary toxicity. In addition, research has been done evaluating mechanisms of resistance of tumor cells to chemotherapeutic agents and compounds are being engineered to specifically block these pathways. The ultimate goal is the development of a compound that specifically targets a chromosomal abnormality, leaving healthy cells free of toxic effects and dramatically improving the quality of life of cancer patients.

## REFERENCES

1. Papac RJ: Origins of cancer therapy. *Yale J Biol Med* 74:391–398, 2001.

2. Gilman A, Philips FS: The biological actions and therapeutic applications of the B-chloroethyl amines and sulfides. *Science* 103:409–415, 1946.

3. Gilman A: The initial clinical trial of nitrogen mustard. *Am J Surg* 105:574–578, 1961.

4. Hall AG, Tilby MJ: Mechanisms of action of, and modes of resistance to, alkylating agents used in the treatment of hematological malignancies. *Blood Rev* 6(3):163–173, 1992.

5. Chabner BA, Ryan DP, Paz-Ares L, Garcia-Carbonero R, Calabresi P: Chemotherapy of neoplastic diseases. In: Hardman JG, Limbird LE, Gilman AG (eds.) *Goodman & Gillman's The Pharmacologic Basis of Therapeutics*, 10th edn. New York: McGraw-Hill; 2001:1381–1460.

6. Levine EG, Bloomfield CD: Leukemias and myelodysplastic syndromes secondary to, drug, radiation, and environmental exposure. *Semin Oncol* 19:47–84, 1992.

7. Lacy CF, Armstrong LL, Goldman MP, Lance LL (eds.): Mechlorethamine. In: *Drug Information Handbook*. Hudson: Lexi-comp, Inc.; 1999:627–629.

8. Lacy CF, Armstrong LL, Goldman MP, Lance LL (eds.): Cyclophosphamide. In: *Drug Information Handbook*. Hudson: Lexi-comp, Inc.; 1999:266–268.

9. Stillwell TJ, Benson RC Jr: Cyclophosphamide-induced hemorrhagic cystitis: a review of 100 patients. *Cancer* 61(3):451–457, 1988.

10. Lacy CF, Armstrong LL, Goldman MP, Lance LL (eds.): Melphalan. In: *Drug Information Handbook*. Hudson: Lexi-comp, Inc.; 1999:634–636.

11. Lacy CF, Armstrong LL, Goldman MP, Lance LL, (eds.): Chlorambucil. In: *Drug Information Handbook*. Hudson: Lexi-comp, Inc.; 1999:206–207.

12. Buggia I, Locatelli F, Regazzi MB, Zecca M: Busulfan. *Ann Pharmacother* 28:1055–1062, 1994.

13. Kreisman H, Wolkove N: Pulmonary toxicity of antineoplastic therapy. *Semin Oncol* 19:508–520, 1992.

14. Lacy CF, Armstrong LL, Goldman MP, Lance LL (eds.): Carmustine. In: *Drug Information Handbook*. Hudson: Lexi-comp, Inc.; 1999:172–173.

15. Lacy CF, Armstrong LL, Goldman MP, Lance LL (eds.): Procarbazine. In: *Drug Information Handbook*. Hudson: Lexi-comp, Inc.; 1999:847–848.

16. Lacy CF, Armstrong LL, Goldman MP, Lance LL (eds.): Dacarbazine. In: *Drug Information Handbook*. Hudson: Lexi-comp, Inc.; 1999:276–277.

17. Fleming RA: An overview of cyclophosphamide and ifosfamide pharmacology. *Pharmacotherapy* 17(5, pt 2):146S–154S, 1997.

18. Al-Rawithi S, El-Yazigi A, Ernst P, Al-Fiar F, Nicholls PJ: Urinary excretion and pharmacokinetics of acrolein and its parent drug cyclophosphamide in bone marrow transplant patients. *Bone Marrow Transplant* 22:485–490, 1998.

19. Valley AW, Balmer CM: Oncologic disorders. In: DiPiro JT, Talbert RL, Yee GC, Matzke GR, Wells BG, Posey LM (eds.) *Pharmacotherapy: A Pathophysiologic Approach*, 4th ed. Stamford: Appleton & Lange; 1999:1957–2220.

20. Gandhi V, Plunkett W: Modulatory activity of 2′,2′-difluorodeoxycytidine on the phosphorylation and cytotoxicity of arabinosyl nucleosides. *Cancer Res* 50:3675–3680, 1990.

21. Chu E, DeVita VT: Fludarabine In: *Physicians' Cancer Chemotherapy Drug Manual* 2003. Sudbury: Jones and Bartlett; 2003:171–174.

22. Johnson SA: Clinical pharmacokinetics of nucleoside analogues: focus on haematological malignancies *Clin Pharmacokinet* 39(1):5–26, 2000.

23. Helman DL, Jr, Byrd JC, Ales NC, Shorr AF: Fludarabine-related pulmonary toxicity: a distinct clinical entity in chronic lymphoproliferative syndromes. *Chest* 122(3):785–790, 2002.

24. Chu E, DeVita VT: Mercaptopurine. In: *Physicians' Cancer Chemotherapy Drug Manual* 2003. Sudbury: Jones and Bartlett; 2003:251–254.

25. Sandler A, Ettinger DS: Gemcitabine: single-agent and combination therapy in non-small cell lung cancer. *Oncologist* 4(3):241–251, 1999.

26. Elgemeie GH: Thioguanine, mercaptopurine: their analogues and nucleosides as antimetabolites. *Curr Pharmaceut Design* 9(31):2627–2642, 2003.

27. Lacy CF, Armstrong LL, Goldman MP, Lance LL (eds.): Cytarabine. In: *Drug Information Handbook*. Hudson: Lexi-comp, Inc.; 1999:273–275.

28. Chu E, DeVita VT: Cytarabine: In: *Physicians' Cancer Chemotherapy Drug Manual* 2003. Sudbury: Jones and Bartlett; 100–105, 2003.

29. Touroutoglu N, Gravel D, Raber MN, et al.: Clinical results of a pharmacodynamically based strategy for higher dosing for gemcitabine in patients with solid tumors. *Ann Oncol* 9:1003–1008, 1999.

30. Tempero M, Plunkett W, Ruiz van Haperen V, et al.: Randomized phase II trial of dose intense gemcitabine by standard infusion vs. fixed dose rate in metastatic pancreatic adenocarcinoma. *Proc Am Assoc Clin Oncol* 18:273a, 1999. [Abstract 1048]

31. Chu E, DeVita VT: Gemcitabine: In: *Physicians' Cancer Chemotherapy Drug Manual* 2003. Sudbury: Jones and Bartlett; 189–192, 2003.

32. Christman JK: 5-Azacytidine and 5-aza-2′-deoxycytidine as inhibitors of DNA methylation: mechanistic studies and their implications for cancer therapy. *Oncogene* 21:5483–5495, 2002.

33. Wijermans P, Lubbert M, Verhoef G, et al.: Low-dose 5-aza-2-deoxycytidine, a DNA hypomethylating agent, for the treatment of high-risk myelodysplastic syndrome: a multicenter phase II study in elderly patients. *J Clin Oncol* 18:956–962, 2000.

34. Byrd JC, Ruppert AS, Mrozek K, et al.: Repetitive cycles of high-dose cytarabine benefit patients with acute myeloid leukemia and inv(16)(p13q22) or t(16;16)(p13;q22): results from CALGB 8461. *J Clin Oncol* 22(6):1087–1094, 2004.

35. Galmarini CM, Mackey JR, Dumontet C: Nucleoside analogues: mechanisms of drug resistance and reversal strategies. *Leukemia* 15(6):875–890, 2001.

36. Smith GA, Damon LE, Rugo HS, et al.: High-dose cytarabine dose modification reduces the incidence of neurotoxicity in patients with renal insufficiency. *J Clin Oncol* 15(2):833–839, 1997.

37. Mayer RJ, Davis RB, Schiffer CA, et al.: Intensive post-remission chemotherapy in adults with acute myeloid leukemia. *NEJM* 331(14):896–903, 1994.

38. Thomas A, Steward WP: Gemcitabine–a major advance? *Ann Oncol* 9(12):1265–1267, 1998.

39. Cortes-Funes H, Martin C, Abratt R, et al.: Safety profile of gemcitabine, a novel anticancer agent, in non-small cell lung cancer. *Anti-Cancer Drugs* 8:582–587, 1997.

40. Nabhan C, Gartenhaus RB, Tallman MS: Purine nucleoside analogues and combination therapies in B-cell chronic lymphocytic leukemia: dawn of a new era. *Leuk Res* 28(5):429–442, 2004.

41. Robak T, Kasznicki M: Alkylating agents and nucleoside analogues in the treatment of B-cell chronic lymphocytic leukemia. *Leukemia* 16(6):1015–1027, 2002.

42. Johnson SA: Clinical pharmacokinetics of nucleoside analogues: focus on haematological malignances. *Clin Pharmacokinet* 39(1):5–26, 2000.

43. Product Information: Fludara(R), fludarabine phosphate. Berlex Laboratories, Richmond, CA, USA, (revised 12/2001) reviewed 5/2002.

44. Skeel RT: *Handbook of Cancer Chemotherapy*, 3rd ed. Boston, MA: Little, Brown and Company; 1991.

45. Lacy CF, Armstrong LL, Goldman MP, Lance LL (eds.): Doxorubicin. In: *Drug Information Handbook*. Hudson: Lexi-comp, Inc.; 1999:343–345.

46. Product Information: Adriamycin RDF(R), Adriamycin PFS(R), doxorubicin. Pharmacia & Upjohn, Kalamazoo, MI, (PI revised 5/99) reviewed 3/2000.

47. Product Information: Cerubidine(R), daunorubicin. Ben Venue Laboratories, Bedford, OH, USA, 1999.

48. Lacy CF, Armstrong LL, Goldman MP, Lance LL (eds.): Daunorubicin. In: *Drug Information Handbook*. Hudson: Lexi-comp, Inc.; 1999: 285–287.

49. Anderlini P, Benjamin RS, Wong FC, et al.: Idarubicin cardiotoxicity: a retrospective study in acute myeloid leukemia and myelodysplasia. *J Clin Oncol* 13:2827–2834, 1995.

50. Lacy CF, Armstrong LL, Goldman MP, Lance LL (eds.): Idarubicin. In: *Drug Information Handbook*. Hudson: Lexi-comp, Inc.; 1999:522–523.

51. Product information: Idamycin (R), idarubicin hydrochloride for injection, USP. Pharmacia & Upjohn Company, Kalamazoo, MI, (PI revised 8/2000) reviewed 3/2003.

52. Unverferth DV, Bashore TM, Magorien RD, et al.: Histologic and functional characteristics of human heart after mitoxantrone therapy. *Cancer Treat Symp* 3:47–53, 1984.

53. Coleman RE, Maisey MN, Knight RK, et al.: Mitoxantrone in advanced breast cancer—a phase II study with special attention to cardiotoxicity. *Eur J Cancer Clin Oncol* 20:771–776, 1984.

54. Stuart-Harris R, Pearson M, Smith IE. Cardiotoxicity associated with mitoxantrone. *Lancet* 2:219–220, 1984.

55. Clark GM, Tokaz LK, Von Hoff DD, et al.: Cardiotoxicity in patients treated with mitoxantrone on Southwest Oncology Group Phase II Protocols. *Cancer Treat Symp* 3:25–30, 1984.

56. Unverferth DV, Unverferth BJ, Balcerzak, et al.: Cardiac evaluation of mitoxantrone. *Cancer Treat Rep* 67:343–50, 1983.

57. Neidhart J, Stanbus A, Young D, et al.: Pharmacokinetic studies of dihydroxyanthracenedione with clinical correlations. *Proc Am Assoc Cancer Res* 22:363, 1981.

58. Minotti G, Menna P, Salvatorelli E, Cairo G, Gianni L: Anthracyclines: molecular advances and pharmacologic developments in antitumor activity and cardiotoxicity. *Pharmacol Rev* 56:185–229, 2004.

59. Danesi R, Fogli S, Gennari A, Conte P, Del Tacca M: Pharmacokinetic-pharmacodynamic relationships of the anthracycline anticancer drugs. *Clin Pharmacokinet* 41(6):431–444, 2002.

60. Thomas X, Le QH, Fiere D: Anthracycline-related toxicity requiring cardiac transplantation in long-term disease-free survivors with acute promyelocytic leukemia. *Ann Hematol* 81(9):504–507, 2002.

61. Hecht SM: Bleomycin: new perspectives on mechanism of action. *J Nat Prod* 63(1):158–168, 2000.

62. Aouida M, Page N, Ledue A, Peter M, Ramotar D: A genome-wide screen in *Saccharomyces cerevisiae* reveals altered transport as a mechanism of resistance to the anticancer drug bleomycin. *Cancer Res* 64(3):1102–1109, 2004.

63. Jordan MA: Mechanism of action of antitumor drugs that interact with microtubules and tubulin. *Curr Med Chem Anti-Cancer Agents* 2(1):1–17, 2002.

64. Jordan MA, Wilson L: Microtubules as a target for anticancer drugs. *Nat Rev Cancer* 4(4):253–265, 2004.

65. Hadfield JA, Ducki S, Hirst N, McGown AT: Tubulin and microtubules as targets for anticancer drugs. *Prog Cell Cycle Res* 5:309–325, 2003.

66. Alcaraz A, Rey C, Concha A, Medina A: Intrathecal vincristine: fatal myeloencephalopathy despite cerebrospinal fluid perfusion. *J Toxicol Clin Toxicol* 40(5):557–561, 2002.

67. Handke KR: Etoposide pharmacology. *Semin Oncol* 19(6, suppl 13):3–9, 1992.

68. Clark PI, Slevin ML: The clinical pharmacology of etoposide and teniposide. *Clin Pharmacokinet* 12(4):223–252, 1987.

69. Slevin ML, Clark PI, Joel SP, et al.: A randomized trial to evaluate the effect of schedule on the activity of etoposide in small cell lung cancer. *J Clin Oncol* 7:1333–1340, 1989.

70. Toffoli G, Corona G, Basso B, Boiocchi M: Pharmacokinetic optimization of treatment with oral etoposide. *Clin Pharmacokinet* 43(7):441–466, 2004.

71. Bennett WM, Aronoff GR, Golper TA, et al.: *Drug Prescribing in Renal Failure*. Philadelphia, PA: American College of Physicians; 1987.

72. Product Information: Vepesid(R), etoposide. Bristol Laboratories, Princeton, NJ, (PI revised 9/1998) reviewed 6/2000.

73. Ettinger LJ, Ettinger AG, Avramis VI, et al.: Acute lymphoblastic leukemia: a guide to asparaginase and pegaspargase therapy. *BioDrugs* 7:30–39, 1997.

74. Lacy CF, Armstrong LL, Goldman MP, Lance LL (eds.): Asparaginase. In: *Drug Information Handbook*. Hudson: Lexi-comp, Inc.; 1999:88–90.

75. Shepherd GM: Hypersensitivity reactions to chemotherapeutic drugs. *Clin Rev Allergy Immunol* 24(3):253–262, 2003.

76. Feinberg WM, Swenson MR: Cerebrovascular complications of L-asparaginase therapy. *Neurology* 38:127–133, 1988.

77. Gugliotta L, Mazzucconi M, Leone G, et al.: Incidence of thrombotic complications in adult patients with acute lymphoblastic leukaemia receiving L-asparaginase during induction therapy: a retrospective study. *Eur J Haematol* 49:63–66, 1992.

78. Sutor AH, Mall V, Thomas KB: Bleeding and thrombosis in children with acute lymphoblastic leukaemia, treated

according to the ALL-BFM-90 protocol. *Klin Padiatr* 211(4):201–204, 1999.

79. Wilmink T, Frick TW: Drug-induced pancreatitis. *Drug Saf* 14(6):406–423, 1996.

80. Lacy CF, Armstrong LL, Goldman MP, Lance LL (eds.): Hydroxyurea. In: *Drug Information Handbook*. Hudson: Lexi-comp, Inc.; 1999:515–516.

81. Gottesman MM: Mechanisms of cancer drug resistance. *Annu Rev Med* 53:615–627, 2002.

82. Funato T, Satou J, Nishiyama Y, et al.: In vitro leukemia cell models of Ara-C resistance. *Leuk Res* 24(6):535–541, 2000.

83. Arcamone F, Animati F, Berettoni M, et al.: Doxorubicin disaccharide analogue: apoptosis-related improvement of efficacy *in vivo. J Natl Cancer Inst* 89(16):1217–1223, 1997.

84. Dumontet C, Sikic BL: Mechanisms of action of and resistance to antitubulin agents: microtubule dynamics, drug transport, and cell death. *J Clin Oncol* 17(3):1061–1070, 1999.

# Chapter 102

# BIOLOGICAL RESPONSE MODIFYING AGENTS IN THE TREATMENT OF HEMATOLOGIC MALIGNANCIES

*Christopher J. Lowe and Jennifer Fisher Lowe*

*Drugs can only repress symptoms: they cannot eradicate disease. The true remedy for all disease is nature's remedy . . . There is at bottom only one genuine scientific treatment for all diseases, and that is to stimulate the phagocytes. Stimulate the phagocytes. Drugs are a delusion*

*Sir Bloomfield Bonington (George Bernard Shaw—The Doctor's Dilemma, 1906)*

Sir Bloomfield Bonington's views on medicine are not completely fictitious, as numerous investigators have attempted to harness and employ nature's remedy in the treatment of various diseases. In the early 1900s, an orthopedic surgeon by the name of William Coley investigated the association of febrile illnesses with spontaneous tumor regression.[1] This unusual therapeutic relationship prompted him to attempt treating sarcomas by infecting patients with bacterial infections with the hope of inducing high fevers. Obvious problems ensued with this approach and so he modified the therapy to be less pathologic. In place of inducing a true infection, he attempted to elicit the febrile state with a vaccine containing two killed bacteria: *Streptococcus pyogenes* and *Serraria marcescens*. Coley's vaccine became widely used and was eventually endorsed by the American Medical Association in 1936.[1]

This is an early example of modifying the human body's defenses to serve as a therapeutic intervention. This chapter describes current therapeutic modalities, which like Dr. Coley's vaccine manipulate the function of the human body with the intent of curing disease.

## TYROSINE KINASE INHIBITORS

The analysis of the human genome has revealed 518 putative protein kinase genes.[2,3] Of these genes, a subset of approximately 90 are responsible for protein tyrosine kinases.[2,3] Various protein tyrosine kinases have been implicated in the pathophysiology of malignant conditions. Increased activity or deregulation of these kinases results in alterations in normal downstream cellular signaling. Examples of such processes include the bcr-abl fusion protein in chronic myeloid leukemia and HER-2 overexpression in breast cancer.

Recently, numerous targeting methodologies have been employed to inhibit specific tyrosine kinases in various malignancies. The most promising binding site for such inhibitors has been the adenosine triphosphate (ATP) complex binding site. Although a consistent structure within various tyrosine kinases, minor nuances in this catalytic domain configuration has allowed the development of highly selective inhibitors.[4]

### IMATINIB (STI-571, GLEEVEC)

Historically, chronic myelogenous leukemia (CML) was treated with agents that had little effect on overall survival (hydroxyurea and busulfan) or induced such toxicity that effective doses were rarely maintained (interferon). Imatinib, a phenylaminopyrimidine derivative, is a selective tyrosine kinase inhibitor used in the treatment of Philadelphia chromosome positive leukemia. This orally administered agent represented a breakthrough in the therapy of CML, and more recently has been integrated into Philadelphia chromosome positive acute lymphoblastic leukemia (ALL) treatment regimens.

Imatinib's ability to competitively inhibit the ATP binding site of the bcr-abl tyrosine kinase prevents phosphorylation of proteins involved in signal transduction.[5] By inhibiting the aberrant tyrosine kinase, imatinib halts cellular proliferation and tumor formation by bcr-abl expressing cells and decreases CML colony growth without inhibiting normal colony growth.[6,7] This inhibition is accomplished not only by the parent compound, but also by the active *N*-demethylated piperazine metabolite.

In addition to the pharmacological activity described above, the drug has exhibited the ability to inhibit the tyrosine kinase activity of c-kit, platelet-derived growth factor (PDGF), and stem cell factor (SCF). The former has led to its utility in gastrointestinal stromal tumor therapy.[8] Imatinib also inhibits tyrosine kinase activity of abl in normal cells, although this is not considered clinically relevant.[5]

While a large number of patients have experienced clinical benefit from receiving imatinib, success has not been uniform. Some patients have exhibited de novo resistance, while others have developed resistant disease after an initial favorable response. This resistance may be multifactorial, with possible variables including gene and protein amplification, mutations in the protein kinase, binding of imatinib to proteins in the plasma, and additional oncogenic mutations that may bestow an additional growth advantage on the cells.[9–11]

## Pharmacokinetics/metabolism

Oral imatinib is well absorbed, with a bioavailability of nearly 100%.[12] Peak plasma concentration occurs within 4 h of administration, regardless of whether or not the dose is taken with food.[13] Following oral administration, the elimination half-lives of imatinib and its major active metabolite are approximately 18 and 40 h, respectively.[13] Repeat dosing does not have a significant impact on the drug's pharmacokinetics and accumulation is 1.5 to 2.5-fold with daily administration.[12,13] In-vitro models have established that at clinically relevant concentrations, imatinib is approximately 95% protein bound, primarily to albumin and $\alpha_1$-acid glycoprotein.[12] Hepatic enzymes, predominantly the cytochrome P450-3A4 isoenzyme, are responsible for the drug's metabolism.[13] Other cytochrome enzymes, such as CYP1A2, CYP2D6, CYP 2C9, and CYP 2C19, also contribute to imatinib's degradation.[13] Because many other medications can affect this metabolic system, imatinib is susceptible to alterations in kinetics/dynamics via cytochrome-based drug–drug interactions (Table 102.1) Most of the oral dose is eliminated via the feces and only 5% is excreted unchanged through the urine.[13]

| Table 102.1 Imatinib CYP450 mediated drug–drug interactions[13] | |
| --- | --- |
| Interacting medication | Result |
| Alfuzosin | Imatinib's enzyme inhibition results in increased alfuzosin exposure |
| Aprepitant | Enzyme inhibition by aprepitant may result in elevated plasma concentrations of imatinib |
| Carbamazepine | Significant decrease in exposure to imatinib may occur when coadministered with the enzyme inducer carbamazepine |
| Clarithromycin | Clarithromycin may decrease the metabolism and increase concentrations of imatinib |
| Cyclosporine | Plasma concentrations of cyclosporine may be altered when coadministered with imatinib |
| Dexamethasone | Significant decrease in exposure to imatinib may occur when coadministered with dexamethasone |
| Eletriptan | Increased exposure to eletriptan may be expected when eletriptan is used concomitantly with imatinib |
| Erythromycin | Erythromycin may decrease the metabolism and increase concentrations of imatinib |
| Itraconazole, ketoconazole, voriconazole | Azole antifungals may decrease the metabolism and increase concentrations of imatinib |
| Phenobarbital | Significant decrease in exposure to imatinib may occur when coadministered with the enzyme inducer phenobarbital |
| Phenytoin | Significant decrease in exposure to imatinib may occur when coadministered with the enzyme inducer phenytoin |
| Rifabutin, rifampin | Imatinib is susceptible to significantly increased clearance when coadministered with enzyme inducers such as rifampin and rifabutin |
| Simvastatin | Plasma concentrations of simvastatin may be increased when coadministered with imatinib |
| St. John's Wort | Concomitant use of imatinib and St. John's Wort resulted in significantly increased clearance of imatinib |
| Warfarin | Concurrent treatment with imatinib and warfarin may increase the bioavailability of warfarin, sthereby increasing the risk of bleeding |

## Toxicity

The majority of patients who received imatinib in clinical studies did experience side effects, but most of these effects were mild or moderate in severity.[12] Approximately 4% of patients discontinue therapy due to toxicity.[13] The most common side effects are nausea, vomiting, edema, muscle cramps/pain, diarrhea, and rash. Nausea can be minimized if the dose is taken with food and/or a large glass of water.[13] Edema most commonly manifests in the periorbital area or in the lower extremities and is usually ameliorated with diuretics or other supportive care measures.[13,14] A small percent of patients experience more severe forms of fluid retention (pleural/pericardial effusions, pulmonary edema, ascites, and cerebral edema) and may require interruptions in therapy.[14] This is usually dose-related and more common in the elderly and those in blast crisis and accelerated phase CML.[13] Skin rashes, which vary greatly in appearance and severity, are commonly controlled with antihistamines or steroids. These topical reactions can be quite severe and are actually the most common reason for termination of imatinib therapy.[14]

Two additional adverse effects, which occur with lower frequencies but have noteworthy clinical significance, are hepatic and hematological toxicity. Significant liver dysfunction occurs in fewer than 5% of patients and is managed with dose reductions or temporary interruptions in therapy.[13] Therefore, liver function tests should be monitored routinely throughout the duration of imatinib therapy.[14] Myelosuppression is the most common Grade 3 or 4 adverse event observed in patients being treated with imatinib.[15] Marrow suppression may represent a beneficial therapeutic effect, but may also be due to toxicity to normal progenitor cells.[14] Neutropenia and thrombocytopenia, the most common manifestations of the marrow suppression, are more common in patients with advanced disease. Colony stimulating factors (filgrastim) have been successfully employed to assist neutrophil recovery and facilitate more sustained administration of imatinib.[15]

## INTERFERONS

Discovered in 1957 and named after their ability to *interfere* with viral replication, interferons are cellular glycoproteins with numerous biologic activities.[16] In 1981, the first recombinant DNA-derived interferon was successfully expressed in bacteria and purified in large quantities for clinical study.[16,17] The naturally occurring proteins have since been found to possess antiviral, antiproliferative, and immunomodulating properties.[18]

There are five major species of interferon: alpha, beta, gamma, omega, and tau.[19] Three of these (alpha, beta, and gamma) have been approved by the U.S. Food and Drug Administration (FDA) for a total of 11 disease states (Table 102.2).

### INTERFERON ALPHA

Interferon-α-2a is produced by recombinant DNA technology–combining an *Escherichia coli* start codon with the DNA sequence for human interferon-α-2a. The resulting molecule is nearly identical to naturally occurring interferon-α, with the exceptions being the addition of an N-terminal methionine residue and the lack of carbohydrate side chains.[18]

This class of drugs, because of its antiproliferative and immunomodulatory capabilities, has found its place in the treatment of various malignancies. Specifically, interferon-α has exhibited clinical activity in multiple tumor types. Drug effect has been observed in acute and chronic leukemia, lymphomas, and multiple myeloma.[20–23]

The precise mechanism of action of interferons is not fully understood. Unlike traditional antineoplastic agents that exert their activity directly from their cytotoxic interactions on cancer cells, interferon's benefits result from a complex cascade of biologic modulation and drug-induced antiproliferation. The binding of interferon to the cell surface elicits alterations in gene transcription and translation.[24] Influences such as these on the activities of natural killer cells and macrophages appear to be the most noteworthy.[25]

Interferon's ability to inhibit cellular proliferation affects both normal and malignant cells. Although the mechanism is not completely understood, interferon-induced prolongation of the cell cycle is principally responsible for the antiproliferative effects.[24] This activity appears to be concentration-dependent and occur primarily while the tumor cells are in phases $G_0$ and $G_1$.[26,27] Additionally, these effects appear to be reversible since normal cellular growth resumes upon cessation of interferon exposure.[24]

| Table 102.2 | Therapeutic indications[25] |
| --- | --- |
| Drug | FDA approved indication |
| Interferon-α | Chronic myelogenous leukemia, condyloma acuminata, follicular lymphoma, hairy cell leukemia, chronic hepatitis B (adult and pediatric), chronic hepatitis C, Kaposi's sarcoma, malignant melanoma |
| Interferon-β | Multiple sclerosis |
| Interferon-γ | Chronic granulomatous disease |

## Pharmacokinetics/metabolism

Interferonα is supplied as a clear liquid for injection. Bioavailability is greater than 80% upon subcutaneous or intramuscular injection.[28] Interferonα, both recombinant and naturally occurring, is widely distributed in the body (excluding the central nervous system), with highest concentrations occurring in the spleen, kidney, liver, and lung.[24,28] The metabolism of recombinant interferon-α-2a is consistent with that of alpha interferons in general.[24] Alpha-interferons undergo renal filtration and extensive proteolytic degradation at the brush border or in the lysosomes of the tubular epithelium during reabsorption, resulting in a half life of approximately 5 h.[28] Because of the unique mechanism of metabolism, it has been suggested that interferon-α may accumulate in patients with impaired renal function, but this is controversial.[24] Interferon-α may not be removed by hemodialysis.[29]

## Toxicity

The side effect profile of interferon-α is well documented in the literature. Uniformly, with the first dose of interferon, patients experience a flu-like syndrome consisting of fever, chills/rigors, tachycardia, nausea, vomiting, malaise, and headaches.[17,24,25,28] Although the presence of these side effects is relatively consistent, the severity can be affected by variables such as dose, route of administration, and treatment schedule.[17] As a result of the cytokines released (IL-2, IL-6, TNF-α) in response to interferon administration, the patient's body attempts to generate heat via shivering and vasoconstriction. The onset of this fever, which often reaches 38–40°C, usually occurs within 4 h of drug administration and may persist for up to 8 h.[17,24] This reaction is frequently followed by a period of diaphoresis.[25] As a preventative measure to attenuate this constellation of symptoms, patients may be premedicated with acetaminophen or nonsteroidal anti-inflammatory drugs. These symptoms will likely diminish over time and may resolve with continued therapy; however, tolerance may be lost if therapy is delayed for more than one day. [17,24]

On the other hand, fatigue continues and often worsens throughout therapy. Considered the most common dose-limiting toxicity, fatigue is often described as a feeling of lassitude, weakness, tiredness, or lack of motivation. This may manifest itself as job absenteeism, social withdrawal, increased sleeping, and potentially a decrease in performance status.[17,24,25] Intermittent and/or evening dosing schedules may diminish the impact of this significant side effect.[24,25]

Laboratory abnormalities described with the use of interferon-α include neutropenia and elevated liver enzymes that require dose modifications to maintain safety. Other side effects include depression, myalgias/arthralgias, gastrointestinal toxicity, and CNS depression.[28]

# RETINOIDS

The therapeutic potential of vitamins has been evaluated in cancer trials for many years. A correlation between retinol (vitamin A) and cancer was first noted in the 1920s, when experimentally induced vitamin-A deficiency led to preneoplastic lesions and ultimately neoplasms.[30] Retinoids, naturally occurring and synthetic analogues of retinol, modulate differentiation, inhibit growth, and induce apoptosis in a wide variety of cancer cell lines. This is accomplished through interaction with two types of nuclear receptors, retinoic acid receptors (RARs) and retinoic X receptors (RXRs).[31,32] Dysregulation of retinoid metabolism has been implicated in carcinogenesis, and the therapeutic administration of retinoids is beneficial in certain cases.[33] The ability of retinoids to function as differentiating agents has lead to unique opportunities in the treatment of acute promyelocytic leukemia (APL).

## TRETINOIN (VESANOID, ALL-TRANS-RETINOIC ACID, ATRA)

APL is characterized by the specific chromosomal translocation t(15;17). This translocation fuses the promyelocytic leukemia (PML) gene located on chromosome 15 to the retinoic acid receptor α (RAR-α) gene positioned on chromosome 17, resulting in the formation of a chimeric protein, PML/RAR-α.[34] The PML/RAR-α fusion protein, which is leukemogenic, occurs in more than 99.9% of cases of APL. This protein causes an arrest of maturation at the promyelocyte stage of myeloid-cell development and accumulation of abnormal promyelocytes in the bone marrow.[35] Tretinoin binds to RAR-α on the surface of malignant promyelocytes. This leads to degradation of the PML/RAR-α fusion protein, resulting in the differentiation of malignant cells into mature myeloid cells that are then incapable of further proliferation.[36] The use of tretinoin has significantly improved the outcome of APL patients.[37–41]

## Pharmacokinetics/metabolism

Tretinoin, as an oral preparation, is well absorbed into systemic circulation, with a peak plasma concentration between 1 and 2 hours after oral administration.[42] Food increases the bioavailability of tretinoin; however, the clinical significance of this is unknown. The activity of intravenous liposomal tretinoin has been evaluated, but demonstrated no clear advantage when compared with standard oral tretinoin.[43] The drug undergoes hepatic metabolism via the cytochrome P450 system. The degradation of the parent compound results in the formation of four identified metabolites: 13-cis retinoic acid, 4-oxo trans retinoic acid, 4-oxo cis retinoic acid, and 4-oxo trans retinoic acid glucuronide.[42] Tretinoin acts as both an inhibitor and a substrate of the cytochrome P450 enzyme and therefore the product is susceptible to potential drug interactions. Tretinoin is greater than 95% protein-bound, predominantly to albumin. The drug is eliminated via both the urine and the feces, although no dosage adjustments are required for any organ dysfunction. The terminal half-life is approximately 0.5–2 h following initial dosing in patients with APL.[42]

## Toxicity

Tretinoin does not elicit the usual toxicities associated with cytotoxic chemotherapy administration. It is neither immunosuppressive nor myelosuppressive. There are, however, two serious and specific complications that can result from tretinoin treatment of APL: hyperleukocytosis (40%) and retinoic acid syndrome (25%).[42] Hyperleukocytosis is thought to be due to the increased amount of circulating mature cells that have undergone differentiation, and more commonly occurs in patients who present with an initial high white blood cell count ($>5 \times 10^9$/L) at diagnosis. Hyperleukocytosis may precede the development of the second complication, retinoic acid syndrome. This syndrome is characterized by fever, dyspnea, weight gain, diffuse pulmonary infiltrates on chest X-ray, and pleural or pericardial effusions.[44] The syndrome generally occurs during the first month of treatment and may commence following the initial dose of tretinoin. The management of the syndrome includes the administration of high-dose steroids and appropriate supportive care measures. Treatment with dexamethasone (10 mg intravenously administered every 12 h for 3 days or until resolution of symptoms) should be initiated without delay at the first suspicion of symptoms. Tretinoin can be restarted in most cases once the syndrome has resolved.[45]

Virtually all patients experience some degree of vitamin A toxicity, including headache, fever, weakness, and fatigue.[42] These adverse effects are seldom permanent or irreversible, nor do they usually require interruption of therapy. Other common adverse drug reactions include flushing, hypotension, increase in serum cholesterol and triglycerides, and gastrointestinal toxicity such as abdominal pain, constipation, and diarrhea.[42]

**Table 102.3** Biological response modifying agents[13,28,42,48,52,61,64]

| Drug | Dosing | Dosage form | Common side effects |
|---|---|---|---|
| Imatinib (Gleevec®) | CML: 400–600 mg PO QD<br>ALL: 400–800 mg PO QD | 100 and 400 mg capsules | Fluid retention, muscle cramps, nausea/vomiting, myelosuppression |
| Interferon-α 2a (Roferon® A) | CML: 9 million IU SQ/IM QD<br>Hairy cell leukemia:<br>3 million IU SQ/IM QD | Prefilled syringes:<br>3 million IU/0.5 ml,<br>6 million IU/0.5 ml,<br>9 million IU/0.5 ml | Flu-like symptoms, fatigue, injection site reaction, depression, nausea, vomiting |
| Interferon-α-2b (Intron® A) | Hairy cell leukemia:<br>2 million IU/m² SQ/IM,<br>three times/week<br>Follicular lymphoma:<br>5 million IU SQ,<br>three times/week | Multidose prefilled pens:<br>18 million IU pen, six<br>3 million IU doses/pen<br>30 million IU pen, six<br>5 million IU doses/pen<br>60 million IU pen, six<br>10 million IU doses/pen<br>Vials (powder):<br>10 million IU/vial<br>18 million IU/vial<br>50 million IU/vial<br>Vials (solution):<br>10 million IU/vial<br>18 million IU/vial<br>25 million IU/vial | Flu-like symptoms, fatigue, injection site reaction, depression, nausea, vomiting, sarcoidosis |
| Tretinoin (Vesanoid®) | 45 mg/m²/day PO<br>(divided twice daily) | 10 mg capsules | Headache, elevated liver function tests, leukocytosis, APL syndrome |
| Bexarotene (Targretin®) | Oral: 300 mg/m² PO QD<br>Topical: apply 1% gel every other day for 1 week then at weekly intervals increase to once daily, then twice daily, then three times daily, and finally four times daily (as tolerated) | 75 mg capsules<br>1% gel (60g tube) | Oral: rash, hypercholesteremia, hyperlipidemia,<br>Topical: pruritus, rash |
| Arsenic Trioxide (Trisenox™) | 0.15 mg/kg IV QD for a maximum of 60 days (administer over 1 hour) | 1 mg/10 ml ampule | Headache, nausea, fatigue, leukocytosis, APL syndrome, cardiac abnormalities |

### BEXAROTENE (TARGRETIN)

In 1994, a new family of intracellular receptors, the retinoid X receptors (RXRs) was described.[46] RXRs can form heterodimers with various receptor partners, such a retinoic acid receptor, vitamin D receptor, thyroid receptor, and peroxisome proliferator activator receptors. Bexarotene, available for both topical and oral use, is an RXR ligand that selectively binds and activates RXR subtypes (RXRα, RXRβ, RXRγ). Once activated, these receptors function as transcription factors regulating the expression of genes that control apoptosis, cellular differentiation, and proliferation.[47–49] The capsules are indicated for the treatment of topical manifestations of cutaneous T-cell lymphoma in patients who are refractory to at least one prior systemic therapy, while the 1% gel is indicated for the topical treatment of cutaneous lesions (Stage IA and IB) who have refractory or persistent disease after other therapies or who have not tolerated other therapies.[50–54] Oral bexarotene is also under investigation for use in AIDS-related Kaposi's sarcoma, diabetes mellitus, lymphomatoid papulosis, psoriasis, and solid tumors such as breast, non-small cell lung cancer, and renal cell carcinoma.

### Pharmacokinetics/metabolism

Bexarotene is well absorbed by the gastrointestinal tract, with peak plasma levels occurring 2–4 h after oral administration and an initial response expected between 8 and 26 weeks.[48] Absorption is significantly increased after a fat-containing meal. Bexarotene is highly protein bound (>99%). Extensive metabolism occurs hepatically via the CYP3A4 isoenzyme, and the drug is primarily eliminated through the hepatobiliary system and in the feces, with less than 1% of the drug is excreted in urine. The elimination half-life is approximately 7 h.[48]

### Toxicity

Bexarotene's use is commonly associated with reversible hypertriglyceridemia (80%) and hypercholesterolemia (32%).[48] The antihyperlipidemic medications that are most effective for reversing this hypertriglyceridemia are atorvastatin and fenofibrate.[50] The incidence of hypothyroidism is 30% with thyroid function tests returning to baseline as early as eight days after discontinuation.[48,55] Dose-related leukopenia has also been reported. The most common symptomatic side effects reported are fatigue/lethargy, headache, asthenia, rash, nausea, abdominal pain, infection, peripheral edema, dry skin, cataracts, and sensitivity to sunlight. Bexarotene is contraindicated in pregnancy, being classified as category X.[48]

## MISCELLANEOUS

### ARSENIC TRIOXIDE (TRISENOX, ATO)

Although arsenic's accolades primarily revolve around its reputation as an almond-flavored poison, as it was depicted in Frank Capra's 1944 film *Arsenic and Old Lace*, it has an older and more admirable history as a medicinal agent. In the eighteenth century, Thomas Fowler compounded a potassium-bicarbonate-based solution of arsenic trioxide ($As_2O_3$) that was used empirically to treat a variety of diseases.[56] In 1910, Nobel prize winner Paul Ehrlich created the organic arsenical compound salvarsan that was best known as the "magic bullet" for syphilis, but also found use in treating hypertension, ulcers, heartburn, and chronic rheumatism.[57] With evolutions in medicine and the concerns for toxicity, arsenic's use declined over time. In the late 1970s, observational studies preformed in China reported the effectiveness of arsenic trioxide as part of a treatment regimen for APL.[58] These results have since been confirmed in trials in the United States, leading to FDA approval in September 2000.[59–61]

Similar to tretinoin, arsenic has been shown to cause degradation of PML-RAR-α, promoting cellular differentiation.[62] However, arsenic acts primary on the PML gene and restores the cell's apoptotic ability, while tretinoin targets the RAR-α gene and reverses the differentiation arrest. Yet, the degradation of PML-RAR-α may not be the sole mechanism of action.[62] Arsenic is thought to also act through the intracellular environment to influence apoptosis, differentiation, growth arrest, and angiogenesis.

The multiple mechanisms of actions suggest that arsenic may have antitumor activity in other hematological malignancies, such as multiple myeloma, the

| Table 102.4 Dosing adjustments[13, 28, 64] | |
|---|---|
| Drug | Necessary dosing adjustment |
| Imatinib (Gleevec®) | Discontinue if liver transaminases are >5 times upper limit of normal or bilirubin is >3 times upper limit of normal. May resume at a reduced dose once transaminase level is <2.5 times upper limit of normal and/or bilirubin is <1.5 times upper limit of normal. Neutropenia may also necessitate dose reductions. |
| Interferon-α-2a (Roferon®-A) | Dose reductions of 50% or withholding individual doses may be needed when severe adverse events occur. |
| Interferon-α-2b (Intron®-A) | Dose reductions of 50% or withholding individual doses may be needed when severe adverse events occur. Administration should be withheld for a neutrophil count <1000/mm³, or a platelet count <50,000/mm³. |

myelodysplasic syndromes, and a variety of solid tumors.[63] Most of the available data is preliminary and published in abstract form, and therefore must be interpreted with caution. Arsenic's use continues to be explored, and novel combination strategies are being studied to expand its potential use.

## Pharmacokinetics/metabolism

Arsenic is administered solely by the intravenous route. Oral formulations are no longer used due to the high occurrence of severe gastrointestinal toxicity.[58] After intravenous injection, peak levels are achieved 4 h from the end of the infusion. Arsenic is metabolized by methylation in the liver and excreted primarily in the bile. Arsenic is preferentially distributed in tissues containing significant amounts of sulfhydryl group-containing proteins; mainly in the liver, kidneys, heart, lung, hair, and nails.[61] The drug is rapidly eliminated with an half-life of 12 h.[61]

## Toxicity

There are several adverse events associated with arsenic trioxide that warrant careful monitoring and management. The most common non-life-threatening adverse events are nausea, rash, fatigue, neuropathy, fever, headache, vomiting, diarrhea, tachycardia, and hypokalemia. More serious complications include the APL differentiation syndrome, and QT prolongation.[60,61] Most of the toxicities are manageable, reversible, more common during induction therapy and do not require discontinuation.

APL differentiation syndrome, characterized by fever, dyspnea, weight gain, pulmonary infiltrates, and pleural or pericardial effusions, with or without leukocytosis, occurred in 23% of APL patients.[60] This syndrome can be fatal and is treated immediately with intravenous dexamethasone (10 mg twice daily for 3 days or until signs have abated).[61]

Arsenic can cause QT prolongation (potentially leading to a torsade de pointes ventricular arrhythmia) and complete atrioventricular block. Prior to patients receiving arsenic, a 12-lead electrocardiogram should be performed and serum electrolytes (potassium and magnesium) should be assessed and replaced aggressively if indicated. If the absolute QT interval is greater than 500 msec, the drug should be discontinued.[61]

## REFERENCES

1. Hoption Cann SA, Van Netten JP, Van Netten C: Dr. William Coley and tumour regression: a place in history or in the future. *Postgrad Med J* 79:672–679, 2003.
2. Manning G, Whyte DB, Martinez R, Hunter T, Sudarsanam: The protein kinase complement of the human genome. *Science* 298:1912–1934, 2002.
3. Uckun FM, Mao C: Tyrosine kinases as new molecular targets in the treatment of inflammatory disorders and leukemia. *Curr Pharml Des* 10:1083–1091, 2004.
4. Madhusudan S, Ganesan TS: Tyrosine kinase inhibitors in cancer therapy. *Clinl Biochem* 37:618–635, 2004.
5. Goldman JM, Melo JV: Targeting the BCR-ABL tyrosine kinase in chronic myeloid leukemia. *N Engl J Med* 344:1084–1086, 2001.
6. Druker BJ, Tamura S, Buchdunger E, et al.: Effects of a selective inhibitor of the Abl tyrosine kinase on the growth of Bcr-Abl positive cells. *Nat Med* 2:561–566, 1996.
7. Holtz MS, Slovak ML, Zhang F, Sawyers CL, Forman SJ, Bhatia R: Imatinib mesylate (STI571) inhibits growth of primitive malignant progenitors in chronic myelogenous leukemia through reversal of abnormally increased proliferation. *Blood* 99:3792–3800, 2002.
8. Demetri GD, von Mehren M, Blanke CD, et al.: Efficacy and safety of imatinib mesylate in advanced gastrointestinal stromal tumors. *N Engl J Med* 347:472–480, 2002.
9. Druker BJ, Talpaz M, Resta DJ, et al.: Efficacy and safety of a specific inhibitor of the bcr-abl tyrosine kinase in chronic myeloid leukemia. *N Engl J Med* 344:1031–1037, 2001.
10. Gorre ME, Mohammed M, Ellwood K, et al.: Clinical resistance to STI-571 cancer therapy caused by BCR-ABL gene mutation or amplification. *Science* 293:876–880, 2001.
11. Gambacorti-Passerini C, Barni R, le Coutre P, et al.: Role of alpha1 acid glycoprotein in the in vivo resistance of human bcr-abl + leukemic cells to the abl inhibitor ST1571. *J Natl Cancer Inst* 92:1641–1650, 2000.
12. Lyseng-Williamson K, Jarvis B: Imatinib. *Drugs* 61:1765–1774, 2001.
13. Product information: Gleevec®, imatinib. Novartis, East Hanover, NJ, (PI revised 3/2005) reviewed 6/2005.
14. Deininger MW, Druker BJ: Specific trageted therapy of chronic myelogenous leukemia with imatinib. *Pharmacol Rev* 55:410–423, 2003.
15. Quintas_Cardama A, Kantarjian H, O'Brien S, et al.: Granulocyte-colony-stimulating factor (filgrastim) may overcome imatinib-induced neutropenia in patients with chronic-phase chronic myelogenous leukemia. *Cancer* 100:2592–2597, 2004.
16. Lindenmann IA: Virus interference, I: The interferon. *Proc Royal Soc London* 147:258–267, 1957.
17. Quesada JR, Talpaz M, Rios A, Kurzrock R, Gutterman JU: Clinical toxicity of interferons in cancer patients: a review. *J Clin Oncol* 4:234–243, 1986.
18. Gutterman JU, Fine S, Quesada J, et al.: Recombinant leukocyte a interferon: pharmacokinetics, single-dose tolerance, and biologic effects in cancer patients. *Ann Intern Med* 95:549–556, 1982.
19. Viscomi G: Structure-activity of type I interferons *Biotherapy* 10:59–86, 1997.
20. Rigby WF, Ball ED, Guyre PM, Fanger MW: The effects of recombinant-DNA-derived interferons on the growth of myeloid progenitor cells. *Blood* 65:858–861, 1985.
21. Ochs J, Abromowitch M, Rudnick S, Murphy SB: Phase I-II study of recombinant alpha-2 interferon against advanced leukemia and lymphoma in children. *J Clin Oncol* 4:883–887, 1986.

22. Leandersson T, Lundgren E: Antiproliferative effect of interferon on a Burkitt's lymphoma cell line. *Exp Cell Res* 130:421–426, 1980.

23. Oken MM, Kyle RA: Strategies for combining interferon with chemotherapy for the treatment of multiple myeloma. *Semin Oncol* 18:30–32, 1991.

24. McEvoy GK, Miller J, Snow EK, eds.: Interferon alpha. In: *AHFS Drug Information*. Bethesda, MD: American Society of Health-System Pharmacists; 2004, 1033–1055.

25. Cuaron L, Thompson J: The Interferons. In: Trahan-Rieger P (ed.) *Biotherapy—A Comprehensive Overview*, 2nd edn. Sudbury, MA: Jones and Bartlet; 2001, 125–191

26. Qin XQ, Runkel L, Deck C, DeDios C, Barsoum J: Interferon-beta induces S phase accumulation selectively in human transformed cells. *J Interferon Cytokine Res* 17:355–367, 1997.

27. Balkwill FR, Moodie EM, Freedman V, Fantes KH: Human interferon inhibits the growth of established human breast tumours in the nude mouse. *Intl J Cancer* 30:231–235, 1982.

28. Product information: Roferon-A®, interferon alpha-2a. Hoffmann-La Roche, Inc, Nutley, NJ, (PI revised 3/2005) reviewed 6/2005.

29. Hirsch MS, Tolkoff-Rubin NE, Kelly AP: Pharmacokinetics of human and recombinant leukocyte interferon in patients with chronic renal failure who are undergoing hemodialysis. *J Infect Dis* 148:335, 1983.

30. Bollag W: Retinoids in oncology: experimental and clinical aspects. *Pure Appl Chem* 66:995–1002, 1994.

31. Smith MA, Parkinson DR, Cheson BD, et al.: Retinoids in cancer therapy. *J Clin Oncol* 10:839–863, 1992.

32. Hansen LA, Sigman CC, Andreola F, et al.: Retinoids in chemoprevention and differentiation therapy. *Carcinogenesis* 21:1271–1279, 2000.

33. Lotan R: Retinoids and apoptosis: implications for cancer chemoprevention and therapy. *J Natl Cancer Inst* 87:1655, 1995.

34. Miller WH Jr, Warrell RP Jr, Frankel SR, et al.: Novel retinoic acid receptor-α transcripts in acute promyelocytic leukemia responsive to all-trans-retinoic acid. *J Natl Cancer Inst* 32:1932–1933, 1990.

35. Warrell RP Jr, The H, Wang ZY, Degos L: Acute promyelocytic leukemia. *N Engl J Med* 329:177–189, 1993.

36. Melnick A, Licht JD: Deconstructing a disease: RARalpha, its fusion partners, and their roles in the pathogenesis of acute promyelocytic leukemia. *Blood* 93:3167–3215, 1999.

37. Tallman MS, Anderson JW, Schiffer CA, et al.: All-trans-retinoic acid in acute promyelocytic leukemia: long-term outcome and prognostic factor analysis from the North American Intergroup protocol. *Blood* 100:4298–4302, 2002.

38. Sanz M, Martin G, Gonzalez M, et al.: Risk-adapted treatment of acute promyelocytic leukemia with all-trans-retinoic acid and anthracycline monochemotherapy: a multicenter study by the PETHEMA group. *Blood* 103:1237–1243, 2004.

39. Sanz M, Martin G, Rayon C, et al.: A modified AIDA protocol with anthracycline-based consolidation results in high antileukemic efficacy and reduced toxicity in newly diagnosed PML/RARα-positive acute promyelocytic leukemia. *Blood* 94:3015–3021, 1999.

40. Fenaux P, Chastand C, Sanz MA, et al.: A randomized comparison of ATRA followed by chemotherapy and ATRA plus chemotherapy, and the role of maintenance therapy in newly diagnosed acute promyelocytic leukemia. *Blood* 94:1192–1200, 1999.

41. Mandelli F, Diverio D, Avvisati G, et al. :Molecular remission in PML/RARα-positive acute promyelocytic leukemia by combined all-trans-retinoic acid and idarubicin (AIDA) therapy. *Blood* 90:1014–1021, 1997.

42. Product information: Vesanoid® tretinoin. Roche, Nutley, NJ, (PI revised 10/2004) reviewed 6/2005.

43. Douer D, Estey E, Santillana S, et al.: Treatment of newly diagnosed and relapsed acute promyelocytic leukemia with intravenous liposomal all-trans retinoic acid. *Blood* 97:73–80, 2001.

44. Tallman MS; Andersen JW; Schiffer CA, et al.: Clinical description of 44 patients with acute promyelocytic leukemia who developed the retinoic acid syndrome. *Blood* 95:90–95, 2000.

45. De Botton S; Dombret H; Sanz M, et al.: Incidence, clinical features, and outcome of all trans-retinoic acid syndrome in 413 cases of newly diagnosed acute promyelocytic leukemia. The European APL Group. *Blood* 92:2712–2718, 1998.

46. Boehm M, Zhang L, Badea B, et al.: Synthesis and structure-activity relationships of novel retinoid X receptor-selective-retinoids. *J Med Chem* 37:2930–2942, 1994.

47. Miller V, Benedetti F, Rigas J, et al.: Initial clinical trial of a selective retinoids X receptor ligand, LGD1069. *J Clin Oncol* 15:790–795, 1997.

48. Package Insert. Targetrin capsules (bexarotene). Ligand Pharmaceuticals, San Diego, CA, March 2003.

49. Kizaki M, Dawson MI, Heyman R, et al.: Effects of novel retinoid X receptor-selective ligands on myeloid leukemic differentiation and proliferation in vitro. *Blood* 87:1977–1984, 1996.

50. Duvic M, Hymes K, Heald P, et al.: Bexarotene is effective and safe for treatment of refractory advanced-stage cutaneous T-cell lymphoma: multinational phase II-III trial results. *J Clinl Oncol* 19:2456–2471, 2001.

51. Duvic M, Martin AG, Kim Y, et al.: Phase II and III clinical trial of oral bexarotene (targetrin capsules) for the treatment of refractory or persistent early-stage cutaneous T-cell lymphoma. *Arch Dermatol* 137:581–593, 2001a.

52. Package Insert. Targetrin gel (bexarotene). Ligand Pharmaceuticals, San Diego, CA, January 2001.

53. Breneman D, Duvic M, Kuzel T, et al.: Efficacy and safety of bexarotene gel in patients with previously untreated CTCL [Poster]. Presented at the Annual Meeting of the American Academy of Dermatology, Washington, DC, March 2001.

54. Duvic M, Martin A, Kim Y, et al.: Phase II-III clinical trial of bexarotene capsules demonstrated efficacy and safety for patients with refractory or persistent early stage CTCL [Abstract 231]. Poster presented at the 58th Annual Meeting of the American Academy of Deermatology, San Francisco, March 10–15, 2000.

55. Sherman S, Gopal J, Hugen B, et al.: Central hypothyroidsim associated with retinoid X receptor-selective ligands. *N Engl J Med* 340:1075–1079, 1999.

56. Kwong YL, Todd D: Delicious poison: arsenic trioxide for the treatment of leukemia [Letter]. *Blood* 89:3487–3488, 1997.

57. Antman KH: Introduction: the history of arsenic trioxide in cancer therapy. *Oncologist* 6(suppl 2): 1–2, 2001.

58. Shen Z-X, Chen G-O, Ni J-H, et al.: Use of arsenic trioxide (As203) in the treatment of acute promyelocytic leukemia (APL): II. Clinical efficacy and pharmacokinetics in relapse patients. *Blood* 89:3354–3360, 1997.

59. Soignet SL, Maslak P, Wang Z-G, et al.: Complete remission after treatment of acute promyelocytic leukemia with arsenic trioxide. *N Engl J Med* 339:1341–1348, 1998.

60. Soignet SL, Frankel SR, Douer D, et al.: United States multicenter study of arsenic trioxide in relapsed acute promyelocytic leukemia. *J Clin Oncol* 19:3852–3860, 2001.

61. Product information: Trisenox™, arsenic trioxide. Cell Therapeutics, Inc., Seattle, WA, (PI revised 3/2000) reviewed 6/2005.

62. Davison K, Mann KK, Miller WH: Arsenic trioxide: mechanisms of action. *Semin Hematol* 39(suppl 2): 3–7, 2002.

63. Murgo AJ: Clinical trials of arsenic trioxide in hematologic and solid tumors: overview of the National Cancer Institute Cooperative Research and Development studies. *Oncologist* 6(suppl 2): 22–28, 2001.

64. Product information: Intron-A®, interferon alpha-2b. Schering Corporation, Kenilworth, NJ, (PI revised 3/2004) reviewed 6/2005.

# Chapter 103

# PHARMACOLOGY OF MONOCLONAL ANTIBODIES

*Jennifer L. Shamp*

## HISTORY

Currently, dynamic changes are taking place in the field of oncology. Remarkable advances have been made in elucidating the complex mechanisms of cellular signaling and malignant transformation, providing unique targets for therapy. Monoclonal antibodies (MoAbs) represent a subset of these newer, targeted therapies. MoAbs are designed to target specific surface proteins found on tumor cells, thus selecting malignant cellular clones for destruction while sparing healthy cells. This streamlined approach offers significant advantages over traditional chemotherapy, where healthy cells are often sacrificed in order to eradicate malignant cells. Recent improvements in technology and laboratory methods have enhanced the effectiveness of MoAbs, making them more amenable to clinical use.

Interestingly, while most of the currently available MoAbs have entered the marketplace in the past decade, the notion of antibody therapy has been around for years. Conceptually dating back to the nineteenth century, the initial idea of "serotherapy" was developed by Behring through his work with tetanus toxin. He discovered that immunizing toxin-naïve animals with serum from animals exposed to tetanus toxin provided a protective effect against lethal doses of tetanus. Thus, he concluded that some form of antitoxin develops upon exposure to lower doses of toxin, providing future protection against the disease.[1] Rapidly building on this concept of a "magic bullet," Hericourt and Richet prepared an "antiserum" to extracts of osteogenic sarcoma, which they used to treat patients with the disease. In 1953, Pressman and Korngold showed that antibodies could specifically target tumor cells, thus renewing interest in using immunotherapy for the treatment of cancer.[2] Another breakthrough occurred in 1968, when Porter and Edelman identified the "antitoxin," or Y-shaped immunoglobulin structure well-known today.[3] Finally, in 1975, the Nobel prize-winning publication by Kohler and Milstein described a realistic methodology for the creation of compounds that specifically select and bind to cancer cells. Their "hybridoma" cell lines were created from animals repeatedly immunized with target antigen. Subsequently, the B lymphocytes of these animals were isolated and immortalized, and the ability to produce specifically targeted antibodies was retained.[4] Thus began the serious evaluation of MoAbs as potential therapeutic agents in the treatment of cancer.

Three types of MoAbs have emerged, representing three distinct therapeutic strategies: unconjugated MoAbs, immunotoxin-conjugated MoAbs, and radionuclide-conjugated MoAbs.[1] The unconjugated MoAbs represent the simplest form of therapy, where the antibody itself achieves cell death through stimulation of host immune effector mechanisms. The conjugated MoAbs, on the other hand, are covalently linked to either a toxin or a radioisotope. The release of the toxin/radioisotope upon direct delivery to the targeted cell accounts for the cytotoxicity of these compounds.[5]

## UNCONJUGATED MOABS

### PHARMACOLOGY

The unconjugated MoAb is a structurally complex macromolecule comprising an immunoglobulin with a constant region (Fc) and a variable region (Fab) that is engineered to target a specific cell surface marker. Ideally, cell surface markers would be found solely on malignant clones; unfortunately, a cell surface marker of this type has not yet been discovered. Thus, these cell surface proteins are found not only on malignant cells, but on healthy lymphoid or myeloid cell lines as well. These agents bind to the targeted cell surface protein and form an antigen–MoAb complex, which then allows the exposed Fc fragment of the drug to activate host effector mechanisms.[5] Cellular destruction can occur via two pathways: (1) complement-mediated cytotoxicity (CMC), which involves activation of complement C1q on the Fc region, leading to the formation of a membrane-attack complex that lyses the target cell and (2) antibody-dependent cellular cytotoxicity (ADCC), which occurs through binding of Fc region receptors to natural killer cells, monocytes, and macrophages, leading to opsonization of the target. Because host effector mechanisms require activation by Fc region receptors located on cell surfaces, these molecules cannot be internalized, but must remain on the cell surface in order to function.[1,5] The immunoglobulin isotypes vary in their ability to activate these cellular functions. The IgG1 subclass is thought to be the most effective in stimulating ADCC and CMC functions in humans.[6]

### THERAPEUTIC CHALLENGES

Between 1975 and the early 1990s, researchers in MoAb therapy suffered a variety of setbacks and challenges. Patients treated with the agents in clinical settings did not show dramatic responses. The initial murine products were hindered by the development of HAMA (human anti-mouse antibodies); host antibodies identified murine protein fragments as foreign, subsequently inactivating the compounds after repeated administration.[1] This was further complicated by allergic-type reactions and even anaphylaxis. Other potential reasons for the limited success of these compounds included short drug half-lives, inadequate recruitment of the patients' immune effector cells, lack of specificity of tumor antigens, internalization of the target antigen by tumor cells, and inadequate quantities of antibody administered.[1] With the advancement of technology and laboratory techniques involved in the production of antibodies, as well as clinical research in genomics and cellular-signaling pathways, the development of therapeutic MoAbs has improved significantly in the past 15 years. Production of humanized and human chimeric antibodies, as well as clinical advances in identification of antigenic receptors, has resulted in the FDA approval of 17 MoAbs since 1986. Eight of these compounds received approval for cancer indications (Table 103.1).

### APPROVED COMPOUNDS

#### Rituximab (Rituxan)

Rituximab, the most extensively studied MoAb to date, is a chimeric human/mouse IgG1-κ MoAb designed to target cell surface protein CD20. Rituximab consists of murine variable regions from the parent 2B8 MoAb grafted onto a human IgG1 constant-region backbone.[5] The cell surface protein CD20 offers an ideal target, as it is expressed on >95% normal B lymphocytes and B-cell lymphomas, but not stem cells or plasma cells. Additionally, CD20 is not shed or internalized upon antibody binding; thus, the antibody-CD20 complex remains on the surface of the cell, available to bind and stimulate ADCC and CMC.[8] In addition to ADCC and CMC, rituximab achieves therapeutic activity by direct induction of calcium influx

**Table 103.1** Monoclonal antibodies currently approved for the treatment of hematologic and oncologic malignancies[7]

| Monoclonal antibody | Target antigen | Clinical uses | FDA approval |
|---|---|---|---|
| Rituximab (Rituxan®) | CD20 | B-cell lymphomas, CLL | 1997 |
| Trastuzumab (Herceptin®) | HER2/neu | Breast cancer | 1998 |
| Gemtuzumab (Mylotarg®) | CD33 | AML, APL | 2000 |
| Alemtuzumab (Campath®) | CD52 | B-cell CLL | 2001 |
| ⁹⁰Y-ibritumomab (Zevalin®) | CD20 | B-cell lymphoma | 2002 |
| ¹³¹I-tositumomab (Bexxar®) | CD20 | B-cell lymphoma | 2003 |
| Bevacizumab (Avastin®) | VEGFR | Colorectal cancer | 2004 |
| Cetuximab (Erbitux®) | EGFR | Colorectal cancer | 2004 |

and apoptosis.[5,8] Rapid depletion of CD20+ B lymphocytes from blood, bone marrow, and lymph nodes lasting 3–6 months is observed following administration of rituximab.[1] Full recovery is typically achieved after 9–12 months.[9] However, during this time, T lymphocyte and IgG levels remain constant, even though B lymphocyte and IgM levels drop. In essence, humoral immunity remains intact and patients do not experience an increased risk of infection during this time.[1,5]

*Clinical trials* Original phase I studies of rituximab used single doses escalating up to 375 mg/m². The trials were actually stopped before any dose-limiting toxicity was reached, illustrating the favorable side effect profile of the drug. While some patients received more than 1000 mg of rituximab, adverse effects were mild and typically reversible. These consisted mainly of infusion-related effects such as fever, asthenia, chills, nausea, vomiting, rash, and urticaria.[10] Adverse effects were most common with initial doses and typically subsided with subsequent drug exposure. Further studies evaluated rituximab for a variety of indications, beginning with relapsed low-grade and follicular non-Hodgkin's lymphoma.[11] A pivotal trial evaluated weekly rituximab 375 mg/m² for 4 weeks in a population of patients with a median of two prior relapses. Response rates were impressive, with 48% of patients achieving partial responses and 6% achieving complete responses.[12] Rituximab has been studied in combination with traditional chemotherapy as well. A second pivotal trial compared CHOP alone to CHOP plus rituximab in patients between 60 and 80 years of age with previously untreated diffuse large B-cell lymphoma. The rituximab arm had no significant increase in adverse events compared to the control arm, but showed significantly higher rates of event-free and overall survival.[13] Use of rituximab has now expanded to other B-cell malignancies, including chronic lymphocytic leukemia and small lymphocytic lymphoma.[8] Dose intensification protocols have been evaluated with the goal of improving response rates in these disease states; however, the exact role of rituximab in these malignancies remains to be defined.[14]

*Pharmacokinetics* The pharmacokinetic profile of rituximab exhibits significant interpatient variability. Serum concentrations can fluctuate up to fivefold between patients; in addition, with each successive dose of drug, an individual's serum concentration increases significantly. In one pharmacokinetic study, median values for peak serum levels essentially doubled from the first to the fourth dose.[15] Rituximab serum half-life follows the same pattern, increasing 2.7-fold between the first and fourth doses (ranging from 3.2 to 8.6 days). This increase in half-life supports the theory that rituximab undergoes lymphocyte-mediated clearance. Fluctuating plasma concentration values may correspond to circulating CD20+ lymphocyte numbers, as well as CD20+ receptor saturation, suggesting that clearance is dependent on the amount of CD20+ cells present.[9,14]

*Adverse effects* Rituximab is fairly well tolerated, with the majority of adverse effects being infusion-related. In one pivotal trial, adverse events were reported in 84% patients; however, <5% of these were considered severe (grade 3 or 4 based on NCI–CTC criteria). Additionally, these adverse reactions were typically limited to the first dose; 55% of patients reported no adverse effects with subsequent doses.[12] These reactions appear to correspond to clearance of CD20+ lymphocytes, and are most severe upon initial exposure to the drug.[9] Patients at highest risk include those with circulating malignant lymphocyte counts >25,000/mm³ as well as patients with bulky disease (lesions ≥10 cm). Premedication with acetaminophen and antihistamines reduces the commonly experienced fever, chills, and malaise; in the rare cases where bronchospasm, angioedema, or hypotension occurs, stopping the infusion and providing supportive care usually resolves the reaction.[9]

## Alemtuzumab (Campath-1H)

Alemtuzumab, the end result of two decades' worth of research and development, is a humanized rat IgG-1 antibody directed against cell surface marker CD52.[1] Initially, alemtuzumab was developed as a rat IgM antibody and used for in vitro T-cell depletion prior to stem cell transplantation. While in vitro Campath-1M was successful, trials evaluating systemic use in lymphoma patients demonstrated disappointing results. This was thought to be due to the IgM component of the compound ineffectively stimulating ADCC. Thus, Campath-1G was developed, an IgG2b antibody. Initially more successful against lymphoma and bone marrow cells, Campath-1G encountered problems when patients quickly developed HAMA as a result of the murine nature of the drug.[16] Finally, a humanized rat IgG-1 antibody was developed, known as Campath-1H or alemtuzumab. The CD52 surface protein is expressed on most lymphocytes (both B and T cells), monocytes, macrophages and eosinophils, as well as cells lining the distal epididymis, vas deferens, and seminal vesicles in the male reproductive tract; however, it is not found on erythrocytes, platelets, or stem cells.[8] In addition, while CD52 is highly expressed in some forms of CLL, NHL, and ALL, it is not shed or internalized, making it an excellent MoAb target.[8] Once alemtuzumab binds to the CD52 receptor, cellular cytotoxicity is achieved through ADCC, CMC, and direct apoptosis.[17]

*Clinical trials* Alemtuzumab is currently indicated for the treatment of fludarabine-refractory B-cell CLL. Three major studies have assessed alemtuzumab in this population.[18–20] The largest of these studies was an international collaboration between centers in the United States and Europe; this study evaluated 12 weeks of intravenous alemtuzumab in 92 fludarabine-resistant patients, of which 76% had Rai stage II or IV disease.[20] The overall response rate was 33%, with 2% CR. Median survival was 16 months. Patients with bulky lymphadenopathy were less likely to respond, possibly indicating poor tumor penetration of alemtuzumab.[8,20] Toxicity was moderate and consisted mainly of infectious problems (55% patients) as well as infusion-related reactions. Rai et al. supported these findings with a study evaluating 24 poor-prognosis, fludarabine-treated chronic lymphocytic leukemia patients.[19] After up to 16 weeks of treatment with alemtuzumab (target dose 30 mg three times weekly), the overall response rate was 33%. Median time to progression was 19.6 months. Because of the high incidence of infusion-related reactions encountered during intravenous infusion of alemtuzumab, subcutaneous use has emerged as a potential alternative route of administration. Another trial evaluated subcutaneous alemtuzumab in 41 patients with advanced, previously untreated CLL.[21] An overall response rate of 87% was achieved, with 19% CR. While injection site reactions were seen in 90% patients, these were grades 1–2 in severity. The infusion reactions generally encountered with intravenous dosing were absent, aside from some patients experiencing rigors.[21,22]

Alemtuzumab has demonstrated some activity in other hematologic malignancies as well, including T-cell PLL and low-grade lymphomas.[23–25] An encouraging study by Pawson et al. evaluated 15 patients with refractory T-cell prolymphocytic leukemia, most of whom had failed prior treatment with pentostatin. The response rate was 73%, with 60% patients achieving CR.[23] These results were subsequently verified in other studies with T-cell lymphoma patients; response rates have consistently remained above 50% even in heavily pretreated populations.[24,25]

Combination therapy with alemtuzumab has recently been explored; one study evaluated six patients with refractory disease who were treated with fludarabine and alemtuzumab concurrently.[26] Five patients responded, with one patient achieving a complete response. Additionally, sequential therapy with fludarabine followed by alemtuzumab has been studied; this combination, while associated with significant rates of infectious complications (12 of 57 patients developed grade 3 or 4 infections during or after alemtuzumab treatment), patients who completed therapy showed significant response rates. Thirty-six of 57 patients enrolled finished both the fludarabine and alemtuzumab phases of treatment; this group achieved an overall response rate of 92%, with 42% CR.[27] Longer follow up and additional studies will help to fully elucidate the role of combination therapy with alemtuzumab.

***Administration and pharmacokinetics*** Alemtuzumab is typically administered in a gradual dose-escalation fashion, which helps reduce the severity of infusion-related reactions that occur upon first exposure to the compound. The initial recommended dose of alemtuzumab is 3 mg infused over 2 h on day 1, followed by 10 mg on day 2, and if tolerated, 30 mg thrice weekly. Treatment is generally continued for 4–12 weeks as tolerated. With maintenance dosing, peak levels of alemtuzumab reach steady state after approximately 6 weeks, at which point the drug half-life is 12 days.[28]

***Adverse effects*** Adverse effects associated with alemtuzumab consist mainly of infusion-related reactions, infectious complications, and hematologic toxicity. Acute infusion toxicities are quite common, seen in 90% of patients in a large trial by Keating et al.[20] Rigors, fever, nausea, vomiting, and rash are often seen with initial infusions; however, these typically decrease with subsequent drug exposure.[22] Rarely, hypotension and dyspnea are encountered.[8] Premedication with acetaminophen and antihistamines is recommended to reduce this possibility. Infectious complications have been problematic as well; opportunistic infections, CMV reactivation, HSV infection, PCP, candidiasis, and septicemia have all been reported.[20] Currently, antibacterial and antiviral prophylaxis is recommended in order to prevent these complications. Lymphocyte counts drop rapidly after alemtuzumab treatment, resulting in a severe and prolonged lymphopenia. Myelosuppression, on the other hand, consisting of anemia, neutropenia, and thrombocytopenia, is typically moderate and transient.[8,20]

## IMMUNOTOXINS

### PHARMACOLOGY

The immunotoxin-conjugated MoAbs, or ITs, are fusion proteins that consist of MoAbs covalently linked to protein toxins. These highly potent toxins are typically derived from plant, bacterial, or fungal sources and possess the ability to disrupt protein synthesis through a series of catalytic enzymatic reactions at very small concentrations.[1] The most technically challenging of all MoAbs to design and deliver, immunotoxins are genetically engineered to retain their cytotoxic potency, while their tissue-binding domains are truncated in order to allow for MoAb-directed targeting of specific cell surface proteins. This minimizes binding of the toxin to healthy cells, while selectively targeting malignant clones.[29] In order for the toxin to exert its effect, it must undergo internalization by the cell, rather than remaining on the cell surface as with unconjugated MoAbs. This allows the toxin to gain access to critical intracellular functions located within the cytosol. Receptor-mediated endocytosis occurs once the compound binds to the cell surface. Upon entering a cell, the toxin is carried by clathrin-coated vesicles to either acidic endosomes (bacterial toxins) or neutral *trans*-Golgi (plant toxins), where interruption of protein synthesis occurs. Both plant and bacterial toxins disrupt the elongation step of protein synthesis, through enzymatic alteration of either elongation factor 2 or its binding site.[30] Toxins that have been used in this manner include ricin, abrin, diphtheriatoxin, and pseudomonas toxin. A variety of compounds are currently in clinical development (Table 103.2).

### THERAPEUTIC CHALLENGES

The majority of literature evaluating immunotoxins consists of data from phase I trials. While these studies have collectively shown that therapeutic serum levels of toxin can be achieved with acceptable toxicity, much research remains to be done. The compounds have been plagued with high toxicity profiles and low response rates.[30] Many different MoAb-toxin combinations have been studied and the adverse effect profile has remained surprisingly consistent. Most of the phase I dose-escalation trials have been limited by the development of a vascular leak syndrome; peripheral edema, pulmonary edema, weight gain, hypoalbuminemia, hypotension, and pericardial effusions are thought to be due to toxin-mediated endothelial damage.[5,30] Hypersensitivity reactions are common as well, along with fever, malaise, and nausea. Further complicating these hypersensitivity responses is the fact that patients can react to one or both components of the

| Table 103.2 | Immunotoxins currently under investigation for hematologic malignancies[31,32] | | |
|---|---|---|---|
| Compound | Target | Toxin | Clinical use |
| DAB389-IL2 (**Ontak**) | Interleukin 2 receptor | Diptheria toxin | Cutaneous T-cell lymphoma |
| Anti-TAC (Fv)-PE38 (**LMB-2**) | CD25 | Pseudomonas toxin | B-cell lymphomas, T-cell lymphomas, and Hodgkin's disease |
| RFT5-dgA | CD25 | Ricin | Hodgkin's disease |
| RFB4-dgA | CD22 | Ricin | Non-Hodgkin's lymphoma, B-CLL |
| HD37-dgA | CD19 | Ricin | Relapsed B-cell non-Hodgkin's lymphoma |
| RFB4(dsFv)-PE38 (**BL22**) | CD22 | Pseudomonas toxin | B-cell lymphomas, B-CLL, hairy cell leukemia |
| Anti-CD7-dgA | CD7 | Ricin | T-cell non-Hodgkin's lymphoma |
| DT-Anti-Tac(Fv) | CD25 | Diptheria toxin | Leukemias, lymphomas |
| B3-Lys-PE38 | Lewis Y | Pseudomonas | Carcinoma |
| B3(Fv)-PE38 | | toxin | |
| B3(dsFv)-PE38 | | | |
| BR96(sFv)-PE40 | | | |
| e23(Fv)-PE38 | ErbB2/HER2 | Pseudomonas toxin | Breast cancer |
| FRP5(scFv)-ETA | | | |
| MR1(Fv)-PE38 | Mutant EGF-R | Pseudomonas toxin | Liver, brain tumors |
| SS1(Fv)-PE38 | Mesothelin | Pseudomonas toxin | Ovarian cancer |

Fv, antigen recognition site on the monoclonal antibody; IL2, interleukin 2; toxins include PE38 (truncated pseudomonas exotoxin), DAB$_{389}$ (truncated diphtheria toxin), and dgA (deglycosylated ricin A chain).

compound. HAMA and antitoxin responses have been documented, which limits the ability to retreat patients because of neutralizing antibodies that render the compounds ineffective.[5] Other factors contributing to the limited activity of immunotoxins include minimal penetration of bulky tumor sites, particularly in non-Hodgkin's lymphoma and Hodgkin's disease.[30,33]

### APPROVED COMPOUNDS
### Gemtuzumab ozogamicin (Mylotarg)

Gemtuzumab ozogamicin (GO) is one of the first clinically available immunoconjugates, approved in 2000 for the treatment of relapsed AML in patients ≥60 years of age with CD33-positive disease. The compound consists of a humanized MoAb to CD33 linked to two molecules of the enediyne antitumor antibiotic *n*-acetyl-γ-calicheamicin.[28] Calicheamicin is a cytotoxic natural product isolated from *Micromonospora echinospora* that is at least 1000 times more potent than conventional chemotherapy agents such as doxorubicin.[34] The cell surface protein CD33 is expressed by most hematopoietic cells; in fact, this protein is not found outside of the hematopoietic system. As such, it is an excellent target for new therapies in hematologic malignancies. Immature and mature myeloid cells as well as erythroid, megakaryocytic, and multipotent progenitor cells express CD33. More importantly,

leukemic blasts in approximately 90% of patients with AML express this marker.[28] Once GO binds to CD33 receptors, it forms an antibody–calicheamicin complex on the cell. This complex rapidly undergoes endocytosis, where lysosomal enzymes then cleave the covalent bond between the MoAb and calicheamicin, liberating the calicheamicin toxin inside the cell. The enediyne component of calicheamicin is responsible for much of its toxicity; this reactive portion of the molecule produces cytotoxic biradicals upon aromatization, which leads to phosphodiester DNA strand breaks. After calicheamicin binds to the DNA duplex minor groove, double-strand breaks in the oligopyrimidine and oligopurine tracts occur; this positions the enediyne ring to abstract hydrogen atoms from neighboring strands.[34]

*Clinical trials* Results of phase I studies evaluating GO in patients with relapsed AML showed that two doses of 9 mg/m$^2$ resulted in >75% saturation of CD33 antigen on peripheral blood mononuclear cells.[35] This subsequently became the recommended dose for phase II trials. A series of three phase II trials enrolled a total of 142 patients with untreated, relapsed AML. The data was compiled and published in one report.[36] The median age was 61, and the median length of first CR was 11.1 months; 109 patients (77%) received two doses of drug and 5 (3%) received 3 doses; the overall response rate was 28% in patients whose initial responses lasted < 1 year and 32% in patients whose original responses lasted > 1 year. There were 23 complete responses (16%) and 19 CR$_p$s (complete response without full platelet recovery, >100,000/l). No significant difference in response rates or overall survival was seen based on age or cytogenetic profiles. Toxicities consisting of fever, rigors, hypotension, and other infusion-related events were common (grade 3 or 4 infusion reactions occurred in 34% patients during the first dose, but only 12% during the second dose). Other significant grade 3/4 adverse effects included thrombocytopenia (99%), neutropenia (97%), hyperbilirubinemia (23%), and infections (28%). Based on these studies, the FDA granted GO conditional approval as single-agent therapy for CD33-positive, relapsed AML in patients >60 years of age who are not candidates for other chemotherapy. This approval was contingent upon ongoing studies evaluating the role of GO in recurrent AML as well as the comparison of GO with chemotherapy versus chemotherapy alone.[28]

A variety of studies further evaluating GO have been conducted[37,38]; Nabhan et al. published a trial evaluating GO as initial AML treatment in 12 patients who were >65 years old. The overall response rate was 27%. Treatment was fairly well tolerated; however 100% patients experienced grade 3 or 4 neutropenia and/or thrombocytopenia.[37] Five patients experienced elevations in LFTs, notably bilirubin, although none of these were considered grade 3 or 4. No evidence of hepatic venoocclusive disease (VOD) was reported.

Additionally, GO has been evaluated in combination with other chemotherapeutic agents.[39] Piccaluga et al. evaluated nine patients with a median age of 63 years (five with untreated AML and four with relapsed AML). Patients received GO 6 mg/m$^2$ on day 1 and 4 mg/m$^2$ on day 8 concurrently with cytarabine 100 mg/m$^2$/day continuous infusion days 1–7. Three of five patients with untreated disease achieved CR, along with two of four patients with relapsed AML. Median overall survival was 6 months. The most common adverse effect was myelosuppression; again, 100% patients experienced grade 3 or 4 neutropenia and/or thrombocytopenia. Infusion-related reactions were documented in two patients; transaminase elevations were encountered as well, with ALT/AST elevations occurring in seven patients (grade 3 in two cases), hyperbilirubinemia in three patients, and alkaline phosphatase elevation in seven cases.[39] The most concerning adverse event was grade 3/4 bleeding, which occurred in four patients.

Other combination regimens with different agents, including cytarabine, daunorubicin, topotecan, idarubicin, cyclosporine, fludarabine, troxacitabine, and anti BCL-2 antisense are currently under investigation or being published. A trial with topotecan, Go, and cytarabine was moderately effective but associated with significant toxicity.[40] Additionally, 2 of 14 patients included in this study developed hepatic VOD. This seems to be a major toxicity of concern with GO combination regimens. More data is needed before GO can be recommended in conjunction with other chemotherapy agents.

***Administration/pharmacokinetics*** Gemtuzumab is administered as an intravenous infusion over 2 h. A full course of treatment consists of two doses of 9 mg/m$^2$, given 14 days apart.[28] Pretreatment with antihistamines and/or corticosteroids is recommended in order to reduce infusion-related reactions. Elimination half-life of the drug is fairly long; median half-life of the antibody component is 72.4 h, while median half-life of the calicheamicin component is 45.1 h.[28] Increased median plasma concentrations are observed following a second dose; this indicates reduced tumor burden and lesser clearance by CD33+ blast cells as compared to the first dose.[41]

***Adverse effects*** GO is associated with a variety of adverse effects, mainly consisting of infusion-related reactions, hepatotoxicity, and myelosuppression.[34] The infusion-related events are similar to those associated with other MoAbs and include fever, rigors, hypotension, dyspnea, nausea, emesis, and headache. Premedication with corticosteroids may reduce this complication. Myelosuppression is profound and prolonged; counts typically nadir at 7–14 days and recover at 28–35 days.[36] In some cases, recovery may take even longer; in fact, some patients never achieve full recovery of platelet counts; thus, the development of the response denoted CRp (<100,000/mm$^3$). Hepatotoxicity associated with GO therapy is another recognized adverse effect. Typically, this consists of transient hyperbilirubinemia and/or transaminitis that is of little clinical significance. The average onset is within 8 days, and duration is 20 days.[36] A more concerning manifestation of hepatotoxicity is hepatic veno-occlusive disease (VOD). This seems to be more common when GO is used in combination with other chemotherapy or after stem cell transplant.[34] When GO is used in the approved single-agent manner, VOD incidence is approximately 1–5%. However, when GO is used in combination therapy, VOD risk increases to 5–12%.[34] This adverse effect is unpredictable and does not correlate to age, gender, underlying disease (MDS versus AML), baseline renal or hepatic function, alcoholism, or hepatitis history.[34] It has been postulated that premedication with acetaminophen may increase the risk of VOD by interfering with glutathione oxidation-reduction reactions, leaving sinusoidal endothelial cells susceptible to attack by calicheamicin-generated free radicals. Until the exact mechanism of VOD development is discovered, it is recommended to avoid premedication with acetaminophen prior to GO treatment.[28,42] VOD remains a significant concern with GO therapy and more data is needed to determine the risks and benefits of treatment with this agent.

## RADIOIMMUNOCONJUGATES

### PHARMACOLOGY

The radiolabeled MoAbs consist of a MoAb coupled with a radionuclide. This therapeutic modality was developed to act as a "guided missle"; the MoAb delivers ionizing radiation solely to cells that express the antigenic determinant to which the antibody was originally developed. Thus, healthy cells are spared from the toxic effects of the radiation. Hematologic malignancies are ideal candidates for this type of treatment because they are known to be exquisitely radiosensitive.[5,43] Radiolabeled MoAbs offer certain advantages over other MoAbs: They do not depend on host effector mechanisms or cellular internalization transport mechanisms to exert their toxic effects; rather, they emit continuous, decreasing, low-dose-rate irradiation in the form of electrons, or β⁻ particles, that are discharged over 1–5 mm.[43] These particles induce lethal DNA damage to antigen-positive cells as well as neighboring cells in close proximity to target cells.[5,44] This can be advantageous when treating physically inaccessible, bulky tumors. Two major radionuclides are currently used in radioimmunoconjugate synthesis: $^{131}$I and $^{90}$Y. These two radionuclides differ slightly in terms of radiation and half-life. $^{131}$I emits not only β⁻ particles, but also a high degree of γ radiation. The half-life of $^{131}$I is 193 h. In contrast, $^{90}$Y emits only β⁻ particles and has a much shorter half-life of 64 h.[5] However, $^{90}$Y emits higher energy particles that actually penetrate deeper into tissue. Theoretically, this may be advantageous when treating larger, more bulky tumors. On the other hand, $^{90}$Y is less readily available and more expensive than $^{131}$I. In addition to the DNA damage induced by the radionuclide, there is some evidence to suggest that the antibody itself stimulates host immune effector mechanisms, which may account for some of the activity of these radioimmunoconjugates in non-Hodgkin's lymphoma.[44]

### THERAPEUTIC CHALLENGES

Some challenges have been encountered with radioimmunoconjugates as well. Tumor bulk, location, and burden vary greatly among patients and can significantly affect the distribution of the drug. Complex and meticulous dosimetry studies using trace-labeled radioimmunoconjugates must be conducted with each patient prior to initiating therapy. This determines where the highest concentration of radiation will be delivered; ideally, tumor sites receive the largest dose, while healthy organ and tissue sites are exposed to smaller doses.[5] If dosimetry studies show unfavorable distribution of radiation, patients do not receive adequate therapy. Other issues hindering the success of

these compounds include large tumor burden, which prevents access of the radionuclide to the site; shedding of the antigen and circulating tumor cells, both of which deplete drug from the circulation; and nonspecific binding of the compound by normal host tissues, subsequently enhancing the toxicity.[5] Some adverse effects encountered with these agents are similar to those experienced with other MoAbs, such as fever, chills, rash, nausea, and other infusion reactions as well as potential development of HAMA. Of particular concern is the myelosuppression, especially thrombocytopenia, seen with these compounds.[45,46] While considerable patient variability exists, peripheral blood counts typically nadir at 3–4 weeks and stay low for up to 16 weeks after treatment. Bone marrow involvement, prior radiation, and chemotherapy exposure can enhance this effect.[43]

### APPROVED COMPOUNDS

#### $^{90}$Y-Ibritumomab tiuxetan (Zevalin)

$^{90}$Y-Ibritumomab tiuxetan is a radioimmunoconjugate comprising a murine-derived MoAb, targeting cell surface protein CD20, bound to the radionuclide $^{90}$Y. The cell surface protein CD20 is expressed on >95% normal B lymphocytes and B-cell lymphomas, yet not stem cells. Additionally, CD20 is not internalized upon antibody binding; thus, the antibody-CD20 complex remains on the surface of the cell, available to bind and stimulate antibody-dependent and complement-mediated cytotoxicity.[47] The bridge between the Fc portion of the MoAb and the $^{90}$Y isotopes is achieved through the linking compound tiuxetan. Isotopes are electrostatically chelated to tiuxetan, which is then attached to exposed amino acids in the antibody by very stable thiourea covalent bonds. Upon selective binding of the compound to CD20 receptors, $^{90}$Y emits β-radiation that is discharged over 1–5 mm, damaging the DNA of B lymphocytes and immediately surrounding cells.[43] In addition, it is thought that some contributory activity of the drug is derived from CMC and effector cell mechanisms induced by the MoAb component. Because the half-life of this compound is relatively short (64 h) and $^{90}$Y does not emit γ-rays, ibritumomab tiuxetan is considered the safer of the approved radioimmunoconjugates.[28,43]

***Administration and pharmacokinetics*** Treatment with ibritumomab tiuxetan can be divided into two phases 1-week apart: a "cold" phase and a "hot" phase. The cold phase consists of delivery of an imaging agent, $^{111}$In, which lacks therapeutic β-emissions but does emit γ-radiation for imaging. This serves to map the distribution and uptake of the drug. In addition, rituximab is administered with the goal of clearing circulating CD20+ B lymphocytes from the circulation. This dose of rituximab is repeated in 1–2 weeks, again clearing the bloodstream of circulating CD20+ lymphocytes in order to better facilitate uptake of radiolabeled drug into the tumor mass.[43] Administering therapeutic radiolabeled drug without first priming the system with cold anti-CD20 antibody merely results in uptake of drug by circulating B lymphocytes and the reticuloendothelial system.[28] By initially binding up circulating B lymphocytes, as well as tumor cells on the periphery of the mass, drug penetration of the tumor is enhanced. Additionally, the unlabeled anti-CD20 antibody also stimulates immune effector cells and leads to more effective tumor kill.[43]

*Adverse effects*  The major adverse effect associated with ibritumomab tiuxetan is myelosuppression, consisting mainly of neutropenia and thrombocytopenia.[45,46] Because of this, several parameters must be met before patients can be treated with this agent. Qualifications for therapy include <25% lymphoma involvement of bone marrow, platelet count >100,000 cells/mm$^3$, and no history of hypocellular marrow or failed stem cell collection.[28] The average time to neutrophil nadir is 62 days, while platelets typically nadir around day 53. Cells recover after approximately 22–35 days.[43] Additional adverse effects include those seen with other anti-CD20 agents, such as fever, hypotension, chills, skin rash, and rarely nausea and vomiting.[45]

### $^{131}$I Tositumomab (Bexxar)

$^{131}$I tositumomab is a radioimmunoconjugate comprising a murine anti-CD20 MoAb covalently linked through tyrosine amino acids in the immunoglobulin protein to iodine-131. Tositumomab does not require a linker due to direct covalent bonding between the MoAb and the radionuclide. $^{131}$I is more readily available than $^{90}$Y and is relatively inexpensive. However, $^{131}$I emits both β- and γ-irradiation, necessitating special radiation precautions for patients receiving this compound. Dehalogenation (cleaving of the radionuclide from the compound) can occur as well; this results in potential uptake of free iodine by the thyroid and stomach. Oral thyroid blockade is recommended beginning 24 h before therapy and continuing for 14 days in order to prevent iodine uptake and subsequent hypothyroidism.[47] The rate of dehalogenation varies significantly among patients, resulting in fluctuating rates of urinary clearance. Thus, dosimetry calculations incorporating total-body distribution and tissue uptake must be completed for each patient. Doing this enables maximal tumor targeting while minimizing toxic effects to normal tissues.[43] Because $^{131}$I emits γ-radiation as well, it can be used as the tracer agent for the cold phase of treatment. Thus, the imaging agent is the same $^{131}$I tositumomab, used at a lower dose. Unlabeled tositumomab is also used as the cold antibody to deplete the CD20+ B-lymphocyte "sinks," resulting in a higher dose of drug delivered to the tumor.[47]

*Pharmacokinetics*  The half-life of $^{131}$I tositumomab is approximately 8 days, but varies somewhat among individuals because of fluctuating clearance rates of the compound.[1] The major dose-limiting toxicity of $^{131}$I tositumomab is myelosuppression, similar to that seen with $^{90}$Y ibritumomab. Therefore, patients must have <25% lymphoma involvement of bone marrow, platelet count >100,000 cells/mm$^3$, and no history of hypocellular marrow or failed stem-cell collection in order to receive drug.[28] Other acute toxicities include infusion-related effects such as nausea, vomiting, skin rash, hypotension, fever, and chills.[45] It is thought that these effects are related to the clearance of CD20+ cells.

### INVESTIGATIONAL AGENTS

Numerous conjugated and unconjugated MoAbs are currently under development for the treatment of hematologic malignancies (Table 103.3). This area of research is expanding, with technological advancements rapidly increasing the spectrum of use beyond the current scope. The lymphomas and leukemias are subjects of many clinical trials, from identification of cellular surface proteins and genetic mutations to targeting specific antibodies, cell signaling pathways, and cytokines. Combination MoAb therapy is another avenue that is being explored.[58]

### Epratuzumab (LL2)

Epratuzumab is a humanized IgG1-κ MoAb targeted to cell surface protein CD22 This compound was initially developed in murine form and later genetically engineered to a humanized form. CD22 is mainly expressed on B lymphocytes and has been found in 60–80% of B-cell malignancies.[59] Because of its specificity for B lymphocytes, and relative lack of toxicity toward other cell lines, epratuzumab is considered an attractive agent for use in heavily pretreated lymphoma populations. Both human and murine forms are currently being investigated. Additionally, cold antibody, as well as radiolabeled ($^{131}$I and $^{90}$Yttrium) compounds, are being evaluated. Epratuzumab is rapidly internalized upon binding to CD22-expressing cells, and the main mechanism of toxicity is thought to be ADCC; CMC and direct apoptosis have not been observed in in vitro studies.[60]

Epratuzumab has been studied in relapsed and refractory B-cell malignancies. The compound was administered intravenously, with doses ranging from 120 to 1000 mg/m$^2$/week in phase I studies.[61] Premedication with acetaminophen and diphenhydramine was included to minimize infusion reactions. Patients tolerated treatment well, as most infusion reactions were considered grade 1 and no dose-limiting toxicity was reached. In this initial treatment-refractory group of 40 patients, 3 CRs and 6 PRs were observed.[61] Combination therapy with epratuzumab has also been evaluated.[58] In fact, the first trial of combination MoAb therapy included this agent. Epratuzumab and rituximab target two distinct cell

**Table 103.3** Monoclonal antibodies under investigation for hematologic malignancies

| Compound | Target | Cellular expression | Investigational hematologic uses | Approved clinical uses |
|---|---|---|---|---|
| Infliximab (Remicade®) | TNF-α | Numerous cell lines, including macrophages, are activated by TNF-α[48] | Steroid-refractory GVHD[49] | Rheumatoid arthritis, Crohn's disease[48] |
| Basiliximab (Simulect®) | CD25 | Activated T-lymphocytes[50] | Steroid-refractory GVHD[51] | Transplant rejection |
| Daclizumab (Zenapax®) | CD25 | Activated T-lymphocytes | Steroid-refractory GVHD[52] | Transplant rejection |
| Bevacizumab (Avastin®) | VEGFR | Overexpressed in a variety of malignancies[53] | Refractory AML[54] | Colorectal cancer |
| Epratuzumab (LL2) | CD22 | B lymphocytes | B-cell lymphomas, follicular NHL[22] | [a]Investigational |
| Apolizumab (HU1D10) | HLA-DR | B lymphocytes | B-cell malignancies, relapsed NHL | [a]Investigational |
| Lumiliximab (IDEC-125) | CD23 | IgE, CLL cells[22,55,56] | Relapsed CLL | [a]Allergic asthma |
| EB10 | FLT-3 (FMS-like tyrosine kinase 3) | 90% AML leukemic blasts[57] | AML | [a]Investigational |
| SGN-30 | CD30 | Activated T lymphocytes, activated B lymphocytes, and activated NK cells[58] | Hodgkin's disease | [a]Anaplastic large cell lymphoma |

[a]Agents currently in clinical trials, not yet FDA approved.

surface proteins and therefore may act synergistically. Preliminary results show that combination therapy has been well-tolerated, with most patients demonstrating objective responses.[58] It remains to be seen whether initial results will be confirmed upon further evaluation. However, combination therapy is an exciting therapeutic avenue to explore, potentially offering improved efficacy by targeting two different cell surface proteins.

### Apolizumab(HU1D10)

Apolizumab is another humanized IgG1MoAb currently under investigation. This compound is designed to target the antigenic determinant 1D10, which binds to the β chain variant of human leukocyte antigen-DR (HLA-DR). This 1D10 antigenic determinant is expressed primarily by lymphocytes, macrophages, and mesenchymal dendritic cells.[62] While it is found on normal B lymphocytes, monocytes, and dendritic cells, it is also expressed on a proportion of NHL and CLL cells.[63] A recent study evaluated flow cytometry immunophenotyping of lymphoid malignancies in 105 patients <21 years of age. Results showed that 87/87 (100%) patients with pre-B cell ALL expressed HLA-DR and 3/3 (100%) patients with Burkitt lymphoma expressed this

antigen. However, only 2 out of 11 (18%) patients with T-cell malignancies exhibited a positive result for HLA-DR.[64] Thus, HU1D10 targets an important cell surface protein expressed in leukemias and lymphomas of B-cell origin. HU1D10 stimulates CMC, ADCC, and caspase-independent, direct apoptosis of cells expressing 1D10 antigen.[62,63] A few phase I studies are currently evaluating patients with relapsed B-cell lymphomas; preliminary results indicate manageable toxicity, consisting mainly of grade 1–2 adverse effects.[65–67] In one study, three of six patients with follicular lymphoma treated with 4 weekly infusions exhibited partial responses. These responses were delayed in nature, occurring at a median of 106 days and improving up to 400 days after treatment.[66] Authors suggest a unique mechanism of action due to this pattern of response, and further studies may help clarify the activity of HU1D10, including a potential role in combination therapy.

## CONCLUSIONS

After many long and arduous years of research and development, MoAbs are finally beginning to play a pivotal role not only in cancer therapeutics, but in other disease states as well. Laboratory techniques enabling the chimerization or humanization of antibodies has resulted in significant improvement in the tolerability of these compounds. Additionally, advancements in bioreactor capabilities have enabled companies to meet commercial demands for these products. Developments in recombinant technology involving linkers, toxins, and radiolabeled isotopes will lead to the availability of more MoAbs for routine clinical use. Future studies will center on genomics, and genetic mutations found within cells that affect cellular signaling pathways. Detailed knowledge of these pathways will allow for combination regimens that concurrently target multiple areas in the malignant transformation of a cell. This opens the door for highly explicit treatment regimens that minimize toxicity to healthy cells, while maximizing toxicity to malignant clones.

## REFERENCES

1. Stern M, Herrmann R: Overview of monoclonal antibodies in cancer therapy: present and promise. *Crit Rev Oncol/Hematol* 54:11–29, 2005.
2. Pressman D, Korngold L: The in vivo localization of anti-Wegner osteogenic sarcoma antibody. *Cancer* 6:619–623, 1953.
3. Porter RR: The structure of antibodies. *Sci Am* 217(4): 81–87, 1967.
4. Kohler G, Milstein C: Continuous cultures of fused cells secreting antibody of predefined specificity. *Nature* 256(5517): 495–497, 1975.
5. Multani PS, Grossbard ML: Monoclonal antibody-based therapies for hematologic malignancies. *J Clin Oncol* 16:3691–3710, 1998.
6. Qu Z, Griffiths GL, Wegener WA, et al.: Development of humanized antibodies as cancer therapeutics. *Methods* 36:84–95, 2005.
7. http://www.fda.gov/cder/biologics/biologics_table.htm.
8. Lui NS, O'Brien S: Monoclonal antibodies in the treatment of chronic lymphocytic leukemia. *Med Oncol* 21(4):297–304, 2004.
9. Plosker GL, Figgitt DP: Rituximab: a review of its use in non-Hodgkin's lymphoma and chronic lymphocytic leukaemia. *Drugs* 63(8):803–843, 2003.
10. Maloney DG, Grillo-Lopez AJ, Bodkin DJ, et al.: IDEC-C2B8: Results of a phase i multiple-dose trial in patients with relapsed non-Hodgkins lymphoma. *J Clin Oncol* 15(10):3266–3274, 1997.
11. Czuczman M, Grillo-Lopez AJ, McLaughlin P, et al.: IDEC-C2B8 clears bcl-2 (t14;18) in patients with relapsed low-grade or follicular lymphoma. *Proc Am Assoc Can Res* 38:A565, 1997.
12. McLaughlin P, Grillo-Lopez AJ, Link BK, et al.: Rituximab chimeric anti-CD20 monoclonal antibody therapy for relapsed indolent lymphoma: half of patients respond to a four-dose treatment program. *J Clin Oncol* 16:2825–2833, 1998.
13. Coiffier B, Lepage E, Briere J, et al.: CHOP chemotherapy plus rituximab compared with CHOP alone in elderly patients with diffuse large B-cell lymphoma. *NEJM* 24(346)235–242, 2002.
14. Byrd JC, Murphy T, Howard RS, et al.: Rituximab using a thrice weekly dosing schedule in B-cell chronic lymphocytic leukemia and small lymphocytic lymphoma demonstrates clinical activity and acceptable toxicity. *J Clin Oncol* 19:2153–2164, 2001.
15. Berinstein NL, Grillo-Lopez AJ, White CA ,et al.: Association of serum rituximab (IDEC-C2B8) concentration and anti-tumor response in the treatment of recurrent low-grade or follicular non-Hodgkin's lymphoma. *Ann Oncol* 9:995–1001, 1998.
16. Dyer MJ, Hale G, Hayhoe FG, Waldmann H: Effects of Campath-1 antibodies in vivo in patients with lymphoid malignancies: influence of antibody isotype. *Blood* 73(6):1431–1439, 1989.
17. Greenwood J, Gorman SD, Routledge EG, Lloyd IS, Waldmann H: Engineering multiple-domain forms of the therapeutic antibody CAMPATH-1H: effects on complement lysis. *Ther Immunol* 1:247–255, 1994.
18. Osterborg A, Dyer MJS, Bunjes D, et al.: Phase II multicenter study of human CD52 antibody in previously treated chronic lymphocytic leukemia. *J Clin Oncol* 15:1567–1574, 1997.
19. Rai KR, Freter CE, Mercier RJ, et al.: Alemtuzumab in previously treated chronic lymphocytic leukemia patients who also had received fludarabine therapy. *J Clin Oncol* 20:3891–3897, 2002.
20. Keating MJ, Flinn I, Jain V, et al.: Therapeutic role of alemtuzumab (CAMPATH-1H) in patients who have failed fludarabine: results of a large international study. *Blood* 99:3554–3561, 2002.
21. Lundin J, Kimby E, Bjorkholm M, et al.: Phase II trial of subcutaneous anti-CD52 monoclonal antibody alemtuzumab (CAMPATH-1H) as first-line treatment for patients with B-cell chronic lymphocytic leukemia (B-CLL). *Blood* 100:768–773, 2002.
22. Mavromatis B, Cheson BD: Monoclonal antibody therapy of chronic lymphocytic leukemia. *J Clin Oncol* 21(9):1874–1881, 2003.
23. Pawson R, Dyer MJS, Barge R, et al.: Treatment of T-cell prolymphocytic leukemia with human CD52 antibody. *J Clin Oncol* 15:2667–2672, 1997.
24. Keating MJ, Cazin B, Coutre S, et al.: Campath-1H treatment of T-cell prolymphocytic leukemia in patients for whom at least one prior chemotherapy regimen has failed. *J Clin Oncol* 20:205–213, 2002.
25. Dearden CE, Matutes E, Cazin B, et al.: High remission rate in T-cell prolymphocytic leukemia with CAMPATH-1H. *Blood* 98:1721–1726, 2001.
26. Kennedy B, Rawstron A, Carter C, et al.: CAMPATH-1H and fludarabine in combination are highly active in refractory chronic lymphocytic leukemia. *Blood* 99: 2245–2247, 2002.
27. Rai KR, Byrd JC, Peterson B, et al.: A phase II trial of fludarabine followed by alemtuzumab (CAMPATH-1H) in previously untreated chronic lymphocytic leukemia

(CLL) patients with active disease; Cancer and Leukemia Group B (CALGB) Study 19901. *Blood* 100:205a, 2002. [Abstract 772]

28. Cersosimo RJ: Monoclonal antibodies in the treatment of cancer, Part 2. *Am J Health Syst Pharm* 60(16): 1631–1641, 2003.

29. Krietman RJ: Toxin-labeled monoclonal antibodies. *Curr Pharm Biotechnol* 2(4):313–325, 2001.

30. Hertler AA, Frankel AE. Immunotoxins: a clinical review of their use in the treatment of malignancies. *J Clin Oncol* 7(12):1932–1942, 1989.

31. Krietman RJ: Toxin-labeled monoclonal antibodies. *Curr Pharmaceut Biotechnol* 2; 313–325, 2001.

32. Revital N, Cohen C, Denkberg G, Segal D, Reiter Y: Antibody engineering for targeted therapy of cancer: recombinant Fv-immunotoxins. *Curr Pharmaceut Biotechnol* 2, 19–46, 2001.

33. Kreitman RJ: Recombinant immunotoxins for the treatment of hematological malignancies. *Expert Opin Biol Ther* 4(7):1115–1128, 2004.

34. Giles F, Estey E, O'Brien S: Gemtuzumab ozogamicin in the treatment of acute myeloid leukemia. *Cancer* 98(10):2095–2104, 2003.

35. Nabhan C, Tallman MS: Early phase I/II trials with gemtuzumab ozogamicin (Mylotarg) in acute myeloid leukemia. *Clin Lymphoma* 2(suppl 1):S19–S23, 2002.

36. Sievers EL, Larson RA, Stadtmauer EA, et al.: Efficacy and safety of gemtuzumab ozogamicin in patients with CD33 positive acute myeloid leukemia in first relapse. *J Clin Oncol* 19:3244–3254, 2001.

37. Nabhan C, Rundhaugen LM, Riley MB, et al. :Phase II pilot trial of gemtuzumab ozogamicin (GO) as first line therapy in acute myeloid leukemia patients age 65 or older. *Leuk Res.* (1):53–57, 2005.

38. Larson RA, Boogaerts M, Estey E, et al.: Antibody-targeted chemotherapy of older patients with acute myeloid leukemia in first relapse using Mylotarg (gemtuzumab ozogamicin). *Leukemia* 16:1627–1636, 2002.

39. Piccaluga PP, Martinelli G, Rondoni M, et al.: First experience with gemtuzumab ozogamicin plus cytarabine as continuous infusion for elderly acute myeloid leukemia patients. *Leuk Res* 28(9); 987–990, 2004.

40. Cortes J, Tsimberidou AM, Alvarez R, et al.: Mylotarg combined with topotecan and cytarabine in patients with refractory acute mylogenous leukemia. *Cancer Chemother Pharmacol* 50(6); 497–500, 2002.

41. Dowell JA, Korth-Bradley J, Liu H, King SP, Berger MS: Pharmacokinetics of gemtuzumab ozogamicin, an antibody-targeted chemotherapy agent for the treatment of patients with acute myeloid leukemia in first relapse. *J Clin Pharmacol* 41(11):1206–1214, 2001.

42. Gordon LI: Gemtuzumab ozogamicin (Mylotarg) and hepatic veno-occlusive disease: take two acetaminophen, and . . . *Bone Marrow Transplant* 28:811–812. Editorial, 2001.

43. Dillman RO: Radiolabeled Anti-CD20 monoclonal antibodies for the treatment of B-cell lymphoma. *J Clin Oncol* 20(16); 3545–3557, 2002.

44. Goldenberg DM: The role of radiolabeled antibodies in the treatment of non-Hodgkin's lymphoma: the coming of age of radioimmunotherapy. *Crit Rev Oncol* (39); 195–201, 2001.

45. Leonard JP, Frenette G, Dillman RO, et al.: Interim safety and efficacy results of Bexxar™ in a large multicenter expanded access study. *Blood* 98:133a, 2001. [Abstract 559]

46. Witzig TE, White CA, Gordon LI, et al.: Zevalin radioimmunotherapy can be safely administered to patients with relapsed or refractory B cell non-Hodgkin's lymphoma. *Blood* 98:606a, 2001. [Abstract 2539]

47. Davies AJ: Tositumomab and iodine [131I] tositumomab in the management of follicular lymphoma. An oncologist's view. *Q J Nucl Med Mol Imaging* 48(4):305–316, 2004.

48. Jacobsohn DA, Vogelsang GB: Anti-cytokine therapy for the treatment of graft-versus-host disease. *Curr Pharm Des* 10(11):1195–1205, 2004.

49. Ross WA: Treatment of gastrointestinal acute graft-versus-host disease. *Curr Treat Options Gastroenterol* 8(3):249–258, 2005.

50. Kapic E, Becic F, Kusturica J: Basiliximab, mechanism of action and pharmacological properties. *Med Arh* 58(6):373–376, 2004.

51. Ji SQ, Chen HR, Yan HM, et al.: Anti-CD25 monoclonal antibody (basiliximab) for prevention of graft-versus-host disease after haploidentical bone marrow transplantation for hematological malignancies. *Bone Marrow Transplant* 36(4):349–354, 2005.

52. Wolff D, Roessler V, Steiner B, et al.: Treatment of steroid-resistant acute graft-versus-host disease with daclizumab and etanercept. *Bone Marrow Transplant* 35(10):1003–1010, 2005.

53. Richter M, Zhang H: Receptor-targeted cancer therapy. *DNA Cell Biol* 24(5):271–282, 2005.

54. Karp JE, Gojo I, Gocke CD, et al.: Timed sequential therapy (TSTO of relapsed and refractory adult acute myelogenous leukemia (AML) with the anti-vascular endothelial growth factor (VEGF) monoclonal antibody bevacizumab. *Blood* 100:198a, 2002. [Abstract 744].

55. Rosenwasser LJ, Busse WW, Lizambri RG, Olejnik TA, Totoritis MC: Allergic asthma and an anti-CD23 mAb (IDEC-152): results of a phase I, single-dose, dose-escalating clinical trial. *J Allergy Clin Immunol* 112(3):563–570, 2003.

56. Reichert JM: Technology evaluation: lumiliximab, Biogen Idec. *Curr Opin Mol Ther* 6(6):675–683, 2004.

57. Williams B, Atkins A, Zhang H, et al.: Cell-based selection of internalizing fully human antagonistic antibodies directed against FLT3 for suppression of leukemia cell growth. *Leukemia* 19(8):1432–1438, 2005.

58. Leonard JP, Coleman M, Matthews JC, et al.: Epratuzumab (anti-CD22) and rituximab (anti-CD20) combination immunotherapy for non-Hodgkin's lymphoma: preliminary response data. *Proc. Am Soc. Clin. Oncol* 266a, 2002.

59. Coleman M, Goldenberg DM, Siegel AB, et al.: Epratuzumab: targeting B-cell malignancies through CD22. *Clin Cancer Res* 9(suppl):3991s–3994s, 2003.

60. Carnahan J, Wang P, Kendall R, et al.: Epratuzumab, a humanized monoclonal antibody targeting CD22: characterization of in vitro properties. *Clin Cancer Res* 9:3982S–3990S, 2003.

61. Leonard JP, Coleman M, Ketas JC, et al.: Phase I/II trial of Epratuzumab (humanized anti-CD22 antibody) in indolent non-Hodgkin's lymphoma. *J Clin Oncol* 21(16):3051–3059, 2003.

62. Shi JD, Bullock C, Hall WC, et al.: In vivo pharmacodynamic effects of Hu1D10 (remitogen), a humanized antibody reactive against a polymorphic determinant of HLA-DR expressed on B cells. *Leuk Lymphoma* 43(6):1303–1312, 2002.

63. Mone AP, Huang P, Pelicano H, et al.: Hu1D10 induces apoptosis concurrent with activation of the AKT survival pathway in human chronic lymphocytic leukemia cells. *Blood* 103(5):1846–1854, 2004.

64. Lones M, Kirov I: Cell surface targets for monoclonal antibody therapy in lymphoid neoplasms of children and adolescents. *Proc Am Soc Hematol* 104:4544, 2004.

65. Link BK, Wang H, Byrd J, et al. :Phase I trial of humanized 1D10 (Hu1D10) monoclonal antibody targeting class II molecules in patients with relapsed lymphoma [abstract]. *Proc Am Soc Clin Oncol* 19:24a, 2000.

66. Link BK, Wang H, Byrd JC, et al.: Phase I study of Hu1D10 monoclonal antibody in patients with B-cell lymphoma. In *2001 ASCO Annual Meeting*, Abstract No. 1135, 2001.

67. Abhyankar VV, Lucas MS, Stock W, et al.: Phase I study of escalated thrice weekly dosing of Hu1D10 in chronic lymphocytic leukemia/small lymphocytic lymphoma (CLL/SLL): minimal toxicity and early observation of in vivo tumor cell apoptosis. *Proc Am Soc Clin Oncol* 1069, 2002.

# Chapter 104

# BLOOD PRODUCT TRANSFUSIONS IN THE HEMATOLOGIC MALIGNANCIES

*Ronald E. Domen*

## INTRODUCTION

Blood transfusion support is critical for patients with hematologic malignancies undergoing aggressive treatment regimens. Stem cell transplantation, as well as other chemotherapy treatment protocols for the hematologic malignancies, is associated with periods of prolonged pancytopenia, i.e., "iatrogenic aplastic anemia," that require the ready availability of specialized blood transfusion support. Such blood banking and transfusion medicine expertise is typically available only in facilities that support the highly specialized treatment of these complicated patients. Although the primary treatment of patients with hematologic malignancies may be performed at specialized or academic medical centers located away from the patient's home, it is often the patient's local or community hospital that is called upon to transfuse blood products in specific or emergent situations after the patient has been discharged home. Although convenient for the patient, the local hospital may not be prepared to address complicated transfusion issues. The need for specialized transfusion support in the hematologic malignancies often continues well beyond the patient's immediate hospitalization and treatment, and not occasionally for the life of the patient.

Transfusion of any blood product involves the risk of an adverse reaction, including disease transmission. Therefore, it is important that a patient who requires a transfusion be transfused only when necessary and only with the specific, indicated blood component. This chapter will consider important topics related to blood product transfusion that have relevancy to any physician who may be called upon to treat patients with hematologic malignancies. In addition, the issue of transfusion in palliative care and the hospice setting will be briefly examined.

## RED BLOOD CELL TRANSFUSION

Anemia is a common complication in patients with hematologic malignancies. The symptoms of anemia in any given patient can be variable, depending on several, often independent factors: the hemoglobin level, the rapidity of the development of the anemia, the patient's age, and the presence of underlying disease.[1] In general, red blood cell transfusion is indicated to relieve or prevent the signs and symptoms of hypoxemia. Ideally, the decision to transfuse should be individualized and appropriate for each patient and his or her disease process.[1–3] Anemia is usually not associated with significant symptoms until the hemoglobin concentration is less than 7 or 8 g/dL. Symptoms are also related to the rapidity of the fall in hemoglobin concentration and the patient's ability to maintain a normal blood volume. In general, red cell transfusion is usually not indicated when the hemoglobin concentration is >10 g/dL, but it is usually indicated when the hemoglobin concentration is <7 g/dL.[1–3]

Guidelines for the appropriate use of red cell transfusions have been developed and published by several physician groups.[4-6] Common general principles include the following: (1) the cause of anemia should be determined prior to transfusion, if possible, and appropriate specific or alternative therapy instituted (e.g., iron for anemia secondary to iron deficiency, vitamin $B_{12}$ for anemia secondary to vitamin $B_{12}$ deficiency, etc.); (2) clinical judgment for the need for transfusion should be used rather than a universal or automatic "trigger" hemoglobin level for transfusion; (3) a determination and assessment of those symptoms that are to be alleviated should be made; (4) an assessment of the patient's intravascular blood volume should be done and any volume deficiency restored with crystalloid or colloid solutions; (5) patients with underlying cardiovascular or respiratory diseases may need to maintain a hemoglobin concentration >10 g/dL; and (6) the risks and benefits of the transfusion should be discussed with the patient (i.e., informed consent).

Providing compatible red blood cells for transfusion to patients with cancer who have not undergone stem cell transplantation is usually not significantly different than transfusion for any other patient with anemia. The usual principles of specimen collection, serum antibody screening, and crossmatching apply. In general, approximately 3% of all patients transfused with red cells will form an alloantibody to one or more of the foreign red cell antigens.[7] However, approximately 25% of alloantibodies will decrease in titer over time and may no longer be detectable in routine serological tests.[8] If the patient should again be challenged by the specific foreign antigen, an anamnestic response and subsequent hemolytic transfusion reaction may result. Although patients with hematologic malignancies may be immunosuppressed, they may still form red cell alloantibodies following transfusion.

The patient who has undergone an ABO incompatible hematopoietic stem cell transplantation presents unique challenges in providing compatible transfusion support. Approximately 30–40% of patients undergoing an allogeneic hematopoietic stem cell transplantation will receive an ABO incompatible graft from their donors.[9–11] A major ABO mismatch between the donor and recipient is present when a foreign ABO antigen is introduced into the patient. A typical example would be, a group O recipient receiving a transplant from a group A, B, or AB donor.[9,10] In a major ABO mismatch, the recipient has preformed circulating anti-A and/or anti-B isohemagglutinin that could potentially react with newly introduced ABO antigen on the stem cells or on contaminating donor red blood cells. The production of anti-A and/or anti-B may continue for several months following the transplant.[9,10,12–14] Red cells used for transfusion must, therefore, be compatible with both the donor and the recipient. Group O red cells can be given to all major ABO-incompatible recipients in order to avoid confusion.

A minor ABO mismatch involves the introduction of foreign anti-A and/or anti-B isohemagglutinins or lymphocytes capable of producing anti-A or anti-B after engraftment.[9–11] An example is a group A recipient who receives group O or B stem cells (or a group B recipient who receives group O or A stem cells, or a group AB recipient who receives group O, A, or B donor stem cells).

Combined major and minor ABO mismatch occurs when a group A recipient receives group B cells, or when a group B recipient receives group A stem cells.[9,10] In addition, other antigen mismatches (e.g., in the Rh system) may be important in certain clinical situations.[15,16] Passenger lymphocytes from the donor graft may also produce non-ABO antibodies, with resulting immune hemolysis.[15–17]

Major, minor, and combined major and minor ABO mismatched stem cell transplantation can be associated with acute or delayed hemolysis following transfusion of donor cells.[9,10] Acute hemolysis following a major ABO mismatched transplantation can generally be avoided by removing the incompatible red cells prior to transfusion of the graft. Immune hemolysis complicates approximately 10–15% of minor ABO incompatible stem cell transplants.[11] Delayed immune hemolysis can be seen following minor ABO incompatibility, when the transplanted passenger lymphocytes recognize the recipient's A or B antigen as foreign and actively produce anti-A or anti-B. This scenario is more likely to occur when the donor is group O and the recipient is group A or B and is characterized by the onset of immune hemolysis approximately 7–10 days after transplantation. The risk of immune hemolysis following minor ABO incompatibility appears to increase when the donor is unrelated or when cyclosporin is the sole agent used to prevent graft-versus-host disease (GVHD). While the majority of cases of immune hemolysis following minor ABO incompatibility are self-limited and last for 2 weeks or less, rare cases of severe hemolysis following minor ABO incompatibility have been fatal.[11] As noted above, non-ABO antibodies may also be produced by passenger lymphocytes and result in clinically significant immune hemolysis. Guidelines for blood product selection in the stem cell transplant setting are shown in Table 104.1.

Stem cell transplant patients can also suffer acute or delayed hemolytic transfusion reactions secondary to the usual causes for this adverse reaction (e.g., misidentification of blood crossmatching specimens, patient identification errors, laboratory testing errors, etc.) and it should not be assumed that hemolysis is simply secondary to the engraftment of an ABO mismatched bone marrow.[10] Other causes for hemolysis, such as thrombotic thrombocytopenic purpura (TTP), can also complicate the clinical course of patients with hematologic malignancy or stem cell transplantation.

## PLATELET TRANSFUSION

As early as 1910, platelet transfusions were shown to have a beneficial effect in bleeding patients.[18] In the 1960s, the development of plastic blood collection and storage bags allowed the ready concentration and storage of platelets. In 1964, investigators at the National Cancer Institute reported the efficacy of platelet transfusions in patients undergoing therapy for leukemia.[18]

Thrombocytopenia or decreased platelet function are common complications in patients with hematologic malignancies. Patients with decreased platelet number or function are at increased risk for hemorrhage. The normal lifespan of a platelet is approximately 9.5–10.5 days and approximately 4–5 days for the transfused platelet.[10,19,20] The splenic pool accounts

**Table 104.1**   Transfusion support for patients undergoing ABO-mismatched allogeneic HPC transplanation[10]

| | | | Phase I | | | Phase II | | | Phase III |
|---|---|---|---|---|---|---|---|---|---|
| Recipient | Donor | Mismatch type | All components | RBCs | First choice platelets | Next choice platelets[a] | FFP | All components | |
| A | O | Minor | Recipient | O | A | AB; B; O | A, AB | Donor | |
| B | O | Minor | Recipient | O | B | AB; A; O | B, AB | Donor | |
| AB | O | Minor | Recipient | O | AB | A; B; O | AB | Donor | |
| AB | A | Minor | Recipient | A | AB | A; B; O | AB | Donor | |
| AB | B | Minor | Recipient | B | AB | B; A; O | AB | Donor | |
| O | A | Major | Recipient | O | A | AB; B; O | A, AB | Donor | |
| O | B | Major | Recipient | O | B | AB; A; O | B, AB | Donor | |
| O | AB | Major | Recipient | O | AB | A; B; O | AB | Donor | |
| A | AB | Major | Recipient | A | AB | A; B; O | AB | Donor | |
| B | AB | Major | Recipient | B | AB | B; A; O | AB | Donor | |
| A | B | Minor & major | Recipient | O | AB | A; B; O | AB | Donor | |
| B | A | Minor & major | Recipient | O | AB | B; A; O | AB | Donor | |

[a]Platelet concentrates should be selected in the order presented.[10]

HPC = hematopoietic progenitor (stem) cell; Phase I = from the time when the patient/recipient is prepared for HPC transplantation; Phase II = from the initiation of myeloablativle therapy until (1) for RBC – DAT is negative and antidonor isohemagglutinins are no longer detectable (i.e., the reverse typing is donor type) and (2) for FFPs – recipients erythrocytes are no longer detectable (i.e., the forward typing is consistent with donor's ABO group); Phase III = after the forward and reverse type of the patient are consistent with donor's ABO group. Beginning from Phase I all cellular components should be irradiated and leukocyte reduced. (*From Ref 10, used with permission.*)

for approximately 30–35% of the total body platelet mass.[19,20] However, platelet lifespan decreases with increasing thrombocytopenia.[21] A number of conditions in the patient with hematologic malignancy can potentially alter platelet numbers or function and can be associated with hemorrhage (Table 104.2). Platelets are generally indicated in bleeding patients with thrombocytopenia and/or platelet dysfunction. Platelet transfusion is generally not indicated in platelet-consumptive states (e.g., ITP or TTP) unless life-threatening bleeding is present.[19,21–23]

Assuming a steady-state condition, there is a fairly direct linear relationship between the platelet count and the bleeding time as the platelet count decreases below 100,000/μL.[21] Serious spontaneous hemorrhage usually does not occur until the platelet count falls below 10,000/μL, and this threshold is used by many physicians for the prophylactic administration of platelets.[24,25] Indeed, otherwise stable thrombocytopenic patients can probably tolerate platelets counts in the 5000–10,000/μL range.[22,23] A higher platelet transfusion "trigger" may be considered in those patients with underlying complications of fever or infection, other coagulation defects (e.g., hypofibrinogenemia), intracranial pathology, or other conditions that affect platelet function or number.[19,22,23] Higher platelet counts are also warranted in those thrombocytopenic patients undergoing invasive procedures or

surgery. A platelet count of 50,000/μL is generally felt to be adequate for many surgeries, and a count in the 30,000–40,000/μL range is probably adequate for needle biopsies.[19–23,26] However, only minimal evidence-based data is available as to what constitutes an optimal platelet count for various invasive procedures.

Platelet components for transfusion are prepared by two primary methods: platelet concentrates (random platelets) or platelets pheresis (apheresis platelets).[10,27] A single platelet concentrate is the unit of platelets obtained from an individual unit of randomly donated whole blood. A platelet concentrate contains at least $5.5 \times 10^{10}$ platelets suspended in 40–70 mL of plasma. The approximate dose for platelet concentrates is 1 unit/ 10 kg of patient body weight. Thus, in the adult patient, the usual transfusable dose would be 4–6 units pooled as a single unit. As each platelet concentrate in a pooled product comes from an individual donor, each pooled transfusion exposes the recipient to that number of donors. Although the risk of transfusion-transmitted infection bears some relationship to the number of donor exposures, the increasing efficacy of donor screening and testing has decreased concerns in this area. Apheresis platelets are collected using cell separator technology, and 1 unit of apheresis platelets contains $\geq 3.0 \times 10^{11}$ platelets suspended in 100–500 mL of plasma. Thus, in the adult patient, a unit of apheresis platelets contains one transfusable dose of platelets.

**Table 104.2   Causes of thrombocytopenia and hemorrhage in patients with hematologic malignancies**

*Decreased platelet production*
Bone marrow injury or failure
  Chemotherapy/drugs
  Radiation
  Infection
  Infiltration by carcinoma, leukemia, or lymphoma
  Marrow fibrosis
  Aplastic anemia
  Hereditary quantitative disorders (e.g., May–Hegglin anomaly, Wiskott–Aldrich syndrome)

Nutritional deficiencies
  Vitamin $B_{12}$ deficiency
  Folic acid deficiency
  Iron deficiency

*Accelerated platelet destruction*
Immune causes
  Autoantibody
    Immune/idiopathic thrombocytopenic purpura (ITP)
    Drug-related (e.g., quinidine, heparin)
  Alloantibody
    Anti-HLA antibodies
    Anti-platelet antibodies
    Post-ransfusion purpura (PTP)

Nonimmune causes
  Disseminated intravascular coagulopathy (DIC)
  Thrombotic thrombocytopenic purpura (TTP)
  Hemolytic-uremic Syndrome (HUS)
  Hemorrhage
  Infection

*Impaired platelet function*
Hereditary qualitative disorders (e.g., von Willebrand disease, Bernard—Soulier syndrome, Gray platelet syndrome)
Paraproteinemia (e.g., marcroglobulinemia, multiple myeloma)
Hepatic and/or renal failure

Drugs
*Disordered platelet distribution*
Splenomegaly
Massive transfusion

Both preparations of platelets are stored at room temperature (20–24°C) for up to 5 days after collection. Room temperature storage has been shown to be conducive to the potential growth of contaminating bacteria and this complication has prompted blood banks to recently institute bacterial surveillance systems for platelets.[28] Transfusion-transmitted bacterial infection should be considered in any patient who develops fever during a platelet transfusion, and appropriate cultures from the platelet product and the patient should be obtained.[29] Novel platelet products, such as frozen platelets, cold-stored liquid platelets, and lyophilized platelets are in various stages of research and development.[30]

The response to platelet transfusion will depend on the patient's clinical status and can be assessed by (1) whether or not bleeding stops following transfusion and/or (2) measuring the posttransfusion platelet increment 10–60 min after transfusion. The corrected count increment (CCI) is one accurate measure of patient response to platelet transfusion.[10,20,26] The CCI is calculated as follows:

$$CCI = (\text{posttransfusion count } [\mu L] - \text{pretransfusion count } [\mu L]) \times BSA(m^2)/(\text{platelets transfused } (\times 10^{11})),$$

where BSA is the patient's body surface area $(m^2)$. The CCI is generally >7500 at 10-60 min after transfusion and >4500 at 24 h. The predicted platelet count increment (PPCI) and the percent platelet recovery (PPR) are also measures that have been used to evaluate the expected response to platelet transfusion.[10,20,21,26] Others have more simply defined a poor response to prophylactic platelet transfusion as a failure to increase the platelet count above the "trigger" count prior to the transfusion.[22,23]

Platelet refractoriness is defined as the repeated failure (two or more times) to achieve a satisfactory response to platelet transfusions.[22,23] Some authors have used two consecutive failures to achieve a satisfactory response as indicative of refractoriness, while others have used two to three failures (not necessarily consecutive) over a 2-week period. A number of immune and nonimmune factors can contribute to decreased platelet increments following transfusions (Table 104.2).[19,22,23,31] The primary immune cause of platelet refractoriness is HLA alloimmunization, but its incidence has declined in recent years primarily due to the recognition that leukocyte reduction of blood components helps to prevent HLA alloimmunization. Nonimmune causes of platelet refractoriness, such as infection and splenomegaly, are important reasons associated with decreased platelet survival following transfusion. The Trial to Reduce Alloimmunization to Platelets (TRAP) Study Group found that for patients with AML, the incidence of HLA alloimmunization was 33% in those who had never been pregnant and 62% in those who had been pregnant.[32] In patients who received leukocyte-reduced blood components, the incidence of HLA alloimmunization was 9% and 32%, respectively.[32]

The management of patients refractory to platelet transfusion can present many challenges.[26] Platelets expressing HLA class I antigens and antibodies to these antigens is one of the primary causes of immune-mediated platelet refractoriness. While HLA matching between the donor and the recipient has been the traditional approach to selecting platelets for alloimmunized patients, other methods, such as platelet crossmatching, have shown efficacy.[26] Blood centers or blood banks that have established standardized platelet crossmatch techniques and procedures can often supply compatible apheresis platelets from their inventory in relatively short periods of time. As blood group A and B antigens are also expressed on platelets, ABO matching of platelets should also be considered in the patient who is refractory.[26,33–35] In addition, anecdotal experience supports a trial of random, pooled platelet concentrates for the patient who has been receiving only apheresis platelets. A random mix of HLA types in a pooled platelet concentrate might "bypass" the patient's HLA antibodies. Other approaches to platelet refractoriness, such as the use of intravenous immunoglobulin (IVIG), intravenous Rh-immune globulin, or continuous platelet drips have not been supported by controlled studies.[26] While there is no definitive or standardized approach to managing platelet refractoriness, our approach is presented in Figure 104.1.

## SPECIALIZED BLOOD COMPONENTS

### LEUKOCYTE-REDUCED BLOOD COMPONENTS

There are three main indications for using red blood cell and platelet components that are leukocyte-reduced: (1) to decrease or prevent the occurrence of febrile, nonhemolytic transfusion reactions, (2) to reduce the incidence of HLA alloimmunization, and (3) to prevent or reduce the risk of transfusion-transmitted

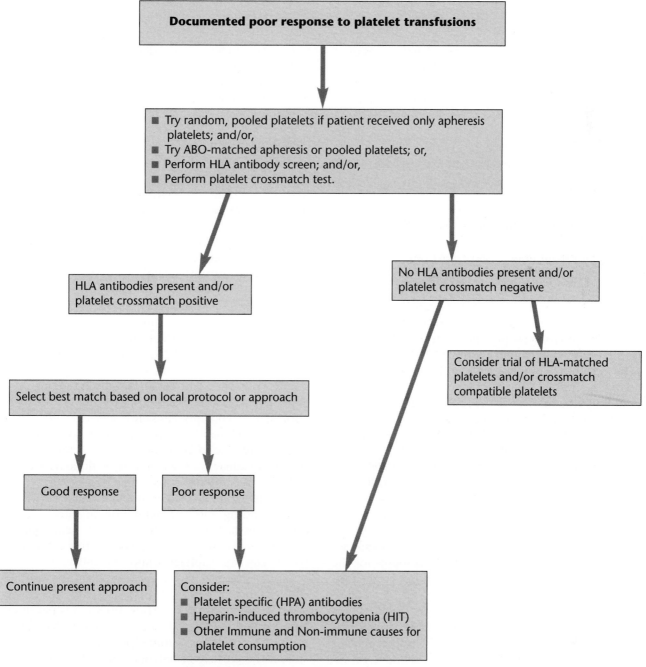

**Figure 104.1** *Algorithm for evaluation of platelet refractoriness*

cytomegalovirus (TT-CMV) infection.[22,23] Other clinical uses of leukocyte-reduced blood components, such as reducing transfusion-related immunomodulation, or reducing other transfusion-transmitted infections (e.g., EBV, HHV-8, HTLV-I/II, etc.), should be considered experimental until additional studies are performed. Leukocyte reduction has not been shown to prevent transfusion-associated GVHD (TA-GVHD; see below).[36,37]

A unit of whole blood contains approximately $\geq 1$–$10 \times 10^9$ white blood cells.[10] Leukocyte reduction can be performed during or shortly after collection (prestorage leukocyte reduction), in the laboratory prior to issuing of the blood component (poststorage leukocyte reduction), or at the bedside. The first two methods are preferable, as bedside leukocyte reduction lacks proper quality control measures to achieve uniform leukocyte reduction.[38] Red blood cells and platelets (pooled platelets and apheresis platelets) are considered to be leukocyte-reduced if the residual leukocyte count is $<5 \times 10^6$. In addition to the use of specialized filters to achieve leukocyte reduction, apheresis platelets can also be considered leukocyte-reduced if the residual leukocyte count is $<5 \times 10^6$ at the time of collection.

Some blood centers in the United States, as well as a number of countries, have promoted and instituted universal leukocyte reduction of all blood components for all patients.

### Leukocyte reduction for febrile, nonhemolytic transfusion reactions

Febrile, nonhemolytic (FNH) transfusion reaction is one of the most frequent adverse reactions related to transfusion.[39] In addition to a rise in temperature ($\geq 1°C$), FNH transfusion reactions can be associated with chills, rigors, headaches, nausea, and/or vomiting.[39] Symptoms typically appear during the transfusion, but may not manifest until 1–2 h later. Usually, FNH transfusion reactions are not life-threatening, but can be associated with increased patient discomfort requiring the administration of additional medications. In addition, fever can also be a manifestation of more severe transfusion reactions (e.g., hemolytic transfusion reactions or bacterial contamination).

Leukocyte reduction for the prevention of FNH reactions is more effective in the case of red blood cell transfusions and less effective for platelet transfusions.[39–42] FNH transfusion reactions can have multiple causes related to both recipient and donor factors, but in the case of platelets, the release of inflammatory cytokines by leukocytes during storage probably accounts for the majority of reactions. Prestorage leukocyte reduction helps to further decrease the incidence of platelet-related FNH reactions by decreasing the passive accumulation of cytokines released by white cells. IL-1α is one of the primary cytokines felt to be responsible for FNH reactions following platelet transfusion. TNFα, IL-6, and IL-8 have also been shown to accumulate in plasma during platelet storage, but the role played by these cytokines in contributing to FNH reactions is unclear.[39,43]

There is suggestive evidence that some severe hypotensive reactions following the transfusion of leukocyte-reduced blood components may be related to the infusion of bradykinin.[39,43] It is speculated that bradykinin is generated during the filtration process when certain leukocyte-depletion filters are used. These hypotensive reactions may be enhanced if the recipient, or the donor, is taking angiotensin converting enzyme (ACE) inhibitor medications.[39,43]

### HLA alloimmunization and leukocyte reduction

A number of studies have been performed that demonstrate the efficacy of leukocyte reduction to prevent HLA alloimmunization.[32,44-48] As platelets have HLA class I antigens, leukocyte reduction has been shown to decrease the incidence of refractoriness to platelet transfusion (see above). There does not appear to be any significant effect of leukocyte reduction on the incidence of platelet refractoriness secondary to platelet-specific antibody. All patients who are potential candidates for stem cell transplantation should receive leukocyte-reduced blood transfusions to minimize the formation of HLA antibodies. In our institution, as in many others, all patients with hematologic and solid tumor malignancies routinely receive leukocyte-reduced blood products from the time of initial diagnosis.

### CMV "safe" blood components and leukocyte reduction

Transfusion-transmitted CMV (TT-CMV) infection was first described in 1966. The incidence of CMV seropositivity in the blood donor population ranges from 60% to 80% or higher, depending on the geographic area. Prior to the advent of current leukocyte-reduction filters, providing CMV "safe" blood products required the collection of blood from CMV-seronegative blood donors. However, despite seronegativity, some donors may still be able to transmit CMV (approximately 4% of seronegative blood products are associated with a risk of TT-CMV), and maintaining a separate inventory of CMV-seronegative blood is problematical.[49,50] Some blood centers no longer routinely test blood donors for CMV.

Following primary infection, CMV remains latent in various white blood cell populations, but periodic viral shedding and/or reactivation of infection may occur. Sites of latency include CD34+ hematopoietic progenitor (stem) cells, CD33+ progenitor cells, monocytes (macrophages), and probably granulocytes. Monocytes appear to be one of the primary sites of CMV latency.[50–53] In healthy, CMV-seropositive blood donors, approximately 0.004–0.12% of peripheral blood mononuclear cells are latently infected.[52] Over the years, a growing number of studies have demonstrated the efficacy of leukocyte reduction in making blood components CMV "safe" for the prevention of

TT-CMV in hematologic and stem cell transplant patients.[51–60] However, some studies question the efficacy of leukocyte reduction in preventing TT-CMV.[61] Improved methods to monitor and detect CMV antigenemia and infection in the immunosuppressed patient have led to early detection and treatment of infection.[62,63] In addition, emerging data indicates that other factors, such as the seropositive stem cell transplant recipient, the degree of immunosuppression, and the stage of acute GVHD put the recipient at greater risk for CMV infection/disease because of reactivation of latent virus, rather than through the acquisition of new infection through blood transfusion.[64–66]

While specific data is lacking, a number of institutions have used leukocyte reduction as the sole method for providing CMV-safe blood components. The only cellular blood component that cannot be leukocyte-reduced is granulocytes. If CMV status of the donor is important in those rare instances when granulocyte transfusions are considered for the infected patient with a hematologic malignancy, consideration should be given to test the donor for CMV (see below).

### IRRADIATION OF BLOOD COMPONENTS

TA-GVHD is a rare, potentially lethal disorder caused by the engraftment and proliferation of donor lymphocytes in the transfusion recipient.[36,67] Viable donor lymphocytes in the transfused blood component recognize the HLA antigens of the recipient and mount an immune response. TA-GVHD was first reported almost four decades ago and, to date, over 200 cases of TA-GVHD have been reported. The true incidence is unknown, as it is thought that many patients with TA-GVHD go unrecognized and additional cases are underreported, but it is estimated that TA-GVHD occurs in 0.1–1.0% of patients with hematologic malignancies.[67,68] While TA-GVHD occurs more commonly in immunocomprised patients, numerous cases have occurred in immunocompetent patients.

TA-GVHD can be prevented by gamma irradiation of blood components prior to transfusion. The standard dose of irradiation is 2500 cGy (25 Gy or 2500 rad) targeted to the central portion of the container, and a minimum of 1500 cGy targeted to all other areas of the component. The maximum dose should not exceed 5000 cGy.[67,68] The only indication for the irradiation of blood is to prevent TA-GVHD. Those at risk for TA-GVHD are still being defined, but most authorities would agree that the patient groups listed in Table 104.3 should receive irradiated blood components.[67–70] Some hospitals have opted to simply irradiate their entire blood supply in order to avoid this complication of transfusion.

All cellular blood products have been implicated in causing TA-GVHD. The clinical presentation of TA-GVHD generally includes fever, rash, diarrhea, and evidence of liver dysfunction.[67,68] Fever is often the presenting sign and may occur as early as 4 days

**Table 104.3    Patients at risk for TA-GVHD who should receive irradiated blood products[67–70]**

**Significant risk**
Patients undergoing hematopoietic stem cell transplantation (allogeneic or autologous)
Recipients of a stem cell transplant (allogeneic or autologous)
Congenital immunodeficiency syndromes
Intrauterine transfusions
Exchange transfusions in neonates
Patients receiving HLA-matched platelet transfusions or donors known to be haplotype-homozygous
Patients with Hodgkin's lymphoma
Transfusions from biologic (blood) relatives
Chronic lymphocytic leukemia treated with highly immunosuppressive purine analogues (e.g., fludarabine)

**Possible/probable risk**
Other hematologic malignancies (e.g., acute leukemia, non-Hodgkin's lymphoma)
Immunosuppressed patients with solid tumors receiving immunosuppressive and myeloblative thrapy (e.g., neuroblastoma, rhabdomyosarcoma, glioblastoma, immunoblastic sarcoma)
Immunosuppressed solid organ transplant recipients
Premature neonates
Recipient-donor pairs from genetically homogeneous populations (e.g., Japan)

**No defined risk**
Patients with acquired immunodeficiency syndrome (AIDS)
Full-term, healthy neonates
Patients receiving immunosuppressive medications

posttransfusion. Pancytopenia (particularly leukopenia and thrombocytopenia) develops late in the course (median 16 days).[67,68] Infection or hemorrhage are the most common causes of death, occurring within 3 weeks of onset.[67,68] Treatment is rarely effective, and the mortality rate is >90%.[67,68] In our institution, as in many others, patients with hematologic malignancies, as well as those who have undergone stem cell transplantation, routinely receive irradiated blood products from the time of initial diagnosis.

### WASHED AND VOLUME-REDUCED BLOOD COMPONENTS

The typical unit of red blood cells for transfusion is already volume-reduced (i.e., low volume or "packed"). Platelets can also be volume-reduced prior to transfusion if there is a clinical need to limit the patient's intake of fluids.[10]

The washing of red cells and platelets is typically performed with 0.9% sodium chloride (normal saline). Washing effectively removes most of the plasma in the unit of red cells or platelets. Limiting a patient's exposure to donor plasma may be indicated for the recipient who is IgA-deficient and in whom there is concern about exposure to IgA-containing plasma, or if the plasma contains a specific protein or antibody that might be detrimental to the recipient.[71,72] A patient known to have anaphylactic/anaphylactoid reactions to allogeneic plasma may also be a candidate for washed blood components.[71,72] In the case of red blood cells, if there are clinical concerns about the recipient receiving potassium, washing may also be indicated to remove potassium that has accumulated in the plasma during storage or following irradiation. Both red cells and platelets are typically lost during the washing process. Washing is not effective in removing infectious agents, and thus does not decrease the potential for transfusion-transmitted infection. Washing is also not effective in removing significant numbers of white blood cells (i.e., for rendering a component leukocyte-reduced).[10]

## GRANULOCYTE TRANSFUSION

Infection remains one of the leading causes of death in the hematologic malignancies, and the transfusion of granulocytes to the neutropenic, infected patient has been attempted with varying levels of success as a therapeutic adjunct.[73–77] Typically, granulocytes are collected from normal donors by apheresis techniques using hydroxyethyl starch (HES) following corticosteroid administration.[10,73,74] Corticosteroid administration to the normal donor enhances the number of granulocytes collected, and HES is a red cell sedimenting agent that promotes separation of the granulocytes from contaminating red cells during collection. The final product should contain at least $1 \times 10^{10}$ granulocytes.[10] Granulocytes should be maintained at 20–24°C without agitation, and must be transfused within 24 h of collection. Once initiated, a course of granulocyte transfusion therapy should be continued at least daily for 4–5 days. Granulocytes should be administered through a standard blood infusion set, but leukocyte-reduction filters are contraindicated. If a CMV-safe granulocyte product is desired then the donor's CMV status must be determined, although the importance of testing the donor for CMV has been questioned by some.[78,79] Granulocytes contain significant amounts of contaminating red blood cells and should thus be ABO and Rh compatible with the recipient. If the recipient also has red cell alloantibodies, then the donor's red cells should be negative for the corresponding antigen(s). If necessary, granulocytes can be irradiated prior to administration.

The indications for granulocyte transfusion typically include patients who have (1) a polymorphonuclear leukocyte (PMN) count <500/μL, (2) a documented infection, and (3) are unresponsive to antibiotic therapy (generally for at least 48 h).[73,74,77] It is also expected that the patient, and his or her bone marrow, will recover once the infection is controlled. Most patients will experience FNH transfusion reactions during or following granulocyte transfusion. In addition, a significant percentage of recipients will develop antileukocyte antibodies following repeated granulocyte transfusions. Pulmonary reactions (e.g., infiltrates, hypoxia, or dyspnea) are also commonly seen after granulocyte transfusions.[73,74,77] These reactions can often be treated symptomatically, but more severe adverse reactions, such as transfusion-related acute lung injury (TRALI), can also be seen.[80] Although not commonly reported following granulocyte transfusion, TRALI can cause significant morbidity and mortality. The administration of amphotericin B in close proximity to granulocyte transfusions has been reported to cause pulmonary reactions.[73,77] This has been disputed but, when feasible, separating the administration of both by several hours seems prudent.

The prophylactic use of granulocytes has not been supported by most randomized studies in the literature.[73–77] In addition, not all types of infection respond equally to a course of granulocyte transfusion therapy. For example, fungal infections appear to be less responsive than bacterial infections.[73–77] Because of the conflicting data on efficacy, the use of granulocytes has decreased over the years. More recent studies have focused on the number of granulocytes collected from donors. With the ready availability of granulocyte colony-stimulating factor (G-CSF), increased interest has been directed towards using G-CSF, with or without concurrent dexamethasone administration, to stimulate the formation and collection of larger numbers of PMNs in donors.[81-83] Several studies have demonstrated the feasibility of collecting large numbers of PMN's from normal donors, but the efficacy of granulocytes collected in this manner remains to be proven.[84] In addition, the side effects associated with G-CSF administration has raised ethical concerns of its usage in otherwise healthy donors.[85] The use of G-CSF in normal donors should only be performed as part of formal research protocols, and a national donor registry should be established to collect safety and efficacy data.[85]

## TRANSFUSION IN PALLIATIVE CARE

There are relatively few studies related to transfusion therapy in the palliative care and hospice settings, although anemia and its associated symptoms may be evident in these patients. Although bleeding may be an indication for transfusion, the relief of symptoms related to anemia, such as weakness or shortness of breath, are probably more common in this setting.[86] Fatigue and mood disturbances are common in patients with advanced cancer.[87] Anemia, and related nutritional deficiencies (e.g., iron deficiency), have been shown to be contributory factors to causing fatigue, impaired cognitive function, poor concentration, memory problems, and other related symptoms.[87–91] Transfusion, with or without erythropoietin, can be considered for these quality of life issues for patients in the terminal stages of cancer, rather than for any possible prolongation of life when, quality may not be significantly altered.[92-94] Transfusions can be administered in the patient's home as well as in conventional care settings; however, home transfusion therapy requires greater commitment and communication between care givers in order to provide safe and efficient transfusion therapy.[95-98] Home transfusion therapy, and transfusion in the hospice setting, has been well-received by those patients unable or unwilling to travel to the hospital or infusion unit.[99-101] If palliative care initiatives for adult and pediatric patients are to be performed in the home, then transfusion therapy should be given consideration in this setting. Adverse reactions to transfusions should be handled with the same due diligence as in any other conventional care setting in order to guard against and prevent any increased morbidity and mortality.[97-101]

## SUMMARY

The use of specialized blood products in patients with hematologic malignancies is an important part of the therapeutic and supportive care of these patients. While the indications for red cell transfusion are essentially the same for any patient who has anemia, platelets and other specialized components have unique requirements in this group of patients. The ready availability of leukocyte-reduced and/or irradiated blood components are essential elements for optimal patient care. Close cooperation and consultation between the treating physicians and the transfusion service are critical, as these patients can present many transfusion-related challenges. Transfusion medicine specialists should be readily available for consultation.

## REFERENCES

1. Stehling L, Simon TL: The red blood cell transfusion trigger: physiology and clinical studies. *Arch Pathol Lab Med* 118:429–434, 1994.
2. Rossi EC: Red cell transfusion therapy in chronic anemias. *Hematol Oncol Clin North Am* 8:1045–1052, 1994.
3. Welch HG, Meehan KR, Goodnough LT: Prudent strategies for elective red blood cell transfusion. *Ann Intern Med* 116:393–402, 1992.
4. American College of Physicians. Practice strategies for elective red blood cell transfusion. *Ann Intern Med* 116:403–406, 1992.
5. A Report by the American Society of Anesthesiologists Task Force on Blood Component Therapy. Practice guidelines for blood component therapy. *Anesthesiology* 84:732–747, 1996.
6. British Committee for Standards in Haematology. Guidelines for the clinical use of red cell transfusions. *Br J Haematol* 113:24–31, 2001.
7. Hoeltge GA, Domen RE, Rybicki LA, Schaffer PA: Multiple red cell transfusions and alloimmunization: experience with 6996 antibodies detected in a total of 159, 262 patients from 1985 to 1993. *Arch Pathol Lab Med* 119:42–45, 1995.
8. Schonewille H, Haak HL, van Zijl AM: RBC antibody persistence. *Transfusion* 40:1127–1131, 2000.
9. Friedberg RC: Transfusion therapy in the patient undergoing hematopoietic stem cell transplantation. *Hematol Oncol Clin of North Am* 8:1105–1116, 1994.
10. Brecher ME (ed.): *Technical Manual*, 14th edn. Bethesda, MD: AABB Press; 2002.
11. Bolan CD, Childs RW, Procter JL, Barrett AJ, Leitman SF: Massive immune haemolysis after allogeneic peripheral blood stem cell transplantation with minor ABO incompatibility. *Br J Haematol* 112:787–795, 2001.
12. Sniecinski IJ, Petz LD, Oien L, Blume KG: Immunohematologic problems arising from ABO incompatible bone marrow transplantation. *Transplant Proceed* 19:4609–4611, 1987.
13. Sniecinski IJ, Oien L, Petz LD, Blume KG: Immunohematologic consequences of major ABO-mismatched bone marrow transplantation. *Transplantation* 45:530–534, 1988.

14. Lee JH, Lee JH, Choi SJ, et al.: Changes in isoagglutinin titres after ABO-incompatible allogeneic stem cell transplantation. *Br J Haematol* 120:702–710, 2003.
15. de la Rubia J, Arriaga F, Andreu R, et al.: Development of non-ABO RBC alloantibodies in patients undergoing allogeneic HPC transplantation: is ABO incompatibility a predisposing factor? *Transfusion* 41:106–110, 2001.
16. Sokol RJ, Stamps R, Booker DJ, et al.: Posttransplant immune-mediated hemolysis. *Transfusion* 42:198–204, 2002.
17. Mytilineos ALJ, Voso MT, Weber-Nordt R, Liebisch P, Lensing C, Schraven B: Passenger lymphocyte syndrome with severe hemolytic anemia due to an anti-Jka after allogeneic PBPC transplantation. *Transfusion* 40:632–636, 2000.
18. Slichter SJ: Controversies in platelet transfusion therapy. *Ann Rev Med* 31:509–540, 1980.
19. Hussein MA, Hoeltge GA: Platelet transfusion therapy for medical and surgical patients. *Clev Clin J Med* 63:245–250, 1996.
20. Davis KB, Slichter SJ, Corash L: Corrected count increment and percent platelet recovery as measures of posttransfusion platelet response: problems and a solution. *Transfusion* 39:586–592, 1999.
21. Slichter SJ: Platelet transfusion therapy. *Hematol Oncol Clin North Am* 4:291–311, 1990.
22. Schiffer CA, Anderson KC, Bennett CL, et al.: Platelet transfusion for patients with cancer: clinical practice guidelines of the American Society of Clinical Oncology. *J Clin Oncol* 19:1519–1538, 2001.
23. British Committee for Standards in Haematology, Blood Transfusion Task Force. Guidelines for the use of platelet transfusions. *Br J Haematol* 122:10–23, 2003.
24. Wandt H, Frank M, Ehninger G, et al.: Safety and cost effectiveness of a $10 \times 10^9/L$ trigger for prophylactic platelet transfusions compared with the traditional $20 \times 10^9/L$ trigger: a prospective comparative trial in 105 patients with acute myeloid leukemia. Blood 91: 3601–3606, 1998.
25. Lawrence JB, Yomtovian RA, Hammons T, et al.: Lowering the prophylactic platelet transfusion threshold: a prospective analysis. *Leuk Lymphoma* 41:67–76, 2001.

26. Sacher RA, Kickler TS, Schiffer CA, Sherman LA, Bracey AW, Shulman IA: Management of patients refractory to platelet transfusion. *Arch Pathol Lab Med* 127:409–414, 2003.

27. Silberman S: Platelets: preparations, transfusion, modifications, and substitutes. *Arch Pathol Lab Med* 123:889–894, 1999.

28. Burns KH, Werch JB: Bacterial contamination of platelet units: a case report and literature survey with review of upcoming American Association of Blood Banks requirements. *Arch Pathol Lab Med* 128:279–281, 2004.

29. Sazama K, DeChristopher PJ, Dodd R, et al.: Practice parameter for the recognition, management, and prevention of adverse consequences of blood transfusion. *Arch Pathol Lab Med* 124:61–70, 2000.

30. Blajchman MA: Novel treatment modalities: new platelet preparations and substitutes. *Br J Haematol* 114:496–505, 2001.

31. Doughty HA, Murphy MF, Metcalfe P, Rohatiner AZS, Lister TA, Waters AH: Relative importance of immune and non-immune causes of platelet refractoriness. *Vox Sang* 66:200–205, 1994.

32. The Trial to Reduce Alloimmunization to Platelets Study Group. Leukocyte reduction and ultraviolet B irradiation of platelets to prevent alloimmunization and refractoriness to platelet transfusions. *N Engl J Med* 337:1861–1869, 1997.

33. Ogasawara K, Ueki J, Takenaka M, Furihata K: Study on the expression of ABH antigens on platelets. *Blood* 82:993–999, 1993.

34. Curtis BR, Edwards JT, Hessner MJ, Klein JP, Aster RH: Blood group A and B antigens are strongly expressed on platelets of some individuals. *Blood* 96:1574–1581, 2000.

35. Heal JM, Blumberg N, Masel D: An evaluation of cross-matching, HLA, and ABO matching for platelet transfusions to refractory patients. *Blood* 70:23–30, 1987.

36. Anderson KC, Weinstein HJ: Transfusion-associated graft-versus-host disease. *N Engl J Med* 323:315–321, 1990.

37. Hayashi H, Nishiuchi T, Tamura H, Takeda K: Transfusion-associated graft-versus-host disease caused by leukocyte-filtered stored blood. *Anesthesiology* 79:1419–1421, 1993.

38. Williamson LM, Wimperis JZ, Williamson P, et al.: Bedside filtration of blood products in the prevention of HLA alloimmunization – a prospective randomized study. *Blood* 83:3028–3035, 1994.

39. Heddle NM, Kelton JG: Febrile nonhemolytic transfusion reactions. In: Popovsky MA (ed.) Transfusion Reactions, 2nd edn. *Bethesda,* MD: AABB Press; 2001:45–82.

40. Heddle NM, Klama LN, Griffith L, Roberts R, Shukla G, Kelton JG: A prospective study to identify the risk factors associated with acute reactions to platelet and red cell transfusions. *Transfusion* 33:794–797, 1993.

41. Heddle NM, Klama L, Meyer R, et al.: A randomized controlled trial comparing plasma removal with white cell reduction to prevent reactions to platelets. *Transfusion* 39:231–238, 1999.

42. Enright H, Davis K, Gernsheimer T, McCullough JJ, Woodson R, Slichter SJ: Factors influencing moderate to severe reactions to PLT transfusions: experience of the TRAP multicenter clinical trial. *Transfusion* 43:1545–1552, 2003.

43. Roback JD, Hillyer CD: Adverse reactions to platelet transfusions. In: Kickler TS, Herman JH (eds.) *Current Issues in Platelet Transfusion Therapy and Platelet Alloimmunity.* Bethesda, MD: AABB Press; 1999:247–285.

44. Gmur J, von Felten A, Osterwalder B, et al.: Delayed alloimmunization using random single donor platelet transfusions: a prospective study in thrombocytopenic patients with acute leukemia. *Blood* 62:473–479, 1983.

45. van Marwijk Kooy M, van Prooijen HC, Moes M, Bosma-Stants I, Akkerman JWN: Use of leukocyte-depleted platelet concentrates for the prevention of refractoriness and primary HLA alloimmunization: a prospective, randomized trail. *Blood* 77:201–205, 1991.

46. Freidberg RC, Donnelly SF, Boyd JC, Gray LS, Mintz PD: Clinical and blood bank factors in the management of platelet refarctoriness and alloimmunization. *Blood* 81:3428–3434, 1993.

47. Ishida A, Handa M, Wakui M, Okamoto S, Kamakura M, Ikeda Y: Clinical factors influencing posttransfusion platelet increment in patients undergoing hematopoietic progenitor cell transplantation–a prospective analysis. *Transfusion* 38:839–847, 1998.

48. Seftel MD, Growe GH, Petraszko T, et al.: Universal prestorage leukoreduction in Canada decreases platelet alloimmunization and refractoriness. *Blood* 103:333–339, 2004.

49. Bowden RA: Transfusion-transmitted cytomegalovirus infection. *Hematol Oncol Clin North Am* 9:155–166, 1995.

50. Larsson S, Soderberg-Naucler C, Wang FZ, Moller E: Cytomegalovirus DNA can be detected in peripheral blood mononuclear cells from all seropositive and most seronegative health blood donors over time. *Transfusion* 38:271–278, 1998.

51. Pamphilon DH, Rider JR, Barbara JAJ, Williamson LM: Prevention of transfusion-transmitted cytomegalovirus infection. *Transfusion Med* 9:115–123, 1999.

52. Roback JD: CMV and blood transfusions. *Rev Med Virol* 12:211–219, 2002.

53. Ljungman P: Risk of cytomegalovirus transmission by blood products to immunocompromised patients and means for reduction. *Br J Haematol* 125:107–116, 2004.

54. Strauss RG: Leukocyte-reduction to prevent transfusion-transmitted cytomegalovirus infections. *Pediatr Transplant* 3(suppl 1):19–22, 1999.

55. Ljungman P, Larsson K, Kumlien G, et al.: Leukocyte depleted, unscreened blood products give a low risk for CMV infection and disease in CMV seronegative allogeneic stem cell transplant recipients with seronegative stem cell donors. *Scand J Infect Dis* 34:347–350, 2002.

56. Narvios AB, Przepiorka D, Tarrand J, Chan KW, Champlin R, Lichtiger B: Transfusion support using filtered unscreened blood products for cytomegalovirus-negative allogeneic marrow transplant recipients. *Bone Marrow Transplant* 22:575–577, 1998.

57. Narvios AB, Lichtiger B: Bedside leukoreduction of cellular blood components in preventing cytomegalovirus transmission in allogeneic bone marrow transplant recipients: a retrospective study. *Haematologica* 86:749–752, 2001.

58. Bowden RA, Slichter SJ, Sayers M, et al.: A comparison of filtered leukocyte-reduced and cytomegalovirus (CMV) seronegative blood products for the prevention of transfusion-associated CMV infection after marrow transplant. *Blood* 86:3598–3603, 1995.

59. Blajchman MA, Goldman M, Freedman JJ, Sher GD: Proceedings of a consensus conference: prevention of post-transfusion CMV in the era of universal leukoreduction. *Transfusion Med Rev* 15:1–20, 2001.

60. Visconti MR, Pennington J, Garner SF, Allain JP, Williamson LM: Assessment of removal of human cytomegalovirus from blood components by leukocyte depletion filters using real-time quantitative PCR. *Blood* 103:1137–1139, 2004.

61. Nichols WG, Price TH, Corey L, Boeckh M: Transfusion-transmitted cytomegalovirus infection after receipt of leukoreduced blood products. *Blood* 101:4195–4200, 2003.

62. Avery RK, Adal KA, Bolwell BJ: A survey of allogeneic bone marrow transplant programs in the United States regarding cytomegalovirus prophylaxis and pre-emptive therapy. *Bone Marrow Transplant* 26:763–767, 2000.

63. Meijer E, Boland GJ, Verdonck LF: Prevention of cytomegalovirus disease in recipients of allogeneic stem cell transplants. *Clin Microbiol Rev* 16:647–657, 2003.

64. Ljungman P, Brand R, Einsele H, Frassoni F, Niederwieser D, Cordonnier C: Donor CMV serologic status and outcome of CMV-seropositive recipients after unrelated donor stem cell transplantation: an EBMT megafile analysis. *Blood* 102:4255–4260, 2003.

65. Lin TS, Zahrieh D, Weller E, Alyea EP, Antin JH, Soiffer RJ: Risk factors for cytomegalovirus reactivation after CD6+ T-cell-depleted allogeneic bone marrow transplantation. *Transplantation* 74:49–54, 2002.

66. Chakrabarti S, Milligan DW, Brown J, Osman H, Vipond IB, Pamphilon DH, Marks DI: Influence of cytomgalovirus (CMV) sero-positivity on CMV infection, lymphocyte recovery and non-CMV infections following T-cell-depleted allogeneic stem cell transplantation: a comparison between two T-cell depletion regimens. *Bone Marrow Transplant* 33:197–204, 2004.

67. Webb IJ, Anderson KC: Transfusion-associated graft-vs-host disease. In: Popovsky MA (ed.) Transfusion Reactions, 2nd edn. *Bethesda,* MD: AABB Press; 2001:171–186.

68. Schroeder ML: Transfusion-associated graft-versus-host disease. *Br J Haematol* 117:275-287, 2002.

69. Przepiorka D, LeParc GF, Stovall MA, Werch J, Lichtiger B. Use of irradiated blood components: practice parameter. *Am J Clin Pathol* 106:6–11, 1996.

70. Reed W, Fiebig EW, Lee TH, Busch MP: Microchimerism and graft-versus-host disease. In: Hillyer CD, Silberstein LE, Ness PM, Anderson KC, Roush KS (eds.) *Blood Banking and Transfusion Medicine: Basic Principles & Practice*. Philadelphia: Churchill Livingstone; 2003:421–430.

71. Vamvakas EC, Pineda AA: Allergic and anaphylactic reactions. In: Popovsky MA (ed.) Transfusion Reactions, 2nd edn. *Bethesda,* MD: AABB Press; 2001:83–127.

72. Domen RE, Hoeltge GA: Allergic transfusion reactions: an evaluation of 273 consecutive reactions. *Arch Pathol Lab Med* 127:316–320, 2003.

73. Yeghen T, Devereux S: Granulocyte transfusion: a review. *Vox Sang* 81:87–92, 2001.

74. Strauss RG: Granulocyte transfusion therapy. *Hematol Oncol Clin North Am* 8:1159-1166, 1994.

75. Vamvakas EC, Pineda AA: Determinants of the efficacy of prophylactic granulocyte transfusions: a meta-analysis. *J Clin Apheresis* 12:74–81, 1997.

76. Vamvakas EC, Pineda AA: Meta-analysis of clinical studies of the efficacy of granulocyte transfusions in the treatment of bacterial sepsis. *J Clin Apheresis* 11:1–9, 1996.

77. Hubel K, Dale DC, Engert A, Liles WC: Current status of granulocyte (neutrophil) transfusion therapy for infectious diseases. *J Infect Dis* 183:321–328, 2001.

78. Vij R, DiPersio JF, Venkatraman P, et al.: Donor CMV serostatus has no impact on CMV viremia or disease when prophylactic granulocyte transfusions are given following allogeneic peripheral blood stem cell transplantation. *Blood* 101:2067–2069, 2003.

79. Narvios A, Pena E, Han XY, Lichtiger B: Cytomegalovirus infection in cancer patients receiving granulocyte transfusions. *Blood* 99:390–391, 2002.

80. Sachs UJ, Bux J. TRALI after the transfusion of cross-match-positive granulocytes. *Transfusion* 43:1683–1686, 2003.

81. Stroncek DF, Yau YY, Oblitas J, Leitman SF: Administration of G-CSF plus dexamethasone produces greater granulocyte concentrate yields while causing no more donor toxicity than G-CSF alone. *Transfusion* 41:1037–1044, 2001.

82. Heuft HG, Goudeva L, Sel S, Blasczyk R: Equivalent mobilization and collection of granulocytes for transfusion after administration of glycosylated G-CSF (3 µg/kg) plus dexamethasone versus glycosylated G-CSF (12 µg/kg) alone. *Transfusion* 42:928–934, 2002.

83. Heuft HG, Goudeva L, Blasczyk R: A comparative study of adverse reactions occurring after administration of glycoslyated granulocyte colony stimulating factor and/or dexamethasone for mobilization of neutrophils in healthy donors. *Ann Hematol* 83:279–285, 2004.

84. Bashir S, Cardigan R: Granulocyte concentrates: how can we assess their quality? *Transfusion Med* 13:245–257, 2003.

85. Volk EE, Domen RE, Smith ML: An examination of ethical issues raised in the pretreatment of normal volunteer granulocyte donors with granulocyte colony-stimulating factor. *Arch Pathol Lab Med* 123:508–513, 1999.

86. Gleeson C, Spencer D: Blood transfusion and its benefits in palliative care. *Palliative Med* 9:307–313, 1995.

87. Barnes EA, Bruera E: Fatigue in patients with advanced cancer: a review. *Int J Gynecol Cancer* 12:424–428, 2002.

88. Weiskopf RB, Kramer JH, Viele M, et al.: Acute severe isovolemic anemia impairs cognitive function and memory in humans. *Anesthesiology* 1646–1652, 2000.

89. Cunningham RS: Anemia in the oncology patient: cognitive function and cancer. *Cancer Nurs* 26(suppl 6): 38S–42S, 2003.

90. Halterman JS, Kaczorowski JM, Aligne CA, Auinger P, Szilagyi PG: Iron deficiency and cognitive achievement among school-aged children and adolescents in the United States. *Pediatrics* 107:1381–1386, 2001.

91. Lipschitz D: Medical and functional consequences of anemia in the elderly. *J Am Geriatr Soc* 51(suppl 3): S10–S13, 2003.

92. Stone P, Kurowska A, Tookman A: Blood transfusion in palliative care. *Palliative Med* 10:166, 1996.

93. Chiu TY, Hu WY, Cheng SY, Chen CY: Ethical dilemmas in palliative care: a study in Taiwan. *J Med Ethics* 26:353–357, 2000.

94. Monti M, Castellani L, Berlusconi A, Cunietti E: Use of red blood cell transfusions in terminally ill cancer patients admitted to a palliative care unit. *J Pain Symptom Manage* 12:18–22, 1996.

95. Wachtel TJ, Mor V: The use of transfusion in terminal cancer patients: hospice versus conventional care setting. *Transfusion* 25:278–279, 1985.

96. Glass E: Different approaches to transfusion practices used in hospice care. *Oncol Nurs Forum* 23:117–118, 1996.

97. Singer Y, Shvartzman P: The feasibility and advisability of administering home blood transfusions to the terminally ill patient. *J Palliative Care* 14:46–48, 1998.

98. Craig JIO, Milligan P, Cairns J, McClelland DBL, Parker AC: Nurse practitioner support for transfusion in patients with haematological disorders in hospital and at home. *Transfusion Med* 9:31–36, 1999.

99. Benson K, Balducci L, Milo KM, Heckel L, Lyman GH. Patients' attitudes regarding out-of-hospital blood transfusion. *Transfusion* 36:140–143, 1996.

100. Thompson HW, McKelvey J: Home blood transfusion therapy: a home health agency's 5-year experience. *Transfusion* 35:453, 1995.

101. Stockelberg D, Lehtola P, Noren I: Palliative treatment at home for patients with haematological disorders. *Support Care Cancer* 5:506–508, 1997.

# Chapter 105

# GROWTH FACTOR SUPPORT IN HEMATOLOGIC MALIGNANCIES

*George Somlo*

## HEMATOPOIETIC GROWTH FACTORS

Over the preceding decades, a variety of hematopoietic growth factors—glycoproteins by their chemical structure—have been identified. Following purification, cloning, and manufacturing of recombinant forms of these glycoproteins, their potential use in clinical practice has been tested extensively. Native growth factors and their recombinant derivatives target cytokine type receptors and facilitate growth and differentiation of multilineage and late-stage cell types.

Two groups of myeloid growth factors currently available for clinical use are recombinant human granulocyte colony-stimulating factor (G-CSF) and granulocyte-macrophage colony-stimulating factor (GM-CSF). These factors differ in their specific roles as well as in their hematopoietic targets. G-CSF stimulates cells of multilineage potential and enhances late-stage differentiation of neutrophils. GM-CSF also effects multilineage proliferation and acts synergistically with G-CSF in its effect on neutrophils. In addition, it supports development of mixed neutrophil, eosinophil, and macrophage colonies.[1,2] Two recombinant G-CSF products are currently in the market: lenograstim—expressed in yeast—is available outside the United States, while filgrastim—expressed in *Escherichia coli*—is in use within the United States. Recently, a pegylated version of filgrastim, characterized by a much-prolonged half-life, has been successfully tested and approved as a potential alternative to filgrastim. Out of the two GM-CSF preparations in use, sargramostim is expressed in yeast, while molgramostim is bacteria-derived. Sargramostim is in clinical use in the United States.

Recombinant human erythropoietin is the primary regulatory growth factor of erythropoiesis. Erythropoietin is responsible for the differentiating and maturation process in later phases of red cell development. Epoetin alpha and its glycosylated modified form darbepoetin alpha (with a resulting longer half-life) are clinically used in the United States, while epoetin beta is used elsewhere.[3-5]

The primary regulator of thrombopoiesis is thrombopoietin. While this glycoprotein does have an effect on multilineage progenitors, there is substantial homology between this growth factor and erythropoietin, e.g., it is unique by its functional ability in stimulating megakaryocyte progenitor colony growth and differentiation. Lack of expression of the receptor for this growth factor will result in substantially reduced thrombocyte counts, but, albeit in reduced number, functional platelets will still be present, suggesting that other factors might play a role in the growth, differentiation, and maturation of the megakaryocyte lineage. Recombinant thrombopoietin will lead to an increase in megakaryocyte and platelet counts, but, due to its relatively late onset of effects (10–14 days), and pending further evaluation of safety of specific recombinant thrombopoietin products following administration, identification of its potential clinical benefits await validation in future clinical trials.[6,7]

Platelet release is also facilitated by interleukin-11 (IL-11), possibly through a synergistic effect with other cytokines, including thrombopoietin. IL-11 is associated with a number of side effects, and its role as well as the appropriate dosing in hematologic malignancies has yet to be established adequately.[8,9]

## GENERAL INDICATIONS FOR PRESCRIBING GROWTH FACTORS

### NEUTROPENIA

The most significant risk from severe and/or prolonged myelosuppression is febrile neutropenia. Majority of patients with leukemias, myelodysplasias, and advanced stages of lymphomas and myeloma are already immunocompromised; hence, they are at high risk for developing febrile neutropenias.

### PRIMARY PROPHYLAXIS

This term describes the application of growth factors for the purpose of preventing febrile neutropenia in untreated patients. According to guidelines developed by the American Society of Clinical Oncology (ASCO),[10] such prophylaxis is warranted in the setting of treating high-risk patients with chemotherpy regimens associated with at least a 20% likelihood of febrile neutropenia. Most patients in need of intense combination of chemotherapy for newly diagnosed or relapsed leukemia or lymphoma are at high risk for febrile neutropenic complications, either because of disease-related cytopenia, age, poor performance-status, immune-deficiency, or due to myelosuppression caused by therapy. Most patients suffering from hematologic malignancies should be considered candidates for growth factor support even under the current guidelines, based on conclusions from randomized or well-conducted controlled studies in virtually every disease category and with differing treatment modalities. Debate, however, exists about the use of primary prophylaxis growth factor support in patients with acute myeloid leukemia or advanced myelodysplastic syndrome.

### SECONDARY PROPHYLAXIS

In patients who have experienced febrile neutropenia following chemotherapy, chances of a repeat incidence can be avoided by either dose reduction, delay in treatment, or by administration of growth factors. While not all patients who have developed febrile neutropenia with the first cycle of chemotherapy will develop it during subsequent cycles, appropriate actions are needed to avoid potentially fatal future episodes. Recent data with dose-dense, growth factor-supported regimens in patients with malignant lymphomas suggest that prescribing the full planned dose without delay translates into clinical benefits. While dose-dense/intense chemotherapy mandates the use of growth factors, considering that timely administration of chemotherapy is of therapeutic importance, administration of growth factors in general is an important ancillary tool and should be preferred to the strategy of dose adjustment or delay of therapy.[11]

### ANEMIA

Patients with hematologic malignancies frequently present with anemia and are likely to face worsening of this condition while undergoing induction therapy, as well as repetitive consolidation, or maintenance therapy. While acute reversal of anemias still requires blood transfusions, epoetin alpha and beta are now available to treat both disease and treatment-related anemias. Current guidelines developed by ASCO recommend use of erythropoietin for patients with a hemoglobin of less than 10 g/dL in the setting of treated or untreated myelodysplasia. Either treatment-related or disease-associated anemia can also be alleviated by the judicious use of erythropoietin.[4]

### THROMBOCYTOPENIA

Hematologic malignancies frequently present with symptoms due to absolute and/or functional thrombocytopenia. Currently, platelet transfusion remains the only proven method leading to rapid rise in platelet counts. The exact role and optimal dosing of the only approved platelet-lineage specific agent, IL-11, either in the prevention of the need for platelet transfusion or as a facilitator of platelet recovery, is unclear.[8,9] Advanced clinical studies of thrombopoietin-like agents in patients with autoimmune thrombocytopenia are in progress .

## GROWTH FACTORS IN SPECIFIC HEMATOLOGIC DISEASES

### ACUTE MYELOID LEUKEMIA

The majority of patients undergoing remission induction and subsequent postremission therapy for acute myeloid leukemias will suffer from neutropenic fever. Given that their general health is frequently compromised by the time the diagnosis is made, whenever such patients develop this complication, prolonged hospitalization and antibiotic therapy are the likely consequences. Bacterial and fungal infections are significant causes for morbidity and mortality following administration of intensive induction or consolidation chemotherapy. Concerns over the routine use of growth factors have been based on the theoretical possibility that such factors may stimulate growth of clonogenic leukemia cells. Additionally, by enhancing proliferation and rendering the nonclonal, healthy hematopoietic progenitors prime targets to cytotoxic agents, prolonged cytopenia could become an unintended result.

Over the past decade, several randomized, placebo-controlled trials of growth factor administration after induction chemotherapy, generally in older patients with newly diagnosed acute myeloid leukemia, demonstrated a significant reduction, by 2–6 days, in the time period required to reach an absolute neutrophil count more than $0.5 \times 10^9$/L. Similarly, duration of antibiotic use and hospitalization were significantly reduced in many studies. When growth factors were prescribed within 1–3 days from completion of remission induction therapy, neither the time of initiating them, nor the degree of marrow suppression seemed to have an effect on outcome.[12–23] The concept of priming leukemia cells is based on the assumption that changes in the cell cycle may increase sensitivity to specific agents used for remission induction, specifically to Ara C. Several trials prescribed CSF prior to therapy, but none of them suggested any benefit associated with this approach.[24,25] One study evaluating the addition of G-CSF, both with or without all-trans retinoic acid (ATRA), to chemotherapy revealed an increased complete response rate but no improvement in survival.[21] Only two trials demonstrated either improved disease-free or overall survival.[13,19] Similarly, following consolidation therapy, two studies demonstrated a significant decrease in the duration of absolute neutropenia and use of antibiotic therapy, without any effect on survival.[15,20]

In general, these trials did not reveal evidence suggesting stimulation of either leukemic growth or drug resistance, and majority of studies did not reveal therapeutic benefits in terms of complete response rate or overall survival. There were no studies comparing the effect of G-CSF to GM-CSF in the setting of postinduction or postconsolidation support.

### CHRONIC MYELOID LEUKEMIA

Grade 3 or 4 neutropenia had been observed in 13% patients with chronic myelogenous leukemia (CML), treated on a phase III randomized trial with imatinib. Imatinib does not affect the Philadelphia chromosome negative normal hematopoietic progenitors, and while G-CSF and GM-CSF have been tested without adverse consequences in a phase II trial of this agent, the standard recommendation is to withhold and subsequently restart the therapy, rather than prescribing growth factors.[26]

### MYELODYSPLASTIC SYNDROME

GM-CSF and G-CSF increase the neutrophil count in patients with severe neutropenia secondary to myelodysplasia. Both neutrophil and eosinophil counts increase following administration of GM-CSF.[27] Randomized studies demonstrated a decrease in the duration of neutropenia and improved treatment response associated with the use of G-CSF in patients receiving chemotherapy, or subsequent chemotherapeutic intervention.[21,28,29] There was no evidence of any effect on duration of response or survival, although in one study higher remission rates and reduced infection rates allowed consideration of allogeneic transplantation in a greater number of patients.[29] There was no evidence of transformation to leukemia in either in these studies, in spite of theoretical risk to the contrary. However, prolonged administration of G-CSF in patients having more than 5% myeloblast counts is not recommended due to the potential risk of facilitating disease progression.

The use of erythropoietin is based on a relatively small, randomized placebo-controlled trial in low risk (refractory anemia without ring sideroblasts) myelodysplasia. A fixed erythropoietin dose of 1050 U/kg per week led to an increase of hemoglobin by 1–2 g/dL of hemoglobin in 50% of low-risk patients, versus 6% in the control group.[30] The addition of G-CSF or GM-CSF to erythropoietin may also have a synergistic effect on erythropoietic differentiation and response. In at least one study, administration of both G-CSF and erythropoietin was required in order to generate and maintain an erythrocyte response.[31] A predictive model based on serum epo level and prior transfusion requirements has been developed to guide the use of combination of G-CSF and erythropoietin in patients with myelodysplasia.[32]

### ACUTE LYMPHOCYTIC LEUKEMIA

The effect of G-CSF both in the setting of remission induction and consolidation therapy has been tested in prospective trials, most of which were randomized. These trials were carried out in adults and children, both during remission induction and consolidation therapy. In the larger studies, duration of neutropenia was shortened by 5–8 days.[33–39] At least in one acute lymphocytic leukemia trial conducted in adults, a trend toward increased complete response rate was also observed, but without improvement in survival.[33] In general, there was no improvement in relapse-free or overall survival in any of the randomized trials using posttreatment G-CSF.

All of these studies demonstrated a decrease in the duration of neutropenia following the use of growth factors. The majority of studies also revealed decreased hospitalization, antibiotic use, and decrease in documented infections.[39]

Administration of G-CSF allowed for timely delivery and intensification of the planned chemotherapy cycles. Hence, G-CSF is recommended both following remission induction therapy, and consolidation, with an expectation to reduce the duration of absolute neutropenia by approximately 1 week, and in order to allow maintenance of dose intensity.

### CHRONIC LYMPHOCYTIC LEUKEMIA

Single-agent therapy does not usually mandate the use of growth factors in patients treated for chronic lymphocytic leukemias. More intense attempts of induction with combination regimens are likely to generate a higher incidence of grade 3 or 4 neutropenias. While randomized trials are unavailable, in a recent study administration of FAND (Fludarabine, Ara C, mitoxantrone, and dexamethasone) resulted in an incidence of more than 60% grade 3 or 4 absolute neutropenia. This study suggested that the incidence of severe neutropenia-associated pneumonias might have been reduced in patients supported by G-CSF prophylaxis, in contrast to an earlier cohort of patients treated on the same study but without administration of G-CSF.[40] One randomized trial that included patients with chronic lymphocytic leukemia suggested a benefit in terms of reduced need of red cell transfusion in patients who were given erythropoietin. General recommendations of erythropoietin use for the treatment of postchemotherapy anemias, according to ASCO guidelines, do apply to this category of malignancies. Erythropoietin may be beneficial for patients who are receiving supportive care only. though these guidelines do not address this specific clinical scenario.[41]

## LYMPHOMA AND MULTIPLE MYELOMA

Both G-CSF and GM-CSF have been tested in prospective, randomized trials in patients with lymphomas, in an effort to reduce morbidity and mortality associated with infectious complications, and to potentially improve response rates and therapeutic outcome. Results of an updated meta-analysis of 12 prospective, randomized, controlled (placebo or no prophylaxis) trials have recently been published. The findings support the use of G-CSF/GM-CSF, especially in older patients who are receiving treatment for non-Hodgkin's lymphoma. In the meta-analysis, the relative risk of febrile neutropenia (RR 0.74) and infection (0.74) were both reduced. Other potential study endpoints, such as antibiotic use, infection-related mortality, and overall outcome, were not affected.[42]

Recently, a pegylated, longer-acting version of G-CSF had been tested in a phase II randomized trial of patients receiving salvage chemotherapy for refractory non-Hodgkin's or Hodgkin's lymphomas. Chemotherapy consisting of ESHAP (etoposide, cisplatin, ARA-C and methylprednisolone) was followed by administration of filgrastim daily single dose of 5 μg/kg versus pegfilgrastim given once 100 μg/kg. The incidence and duration of grade 4 neutropenias were similar between the two groups, revealing equivalent effects of single administration of the pegylated compound versus a median of 11 injections of filgrastim.[43]

The concept of dose-dense chemotherapy is based on the assumption that, although rapid reduction of tumor mass promotes faster tumor regrowth, sensitivity to the effects of chemotherapy agents may also increase during such periods.[44] Hence, the goal of this therapeutic strategy is to deliver chemotherapy in the shortest possible interval. To test this theory, the German High-Grade Lymphoma Study Group compared six cycles of CHOP (cyclophosphamide, doxorubicin, Vincristine, and prednisone) given either every 21 days, or every 14 days (this latter schedule was supported with G-CSF). These investigators also attempted to answer whether the addition of etoposide to CHOP would result in improved outcome. Based on this 2 × 2 factorial design, two parallel studies (in patients aged 60 or less vs patients aged over 60 years) were carried out. Patients receiving CHOP every 2 weeks were prescribed G-CSF for 10 days, starting on day 4, based on the expected high incidence of significant neutropenia. In patients aged over 60 years, complete response rates were higher (76.1% vs 60.1%) and relative risk reduction for event-free and overall survival was significantly greater (0.66, $p = 0.003$; 0.58, $p < 0.001$) in those treated on the dose-dense, every 2-week schedule. The addition of etoposide was associated with increased toxicity and no obvious benefit. Hence, further trials to expand and confirm the role of dose-dense delivery of CHOP are ongoing, and these studies are also incorporating rituximab into the treatment arms.[11] The ASCO growth factor guidelines regarding both primary and secondary prophylaxis of neutropenia and, similarly, guidelines regarding chemotherapy-associated anemia, apply to patients with multiple myeloma.[4,10] Evaluation of epoetin beta in a randomized, double-blind, controlled study in transfusion-dependent patients with multiple myeloma (the study also included patients with chronic lymphocytic leukemia and low-grade malignant lymphoma) revealed that transfusion-free and severe anemia-free survival were significantly better, with a risk reduction of 43% and 51%, respectively, in patients receiving epoietin beta at a dose of 150 IU/kg three times a week for a period of 16 weeks, versus control. Approximately 2/3 of patients receiving epoietin beta responded, versus 27% in the placebo group. Quality of life was also significantly improved and correlated with a rise of ≥2 g/dL of hemoglobin.[41]

## AUTOLOGOUS AND ALLOGENEIC STEM CELL TRANSPLANTATION

### AUTOLOGOUS STEM CELL TRANSPLANTATION AND SUBSEQUENT GROWTH FACTOR SUPPORT

Randomized trials of G-CSF versus control following autologous peripheral blood and stem cell transplantation have documented a benefit from prescribing G-CSF, in terms of decreased duration of neutropenia and hospitalization. In general, patients treated with autologous transplantation do experience shortened periods of neutropenia and reduced duration of hospitalization after receiving filgrastim ranging from 5 to 30 μg/kg per day, or two different dose schedules of lenograstim.[45–48] As illustrated by the wide range of prescribed doses of G-CSF and lenograstim, the optimal dose and timing/duration of administration is still unclear in the postautologous recovery phase.[47] A non-randomized study suggested a benefit in terms of decreased duration of hospitalization, neutrophil recovery, and cost savings, when G-CSF was initiated on the day immediately after peripheral blood progenitor cell reinfusion, in comparison to starting this therapy 4 days later.[49] These findings have not been supported in other randomized studies regardless of whether administration of G-CSF began on day 1 versus 7, or 3 versus 5 days after reinfusion of stem cells.[50,51]

Not all growth factors are created equal: GM-CSF support following reinfusion of primed peripheral blood progenitor cells did not result in any benefit in one placebo-controlled trial.[52]

Myeloablative therapy will induce severe anemia necessitating transfusion of virtually all patients undergoing autologous transplantation. Earlier data suggested that administration of erythropoietin, when given both prior to ablative therapy and when resumed subsequently on day 1, failed to decrease the number of red blood cell transfusions in comparison to placebo.[53] Recently, the effects of erythropoietin, administered at a dose of 500 units/kg per week starting from day 30 after transplantation, to a cohort of patients treated for malignant lymphoma or myeloma were assessed. In a retrospective analysis, mean hemoglobin levels were substantially better: only 2 of 41 patients in the treatment group versus 12 of 45 patients in a previously treated "control" group without erythropoietin support experienced hemoglobin levels less than 9 g/dL.[54] The potential benefit of such delayed administration, as well as pilot data demonstrating a protective effect in multiple myeloma patients in whom erythropoietin is provided prior to the second phase of a tandem transplant, needs to be confirmed in a prospective randomized fashion.[55] The effect of erythropoietin has also been evaluated in patients with lymphomas undergoing intense salvage therapy followed by consolidation. When epoetin beta was prescribed at a dose of 10,000 IE thrice a week during the entire course of two cycles of DHAP (dexamethasone, ARA-C, and cisplatin), followed by further intensification and peripheral blood progenitor cell collection and BEAM (carmustine, etoposide, melphalan, and ARA-C) therapy, the number of red cell transfusion required (4.5 vs 8.3) and mean hemoglobin levels during the course of therapy were all favorably affected by growth factor therapy.[5]

### ALLOGENEIC STEM CELL AND STEM CELL TRANSPLANTATION FOLLOWED BY GROWTH FACTORS

In the early posttransplant phase, neutropenia-associated infectious complications are one of the most significant treatment-related toxicities. Infusions of primed peripheral blood progenitor cell and stem cell transplantations from HLA-matched siblings have shortened the duration of neutropenia. A benefit in terms of accelerated neutrophil recovery has been described in trials involving patients who were recipients of allogeneic peripheral blood progenitor cells and growth-factor support (G-CSF).[56] In a subsequent randomized trial in T-cell depleted allogeneic blood progenitor recipients treated with or without posttransplantation growth factor support, there was no difference in the degree of immune reconstitution and no statistically significant difference in treatment outcome as measured by relapse, infections, or incidence of chronic graft versus host disease.[57]

Use of growth factors following allogeneic stem cell transplantation is not without side effects. There is a potential for delay in platelet recovery after using GM-CSF in the posttransplantation setting.[58] A recent retrospective analysis suggested that recipients of stem cell transplantations should not receive G-CSF support in the immediate posttransplantation period. In the study, patients with acute myelogenous leukemia (1789 patients transplanted with HLA-matched sibling bone marrow and 434 patients transplanted with peripheral blood progenitor cells) were analyzed. Twenty-eight percent of bone marrow recipients and 40% of peripheral blood progenitor cell recipients received G-CSF during the first 2 weeks following transplantation.

While neutrophil recovery was faster, platelet engraftment did take longer, and the incidence of acute grades II–IV graft versus host disease was also higher (50% vs 39%, $p = 0.007$) in recipients of bone marrow who also received G-CSF support. The incidence of chronic graft versus host disease, as well as transplant-related mortality and leukemia-free and overall survival were also adversely affected. No such adverse effects were noted in recipients of peripheral blood progenitor cells regardless of whether they received growth factor support.[59]

## CONCLUSIONS

*Granulocyte growth factors* can be given safely both as primary and secondary prophylaxis to the majority of patients with hematologic malignancies.

G-CSF administration in acute myeloid and lymphoid leukemias, chronic lymphocytic leukemia, myelodysplasia, lymphomas, and in the postperipheral blood progenitor phase in all of these disease categories, and in myeloma, has lead to shortened duration of myelosuppression and subsequent decrease in morbidity due to reduction in the incidence of febrile neutropenias and other infectious complications. Survival, however, has not been reliably affected.

G-CSF is also indicated and should be prescribed in the specific situation when dose-dense/intense therapy is of potential benefit to the patient; e.g., when treating older lymphoma patients on a biweekly schedule with CHOP. While the optimal timing, dose, and duration are still not well established in most clinical situations, administration of 5 µg/kg of G-CSF and, if chosen, 250 µg/kg of GM-CSF are recommended, starting within 1–5 days after completion of therapy.[10] Pegylated G-CSF has been found to be equally efficacious and safe as G-CSF in the setting of treating lymphomas with a standard regimen. However, further evaluation of pegfilgrastim is required to confirm safety and efficacy during induction and dose/dense consolidation therapy for leukemias, and in combination with dose/dense treatment regimens. Further evaluation is also needed in the pre- and posttransplantation settings.

*Administration of erythropoietin* is justified in early phases of myelodysplasias and during repetitive administration of chemotherapy cycles for patients with lymphomas in order to increase hemoglobin values, avoid transfusions, and ameliorate anemia-associated fatigue and improve quality of life. The optimal dose and frequency are still unknown, but the effects of erythropoietin prescribed to lymphoma patients at doses of 10,000 U thrice a week were equivalent to a dose of 30,000 U, given every 3 weeks, in one randomized trial. Darbepoetin alpha had been tested in patients with lymphoproliferative diseases and was found to be effective at ranges 1–4.5 g/kg per week in comparison to placebo. Patients with multiple myeloma, chronic lymphocytic leukemia, and lymphomas may benefit from administration of erythropoietin when they are experiencing symptoms related to low hemoglobin, and/or are transfusion dependent. Further studies are required to establish the role of erythropoietin and darbepoetin alpha in acute leukemias and, while preliminary data are encouraging, additional trials are needed in the peri- and posttransplantation settings.

## REFERENCES

1. Lieschke GJ, Burgess AW: Granulocyte colony-stimulating factor and granulocyte-macrophage colony-stimulating factor. *N Engl J Med* 327:28–35, 1992.
2. Lieschke GJ, Burgess AW: Granulocyte colony-stimulating factor and granulocyte-macrophage colony-stimulating factor. *N Engl J Med* 327:99–106, 1992.
3. Egrie JC, Browne JK: Development and characterization of novel erythropoiesis stimulating protein (NESP). *Br J Cancer* 84(suppl 1):3–10, 2001.
4. Rizzo JD, Lichtin AE, Woolf SH, et al.: Use of Epoetin in patients with cancer: evidence-based clinical practice guidelines of the American Society of Clinical Oncology and the American Society of Hematology. *J Clin Oncol* 20:4083–4107, 2002.
5. Glossmann JP, Engert A, Wassmer G, et al.: Recombinant human erythropoietin, epoetin beta, in patients with relapsed lymphoma treated with aggressive sequential salvage chemotherapy—results of a randomized trial. *Ann Hematol* 82:469–475, 2003.
6. Kaushansky K: Thrombopoietin: from theory to reality. *Int J Hematol* 76(suppl 1):343–345, 2002.
7. Nash RA, Kurzrock R, DiPersio J, et al.: A phase I trial of recombinant human thrombopoietin in patients with delayed platelet recovery after hematopoietic stem cell transplantation. *Biol Blood Marrow Transplant* 6:25–34, 2000.
8. Tepler I, Elias L, Smith JW, et al: A randomized placebo-controlled trial of recombinant human interleukin-11 in cancer patients with severe thrombocytopenia due to chemotherapy. *Blood* 87:3607–3614, 1996.
9. Kurzrock R, Cortes J, Thomas DA, et al.: Pilot study of low-dose interleukin-11 in patients with bone marrow failure. *J Clin Oncol* 19:4165–4172, 2001.
10. Smith TJ, Khatcheressian J, Lyman GH, et al.: 2006 update of recommendations of the use of white blood cell growth factors: an evidence-based clinical practice guideline. *J clin Oncol* 24:187–205, 2006.
11. Pfreundschuh M, Trumper L, Kloess M, et al.: Two-weekly or 3-weekly CHOP chemotherapy with or without etoposide for the treatment of elderly patients with aggressive lymphomas: results of the NHL-B2 trial of the DSHNHL. *Blood* 104:634–641, 2004.
12. Dombret H, Chastang C, Fenaux P, et al.: A controlled study of recombinant human granulocyte colony-stimulating factor in elderly patients after treatment for acute myelogenous leukemia. *N Eng J Med* 332: 1678–1683, 1995.
13. Rowe JM, Andersen JW, Mazza JJ, et al.: A randomized placebo-controlled phase III study of granulocyte-macrophage colony-stimulating factor in adult patients (>55 to 70 years of age) with acute myelogenous leukemia: a study of the Eastern Cooperative Oncology Group (E1490). *Blood* 86:457–462, 1995.
14. Stone RM, Berg DT, George SL, et al.: Granulocyte-macrophage colony-stimulating factor after initial chemotherapy for elderly patients with primary acute myelogenous leukemia, Cancer and Leukemia Group B. *N Engl J Med* 332:1671–1677, 1995.
15. Heil G, Hoelzer D. Sanz MA, et al.: A randomized, double-blind, placebo-controlled, phase III study of filgastim in remission induction and consolidation therapy for adults with de novo acute myeloid leukemia. The International Acute Myeloid Leukemia Study Group. *Blood* 90:4710–4718, 1997.
16. Godwin JE, Kopecky KJ, Head DR, et al: A double-blind placebo-controlled trial of granulocyte colony-stimulating factor in elderly patients with previously untreated acute myeloid leukemia: a Southwest oncology group study (9031). *Blood* 91:3607–3615, 1998.
17. Lowenberg B, Boogaerts MA, Daenen SM, et al.: Value of different modalities of granulocyte-macrophage colony-stimulating factor applied during or after induction therapy of acute myeloid leukemia. *J Clin Oncol* 15:3496–3506, 1997.
18. Zittoun R, Suciu S, Mandelli F, et al.: Granulocyte-macrophage colony-stimulating factor associated with induction treatment of acute myelogenous leukemia: a randomized trial by the European Organization for Research and Treatment of Cancer Leukemia Cooperative Group. *J Clin Oncol* 14:2150–2159, 1996.
19. Witz F, Sadoun A, Perrin MC, et al.: A placebo-controlled study of recombinant human granulocyte-macrophage colony-stimulating factor administered during and after induction treatment for de novo acute myelogenous leukemia in elderly patients. Groupe Ouest Est Leucemies Aigues Myeloblastiques (GOELAM). *Blood* 91:2722–2730, 1998.
20. Harousseau JL, Witz B, Lioure B, et al.: Granulocyte colony-stimulating factor after intensive consolidation chemotherapy in acute myeloid leukemia: results of a randomized trial of the Groupe Ouest-Est Leucemies Aigues Myeloblastiques. *J Clin Oncol* 18:780–787, 2000.
21. Estey EH, Thall PF, Pierce S, et at.: Randomized phase II study of fludarabine + cytosine arabinoside + idarubicin +/− all-trans retinoic acid +/− granulocyte colony-stimulating factor in poor prognosis newly diagnosed acute myeloid leukemia and myelodysplastic syndrome. *Blood* 93:2478–2484, 1999.
22. Uyl-de Groot CA, Lowenberg B, Vellenga E, et al.: Cost-effectiveness and quality-of-life assessment of GM-CSF as an adjunct to intensive remission induction

chemotherapy in elderly patients with acute myeloid leukemia. *Br J Haematol* 100:625–636, 1998.

23. Usuki K, Urabe A, Masaoka T, et al.: Efficacy of granulocyte colony-stimulating factor in the treatment of acute myelogenous leukaemia: a multicentre randomized study. *Br J Haematol* 116:103–112, 2002.

24. Ohno R, Naoe T, Kanamaru A, et al.: A double-blind controlled study of granulocyte colony-stimulating factor started two days before induction chemotherapy in refractory acute myeloid leukemia. Kohseisho Leukemia Study Group. *Blood* 83:2086–2092, 1994.

25. Lowenberg B, van Putten W, Theobald W, et al.: Effect of priming with granulocyte colony-stimulating factor on the outcome of chemotherapy for acute myeloid leukemia. *N Engl J Med* 349:743–752, 2003.

26. Deininger MWN, O'Brien SG, O'Brien, et al.: Practical management of patients with chronic myeloid leukemia receiving imatinib. *J Clin Oncol* 21:1637–1647, 2003.

27. Yoshida Y, Nakahata T, Shibata A, et al.: Effects of long-term treatment with recombinant human granulocyte-macrophage colony-stimulating factor in patients with myelodysplastic syndrome. *Leuk Lymphoma* 18:457–463, 1995.

28. Ossenkoppele GJ, van der Holt B, Verhoef GE, et al.: A randomized study of granulocyte colony-stimulating factor applied during and after chemotherapy in patients with poor risk myelodysplastic syndromes: a report from the HOVON Cooperative Group. Dutch-Belgian Hemato-Oncology Cooperative Group. *Leukemia* 13:1207–1213, 1999.

29. Bernasconi C, Alessandrino EP, Bernasconi P, et al.: Randomized clinical study comparing aggressive chemotherapy with or without G-CSF support for high-risk myelodysplastic syndromes or secondary acute myeloid leukaemia evolving from MDS. *Br J Haematol* 102:678–683, 1998.

30. Anonymous: A randomized double-blind placebo-controlled study with subcutaneous recombinant human erythropoietin in patients with low-risk myelodysplastic syndromes: Italian Cooperative Study Group for rHuEpo in Myelodysplastic Syndromes. *Br J Haematol* 103: 1070–1074, 1998.

31. Negrin RS, Stein R, Doherty K, et al.: Maintenance treatment of the anemia of myelodysplastic syndromes with recombinant human granulocyte colony-stimulating factor and erythropoietin: evidence for *in vivo* synergy. Blood 87:4076–4081, 1996.

32. Hellstrom-Lindberg E, Negrin R, Stein R, et al.: Erythroid response to treatment with G-CSF plus erythropoietin for the anaemia of patients with myelodysplastic syndromes: proposal for a predictive model. *Br J Haematol* 99:344–351, 1997.

33. Larson RA, Dodge RK, Linker CA, et al.: A randomized controlled trial of filgrastim during remission induction and consolidation chemotherapy for adults with acute lymphoblastic leukemia: CALGB study 9111. *Blood* 92:1556–1564, 1998.

34. Ottmann OG, Hoelzer D, Gracien E, et al.: Concomitant granulocyte colony-stimulating factor and induction chemoradiotherapy in adult acute lymphoblastic leukemia: a randomized phase III trial. *Blood* 86:444–450, 1995.

35. Welte K, Reiter A, Mempel K, et al.: A randomized phase-III study of the efficacy of granulocyte colony-stimulating factor in children with high-risk acute lymphoblastic leukemia. Berlin-Frankfurt-Munster Study Group. *Blood* 87:3143–3150, 1996.

36. Geissler K, Koller E, Hubmann E, et al.: Granulocyte colony-stimulating factor as an adjunct to induction chemotherapy for adult acute lymphoblastic leukemia—a randomized phase-III study. *Blood* 90:590–596, 1997.

37. Scherrer R, Geissler K, Kyrle PA, et al.: Granulocyte colony-stimulating factor (G-CSF) as an adjunct to induction chemotherapy of adult acute lymphoblastic leukemia (ALL). *Ann Hematol* 66:283–289, 1993.

38. Laver J, Amylon M, Desai S, et al.: Randomized trial of r-metHu granulocyte colony-stimulating factor in an intensive treatment for T-cell leukemia and advanced-stage lymphoblastic lymphoma of childhood: a Pediatric Oncology Group pilot study. *J Clin Oncol* 16:522–526, 1998.

39. Heath JA, Steinherz PG, Altman A, et al.: Human granulocyte colony-stimulating factor in children with high-risk acute lymphoblastic leukemia: a Children's Cancer Group Study. *J Clin Oncol* 21:1612–1617, 2003.

40. Mauro FR, Foa R, Meloni G, et al.: Fludarabine, ara-C, novantrone and dexamethasone (FAND) in previously treated chronic lymphocytic leukemia patients. *Haematologica* 87:926–933, 2002.

41. Osterborg A, Brandberg Y, Molostova V, et al.: Randomized, double-blind, placebo-controlled trial of recombinant human erythropoietin, epoetin beta, in hematologic malignancies. *J Clin Oncol* 20:2486–2494, 2002.

42. Bohlius J, Reiser M, Schwarzer G, et al.: Granulopoiesis-stimulating factors to prevent adverse effects in the treatment of malignant lymphoma. *Cochrane Datebase Syst Rev* (3):CD003189, 2004.

43. Vose JM, Crump M, Lazarus C, et al.: Randomized, multicenter, open-label study of pegfilgrastim compared with daily filgrastim after chemotherapy for lymphoma. *J Clin Oncol* 21:514–519, 2003.

44. Norton L: Evolving concepts in the systemic drug therapy of breast cancer. *Semin Oncol* 24:S10-13-S10-10, 1997.

45. Nademanee A, Sniecinski I, Schmidt GM, et al.: High-dose therapy followed by autologous peripheral-blood stem-cell transplantation for patients with Hodgkin's disease and non-Hodgkin's lymphoma using unprimed and granulocyte colony-stimulating factor-mobilized peripheral-blood stem cells. *J Clin Oncol* 12:2176–2186, 1994.

46. Klumpp TR, Mangan KF, Goldbert SL, et al.: Granulocyte colony-stimulating factor accelerates neutrophil engraftment following peripheral-blood stem-cell transplantation: a prospective, randomized trial. *J Clin Oncol* 13:1323–1327, 1995.

47. Suh C, Kim HG, Kim SH, et al.: Low-dose lenograstim to enhance engraftment after autologous stem cell transplantation: a prospective randomized evaluation of two different fixed doses. *Transfusion* 44:533–538, 2004.

48. Schmitz N, Dreger P, Zander AR, et al.: Results of a randomized, controlled, multicentre study of recombinant human granulocyte colony-stimulating factor (filgrastim) in patients with Hodgkin's disease and

non-Hodgkin's lymphoma undergoing autologous bone marrow transplantation. *Bone Marrow Transplant* 15:261–266, 1995.

49. Colby C, McAfee SL, Finkelstein, et al.: Early vs. delayed administration of G-CSF following autologous peripheral blood stem cell transplantation. *Bone Marrow Transplant* 21:1005–1010, 1998.

50. Bence-Bruckler I, Bredeson C, Atkins H, et al.: A randomized trial of granulocyte colony-stimulating factor (Neupogen) starting day 1 vs. day 7 post-autologous stem cell transplantation. *Bone Marrow Transplant* 10:965–969, 1998.

51. Bolwell BJ, Pohlman B, Andresen S, et al.: Delayed G-CSF after autologous progenitor cell transplantation: a prospective randomized trial. *Bone Marrow Transplant* 21:369–373, 1998.

52. Chao NJ, Schriber JR, Long GD, et al.: A randomized study of erythropoietin and granulocyte colony-stimulating factor (G-CSF) vs. placebo and G-CSF for patients with Hodgkin's and non-Hodgkin's lymphoma undergoing autologous bone marrow transplantation. *Blood* 83:2823–2828, 1994.

53. Chao NJ, Schriber JR, Grimes K, et al.: Granulocyte colony-stimulating factor 'mobilized' peripheral blood progenitor cells accelerate granulocyte and platelet recovery after high-dose chemotherapy. *Blood* 81:2031–2035, 1993.

54. Baron F, Frere P, Fillet G, et al.: Recombinant human erythropoietin therapy is very effective after an autologous peripheral blood stem cell transplant when started soon after engraftment. *Clin Cancer Research* 9:5566–5572, 2003.

55. Baron F, Frere P, Fillet G, et al.: Tandem high-dose therapy (HDT) for multiple myeloma: recombinant human erythropoietin therapy given between first and second HDT allows second peripheral blood stem cell transplantation without red blood cell transfusion. *Br J Haematol* 123:103–105, 2003.

56. Bishop MR, Tarantolo SR, Geller RB, et al.: A randomized, double-blind trial of filgrastim (granulocyte colony-stimulating factor) vs. placebo following allogeneic blood stem cell transplantation. *Blood* 96:80–85, 2000.

57. Joshi SS, Bishop MR, Lynch JC, et al.: Immunological and clinical effects of post-transplant G-CSF vs. placebo in T-cell replete allogeneic blood transplant patients: results from a randomized double-blind study. *Cytotherapy* 5:542–552, 2003.

58. Powles R, Smith C, Milan S, et al.: Human recombinant GM-CSF in allogeneic bone marrow transplantation for leukemia: double-blind placebo-controlled trial. *Lancet* 336:1417–1420, 1990.

59. Ringden O, Labopin M, Gorin NC, et al.: Treatment with granulocyte colony-stimulating factor after allogeneic bone marrow transplantation for acute leukemia increases the risk of graft-versus-host disease and death: a study from the Acute Leukemia Working Party of the European Group for Blood and Marrow Transplantation. *J Clin Oncol* 22:416–423, 2004.

# Chapter 106

# TREATMENT APPROACH TO PREGNANT WOMEN

*Revathi Suppiah, Joanna Brell, and Matt E. Kalaycio*

The hematologic malignancies are uncommon disorders in reproductive-age women. Cancer complicates 1 in 1000 pregnancies.[1] The most frequently occurring tumor in pregnancy is cervical cancer, followed by breast cancer, melanoma, ovarian cancer, thyroid cancer, leukemia, and lymphoma.[2] The incidence of leukemia during pregnancy is estimated to be 1 per 75,000 pregnancies.[3] Pregnancy per se does not increase the risk of malignancy.

Cancer is the leading cause of death among women aged 35–54 years,[4] and as childbearing increases among older females, the incidence of pregnancies complicated by malignancy is likely to increase. Depending on the type of malignancy and stage of diagnosis, postponing chemotherapy until after delivery may not be feasible. This is often the case in acute leukemia.[5] The use of chemotherapy during the second and third trimester has been reported with good outcomes. Despite the emotionally and physically demanding therapy, pregnant patients with leukemia have successfully delivered healthy term infants either before, during, or after chemotherapy.

## MATERNAL PHYSIOLOGIC CHANGES WITH PREGNANCY

Several normal adaptive changes occur in the hematologic environment during pregnancy. Plasma volume increases by about 50% with only a 20–50% rise in red cell mass, resulting in a normocytic anemia.[6] Inadequate hematopoiesis can result if iron and folate stores are not supplemented in advance. The normocytic anemia often becomes microcytic if iron metabolism cannot keep pace with fetal demand despite supplementation.

Leukocytosis occurs during pregnancy, most likely due to increased levels of endogenous steroids. By the third trimester, white blood cell (WBC) may reach as high as 12,000/μL and up to 20,000–30,000/μL during labor.[7] Platelet counts in the low normal range may be seen during gestation (gestational thrombocytopenia).[6] Immune thrombocytopenic purpura occurs more often in young women; any platelet count that acutely drops or is less than 50,000/μL must be investigated.

The physiologic changes occurring with pregnancy can directly affect the dosing and toxicity of chemotherapeutic agents. The increase in renal blood flow, glomerular filtration rate, and creatinine clearance may increase the clearance of drugs excreted by the kidneys. Amniotic fluid may act as a physiologic third space, and thereby may enhance the toxicity of agents by delaying elimination. The physiologic increase in body water with the increase in plasma volume may change the volume of drug distribution.

## INTERACTIONS BETWEEN PREGNANCY, LEUKEMIA, AND MATERNAL/FETAL OUTCOME

### IMPACT OF PREGNANCY ON LEUKEMIA

Pregnancy has not been shown to have any consequence on the development, response to treatment, duration of response, or overall survival of acute leukemia.[1,8] The complete response rates of 76–77% reported by Reynoso et al. in both pregnant acute myelogenous leukemia (AML) and acute lymphoblastic leukemia (ALL) patients are consistent with those of nonpregnant patients.[8] Acute leukemia is fatal if untreated. In all patients, untreated acute leukemia has an overall survival from 2 weeks to 3 months, with deaths most commonly resulting from infection or hemorrhage. Patients not receiving leukemia therapy prior to labor and delivery had approximately 60% perinatal mortality rate in the 1960s–1970s.[9] Many of the maternal deaths in leukemic patients during labor and delivery appear to occur in women with either untreated acute leukemia or with disease unresponsive to therapy.[8]

In the early stages of chronic leukemias, treatment is not essential. If adequate hematologic parameters are maintained without significant bleeding or infection, uncomplicated gestation and delivery can take place with sufficient prenatal care. Leukapheresis may be performed if cytoreduction is necessary.

Acute leukemias, however, are more aggressive and patients require therapy for disease control almost immediately upon diagnosis. There are a few reports of pregnant patients not receiving chemotherapy for acute leukemia. Some patients were diagnosed at delivery or in the last few weeks of gestation and had labor induced before beginning the treatment.[10] Catanzarite and Ferguson reviewed fetal outcomes in untreated acute leukemic patients.[11]

Four patients diagnosed close to delivery (induced or spontaneous deliveries), between 37 and 42 weeks of gestation—all healthy infants

One patient diagnosed at 14 weeks—elective abortion with retained placenta and maternal death from hemorrhage

One patient diagnosed at 28 weeks—intrauterine death, maternal demise from intracerebral hemorrhage at 30 weeks

One patient diagnosed 1 month prior to conception—disseminated intravascular coagulation (DIC) at 34 weeks with fetal demise within 24 hours

Five of the seven patients died 33 days or less after diagnosis, primarily from hemorrhage and/or infection.[11] These examples emphasize the need for early intervention in acute leukemia; pregnant patients require the same aggressive approach as nonpregnant leukemics to attain a goal of complete remission.

### PLACENTAL FUNCTION

The placenta separates maternal and fetal circulatory systems and regulates transport between the two systems. Transport occurs via the placental membrane, which is composed of fetal tissue.[12] Maternal arterial blood is driven by the blood pressure into the intervillous spaces. Fetal blood is confined to the villous vascular system. Substances cross by simple diffusion, facilitated diffusion, active transport, or pinocytosis. Placental membrane interruptions can occur, especially toward the end of gestation, due to thinning of the membrane with time. The fetal capillary system also becomes progressively more exposed to the intervillous spaces.

Several substances can easily transfer across this membrane, including most nutrients, waste products, proteins such as immunoglobin G antibodies, certain hormones, viruses, and water-soluble vitamins.[9] Substances that are lipid-soluble, less plasma protein-bound, nonionized, or of low molecular weight are capable of crossing the placenta; most chemotherapeutic agents have similar qualities.[9]

In a retrospective review by Germann et al.,[13] 160 patient pregnancies exposed to anthracyclines were analyzed. Fetal outcome was normal in 73% cases. After intravenous injection of anthracyclines, only barely detectable concentrations were detected in the fetus. Table 106.1 illustrates the results of two studies of anthracycline concentrations in fetal tissues, amniotic fluid, and placenta.[13,14]

Transplacental studies have resulted in conflicting data. Roboz et al.[15] reported that doxorubicin was undetectable in amniotic fluid at 4 and 16 hours post-maternal intravenous administration; this nonexistence in the amniotic fluid cannot exclude transplacental passage. D'Incalci et al.[16] detected doxorubicin in fetal liver, kidney, and lung after elective termination; no levels were found in the amniotic fluid, fetal brain, or gastrointestinal tract 15 hours after administration. The fetal heart was not assessed.

Using liquid chromatography, Karp et al.[17] illustrated that doxorubicin concentrations were greatest in placental tissue, with none in cord tissue or blood in a healthy infant born 48 hours after therapy. A doxorubicin metabolite was detected in the cord, placental tissue, and neonatal spleen in a stillborn baby delivered 36 hours after maternal intravenous therapy.

At the time of delivery in a woman with acute promyelocytic leukemia (APL) undergoing therapy with all-trans retinoic acid (ATRA), its levels were measured in her venous blood and in the neonate's umbilical artery, vein, and peripheral blood.[18] Maternal ATRA levels were detectable at 2 and 4 hours after

| | | | | | | Time interval between infusion and | | |
| Ref. | Maternal cancer | Time of therapy (weeks) | Treatment | Dose | Fetal outcome | measurements (hours) | Measurements in fetal tissues | Results |
|------|-----------------|-------------------------|-----------|------|---------------|---------------------|------------------------------|---------|
| 13 | AML-FAB 3 | 29–30 | Daunorubicin | 45 mgm$^2$ daily for 3 days | Fetal death | 48 | Liver Kidney Lung Skin Heart | 0.015 ng/mL 0.02 ng/mL 0.02 ng/mL ND; LD 1.5 ng/100 mg ND |
| 14 | Breast cancer | 32–35 | Doxorubicin | 20 mg/m$^2$ | Normal child | 96 | Amniotic fluid only | ND; LD 0.2 ng/mL |

**Table 106.1** Transplacental passage of anthracyclines in vivo

FAB, French American British classification; ND, not detectable; LD, limit of quantification.

the last dose; no neonatal levels were found at 2 or 4 hours.

Although there are inconsistent data regarding the passage of chemotherapeutic agents across the placenta, it is assumed that virtually all chemotherapeutic agents do cross and other factors, such as fetal metabolism, may be the major determinant of teratogenicity.

### PASSAGE OF LEUKEMIC CELLS TO THE FETUS

Maternal cancer cells can metastasize to the placenta, and occasionally to the fetus. Read and Platzer[19] reported on 44 pregnant patients with various malignancies. They found six cases of acute leukemia involving the placenta or fetus, three patients with AML with only placental involvement (fetus not assessed in one instance), one ALL patient with placental involvement but not fetal, and two ALL patients with the placenta not examined, but ALL diagnosed in those fetuses.

Dildy et al.[20] published a review on maternal malignancies metastatic to the products of conception. Out of 53 patients, there were 8 cases of either leukemia or lymphoma detected in the placental tissue. Four of these included fetal involvement.

Another case involved a patient diagnosed with acute monocytic leukemia one day after delivery of a healthy male infant; subsequently at 20 months of age, the child was diagnosed with acute monocytic leukemia.[21] The histochemical staining and immunophenotyping of the mother and child's leukemic cells were identical. The child's bone marrow cytogenetic karyotype was 40% 46 XY, but the remaining 60% was 46 XX and most likely originated from his mother. The child had no other cytogenetic anomalies and both mother and child were in complete remission when last assessed.[21]

### DIAGNOSIS IN PREGNANCY

### PRENATAL CARE

Prenatal care provides a thorough medical monitoring system for young women. This includes a complete blood count (CBC) at the patient's first presentation; any abnormalities other than the expected hematopoietic changes should be further investigated, including bone marrow aspirate and biopsy. A repeat hemoglobin/hematocrit should be performed between 26 and 28 weeks of gestation and again at 32–36 weeks, with further testing according to abnormal results.[10]

The symptoms of leukemia in general are nonspecific: fatigue, dyspnea, fever, chills, and generalized malaise. Signs may include bleeding, bruising, petechiae, or infections that point to hematologic dysfunction. Pregnant patients should seek medical attention with any of these problems, as the symptoms of acute leukemia will only worsen with time. The diagnosis of any type of malignancy during pregnancy can be challenging as constitutional symptoms are often attributed to a normal pregnancy.

### DIAGNOSTIC WORK-UP

If there is any suspicion of marrow dysfunction based on the blood counts, peripheral blood smear, or presence of circulating leukemic blasts, then a bone marrow biopsy and aspirate should be performed. Bone marrow evaluation at any gestational age is safe; only local anesthesia is used and the patients can maintain a lateral decubitus position for an estimated 20-minute procedure. If a pregnant woman is diagnosed with acute leukemia, a multilumen central venous catheter is often required due to frequent blood draws, transfusions, chemotherapy infusions, and antibiotic use. Catheter placement can be safely performed by a general surgeon or interventional radiologist. Fluoroscopy is often used for guidance during placement, but can be avoided or used sparingly with pelvic shielding. Measurement of left ventricular ejection fraction is recommended prior to initiation of therapy, as anthracyclines are cardiotoxic. Multigated acquisition scans are often used, but in pregnant patients an echocardiogram can be performed to avoid radiation exposure. Computed tomography (CT) scans of the abdomen and pelvis are not critical for treatment or prognosis, and therefore are not required in the workup of a pregnant leukemic patient. In summary, there is minimal fetal risk in the maternal diagnostic workup for acute leukemias and in preparation for therapy.

### PHARMACOKINETICS WITH PREGNANCY

Maternal changes occur during pregnancy that can affect the metabolism of drugs.[9] These include:

Increased plasma volume, which in turn can increase the volume for drug dilution

Decreased albumin and increased plasma proteins due to estrogen, which can affect ratios of free and bound drugs

Increased renal blood flow and glomerular filtration rate, with subsequent influence on excretion of drugs

Increased activity of hepatic mixed function oxidases, thereby directly altering drug metabolism

Decreased gastric emptying, leading to interference with drug absorption

Fetal pharmacokinetics are not well established. The length of exposure to possible teratogens is an important factor; metabolites of maternal medications can be eliminated by the fetus into the amniotic fluid with subsequent fetal ingestion, gastrointestinal absorption, and elimination, thereby continuing the cycle.[9] Depending on the efficacy of these various processes and the types of drugs and their metabolites, there may be enhanced or diminished fetal exposure to medications. There is no data to conclude that amniotic fluid functions as a third-space compartment or if this could affect the dosing of medications during pregnancy. There is also no evidence to suggest that doses of chemotherapeutic agents should be altered to account for the new metabolic function in the mother.

## TERATOGENICITY OF CHEMOTHERAPEUTIC AGENTS

All chemotherapeutic agents are theoretically teratogenic and mutagenic. Fetal malformation, intrauterine growth retardation (IUGR), spontaneous abortion, and fetal death may occur. The teratogenicity of any particular drug depends on the timing of exposure, the total dose, and the drug characteristics on placental transfer. Drugs with high lipid solubility, low molecular weight, and decreased plasma protein binding have greater tendency for placental transfer from mother to fetus.

Chemotherapeutic agents cause cell death through several different mechanisms. They act on rapidly proliferating cells and thereby are potentially harmful to fetal tissues. Normal fetal cells undergo rapid growth with multiple cell divisions during the first trimester, especially during organogenesis (2–11 weeks of gestation). With the exception of brain and gonadal tissues, organogenesis is accomplished by 12 weeks of gestation. Therefore, if chemotherapy is administered during the first trimester, there is a high risk of fetal death due to immaturity of all fetal tissues.[9,22] During organogenesis, drug-induced teratogenesis can also manifest with major or minor abnormalities of organ systems without fetal death.

If chemotherapy causes severe damage early in gestation, spontaneous abortion often occurs. If sublethal damage occurs during organogenesis, malformation can result. Once organ development is complete, the rate of cell division decreases and the rate of cell injury and congenital malformations due to chemotherapy equals the risk in the general population (3%).[23,24] Although the available data suggests that chemotherapy administration after organogenesis does not appear to cause significant teratogenicity, one needs to take into account that central nervous system development is not complete and fetal growth and development may still be affected.

Doll et al.[9] reported on 139 cancer patients treated with various chemotherapeutic agents during the first trimester; the rate of fetal malformations was 17%. In 45 of these patients exposed to two or more agents concurrently, 16% had infants with malformations. If patients who received folate antagonists and radiation therapy were excluded, the malformation rate dropped to 6%.

The Toronto Leukemia Study Group reported that one-third of all infants exposed to chemotherapy in utero had pancytopenia at birth.[25] Aviles and Niz[26] reported on 17 infants delivered to mothers with acute leukemia treated during pregnancy. They concluded that chemotherapy did not have a major impact on later development. Garber[27] also reported on 43 children

born to mothers with hematologic malignancies who underwent chemotherapy during pregnancy. Nineteen of the mothers received treatment during the first trimester. No physical, neurologic, psychologic, hematologic, or cytogenetic defects were detected.

Cytarabine is a significant chemotherapeutic agent in leukemia. Wagner et al.[28] treated a patient for ALL, with relapse of disease on maintenance therapy, who acquired a second complete remission. The patient was on maintenance therapy with cytarabine when she conceived. Her three cytarabine cycles may have coincided with normal limb bud development, as her infant had a malformed right hand and bilateral femur, tibiofibular and foot defects, as well as bilateral external ear abnormalities.[28]

Another woman with AML conceived while undergoing treatment with cytarabine and oral thioguanine.[29] She continued this treatment until her term delivery. The neonate had upper and lower distal limb abnormalities, especially of his hands. The patient was continued on the same medications and again conceived 2–4 weeks after her last dose of chemotherapy. This infant was born without any abnormalities.[29]

Caligiuri and Mayer[23] reported on leukemic pregnant patients treated with cytarabine as either a single agent or in combination. Eighteen of these women gave birth to normal offsprings, and five pregnancies ended in elective abortions. Another AML patient was 20 weeks pregnant when treated with cytarabine and daunorubicin; she received reinduction with mitoxantrone and cytarabine. She subsequently underwent consolidation therapy with one cycle of cytarabine and idarubicin between weeks 29 and 30. Two days later she delivered a stillborn but phenotypically normal infant.[30]

The use of anthracyclines with combination chemotherapy has been reported by Turchi and Villasis in 20 pregnant patients.[31] Among the 20 patients treated, no fetal malformations resulted, but there was one maternal-fetal death, one therapeutic abortion, one spontaneous abortion, and four neonatal problems (marrow hypoplasia, pneumothorax, sepsis, and polycythemia) that all resolved.[31] In the infant who developed polycythemia, the maternal course was complicated by relapsed null-cell ALL on maintenance folate antimetabolites, requiring reinduction chemotherapy, pulmonary infiltrates requiring mechanical ventilation, and prolonged bone marrow aplasia. The infant was born at 36 weeks' gestation, weighed 2400 g, and polycythemia resolved with normal marrow function.[32]

APL has been reported in approximately 10% of cases of leukemia in pregnancy, similar to the percentage in nonpregnant leukemic patients. In 1995, Hoffman et al.[33] published a case report and a review of the English literature that compiled 24 cases of APL occurring in pregnant patients. Ten of these patients received an anthracycline with or without cytarabine or another agent for induction therapy. Three fetuses were exposed in the first trimester, with one spontaneous abortion, and five were exposed in the second trimester; the seven live neonates were normal. Two patients were treated in the third trimester, with one intrauterine death at 29 weeks' gestation.[33]

Requena et al.[34] described two patients with APL treated with cytarabine, thioguanine, daunorubicin, and mitoxantrone during the second trimester. Both women delivered normal neonates, though one infant was intubated for a total of 7 minutes. Takatsuki et al.[35] evaluated two APL patients who were both given a non-ATRA chemotherapy regimen. One patient received combination chemotherapy with daunorubicin at 14 weeks, when she presented with APL and DIC; intrauterine fetal death occurred (IUFD) at 19 weeks. The other patient was diagnosed with APL and DIC at 29 weeks of gestation. Combination chemotherapy including daunorubicin produced a complete remission, and the patient successfully delivered a normal infant.[35]

The advent of ATRA brought unknown risks to pregnant patients with APL. Another vitamin A derivative, 13-*cis*-retinoic acid, causes a specific retinoic embryopathy when taken in the first trimester.[3] Therefore, ATRA would be suspected of causing a similar set of deformities. Three of the patients described by Hoffman et al.[33] received ATRA between gestational weeks 30 and 32; they delivered a total of four normal, but premature, neonates. One patient was diagnosed with relapsed APL in the first trimester and treated with ATRA. Her infant was premature, but healthy at 15 months of age[33] Giagounidis et al.[36] reviewed 13 cases of APL in pregnancy treated with ATRA and did not find any fetal malformations attributed to ATRA. Several reports of fetal outcomes of pregnant patients who received ATRA are illustrated in Table 106.2.[37–47]

With the exception of the folate antimetabolites, teratogenicity cannot be completely attributed to one single

**Table 106.2** Pregnancy outcomes of 11 patients with APL who received ATRA during gestation

| Ref. | Week treated | Response | Other agents administered | DIC | Week delivered; outcome |
|---|---|---|---|---|---|
| 37 | At 23 weeks, for 35 days | CR | None | Yes; clinically mild, but excess perinatal hemorrhage | 32 weeks; normal twins |
| 38 | At 26 weeks, for 30 days | CR | None | Yes | 30 weeks; normal, but cardiac arrest (recovered) |
| 39 | At 28 weeks, for 30 days | CR | None | Yes | 32 weeks; normal |
| 40 | At 6 weeks, for 4 weeks | CR, then relapsed at 30 weeks | Prednisone | Yes | 32 weeks; normal, RDS (resolved) |
| 41 | At 14 weeks, for 60 days | CR | rhG-CSF, rhEPO | No; Jehovah's Witness | 40 weeks; normal |
| 42 | At 34 weeks, for 4 weeks | CR | None | Yes; received blood products | 38 weeks; normal |
| 43 | At 29 weeks, for 1 day; labor began 24–36 hours later | NR | None | No; no bleeding complications | Postnatal death; bilateral renal agenesis before APL diagnosed |
| 44 | At 30 weeks, for 2 weeks | CR | Daunorubicin, steroids day of delivery | Yes | 32 weeks; fetal distress, normal |
| 45 | At 30 weeks, for 38 days | CR | None | No | 33 weeks; atrial arrhythmia 2 days before delivery up to 1 day after birth; otherwise normal |
| 46 | At 24 weeks, until delivery | CR | daunorubicin, IV heparin | yes; received multiple blood products | 33 weeks; small intracranial hemorrhages by imaging |
| 47 | At 28 weeks, for 4 weeks | CR | none | no | 29 weeks; normal |

Reprinted with permission from Brell J, Kalaycio M.
CR, complete remission; NR, no response; RDS, respiratory distress syndrome; rhG-CSF, recombinant human granulocyte colony-stimulating factor; rhEPO, recombinant human erythropoietin; IV, intravenous.

chemotherapeutic agent when combination chemotherapy is administered with various other agents such as antiemetics, antibiotics, antifungals, antivirals, premedications, and blood products. The majority of leukemic patients and neonates survive gestation, labor, and delivery without major complications. Conventional chemotherapy to treat leukemia during pregnancy is not associated with a marked increase in the rate of malformation or long-term sequelae.[23,26]

## TREATMENT OF SPECIFIC HEMATOLOGIC MALIGNANCIES

### OVERVIEW

The diagnosis of a life-threatening disorder during pregnancy is a formidable challenge for both the patient and the physician. All risks, benefits, and alternatives for the patient and fetus must be discussed in detail. The patient should understand that no outcome can be guaranteed, but the available data should be presented to her in a comprehensive manner. Conclusions regarding the complexity of the decision to treat and continue the pregnancy should be reached by the consensus of the patient, patient's family, and physician. Unfortunately, there are no large prospective studies that address chemotherapy administration during pregnancy, and subsequently physicians are forced to formulate treatment regimens based on small retrospective studies and case reports.

### ACUTE LEUKEMIAS

Leukemia itself can adversely affect perinatal outcome. Spontaneous abortion, prematurity, IUGR, and death have been associated with maternal leukemia. The earlier the diagnosis of leukemia during pregnancy, the higher the perinatal mortality. Adverse factors include maternal anemia, DIC, or leukemic cells affecting blood flow, nutrient exchange, and oxygen delivery in the intervillous spaces of the placenta. Acute leukemia is a hematologic urgency and requires treatment without delay. Chemotherapy at full doses can be safely administered, even during the first trimester, if cure of the hematologic malignancy is considered reasonable.[48–50] However, great concerns remain about the teratogenic and mutagenic effects on the fetus during organogenesis.

Management of acute leukemias is based on the stage of pregnancy at the time of diagnosis of the malignancy. In the first trimester, the patient should be offered the option of termination due to concerns of the 10–20% risk of teratogenicity with chemotherapy during organogenesis[51,52]; if abortion is declined, then the patient should be treated. Patients diagnosed with leukemia after the first trimester should undergo prompt chemotherapy.

Caliguiri and Mayer compiled 72 cases of new-onset leukemia diagnosed with or during pregnancy.[23] AML was diagnosed in 44 patients, ALL in 20, chronic myelogenous leukemia (CML) accounted for five cases (four in chronic phase), hairy-cell leukemia (HCL) in one instance, and two cases were not specified. They reported on 58 patients who were administered chemotherapy while pregnant; only eight cases were not given cytarabine, or an anthracycline, or both. As the time of the first exposure to chemotherapy advanced from first to third trimester, the number of spontaneous abortions and stillbirths decreased, with most neonates born normal regardless of premature or term birth. There were no congenital defects reported in patients undergoing chemotherapy during the first trimester. There were no perinatal deaths; overall fetal survival was 84% (49 of 58 fetuses).[23]

Catanzarite and Ferguson[11] reviewed records on pregnancy and acute leukemia. They collected outcomes on 39 fetuses first exposed to chemotherapy during gestation, ranging from conception to the third trimester. A total of 31 patients received induction chemotherapy for AML (24 patients) or ALL (seven patients) during their pregnancy. Eight patients conceived while on maintenance therapy. Twenty infants were delivered at term and 12 were premature. There were a total of three therapeutic abortions, two perinatal deaths (at 21 days and 3 months of life, both from infection with no evidence of leukemia), and two intrauterine deaths (at 24 and 30 weeks), for a fetal survival of 32/39 or 82%. There were no malformations recorded.[11]

In a recent review by Ali et al.,[53] 10 pregnancies in 8 patients with acute leukemia were discussed. Six of the patients had AML and two had ALL. Three of the pregnancies were diagnosed when the leukemia was in remission, six at the time of leukemia diagnosis, and one at the time of relapse. In this case series, five of the eight pregnant women died from their malignancy. Only 1 child survived from the 10 pregnancies, and this child was not exposed to any chemotherapeutic agents.[53] Table 106.3 illustrates the maternal and fetal data of the eight cases.

Hansen et al. published a case of a 24-year-old patient diagnosed with ALL at 24 weeks of gestation.[54] The patient began course one of induction chemotherapy at 26 weeks with cyclophosphamide, daunorubicin, vincristine, prednisone, and L-asparaginase. At 30 weeks gestation, she was started on intensification therapy with methotrexate, cyclophosphamide, 6-mercaptopurine, vincristine, and L-asparaginase. This course of chemotherapy was repeated at 34 weeks. Two days later, she had a normal spontaneous vaginal delivery with a normal infant, but with mild meconium aspiration. Serial abdominal ultrasounds throughout pregnancy revealed gradual decline in the rate of fetal growth, with recurrent, transient oligohydramnios, yet uterine artery doppler and fetal heart rate testing remained normal.[54]

Children and adults who undergo treatment with anthracyclines are at risk for dose-related cardiotoxicity.[55]

**Table 106.3** Summary of eight patients with acute leukemia during pregnancy

| Case | Age (year) | Pregnancy | AML subtype | Leukemia status | Period of pregnancy, status of fetus | Treatment during pregnancy | Outcome of pregnancy | Condition of patient |
|---|---|---|---|---|---|---|---|---|
| 1 | 23 | 1 | AML-M$_4$ | Active disease | 8 weeks, alive | — | Spontaneous abortion | Died during CT |
| 2 | 25 | 2<br>3 | ALL-L$_1$, B cell<br>ALL-L$_1$, B cell | Active disease<br>4th year of CR | 24 weeks, dead fetus<br>8 weeks, alive | —<br> | Therapeutic abortion<br>Alive baby, normal | CR<br>CR, still alive |
| 3 | 21 | 4<br>5 | ALL-L$_2$, B cell<br>ALL-L$_2$, B cell | 12th mon. of CR.<br>Relapse, active disease (31st month of CR) | 12 weeks, alive<br>8 weeks, alive | —<br>— | Spontaneous abortion<br>Therapeutic abortion | CR Died during CT |
| 4 | 37 | 6 | AML-M$_3$ | Active disease | 26 weeks, alive | Daunorubicin, cytarabine | Spontaneous abortion in 1st wk of CT | Died during CT |
| 5 | 29 | 7 | AML-M$_4$ | Active disease | 24 weeks, alive | Daunorubicin, cytarabine | IUD during CT, therapeutic abortion | Died during CT |
| 6 | 24 | 8 | AML-M$_1$ | 6th month of CR, relapse at 12th week of gestation | 8 weeks, alive | — | Therapeutic abortion | Died during CT |
| 7 | 20 | 9 | AML-M$_3$ | Active disease | 19 weeks, dead fetus | — | Therapeutic abortion | Still in 1st CR |
| 8 | 21 | 10 | AML-M$_4$ | Active disease | 12 weeks, alive | — | Therapeutic abortion | Still in 1st CR |

Reprinted with permission from Ali R. et al.
CR, complete remission; IUD, intrauterine death; CT, chemotherapy.

This toxicity is related to free-radical damage to myocardial fibers.[56] Whether anthracycline exposure to the developing fetus in utero is cardiotoxic is unknown. Meyer-Wittkopf et al.[57] performed fetal echocardiograms every 2 weeks from week 24 in a patient undergoing treatment for breast cancer with doxorubicin and cyclophosphamide. No differences in systolic function were discovered between exposed and unexposed fetuses. Echocardiograms of up to 2 years of age revealed no myocardial damage.[57] Three cases of neonatal cardiac effects after in utero exposure to anthracyclines have been reported.[56,58,59] One had been exposed to both doxorubicin and pelvic irradiation and subsequently developed only one coronary artery.[58] Two developed right-sided cardiomyopathy after second trimester exposure to idarubicin with tretinoin or with vincristine, daunorubicin, and cyclophosphamide.[56,59]

Idarubicin is more lipophilic and therefore has increased propensity for placental transfer. It may also have a higher affinity for DNA. An IUFD has been reported 2 days after idarubicin was given for consolidation therapy for AML.[30] Epirubicin, another anthracycline, was used to treat 13 women in two studies. Twenty-three percent of fetuses exposed to epirubicin died either as fetuses or as neonates.[60,61]

### MYELODYSPLASTIC SYNDROMES

Siddiqui et al.[62] described five women diagnosed with myelodysplastic syndromes (MDS) during pregnancy from 1982 to 1987 (see Table 106.4). Steensma et al.[63] identified all patients at the Mayo Clinic with MDS and pregnancy seen between 1976 and 2000. A total of seven pregnancies were discovered, occurring in four patients with MDS between 1983 and 2000. In three of the four patients, MDS was suspected after an initial CBC for routine prenatal care. Patients were between 21 and 42 years of age. After bone marrow evaluation, all patients had refractory anemia except one with refractory anemia with excess blasts (RAEB). Three patients, including the RAEB patient, delivered normal term

| Table 106.4 | Myelodysplasia associated with pregnancy | | | |
|---|---|---|---|---|
| Maternal age (year) | Gestational week | Subclass; course or therapy | Pregnancy outcome | Maternal outcome |
| 22 | 16 | RAEB; septic endometritis | Therapeutic abortion | AML by 4th month; expired after 2 years |
| 31 | 12 | RA; no CBC changes after abortion | Therapeutic abortion | Expired 1 month after MRD-BMT |
| 32 | 20 | RA; transfusional support | Healthy, term infant | AML in 5th month, increased platelets postpartum; expired |
| 31 | 30 | RAEB; no treatment | Down syndrome infant at 36 week | AML after 2 years; expired |
| 31 | Unknown | Unknown | Low birth weight infant | Postpartum AML; expired |

Reprinted with permission from Siddiqui T. et al.
CR, complete response; MRD-BMT, matched related donor-bone marrow transplant; RA, refractory anemia.

infants. The other patient developed spontaneous abortion. Only one patient required therapy for MDS due to rapid progression into acute leukemia; she was treated with idarubicin and cytarabine at 30 weeks gestation without remission, and treated again with same agents successfully prior to delivery. She delivered a healthy infant and subsequently underwent a matched unrelated allogeneic stem cell transplantation 2 months postpartum and remained in remission.[63]

Although only a handful of cases of MDS with pregnancy have been reported, the relative indolence of MDS suggests that termination of pregnancy should only be a consideration seldom. In most patients, disease-specific therapy can be postponed until after delivery, but patients in the high-risk International Prognostic Scoring System (IPSS) may require cytotoxic therapy during pregnancy.[63]

## CHRONIC MYELOGENOUS LEUKEMIA

Unlike acute leukemias, chronic leukemias often do not require urgent therapy. With observation and supportive care alone, many pregnancies can be completed successfully without complications. Cytotoxic chemotherapy can often be delayed until after delivery if a patient remains in the chronic phase.

Cytotoxic agents (interferon, hydroxyurea, imatinib mesylate) and leukapheresis have been used in pregnant CML patients. Interferon (IFN) is not teratogenic and has no known adverse effects on pregnancy.[9,64,65] The use of imatinib has recently been reported in one pregnant patient.[66]

There have been a few cases of use of hydroxyurea in pregnant patients[67-71]; the majority of these patients conceived while on therapy, and the fetuses were exposed to the drug throughout the gestational period. Both maternal and fetal outcomes were uncomplicated in these cases.

The first report of a patient conceiving while on IFN for CML was published in 1991. IFN, 4 million units subcutaneously administered every other day,

controlled blood counts, and the patient delivered a healthy infant at term.[64] Another patient on IFN therapy for approximately 2 years for chronic phase CML became pregnant. Therapy was continued and she delivered a normal term infant.[72] No adverse fetal effects from IFN have been reported.

Imatinib has an excellent safety profile, but in toxicology studies it has been shown to induce abortions and can be teratogenic at high concentrations in animals.[73] Therefore, pregnancy is considered a contraindication for the use of imatinib and contraception is recommended while on this therapy. The first case of pregnancy conceived while on imatinib was reported by Heartin et al.[66] A 34-year-old woman with Philadelphia positive chronic phase CML was started on leukapheresis and hydroxyurea. She achieved complete hematologic remission within 4 weeks. After two negative pregnancy tests, she was treated with imatinib 400 mg daily. Despite appropriate contraception counseling, the patient became pregnant after 25 days of treatment and ultrasound confirmed a viable fetus of 7 weeks. Imatinib was discontinued immediately, but the fetus had been exposed to imatinib during the crucial period of embryogenesis between approximately days 8 and 33 of gestation. The patient required hydroxyurea at 29 weeks of gestation due to a WBC of 82,000/$\mu$L and platelets of 529,000/$\mu$L. Labor was induced at 38 weeks of pregnancy, and a healthy baby girl was delivered. At 6 weeks postpartum, hydroxyurea was stopped and imatinib was resumed. Six months after imatinib therapy, she attained a major complete cytogenetic response and maintained the response for at least 24 months. This was the first reported case of a pregnant woman exposed to imatinib. Although the pregnancy was uneventful for both mother and child, there is not yet enough data to support the use of imatinib in pregnant patients. The recommendation of barrier contraceptive use in women of child-bearing age while undergoing treatment with imatinib is still enforced. However, this case report suggests that if and when patients inadvertently conceive while on imatinib, the pregnancy can evolve uneventfully and successfully with adequate care and monitoring.

### CHRONIC LYMPHOCYTIC LEUKEMIA

The incidence of chronic lymphocytic leukemia (CLL) during pregnancy is rare, as this malignancy affects mainly the older population, with a median age of approximately 70 years, and it affects men twice as often as women. Only 10–15% of patients are under the age of 50 years.[74] The management of CLL in the pregnant patient is challenging due to lack of data. Information regarding the effects of various chemotherapeutic agents on the developing fetus is derived solely from reports describing teratogenic and mutagenic effects in animal experiments, and case reports on pregnancy outcomes complicated by various other malignancies. Only four cases of pregnancy and CLL have been described.[75-78]

The natural course of CLL can be highly variable, and chemotherapy is often not indicated if the disease is in an early and stable stage, as there is no data to support improvement in survival with early intervention.[79] Therefore, CLL may not require treatment immediately because it has a relatively indolent course, but it can carry a risk of leukostasis, as well as risk of placental insufficiency, IUGR, increased fetal prematurity, and increased mortality.[80] Leukapheresis has been successfully used in both acute and chronic leukemias for rapid reduction of high WBC counts in patients with symptoms of increased viscosity. This form of treatment provides a temporary alternative to chemotherapy for the pregnant patient with signs/symptoms of leukostasis.[81-83]

In a case reported by Chrisomalis et al.,[75] a 30-year-old woman with CLL experienced repeated infections during pregnancy that were treated successfully with antibiotics. She was not treated for the CLL, as she was asymptomatic. In addition to her bone marrow, the intervillous spaces of the placenta were filled with mature-appearing lymphocytes consistent with CLL. The patient delivered a healthy newborn, and the patient and baby remained in good health 1 year after delivery.[75] Welsh et al.[76] reported a 22-year-old patient with CLL diagnosed at 35 weeks gestation with a WBC count of 45,400/µL. She delivered a healthy infant at term. Four months following delivery, her WBC count decreased to 10,300/µL without therapy. She continued to have a high percentage of monoclonal lymphocytes, but the absolute number decreased. The authors concluded that this represents an apparent spontaneous "clinical" but not "clonal" regression.[76]

Ali et al. published a case of a 30-year-old woman who presented with anemia and cervical lymphadenopathy in the 17th week of gestation.[78] Based on clinical findings, and microscopic analysis of her peripheral blood and bone marrow, she was diagnosed

as having stage IV B-cell CLL. The patient underwent three courses of leukapheresis at the 25th, 30th, and 38th weeks of gestation to maintain the WBC count below 100,000/µL. Therapeutic pheresis was well tolerated by the mother and fetus, and no complications were identified. A healthy baby was born at term without anatomical or hematologic abnormalities.

There have been no reports on the use of purine analogues in pregnancy.

Targeted therapy with an anti-CD52 or anti-CD20 monoclonal antibody has been used in untreated CLL patients and in those with progressive disease after fludarabine treatment.[84,85] Rituximab is one such anti-CD20 monoclonal antibody, and there exists little evidence for its safety during pregnancy. One report on rituximab and pregnancy has been published in a non-Hodgkin's lymphoma patient. A 29-year-old female with stage IIA bulky CD20+ diffuse large B-cell lymphoma was treated with rituximab during 21 weeks of gestation. She received four cycles of therapy along with doxorubicin, vincristine, and oral prednisolone. The patient developed a very good partial remission and subsequently delivered a healthy term infant by Cesarean section. The child developed normally, and a normal peripheral B-cell population was detected at 4 months.[86]

### HAIRY-CELL LEUKEMIA

HCL is a rare hematologic malignancy of older men, with a median age of 50–55 years. It has a generally favorable prognosis, with excellent treatment response to nucleoside analogs. HCL has been reported in a few pregnant women.[64,87-89] Two pregnant patients diagnosed with HCL received IFN during second and third trimesters of pregnancy. No side effects were reported, and both delivered healthy infants at term.[64] In another patient, treatment was deferred until after delivery, although the patient required a splenectomy at 16 weeks. She subsequently delivered at term without complications.[88] Another report described a woman found to have HCL and massive splenomegaly late in the second trimester. Due to pancytopenia (WBC 4000/µL, platelet count 65,000/µL, hematocrit 28.6%), she underwent splenectomy with resolution of thrombocytopenia and normal progression of pregnancy successfully.[89]

### ADULT T-CELL LEUKEMIA-LYMPHOMA

Human T-cell lymphotrophic virus type I (HTLV-I), the causative agent in adult T-cell leukemia-lymphoma, is uncommon in the United States. A case report of adult T-cell leukemia-lymphoma during pregnancy has been published.[90] A 23-year-old female was admitted with a 1-week history of sore throat, fever, and fatigue during the 26th week of gestation. The WBC was 55,900/µL with 74% unclassified cells. Flow cytometry revealed increased numbers of CD3+, CD4+, and CD3-CD25+ T cells in her blood, and her bone marrow demonstrated 34% atypical, intermediate-size lymphocytes. IgG anti-HTLV-I or HTLV-II antibodies were present and HTLV-I was detected by a polymerase chain reaction assay. The patient was treated with hydroxyurea and CHOP (cyclophosphamide, doxorubicin, vincristine, and prednisone) with a subsequent drop in her WBC to 12,700/μL. On the eighth day of admission, a healthy infant was delivered by cesarean section.[90]

## SUMMARY

Despite the retrospective and often anecdotal nature of the available data on pregnancy and leukemia, several principles of management can be inferred:

1. If possible, chemotherapy should be avoided during the first trimester; use of chemotherapy after the first trimester appears to be safe.
2. Patients with acute leukemia require chemotherapy as soon as feasible regardless of trimester to avoid poor maternal outcomes.
3. Once a decision to treat has been made, chemotherapy should be given at full doses and on schedule to maximize efficacy.
4. A multidisciplinary team including specialists in oncology, obstetrics, perinatology, and neonatology is necessary to coordinate care, improve the chance of cure in the mother, and minimize neonatal harm.

Beyond these basic tenets, treatment should be individualized with other proper obstetric care and monitoring to maximize the potential for favorable outcomes.

## REFERENCES

1. Potter JF, Schoeneman M: Metastasis of maternal cancer to the placenta and fetus. *Cancer* 25:380–88, 1970.
2. Buekers TE, Lallas TA: Chemotherapy in pregnancy. *Obstet Gynecol Clin North Am* 25:323–32, 1998.
3. Lichtman MA, Liesveld JL: Acute myelogenous leukemia. In: Beutler E, Coller BS, Kipps TJ, Seligsohn U (eds.): *Williams Hematology*, 6th ed. New York: McGraw-Hill; 2001:1047.
4. Antonelli NM, Dotters DJ, Katz VL, et al.: Cancer in pregnancy: a review of the literature, part I. *Obstet Gynecol Sur* 51:125–134, 1996.
5. Donegan WL: Cancer and pregnancy. *CA Cancer J Clin* 33:194–214, 1983.
6. Duffy TP: Hematologic aspects of pregnancy. In: Hoffman R, Benz EJ, Shattil SJ, Furie B, Cohen HJ, Silberstein LE (eds.): *Hematology*, 2nd ed. New York: Churchill Livingstone; 1995:2117.
7. Peck TM, Arias F: Hematologic changes associated with pregnancy. *Clin Obstet Gynecol* 22:785, 1979.
8. Cartwright RA, Staines A: Acute leukemias. *Baillieres Clin Haematol* 5:1, 1992.
9. Doll DC, Ringenberg QS, Yarbro JW: Antineoplastic agents and pregnancy. *Semin Oncol* 16:337, 1989.
10. American Academy of Pediatrics and American College of Obstetricians and Gynecologists. *Guidelines for perinatal care*, 4th ed. Elk Grove Village, IL: 1997:67.
11. Catanzarite VA, Ferguson JE: Acute leukemia and pregnancy: a review of mangament and outcome, 1972–1982. *Obstet Gynecol Surv* 39:663, 1984.
12. Moore KL. *The developing human: Clinically Oriented Embryology*, 4th ed. Philadelphia, PA: WB Saunders; 1988:38.
13. Germann N, Goffinet F, Goldwasser F: Anthracyclines during pregnancy: embryo-fetal outcomes in 160 patients. *Ann Oncol* 15:146–150, 2004.
14. Murray CL, Reichert JA, Anderson J, et al.: Multimodal cancer therapy for breast cancer in the first trimester of pregnancy. *J Am Med Assoc* 252:2607–2608, 1984.
15. Roboz J, Gleicher N, Wuk K, et al.: Does doxorubicin cross the placenta? *Lancet* 2:1382–83, 1979.
16. d'Incalci M, Broggini M, Buscaglia M, et al.: Transplacental passage of doxorubicin. *Lancet* 75:8314–8315, 1983.
17. Karp GI, von Oeyen P, Valone F, et al.: Doxorubicin in pregnancy: possible transplacental passage. *Cancer Treat Rep* 67:773–777, 1983.
18. Terada Y, Shindo Y, Endoh A, et al.: Fetal arrhythmia during treatment of pregnancy-associated acute promyelocytic leukemia with all-trans retinoic acid and favorable outcome. *Leukemia* 11:454, 1997.
19. Read EJ, Platzer PB: Placental metastasis from maternal carcinoma of the lung. *Obstet Gynecol* 58:387–391, 1981.
20. Dildy GA, Moise KJ, Carpenter RJ, et al.: Maternal malignancy metastatic to the products of conception: A review. *Obstet Gynecol Surv* 44:535–540, 1989.
21. Honore LH, Brown LB: Intervillous placental metastasis with maternal myeloid leukemia (letter). *Arch Pathol Lab Med* 114:450, 1990.
22. Zemlickis D, Lishner M, Degendorfer P, et al.: Fetal outcome after in utero exposure to cancer chemotherapy. *Arch Intern Med* 152:573–576, 1992.
23. Caligiuri MA, Mayer RJ: Pregnancy and leukemia. *Semin Oncol* 16:388, 1989.
24. Kalter H, Warkany J: Congenital malformations: etiologic factors and their role in prevention (first of two parts). *N Engl J Med* 308:424, 1983.
25. Reynoso EE, Shepherd FA, Messner HA, et al.: Acute leukemia during pregnancy: the Toronto Leukemia Study Group experience with long-term follow-up of children exposed in utero to chemotherapeutic agents. *J Clin Oncol* 5:1098, 1987.
26. Aviles A, Niz J: Long-term follow-up of children born to mothers with acute leukemia during pregnancy. *Med Pediatr Oncol* 16:3, 1988.
27. Garber JE: Long-term follow-up of children exposed in utero to antineoplastic agents. *Semin Oncol* 16:437, 1989.
28. Wagner VM, Hill JS, Weaver D, et al.: Congenital abnormalities in baby born to cytarabine-treated mother. *Lancet* 2:98, 1990.
29. Schafer AI: Teratogenetic effects of antileukemic chemotherapy. *Arch Intern Med* 141:514, 1981.

30. Reynoso EE, Huerta F: Acute leukemia and pregnancy: fatal fetal outcome after exposure to idarubicin during the second trimester. *Acta Oncol* 33:709, 1994.

31. Turchi JJ, Villasis C: Anthracyclines in the treatment of malignancy in pregnancy. *Cancer* 61:435, 1988.

32. Dara P, Slater LM, Armentrout SA: Successful pregnancy during chemotherapy for acute leukemia. *Cancer* 47:845, 1981.

33. Hoffman MA, Wiernik PH, Kleiner GJ: Acute promyelocytic leukemia and pregnancy: a case report. *Cancer* 76:2237–2241, 1995.

34. Requena A, Velasco JG, Pinilla J, et al.: Acute leukemia during pregnancy: obstetric management and perinatal outcome of two cases. *Eur J Obstet Gynecol Reprod Biol* 63:139–141, 1995.

35. Takatsuki H, Abe Y, Goto T, et al: Two cases of acute promyelocytic leukemia in pregnancy and the effect of anthracyclines on fetal development. *Rinsho Ketsueki* 33:1736–1740, 1992. Abstract.

36. Guigounidis AA, Beckmann MW, Giagounidis AS, et al.: Acute promyelocytic leukemia and pregnancy. *Eur J Haematol* 64:267–271, 2000.

37. Stentoft J, Nielson L, Hvidman LE: All-trans retinoic acid in acute promyelocytic leukemia in late pregnancy. *Leukemia* 8:1585–1588, 1994.

38. Harrison P, Chipping P, Fothergill GA: Successful use of all-trans retinoic acid in acute promyelocytic leukemia presenting during the second trimester of pregnancy. *Br J Haematol* 86:681–682, 1994.

39. Watanabe R, Okamoto S, Moriki T, et al.: Treatment of acute promyelocytic leukemia with all-trans retinoic acid during the first trimester of pregnancy (letter). *Am J Hematol* 48:210–211, 1995.

40. Simone MD, Stasi R, Venditti A, et al.: All-trans retinoic acid (ATRA) administration during pregnancy in relapsed acute promyelocytic leukemia (letter). *Leukemia* 9:1412–1413, 1995.

41. Lin CP, Huang MJ, Liu HJ, et al.: Successful treatment of acute promyelocytic leukemia in a pregnant Jehovah's Witness with all-trans retinoic acid, rhG-CSF, and erythropoietin (letter). *Am J Hematol* 51:251–252, 1996.

42. Lipovsky MM, Biesma DH, Christiaens GC, et al.: Successful treatment of acute promyelocytic leukemia with all-trans retinoic acid during late pregnancy. *Br J Hematol* 94:699–701, 1996.

43. Sham RL: All-trans retinoic acid-induced labor in a patient with acute promyelocytic leukemia (letter). *Am J Hematol* 53:145, 1996.

44. Nakamura K, Dan K, Iwakiri R, et al.: Successful treatment of acute promyelocytic leukemia in pregnancy with all-trans retinoic acid (letter). *Ann Hematol* 71:263–264, 1995.

45. Terada Y, Shindo T, Endoh A, et al.: Fetal arrhythmia during treatment of pregnancy-associated acute promyelocytic leukemia with all-trans retinoic acid and favorable outcome (letter). *Leukemia* 11:454–455, 1997.

46. Incerpi MH, Miller DA, Posen R, et al.: All-trans retinoic acid for the treatment of acute promyelocytic leukemia in pregnancy. *Obstet Gynecol* 89:826–828, 1997.

47. Tsuda H, Doi H, Inada T, et al.: Successful treatment of acute promyelocytic leukemia in a pregnant women by using all-trans retinoic acid. *Rinsho Ketsueki* 35:717–719, 1994. Abstract.

48. Aviles A, Neri N: Hematological malignancies and pregnancy: a final report of 84 children who received chemotherapy in utero. *Clin Lymphoma* 2:173–177, 2001.

49. Aviles A, Diaz-Maqueo JC, Talavera A, et al.: Growth and development of children of mothers treated with chemotherapy during pregnancy: current status of 43 children. *Am J Hematol* 36:243–248, 1991.

50. Pizzuto J, Aviles A, Noriega L, et al.: Treatment of acute leukemia during pregnancy: presentation of nine cases. *Cancer Treat Rep* 64:679–683, 1980.

51. Feliu J, Suarez S, Ordonez A, et al.: Acute leukemia and pregnancy. *Cancer* 61:580–584, 1988.

52. Buekers TE, Lallas TA.: Chemotherapy in pregnancy. *Obstet Gynecol Clin North Am* 25:323–329, 1998.

53. Ali R, Ozkalemkas F, Ozcelik, et al.: Maternal and fetal outcomes in pregnancy complicated with acute leukemia: a single institutional experience with 10 pregnancies at 16 years. *Leukemia Res* 27:381–385, 2003.

54. Hansen WF, Fretz P, Hunter SK, et al.: Leukemia in pregnancy and fetal response to multiagent chemotherapy. *Obstet Gynecol* 97(5):809–812, 2001.

55. Lipshultz SE, Colan SD, Gelber RD, et al.: Late cardiac effects of doxorubicin therapy for acute lymphoblastic leukemia in childhood. *N Engl J Med* 324:808–815, 1991.

56. Siu BL, Alonzo MR, Vargo TA, et al.: Transient dilated cardiomyopathy in a newborn exposed to idarubicin and all-trans-retinoic acid (ATRA) early in the second trimester of pregnancy. *Int J Gynecol Cancer* 12:399–402, 2002.

57. Meyer-Wittkopf M, Barth H, Emons G, et al.: Fetal cardiac effects of doxorubicin therapy for carcinoma of the breast during pregnancy; case report and review of the literature. *Ultrasound Obstet Gynecol* 18:62–66, 2001.

58. Cardonick E, Iacobucci A: Use of chemotherapy during human pregnancy. *Lancet Oncol* 5:283–291, 2004.

59. Achtari C, Hohlfeld P: Cardiotoxic transplacental effect of idarubicin administered during the second trimester of pregnancy. *Am J Obstet Gynecol* 183:511–512, 2000.

60. Peres RM, Sanseverino MT, Guimaraes JL, et al.: Assessment of fetal risk associated with exposure to cancer chemotherapy during pregnancy: a multicenter study. *Braz J Med Biol Res* 34:1551–1559, 2001.

61. Giacalone PL, Laffargue F, Benos P: Chemotherapy for breast carcinoma during pregnancy: a French national survey. *Cancer* 86:2266–2272, 1999.

62. Siddiqui T, Elfenbein GJ, Noyes WD, et al.: Myelodysplastic syndromes presenting in pregnancy. *Cancer* 66:377, 1990.

63. Steensma DP, Tefferi A: Myelodysplastic syndrome and pregnancy: the Mayo Clinic Experience. *Leuk Lymphoma* 42:1229–1234, 2001.

64. Baer MR, Ozer H, Foon KA: Interferon alpha therapy during pregnancy in chronic myelogenous leukemia and hairy cell leukemia. *Br J Haematol* 81:167–169, 1992.

65. Mubarak AA, Kakil IR, Awidi A, et al.: Normal outcome of pregnancy in chronic myeloid leukemia treated with interferon alpha in the 1st trimester: report of 3 cases and review of the literature. *Am J Hematol* 69:115–118, 2002.

66. Heartin E, Walkinshaw, Clark RE: Successful outcome of pregnancy in chronic myeloid leukemia treated with imatinib (letter to the editor). *Leuk Lymphoma* 45(6):1307–1308, 2004.

67. Delmer A, Rio B, Bauduer F, et al.: Pregnancy during myelosuppressive treatment for chronic myelogenous leukaemia (letter). *Br J Haematol* 82:783–784, 1992.

68. Patel M, Dukes IA, Hull JC: Use of hydroxyurea in chronic myeloid leukemia during pregnancy: a case report. *Am J Obstet Gynecol* 165:565–566, 1991.

69. Jackson N, Shukri A, Ali K: Hydroxyurea treatment for chronic myeloid leukaemia during pregnancy. *Br J Haematol* 85:203–204, 1993.

70. Tertian G, Tchernia G, Papiernik E, et al.: Hydroxyurea and pregnancy (letter). *Am J Obstet Gynecol* 166:868, 1992.

71. Fitzgerald JM, McCann SR: The combination of hydroxyurea and leukapheresis in the treament of chronic myeloid leukemia in pregnancy. *Clin Lab Haematol* 15:63–65, 1993.

72. Reichel RP, Linkesch W, Schetitska D: Therapy with recombinant interferon alpha-2c during unexpected pregnancy in a patient with chronic myeloid leukemia. *Br J Haematol* 82:472, 1992.

73. Druker BJ, Lydon NB: Lessons learned from the development of an Abl tyrosine kinase inhibitor for chronic myelogenous leukemia. *J Clin Invest* 105:3–7, 2000.

74. de Lima M, O'Brien S, Lerner S, et al.: Chronic lymphocytic leukemia in the young patient. *Semin Oncol* 25:107–116, 1998.

75. Chrisomalis L, Baxi LV, Heller D: Chronic lymphocytic leukemia in pregnancy. *Am J Obstet Gynecol* 175:1381–1382, 1996.

76. Welsh TM, Thompson J, Lim S: Chronic lymphocytic leukemia in pregnancy. *Leukemia* 14:155, 2000.

77. Gurman G: Pregnancy and successful labor in the course of chronic lymphocytic leukemia. *Am J Hematol* 71:208–210, 2002.

78. Ali R, Ozkalemkas F, Ozkocaman V, et al.: Successful labor in the course of chronic lymphocytic leukemia and management of CLL during pregnancy with leukapheresis. *Ann Hematol* 83:61–63, 2004.

79. Cheson BD, Bennett JM, Rai KR, et al.: Guidelines for clinical protocols for chronic lympocytic leukemia: recommendations of the National Cancer Institute-sponsored working group. *Am J Hematol* 29:152, 1988.

80. Juarez S, Cuadrado-Pastor JM, Feliu J, et al.: Association of leukemia and pregnancy: clinical and obstetric aspects. *Am J Clin Oncol* 11:159–165, 1988.

81. Hester J: Therapeutic cell depletion. In: Mcleod BC, Price TH, Drew MJ (eds.): *Apheresis: Principles and Practice.* Bethesda, MD: AABB Press; 1997:251.

82. Fitzgerald D, Rowe JM, Heal J: Leukapheresis for control of chronic myelogenous leukemia during pregnancy. *Am J Hematol* 22:213–218, 1986.

83. Strobl FJ, Boelkerding KV, Smith EP: Management of chronic myeloid leukemia during pregnancy with leukapheresis. *J Clin Apheresis* 14:42–44, 1999.

84. Flynn JM, Byrd JC: Campath-1H monoclonal antibody therapy. *Curr Opin Oncol* 12:574–581, 2000.

85. Francesca R, Mauro, Foa R, et al.: Autoimmune hemolytic anemia in chronic lymphocytic leukemia: clinical, therapeutic, and prognostic features. *Blood* 95:2786–2792, 2000.

86. Herold M, Schnohr S, Bittrich H: Efficacy and safety of a combined rituximab chemotherapy during pregnancy (letter to the editor). *J Clin Oncol* 19(14):3439, 2001.

87. Williams JK: Hairy cell leukemia in pregnancy: a case report. *Am J Obstet Gynecol* 156:210, 1987.

88. Alothman A, Sparling TG: Managing hairy cell leukemia in pregnancy. *Ann Intern Med* 120:1048, 1994.

89. Stiles GM, Stanco LM, Saven A, et al.: Splenectomy for hairy cell leukemia in pregnancy. *J Perinatol* 18(3):200–201, 1998.

90. Safdar A, Johnson N, Gonzalez F, et al.: Adult T-cell leukemia-lymphoma during pregnancy (letter to the editor). *N Engl J Med* 346(25):2014–2015, 2002.

# Chapter 107

# TUMOR LYSIS SYNDROME, DISSEMINATED INTRAVASCULAR COAGULOPATHY, AND OTHER NON-INFECTIOUS COMPLICATIONS OF LEUKEMIA AND LYMPHOMA

*Rajesh Kukunoor and Mikkael A. Sekeres*

## INTRODUCTION

A multitude of complications are known to occur during the treatment of leukemia and lymphoma. This chapter will summarize some of the more common, yet unique syndromes that carry serious implications of morbidity and mortality if not recognized and treated early.

## TUMOR LYSIS SYNDROME

A constellation of metabolic abnormalities seen in tumors with rapid cell turnover, often as a consequence of treatment, is termed tumor lysis syndrome (TLS). It results from the lysis of predominantly malignant cells, releasing their contents into the systemic circulation at a rate that exceeds the elimination capacity of the kidneys. Hyperuricemia is central to the pathogenesis and diagnosis of this disorder.

### PURINE METABOLISM

Leukemic cell lysis results in releasing purines into the extracellular space. Through a process of deamination, these purines are converted to xanthine and hypoxanthine. The oxidation of xanthine and hypoxanthine by xanthine oxidase leads to the formation of uric acid, which is eventually converted to allantoin by urate oxidase. Inhibition of these enzymatic pathways forms the basis for the treatment of hyperuricemia in TLS.

### RISK FACTORS FOR THE DEVELOPMENT OF TLS

A large tumor burden with rapid cell turnover, elevated LDH, preexisting hyperuricemia, sensitivity of tumors to chemotherapy, and abnormal baseline renal function, predispose to an increased risk of TLS.[1] Tumor cell type is also an important determinant in assessing risk. TLS is most frequently encountered in aggressive lymphomas, especially the Burkitt's type.[2-7] Among the other hematological malignancies, T-cell ALL has the highest risk of TLS,[8] followed by chronic leukemias[9-11] and other indolent lymphomas.[12,13] Most often, TLS is observed in the setting of systemic chemotherapy, but spontaneous occurrences are reported.[2,13] In addition, TLS can occur in response to a variety of other therapies, such as corticosteroids,[3,4,12,14] intrathecal methotrexate,[15-17] tamoxifen, total body radiation,[18] imatinib mesylate,[19] and monoclonal antibodies such as rituximab[6,20] and gemtuzumab ozogamicin.[21]

### DIAGNOSIS AND CLINICAL FEATURES

The diagnosis of TLS is based on the demonstration of characteristic metabolic abnormalities, including hyperuricemia, hyperkalemia (or, rarely, hypokalemia), hyperphosphatemia, and hypocalcemia.

#### Hyperuriciemia

Increased uric acid levels predispose to uric acid crystal deposition in renal tubules leading to oliguric renal failure.[22] Nausea, vomiting, hematuria, oliguria, and anuria requiring dialysis can be encountered. Occasionally, hyperuricemia results in crystal deposition in joints (gouty arthritis) and can present as arthralgias or monoarthritis.

### Hyperphosphatemia and hypocalcemia

Leukemic cells may contain four times the amount of inorganic and organic phosphorous as noncancerous cells.[23] Cell lysis causes extracellular release of this phosphorous, which in turn binds to calcium, with subsequent hypocalcemia. Precipitation of calcium phosphate crystals in renal tubules may further contribute to renal failure. Severe hypocalcemia can be associated with hypotension, QT prolongation, and arrythmias. Neurologic manifestations can include tetany, carpopedal spasm, paraesthesias, and laryngospasm.[24]

### Hyperkalemia

Leukemic cells lysed by induction chemotherapy also release potassium into the extracellular space. This becomes a concern especially in the setting of inadequate renal clearance, when serum potassium concentration can rise to dangerous levels and result in cardiac arrest.[25] Hypokalemia may occur in the setting of acute monoblastic leukemia in which lysozyme release acts at the level of kidneys to cause potassium depletion.

### MANAGEMENT

Identification of patients at risk and institution of appropriate prophylactic measures are essential for the management of TLS. The cornerstones of therapy include aggressive hydration, maintenance of adequate urinary output (with gentle diuresis, if necessary), urinary alkalinization, frequent monitoring of electrolytes, and specific treatment of individual metabolic abnormalities.

### Hyperkalemia

Several approaches for the treatment of hyperkalemia are available. Methods that reduce serum potassium level through excretion, rather than via intracellular shifts, are preferred. Elimination of potassium in infusions, use of cation exchange resins such as sodium polystyrene sulfonate, loop diuretics (especially in the fluid overloaded patient), and hemodialysis (in severe cases)[26] are reasonable strategies.

### Hyperphosphatemia and hypocalcemia

Reduction of serum phosphate levels with oral phosphate binders, such as aluminum hydroxide, is usually effective. Spontaneous correction of serum calcium levels is noted when hyperphosphatemia is adequately managed. In cases of severe symptomatic hypocalcemia, cautious repletion with calcium chloride or gluconate can be undertaken. Overzealous intravenous calcium replacement should be avoided, as this can promote metastatic calcifications.[27,28]

### Hyperuricemia

Treatment of hyperuricemia should focus on measures that prevent uric acid formation and precipitation,

and augment uric acid metabolism to allantoin. Allopurinol 300 mg/day is used prophylactically to prevent uric acid synthesis from purines released as a result of leukemic cell lysis, through inhibition of xanthine oxidase. Alkalinization of urine with sodium bicarbonate infusions to a target urinary pH of 7.0 is effective in preventing uric acid deposition in the renal tubules. However, overaggressive alkalinization could foster calcium phosphate precipitation, and therefore should be done with care.[27]

Urate oxidase metabolizes uric acid to allantoin, which is 5- to 10-fold more soluble than uric acid[29] and is readily excreted by the kidneys.[30] Recombinant urate oxidase (rasburicase) has been recently approved for the treatment of hyperuricemia in pediatric patients with acute leukemia. It is extremely effective in reducing serum uric acid to low levels within a few hours of administration,[31] but is used in severe cases that have failed traditional prophylactic methods, and in whom the probability of acute renal failure is very high. This therapy is initiated only when a patient's uric acid rises to $\geq 14$.

## DISSEMINATED INTRAVASCULAR COAGULOPATHY

Among the thrombo-hemorrhagic complications of hematologic neoplasia, disseminated intravascular coagulation (DIC) remains one of the most common and life-threatening disorders. DIC is not a disease in itself, but represents a syndrome characterized by excess thrombin generation, usually triggered by an underlying condition.

### PATHOGENESIS

Though it is well known that DIC can accompany any kind of leukemia, it is most commonly observed in patients with acute promyelocytic leukemia (APL). The development of DIC in leukemia is related to several mechanisms, including release of procoagulant factors, fibrinolytic substances, and inflammatory cytokines, and the interaction of the leukemia cells with the vascular endothelium, macrophages, and platelets.

Tissue factor (TF)[32, 33] and cancer procoagulant (CP)[34] are expressed in all leukemic cell types, with greatest expression seen in APL. Differentiation of leukemic blasts to more mature forms by all-*trans* retinoic acid (ATRA) is associated both with loss of expression of CP,[35] and with decreased expression of TF,[36] regardless of the degree of cellular differentiation.[37] Fibrinolytics, such as u-PA and t-PA,[38,39] and the proteases elastase and chymotrypsin have been identified in leukemic blasts. These enzymes may be responsible for the proteolytic cleavage of clotting factors,[40] $\alpha$2 antiplasmin and fibrinogen.[41] In addition, the overexpression of annexin II, a fibrinolytic receptor protein on the surface of APL cells, correlates with both the clinical manifestation of bleeding and the in vitro ability of the promyelocytic cell lines to generate plasmid.[42]

There is some evidence that induction chemotherapy itself transiently worsens the coagulopathy of APL. Postulated mechanisms for this phenomenon include release of procoagulants from lysis of tumor cells, vascular endothelial damage by chemotherapy, induction of leukemic blast and monocyte tissue factor, and decrease in naturally occurring anticoagulants, such as antithrombin, and protein C and S.[43]

### MANAGEMENT OF DIC

Supportive care and treatment of the underlying cause are the cornerstones of therapy of DIC. Platelet transfusions represent an important aspect of managing patients with DIC in the setting of APL. The risk of bleeding is significantly decreased by prophylactic platelet transfusions coupled with the urgent institution of chemotherapy to counteract the coagulopathy.[44,45] In one study, giving prophylactic platelet transfusions to keep platelet count $>30 \times 10^9/L$ and no heparin was associated with a higher response rate to induction chemotherapy.[46] The role of heparin therapy in the treatment of DIC associated with APL is uncertain. The rationale for the use of heparin is to decrease the consumption of clotting factors and platelets and to reduce intravascular fibrin formation and thrombus deposition in the microvasculature. Several small retrospective uncontrolled studies support the use of heparin in this setting.[47] However, another large retrospective study showed no benefit with respect to early hemorrhagic deaths, CR rate, or overall survival in patients treated with heparin compared with supportive care only.[48]

Differentiation therapy with ATRA is also known to alter the clinical course of the coagulopathy of APL. Falanga et al.[49] noted a steep decline in all markers of fibrin degradation and clotting activation after therapy with ATRA. ATRA is also thought to exert this effect by inhibiting secretion of TNF-α and IL1-β; inhibiting TF expression on monocytes, and by stimulating t-PA production.[50] Randomized clinical trials have not only demonstrated an increase in CR rate and a reduction in the rate of early hemorrhagic deaths in patients treated with concurrent ATRA plus chemotherapy.[51]

## HYPERLEUKOCYTOSIS AND LEUKOSTASIS

The majority of patients with acute leukemia present with non-specific symptoms such as fatigue, weight loss, and fevers. Approximately 5–30% of adult patients with acute leukemia will have a more dramatic presentation related to an extraordinarily high leukocyte count, usually greater than 100,000/mm³. About 5–18% patients with adult AML[52,53] present with hyperleukocytosis, with a majority of them having symptoms referable to leukostasis.[54] Even though hyperleukocytosis is

generally considered to have a negative impact on prognosis,[53,55] its independent prognostic value in AML is controversial due to its close association with other established markers of unfavorable disease such as age, karyotype, CNS involvement, and antecedent hematological disorders.

The incidence of hyperleukocytosis in ALL is 10–30%. Hyperleukocytosis is a well-established negative prognostic factor for pediatric and adult ALL. Interestingly, in ALL, hyperleukocytosis rarely results in leukostasis. T-cell ALL, male sex, 11q23 rearrangements, and Ph+ ALL are all associated with a higher incidence of hyperleukocytosis. The major consequence of an increased WBC count is leukostasis, which is sludging of the microcirculation with leukemic blasts. Leukemic blasts can also form microaggregates and white, bland thrombi in these small vessels, leading to further impairment in flow. Direct endothelial damage and bleeding can occur as a result of local hypoxemia that is exacerbated by the high metabolic activity of the dividing blasts. Pathological examination frequently reveals end-organ infiltration with leukemic blasts. This is a consequence of direct endothelial damage mediated by soluble cytokines released during the interaction between leukemic blasts and the endothelium, with subsequent migration of these blasts into the perivascular space. There is emerging evidence that the differential expression of certain adhesion molecules on the vascular endothelium of AML patients may facilitate interaction of the leukemic blast with the vascular endothelium, with subsequent migration.[56] The pulmonary and cerebral vascular beds are the most clinically relevant targets of leukostasis. Cerebral involvement can range from subtle confusion and somnolence to frank intracerebral bleeding and coma. Early pulmonary involvement is signaled by mild dyspnea and respiratory alkalosis. Without treatment, this can progress to respiratory failure requiring mechanical ventilation. Typical chest X-ray findings include diffuse interstitial or alveolar infiltrates, but can be normal in the early stages.

Pulmonary leukostasis was found to be the single worst prognostic factor in patients with AML.[57] Fever is almost always present at presentation, and usually is not related to infection. Spurious hypoxemia can be related to increased consumption of oxygen by the blasts in the blood collection tube, and can be avoided by immediate transportation of an arterial blood gas sample on ice.

The short-term prognosis for patients with AML with hyperleukocytosis remains poor. As predictive factors for leukostasis lack a high degree of specificity, aggressive supportive care and prompt cytoreduction are essential. At our center, we use hydroxyurea,[58,59] 1–3 grams orally every 6 hours in combination with emergent leukapheresis for patients presenting with WBC counts >100,000/mm³ or signs or symptoms indicative of leukostasis in AML. In ALL, the threshold to initiate leukapheresis is higher; usually >200,000/mm³ in many centers. In addition to clearing circulating blasts, leukapheresis is thought to improve the coagulopathy that may be present in these patients by replacement with fresh frozen plasma, thereby reducing the risk of hemorrhage. However, leukapheresis has never been shown convincingly to reduce the risk of developing clinically significant leukostasis or reducing early mortality.[60] Though there are scanty reports in the literature regarding the use of cranial irradiation,[61] it has been largely abandoned as a therapeutic modality due to toxicity, inconvenience, and lack of efficacy data.

## DIFFERENTIATION SYNDROME

The incorporation of ATRA into the treatment paradigm of acute promyelocytic leukemia has significantly improved the cure rate of this disorder. ATRA causes differentiation of the malignant phenotype into a more mature myeloid cell.[62,63] Treatment with ATRA is generally well tolerated, but a distinct clinical syndrome has been described in treated patients. Termed variably as differentiation syndrome or the retinoic acid syndrome (RAS), it was first formally described by Frankel et al. in 1992.[64] The differentiation syndrome can also occur in the setting of therapy with arsenic trioxide.

The differentiation syndrome occurs with an incidence of 6–26% in most large series.[65,66] The incidence seems to be somewhat increased (26%)[66] in patients treated with ATRA monotherapy, compared to 10% when combined with cytotoxic chemotherapy.[67] Concurrent versus sequential administration of ATRA does not appear to alter the incidence of this syndrome. Median time to onset of symptoms is 10–12 days, but can range from 2 to 47 days.[66] Typical findings include leukocytosis, fever, weight gain, dyspnea, and alreolas infiltrates on radiological examination of the chest.

### PATHOPHYSIOLOGY

Several mechanisms have been postulated to explain the pathogenesis of the differentiation syndrome. Molecules such as cathepsin G that are known to increase capillary permeability, and cell surface adhesion molecules such as CD15s and the integrins (CD 11a and CD11b) are implicated in the pathogenesis of this syndrome.[68] Increased expression of IL-1 on the APL cell induces ICAM-1 and VCAM-1 expression on the vascular endothelium, which in turn enhances leukemic cell binding to the endothelium.[69] Cytokines, including TNF-α, IL-6, and IL-1β, may contribute by promoting leukocyte activation.[70,71]

### PROPHYLAXIS AND TREATMENT

Prophylactic administration of prednisolone in APL patients with WBC counts rising above 10,000/ml on treatment with ATRA prevented pulmonary toxicity despite WBC counts as high as 100,000/ml.[72] This is a promising strategy, but needs to be evaluated in a larger prospective trial.

In an attempt to decrease the incidence of the differentiation syndrome, several dose modifications of ATRA have been tried. ATRA at a dose of 25 mg/m²/d did not decrease the incidence of the syndrome, but appeared to have similar efficacy as the standard dosage of 45 mg/m²/d.[73] In another small study, an even lower dose of ATRA at 15–20 mg/m²/d had a lower incidence of the differentiation syndrome without compromising efficacy.[74] These strategies, however, need confirmation in larger trials.

Recognition of the clinical syndrome and prompt initiation of therapy with intravenous dexamethasone 10 mg every 12 hours for three days at the first sign of fever, dyspnea, unexplained weight gain, or pulmonary infiltrates is of utmost importance. Treatment with ATRA can be continued in mild cases of the differentiation syndrome with good outcomes.[66] However, ATRA should be discontinued in moderate to severe cases and may be resumed once symptoms resolve. If ATRA is resumed, close monitoring is required, as the syndrome can recur despite prophylaxis with steroids. ATRA does not appear to cause the syndrome when used in the maintenance phase. With early and aggressive treatment, the mortality of RAS in most large series is about 1%.[66]

## NEUTROPENIC ENTEROCOLITIS

Neutropenic enterocolitis (NE), or typhlitis, is a relatively frequent gastrointestinal complication encountered in patients with prolonged neutropenia, usually in the setting of post-induction therapy for acute leukemia. Its incidence ranges between 2.6 and 12%,[75,76] depending on clinical diagnoses versus autopsy findings. It can also occur after prolonged neutropenia, as occurs with bone marrow transplantation.[77] It is encountered after induction therapy for acute leukemias in approximately 3–7%[78,79] of patients, and only rarely with chronic leukemias.[80] Occasionally, NE is reported in non-neoplastic conditions, such as HIV infections.[81] Although typhlitis is predominantly seen in patients with prolonged neutropenia after aggressive chemotherapy for leukemia, it can occasionally be the presenting feature of the disease.[82,83]

### PATHOGENESIS

The parts of the gastrointestinal tract that are most commonly affected by NE include the cecum, ascending colon, and terminal ileum. Macroscopic changes include bowel wall edema, mucosal ulcerations, serosal ecchymoses, and fibrinous plaques. Histopathological examination reveals transmural necrotizing inflammation, mucosal leukemic cell infiltration, ischemic and hemorrhagic necrosis, microvascular thrombosis, bacterial infiltrates with absence of an inflammatory response, and mucosal pseudomembranes.[80]

The factors implicated in the pathogenesis of NE are: prolonged neutropenia and an immunocompromised state; bowel ischemia worsened by anemia; leukemic infiltration of bowel wall; bacterial translocation to pockets of necrosis caused by rapid regression of the bowel wall; intramural hemorrhage secondary to thrombocytopenia; shift in bacterial flora due to antibiotic usage; nosocomial colonization by hospital flora; drug induced paralytic ileus (vincristine); and cytarabine induced mucosal damage.

The most common bacterial pathogens involved are gram negative gut flora such as *E. coli*, *Enterococcus*, *Enterobacter* and the *Clostridium* species. Septic shock can ensue and is associated with a high mortality.

The symptom complex of fever, abdominal pain or tenderness, and diarrhea in a patient with prolonged neutropenia after aggressive chemotherapy may suffice for a clinical diagnosis of NE.[84] Surgical consultation is frequently obtained, although surgical intervention is required less often. The most common finding on plain X-ray of the abdomen is ileus, and is present in 85% of cases. Ultrasound of the RLQ is sensitive, and may show bowel wall thickening.[85,86] CT scan may reveal a RLQ infiltrative mass, pericecal fluid, and pericecal fat standing suggestive of inflammation.[87] Histological confirmation of the diagnosis is not required.

Management of the patient with NE should be individualized. Aggressive supportive care measures including broad gram negative and anaerobic coverage, adequate fluid and electrolyte balance, and adherence to strict neutropenic precautions are imperative. Surgical intervention is required in cases of perforation or peritonitis, persistent GI bleeding despite resolution of neutropenia and thrombocytopenia, or clinical deterioration suggesting septic shock.[88] Barring a few reports,[89] there is no convincing data to support the routine use of growth factors in the treatment of this disorder. Complications arising as a consequence of NE include: fistula formation, bowel perforation, bowel stenosis, prolonged ileus, massive GI bleeding, bacteremia with metastatic abscesses (hepatosplenic), acute colonic pseudoobstruction (Ogilvie's syndrome), and frank septic shock.[90]

## PARANEOPLASTIC SYNDROMES

Several paraneoplastic manifestations are associated with the hematological malignancies, particularly the lymphomas. In several instances, autoimmune disorders such as Sjogren's disease, rheumatoid arthritis, SLE, and autoimmune thyroiditis precede the development of the lymphoma by several years. While tests supporting a diagnosis of autoimmune phenomena such as platelet antibodies, direct antiglobulin tests, antineutrophil and antipholspholipid antibodies are positive in approximately 40% patients with NHL, clinically relevant problems are seen in a minority of patients (<10%).[91]

## HEMATOLOGIC SYNDROMES

Warm autoimmune hemolytic anemia (AIHA) and occasionally cold antibody-mediated hemolysis is seen most commonly in association with CLL,[92] but 3–5% patients with NHL[93] and 1–2% with HD also develop this complication.[94] Fludarabine associated hemolytic anemia is also observed in patients with CLL and occasionally in NHL. In a study of patients with NHL, AIHA was associated with female sex, poorer response rate to treatment, a higher incidence of monoclonal gammopathy, and inferior overall survival when compared to patients without AIHA.[93] AIHA associated with lymphoma usually parallels the disease course and sometimes heralds the onset of relapsing disease. In contrast, autoimmune thrombocytopenia is seen more commonly with HD than with NHL. Unlike AIHA, when ITP recurs, it is seldom associated with a relapse. Treatment is the same as for de novo cases, and accompanies therapy for the underlying malignancy.

Several paraneoplastic coagulopathies resulting in bleeding diatheses, mediated by the secreted paraprotein, are well described in the lymphoproliferative disorders. Acquired factor VIII[95,96] and factor X inhibitors, acquired von Willebrand's disease,[97,98] and rarely acquired Glanzmann's thrombasthenia[99] have all been reported. Conversely, thrombosis as a result of anticardiolipin and anti-beta 2 glycoprotein-I antibodies is also reported in patients with NHL.[100]

Eosinophilic syndrome with organ infiltration has been observed with HD and T-cell lymphoma. IL-5 is the principle cytokine that is believed to mediate this process.[101,102] Other rarer paraneoplastic hematologic syndromes associated with the lymphomas include hemophagocytic syndrome,[103] autoimmune neutropenia,[104] pure red cell aplasia,[105] and amegakaryocytic thrombocytopenic purpura.[106]

## RENAL SYNDROMES

A variety of renal syndromes have been observed in association with hematological neoplasms. Notably, nephrotic range proteinuria precedes the diagnosis of HD in many cases. A renal biopsy most commonly reveals minimal change disease.[107] Unlike other paraneoplastic manifestations, this condition responds well to the treatment of the underlying malignancy; recurrence of proteinuria is an ominous sign and usually indicates relapsing disease. Renal amyloidosis is well described in the advanced stages of HD.[108] In contrast, renal disease in NHL is more heterogenous and often presents with renal dysfunction along with proteinuria. Membranoproliferative glomerulonephritis and crescentic glomerulonephritis are somewhat more common, though a variety of other histopathologies have been reported.[109,110] Treatment of the lymphoma usually results in improvement of renal function.

## DERMATOLOGIC SYNDROMES

Paraneoplastic pemphigus is a severe dermatologic syndrome that is most commonly associated with NHL,[111] but can also be seen in the course of CLL, multiple myeloma, Waldenstrom's macroglobulinemia, HD, and other solid tumors. It presents as painful mucocutaneous erosions of the lips, oropharynx, and skin. In paraneoplastic pemphigus, the antibodies target the plakin proteins of desmosomes that are found in all epithelial tissues, including the respiratory tract.[112,113] As a consequence, bronchiolitis obliterans with respiratory failure may develop in about 30% of these patients. Immunosuppressive therapy with cyclosporine and rituximab,[114,115] in some cases, has been associated with good responses to the skin and mucosal lesions, but does not seem to alter the eventual outcome, even when good control of the underlying neoplasm is achieved. Nousari et al.[113] noted a mortality rate of greater than 90% in 84 patients with paraneoplastic pemphigus, the leading cause of death in the absence of respiratory failure being infection.[114] Sweet's syndrome is a prototype of the neutrophilic dermatoses and is found more often with AML, but is also reported in NHL, HD, and a variety of other hematological malignancies.[116,117] It manifests with an acute onset of fever, leukocytosis, and cutaneous plaques which show dermal infiltration with neutrophils.

T-cell lymphoma and HD can rarely be associated with eosinophilic fasciitis, which presents with painful sclerotic lesions on the extremities and trunk.[118–120] Treatment with corticosteroids has modest results, but as with any other paraneoplastic manifestation, control of the underlying malignancy is crucial. Other conditions that have been rarely associated with lymphoma are pyoderma gangrenosum,[121] Bazex syndrome,[122] granuloma annulare,[123] and molluscum contagiosum.[124]

## NEUROLOGIC SYNDROMES

Paraneoplastic manifestations of the central nervous system, while being quite rare, tend to occur more commonly in the course of HD than with any other hematological neoplasm. Paraneoplastic cerebellar degeneration (PCD) and paraneoplastic limbic encephalitis (PLE) are two distinct syndromes that deserve mention. HD is the most common hematologic malignancy associated

with PCD,[125] which occurs in about 0.5% of patients with HD.[126] It has been reported in all phases of the disease and is characterized by the symptom complex of dysarthria, nystagmus, ataxia, and intention tremor. The pathogenesis involves Purkinje cell destruction in the cerebellum by antineuronal antibodies such as anti-Tr antibodies[127,128] and anti-mGluR1 antibodies[129] in HD. PLE is more infrequent than PCD, and HD accounts for 4–7% of this rare disorder.[130] While anti-Hu and anti-Ta antibodies have been described in patients with PLE in the context of other solid tumors, no specific antibodies have been identified in patients with PLE in the setting of HD. Personality changes, depression, memory loss, cognitive impairment, and occasionally psychosis are the predominant clinical manifestations. Prognosis is poor, and neurological improvement is rare.

As a group, peripheral neuropathy is probably the most common paraneoplastic manifestation of hematological malignancies, most often occurring in patients with lymphoma. In the majority of cases, these neuropathies tend to be a direct consequence of the cancer (nerve compression by tumor, immunoglobulin deposition, or treatment toxicity) rather than paraneoplastic. However, when it occurs, paraneoplastic neuropathy can manifest either as an indolent process, as in chronic inflammatory demyelinating polyneuropathy, or in a more acute fashion as Guillain-Barre syndrome.[131–133] In patients who have high monoclonal paraprotein IgM in the setting of either Waldenstrom's macroglobulinemia, multiple myeloma, or occasionally NHL, a debilitating peripheral neuropathy can develop as a consequence of anti-myelin associated glycoprotein antibodies (anti-MAG antibodies).[134] A variety of therapies have been used with limited success in the treatment of these neuropathies and include IVIg, plasmapheresis, corticosteroids, cyclophosphamide, fludarabine, interferon, and rituximab.

## MISCELLANEOUS

Nonbacterial or marantic endocarditis was noted in 19% of asymptomatic patients with HD or NHL.[135] The thrombotic rate was also increased in these patients, suggesting a hypercoagulable state.

Hypercalcemia occurs in 0.3–0.4% of patients with lymphoma.[136] While it is more common with adult T-cell leukemia/lymphoma, it can also be seen with HD and B-cell NHL. A variety of mechanisms, including parathyroid hormone-related peptide, Il-6, TNF,[137] prostaglandins, and elevated levels of vitamin $D_3$,[138] have been postulated as being etiologic. Therapy is similar to that used for other forms of hypercalcemia.

Another rare disorder is recurrent angioedema of the face, larynx, extremities, and occasionally scrotum due to acquired C1 esterase-inhibitor deficiency.[139] It is usually associated with indolent B-cell lymphoproliferative disorders, commonly with lymphoplasmacytoid differentiation and paraprotein secretion, and can precede the diagnosis of lymphoma by several years.[140] Laboratory testing reveals low C1 esterase-inhibitor activity, low C4 and C3, and low C1q levels.

Rare cases of cholestatic jaundice without evidence of intrahepatic disease may occur in NHL and HD.[141,142] The so-called "vanishing duct" syndrome, characterized by extrahepatic obstruction without intrahepatic ductal dilatation, eventually culminates in hepatic failure and carries a poor prognosis.[143,144] There are several case reports of vasculitis associated with lymphoproliferative disease, including Wegener's granulomatosis and Churg-Strauss disease, temporal arteritis, and cryoglobulinemia.

## THROMBOCYTOPENIA

A low platelet count often is present in a person with acute leukemia, either from bone marrow replacement or from the bone marrow suppressive effects of the leukemia itself; from platelet consumption as a sequela of the disease or infection; or from the myelosuppressive effects of antileukemic chemotherapy. The incidence of serious spontaneous hemorrhage increases when the platelet count falls below $10,000/mm^3$, and this should be the threshold for platelet transfusions in the absence of bleeding. Using a platelet count of $10,000/mm^3$, as opposed to a count of $20,000/mm^3$, results in a similar incidence of bleeding complications and a 21.5% reduction in platelet use.[145]

## REFERENCES

1. Jeha S: Tumor lysis syndrome. *Semin Hematol* 38 (4 Suppl 10):4–8, 2001.
2. Jasek AM, Day HJ: Acute spontaneous tumor lysis syndrome. *Am J Hematol* 47(2):129–131, 1994.
3. Dhingra K, Newcom SR: Acute tumor lysis syndrome in non-Hodgkin lymphoma induced by dexamethasone. *Am J Hematol* 29(2):115–116, 1988.
4. Malik IA, Abubakar S, Alam F, Khan A: Dexamethasone-induced tumor lysis syndrome in high-grade non-Hodgkin's lymphoma. *South Med J* 87(3):409–411, 1994.
5. Cohen LF, Balow JE, Magrath IT, Poplack DG, Ziegler JL: Acute tumor lysis syndrome. A review of 37 patients with Burkitt's lymphoma. *Am J Med* 68(4):486–491, 1980.
6. Yang H, Rosove MH, Figlin RA: Tumor lysis syndrome occurring after the administration of rituximab in lymphoproliferative disorders: high-grade non-Hodgkin's lymphoma and chronic lymphocytic leukemia. *Am J Hematol* 62(4):247–250, 1999.
7. Hande KR, Garrow GC: Acute tumor lysis syndrome in patients with high-grade non-Hodgkin's lymphoma. *Am J Med* 94(2):133–139, 1993.
8. Chasty RC, Liu-Yin JA: Acute tumour lysis syndrome. *Br J Hosp Med* 49(7):488–492, 1993.
9. Przepiorka D, Gonzales-Chambers R: Acute tumor lysis syndrome in a patient with chronic myelogenous leukemia in blast crisis: role of high-dose Ara-C. *Bone Marrow Transplant* 6(4):281–282, 1990.
10. McCroskey RD, Mosher DF, Spencer CD, Prendergast E, Longo WL: Acute tumor lysis syndrome and treatment response in patients treated for refractory chronic lymphocytic leukemia with short-course, high-dose cytosine arabinoside, cisplatin, and etoposide. *Cancer* 66(2):246–250, 1990.
11. List AF, Kummet TD, Adams JD, Chun HG: Tumor lysis syndrome complicating treatment of chronic lymphocytic leukemia with fludarabine phosphate. *Am J Med* 89(3):388–390, 1990.
12. Sparano J, Ramirez M, Wiernik PH: Increasing recognition of corticosteroid-induced tumor lysis syndrome in non-Hodgkin's lymphoma. *Cancer* 65(5):1072–1073, 1990.
13. Boccia RV, Longo DL, Lieber ML, Jaffe ES, Fisher RI: Multiple recurrences of acute tumor lysis syndrome in an indolent non-Hodgkin's lymphoma. *Cancer* 56(9):2295–2297, 1985.
14. Vaisban E, Zaina A, Braester A, Manaster J, Horn Y: Acute tumor lysis syndrome induced by high-dose corticosteroids in a patient with chronic lymphatic leukemia. *Ann Hematol* 80(5):314–315, 2001.
15. Simmons ED, Somberg KA: Acute tumor lysis syndrome after intrathecal methotrexate administration. *Cancer* 67(8):2062–2065, 1991.
16. Benekli M, Gullu IH, Savas MC, et al.: Acute tumor lysis syndrome following intrathecal methotrexate. *Leuk Lymphoma* 22(3–4):361–363, 1996.
17. Fleming DR, Doukas MA: Acute tumor lysis syndrome in hematologic malignancies. *Leuk Lymphoma* 8(4–5):315–318, 1992.
18. Fleming DR, Henslee-Downey PJ, Coffey CW: Radiation induced acute tumor lysis syndrome in the bone marrow transplant setting. *Bone Marrow Transplant* 8(3):235–236, 1991.
19. Dann EJ, Fineman R, Rowe JM: Tumor lysis syndrome after STI571 in Philadelphia chromosome-positive acute lymphoblastic leukemia. *J Clin Oncol* 20(1): 354–355, 2002.
20. Jensen M, Winkler U, Manzke O, Diehl V, Engert A: Rapid tumor lysis in a patient with B-cell chronic lymphocytic leukemia and lymphocytosis treated with an anti-CD20 monoclonal antibody (IDEC-C2B8, rituximab). *Ann Hematol* 77(1–2):89–91, 1998.
21. Bross PF, Beitz J, Chen G, et al.: Approval summary: gemtuzumab ozogamicin in relapsed acute myeloid leukemia. *Clin Cancer Res* 7(6):1490–1496, 2001.
22. Jones DP, Mahmoud H, Chesney RW: Tumor lysis syndrome: pathogenesis and management. *Pediatr Nephrol* 9(2):206–212, 1995.
23. Zusman J, Brown DM, Nesbit ME: Hyperphosphatemia, hyperphosphaturia and hypocalcemia in acute

lymphoblastic leukemia. *N Engl J Med* 289(25): 1335–1340, 1973.

24. Lawrence J: Critical care issues in the patient with hematologic malignancy. *Semin Oncol Nurs* 10(3): 198–207, 1994.

25. Wilson D, Stewart A, Szwed J, Einhorn LH: Cardiac arrest due to hyperkalemia following therapy for acute lymphoblastic leukemia. *Cancer* 39(5):2290–2293, 1977.

26. Arrambide K, Toto RD: Tumor lysis syndrome. *Semin Nephrol* 13(3):273–280, 1993.

27. Flombaum CD: Metabolic emergencies in the cancer patient. *Semin Oncol* 27(3):322–334, 2000.

28. Ezzone SA: Tumor lysis syndrome. *Semin Oncol Nurs* 15(3):202–208, 1999.

29. Pui CH, Relling MV, Lascombes F, et al.: Urate oxidase in prevention and treatment of hyperuricemia associated with lymphoid malignancies. *Leukemia* 11(11): 1813–1816, 1997.

30. Brogard JM, Coumaros D, Franckhauser J, Stahl A, Stahl J: Enzymatic uricolysis: a study of the effect of a fungal urate-oxydase. *Rev Eur Etud Clin Biol* 17(9):890–895, 1972.

31. Pui CH, Mahmoud HH, Wiley JM, et al.: Recombinant urate oxidase for the prophylaxis or treatment of hyperuricemia in patients With leukemia or lymphoma. *J Clin Oncol* 19(3):697–704, 2001.

32. Bauer KA, Conway EM, Bach R, Konigsberg WH, Griffin JD, Demetri G: Tissue factor gene expression in acute myeloblastic leukemia. *Thromb Res* 56(3):425–430, 1989.

33. Gouault Heilmann M, Chardon E, Sultan C, Josso F: The procoagulant factor of leukaemic promyelocytes: demonstration of immunologic cross reactivity with human brain tissue factor. *Br J Haematol* 30(2):151–158, 1975.

34. Falanga A, Alessio MG, Donati MB, Barbui T: A new procoagulant in acute leukemia. *Blood* 71(4):870–875, 1988.

35. Falanga A, Consonni R, Marchetti M, et al.: Cancer procoagulant in the human promyelocytic cell line NB4 and its modulation by all-trans-retinoic acid. *Leukemia* 8(1):156–159, 1994.

36. De Stefano V, Teofili L, Sica S, et al.: Effect of all-trans retinoic acid on procoagulant and fibrinolytic activities of cultured blast cells from patients with acute promyelocytic leukemia. *Blood* 86(9):3535–3541, 1995.

37. Falanga A, Consonni R, Marchetti M, et al.: Cancer procoagulant and tissue factor are differently modulated by all-trans-retinoic acid in acute promyelocytic leukemia cells. *Blood* 92(1):143–151, 1998.

38. Francis RB, Jr., Seyfert U: Tissue plasminogen activator antigen and activity in disseminated intravascular coagulation: clinicopathologic correlations. *J Lab Clin Med* 110(5):541–547, 1987.

39. Bennett B, Booth NA, Croll A, Dawson AA: The bleeding disorder in acute promyelocytic leukaemia: fibrinolysis due to u-PA rather than defibrination. *Br J Haematol* 71(4):511–517, 1989.

40. Schmidt W, Egbring R, Havemann K: Effect of elastase-like and chymotrypsin-like neutral proteases from human granulocytes on isolated clotting factors. *Thromb Res* 6(4):315–329, 1975.

41. Sterrenberg L, Nieuwenhuizen W, Hermans J: Purification and partial characterization of a D-like fragment from human fibrinogen, produced by human leukocyte elastase. *Biochim Biophys Acta* 755(2): 300–306, 2002.

42. Kim J, Hajjar KA: Annexin II: a plasminogen-plasminogen activator co-receptor. *Front Biosci* 7:d341–348, 2002.

43. Barbui T, Falanga A: Disseminated intravascular coagulation in acute leukemia. *Semin Thromb Hemost* 27(6):593–604, 1996.

44. Goldberg MA, Ginsburg D, Mayer RJ, et al.: Is heparin administration necessary during induction chemotherapy for patients with acute promyelocytic leukemia? *Blood* 69(1):187–191, 1987.

45. Kantarjian HM, Keating MJ, Walters RS, et al.: Acute promyelocytic leukemia. M.D. Anderson Hospital experience. *Am J Med* 80(5):789–797, 1986.

46. Bassan R, Battista R, Viero P, et al.: Short-term treatment for adult hypergranular and microgranular acute promyelocytic leukemia. *Leukemia* 9(2):238–243, 1995.

47. Tallman MS, Kwaan HC: Reassessing the hemostatic disorder associated with acute promyelocytic leukemia. *Blood* 79(3):543–553, 1992.

48. Rodeghiero F, Avvisati G, Castaman G, Barbui T, Mandelli F: Early deaths and anti-hemorrhagic treatments in acute promyelocytic leukemia. A GIMEMA retrospective study in 268 consecutive patients. *Blood* 75(11):2112–2117, 1990.

49. Falanga A, Iacoviello L, Evangelista V, et al.: Loss of blast cell procoagulant activity and improvement of hemostatic variables in patients with acute promyelocytic leukemia administered all-trans-retinoic acid. *Blood* 86(3):1072–1081, 1995.

50. Kooistra T, Opdenberg JP, Toet K, et al.: Stimulation of tissue-type plasminogen activator synthesis by retinoids in cultured human endothelial cells and rat tissues in vivo. *Thromb Haemost* 65(5):565–572, 1991.

51. Fenaux P, Chastang C, Chevret S, et al.: A randomized comparison of all transretinoic acid (ATRA) followed by chemotherapy and ATRA plus chemotherapy and the role of maintenance therapy in newly diagnosed acute promyelocytic leukemia. The European APL Group. *Blood* 94(4):1192–1200, 1999.

52. Hug V, Keating M, McCredie K, Hester J, Bodey GP, Freireich EJ: Clinical course and response to treatment of patients with acute myelogenous leukemia presenting with a high leukocyte count. *Cancer* 52(5):773–779, 1983.

53. Dutcher JP, Schiffer CA, Wiernik PH: Hyperleukocytosis in adult acute nonlymphocytic leukemia: impact on remission rate and duration, and survival. *J Clin Oncol* 5(9):1364–1372, 1987.

54. Lichtman MA, Heal J, Rowe JM: Hyperleukocytic leukaemia: rheological and clinical features and management. *Baillieres Clin Haematol* 1(3):725–746, 1987.

55. Slovak ML, Kopecky KJ, Wolman SR, et al.: Cytogenetic correlation with disease status and treatment outcome in advanced stage leukemia post bone marrow transplantation: a Southwest Oncology Group study (SWOG-8612). *Leuk Res* 19(6):381–388, 1995.

56. Stucki A, Cordey A, Monai N, Schapira M, Spertini O: Activation of vascular endothelial cells by leukemic blast cells: a mechanism of leukostasis. *Blood* 86:435a, 1995.

57. Lester TJ, Johnson JW, Cuttner J: Pulmonary leukostasis as the single worst prognostic factor in patients with acute myelocytic leukemia and hyperleukocytosis. *Am J Med* 79(1):43–48, 1985.

58. Schwartz JH, Cannellos GP: Hydroxyurea in the management of the hematologic complications of chronic granulocytic leukemia. *Blood* 46(1):11–16, 1975

59. Grund FM, Armitage JO, Burns P: Hydroxyurea in the prevention of the effects of leukostasis in acute leukemia. *Arch Intern Med* 137(9):1246–1247, 1977.

60. Porcu P, Danielson CF, Orazi A, Heerema NA, Gabig TG, McCarthy LJ: Therapeutic leukapheresis in hyperleucocytic leukaemias: lack of correlation between degree of cytoreduction and early mortality rate. *Br J Haematol* 98(2):433–436, 1997.

61. Flasshove M, Schuette J, Sauerwein W, Hoeffken K, Seeber S: Pulmonary and cerebral irradiation for hyperleukocytosis in acute myelomonocytic leukemia. *Leukemia* 8(10):1792, 1994.

62. Castaigne S, Chomienne C, Daniel MT, et al.: All-trans retinoic acid as a differentiation therapy for acute promyelocytic leukemia. I. Clinical results. *Blood* 76(9):1704–1709, 1990.

63. Huang ME, Ye YC, Chen SR, et al.: Use of all-trans retinoic acid in the treatment of acute promyelocytic leukemia. *Blood* 72(2):567–572, 1988.

64. Frankel SR, Eardley A, Lauwers G, Weiss M, Warrell RP Jr: The "retinoic acid syndrome" in acute promyelocytic leukemia. *Ann Intern Med* 117(4):292–296, 1992.

65. De Botton S, Dombret H, Sanz M, et al.: Incidence, clinical features, and outcome of all trans-retinoic acid syndrome in 413 cases of newly diagnosed acute promyelocytic leukemia. The European APL Group. *Blood* 92(8):2712–2718, 1998.

66. Tallman MS, Andersen JW, Schiffer CA, et al.: Clinical description of 44 patients with acute promyelocytic leukemia who developed the retinoic acid syndrome. *Blood* 95(1):90–95, 2000.

67. Avvisati G, Lo Coco F, Diverio D, et al.: AIDA (all-trans retinoic acid + idarubicin) in newly diagnosed acute promyelocytic leukemia: a Gruppo Italiano Malattie Ematologiche Maligne dell'Adulto (GIMEMA) pilot study. *Blood* 88(4):1390–1398, 1996.

68. Seale J, Delva L, Renesto P, et al.: All-trans retinoic acid rapidly decreases cathepsin G synthesis and mRNA expression in acute promyelocytic leukemia. *Leukemia* 10(1):95–101, 1996.

69. Marchetti M, Falanga A, Giovanelli S, Oldani E, Barbui T: All-trans-retinoic acid increases adhesion to endothelium of the human promyelocytic leukaemia cell line NB4. *Br J Haematol* 93(2):360–366, 1996

70. Dubois C, Schlageter MH, de Gentile A, Balitrand N, Toubert ME, Krawice I, Fenaux P, Castaigne S, Najean Y, Degos L, et al.: Modulation of IL-8, IL-1 beta, and G-CSF secretion by all-trans retinoic acid in acute promyelocytic leukemia. *Leukemia* 8(10):1750–1757, 1994.

71. Di Noto R, Schiavone EM, Ferrara F, Manzo C, Lo Pardo C, Del Vecchio L: All-trans retinoic acid promotes a differential regulation of adhesion molecules on acute myeloid leukaemia blast cells. *Br J Haematol* 88(2): 247–255, 1994.

72. Wiley JS, Firkin FC: Reduction of pulmonary toxicity by prednisolone prophylaxis during all-trans retinoic acid treatment of acute promyelocytic leukemia. Australian Leukaemia Study Group. *Leukemia* 9(5):774–778, 1995.

73. Castaigne S, Lefebvre P, Chomienne C, Suc E, Rigal-Huguet F, Gardin C, Delmer A, Archimbaud E, Tilly H, Janvier M, et al.: Effectiveness and pharmacokinetics of low-dose all-trans retinoic acid (25 mg/m$^2$) in acute promyelocytic leukemia. *Blood* 82(12):3560–3563, 1993.

74. Chen GQ, Shen ZX, Wu F, et al.: Pharmacokinetics and efficacy of low-dose all-trans retinoic acid in the treatment of acute promyelocytic leukemia. *Leukemia* 10(5):825–828, 1996.

75. Mower WJ, Hawkins JA, Nelson EW: Neutropenic enterocolitis in adults with acute leukemia. *Arch Surg* 121(5):571–574, 1986.

76. Steinberg D, Gold J, Brodin A: Necrotizing enterocolitis in leukemia. *Arch Intern Med* 131(4):538–544, 1973.

77. Avigan D, Richardson P, Elias A, et al.: Neutropenic enterocolitis as a complication of high dose chemotherapy with stem cell rescue in patients with solid tumors: a case series with a review of the literature. *Cancer* 83(3):409–414, 1998.

78. Gorschluter M, Glasmacher A, Hahn C, et al.: Severe abdominal infections in neutropenic patients. *Cancer Invest* 19(7):669–677, 2001.

79. Dietrich CF, Brunner V, Lembcke B: Intestinal ultrasound in rare small and large intestinal diseases. *Z Gastroenterol* 36(11):955–970, 1998.

80. Buyukasik Y, Ozcebe OI, Haznedaroglu IC, et al.: Neutropenic enterocolitis in adult leukemias. *Int J Hematol* 66(1):47–55, 1997.

81. Till M, Lee N, Soper WD, Murphy RL: Typhlitis in patients with HIV-1 infection. *Ann Intern Med* 116 (12 Pt 1): 998–1000, 1992.

82. Ahsan N, Sun CC, Di John D: Acute ileotyphlitis as presenting manifestation of acute myelogenous leukemia. *Am J Clin Pathol* 89(3):407–409, 1988.

83. Kaste SC, Flynn PM, Furman WL: Acute lymphoblastic leukemia presenting with typhlitis. *Med Pediatr Oncol* 28(3):209–212, 1997.

84. Wade DS, Nava HR, Douglass HO Jr: Neutropenic enterocolitis. Clinical diagnosis and treatment. *Cancer* 69(1):17–23, 1992.

85. Gootenberg JE, Abbondanzo SL: Rapid diagnosis of neutropenic enterocolitis (typhlitis) by ultrasonography. *Am J Pediatr Hematol Oncol* 9(3):222–227, 1987.

86. Teefey SA, Montana MA, Goldfogel GA, Shuman WP: Sonographic diagnosis of neutropenic typhlitis. *AJR Am J Roentgenol* 149(4):731–733, 1987.

87. Adams GW, Rauch RF, Kelvin FM, Silverman PM, Korobkin M: CT detection of typhlitis. *J Comput Assist Tomogr* 9(2):363–365, 1985.

88. Shamberger RC, Weinstein HJ, Delorey MJ, Levey RH: The medical and surgical management of typhlitis in children with acute nonlymphocytic (myelogenous) leukemia. *Cancer* 57(3):603–609, 1986.

89. Hanada T, Ono I, Hirano C, Kurosaki Y: Successful treatment of neutropenic enterocolitis with recombinant granulocyte colony stimulating factor in a child with acute lymphocytic leukaemia. *Eur J Pediatr* 149(11):811–812, 1990.

90. Wach M, Dmoszynska A, Wasik-Szczepanek E, Pozarowski A, Drop A, Szczepanek D: Neutropenic

enterocolitis: a serious complication during the treatment of acute leukemias. *Ann Hematol* 83(8):522–526, 2004.

91. Timuragaoglu A, Duman A, Ongut G, Saka O, Karadogan I: The significance of autoantibodies in non-Hodgkin's lymphoma. *Leuk Lymphoma* 40(1–2):119–122, 2000.

92. Mauro FR, Foa R, Cerretti R, et al.: Autoimmune hemolytic anemia in chronic lymphocytic leukemia: clinical, therapeutic, and prognostic features. *Blood* 95(9):2786–2792, 2000.

93. Sallah S, Sigounas G, Vos P, Wan JY, Nguyen NP: Autoimmune hemolytic anemia in patients with non-Hodgkin's lymphoma: characteristics and significance. *Ann Oncol* 11(12):1571–1577, 2000.

94. Xiros N, Binder T, Anger B, Bohlke J, Heimpel H: Idiopathic thrombocytopenic purpura and autoimmune hemolytic anemia in Hodgkin's disease. *Eur J Haematol* 40(5):437–441, 1988.

95. Gesierich W, Munker R, Geiersberger U, Pohlmann H, Brack N, Hartenstein R: Spontaneous bleeding in a patient with malignant lymphoma: a case of acquired hemophilia. *Onkologie* 23(6):584–588, 2000.

96. Tiplady CW, Hamilton PJ, Galloway MJ: Acquired haemophilia complicating the remission of a patient with high grade non-Hodgkin's lymphoma treated by fludarabine. *Clin Lab Haematol* 22(3):163–165, 2000.

97. Hunault-Berger M, Rachieru P, Ternisien C, et al.: Acquired von Willebrand disease and lymphoproliferative syndromes. *Presse Med* 30(5):209–212, 2001.

98. Rao KP, Kizer J, Jones TJ, Anunciado A, Pepkowitz SH, Lazarchick J: Acquired von Willebrand's syndrome associated with an extranodal pulmonary lymphoma. *Arch Pathol Lab Med* 112(1):47–50, 1988.

99. Malik U, Dutcher JP, Oleksowicz L: Acquired Glanzmann's thrombasthenia associated with Hodgkin's lymphoma: a case report and review of the literature. *Cancer* 82(9):1764–1768, 1998.

100. Genvresse I, Buttgereit F, Spath-Schwalbe E, Ziemer S, Eucker J, Possinger K: Arterial thrombosis associated with anticardiolipin and anti-beta2-glycoprotein-I antibodies in patients with non-Hodgkin's lymphoma: a report of two cases. *Eur J Haematol* 65(5):344–347, 2000.

101. Di Biagio E, Sanchez-Borges M, Desenne JJ, Suarez-Chacon R, Somoza R, Acquatella G: Eosinophilia in Hodgkin's disease: a role for interleukin 5. *Int Arch Allergy Immunol* 110(3):244–251, 1996.

102. Gallamini A, Carbone A, Lista P, et al.: Intestinal T-cell lymphoma with massive tissue and blood eosinophilia mediated by IL-5. *Leuk Lymphoma* 17(1–2):155–161, 1995.

103. Kojima H, Takei N, Mukai Y, et al.: Hemophagocytic syndrome as the primary clinical symptom of Hodgkin's disease. *Ann Hematol* 82(1):53–56, 2003.

104. Gordon BG, Kiwanuka J, Kadushin J: Autoimmune neutropenia and Hodgkin's disease: successful treatment with intravenous gammaglobulin. *Am J Pediatr Hematol Oncol* 13(2):164–167, 1991.

105. Reid TJ, IIIrd, Mullaney M, Burrell LM, Redmond J, IIIrd, Mangan KF: Pure red cell aplasia after chemotherapy for Hodgkin's lymphoma: in vitro evidence for T cell mediated suppression of erythropoiesis and response to sequential cyclosporin and erythropoietin. *Am J Hematol* 46(1):48–53, 1994.

106. Lugassy G: Non-Hodgkin's lymphoma presenting with amegakaryocytic thrombocytopenic purpura. *Ann Hematol* 73(1):41–42, 1996.

107. Da'as N, Polliack A, Cohen Y, et al.: Kidney involvement and renal manifestations in non-Hodgkin's lymphoma and lymphocytic leukemia: a retrospective study in 700 patients. *Eur J Haematol* 67(3):158–164, 2001.

108. Ronco PM: Paraneoplastic glomerulopathies: new insights into an old entity. *Kidney Int* 56(1):355–377, 1999.

109. Dabbs DJ, Striker LM, Mignon F, Striker G: Glomerular lesions in lymphomas and leukemias. *Am J Med* 80(1):63–70, 1986.

110. Rault R, Holley JL, Banner BF, el-Shahawy M: Glomerulonephritis and non-Hodgkin's lymphoma: a report of two cases and review of the literature. *Am J Kidney Dis* 20(1):84–89, 1992.

111. Anhalt GJ, Kim SC, Stanley JR, Korman NJ, Jabs DA, Kory M, Izumi H, Ratrie H, 3rd, Mutasim D, Ariss-Abdo L, et al.: Paraneoplastic pemphigus. An autoimmune mucocutaneous disease associated with neoplasia. *N Engl J Med* 323(25):1729–1735, 1990.

112. Schlesinger T, McCarron K, Camisa C, Anhalt G: Paraneoplastic pemphigus occurring in a patient with B-cell non-Hodgkin's lymphoma. *Cutis* 61(2):94–96, 1998.

113. Nousari HC, Deterding R, Wojtczack H, Aho S, Uitto J, Hashimoto T, Anhalt GJ: The mechanism of respiratory failure in paraneoplastic pemphigus. *N Engl J Med* 340(18):1406–1410, 1999.

114. Heizmann M, Itin P, Wernli M, Borradori L, Bargetzi MJ: Successful treatment of paraneoplastic pemphigus in follicular NHL with rituximab: report of a case and review of treatment for paraneoplastic pemphigus in NHL and CLL. *Am J Hematol* 66(2):142–144, 2001.

115. Gergely L, Varoczy L, Vadasz G, Remenyik E, Illes A: Successful treatment of B cell chronic lymphocytic leukemia-associated severe paraneoplastic pemphigus with cyclosporin A. *Acta Haematol* 109(4):202–205, 2003.

116. Gille J, Spieth K, Kaufmann R: Sweet's syndrome as initial presentation of diffuse large B-cell lymphoma. *J Am Acad Dermatol* 46(2 Suppl Case Reports):S11–13, 2002.

117. Suvajdzic N, Dimcic Z, Cvijetic O, Colovic M: Sweet's syndrome associated with Hodgkin's disease. *Haematologia* (Budap) 29(2):157–158, 1998.

118. Chan LS, Hanson CA, Cooper KD: Concurrent eosinophilic fasciitis and cutaneous T-cell lymphoma. Eosinophilic fasciitis as a paraneoplastic syndrome of T-cell malignant neoplasms? *Arch Dermatol* 127(6): 862–865, 1991.

119. Vassallo C, Ciocca O, Arcaini L, et al.: Eosinophilic folliculitis occurring in a patient affected by Hodgkin lymphoma. *Int J Dermatol* 41(5):298–300, 2002.

120. Kim H, Kim MO, Ahn MJ, et al.: Eosinophilic fasciitis preceding relapse of peripheral T-cell lymphoma. *J Korean Med Sci* 15(3):346–350, 2000.

121. Allen LE, Heaton ND, Hurst PA: Pyoderma gangrenosum–an association with Hodgkin's disease. *Clin Exp Dermatol* 16(2):151, 1991.

122. Lucker GP, Steijlen PM: Acrokeratosis paraneoplastica (Bazex syndrome) occurring with acquired ichthyosis in Hodgkin's disease. *Br J Dermatol* 133(2):322–325, 1995.

123. Ono H, Yokozeki H, Katayama I, Nishioka K: Granuloma annulare in a patient with malignant lymphoma. *Dermatology* 195(1):46–47, 1997.

124. Arnold J, Berens N, Brocker EB, Goebeler M: Recurrent angio-oedema and solitary molluscum contagiosum as presenting signs of non-Hodgkin's B-cell lymphoma. *Br J Dermatol* 146(2):343–344, 2002.

125. Hammack J, Kotanides H, Rosenblum MK, Posner JB: Paraneoplastic cerebellar degeneration. II. Clinical and immunologic findings in 21 patients with Hodgkin's disease. *Neurology* 42(10):1938–1943, 1992.

126. Spyridonidis A, Fischer KG, Glocker FX, Fetscher S, Klisch J, Behringer D: Paraneoplastic cerebellar degeneration and nephrotic syndrome preceding Hodgkin's disease: case report and review of the literature. *Eur J Haematol* 68(5):318–321, 2002.

127. Graus F, Dalmau J, Valldeoriola F, et al.: Immunological characterization of a neuronal antibody (anti-Tr) associated with paraneoplastic cerebellar degeneration and Hodgkin's disease. *J Neuroimmunol* 74(1–2):55–61, 1997.

128. Bernal F, Shams'ili S, Rojas I, et al.: Anti-Tr antibodies as markers of paraneoplastic cerebellar degeneration and Hodgkin's disease. *Neurology* 60(2):230–234, 2003.

129. Sillevis Smitt P, Kinoshita A, De Leeuw B, et al.: Paraneoplastic cerebellar ataxia due to autoantibodies against a glutamate receptor. *N Engl J Med* 342(1):21–27, 2000.

130. Gultekin SH, Rosenfeld MR, Voltz R, Eichen J, Posner JB, Dalmau J: Paraneoplastic limbic encephalitis: neurological symptoms, immunological findings and tumour association in 50 patients. *Brain* 123 (Pt 7):1481–1494, 2000.

131. Hughes RA, Britton T, Richards M: Effects of lymphoma on the peripheral nervous system. *J R Soc Med* 87(9):526–530, 1994.

132. Vallat JM, De Mascarel HA, Bordessoule D, et al.: Non-Hodgkin malignant lymphomas and peripheral neuropathies-13 cases. *Brain* 118 ( Pt 5):1233–1245, 1995.

133. Re D, Schwenk A, Hegener P, Bamborschke S, Diehl V, Tesch H.:Guillain-Barre syndrome in a patient with non-Hodgkin's lymphoma. *Ann Oncol* 11(2):217–220, 2000.

134. Gorson KC, Ropper AH, Weinberg DH, Weinstein R: Treatment experience in patients with anti-myelin-associated glycoprotein neuropathy. *Muscle Nerve* 24(6):778–786, 2001.

135. Edoute Y, Haim N, Rinkevich D, Brenner B, Reisner SA: Cardiac valvular vegetations in cancer patients: a prospective echocardiographic study of 200 patients. *Am J Med* 102(3):252–258, 1997.

136. Muggia FM: Overview of cancer-related hypercalcemia: epidemiology and etiology. *Semin Oncol* 17(2 Suppl 5):3–9, 1990.

137. Daroszewska A, Bucknall RC, Chu P, Fraser WD: Severe hypercalcaemia in B-cell lymphoma: combined effects of PTH-rP, IL-6 and TNF. *Postgrad Med J* 75(889):672–674, 1999.

138. Seymour JF, Gagel RF: Calcitriol: the major humoral mediator of hypercalcemia in Hodgkin's disease and non-Hodgkin's lymphomas. *Blood* 82(5):1383–1394, 1993.

139. Bain BJ, Catovsky D, Ewan PW: Acquired angioedema as the presenting feature of lymphoproliferative disorders of mature B-lymphocytes. *Cancer* 72(11):3318–3322, 1993.

140. Geha RS, Quinti I, Austen KF, Cicardi M, Sheffer A, Rosen FS: Acquired C1-inhibitor deficiency associated with antiidiotypic antibody to monoclonal immunoglobulins. *N Engl J Med* 312(9):534–540, 1985.

141. Yalcin S, Aybar B, Ertekin C, Guloglu R: Use of a modified occlusal bite guard to treat self-induced traumatic macroglossia (two case reports). *Ulus Travma Derg* 7(1):70–73, 2001.

142. Watterson J, Priest JR: Jaundice as a paraneoplastic phenomenon in a T-cell lymphoma. *Gastroenterology* 97(5):1319–1322, 1989.

143. Yusuf MA, Elias E, Hubscher SG: Jaundice caused by the vanishing bile duct syndrome in a child with Hodgkin lymphoma. *J Pediatr Hematol Oncol* 22(2):154–157, 2000.

144. Rossini MS, Lorand-Metze I, Oliveira GB, Souza CA: Vanishing bile duct syndrome in Hodgkin's disease: case report. *Sao Paulo Med J* 118(5):154–157, 2000.

145. Rebulla P, Finazzi G, Marangoni F, et al.: The threshold for prophylactic platelet transfusions in adults with acute myeloid leukemia. Gruppo Italiano Malattie Ematologiche Maligne dell'Adulto. *N Engl J Med* 337(26):1870–1875, 1997.

# Chapter 108

# FERTILITY ISSUES IN THE HEMATOLOGIC MALIGNANCIES

*Ashok Agarwal and Tamer M. Said*

## INTRODUCTION

Young adults diagnosed with cancer are living longer than ever due to improved treatment regimens. The 5-year survival rate for certain subtypes of leukemia and Hodgkin's and non-Hodgkin's diseases, for example, has dramatically increased to 75%–90%.[1] However, the neoplastic disease per se and/or its treatment commonly impair fertility, leaving many patients unable to bear healthy, biological children.

Hematologic malignancies, in particular, can adversely affect fertility in a number of ways. Since these diseases generally involve the hypothalamus and pituitary, they can directly affect gonadotropin secretion, resulting in secondary hypogonadism and, hence, defective sperm formation and infertility. In addition, chemotherapy and radiation therapy—both being used to treat hematologic malignancies—are toxic to the male and female gonads. Even if fertility does not decline as a result of therapy or returns naturally, patients can still be rendered sterile by cytotoxic therapy, as these drugs can cause genetic mutations in germ cells.[2] Similarly, any cytotoxic therapy administered to pregnant women has the potential for serious teratogenic consequences on the fetus (see Chapter 106).

## IMPACT OF MALIGNANCY ON THE REPRODUCTIVE SYSTEM

In the past, infertility associated with malignant disease was considered a side effect of the drugs and radiation used during the course of treatment. However, this view is changing due to strong evidence that decreased fertility sometimes exists before the treatment starts. In a study conducted on 158 male patients with Hodgkin lymphoma,[3] severe damage to fertility was observed in 21% cases before treatment. The decrease in fertility was most prominent in patients with an elevated erythrocyte sedimentation rate (ESR) and in those with advanced disease. In another study, semen analysis showed that 70% of male patients with Hodgkin lymphoma had reduced fertility before therapy.[4]

The effect of Hodgkin lymphoma on testicular function does not involve local tumor or metastasis. Instead, the disease may lead to structural abnormalities in the testicular parenchyma, such as tubular hyalinization.[5] These changes may be caused by an immune-mediated disorder that alters the balance between distinct subpopulations of lymphocytes, which normally inhibit or stimulate the production of spermatozoa. However, this hypothesis requires further testing.[6] In addition, cytokines (e.g., interleukins and tumor necrosis factor) that are secreted by tumor tissue may be partly responsible for the impaired testicular function seen in patients with Hodgkin's disease.[7]

In general, malignancy is associated with an increased catabolic state and malnutrition. Therefore, most patients experience weight loss and decreased reproductive capacity. In addition, hypothalamic dysfunction can occur and pituitary gonadotropin levels can fall, thus affecting the fertility.[8] Stress hormones may further reduce fertility by leading to a rise in prolactin and endogenous opiate secretion, which in turn suppress gonadotropins.[9]

## GONADAL TOXICITY FOLLOWING MALIGNANCY TREATMENT

In addition to Hodgkin and non-Hodgkin's lymphoma, acute lymphocytic leukemia and acute myeloid leukemia are among the most common neoplastic disorders during the reproductive years.[10] As the mortality rate decreases and the survival rate increases, the consequences of cancer treatment vis-a-vis impaired fertility are more frequently encountered.

### SUSCEPTIBILITY OF THE MALE GONAD TO CANCER TREATMENT

**Testicular architecture**

Chemotherapeutic agents enter testis via blood vessel plexus in the interstitial region. Although the Sertoli cells usually maintain a protective barrier between the blood and the testicular germ cells, many chemotherapeutic drugs can severely interrupt the integrity of this barrier.

Germ cells that do actively differentiate are more susceptible to cytotoxic injury, resulting in necrosis, whereas testicular somatic cells are affected only in function. As a result, cytotoxic therapy can deplete germ cells to the point where the seminiferous tubules contain only Sertoli cells. The depletion occurs in a time-dependant manner because late-stage germ cells (spermatocytes onward) are relatively more resistant. However, studies in rodents revealed that these late-stage cells are susceptible to mutagenesis, and any mutations in their DNA can be passed on to the next generation.[11] Surviving stem cells can remain in the testis, but will fail to differentiate into mature spermatozoa for several years after cytotoxic abuse. The eventual recovery of sperm production depends on the survival of the spermatogonial stem cells, as well as on their ability to differentiate.[12]

The effects of cancer therapy on testicular architecture vary with the patient's age and pubertal status. It was initially thought that the testicles of pre- and peripubertal males were less vulnerable to toxic effects induced by treatment. However, it is now clear that these patients experience as much testicular structure damage following chemo/radiotherapy as adults.[13]

### Hormonal imbalances

The loss of germ cells exerts secondary effects on the hypothalamic-pituitary-gonadal axis. Germinal aplasia reduces the size of the testes. Consequently, testicular blood flow decreases, thus reducing the testosterone levels in the circulation.[14] Because testosterone is a negative regulator of luteinizing hormone (LH), which is secreted by the pituitary, and LH is the primary stimulator of testosterone synthesis by the Leydig cells, LH increases to maintain constant serum testosterone levels. In addition, inhibin secretion by the Sertoli cells declines and, as inhibin limits follicle-stimulating hormone (FSH) secretion by the pituitary, serum FSH levels tend to rise.

### SUSCEPTIBILITY OF THE FEMALE GONAD TO CANCER TREATMENT

### Ovarian architecture

Histological sections of ovaries exposed to cytotoxic drugs show a spectrum of changes, ranging from reduced number of follicles to no follicles and fibrosis.[15] The exact incidence of premature ovarian failure (POF) after chemotherapy is difficult to establish because there are many contributing factors. Depending on the type of chemotherapy regimen used, the incidence of amenorrhea ranges from 0% to 100%.[16] Cytotoxic drugs may impair follicular maturation and/or deplete primordial follicles.[15,17] Temporary amenorrhea occurs when cytotoxic drugs destroy maturing follicles,

whereas permanent amenorrhea or POF occurs when all primordial follicles are destroyed. The close structural and functional relationship between the oocyte and the hormone secreting-granulosa cells makes it difficult to identify an exact target for cytotoxic drugs. The destruction of one leads to the demise of the other.

### Hormonal imbalances

Unlike male germ cells, female germ cells proliferate only during prenatal life; after birth, these progressively decrease in number due to apoptosis, and ovulation. Germ cells inside the female gonad do not proliferate, whereas the somatic cells do. Radiation and chemotherapy induce oocytes to undergo apoptosis, which reduces the number of germ cells,[18] resulting in estrogen insufficiency. Therefore, when follicles are destroyed by cytotoxic therapy, the frequency of menses decreases and amenorrhea commonly occurs. Irreversible ovarian failure and menopause occur if the number of follicles falls below that is required for menstrual cyclicity.

### EFFECT OF MALIGNANCY TREATMENT ON FERTILITY

Post-treatment of Hodgkin's lymphoma in men with chemotherapy results in testicular germ cell aplasia and decreased libido.[5] The seminiferous epithelium inside the testes is most sensitive to the detrimental effects of chemotherapy. Therefore, after treatment with gonadotoxic agents, patients may be rendered oligozoospermic or azoospermic. Because testosterone production by the Leydig cells remains unaffected, patients still develop normal secondary sexual characteristics.[19] However, treatment with high, cumulative doses of gonadotoxic chemotherapy can lead to Leydig cell dysfunction.

Doses as low as 0.1 Gy to 1.2 Gy can have detectable effects on spermatogenesis in adult males, with doses over 4 Gy causing more permanent effects.[20] Somatic cells are more resistant to chemotherapy and radiation-induced damage than are germ cells. Indeed, Leydig cell dysfunction is not observed until doses of 20 Gy are administered to the prepubertal boy and up to 30 Gy in sexually mature males.[21] Testosterone production is therefore relatively preserved below these doses. Thus, many patients develop normal secondary sexual characteristics despite a severe impairment of spermatogenesis.

Young patients with a hematological malignancy are often treated with bone marrow transplantation (BMT).[22] During BMT, patients may be given alkylating agents and receive total body irradiation for conditioning, both of which result in POF, hormonal disturbances, and eventually, infertility.[23] Long-term female survivors treated with total body irradiation and BMT are at risk for ovarian follicular depletion and impaired uterine growth and blood flow, in addition to early pregnancy loss and premature labor if pregnancy is achieved.[24] Because women aged above 30 years face a higher incidence of POF following chemotherapy, their treatment regimens should contain fewer alkylating agents.[25]

A study that documented the late effects associated with treatment of early Hodgkin's lymphoma revealed that 43/191 men and 16/149 women had sought medical advice for infertility, while 57/191 men and 54/149 women were able to parent children. In addition, sexual activity was disrupted in 25.8% of cases.[26]

### TRANSMISSION OF GENETIC MATERIAL

Radiation and several alkylating agents can produce single-gene mutations and chromosomal translocations in spermatogonia.[27] The persistence of a mutation depends mainly on its location. Mutations that occur early in stem spermatogonia will produce mutation-carrying sperm for the lifetime of the male, whereas those occurring in later stages of spermatogenesis will only lead to a mutation-carrying sperm for a few months.[11] Meiotic and post-meiotic germ cells are more susceptible to mutations than are stem spermatogonia. Therefore, the mutational risks are highest when a pregnancy occurs within one spermatogenic cycle after the male is exposed to the damaging agent.[11] In females, most alkylating agents and a variety of other chemotherapeutic drugs induce chromosome aberrations or other mutations in developing oocytes that result in embryonic death.[27]

Although sperm DNA integrity can vary greatly among cancer patients, patients with Hodgkin's and non-Hodgkin's diseases generally have a significantly higher prevalence of DNA damage than healthy men.[28] Sperm DNA damage can be assessed with a variety of techniques,[29] but none can definitively determine whether the mutations will be passed onto any offspring.

## POTENTIAL FOR FERTILITY FOLLOWING MALIGNANCY TREATMENT

### RESTORATION OF FERTILITY

Sperm quality may naturally improve after cancer treatment. However, some defects may persist. The incidence of infertility in men who have recovered sperm production following cytotoxic therapy is generally not higher than that of the general population. An interesting case report[30] has documented paternity following bone marrow conditioning and transplantation in a patient with acute myeloid leukemia. For the first time, the preservation of fertile sperm was seen despite the use of chemotherapy. Cancer patients with sperm counts below normal (oligozoospermic) are still capable of having children.[31] Similarly, infertile women who have menstrual dysfunction following cytotoxic therapy may be treated for menstrual dysfunction and infertility in a manner similar to that of

the general population. However, the risk of an adverse pregnancy outcome is higher in these women, and they may require closer observation.[32]

### ASSISTED REPRODUCTIVE TECHNIQUES

The reproductive capacity of individuals undergoing malignancy treatment can be preserved by cryopreserving the gametes and using assisted reproductive techniques (ART) when pregnancy is desired.[33] When non-cryopreserved spermatozoa are used in combination with intrauterine insemination (IUI), in vitro fertilization (IVF), and intracytoplasmic sperm injection (ICSI), clinical pregnancy rates of 30–40% per cycle and delivery rates of 30% can be expected at most reproductive clinics. On the other hand, cryopreserved sperm from cancer patients results in complete pregnancies in only 18% of cycles.[34] Similarly, autologous cryopreserved embryos from in vitro-fertilized oocytes can be successfully implanted after cytotoxic therapy if the patient can undergo ovarian hyperstimulation before therapy.[35]

Men who remain azoospermic long after chemotherapy may benefit from testicular sperm extraction (TESE) combined with intracytoplasmic sperm injection (ICSI). The potential for sperm retrieval is not clearly affected by the chemotherapy regimen or by the disease treated.[36] Therefore, men should not be considered sterile despite prolonged non-obstructive azoospermia after undergoing chemotherapy.

## OPTIONS FOR FERTILITY PRESERVATION

### SEMEN CRYOPRESERVATION

With the advancement of ART, all men diagnosed with cancer should be offered the option of semen cryobanking, a procedure that provides the only reasonable chance of establishing pregnancy after therapy.[37] Semen cryopreservation is a widely available and inexpensive option (< $1000) that yields good results.

Patients diagnosed with cancer used to be considered poor candidates for sperm cryopreservation because they present with disease-induced suboptimal semen quality and cryosensitivity. Men with Hodgkin's lymphoma have pre-freeze and post-thaw sperm quality that is below normal.[38,39] However, as a general rule, there is no cancer group for which sperm cannot be retrieved and stored.[40] Even the absence of spermatozoa in semen should not prevent physicians from attempting to preserve a patient's fertility. In many cancer patients who suffer from azoospermia before treatment, testicular sperm extraction "Onco-tese" may be successfully attempted (unilateral or bilateral), and the retrieved sperms may be cryopreserved for future use.[41]

Almost 40% of patients who cryopreserve their semen may have a healthy live birth using ART.[33] Based on the experience at the Cleveland Clinic in the last two decades, the percentage decline in semen quality (from pre-freeze to post-thaw) in patients with cancer shows a similar trend that of normal donors. This suggests that the effect of cryodamage on spermatozoa from patients with cancer is similar to that of normal donors.[42,43] Cryopreserving semen after the start of therapy can adversely affect their chromosomal structure, causing de novo mutations, but should still be attempted if the imperativeness of starting therapy outweighs the chance for cryopreservation, as viable sperm may still be recovered. Therefore, it is crucial to cryopreserve sperm before chemotherapy or radiotherapy and also to advocate the use of contraception during therapy and for 6 months after.

Only a small percentage of patients (< 10%) who bank their spermatozoa before chemotherapy or radiotherapy return for assisted reproduction.[44–46] This finding may be explained by several reasons: recovery or waiting for possible resumption of spermatogenesis, short period from original illness, anxiety regarding potential risks for the children, and uncertainty about long-term health and, therefore, suitability to be parents.[42] However, trends have started to change, and awareness of sperm banking has increased over the past 4 to 5 years, coinciding with the advent of ICSI.

In males with cancer, the extent of sperm DNA damage plays an important role in determining how semen should be cryopreserved before therapy begins. Specimens with high sperm concentration and motility and low levels of DNA damage can be preserved in relatively large aliquots suitable for IUI. If a single specimen of good quality is available, then it should be preserved in multiple small aliquots suitable for IVF or ICSI.[28]

### TESTICULAR TISSUE HARVESTING

Although spermatogenesis does not occur in prepubertal testes, and prepubertal testes do not produce mature spermatozoa, these do contain the diploid stem germ cells from which haploid spermatozoa can be derived. Therefore, testicular tissue can be harvested from a biopsy and stored either as a tissue section or as isolated germ cells, before cancer therapy. Following cure and on entering adulthood, this tissue can be thawed and used to produce offspring in either of the two ways: the stored germ cells can be re-implanted into the patient's own testes to restore natural fertility, a procedure known as germ cell transplantation, or the stored stem cells can be matured in vitro until they are able to achieve fertilization via ICSI.[47] Although these two measures have been the subject of intensive research in the last decade, further refinements in the protocols may still be needed before they can be used routinely in clinical practice.

### Germ cell transplantation

Germ cells isolated from the testes of donor male mice can repopulate immunologically compatible testes when injected into the seminiferous tubules of recipient animals; the recipients show normal morphological features characteristic of the donor species.[48] Similarly, mouse germ cells transplanted into the testes of infertile mice colonize the recipient seminiferous tubules and initiate donor spermatogenesis in more than 70% of recipients.[49] The most striking result of these experiments was that healthy offspring (by mating) were produced from spermatozoa generated within the recipient testes by donor germ cells.

Establishing a successful method for testicular stem cell transplantation of frozen, thawed testicular cells would be of immense benefit to boys with childhood cancer undergoing sterilizing treatment. It is possible to reinitiate spermatogenesis after cryopreservation of testicular germ cell suspensions. Although cell survival is acceptable, current protocols need further improvement.[50] Male germ cells obtained before chemotherapy can be frozen and, after thawing, can be transplanted into animals to maintain the entire genetic information of the donor for a limited period.

Before stem cell transplantation can be considered for preserving the fertility of pre-pubertal boys, two issues must be carefully examined.[51] First, the testis biopsy taken from the cancer patient may contain malignant cells. These cells must be removed from the cell suspension because studies in rats have shown that one single malignant cell can reintroduce the disease. Second, the cell suspension consists of all testicular cells, and the proportion of spermatogonial stem cells is low (estimated at 1/5000).[52]

### In vitro maturation

In vitro germ cell maturation would be particularly useful in patients who have received extremely gonadotoxic therapy and in whom the supporting Sertoli cells would be unable to support spermatogenesis. Mouse spermatogonial stem cells can survive up to 4 months in culture and retain their ability to commence spermatogenesis following transplantation into a recipient.[53] However, it appears that current methods for in vitro maturation of diploid stem cells into haploid spermatozoa are not well developed. Ongoing research may improve their feasibility.

### OOCYTE CRYOPRESERVATION

Although successful fertilization and embryonic cleavage have been reported after injection of cryopreserved thawed oocytes, the pregnancy rate is not high enough to justify its routine use in clinical practice.[54] The main reason for poor outcomes after oocyte cryopreservation is related to the oocyte's structural complexity. Oocyte subcellular organelles are far more complex and perhaps more sensitive to thermal injury than preimplantation embryos. Oocyte donation may be considered in cases characterized by complete ovarian follicular depletion. However, the presence of other factors, such as uterine impairment, would be of major concern. In addition, complications during pregnancy and pre-term deliveries would be expected in these cases.[55]

## OVARIAN TISSUE CRYOPRESERVATION

Ovarian tissue banking in humans is being considered to restore fertility in patients who lose ovarian function because of chemotherapy or radiotherapy.[56] Ovarian tissue cryopreservation and transplantation was first examined in rodent studies and then in sheep and human ovarian xenograft studies.[57] However, no pregnancies have been reported in humans from the use of cryopreserved ovarian tissue. Although promising, there is a theoretical risk that malignant stem cells will be reimplanted along with the thawed cryopreserved ovary.[58,59] With the publication of promising data from humans, ovarian tissue cryopreservation from selected patients before cancer treatment and in those requiring oophorectomy may be advocated. However, this option is currently under experimental evaluation, and few centers offer this to patients.

## EMBRYO CRYOPRESERVATION

Embryo cryopreservation was introduced to maximize the chances of conception during a single menstrual cycle. Cryopreservation of preimplantation embryos is currently an integral part of patient care in clinical practice. This option may not be socially acceptable in prepubertal females and adolescents. However, acceptable, long-term data are available about the outcome of children born from these procedures.[60]

## CHOICE OF CYTOTOXIC REGIMENS

Currently, treatment regimens for hematologic malignancy include a variety of chemotherapeutic agents, all of which affect reproductive functions differently. For young patients, agents with minimal toxicity but maximal therapeutic effect are selected. For example, NOVP (Novantrone (mitoxantrone), Oncovin (vincristine), Vinblastine, Prednisone) may be preferred over MOPP (nitrogen mustard, vincristine, procarbazine, and prednisone) for the treatment of Hodgkin's lymphoma. Although NOVP markedly affects spermatogenesis, sperm production recovers rapidly after treatment, usually within 3 to 4 months. This rapid recovery is due to the fact that NOVP chemotherapy damages spermatogenic germ cells rather than inhibiting stem cells.[61]

Similarly, ABVD (adriamycin, bleomycin, vinblastine, and dacarbazine) is used to treat Hodgkin's disease instead of MOPP because the former dramatically reduces gonadal toxicity.[62] VAPEC-B (adriamycin, cyclophosphamide, etoposide, vincristine, bleomycin, and prednisolone), which is used in the treatment of non-Hodgkin's lymphoma, minimizes the dose of cyclophosphamide and therefore results in less gonadal failure than CHOP-Bleo (cyclophosphamide, adriamycin, Oncovin (vincristine), prednisone, bleomycin).[63]

## GONADAL SHIELDING

The gonads must be outside the field of radiation or shielded from the direct radiation beam unless they are being irradiated directly as a result of actual or potential neoplastic involvement. Although gonadal shields can reduce the amount of radiation two- to fivefold, some radiation may still reach the gonads. For example, the gonads typically receive 2 to 3 Gy with an inverted Y-field, which is used for Hodgkin's disease.[64] To minimize ovarian exposure, oophoropexy may be performed to relocate the ovaries away from the direct beam.[65,66] Laparoscopic oophorpexy may be of benefit in cases of Hodgkin's disease, if performed before pelvic irradiation.[67]

## MEDICAL TREATMENT

### Hormones

When testosterone suppressors such as gonadal steroids, GnRH analogs, and antiandrogens were used before and during cytotoxic therapy in male rats, they enhanced the recovery of spermatogenesis and fertility.[68] These suppressors may work by enhancing the potential of the somatic cells in the testis to support the recovery of spermatogenesis.[69] For a while, it was assumed that recovery of stem spermatogonia cells could possibly be stimulated after prolonged periods of iatrogenic azoospermia, but research does not support this theory. Hormone treatment given before and during cytotoxic therapy was found to protect spermatogenesis in only one of eight clinical trials.[40]

Gonadotropin-releasing hormone (GnRH) agonists may protect ovarian function from the effects of cyclophosphamide[71] by decreasing the recruitment of primordial follicles. Strong evidence supports the use of GnRH agonistic analogues to minimize the gonadotoxic effect of chemotherapy because they induce a pre-pubertal milieu.[59,72] However, the feasibility of using oral contraceptives or GnRH agonists to protect women against ovarian damage has not been established.[73] Another hormone, medroxyprogesterone, helps protect primordial follicles from the acute toxic effects of chemotherapy. Nevertheless, the quality of the follicles will be impaired, and many will undergo atresia, resulting in a shortened fertility period.[74]

Hormone replacement therapy (HRT) should be considered in young pre-menopausal women who have developed ovarian failure due to malignancy or cancer treatment.[75] Even with the use of HRT, though, uterine size can decrease by 40%.[24] Importantly, any residual ovarian function remaining after chemotherapy is considered a good prognostic sign because the ovaries may be stimulated with steroid hormones and/or gonadotropins.[76]

### Anti-apoptotic drugs

Oocytes exposed to chemotherapeutic agents in vitro undergo various changes leading to apoptosis.[77] Because a series of specific signaling events are activated in the cell that is bound for apoptosis, inhibiting these signaling events could potentially stop the apoptotic process and protect the patient from POF. Sphingosine-1-phosphate is an example of an apoptotic inhibitor. The oocytes of mice that had been treated with sphingosine-1-phosphate therapy resisted apoptosis that was induced by doxorubicin.[78] This concept offers a promising experimental alternative to guard against apoptosis. With the eventual identification of the molecular and genetic framework of chemotherapy-induced germ cell death, apoptotic inhibitors may some day play a role in preventing oocyte loss.

## ETHICAL AND LEGAL ISSUES

Options for future fertility following cancer treatment must be considered in the patient's best interests. Thus, the advantages of any intervention or of an active decision not to intervene must outweigh any disadvantages, both in the short and long term. Any intervention intended to preserve fertility must have a sound evidence base as well as moral provenance. It should neither raise unrealistic expectations, nor have long term adverse effects on the patient or his or her offspring.[79]

Informed consent should be given voluntarily by a competent person. However, in view of the complexity of the issues surrounding fertility preservation, the anxieties of both patients and their families at the time of diagnosis, and the limited time for discussion due to the urgency of commencing treatment, the validity of such consent may be impaired. The first stage of consent is for the collection and storage of the germinal tissue or gametes. The second stage is for use of the collected material for fertilization. In addition, it is important to consider what will happen to stored cells in the event of divorce or the patient's death. While some would advocate destruction of the tissue in the latter situation, others have suggested allowing the parents to donate the tissue for research purposes.[80]

## SUMMARY

Patients with hematologic malignancies have impaired fertility indirectly as a result of necessary cytotoxic treatment regimens. The deterioration in fertility potential may be temporary or permanent. However, the decreasing mortality rate and the increasing survival rate as a result of effective treatment have made fertility issues more frequently encountered.

A variety of measures may be used to minimize the deleterious effects of malignancy and its treatment on the human fertility potential. Moreover, assisted reproductive techniques in combination with our rapidly evolving understanding of cryobiology offer encouraging measures to preserve productiveness following malignancy treatment. These measures should be considered in young adults, and patients should be counseled regarding the pros and cons of each of the available options for fertility preservation.

## REFERENCES

1. Meirow D, Nugent D: The effects of radiotherapy and chemotherapy on female reproduction. *Hum Reprod Update* 7:535, 2001.
2. Agarwal A, Allamaneni SS: Disruption of spermatogenesis by the cancer disease process. *J Natl Cancer Inst* 34:9–11, 2005.
3. Rueffer U, Breuer K, Josting A, et al.: Male gonadal dysfunction in patients with Hodgkin's disease prior to treatment. *Ann Oncol* 12:1307, 2001.
4. Viviani S, Ragni G, Santoro A, et al.: Testicular dysfunction in Hodgkin's disease before and after treatment. *Eur J Cancer* 27:1389, 1991.
5. Chapman R, Sutcliffe S, Malpas J: Male gonadal dysfunction in Hodgkin's disease. A prospective study. *JAMA* 245:1323, 1981.
6. Barr R, Clark D, Booth J: Dyspermia in men with localized Hodgkin's disease. A potentially reversible, immune-mediated disorder. *Med Hypotheses* 40:165, 1993.
7. Marmor D, Elefant E, Dauchez C, Roux C: Semen analysis in Hodgkin's disease before the onset of treatment. *Cancer* 57:1986–1987, 1986.
8. Vigersky R, Andersen A, Thompson R, Loriaux D: Hypothalamic dysfunction in secondary amenorrhea associated with simple weight loss. *N Engl J Med* 297: 1141, 1977.
9. Schenker J, Meirow D, Schenker E: Stress and human reproduction. *Eur J Obstet Gynecol Reprod Biol* 45:1, 1992.
10. Meirow D, Schenker J: Cancer and male infertility. *Hum Reprod* 10:2017, 1995.
11. Meistrich M: Potential genetic risks of using semen collected during chemotherapy. *Hum Reprod* 8:8, 1993.
12. Meistrich M, Wilson G, Brown B, da Cunha M, Lipshultz L: Impact of cyclophosphamide on long-term reduction in sperm count in men treated with combination chemotherapy for Ewing's and soft tissue sarcomas. Cancer 70:2703, 1992.
13. Puscheck E, Philip P, Jeyendran R: Male fertility preservation and cancer treatment. *Cancer Treat Rev* 30:173, 2004.
14. Wang J, KAA G, Setchell B: Changes in testicular blood flow and testosterone production during aspermatogenesis after irradiation. *J Endocrinol* 98:35, 1983.
15. Warne G, Fairley K, Hobbs J, Martin F: Cyclophosphamide-induced ovarian failure. *N Engl J Med* 289:1159, 1973.
16. Bines J, Oleske D, Cobleigh M: Ovarian function in premenopausal women treated with adjuvant chemotherapy for breast cancer. *J Clin Oncol* 14:1718, 1996.
17. Gradishar W, Schilsky R: Ovarian function following radiation and chemotherapy for cancer. *Semin Oncol* 16:425, 1989.

18. Tilly J, Kolesnick R: Sphingolipids, apoptosis, cancer treatments and the ovary: investigating a crime against female fertility. *Biochim Biophys Acta* 1585:135, 2002.

19. Thomson A, Campbell A, Irvine D, Anderson R, Kelnar C, Wallace W: Semen quality and spermatozoal DNA integrity in survivors of childhood cancer: a case-control study. *Lancet* 360:361, 2002.

20. Centola G, Keller J, Henzler M, Rubin P: Effect of low-dose testicular irradiation on sperm count and fertility in patients with testicular seminoma. *J Androl* 15:608, 1994.

21. Shalet S, Tsatsoulis A, Whitehead E, Read G: Vulnerability of the human Leydig cell to radiation damage is dependent upon age. *J Endocrinol* 120:161, 1989.

22. O'Reilly R: Allogenic bone marrow transplantation: current status and future directions. *Blood* 62:941, 1983.

23. Hinterberger-Fischer M, Kier P, Kalhs P, et al.: Fertility, pregnancies and offspring complications after bone marrow transplantation. *Bone Marrow Transplant* 7:5, 1991.

24. Critchley H, Bath L, Wallace W: Radiation damage to the uterus—review of the effects of treatment of childhood cancer. *Hum Fertil (Camb)* 5:61, 2002.

25. Franchi-Rezgui P, Rousselot P, Espie M, et al.: Fertility in young women after chemotherapy with alkylating agents for Hodgkin and non-Hodgkin lymphomas. *Hematol J*:116, 2003.

26. Brierley J, Rathmell A, Gospodarowicz M, et al.: Late effects of treatment for early-stage Hodgkin's disease. *Br J Cancer* 77:1300, 1998.

27. Witt K, Bishop J: Mutagenicity of anticancer drugs in mammalian germ cells. *Mutat Res* 355:209, 1996.

28. Kobayashi H, Larson K, Sharma R, et al.: DNA damage in patients with untreated cancer as measured by the sperm chromatin structure assay. *Fertil Steril* 75:469, 2001.

29. Agarwal A, Said T: Role of sperm chromatin abnormalities and DNA damage in male infertility. *Hum Reprod Update* 9:331, 2003.

30. Check M, Brown T, Check J: Recovery of spermatogenesis and successful conception after bone marrow transplant for acute leukaemia: case report. *Hum Reprod* 15:83, 2000.

31. Marmor D, Duyck F: Male reproductive potential after MOPP therapy for Hodgkin's disease: a long-term survey. *Andrologia* 27:99, 1995.

32. Critchley H: Factors of importance for implantation and problems after treatment for childhood cancer. *Med Pediatr Oncol* 33:9, 1999.

33. Agarwal A, Ranganathan P, Kattal N, et al.: Fertility after cancer: a prospective review of assisted reproductive outcome with banked semen specimens. *Fertil Steril* 81:342, 2004.

34. Ginsburg E, Yanushpolsky E, Jackson K: In vitro fertilization for cancer patients and survivors. *Fertil Steril* 75:705, 2001.

35. Lipton J, Virro M, Solow H: Successful pregnancy after allogeneic bone marrow transplant with embryos isolated before transplant. *J Clin Oncol* 15:3347, 1997.

36. Chan P, Palermo G, Veeck L, Rosenwaks Z, Schlegel P: Testicular sperm extraction combined with intracytoplasmic sperm injection in the treatment of men with persistent azoospermia postchemotherapy. *Cancer* 92:1632, 2001.

37. Sanger W, Olson J, Sherman J: Semen cryobanking for men with cancer—criteria change. *Fertil Steril* 58:1024, 1992.

38. Reed E, Sanger W, Armitage J: Results of semen cryopreservation in young men with testicular carcinoma and lymphoma. *J Clin Oncol* 4:537, 1986.

39. Agarwal A, Newton R: The effect of cancer on semen quality after cryopreservation of sperm. *Andrologia* 23:329, 1991.

40. Bahadur G, Ling K, Hart R, et al.: Semen quality and cryopreservation in adolescent cancer patients. *Hum Reprod* 17:3157, 2002.

41. Schrader M, Muller M, Sofikitis N, et al.: "Onco-tese": testicular sperm extraction in azoospermic cancer patients before chemotherapy-new guidelines? *Urology* 61:421, 2003.

42. Hallak J, Sharma R, Thomas A, Jr., Agarwal A: Why cancer patients request disposal of cryopreserved semen specimens posttherapy: a retrospective study. *Fertil Steril* 69:889, 1998.

43. Agarwal A: Semen banking in patients with cancer: 20-year experience. *Int J Androl* 23:16, 2000.

44. Audrins P, Holden C, MacLachlan R, Kovas G: Semen storage for special purposes at Monash IVF from 1977 to 1997. *Fertil Steril* 72:179, 1999.

45. Schover L, Rybicki L, Martin B, Bringeisen K: Having children after cancer. A pilot survey of survivors' attitudes and experiences. *Cancer* 86:697, 1999.

46. Lass A, Akagbosu F, Brinsden P: Sperm banking and assisted reproduction treatment for couples following cancer treatment of the male partner. *Hum Reprod Update* 7:370, 2001.

47. Brougham M, Kelnar C, Sharpe R, Wallace W: Male fertility following childhood cancer: current concepts and future therapies. *Asian J Androl* 5:325, 2003.

48. Brinster R, Avarbock M: Germline transmission of donor haplotype following spermatogonial transplantation. *Proc Natl Acad Sci USA* 91:11303, 1994.

49. Brinster R, Zimmermann J: Spermatogenesis following male germ-cell transplantation. *Proc Natl Acad Sci USA* 91:11298, 1994.

50. Frederickx V, Michiels A, Goossens E, et al.: Recovery, survival and functional evaluation by transplantation of frozen-thawed mouse germ cells. *Hum Reprod* 19:948, 2004.

51. Aslam I, Fishel S, Moore H, Dowell K, Thornton S: Fertility preservation of boys undergoing anti-cancer therapy: a review of the existing situation and prospects for the future. *Hum Reprod.* 15:2154, 2000.

52. Jahnukainen K, Hou M, Petersen C, Setchell B, Soder O: Intratesticular transplantation of testicular cells from leukemic rats causes transmission of leukemia. *Cancer Res* 61:706, 2001.

53. Nagano M, Avarbock M, Leonida E, Brinster C, Brinster R: Culture of mouse spermatogonial stem cells. *Tissue Cell* 30:389, 1998.

54. Gook D, Osborn S, Bourne H, Johnston W: Fertilization of human oocytes following cryopreservation; normal karyotypes and absence of stray chromosomes. *Hum Reprod* 9:684, 1994.

55. Larsen E, Loft A, Holm K, Muller J, Brocks V, Andersen A: Oocyte donation in women cured of cancer with bone marrow transplantation including total body irradiation in adolescence. *Hum Reprod* 15:1505, 2000.

56. Falcone T, Attaran M, Bedaiwy MA, Goldberg JM: Ovarian function preservation in the cancer patient. *Fertil Steril* 81:243, 2004.

57. Oktay K: Ovarian tissue cryopreservation and transplantation: preliminary findings and implications for cancer patients. *Hum Reprod Update* 7:526, 2001.

58. Kim S, Radford J, Harris M, et al.: Ovarian tissue harvested from lymphoma patients to preserve fertility may be safe for autotransplantation. *Hum Reprod* 16:2056, 2001.

59. Blumenfeld Z: Preservation of fertility and ovarian function and minimalization of chemotherapy associated gonadotoxicity and premature ovarian failure: the role of inhibin-A and -B as markers. *Mol Cell Endocrinol* 187:93, 2002.

60. Meniru G, Craft I: In vitro fertilization and embryo cryopreservation prior to hysterectomy for cervical cancer. *Int J Gynaecol Obstet* 56:69, 1997

61. Meistrich ML, Wilson G, Mathur K, et al.: Rapid recovery of spermatogenesis after mitoxantrone, vincristine, vinblastine, and prednisone chemotherapy for Hodgkin's disease. *J Clin Oncol* 15:3488, 1997.

62. Viviani S, Santoro A, Ragni G, Bonfante V, Bestetti O, Bonadonna G: Gonadal toxicity after combination chemotherapy for Hodgkin's disease. Comparative results of MOPP vs. ABVD. *Eur J Cancer Clin Onc* 21:601, 1985.

63. Radford J, Clark S, Crowther D, Chalet S: Male fertility after VAPEC-B chemotherapy for Hodgkin's disease and non-Hodgkin's lymphoma. *Br J Cancer* 69:379, 1994.

64. Bieri S, Rouzaud M, Miralbell R: Seminoma of the testis: is scrotal shielding necessary when radiotherapy is limited to the para-aortic nodes. *Radiother Oncol* 50:349, 1999.

65. Ortin T, Shostak C, Donaldson S: Gonadal status and reproductive function following treatment for Hodgkin's disease in childhood: the Stanford experience. *Int J Radiat Oncol Biol Phys* 19: 873, 1990.

66. Morice P, Juncker L, Rey A, El-Hassan J, Haie-Meder C, Castaigne D: Ovarian transposition for patients with cervical carcinoma treated by radiosurgical combination. *Fertil Steril* 74:743, 2000.

67. Williams R, Littell R, Mendenhall N: Laparoscopic oophoropexy and ovarian function in the treatment of Hodgkin disease. *Cancer* 86:2138, 1999.

68. Meistrich M, Shetty G: Suppression of testosterone stimulates recovery of spermatogenesis after cancer treatment. *Int J Androl* 26:141, 2003.

69. Meistrich M, Wilson G, Kangasniemi M, Huhtaniemi I: Mechanism of protection of rat spermatogenesis by hormonal pretreatment: stimulation of spermatogonial differentiation after irradiation. *J Androl* 21: 464, 2000.

70. Masala A, Faedda R, Alagna S, Satta A, et al.: Use of testosterone to prevent cyclophosphamide-induced azoospermia. *Ann Intern Med* 126:292, 1997.

71. Ataya K, Rao L, Lawrence E, Kimmel R: Luteinizing hormone-releasing hormone agonist inhibits cyclophosphamide-induced ovarian follicular depletion in rhesus monkeys. *Biol Reprod* 52:365, 1995.

72. Blumenfeld Z, Dann E, Avivi I, Epelbaum R, Rowe J: Fertility after treatment for Hodgkin's disease. *Ann Oncol* 13:138, 2002.

73. Waxman J, Ahmed R, Smith D, et al.: Failure to preserve fertility in patients with Hodgkin's disease. *Cancer Chemother Pharmacol* 19:159, 1987.

74. Familiari G, Caggiati A, Nottola S, Ermini M, Di Benedetto M, Motta P: Ultrastructure of human ovarian primordial follicles after combination chemotherapy for Hodgkin's disease. *Hum Reprod* 8:2080, 1993.

75. Mulder JE: Benefits and risks of hormone replacement therapy in young adult cancer survivors with gonadal failure. *Med Pediatr Oncol* 33:46, 1999.

76. Chatterjee R, Goldstone A: Gonadal damage and effects on fertility in adult patients with haematological malignancy undergoing stem cell transplantation. *Bone Marrow Transplant* 17:5, 1996.

77. Tilly J: Molecular and genetic basis of normal and toxicant-induced apoptosis in female germ cells. *Toxicol Lett* 102–103:497, 1998.

78. Morita Y, Perez G, Paris F, et al.: Oocyte apoptosis is suppressed by disruption of the acid sphingomyelinase gene or by sphingosine-1-phosphate therapy. *Nat Med* 6:1109, 2000.

79. Grundy R, Larcher V, Gosden R, et al.: Fertility preservation for children treated for cancer (2): ethics of consent for gamete storage and experimentation. *Arch Dis Child* 84:360, 2001.

80. Wallace W, Walker D: Conference consensus statement: ethical and research dilemmas for fertility preservation in children treated for cancer. *Hum Fertil (Camb)* 4:69, 2001.

# Chapter 109

# PALLIATION OF SYMPTOMS ASSOCIATED WITH HEMATOLOGIC MALIGNANCIES

*Mellar P. Davis*

## INTRODUCTION

Patients presenting with hematologic malignancies experience multiple symptoms while also confronting the emotional distress of a newly diagnosed life-threatening illness. Most will notice reduced physical functioning prior to admission. Many will also note a change in their role within the family structure as they become more dependent because of the symptoms. Overall quality of life is significantly impaired compared to the age-matched normal population.[1] Pain and fatigue will improve with successful treatment and approximate the normal population at 3 months. However, physical and role (social) functioning within the family remains substantially below premorbid levels despite successful therapy.[1] Other symptoms at diagnoses include fever from infections, bleeding, and weight loss.[2] Weight loss is particularly evident in patients with myeloma and amyloid or in individuals who have primary amyloidosis.[3] Little is written about the presenting symptoms associated with acute leukemia. Some of the reported symptoms include fatigue, fever, bleeding, and pain. The pain from acute leukemia is more generalized than the pain that occurs with myeloma, and more frequently centered in the chest.[4]

Symptoms near the end of life for hematologic malignancies in general are protean. Dyspnea occurs due to cardiac insufficiency (perhaps from comorbidities, anthracycline toxicity, or radiation), fevers from infections, and hyperleukocytosis, which can cause neurologic deficits and hypoxemia. Lymphangitic tumor infiltration with pain and shortness of breath, pulmonary fibrosis, mediastinal adenopathy with atelectasis, pleural effusion, and growing tumor masses add to dyspnea, pain, and debility.[5] Fevers occur in 40% of acute leukemia patients near the end of life. Severe pain is present in 27%. Abdominal pain is present in 60%, bone pain in 30%, and thoracic pain in 10%.[5] Clinical evidence of bleeding occurs in 20%, excluding ecchymosis

and petechiae. Delirium will be present in at least 25%, with the incidence steadily rising as death approaches. Mucositis will be a major problem in 9%.[5]

Chemotherapy will be given to 46% as palliation in the terminal phase, either for hyperleukocytosis or painful compressive lymphadenopathy. Many will receive short courses of radiation for the same reason. Antibiotics will be prescribed in nearly half. Blood transfusions, particularly red blood cells, will be given to 40% in the terminal phase of their illness.[5] Patients will be on opioids (27% of patients), steroids (40%), and benzodiazepines (90%), all of which will be necessary to palliate symptoms but will also increase the risk of delirium. A Do Not Resuscitate (DNR) order will be written in only 38% despite the fact that deaths are anticipated in nearly 80%.[5]

Many patients with acute leukemia in the terminal phase will have clinically evident (wet) bleeding (44%), fever with infections (71%), and bone pain (76%).[4] One quarter will have oral pain and dysphagia and over one-third of patients will have problems with nausea and vomiting.[4] Such symptoms will preclude oral opioids for pain control. Many patients will have central lines for parenteral infusion, while a minority without venous access will be given subcutaneous opioids.[4] Rectal administration of medications, commonly used in hospice, is avoided because of the risk of infections and bleeding. As a result, the versatility of palliative medications is limited by the disease process.

Unadjusted survival for leukemia and lymphoma patients entering hospice programs is much shorter than that for the patients with solid tumors. In 1996, the median survival for patients with hematologic malignancies after hospice enrollment was 23 days, and 20% died within 7 days.[6]

Patients with hematologic malignancies have a greater chance of dying within the hospital compared to patients with solid tumors[7]. In South Australia, all leukemia patients died in the hospital and few received palliative consults for managing symptoms at the end of life.[7] On average, the risk of dying within a hospital is four times that of solid tumor patients. Patients with hematologic malignancies have the lowest enrollment in hospice programs per disease category.[8] This may in part be because of the reluctance of hospice programs to administer blood transfusions, a treatment considered palliative by most physicians specializing in the hematologic malignancies.

## SYMPTOMS AND MANAGEMENT

### LOCAL SYMPTOMS
### Pain

Pain will be experienced by most patients with advanced cancers, and hematologic malignancies are no exceptions.[9] Myeloma pain is well localized, whereas acute leukemia often is associated with more generalized pain, as previously discussed. Neuropathic pain will occur in myeloma because of the development of amyloid, spinal cord compression, leptomeningeal metastases, or due to myelin-associated monoclonal proteins.[10] As a general rule, two-thirds of the pain syndromes in cancer patients are directly related to cancer and one-third are related to treatment. However, many of the chemotherapy agents used to treat hematologic malignancies produce neuropathic pain (e.g., thalidomide, now popular in the treatment of myeloma). Mucositis is treatment related, and is a major cause of pain during induction chemotherapy and periods of myelosuppression. This is particularly true for high-dose antimetabolites such as methotrexate or cytosine arabinoside, and high-dose melphalan used as preparation for stem cell transplantation (SCT) in myeloma. Graft-versus-host disease will produce a mucositis and oral pain, which can persist.

Pain intensity is easily "quantified" by using unidimensional pain scales such as the visual analogue scale, the numerical scale, and the category scale.[9,11] Older patients are usually able to complete a category scale by rating pain as none, mild, moderate, or severe. Either the category scale or even a pictorial face scale can be used by those with moderate cognitive impairment.[9] Pain intensity is influenced by mood, perceived meaning of pain, and psychological state (depression, delirium, or anxiety), and is not the same as nociception. Pain syndromes that are resistant to opioids include neuropathic pain, cutaneous pain, incident flares of pain, and colic.[9,12]

The evaluation of pain by most physicians is suboptimal.[13–15] Assessment requires a good pain history, which requires evaluating pain intensity, location, radiation, palliative factors, and referral, as well as response to prior treatments. In addition, the physician should understand the influence of pain on daily activities (pain interference). Multidimensional pain tools such as the Brief Pain Inventory are available for this purpose.[16]

As pain is a multidimensional experience, treatment should include both nonpharmacologic and pharmacologic therapies.[9] The reduction of anxiety, depression, and delirium with supportive psychotherapy, cognitive behavioral therapy, and medications will increase pain thresholds and reduce pain intensity. Surgery and orthodontics, as well as radiation therapy, should be considered as complementary to pharmacologic therapy.

Most patients with cancer actually have several pains. Most have chronic pain with transient flares of acute pain.[17] In approximately one-third, neuropathic pain will be prominent, though many will have a mixed pattern of neuropathic and nociceptive pain.[18] Both the type of pain, pain intensity, and the temporal nature of pain govern the analgesic dosing strategy. Therapy needs to be individualized.[19,20] Opioids should be used for moderate to severe pain.[19,20] Eighty percent of patients with severe pain will have pain controlled by morphine or other potent opioids. Opioid titration to response is a cardinal principle of treatment. An effective drug will be ineffective if underdosed; potent opioids do not have a ceiling dose. Twenty percent of patients will require a complex approach to pain management of opioid (route) conversion, opioid rotation to an alternative opioid, opioid sparing (by adding an adjuvant analgesic), or maintenance of opioid dosing with simultaneous treatment of opioid side effects (particularly in those who are actively dying).[9,21,22] Most mistakes in dosing occur with (1) failure to give around-the-clock doses; (2) failure to provide breakthrough doses for transient flares of pain; (3) failure to titrate to response; (4) combining different opioids at less than optimal levels; (5) failure to use adjuvant analgesics effectively; and (6) failure to recognize and treat opioid side effects and proactively prevent constipation with laxatives.[23]

Several factors play a role in opioid choices: efficacy, versatility, drug interaction, therapeutic index, availability, cost, and organ function. Opioid agonist/antagonists, nalbuphine, butorphanol, and meperidine should not be used.[9,21] The most common potent opioids in the first-line treatment of cancer pain are morphine and methadone, fentanyl, hydromorphone, and oxycodone if limiting side effects occur with morphine.[24–28] Low doses of a potent opioid can be substituted for "weak" opioids (by World Health Organization classification). Choices will depend upon the patient's previous opioid experience, comorbidities (renal and hepatic function), and comedications. The type of pain does not play a particularly strong role in the choice of opioids.

Principles to opioid dosing include titration to response, around-the-clock dosing, provision for rescue doses for transient flares of pain, use of sustained release formulations to improve compliance, proactive treatment of constipation with stool softeners and laxatives, and individualized dosing to pain pattern.

Dose titration is based upon the percentage of baseline dose. Baseline dose should be increased 100% for pain levels that persist between 7 and 10 on a numerical scale (in which 0 indicates no pain and 10 represents the worst pain imaginable) and 50% for pain levels of 5–6.[21]

Rescue doses are either 100% of the four-hourly dose, 25–50% of the four-hourly dose, or 5–15% of the total opioid daily dose.[19,21] Both breakthrough pain and "end of dose failure" pain are a result of suboptimal around-the-clock dosing, and the around-the-clock dose should be increased in order to improve pain and reduce the number of pain flares during the day. Incident pain should be titrated separately and not added to the around-the-clock dose of opioids.

Opioid rotation will successfully manage pain in those who are experiencing dose-limiting side effects with opioids (cognitive failure, visual hallucinations, myoclonus, or intractable nausea and vomiting) and poorly controlled pain.[22] Non-cross-tolerance between potent opioids is a clinical feature that allows for opioid rotation. Non-cross-tolerance is related to genetic differences in opioid receptors and differences in receptor conformations induced by the opioid binding to the receptor. Differences in multiple opioid subtypes and G-protein interactions also contribute to non-cross-tolerance.[9,22,29] In order to rotate or switch an opioid it is necessary to understand opioid equivalents (Table 109.1).

Rotations for reasons of uncontrolled pain should be at equivalent doses and rotations for reasons of side effects should be at 50–75% of equivalent doses.[21] Converting from oral to rectal route should be done at equivalent doses. Converting the same opioid from oral to parenteral should be 3:1 for morphine, 2:1 for oxycodone (if parenteral oxycodone is available), 2:1 for methadone, and 5:1 for hydromorphone (though some use 2:1 for hydromorphone).

Adjuvant analgesics improve the opioid therapeutic index either by blocking opioid tolerance (which occurs with N-methyl-D-aspartate receptor antagonists) or by facilitating opioid analgesia, as occurs through tricyclic antidepressants (and enhanced monoamine release). Adjuvants are used for three reasons (1) a pain pathophysiology that is less responsive to opioids, such as neuropathic pain; (2) when opioid side effects occur and adjuvants allow for reduced opioid doses; and (3) to diagnose a complex pain syndrome.[21] (Table 109.2).

As mentioned previously, supportive psychotherapy, surgery, radiation therapy, and orthotics are an important part of pain management in cancer patients. Kyphoplasty, as an example, has been found to effectively reduce the mechanical back pain associated with myeloma and osteolytic vertebral compression fractures.[30]

## Nausea and vomiting

Nausea is common with uncontrolled infections, elevated intracranial pressure, certain medications, abdominal radiation, chemotherapy, and advanced cancer independent of treatment.[31,32]

| Table 109.1 | Opiod equivalents | |
|---|---|---|
| Opioid | Potency ratio compared to morphine | Available routes |
| Fentanyl | 70–100:1 (oral morphine to parenteral fentanyl) | IV/SC/ED/IT |
| Methadone | 4–12:1 | PO/PR/SC/IV |
| Oxycodone | 1–1.5:1 | PO/PR |
| Hydromorphone | 4–6:1 | PO/PR/SC/IV/ED/IT |
| Morphine | 1:1 | PO/PR/SC/IV/ED/IT |

PO, by mouth; PR, by rectum; SC, subcutaneous; IV, intravenous; ED, epidural; IT – Intrathecal.

| Table 109.2 | Adjuvant analgesics |
|---|---|
| Drug | Dose |
| Anti-seizure medications | Gabapentin 100 mg TID up to 3600 mg/day<br>Valproic acid 250–500 mg at night up to 150 mg/day<br>Carbamazepine 100 mg BID up to 1200 mg/day |
| Tricyclic antidepressants | Amitriptyline 10–25 mg at night up to 150 mg/day<br>Desipramine 10–25 mg at night up to 150 mg/day<br>Nortriptyline 10–25 mg at night up to 150 mg/night |
| Nonsteroidal anti-inflammatory drugs | Ibuprofen 200 mg BID up to 800 mg 3 times daily<br>Naprogen 250 mg twice daily up to 500 mg 3 times daily |
| Corticosteroids | Dexamethasone 2–4 mg daily up to 16 mg daily<br>Prednisone 10 mg daily up to 60 mg per day |
| Miscellaneous | |
| Mexiletine | 150 mg twice daily up to 450 mg twice daily |
| Clonazepam | 0.5 mg twice daily up to 20 mg/day |
| Lidocaine Trandermal Patch 5% | 1–3 daily over 12 h |
| Pamidionate | 90 mg IV monthly |
| Zolendronate | 4 mg monthly |

The frequency and severity of chemotherapy-induced nausea and vomiting (CINV) depends upon the type of chemotherapy, the dose, patient risk factors (for example, females and nonusers of alcohol are at higher risk), and the type of antiemetic regimen. CINV and nausea in general are major concerns that patients have with chemotherapy, and a major factor contributing to noncompliance.[33]

In the 1980s, high-dose metoclopramide was found to be effective in preventing CINV from highly emetogenic chemotherapy (principally cisplatin). In the 1990s, serotonin receptor antagonists were found to dramatically reduce acute CINV and were better tolerated than high-dose metoclopramide.[33] As a result of their increased use, along with the use of corticosteroids, delayed (after 24 h) CINV became more prevalent. Delayed nausea and vomiting is experienced by 60% of the patients, whereas acute nausea and vomiting is experienced by 26% despite the use of 5-HT$_3$ receptor antagonists and corticosteroids.[34] Though corticosteroids and 5-HT$_3$ receptor antagonists are more effective in reducing vomiting than nausea, patients actually fear nausea more than vomiting.

Physicians are generally compliant with guidelines for prophylaxis of acute CINV based upon the emetogenic potential of individual chemotherapy protocols, but poorly follow the recommendations for preventing delayed CINV.[34] Such recommendations include dexamethasone and either metoclopramide or a 5-HT$_3$ receptor antagonist for 4 days postchemotherapy in highly emetogenic or moderately emetogenic chemotherapy.

Serotonin receptor antagonists reduce nausea and vomiting associated with radiation, total body radiation, and high-dose chemotherapy as preparation for SCT, but do not particularly prevent delayed nausea and vomiting from total body radiation or with SCT. Serotonin plays a minor role in delayed nausea and vomiting associated with highly emetogenic chemotherapy, total body radiation, and transplant. Substance P may actually be the more important neurotransmitter.[35,36]

Responses among the various 5-HT$_3$ receptor antagonists tend to be equivalent. Palonosetron, however, has been found to reduce delayed CINV compared to first generation 5-HT$_3$ antagonists, probably due to its long half-life.[37-39]

The addition of aprepitant, a neurokinin 1 receptor antagonist, to dexamethasone plus a 5-HT$_3$ receptor antagonist improves both acute and delayed CINV relative to dexamethasone and a first generation 5-HT$_3$ antagonist.[40,41] However, the three-drug regimen has been reported to be effective only in cisplatin or highly emetogenic regimens, whereas palonosetron is approved for moderately emetogenic chemotherapy.[39] Initial trials of palonosetron- and aprepitant-containing regimens were not compared to regimens that included dexamethasone for delayed CINV. Combinations of palonosetron, dexamethasone, and aprepitant have been recommended for moderate to highly emetogenic chemotherapy, including protocols containing cyclophosphamide, doxorubicin, and carboplatin in high doses, though this prophylactic regimen needs to be tested clinically.[39] Finally, at least in a small group of patients receiving moderate to highly emetogenic chemotherapy, the atypical neuroleptic, olanzapine, plus dexamethasone was found to prevent delayed nausea and vomiting, and this may be a reasonable regimen for those who have extrapyramidal reactions to metoclopramide or standard neuroleptics.[37]

## Mucositis

Mucositis can be dose limiting to chemotherapy or radiation. This can be the worst experience a patient has during high-dose chemotherapy or SCT.[42] Mucositis can be quite painful, and it can accelerate nutritional depletion, prolong hospital stays, and increase medical expenditures associated with treatment. Pain severity follows the degree of observable mucositis. The peak pain severity and observable mucositis also correlate with dysphagia. Pain severity and objective mucositis are used in the National Cancer Institute Common Toxicity Criteria (Table 109.3).[43] Mucositis is also a common portal of entry for bacteria, particularly in myelosuppressed patients, and can lead to bacterial infections.[42] It is the major factor associated with sepsis in SCT patients.

Factors that predispose to mucositis are the duration of chemotherapy (more than dose), diurnal variation in chemotherapy exposure, drug type (greatest with antimetabolites), and combinations of chemotherapy with radiation.[42] Patient factors include poor oral hygiene, preexisting xerostomia, hepatic and renal dysfunction, impaired DNA repair capability, poor nutritional status, and pleural or peritoneal effusions (which act as reservoirs for antimetabolites).[42,44,45]

***Treatment of mucositis*** Treatment regimens can be categorized into those which minimize chemotherapy contact with oral mucosa, modify mucosal epithelium proliferation, reduce the inflammatory or infectious complications, and reduce pain[42] (Table 109.4).

---

**Table 109.3** National Cancer Institute common toxicity criteria for myeloablative chemotherapy[43]

0 = No mucositis

1 = Painless ulcer, errythema, or mild soreness in the absence of lesions

2 = Painful errythema, edema, or ulcers but the pain is such that patients can swallow

3 = Painful errythema, edema, or ulcers that prevent swallowing or necessitate hydrate or parenteral nutrition

4 = Severe ulceration which requires prophylactic intubation or results in aspiration pneumonia

| Table 109.4 | Therapies for oral mucositis |
|---|---|

**Treatment therapies that alter drug contact with mucosal surface**
  Allopurinal
  Cryotherapy
  Propantheline (etoposide)
  Amifostine
  Leucovorin (methotrexate)

**Therapies that modify mucosal epithelial proliferation**
  Beta carotene
  Tretinoin
  G-CSF
  GM-CSF
  TGF-B
  EGF
  Keratinocyte growth factor

**Therapies that reduce potential infections and inflammatory complications**
  Chlorohexidine
  Benzydamine
  Pentoxifylline
  Chamomile
  Thalidomide
  Sucralfate
  Tocopherol
  Glucocorticocoids
  Providone Iodine
  5–Aminosalicylate
  Antibacterial agents
  Antifungal agents
  Antiviral agents
**Therapies to reduce the pain of mucositis**
  Topical disphenhydramine
  Viscous lidocaine
  Dyclonine HCL
  Low energy helium neon laser
  Opioids

Preventive measures are generally unproven or marginally helpful.[46–49] No particular agent is uniformly efficacious and accepted as a standard of care. There are a large number of management practices but little evidence to base recommendations.[45]

Mucosal and dental health should be evaluated before treatment. Periodontal evaluation, and if necessary radiographic examinations (panorex), should be done prior to considering high-dose chemotherapy, SCT, or radiation therapy. Dental prosthetics should be checked for proper fitting. Restoration procedures should be done 3 weeks before mucotoxic therapy.[42] Cultures for herpes simplex may be helpful if prolonged neutropenia is anticipated or if mucositis is prolonged. Xerostomia should be treated to avoid prolonged chemotherapy contact with oral mucosal surfaces. Drugs associated with xerostomia, such as tricyclic antidepressants, should be avoided during chemotherapy or SCT. Saliva substitutes, sodium bicarbonate, milk, or sugarless gum may act as a saliva

"wash" to reduce or dilute oral chemotherapy concentrations. Fluoride (stannous fluoride) will reduce dental caries and calcium phosphate oral rinses maintain enamel.[42] Brushing with a soft brush and flossing should be encouraged except during radiation or myeloablative chemotherapy. Foam brushes should be used during mylosuppression. Removable prosthetics should not be worn except at meal times.[42] Hot, spicy, coarse foods, fruits, and beverages with high-acid content or alcohol should be avoided. Smoking should be discouraged.[42]

## GENERALIZED SYMPTOMS
### Fatigue

Fatigue is the most prevalent and one of the most important untreated cancer symptoms.[50–54] (Table 109.5). Fatigue is of primary importance to quality of life. There is a large discrepancy between the known importance of fatigue to quality of life and discussions and treatment of fatigue by physicians. Most oncologists believe that pain affects their patients to a greater extent than fatigue, whereas most patients feel that fatigue affects their lives to a greater extent than pain.[55] Even though nearly 80% of physicians believe that fatigue is both overlooked and undertreated, 74% of patients believe that fatigue must simply be endured without any recourse to treatment.[55] Half or more of patients do not discuss fatigue with their hematologist/oncologist and only 27% receive any recommendations about treatment.[55] Unfortunately, the most common information physicians impart to patients regarding fatigue are (1) nothing can be done (told to patients 40% of the time) or (2) increase time spent resting (37% of the time), both of which are poor advice.[50,51] Other advice includes taking multivitamins or modifying diet, which again is a poor advice,[53] particularly when considering that fatigue can persist for years in cancer survivors.[53,56]

Fatigue has a multifaceted character similar to pain. This includes a physical, affective, and cognitive dimension. Patients with fatigue will complain of a lack of energy, weakness, somnolence, and inability to concentrate.[57,59] Cancer fatigue does not usually improve with rest and is unlike fatigue in individuals without cancer.[53] Fatigue is frequently accompanied by loss of emotional control (90%), a feeling of isolation (74%), and dejection (72%).[53]

| Table 109.5 | Fatigue prevalance |
|---|---|

Normal population, 13–23%
At diagnosis of cancer, 50%
With bone metastasis, 75%
During chemotherapy or radiation, 60–96%

Assessment for fatigue can be done using following three questions:

1. Do you feel or have you felt unusually tired?
2. If you are fatigued can you indicate how tired you are using a numerical scale of 0 (no fatigue) to 10 (the greatest degree of fatigue imaginable)?
3. How much does your fatigue impact your daily life?.[57]

The National Capital Comprehensive Cancer Network has established that the patients who rate the severity of fatigue >4 require detailed assessment and treatment.[52,57,60]

The NCCN recommends focusing on following five factors that may influence fatigue: pain, emotional distress, insomnia and sleep hygiene, anemia, and hypothyroidism. In addition, comorbidities such as infection, poor nutritional status, and metabolic abnormalities should be considered.[53,60]

The treatment of fatigue requires an understanding of associative causes, and intervention when possible. These include elimination of nonessential central-acting (sedative) medications, treatment of insomnia, transfusion of blood for anemia, correction of electrolyte and endocrine abnormalities, treatment of pain, treatment of depression, prevention of deconditioning with moderate exercise, and treatment of hypothyroidism.[57,61]

The nonpharmacologic management of fatigue includes education centered on energy conserving techniques and stress reduction. Tasks should be spread out over a longer period of time during the day.[62] A diary of activities may help patients cope with their fatigue and adjust activities to their fatigue level.[62] Low-intensity, short-interval exercises should be encouraged.[60,62] Rhythmic or repetitive movements, as with walking, cycling, or swimming, will gradually increase stamina.[57] There is an added psychological benefit to exercise.[63,64] Restorative activities such as gardening, quiet times (spiritual or meditation), volunteer activities, and walking in a natural environment can reduce cancer fatigue.[62] Stress can be reduced by massage, visual imagery, biofeedback, and laughter.[53,59,60,62] Education about sleep hygiene and a concerted effort to improve nutrition are considerations. Both pharamacologic and nonpharmacologic therapies should be used together (Table 109.6).

### Depression

Approximately 80% and certainly more than 50% of psychologic and psychiatric morbidity associated with advanced malignancies goes unnoticed by physicians.[65–67] Antidepressants account for only 1–5% of the psychotropic medications prescribed by physicians to cancer patients, even though one-third of patients have significant depression. The reasons for under recognition include the absence of biological markers for depression, a lack of training on the part of physi-

| Table 109.6 | Pharmacologic management of fatigue |
|---|---|
| **Anemia (goal is ≥12 gm %)** | |
| Erythropoietin 40,000 iu weekly | |
| Darbepoeitin 200 μg every other week | |
| **Depression** | |
| Methylphenidate 5 mg at 8 am and 5 mg at noon, titrate to 1 mg/kg | |
| Sertraline 50 mg/day up to 200 mg/day | |
| Paroxetine 10 mg/day up to 50 mg/day | |
| Mirtazapine 15 mg at night titrate to 45 mg | |
| Bupropion 100 mg/day up to 450 mg kkg | |
| **Miscellaneous agents** | |
| Modafinil 100 mg at 8 am and noon up to 400 mg/day | |
| Prednisone 20–40 mg daily | |

cians to recognize depression (and delirium), a sense that both depression and cognitive changes are "appropriate" and normal for advanced cancer, the inappropriateness of screening instruments developed in noncancer populations for cancer patients, overlapping neurovegetive signs associated with cancer and depression (i.e., anorexia, cachexia, insomnia), and time constraints or lack of interest.[65,67]

Physicians should screen patients for depression as depression will make it difficult to treat other symptoms and other symptoms may improve with resolution of depression. The depressed patient may not be compliant with medications. Depression is a major cause of symptom distress in advanced malignancies and is a primary reason for the desire for death at the end of life.[66,68] Depression reduces pleasure, meaning, and social connections. It reduces the ability to do the work of separating and saying goodbye and is a major cause of anguish among family members.[67]

Screening tools aid in detecting depression, especially for physicians who are not psychiatrically astute (Table 109.7). Screening tools that are sensitive to cancer-associated depression are not dependent upon neurovegetive symptoms to diagnose depression. Screening tools that probe for helplessness, hopelessness, worthlessness, and anhedonia are, on the other hand, more discriminating in cancer.[70] In addition, patient scores on these self-rated depression scales rarely change over time in untreated patients, with little week-to-week variation,[70] indicating good intrasubject reliability.

The diagnosis of depression is fairly reliable when dysphoria and/or anhedonia are present for at least 2

| Table 109.7 | Depression screening tools[69] |
|---|---|
| Hospital Anxiety and Depression Scale | |
| Beck Depression Scale | |
| Edinburgh Post Natal Depression Scale (adapted for cancer) | |

**Table 109.8** Factors associated with an increased risk for depression[71,72]

Women
Young age
Premorbid history of depression
Lack of social support
Poor functional status
Uncontrolled pain
Certain cancers (pancreatic cancer)
Medications (calcium channel blockers, clonidine, NSAIDS, corticosteroids, propanolol, metoclopramide, benzodiazepines, haloperidol, macrolides, fluoroquinolones, opioids)
Advanced cancers

weeks and are accompanied by at least two of the following four symptoms: depressed mood, weight loss or gain, insomnia/hypersomnia, agitation or psychomotor retardation, fatigue or lack of energy, depreciation or guilt of feelings, and difficulty concentrating (DSM-IV criteria).[71] The Endicott modification of the DSM-IV criteria for cancer patients exchanges fearfulness and depressed appearance for appetite/weight loss; social withdrawal and reduced talkativeness for insomnia or hypersomnia; brooding, self-pity, and pessimism for lack of energy and fatigue; and anhedonia for diminished concentration.[69,72]

A list of factors associated with an increased risk for depression can be found on Table 109.8.

***Treatment*** Treatment is divided into nonpharmacologic and pharmacologic approaches. Nonpharmacologic therapy includes individual psychotherapy, cognitive-behavioral techniques, and supportive psychotherapy. Psychotherapy and pharmacotherapy are complementary and should be used together.[72] Responses occur in a graded fashion with improvement in sleep first, followed by increased activities and mood.[71]

Treatment of the underlying cause should be initiated before beginning antidepressants (Table 109.9).[71] Most antidepressants in cancer are prescribed too late and in too low a dose.[66,72,73]

The choice of medical therapy is in part determined by survival. Tricyclic antidepressants and selective serotonin receptive inhibitors can be started if life expectancy is

months and methylphenidate can be started if survival is expected to be short.[72,74] The patient should be screened for medical causes of depression (Table 109.9).

### Delirium

Cancer patients are prone to delirium. They are usually elderly, malnourished, frequently dehydrated, have multisystem impairment, are immobile, and often have sensory deprivation due to hearing loss or vision loss.[75] Delirium is one of the most frequent neuropsychiatric complications of cancer.[76,77] Delirium is missed by physicians in 32–67% of patients, and is largely untreated.[75] The symptoms of delirium are most commonly misconstrued as anxiety, debility, or depression as a normal part of the illness.[78,79] Because symptom severity changes with time and fluctuates during the day, it can be missed in a single encounter. Physicians are frequently untrained in recognizing and treating delirium.[77] The frequency of delirium in advanced cancer ranges between 25 and 40% and between 45 and 85% in those who are terminally ill.[78–80] Delirium, if untreated (or irreversible), leads to self-injury (e.g., through falls, pulling out lines, inadequate self-care, and reduced compliance) as well as secondary medical problems such as decubitus ulcers and aspiration pneumonia.[78,79] Delirium confers a relative risk for mortality of 6.2 during hospitalization compared to individuals who are not delirious. Risk factors for delirium include a previous brain insult such as a cerebral vascular accident or head injury, brain radiation or intrathecal chemotherapy, central nervous system tumor involvement, bone metastases, a previous confusional state or dementia, alcohol abuse, corticosteroids, cytotoxic therapy within the last month, the use of benzodiazepines and opioids, dehydration, visual and hearing impairment, elevated temperature, abnormal liver function tests, abnormal calcium, phosphorus, or sodium, or a low albumin.[81] Patients with malignancies are almost uniformly exposed to polypharmacy and a significant portion have either brain metastases or leptomeningeal implants (Table 109.10). Comorbidities such as heart failure will further predispose these individuals to the development of delirium.[77–80] Delirium typically evolves from multiple factors, often a combination of medications, infection, and organ failure.[80,82] Approximately 25% of the patients will have cranial lesions at the time of their delirium.[78,79] Patients with advanced cancer frequently have elevated proinflammatory cytokines such as IL-1,

**Table 109.9** Medical causes for depression[71]

Hypercalcemia
Brain metastases
Whole brain radiation
Poor nutrition
Electrolyte disturbances
Adrenal gland dysfunction
Paraneoplastic

**Table 109.10** Causes of delirium by frequency[82]

| | |
|---|---|
| Opioids, anticholingerics, benzodiazepines | 53% |
| Infection | 46% |
| Recent surgery | 32% |
| Structural brain lesion | 15% |
| Multiple causes | 67% |

TNFα, and IL-6, which stimulate microglial IL-1 and TNFα, resulting in insomnia, depression, and delirium.[83] Delirium risk increases with the number of risk factors. Unusual causes for delirium in cancer are nonconvulsive status epilepticus most frequently related to brain metastases, a previous stroke, or a metabolic abnormality.[84–86]

Delirium occurs during transplantation more frequently with older age, female gender, acute leukemia or solid tumors, a history of alcohol abuse, and total body radiation.[78,79] SCT patients have an incidence of delirium that approximates 50%. High-risk individuals are those with pretransplant hepatic and renal dysfunction, poor performance status, and preexisting cognitive deficits. The median duration of each delirium episode is 8 days. The peak incidence occurs in the second or third week.

The DSM-IV criteria for delirium involves the following four clinical factors: disturbances in consciousness, changes in cognition (memory, language, or perception), acute and fluctuating course, and occurring in conjunction with a serious medical illness.[78] (Table 109.11). Changes in sleep–wake cycles commonly occur (e.g., the Sundown syndrome). Delirium can be hyperalert, hypoalert, or mixed.[77] (Table 109.10). The hypoalert subtype is frequently under recognized and often does not prompt a response by physicians, but actually has the worst outlook.[75] These individuals are usually not "problem" patients compared to individuals with hyperalert delirium. Their delirium can be misinterpreted as fatigue or somnolence.[78] The differential diagnosis of delirium includes dementia, unipolar or bipolar affective disorders, psychosis (schizophrenia), or substance toxicity or withdrawal.[78]

Multiple screening tools for delirium are available (Table 109.12). The most well-known screening tool is the Mini-Mental State Examination Scale (MMSES), which is not as sensitive to delirium as other screening tools because of its emphasis on short-term memory and concentration. The MMSES requires a minimum of an eighth-grade education.[78] The Confusion Assessment Method and the Memorial Delirium Assessment Scale may be more apropos in this population.

Preventing delirium involves targeting six factors: (1) minimizing cognitive impairment (limiting polypharmacy, particularly anticholinergics and benzodiazepines); (2) preventing sleep deprivation; (3) minimizing immobility; (4) improving visual impairment; (5) improving hearing impairment; and (6) proactively

| Table 109.12 | Delirium scales |
| --- | --- |
| Mini-Mental State Examination | |
| Bedside Delirium Scale | |
| Confusion Assessment Method | |
| Memorial Delirium Assessment Scale | |
| Delirium Rating Scale | |
| Delirium Symptom Interview | |

treating dehydration.[87,88] Reversible factors for the treatment of delirium are outlined in Table 109.12. Once delirium has occurred, preventive interventions will have little impact on decreasing the delirium severity or relapse.[87,88]

The initial treatment for delirium is to reverse the underlying cause. Opioid rotation is usually effective if delirium is due to opioid neurotoxicity. Discontinue psychotropics (tricyclic antidepressants, benzodiazepines) as well as anticholinergics, if possible. Treat hypercalcemia, hyponatremia, hypomagnesemia, and infections. Nonconvulsive status epilepticus requires an EEG for detection, and the treatment of choice is either antiseizure medication or benzodiazepines, and not neuroleptics.[84]

Neuroleptics are the drug of choice for delirium (Table 109.13). There are only two randomized controlled trials of neuroleptics in advanced cancer. Haloperidol and chlorpromazine, but not lorazepam (as a single agent), were beneficial in the management of delirium. Three nonrandomized trials found olanzapine and mianserin (the parent compound for mirtazapine) efficacious in resolving delirium.[87] The peak response will occur in 5–7 days after initial therapy.[89] Patients who have developed extrapyramidal reactions to haloperidol can be safely treated with olanzapine.[90] High doses of haloperidol (over 5 mg as a single dose) will rapidly reduce agitation and paranoia, but also can induce a prolong QTc interval and predispose patients to a rhythm disturbance.[91] Lorazepam or other benzodiazepines reduce agitation, but will not improve orientation, concentration, or organizational skills. Benzodiazepines are the treatment of choice for delirium associated with alcohol withdrawal.[80,92] Other agents that are useful in treating delirium are gabapentin and valproic acid.[77] Neuroleptics can be

| Table 109.11 | Presentation of delirium[82] | |
| --- | --- | --- |
| Lethargy or coma | | 61% |
| Agitation | | 44% |
| Disorientation | | 83% |
| Lateralizing signs | | 41% |
| Delusions or hallucinations | | 28% |
| Seizures | | 9% |

| Table 109.13 | Pharmacologic management of delirium |
| --- | --- |
| Haloperidol | 1–2mg IV/SC/PO q 2–4 hours as needed up to 20 mg per day |
| Resperidol | 0.5 mg twice daily to 1mg twice daily up to 4 mg per day |
| Olanzapine | 2.5–5.0 mg twice daily up to 20 mg per day |
| Quetiapine | 25 mg twice daily up to 100 mg twice day |

safely discontinued 7–10 days after the return to baseline cognitive function.[89]

Responses (in terms of resolution of delirium) with neuroleptics range between 30 and 50%.[77,93] Delirium associated with hypoxemia, metabolic abnormalities, and infections tend to be irreversible with medications. Twenty-five percent of delirious patients will die within 30 days of the onset of delirium, and only one-third who sustain a delirium episode recover enough function to be able to be discharged home.[93]

## HOSPICE TRANSITION AND HEMATOLOGIC MALIGNANCIES

Hematologic malignancies are poorly represented in hospice populations. There are several reasons for this. Patients continue to receive palliative therapies including blood transfusion, platelet transfusions, and recombinant erythropoietin which hospices (because of capitated reimbursement) cannot afford and thus do not support. It is hard to not give antibiotics or blood product transfusions while a patient remains hospitalized. Thus, transfusions are usually continued until the patient's performance score is so poor that he or she cannot attend an outpatient clinic and there may not be time to refer to hospice. Radiation for the relief of bone pain in myeloma and soft tissue pain in lymphoma is expensive. Some hospices cannot afford even single-fraction radiation. In addition, a significant number of myeloma patients, as well as patients with amyloid, will be on dialysis, which precludes hospice care due to financial constraints. Newer targeted specific agents, including monoclonal antibodies, proteasome inhibitors, and thalidomide, are palliative but expensive and delay hospice transfers, again for cost reasons.

Prior to each change in treatment and with each relapse, the goals of care (and therapy) should be reviewed with the patient. The understanding by the patient as to the intent of treatment, and what is meant by "treatment," can be widely divergent. Patients may believe they are receiving curative therapy while physicians have palliation and disease maintenance in mind. Discussions about advanced directives are important early in the course of disease, particularly for chronic leukemias, myeloma, and amyloid. This is sometimes difficult for physicians, as they recognize that patients assume by such conversations that they are terminally ill. Advanced directives should be portrayed as an extension of autonomy in the face of an unpredictable disease course ("hoping for the best but planning for the worst," which is a good way of introducing the subject).

Hope can be fostered in those with advanced or incurable hematologic malignancies. Patients should be taught that they can live with their illness rather than die from their disease. Hope can be defined in increments that are achievable: hope to have symptoms relieved, hope to have a series of better days, hope to live to an important date, hope to have life closure. Inquiry into prognosis is a teachable moment. It is better that patients and families see what is evolving than physicians foretell the date of death. Patients and families value knowledge concerning the symptoms and signs of the dying process. Quantifying life expectancy as an answer to prognosis does not equip the patient or family to understand the dying process, nor discern its presence. Physicians are also usually overly optimistic regarding the time a patient has left. Prognostication by physicians, if taken by families as "the gospel," results in sociologic death as the predicted hour approaches. "Foreseeing" the dying process rather than foretelling life expectancy is the better way of handling questions about prognosis. On the other hand, a relative timetable may help patients with closure and estate planning, and so a general answer as "days to weeks" or "weeks to months" or "months to years" may suffice.

It is important to nurture spirituality throughout the course of illness, but even more so near the end of life. Rituals help move the center of hope from this life to the afterlife.[94] Many religious traditions have sacraments particular to the afterlife. These rituals become a physical sign for preparedness and belief and can help transition family and friends who are reluctant to "give up the fight" at the end of life care.[95–97]

## MANAGING THE ACTIVELY DYING

Dying patients require symptom management, physical expressions of love, the presence of significant others, truth telling, and dignity through meticulous maintenance of personal hygiene.[98,99] Patients should not be subject to venipuncture and procedures for curiosity sake when the goals of care are "comfort." Family education, frequent visits, and intensive low-technology care are other elements to good end of life care. Symptoms change during the course of illness. At the end, pain, delirium, nausea, vomiting, and secretions are the important symptoms to control.[99–101] Opioids should be maintained despite changing mentation. Families often mistake the dying process for drug toxicity and need to understand the difference. Terminal agitation or restlessness may arise from a full rectum or bladder, poorly controlled pain, or delirium. Patients should be examined for fecal impaction and a distended bladder, and measures should be taken to relieve either one if present. As patients become more nonverbal, the therapeutic decision regarding terminal agitation is between adjusting the opioid or the neuroleptic. Families may be helpful in deciphering pain behaviors. However, in the end it is a trial of one or the other.[99–101] We have used chlorpromazine for terminal delirium, while others have used a combination of haloperidol and a benzodiazepine, usually lorazepam or midazolam. Both chlorapromazine and haloperidol treat nausea and vomiting. Individual doses of chlorapromazine are 12.5–25 mg parenteral or per rectum titrated to response. Doses may range from 25 to 200 mg every 4–6 h. Secretions respond to antimuscarinics. Once secretions are clinically evident, antimuscarinics should be given around the clock, with dosing similar to opioids in pain management. Glycopyrrolate 0.1–0.2 mg intravenous or subcutaneous every 4–6 h is a reasonable choice. Terminal sedation is occasionally necessary for refractory delirium or dyspnea. Phenobarbital 100 mg intravenous or subcutaneous every 8 h up to 1200 mg over 24 h has been our choice for sedation.

## SUMMARY

Hematologic malignancies have a cluster of symptoms that differ in degree from solid tumors. Fatigue, depression, delirium, treatment-related mucositis, and treatment-related pain are common symptoms. These symptoms can occur at early stages of disease, can persist through remission, and will require both nonpharmacologic and pharmacologic management. Involvement of palliative therapy early in the course of disease can minimize suffering from multiple symptoms while the patient undergoes disease-modifying antitumor therapy.

## REFERENCES

1. Gulbrandsen N, Hjermstad MJ, Wisloff F: Interpretation of quality of life scores in multiple myeloma by comparison with a reference population and assessment of the clinical importance of score differences. *Eur J Haematol* 72:172–180, 2004.
2. Riccardi A, Gobbi PG, Bertoloni D, et al: Changing clinical presentation of multiple myeloma. *Eur J Cancer* 27(11):1401–1405, 1991.
3. Kyle RA: Clinical aspects of multiple myeloma and related disorders including amyloidosis. *Pathologie et Biologie* 47(2):148–157, 1999.
4. Stalfelt AM, Brodin H, Pettersson, et al: The final phase in acute myeloid leukaemia (AML) A study on bleeding, infection and pain. *Leukemia Research* 27:481–488, 2003.
5. Beguin C, France FR, Ninane J: Systematic analysis of in-patients' circumstances and causes of death: a tool to improve quality of care. *Intl J Qual Health Care* 9(6):427–433, 1997.
6. Christakis NA, Escarce JJ: Survival of medicare patients after enrollment in hospice programs. *N Engl J Med* 335:172–178, 1996.
7. Maddocks I, Bentley L, Sheedy J: Quality of life issues in patients dying from haematological diseases. *Ann Acad Med Singapore* 23(2):244–248, 1994.
8. Bruera E, Russell N, Sweeney C, et al: Place of death and its predictors for local patients registered at a comprehensive cancer center. *JCO* 20(8):2127–2133.
9. Bruera E, Kim HN: Cancer pain. *JAMA* 290(18): 2476–2479, 2003.
10. Dimopoulos MA, Papadimitriou C, Sakarellou N, et al: Complications and supportive therapy of multiple myeloma. *Baillieres Clin Haematology* 8(4):845–852, 1995.
11. Management of cancer pain: Evidence report/technology assessment: Number 35. http//www.ahrq.gov/clinic/epcsums/canpainsum.htm.
12. Portenoy RK, Payne D, Jacobsen P: Breakthrough pain: characteristics and impact in patients with cancer pain. *Pain* 81(1/2):129–134, 1999.
13. Cleeland CS, Janjan NA, Scott CB, et al: Cancer pain management by radiotherapists: a survey of radiation therapy oncology group physicians. *Int J Radiat Onc Biol Phys* 47(1):203–208, 2000.

14. Von Roenn JH, Cleeland CS, Gonin R, et al: Physician attitudes and practice in cancer pain management. A survey from the Eastern Cooperative Oncology Group. *Ann Intern Med* 119(2):121–126, 1993.
15. Shvartzman P, Friger M, Shani A, et al: Pain control in ambulatory cancer patientes – can we do better? *J Pain Symptom Management* 26(2):716–722, 2003.
16. Cleeland CS, Ryan KM: Pain assessment: global use of the Brief Pain Inventory. *Ann Acad Med Singapore* 23(2):129–138, 1994.
17. Twycross R, Harcourt J, Bergl S: A survey of pain in patients with advanced cancer. *J Pain Symptom Management* 12(5):273–282, 1996.
18. Twycross R: Cancer pain classification. *Acta Anaesthesiol Scand* 41(1 Pt 2):141–145, 1997.
19. Hanks GW, Conno F, Cherny N, et al: Morphine and alternative opioids in cancer pain: the EAPC recommendations. *Br J Can* 84(5):587–593, 2001.
20. Walsh D: Pharmacological management of cancer pain. *Sem Onc* 27(1):45–63, 2000.
21. Cherny N, Ripamonti C, Pereira J, et al: Strategies to manage the adverse effects of oral morphine: an evidence-based report. *JCO* 19(9):2542–2554, 2001.
22. Mercadante S: Opioid rotation for cancer pain. *Cancer* 86:1856–1866, 1999.
23. Kochhar R, LeGrand, SB, Walsh D, et al: Opioids in cancer pain: common dosing errors. *Oncology* 17(4):571–575, 2003.
24. Davis MP, Walsh D: Methadone for relief of cancer pain: a review of pharmacokinetics, pharmacodynamics, drug interactions and protocols of administration. *Supportive Care Cancer* 9:73-83, 2001.
25. Davis MP, Varga J, Dickerson D, et al: Normal-release and controlled-release oxycodone: pharmacokinetics, pharmacodynamics, and controversy. *Supportive Care Cancer* 11:84–92, 2003.
26. Donnelly S, Davis MP, Walsh D, et al: Morphine in cancer pain management: a practical guide. *Supportive Care Cancer* 10:13–35, 2002.
27. Menten J, Desmedt M, Lossignol D, et al: Longitudinal follow-up of TTS-fentanyl use in patients with cancer-related pain: results of a compassionate-use study with special focus on elderly patients. *Curr Med Res Opin* 18(8):488–498, 2002.

28. Sarhill N, Walsh D, Nelson KA: Hydromorphone: pharmacology and clinical applications in cancer patients. *Supportive Care Cancer* 9:84–96, 2001.

29. Pasternak GW: Insights into mu opioid pharmacology. The role of mu opioid receptor subtypes. *Life Sci* 68:2213–2219, 2001.

30. Dudeney S, Lieberman IH, Reinhardt M-K, et al: Kyphoplasty in the treatment of osteolytic vertebral compression fractures as a result of multiple myeloma. *JCO* 20(9):2382–2387, 2002.

31. Saito R, Takano Y, Kamiya H: Roles of substance P and KK$_1$ receptor in the brainstem in the development of emesis. *J Pharm Sci* 91:87–94, 2003.

32. Koga T, Fukuda H: Descending pathway from the central pattern generator of vomiting. *Neuroreport* 8(11):2587–2590, 1997.

33. Martin CG, Rubenstein EB, Elting LS, et al: Measuring chemotherapy-Induced nausea and emesis. *Cancer* 98:645–655, 2003.

34. Ihbe-Heffinger A, Ehlken B, Bernard R, et al: The impact of delayed chemotherapy-induced nausea and vomiting on patients, health resource utilization and costs in German cancer centers. *Ann Onc* 15:526–536, 2004.

35. Spitzer TR, Grunberg SM, Dicato MA: Antiemetic strategies for high-dose chemoradiotherapy-induced nausea and vomiting. *SCC* 6:233–236, 1998.

36. Chevalier-Evain V, Bonneterre J, Adenis A, et al: Loss of efficacy of ondansetron-dexamethasone during success courses in female patients receiving high-dose cisplatin. *Bull Cancer* 81(3):219–222, 1994.

37. Navari RM: Pathogenesis-Based treatment of chemotherapy-induced nausea and vomiting – two new agents. *Supp Onc* 1(2):89–103.

38. Bonneterre J, Hecquet B: Granisetron (IV) compared with ondansetron (IV plus oral) in prevention of nausea and vomiting induced by moderately-emetogenic chemotherapy. A cross-over study. *Bull Cancer* 82(12):1038–1043, 1995.

39. Lonback MK: Why do we need another antiemetic? Just ask. *JCO* 21(22):4077–4080, 2003.

40. De Wit R, Herrstedt J, Rapoport B, et al: Addition of the oral NK1 antagonist aprepitant to standard antiemetics provides protection against nausea and vomiting during multiple cycles of cisplatin-based chemotherapy. *JCO* 21(22):4105–4111, 2003.

41. Hesketh PJ, Grunberg SM, Gralla RJ, et al: The oral neurokinin-1 antagonist aprepitant for the prevention of chemotherapy-induced nausea and vomiting: a multinational, randomized, double-blind, placebo-controlled trial in patients receiving high-dose cisplatin- the Aprepitant Protocol 052 study group. *JCO* 21(22):4112–4119, 2003.

42. Knox JJ, Puodziunas ALV, Feld R: Chemotherapy-Induced oral mucosistis. *Drugs Aging* 17(4):257–267, 2000.

43. Cella D, Pulliam J, Fuchs H, et al: Evaluation of pain associated with oral mucositis during the acute period after administration of high-dose chemotherapy. *Cancer* 98:406–412, 2003.

44. Kostler WJ, Hejna M, Wenzel C, et al: Oral mucositis complicating chemotherapy and/or radiotherapy: options for prevention and treatment. *CA Can J Clin* 51:290–315, 2001.

45. Plevova P: Prevention and treatment of chemotherapy and radiotherapy induced oral mucositis: a review. *Oral Onc* 35:453–470, 1999.

46. Clarkson JE, Worthington HV, Eden OB: Interventions for preventing oral mucositis for patients with cancer receiving treatment. *Cochrane Database Syst Rev* 3:CD000978, 2003.

47. Worthington HV, Clarkson JE: Prevention of oral mucositis and oral candidiasis for patients with cancer treated with chemotherapy: cochrane systematic review. *J Dent Educ* 66(8):903–911, 2002.

48. Worthington HV, Clarkson JE, Eden OB: Interventions for treating oral mucositis for patients with cancer receiving treatment. *Cochrane Database Syst Rev* 1:CD001973, 2002.

49. Donnelly JP, Bellm LA, Epstein JB, et al: Antimicrobial therapy to prevent or treat oral mucositis. *Lancet* 3:405–412, 2003.

50. Curt GA: Fatigue in cancer. *Br Med J* 322:1560, 2001.

51. Curt GA, Breitbart W, Cella D, et al: Impact of cancer-related fatigue on the lives of patients: new findings from the fatigue coalition. *Oncology* 5:353–360, 2000.

52. Curt GA: The impact of fatigue on quality of life in oncology patients. *Sem Hematol* 37(4 suppl 6):14–17.

53. Stasi R, Abriani L, Beccaglia P, et al: Cancer-related fatigue Evolving concepts in evaluation and treatment. *Cancer* 98:1786–1801, 2003.

54. Respini D, Jacobsen PB, Thors C, et al: The prevalence and correlates of fatigue in older cancer patients. *Crit Rev Onc-Hema* 47(3):273–279.

55. Vogelzang NJ, Breitbart W, Cella D, et al: Patient, caregiver, and oncologist perceptions of cancer-related fatigue: results of a tripart assessment survey. The Fatigue Coalition. *Sem Hema* 34(3, suppl 2):4–12, 1997.

56. Langeveld N, Ubbink M, Smets E: 'I don't have any energy': the experience of fatigue in young adult survivors of childhood cancer. *Eur J Onc Nurs* 4(1):20–28, 2000.

57. Portenoy RK, Itri L: Cancer-related fatigue: guidelines for evaluation and management. *Oncologist* 4:1–10, 1999.

58. Berger A: Treating fatigue in cancer patients. *Oncologist* 8(suppl 1):10–14, 2003.

59. Barnes EA, Bruera E: Fatigue in patients with advanced cancer: A review. *Int J Gyn Can* 12:424-428, 2002.

60. Mock V: Fatigue management: evidence and guidelines for practice. *Cancer* 92(6, suppl):1699–1707, 2001.

61. Tralongo P, Respini D, Ferra AF: Fatigue and aging. *Crit Rev Onc-Hema* 48(suppl):S57–S64, 2003.

62. Escalante CP: Treatment of cancer-related fatigue: an update. *SCC* 11:79–83, 2003.

63. Penedo FJ, Schneiderman N, Dahn JR, et al: Physical activity interventions in the elderly: cancer and comorbidity. *Cancer Invest* 22(1):51–67, 2004.

64. Irwin ML, Ainsworth BE: Physical activity interventions following cancer diagnosis: methodologic challenges to delivery and assessment. *Cancer Invest* 22(1):30–50, 2004.

65. Lloyd-Williams M: Difficulties in diagnosing and treating depression in the terminally ill cancer patient. *Postgrad Med J* 76(899):555–558, 2000.

66. Maguire P: The use of antidepressants in patients with advanced cancer. *SCC* 8:265–267, 2000.

67. Block SD: Assessing and managing depression in the terminally ill patient. *Ann Int Med* 132(3):209–218, 2000.

68. Tiernan E, Casey P, O'Boyle C, et al: Relations between desire for early death, depressive symptoms and antidepressant prescribing in terminally ill patients with cancer. *J Roy Soc Med* 95:386–390, 2002.

69. Lloyd-Williams M: Screening for depression in palliative care patients: a review. *Eur J Can Care* 10:31–5, 2001.

70. Lloyd-Williams M, Riddleston H: The stability of depression scores in patients who are receiving palliative care. *JPSM* 24(6):593–597, 2002.

71. Berney A, Stiefel F, Mazzocato, et al: Psychopharmacology in supportive care of cancer: a review for the clinician. *SCC* 8:278–286, 2000.

72. Pessin H, Potash M, Breitbart W: Diagnosis, assessment, and treatment of depression in palliative care. In: Lloyd-Williams M (ed.) *Psychosocial Issues in Palliative Care*, 1st edn. Oxford, Oxford University Press; 2003.

73. Sharpe M, Strong V, Allen K, et al: Major depression in outpatients attending a regional cancer centre: screening and unmet treatment needs. *Br J Can* 90:314–320, 2004.

74. Lloyd-Williams M, Friedman T, Rudd N: A survey of antidepressant prescribing in the terminally ill. *Pall Med* 13:243–248, 1999.

75. Inouye SK: Prevention of delirium in hospitalized older patients: risk factors and targeted strategies. *Ann Med* 32(4):257–263, 2000.

76. Pereira J, Bruera E: Depression with psychomotor retardation: diagnostic challenges and the use of psychostimulants. *J Pall Med* 4(1):15–21, 2001.

77. Bruera E, Neumann CM: The uses of psychotropics in symptom management in advanced cancer. *Psyco-Onc* 7:346–358, 1998.

78. Fann JR, Roth-Roemer S, Burington BE, et al: Delirium in patients undergoing hematopoietic stem cell transplantation: Incidence and pretransplantation risk factors. *Cancer* 95:1971–1981, 2002.

79. Fann JR, Sullivan AK: Delirium in the course of cancer treatment. *Sem Clin Neuropsychiatry* 8(4):217–228, 2003.

80. Brown TM, Boyle MF: ABC of psychological medicine Delirium. *Br Med J* 325:644–647, 2002.

81. Ljubisavljevic V, Kelly B: Risk factors for development of delirium among oncology patients. *Gen Hosp Psych* 25:345–352, 2003.

82. Tuma R, DeAngelis LM: Alttertered mental status in patients with cancer. *Arch Neurol* 57(12):1727–1731, 2000.

83. Dunlop RJ, Campbell CW: Cytokines and advanced cancer. *JPSM* 20(3):214–232, 2000.

84. Walker MC: Diagnosis and treatment of nonconvulsive status epilepticus. *CNS Drugs* 15(12):931–939, 2001.

85. Martinez-Rodriguez JE, Barriga FJ, Santamaria J, et al: Nonconvulsive status epilepticus associated with cephalosporins in patients with renal failure. *Am J Med* 111(2):115–119, 2001.

86. Markand ON: Pearls, perils, and pitfalls in the use of the electroencephalogram. *Sem Neurol* 23(1):7–46, 2003.

87. Inouye SK, Bogardus ST Jr, Charpentier PA, et al: A multicomponent intervention to prevent delirium in hospitalized older patients. *NEJM* 340(9):669–676, 1999.

88. Weber JB, Coverdale, JH, Kunik ME: Delirium: current trends in prevention and treatment. *Int Med J* 34:115–121, 2004.

89. Schwartz TL, Masand PS: The role of atypical antipsychotics in the treatment of delirium. *Psychosomatics* 43(3):171–174, 2002.

90. Passik SC, Cooper M: Complicated delirium in a cancer patient successfully treated with olanzapine. *JPSM* 17:219–223, 1999.

91. Seneff MG, Mathews RA: Use of haloperidol infusions to control delirium in critically ill adults. *Ann Pharm* 29(7/8):690–693, 1995.

92. Meagher DJ: Delirium: optimising management. *Br Med J* 322:144–149, 2001.

93. Lawlor PG, Gagnon B, Mancini I, et al: Occurrence, causes, and outcome of delirium in patients with advanced cancer: a prospective study. *Arch Int Med* 160(6):786–794, 2000.

94. McClain CS, Rosenfeld B, Breitbart W: Effect of spiritual well-being on end-of-life despair in terminally ill cancer patients. *Lancet* 361:1603–1607, 2003.

95. Clark PA, Drain M, Malone MP: Addressing patients' emotional and spiritual needs. *Jt Comm J Qual Saf* 29(12):659–670, 2003.

96. Lunn JS: Spiritual care in multi-religious context. *J Pall Care Pharm* 17(3/4):153–166, 2003.

97. Keeley Maureen P: Final conversations: survivors' memorable messages concerning religious faith and spirituality. *Health Comm* 16(1):87–104.

98. Proulx K, Jacelon C: Dying with dignity: the good patient versus the good death. *Am J Hosp Pall Care* 21(2):116–120.

99. Davis MP, Frandsen J, Dickerson D, et al: Prescribing for the dying patient: principles and practice. *JTO* 1(1):32–45, 2002.

100. Nelson KA, Walsh D, Behrens C, et al: The dying cancer patient. *Sem Onc* 27(1):84–89, 2000.

101. Ellershaw J, Ward C: Care of the dying patient: the last hours or days of life. *Br Med J* 326:30–34, 2003.

# INDEX

**A**

Abelson oncogene *(c-abl)*, 103
absolute neutrophil count (ANC), 440
ABVD regimen, 774–775
acquired immunodeficiency syndrome, 837
acute basophilic leukemia, 27
acute erythroleukemia, 33
acute lymphoblastic leukemia
  in adults, treatment of
    age-stratified therapy, 135–136
    background, 127
    prognostic factors and risk stratification, 127–128
    risk-adapted therapy, 132–135
    supportive care, 136–137
    treatment algorithm, 137
    treatment strategies, 129–132
  classification, 106–108
  clinical features of, 121–123
  complete remission in, 143–145
  cytogenetic aberrations, 111–115
  diagnosis of, 123–124
  epidemiology, 104
  follow-up of, 145–147
  genetic mutation, 104–105
  molecular aberrations, 115–116
  morphology, 111
  polymorphisms in, 116
  prognostic factors, 145
  relapsed or refractory, treatment of
    chemotherapy strategies, 152
    CNS relapse, 154
    Philadelphia-chromosome positive disease, 153–154
    prognostic features, 151–152
    stem cell transplantation, 152–153
    therapies for, 154
  risk factors, 105–106
acute megakaryoblastic leukemia (AMKL), 10
acute megakaryocytic leukemia, 27
acute monoblastic leukemia, 32
acute myelocytic leukemia. *See* acute myeloid leukemia
acute myelogenous leukemia. *See* acute myeloid leukemia
acute myeloid leukemia
  classification, 4–5
  clinical features associated with specific subtypes and/or
    cytogenetic abnormalitites, 27–28
  clinical features in, 25–27
  clinical work up of, 35–36
  comparison of older and young adults, 52
  conditions associated with incidence of, 2
  criteria for a morphologic CR in, 84
  cytogenetics, 10–18
  diagnosis of, 28–34
  entities of, 35

  epidemiology and risk factors, 1–4
  epigenetic changes of, 20–21
  FAB classification of, 34–35
  follow up, 87–88
  history of, 25
  molecular genetics, 18–20
  in older adults, treatment of
    disease features, 51–52
    indications for treatment, 52–53
    response to therapy, 52
    treatment options, 53–59
  pathology, 9–10
  in patients less than 60, treatment of
    diagnosis and classification, 41–42
    treatment strategies, 42–47
  prognosis of
    age factors, 84–85
    antecedent hematologic disorders, 85
    biologic features, 85–87
    other clinical features, 85
    prior cytotoxic therapy, 85
  prospective phase II studies of chemotherapy for, in first relapse,
    93
  relapsed or refractory, treatment of
    combination chemotherapy for patients in first relapse, 92–94
    definition ion, 91–92
    frontiers in, 96–98
    hematopoictic cell transplantation, 94–96
  remission induction therapy, 53–57
  risk groups in, 86
  with t(8;21)(q22;q22), 31
  with t(15;17)(q22;q21), 32
  trials of biologic assignments, 345–346
  WHO classification of, 11–15, 34–35
acute promyelocytic leukemia, 41
  allogeneic stem cell transplantation for, 348
  outcomes of ATRA therapy, 65, 69
  treatment of, 45
    prognostic factors, 63
    role of ARA-C, 67–68
    therapeutic monitoring, 63–64
    treatment of, in older adults, 68–69
    treatment of newly diagnosed, 64–67
    treatment of relapsed, 69–70
agnogenic myeloid metaplasia (AMM), 475
Airlie House meeting, agenda of, 505
alemtuzumab, 304, 602
alkylating agents, 481
alkyl sulfonates, 1089
allogeneic hematopoietic stem cell transplantation
  for nonmyeloablative conditioning regimen
    aims of, 1025–1026
    chimerism evalauation and engraftment kinetics, 1031–1032

allogeneic hematopoietic cell transplantation (*continued*)
    in DLA-identical transplant model, 1026–1027
    graft vs host disease, 1032–1033
    immune reconstitution and infections, 1033–1034
    preliminary results with conditioning regimen, 1034–1035
    reduced-intensity or truly nonmyeloablative conditioning
        regimens, 1028–1031
    toxicity, 1032
allogeneic stem cell transplantation, 47, 498, 718. *See also*
    multiple myeloma (MM)
  for ALL
    for advanced patients, 341
    for any patient, 338–340
    in combination with imatinib, 341
    with non-myeloblative or reduced intensity conditioning
        regimes, 341–342
  for AML
    acute promyctocytic leukemia, 348
    for advanced AML patients, 344–347
    in first complete remission, 342–344
    with non-myeloblative regimes, 347
    stem cell source, 348
    therapy of relapse after, 347–348
    transplantation for secondary, 348
  in aplastic anemia
    alternative donor sources, 420–421
    conditioning regimen, 419–420
    cytokine mobilized PBSC *versus* bone marrow, 420
    effects of age on outcome, 419
  in myelodysplastic syndrome
    effect of IPSS scores on outcome, 416
    effect of time to transplant from diagnosis, 416
    effect on age on outcome, 415–416
    peripheral blood *versus* bone marrow as source of stem
        cell, 418
    role of alternate donor sources, 418
    role of induction chemotherapy prior to, 416–417
allopurinol, 36, 42
allosensitization, 488
all-*trans*-retinoic acid (ATRA), 28, 45, 63–65
alpha-naphthyl acetate (ANA), 10
alpha-naphthyl butyrate, 10
AMD 3100, 1006
ε-aminocaproic acid, 65
aminothiols, 441
AML. *See* acute myeloid leukemia
*AML1(RUNX1)-ETO(CBFA2T1)* fusion gene, 10–11
amyloidosis
  clinical features, 956–957
  diagnosis of, 957–958
  evaluation of response, 958
  molecular pathogenesis, 955–956
  principles of therapy, 958
  prognostic factors of, 958
  specific therapy for, 959–960
  supportive care, 958–959
anagrelide, 471
anaplastic large cell lymphoma (ALCL), 505, 522–523
anaplastic lymphoma kinase (ALK), 510
androgens, 479
anemia, 467, 475, 487, 489, 494, 963–964
angioimmunoblastic T-cell lymphoma (AITL), 523
ankylosing spondylitis, 2
antecedent hematologic disorders, 85
anthracenediones, 53
anthracycline, 42, 53
anthracycline antibiotic idarubicin, 489
antibacterial therapy, for neutropenic patients
  antiviral therapy, 315
  beta-lactum plus aminoglycoside therapy, 315
  change of therapy, 315
  hypogamma globulinemia, 318
  oral therapy, 316

  outpatient and home IV antibiotic therapy, 316
  pneumocystis prophylaxis, 318
  stopping of antimicrobial therapy, 315–316
  timing of gram-positive therapy, 315
anti-CD45 radiolabeled antibodies, 78
antifungal therapy, for neutropenic patients
  closteridium difficile colitis, 318
  randomized trials and meta analysis of, 317
  rash, 318
  renal dysfunction, 317
  timing of, 316
antiglycophorin A (erythroid), 33
antihemoglobin A (erythroid), 33
antithrombotic therapy, 471
APL. *See* acute promyelocytic leukemia
aplastic anemia
  allogeneic stem cell tranplantation for, 419–421
  clinical features of, 401–404
  complications in, 406–409
  epidemiology and demographics of, 397
  history of, 397
  pathophysiology, 397–401
  prognosis of, 406–409
  therapies for, 404–406
APL differentiation syndrome, 66
ara-C-based chemotherapy, 45, 67–68
ara-C-based consolidation regimen, 45
arsenic trioxide, 46, 67, 662–664, 1110–1111
asoblimersen, 47
ataxia-telangiectasia, 1, 9
ATRA-based therapy, 65
atypical chronic myelogenous leukemia, 456
  treatment of
    allogeneic stem cell transplantation, 495–496
    combination chemotherapy, 495
    cytoreductive agents, 495
    interferon α, 495
auer bodies or rods, 31
autoimmune disease
  acquired angioedema, 256
  autoimmune hemolytic anemia, 255
  blistering skin diseases, 256–257
  glomerulonephritis, 256
  immune thrombocytopenia, 255
  mechanisms of, in CLL
    autoimmunity triggered by treatment, 257–258
    secretion of autoantibody by tumor cells, 257
  nephrotic syndrome, 256
  pure red cell aplasia, 255–256
  treatment of
    acquired angioedema, 258
    autoimmune hemolytic anemia, 258–259
    autoimmune thrombocytopenia, 259
    paraneoplastic pemphigus, 259
    pure red cell aplasia, 259
    rapidly progressive glomerulonephritis, 259
autologous stem cell transplantation, 658, 717–718, 877
  for acute lymphoblastic leukemia
    clinical trial results of, 330–331
    high dose regimes, 330
    in-vitro HSC purging, 329–330
    rationale in using, 329
  for acute myelogenous leukemia, 321–329
    clinical trial results, 324–328
    methods of stem cell therapy, 322–32
    prognostic factors, 322
    rationale for using, 321–322
  in chronic lymphocytic leukemia, 359–360
  for chronic myelogenous leukemia
    clinical trial results, 331–332
    rationale, 331
  in CML, 359
  history of, 321

for lymphoma, 3
in MMM, 476
5-azacytidine, 76, 489–490
5-aza-2'-deoxycytidine, 490

**B**

BAALC gene expression, in AML patients, 20
B-and T-cell image in acute lymphoblastic leukemia, 107–108
B-cell lymphomas, 513
    approaches to treatment of, 550
    Burkitt lymphomas, 520
    diagnosis and initial evaluation, 543–544
    diffuse large B-cell lymphomas, 507, 509, 519–520
    follicular lymphoma, 509, 515–516
    initial presentation, 543
    initial therapy of localized DLBLL, 546–550
    lymphomatoid granulomatosis, 520–521
    lymphoplasmacytic lymphoma, 518–519
    mantle cell lymphoma, 514–515
    mucosa-associated lymphoid tissue lymphomas, 516–517
    nodal marginal zone lymphomas, 518
    pathologic and prognostic features, 544–545
    primary effusion lymphoma, 521
    of primary mediastinal, 530–551
    relapsed and refractory DLBCL, treatment of, 551
    small lymphocytic lymphoma, 513–514
    splenic marginal zone lymphoma, 517–518
Bcl-2 compound, 97
BCNU, 3
BCR/ABL-negative CML, 494
BCR/ABL-positive disease, 495
BCR/ABL translocation, 488, 494
BEACOPP regimens, 775
bendamustine, 536
benzolystaurosporine, 97
bestrabucil, 662
bevacizumab, 441
bexarotene, 1110
bilineage leukemia, 35
blastic NK-cell lymphoma, 526
blood transfusion products
    granulocyte transfusion, 1134
    platelet transfusion, 1128–1131
    red blood cell transfusion, 1127–1128
    specialized blood components, 1131–1134
    transfusion in palliative care, 1134–1135
Bloom syndrome, 1, 9
bone marrow
    aplastic anemia and stem cell failure, 401, 403
    biology, 51
    biopsy, 87, 466
    multiple myeloma and related disorders, 860–861
    myelodysplastic syndromes and, 377, 426
    myeloma cells and, 865
bone marrow plasma cell labeling index (PCLI), 917
bone marrow transplantation. *See also* allogeneic stem cell
            transplantation; autologous stem cell transplantation;
            hematopoietic stem cell transplantation (HSCT);
            stem cell transplantation
    aplastic anemia and, 405
    chronic leukemia and, 361
    cytokine mobilized PBSC *versus*, 420
    peripheral blood *versus* bone marrow as source of
            stem cell, 418
bortezomib, 536, 728, 879
Burkitt-like lymphoma, 509, 520
    autologous hematopoietic cell transplantation for, 680–681
    clinical features, 570
    frequency of occurence, 569–570
    pathology and pathogenesis, 570–571
    stem cell transplantation, 573
    treatment of, 571–572
busulfan, 3, 95, 488, 495, 1089

**C**

cancer chemotherapy, 1089
Cancer Therapy scale, 53
carboplatinum, 492
CBF mutations, in AML patients, 20
*CBFB-MYH11* gene, 10–11
CC-5013, 880
*CCAAT/enhancer-binding protein α (CEBPA)* gene, 16
CCNU, 3
CD13 antigen marker, 33
CD33 antigen marker, 33, 46, 94
CD2 expression, 63
CD34 expression, 63
CD56 expression, 63, 66
CEBPA mutations, in AML patients, 18–19
CEP-701, 97
chemotherapeutic agents
    alkylating agents, 1089–1092
    antimetabolites, 1092–1095
        folic acid analog, 1096–1097
        selected nucleoside analogs, 1095–1096
    antitumor antibiotics, 1097–1099
    other agents, 1100–1101
    podophyllotoxin derivatives, 1099–1100
    vinca alkaloids, 1099
chemotherapy with all *trans*-retinoic acid, 45
chlorambucil, 3
2-chlorodeoxyadenosine, 481
chromatin, dispersion of, 526
chromosome 8 abnormalities, 26
chronic and smouldering ATL, 657, 660
chronic eosinophilic leukemia
    diagnostic and treatment approach, 496
    management of, 496–498
chronic lymphocytic leukemia
    abnormal reactions to insect bites, 259
    aggressive transformation in
        prolymphocytoid transformation, 253–254
        Richter's syndrome, 251–253
        transformation to acute leukemia, 254
    autologous stem cell transplantation in, 360
    B-cell, 282
    bendamustine treatment, 248
    biology of, 220–221
    CD5⁺B cells, role of, 214
    chemotherapy plus monoclonal antibodies treatment, 245
        fludarabine plus rituximab, 245–246
        fludarabine plus rituximab plus cyclophosphamide, 246
    chemotherapy treatment
        chlorambucil versus fludarabine, 245
        fludarabine versus fludarabine plus cyclophosphamide, 245
    clinical presentation of, 224
    consolidation therapy to eliminate minimal residual disease, 246
    criteria for diagnosis, 224
    cytology/histopathology, 214–216
    differential diagnosis, 224
    epidemiology of, 223–224
    evaluations of patients with, 227–228
    familial clustering of xases of, 213–214
    follow-up of, 240
    genome-wide GEP of, 220
    hypercalcemia, 259
    *IG* translocations in, 219
    *IGHV* gene and *BCL6* mutation in, 219–220
    immune defects in, 228–229
    immunophenotype of, 216–218
    laboratory findings, 226
    myeloblative allogeneic stem cell transplantation, 360–361
    neurologic aomplications, 259
    non-myeloblative allogeneic stem cell transplantation, 361
    paraneoplasticcomplications, 254–259
    physical findings, 225
    prognosis, 238–240

chronic lymphocytic leukemia (*continued*)
  response criteria for, 237–238
  role of clonal lymphocytes, 214
  RS3PE, 260
  staging, 226–227
  symptoms in, 225
  treatment and treatment approach for
    cytotonic therapy, 233–235
    influence of biologic and cytogenetic prognostic markers, 235–236
    treatment approach, 236
    on a wait and watch policy, 233
chronic myeloid leukemia
  accelerated phase or blast crisis, treatment of
    allogeneic hematopoietic stem cell transplantaion therapy, 192–193
    chemotherapy, 191
    cytarabine-based combination approach, 191
    management of lymphoid blast phase, 192
    with single agent therapy, 191–192
    using imatinib mesylate, 189–191
  approaches to patients, 358–359
  autologous transplantation, 359
  blastic phase in, 164
  chronic phase, treatment of
    with IFN-α, 177–178
    recommendations, 183–184
    stem cell transplantation, 178
    using imatinib mesylate, 179–182
  classification, 160
  cytogenetic remission of, 195
  cytogenetics of, 164–166
  epidemiology, 160
  follow-up of patients with, 198–199
  hematologic remission of, 195
  matched sibling transplants, 355–356
  molecular pathogenesis, 166–171
  molecular remission of, 195–196
  morphology, 163–164
  myeloblative allogeneic transplantation in, 355
    prognostic factors, 356–358
    from unrelated donors, 356
  prognosis of, 196–198
  reduced-intensity stem cell transplantation, 359
  relapse management, 359
  relapsed or refractory, treatment of
    with imatinib mesylate, 203–207
    immunotherapy, 207–209
  risk factors, 160
chronic myelomonocytic leukemia
  pretreatment evaluation of, 487–488
  prognosis of, 487
  treatment options
    agents targeting fusion RTKs, 490–491
    allogeneic stem cell transplantation, 493–494
    chemotherapy with regimens, 491–493
    established single-agent oral chemotherapy, 488–489
    farnesyltransferase inhibitors, 491
    hypomethylating agents, 490
    other antiahgiogenic and immunomodulating agents, 491
    other chemotherapeutic agents, 489
    supportive care, 488
    topiosomerase I inhibitors, 489–490
chronic myelomonocytic leukemia (CMML), 455
chronic myeloproliferative diseases
  agnogenic myeloid metaplasia (AMM), 466–467
  chronic eosinophilic leukemia/hyper eosinophilic syndrome, 454
  chronic idiopathic MF
    cytogenetics, 453
    molecular biology, 453–454
    pathology, 453
  chronic idiopathic myelofibrosis (CIMF)
    autologous stem cell transplant in MMM, 476

    clinical presentation, 475
    constitutional symptoms of, 476
    cytopenias of, 475–476
    myeloproliferative symptoms, 475
    non myelopblastive stem cell transplantatation in MMM, 476
    prognosis of, 476
  chronic MPD, unclassifiable, 455
  chronic myeloid leukemia, 461–462
  chronic neutrophilic leukemia, 455
  classification, 445–446
  epidemiology, 446–447
  essential thrombocythemia (ET), 464–466
    criteria for diagnosis of, 471–472
    cytogenetics, 452
    incidence and clinical presentation of, 471
    laboratory findings, 472
    molecular biology, 452–453
    pathology, 452
    treatment of, 472–473
  mastocytosis, 455
  myelofibrosis with myeloid metaplasia (MMM), 466–467
  myeloproliferative/myelodysplastic disorders, 455
  myeloproliferative/myelodysplastic unclassified, 456
  polycythemia vera (PV), 462–464
    cytogenetics, 451
    diagnosis, 469–470
    incidence and clinical presentation, 467
    molecular biology, 451
    pathology of, 451
    survival, 469
    treatment of, 470–471
  risk factors, 447
chronic idiopathic myelofibrosis
  leukemia transformation of MMM, 482
  medical surgical and radiotherapeutic options in, 476
  nonsplenic extramedullary hematopoiesis, 481
  therapeutic management of MMM, 483
  therapy of constitutional symptoms, 481–482
  therapy of cytopenias, 478–480
  therapy of myeloproliferative symptoms, 480–481
cladribine, 489, 662
clofarabine, 76
clonal bone marrow disorder, 487
clonal hematopoietic stem disorder, 475
CNS leukemia, 26
coagulopathy, 28
collagen deposition, 475
complete remission
  in ALL, 143–145
  in AML, 83–84
complex karyotype category, 10
computed tomography (CT), 823
core-binding factor (CBF), 16
corticosteroids, 497
CpG island hypermethylation, in AML, 21
C-reactive protein (CRP), 917
CT53518, 97
cutaneous follicle center lymphoma, 509
cyclophosphamide, 3, 75
cyclosporine, 94
cyclosporine A, 47, 56
cytarabine, 17, 43, 52, 91, 93, 489, 491–492
cytopenias, 475–476
*cytoplasmic (BAALC) gene*, 16
cytotoxic therapy, 488
cytotoxic T-lymphocytes, 526

**D**
danazol, 479
daunorubicin, 42–43, 47, 54, 56–57, 59, 64, 491
decitabine, 76, 489–490
denileukin diftitox, 602, 723–724
2-deoxycytidine analogs, 490

depsipeptide, 97
dermatologic syndromes, 1164
dexamethasone, 876
diabetes insipidus, 28
differentiation syndrome, 1162
diffuse large B-cell lymphoma (DLBCL), 507, 509, 519–520
  prognosis and prognostic factors of, 705–707
disseminated intravascular coagulation (DIC), 1160–1161
donor lymphocyte infusions (DLI), 96
Down syndrome, 1, 9
Durie–Salmon staging system, 917
dyskaratosis congenita, 1

**E**
electron microscopy, 281
enteropathy-type T-cell lymphoma (ETL), 523
Epstein-Barr virus, 734
Epstein–Barr virus (EBV) reactivation, 105
erythrocyte transfusions, 478
erythroid cells, 1
erythroleukemia, 27
erythropoietin, 479, 488
essential thrombocythemia (ET)
  criteria for diagnosis of, 471–472
  cytogenetics, 452
  incidence and clinical presentation, 471
  laboratory findings, 472
  molecular biology, 452–453
  pathology, 452
  treatment of, 472–473
ethylenimines, 1089
etoposide, 94, 488
event-free survival (EFS), of patients, 64
external beam radiotherapy (XRT), 481
extramedullary hematopoiesis, 466, 475
extranodal NK/T-cell lymphoma of nasal type, 523–524

**F**
Fanconi anemia, 1, 9
farnesyltransferase inhibitors, 97, 491
farnesyltransferase inhibitor tipifarnib, 481
fibronectin, 475
FLT3 inhibitors, 47
FLT3 mutations, 46
  in AML patients, 19–20
FLT3 transmembrane tyrosine kinase, 46
fludarabine, 93, 95, 492, 662
fluorescence in situ hybridization (FISH) techniques, 17, 34, 104
18-fluoro-2-deoxyglucose positron emission tomography
  detection technique, 824–825
  early response evaluation, 827
  limitations of, 827–828
  prognosis in SCT, 827
  response assessment, 826–827
  staging, 825–826
fms-like tyrosine kinase 3 (FLT3), 34
follicular lymphoma, 509, 515–516
  agents for treating
    antisence oligonucleotides, 536
    other drugs in, 536
    stem cell transplantation, 536–537
    vaccines, 536
  autologous hematopoietic cell transplantation for, 677–679
  classification and prognosis, 531
  conventional therapy for, 716
  histological transformation of, 537
  monoclonal antibody therapy for, 716
  prognosis and prognostic factors of, 705–707
  therapy, 531–536
  transplantation in, 716–718

**G**
G3139, 536
gallium-67 citrate, 823–824
Ga-67 scintigraphy, 823–824
GATA1 mutations, in AML patients, 19
Gaucher's disease and gammopathy, 837
gemtuzumab ozogamicin, 46, 57, 67, 94, 97
gene therapy, for x-linked severe combined immunodeficiency syndrome, 105
G6PD deficiency, 26
graft-*versus*-host disease (GVHD), 95–96, 98
  cellular modulation and separation of, 1055–1056
  clinical presentation and pathophysiology of acute GVHD, 1051–1053
  prevention of, 1053–1055
  treatment of, 1056–1057
granulocyte-colony-stimulating factor, 488
granulocyte-macrophage colony-stimulating factor, 488
granulocytic cells, 1
granulocytic sarcomas, 25–26

**H**
hairy cell leukemia
  BL22 therapy, 306–307
  cell and molecular biology of, 269–272
  classification of, 267
  clinical features of, 277–278
  criteria for response assessment in, 295
  cytochemistry, 279
  cytogenetics of, 275
  differential diagnosis of, 281–282
  epidemiology, 265
  follow-up of, 298
  gene profile of, 281
  histopathology, 278–279
  immunohistochemistry, 280–281
  immunophenotypic profile of, 279–280
  indications for treatment, 285
  initial treatment approach
    2-chlorodeoxyadenosine, 285–289, 296
    2-deoxycoformycin, 289–290, 296
    interferon, 291–292, 295–297
    splenectomy, 290–291, 295
  LMB-2 therapy, 304–305
  monoclonal antibody therapy of
    with alemtuzumab, 304
    rituximab, 302–304
  natural history of, 295
  pathology of, 272–274
  prognosis of, 296–298
  risk factors, 265–266
  risk of second malignancies, 266
  treatment of relapsed or refractory
    with fludarabine for purine analogy-resistant, 302
    with interferon in purine analogy-resistant, 302
    nonstandard biologic therapy vs additional purine analogy therapy, 302
    with salvage splenectomy, 301
hematologic malignancies, fertility issues in
  ethical and legal issues on, 1176
  gonadal toxicity following malignancy treatment, 1171–1173
  impact of malignancy on reproductive system, 1171
  options for fertility preservation, 1173–1176
  potential for fertility following malignancy treatment, 1173
hematologic syndromes, 1163
hematopoietic growth factors (HGF), 57
  allogeneic stem cell transplantation, 1142–1143
  autologous stem cell transplantation, 1142–1143
  general indications for prescribing, 1139–1140
  in specific hematologic diseases, 1140–1142

hematopoietic stem cell transplantation (HSCT) , 44–45, 94–96
    clinical decisions, 976
    clinical efficacy of, 979–980
    conditioning regimens for, 979
    history of, 975–976
    types of
        allogeneic, 976–978
        autologous, 978–979
        syngeneic, 978
hemophagocytic syndrome, 526
hemorrhagic episodes, 478
hepatitis C virus, 837
hepatosplenic T-cell lymphoma (HSTL), 524
hepatosplenomegaly, 475, 495
herbal medicines, 59
Hickman catheter, 36
histone deacetylase (HDAC) inhibitors, 76
HIV-related lymphomas
    AIDS-related systemic lymphoma
        clinical presentation of, 632
        epidemiology of, 631–632
        outcomes with HAART, 635–636
        predictors of, 632
        treatment of, 632–635
    HIV-associated Hodgkin's disease
        clinical presentation of, 638
        epidemiology, 637–638
        treatment of, 638–639
    HIV-associated multicentric Castleman's disease
        clinical features, 639
        treatment of, 639–640
    primary cerebral lymphoma
        clinical presentation and differential diagnosis, 636–637
        epidemiology, 636
        treatment of, 637
Hodgkin's disease (HD)
    association with rheumatologic conditions treated with
        methotrexate, 735
    epidemiology, 733
    autologous stem cell transplantation for
        and criteria of chemosensitive disease, 793–794
        in patients with primary refractory disease, 794–795
        and pre-cytoreductive radiation therapy, 797–798
        survival rate in relapsed and primary refractory HL, 795–796
        use of consolidated radiation therapy, 796–797
        use of radiation therapy in, 796
    cell of origin and evidence of disrupted B-cell transcription factor,
        751
    classical form of, 752–755
        clinical features of, 759–761
        diagnostic evaluation, 761–762
        epidemiology, 759
        principles of therapy for stages III and IV, 772–778
        staging of, 762–764
        standard principles of therapy, for stage I and II, 767–771
    classification of, 751–752
    definition and use of prognostic factors, 739–740
    follow-up care
        after initial treatment, 801–802
        for long-term complications of, 802–804
    limits of prognostic factors, 745–746
    lymphocyte-predominant
        clinical features, 764
        diagnostic evaluation, 764
        epidemiology, 764
        staging of, 764
    nodular lymphocyte predominant, 755–756
        clinical features and prognosis of, 783–786
        guidelines and recommendations for treatment of, 789
        pathology of, 783
        treatment of advanced stage of, 788–789
        treatment of early stage of, 786–788
    prognostic factors, 740–741

prognostic indices or scores, 741–745
treatment of relapsed or refractory
    after radiation therapy, 807–808
    with monoclonal antibodies, 810–811
    recurrent/ resistant disease after initial chemotherapy, 808–810
use of prognostic factors, 746–747
    history of, 733
    and viruses, 734
hospice services, 59
human leukocyte antigen matching, principles of
    HLA genetic organization, 985
    polymorphism of HLA genes, 989–990
    stem cell transplantation in relation to donors, 991–992
    stem cell transplantation in relation to unrelated donors, 992–996
    structure and function, 985–988
human T-cell lymphotropic virus type 1, 837
hydration, 36
hydroxyurea, 52, 59, 470, 480, 488–489, 493, 495, 497
hypercalcemia, 964
hypereosinophilic syndrome
    diagnostic and treatment approach, 496
    management of, 496–498
hyperleukocytosis, 26, 1161–1162
hyperviscosity syndrome (HVS)
    clinical findings, 938–939
    pathophysiology, 937–938
    treatment of, 939–940
hypokalemia, 28

**I**
idarubicin, 42–43, 54, 64, 491–492
imatinib, 491
imatinib mesylate, 490, 497
immunoglobulin gene *IgH,* 107
immunohistochemistry, 33
immunophenotyping, 33
indolent lymphoproliferative disorders, 489
induction chemotherapy, 42–43
induction therapy, 65–66
infliximab, 441
interferon, 291–292, 295–297, 1107–1108
interferon α, 470–471, 497
intermediate chromosomal abnormalities, 45
internal tandem duplication (ITD), 46, 63
International Agency for Research on Cancer (IARC), 3
International Prognostic Index (IPI), 506, 743–744
International Prognostic Scoring System, 490
International Workshop on Chronic Lymphocytic Leukemia
    (IWCLL), 237
inv(16)(p13q22)/ t(16;16)(p13;q22), 10–11
irinotecan hydrochloride (CPT-11), 664

**J**
juvenile myelomonocytic leukemia, 456

**K**
Kaposi's sarcoma-associated herpesvirus, 837
KIT mutations, in AML patients, 19–20
Klinefelter syndrome, 9
Kostmann granulocytic leukemia, 9

**L**
lactate dehydrogenase (LDH) concentrations, 488
lenalidomide, 481
lenalidomide (Revlimid), 440
leukemia
    acute lymphoblastic. *See* acute lymphoblastic leukemia
    acute myeloid. *See* acute myeloid leukemia
    acute promyelocytic. *See* acute promyelocytic leukemia
    choice of antimicrobial therapy, 315–318
    chronic lymphocytic. *See* chronic lymphohcytic leukemia
    and cigarette smoking, 3
    clinical presentation of neutropenic patients, 312–315

core-binding factor, 16
cosmic radiation exposure, 2
environmental factors responsible for, 2
excess relative risk (ERR) of, 2
exposure to nuclear explosions and, 2
familial acute, 1
in females, 1
hairy cell. *See* hairy cell leukemia
in identical twins, 1
infection control, 318–319
life span study (LSS) of atomic bomb survivors, 2
in males, 1
management of fever in neutropenic patients, 311–312
microbiology of infection in neutropenic patients, 312
and use of hair dyes, 3
vaccines for, 47
leukocytosis, 475
leukoerythroblastic, 466
leukostasis, 1161–1162
Lille criteria modeled median survival, in MMM patients, 476
liposomal daunorubicin, 492
lonafarnib, 491
lovastatin, 97
lymphoblasts, 31
Lymphoma Classification Project, 508
lymphoma
    AIDS-related systemic, 632
    anaplastic large cell lymphoma (ALCL), 505, 522–523
    anaplastic lymphoma kinase (ALK), 510
    angioimmunoblastic T-cell lymphoma (AITL), 523
    autologous stem cell transplantation for, 3
    B-cell. *See* B-cell lymphomas
    blastic NK-cell, 526
    Burkitt, 520
    Burkitt-like, 509, 520
    cutaneous follicle center, 509
    diffuse large B-cell lymphoma (DLBCL), 507, 509, 519–520, 705
    enteropathy-type T-cell lymphoma (ETL), 523
    extranodal NK/T-cell lymphoma of nasal type, 523–524
    follicular, 509, 515–516
    hepatosplenic T-cell lymphoma (HSTL), 524
    HIV-related. *See* HIV-related lymphomas
    HIV-associated Hodgkin's disease, 637
    HIV-associated multicentric Castleman's disease, 639
    immunophenotype of, 505
    lymphoplasmacytic, 518–519
    mantle cell, 504, 514–515, 555, 557–561, 675–676
    marginal zone. *See* marginal zone lymphomas
    mature T-cell non-Hodgkin's lymphoma, 613–624
    mucosa-associated lymphoid tissue, 508, 516–517
    NK-cell lymphoma, 504, 510
    nodal marginal zone, 518
    non-Hodgkin's. *See* non-Hodgkin's lymphoma
    peripheral T-cell lymphoma, 521–522, 679–680
    precursor B-cell and T-cell lymphoblastic, 565–569
    primary central nervous system. *See* primary central nervous
        system lymphoma
    primary cerebral, 636, 637
    primary cutaneous B-cell lymphoma, 602
    primary cutaneous T-cell lymphoma, 603, 605, 607
    primary effusion, 521
    small lymphocytic, 513–514
    splenic marginal zone, 282, 517–518
    subcutaneous panniculitis-like T-cell lymphoma (SPTCL), 526
    T-cell. *See* T-cell lymphomas
lymphomatoid granulomatosis (LYG), 520–521
lymphoplasmacytic lymphoma (LPL), 518–519

**M**
macrophage colony-stimulating factor receptor *(M-CSFR),* 16
magnetic resonance imaging (MRI), 823
mantle cell lymphoma (MCL), 504, 514–515
    autologous hematopoietic cell transplantation for, 675–676

histology, 555
immunophenotypes of, 555–557
prognostic factors, 557
treatment approaches to, 557–561
MAP/ERK kinase, 97
marginal zone lymphomas, 509
    extra nodal
        clinical features, 579
        diagnosis and staging of gastric type, 579
        epidemiology and etiology, 578
        genetic abnormalities, 578–579
        pathology, 577–578
        treatment of, 579–581
    of mucosa associated lymphoid tissue, 509
    nodal marginal zone lymphoma
        clinical features, 582–583
        genetic abnormalities, 582
        pathology, 582
        treatment of, 583
    splenic marginal zone
        clinical features, 582
        genetic abnormalities, 581–582
        pathology, 581
        treatment of, 582
marrow donor program, 985
marrow erythroblasts, 31
matrix metalloprotease inhibitors (MMPIS), 441
mature B-cell leukemias, 509
mature T-cell non-Hodgkin's lymphoma
    classification and clinicopathological features
        predominantly extranodal group, 616
        predominantly leukemic group, 613–614
        predominantly nodal group, 614–615
    prognostic factors, 617–618
    treatment modalities
        campath-IH, 624
        CD52 antibody, 624
        conventional chemotherapy, 618–620
        gem citabine therapy, 623–624
        high-dose chemotherapy/stem cell transplantation, 620–621
        purine analogs, 621–623
May–Grünwald–Giemsa stains, 9
Mayo Clinic experience, 481
MD Anderson Prognostic Score (MDAPS), 488
MDX-060, 811
mechlorethamine, 3
megakaryoblasts, 31
megakaryocytes, 466
megakaryocytic lineage cells, 1
melphalan, 481, 874–876
menorrhagia, 2
M4eo, 27, 31
6-mercaptopurine, 66, 488
metamyelocytes, 475
methotrexate (MTX), 66
mevastatin, 97
$\beta_2$-microglobulin, 488, 918
minimal residual disease (MRD), 237
mitoxantrone, 44, 57, 93–94, 491
modifying agents, treating hematologic malignancies
    arsenic trioxide, 1110–1111
    interferons, 1107–1108
    retinoids, 1108–1110
    tyrosine kinase inhibitors, 1105–1107
monoclonal antibodies
    immunotoxins, 1118–1121
    radioimmunoconjugates, 1121–1123
    unconjgated MoAbs, 1115–1118
monoclonal gammopathy of undetermined significance (MGUS)
    clinical and laboratory features, 945–946
    diagnosis, 944–945
    differential diagnosis, 947–949
    disease associations, 949–950

monoclonal gammopathy of undetermined significance
        (MGUS) (continued)
    disease variants, 950
    epidemiology, 943–944
    management of, 950–951
    risk factors for progression, 946–947
monocyte/macrophage cells, 1
MOPP/ABV hybrid regimen, 775
MOPP chemotherapy, 773–774
morphology, 505
MSH2 protein, 52
mucosa-associated lymphoid tissue (MALT) lymphomas, 508,
        516–517
multiple myeloma (MM)
    allogeneic stem cell transplantation for
        clinical trial results of, 902–903
        conditioning regimens, role of, 903–904
        induction of GvM, 906–907
        monitoring of patients after, 902
        myeloablative allogeneic peripheral blood transplants, 904
        nonmyeloablative stem cell transplantation (NST), 907
        prognostic factors of, 904
        and standard therapy, 905–906
        syngeneic transplantation, 904
        targets of GvM effect, 907–908
        treatment related to toxicity and GvHD, 903
        vs autologous stem cell transplantation, 904–906
        vs graft effects, 906
    clinical evaluation of, 865–866
    clinical manifestations and pathophysiology
        blood chemistries, 861
        bone and bone marrow changes, 860–861
        extramedullary plasmacytoma, 865
        hemostasis defects, 861
        hyperviscosity syndrome, 864
        meningeal myelomatosis, 863
        myeloma bone disease and hypercalcemia, 861
        myeloma renal disease, 861
        neurologic dysfunctions, 862
        peripheral neuropathies, 863–864
        solitary plasmacytoma of bone, 865
        spinal cord injuries, 862–863
        systemic amyloidosis, 864
        tubular dysfunction, 861–862
    cytogenetic abnormalities in, 850–853
    development of plasma cells, 849–850
    differential diagnosis, 867
    epidemiology
        gender effects, 834
        racial difference and incidence, 834–835
        time trends, 833
    etiology, 836–839
    genetic and molecular factors, 839–840
    initial treatment approach of
        conventional regimens, 874–877
        newer regimens, 878–880
        supportive care, 881–882
        therapy duration, 880
    and life style changes, 839
    microenvironment factors, 853–854
    morphology of, 847–849
    occupational hazards and incidence, 838
    origin of malignant plasma cell, 850
    prognostic factors, 916–922
    remission criteria, 913–916
    skeletal complications of, 967–970
    symptoms of, 859–860
    thromboembolic events, 970
    treatment of infectious complications, 965–967
    treatment of relapsed or refractory form of
        with arsenic trioxide, 931–932
        biology of multiple myeloma, 927–928
        drug resistance mechanisms, 928

    other drugs, 932
    with proteasome inhibitor, 928–929
    salvage therapies, 932–933
    with thalidomide, 929–931
    transplantation, 932
    variants of
        extramedullary plasmacytoma, 891–892
        immunoglobulin D myeloma, 897–902
        multiple solitary plasmacytomas, 892
        nonsecretory myeloma, 896–897
        plasma cell leukemia (PCL), 892–894
        POEMS syndrome, 894–896
        smoldering multiple myeloma, 894
        solitary plasmacytoma of bone, 889–891
mycosis fungoides (MF), 524–525
myeloablative allogeneic stem cell transplant
    in chronic lymphocytic leukemia, 360–361
    in chronic myeloid leukemia, 355
        prognostic factors, 356–358
        from unrelated donors, 356
    in MMM, 476
myeloablative stem cell transplantation, 658, 660
myelodysplastic syndromes (MDS), 51
    apoptosis in, 370
    clinical features of, 377
    cytogenetic abnormalities in, 369–370
    diagnosis of, 380
        dielemmas in, 380–381
    evidence of clonality, 368
    follow-up of, 431
    gene alterations, 368
    hematologic laboratory findings, 377–380
    high risk, 435
    international risk classification of, 430
    low risk, treatment of
        angiogenesis, 439
        angiogenesis agents, 440–441
        cytoprotective agents, 441–442
        immuno modulation, 442
        vitamin D, 441
    micro array analysis in, 369
    micro environment in, 371
    pathogenesis model, 367
    pathology of, 371–372
    phase, 3
    prognosis of, 427–430
    relaspsed or refractory, treatment of
        with arsenic trioxide, 438
        with DNA methyltransferase inhibitors,
            435–436
        with DNA topoisomerase I inhibitors, 438
        with franesyltransferase inhibitors (FTIS), 437
        with histone deacetylase inhibitors, 436
        with proteosome inhibitors, 438
        with tyrosine kinase receptor inhibitors (RTKC),
            437–438
    response criteria with, 425–427
    treatment of early
        allogeneic stem cell transplantation for, 415–419
        comprehensive strategies for, 392–393
        high-intensity therapy
        low-intensity therapy, 386–392
        other options, 392
        supportive care of, 385–386
myelofibrosis with myeloid metaplasia (MMM), 475
myeloperoxidase (myeloid), 33
myeloproliferative disorder, 5
myeloproliferative hypereosinophilic diseases, 454
myelosuppression, 470


N
nandrolone, 479
National Cancer Institute–Working Group (NCI-WG), 237

National Comprehensive Cancer Network, 87
natural killer cell acute leukemia, 27–28
neoangiogenesis, 475
neutropenic enterocolitis (NE), 1162–1163
nitrogen mustard derivatives, 1089
9-nitro-20-(S)-camptothecin, 490
nitrosoureas, 1089
NK-cell lymphoma, 504, 510
nodal marginal zone lymphoma, 518
non-Hodgkin's lymphoma
  allogeneic hematopoietic stem cell transplantation
    in aggressive NHL patients, 690
    concept of reduced-conditioning of, 694–695
    donor lymphocytes infusions, 696
    in failed auto PBSCT, 690
    in follicular NHL patients, 690
    rationale for, 690
    therapy for specific subtypes of, 695–696
    using reduced-conditioning of, 695
    vs autologous SCT, 693–694
  assessment of molecular response and minimal residual disease,
    704–705
  autologous hematopoietic cell transplantation for
    Burkitt's lymphoma, 680–681
    follicular NHL, 677–679
    mantle cell lymphoma, 675–677
    peripheral T-cell lymphoma, 679–680
    posttransplant consolidation and maintenance therapy,
      681–682
    risks after autografting, 682–683
  follow up of, 708–709
  histopathological reproductibility and clinical relevance of,
    507–508
  prognosis and prognostic factors of
    of diffuse large B-cell lymphoma, 705–706
    of follicular lymphoma, 707–708
  relative frequency of different lymphomas, 508
  revised European American classification, 504
  standard response criteria in, 701–703
  therapies for
    antisense oligonucleotide therapy, 726–727
    fusion toxins, 723–724
    gallium nitrate therapy, 727–728
    histone deacetylase inhibitors, 728
    monoclonal antibody therapy for, 723
    proteosome inhibitors, 728
    radiolabeled antibody therapy, 724–726
    tumor vaccines, 728–729
  treatment approach to high-grade
    of Burkitt's lymphoma, 569–573
    precursor B-cell and T-cell lymphoblastic lymphoma, 565–569
  treatment of transformed
    clinical findings and outcomes, 712–714
    conventional therapy for follicular lymphomas, 715–716
    etiology of transformation, 714–715
    incidence of histologic transformation, 711–713
    monoclonal antibody therapy for follicular lymphomas, 716
    of Richter's syndrome, 718–719
    risk factors, 712
    transplantation in follicular lymphomas, 716–718
  use of functional imaging in response assessment in, 703–704
  WHO classification, 504–505
    basis of real and WHO classification, 505–506
    issue relating to individual entities in, 508–510
    structure of, 506–507
    updating of, 508
nonlymphoid hematopoietic progenitors, 1
nonmyeloablative allogeneic stem cell transplantations, 59
nonmyeloablative stem cell transplantation, 661
  in MMM, 476
nonspecific esterase (monocytic), 33
nonspecific esterase (NSE), 10
NPM gene, 87

**O**
operating characteristics (OCs), 79
oral antimetabolite therapy, 45
oral chemotherapy, 488
oral vascular endothelial growth factor inhibitor PTK787, 481
osteosclerosis, 475
osteosclerotic and osteolytic lesions, 27
otosclerosis, 466
oxymethalone, 479

**P**
paraneoplastic syndromes, 1163
pentostatin, 662
peptic ulcer disease, 2
periodic acid—Schiff (PAS) (erythroid), 33
peripheral T-cell lymphoma
  autologous hematopoietic cell transplantation for, 679–698
  unspecified (PTCLU), 521–522
p-glycoprotein efflux pump, 56
p-glycoprotein (gp170) chemotherapy efflux pump, 51
phenylbutyrate, 97
Philadelphia chromosome, t(9;22), 35
phlebotomies, 470
PI-3 kinase, 97
PKC412, 78, 97
PML-RARA gene, 10–11
  expression, in AML, 20
Pneumocystis carinii pneumonia, 67
polyclonal hairy B-cell lymphoproliferative disorder, 282
polycythemia vera (PV), 462–464
  cytogenetics, 451
  diagnosis of, 469–470
  incidence and clinical presentation, 469
  molecular biology, 451
  pathology of, 451
  survival, 469
  treatment of, 470–471
polymerase chain reaction (PCR), 238, 488
postpolycythemic myeloid metaplasia (PPMM), 475
postremission chemotherapy, 43–44, 57–59
postremission therapy, 43–44
postthrombocythemic (PTMM), 475
posttransplant lymphoproliferative disorders
  clinical features, 647
  evaluation, 647–650
  incidence and risk factors, 646–647
  management of
    adoptive immunotherapy, 653
    anti-B cell therapy, 651–652
    anti-interleukin 6 therapy, 653
    antiviral therapy, 653–654
    arginine butyrate, 653
    chemotherapy, 652–653
    decreasing immunosuppressive therapy, 650–651
    interferon alpha therapy, 654
    rapamycin, 652
  pathophysiology, 645–646
precursor B-cell and T-cell lymphoblastic lymphoma
  clinical features, 565–566
  frequency of occurence, 565
  pathology and pathogenesis, 566
  prognostic factors, 566–567
  radiation therapy, 567
  stem cell transplantation, 567–569
  treatment of, 567
precursor cell tumors, 508
prednisone, 3
pregnant women, treatment approach to
  diagnosis of, 1149
  impact of pregnancy on leukemia, 1147–1148
  passage of leukemic cells to fetus, 1149
  pharmacokinetics with, 1149–1150
  physiological changes with pregnancy, 1147

pregnant women, treatment approach to (*continued*)
  placental function, 1148–1149
  teratogenicity of chemotherapeutic agents, 1150–1152
  treatment of specific hematologic malignancies
    acute leukemias, 1152–1153
    chronic lymphocytic leukemia, 1155
    chronic myelogenous leukemia, 1154–1155
    hairy-cell leukemia, 1155
    human T-cell lymphotrophic virus type I, 1155–1156
    myelodysplastic syndromes (MDS), 1153–1154
primary central nervous system lymphoma
  clinical characteristics, 589–591
  definition of, 589
  epidemiology, 589
  pathology, 589
  primary treatment
    chemotherapy alone, 594–596
    chemotherapy in combination with WBXRT, 592–594
    corticosteroids, 591
    neurotoxicity, 594
    surgery, 591
    whole brain irradiation, 591–592
  relapsed or refractory, treatment of, 596–597
  special therapeutic circumstances
    intraocular lymphoma, 596
    leptomeningeal lymphoma, 596
    special lymphoma, 596
primary cutaneous B-cell lymphoma, treatment of
  chemotherapy, 602–603
  peripheral stem cell transplantation, 603
  radiation therapy, 601–602
  recommended treatment approaches for, 603
  surgery, 602
primary cutaneous CD30 positive lymphoproliferative disorders, 525–526
primary cutaneous T-cell lymphoma, treatment of
  of advanced stage mycosis fungoides/Sézary syndrome, 605
  biologic response modifiers, 605
  of CD30 positive lymphoproliferative disorders, 607
  early stage mycosis fungoides, 603–604
  extra corporeal photochemotherapy, 606
  interferon-alpha therapy, 605–606
  peripheral stem cell transplantation, 607
  phototherapy/ photochemotherapy, 604
  recommended treatment approaches, 604–605
  retinoids, 606
  of small and medium pleomorphic
    T-cell lymphoma, 607
  systemic chemotherapy, 605
  topical chemotherapy, 604
  topical retinoid application, 604
  topical steroids, 604
  total skin electron beam therapy, 604
  trageted modalities, 606
primary effusion lymphoma, 521
primary induction failure, 91
procarbazine, 3
promyelocytes, 31
prophylactic platelet transfusions, 488
proteoglycans, 475
PSC 833, 56
PTK787, 76
purine nucleosides, 296–297

**Q**
11q23 gene, 35
quality of life measurements, 77

**R**
R115977, 78, 97
*RAB5EP/PDGFRβ* fusion gene, 490
RAS mutations, in AML patients, 20
receptor tyrosine kinases (RTKs), 487

reduced-intensity stem cell transplantation in CML, 359
Reed-Sternberg cells, 752, 810
refractory anemia with excess blasts in
    transformation (RAEBt), 490
refractory anemia with excess blasts (RAEB), 490
Reike, 59
relapsed leukemia, 45–46
remission induction therapy, in AML, 53–59, 83
  additional induction agents, 56–57
  anthracenediones, 54–56
  anthracyclines, 54–56
  gemtuzumab ozogamicin, 57
  post-remission stem cell transplantation, 59
  post remission therapy, 57–59
  protracted post-remission therapy, 59
  varying doses of anthracyclines, 56
renal insufficiency, 964–965
renal syndromes, 1163–1164
reticulin fibrosis, 475
*retinoic acid receptor* α (RARA) gene, 17
retinoic acid receptor α (PAPA)γενε, 63
retinoids, 1108–1110
reverse transcriptase polymerase chain reaction (RT-PCR)
    techniques, 84
reverse transcription polymerase chain reaction (RT-PCR),
    9, 104
rheumatoid arthritis, 2, 837
Richter's syndrome, 718–719
rituximab, 304, 723
Romanowsky stains, 9
Royal Marsden criteria, 35
RUNXI mutations, in AML patients, 19

**S**
SAHA, 76
salvage therapy, 69, 92, 95
Schwachman syndrome, 1, 9
secondary AML/MDS treatment of
  clinical trials of investigational agents, 78–80
  general issues, 73–75
  investigational approaches, 75–78
secondary leukemias, 27
second malignancies
  of acute myeloid leukemia, 817–819
  incidence and risk factors, 815–817
  of myelodysplastic syndrome (MDS), 817–819
  prevention of, 819
  secondary AML, 52
  strategies for screening, 819
Sezary syndrome, 497
signal transduction pathways, in AML patients, 19
small lymphocytic lymphoma (SLL), 513–514
sobuzoxane (MST-16), 664
soluble interleukin-2 receptor, 298
splenectomy, 290–291, 295, 297
splenic marginal zone lymphoma (SMZL), 282, 506, 509, 517–518
splenic radiation, 481
splenomegaly, 466, 470, 479–481, 488, 495
standard chemotherapy (SCH), 73
Stanford V regimens, 775
stem cell mobilization
  clinical significance of, 1007–1008
  factors affecting, 1007
  mechanism of, 1001–1002
  methods of, 1001–1006
  mobilization of allogeneic stem cells, 1008
  optimal time for, 1006
  parameters in, 1002–1003
  strategies for, 1006
  target and threshold, 1007
stem cell transplantation
  infectious complications following
    early engraftment period, 1068–1071

late engraftment period, 1071–1073
preengraftment period, 1064–1068
pretransplant evaluation, 1063–1064
noninfectious complications following
regimen-related toxicity, 1077–1080
renal dysfunction, 1080–1082
for solid tumors and nonmalignant conditions
adult small round-cell tumors, 1017
adult soft-tissue sarcoma, 1017
allogeneic transplants for solid tumors, 1019
for amyloidosis, 1019–1020
brain tumors, 1016–1017
breast cancer, 1013–1015
germ cell cancer, 1017–1019
melanoma, 1016
for ovarian carcinoma, 1015–1016
smallcell lung cancer, 1016
SU5416, 76, 97
SU11248, 97
subcutaneous panniculitis-like T-cell lymphoma (SPTCL), 526
Sudan black B (SBB), 10
Surveillance, epidemiology, and end-results (SEER) data, 1
systematic mastocytosis, 282

**T**
T-cell and NK cell malignancies
anaplastic lymphoma large cell, 522–523
angioimmunoblastic T-cell lymphomas, 523
blastic NK-cell lymphomas, 526
enteropathy-type T-cell lymphomas, 523
extranodal of nasal type, 523–524
hepatosplenic T-cell lymphomas, 524
mycosis fungoides/Sézary syndrome, 524–525
peripheral T-cell lymphoma unspecified, 521–522
primary cutaneous CD30 positive type, 525–526
subcutaneous panniculitis like, 526
T-cell lymphomas, 497, 510
treatment approach to adult related
arsenic trioxide, 662–664
chemotherapy, 657
monoclonal antibodies, 664
nucleoside analogs, 662
retroviral and immunomodulatory agents, 662
stem cell transplantation, 658–662

supportive care, 665
toposiomerase inhibitors, 664
tenofovir, 662
thalidomide, 440, 479, 491, 876
therapeutic touch, 59
thorotrast, 2
thrombocytopenia, 476, 478, 487–489, 494
thrombocytosis, 28, 475
tipifarnib, 491
topoisomerase I inhibitors, 489–490
topoisomerase II inhibitors, 3, 5, 9, 664
topotecan, 489, 492–493
t(5;12)(q33;p13) gene, 490
t(5;10)(q33;q22), 490
t(15;17)(q22;q12-21), 10
t(8;21)(q22;q22)/*AML1(RUNX1)- ETO(CBFA2T1)*, 16–17
t(8;21)(q22;q22) gene, 10–11
tranexamic acid, 65
trapoxin, 97
treatment-related mortality (TRM), 73
triazenes, 1089
trichostatin, 97
tumor lysis syndrome (TLS), 26–27, 42, 1159–1160
tumor necrosis factor α (TNF-α), 482
tyrosine kinase inhibitors, 1105–1107

**U**
umbilical cord blood (UCB) transplantation
biologic characterization and immune reconstitution, 1041–1042
clinical data on outcomes of, 1042–1047
future research, 1047
UCB banking, 1039–1041

**V**
VAD, 876
vincristine, 3

**W**
Wright–Giesma stain, 28, 32

**Z**
zalcitabine, 662
zaragozic acid, 97
zidovudine, 662